KT-487-972

# TEXTBOOK OF VETERINARY ANATOMY

## THIRD EDITION

K. M. Dyce, D.V.M.&S., B.Sc., M.R.C.V.S.
Professor Emeritus of Veterinary Anatomy
Royal (Dick) School of Veterinary Studies
University of Edinburgh,
Edinburgh, Scotland

W. O. Sack, D.V.M., Ph.D., Dr. med. vet.
Professor Emeritus of Veterinary Anatomy
College of Veterinary Medicine
Cornell University,
Ithaca, New York

C. J. G. Wensing, D.V.M., Ph.D.
Professor of Veterinary Anatomy and Embryology
School of Veterinary Medicine,
State University Utrecht,
The Netherlands

**Saunders**
*An Imprint of Elsevier*

**SAUNDERS**
*An Imprint of Elsevier*

The Curtis Center
Independence Square West
Philadelphia, Pennsylvania 19106

**Copyright © 2002, 1996, 1987 Elsevier (USA). All rights reserved.**

No part of this publication may be reproduced or transmitted in any form or by any means, electronic or mechanical, including photocopy, recording, or any information storage and retrieval system, without permission in writing from the publisher (Saunders, The Curtis Center, Independence Square West, Philadelphia, PA 19106-3399).

Permissions may be sought directly from Elsevier's Health Sciences Rights Department in Philadelphia, PA, USA: phone: (+1) 215 239 3804, fax: (+1) 215 239 3805, e-mail: healthpermissions@elsevier.com. You may also complete your request on-line via the Elsevier homepage (http://www.elsevier.com), by selecting 'Customer Support' and then 'Obtaining Permissions'.

## NOTICE

Veterinary Medicine is an ever-changing field. Standard safety precautions must be followed, but as new research and clinical experience broaden our knowledge, changes in treatment and drug therapy may become necessary or appropriate. Readers are advised to check the most current product information provided by the manufacturer of each drug to be administered to verify the recommended dose, the method and duration of administration, and contraindications. It is the responsibility of the treating veterinarian, relying on experience, and knowledge of the animal, to determine dosages and the best treatment for each individual animal. Neither the Publisher nor the editor assumes any liability for any injury and/or damage to animals or property arising from this publication.

THE PUBLISHER

**Library of Congress Cataloging-in-Publication Data**

Dyce, K. M. (Keith M.)
Textbook of veterinary anatomy/K.M. Dyce, W.O. Sack, C.J.G. Wensing—3rd ed.

p. cm.

ISBN-13: 978-0-7216-8966-1 ISBN-10: 0-7216-8966-3

1. Veterinary anatomy. I. Sack, W. O. (Wolfgang O.) II. Wensing, Cornelis Johannes Gerardus. III. Title.

SF761.D93 2002

636.089'1—dc21 2001049546

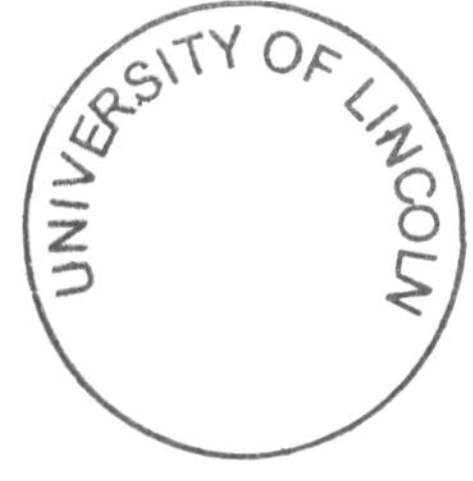


*Acquisitions Editor:* Ray Kersey
*Developmental Editor:* Denise LeMelledo
*Project Manager:* Robin E. Davis

ISBN-13: 978-0-7216-8966-1
ISBN-10: 0-7216-8966-3

Printed in the United States of America.

Last digit is the print number: 9 8 7 6 5

# PREFACE TO THE THIRD EDITION

The call for a new edition gave us an opportunity to incorporate new material in both text and figures. Among the latter, the most prominent change consists in the substantial revision, and considerable increase in number, of the color plates; these, in addition to illustrating many aspects of gross anatomy, now provide a selection of photomicrographs. The text figures include a wider range depicting normal structures by means of the newer imaging techniques; apart from their intrinsic interest, they may gently introduce the junior student to the potential of these increasingly important diagnostic aids. Neither the microscopic nor the imaging set of figures professes to provide systematic coverage of its field. The other new figures are more diverse but, though less easily categorized, mostly share a common purpose—the reaffirmation of the relevance of anatomy to other disciplines, both preclinical and clinical.

Major changes to the text include an expanded consideration of life in utero, and various passages relating anatomy to function. Together with numerous lesser additions, these threatened to enlarge our book unduly, and some compensation has been sought by shortening certain chapters. We believe this action justified by the diminished attention that is now commonly afforded to the treatment of individual farm animals under prevailing economic conditions. Because these conditions do not operate everywhere with equal force, we judged it premature to shorten any chapter very drastically.

In previous editions we acknowledged the many colleagues to whom we were, and to whom we of course remain, indebted. We must now add substantially to these lists. Our recent benefactors include: at State University Utrecht, Dr. Katja Teerds, who made the major contribution of the figures illustrating microscopic anatomy together with associated text, and Dr. George Voorhout, Dr. Rosalinde van der Vlugt-Meijer, and Aart van der Woude, who supplied many new radiographic, CT, and MRI images, and Drs. M.A.M. Taverne and C. van Vorstenbosch, who supplied SEM and ultrasonagraphic images; at the University of Ghent, Dr. S. Muylle, who made available photographs of equine incisors of known age; at Cornell University, Dr. Alexander deLahunta, Dr. William E. Hornbuckle, and Dr. Robin D. Gleed, whose counsel we often sought on physiological and clinical matters, and Dr. Peter V. Scrivani, who supplied radiographic and CT images and advised upon their interpretation; and at Virginia Technical and State University, Dr. Bonnie J. Smith, who supplied radiographic and other images and made suggestions for the revision of the avian chapter. Other colleagues at various centers supplied and generously allowed us to reproduce illustrations of their work; their individual contributions are acknowledged on pages ix–xii.

We cannot adequately express how much we owe to the technical staff of the Veterinary Anatomy Department in Utrecht, in particular to Henk van Dijk and Wim Kersten, who prepared the dissections depicted in many color plates or used in the production of drawings; to Harry Otter and Onno van Veen, who contributed substantially to the development of the color plates; and to Henk Halsema, who made new, and adapted certain existing, drawings.

We are indebted to Professor Heugshik S. Lee and his colleagues at Seoul University and elsewhere, who translated our book into Korean—the fifth translation of our work. Finally, we thank Mr. Ray Kersey and his colleagues at W.B. Saunders for their support, which has lightened our burden at all stages of this revision.

K. M. Dyce
W. O. Sack
C. J. G. Wensing

# PREFACE TO THE FIRST EDITION

What one does not understand one does not possess.

*—Goethe*

A few words in explanation of the purpose and arrangement of this book may not be out of place. It is intended to meet the needs of the veterinary student, providing first that general knowledge of mammalian structure that is indispensable to the understanding of the other basic sciences, and secondly the more detailed information that is directly applicable to the practice of veterinary medicine. Though we shall naturally be pleased if others find our book useful, we have regarded the interest of the student reader as paramount.

The dual role of anatomy determined the division of the book into two parts. The first part comprises ten chapters, one a general introduction, the others devoted to the various body systems. For these we have taken as our model the dog, the animal best suited to this purpose by its relatively unspecialized anatomy and its widespread use as the initial dissection subject. We allude to the salient differences found in other domesticated species but do not dwell upon them at this time when our concern is to emphasize general concepts and function rather than specific details. The remarks on development are intended to elucidate the broad features of adult anatomy and do not profess to provide a complete account of this branch of our subject. Since these chapters deal largely with elementary, well-established, and noncontroversial matters, we decided that it would be an affectation to embellish them with references to the literature.

The second part of the book presupposes a working knowledge of the first. It consists of several series of chapters, each series dealing with the regional anatomy of a particular species—or group of species since we have accommodated the cat with the dog, the small ruminants with cattle. This part seeks to emphasize those features and topics that have direct relevance to clinical work. Though the several chapters that deal with the same region of the body of different animals follow a common plan, they do so only loosely; we have expanded, curtailed, and diversified the accounts according to our perceptions of contemporary clinical concern with different species, and occasionally according to the availability of relevant information. This method of proceeding results in some repetition, but we hope compensation will be found in the independence of these chapters, which can be read or consulted in any order and without reference to each other. Finally, there is a single chapter on systematic avian anatomy in which the main subject is the chicken, although some attention is given to cagebirds and other species of veterinary importance. Since the chapters of this second part deal with matters of immediate practical concern we have furnished them with a selection of references for the benefit of those who may wish to inform themselves more fully.

Inevitably, the principal difficulty we encountered when writing this book lay in the selection of appropriate material from the vast array. Since in most schools, courses of anatomy have been progressively, and sometimes savagely, shortened in recent years, there is an obligation to identify and retain "core" material while rigorously pruning matters of more peripheral concern. Alas, there neither is nor can be a unanimous view of what constitutes the "core" while the continuing development and increasing specialization of veterinary medicine attach significance to many details that formerly lacked importance. The reconciliation of these opposing pressures places both teachers and authors in a dilemma from which there is no clear route of escape, and, though we hope we have chosen wisely, we anticipate that some colleagues will reproach us for being overtimid in our culling while others will be as ready to judge us overbold. Readers who take the former view may find that the subdivision of the text enables them to skim or skip judiciously; those more demanding may find some consolation in the references. We hope both groups of readers will welcome the digressions from the conventional stuff of anatomy with which we have sought to make the account more interesting—for it would be folly to deny that anatomical description does not always make the most lively reading.

While each of us has been responsible for the initial draft of portions of the text, the final version represents the consensus of our views. We like to think that there has been advantage in our having gained experience in a variety of schools and we have sought to avoid tailoring the text to fit any particular course too closely. Problems of nomenclature receive some attention in Chapter One, but it may be well to state here that we have consistently employed anglicized versions of the terms contained in the most recent (1983) version of the *Nomina Anatomica Veterinaria.*

Such have been our intentions. Whether they were well conceived or have been properly put into effect we must leave to the judgment of each reader.

K. M. Dyce
W. O. Sack
C. J. G. Wensing

# SOURCES OF NONORIGINAL ILLUSTRATIONS

**Figure 1–3:** After Feeney, D.A., T.F. Fletcher, and R.M. Hardy: Atlas of correlative imaging anatomy of the normal dog. Philadelphia, W.B. Saunders, 1991.

**Figure 1–5/*A*:** Courtesy Dr. J.S. Boyd, Glasgow University.

**Figures 1–5/*B*, 22–17:** Courtesy Dr. B.A. Ball, Cornell University.

**Figure 1–12:** After Dawkins, M.J.R. and D. Hull: The production of heat by fat. Scient. Am. 213:62–67, 1965.

**Figures 1–14/*A*, 1–20/*A*, 1–22/*A*, 2–13, 2–22, 2–23, 2–24, 2–27, 2–39, 2–50, 2–51, 3–63, 5–21, 11–28, 12–7, 12–8, 15–9, 16–2, 16–6, 16–12, 17–6, 23–3, 32–6,** drawn by D.S. Geary. Courtesy Dr. A. Horowitz, Oregon State University; and from Horowitz, A.: Guide for the Laboratory Examination of the Anatomy of the Horse. Columbus, The University of Ohio, Dept. of Veterinary Anatomy, 1965 [Published by the author.]; and Horowitz, A.: The Fundamental Principles of Anatomy: Dissection of the Dog. Saskatoon, University of Saskatchewan, 1970. [Published by the author.]

**Figure 1–15:** After Brookes, M., A.C. Elkin, R.G. Harrison, and C.B. Heald: A new concept of capillary circulation in bone cortex. Lancet 1:1078–1081, 1961.

**Figure 1–20/*C*:** Courtesy Dr. K.-D. Budras, Berlin.

**Figures 2–15, 2–61/*A*,*B*, 17–5, 34–8:** After Taylor, J.A.: Regional and Applied Anatomy of the Domestic Animals. Edinburgh, Oliver & Boyd, 1970.

**Figures 2–25/*B*, 15–8/*C*:** Courtesy Dr. Rijnberk, State University Utrecht.

**Figure 2–26:** After Bradley, O.C.: Topographical Anatomy of the Dog, 6th ed. Edinburgh, Oliver & Boyd, 1959.

**Figures 2–37, 3–26, 5–33, 18–3/*B*, 18–36:** Based on (2–37, 5–33, 18–3/*B*, 18–36) and with permission (3–26) from Nickel, R., A. Schummer, and E. Seiferle: Lehrbuch der Anatomie der Haustiere. Berlin, Paul Parey, 1962, 1987.

**Figure 3–31:** Courtesy Dr. D.V. Rendano, Cornell University.

**Figures 3–38, 10–16, 10–17:** Redrawn from Ellenberger, W., and H. Baum: Handbuch der vergleichenden Anatomie der Haustiere, 18th ed. Berlin, Springer, 1974.

**Figure 3–44:** Courtesy Dr. F. Preuss, Berlin.

**Figures 4–3/*B*, 11–6/*B*, 11–24, 11–26, 13–8/*B*, 14–6/*B*, 14–12/*B*, 14–20/*B*, 18–27/*B*, 23–22, 23–24/*A*:** Courtesy Dr. Peter V. Scrivani, Cornell University.

**Figures 4–10, 4–17:** After Nickel, R., A. Schummer, E. Seiferle, and W.O. Sack: The Viscera of the Domestic Mammals, 2nd ed. New York, Springer Verlag, 1979.

**Figure 7–2:** Redrawn after Noden, D.M., and A. deLahunta: The Embryology of Domestic Animals. Baltimore, Williams & Wilkins, 1985.

**Figure 7–22:** Redrawn after Moore, K.L.: The Developing Human: Clinically Oriented Embryology, 5th ed. Philadelphia, W.B. Saunders, 1993.

**Figure 7–25:** Courtesy v. d. Linde-Sipman, State University Utrecht.

**Figures 7–36, 7–40:** After Simoens, P., N.E. de Vos: Angiology. *In* O. Schaller (ed): Illustrated Veterinary Anatomical Nomenclature. Kinderhook, NY, IBD Ltd., 1992.

**Figure 7–39:** Based on Evans, H.E., and A. deLahunta: Miller's Guide to the Dissection of the Dog, 3rd ed. Philadelphia, W.B. Saunders, 1988.

**Figures 7–40, 7–41, 7–43:** After Budras, K.-D., and W. Fricke: Atlas der Anatomie des Hundes, Kompendium für Tierärzte und Studierende. Hannover, Schlütersche Verlagsanstalt, 1993.

**Figures 7–49, 7–50:** Based on Frewein, J., and B. Vollmerhaus (eds.): Anatomie von Hund und Katze. Berlin, Blackwell, 1994.

**Figures 7–51, 7–55:** After Baum, H.: Das Lymphgefässsystem des Hundes. Berlin, Hirschwald Verlag, 1918.

**Figure 7–56:** Based on Vollmerhaus, B.: *In* Nickel, R., A. Schummer, and E. Seiferle (eds.): The Anatomy of the Domestic Animals, Vol. 3. Berlin, Paul Parey Verlag, 1981.

**Figure 7–58:** After Steger, G.: Zur Biologie der Milz der Haussäugetiere. Dtsch. Tierärztl. Wochenschr. 39:609–614, 1939.

**Figures 8–12, 8–25:** Based on Romer, A.S.: The Vertebrate Body, 3rd ed. Philadelphia, W. B. Saunders, 1962.

**Figure 8–61:** From DeLahunta, A.: Veterinary Neuroanatomy and Clinical Neurology, 2nd ed. Philadelphia, W.B. Saunders, 1983.

**Figure 8–77:** Redrawn from Mizeres, N.J.: The anatomy of the autonomic nervous system in the dog. Am. J. Anat. 96:285–318, 1955.

**Figure 9–18:** Courtesy Dr. P. Simoens, Gent.

**Figure 9–27/*A*,*B*:** After Kratzing, J.: The structure of the vomeronasal organ in the sheep. J. Anat. 108:247–260, 1971.

**Figures 9–27/*C*, 23–2:** Courtesy C.A. Collyer, Cornell University.

**Figure 10–10/*A*:** Courtesy Dr. A. von Rotz, Bern.

**Figures 11–4/*B*, 11–6/*C*, 16–10/*E*,*F*, 17–8/*B*:** Courtesy Dr. Cordula Poulsen Nautrup, Hannover.

**Figure 11–10:** Courtesy Dr. Venker van Haagen, Utrecht.

**Figures 11–11, 11–25:** Redrawn from DeLahunta, A., and R.E. Habel: Applied Veterinary Anatomy. Philadelphia, W.B. Saunders, 1986.

**Figures 11–17/*B*, 15–2, 15–16, 16–3/*C*,*D*, 16–7/*C*,*D*, 16–10/*C*,*D*, 17–1/*C*,*D*, 18–6, 18–26, 23–7, 23–10, 23–13:** Courtesy Dr. Nathan Dykes, Cornell University.

**Figures 11–19, 13–13, 14–9/*A*, 15–19/*B*, 17–3/*D*, 17–7/*C*,*D*, 39–16/*B*:** Courtesy Dr. Bonnie J. Smith, Virginia Technical and State University.

**Figures 13–2, 14–1, 14–2:** After Marthen, G.: Über die Arterien der Körperward des Hundes. Morph. Jahrb. 84:187–219, 1939.

**Figure 15–13:** After Vaerst, L.: Über die Blutversorgung des Hundepenis. Morph. Jahrb. 81:307–352, 1938.

**Figure 15–17:** Redrawn from Christensen, G.C.: Angioarchitecture of the canine penis and the process of erection. Am. J. Anat. 95:227–262, 1954.

**Figures 16–11, 17–9:** Courtesy Dr. R.L. Kitchell, University of California, Davis.

**Figure 18–8:** Courtesy Drs. H.N. Engel and L.L. Blythe, Oregon State University.

**Figures 18–20, 18–21:** Courtesy Dr. I. Kassianoff, Hannover.

**Figure 18–28:** Courtesy Dr. R.P. Hackett, Cornell University.

**Figure 18–30:** Courtesy Dr. Patrick H. McCarthy, University of Sydney.

**Figure 20–4:** After Popesko, P.: Atlas of Topographic Anatomy of the Domestic Animals, Vol. 2: Thoracic and Abdominal Cavities. Philadelphia, W.B. Saunders, 1971.

**Figures 21–15, 21–17, 21–21, 22–25, 23–33, 23–38/*A*, 24–15/*A*:** From (and based on) Schmaltz, R.: Atlas der Anatomie des Pferdes. Vol. 4, Die Eingeweide. Berlin, Paul Parey, 1927; and Schmaltz, R.: Atlas der Anatomie des Pferdes, 3rd ed, Vol. 1. Berlin und Hamburg, Paul Parey, 1911.

**Figures 22–4, 23–9, 23–44:** Modified from Hopkins, G.S.: Guide to the dissection and study of the blood vessels and nerves of the horse, 3rd ed. Ithaca, NY, [Published by the author], 1937.

**Figure 22–13:** Courtesy Dr. R.B. Hillman, Cornell University.

**Figure 23–1:** After Blythe, L.L., and R.L. Kitchell: Electrophysiologic studies of the thoracic limb of the horse. Am. J. Vet. Res. 43:1511–1524, 1982.

**Figure 23–4:** After Ellenberger, W., H. Dittrich, and H. Baum: Atlas of Animal Anatomy for Artists. New York, Dover Publications, 1956.

**Figure 23–14/*B*:** Courtesy Dr. Alan J. Nixon, Cornell University.

**Figures 23–16, 24–4, 24–10/*A*:** After B. Vollmerhaus, München.

**Figure 23–35/*B*:** Courtesy Dr. Natalie Crevier-Denoix, École National Vétérinaire Alfort.

**Figure 23–37:** Courtesy Dr. H. Brugalla, Berlin.

**Figure 24–18:** After Pohlmeyer, K. and R. Redecker: Die für die Klinik bedeutsamen Nerven an den Gliedmassen des Pferdes einschliesslich möglicher Varianten. Deutsche Tierärztl. Wschr. 81:501–505, 1974.

**Figures 25–27, 28–23, 32–15/*A*, 32–16, 33–9/*A*, 33–12/*A*:** Courtesy Dr. J.E. Smallwood, North Carolina State University.

**Figures 25–29, 26–1/*B*, 33–3, 33–10:** Courtesy Dr. Ceferino Maala, University of the Philippines.

**Figures 28–13, 28–16:** Courtesy Dr. Reinhold R. Hofmann, Berlin.

**Figure 28–19:** After Lagerlöf, N.: Investigations of the topography of the abdominal organs in cattle, and some clinical observations and remarks in connection with the subject. Skand. Vet. 19:1–96, 1929.

**Figure 28–22:** After Christ, H.: Nervus Vagus und die Nervengeflechte der Vormägen der Wiederkäuer. Z. Zellforsch. 11:342–374, 1930.

**Figure 29–4:** Redrawn from Habel, R.E.: Guide to the Dissection of Domestic Ruminants, 3rd ed. Ithaca, NY, [Published by the author], 1983.

**Figure 29–5:** From Habel, R.E.: A source of error in the bovine pudendal nerve block. JAVMA 128:16–17, 1956.

**Figure 29–24:** Courtesy Dr. J.R. Hill, Cornell University.

**Figure 31–7:** Courtesy Jeanne Peter, Zürich.

**Figure 32–1:** Courtesy Drs. Alan D. McCauley, veterinary practitioner, and Francis H. Fox, Cornell University.

**Figures 34–1, 34–5, 34–15, 36–1, 36–7:** Drawn by Bud Kramer and D.S. Geary. From Sack, W.O. (ed.): Horowitz/Kramer Atlas of the Musculoskeletal Anatomy of the Pig. Ithaca, NY, Veterinary Textbooks, 1982.

**Figure 34–14:** After Saar, L.I., and R. Getty: The interrelationship of the lymph vessel connections of the lymph nodes of the head, neck, and shoulder regions of swine. Am. J. Vet. Res. 25:618–636, 1964.

**Figure 35–6:** Modified after Baum, H., and H. Grau: Das Lymphgefässsystem des Schweines. Berlin, Paul Parey, 1938.

**Figure 37–9:** After Mollerus, F.W.: Zur funktionellen Anatomie des Eberpenis. Berlin (FU), Vet. Diss., 1967.

**Figure 37–10/*B,C*:** After Meyen, J.: Neue Untersuchungen zur Funktion des Präputialbeutels des Schweines. Zentralbl. Vet. Med. 5:475–492, 1958.

**Figures 39–2, 39–4:** After Lucas, A.M., and P.R. Stettenheim: Avian Anatomy: Integument, Parts I and II. Agriculture Handbook 362. Washington, D.C., U.S. Government Printing Office, 1972.

**Figure 39–20:** Courtesy Dr. Fentener van Vlissingen, Barneveld.

**Figure 39–21/*C*:** After King, A.S., and J. McLelland: Birds—their structure and function, 2nd ed. London, Baillière Tindall, 1984.

**Figure 39–22:** After Komarek, V.: Die Männliche Kloake der Entenvögel. Anat. Anz. 124:434–442, 1969.

**Color Plate 2/*G*:** Courtesy Dr. C. van Vorstenbosch, Utrecht.

**Color Plates 3/*A–C*, 23/*A,B,D,E*, 24/*E*:** Courtesy Dr. M.M. Sloet van Oldenruitenberg-Oosterbaan, Utrecht.

**Color Plates 6/*A*, 23/*D*, 29/*E*:** Courtesy Dr. B. Colenbrander, Utrecht.

**Color Plate 8/*E*:** Courtesy Dr. Douglas F. Antczak, Cornell University.

**Color Plate 10/*A*:** Courtesy Dr. J.M. Fentener van Vlissingen, Barneveld.

**Color Plates 10/*C*, 17/*E,G,H*, 20/*G*:** Courtesy Mr. M. Gaus, Lelystad.

**Color Plates 13/*C,D,G*, 17/*A,B*:** Courtesy Dr. J. Ruberte, Barcelona.

**Color Plates 14/*A–I*, 18/*C,E,F*:** Courtesy Drs. Stades and Bouve, Utrecht.

**Color Plates 16/*E,F,G*, 17/*C,D*:** Courtesy Dr. A.J. Venker van Haagen, Utrecht.

**Color Plates 21 and 22:** Courtesy Dr. Sofie Muylle, Gent.

**Color Plate 23/*C*:** Courtesy Dr. Keith E. Baptiste, Copenhagen.

**Color Plates 24/*I*, 27/*G*:** Courtesy Dr. G.C. van der Weyden, Utrecht.

**Color Plate 24/*J*:** Courtesy Dr. L. de Shaepdrijver, Gent.

**Color Plate 29/*B*:** Courtesy Dr. Claude Pavaux, Toulouse.

**Color Plate 30/*A*:** Courtesy Dr. G.H. Wentink, Arnhem.

**Color Plate 31/*A–D*:** Courtesy Dr. M. Frankenhuis, Amsterdam Zoo.

# CONTENTS

## HORSE



## RUMINANTS



## PIG



## AVIAN

# CHAPTER 1

# Some Basic Facts and Concepts

## THE SCOPE OF ANATOMY

Anatomy is the branch of knowledge concerned with the form, the disposition, and the structure of the tissues and organs that compose the body. The word, which is of Greek origin, literally means "cutting apart," and the dissection of the dead is its traditional, as it remains its primary, method. However, anatomists have long used a host of other techniques to supplement the knowledge of *gross anatomy* that is obtained by use of the scalpel. Details invisible to the naked eye are revealed by light and electron microscopy and constitute the subdivision known as *microscopic anatomy*. The discipline is also extended by the study of the stages through which the organism evolves from conception through birth, youth, and maturity to old age; this study, known as *developmental anatomy,* is rather broader in scope than is classic embryology, which confines its attention to the unborn. Few anatomists are now satisfied by the mere description of the body and its parts, and most seek to understand the relationships between structure and function. The study of these relationships clearly merges into physiology, biochemistry, and other life sciences; it can be described as functional anatomy, but we prefer to regard a functional approach as an attitude that should pervade all branches rather than one constituting a quasi-independent study.

This book is mainly concerned with gross anatomy, a limitation justified by the general practice of presenting microscopic and developmental anatomy in separate courses. Nonetheless, we have allowed ourselves to draw on microscopic and developmental aspects when this has seemed helpful in promoting an understanding of gross anatomy or as a means of enlivening what would otherwise be a rather dry account.

The information obtained by dissection can be arranged and organized in two principal and complementary ways. In the first, *systematic anatomy,* attention is successively directed to groups of organs that are so closely related in their activities that they constitute body systems with an evident common function—the digestive system, the cardiovascular system, and so forth. Systematic anatomy lends itself to a comparative approach; readily combines gross, microscopic, developmental, and functional aspects; and provides the basis for the study of the other medical sciences. Moreover, for the beginner it is easier to understand than regional anatomy. It is the approach employed in Chapters 2 through 10.

The alternative approach, *regional anatomy,* is used in the second and larger part of this book. Regional (or topographical) anatomy is directly concerned with the form and relationships of all the organs present in particular parts or regions of the body. It pays less attention to structure and function, other than the simpler mechanical functions, than does systematic anatomy but obtains a compensating importance from its immediate application to clinical work. Because matters of detail that may lack theoretical interest are often relevant to the clinician, it is necessary to give separate consideration to the regional anatomy of the different species. Regional anatomy is one of the foundations of clinical practice, and different aspects pursued with particular aims are sometimes known as *surface, applied, surgical,* and *radiological anatomy*—terms whose connotations overlap but do not require definition.

## THE LANGUAGE OF ANATOMY

Anatomical language must be precise and unambiguous. In an ideal world each term would have a single meaning, each structure a single name. Unhappily, there has long been an alarming superfluity of terms and much inconsistency in their use. In the hope of reducing this confusion, an internationally agreed-upon vocabulary—*Nomina Anatomica Veterinaria* (NAV)*—was introduced

*There is a separate but similar vocabulary *(Nomina Anatomica Avium)* that is concerned with the anatomy of birds.

in 1968 and has since obtained wide acceptance. It is revised periodically, most recently in 1994, and we have tried to use it consistently throughout this work. Occasionally we have included a second, older, and unofficial alternative when such a term appears to be so deeply rooted in clinical usage that it is unlikely to be eliminated by edict. The terms of the NAV are in Latin, but it is permissible to translate them into vernacular equivalents and is usual in English-speaking countries to do so. We have given preference to translations that so closely resemble the original Latin that the equivalence is immediately recognizable. We therefore give the Latin name only when the translation could be in doubt and then only at the first reference to the structure. No handy English equivalents exist for some official terms; in these cases it is conventional to use the Latin terms, perhaps in abbreviated form, as though they were English words or phrases. The resulting mixture of languages is jarring but not easily avoided, particularly when describing groups of muscles. The names, whether in Latin or in English, are intended to be informative and an aid to comprehension. It is more sensible to look up any whose meaning is not self-evident in an anatomical or medical dictionary than to use them "parrot fashion."

The names that are given to particular structures will be encountered gradually, but the terms that indicate position and direction must be mastered at once. These official terms are more precise than the common alternatives because they retain their relevance regardless of the actual posture of the subject. They are defined in the following list, and their use is illustrated in Figure 1–1. We have not thought it sensible to use them pedantically when there is no reasonable prospect of misunderstanding. When we use common terms (above, behind, and so forth), we always have in mind a standard anatomical position, which, for a quadruped, is that in which the animal stands square and alert. This differs from the human anatomical position and difficulties with terminology will be encountered when consulting books that refer primarily to the human body. Medical anatomists make much use of the terms anterior and posterior, superior and inferior, all of which have very different connotations when applied to quadrupeds. These terms are therefore best avoided except for a few specific applications to the anatomy of the head.

The principal recommended terms of position and direction are arranged in pairs, and it should be emphasized that they refer to relative, not absolute, position. Most of these adjectives form corresponding adverbs by the addition of the suffix *-ly.*

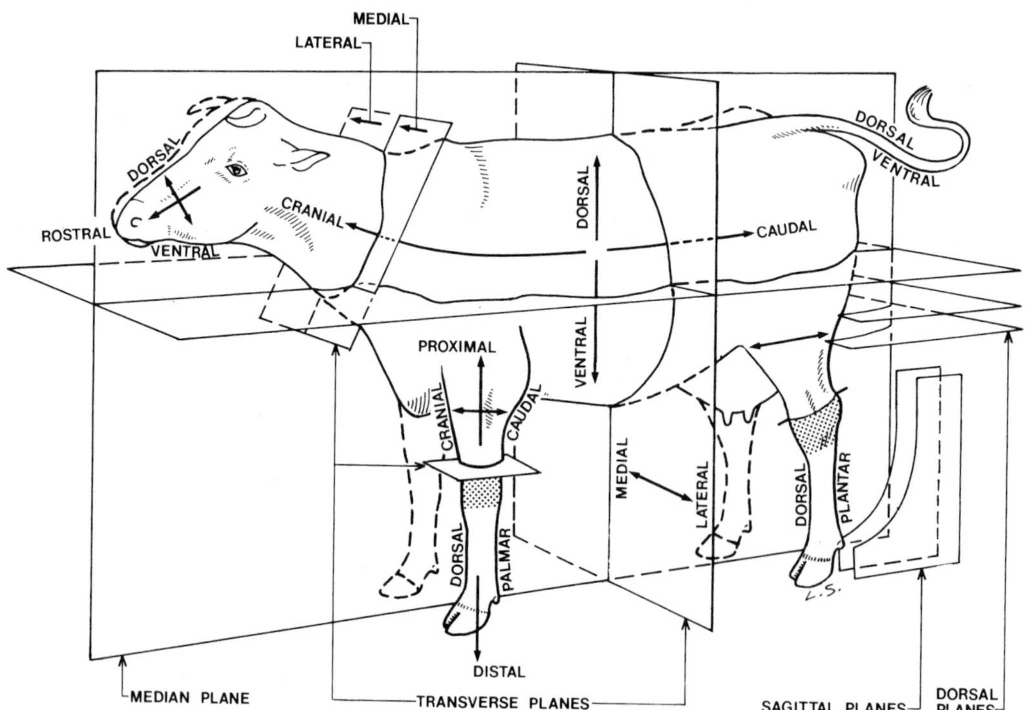


**Figure 1–1.** Directional terms and planes of the animal body. The stippled areas represent the carpus and tarsus on fore- and hindlimbs, respectively.

*Dorsal* structures (or positions) lie toward the back (dorsum) of the trunk or, by extension, toward the corresponding surface of the head or tail.

*Ventral* structures lie toward the belly (venter) or the corresponding surface of the head or tail.

*Cranial* structures lie toward the head (cranium, literally skull), *caudal* ones toward the tail (cauda). Within the head, structures toward the muzzle (rostrum) are said to be *rostral;* caudal remains appropriate.

*Medial* structures lie toward the median plane (medianus, in the middle) that divides the body into symmetrical right and left "halves."

*Lateral* structures lie toward the side (latus, flank) of the animal.

Different conventions apply within the limbs. Structures that lie toward the junction with the body are *proximal* (proximus, near), whereas those at a greater distance are *distal* (distantia, distance). Within the proximal part of the limb (which is defined for this purpose as extending to the proximal limit of the carpus [wrist] or tarsus [hock, ankle]), structures that lie toward the "front" are said to be *cranial,* those that lie toward the "rear," *caudal.* Within the remaining distal part of the limb, structures toward the "front" are *dorsal* (dorsum, back of the hand), and those toward the "rear" are *palmar* (palma, palm of the hand) in the forelimb, *plantar* (planta, sole of the foot) in the hindlimb. Additional terms may be applied to the anatomy of the digits. *Axial* structures lie close to the axis of a central digit, close to the axis of the limb if this passes between two digits; *abaxial* (ab, away from) positions are at a distance from the reference axis.

The terms *external* and *internal, superficial* and *deep* (profundus) hardly require explanation or definition.

Sometimes it is necessary to refer to a section through the body or a part of it (Fig. 1–1). The *median plane* divides the body into symmetrical right and left "halves." Any plane parallel to this is a *sagittal plane,* with those close to the median sometimes being termed *paramedian planes.* A *dorsal plane* sections the trunk or other part parallel to the dorsal surface. A *transverse plane* transects the trunk, head, limb, or other appendage perpendicular to its own long axis.

# AN INTRODUCTION TO REGIONAL ANATOMY

Although the first nine chapters that follow deal with systematic anatomy, those readers who are about to begin a laboratory course will find that they require an elementary knowledge of several systems at once. It is the principal purpose of the remainder of this chapter to supply that background. But first some remarks on the benefits of devoting some attention to the live animal.

## Study of the Live Animal

Regional anatomy is most conveniently studied by the dissection of the embalmed cadaver. This has obvious limitations, however, if the goal is knowledge of the anatomy of the living. When embalmed, organs are uncharacteristically inert and greatly changed in color and consistency from their living state. The impressions gained in the dissection room must therefore be modified and corrected by frequent reference to fresh material and by observation of surgical operations whenever possible. Since most of those who study the anatomy of domestic animals do so with a future professional career in mind, they will find it both stimulating and advantageous to learn how to apply the simpler methods of clinical examination to normal animals at this stage in their training. Students in some departments receive elementary instruction in these methods; others must create their own opportunities, perhaps by enlisting the assistance of senior student colleagues. They will find a little direct experience to be far more rewarding than much unsupported reading. We merely list some methods and rely on our colleagues in the clinics to provide more adequate guidance.

The simplest method is *observation* of the contours, the proportions, and the posture of the body. Bony projections provide the clearest landmarks, but superficial muscles and blood vessels are also useful, if less striking; reference to these landmarks allows the positions of other structures to be deduced from their known relationships. Little experience is required to reveal the importance of breed, age, sex, and individual variation, or to show that although some landmarks are fixed and reliable, others are prone to move. Some (e.g., the costal arch) move with each respiration, whereas other features change more gradually, for example, becoming more or less prominent or shifting in position with the deposition or depletion of fat or with the advance of pregnancy.

Structures that are not directly visible may be identified by touch, by gentle or firmer *palpation* as circumstances require. Bones may be identified by their rigidity, muscles by their contraction, arteries by pulsation, veins by swelling when the blood flow is interrupted by pressure, and lymph nodes and internal organs by their size, configuration, and consistency. But variation is great and is affected by many factors that make it difficult to know whether one should expect to be able to identify certain organs in all normal subjects—another useful lesson. Palpation through the skin can be supplemented by digital or manual exploration per rectum and per vaginam.

Certain organs may be identified by *percussion* to elicit resonance when the overlying skin is struck a sharp blow (in a prescribed fashion). Different materials produce different notes; that from a gas-filled organ is more resonant than the duller one elicited from an organ that is solid or filled with fluid. The normal activities of certain organs produce sounds continuously or intermittently. Although the lungs and heart (not forgetting the fetal heart) are the prime examples of organs whose position can be determined by *auscultation,* the movement of blood within vessels or of gas or ingesta within the stomach or intestines can also be a useful source of anatomical information. It must not be forgotten when applying these two techniques that the vagaries of sound conduction through materials of different densities may provide a distorted indication of the position and dimensions of the source.

The study of the anatomy of the live animal can be enlarged by other methods whose exercise requires considerable training and more elaborate apparatus than the simple stethoscope. These additional procedures have provided a variety of new illustrations scattered through later chapters but, while some elementary knowledge of how these illustrations were obtained may assist their appreciation, detailed consideration of the various technologies involved is clearly beyond the scope of this book.*

Many parts and cavities that are normally out of sight can be brought into view by the use of various instruments. Perhaps the most familiar of these are the ophthalmoscope, used to study the fundus of the eye, and the otoscope, used to explore the external ear canal. Other instruments, for which the generic title "endoscope" is available, may be introduced into natural orifices and advanced to allow inspection of deeper parts, such as the nasal cavity, bronchial tree, or gastric lumen. These examples of *endoscopy* are noninvasive but other examinations require preparatory surgery. Among these are arthroscopy, the inspection of the interior of synovial joints, and laparoscopy, the technique in which an endoscope is passed into the peritoneal cavity through a small opening in the abdominal wall. This last technique may be employed for diagnostic purposes or for the visual control of ("keyhole") surgery using instruments introduced through separate portals. For both purposes moderate inflation of the abdomen creates the necessary viewing chamber.

Early endoscopes were rigid, which limited their utility, but the modern fiber-optic version is flexible and can negotiate bends while its tip may be turned, under remote control, to widen the field that may be scrutinized. The essential components of the fiber-optic instrument are two bundles of glass fibers. Such fibers, when suitably prepared and coated, conduct light from one end to the other without significant leakage to the side. One bundle is used to convey light distally, from an external source to the region to be viewed; the component fibers can be relatively coarse and randomly arranged. The second bundle conveys the image and is composed of finer fibers that maintain fixed positions in relation to each other. The image is composed of very many tiny units, each corresponding to an individual fiber, and is presented to the eye (or to a camera or video system) at the proximal end of the instrument.

*Radiographic anatomy* has for some time been an indispensable component of every course of anatomy influenced by clinical considerations. Most departments routinely display previously prepared radiographs and, while students are unlikely to be involved in their production, it is prudent to remind them that considerable risks are associated with x-radiation, risks that must always be assessed for those conducting and those subjected to these procedures.

X-rays are produced by bombarding with electrons a tungsten target (focus) housed within a shielded tube. Only a narrow x-ray beam is permitted to escape and this is directed toward the relevant region of the subject. The passage of the rays through the body is affected by the tissues they encounter; tissues substantially composed of elements of high atomic weight tend to scatter or absorb the rays; tissues substantially composed of elements of low atomic weight have proportionately less effect. Bone with its calcium content clearly belongs to the first (radiopaque) category while soft tissues generally belong to the second (radiolucent) category. Those rays that succeed in passing through the subject are allowed to impinge upon a sensitive film (or other detector) which

*Readers desiring more detailed information will find the following titles helpful: Burk, R.L., and N. Ackerman: Small Animal Radiology and Ultrasonography, 2nd ed. Philadelphia, W.B. Saunders Company, 1996; Feeney, D.A., T.F. Fletcher, and R.M. Hardy: Atlas of Correlative Imaging: Anatomy of the Normal Dog. Philadelphia, W.B. Saunders Company, 1991; Nyland, T.G., and J.S. Mattoon: Veterinary Diagnostic Ultrasound. Philadelphia, W.B. Saunders Company, 1995; Thrall, D.E. (ed.): Textbook of Veterinary Diagnostic Radiology, 3rd ed. Philadelphia, W.B. Saunders Company, 1998.

responds to the radiation received. When the film is developed those areas that were overlain by soft tissues (or gas-filled spaces) appear dark, even black, while those areas that were overlain by bone (or other radiopaque material) appear lighter, even white. The distinction between tissues of similar radiodensity may be enhanced by introducing an appropriate contrast agent to coat a surface or fill a space. Specific methods, utilizing various materials, are available to depict such different features as the gastric lumen, urinary tract, and subarachnoid space.

Radiographic views are appropriately identified by reference to the direction taken by the x-ray beam in its passage through the subject. Thus a radiograph of a supine animal, presenting its belly toward the x-ray source, is described as a ventrodorsal film; that obtained with the animal turned over, with its belly now facing the film, is described as a dorsoventral film. The convention provides little scope for confusion but occasionally produces an awkward term, such as dorsolateral-plantaromedial which specifies a particular, oblique view of the hock.

Awareness of certain general principles will help in the avoidance of some common misinterpretations: the image of any structure is always magnified to the degree determined by the ratio focus-film : focus-object; the divergence of the x-rays produces an apparent shift in position of any object not directly below the focus. Two simple diagrams (Fig. 1–2) will make these points clear. A less easily resolved difficulty results from the superimposition of the images of structures that lie over each other. An ingenious, only partly successful, solution to this problem was sought in the coordinated movement—in opposite directions—of tube and film during the period of the exposure (Fig. 1–3/*A*). In this technique, known as tomography, the axis about which tube and film travel coincides with the plane of the horizontal slice of the subject that is of current interest. Structures contained within this slice remain more or less in focus throughout the exposure,

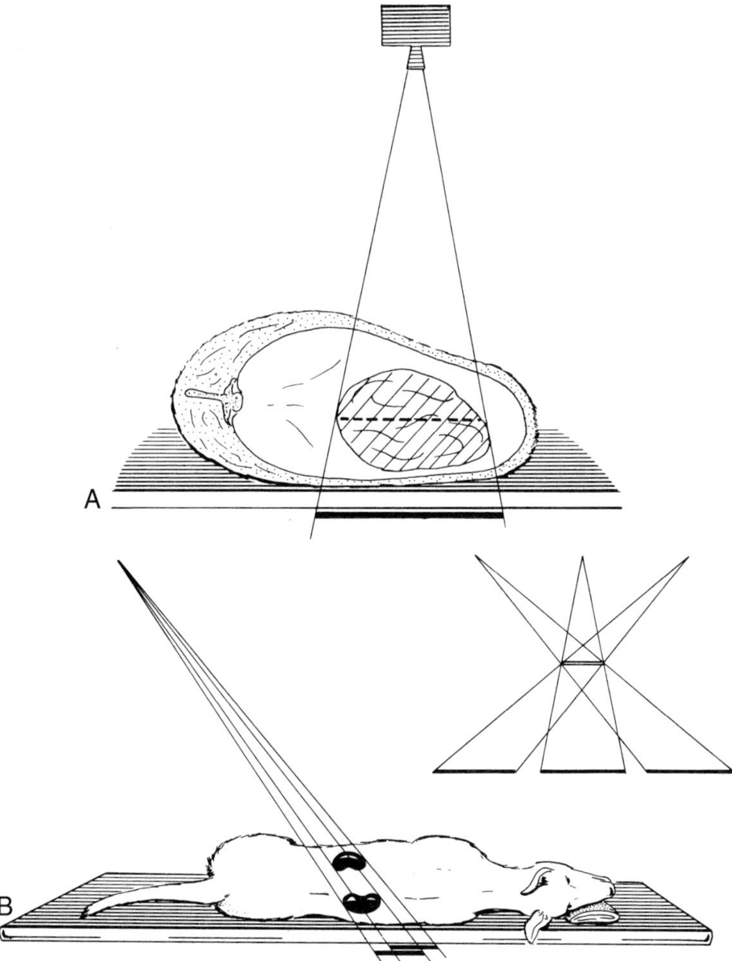


**Figure 1–2.** *A*, Schematic drawing illustrating the magnifying effect caused by the divergence of the x-rays. *B*, Schematic drawing illustrating the apparent shift in position of an organ that is not directly below the focus.

while the images produced by structures at other levels are blurred or subsumed within the general background. Such tomograms never found much employment in veterinary radiology. The more recently developed and more sophisticated technique known as *computed tomography* (CT) has a different basis but retains the aim of clearly depicting the parts within one particular body slice while excluding extraneous images. Despite the considerable cost of the apparatus, and its limited suitability for use with large animals, the technique is now widely offered by veterinary referral centers.

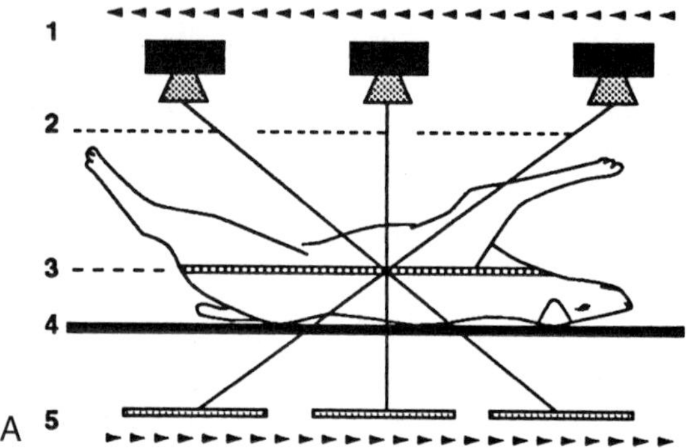


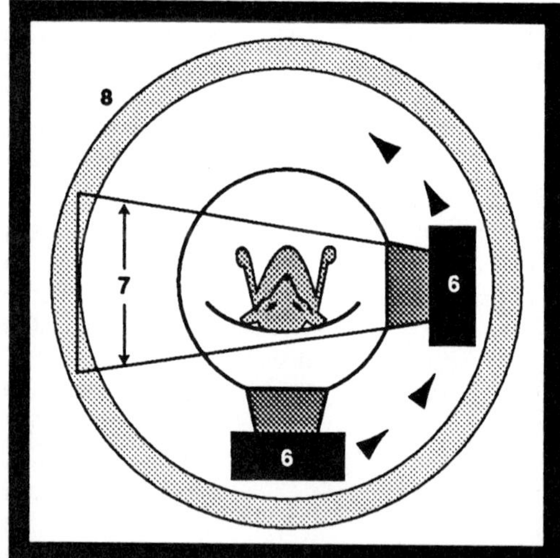


**Figure 1–3.** Diagrams of a basic (noncomputed) x-ray tomographic apparatus *(A),* and of a fourth-generation computed tomographic (CT) scanner *(B).*

1, Movement of x-ray source during exposure; 2, lines indicating mechanical connection between x-ray source and radiation detector (i.e., film); 3, plane of focus; 4, supine patient on stationary table; 5, movement (in the opposite direction) of detector during exposure; 6, movement of x-ray source around stationary patient; 7, x-ray beam during exposure; 8, ring of fixed detectors surrounding the rotating x-ray tube mechanism.

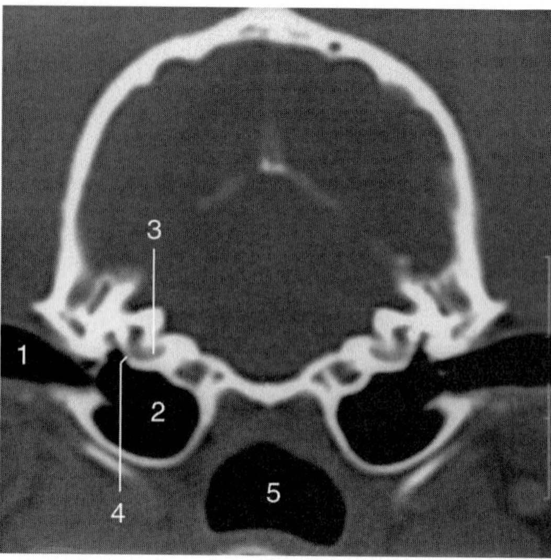


**Figure 1–4.** Transverse image of a 2-mm-thick computed tomographic slice of the canine tympanic bullae and petrous temporal bones. (Bone settings were used.)

1, External acoustic meatus; 2, tympanic bulla; 3, cochlea; 4, round window; 5, nasopharynx.

In the modern CT scanner, the x-ray source is moved in a circle, centered upon the longitudinal axis of the subject, during the procedure which takes from one to several seconds for its completion (*/B*). During this time the movement of the tube is repeatedly arrested but for very short periods; during each of these a burst of radiation is directed through the subject along a different radius. The beams that penetrate the selected, very narrow, slice of the subject impinge upon a series of discrete detectors or, in some designs, upon portions of a continuous circumferential detector, and are photomultiplied. The procedure completed, these records are analyzed, compared, and combined according to complex formulae (algorithms*); from these computations there is constructed a single cross-sectional image in which are represented the forms, the locations, and the comparative radiodensities of all the tissues within the selected body slice (Fig. 1–4). In more complex settings, multiple overlapping or adjacent slices can be imaged in an extended, continuous process. With the amount of information the extended process supplies it is possible by even more elaborate computation to construct images in other than transverse planes. The data may also be manipulated to enhance subtle differences in contrast presented by tissues of very similar radiodensity.

---

*Algorithms generate solutions to complex problems, solutions that while not absolutely accurate are yet sufficiently precise for practical purposes.

Computed tomography is of course not free from all drawbacks: subjects must be strictly immobilized during the relatively lengthy exposure procedure; the total radiation dose may be quite considerable, even though individual exposures are very short and the resulting images amplified; artifacts may produce deceptive images; current apparatus designed for medical use is suitable for small animals but must be adapted for application with large animals and is then limited to the investigation of the head and limbs. One by-product of CT is the revival of interest in cross-sectional anatomy, an approach to the discipline until recently regarded as irretrievably passé but now clearly indispensable for CT interpretation.

Familiarity with cross-sectional anatomy is also required for the practice of *ultrasonography.* This technique depends upon the capacity of a piezoelectric crystal to convert electrical energy into sound waves, and vice versa. When stimulated, a suitably housed crystal transducer, coupled to the appropriate area of skin, directs a narrow beam of sound waves of uniform frequency into the body. The waves are propagated through the tissues with decaying intensity, and with a fraction directed back toward their source at each encounter with an interface between tissues offering different resistance (acoustical impedance). Reconverted into electrical energy, the echoes generate a visible image on a screen. This image, which can be "frozen" or recorded in various ways, represents the thin body slice directly below the transducer. The sound wave is not produced continuously but in very short bursts, perhaps lasting for no more than one-millionth part of a second. The longer silences that alternate with these bursts allow the time necessary for the receipt of echoes bounced back from interfaces at different depths.

The frequency and the wavelength of sound waves are inversely related. The first parameter determines the depth to which waves will penetrate, the second the resolution that may be obtained—the detail that may be distinguished. Since waves of high frequency penetrate less deeply but record more detail, a compromise is involved when selecting the appropriate crystal to deploy for a specific examination—for several crystals are normally to hand, each with its own inherent and invariable oscillation frequency. The maximum depth from which it is possible to obtain useful images is about 25 cm and this limits the application of ultrasonography in horses and cattle. In these large species its use is more or less restricted to the examination of the distal parts of the limbs and to pregnancy diagnosis (when the transducer may be applied to the rectal mucosa). Ultrasonography is also widely used in the diagnosis of pregnancy in sows (although here a transabdominal approach is employed).

Water, blood, and most soft tissues offer very similar acoustical impedance, and interfaces between these substances are at best only moderately reflective—they are hypoechoic in ultrasonographers' jargon. In contrast, the difference in impedance between soft tissue and bone, or between soft tissue and a gas-filled cavity, is very large and the reflection of sound waves is almost total—the interface is hyperechoic. This makes it impossible to image tissues and organs that, like the brain within the skull, lie deep to bone; such parts are said to be within acoustical shadow. Conversely, a distended bladder, or other large volume of uniform impedance, may be used as a window through which deeper structures may be approached.

There are many differences in transducer design and usage. Some transducers contain multiple crystals arranged in line; when these are activated sequentially, the resulting image is rectangular and represents the thin slice of tissue situated deep to the transducer. More often a single crystal is employed but so arranged that the narrow beam that it generates swings repetitively in an arc, producing a wedge- or sector-shaped image (Fig. 1–5). In these B (or brightness) settings the image represents a cross section through the field surveyed. In the alternative M (or motion) setting the beam is only emitted at one fixed point in the crystal's oscillation and the recording is therefore limited to the structures penetrated along a single axis; if the parts are moving, successive images reveal their changing shapes, changes emphasized if successive images are recorded side by side. M-mode recordings are especially useful for demonstrating the movements of the walls of the heart chambers and valves.

Ultrasonograms are, in general, less easy for the novice to interpret than radiographs. Reverberations occur when the waves bounce back and forth, often because of defective coupling of the transducer to the skin, and this may produce what appear to be multiple parallel interfaces within an organ. Small interfaces between the parenchyma and fibrous scaffolding of certain tissues produce diffuse scattering, a stippled effect. Despite these (and other) drawbacks, ultrasonography possesses very considerable advantages, not the least being its freedom from the risks inescapably associated with ionizing radiation.

*Magnetic resonance imaging* (MRI) requires less extensive consideration since the expense of the installation and operation of the equipment make it presently available in only a few veterinary

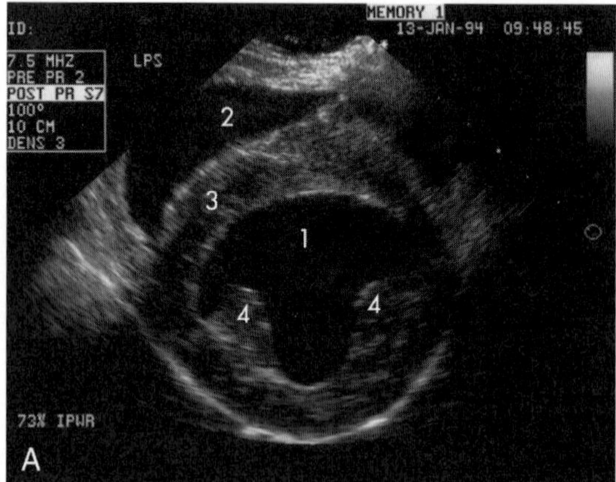


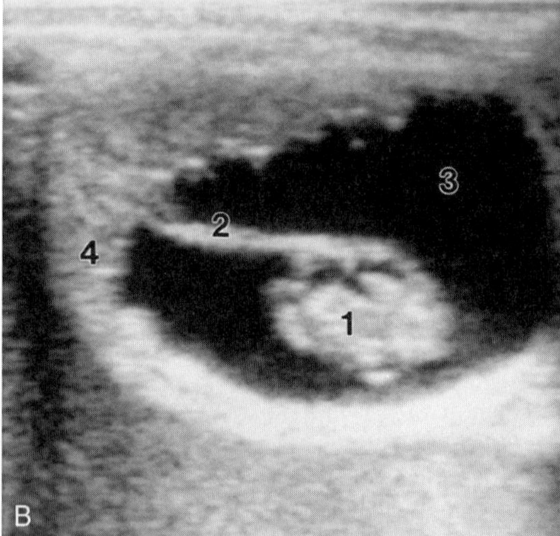


**Figure 1–5.** *A*, Ultrasonographic transverse (short-axis) view of the canine heart.

1, Left ventricle; 2, right ventricle; 3, septum; 4, papillary muscles.

*B*, Ultrasonographic view of a 42-day-old equine embryo.

1, Embryo, about 2 cm in length; 2, umbilical cord; 3, allantoic fluid; 4, uterine wall.

centers. The theoretical basis of MRI lies in changes in the structure of hydrogen atoms induced by strong magnetic fields and radio waves. Weak radio signals are subsequently produced when the subatomic structure returns to its normal configuration. These signals may be amplified and their origins within the body precisely fixed in three dimensions. Since different tissues contain different concentrations of hydrogen atoms, their different responses can be used for their distinction. Tissues, such as fat, that are rich in hydrogen produce bright images in contrast to the black images of hydrogen-poor tissues such as bone (Fig. 1–6). Extremely high resolution is possible. There appear to be no health risks associated with the MRI scanner. Both CT and MRI are especially useful in the study of intracranial structures.

## Skin

The skin covers the body and protects it against injury; it plays an important part in temperature control and enables the animal to respond to various external stimuli by virtue of its many nerve endings. There are numerous local modifications of skin (Chapter 10), but at present we are concerned only with its more general properties.

The skin varies greatly in thickness and flexibility, both among species and locally. It is naturally thicker in larger animals (though not in constant

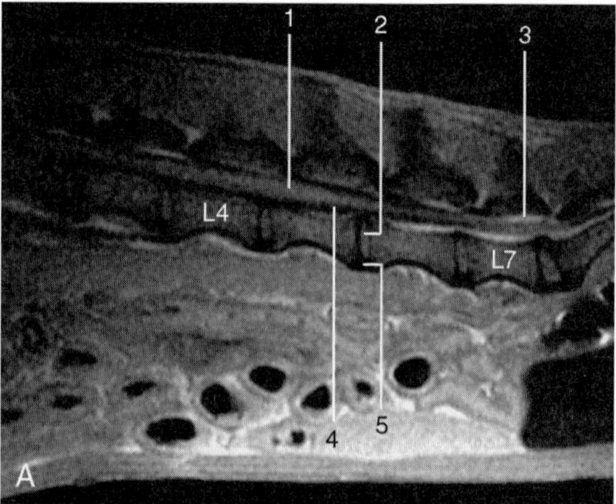


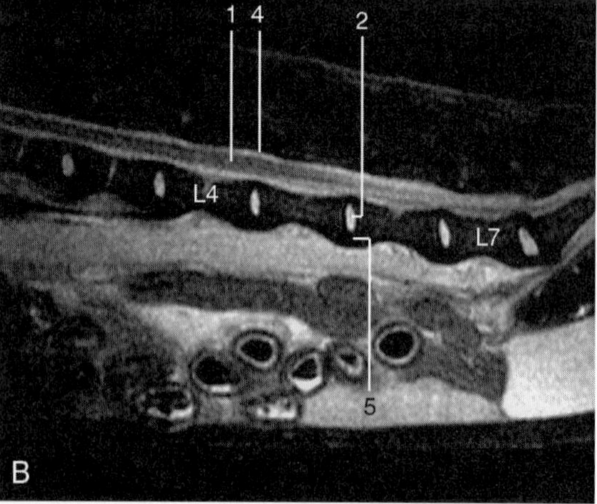


**Figure 1–6.** Midsagittal images of 3-mm-thick spine-echo magnetic resonance slices of the canine lumbar vertebral column. *A*, T1-weighted (fat appears white, fluids dark). *B*, T2-weighted (fluids appear white, fat darker than on T1-weighted images).

1, Spinal cord; 2, nucleus pulposus; 3, epidural fat; 4, cerebrospinal fluid; 5, annulus fibrosus.

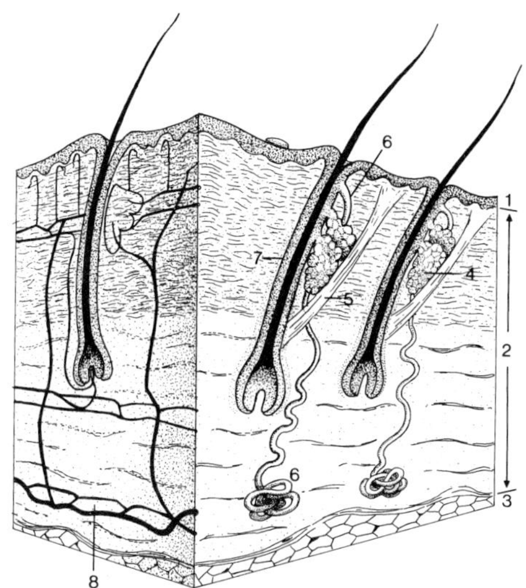


**Figure 1–7.** A block of skin.

1, Epidermis; 2, dermis; 3, subcutis; 4, sebaceous gland; 5, arrector pili muscle; 6, sweat gland; 7, hair follicle; 8, arterial networks.

proportion to their size) and in more exposed areas; these inequalities are obviously important to the surgeon. Although the skin is generally closely molded to the underlying structures, it appears redundant in some areas, forming folds and creases; some folding allows for change in posture, some is an adaptation to increase the area through which heat may be dissipated to the environment, and some is no more than the expression of breeders' whims, grotesquely illustrated by the Shar-Pei breed of dog.

Skin consists of two layers, an outer epidermis and an inner dermis, and in most situations it rests on a looser connective tissue variously known as the subcutis, hypodermis, or superficial fascia (Fig. 1–7). The epidermis is a stratified squamous epithelium whose thickness is adapted to the treatment it receives; it responds to rough usage, as exemplified by the footpads of dogs and cats. Numerous modifications of this layer exist, the most common being the occurrence of sweat and sebaceous glands and of hair. Sweat glands are most important as a provision for heat loss by surface evaporation but also play a subsidiary role in the excretion of waste. The sebaceous glands produce an oily secretion that waterproofs the surface and provides certain relatively naked areas, such as the groin of horses, with a characteristic sheen. Both types of gland are usually widely, though not ubiquitously, spread. The haircoat, which is a uniquely mammalian feature, is a mechanical protection and a thermal insulator, the latter property depending on the entrapment of air within the pile. The haircoat is usually widespread. Among the more familiar species, only the human and the pig are relatively naked, although naked individuals may appear in other species and as occasional "sports," the origin, for example, of the Sphynx breed of cat. Some aquatic mammals, such as whales, are wholly naked.

The dermis, which consists essentially of felted connective tissue fibers, is the raw material of leather. It is secured to the epidermis by interlocking papillae, which are most pronounced where normal wear might risk separation. In most situations, the skin moves easily over the underlying tissues, and this looseness facilitates the flaying of a carcass. It is more tightly bound down in a few places where it grades into a tougher-than-usual underlying fascia; good examples of this binding are provided by the scrotum and the lips. Some risk of pressure injury is present where the dermis is molded over bony prominences, and synovial bursae (p. 25) often develop adventitiously in such sites. Unlike the epidermis, the dermis is well supplied with blood vessels (Fig. 1–7) and cutaneous nerves.

The superficial fascia is considered in the following section.

## Fascia and Fat

The connective tissue that separates and surrounds the more obviously important structures is generically known as *fascia,* a term of rather elastic usage; many of its larger accumulations, particularly those of a sheetlike nature, have specific names. This tissue frequently receives scant notice from the dissector, which is unwise, since it has significant functions to perform. Moreover, fascia is encountered in surgery, when it is necessary to predict its nature and extent in different situations.

The *superficial fascia* (subcutis) is a loose (areolar) tissue extensively spread below the skin of animals that possess a hairy coat. A similar tissue surrounds many deeper organs, and in both situations, the loose fascia allows neighboring structures to change in shape and to move easily against each other. Its looseness varies with the amount of fluid it contains and may provide an indication of ill health. The superficial fascia is one of the principal sites for the storage of fat. In naked species, the fat forms a continuous layer, the panniculus adiposus.

The *deep fascia* is generally organized into much tougher fibrous sheets. A layer beneath the superficial fascia extends over most of the body and fuses to bony prominences. In many places it detaches septa that penetrate between the muscles,

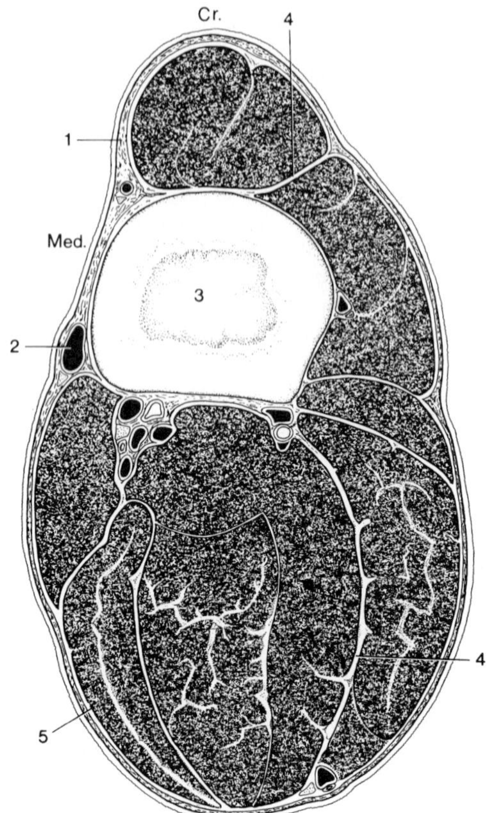


**Figure 1–8.** Osteofascial compartments in the forearm of a horse.

1, Superficial fascia; 2, cephalic vein; 3, radius; 4, septa of deep fascia enclosing individual muscles or groups of muscles; 5, deep fascia. (In transverse sections of the limbs, cranial [Cr.] and medial [Med.] are identified.)

enclosing them individually or in groups (Fig. 1–8); sometimes the periosteum, the fibrous covering of the bones, participates in outlining the enclosures. This division into fascial or osteofascial compartments is very prominent in the forearm and leg and plays a part in the circulation, assisting the return of blood and lymph to the heart. Muscles thicken when they contract, and when they are contained within unyielding walls they compress any other structures that share the space. If these are valved tubes (veins and lymphatic vessels), their contents are squeezed in one direction, toward the heart. Because of this, muscular paralysis or prolonged inactivity may lead to stasis of blood or lymph flow. Arteries and nerves whose functions would not be assisted by compression often travel in small tunnels within the septa.

More specific functions can be assigned to localized thickenings (retinacula: tethers) of deep fascia, which hold tendons in place and sometimes provide pulleys around which the tendons wind to change direction. Good examples are provided by the retinacula on the dorsal aspect of the hock and the palmar aspect of the digits (Fig. 1–9/9).

Since dense fascia is relatively impermeable, it determines the direction taken by spreading fluids, such as pus, which sometimes tracks below a fascial sheet before breaking through far from its source. This is one reason why some knowledge of the deep fascia is useful to the surgeon. Its toughness enables it to hold sutures securely while it also provides cleavage planes, which allow relatively bloodless access to deeper parts during surgery.

Most deposits of *fat* (adipose tissue) may be regarded primarily as food reserves. Small amounts of fat are widely distributed, but the bulk is con-

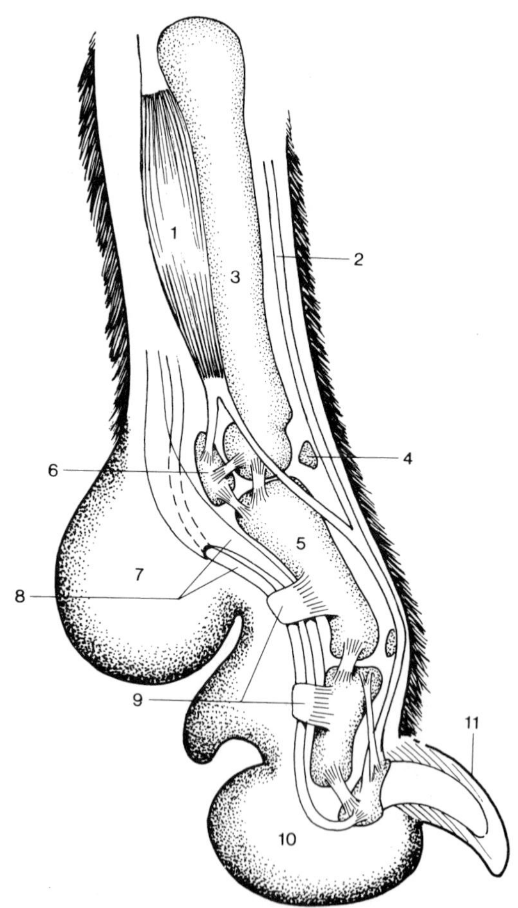


**Figure 1–9.** Axial section of a dog's paw; the metacarpal pad (7) is in contact with the ground during standing.

1, Interosseous; 2, extensor tendon; 3, metacarpal bone; 4, dorsal sesamoid bone; 5, proximal phalanx; 6, proximal sesamoid bone; 7, metacarpal pad; 8, flexor tendons; 9, retinacula; 10, digital pad; 11, claw.

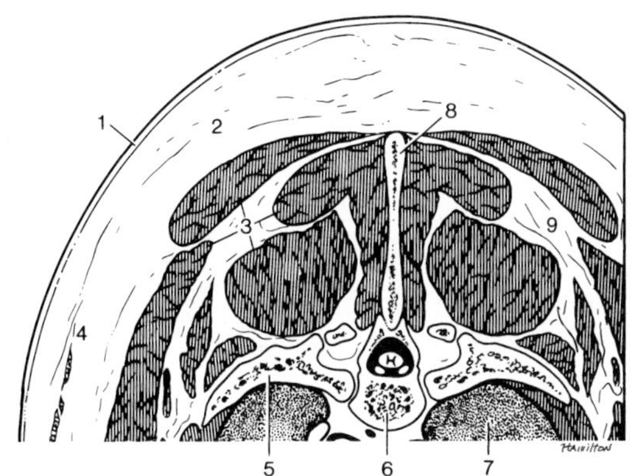


**Figure 1–10.** Transverse section of the back of a pig.

1, Skin; 2, fat (panniculus adiposus) associated with the superficial fascia; 3, back muscles; 4, cutaneous muscle enclosed within superficial fascia; 5, rib; 6, thoracic vertebra 5; 7, lung; 8, spinous process of vertebra; 9, additional fat deposited between muscles.

tained in three or four places: in the superficial fascia (Fig. 1–10/2); between and within muscles; below the peritoneum (the delicate membrane lining the abdominal cavity); and in the marrow cavities of long bones. Subcutaneous fat deposits help mold the body contours and often show specific and sexual differences in localization and development. Animals that are adapted to torrid habitats often develop localized depots (e.g., humped zebu cattle, camels, fat-tailed sheep), since a more even distribution might interfere with heat loss to the environment. Some of the differences in the body form of men and women that become accentuated at puberty are produced by the deposition of fat in the breasts and over the hips and lower abdomen of girls. In many male animals, much fat is deposited in the tissues of the dorsal part of the neck—the thickened crest of stallions is a good example.

Some fat deposits, like that enclosed within a fibrous lattice in the footpad of the dog, function as mechanical buffers (Fig. 1–9/7,10). Fat with a mechanical function is usually resistant to mobilization in starvation.

Differences in the chemical and physical nature of fat can be pronounced but may reflect diet as much as specific genetic factors. It is certainly often useful, when required to determine the origin of a specimen, to know that the fat of horses and of Channel Island breeds of cattle is yellow, that of sheep hard and white, and that of pigs soft and grayish. It should also be remembered that fat at body temperature is softer (semifluid) than that exposed in a colder environment. Certain procedures—liposuction and lipofixation—employed by the cosmetic surgeon depend on this fortunate circumstance.

All these remarks refer to the common sort of fat. A second variety, *brown fat,* is of much more restricted distribution in time and place. Brown fat differs in structure (Fig. 1–11) and function as well as in color. In domestic species it is especially found during the fetal and neonatal periods; in wild species it is especially prominent in those that hibernate (Fig. 1–12). It provides both groups with a readily available source of heat, equally useful in newborn animals with imperfect thermoregulation and in hibernators required to awaken rapidly from the deep winter sleep.

## Bones

The primary functions of the skeleton are to support the body, to provide the system of levers used in locomotion, and to protect soft parts. Therefore, biomechanical factors are most important in shaping the bones and in determining their microscopic design. The major skeletal tissue, bone, has a secondary role in mineral homeostasis, supplying a reserve of calcium, phosphate, and other ions.

### *The Classification of Bones*

Bones may be classified in various ways. A topographical classification recognizes a cranial skeleton (of the head) and a postcranial skeleton consisting of two divisions: the axial skeleton of the trunk and the appendicular skeleton of the limbs. A second classification based on ontogeny distinguishes the somatic skeleton, formed in the body wall, from the visceral skeleton, derived from the pharyngeal (branchial) arches. A third system is also based on development and distinguishes

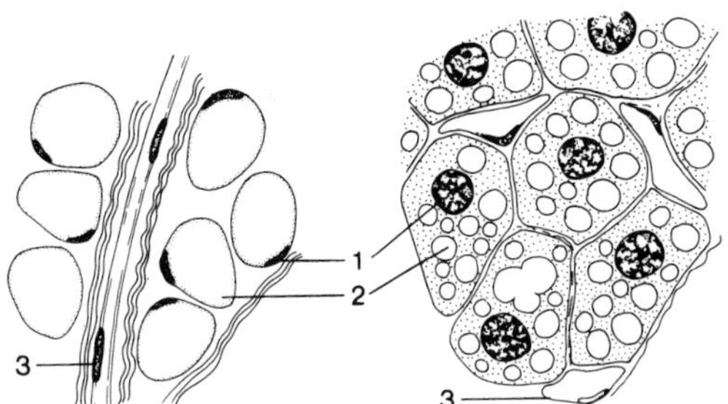


**Figure 1–11.** Fat cells of white *(left)* and brown *(right)* fat. In white fat a single large fat vacuole displaces the cytoplasm and the nucleus to the periphery of the cell. The small fat vacuoles are evenly distributed in the cells of brown fat.

1, Nuclei; 2, fat vacuoles; 3, capillaries.

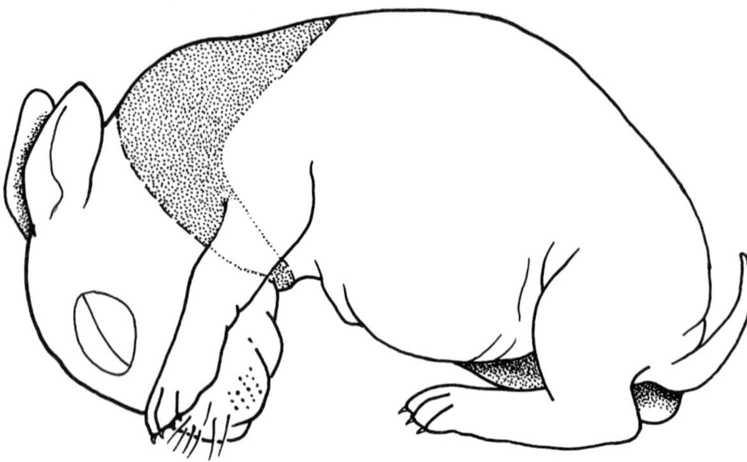

**Figure 1–12.** The distribution of brown fat in the newborn rabbit, concentrated around the neck and between the shoulder blades.

parts preformed in cartilage (and later largely replaced by bone) from those that ossify directly in fibrous connective tissue. This classification reflects the phylogeny, since bones that develop in membrane are homologous with dermal bones of lower vertebrates.

Individual bones are classified by shape according to a rather naive system (Fig. 1–13). *Long bones,* which are typical of the limbs, are broadly cylindrical and are clearly adapted to perform as levers. It is perhaps more important to know that they develop from at least three centers of ossification: one for the shaft (diaphysis), and one for each extremity (epiphysis) (p. 72).

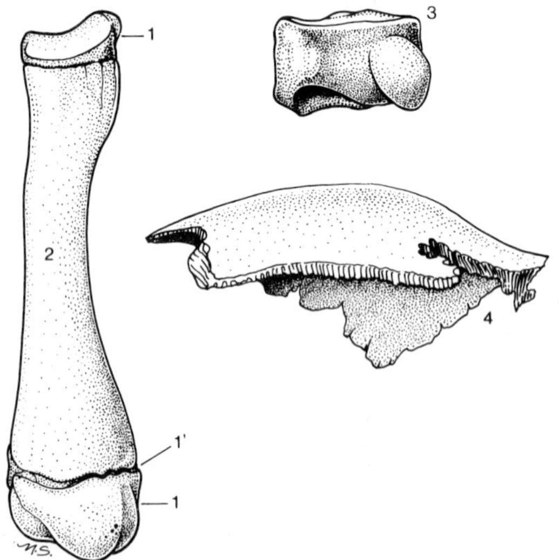


**Figure 1–13.** Long, short, and flat bones.

1, Proximal and distal epiphyses; 1′, epiphysial cartilage; 2, diaphysis of a young dog's radius; 3, carpal bone of a horse; 4, parietal bone from the skull of a dog.

*Short bones* have no dimension that greatly exceeds the others. Many are grouped together at the carpus and tarsus, where the multiplication of articulations makes provision for complex movements and may also diminish concussion. The majority of short bones develop from a single center of ossification; replication of centers generally indicates that the bone represents the fusion of elements distinct in ancestral forms.

*Flat bones* are expanded in two directions. The category includes the scapula, the bones of the pelvic girdle, and many of those of the skull. Their broad surfaces afford attachment to large muscle masses and protection to underlying soft parts.

The remaining bones are too irregular in form to be grouped in clearly defined categories. Neither flat nor irregular bones exhibit uniformity in development.

## The Organization of a Long Bone

Many features of bone construction are conveniently approached through the examination of a longitudinal section of a long bone (Fig. 1–14)/*A*). The form of the bone is determined by a sheath or *cortex* of solid (compact) bone that is composed of thin lamellae arranged mainly in series of concentric tubes about small central canals. Each such system is known as an osteone (/*B*). The cortex is thick toward the middle of the shaft but thins as it flares toward each extremity, over which it continues as a crust. The external surface is smooth except where irregularities serve as the attachment sites of muscles or ligaments; these irregularities may be raised or depressed and in both cases permit a concentration of the attachment. These features are generally most pronounced in larger, older males. They are given a variety of descriptive

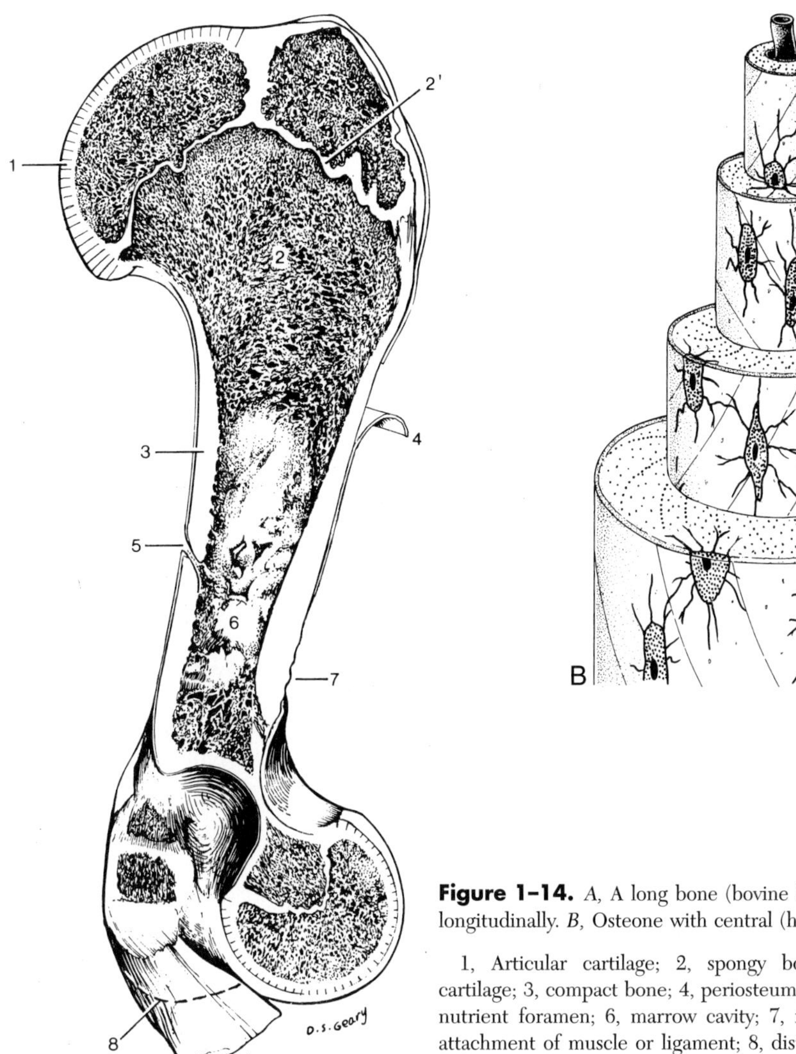


**Figure 1–14.** *A,* A long bone (bovine humerus) sectioned longitudinally. *B,* Osteone with central (haversian) canal.

1, Articular cartilage; 2, spongy bone; 2′, epiphysial cartilage; 3, compact bone; 4, periosteum, partly reflected; 5, nutrient foramen; 6, marrow cavity; 7, roughened area for attachment of muscle or ligament; 8, distal extent of medial epicondyle; 9, tendon of origin of carpal and digital flexors.

names of conventional significance; most elevations are known as lines, crests, tubercles, tuberosities, or spines; most depressions, as fossae or grooves (sulci).

The inner surface of the shaft bounds a central medullary (marrow) cavity and is rough; the irregularities are low, indiscriminate, and without apparent significance.

The extremities are occupied by cancellous or *spongy bone,* which forms a three-dimensional lattice of interlacing spicules, plates, and tubes of varying density.

The medullary cavity and the interstitial spaces of the spongy bone are occupied by *bone marrow,* which occurs in two intergrading forms. Red bone marrow is a richly vascularized, gelatinous tissue with hemopoietic properties; it produces the red and granular white corpuscles of the blood. Although all marrow is of this type in the young animal, most is later infiltrated with fat and converted into waxy yellow marrow whose hemopoietic potential is dormant. It is the marrow in the larger spaces that first becomes inactive, then that of the spongy bone of the distal limb bones, until finally active marrow is confined to the proximal extremities of the humerus and femur, the bones of the limb girdles, and those of the axial skeleton. The chronology of these events for domestic animals is uncertain.

The parts that articulate with neighboring bones are smooth. These articular surfaces are more extensive than are the areas in contact in any position of the joint to make provision for a range of movement. They are clothed in hyaline *articular cartilage,* which, for present purposes, may be regarded as a residue of the cartilaginous model

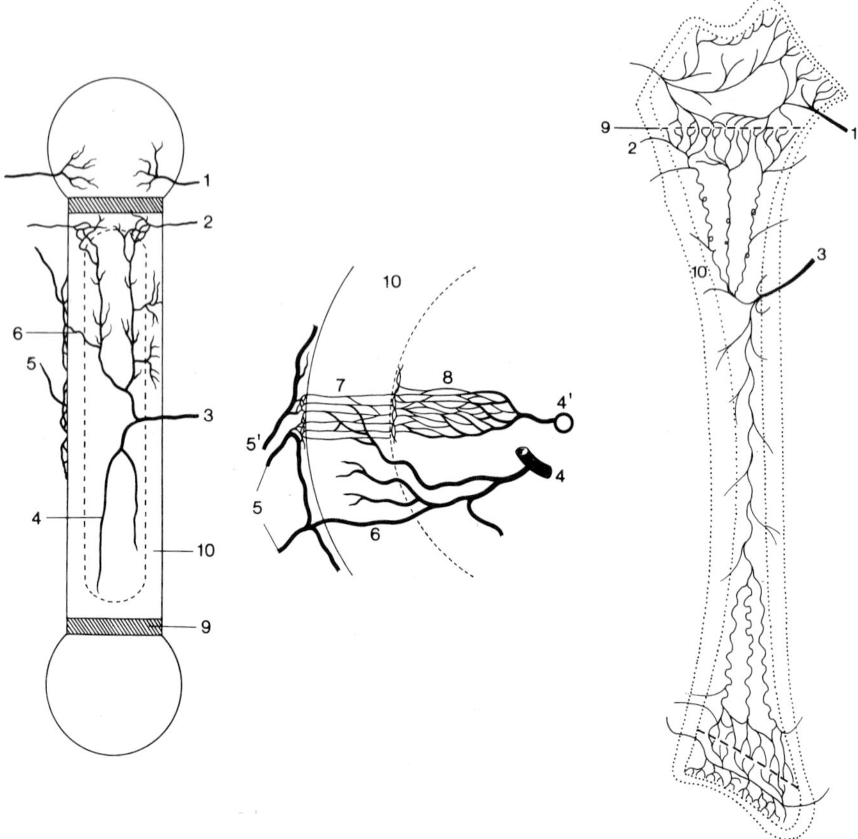


**Figure 1–15.** The blood supply of a long bone, schematic. The supply of the cortex is shown (enlarged) in the center.

1, Epiphysial arteries; 2, metaphysial arteries; 3, nutrient artery; 4, 4′, artery and vein of the bone marrow; 5, periosteal arteries; 5′, periosteal vein; 6, anastomosis between periosteal and bone marrow arteries; 7, capillaries of the cortex; 8, sinusoids in the bone marrow; 9, growth cartilage; 10, cortex.

from which the bone developed. The cartilage is not uniform in structure; it is calcified in its deepest layer, which is firmly attached to the underlying cortex, and becomes fibrous toward the periphery, where it blends with the periosteum and joint capsule.

A tough fibrous membrane, the *periosteum,* ensheathes the remainder of the outer surface, from which it can be readily stripped, except where it is penetrated by tendons and ligaments proceeding to anchor in the compacta. Its appearance is rather misleading, since the deeper layer is cellular and even in adults retains the bone-forming capacity that it exercised during development (p. 72). This osteogenic function is reactivated in the healing of a fracture.

Bones have a generous *blood supply,* perhaps amounting to 5% to 10% of the cardiac output. Several sets of vessels exist; the so-called nutrient artery, though generally the largest single source, probably contributes less than do the others in the aggregate. The nutrient artery penetrates toward the middle of the shaft in a position that is fairly constant for each bone. It is usually directed toward one extremity, and the foramen through which it passes may simulate an oblique fracture when depicted in radiographs. The artery divides into two divergent branches within the marrow; these and the later divisions pursue very tortuous courses, which may have the purpose of reducing the pressure within the vessels of the delicate marrow (Fig. 1–15). The smaller branches supply the sinusoids of the marrow tissue and also the arterioles and capillaries that permeate a system of tiny central channels (haversian canals) within the osteones of compact bone. A further supply to the cortex arises from the medullary sinusoids. Branches of the nutrient artery that reach the metaphysial region (the part of the shaft adjacent to the epiphysis) anastomose there with branches of metaphysial and epiphysial vessels that enter the bone toward its extremity. The central region of this part of the shaft probably relies mainly on the nutrient artery, the peripheral part on metaphysial arteries. The anastomoses are of varying efficiency, but the collateral circulation is generally sufficient to allow a bone to survive deprivation of part of its usual supply when fractured. One technique (intramedullary pinning) employed in fracture repair is possibly even more damaging to the vessels than is the initial injury, and its success serves to emphasize the value of the anastomoses. Some authors have described an additional supply entering the cortex from numerous small periosteal arteries. The weight of opinion denies their presence in healthy young bones.

The main drainage of the marrow is effected by large, thin-walled veins that accompany the major arteries and emerge through the nutrient, epiphysial, and metaphysial foramina. The capillaries within cortical tissue drain into venules within the periosteum. The normal cortical circulation is therefore centrifugal—from within outward. No lymphatic vessels are present within bone, although infections of bone may spread to the lymphatics that drain neighboring tissues.

One important difference is exhibited by the circulation in young growing bones. In these, the circulation within the epiphyses forms separate and independent compartments, since (with few exceptions) arteries do not penetrate the growth (epiphysial) cartilage.

Nerves accompany the larger vessels, and their branches are to be found within the central canals of the osteones. Some (vasomotor) fibers pass to the vessels, some are sensory to the bone tissues (especially the periosteum), and the destination of others remains unclear. It is no longer believed that nerves exert a trophic influence on bone. The skeletal atrophy that follows section of peripheral nerve trunks is believed to be secondary to local muscular paralysis; it is the immobilization that promotes wastage.

## Biomechanical Aspects

It has long been conventional to explain the tubular construction of long bones by drawing the comparison with a loaded beam of some stiff, homogeneous material supported at both ends (Fig. 1–16). In this construction the tensile forces that

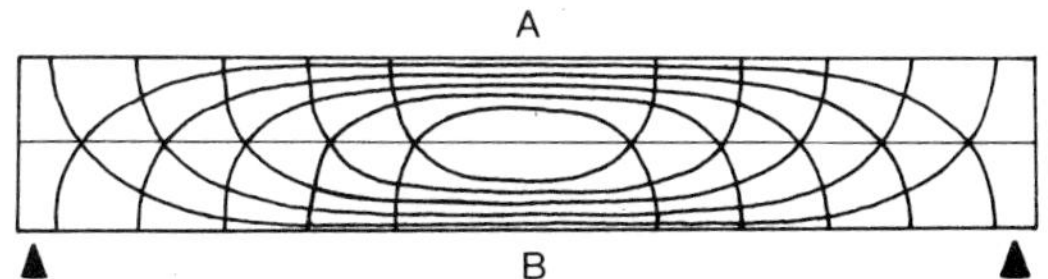


**Figure 1–16.** Pattern of compressive *(A)* and tensile *(B)* stress lines in a beam supported at both ends. The greatest stresses (closeness of lines) occur in the middle of the beam toward the surfaces.

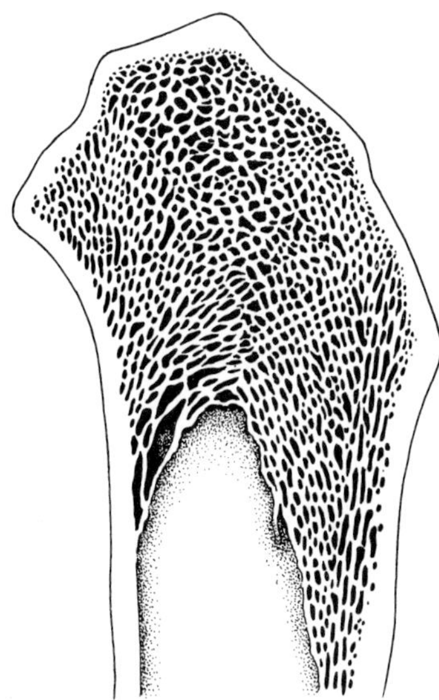

**Figure 1–17.** Proximal end of the tibia of a horse, sectioned sagitally, as an example of the architecture of spongy bone.

tend to disrupt the material are concentrated toward the lower surface while the compressive forces that tend to crush and compact the material are concentrated toward the upper surface. These forces tend to neutralize each other along, and close to, the axis and the material here is more or less redundant. It can be dispensed with or replaced by some weaker but lighter material—as in a long bone. The analogy is not exact—for a start, bone is a composite material—but useful as a first approach. The diagram shows that the lines of principal compressive and tensile stress intersect in orthogonal fashion toward the extremities of the model; the spongy architecture of a bone closely mimics the theoretical pattern. Indeed, the pattern of trabecular bone has been described as the crystallization of the lines of stress, an attractive if faulty metaphor. Since the more detailed analysis of the spongy architecture (Fig. 1–17) introduces matters that are both complicated and controversial, it is probably wiser to leave discussion to the specialist, noting only that a relationship exists between architecture and mechanics and that, over time, the architecture adjusts to changes in the direction and magnitude of applied forces.

Compact bone is a plastic, composite material of considerable strength, capable of sustaining and recovering from considerable deformation. When bent, the lamellae and osteones of which compact bone is constructed first shear past each other; if bent too far, a crack appears at right angles to the line of shear and then quickly spreads to create a brittle fracture. Most fractures are caused by excessive bending, which stresses both aspects of the bone approximately equally. Since the side under tensile stress generally fails first, this indicates that compact bone is better able to resist compression. However, spongy bone is commonly crushed and impacted by compression.

### Some Specialized Varieties of Bones

Bones are often found within tendons (rarely within ligaments) where they change direction over prominences that would expose them to excessive pressure and friction. These bones, known as *sesamoid bones,* form regular synovial joints with the major bones with which they are in contact. In addition to preventing tendon wear, a sesamoid bone displaces the tendon farther from the axis of the adjacent joint and so serves to increase the leverage exerted by the muscle. The best-known example is the patella (kneecap) that forms in the principal muscle that extends the stifle joint (the name given to the knee of quadrupeds) (see Figs. 2–61 and 17–3). In the dog, smaller sesamoids also develop in muscles behind the stifle, in the tendons passing behind the metacarpophalangeal joints (at the bases of the digits), and in the extensor tendons within the digits (Fig. 1–9). The chief practical importance of these and other lesser sesamoids lies in the risk of their being wrongly identified as chip fractures when they are depicted in radiographs. In large animals one or more additional sesamoids form dorsal to the deep flexor tendon shortly before its insertion on the distal phalanx (or phalanges). In the dog the reaction is limited to the development of a nubbin of cartilage in each branch of the tendon.

Although sesamoids are a device to protect tendons from injury, the major sesamoids develop in the embryo before movement is possible, and their origin must therefore be genetically determined. They do not re-form after extirpation when the limb is immobilized but only if movement is allowed; this indicates that they can also develop in reaction to an appropriate stimulus in the lifetime of the animal.

*Splanchnic bones* develop in soft organs, remote from the rest of the skeleton. The most familiar, indeed the only significant, examples in veterinary anatomy are the os penis (and the female equivalent, os clitoridis) of the dog and cat, and the ossa cordis found in the heart, of ruminants especially.

Certain bones are excavated to contain air spaces. In mammals, these *pneumatic bones* are confined to the skull and contain the paranasal sinuses, which communicate with the nasal cavities. The sinuses principally develop after birth, when outgrowths of the nasal mucosa invade certain skull bones and replace the diplöe, the spongy bone between the outer and inner layers ("tables") of compacta. The separation of the tables can be very considerable and can lead to a remarkable postnatal remodeling of the skull, best exhibited by cattle and pigs. The postcranial skeleton of birds develops an extensive system of air-filled cavities in communication with the respiratory organs.

## Joints

Bones meet each other at joints or articulations, some of which are designed to unite the bones firmly and others to allow free movement. Because of this, and because of differences in development, enormous variation in joint structure exists, which makes it extremely difficult to devise a suitable classification. Periodic revisions of terminology have seen new categories defined and former categories merged or renamed so that some confusion now exists, with many superfluous terms in circulation. The current official system recognizes three major categories, namely, fibrous joints, in which the bones are united by dense connective tissues; cartilaginous joints, in which the bones are united by cartilage; and synovial joints, in which a fluid-filled cavity intervenes between the bones. It is obvious that most joints of the first and second categories must be relatively immovable or even rigid; these classes were formerly together known as *synarthroses.* In contrast, most joints of the third category are freely movable; they were formerly termed *diarthroses.* Both of these terms, although obsolete, are likely to be encountered.

### Fibrous Joints

Most fibrous joints occur in the skull and are known as *sutures* (Fig. 1–18). The narrow strips of fibrous tissue that outline and unite the margins of the bones represent the surviving part of the originally continuous membrane in which the separate ossification centers appeared. Sutures play an important role in the young animal, allowing for the growth of the skull through the extension of individual bones at their margins while proliferation of the membrane continues. Sutures are gradually eliminated when ossification extends across the membrane after it has ceased to grow. This is a slow and uneven process that is not complete even in the aged. The gradual modification of the sutural pattern is used in anthropology and forensic medicine as a guide—though not a very reliable one—to the age of the individual. Although movement between the bones of the

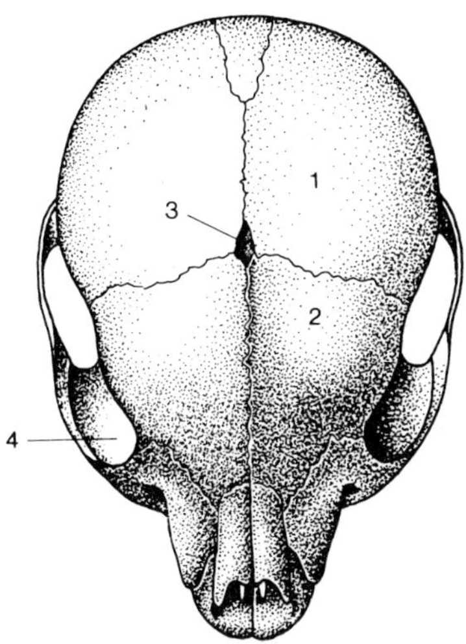


**Figure 1–18.** Sutures between the bones of a puppy's skull.

1, Parietal bone; 2, frontal bone; 3, fontanelle (fonticulus); 4, orbit.

adult skull is neither required nor allowed, the wider sutures of the fetal skull allow some useful passive deformation during birth in some species, including primates.

The other fibrous joints are known as *syndesmoses.* In these, facing areas of two bones are joined by connective tissue ligaments. In some syndesmoses relatively broad areas of bone are united by short ligaments, and movement is inevitably very limited; examples are the joints between the major and minor bones of the horse's metacarpus. In others the ligaments are longer and their attachments narrower so that more appreciable movement is possible; an example is the joint between the shafts of the radius and ulna in the forearm of the dog.

The attachment of a tooth to the bone of its socket may be included among the fibrous joints under the name *gomphosis.*

## Cartilaginous Joints

Most cartilaginous joints are known as *synchondroses.* These include the joints between the epiphyses and diaphyses of juvenile long bones and the corresponding joints of the base of the skull. Most are temporary and disappear after growth has ceased, when the cartilage is replaced by bone. The few permanent synchondroses include the joint between the skull and hyoid apparatus (p. 66), which allows appreciable movement in some species.

In the more complicated *symphysis* the articulating bones are divided by a succession of tissues; usually cartilage covers the bones with fibrocartilage or fibrous tissue in the middle. The category includes the joints between the symmetrical halves of the mandible (in those species, such as the dog, cat, and ruminants, in which fusion is not complete) and of the pelvic girdle, and the joints between, the bodies of successive vertebrae (Fig. 1–19). Each of these joints presents its own, sometimes specifically variable, features that are best considered later.

## Synovial Joints

**Structure.** In synovial joints the articulating bones are separated by a fluid-filled space, the joint cavity (Fig. 1–20). The boundaries of the space are completed by a sleeve of delicate connective tissue, the synovial membrane. This is attached around the periphery of the articular surfaces, which are clothed with thin layers of cartilage. No other essential features exist. However, in most synovial joints the synovial membrane is strengthened externally by a fibrous capsule, and additional fibrous bands (ligaments) are strategically placed to join the bones and to restrict movement to the required directions and extents. Each of these components is described in the detail made necessary by the prevalence of joint injuries and pathology in domestic animals. It may be stated with confidence that no branch of anatomy better rewards study.

The *articular surface* is clothed with articular cartilage that is generally of the hyaline variety, although fibrocartilage or even dense fibrous tissue is substituted in a few locations. The cartilage is only a millimeter or so thick in the joints of the dog but may be several millimeters thick in the larger joints of horses and cattle. It accentuates the curvature of the underlying bone, being thickest in the center of convex surfaces and about the periphery of concave ones. It is a pliant material that is translucent and glassy in appear-

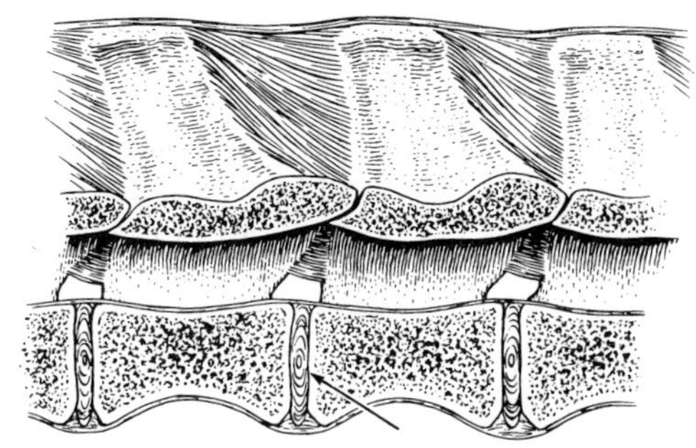

**Figure 1–19.** Intervertebral disc *(arrow)* joining bodies of adjacent vertebrae.

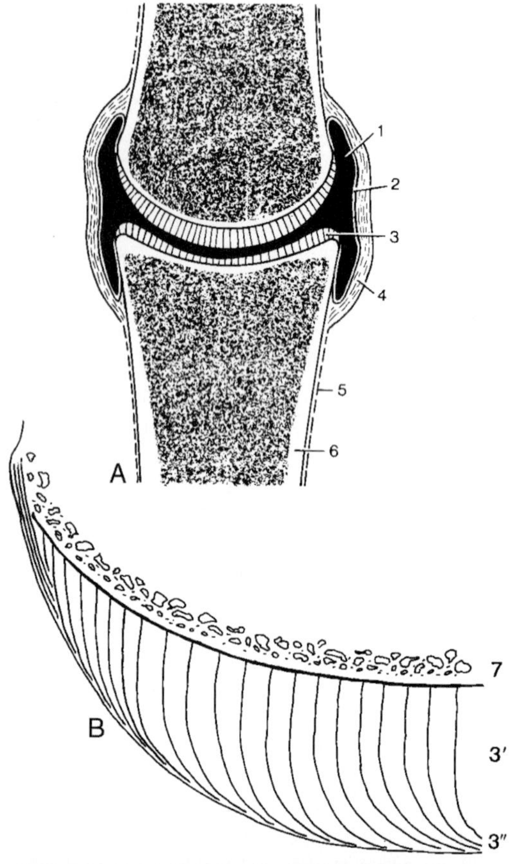


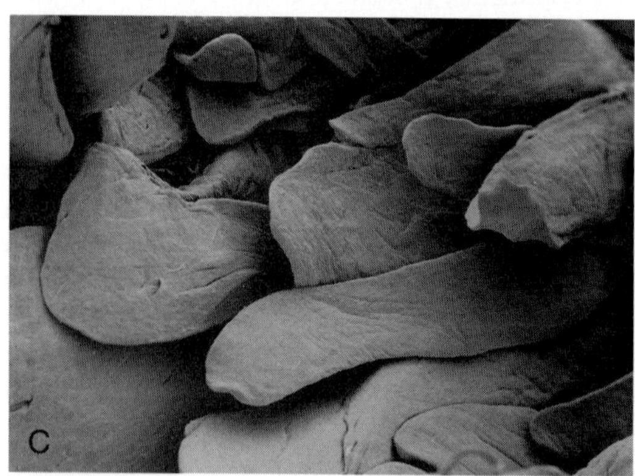


**Figure 1–20.** *A,* A synovial joint in section. *B,* Segment of articular cartilage showing fiber pattern (both schematic). *C,* Scanning electron micrograph of villi projecting from the synovial membrane of the equine fetlock joint; greatly enlarged.

1, Joint cavity; 2, synovial membrane; 3, articular cartilage; 3′, 3″, radial and tangential zones of articular cartilage; 4, fibrous layer of joint capsule; 5, periosteum; 6, compact bone; 7, subchondral bone.

ance and, while generally white with a blue or pink tinge in young animals, it becomes yellowish with age, a change indicating a loss of elasticity. The surface is smooth to the touch and to the naked eye, though quite irregular when seen at low magnification.

The cartilage has a complex structure in which fine fibers within its matrix pass from the underlying bone to the surface, where they bend to lie closely together (Fig. 1–20/*B*,3′,3″). Since splitting of the cartilage, common in joint disease, tends to follow the fiber course, superficial lesions lead to tangential flaking, whereas those that extend more deeply create more or less vertical cracks.

Articular cartilage is insensitive and avascular. The insensitivity explains why joint lesions may progress far before the patient becomes aware of their existence. The oxygen and nutritive requirements are met by diffusion from three sources: fluid within the joint cavity, vessels in the tissues at the periphery of the cartilage, and vessels in the subjacent marrow spaces. Diffusion is assisted by the porosity of the cartilage matrix, which soaks up and releases fluid as the cartilage is alternately unloaded and compressed during movements of the joint.

Certain large articular cartilages are interrupted by depressed areas that may indent the periphery or appear as islands. These naked areas (synovial fossae) are clothed by a thin connective tissue resting on the underlying bone; they are sometimes interpreted by the unwary as pathological lesions. Their significance is disputed, but the constancy of their occurrence as well as frequent coincidence in opposing bones in certain positions of the joint has led to the speculation that they assist in spreading synovia.*

The *synovial membrane,* which completes the lining of the joint, is a glistening pink connective tissue sheet. It may be left entirely unsupported, may rest directly on a tough outer fibrous capsule, or may be separated from this by the interposition of pads of fat; all three arrangements may occur in different regions of the same joint. The membrane may pouch where it is unsupported, and these diverticula may extend quite far, a point of potential significance because it explains how joints may be entered by apparently remote wounds. The inner surface of the membrane carries many projections of various sizes and degrees of

**Synovial fossae* are present in the horse and in cattle among domestic mammals. Though not quite constant, they appear in the majority of animals and are always bilateral in the limbs. They appear as early as 10 days after birth in foals. In the horse, opposing synovial fossae are found at the shoulder, elbow, carpal, tarsocrural, and talocalcaneal joints. Single fossae are present in the fetlock joints (of both fore- and hindlimbs), on the acetabulum, and on the atlantal surface of the atlantoaxial joint. In cattle more or less distinct synovial fossae may be present in all limb joints, other than the shoulder and hip. They also may be present at the atlanto-occipital and atlantoaxial joints.

permanency, which greatly increase its surface area (Fig. 1–20/*C*). Unlike mucous membranes, the synovial membrane has no continuous covering of cells; the more cellular parts, limited to relatively protected situations, are responsible for the production of the lubricant component (aminoglycans) of the synovial fluid. The other components are derived from the blood plasma. The membrane is both vascular and sensitive.

*Synovia,* the fluid within the cavity, obtains its name from its resemblance to egg white. It is a viscous, glairy fluid, whose color ranges from pale straw to medium brown. It is usually said to be present in very small amounts but is in fact quite copious in the larger joints; as much as 20 to 40 mL can sometimes be aspirated from limb joints of horses and cattle. The quantity is greatest in animals permitted free exercise.

Synovia has both lubricant and nutritive functions. The ways in which it acts as a lubricant are disputed, but it is certainly very efficient, the friction being such that virtually no wear occurs in healthy joints. The fluid helps to nourish the articular cartilage, any intra-articular structures, and possibly the surface layer of the synovial membrane itself.

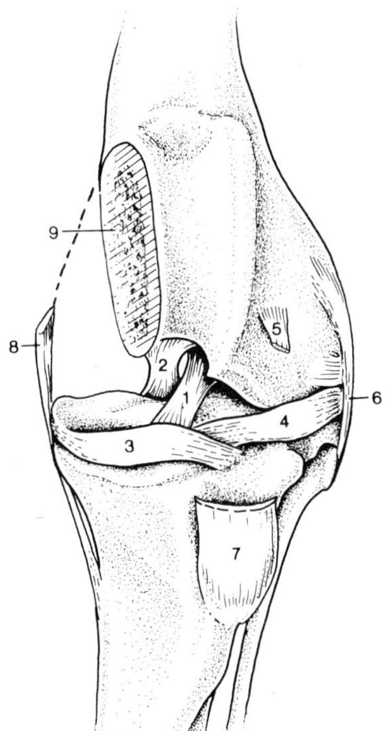


**Figure 1–21.** Cranial view of left stifle joint of the dog, resected to show intra- (1, 2) and extracapsular (6, 8) ligaments.

1, Cranial cruciate ligament; 2, caudal cruciate ligament; 3, medial meniscus; 4, lateral meniscus; 5, tendon of origin of long digital extensor; 6, lateral collateral ligament; 7, patellar ligament; 8, medial collateral ligament; 9, medial condyle, partly removed.

An outer *fibrous layer* usually completes the capsule. It attaches around the margins of the articular surfaces and presents local thickenings, which are named individually as *ligaments* when well developed and discrete. Some, of which the cruciate ligaments of the stifle are good examples, appear to run within the joint cavity from bone to bone. Such ligaments are sometimes designated *intracapsular* to distinguish them from the majority in peripheral and clearly extracapsular positions; but they are actually excluded from the cavity by a covering of synovial membrane (Fig. 1–21). The fibrous layer and ligaments are supplied with proprioceptive nerve endings that register the position and the rate of change in position of the joint; other receptors register pain.

A few joints possess *discs* or *menisci* that are truly intracapsular (Fig. 1–22*A,B*). A disc, such as occurs in the temporomandibular joint formed between the mandible and the skull, fuses with the synovial membrane around its periphery and so divides the cavity into upper and lower compartments. Paired menisci, which are semilunar as the name suggests, are found within the stifle joint. They are attached only around their convex borders and therefore divide the cavity incompletely. Both of these structures are composed of hyaline cartilage, fibrocartilage, and fibrous tissue in proportions that vary with the part, the species, and the age. Menisci and discs provide congruence of incompatible articulating surfaces, but this can hardly explain their presence because congruence is achieved at other joints more simply. The most probable alternative explanation regards them as a means of resolving complicated movements into simpler components that are assigned to different levels of the articulation. Thus, in the temporomandibular joint the hinge movement involved in opening the mouth occurs at the lower level (between the disc and the mandible), while the translatory movements that protrude, retract, or slide the lower jaw sideways occur at the upper level (between the disc and the skull).

An *articular labrum* is a fibrocartilaginous lip or rim placed around the circumference of certain concave articular surfaces, including the acetabulum (the deep socket at the hip). A labrum serves to extend and deepen the articular surface, increasing the load-bearing area and helping to spread the synovial fluid. Since a labrum is deformable, it allows the surface to adapt to disparities in the curvature of the bone with which it comes in contact.

*Synovial pads* or cushions are formed where fat masses are included between the synovial and

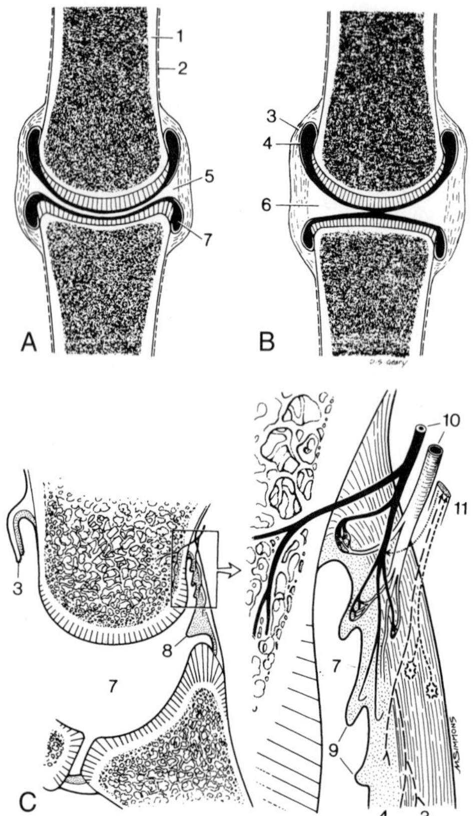


**Figure 1–22.** *A,* Synovial joint with articular disc. *B,* Synovial joint with meniscus. *C,* Blood and nerve supply of a joint.

1, Compact bone; 2, periosteum; 3, fibrous layer of joint capsule; 4, synovial membrane; 5, articular disc; 6, meniscus; 7, joint cavity; 8, synovial fold; 9, synovial villi; 10, blood vessels supplying epiphysis and joint capsule; 11, nerve with efferent fibers for blood vessels and pain and proprioceptive afferent fibers.

fibrous layers of the joint capsule. They are sometimes interpreted as swabs that spread the synovia over the surface, but their main purpose is to allow the synovial membrane to accommodate its shape to the part of the bone with which it is momentarily in contact.

**Movements.** Although many joint movements appear to be complicated, they can always be resolved into simple components. Moreover, many activities are the result of coordinated movement at several neighboring joints; the sum of changes can be considerable when the movement at each individual joint is modest.

The simplest type of movement is described as *translation.* In its pure form, translation consists in one flat surface sliding over another while the bodies to which the surfaces belong maintain their original orientation. True translatory movements probably never occur because the prerequisites are perfectly flat surfaces and the absence of spin. Nonetheless, a category of joint (plane joint) is defined in which movement is supposed to be of this kind. These joints have small articular surfaces that appear flat at first scrutiny; in reality, articular surfaces are always curved.

All other movements involve angular change. In some, the moving bone turns (spins) about an axis perpendicular to its articular surface, a movement described as *rotation.* Rotation can always be reversed, and it is therefore necessary to specify its direction. According to convention, an internal rotation of a limb carries the cranial surface medially (Fig. 1–23/4); an external rotation carries this surface laterally (/5).

Other movements involve the moving bone turning about an axis parallel to its articular surface in a pendular or rolling movement (Fig. 1–24/3); this is a slide between curved surfaces and may be described as a *swing.* Most swings are accompanied by some rotation, although this often goes undetected.

Pendular movements in sagittal planes predominate in the joints of the limbs and are known as flexion and extension. *Flexion* reduces the angle between the two segments of the limb. The opposite movement of *extension* opens the angle and brings the two segments more closely into alignment (Fig. 1–24). However, the movement at some joints ranges from one flexed position

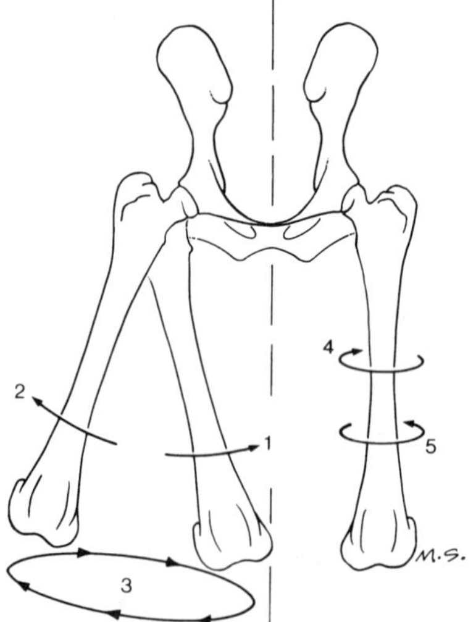


**Figure 1–23.** Limb movements illustrated by the femurs of the dog, cranial view.

1, Adduction; 2, abduction; 3, circumduction; 4, inward rotation; 5, outward rotation.

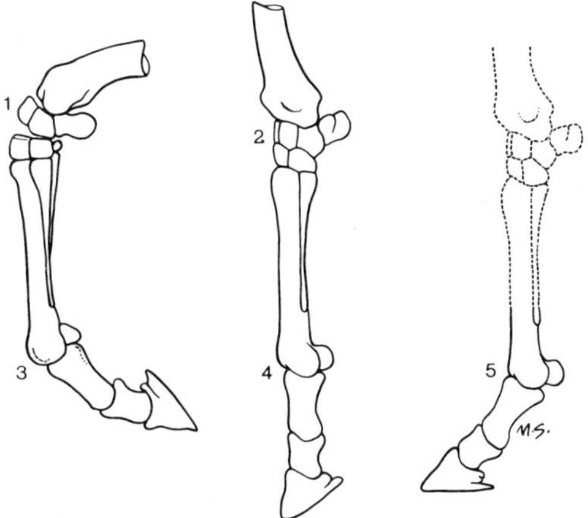


**Figure 1–24.** Flexion, extension, and overextension illustrated by the distal part of the horse's forelimb.

1, Flexed carpal joint; 2, extended carpal joint; 3, flexed fetlock joint; 4, extended fetlock joint; 5, overextended fetlock joint.

through full extension (180 degrees) to a second flexed position at the other limit. The fetlock joint of the horse is a good example of a joint with such a wide range of movement. In such cases the two terminal positions may be distinguished as overextension (or dorsal flexion), the posture of the animal standing at rest, and (palmar) flexion, the posture when the foot is passively raised. Figure 1–24 may make this rather confusing distinction plain.

Adduction and abduction are pendular movements in transverse planes (Fig. 1–23/1,2). *Adduction* carries the moving part toward the median plane, and *abduction* carries it farther from this plane. When applied to the digits, adduction and abduction describe movement with reference to the axis of the limb and indicate the convergence or the spread of the digits, respectively.

The combination of flexion and extension, adduction and abduction, allows the extremity of the limb to describe a circle or ellipse, a movement known as *circumduction.*

Limitations are placed on the movements of all joints. Several potentially limiting factors exist, and it is not easy to determine their relative importance. The shape of the articular surfaces is obviously relevant. A degree of incongruence is required to maintain a wedge of the lubricant synovia between the surfaces. This wedge is reduced when the radius of curvature of the convex surface increases toward its margin to approximate to the radius of curvature of the opposing concave surface. The surfaces thus become congruent in the closely packed terminal position, and further movement is checked by their being squeezed together.

Tension in extracapsular ligaments can certainly arrest movement, although it is uncertain whether this method of braking is required in normal circumstances. Some ligaments appear to be moderately taut throughout the normal range of movement, whereas others are generally slack and become taut only when movement threatens to go beyond the normal limit.

In some situations, contact between extra-articular structures may be of importance; the olecranon obviously prevents forceful overextension of the elbow, and apposition of the caudal muscles of the thigh and calf prevents overflexion of the human knee. Tension in muscles and other soft structures in the neighborhood of a joint may first decelerate and then arrest movement; inability to stretch beyond a certain limit—passive insufficiency—of the muscles of the caudal aspect of the human thigh prohibits many people from "touching their toes." The contraction of muscles that oppose a given movement may be the most important factor; its significance is discussed in the following section.

**Classification.** Synovial joints may be classified according to numerical and geometrical criteria. The numerical system distinguishes simple joints with one pair of articular surfaces and composite joints in which more than two opposing surfaces are involved and in which movement occurs at more than one level within a shared capsule. The shoulder joint illustrates the first and the carpal joint the second variety.

There are seven categories in the current version of the geometrical system. One, the *plane joint* (Fig. 1–25/*A*), has already been mentioned (p. 20).

The *hinge joint* (ginglymus; /*B*) has one articular surface shaped like a segment of a cylinder and the other excavated to receive it. Pendular movement is possible in one plane only; prohibition of other movements may be reinforced by stout collateral (one to each side) ligaments and possibly by the development of matching ridges and grooves on the articular surfaces. The elbow joint between the humerus and bones of the forearm is an example.

The *pivot joint* (articulatio trochoidea; /*C*) comprises a peg fitted within a ring. Movement takes place about the long axis of the peg. In some joints (e.g., the proximal radioulnar joint) the peg rotates within the fixed ring; in others (e.g., the atlantoaxial joint between the first two vertebrae) the ring rotates about the fixed peg.

The *condylar joint* (/*D*) is formed by two knuckle-shaped condyles that engage with corresponding concave surfaces. The two complexes may be close together, as in the femorotibial joint, or widely separate and provided with independent

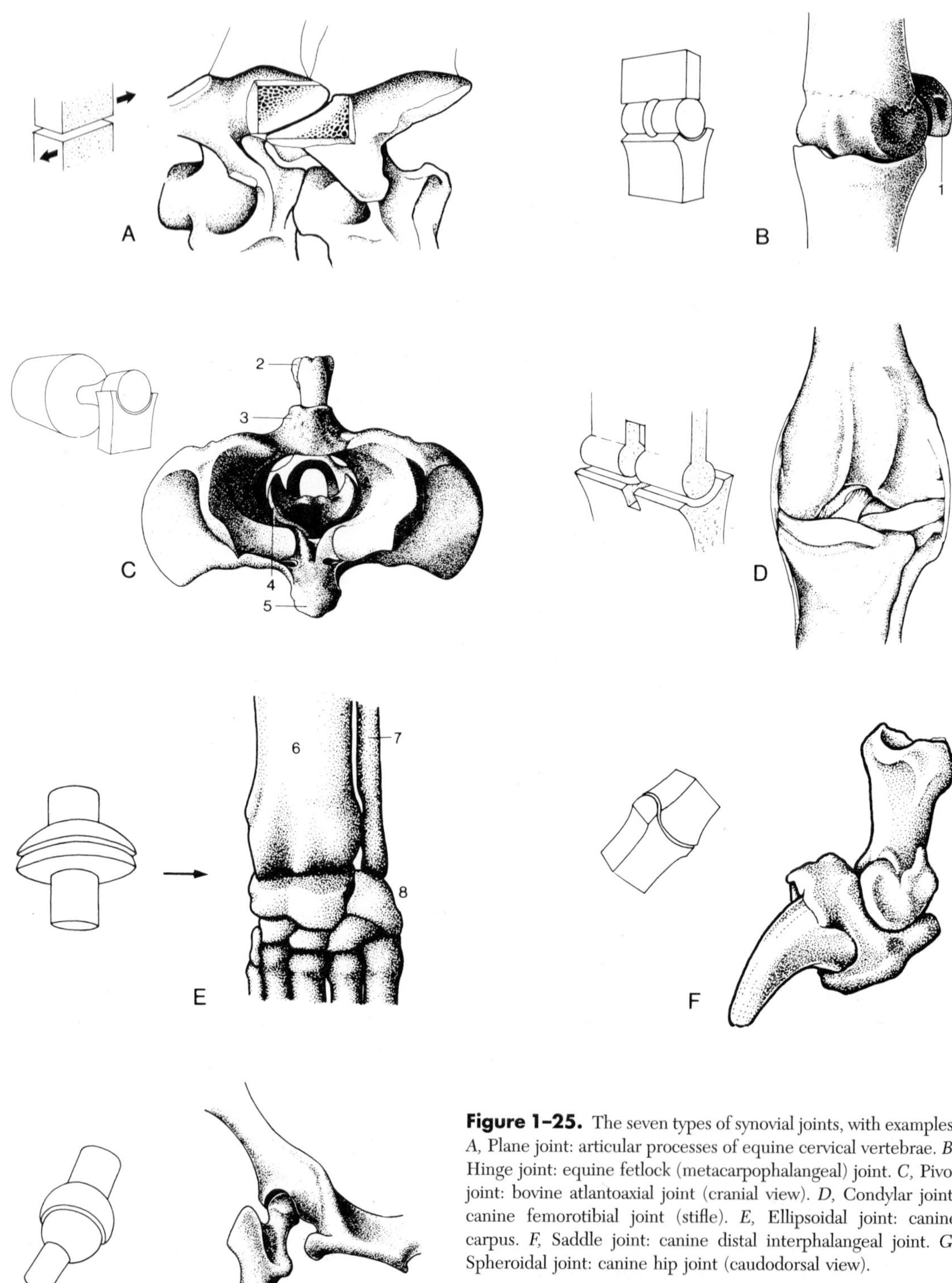


**Figure 1–25.** The seven types of synovial joints, with examples. *A,* Plane joint: articular processes of equine cervical vertebrae. *B,* Hinge joint: equine fetlock (metacarpophalangeal) joint. *C,* Pivot joint: bovine atlantoaxial joint (cranial view). *D,* Condylar joint: canine femorotibial joint (stifle). *E,* Ellipsoidal joint: canine carpus. *F,* Saddle joint: canine distal interphalangeal joint. *G,* Spheroidal joint: canine hip joint (caudodorsal view).

1, Proximal sesamoid bone; 2, spine of axis; 3, dorsal arch of atlas; 4, dens of axis; 5, ventral arch of atlas; 6, radius; 7, ulna; 8, proximal row of carpal bones.

joint capsules, as are the twin articulations of the mandible. In each case the whole arrangement is regarded as constituting a single condylar joint. Movement is primarily uniaxial, about a transverse axis common to the two condyles; certain amounts of rotation and of slide are also permitted.

The *ellipsoidal joint (/E)* presents an ovoid convex surface that fits into a corresponding concavity. Movements are principally in two planes at right angles to each other (flexion-extension; adduction-abduction), but a small amount of rotation may be possible. The radiocarpal joint of the dog is of this variety.

The *saddle joint* (articulatio sellaris; */F*) combines two surfaces, each maximally convex in one direction, maximally concave in a second direction at right angles to the first. These are also biaxial joints, allowing flexion-extension and adduction-abduction but with a certain amount of rotation permitted or imposed by the geometry of the surfaces. An example is the distal interphalangeal joint of the dog.

The ball-and-socket or *spheroidal joint (/G)* consists of a portion of a sphere received within a corresponding cup. This multiaxial joint enjoys the greatest versatility of movement. The hip joint is the best example; the human shoulder joint also conforms closely to the pattern, but the shoulder of domestic species largely restricts its movement to flexion and extension.

It must be emphasized that anatomical joints correspond very imperfectly to the theoretical models. Sometimes the departure from the ideal can be sufficiently large to make it a matter of controversy which category best accommodates a particular articulation.

## Muscles

Most movements of the animal body and its parts are caused by muscular contraction. The exceptions are those caused by gravity or other external forces and those, trivial in magnitude though not in importance, produced at the cellular level by cilia and flagella. Muscle is also used to prevent movement, stabilizing joints to prevent their collapse under a load and maintaining continence of bladder and bowel. A subsidiary function of the skeletal muscles is to generate heat by shivering, involuntary tremors initiated by exposure to cold.

There are three varieties of muscle tissue, but two, the specialized (cardiac) muscle that forms the bulk of the heart, and the smooth (visceral) muscle of the blood vessels and viscera (internal organs), are not of present concern. The third variety is generally known as skeletal muscle because it is organized into units that are mostly attached to the bones and used to effect their movements. Skeletal muscle is also known as striated, somatic, or voluntary muscle, but these terms are less acceptable for one reason or another.

### The Organization of Skeletal Muscles

Skeletal muscle is butcher's meat and accounts for about half the weight of an animal carcass (the proportion varies with species, breed, age, sex, and method of husbandry). Each individual muscle is composed of many cells held together by connective tissue. When compared with the common run of cell, these muscle cells are giants, varying from about 10 to 100 μm in diameter and being about 5 or 10 cm in length—with the probability that some are much longer. They are visible to the naked eye when teased apart and are also called muscle fibers because of their size and shape. The whole muscle is invested by a dense connective tissue sheet, the epimysium (Fig. 1–26); below this a looser layer, the perimysium, invests the small bundles (fasciculi) into which the fibers are grouped; finally, each fiber is provided with its own delicate covering, the endomysium. These connective tissue components merge at each end of the muscle "belly" and continue as the tendons by which the muscle makes its attachment. The amount and quality of the connective tissue partly explain variations in the appearance and in the cooking and table

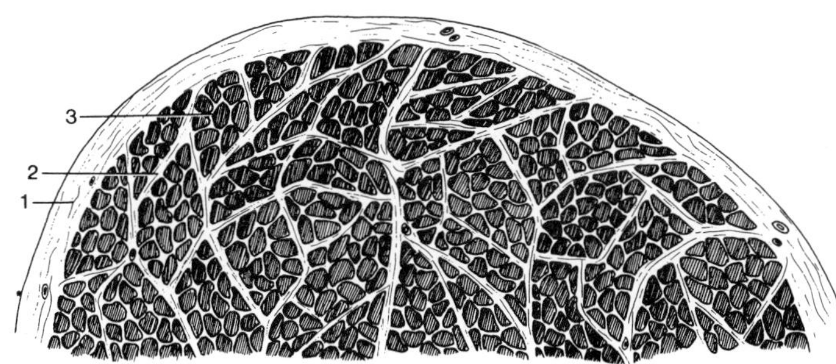


**Figure 1–26.** Transection of a skeletal muscle; the fibrous tissue has been emphasized.

1, Epimysium; 2, perimysium; 3, endomysium.

qualities of different "cuts" of meat (another important factor is the degree of shortening that is allowed by hanging during postmortem rigor). The consumer is willing to pay more for some cuts than for others; much effort has been devoted to breeding animals in which the more desirable muscle groups form a larger part of the carcass, but with limited success (except in a few breeds, e.g., Charolais, Belgian Blue, in which there is a natural tendency for muscular hypertrophy).

**Variations in Muscle Architecture.** The way in which the muscle fibers are arranged within the muscle belly varies greatly, which can be explained by reference to two principles. The shortening (about 50%) that a muscle may demonstrate on contraction is a function of the length of the component fibers. The power that it may develop is a function of the aggregate of their cross-sectional area. The greatest displacement is therefore produced by the so-called strap muscle (Fig. 1–27), in which the fibers run parallel to the long axis and throughout the length of the muscle, which is completed by very short tendons of attachment.

Muscles in which the fibers join the tendons at an angle tend to be strong in relation to their bulk, since more fibers and a greater total cross section can be accommodated. Although muscles of this sort are powerful, they waste a proportion of their strength and of their potential for displacement; only part, corresponding to the cosine of the angle of fiber insertion, is applied along the line of pull. In calculating the power that such muscles develop, it is necessary to substitute for the simple "anatomical" cross section the "physiological" cross section, the complex plane that divides the muscle in such a way that each component fiber is cut transversely. Muscles with angled fibers can be arranged in several categories of increasing complexity of construction: pennate, bipennate, circumpennate, and multipennate (Fig. 1–27).

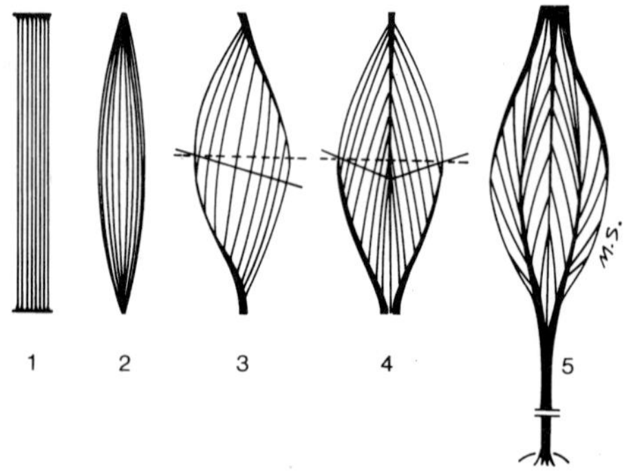


**Figure 1–27.** Architecture of skeletal muscles. The broken lines represent the "anatomical," the solid lines the "physiological" transverse sections.

1, Strap muscle; 2, spindle-shaped muscle; 3, pennate muscle; 4, bipennate muscle; 5, multipennate muscle.

Many limb muscles have a pennate form and, unlike the strap muscles, are provided with long, cordlike tendons that permit the heavy bellies to be placed close to the trunk; since only the light tendons extend to the digits to operate the joints, less energy is required to swing the limb to and fro. Certain muscles of the body wall form thin flat layers that are continued by broad tendon sheets (distinguished as aponeuroses), an arrangement clearly adapted to supporting the abdominal organs. Other muscles arise by two, three, or four separate heads that join in a common tendon, arrangements indicated by inclusion of the descriptive terms biceps (two-headed), triceps, or quadriceps in the muscles' names.

In another less common variety, two or more fleshy units are separated by intermediate tendon forming digastric (two-bellied) or polygastric units. Still other muscles are arranged in rings that surround natural orifices, such as the mouth or anus, and act as sphincters to constrict or close the opening. In all these examples the construction of the muscle is clearly adapted to the functions that it is called upon to perform.

Paired muscles lying against, or originating from, the midline are separated by a connective tissue strip known as a raphe.*

Muscles also vary in appearance according to color which reflects the amount of myoglobin (a pigment related to hemoglobin) within their constituent fibers. The difference, well exemplified by the pale breast and dark leg muscles of the chicken, is generally regarded as reflecting a pale muscle's adaptation for rapid contraction over a short period, a darker muscle's adaptation for slower but sustained activity; the correlation does not always pertain. Most muscles are actually composed of two fiber types in varying proportion; fast twitch fibers that rely upon glycolytic metabolism predominate in dark (red) muscles, slow twitch fibers that obtain their energy from aerobic metabolism predominate in pale (white) muscles. There are many other structural and physiological differences between fibers and the suggestion that there are only these two, sharply distinguished, varieties, though convenient, is a dangerous simplification.

**Tendons.** Muscles always attach by means of connective tissue tendons; when these are so short that they almost evade notice, muscles are loosely

*The term *raphe* denotes a seam suggestive of the union of two (usually symmetrical) parts. The term may also be used of a surface feature, such as the raphe of the scrotum.

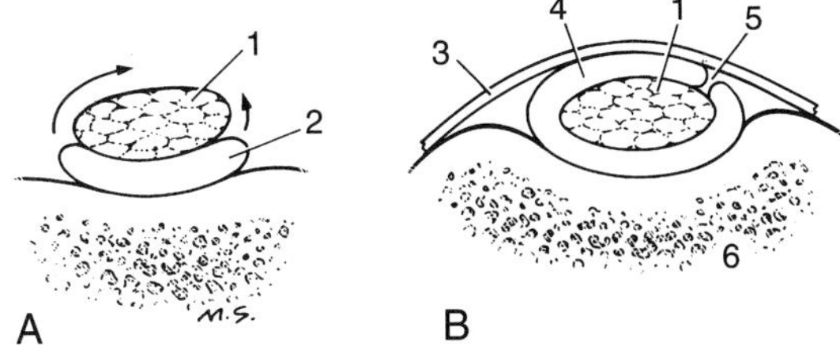


**Figure 1–28.** Sections of a synovial bursa *(A)* and a tendon sheath *(B)*. The bursa permits frictionless movement of a tendon (1) over bone, the sheath movement of a tendon over bone and under a retinaculum, respectively. The arrows show that a tendon sheath may be regarded as a large bursa that has wrapped around a tendon.

1, Tendon; 2, bursa; 3, retinaculum; 4, tendon sheath; 5, mesotendon, through which blood vessels reach the tendon; 6, bone.

said to have direct attachments. Tendons consist almost entirely of collagen bundles in regular arrangement, and they possess great tensile strength. Indeed, excessive tension is more likely to rupture the muscle belly or to detach a fragment of bone at the insertion than to disrupt the tendon itself. Tendons are also more elastic than is commonly supposed and are capable of absorbing and storing energy when stretched. It is not always sufficiently appreciated that the elastic recoil of tendons makes a substantial contribution to locomotion and that a good fraction of the metabolic work performed by many muscles is devoted to stretching tendons so that the stored energy can later be released.

Although they are tough, tendons may be damaged by excessive pressure or friction, particularly when they change direction over bony prominences or are shifted over hard tissues. One form of the protection that they develop in such places, local chondrification or ossification (sesamoid bones), has been mentioned (p. 16). An alternative is provided by the development of fluid-filled cushions at the danger sites. If only one aspect of the tendon is at risk, a bag (bursa synovialis) may be interposed on that side (Fig. 1–28//*A*), if a greater part of the circumference is vulnerable, the cushion wraps around the tendon, enclosing it within a tendon sheath (vagina synovialis; /*B*). The walls of these bursae and sheaths and the fluid they contain resemble the similar components of synovial joints. When the tendon moves, it is the lubricated synovial layers that rub together.

Inflammation of synovial bursae and sheaths is common, and it is necessary to know their positions and extents. This is not difficult, since they occur precisely where they can be seen to be required.

**Blood and Nerve Supply of Muscles.** Muscles receive a relatively generous blood supply from neighboring arteries. Sometimes a single artery enters the muscle belly, and then the well-being of the muscle clearly depends on the integrity of that artery. Often, two or more arteries enter separately, which would appear to be a safer arrangement since the arteries form connections within the flesh. Unfortunately, these connections (anastomoses) are not always sufficient to allow the muscle to survive unscathed an interruption to one of its sources of supply. The intramuscular arteries ramify within the perimysium to open into capillaries that follow the endomysial sheaths of individual fibers.

The veins are satellite to the arteries. Normal activity, when only a fraction of the muscle fibers contract, probably promotes the circulation within the muscle by massaging the capillaries and smaller veins. Mass contractions squeeze these vessels from all sides, stopping the circulation, and are likely to be harmful if sustained.

Tendons have low metabolic needs, are poorly vascularized, and do not hemorrhage when cut. This feature, initially an apparent advantage, has its adverse side: damaged tendons are inevitably slow to heal. Lymphatic vessels are found within the larger connective tissue tracts of the muscle belly.

Most muscles are supplied by a single nerve, but those of the trunk that are formed from several somites (p. 32) retain a multiple innervation. The nerve that enters a muscle, generally in company with the principal vessels, ramifies within the connective tissue septa. It consists of fibers of several types; large alpha motor fibers supply the muscle fibers of the main mass; smaller gamma motor fibers supply modified muscle cells within the muscle spindles buried in the muscle; nonmyelinated vasomotor fibers supply blood vessels; and sensory fibers supply the spindles, tendon organs, and other receptors. The ratio of motor to sensory fibers varies considerably, one among many complications in the determination of motor unit size.

The motor neurons that supply a particular muscle are roughly grouped within the ventral horns of gray matter in the spinal cord (or within motor nuclei of the brainstem). The axon from each neuron branches repeatedly in its passage, both within the nerve trunk and within the intermuscular septa, and ultimately ends in the motor end plates of several or many muscle fibers. The single neuron, as well as the (alpha) fibers it supplies, is known as the motor unit, an important concept since it is the physiological unit of muscular contraction. It is these groups and not individual fibers that are called up or discharged from service when a muscle varies the force of its contraction. The muscle fibers belonging to a unit are intermingled with those of other units and do not correspond with any readily identifiable portion of the muscle—they do not correspond with the fasciculi, as one might suppose. The fibers constituting a motor unit are invariably of a uniform type.

In the human species, the number of fibers within a unit varies from about 5 to 10 in the muscles that move the eyeball, around 200 in the muscles of the fingers, and around 2000 in the muscles of the limbs. The exact figures are not important, but the trend is; the muscles with the smallest units are those capable of the most delicate adjustment. Motor unit size is determined from the innervation ratio, the ratio between the number of fibers within a muscle and the number of motor neurons that supply it.

## Muscle Actions

When a muscle is activated, its fibers attempt to shorten. When shortening occurs, the tension in the muscle may increase, stay the same, or decrease, according to circumstances. When external forces prevent the muscle from shortening, the tension within it increases; such activity is said to be isometric.

The usual activity of most muscles involves changes in the angle of the joint(s) bridged by that muscle. The musculoskeletal system thus operates as a system of levers in which the joints act as fulcra. The mechanical advantages of the arrangement depend on the positions (relative to the fulcrum) of the muscle attachment and the application of the load (Fig. 1–29). Although a muscle attaching close to a fulcrum is less powerful than a comparable muscle attaching at a greater distance, it produces its effect more rapidly; the requirements of speed and power thus conflict. When several muscles are available to move a joint in a particular way, the attachments of some make them more suited to getting the movement started, whereas the attachments of others make them more suited to carrying the movement through to completion.

Bi- or polyarticular muscles (those that cross two or several joints) may be incapable of shortening sufficiently to produce the full range of movement at both or all of the relevant joints at the same time. Such muscles are said to be actively insufficient.

Any muscle that produces a certain effect may be termed an *agonist* or *prime mover;* a muscle capable of actively opposing that movement is termed an *antagonist.* Clearly these terms have force only in relation to a specified movement. Thus, in flexion of the elbow, the brachialis that produces the movement is agonist, and the triceps brachii that opposes the movement is antagonist; in extension of the same joint, however, the triceps is agonist, and the brachialis antagonist. Other muscles may neither facilitate nor directly oppose a movement but may modify the action of the agonist, perhaps by eliminating an unwanted side effect. Such muscles are known as *synergists.* When muscles are employed to stabilize joints rather than to promote their movement, they are known as *fixators.* Fixation or stabilization of a joint often involves the co-contraction of muscles that oppose each other when the joint is moved.

The terms *origin* and *insertion* have been left undefined until now. They are best regarded as having purely conventional meaning, origin denoting the more proximal or central attachment, insertion the more distal or peripheral attachment. Although it is true that in their common employment most muscles draw the insertion toward the origin, the vast majority are able to shorten toward

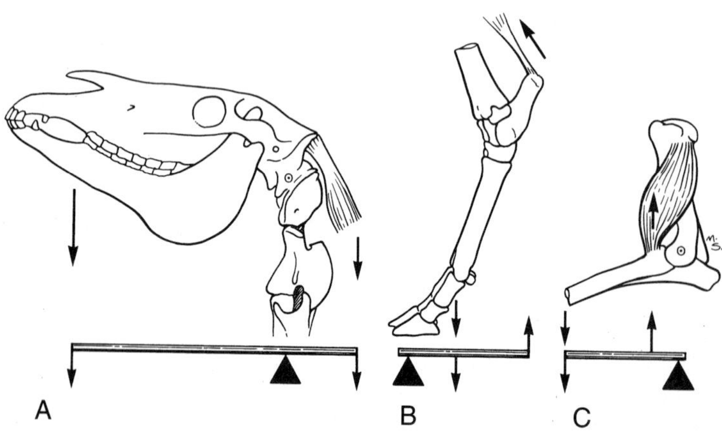


**Figure 1–29.** The action of muscles on the skeleton can be compared to different lever systems. *A,* Support of the head by dorsal neck muscles. *B,* Extension of the hock joint. *C,* Flexion of the elbow joint.

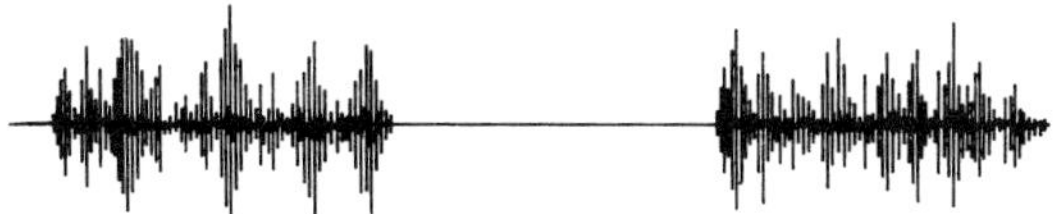

**Figure 1–30.** Record (electromyogram) of electrical activity during muscle contraction.

either extremity; which attachment will maintain its position and which will be drawn toward the other depend on external circumstances. These circumstances must always be taken into account when considering the possible actions of a muscle.

Deductions on muscle action may be made from consideration of the attachments in relation to the axis (axes) of the joint(s). If these deductions are sound, they indicate what a muscle can do—but not how it is habitually used in life. Direct stimulation of a muscle or of its nerve shows what that muscle can do when it acts alone. It does not show how it is used naturally, for often several alternative muscles are available to perform a given movement, and not all are normally used.

The most elegant technique for studying muscle actions is electromyography—the registration of the electrical activity that accompanies muscular contraction. Electrodes are placed over or inserted into the muscles to time the activity and crudely quantify its intensity (Fig. 1–30). The use of this technique has upset many long-held beliefs concerning the actions and use of the muscles of humans; much remains to be investigated where domestic animals are concerned. Even this method demands to be used with caution. It shows when a muscle is active but leaves the experimenter to interpret the activity as agonistic, antagonistic, or a mere adjustment to the alteration in joint angle brought about by other forces.

## Peripheral Blood Vessels

The peripheral blood vessels comprise arteries that lead blood from the heart, veins that return blood to the heart, and capillaries that are the minute connections between the smallest arteries and the smallest veins within the tissues. These vessels are arranged to form two circuits (Fig. 1–31). One, the greater or systemic circulation, arises from the left ventricle, conveys oxygenated (arterial) blood to all organs and parts of the body other than the exchange tissue of the lungs, and then transports the now deoxygenated (venous) blood back to the right atrium; the second, the lesser or pulmonary circulation, conveys deoxygenated blood from the right ventricle to the exchange tissue of the lungs, where it is reoxygenated before being returned to the left atrium by a special set of veins. The systemic and pulmonary circulations together with the chambers of the heart form a single complex course through which the blood circulates endlessly.

### Arteries

In the dissection room, the arteries may be distinguished from other vessels by their white, thick, and relatively rigid walls and their empty lumina (unless filled with an injection mass for the convenience of the dissector). The larger arteries follow a rather constant pattern, but their smaller branches show much variation—so much so that some patterns described in the textbooks, though the most common, may actually occur in only a minority of subjects. When arteries branch, the combined cross-sectional area of the daughter

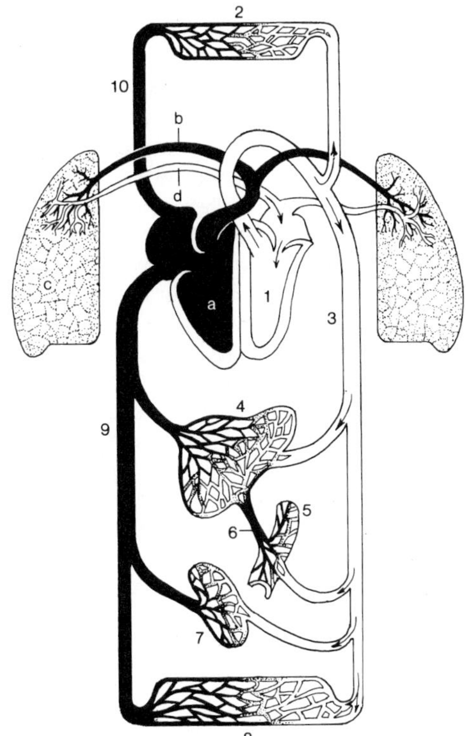


**Figure 1–31.** Schema of the circulation; vessels carrying oxygenated blood are shown in white, those carrying deoxygenated blood in black.

*Systemic circulation:* 1, Left side of the heart; 2, vessels in the cranial part of the body; 3, aorta; 4, liver; 5, intestines; 6, portal vein; 7, kidneys; 8, vessels in the caudal part of the body; 9, caudal vena cava; 10, cranial vena cava. *Pulmonary circulation:* a, Right side of the heart; b, pulmonary artery; c, lung; d, pulmonary vein.

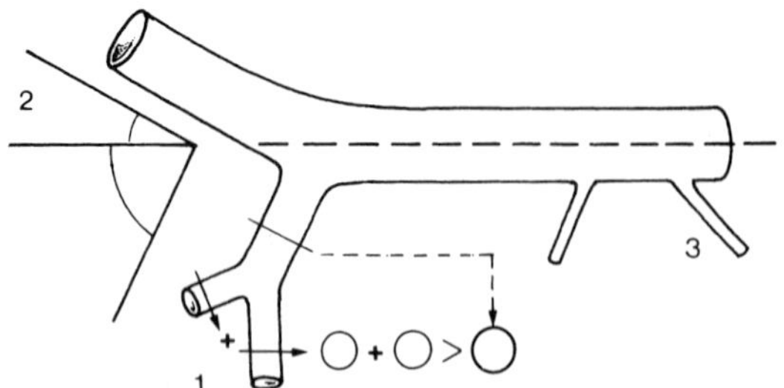


**Figure 1–32.** The branching of the arteries. Note that (1) the sum of the cross-sectional areas of the branches always exceeds that of the parent trunk; (2) large branches leave the trunk at more acute angles than smaller branches; and (3) the smallest branches leave erratically.

vessels always exceeds the cross section of the parent trunk (Fig. 1–32).

A general correspondence exists between the absolute and relative sizes of parent and daughter vessels and the angles at which the latter diverge from the main trunk. Although there are exceptions, larger branches diverge at more acute angles to minimize resistance. Hemodynamic factors are less important where small branches are concerned, and these often follow the shortest routes to their destinations (Fig. 1–32).

Another factor influencing arterial course is a preference for protected situations; this is well illustrated in the limbs, where the major vessels tend to run medially and also to reorient themselves to cross the flexor aspects of successive joints. In comparable fashion, arteries that supply organs that change much in size or position are protected against stretching by taking meandering courses.

Although arteries ultimately discharge into capillary beds, most also have more proximal and more substantial connections with their neighbors. These interarterial connections (anastomoses) provide alternative collateral pathways or bypasses by which a circulation can be maintained when the more direct route is blocked. Collateral circulations operate as soon as a main trunk is obstructed but become more efficient with the passage of time.

The possibility for collateral circulation in different regions and organs has obvious importance to the clinician and the pathologist, and more attention is given to this topic later (p. 235). Meanwhile, this possibility suggests that it may be unnecessary to know the details of all the smaller vessels.

### Veins

In the dissection room, veins are distinguished by their thinner walls, their frequently collapsed appearance, and their capacity, which is invariably greater than that of the associated arteries. They appear blue when filled with clotted blood. Most veins are also distinguished by the presence of valves, which are repeated at intervals along their length; the valves ensure a unidirectional flow and prevent reflux of blood when the circulation stagnates (Fig. 1–33). Each valve consists of two or three semilunar cusps facing each other. Valves are most numerous in veins that are exposed to intermittent changes in external pressure and are wholly lacking in those isolated from such influences. They are thus common in veins running between muscles and absent from those in the vertebral canal and cranial cavity; partly on this account, the veins in the latter site are known by the special term "venous sinuses."

The very largest arteries and veins run separately, but most veins of medium and lesser size accompany the corresponding arteries to which they are said to be satellite. However, they show even more variation than do the arteries and are quite commonly duplicated, further replicated, or arranged in plexus formation.

## Lymphatic Structures

The lymphatic system has two components. The first comprises a system of lymphatic capillaries and larger vessels that return interstitial fluid to the blood stream. The second comprises a variety of widely scattered aggregations of lymphoid tissue, including the many lymph nodes; less discrete lymphoid aggregations, such as tonsils, are not considered until later (p. 250).

### Lymphatic Vessels

A plexus of lymphatic capillaries spread through most tissues collects a fraction of the interstitial fluid, a fraction that is disproportionately important because it includes the protein and other large molecules that are unable to enter the less permeable blood vessels. The greater permeability of the lymphatic capillaries also allows them to take in particulate matter, including microorgan-

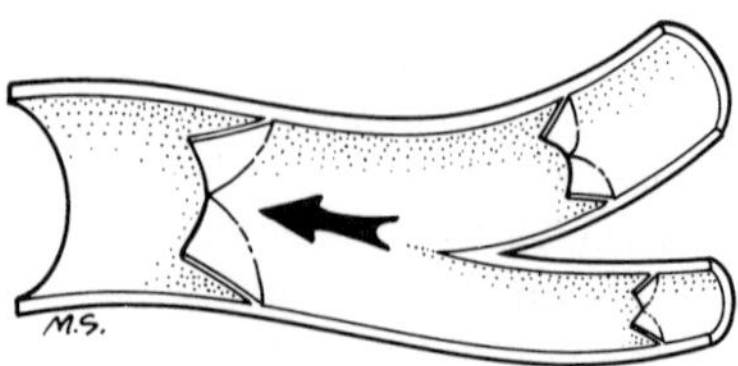


**Figure 1–33.** A branching vein opened to expose valves. The arrow indicates the direction of blood flow.

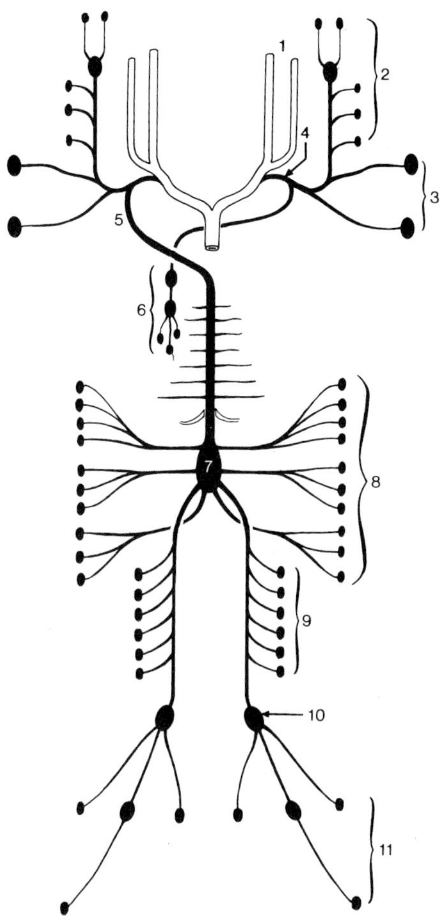


**Figure 1–34.** Generalized schema of the lymph nodes and lymphatic vessels (dorsal view). The top of the diagram represents the neck region.

1, External and internal jugular veins; 2, lymph from the head; 3, lymph from the shoulder and forelimb; 4, tracheal duct; 5, thoracic duct; 6, lymph from the thoracic organs; 7, cisterna chyli; 8, lymph from the abdominal organs; 9, lymph from the lumbar region and kidneys; 10, lymph nodes of the pelvis; 11, lymph from the hindlimb.

isms on occasion. The lymphatic capillaries commence blindly and form plexuses from which larger lymphatic vessels take origin. These larger vessels closely resemble veins in structure but are more delicate. Since the fluid (lymph) they contain is generally pale, they are rarely conspicuous, though easily identified once seen, as closely spaced valves give them a distinctive beaded appearance when they are well filled. The largest vessels take independent courses, but many of smaller size accompany blood vessels and nerves. The lymphatic vascular tree eventually converges on two or three large trunks that open in a rather erratic fashion into major veins at the junction of the neck and thorax (Fig. 1–34).

## Lymph Nodes

Lymph nodes, often incorrectly termed lymph glands, are placed along the lymph pathways in a pattern that shows considerable specific and some individual variation. Groups of neighboring nodes constitute lymphocenters, whose occurrence and drainage territories exhibit greater constancy than is presented by individual nodes. There are important interspecific differences in the lymphocenters; those of the domestic carnivores and ruminants each contain rather few but individually large nodes, particularly in cattle; those of pigs and, more especially, horses each contain a great many small nodes packeted together.

Lymph nodes are firm, smooth-surfaced, and generally ovoid or bean-shaped. Some that are superficial can be identified on palpation through the skin. Naturally, they are more easily found when they are enlarged, and it is therefore a matter of importance to have a clear expectation of which nodes can usually be identified in the healthy animal. Each node is bounded by a capsule, below which runs an open space (subcapsular sinus) into which the afferent vessels open at scattered sites. Branches from the subcapsular sinus lead to a medullary sinus close to the generally indented hilus, where the few efferent vessels emerge (Fig. 1–35/*A;* Plate 12/*G*). The tissue of the node is divided between cortical and medullary regions. The cortex contains the germinal centers in which lymphocytes are continually produced; the medulla consists of looser branching cellular cords; both are supported by a reticular framework containing many phagocytic cells. The organization of the lymph nodes of pigs *(/B)* shows a reversal of the usual flow pattern; the afferent vessels enter together, whereas the efferent vessels have dispersed origins (Plate 12/*E,F*).

With very few exceptions (and these disputed), all lymph passes through at least one node in its passage from the tissues to the blood stream. As it percolates through the node it receives a recruitment of lymphocytes and is also exposed to the activities of the phagocytes. These remove and destroy, or attempt to remove and destroy, particulate matter, including any microorganisms within the lymph. The lymph node thus provides a barrier to the spread of infection and tumors, some varieties of which favor lymphatic pathways for their dissemination. Swelling of a lymph node frequently indicates the existence of a disease process in its drainage territory. It is clear that the role of the lymphatic system in disease is equivocal. On the one hand, lymph flow facilitates the spread of microorganisms or tumor cells; on the other, the intervention of the node provides an opportunity for their containment and destruction. There are obviously weighty reasons why the position, the accessibility, the drainage territory, and the destination of the efferent flow of all major nodes must be familiar to the clinician, the pathologist, and the veterinarian engaged in meat inspection.

## Peripheral Nerves

The central nervous system, the brain and spinal cord, is in two-way communication with virtually all body tissues by means of a system of branching peripheral nerves. These are composed of afferent (sensory) fibers, which convey information to the central nervous system from peripheral receptors, and efferent (motor) fibers, which convey instructions from the central nervous system to peripheral effector organs. The peripheral nerves comprise the 12 pairs of cranial nerves and the considerably larger number of pairs of spinal nerves whose total varies with the vertebral formula. The dog has 8 cervical, 13 thoracic, 7 lumbar, 3 sacral, and about 5 caudal pairs. The present account is restricted to the rather uniform spinal nerves; the cranial nerves differ from these and from one another in many respects that are considered later (p. 305).

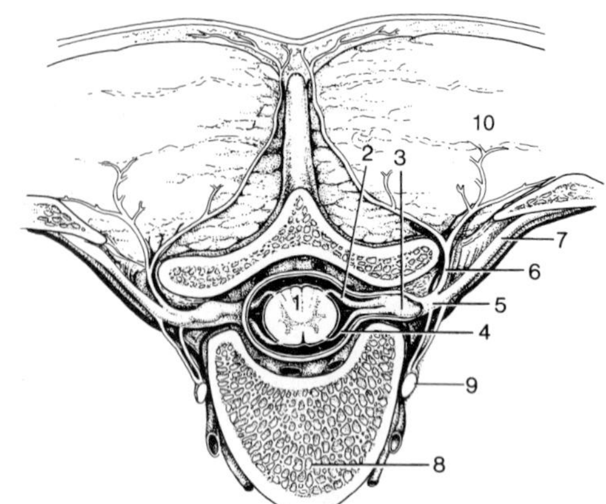


**Figure 1–36.** Transection of the vertebral column to show the formation of a spinal nerve.

1, Spinal cord; 2, dorsal root; 3, spinal ganglion; 4, ventral root; 5, spinal nerve; 6, dorsal branch of spinal nerve; 7, ventral branch of spinal nerve; 8, body of vertebra; 9, sympathetic trunk; 10, epaxial muscles.

The orderly origin of the spinal nerves reveals the segmentation of the spinal cord. Each nerve is formed by the union of two roots (Fig. 1–36). The *dorsal root* is almost exclusively composed of afferent fibers whose cell bodies are clumped together to form a visible swelling, the spinal (dorsal root) ganglion. The central processes enter the cord along a dorsolateral furrow. The peripheral processes extend from the wide variety of exteroceptive, proprioceptive, and enteroceptive endings that respond to external stimuli, changes within the muscles and other locomotor organs, and changes in the internal organs, respectively. The *ventral root* is exclusively composed of efferent fibers emanating from motor neurons within the ventral horn of gray matter and leaving the cord along a ventrolateral strip; they are in passage to the effector organs—muscles and glands.

The dorsal and ventral roots join peripheral to the dorsal root ganglion to form the mixed *spinal nerve* (/5), which leaves the vertebral canal through the appropriate intervertebral foramen. In the cervical region, each nerve emerges cranial to the vertebra of the same numerical designation as the nerve, except the eighth, which emerges between the last cervical and first thoracic vertebrae; in other regions, each nerve emerges caudal to the vertebra of the same numerical designation.

The mixed trunk formed by the union of dorsal and ventral roots divides almost at once into dorsal

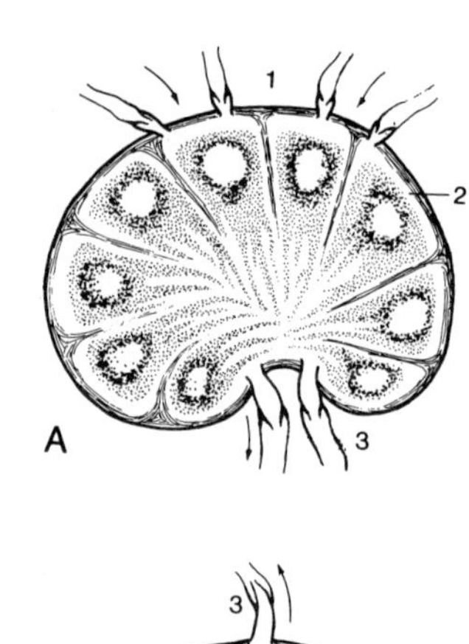


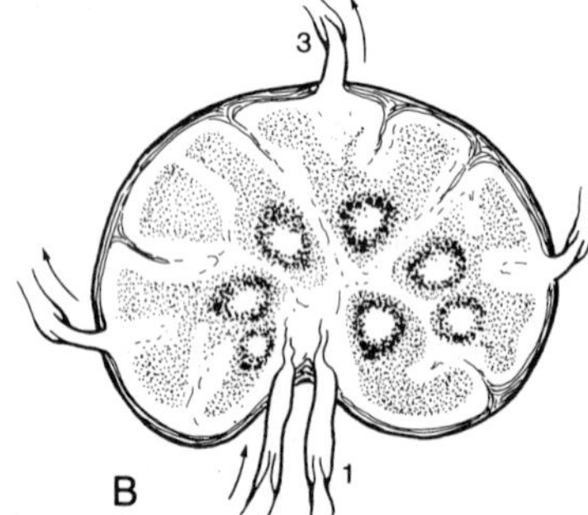


**Figure 1–35.** Structure of a lymph node *(A)* in which the germinal centers (lymph nodules) occupy the cortical region. In the pig *(B)* the germinal centers lie centrally. The arrows indicate the direction of lymph flow.

1, Afferent lymphatics; 2, subcapsular sinus; 3, efferent lymphatics.

and ventral branches (rami). The *dorsal branch* is distributed to dorsal structures: epaxial muscles of the trunk (broadly, those that lie dorsal to the line of transverse processes), and the skin over the back (Fig. 1–37). The much larger *ventral branch* is distributed to hypaxial muscles of the trunk (broadly, those ventral to the transverse processes), the muscles of the limbs (with a few exceptions), and the remaining part of the skin, including that of the limbs. Both dorsal and ventral branches have connections with their neighbors that form continuous dorsal and ventral plexuses. These plexuses are generally neither obvious not important except for enlarged portions of the ventral plexus opposite the origins of the limbs. These, the brachial and lumbosacral plexuses, give rise to the nerves that are distributed to forelimb and hindlimb structures, respectively.

The *brachial plexus* (Fig. 1–38) is usually formed by contributions from the last three cervical and the first two thoracic nerves, the *lumbosacral plexus* by contributions from the last few lumbar and the first two sacral nerves. The limb plexuses allow for regrouping and reassociation of the constituent nerve fibers, and the nerve trunks that emerge distally are each composed of fibers derived from two or three spinal segments; thus the median nerve is composed of fibers from spinal nerves C8 and T1, the femoral nerve of fibers from L4–L6.

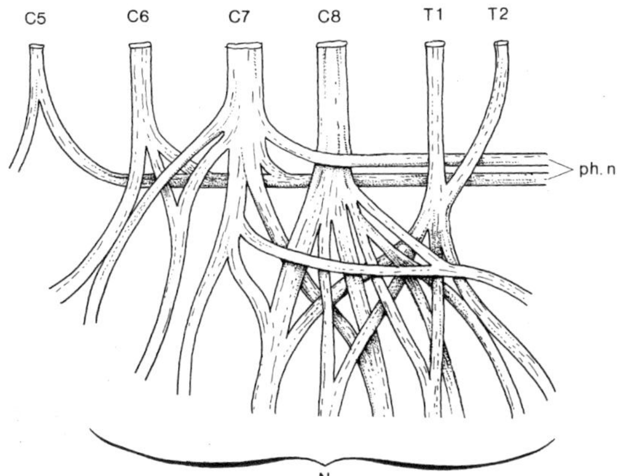


**Figure 1–38.** The brachial plexus. The ventral divisions of the spinal nerves (C6–T2) contributing to the plexus are at the top of the schema, the peripheral branches (N) supplying the forelimb at the bottom. Contributions from C5, C6, and C7 form the phrenic nerve (ph. n.).

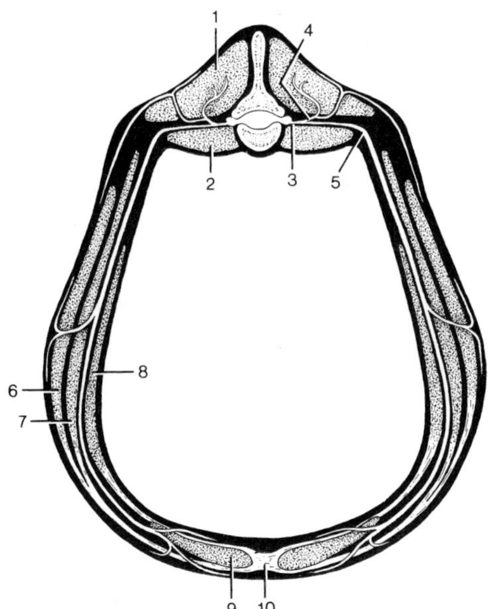


**Figure 1–37.** The distribution of a (lumbar) spinal nerve.

1, Epaxial muscles; 2, sublumbar muscles; 3, spinal nerve; 4, dorsal branch of spinal nerve; 5, ventral branch of spinal nerve; 6, 7, external and internal abdominal oblique muscles; 8, transversus abdominis muscle; 9, rectus abdominis muscle; 10, linea alba.

The courses of the major peripheral trunks must be known to avoid placing the nerves at unnecessary risk during surgery. Their central connections are important in two contexts. First, local anesthetic solutions injected near selected spinal nerves have predictable effects in paralyzing muscles and in depriving skin areas of sensation. Conversely, paralysis of particular muscles or absent or altered sensibility of specific skin areas may point to the precise location of a central lesion.

So far, reference to nerve fibers concerned with the innervation of blood vessels, glands, and internal organs has been avoided. These structures are supplied by the autonomic division of the nervous system, which is described in Chapter 8. For the present, it is sufficient to state that although autonomic fibers are not present in the roots of every spinal nerve, arrangements exist that ensure that each peripheral nerve receives its necessary quota.

CHAPTER 2

# The Locomotor Apparatus

This chapter is concerned with the descriptive anatomy of the bones, joints, and muscles, studies known as *systematic osteology, arthrology,* and *myology.** The accounts of these three classes of organs are grouped according to the major divisions of the body—the trunk, the head, the forelimb, and the hindlimb—since this breaks them into more manageable, and possibly more palatable, fragments. The system has the further advantage of better suiting the needs of any reader who is concurrently engaged in dissection. The descriptions are based on the structures of the dog, and only the most salient comparative features are noted. They omit much that is commonly included in books of systematic anatomy, but many additional details, particularly those that have an applied value, are found in the regional chapters. The introduction to each section mentions those features of development that are likely to be immediately helpful to understanding adult anatomy. These digressions are intended to recapitulate, not to supplant, the descriptions in the standard embryology texts.

## THE TRUNK

### Basic Plan and Development

The trunk is the large part of the carcass that remains after the removal of the head and neck, the tail, and the fore- and hindlimbs; in common speech, it is the body of the animal (Fig. 2–1). It consists of three segments, thorax, abdomen, and pelvis, which are not clearly divided externally. Each is bounded by the body wall, and each contains a cavity, or a potential cavity, since in life the space is more or less obliterated by the close apposition of the walls and contents. The thoracic cavity lies cranial to the diaphragm, a domed sheet of muscle and tendon with a peripheral attachment to the body wall and a free center that bulges cranially. The abdominal cavity lies caudal to the diaphragm and corresponds to the belly. It communicates freely with the pelvic cavity within the enclosure of the bony pelvis (Fig. 2–2).

The *dorsal part of the body wall* that roofs the thoracic, abdominal, and pelvic cavities is known as the back. It is provided by the vertebral column and associated muscles, structures that also extend through the neck and tail. It is therefore convenient, if not entirely appropriate, to consider the vertebrae and associated structures of the neck and tail in this section. The structures of the ventral part of the neck are included with the head.

The neck, back, and tail exhibit a serial repetition of like elements, most notably the vertebrae. This apparent segmentation is, as reference to a young embryo shows (Fig. 2–3), a legacy of the somites, the blocks into which the paraxial mesoderm is segregated to each side of the neural tube and notochord. The appearance in the adult is somewhat misleading; the vertebrae are in fact each formed by contributions from two somites of each side and are therefore more accurately described as intersegmental. Together with the ribs and sternum, they are produced from the medial portions of the somites known as *sclerotomes.* The muscles of the vertebral column are derived from the lateral portions of the somites, the myotomes. Many adult muscles are polysegmental and combine contributions from several or even many myotomes, but certain groups of deeper units retain the unisegmental pattern. Because the vertebrae are intersegmental, even the shortest muscles bridge, and thus can move, the joint between two successive bones.

Each myotome early attracts a single nerve (Fig. 2–3/8) that grows out from the adjacent neural tube; from this it follows that the motor innervation of the muscles is also segmental and that polysegmental muscles will have a multiple innervation. A similar pattern is apparent in the sensory innervation of the skin. It was formerly believed that the connective tissue component of the skin—the dermis—derived exclusively from third portions of the somites, the dermatomes. Cells

**Osteology* derives from *osteon*, Gr. bone; *arthrology* from *arthron*, Gr. joint; and *myology* from *mys*, Gr. muscle. These terms, rather than the Latin equivalents, provide the stems for many medical terms: osteoma, arthrosis, myositis, and so forth. *Syndesmology* is sometimes used as an alternative term for the study of joints.

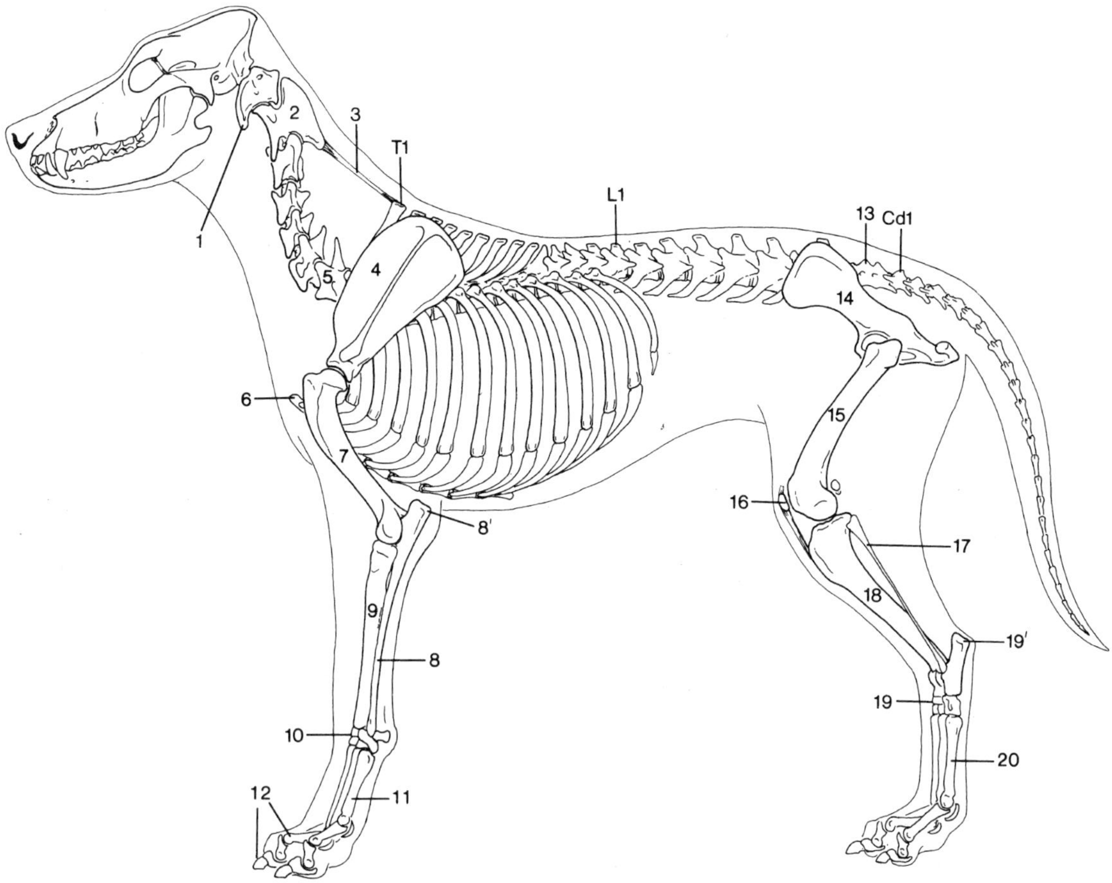

**Figure 2–1.** The skeleton of the dog.

1, Wing of atlas, first cervical vertebra (C1); 2, spine of axis (C2); 3, ligamentum nuchae; 4, scapula; 5, last cervical vertebra (C7); 6, cranial end (manubrium) of sternum; 7, humerus; 8, ulna; 8′, olecranon (point of elbow); 9, radius; 10, carpal bones; 11, metacarpal bones; 12, proximal, middle, and distal phalanges; 13, sacrum; 14, hip bone (os coxae); 15, femur; 16, patella; 17, fibula; 18, tibia; 19, tarsal bones; 19′, calcanean tuber (point of hock); 20, metatarsal bones; T1, L1, and Cd1, first thoracic, lumbar, and caudal (tail) vertebrae.

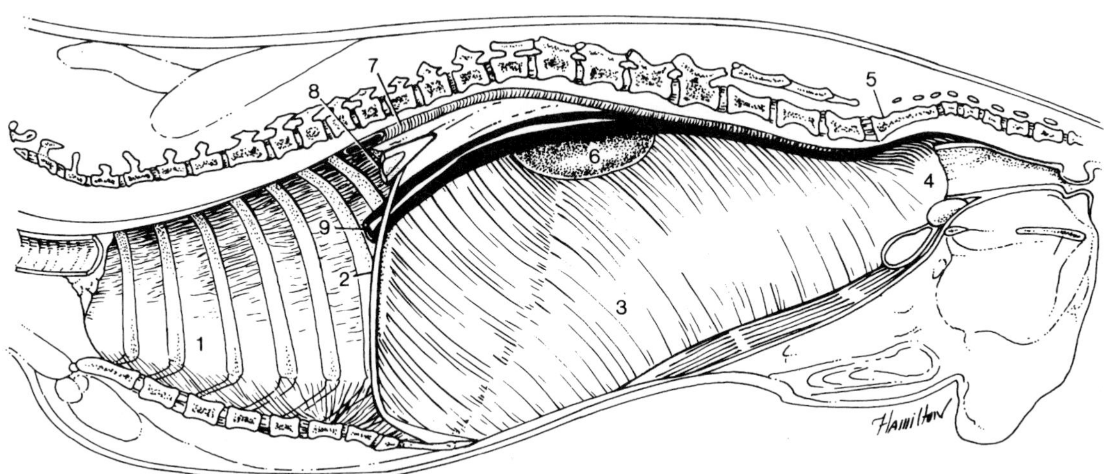


**Figure 2–2.** The thoracic, abdominal, and pelvic cavities of a dog; viewed from the left.

1, Thoracic cavity; 2, diaphragm; 3, abdominal cavity; 4, pelvic cavity; 5, sacrum; 6, right kidney; 7, aorta; 8, esophagus; 9, caudal vena cava.

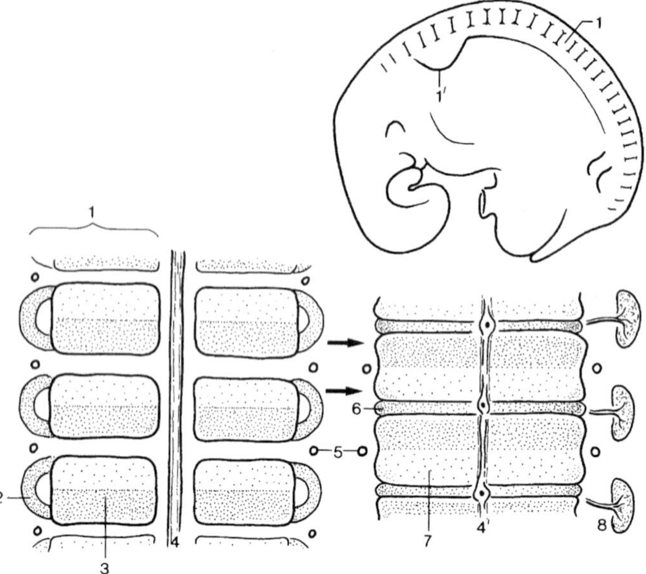


**Figure 2–3.** Segmentation of the paraxial mesoderm shown in a 10-mm bovine embryo *(above)* together with two stages in the development of the vertebrae and related vessels and nerves. The arrows show the formation of each vertebra from two pairs of adjacent somites.

1, Somite; 1′, forelimb bud; 2, myotome; 3, sclerotome; 4, notochord; 4′, notochord giving rise to the nucleus pulposus in the center of the intervertebral disc (6); 5, intersegmental artery; 6, intervertebral disc; 7, body of vertebra; 8, myotome with segmental nerve.

from these were supposed to migrate to underlie specific regions of the surface ectoderm. This ordered pattern of migration is now in question, and it is thought that the dermis may be in part produced through mesenchyme differentiating in situ. Be that as it may, there exists in the adult a segmental innervation of skin (Fig. 2–4) that is very regular in some places and less so in others. The bands of skin that are the provinces of particular pairs of spinal nerves are also known as dermatomes. Many ovelap their neighbors. The associations between these bands and particular sensory nerves develop quite separately from those between the motor nerves and the muscles. The sensory component of the spinal nerve develops from a group of ganglion cells of neural crest origin; central branches of these cells form the dorsal root, which grows into the segment of the neural tube already defined by the outgrowth of the motor root. Together, the dorsal and ventral roots constitute the mixed spinal nerve.

In contrast to the segmental pattern of the nerves, the arteries to the body wall are branches of the aorta that initially pass intersegmentally between the somites (Fig. 2–3/5). Despite this, the arteries and nerves later associate in a way that fails to reflect the different patterns of their origins.

The *lateral and ventral parts of the body wall* are initially unsegmented (Fig. 2–3). The tissues of these parts develop in the somatopleure, which is formed by the association of the ectoderm and the outer of the two sheets into which the lateral plate mesoderm is split. The inner sheet of the lateral mesoderm is, of course, combined with the endoderm to constitute the splanchnopleure or gut wall. The separation of these sheets is achieved by the coalescence of initially scattered spaces to form a continuous cavity (Fig. 2–5/9). The cavity, known as the celom, is afterward divided to yield the pericardial and pleural spaces of the thorax and the peritoneal space of the abdomen and pelvis. The somatopleure is later invaded by cells that migrate ventrally from local somites. Cells that migrate from the sclerotomes of thoracic somites differentiate to form the ribs and sternum. Cells that migrate from the myotomes of both thoracic and abdominal somites differentiate to form the

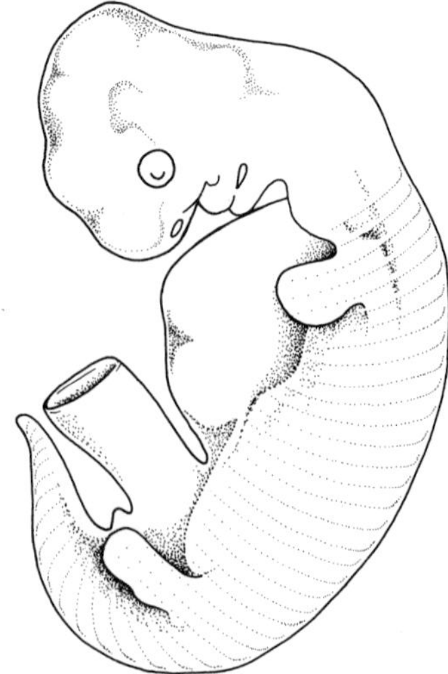

**Figure 2–4.** Embryo with "dermatomes" indicating the segmental innervation of the skin.

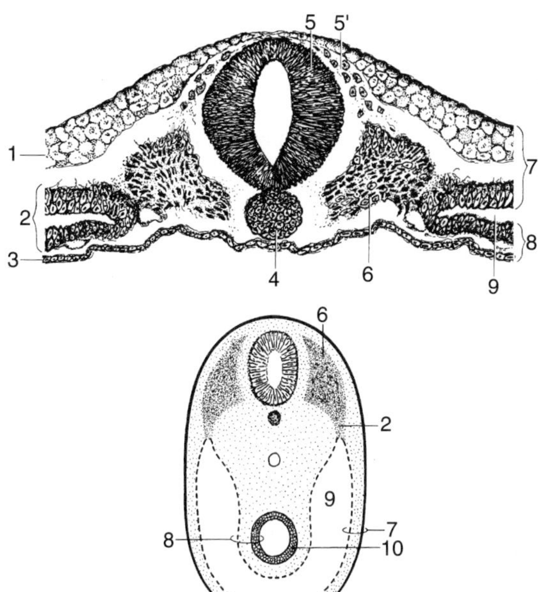


**Figure 2–5.** Transections of an early discoidal embryo *(above)* and of an older ventrally closed one to show the splitting of the lateral mesoderm and the development of the celom.

1, Ectoderm; 2, lateral plate of mesoderm; 3, endoderm; 4, notochord; 5, neural tube; 5′, neural crest cells; 6, somite; 7, somatopleure; 8, splanchnopleure; 9, celom; 10, primitive gut.

muscles of the thoracic and abdominal walls. The presence of the ribs ensures that the thoracic wall retains a segmental pattern, which is almost completely lost by the abdominal wall.

The embryo is still open ventrally while these events are proceeding. The ventral aspect of the body wall closes only in the final stage of the folding (reversal) process (p. 100) that converts the embryonic disc into a more or less cylindrical body. Ventral midline structures including the sternum and the linea alba—the median connective tissue strip of the abdominal floor—are therefore initially represented bilaterally. The umbilical scar—our "bellybutton"—betrays the site of final closure of the body wall.

The clinician's chief interest in the umbilical scar relates to the prevalence of umbilical hernia, a congenital (possibly inherited) defect that frequently occurs in domestic species. Some delay in the closure of the ventral abdominal wall is always necessary to allow for the temporary physiological herniation (p. 145) of a part of the gut into the extraembryonic celom (within the umbilical cord). Normally the herniated loops of intestine are soon drawn back into the abdomen, and narrowing and eventually closure of the peritoneal ring at the junction of the intra- and extraembryonic parts of the celom then follows. This in turn allows the closure of the defect in the mesodermal tissues, so creating the umbilical scar. These processes may be at fault. The intestine may fail to complete its return to the abdomen or, once returned, may make a second escape into the umbilical cord through a persistent peritoneal ring and thus be exposed when the cord is ruptured at birth. More commonly, the peritoneal ring closes, but the overlying tissues remain defective and herniation occurs into a protuberant sac formed by stretching of the peritoneum and covering fasciae and skin. Fortunately, umbilical hernia is usually amenable to simple surgical correction.

## The Skeleton and Joints of the Trunk

### *The Vertebral Column*

The vertebral column (or spine) extends from the skull to the tip of the tail. It consists of a large number of separate bones, the vertebrae, firmly but not rigidly joined together. It serves to stiffen the body axis and thus contributes to the maintenance of posture; by alternate flexion and extension, and sometimes by torsion, it plays a part in progression and other activities. The vertebral column encloses and protects the spinal cord and accessory structures within a central canal; in a more general way it shields the structures of the neck, thorax, abdomen, and pelvis (Fig. 2–1).

Most vertebrae conform to a common pattern on which are superimposed features that distinguish the several regions: cervical (neck), thoracic (back, in the narrow sense), lumbar (loins), sacral (croup), and caudal (tail). The numbers of vertebrae that compose these regions vary among species and also, although to a much smaller extent, individually. They can be represented by a formula: that for the dog is C7, T13, L7, S3, Cd20–23.

A typical vertebra (Fig. 2–6) consists of a massive body surmounted by an arch that completes the enclosure of a vertebral foramen; it is the summation of these foramina that constitutes the vertebral canal. The body, broadly cylindrical, is somewhat flattened on its dorsal surface, which faces into the vertebral canal; it may carry a median crest ventrally. Its extremities are usually curved, the cranial one being convex, the caudal one concave. The arch consists of two upright pedicles, and from each of these a lamina projects medially to meet its fellow and thus complete the ring about the spinal cord. The bases of the pedicles are notched, and when successive bones

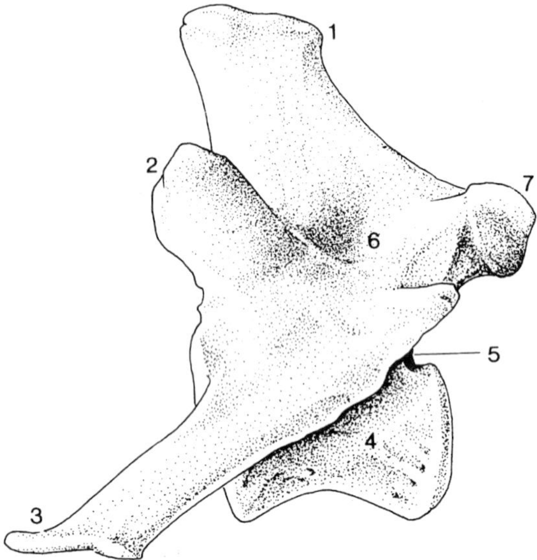


**Figure 2–6.** Lumbar vertebra of the dog, left lateral view.

1, Spinous process; 2, cranial articular process; 3, transverse process; 4, body; 5, caudal vertebral notch; 6, arch; 7, caudal articular process.

articulate, these notches combine to outline intervertebral foramina, openings through which pass both the spinal nerves and the vessels that supply the structures within the vertebral canal. Sometimes an additional lateral vertebral foramen perforates the pedicle next to the intervertebral foramen.

Each vertebra also carries a number of processes. The dorsal or spinous process springs from the union of the laminae and is generally prominent, although its form, its length, and its inclination vary with the region and with the species. Transverse processes project to each side at the junction of the body and the arch; these processes arise at the level of the intervertebral foramina and divide the muscles of the trunk into dorsal and ventral divisions. Synovial joints connect restricted parts of the arches. Sometimes the articular facets hardly rise above the level of their surroundings, but elsewhere, and especially in the caudal thoracic and lumbar region, the facets are carried on articular processes that project cranially and caudally from the dorsal portions of the arches (Fig. 2–6/2,7).

In domestic as in almost all mammals there are seven *cervical vertebrae.* The first two, the atlas and the axis, are much modified to allow free movement of the head and require individual description. The remaining five are more typical.

The atlas is the most unusual of all the vertebrae, since it appears to possess no body but to consist of two lateral masses joined by dorsal and ventral arches (Fig. 2–7/*A*). This form results from the fusion (in early embryonic life) of a component of the atlantal body with the corresponding part of the following bone, the axis. This addition provides the axis with a cranial projection (dens; /*B*,5), which fits into the vertebral foramen of the atlas and serves as a pivot around which the atlas (and the head) may be rotated. A plate of bone, the wing of the atlas (ala atlantis, transverse process), projects laterally from each mass, constituting a landmark that is often visible and always palpable in the living animal. The cranial aspect of the ventral arch and the adjacent areas on the wings carry two deep excavations that receive the occipital condyles of the skull. These facets approach ventrally, and in some species they merge. The caudal aspect of the ventral arch is hollowed transversely to provide an articular surface that engages with the cranial extremity of the axis. An extension (fovea dentis; /*A*,2) of this facet onto the dorsal surface of the ventral arch accommodates the dens. The dorsal arch is perforated by openings that correspond with the transverse and intervertebral foramina of more typical cervical vertebrae; in some species a third (alar) foramen perforates the wing.

The axis is the longest vertebra. Its cranial extremity carries the dens, which is rodlike in carnivores and more spoutlike in some other species. The cranial extremity of the body and the ventral surface of the dens concur in forming a

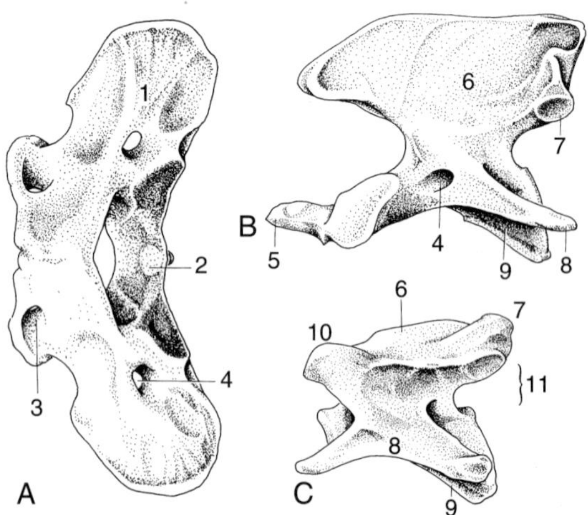


**Figure 2–7.** Cervical vertebrae of the dog; cranial is to the left. *A,* Atlas, dorsal view. *B,* Axis, lateral view. *C,* Fifth vertebra, lateral view.

1, Wing of atlas; 2, fovea dentis; 3, lateral vertebral foramen; 4, transverse foramen; 5, dens; 6, spinous process; 7, caudal articular process; 8, transverse process; 9, body; 10, cranial articular process; 11, position of vertebral foramen.

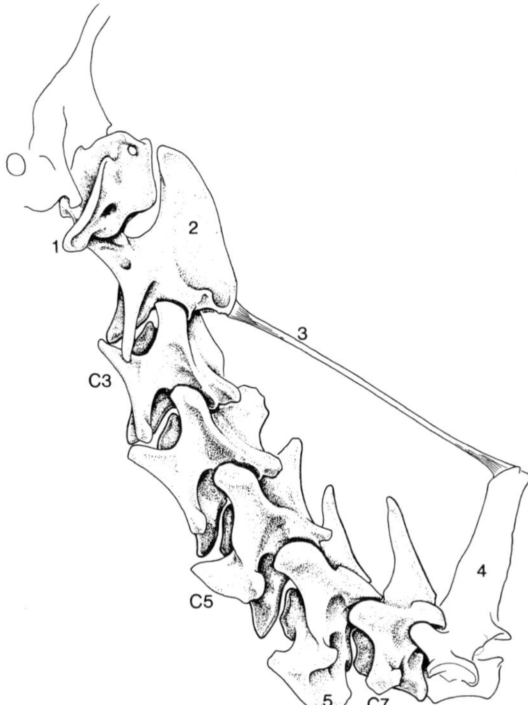


**Figure 2–8.** Nuchal ligament of the dog.

1, Wing of atlas; 2, spinous process of axis; 3, nuchal ligament; 4, spinous process of first thoracic vertebra; 5, platelike extension of transverse process.

single wide articulation for the atlas. Dorsally the dens is roughened for the attachment of ligaments that hold it in place. The arch carries a very high (and in the dog, long) spinous process that bears articular facets at its caudal extremity; these meet corresponding facets on the third cervical vertebra. The transverse processes are large; each is perforated toward its root by a transverse foramen that transmits the vertebral artery, vein, and nerve.

The remaining cervical vertebrae become progressively shorter as the series is followed toward its junction with the thorax. The extremities of the body are more strongly curved than in other regions and slope obliquely. The ventral surface carries a stout crest. The arch is strong and wide, but the spinous process is poorly developed except on the last (but with considerable variation among species). The large transverse process (Fig. 2–7/8) branches into dorsal and ventral tubercles, the latter commonly developing a caudal platelike extension (Fig. 2–8/5). On the third to sixth bones the process is perforated by a transverse foramen through which the vertebral vessels and nerve pass. The articular facets are large and flat but do not rise above the surrounding level. The seventh cervical vertebra, transitional to those of the thoracic region, is distinguished by its taller spinous process, unperforated transverse process, and the presence of facets on the caudal extremity of its body for articulation with the first pair of ribs.

The *thoracic vertebrae* (Fig. 2–9) articulate with the ribs and correspond with these in number. Minor variations in number are not uncommon; they are often compensated by a reciprocal change in the lumbar region that leaves the thoracolumbar total unaffected. All thoracic vertebrae share common features, but serial changes also occur that gradually (and on some points abruptly) distinguish the more cranial from the more caudal bones. Common thoracic features are short bodies with flattened extremities; costal facets, on both extremities for the rib heads and on the transverse processes for the rib tubercles; short, stubby transverse processes; closely fitting arches; very prominent spinous processes; and low articular processes.

Conspicuous serial features are a rapid increase in height of the spinous processes, which reach a maximum a few vertebrae behind the cervicothoracic junction and gradually decline thereafter; progressive simplification of the costal facets, with those on the transverse processes approaching and finally merging with those on the cranial extremity; reduction (and eventual disappearance) of the caudal costal facets; and appearance of an additional (mamillary) process as a projection from the

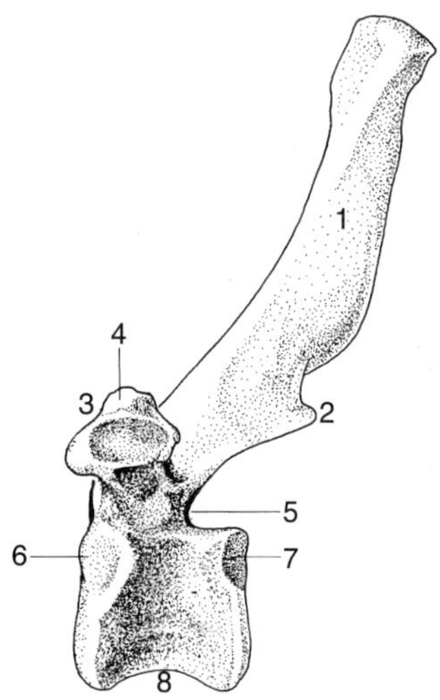


**Figure 2–9.** Thoracic vertebra of the dog; left lateral view. (See also Fig. 2–16.)

1, Spinous process; 2, caudal articular process; 3, transverse process with costal fovea; 4, mamillary process; 5, caudal vertebral notch; 6, 7, costal foveae; 8, body.

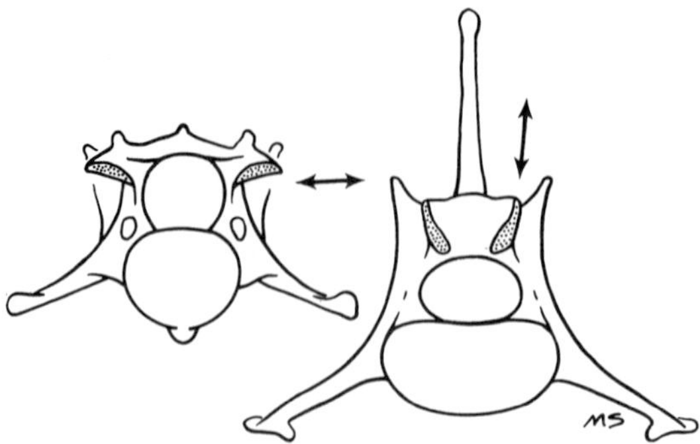

**Figure 2–10.** Contrast the orientation *(arrows)* of the articular surfaces of a cervical *(left)* and a lumbar *(right)* vertebra of the dog, caudal view.

transverse process and its gradual migration to join the cranial articular process. More abrupt changes toward the end of the thoracic series include sudden alteration from a caudodorsal to a craniodorsal orientation of the spinous processes; a change in the character of the articular facets from the cervical to the lumbar pattern (Fig. 2–10). In some species, including the dog, the last members of the thoracic series possess yet other (accessory) processes that spring from the caudal part of the arch to overlap the following bone.

The *lumbar vertebrae* (Fig. 2–11) differ from the thoracic vertebrae in the greater length and more uniform shape of their bodies. Other regional features are absence of the costal facets; a shorter height and generally forward slope of the spinous processes; long, flattened transverse processes that project laterally, sometimes (as in the dog) with a cranioventral inclination; interlocking articular processes; and prominent mamillary, and sometimes also accessory, processes.

Caudal to the loins the vertebral column is continued by the *sacrum,* a single bone formed by the fusion of several vertebrae. The sacrum forms a firm articulation with the pelvic girdle through which the thrust of the hindlimbs is transmitted to the trunk. Usually only one or two of the constituent vertebrae directly participate in the articulation. The more caudal bones project behind this to furnish the greater part of the roof of the pelvic cavity. In some animals (especially pigs) one or more tail vertebrae may be incorporated into the sacrum in later life. In the dog the three sacral vertebrae form a short quadrilateral block (Fig. 2–12).

The sacrum commonly narrows from its cranial to its caudal extremity and is curved along its length to present a smooth, slightly concave face toward the pelvic cavity. In most species the dorsal surface is marked by the appropriate number of spinous processes, although these may be much reduced or even absent (e.g., pig). When present, they may preserve their independence (e.g., dog, horse) or fuse to form a continuous crest (e.g., ruminants). Lateral to this, a lower irregular crest usually marks the site of the articular processes. The margin of the bone is formed by the fused transverse processes and carries toward its cranial extremity the articular surface for the ilium; this is often "ear-shaped," hence the name auricular surface (/2).

The degree of fusion of the sacral vertebrae varies among species; it is least complete in the pig. Even when fusion is total, the composition of the sacrum is betrayed by the number of foramina that mark both surfaces; the dorsal and the ventral branches of the sacral nerves issue separately through these. The junction of the ventral surface with the cranial extremity forms a lip known as the promontory (/1); though often inconspicuous, it is a reference point in obstetrics.

The number of *caudal vertebrae* varies greatly even within a single species. These vertebrae show a progressive simplification in form, and although

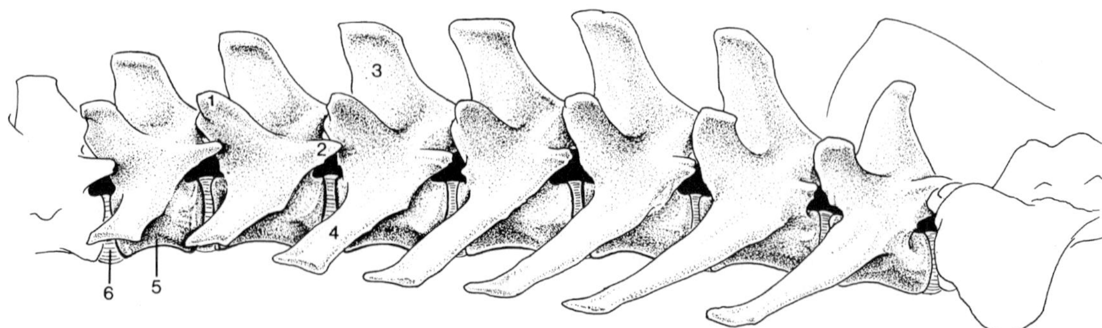


**Figure 2–11.** Lumbar vertebrae of the dog, left lateral view.

1, Mamillary process; 2, accessory process; 3, spinous process; 4, transverse process; 5, body; 6, intervertebral disc.

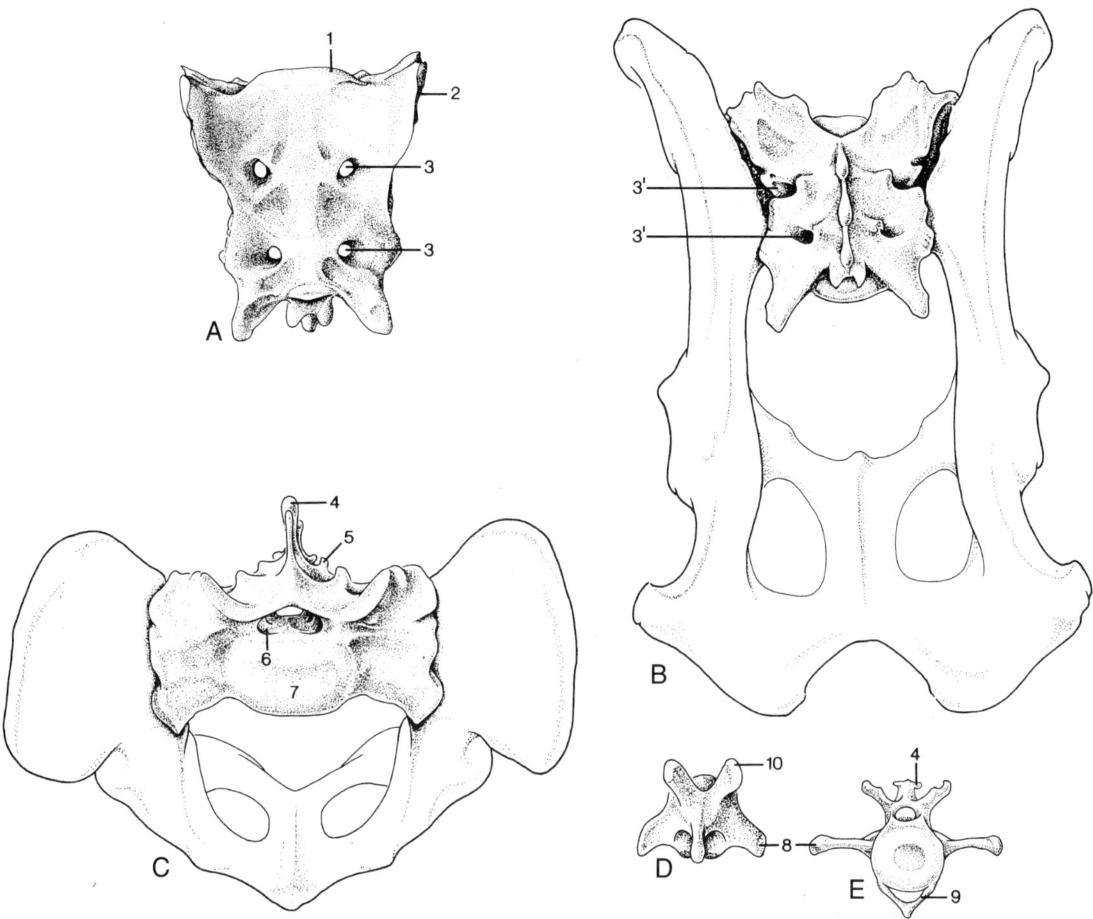


**Figure 2–12.** Canine sacrum and caudal vertebrae. *A,* Sacrum, ventral view. *B,* Sacrum, dorsal view. *C,* Sacrum, cranial view. *D,* Caudal vertebra, dorsal view. *E,* Caudal vertebra, cranial view.

1, Promontory; 2, auricular articular surface; 3, ventral (3′ dorsal) sacral foramina for ventral (3′ dorsal) branches of sacral nerves; 4, spinous process; 5, rudimentary articular process; 6, vertebral canal; 7, body; 8, transverse process; 9, hemal arch, also called chevron; 10, cranial articular process.

the first few resemble miniature lumbar vertebrae, the middle and later members of the series are reduced to simple rods. In addition to the usual features, the more cranial vertebrae of some species provide protection to the main artery of the tail, in the form of ventral (hemal) arches, separate small chevron (V-shaped) bones connected to the undersurfaces of the bodies, or paired ventral (hemal) processes (Fig. 2–12/*E*).

The *contours of the vertebral column* vary with the posture, the species, and the breed. In general, the vertebrae from the caudal thoracic region to the tail head follow a more or less horizontal line. The more cranial thoracic vertebrae slope downward to reach the lowest point at the entrance to the chest, where an abrupt change in direction puts the spine on a course that ascends toward the head. The ventral inclination of the cranial thoracic vertebrae is masked in the live animal by the height of the spinous processes; indeed, in some species, the horse most notably, the spines are so long that the contour of this part of the back is raised to constitute the withers. Except toward the poll, the cervical vertebrae run at some distance from the dorsal skin. This is not apparent in the live subject, and in larger animals it may not be easy to determine even on palpation. The greater part of the tail hangs down in large animals, but its posture is more variable in dogs and cats, being expression of emotion in both species and influenced by breed in the former.

## The Joints of the Vertebral Column

The vertebrae form two sets of joints: one cartilaginous, involving the direct connection of the vertebral bodies, the other synovial, existing between facets carried on the vertebral arches. In addition, certain long ligaments extend over many vertebrae. This pattern is modified in two regions; cranially, allowance is made for the free movement of the head, and in the pelvic region the sacral fusion occurs.

The two joints of the atlas are described first. The *atlanto-occipital joint* (Fig. 2–13) is formed between the condyles of the skull and the corresponding concavities of the atlas. Although the separate right and left articular surfaces converge ventrally, they do not always merge; despite this a single synovial cavity generally exists. The synovial membrane attaches around the occipital and atlantal facets. It is strengthened externally by dorsal and ventral atlanto-occipital membranes, which pass from the arches of the atlas to corresponding parts of the margin of the foramen magnum (Fig. 2–32/12), and by lesser lateral ligaments, which pass between the atlas and adjacent regions of the skull. Despite its odd character, the joint functions as a ginglymus, with movement virtually restricted to flexion and extension in the sagittal plane—the nodding movement that in ourselves conveys agreement.

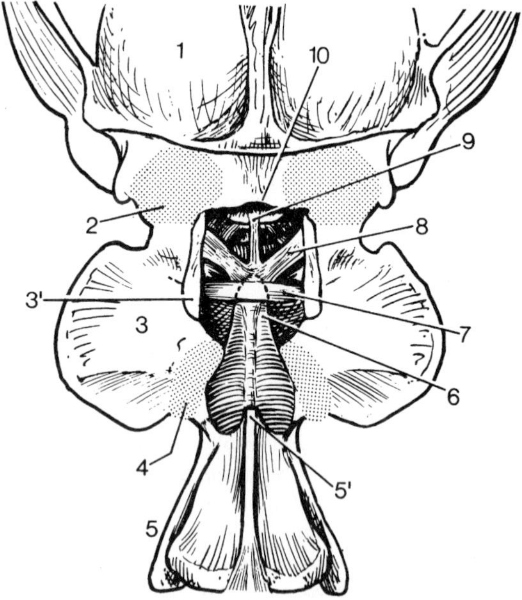


**Figure 2–13.** Canine atlanto-occipital joint, dorsal view; the dorsal arch of the atlas has been removed.

1, Skull; 2, atlanto-occipital joint capsule; 3, wing of atlas; 3′, dorsal arch of atlas, resected; 4, atlantoaxial joint capsule; 5, axis; 5′, spine of axis, its overhanging cranial portion having been removed; 6, dens; 7, transverse ligament of atlas; 8, alar ligaments; 9, apical ligament of dens; 10, dorsal margin of foramen magnum.

The *atlantoaxial joint* is even more peculiar. The extensive articular surfaces of the ventral arch of the atlas and of the body and dens of the axis face into a single synovial cavity. The surfaces are so formed that only limited areas are in contact in any position of the head. This limitation of contact, together with the roomy capsule, allows some versatility of movement, although free excursion is confined to rotation about a longitudinal axis—the head-shaking movement that implies negation. The dorsal atlantoaxial ligament that joins adjacent parts of these vertebrae imposes little restraint. The dens of the axis, which occupies a potentially dangerous position in relation to the spinal cord, is secured by one or more ligaments that strap it to the adjacent part of the upper surface of the ventral atlantal arch and sometimes also to the occipital bone (as in the dog). It is rupture of these ligaments—or fracture of the dens itself—that allows the axis to strike against the cord and procure death in judicial hanging, according to traditional accounts (other forms of cervical fracture or dislocation may be at least as common).

A single description serves for the articulations of most other vertebrae. The *intervertebral articulations* combine symphyses between the bodies and synovial joints between the articular processes. The bodies of adjacent bones are connected through thick but flexible pads, the intervertebral discs, which make an appreciable contribution to the articulated column. They account for about 10% of its length in ungulates, about 16% in dogs, and about 25% in ourselves—proportions that are clearly correlated with different degrees of suppleness of the trunk. The discs are among the organs that most consistently show degenerative changes with advancing age; disc lesions are a common source of back trouble, long recognized in ourselves and in dogs, now also diagnosed in other domestic and even in wild animals. Therefore, their structure has considerable importance, and it may be wise to stress that the details of anatomy and the nature of the troubles that may occur are not the same in ourselves and in quadrupeds.

Each disc consists of two parts, a nucleus pulposus and an anulus fibrosus (Fig. 2–14). The nucleus occupies a slightly eccentric position. In the young animal it consists of an unusual semifluid tissue derived from the embryonic notochord and retains some resemblance to this in structure. It is contained under pressure and escapes if afforded opportunity. The anulus fibrosus consists of encircling bundles of fibrous tissue that pass obliquely from one vertebra to the other, in most species merging with cartilage plates that cap the bones. The orientation of the fibers changes between successive lamellae, of which about a

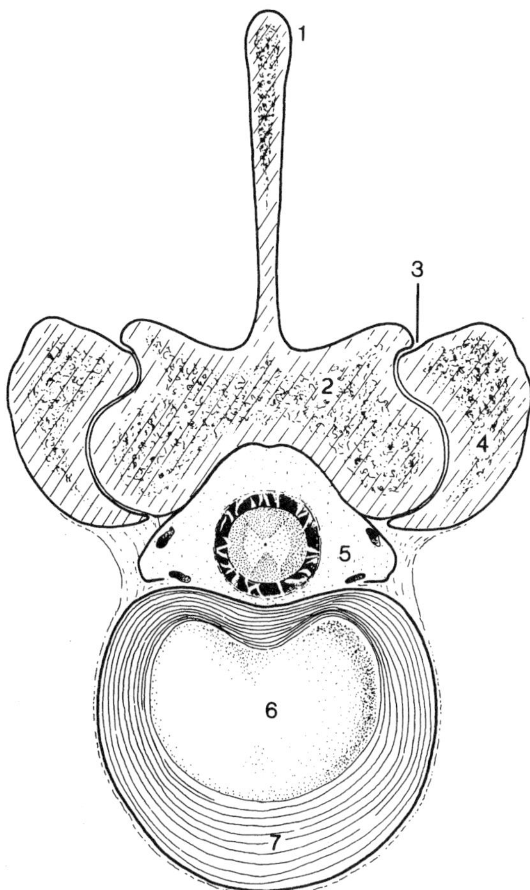


**Figure 2–14.** Bovine lumbar intervertebral disc.

1, Spinous process; 2, lamina; 3, synovial intervertebral joint; 4, articular process of adjacent vertebra; 5, vertebral canal with contents (spinal cord and meninges surrounded by epidural fat); 6, nucleus pulposus; 7, anulus fibrosus.

score exist. The distinction between anulus and nucleus is not always very distinct, particularly in the larger species. Retention of the nucleus within the fibrous ring absorbs shock and spreads over a wider part of the vertebrae the compressive forces to which the column is subjected.

Insidious changes involving both nucleus and anulus commence relatively early in life. Fragmentation of the ring may allow the nucleus to escape, usually in the direction of the vertebral canal, where, directly or indirectly, it may press on the cord. Calcification of the nucleus diminishes the normal resilience and flexibility of the spine. Degenerative changes may affect any disc, but the effects are naturally likely to be most severe when they involve the discs at the most mobile regions; those of the neck and, in large animals, that at the lumbosacral junction are especially susceptible. Most thoracic discs are crossed dorsally by the intercapital ligaments that unite the heads of the right and left ribs (p. 44), and these are alleged to mitigate the effects of disc rupture at these levels.

The joints between the facets on the vertebral arches are conventional synovial joints. The nature and degree of mobility vary with the region and to some extent also with the species. In the cervical and cranial thoracic regions the joint surfaces are arranged tangential to the circumference of a circle centered in the vertebral body (Fig. 2–10); in these regions rotation is possible in addition to the usual flexion and extension. In the caudal thoracic and lumbar regions the surfaces have a radial alignment, and movement is more or less restricted to the median plane. Movement is most free in the neck where the articular surfaces are largest and the capsules most loose. The elastic interarcuate ligaments that fill the dorsal spaces between the arches of successive vertebrae may be regarded as accessory to these joints; their extent is inversely related to the width of the arches. In certain regions interspinous and intertransverse ligaments also exist, but these are of less importance.

Three *long ligaments* extend along substantial portions of the column. A dorsal longitudinal ligament (Fig. 2–15/7) runs along the floor of the vertebral canal from the axis to the sacrum. Narrow over the middle of each vertebral body, it widens where it crosses each intervertebral disc. A ventral longitudinal ligament follows the ventral aspect of the vertebrae from the midthoracic region to the sacrum; more cranially its role is filled by the longus colli muscles. It also widens over and fuses with the intervertebral discs.

A third (supraspinous) common ligament runs over (or to each side of) the summits of the spinous

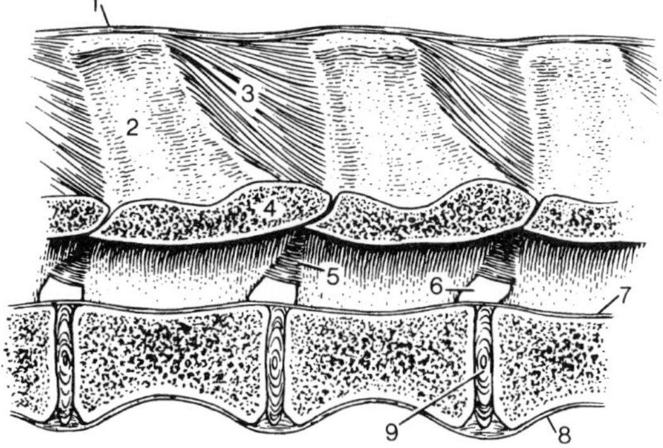


**Figure 2–15.** Ligaments of the vertebral column. Paramedian section of lumbar vertebrae of a dog; viewed from the left.

1, Supraspinous ligament; 2, spinous process; 3, interspinous ligament; 4, arch of vertebra; 5, interarcuate ligament; 6, intervertebral foramen; 7, dorsal longitudinal ligament; 8, ventral longitudinal ligament; 9, intervertebral disc.

processes of the thoracic and lumbar vertebrae. It merges with the tendons of the epaxial muscles so completely that some dispute its independent existence. Except in the pig and cat, a cranial continuation of this ligament leaves the highest spines of the withers and runs by the shortest route to attach to the nuchal surface of the skull or, as in the dog, the spinous process of the axis (Fig. 2–8). This nuchal ligament runs close to the upper contour of the neck, and for most of its length it is well separated from the more ventral course followed by the cervical vertebrae. Unlike the other long ligaments, it is elastic and thus able to accept much of the burden of the head when this is held high without interfering with the animal's ability to lower the head to feed or drink from the ground. There is an obvious correlation between the strength of this ligament and the weight of the head and the length of the lever arm of the neck; the nuchal ligament is therefore much more powerfully developed in the larger species (see Fig. 19–3), in which it is also more complicated in structure.

## The Ribs and Sternum

The thoracic skeleton is completed by the ribs and sternum. The *ribs* (costae) are arranged in pairs and generally articulate with two successive vertebrae, the caudal one being that with the same numerical designation as the rib. Each rib consists of a bony dorsal part, the rib proper, and a cartilaginous ventral part, the costal cartilage (Fig. 2–16/*A*). The two parts meet at a costochondral junction. The dorsal part of the rib articulates with the vertebral column, while the cartilage articulates with the sternum either directly, as do the first eight or so sternal or "true" ribs, or indirectly through connection of the cartilage with that in front, as do the asternal or "false" ribs. In this way, the cartilages of the asternal ribs combine to form the costal arch (Fig. 2–17/*A*,6), the cranial boundary of the flank. The cartilage of the last rib may fail to make contact with its neighbor, and this rib is then said to be "floating."

The dorsal extremity of the rib terminates in a rounded head that carries two facets, one for articulation with the body of each of the two vertebrae with which it is connected. These facets are separated by a rougher area (crest) that makes contact with the intervertebral disc and on most ribs also gives origin to the intercapital ligament. The head is joined to the body of the rib by a short constricted neck whose lower part carries a lateral tubercle. The tubercle bears a third articular facet, which meets that on the transverse process of the more caudal of the associated vertebrae (Fig. 2–16/*B*).

The body of the rib begins beyond the tubercle. It is long, curved in its length, and usually laterally flattened, particularly in the larger species and toward the lower extremity. It is most strongly bent at a region known as the angle (/4), where the lateral surface is roughened for the attachment of the iliocostalis. The cranial and caudal margins of the body are often sharply defined and give attachment to the intercostal muscles that fill the space between successive ribs. The caudal margin may also be grooved to give protection to the neurovascular bundle of the intercostal space.

The costal cartilage is flexible in the young animal, especially if it is long and thin, as in the dog. It becomes more rigid as calcification develops and increases with age. The cartilage either meets the bony rib at an angle (knee, genu) or is itself flexed cranioventrally some way beyond the costochondral junction.

Serial changes are obvious. The first rib is always relatively strong, short, and straight. Its cartilage is also stumpy and articulates with the sternum at a tight joint that fixes the rib; this allows it to act as a firm base toward which the other ribs may be drawn on inspiration. The

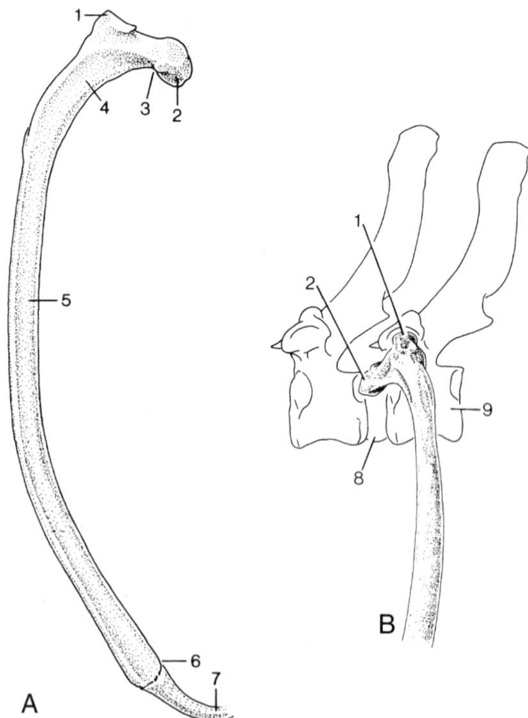


**Figure 2–16.** *A*, Left rib of a dog, caudal view. *B*, Left rib of a dog articulating with two vertebrae, lateral view.

1, Tubercle; 2, head; 3, neck; 4, angle; 5, body; 6, costochondral junction; 7, costal cartilage; 8, intervertebral disc; 9, vertebra of same number as rib.

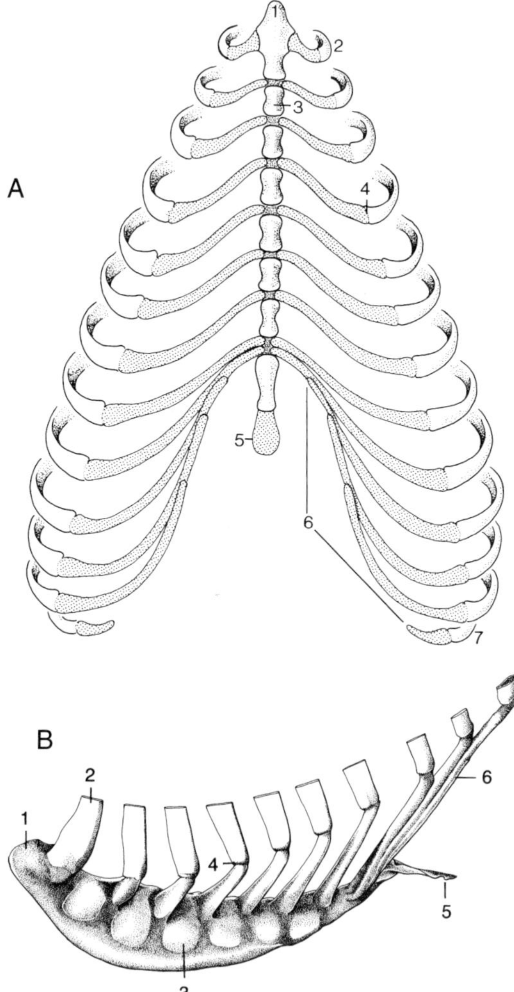


**Figure 2–17.** *A*, Canine and *B*, equine sternum and costal cartilages, ventral and left lateral views.

1, Manubrium; 2, first rib; 3, sternebra; 4, costochondral junction; 5, xiphoid cartilage; 6, costal arch; 7, floating rib.

succeeding ribs increase in length, in curvature, and in caudoventral inclination, most markedly over the caudal part of the thoracic wall, although the very last two or three may again be somewhat shorter. The three articular facets of the upper end approach and eventually merge on the ribs toward the end of the series. The cartilages of the sternal ribs are short and about as thick as the bony ribs; those of the asternal ribs are mostly slender and taper toward their ventral extremities.

The *sternum* is composed of three parts. The most cranial part, known as the manubrium (Fig. 2–17/1), generally projects in front of the first ribs and may be palpated at the root of the neck. It is rodlike in the dog and cat but is laterally compressed in the larger animals. The body of the bone is composed of several segments (sterne-brae), in youth joined by cartilage that is later replaced by bone. It is cylindrical in the dog, wide and flat in ruminants, and carries a ventral keel in the horse (/*B*). Its dorsolateral margin bears a series of depressions in which the extremities of the costal cartilages are lodged. The more cranial of these depressions alternate with the sternebrae, and each receives a single cartilage; the more caudal depressions are crowded more closely together and may receive more than one cartilage. The caudal part of the sternum consists of a flat (xiphoid) cartilage (/5) that projects between the lower parts of the costal arches. It supports the most cranial part of the abdominal floor and gives attachment to the linea alba.

## The Joints of the Thoracic Wall

Most ribs make two separate articulations with the vertebral column. The head participates in a ball-and-socket *costovertebral joint* of unusually restricted mobility. The joint cavity is divided into two compartments by the intercapital ligament (Fig. 2–18/2), which arises from the interarticular crest. This ligament passes through the interverte-bral foramen, crosses the floor of the vertebral canal, and ends by inserting on the corresponding region of the rib of the other side. In its passage it detaches slips that anchor to the intervertebral disc and the adjacent parts of the vertebrae. It passes below the dorsal longitudinal ligament (/6) and offers some protection against protrusion into the vertebral canal of nuclear material from a ruptured disc. An intercapital ligament is not found at the first costovertebral joint or at the last few. Additional short and tight ligaments support the joint dorsally and ventrally.

The *costotransverse joint* in which the tubercle participates is of the sliding variety. It is supported by a ligament that passes between the neck of the rib and the transverse process of the vertebra (/8).

The *costosternal joints* are synovial joints of the pivot variety. The *interchondral joints* of the asternal ribs are syndesmoses of a rather elastic nature. The *intersternal joints* are mostly imperma-nent synchondroses, although in some species the manubrium articulates with the body at a synovial joint.

The movements possible at these joints are discussed with the actions of the muscles of the thoracic wall.

## The Pelvic Girdle

Although the pelvic girdle is formally a part of the hindlimb skeleton, it seems more sensible to treat it here since it is fully integrated into the construction of the trunk. The girdle consists of

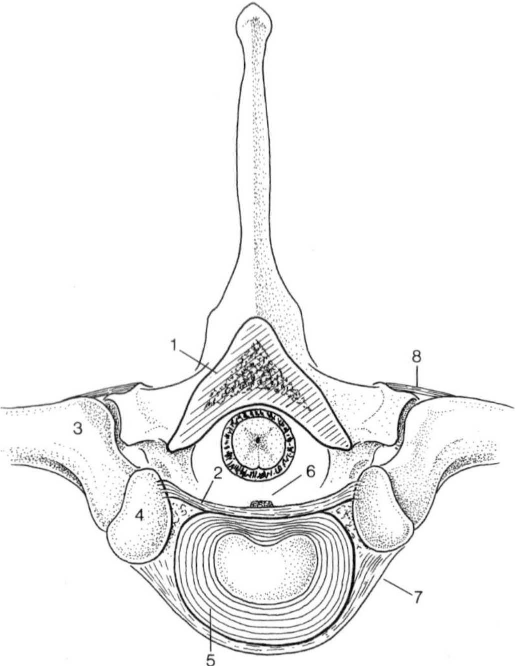


**Figure 2–18.** Costovertebral articulations; transverse section of the vertebral column of the dog (about T8).

1, Lamina of vertebra; 2, intercapital ligament; 3, tubercle of rib; 4, head of rib; 5, intervertebral disc; 6, dorsal longitudinal ligament; 7, costovertebral joint; 8, costotransverse joint covered by costotransverse ligament.

symmetrical halves, the hip bones (ossa coxarum), which meet at the pelvic symphysis ventrally and form firm, though not rigid, articulations with the sacrum dorsally. When augmented by the sacrum and first few tail vertebrae, it forms a ring known as the bony pelvis around the pelvic cavity. The close association with the pelvic organs exposes the girdle to visceral influences of which those related to giving birth are most important; the form of the bony pelvis therefore reflects a compromise between these and the requirements of locomotion and posture.

Each hip bone is composed of three bones that develop from separate ossifications within a single cartilage plate. Though in the young animal strips of cartilage demarcate the boundaries to allow for growth, they disappear once growth is complete. It is therefore artificial to describe the three components—ilium, pubis, and ischium—as separate units; the practice can be justified only by its convenience in facilitating description. The ilium (Fig. 2–19/1) is the craniodorsal part that extends obliquely forward from the hip joint to articulate with the sacrum. The pubis (/6) extends medially from the joint to form the cranial part of the pelvic floor. The ischium (/8) is more caudal and forms the larger part of the floor, though it also sends a branch to the joint. Both pubis and ischium participate in the symphysial joint in domestic species, although only the pubis does so in the human pelvis.

The *ilium* consists of a cranial expansion or wing and a caudal shaft or body. The wing varies much among species; it is oblong with a more or less sagittal orientation in the dog and cat and is triangular and almost vertical in the horse and ruminants (Fig. 2–19). Its margin forms saliences, generally thickened, at certain points. Dorsally (dorsomedially in the larger species), it forms a sacral tuber; this is reduced to two low (cranial and caudal dorsal iliac) spines in the dog and cat (/3) but is prominent in the large animals, in which it is close to the spinous processes of the vertebrae (/3′). Ventrally (ventrolaterally in the larger species), the ilium forms a coxal tuber (/2′, 2); this is also reduced to low (cranial and caudal ventral iliac) spines in the carnivores but is prominent in large species, forming the point of the hip at the dorsocaudal corner of the flank (Fig. 2–20/*B*, 8). Including these projections, the margin of the wing is known as the iliac crest; thickened and convex in carnivores, it is thin and concave in large animals. Some of these features form important landmarks in the living animal.

The lateral (dorsolateral) surface is excavated and largely given over to the origin of the gluteus medius, whose attachment may raise one or more quite prominent ridges. The medial (ventromedial) surface faces toward the body cavity. The ventral part gives origin to the iliacus, while more dorsally it bears the roughened auricular articular surface (Fig. 2–19/*B*,15) for the sacrum. The dorsal border of the wing is cut away at its junction with the shaft, forming the greater sciatic notch (incisura; /4), over which the sciatic nerve runs in passage to the hindlimb.

The shaft of the ilium is robust and columnar. Its caudal extremity contributes to the acetabulum, the deep cavity that receives the head of the femur. Its ventral border is marked by the low arcuate line that serves as part of the arbitrary boundary (“terminal line”; p. 691) between the abdominal and pelvic cavities. Except in the dog, the line carries the psoas tubercle midway along its length; the psoas minor attaches here.

The *pubis* (/6), essentially L-shaped, consists of cranial (acetabular) and caudal (symphysial) branches. The lateral end of the cranial branch contributes to the acetabulum and is known as the body. Its cranial edge, known as the pecten of the pubis, bears the iliopubic eminence and gives attachment to the abdominal muscles. Between them, the two branches account for about half the circumference of the obturator foramen (/7), the large opening in the pelvic floor through which the obturator nerve emerges. The foramen is closed by muscle and membrane in the fresh state.

The *ischium* (/8) consists of a horizontal plate extended cranially by symphysial and acetabular branches, one to each side of the obturator foramen. The extremity of the acetabular branch that contributes to the articular cup is known as the body. The body and the cranial part of this branch are surmounted by a crest, the ischial spine (/5), which also extends onto the caudal part of the ilium. Marked by the origin of the gluteus profundus, it is relatively low in the dog, particularly high in ruminants. The caudolateral corner of the plate forms the ischial tuber (/9); the border between this and the spine is indented by the lesser sciatic notch (/10). The ischial tuber is a horizontal thickening in the dog, a conspicuously triangular swelling in cattle. In most species it is subcutaneous, and it may be a visible landmark. The remaining part of the caudal border forms with its fellow the ischial arch, a notch that is broad and, except in the horse, shallow.

The *acetabulum* is a deep articular cup to which all three bones contribute; an additional small acetabular bone may be found in young animals. The acetabulum is contained by a prominent rim that is interrupted by a notch caudoventrally. It carries a lunate articular surface internally, but the depth of the cup is nonarticular and rough.

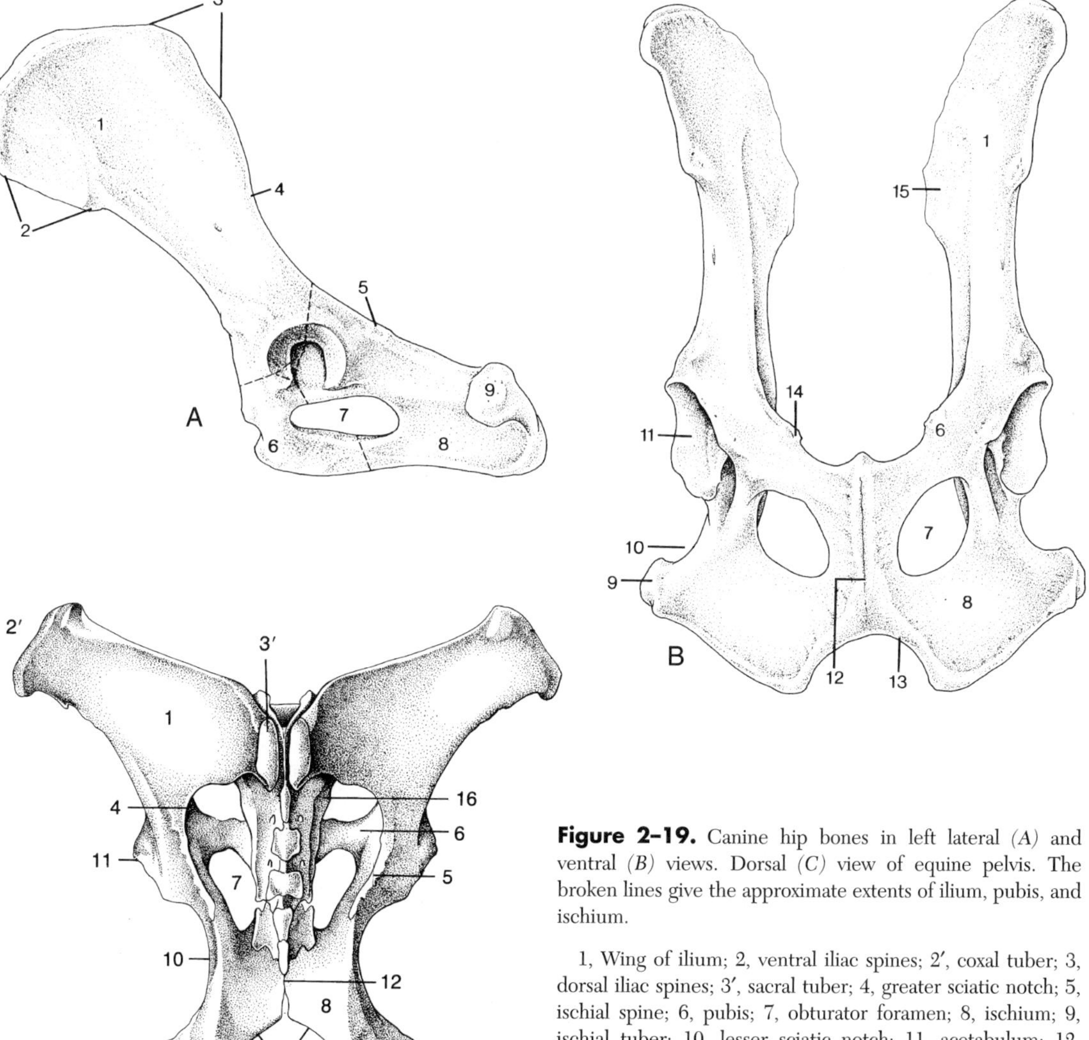


**Figure 2-19.** Canine hip bones in left lateral *(A)* and ventral *(B)* views. Dorsal *(C)* view of equine pelvis. The broken lines give the approximate extents of ilium, pubis, and ischium.

1, Wing of ilium; 2, ventral iliac spines; 2′, coxal tuber; 3, dorsal iliac spines; 3′, sacral tuber; 4, greater sciatic notch; 5, ischial spine; 6, pubis; 7, obturator foramen; 8, ischium; 9, ischial tuber; 10, lesser sciatic notch; 11, acetabulum; 12, pelvic symphysis; 13, ischial arch; 14, iliopubic eminence; 15, auricular articular surface; 16, sacrum.

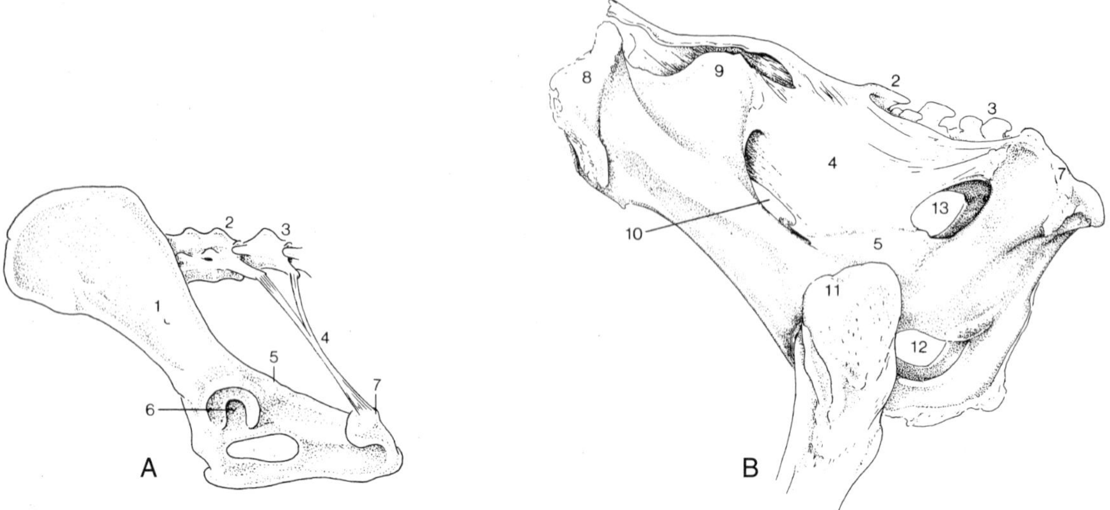


**Figure 2–20.** Canine sacrotuberous ligament *(A)* and bovine sacrosciatic ligament *(B)*, left lateral views.

1, Ilium; 2, sacrum; 3, caudal vertebra(e); 4, sacrotuberous ligament (in *A*), sacrosciatic ligament (in *B*); 5, ischial spine; 6, acetabulum; 7, ischial tuber; 8, coxal tuber; 9, sacral tuber; 10, greater sciatic foramen; 11, greater trochanter; 12, obturator foramen; 13, lesser sciatic foramen.

Species differences in the general form of the *pelvic girdle* are very pronounced. The ilium is most vertical in the larger and heavier species, a conformation that brings the sacroiliac joint, and therefore the weight of the trunk, more nearly above the hip joint (Fig. 2–20/*B*). In smaller species, in which this consideration is of less importance, the ilium is very oblique (Fig. 2–1). This displaces the pelvic floor caudally relative to the vertebral column and increases the effectiveness of the abdominal muscles that flex the column in bounding gaits. Caudal displacement of the ischial tuber also increases the leverage that may be exerted by the hamstring muscles, the powerful extensors of the hip that arise here.

The dimensions of the girdle are most important in species that carry a single large offspring. They are of little significance in polytocous species (those that normally carry a litter), in which the full-term fetuses are relatively small. These aspects of pelvic conformation are discussed in later chapters.

### The Joints and Ligaments of the Pelvic Girdle

The pelvic symphysis is a secondary cartilaginous joint that ossifies with advancing age. The process of ossification is irregular; it commences at different ages and advances at different rates, even in a single species. It is usually more precocious in onset and more advanced at any stage in the pubic than in the ischial part. It is sometimes asserted that in certain domestic species changes can be detected in the tissues of the symphysis (and sacroiliac joint) in advance of parturition. If this is so, and it is not universally accepted, these changes are minor in comparison with those that occur in guinea pigs and many other small animals at this time; in these complete dissolution of the symphysis, which allows the two halves of the girdle to move apart to enlarge the birth passage, may occur.

The *sacroiliac joints* are curious in combining a synovial joint with an adjacent region of extensive fibrous union. The arrangement appears designed to combine firmness of attachment with some shock-absorbent capacity, for these joints are required to transmit the weight of the trunk to the hindlimbs when standing and the thrust of the limbs to the trunk in progression. The sacrum is wedged between the two halves of the pelvic girdle; each sacral wing carries an articular surface that is broadly flat (but irregular in detail) to match the corresponding iliac surface. The joint capsule is tight and is surrounded and supported by short fascicles of connective tissue that join adjacent parts of the two bones. It is a matter of preference whether certain longer sacroiliac ligaments, at a greater distance from the synovial articulation, are to be regarded as components of that joint or as independent structures. They may include long and short dorsal ligaments passing between the wing of the ilium and the spinous processes and other features of the sacrum. A ventral ligament offers more immediate suppot to the joint.

The *sacrotuberous ligament* (Fig. 2–20/4) is of considerably greater interest. In the dog it is a stout rounded cord extending between the caudolateral angle of the sacrum and the lateral part of the ischial tuber; no such ligament is present in the cat. In ungulates it is better named the sacrosciatic ligament, since it is expanded to a broad sheet that largely fills the space between the lateral border of the sacrum and the dorsal border of the ilium and ischium, leaving open two foramina adjacent to the greater and lesser sciatic notches. The caudal edge is palpable in dogs and cattle.

## The Muscles of the Trunk

### The Cutaneous Muscle of the Trunk

The cutaneous muscle of the trunk (Fig. 2–21) varies in relative thickness and extent but generally covers the lateral aspect of the thorax and abdomen with fascicles of a predominately horizontal course. It is contained within the superficial fascia and has as its main function tension and twitching of the skin. In some animals detachments are associated with the prepuce, and in the horse and ox a separate lamella covers the shoulder and arm regions. The innervation comes from the brachial plexus.

### The Muscles of the Vertebral Column

These can be divided into two divisions according to their position and innervation. The epaxial division (Fig. 2–22/*B*,12) is placed dorsal to the line of the transverse processes of the vertebrae and receives its nerve supply from dorsal branches of the spinal nerves. The hypaxial division (/14) lies ventral to the transverse processes and is supplied by the ventral branches of these nerves; it includes the muscles of the thoracic and abdominal walls in addition to those placed closely on the vertebrae. The thoracic and abdominal muscles are considered in later sections.

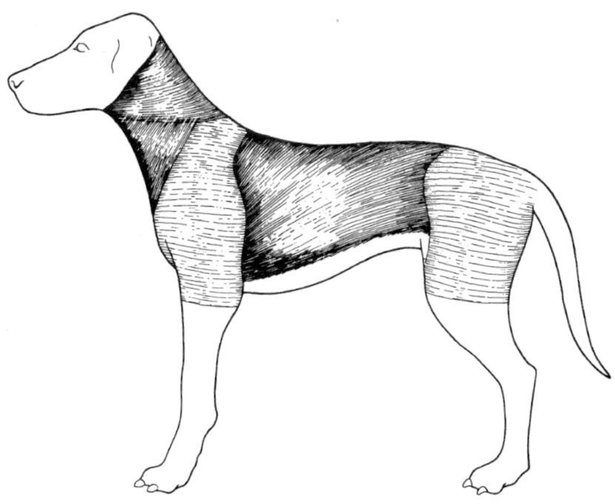

**Figure 2–21** The cutaneous muscle of the dog.

**The Epaxial Muscles.** These are numerous and complicated but fortunately do not require detailed description, since they are rarely of clinical importance, except in the dog (p. 398). The major muscles are arranged in three parallel columns (Fig. 2–22/*C*,19–21), which show some tendency to fuse over the loins and to split into additional units in the neck. They are extensors of the vertebral column, locally or more generally according to their extent, and are relatively more powerful in animals (e.g., dog) that make use of a bounding gait when traveling at speed.

The *lateral column,* the iliocostalis, arises from the ilium and transverse processes of the lumbar vertebrae and inserts on the more cranial lumbar vertebrae and ribs with, in most species, a weaker continuation into the neck. It is composed of many fascicles that overlap; for the most part they span about four vertebrae. Its lateral position makes it also effective in bending the trunk to the side (Fig. 2–23/*B*,17).

The *middle column,* the longissimus (/16) is strongest and can be followed into the neck, even to the head. Some of its more cranial parts are independent to a greater or lesser degree. The caudal attachments—the conventional origin—are from the ilium, the sacrum, and the mamillary processes, while the insertions are to the transverse processes and ribs. The fascicles thus pursue a cranial, lateral, and ventral course, and each bridges several vertebrae; the longest fascicles span the especially mobile thoracolumbar junction. Different parts may be designated longissimus lumborum, longissimus dorsi, longissimus cervicis, longissimus atlantis, and longissimus capitis, but usually the generic term is sufficient. The muscle tends to fuse with its medial and lateral neighbors in the lumbar region.

In addition to the more or less direct continuation, the cervical part of the longissimus is closely associated with the more superficial *splenius* (/*A*,4). This passes from the highest spines of the withers and thoracolumbar fascia to the occipitomastoid region of the skull. It is covered by certain muscles of the thoracic girdle, especially the trapezius and rhomboideus.

The longissimus complex also includes certain small muscles passing between adjacent transverse processes as well as the dorsal (sacrocaudal) muscles of the tail (/14); the latter are fleshy at their origin and are continued by tendons that run the length of the tail.

The *medial column,* the transversospinalis system (Fig. 2–24/2), is the most complex, although

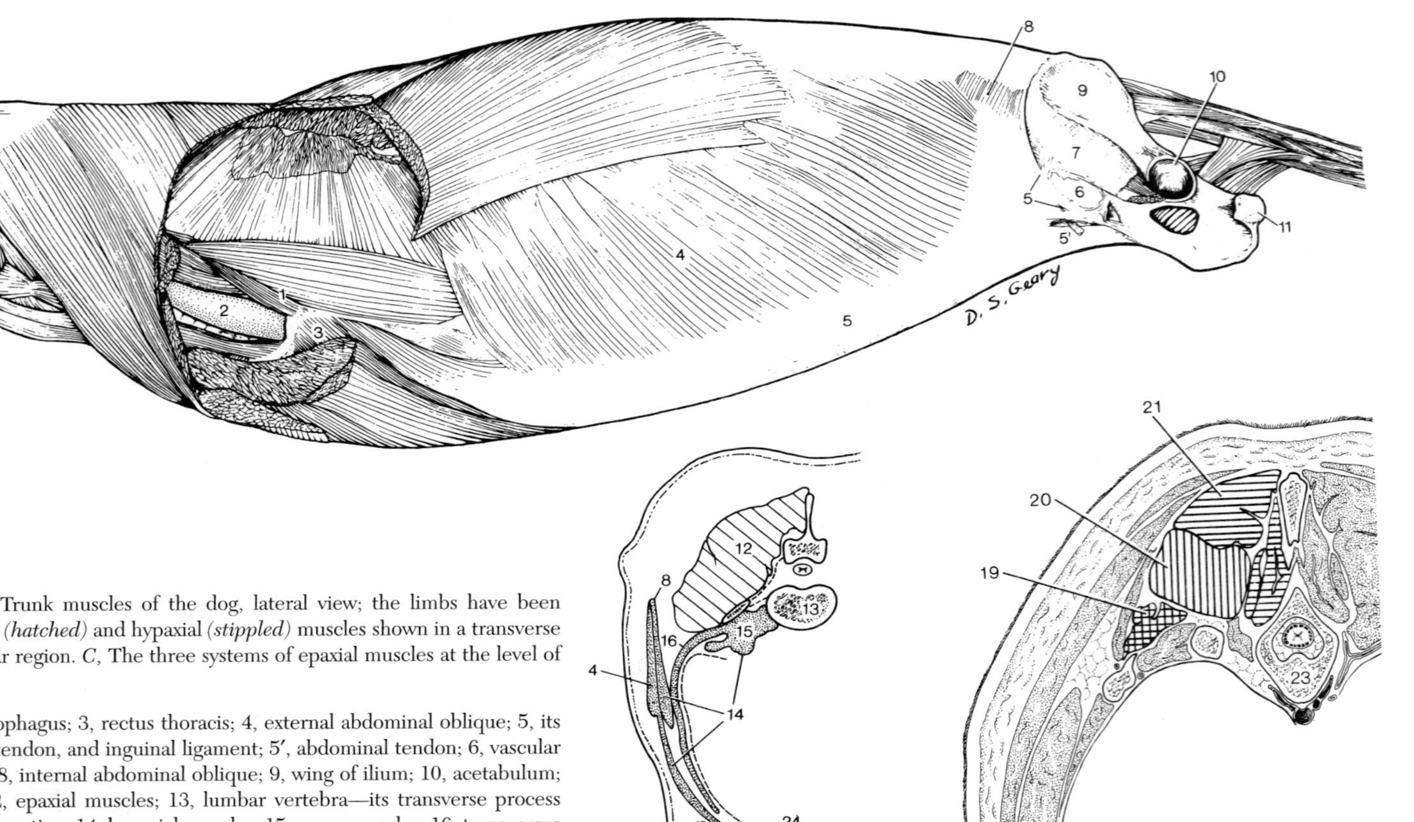


**Figure 2–22.** *A*, Trunk muscles of the dog, lateral view; the limbs have been removed. *B*, Epaxial *(hatched)* and hypaxial *(stippled)* muscles shown in a transverse section of the lumbar region. *C*, The three systems of epaxial muscles at the level of the thorax.

1, Scalenus; 2, esophagus; 3, rectus thoracis; 4, external abdominal oblique; 5, its aponeurosis, pelvic tendon, and inguinal ligament; 5′, abdominal tendon; 6, vascular lacuna; 7, iliopsoas; 8, internal abdominal oblique; 9, wing of ilium; 10, acetabulum; 11, ischial tuber; 12, epaxial muscles; 13, lumbar vertebra—its transverse process appears as detached section; 14, hypaxial muscles; 15, psoas muscles; 16, transversus abdominis; 17, rectus abdominis; 18, flank fold; 19, iliocostalis system *(crosshatched)*; 20, longissimus system *(vertically hatched)*; 21, transversospinalis system *(horizontally hatched)*; 23, thoracic vertebra and ribs; 24, peritoneum.

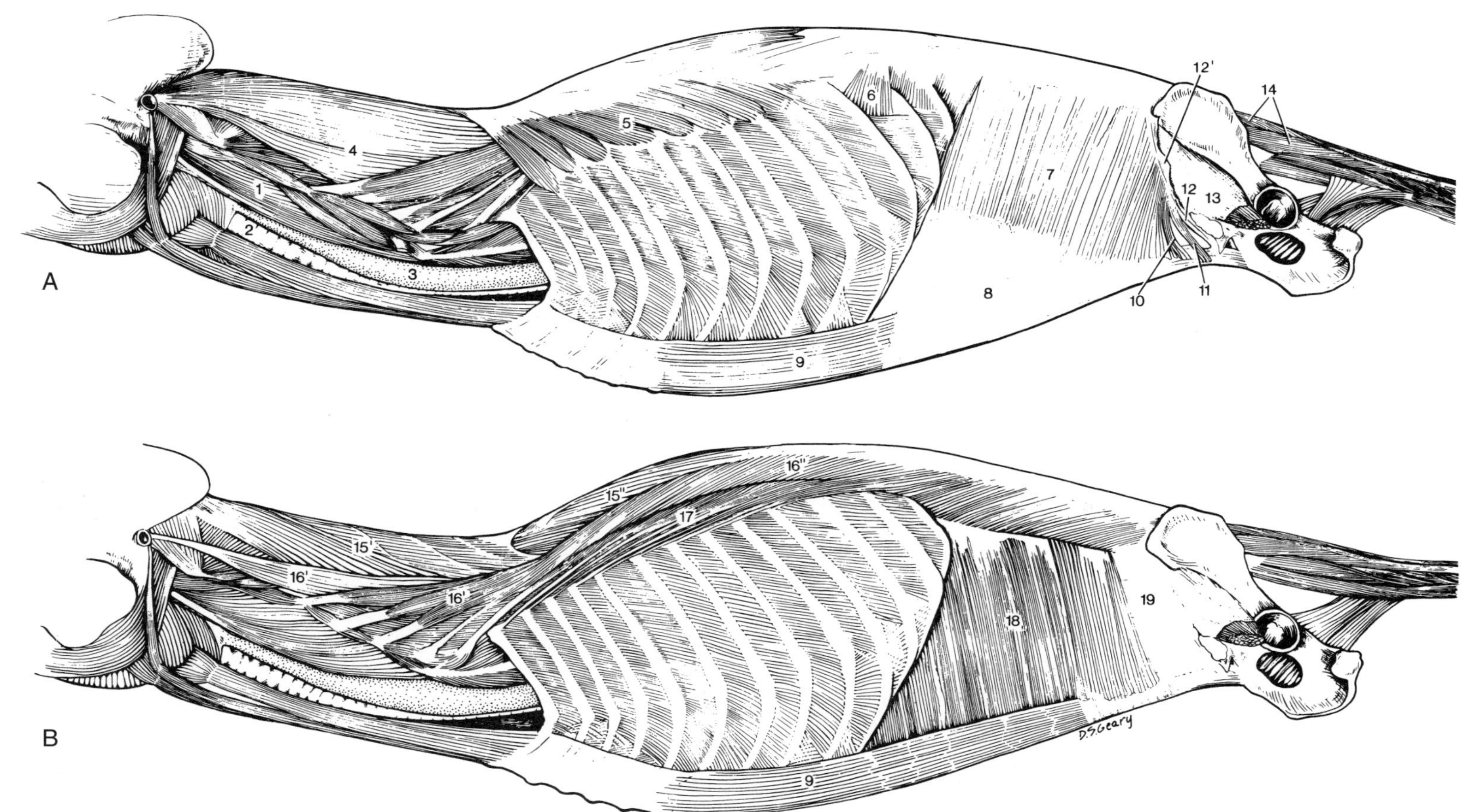


**Figure 2–23.** *A* and *B*, Trunk muscles of the dog, deeper layers.

1, Longus capitis; 2, trachea; 3, esophagus; 4, splenius; 5, 6, serratus dorsalis cranialis and caudalis; 7, internal abdominal oblique; 8, its aponeurosis; 9, rectus abdominis; 10, caudal free border of internal abdominal oblique; 11, cremaster; 12, inguinal ligament; 12′, external abdominal oblique aponeurosis, cut and reflected; 13, iliopsoas; 14, dorsal sacrocaudal muscles; 15, transversospinalis system; 15′, semispinalis capitis; 15″, spinalis et semispinalis; 16, longissimus system; 16′, longissimus capitis and cervicis; 16″, longissimus thoracis; 17, iliocostalis; 18, transversus abdominis; 19, transverse fascia.

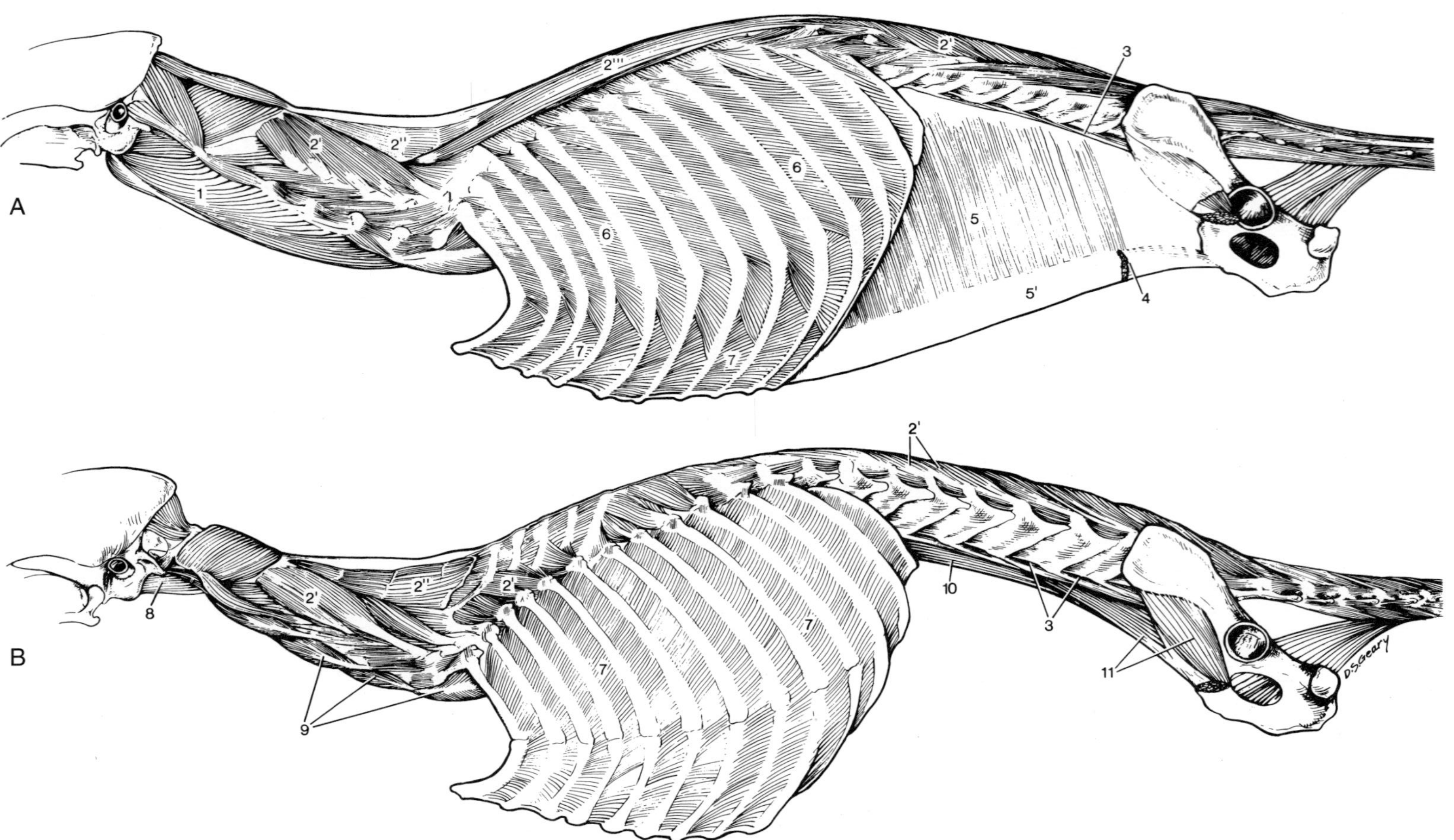


**Figure 2–24.** *A* and *B*, Trunk muscles of the dog, deepest layers.

1, Longus capitis; 2, transversospinalis system; 2′, multifidus; 2″, spinalis cervicis; 2‴, spinalis et semispinalis; 3, quadratus lumborum; 4, rectus abdominis; 5, transversus abdominis; 5′, its aponeurosis; 6, external intercostal muscles; 7, internal intercostal muscles; 8, rectus capitis ventralis; 9, longus colli; 10, psoas minor; 11, iliopsoas (psoas major and iliacus).

the number of discrete units into which it may be divided varies among species. It lies on and between the medial parts of the vertebral arches and the spinous processes. Some fascicles run sagittally; others pursue a cranial, medial, and dorsal course from their caudal origin. The sagittal bundles include small units—often converted into ligaments—passing between adjacent spinous processes as well as larger units that span several vertebrae. The oblique bundles run from mamillary to spinous processes and may be distinguished by name according to whether they span one, two, three, or more joints. The longest fascicles are again concentrated at the middle, most mobile region of the back.

A number of specialized units bridge the joints between the axis, the atlas, and the skull and are responsible for the special movements in this region. Those of the dog are briefly described later (p. 399).

**The Hypaxial Muscles.** These are flexor muscles of the neck or tail. The *longus colli* (/9) runs from the cranial thoracic region to the atlas, covering the ventral surfaces of the vertebral bodies. It has a complex organization, and most of its constituent bundles are relatively short and cross only a few joints; their orientation varies. It is complemented by the *rectus capitis ventralis* (/8), which extends from the atlas to the ventral aspect of the skull, and the *longus capitis* (/1), which lies lateral to the longus colli and extends from the transverse processes of the midcervical vertebrae to the skull. The *scalenus* group occupies a similar position in relation to the caudal cervical vertebrae (Fig. 2–22/1). It passes to the first one or few ribs, which it helps stabilize during inspiration. In some species the scalenus is readily divisible into dorsal, middle, and ventral parts.

The ventral muscles of the tail are close counterparts of the dorsal muscles.

### The Muscles of the Thoracic Wall

The muscles of the thoracic wall are primarily concerned with respiration. Most are inspiratory and enlarge the thoracic cavity, causing air to flow into the lungs. Some are expiratory and diminish the cavity, expelling air. They comprise muscles that fill the spaces between the ribs, certain small units placed lateral to the ribs, and, by far the most important, the diaphragm.

The intercostal muscles are theoretically arranged in three layers that correspond to the layers of the abdominal wall. The *external intercostal* muscles are outermost (Fig. 2–24/6). Each of these muscles is confined to a single intercostal space in which its fibers run caudoventrally from an origin on one rib to a termination on the following rib. They fill the spaces from the upper ends to the costochondral junctions and sometimes beyond these but fail to reach the sternum. The parts between the cartilages are sometimes separately named. The *internal intercostal* muscles (/7) are placed more deeply within the intercostal spaces and run cranioventrally, approximately perpendicular to the course of the external muscles. They do not occupy the most dorsal parts of the spaces, but, as if in compensation, they do reach the margin of the sternum. The third (subcostal) layer is so weak and so inconsistently developed that it may be ignored. The *transversus thoracis* is a triangular sheet that arises from and covers the dorsal surface of the sternum. The apex points cranially, and the muscle splits into slips that run caudolaterally to insert on the sternal ribs close to the costochondral junctions. It is morphologically the equivalent of the ventral part of the transversus abdominis.

Two muscles lie on the lateral surface of the thoracic wall. The *rectus thoracis* (Fig. 2–22/3) is a small quadrilateral sheet placed over the lower ends of the first four ribs in apparent continuation of the rectus abdominis. The *serratus dorsalis* (Fig. 2–23/*A*5,6) lies over the dorsal parts of the ribs. It takes origin from the fascia of the back and inserts on the ribs by a series of slips. The slips of the cranial part of the muscle slope caudoventrally, and those of the caudal part slope cranioventrally, which points to antagonistic functions. The two parts are sometimes quite widely separated. The *scalenus,* mentioned in the preceding section, has an attachment to the first rib; in some species it also passes quite extensively over the rib cage.

The *diaphragm* separates the thoracic and abdominal cavities. It is dome-shaped, being convex in all directions on its cranial surface, and bulges cranially under cover of the ribs to enlarge the abdominal at the expense of the thoracic cavity (Figs. 2–2 and 2-25/*A*). It consists of a heart-shaped (trefoil-shaped in the dog) central tendon (/7) and a muscular periphery that is divisible into portions that arise from the lumbar vertebrae, the caudal ribs, and the sternum.

The central tendon is the most cranial part and forms the vertex. In the neutral position between full inspiration and full expiration it reaches the level of the lower part of the sixth rib (or following space) and is thus only a little behind the plane of the olecranon in an animal standing square. Knowledge of this fact and of the line of the costal attachment is indispensable to appreciation of the extent of the thoracic cavity (Fig. 2–25/*B*).

The powerful lumbar portion of the peripheral muscle consists of left and right crura (/1,2) that

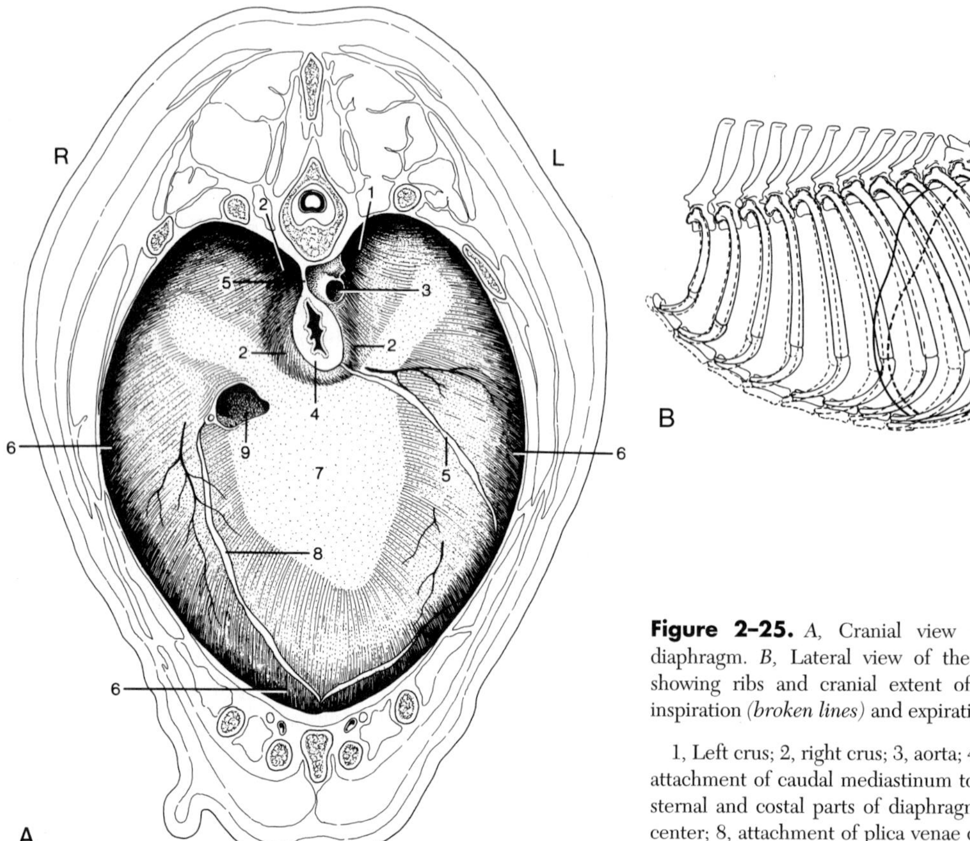


**Figure 2–25.** *A*, Cranial view of the canine diaphragm. *B*, Lateral view of the canine thorax showing ribs and cranial extent of diaphragm in inspiration *(broken lines)* and expiration *(solid lines)*.

1, Left crus; 2, right crus; 3, aorta; 4, esophagus; 5, attachment of caudal mediastinum to diaphragm; 6, sternal and costal parts of diaphragm; 7, tendinous center; 8, attachment of plica venae cavae; 9, caudal vena cava.

arise from the ventral aspect of the first three or four lumbar vertebrae by means of stout tendons. The right crus is considerably the larger and it divides into three branches that radiate ventrally to join the central tendon. The left crus is undivided.

The much thinner costal part arises by serial digitations from the inner surfaces of the ribs and costal cartilages. The most caudal slip, which is also the most dorsal, arises close to the dorsal end of the last rib; those in front arise at successively more ventral levels, with the last costal digitation following the cartilage of the eighth rib to the sternum. A final sternal slip arises from the dorsal surface of the sternum and runs dorsally to meet the tendon, which is thus bordered by muscle on all sides.

The diaphragm has three openings. The most dorsal, the aortic hiatus (/3), is between the lumbar vertebrae and the crural tendons. It transmits the aorta, the azygous vein, and the thoracic duct. The esophageal hiatus (/4) lies more ventrally, between the two medial divisions of the right crus. It transmits the esophagus, the dorsal and ventral vagal trunks that accompany the esophagus, and the vessels that supply it. The third opening, the caval foramen (/9), lies within the central tendon, somewhat dorsal to the vertex and to the right of the median plane. It conveys the caudal vena cava and is of a rather different nature from the other openings since the adventitia of the vessel fuses with the tendon to leave no surrounding space. The margins of the other openings can slide over the structures passing through.

The diaphragm is supplied by the phrenic nerves formed from contributions by ventral branches of caudal cervical nerves (usually C5–C7). Despite the apparently involuntary nature of breathing these are ordinary somatic nerves of mixed composition. The other muscles of the chest wall are supplied by intercostal nerves (ventral branches of thoracic spinal nerves).

**Functional Considerations.** The form and construction of the thorax represent a compromise between the requirements of posture and locomotion and the more specialized needs of respiration. In most domestic mammals the advantages for respiration of a barrel-shaped thorax are largely sacrificed to the easier movement allowed to the scapulae by flattening the cranial part of the rib cage. The potential for movement of the cranial ribs is also reduced in favor of the more rigid construction that provides a stable origin for the muscles that pass between the trunk and the forelimbs.

Respiratory activity is therefore most evident in changes in the form of the caudal part of the rib cage and of the abdomen. All species exhibit both costal and abdominal (i.e., diaphragmatic) modes of breathing, but their relative importance varies with the species, with the prevailing circumstances, and with the individual since breathing pattern is as distinctive as stance or gait. It is commonly stated that in ourselves, about 70% of the air flow is attributable to movements of the diaphragm; the proportion is unlikely to be very different in the domestic species, although such matters have received little attention. It is certainly safe to conclude that normal respiration is always accompanied by contraction of the diaphragm, while involvement of the intercostal and other accessory respiratory muscles is less certain.

The diaphragm contracts against the resistance of the abdominal viscera; for practical purposes these can be regarded as incompressible, and they must be displaced caudally into space provided by relaxation of the abdominal floor and flanks. In the course of this movement the central part of the dome of the diaphragm shifts backward—perhaps half a vertebral length in quiet breathing—while additional thoracic enlargement is obtained through flattening its peripheral parts. Contraction of the sternocostal parts of the diaphragm, which attach to the last ribs, tends to pull these ribs inward in opposition to the outward and forward pull exerted on them by the intercostal muscles. It is a common observation (easily confirmed by watching a sleeping dog) that the last rib may actually be tucked inward during inspiration while its more cranial fellows move outward to broaden the thorax.

The actual movements undertaken by the ribs and the forces that produce them are controversial. The caudal inclination of the lower part of the rib (before it is turned forward by the cartilage) results in the rib performing a movement that is compared with raising a bucket handle. Just how the articular surfaces engage during this movement and where the axes of rotation may be found are matters in dispute; it is clear, however, that the overall effect is to widen while shortening the rib cage. In humans and some quadrupeds (including the dog), a concurrent ventral displacement of the sternum occurs.

A considerable number of the muscles attaching to the ribs and sternum appear from their geometry to be capable of producing the necessary movements. Electromyographic studies, admittedly performed mainly in humans, have shown that little of this potential is actually employed in quiet breathing. During inspiration the superficial layer of intercostal musculature is most consistently engaged, that is, the external intercostals and the interchondral parts of the internal intercostals. The scalenus (and possibly also muscles that pass forward from the manubrium) may assist in fixing the thoracic inlet. Expiration is mainly passive, with the elastic recoil of the lungs being the major force. The muscles of the abdominal wall may contract to reinforce the passive tension in the tendinous parts that raises the viscera and that indirectly helps to restore the diaphragm to its former position. Sometimes the deeper layer of intercostal muscle—the interosseous parts of the internal intercostals and the transversus thoracis—is also engaged.

Contrary to common belief, the diaphragm is not indispensable. Evidence obtained from experimental and clinical subjects (dogs and ruminants) in which both phrenic nerves have been sectioned or paralyzed indicates little obvious loss of respiratory efficiency even under moderate stress. This of course does not deny the diaphragm the major role in normal animals; it confirms that there is an ample reserve of inspiratory muscle.

## *The Muscles of the Abdominal Wall*

The muscles of the abdominal wall are conveniently divided into ventrolateral and dorsal (sublumbar) groups (Fig. 2–22/*B*). The first comprises the muscles of the flanks and abdominal floor, muscles that possess a particular importance since they are encountered and incised in almost all surgical approaches to abdominal organs. Most muscles of the second group properly belong to the girdle division of hindlimb musculature. They are included here because they constitute part of the body wall, namely, the roof of the abdomen to each side of the vertebral column.

**The Ventrolateral Group.** The intrinsic musculature of the flank comprises three broad fleshy sheets superimposed on each other with contrasting orientation of their fibers. Each is continued ventrally by an aponeurotic tendon that proceeds to a principal insertion within a fibrous cord, the linea alba, which runs in the ventral midline from the xiphoid cartilage to the cranial end of the pelvic symphysis (via the prepubic tendon). In so doing, the tendons ensheathe the fourth muscle, the rectus abdominis, which pursues a sagittal course within the abdominal floor directly to the side of the linea alba. The following account is of the basic arrangement. The details vary among species and may have surgical importance, especially in the small species (Fig. 2–26; see also pp. 418, 419).

The outermost *external abdominal oblique* muscle (Fig. 2–22/4) arises from the lateral surfaces of the ribs and from the lumbar fascia. The majority of its fibers run caudoventrally but some radiation is present that allows the most dorsal bundles to follow a more horizontal course. The aponeurosis (/5) that succeeds the fleshy part divides into two parts (tendons) before its insertion. The larger abdominal tendon terminates on the linea alba after passing ventral to the rectus muscle; the smaller pelvic tendon proceeds to attach on the fascia over the iliopsoas and on the pubic brim lateral to the insertion of the rectus (Fig. 2–27/3′,4).

The second muscle, the *internal abdominal oblique* (Fig. 2–23/7), arises mainly from the coxal tuber (or the equivalent region of the ilium) but to

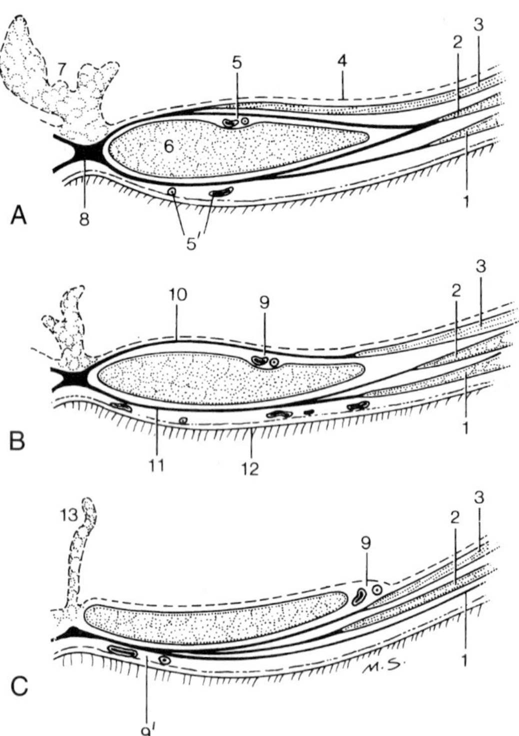


**Figure 2–26.** Rectus sheath of the dog in transverse sections taken cranial *(A)* and caudal *(B)* to the umbilicus and near the pubis *(C)*.

1, External abdominal oblique; 2, internal abdominal oblique; 3, transversus abdominis; 4, peritoneum; 5, cranial epigastric vessels; 5′, cranial superficial epigastric vessels; 6, rectus abdominis; 7, fat-filled falciform ligament; 8, linea alba; 9, caudal epigastric vessels; 9′, caudal superficial epigastric vessels; 10, internal lamina of rectus sheath; 11, external lamina of rectus sheath; 12, skin; 13, median ligament of the bladder.

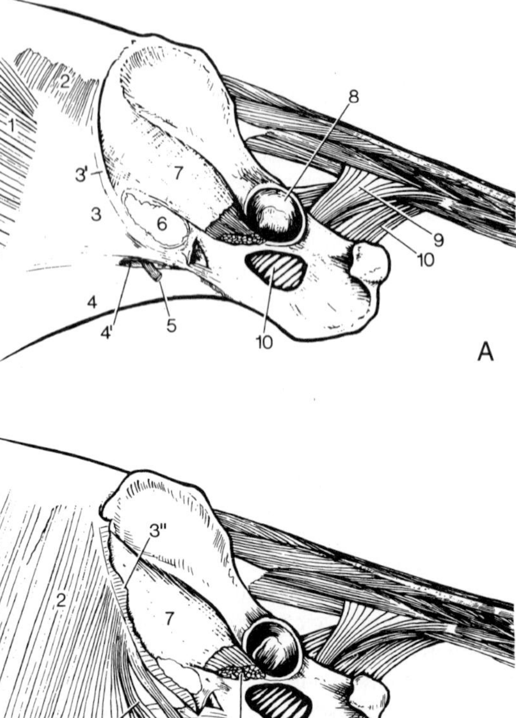


**Figure 2–27.** Inguinal canal and pelvic diaphragm of the dog, left lateral view. The external abdominal oblique muscle, present in *A*, has been removed in *B*.

1, External abdominal oblique; 2, internal abdominal oblique; 2′, free caudal edge of internal oblique, forming border of deep inguinal ring; 3, pelvic tendon of external oblique aponeurosis; 3′, caudal border of 3 (inguinal ligament) ending on 7; 3″, stump of external oblique aponeurosis reflected caudally *(B);* 4, abdominal tendon of external oblique aponeurosis; 4′, superficial inguinal ring; 5, cremaster derived from internal oblique; 6, vascular lacuna; 7, iliac fascia covering iliopsoas; 7′, iliopsoas; 8, acetabulum; 9, coccygeus; 10, levator ani.

lesser extents from the insertion of the pelvic tendon of the external oblique, the thoracolumbar fascia, and the tips of the lumbar transverse processes. This muscle fans out more obviously; its most caudal fascicles pass ventrocaudally, the next group runs more or less transversely in the plane of the coxal tuber, while most pass ventrocranially. Some cranial fascicles insert directly on the last rib, but the bulk are continued by an aponeurosis (/8) that passes ventral to the rectus to reach the linea alba. Toward the midline some interchange of fibers between the aponeuroses of the two oblique muscles usually occurs. The origin from the pelvic tendon allows the muscle a free caudal edge (/10) that is mentioned again shortly in connection with the inguinal canal. A caudal slip (cremaster; /11) detached from the internal oblique passes onto the spermatic cord (p. 187).

The deepest muscle of the flank, the *transversus abdominis* (Fig. 2–24/5), arises from the inner surfaces of the last ribs and the transverse processes of the lumbar vertebrae. Its fibers run more or less transversely and are succeeded by an aponeurosis (/5′) that passes dorsal to the rectus abdominis before terminating on the linea alba. This muscle does not extend caudal to the coxal tuber, and as a result the most caudal portion of the rectus is left uncovered dorsally.

The fourth muscle, the *rectus abdominis* (Fig. 2–23/9), forms a broad band to the side of the linea alba in the abdominal floor. It arises from the ventral surfaces of the rib cartilages and sternum and inserts on the pubic brim by means of a prepubic tendon. The fleshy part, which is widest about the middle of the abdomen, is divided into a series of segments by irregular transverse septa (tendinous intersections) that recall, even if they do not exactly reproduce, its polysegmental origin. The prepubic tendon serves as a common insertion for the abdominal muscles and the linea alba and may incorporate part of the tendons of origin of adductor (pectineus and gracilis) muscles of the thigh.

The *rectus sheath* (vagina musculi recti abdominis), the arrangement of the aponeurotic tendons of the flank muscles about the rectus abdominis, varies in detail among species. In the basic arrangement, the tendons of the two oblique muscles form a layer on the external (ventral) surface of the rectus, while that of the transversus lies against the internal surface; both layers merge with the linea alba to complete the enclosure (see Fig. 2–26 and p. 418 for a fuller description of the rectus sheath in the dog).

The abdominal wall is perforated in the region of the groin by a passage known as the *inguinal canal* (Figs. 2–27 and 21–5). Before or shortly after birth this transmits the testis in its descent toward the scrotum; in the adult male it contains the spermatic cord, consisting of the duct from the testis, and associated structures within an outpouching of the peritoneum. In both sexes it also transmits the external pudendal artery and (usually) vein, efferent vessels from the superficial inguinal lymph nodes, and the genitofemoral nerve—structures associated with the groin.

The term "canal" is misleading because it suggests a roomier passage than actually exists. The canal is a potential flat space between the fleshy part of the internal oblique on the one side and the pelvic tendon of the external oblique aponeurosis on the other (Fig. 2–27/2, 3). The walls are apposed and joined by areolar tissue except where the transmitted structures hold them apart. The slitlike abdominal entrance to the canal (the deep inguinal ring) lies along the free caudal edge of the internal oblique muscle (/2′). The exit from the canal (the superficial inguinal ring; /4′) is contained between the two divisions of the external oblique tendon. (The edges of the superficial inguinal ring are known as medial and lateral crura.) Species differences are mentioned in later chapters and may be of great importance since some explain why the escape of organs into and through the canal (inguinal hernia) occurs more readily in certain animals. Other differences are of immediate relevance to surgery in this area, most obviously in connection with castration, whether of the normal male or of one in which the testis has failed to descend and remains hidden within the abdomen or within the canal itself (a condition known as cryptorchidism).

**Functional Considerations.** Observation and palpation suggest that animals standing quietly make little active use of the abdominal muscles in support of the viscera; the support is obtained from passive tension. Some electromyographic studies have revealed slight though continuous activity in the internal oblique with sporadic bursts in other muscles of the flank. A similar observation in ourselves has provoked the suggestion that the internal oblique muscle guards the entrance to the inguinal canal. Greater activity of the abdominal muscles may occur toward the end of quiet expiration and is more pronounced when breathing is labored, as the muscles then contract to assist the forward recovery of the diaphragm.

When the abdominal muscles are contracted against a fixed diaphragm, the animal is said to "strain." The resulting increase in intra-abdominal pressure reinforces the efforts of visceral muscle to expel urine, feces, or a fetus. The use made of straining varies with the species and conditions. Those animals that adopt a squatting posture for micturition (e.g., goat) or defecation (e.g., dog) obviously use the abdominal muscles to assist expulsion; other species adopt no special posture for these functions and presumably do not require this assistance.

The rigidity of the abdominal wall produced by contraction of these muscles may be used to protect the viscera. This defense is used by a nervous dog when efforts, particularly if unskillful, are made to palpate its abdomen; gentle massage may be necessary to allay the fear before the muscles relax. Abdominal visceral pain may spontaneously provoke local or general contraction with ensuing rigidity, presumably to prevent the organs from sliding against each other.

These muscles are also used in the adjustment of posture and in progression. Acting unilaterally, the muscles of the flank bend the trunk to that side. Acting bilaterally, they may assist in arching the back, a movement of great importance in bounding gaits.

The ventrolateral abdominal muscles are supplied by caudal intercostal nerves and the ventral branches of the lumbar nerves, particularly those more cranial in the series.

**The Sublumbar Muscles.** The *psoas minor* (Fig. 2–24/10) arises from the bodies of the thoracolumbar vertebrae and inserts on the psoas minor tubercle on the ilium. Much tendon is intermingled in the flesh, which supports the contention that the muscle is probably mainly employed to stabilize the vertebral column. It may also rotate the pelvis at the sacroiliac joint.

The *psoas major* and *iliacus* muscles may be regarded as vertebral and pelvic heads of a single muscle (iliopsoas; /11) that terminates on the lesser trochanter of the femur. The psoas major arises from the bodies and ventral surfaces of the transverse processes of the lumbar vertebrae lateral to the psoas minor. The iliacus arises from the ventral aspect of the wing and shaft of the ilium. The tendons of the two heads combine shortly before insertion. The iliopsoas is a flexor of the hip and an outward rotator of the thigh. The psoas head probably also contributes to the stability of the vertebral column.

The *quadratus lumborum* (/3) arises from the last ribs and from the transverse processes of the lumbar vertebrae and inserts on the wing of the sacrum (sometimes also on the ilium). It stabilizes the lumbar portion of the vertebral column.

These muscles are principally innervated by direct twigs from the ventral branches of the last few thoracic and the lumbar nerves. Other twigs detach from named branches of the lumbosacral plexus, principally the femoral nerve.

### *The Muscles of the Pelvic Outlet*

The pelvic outlet is closed about the terminal parts of the digestive and urogenital tracts by a portion of the body wall known as the perineum. The projection of the perineum on the skin outlines the perineal region, which has as its principal features the anus and the vulva (in the female, to which we principally refer here). Since the ventral part of the vulva falls below the level of the pelvic floor, it is usual to enlarge the concept of the perineal region to embrace the whole vulva. Very often the dorsocaudal part of the udder (in animals such as the cow) is also included. Several muscles and fasciae interlace in a node between the anus and the vulva and vestibule, and this formation is properly known as the perineal body or center; however, in clinical, especially obstetrical, literature the perineal body is frequently known simply, though incorrectly, as "the perineum." The three concepts—perineum, perineal region, and perineal body—should be kept distinct. Another potential source of confusion exists. In human anatomy, the structures that occupy the pelvic outlet are said to form a "floor" to the pelvic cavity. In quadrupeds, the "floor" is provided by the pelvic girdle. The difference in posture not only affects the appropriate use of vernacular terms but, more important, also modifies the function of homologous structures. The principal component of the dorsal part of the perineum is the pelvic diaphragm, an arrangement of striated muscles contained between fasciae, which closes about the anorectal junction. A similar but less conspicuous arrangement in the ventral part of the perineum, the urogenital diaphragm, closes about the vestibule.

The *pelvic diaphragm* attaches laterally to the pelvic wall and spreads caudomedially to close about the anal canal. The term "diaphragm" aptly describes the human arrangement, which forms a basin in which the pelvic organs rest. It is less appropriate in domestic species, in which the two "halves" of the diaphragm have more sagittal courses and converge more gently on the anus, the result of the relatively greater length of the pelvic girdle.

The more lateral of the two muscles of the diaphragm, the *coccygeus* (Fig. 2–27/9), is essentially a muscle of the tail. Rhomboidal in outline, it arises from the ischial spine, crosses the sacrotuberous ligament medially, and inserts on and about the transverse processes of the first few tail vertebrae.

The medial muscle, the *levator ani,* is thinner and more extensive and runs more obliquely in a dorsocaudal direction; it is only partly covered by the coccygeus. The two muscles arise close together or by a common tendon in ungulates. In the dog, the levator has a more widely spread origin that continues from the iliac shaft over the cranial ramus of the pubis to follow the pelvic symphysis (/10). The insertion is divided between the fascia and vertebrae of the tail (extending distal to the insertion of the coccygeus), and the fascia about the anus and external anal sphincter. The tail attachment predominates in carnivores, the anal one in ungulates, in which considerable exchange of fascicles with the anal sphincter and constrictor vestibuli muscles occurs.

The coccygeus flexes the tail laterally or, when acting in concert with its fellow, draws the tail ventrally to cover the perineum, an attitude familiar in the nervous dog. The action of the levator is best known from an electromyographic study in the goat, and it is possible that important species differences exist. In the goat it is active whenever the intra-abdominal pressure is raised, presumably to oppose the tendency to displace pelvic organs caudally. Although also involved in other visceral functions, it has a very definite relationship to defecation; it is active prior to the event (when it may fix the position of the anus against the contraction of the smooth muscle of the colon), becomes inactive during the event, and regains activity following the event (when it may restore the parts to their resting positions). The jerky movements of the dog's tail after defecation are probably evidence of levator activity in this species. Both muscles are supplied by ventral branches of the sacral nerves.

The smaller *urogenital diaphragm* (membrana perinei) contains more slender muscles, which are more appropriately described later with the reproductive organs. The fascia of the urogenital diaphragm attaches to the ischial arch and curves cranially, dorsally, and medially to blend with the ventral edge of the pelvic diaphragm and embrace the vestibule. It helps anchor the reproductive tract against a forward drag when the pregnant uterus sinks within the abdomen and against a backward displacement during parturition.

It may now be evident that to each side there is a space that is enclosed by the pelvic girdle but excluded from the pelvic cavity by the pelvic diaphragm. This space is pyramidal and has a cranial apex, a lateral wall furnished by the ischial tuber and sacrotuberous ligament, a medial wall furnished by the pelvic diaphragm, a ventral wall furnished by the pelvic floor, and a base directed toward the skin. It is appropriately known as the *ischiorectal fossa* and is normally occupied by fat (see Fig. 29–12/12). When this fat is depleted, a pronounced sinking of the skin to the side of the anus is apparent (except in the horse and pig, in which the vertebral head of the semimembranosus covers the region).

# THE HEAD AND VENTRAL PART OF THE NECK

## Basic Plan and Development

Even a cursory examination of the head, intact or in sagittal section, shows that it consists of two principal parts. One, the neural part, comprises the brain together with the encasing structures; the other, the facial part, is much larger in most adult mammals and is formed by the jaws and the initial parts of the respiratory and digestive systems. The distinction between neural and facial parts is already plain in embryos at the somite stage (Fig. 2–28).

At this stage of development the dorsal structures predominate, with the size and form of the head largely determined by the brain. The dorsal part is ranged in line with the somites of the trunk but differs in showing no obvious segmentation; the somite series appears to end abruptly behind the brain, but the extension of the notochord to midbrain level maintains a degree of continuity.

The neural part (cranium) of the skull has its primordium in a series of cartilages that form ventral to the brain and are supplemented by cartilaginous capsules enclosing the primitive olfactory organs, eyeballs, and labyrinths of the ears. Later, "dermal bones" appear by ossification within the membrane that covers the brain to the sides and above; ultimately all of these elements fuse with each other and with the bones of the face.

The ventral part of the head—the future face—is much smaller and at this stage blends smoothly with the neck, largely occupied by the heart. It exhibits a quite different patten of segmentation imposed by the pharyngeal arches, serial thickenings of the unsplit mesoderm lateral and ventral to the rostral part of the foregut that becomes the pharynx. It is unclear how many of these arches form; four persist, but one, possibly two, more caudal arches may have a fleeting existence.

The formation, significance, and detailed fate of these arches is not described here; at present it is sufficient to recall that within the core of each arch a cartilage skeleton with an associated musculature innervated by a specific cranial nerve develops. Each arch is also supplied by an arterial loop

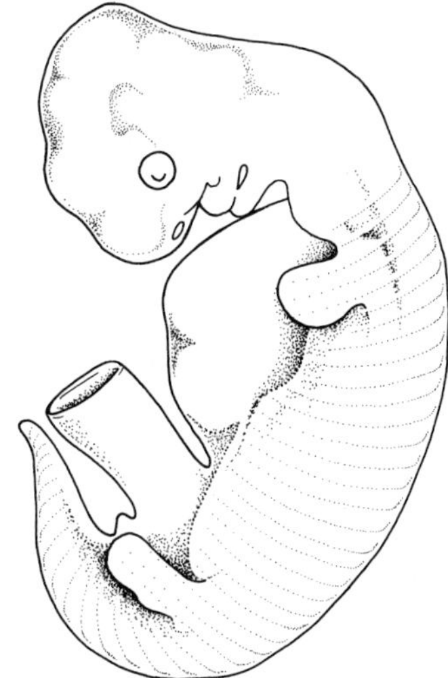

**Figure 2–28.** Pig embryo (1.5 cm) to show dominance of the neural over the facial part of the head at this stage.

connecting the ventral to the dorsal aorta. The structures formed within the various pharyngeal arches are listed in Table 2–1; from this it can be seen that ultimately the cartilaginous parts make only a small contribution to the skeleton of the face. The definitive facial skeleton is mainly provided by dermal bones formed in the connective tissue of the jaws, although certain elements for a time obtain support from cartilaginous precursors such as the cartilage of the first arch and the nasal capsule.

The adult human head in some measure preserves the embryonic plan and proportions, but in most mammals the facial part enlarges disproportionately and comes to lie as much before as below the brain. Despite many qualitative and quantitative differences the basic arrangement is the same in all species. The relationships and topography of the major organs and cavities of the head should be studied before passing on to more detailed matters. Figures 4–2 and 4-3 provide the necessary information.

## The Skull

The complete skeleton of the head comprises the skull,* the mandible or lower jawbone, the hyoid apparatus, the ossicles of the middle ear, and the cartilages of the external ear, nose, and larynx.

The *skull* (in the narrower sense) is a mosaic of many bones, mostly paired but some median and unpaired, that fit closely together to form a single rigid construction. The separate elements, which are named individually, develop from independent centers of ossification and have, for the most part, well established homologies. In the young animal they are separated from each other by narrow strips of fibrous tissue—cartilage in a few situations—and this pattern of joints or sutures makes provision for growth. Once growth has ceased, sutures are no longer necessary and ossification extends into the connective tissue, finally welding the bones together. This process is long-drawn-out, and it may never be completed; the outlines of most bones are therefore discernible even in skulls of old animals. Acquaintance with the names, positions, and approximate extents of the individual bones (Fig. 2–29) is essential since it provides a useful system of reference to regions of the head, but a detailed knowledge of the disarticulated units has little practical value; most readers are better served by an appreciation of the skull as a whole.

Conventional descriptions are based on the views obtained from various directions with the skull resting on a flat surface, even though this may not be its habitual orientation in life. In most views the two distinct portions of the skull are immediately apparent—the caudal part encasing the brain and the rostral part supporting the face. The orbits, the fossae containing the eyeballs, are part of the face but lie at the boundary. In most domestic animals the facial part of the skull is larger than the neural part and is situated mainly in front of this. However, the ratio varies among species and also with breed, age, and individual conformation. The many particular differences make it impossible to provide even a general description of the skull that is valid for all species.

### *The Skull of the Dog*

This initial account is of the skull of an adult dog of average (mesaticephalic) conformation—neither short-headed (brachycephalic) like a Pekingese nor long-headed (dolichocephalic) like a Borzoi. Some salient breed differences are mentioned later (p. 367).

*This term is sometimes used elsewhere in a wider sense to include the mandible and even the hyoid apparatus. Since comtemporary practice is inconsistent, an author's intention must often be deduced from the context.

**Table 2–1.** Derivatives of the Pharyngeal Arches

| Pharyngeal Arch | Skeleton | Muscles | Motor Innervation |
|---|---|---|---|
| First (mandibular) | Mandible (in part); certain ear ossicles (malleus and incus) | Muscles of mastication; mylohyoideus; digastricus (in part); tensor veli palatini; tensor tympani | Mandibular division of trigeminal nerve (V3) |
| Second (hyoid) | Hyoid apparatus (in part); ear ossicle (stapes) | Muscles of facial expression; digastricus (in part); stapedius | Facial nerve (VII) |
| Third | Hyoid apparatus (remaining part) | Stylopharyngeus caudalis; possibly other pharyngeal muscles | Glossopharyngeal nerve (IX) |
| Fourth (and subsequent arches) | Most laryngeal cartilages | Pharyngeal and laryngeal muscles; muscles of accessory nerve field | Vagus nerve (X); (medullary) part of accessory nerve (XI) |

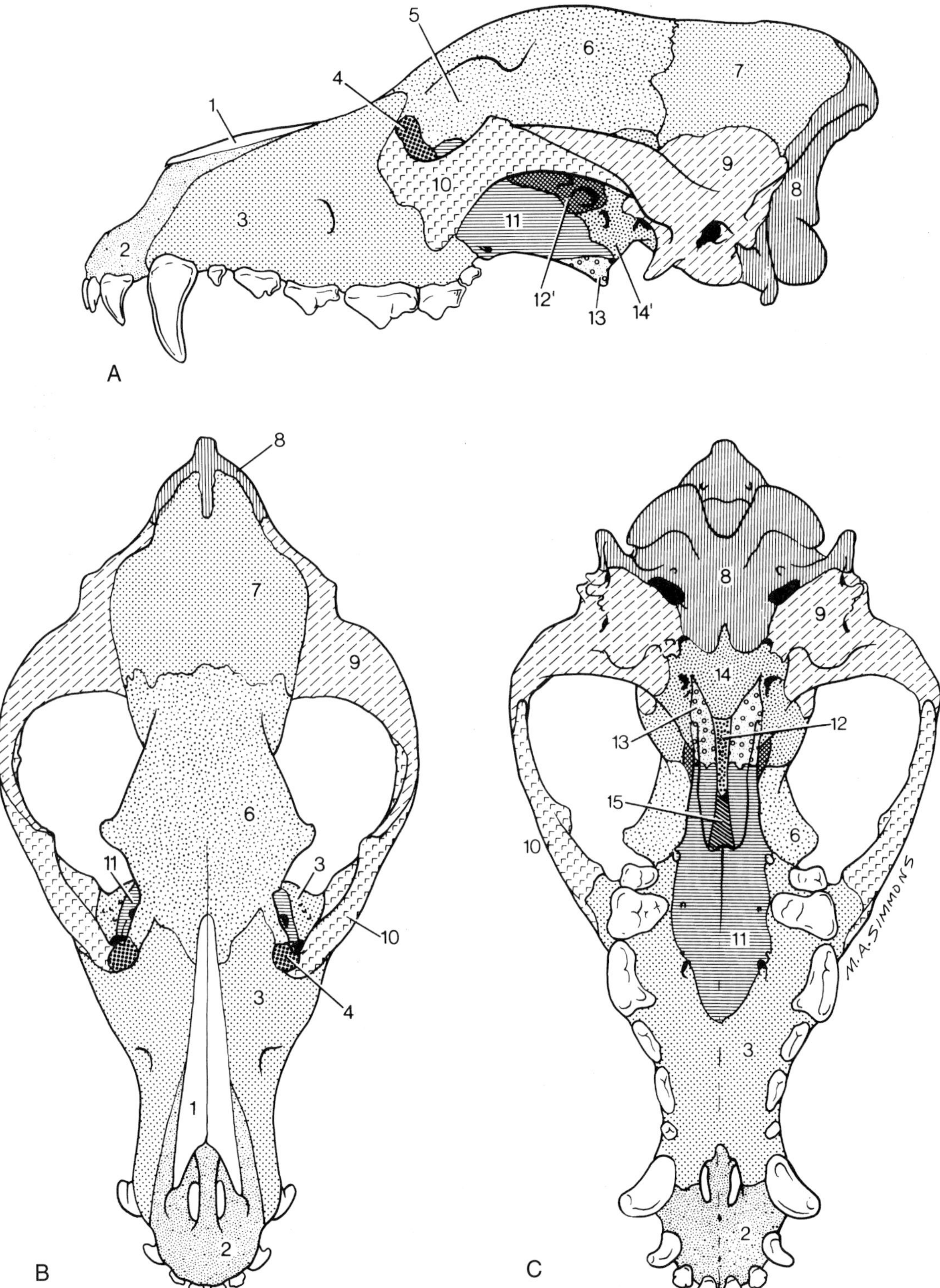


**Figure 2–29.** Lateral *(A)*, dorsal *(B)*, and ventral *(C)* views of the canine skull to show the extents of the cranial bones.

1, Nasal bone; 2, incisive bone; 3, maxilla; 4, lacrimal bone; 5, orbit; 6, frontal bone; 7, parietal bone; 8, occipital bone; 9, temporal bone; 10, zygomatic bone; 11, palatine bone; 12, presphenoid; 12′, wing of presphenoid; 13, pterygoid bone; 14, basisphenoid; 14′, pterygoid process of basisphenoid; 15, vomer.

In *dorsal view* (Fig. 2–30), the ovoid cranium meets the bones of the face where the zygomatic processes (/4′) of the frontal bones project laterally to form the dorsocaudal parts of the orbital walls. The caudal extremity of the cranium is marked by the external occipital protuberance in the midline; its demarcation from the caudal (nuchal) surface is completed by the nuchal crests that extend laterally to each side. The median sagittal crest that extends forward from the occipital protuberance is most prominent in robust, well-muscled animals. All these features are easily palpated in life. The dorsal and lateral surfaces of each half of the cranium blend in a continuous and slightly roughened surface from which the temporalis muscle arises. Rostral to the zygomatic processes of the frontal bones the dorsal surface of the skull dips, sometimes quite markedly, before continuing as the straight and narrow dorsum of the nose. This ends at the wide nasal aperture beyond which the bony skull is prolonged by pliant nasal cartilages.

The orbit is the most prominent feature of the *lateral view* (Fig. 2–31). Behind the orbit, the dorsolateral part of the braincase forms the wall of the temporal fossa (/16). The ventrolateral part is more complicated and presents the zygomatic arch and ear regions. The zygomatic arch (/15) springs free from the braincase and, bowing laterally, passes below the orbit to rejoin the facial part of the skull. It is formed by two bones—the squamous temporal and zygomatic—which meet at an overlapping suture. The ventral surface of the caudal part of this arch carries the articular surface for the mandible, shaped as a transverse gutter in this species; the articular area continues caudal to this onto the rostral surface of a ventral projection, the retroarticular process (/6). The large, smooth dome of the tympanic bulla (/9) (enclosing part of the cavity of the middle ear) and the rough mastoid process lie behind the retroarticular process. Three openings are present in this region of the skull; the retroarticular foramen emits a major vein draining the cranial cavity, the stylomastoid foramen gives passage to the facial nerve, and the external acoustic meatus is in the fresh state closed by a membrane (eardrum) that separates the canal of the external ear from the cavity of the middle ear. The paracondylar process (/11) is conspicuous at the caudal limit of the skull.

The orbit is funnel-shaped and in the macerated state its walls are very incomplete. In life the orbital rim is completed by a ligament (/1) that connects the zygomatic process of the frontal bone to the zygomatic arch. Ventrally the orbital cavity is continuous with the pterygopalatine fossa (/4), but in the fresh state these regions are separated by the periorbita, a dense fascial sheet that completes the definition of the orbit. Two groups of foramina are visible in this region. The caudal group (/5) comprises the optic canal, orbital fissure, and rostral alar foramen. The optic opening, placed at the apex of the conical orbital cavity, is the portal

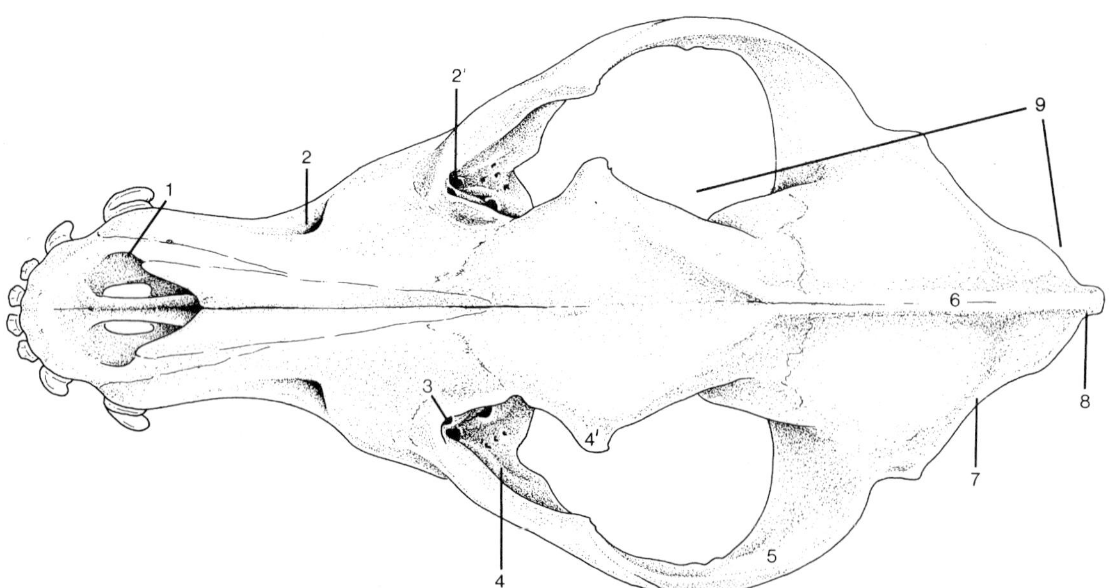


**Figure 2–30.** Dorsal view of canine skull.

1, Nasal aperture; 2, infraorbital foramen; 2′, maxillary foramen; 3, fossa for lacrimal sac; 4, orbit; 4′, zygomatic process of frontal bone; 5, zygomatic arch; 6, external sagittal crest; 7, nuchal crest; 8, external occipital protuberance; 9, cranium.

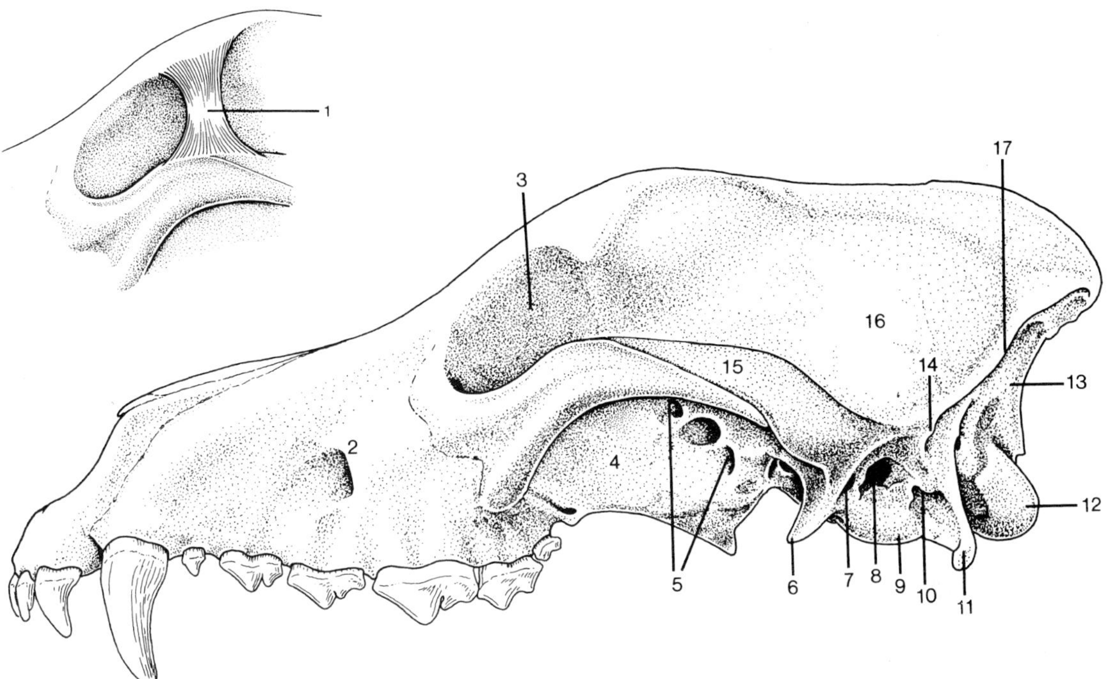


**Figure 2–31.** Lateral view of canine skull.

1, Orbital ligament *(inset)*; 2, infraorbital foramen; 3, orbit; 4, pterygopalatine fossa; 5, optic canal, orbital fissure, and rostral alar foramen; 6, retroarticular process; 7, retroarticular foramen; 8, external acoustic meatus; 9, tympanic bulla; 10, stylomastoid foramen; 11, paracondylar process; 12, occipital condyle; 13, nuchal surface; 14, mastoid process; 15, zygomatic arch; 16, temporal fossa; 17, nuchal crest.

of entry of the optic nerve. The more ventral orbital fissure transmits the nerves (ophthalmic, oculomotor, trochlear, and abducent) that supply ancillary structures of the eye and transmits also the external ophthalmic vein. Most ventrally the rostral alar foramen provides a common opening for the maxillary nerve, passing from the cranial cavity, and the maxillary artery, which transverses a canal (alar canal) in the sphenoid bone.

The rostral group of foramina comprises the maxillary, sphenopalatine, and caudal palatine foramina. The maxillary foramen (Fig. 2–30/2′) leads to the infraorbital canal, the sphenopalatine foramen to the nasal cavity, and the caudal palatine to the palatine canal, which emerges on the hard palate; each opening conveys like-named branches of the maxillary artery and nerve. More dorsally the rostral orbital wall contains the lacrimal fossa for the lacrimal sac (/3); an opening in the depth of the fossa leads to a passage that conveys the nasolacrimal (tear) duct to the nose.

The infraorbital foramen (/2) is the most prominent feature of the lateral aspect of the face and is easily palpable in the live animal; it is the site of emergence of the infraorbital nerve, which continues from the maxillary nerve through the infraorbital canal. Toward the alveolar margin the facial skeleton is molded over the roots of the teeth, most especially over the large root of the canine tooth.

In *ventral view* (Fig. 2–32) three regions of the skull are distinct—the base of the cranium, the choanal region where the nasal cavities open into the pharynx, and the hard palate. The first shows at its caudal limit the ovoid, obliquely oriented occipital condyles that flank the foramen magnum (/12) through which the spinal cord connects with the brain. Rostral to this the median area is generally flat, although midway along its length tubercles are present for the attachment of muscles that flex the head on the neck. The tympanic bulla and paracondylar process occupy much space to each side. The medial aspect of the bulla (/7) meets the occipital bone, and this fusion separates two openings that are confluent in some other species (e.g., horse; Fig. 2–37), namely, the more caudal jugular foramen and the more rostral foramen lacerum (Fig. 2–32/8,6). The glossopharyngeal, vagus, and accessory nerves emerge through the jugular foramen together with a large vein draining the interior of the cranium. Between the jugular foramen and the condyle is the

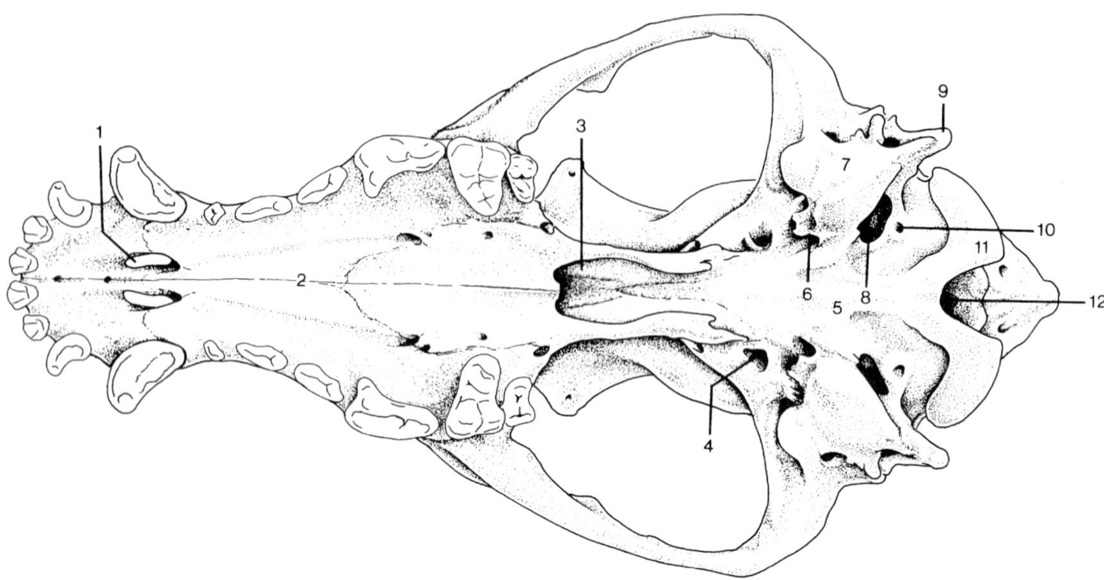


**Figure 2–32.** Ventral view of canine skull.

1, Palatine fissure; 2, hard palate; 3, choanal region; 4, oval foramen; 5, base of cranium; 6, foramen lacerum; 7, tympanic bulla; 8, jugular foramen; 9, paracondylar process; 10, hypoglossal canal; 11, occipital condyle; 12, foramen magnum.

hypoglossal canal, which transmits the hypoglossal nerve.

Lateral to the foramen lacerum small fissures exist for the exit of the chorda tympani (a branch of the facial nerve) and for the communication of the cartilaginous auditory tube with the cavity of the middle ear. Rostral to these is the prominent oval foramen (/4), through which the mandibular nerve emerges.

The openings (choanae) that lead from the nasal cavities to the nasopharynx are the main features of the middle part of the ventral aspect. The choanal region is bounded dorsally by the floor of the cranium and laterally by the thin plates of bone whose outer surfaces were earlier noted as forming the medial walls of the pterygopalatine fossae. The soft palate, which arises from the free margin of the hard palate, in life provides the floor of the space—essentially the first part of the nasopharynx—enclosed by these formations. The palate, which lies rostral to this, is broad behind, narrower in front. It is margined by the alveoli or sockets in which the upper teeth are implanted. Toward its rostral extremity it is perforated by the large bilateral palatine fissures. Several smaller foramina toward the caudal extremity of the palate are rostral openings of the palatine canal.

The *nuchal surface* (Fig. 2–31/13), broadly triangular, is limited dorsally by the external occipital protuberance and the nuchal crests. Its lower part presents the foramen magnum, the occipital condyles, and the paracondylar processes. The remainder of the surface is roughened for the attachment of dorsal muscles of the neck.

The *apex* of the skull is formed by the nasal aperture situated dorsal to the rostral extremities of the jaws that carry the incisor teeth.

The cavities of the skull are described with the respiratory system (Chapter 4), central nervous system (Chapter 8), and ear (Chapter 9).

The lower jaw or *mandible* comprises two halves (Fig. 2–33). In the dog these are firmly but not rigidly united by the connective tissues of the mandibular symphysis. Each half is divided between a body, or horizontal part, and a ramus, or vertical part. The body carries the alveoli of the lower teeth and is laterally compressed. Except at its rostral extremity it diverges from its fellow to bound an intermandibular space. Toward its rostral extremity the lateral surface presents several mental foramina, one generally much larger than the rest; through these emerge the mental branches of the inferior alveolar nerve and vessels. The ramus (/2) is wider but less robust. Its dorsal extremity ends in the high recurved coronoid process, which projects into the temporal fossa and gives attachment to the temporalis muscle, and the lower and more caudal condylar process (/3), which carries an articular head shaped like a portion of a truncated cone. The lower part of the caudal margin of the ramus carries the projecting angular process which enlarges the areas of attachment of the masseter and medial pterygoid muscles. The lateral surface is scooped out to provide a roughened depression where the masseter inserts. The medial surface gives insertion to the pterygoid muscles and also presents the large mandibular foramen (/7) where the inferior alveolar vessels and nerve enter the bone.

The *hyoid apparatus* consists of a series of bony rods, jointed together and forming a means of suspending the tongue and larynx from the skull. The names given to the several parts are shown in Fig. 2–34, which illustrates their arrangement and the attachment of the apparatus as a whole to the temporal region of the skull. The transversely placed basihyoid may be palpated within the intermandibular space; other parts are palpable—indeed their positions are visible—when the walls of the pharynx are inspected through the mouth (see Fig. 11–10).

## Some Comparative Features of the Skull

When equipped with the mandible the *skull of the cat* (Fig. 2–35) appears globular. Several features combine to create this conformation: the rounded cranial capsule, surmounted by a short, often weak sagittal crest, and corresponding closely to the contours of the brain; the very salient convex zygomatic arches; and the relative shortness of the face, which may account for as little as 20% of the total length. Breed differences are more pronounced than sometimes supposed. The skulls of Siamese and similar cats have much longer faces, which often blend smoothly with the cranium without any break (stop) in the dorsal contour. In contrasting types, for example, the Persian, the face is short and shallow and the stop prominent.

The orbital region is distinctive. The orbits are large, face more directly forward than in the dog, and have more complete bony margins. The frontal process of the zygomatic and the zygomatic process of the frontal bone leave only a small gap in the ovoid margin to be closed by the orbital ligament. The zygomatic arch is surprisingly strong where it contributes to the orbital rim. The infraorbital foramen is placed close to the rostroventral part of the orbit where it may be palpated.

On the ventral aspect, the hard palate is short, wide, and carries alveoli for only four cheek teeth. That for the largest ($P^4$) of these teeth is located dangerously close to the orbit, which may become involved in a spreading alveolar abscess. Caudally, the deep gutter of the temporomandibular articulation is bounded by a prominent retroarticular process. The very large tympanic bulla is so salient that it may be palpated between the caudal part of the zygomatic arch and the wing of the atlas.

As in the dog, the two halves of the mandible do

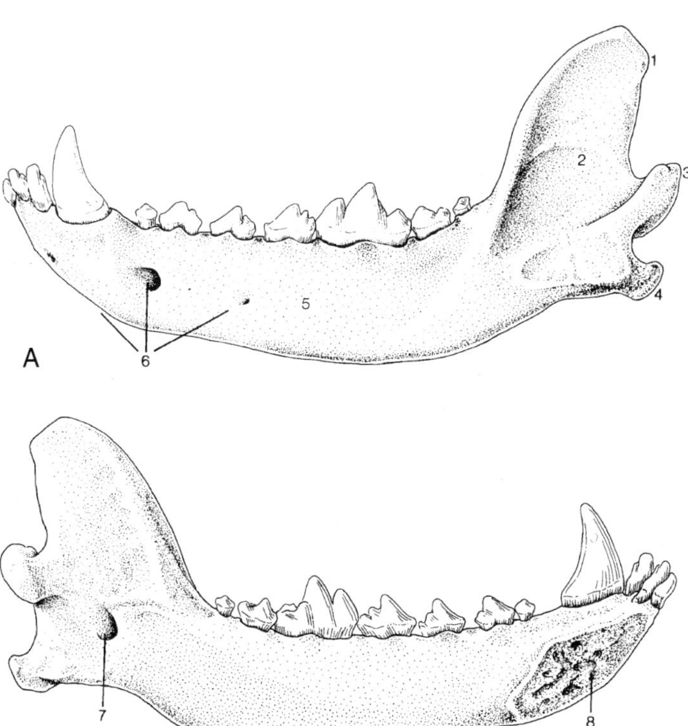


**Figure 2–33.** Lateral *(A)* and medial *(B)* views of the left half of the canine mandible.

1, Coronoid process; 2, vertical part (ramus); 3, condylar process; 4, angular process; 5, horizontal part (body); 6, mental foramina; 7, mandibular foramen; 8, symphysial surface.

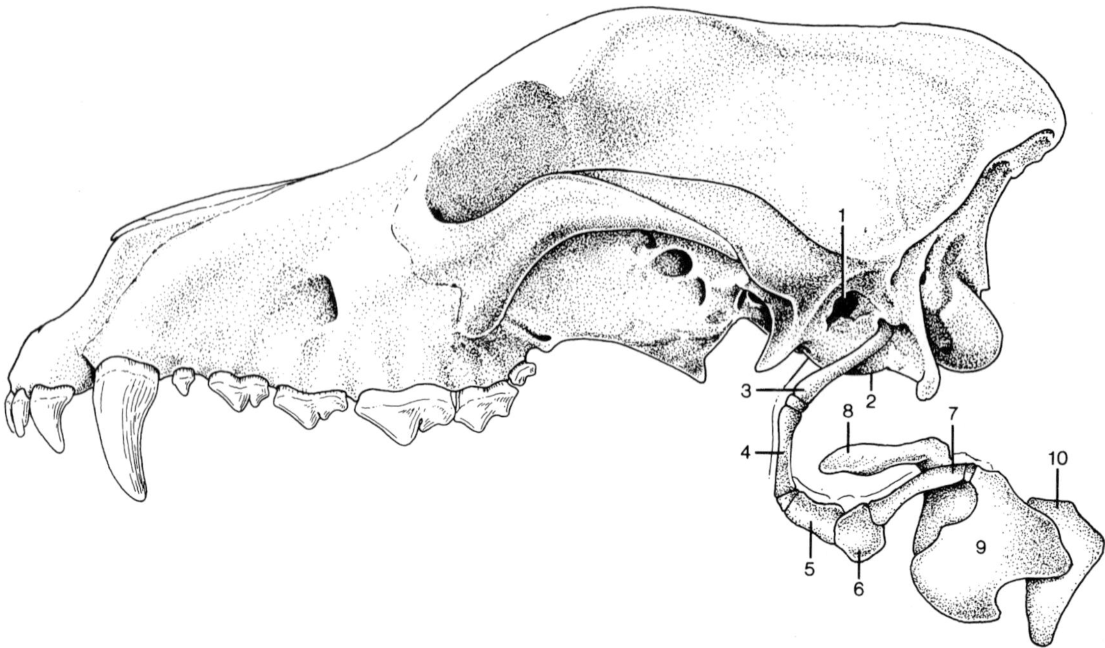


**Figure 2–34.** Hyoid apparatus and larynx suspended from the temporal region of a canine skull.

1, External acoustic meatus; 2, tympanic bulla; 3, stylohyoid; 4, epihyoid; 5, ceratohyoid; 6, basihyoid; 7, thyrohyoid; 8, epiglottic cartilage; 9, thyroid cartilage; 10, cricoid cartilage.

not fuse, even in old age, and a small degree of movement is allowed at the mandibular symphysis. Each half carries sockets for only three cheek teeth.

The *equine skull* (Fig. 2–36) is characterized by a relatively long face, a feature that develops further with increasing size; it is therefore more pronounced in mature than in juvenile animals and in large than in small breeds. The cranium is relatively narrow and generally not unlike that of the dog. The external sagittal crest is weaker. The forehead is wide between the origins of the zygomatic processes of the frontal bones, which bend ventrally to join the zygomatic arches.

The zygomatic arch (/7) is conspicuously strong, even without taking account of the extra support it obtains from the zygomatic process connecting it with the frontal bone. It is not bowed laterally to any extent and on its caudoventral aspect carries a rather complicated articular surface; this comprises a rostral tuber, an intermediate fossa, and a salient retroarticular process (/8). The orbit faces almost

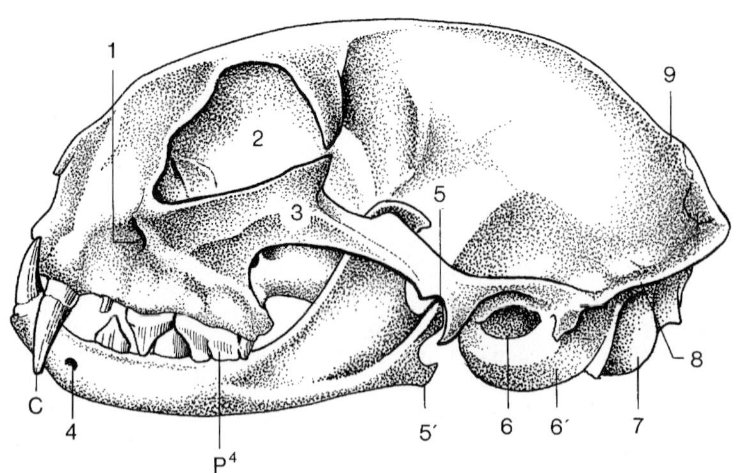


**Figure 2–35.** Feline skull with mandible.

1, Infraorbital foramen; 2, orbit; 3, zygomatic arch; 4, mental foramen; 5, temporomandibular joint; 5′, angular process of mandible; 6, external acoustic meatus; 6′, tympanic bulla; 7, occipital condyle; 8, nuchal crest; 9, sagittal crest; C, canine tooth; $P^4$, upper fourth premolar.

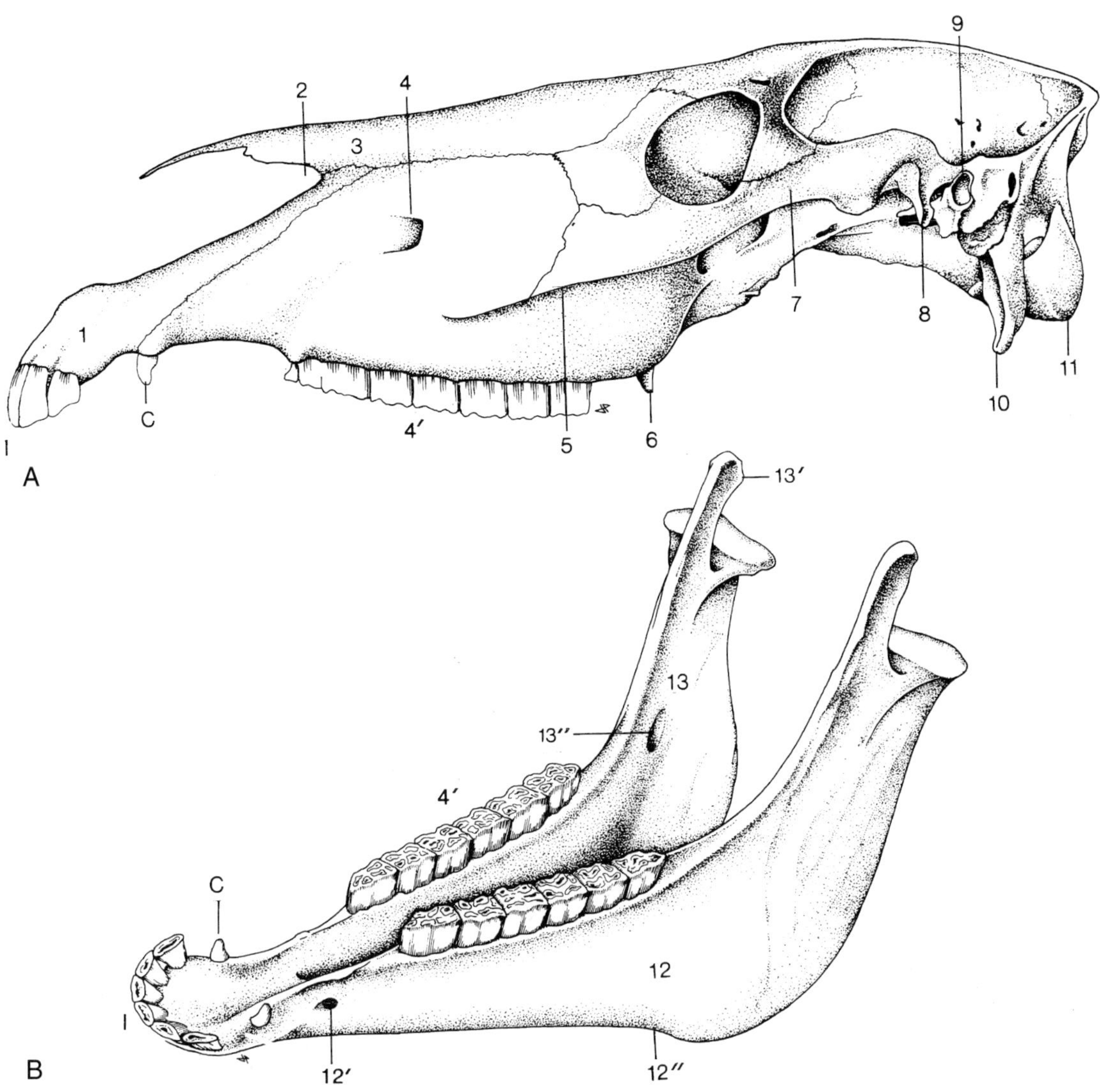


**Figure 2–36.** *A*, Equine skull and *B*, equine mandible.

1, Incisive bone; 2, nasoincisive notch; 3, nasal bone; 4, infraorbital foramen; 4′, cheek teeth; 5, facial crest; 6, hamulus of pterygoid bone; 7, zygomatic arch; 8, retroarticular process; 9, external acoustic meatus; 10, paracondylar process; 11, occipital condyle; 12, horizontal part (body) of mandible; 12′, mental foramen; 12″, vascular notch; 13, vertical part (ramus) of mandible; 13′, coronoid process; 13″, mandibular foramen; I, incisors; C, canine tooth (present only in the male).

laterally and has a complete bony rim. A large maxillary tuberosity appears to continue the alveolar process directly. The zygomatic arch is continued rostrally, beyond the orbit, as a prominent ridge on the lateral surface of the face. This ridge, the facial crest (/5), runs parallel to the dorsal contour of the nose and ends above a septum between the alveoli of the third and fourth cheek teeth in the adult.

A deep (nasoincisive) notch separates the pointed nasal bone from the incisive bone (/1,2,3). This notch and the rostral end of the facial crest are both very easily identified landmarks; they are used as guides to the position of the infraorbital foramen, which lies a little caudal to the middle of the connecting line (/4).

The features visible on ventral view lie more or less on one level. The caudal part of this surface is distinguished by the large and very salient paracondylar processes (/10) and the jagged outlines of the large openings to each side of the occipital bone. Each opening results from the failure of the temporal bone to reach the lateral margin of the occipital bone, which permits the confluence of several foramina that are distinct in the dog. The caudal part is the equivalent of the jugular foramen; the cranial part (foramen lacerum) combines the oval and carotid foramina (Fig. 2–37/7,6). In life the greater part of the large opening is occluded by membrane that leaves barely sufficient passage for the various nerves and vessels. The tympanic bulla is not prominent, but styloid (for the hyoid apparatus) and muscular processes of the temporal bone are well developed.

The choanae lie almost in the plane of the hard palate. The vertical plate of bone that separates the choanal from the pterygopalatine region carries a prominent hamular process (Fig. 2–36/6). The palate is flat and unremarkable. The greater part of its margin is occupied by the alveoli of the incisor and cheek teeth.

A well-marked external occipital protuberance is present on the nuchal surface, midway between the nuchal crest and the dorsal margin of the foramen magnum.

The mandible is massive, and its right and left halves diverge at a relatively small angle (/*B*). The symphysis becomes obliterated quite early, usually about 2 years after birth. The lower margin carries a prominent vascular notch where the facial vessels wind onto the face (/12″). The ramus is high; the coronoid process projects far into the temporal fossa, and the articular process carries the ovoid articular surface well above the occlusal plane of the cheek teeth.

The parts of the hyoid apparatus (see Fig. 4–8) are of different proportions to their counterparts in the dog and are laterally compressed. A substantial lingual process projects from the basihyoid into the root of the tongue.

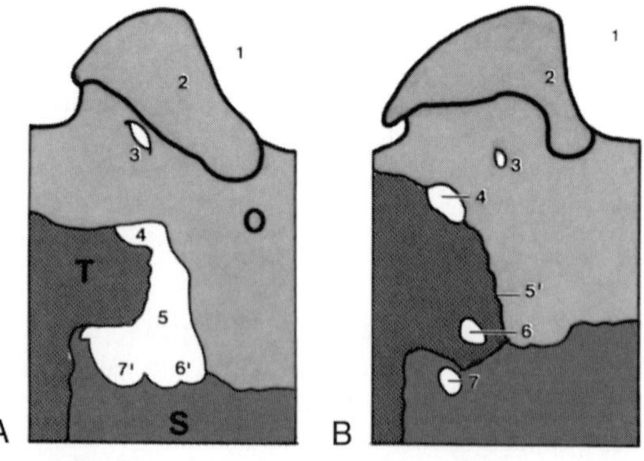


**Figure 2–37.** Left caudolateral parts of the base of the equine *(A)* and canine *(B)* cranium, showing portions of the occipital (O), sphenoid (S), and temporal (T) bones; ventral view (schematic).

1, Foramen magnum; 2, occipital condyle; 3, hypoglossal canal; 4, jugular foramen; 5, foramen lacerum; 5′, petro-occipital suture; 6, carotid canal; 6′, carotid notches; 7, oval foramen; 7′, oval notch.

The *bovine skull* (Fig. 2–38) is relatively short and wide, its general form being pyramidal. Cornual (horn) processes project from the frontal bones of horned breeds where the dorsal, lateral, and nuchal surfaces meet; their size and direction vary greatly with breed, age, and sex. The very wide and flat frontal region is bounded by a prominent temporal line that overhangs the deep temporal fossa and confines this to the lateral aspect of the skull. The forehead continues smoothly into the dorsal contour of the nose.

The principal features of the lateral aspect are the confinement of the temporal fossa and the elevation of the orbital rim above its surroundings. The rim is complete and in its caudal part is formed by the meeting of processes from the zygomatic and frontal bones. There is no facial crest, only a discrete facial tuberosity from which the rostral part of the masseter arises. The infraorbital foramen is directly above the first cheek tooth, rather low toward the palate.

The ventral surface is very uneven, with the cranial base located in a considerably more dorsal plane than the palate. The temporal and occipital bones are separated by a narrow fissure, an arrangement intermediate between the suture of the dog and the wide opening of the horse and pig. The tympanic bulla is prominent and laterally compressed. The choanae are separated by the caudal prolongation of the ventral part of the nasal septum and are enclosed laterally by very extensive plates of bone. The palate, long and narrow, is bounded by high alveolar processes. Of course, no alveoli are present for incisor or canine teeth (lacking in the upper jaws of ruminants).

The mandibular symphysis ossifies late, if at all, in ruminants. In general, the mandible is weaker than that of the horse, a feature very apparent in the body of the bone with its gently convex ventral border. The coronoid process is high and caudally inflected. The articular surface is concave and widened laterally.

The few remarks necessary regarding the skulls of the small ruminants and pig are found on pages 629 and 761, respectively.

## The Joints of the Head

The articulations between the skull and mandible (temporomandibular joints) and that between the two halves of the mandible (mandibular symphysis) are appropriately considered in the following chapter (p. 113) since the teeth, the muscles of mastication, and the joints form a single functional complex.

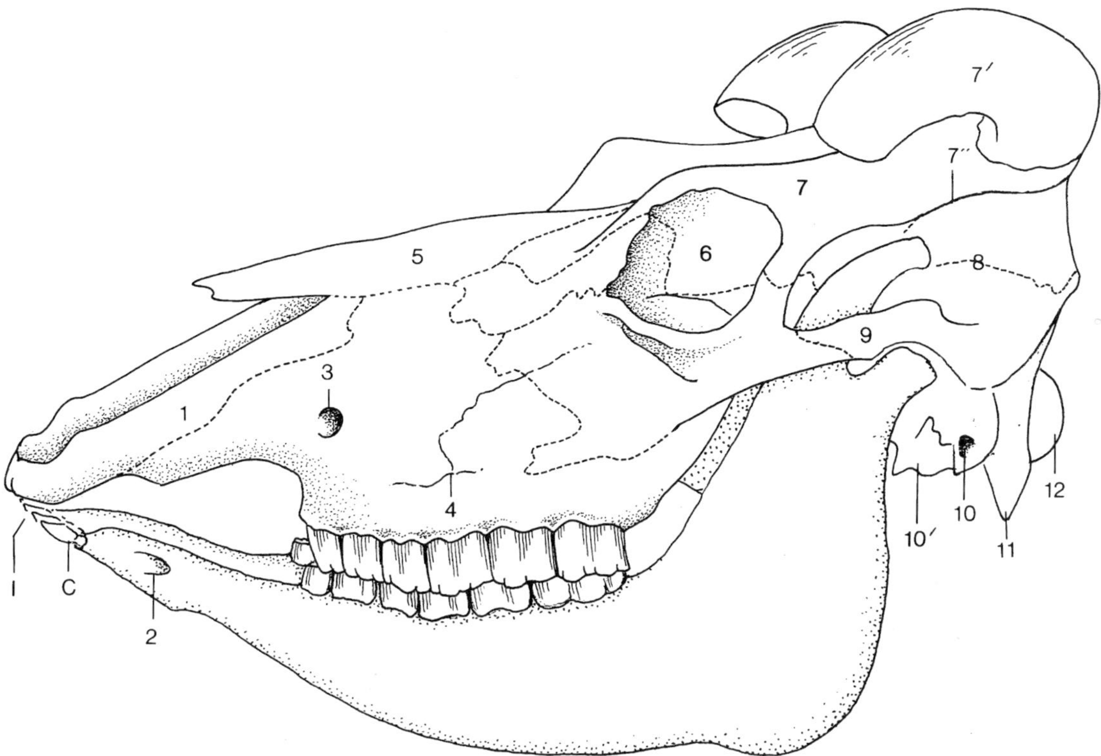


**Figure 2–38.** Bovine skull with mandible.

1, Incisive bone; 2, mental foramen; 3, infraorbital foramen; 4, facial tuberosity; 5, nasal bone; 6, orbit; 7, frontal bone; 7′, horn surrounding cornual process of frontal bone; 7″, temporal line; 8, temporal fossa; 9, zygomatic arch; 10, external acoustic meatus; 10′, tympanic bulla; 11, paracondylar process; 12, occipital condyle; I, incisors; C, canine tooth, incorporated in the row of incisors.

## The Muscles of the Head and Ventral Part of the Neck

The principal groups into which the muscles of the head may be divided are given in Table 2–2, which draws attention to the correspondence between embryological origin, innervation, and function. The functional associations are so well defined and specific that it is both more convenient and more profitable to refer treatment of most groups to other chapters where they are considered together with related organs.

The first four groups take origin in the unsplit mesoderm, which covers the lateral and ventral walls of the pharynx and condenses to form the cores of the pharyngeal arches.

In lower vertebrates the muscles equivalent to the last two groups in Table 2–2 are known to develop from somites that appear to each side of

**Table 2–2.** Source and Innervation of the Principal Muscle Groups of the Head

| Muscle Group | Source | Innervation |
|---|---|---|
| Masticatory musculature | First pharyngeal arch | Mandibular division of trigeminal nerve (V3) |
| Mimetic musculature | Second pharyngeal arch | Facial nerve (VII) |
| Pharyngeal and palatine musculature | Third and fourth pharyngeal arches | Glossopharyngeal (IX) and vagus (X) nerves |
| Laryngeal musculature | Sixth pharyngeal arch | Vagus nerve (X) |
| External ocular musculature | Hypothetical preotic somites | Oculomotor (III), trochlear (IV), and abducent (VI) nerves |
| Lingual musculature | Hypothetical postotic somites | Hypoglossal nerve (XII) |

the hindbrain, some rostral to the otocyst, the primordium of the inner ear, the others caudal to it. A similar origin may be assumed in mammals, although the evidence for the formation of these somites is unconvincing at the least. They are of course somatic muscles with the appropriate type of innervation.

## The Trigeminal Musculature

The muscles of mastication constitute the greater part of the musculature supplied by the mandibular division of the trigeminal nerve, the motor nerve to the first pharyngeal arch. They are described in the chapter on the digestive system (p. 115). The same chapter deals with the digastricus—a composite muscle to which the mandibular field makes a contribution; the mylohyoideus (p. 106), which slings the tongue between the lower jaws; and one (tensor veli palatini) of the muscles of the soft palate (p. 119). The tensor tympani is considered with the middle ear (p. 339).

## The Facial Musculature

The musculature supplied by the facial nerve, the nerve of the second pharyngeal arch, is resolvable into two divisions. The superficial division comprises the cutaneous muscle of the head and neck in addition to many small units that control the posture of the lips, cheeks, nostrils, eyelids, and external ears. The deep division is rather scattered but includes some muscles associated with the hyoid apparatus, a contribution to the digastricus (p. 115), and the stapedius (p. 339) of the middle ear.

**The Superficial Division.** The muscles of this division are conjectured to have their source in an ancestral deep sphincter muscle of the neck, which may be envisaged as arranged in three incomplete overlapping layers. The outermost layer, consisting of transversely disposed fascicles, is reduced to insignificance or is entirely lacking in domestic mammals. A remnant (sphincter colli) survives in the dog. A more substantial portion of the middle layer commonly persists in the form of a sheet of longitudinally disposed fibers that covers the ventral part of the face and extends onto the neck, even reaching the nape in the dog. It is known as the platysma. Detached slips are believed to provide the small muscles that attach to the caudal aspect of the external ear.

The third and deepest layer is again transverse. Although little of it remains in sheet form, it is believed to be the origin of the many discrete muscles of the mammalian face. These are extremely variable among species, but fortunately, few units, and even fewer differences, require detailed notice. Because of their effect on the appearance of the face they are collectively known as the *muscles of facial expression* or *mimetic musculature.*

The principal muscles of the lips and cheeks are the buccinator, orbicularis oris, caninus, levator nasolabialis, levator labii superioris, and depressor labii inferioris (Figs. 2–39 and 11–3). The *buccinator* (Fig. 2–39/5) passes between the margins of the upper and lower jaws and is partly covered by the masseter. It forms the basis of the cheek and acts in opposition to the tongue, preventing food from collecting in the vestibule by returning it to the central cavity of the mouth. The buccal salivary glands are scattered among its fascicles, and discharge of their secretion into the mouth may be assisted by contraction of the muscle. The *orbicularis oris* (/1) surrounds the mouth opening where it is closely attached to the skin and mucosa of the lips. It closes the opening of the mouth by pursing the lips and is important in sucking. The *caninus* (/2) arises ventral to the infraorbital foramen and radiates into the wing of the nostril and the upper lip. It dilates the nostril and, in the dog especially, elevates the corner of the mouth in the snarling gesture. The *levator nasolabialis* (/6) arises over the dorsum of the nose and inserts partly on the wing of the nostril, partly into the lateral part of the upper lip. It is able to dilate the nostril and to elevate and retract the upper lip. The medial part of the upper lip is elevated by the separate *levator labii superioris* (/7). This muscle arises on the lateral aspect of the face and runs dorsorostrally to form with its fellow a common tendon that descends into the lip between the nostrils. A special *depressor labii inferioris* (/4) is present in the lower lip of certain species (excluding the dog and cat). It appears to be a detachment from the buccinator muscle. Other muscles associated with the lips and nostrils do not merit specific mention, although some are identified in various illustrations.

The muscles of the eyelids include one, the levator palpebrae superioris, which is clearly foreign to the facial group since it arises within the orbit and is supplied by the oculomotor nerve. It is described on page 331. The muscles of the lids that are supplied by the facial nerve include a sphincter—the *orbicularis oculi* (/8)—that surrounds the palpebral fissure, the opening between the lids. It is anchored at the medial and lateral commissures and therefore narrows the opening to a horizontal slit when it contracts. Other muscles are present to raise the upper (levator anguli oculi) lid and to depress the lower (malaris) lid, enlarging the eye opening.

The muscles of the external ear are especially numerous but of little account individually. A

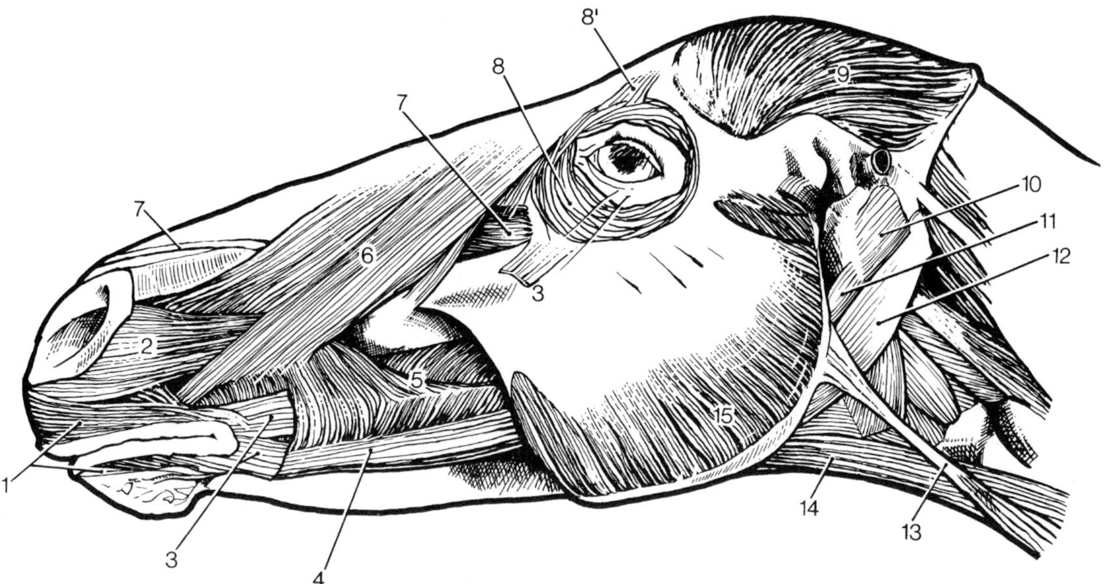


**Figure 2–39.** Superficial muscles of the equine head. The cutaneous muscle has been removed.

1, Orbicularis oris; 2, caninus; 3, stumps of cutaneous muscle; 4, depressor labii inferioris; 5, buccinator; 6, levator nasolabialis; 7, levator labii superioris; 8, orbicularis oculi; 8′, levator anguli oculi medialis; 9, temporalis; 10, occipitohyoideus; 11, stylohyoideus; 12, occipitomandibular part of digastricus; 13, sternocephalicus; 14, combined sterno- and omohyoideus; 15, masseter.

caudal group has already been mentioned. Others converge on the auricle—the skin-covered cartilaginous ear "trumpet"—from medial, rostral, and lateral directions; they lie between the skin and the temporalis muscle and skull and form a thin, incomplete sheet that includes a (scutiform) cartilage plate. The scattered origins and precisely located insertions provide for displacement and rotation of the ear in all directions. One, the *parotidoauricularis,* is of somewhat greater importance since it is encountered in the operation for drainage of infections of the external ear of the dog (p. 385). As its name suggests, it arises from the fascia over the parotid gland and approaches the auricle from the ventrolateral direction.

Besides the individual functions mentioned or implied in the preceding paragraphs these muscles have a collective function in communication, mainly within the species but also between species. Human observers can intuitively, or as the result of experience, interpret many facial gestures of animals—one need only recall the "hangdog" expression of submission, the evident threat conveyed by snarling or laying back the ears, or the quizzical look a dog may adopt. The analysis of the more subtle expressions in terms of specific muscle activity is not yet possible for domestic species.

Paralysis of these muscles is not uncommon following damage to the facial nerve. Since different groups are supplied by branches of the nerve that arise at different levels, the particular pattern of distortions can be a valuable pointer to the location of the nerve lesion (p. 309).

**The Deep Division.** The muscles attaching to the hyoid apparatus are a rather heterogeneous assemblage (Fig. 2–39/10,11). Certain small units are supplied by the facial nerve and elevate the hyoid, in consequence drawing the tongue backward. Although it cannot be denied that these activities have a significance in swallowing, the muscles do not appear to merit description. The digastricus, in part derived from the facial musculature, is described on page 115; the stapedius of the middle ear is described on page 339.

### The Muscles of the Pharynx and Soft Palate

These are considered beginning on page 330.

### The Muscles of the Larynx

These are considered beginning on page 154.

### The External Muscles of the Eyeball

These are considered beginning on page 117.

### The Muscles of the Tongue

These are considered beginning on page 105.

## The Muscles of the Ventral Part of the Neck

The neck connects the head with the trunk and is usually distinguished by its relatively slender construction—although this is hardly true of the pig. It has a generally cylindrical form in the dog and cat but is quite obviously compressed from side to side in the larger animals, in which it deepens considerably toward its junction with the thorax (Fig. 2–40). The core structures of the neck—the cervical vertebrae and the muscles closely applied to them—were described with the trunk (p. 47). Certain superficial muscles are considered under the heading of girdle muscles of the forelimb (p. 83). The present section is therefore concerned only with the ventral part of the neck, a region of considerable clinical importance on account of the numerous visceral, vascular, and nervous structures that traverse it en route between the head and thorax.

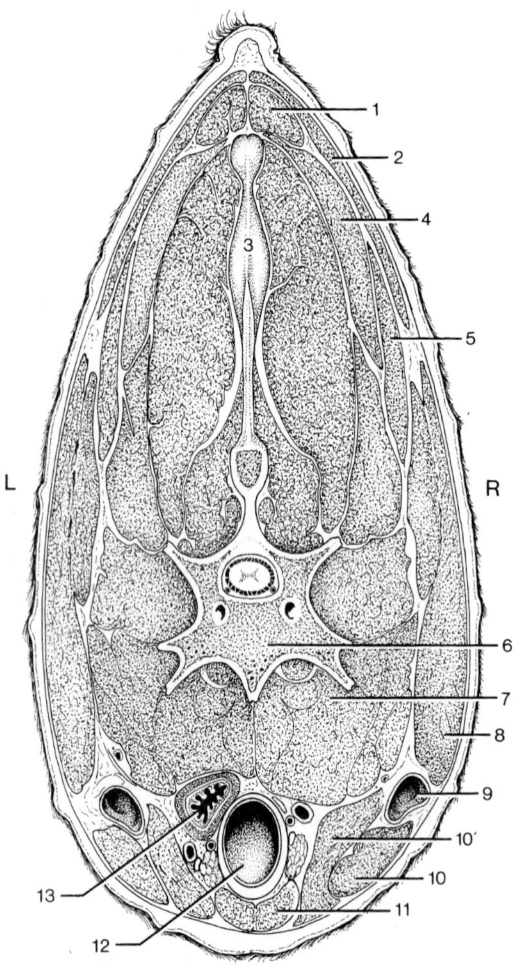


**Figure 2–40.** Transverse section of the bovine neck.

1, Rhomboideus; 2, trapezius; 3, nuchal ligament; 4, splenius; 5, omotransversarius; 6, vertebra; 7, longus colli; 8, brachiocephalicus; 9, external jugular vein in jugular groove; 10, 10′, sternocephalicus, mandibular, and mastoid parts; 11, combined sternohyoideus and sternothyroideus; 12, trachea; 13, esophagus (ventral to it, nerves, blood vessels, and thymus).

These structures—with the important exception of the external jugular veins (/9)—occupy a central visceral space. The roof of this space is provided by the muscles immediately ventral to the vertebrae, namely the longus coli, longus capitis, rectus capitis ventralis, and scalenus (p. 51). The side and ventral walls blend together and are provided by thinner muscles disposed with a sagittal course and joined by stout fasciae.

The cervical part of the *cutaneous muscle* (m. cutaneous colli) is unimportant in the dog and cat. It is much better developed in the ungulates, in which it radiates from a stout origin on the manubrium of the sternum; it thins as it passes cranially and laterally and eventually fades away. In the horse, the cutaneous muscle provides a relatively thick cover to the caudal third or so of the jugular groove.

The straplike *sternocephalicus* (Fig. 2–41/2) is the most ventral of the other muscles. It also arises from the manubrium and is first pressed against its fellow. But as it ascends the neck it diverges laterally toward its insertion, which varies among species but includes one or the other (or both) of the angle of the mandible and the mastoid process of the skull. The divergence of the right and left muscles exposes the upper part of the trachea to palpation through the skin, although a very thin layer of deeper muscle still intervenes. The sternocephalicus is supplied by the ventral branch of the accessory nerve. Unilateral contraction draws the head and neck to that side. Bilateral contraction flexes the head and neck ventrally. In species with a mandibular insertion the sternocephalicus may assist in opening the mouth.

The sternocephalicus forms the ventral border of the jugular groove. The dorsal border of the groove is furnished by the *brachiocephalicus,* described more fully elsewhere (p. 83). The groove is often visible in life, particularly toward the upper part of the neck. It accommodates the external jugular vein (Fig. 2–40/9).

The deeper muscles constitute an infrahyoid group closely integrated in arrangement and function. They provide an incomplete cover to the lateral and ventral aspects of the trachea and insert, directly or indirectly, on the hyoid apparatus, which they stabilize and retract toward the thorax during swallowing. The obvious members of the group are the sternothyroideus, sternohyoideus, and omohyoideus; the thyrohyoideus on the lateral

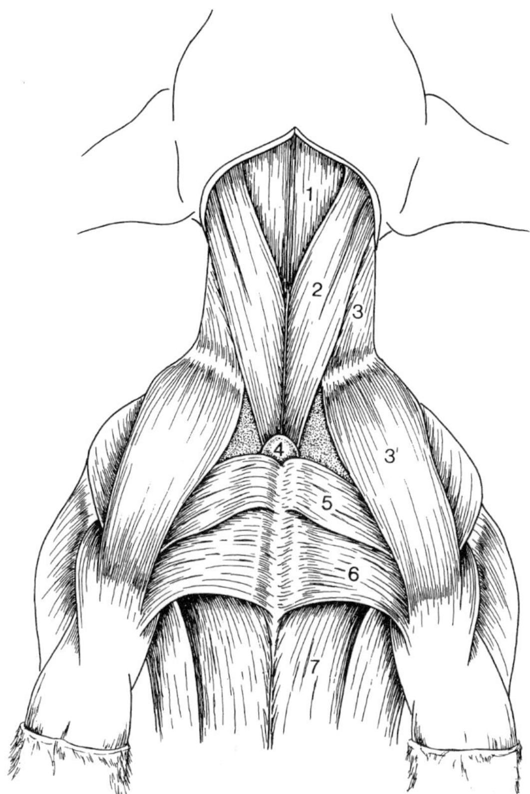


**Figure 2–41.** Ventral muscles of the canine neck and thorax.

1, Combined sternohyoideus and sternothyroideus; 2, sternocephalicus; 3, 3′, brachiocephalicus: cleidocervicalis, cleidobrachialis; 4, manubrium of sternum; 5, pectoralis descendens; 6, pectoralis transversus; 7, pectoralis profundus.

aspect of the larynx may be regarded as a detached member. The nerve supply is mainly, though possibly not entirely, from the first and second cervical nerves.

The *sternothyroideus* and *sternohyoideus* (/11) are very thin ribbon-like muscles that take a common origin from the manubrium of the sternum. The caudal parts of the right and left muscles are not always distinctly divided, and in the middle of the neck they may share a common intermediate tendon from which three or four slips diverge cranially. The sternothyroideus inclines laterally to terminate on the lateral aspect of the thyroid cartilage. The sternohyoideus, not always separable from its fellow, passes beside the midline to insert on the basihyoid.

The *omohyoideus,* lacking in carnivores, is also thin and straplike. Its absence is compensated by the relative enlargement of the other muscles. In the horse it arises from the subscapular fascia, in the ruminants from the deep fascia of the neck; thereafter it edges medially to join the lateral margin of the sternohyoideus beside which it inserts. In the horse it provides a floor to the caudal part of the jugular groove, separating the vein from the structures within the visceral space.

# THE LIMBS

## Basic Plan and Development

Although the fore- and hindlimbs are not homologous, they have a similar organization and segmentation with a remarkably close correspondence of analogous parts. Each first appears as a bud that grows out from the ventrolateral surface of the body of the young embryo at a level corresponding to the origin of the nerves by which it will later be supplied. The bud of the forelimb appears before that of the hindlimb, and its development for some time maintains this advantage—indeed, until after birth in puppies and other animals born in a rather immature state. These animals initially confine their locomotor activities to dragging themselves, using the forelimbs only, toward their dam's teats.

When first formed, a limb bud consists of a mass of mesenchyme, the loose embryonic connective tissue, within an ectodermal covering. The ectoderm becomes the epidermis, including its derivatives; the mesenchyme differentiates to form skeletal tissues, muscles and tendons, fasciae, and blood vessels. Thus it is only the limb nerves that invade from outside; all other structures develop in situ (leaving aside the uncertainty concerning the dermis). The limb bud lengthens, and its free distal part expands to form a flattened hand (foot) plate while the more proximal part acquires a more columnar form. Thickenings corresponding to the digital rays soon appear in the plate and are accentuated when the intervening tissues are reduced. The details of this development naturally vary with the species, for it is only some that retain the primitive pentadactyl (five-digit) pattern and only a few that show a complete separation of digits. It is interesting to note that five digits appear in most species; when evolution has reduced the complement to fewer, the adult condition is usually attained by fetal regression of some digits. Creases formed in the proximal part of the bud soon allow recognition of segments corresponding to the arm and forearm (or thigh and leg) regions of the adult.

The first indication of the future limb skeleton is provided by an axial condensation of the mesoderm to produce a denser core. In the early stages of development—although not always later—a definite proximodistal gradient of differentiation occurs. This establishes and then maintains the girdle elements in advance of those of the arm or thigh, and the latter in advance of more distal parts.

In the next stage of development the mesoderm is locally transformed to create a series of cartilaginous models in the pattern of the adult bones. These precursors soon come to resemble the final forms in broad outline; they remain ensheathed by thin coverings of the unmodified mesoderm, now appropriately known as perichondrium. Dense mesoderm also remains between the cartilages where the joints will develop.

The cartilage models grow mainly by interstitial growth, in which each part expands more or less uniformly to maintain the general form. The next stage involves the replacement of the cartilage by bone tissue—not its transformation into bone, a distinction that deserves to be emphasized. The process does not occur identically or synchronously in different bones, and the remarks that follow concern that hypothetical concept, the "typical long bone."

The initial ossification involves two processes. In one, the perichondrium around the middle of the shaft lays bone down on the cartilage. This process of bone formation is known as intramembranous ossification since it occurs within the connective tissue membrane. Its details must be sought in textbooks of histology. A tubular bony sheath, the periosteal collar, is thus formed about the center of the shaft; it is gradually extended toward each extremity (Fig. 2–42). In the other process, the cartilage of the center of the shaft shows aging or degenerative changes; its cells hypertrophy, come to occupy enlarged lacunae (spaces) in the matrix, and then die, while the matrix becomes impregnated with calcium salts. This central patch of dead cartilage is now invaded by a connective tissue sprout that pushes in from the periosteum (as the perichondrium is now more appropriately known in the region of the collar). The progress of this sprout, which is rather cellular and well vascularized, is facilitated by the spongy texture given to the dead cartilage by the enlarged lacunae. Some of the cells that are carried inward have the capacity to engulf and remove calcified matrix, others the capacity to lay bone down on the surviving framework, while a third group are precursors of marrow cells. The processes of construction and destruction continue in parallel and transform the whole middle portion of the shaft into a parcel of bone known as the primary or diaphysial center of ossification.

Later (much later in some species and mainly after birth in ourselves), similar sprouts from the perichondrium invade the centers of the two extremities; they establish secondary or epiphysial centers of ossification. The secondary centers are not preceded by the formation of any equivalent to the periosteal collar of the shaft. The general stage of development of the long bone at this time is shown in Figure 2–42/8. This reveals that the original cartilage now survives only as two plates, the epiphysial or growth cartilages, that intervene between the primary and secondary centers. These have a special significance since they are responsible for the growth in length of the bone. They are clearly polarized; cell division and matrix expansion are confined to the epiphysial aspect while degeneration, calcification, and replacement occur at the central or diaphysial side. The replacement adds continuously to the length of the diaphysis while the growth of the cartilage continues to shift the epiphyses away from this. The two processes are balanced until finally growth fails to keep pace with replacement; the plate thins and ultimately is

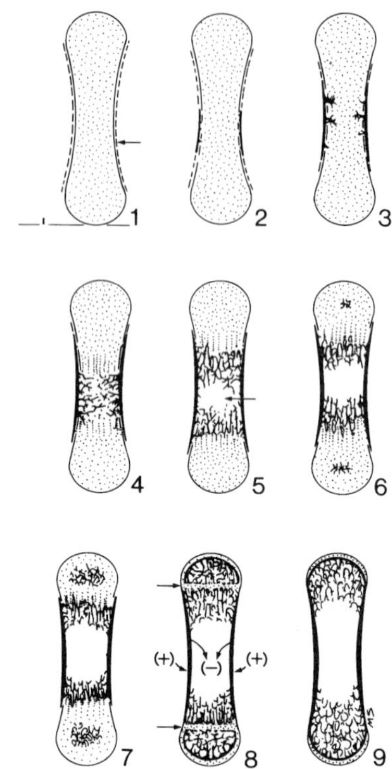


**Figure 2–42.** Development of a long bone, schematic.

1, Cartilage model with perichondral membrane *(arrow);* 2, intramembranous ossification of diaphysis; 3, 4, endochondral (primary) ossification of diaphysis, replaces cartilage; 5, beginning of medullary cavity *(arrow);* 6, epiphysial ossification centers appear; 7, endochondral (secondary) ossification of epiphyses; 8, narrow epiphysial cartilages *(arrows)* separate the diaphysis from epiphyses: these and the articular cartilages are all that remain of the cartilage model (1); note circumferential growth of diaphysis by removal (–) and addition (+) of compact bone; 9, mature bone consisting of articular cartilage, spongy bone, and compact bone; the epiphysial cartilages have disappeared.

quite destroyed; the epiphysis and diaphysis have now fused in one and further longitudinal growth is impossible. Neither the rates of growth nor the times of final disappearance are necessarily the same in the two growth cartilages of a long bone. Meanwhile, however, the bone has also been increasing in its girth, the result of further lamellae being laid in succession on the existing bone within the periosteal sheath. Some of the larger projections on long bones develop from independent centers of ossification and remain separated from the shaft by cartilage growth plates while growth continues. The projections distinguished in this way are known as apophyses.

Little reflection is necessary before deciding that bone growth must be more complicated than this. The form established by the original model would not be maintained by continuous accretion. A simultaneous process of destruction must exist, especially to maintain the shape of the metaphyses (the regions of the shaft adjoining the growth cartilages), to keep surface features in the same relationship to each other, and to establish and then enlarge the medullary cavity. Although we have no space to elaborate on this statement, one point can be made: bone grows by apposition, the deposition of new material on that previously existing. In this it differs from the periosteum, which grows interstitially as though uniformly stretched. The peritoneal sheath therefore shifts relative to the underlying bone, and the consequent drag on the nutrient vessels explains the generally oblique orientation of the adult nutrient foramina. By the time of birth, skeletal development has reached very different stages in different mammalian species. In the precocious ungulates, immediately active after birth, almost all epiphyses are well established at term. This contrasts sharply with the much less mature condition of the canine and, most especially, human neonates, in which many of the secondary ossification centers have yet to appear (Plate 10/*E,F,G*). The individual rate of skeletal development is affected by many factors—inherited, nutritional, and hormonal, the last covering a complex situation in which hormones of hypophysial, thyroid, adrenal, and gonadal origin are involved. It is hardly surprising that abnormality of skeletal development is common.

The important features of the development of joints can be discussed more briefly. The joint tissues derive from the mesoderm left between the cartilaginous primordia of the bones. Spaces that develop in this tissue coalesce to form a single synovial cavity bounded by articular cartilage and synovial membrane. The former is probably produced by delayed chondrification of the mesoderm bordering the cartilaginous models; structural differences suggest that it is not the outer shell of this model left over after completion of epiphysial ossification. The synovial membrane is a more direct transformation of the mesoderm bordering the space. The fibrous part of the capsule and periarticular ligaments develop from more peripheral mesoderm.

It is now generally agreed that the limb muscles develop within the buds; the attractive notion that portions of myotomes migrate into these buds, pulling along the appropriate nerves, has been abandoned. Certain mesenchymal cells outside the denser axial core differentiate into precursor muscle cells (myoblasts); these then increase in number through mitosis while recruitment from the mesenchyme continues. These myoblasts then form myocytes or muscle cells by a maturation in which the nuclei increase in number and migrate to the periphery of the cells. The final number of muscle cells seems, in most species, to be established before birth, perhaps well before birth. The later growth of muscles therefore depends on an increase in the size of existing elements and not on an increase in their number (although a contribution to the bulk is also made by growth of intramuscular connective tissue).

The limb nerves grow in from the ventral rami of certain spinal nerves—generally C6–T2 where the forelimb is concerned and L4–S2 for the hindlimb. The segmental pattern becomes disturbed by the development of the limb plexuses in which fibers from the several ventral rami reassort before combining as the named peripheral trunks. In consequence, all but a few very small muscles are supplied by fibers that lead from neurons in more than one spinal segment. The sensory fibers to the skin arrange themselves so that specific regions are more or less the territory of particular spinal segments. The basis for this has become more difficult to understand now that it is believed that the dermis of the limb skin develops from cells of local origin, not from cells that migrated from particular somites.

Table 2–3 lists in parallel columns the bones of the forelimb skeleton and the parts to which they give support; for comparison, columns for the correspondng bones and parts of the hindlimb (which, it will be recalled, are analogous and not homologous) are also included. A central column gives additional terms, more common in zoological than in veterinary literature, that are common to both limbs; most are not used in this text but may be encountered elsewhere.

Some entries in the first and last columns may include three terms. Those printed in plain type are the technical words used when referring to domestic animals, the terms commonly employed by veterinarians; those italicized are the corresponding words used in human anatomy; and those in brackets are the more elevated Latin terms. Probably the most surprising feature of the table is the apparent absence of vernacular terms for certain regions of animals. The situation is in fact rather better, or rather worse according to one's point of view, than it appears. Many additional vernacular terms are restricted by custom to certain species; for example, the metacarpus of the horse is known as the cannon, but that of the dog is not. A particular difficulty is presented by the lack of handy equivalents to "paw" in description of farm animals; manus and pes are unacceptably pedantic (hence enclosed in brackets), and forefoot and hindfoot are usually (if not entirely logically) preferred; however, to the horse owner the foot generally means only the hoof and its contents. It is impossible to avoid all inconsistency.

In this book we employ the more elevated terms where it seems that vernacular equivalents might be ambiguous, risking the charge of pedantry. It is of course more sensible to use the everyday terms in conversation with laypeople.

## The Skeleton of the Forelimb

### *Pectoral Girdle*

The *scapula,* or shoulder-blade (Fig. 2–43), is a flat bone that lies over the laterally compressed, craniodorsal part of the thorax where it is held in place by an arrangement (synsarcosis) of muscles without forming a conventional articulation with the trunk. It is the basis of the shoulder region, a term that embraces much more than the immediate neighborhood of the shoulder joint. In ungulates, the scapula is extended dorsally by an unossified portion, the scapular cartilage (/*E,*13), which enlarges the area for muscular attachment. The cartilage becomes increasingly calcified and thus more rigid with age.

The bone is roughly triangular, though less so in the dog and cat than in the other domestic species. Its lateral surface is unequally divided by a prominent spine into supraspinous and infraspinous fossae, each occupied by the like-named muscle. The spine extends from the dorsal border almost to the articular angle and may bear a thickening for the insertion of the thoracic part of the trapezius; it is generally palpable through the skin. In all but the horse and pig, it ends in a prominent process (acromion), laterally flattened to form a hamate process in the carnivores (/7′), and furnished with an additional projection (suprahamate process; /7″) in the cat. The medial surface of the bone is largely given over to the origin of the subscapularis, which occupies a shallow fossa; a more dorsal roughened area, where the serratus ventralis attaches, extends onto the cartilage in the larger species.

The caudal border is thickened and almost straight. The thinner and sinuous cranial border is notched toward its distal end for the passage of the suprascapular nerve. The dorsal border is also generally straight and extends between cranial and caudal angles, the latter being thickened and more easily identified on palpation. The ventral or articular angle is joined to the body of the bone by a slightly constricted neck. Its caudal part carries a shallow glenoid cavity (/12) for articulation with the head of the humerus. The cavity, which is somewhat extended in the sagittal direction, faces more or less ventrally. A large muscular process, the supraglenoid tubercle, projects in front of the cavity; it gives origin to the biceps brachii.

The *clavicle* is reduced to a fibrous intersection in the brachiocephalicus. In the dog a nubbin of bone, and in the cat a slender rodlet, is embedded

**Table 2–3.** Terms in Use for the Parts and Bones of the Limbs

| Forelimb | | Terms Common to Both Limbs | Hindlimb | |
|---|---|---|---|---|
| *Body Part* | *Skeleton* | | *Skeleton* | *Body Part* |
| Shoulder region, *shoulder* | Scapula and clavicle | Cingulum (girdle) | Os coxae (hip bone)<br>Ilium<br>Pubis<br>Ischium | Pelvis |
| Arm, *upper arm* (brachium) | Humerus | Stylopodium | Femur (properly os femoris) | Thigh (femur) |
| Forearm (antebrachium) | Radius and ulna | Zeugopodium | Tibia and fibula | Leg (crus) |
| **[Manus]** | | **[Autopodium]** | | **[Pes]** |
| Carpus, *wrist* | Carpal bones | Basipodium | Tarsal bones | Hock, *ankle* (tarsus) |
| Metacarpus | Metacarpal bones | Metapodium | Metatarsal bones | Metatarsus |
| Digit, *finger* | Proximal, middle, and distal phalanges | Acropodium | Proximal, middle, and distal phalanges | Digit, *toe* |

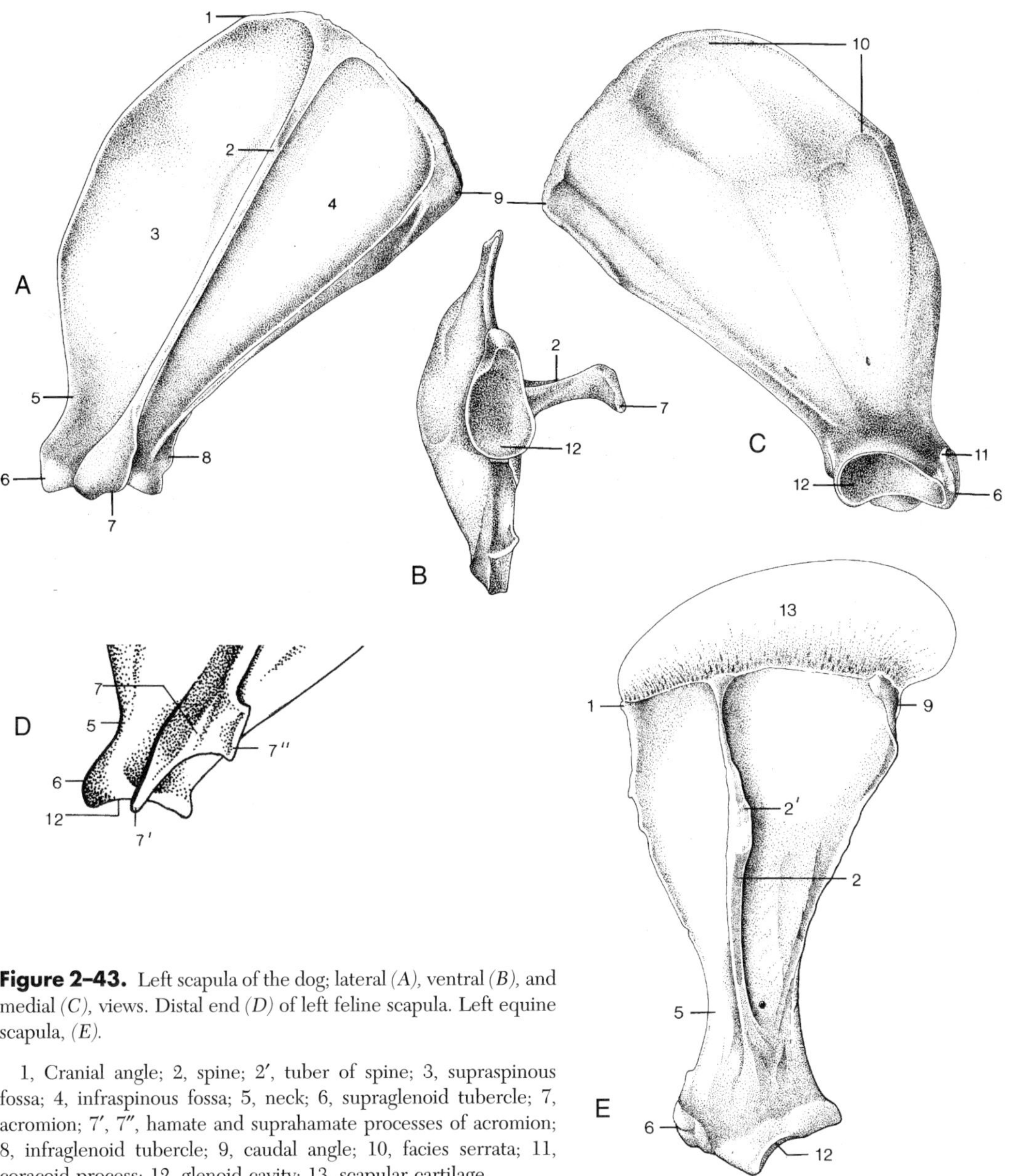


**Figure 2–43.** Left scapula of the dog; lateral *(A)*, ventral *(B)*, and medial *(C)*, views. Distal end *(D)* of left feline scapula. Left equine scapula, *(E)*.

1, Cranial angle; 2, spine; 2′, tuber of spine; 3, supraspinous fossa; 4, infraspinous fossa; 5, neck; 6, supraglenoid tubercle; 7, acromion; 7′, 7″, hamate and suprahamate processes of acromion; 8, infraglenoid tubercle; 9, caudal angle; 10, facies serrata; 11, coracoid process; 12, glenoid cavity; 13, scapular cartilage.

in the intersection; their sole importance lies in the risk of misinterpretation when they are seen in radiographs.

## Skeleton of the Free Appendage

The *humerus* (Fig. 2–44) forms the skeleton of the arm. It is a long bone that lies obliquely against the ventral part of the thorax, more horizontally in the large species than in the small. It is also relatively shorter and more robust in horses and cattle than in the small ruminants and carnivores. The proximal extremity carries a large articular head (/2), facing toward the glenoid cavity of the scapula and thus offset to the shaft to which it is joined by a neck. The head is shaped like a segment of a sphere and is considerably larger than the fossa with which it articulates. Two processes, the greater (lateral) and lesser (medial) tubercles, are placed in front and to the side of the articular area. They are separated by the intertubercular groove (/13) through which the biceps tendon runs. The processes are sometimes more or less equal, as in the horse; more often the lateral one, which forms the basis of the surface feature known as the point of the shoulder, is larger; it is so in the dog. In the horse and in cattle

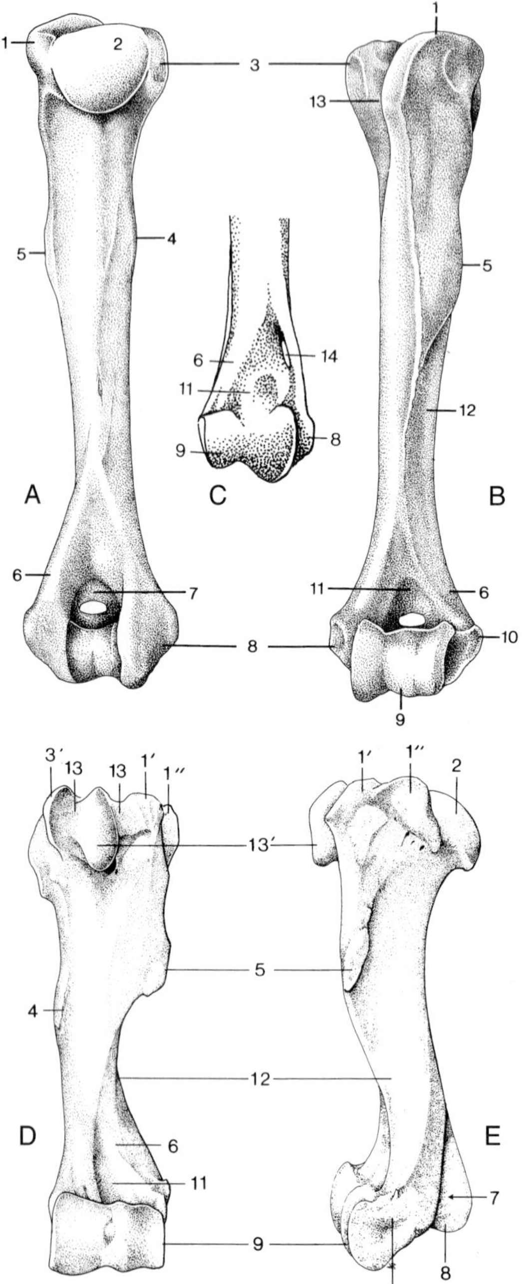


**Figure 2–44.** Left humerus of the dog; caudal *(A)* and cranial *(B)* views. *C,* Distal end of right feline humerus; cranial view. Cranial *(D)* and lateral *(E)* views of left equine humerus.

1, Greater tubercle; 1′, 1″, cranial and caudal parts of greater tubercle; 2, head; 3, lesser tubercle; 3′, cranial part of lesser tubercle; 4, teres (major) tuberosity; 5, deltoid tuberosity; 6, lateral supracondylar crest; 7, olecranon fossa (with supratrochlear foramen in dog); 8, medial epicondyle; 9, condyle; 10, lateral epicondyle; 11, radial fossa; 12, groove for brachialis; 13, intertubercular groove; 13′, intermediate tubercle; 14, supracondylar foramen.

both tubercles are divided into cranial and caudal parts (/1′,1″,3′); the intertubercular groove is also molded by an intermediate tubercle in the horse (/13′). The medial and lateral tubercles give attachment to the muscles that brace and support the shoulder joint, substituting for collateral ligaments.

A twisted appearance is imparted to the shaft by a groove (/12) that spirals over the lateral aspect and carries the brachialis and the radial nerve. Laterally, toward its upper end, the shaft carries the large, easily palpated deltoid tuberosity (/5), which is joined to the greater tubercle by a prominent ridge. A less prominent, gradually subsiding ridge, the crest of the humerus, continues distally beyond the deltoid tuberosity. The medial aspect of the shaft is marked by the much less salient roughening, the teres (major) tuberosity.

The distal extremity bears an articular condyle (/9) that is also set at an angle to the axis of the shaft. In large animals it engages with the radius and has the form of a trochlea. In the dog and cat it is divided into a medial area (trochlea) for the ulna and a lateral area (capitulum) for the radius. In all species the caudal part of the groove of the trochlea is continued proximally into a deep (olecranon) fossa (/7) that receives the anconeal process of the ulna. Two saliences proximal to the articular surface are known as epicondyles. The medial one (/8) is prominent and forms a right-angled, caudally directed projection that gives origin to the flexor muscles of the carpus and digit. The cranial aspect of the lateral epicondyle (/10) gives origin to the extensor muscles of the carpus and digit. To the side, each epicondyle gives origin to the corresponding collateral ligament of the elbow joint. In the dog the floor of the olecranon fossa is perforated by a supratrochlear foramen that opens to a much shallower radial fossa on the cranial aspect of the shaft (/7, 11). In the cat alone, the mediodistal part of the humerus is pierced by a supracondylar foramen (/14) that gives passage to the median nerve and brachial artery.

The *skeleton of the forearm* is provided by two bones, the radius and the ulna (Fig. 2–45). In the standing position they are arranged with the ulna caudal to the radius in the upper part of the forearm but lateral in the lower part. In the primitive condition these bones articulate only at their extremities, leaving an interosseous space between their shafts; rotational movements of the human forearm bones result in turning the hand so that the palm is brought to face forward (supination) or backward (pronation). In most domestic animals the capacity for these movements is reduced or lost, and the two bones are firmly held together by ligaments or by fusion in the prone position. When

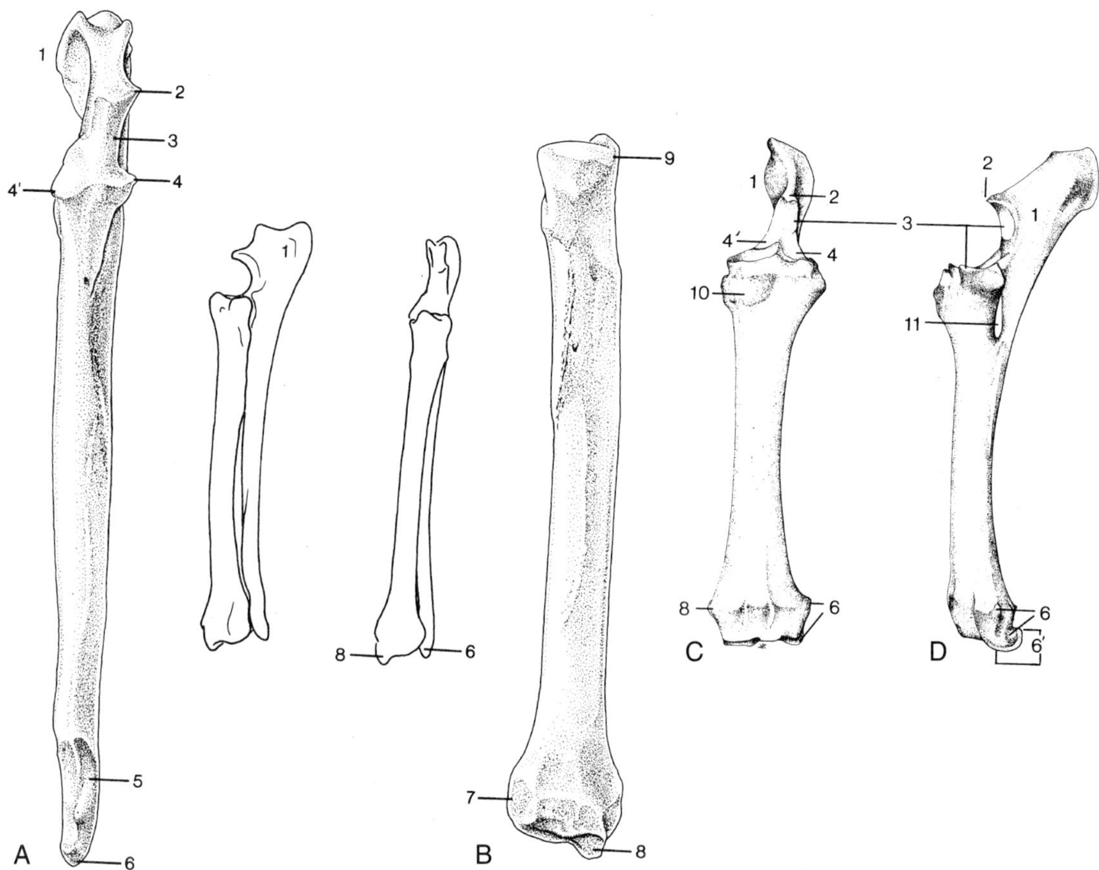


**Figure 2–45.** Left ulna *(A)* and left radius *(B)* of the dog. In sequence from the left: cranial view of the ulna, craniolateral and cranial views of the radius and ulna, and caudal view of the radius alone. Cranial *(C)* and lateral *(D)* views of fused left radius and ulna of the horse.

1, Olecranon; 2, anconeal process; 3, trochlear notch; 4, 4′, lateral and medial coronoid processes; 5, distal articular facet for radius; 6, lateral styloid process (with facet for the ulnar carpal bone in the dog); 6′, distal end of ulna incorporated within radius; 7, articular facet for ulna; 8, medial styloid process; 9, circumferential facet; 10, radial tuberosity; 11, interosseous space.

supination is possible it consists in rotation of the upper extremity of the radius within the embrace of the ulna while the distal extremity is carried in an arc around the ulna.

Clearly, no movement is possible when the bones are fused, the condition prevailing in ungulates and reaching its extreme in the horse, in which only the upper end of the ulna remains distinct (*/D,*1). About 45 degrees of supination is allowed to the dog, somewhat more to the cat. (Rotation at the carpus contributes a substantial extra component to the movement subjectively interpreted as supination.)

The *radius* is a rather simple rodlike bone, usually much stronger than the ulna in ungulates, less dominant in carnivores, in particular the cat. The proximal extremity is transversely widened, though tending to a more circular plan in carnivores, in which some supinatory capacity remains. It articulates with the distal articular surface of the humerus and is shaped to match this. A circumferential facet (*/B,*9) on the caudal part of the extremity articulates with the ulna and is present even when no supination is allowed. The shaft is craniocaudally compressed and slightly bowed in its length. The distal part of the cranial surface is grooved for the passage of the extensor tendons (*/C*), whereas the caudal surface is roughened for muscular attachment. The medial border is subcutaneous and therefore palpable.

The distal extremity of the radius is somewhat expanded. It carries an articular surface that is concave in its cranial part and convex in its caudal part in ungulates; it has a slightly concave ovoid form in carnivores, in which some abduction, adduction, and rotation are allowed to the antebrachiocarpal joint in addition to the major movements of flexion and extension. Medial to the articulation, the radius is prolonged to form a styloid process (/B,8); the corresponding lateral projection is furnished by the ulna, in the horse by the portion of the radius representing the incorporated ulna.

The *ulna* has an unusual appearance, as its shaft is greatly reduced and its proximal extremity is prolonged beyond the articular surface to form the high olecranon, the point of the elbow. This process, which constitutes a very prominent landmark, gives attachment to the triceps. Distal to this, the cranial margin carries the beaklike anconeal process (/2), which fits into the olecranon fossa of the humerus, above an articular notch that engages with the humeral trochlea; yet farther from the extremity, there is a facet for the circumferential articular area of the radius. In the dog the shaft, though slender, runs the full length of the radius from which it is separated by an interosseous space that is bridged by membrane in life. The distal extremity carries a small articular facet for the radius and beyond this is continued as the lateral styloid process (/6), which makes contact with the ulnar carpal bone.

Reduction of the ulna is greatest in the horse in which the shaft tapers to end at midforearm level (/D). The distal part became incorporated within the radius in fetal life (/6′). The ruminants and pig show intermediate conditions. The fusion of the ulna with the radius of course prohibits the movements of supination and pronation in the domestic mammals other than the dog and cat.

The short *carpal bones* articulate in complex fashion. The plan of the primitive carpal skeleton is uncertain, but in domestic species the bones are clearly arranged in two rows (Fig. 2–46). The proximal row comprises (in mediolateral sequence) radial, intermediate, ulnar, and accessory bones; the last appears as an appendage projecting behind the carpus and is a prominent landmark in the live animal. The radial and intermediate carpals fuse in the dog and cat. The elements of the distal row are numbered from one to five (again in mediolateral sequence), although the fifth never appears as a separate bone but is either suppressed or fused with the fourth. The first is also often lacking while the second and third fuse in ruminants. The diagrams illustrate the carpal formulae in different species. Apart from the accessory carpal bone, which is probably a sesamoid by origin, a small sesamoid bone is embedded in the medial tissues of the joint of the dog. Intrinsically unimportant, it can confuse radiographic interpretation by wrongly suggesting a "chip" fracture.

Viewed as a whole, the carpus is convex from side to side on its cranial aspect and flat and very irregular caudally, although in life these irregularities are smoothed by thick ligaments. Most movement occurs at the antebrachiocarpal level, some at the intercarpal, and virtually none at the carpometacarpal level or between neighboring bones in a row. The combined proximal articular surface is the reciprocal of that of the radius (see earlier) and in carnivores has a convex ovoid form.

The primitive pattern for the skeleton of the mammalian *manus* exhibits five more or less equal rays, each consisting of a metacarpal bone and proximal, middle, and distal phalanges in line (Fig. 2–47/A). This pattern has been modified in all domestic species, each of which (not excepting the pig) is to some degree specialized for fast running. Cursorial specialization involves raising the manus (and pes) from the primitive "flatfooted" (planti-

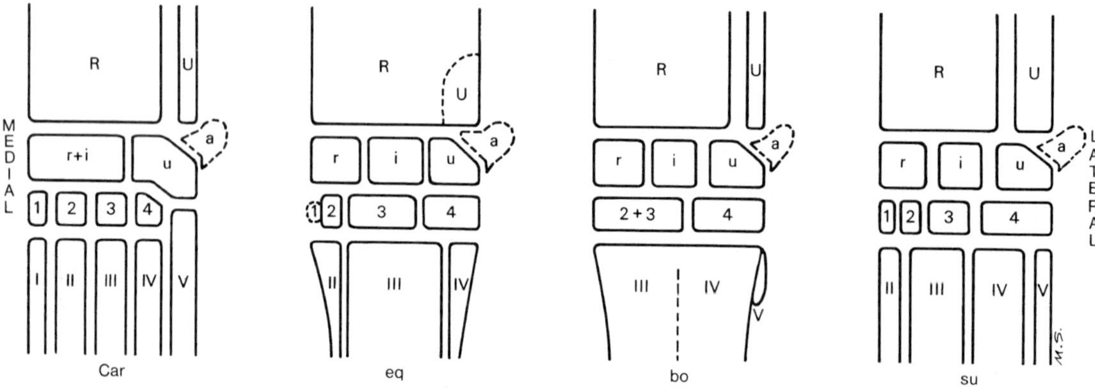


**Figure 2–46.** The bones of the carpal skeleton in the carnivores (Car), horse (eq), cattle (bo), and pig (su), schematic. Roman numerals identify the metacarpal bones; Arabic numerals, the distal carpal bones.

R, Radius; U, ulna; a, accessory carpal bone; i, intermediate carpal bone; r, radial carpal bone; u, ulnar carpal bone.

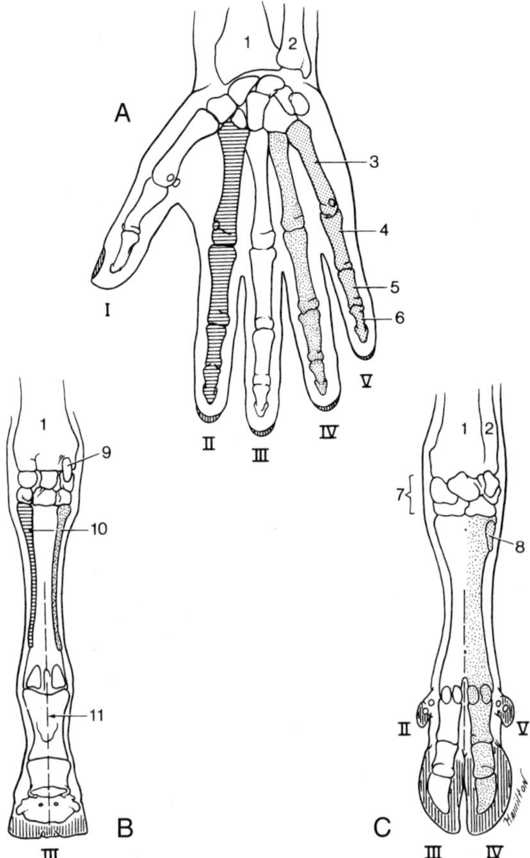


**Figure 2–47.** Right manus (human hand; *A*), of horse *(B)*, and ruminant *(C)*, palmar views. The Roman numerals number the rays.

1, Radius; 2, ulna; 3, metacarpal; 4, 5, 6, proximal, middle, and distal phalanges; 7, carpal bones; 8, rudimentary metacarpal V; 9, accessory carpal bone; 10, rudimentary metacarpals II and IV (medial and lateral splint bones); 11, axis in line with ray III (mesaxonic), in *C* paraxonic.

grade) posture demonstrated by bears (Fig. 2–48). An intermediate stage, the digitigrade posture, has been attained by dogs, which support themselves by the digits only; it culminates in the unguligrade posture attained by ruminants, pigs, and horses, in which only the tips of the digits, protected by hooves (ungulae), give support. The process results in the abaxial digits first losing permanent contact with the ground; a compensating development of the remaining digits enables them to carry an increased proportion of the weight. The process has not progressed very far in the dog and cat, in which only the most medial (first) digit has lost contact and is retained as a nonfunctional dewclaw (Fig. 2–49). The four functional digits are broadly equal, with the axis of the manus passing between the third and fourth digits (a paraxonic position). Pigs have entirely lost the first digit; the second and fifth digits are very much reduced, though each retains a complete skeleton. In ruminants the process has gone further, and although elements of four digits are present, those of the abaxial pair are vestigial; the metacarpal bones of the functional third and fourth digits are fused in a single bone that retains evidence of its composite origin (Fig. 2–47/*C*).

In the horse (/*B*), only the third ray survives in functional form and its axis coincides with that of the limb; the manus is said to be mesaxonic. Remnants of the second and fourth metacarpal bones survive as the splint bones that flank the third metacarpal or cannon bone; they end in nodules, but the assumption that these incorporate greatly reduced elements of all three phalanges of the lost digits is unfounded.

The differences in the metacarpal and digital skeleton are very striking in consequence of these changes, and the short description that follows is amplified in later chapters by details of a species-specific nature.

As the number of *metacarpal bones* is diminished, so the relative stoutness of the surviving members of the series is increased. The single (third) metacarpal bone of the horse (Fig. 2–49,*C*,III) therefore has a particularly strong shaft, whereas the individual metacarpal bones of the dog are relatively much weaker. The dog's bones are also shaped by their mutual contacts; the third and fourth bones are square in section, the flanking second and fifth bones, triangular. Taken as a whole, the metacarpal skeleton of all species is somewhat compressed in the dorsopalmar direction. Each bone has a proximal extremity (base), a shaft, and a distal extremity (caput). The base has

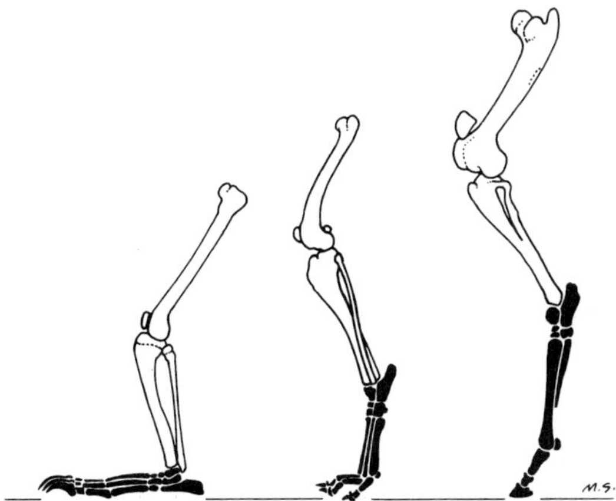

**Figure 2–48.** Hindlimbs of bear, dog, and horse *(from left to right)* illustrating plantigrade, digitigrade, and unguligrade postures.

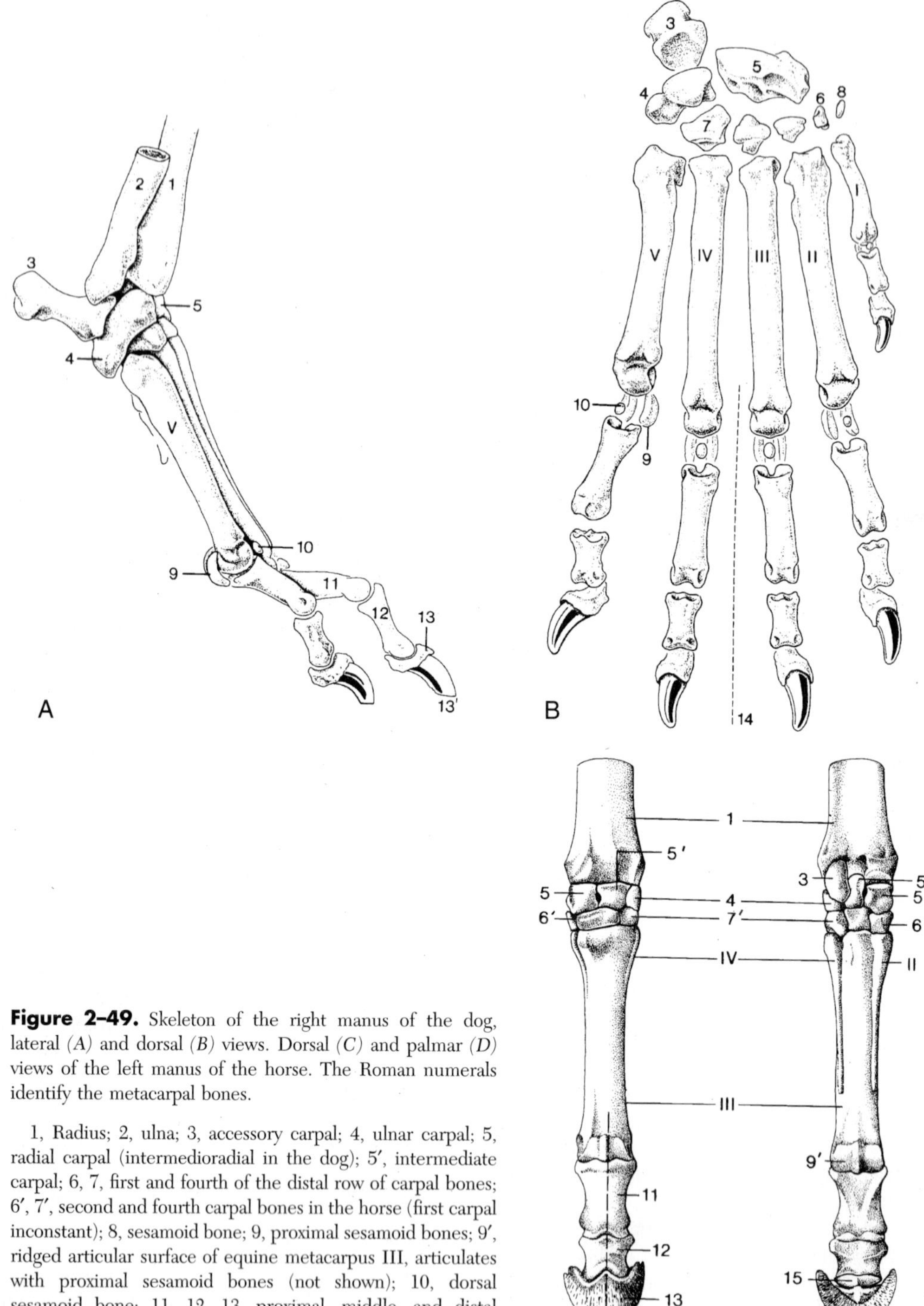


**Figure 2–49.** Skeleton of the right manus of the dog, lateral *(A)* and dorsal *(B)* views. Dorsal *(C)* and palmar *(D)* views of the left manus of the horse. The Roman numerals identify the metacarpal bones.

1, Radius; 2, ulna; 3, accessory carpal; 4, ulnar carpal; 5, radial carpal (intermedioradial in the dog); 5′, intermediate carpal; 6, 7, first and fourth of the distal row of carpal bones; 6′, 7′, second and fourth carpal bones in the horse (first carpal inconstant); 8, sesamoid bone; 9, proximal sesamoid bones; 9′, ridged articular surface of equine metacarpus III, articulates with proximal sesamoid bones (not shown); 10, dorsal sesamoid bone; 11, 12, 13, proximal, middle, and distal phalanges; 13′, claw; 14, axis of manus; 15, distal sesamoid (navicular) bone.

a flattish articular surface for the distal row of carpal bones and may, according to its position in the metacarpal series, have medial and lateral facets where it makes contact with neighbors. The distal extremity articulates with the proximal phalanx by a hemicylindrical surface with a central ridge (/*D*,9′). Various roughenings for ligamentous attachment are present at both extremities.

The *proximal phalanx* is a short cylindrical bone with a proximal extremity adapted to the caput of the metacarpal bone and a distal articulation in the form of a shallow trochlea. Again, the bone may be shaped by its position in the digital series.

The *middle phalanx* is shorter than, but basically very similar to, the first phalanx. The *distal phalanx* corresponds to the form of the hoof or claw in which it is wholly (hoof) or partly (claw) contained. The digital skeleton is completed by paired *proximal sesamoid bones* at the palmar aspect of the metacarpophalangeal joint (*/A*,9) and by a *distal sesamoid bone* (cartilage in the dog) at the palmar aspect of the distal interphalangeal joint (*/D*,15). In the dog small sesamoids also exist within the extensor tendons over the dorsal aspect of the metacarpophalangeal joints.

## The Joints of the Forelimb

The *shoulder joint* (Fig. 2–50/*A*) links the scapula and humerus, and although it has the attributes of the spheroidal variety, sagittal excursions predominate in practice. The glenoid cavity of the scapula is considerably smaller than the head of the humerus. In large animals, both surfaces may be indented peripherally by naked areas (synovial fossae) simulating, to the inexperienced eye, lesions of the cartilage. The joint capsule is roomy and is fused here and there with the tendons of the surrounding muscles, particularly the subscapularis. In all but the horse and ox it sends a prolongation or diverticulum around the tendon of origin of the biceps brachii where this lies within the intertubercular groove. The diverticulum protects the tendon in the manner of a synovial sheath; it is replaced by a discrete intertubercular bursa in the two large species. Although the fibrous layer of the capsule is locally strengthened, it is usual to say that the joint is without pericapsular ligaments. Tendons of immediately adjacent muscles, notably the subscapularis medially and infraspinatus laterally, take the place of ligaments in bracing the joint.

Movement is most free in the sagittal direction, but significant amounts of rotation, abduction, and adduction, and therefore also of circumduction, are possible, particularly in the dog and cat; in these animals a component of the movement interpreted as supination probably occurs at shoulder level.

The *elbow joint* (Fig. 2–50/*B*) combines within a single capsule the hinge joint between the humerus and the radius and ulna and, at least in carnivores, the pivot joint between the proximal extremities of the latter pair of bones. The humeral surface is broadly trochlear, and the lower surface, variously furnished by the radius and ulna, is its reciprocal. Ridging of the surfaces, most pronounced in the larger animals, impedes other than hinge movements. A proximal radioulnar articulation between a circumferential facet on the radius and a corresponding but smaller area on the ulna is present even when more distal fusion precludes the possibility of movement. The joint capsule is surprisingly roomy and, when distended, bulges to each side of the ulna within the olecranon fossa. The strongest ligaments are medial and lateral collateral ligaments, an arrangement predictable in what is basically a hinge joint.

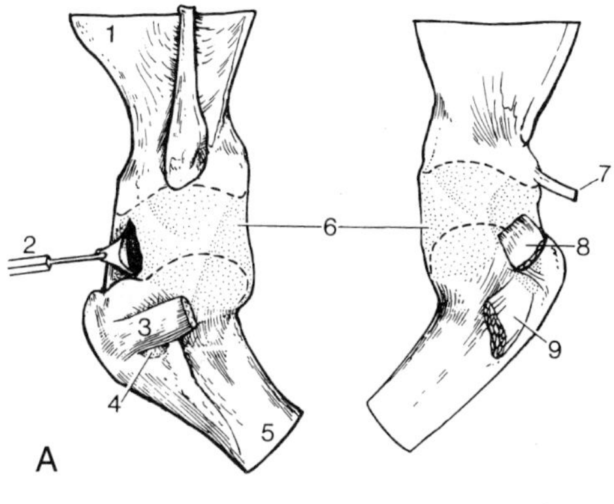


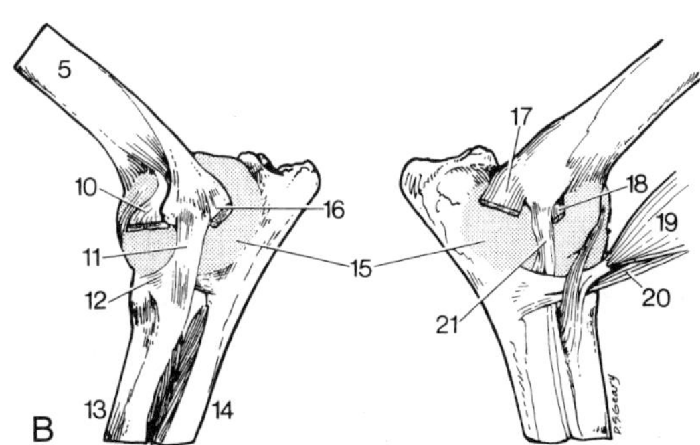


**Figure 2–50.** Left shoulder *(A)* and elbow *(B)* joints of the dog. The drawings on the left are lateral views, those on the right medial.

1, Scapula; 2, joint capsule opened to expose biceps tendon; 3, tendon of infraspinatus; 4, infraspinatus bursa; 5, humerus; 6, joint capsule, stretched by pulling bones apart; 7, tendon of coracobrachialis; 8, tendon of subscapularis, reflected ventrally; 9, biceps tendon emerging from intertubercular groove; 10, stump of extensor carpi radialis and common digital extensor; 11, lateral collateral ligament; 12, annular ligament of radius; 13, radius; 14, ulna; 15, joint capsule; 16, stump of ulnaris lateralis; 17, common stump of carpal and digital flexors; 18, stump of pronator teres; 19, biceps; 20, brachialis; 21, medial collateral ligament.

The lateral of these ligaments is short and thick (/11), and the medial one is longer, more slender, and divisible into two parts (/21)—radial and ulnar in the dog and cat, superficial and deep in the larger animals. An additional oblique ligament is placed over the flexor aspect of the joint of the dog and cat. In these species there is also an annular ligament (/12), extending between the collateral ligaments and completing the enclosure of the head of the radius within an osseoligamentous ring.

In the large species, most notably the horse, the curvature of the humeral surface is not uniform. This feature, combined with the eccentric proximal attachment of the collateral ligaments (see Fig. 23–8), makes the joint more stable in the normal standing position (which approaches but does not reach maximal extension); some effort is required to "unlock" the joint before it can be flexed (p. 575).

The shafts of the radius and ulna are joined by an interosseous membrane that ossifies early in life in ungulates. In the dog and cat the membrane is sufficiently long to allow the limited rotation possible in these species.

The *carpal joint* includes antebrachiocarpal, midcarpal, and carpometacarpal levels of articulation and also a distal radioulnar joint. The antebrachiocarpal and the radioulnar joints share a common joint cavity. The midcarpal and carpometacarpal joint cavities are interconnected. In hoofed species the proximal joint may be regarded as being of the hinge variety (although the form of the surfaces introduces a certain obliquity of movement in ruminants), but in dogs and cats it is more versatile and can be regarded as an ellipsoidal joint, although a poor example of the type. The hinge movement is quite free at the antebrachiocarpal level (horse: ca. 90 degrees). Considerable movement is also possible at the midcarpal level (ca. 45 degrees), but virtually no movement is allowed at the carpometacarpal level. Medial and lateral collateral ligaments are well developed in ungulates but are necessarily much weaker in the dog and cat to allow for some adduction and abduction. On the dorsal aspect, a number of short ligaments join neighboring bones in the same row, and those of the distal row to the metacarpus. More robust ligaments are found on the palmar aspect where a deep ligament (Fig. 2–51/6) covers the entire palmar surface of the skeleton, burying the unevennesses of the bones. A second, superficial, transverse ligament (flexor retinaculum) passes obliquely from the free extremity of the accessory carpal bone to the medial aspect of the carpus (/7), completing the enclosure of a passage behind the carpus. This, the carpal canal, conveys the flexor tendons and other structures continuing into the foot from the forearm. Additional small ligaments (/5) join the accessory bone to the adjacent carpal and metacarpal bones. These palmar ligaments do not interfere with flexion but assist in preventing overextension.

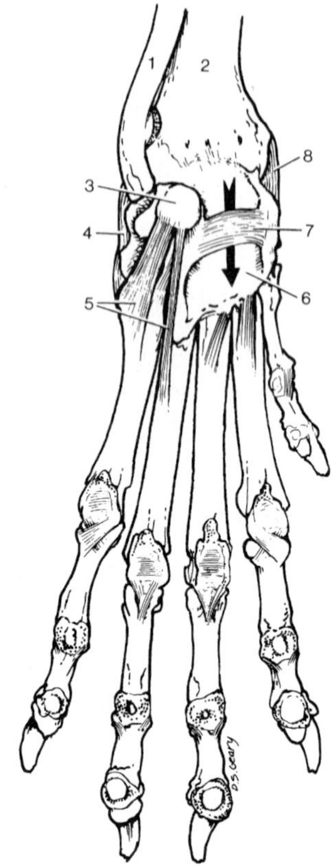


**Figure 2–51.** Left carpal joint of the dog, palmar view.

1, Ulna; 2, radius; 3, accessory carpal; 4, lateral collateral ligament; 5, distal ligaments of accessory carpal; 6, palmar carpal ligament; 7, flexor retinaculum; 8, medial collateral ligament; the arrow is in the carpal canal.

Description of the more distal joints is best deferred because of the marked interspecific variation. These joints are only important in the large species.

## The Muscles of the Forelimb

The muscles of the forelimb comprise the girdle musculature, passing between the trunk and the limb, and the intrinsic musculature.

### Girdle Muscles

The girdle muscles join the forelimb to the trunk, forming a connection known as a synsarcosis that substitutes for a conventional joint. When the animal is standing, some of the muscles of the synsarcosis (the serratus ventralis and pectoralis profundus) sling the body between the forelimbs to which they transmit the weight of the head, neck, and cranial part of the trunk (Fig. 2–52). These and other girdle muscles can also stabilize the scapula against external forces, preventing its displacement or rotation. A good example of this role is supplied by a cat pouncing on a mouse or plaything with forelimbs rigidly braced against the trunk. During progression the same muscles resolve into antagonistic groups that control the swing of the limb; one group advances (protracts) the limb, the other retracts it. In order to understand these actions it is ncessary to appreciate that the scapula may be moved against the chest wall in two different ways. In one, the bone is rotated about a transverse axis located toward its upper end. The position of this axis, which is of course imaginary, is fixed by the balance of opposing muscles, chiefly the rhomboideus and serratus ventralis, which both attach on the dorsal part of the scapula. In the other movement, the whole bone is shifted on the thoracic wall. It is slid downward and forward as the limb is advanced and upward and backward in recovery during retraction. This movement of the scapula, which adds usefully to the length of the stride, is permitted by the looseness of the connective tissue that intervenes between the limb and the trunk where there exists a potential space, the axilla, corresponding to the human armpit. The axilla also gives passage to the nerves and vessels entering the limb from the trunk, and it contains the axillary lymph nodes.

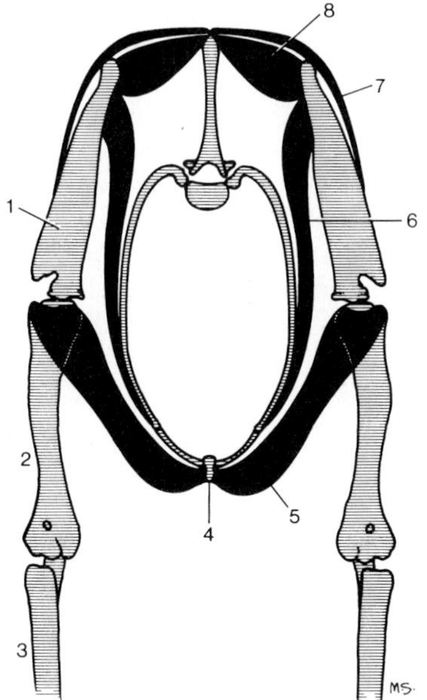


**Figure 2–52.** Muscular suspension of the thorax between the forelimbs (dog).

1, Scapula; 2, humerus; 3, radius and ulna; 4, sternum; 5, pectoralis profundus (ascendens); 6, serratus ventralis; 7, trapezius; 8, rhomboideus.

For the purpose of description, the girdle muscles can be considered in two layers.

**The Superficial Layer.** This consists of a cranial group supplied mostly by the accessory nerve, the latissimus dorsi more caudally, and the two superficial pectoral muscles ventrally. The cranial group comprises the trapezius, omotransversarius, and brachiocephalicus.

The *trapezius* (Fig. 2–53/5,5′) is thin. It takes origin from the mid-dorsal raphe and supraspinous ligament, extending from about the level of the second cervical to that of the ninth thoracic vertebra, and converges to insert on the spine of the scapula. It consists of two fleshy parts, cervical and thoracic, usually separated by an intermediate aponeurosis. The fibers of the cervical part run caudoventrally to attach along the greater part of the length of the scapular spine; those of the thoracic part run cranioventrally to a more confined insertion on the tuberous thickening of the spine. The trapezius may raise the scapula against the trunk and swing the ventral angle of the bone cranially, thus advancing the limb.

The *omotransversarius* (/3) is a narrow muscle that extends between the transverse processes of the atlas (and possibly also the succeeding vertebrae) and the acromion and adjacent part of the scapula. It assists in advancement of the limb.

The *brachiocephalicus* (/2,2′) is more complex, being formed by the union of two elements that are separated by the clavicle in less specialized mammals. In these the caudal part (cleidobrachialis) passes between the clavicle and the humerus and is a component of the deltoideus muscle. The cranial part passes cranially from the clavicle to several attachments in the head and neck. These attachments vary among species and hence a rather bewildering array of names for particular units exists—cleido-occipitalis, cleidomastoideus, and so forth. In domestic species the two parts join in tandem, and the clavicle is generally reduced to a fibrous intersection in the combined muscle at the level of the shoulder joint, although vestigial ossifications are present in the dog and cat (p. 456). Brachiocephalicus is a most appropriate name for the whole complex since it does not specify precise attachments. The brachiocephalicus advances the limb, possibly also extending the shoulder joint, when the cranial attachment is fixed and the limb is free to move; in contrast, when the limb is fixed and the head is free, it draws the head and neck

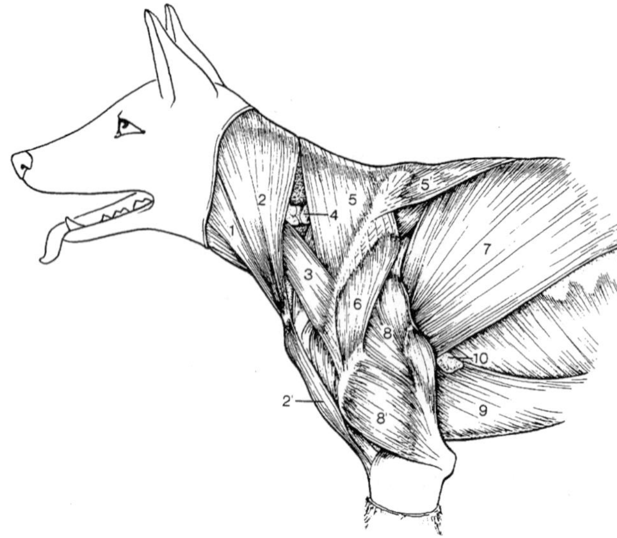


**Figure 2–53.** Superficial muscles of the shoulder and arm.

1, Sternocephalicus; 2, 2′, brachiocephalicus: cleidocervicalis and cleidobrachialis; 3, omotransversarius; 4, superficial cervical lymph node; 5, 5′, cervical and thoracic parts of trapezius; 6, deltoideus; 7, latissimus dorsi; 8, 8′, long and lateral heads of triceps; 9, pectoralis profundus (ascendens); 10, accessory axillary lymph node.

ventrally when acting bilaterally, and toward the side when acting unilaterally.

The muscles supplied by the accessory nerve split from a single primordium in the embryo. However, the caudal part of the brachiocephalicus of deltoid origin retains the appropriate innervation by the axillary nerve.

The *latissimus dorsi* (/7) has a very broad origin from the thoracolumbar fascia and converges to an insertion on the teres tuberosity of the humerus. The most cranial, which are also the most vertical, fibers cover the caudal angle of the scapula and strap it against the chest. The muscle retracts the free limb and may also flex the shoulder joint. On the other hand, when the limb is advanced and the foot firmly planted on the ground, the latissimus may draw the trunk forward. It may be regarded as antagonist to the brachiocephalicus. It is supplied by a local branch (thoracodorsal nerve) of the brachial plexus.

Two *superficial pectoral muscles* (Fig. 2–41/5,6) arise, one behind the other, from the cranial part of the sternum. The cranial muscle (pectoralis descendens) terminates on the crest of the humerus, distal to the deltoid tuberosity. The caudal muscle (pectoralis transversus) descends over the medial aspect of the arm and in the larger species continues distally over the elbow joint, covering the median artery and nerve, to insert into the medial fascia of the forearm. Both muscles adduct the limb, an action that may be understood to embrace the sideways shift of the trunk toward a previously abducted limb. It seems probable that they may also assist protraction or retraction, depending on the initial position of the limb relative to the trunk. They are supplied by local branches (cranial pectoral nerves) from the brachial plexus.

**The Deep Layer.** This comprises the rhomboideus dorsally, the serratus ventralis medially, and the pectoralis profundus ventrally.

The *rhomboideus* (Fig. 2–52/8) takes origin from median connective tissue structures extending from the poll to the withers and lies deep to the trapezius. It always presents cervical and thoracic parts and in carnivores has an additional, capital, part. All attach to the dorsal border and adjacent area on the medial surface of the scapula. Although the fiber courses differ in their relation to the axis of rotation of the scapula, most seem able to draw the dorsal part of the bone cranially, thereby retracting the limb. The muscle may also raise the limb and hold it firmly against the trunk. It is supplied in the dog from the brachial plexus, but in some species it is also supplied by *dorsal* branches of local spinal nerves, which is unusual for a limb muscle.

The *serratus ventralis* (/6) is a large fan-shaped muscle that takes an extensive origin by separate digitations from the fourth cervical vertebra to the tenth rib. The fibers run dorsally to terminate on a well-defined area on the medial aspect of the scapula and scapular cartilage. The direction of the fibers indicates that this muscle must play a large part in supporting the weight of the trunk, and in the larger species it is better adapted to this function by a strong fascial covering and intersections. The cervical portion of the muscle, which inserts craniodorsal to the axis of scapular rotation, can retract the limb; the caudal portion, which inserts caudodorsal to the axis, can advance the limb. When acting unilaterally, the cervical fibers may also draw the neck to that side; when acting bilaterally, they raise the neck. The thoracic part is a potential inspiratory muscle, although it is not normally used in that capacity. The innervation is mainly by a branch (long thoracic nerve) of the brachial plexus.

The *pectoralis profundus* (Fig. 2–53/9) may be considered as having cranial and caudal parts. The cranial part, well formed only in the horse and pig, probably corresponds to the subclavius of other mammals and is now so named officially. Both parts (or muscles) arise from the ventral aspect of the length of the sternum and adjacent cartilages, with the most caudal fibers extendng beyond this onto the abdominal floor. In the horse and pig the subclavius passes dorsally along the leading edge of the scapula, attaching to the supraspinatus (see Fig. 23–5/2). The larger caudal part, also known as the pectoralis ascendens, inserts on the lesser tubercle of the humerus. Both play a role, secondary to that of the serratus ventralis, in slinging the trunk between the forelimbs. They may also act as retractors of the forelimb when this is free. When the limb is advanced and fixed, they draw the trunk forward, toward the limb. The nerves are local branches (caudal pectoral nerves) of the brachial plexus.

## Intrinsic Muscles of the Forelimb

The intrinsic muscles are conveniently grouped by their common location, actions, and innervations.

**Muscles Acting Primarily on the Shoulder Joint.** The muscles acting on the shoulder joint are arranged in lateral, medial, and caudal groups.

The *lateral group* comprises the supra- and infraspinatus, which arise from and fill the corresponding fossae of the scapula. The *supraspinatus* (Fig. 2–54/3) terminates on the summits of both tubercles of the humerus. The *infraspinatus* inserts by a tendon that splits into a shorter deep part, which attaches to the summit, and a longer superficial part, which attaches to the lateral face of the (caudal part of the) greater tubercle; a bursa between the bone and the longer tendon may be the seat of a painful inflammation. Both muscles brace the joint laterally. The supraspinatus tendon passes cranial to the axis of rotation and it may therefore also extend the shoulder. It is sometimes asserted that the infraspinatus tendon passes cranial or caudal to the axis of rotation depending on the actual position of the joint and may then further extend the already extended joint or further flex the already flexed joint; clearly, it is unlikely to be very effective in either role. Both muscles are

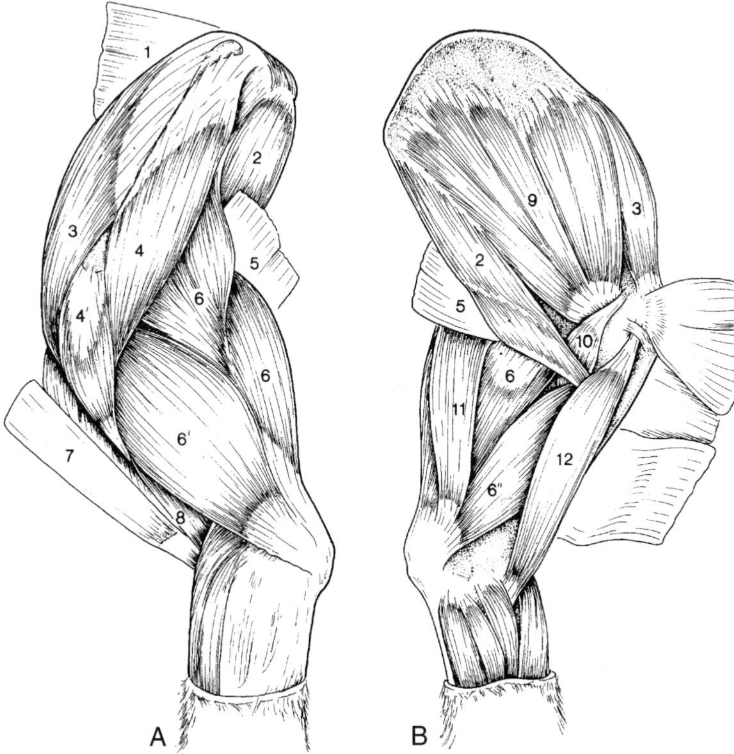


**Figure 2–54.** Intrinsic muscles of the left shoulder and arm of the dog, lateral *(A)* and medial *(B)* views.

1, Rhomboideus; 2, teres major; 3, supraspinatus; 4, 4′, scapular and acromial parts of deltoideus; 5, latissimus dorsi; 6, 6′, 6″, long, lateral, and medial heads of triceps; 7, brachiocephalicus; 8, brachialis; 9, subscapularis; 10, coracobrachialis; 11, tensor fasciae antebrachii; 12, biceps.

supplied by the suprascapular nerve from the brachial plexus.

The *medial group* comprises the subscapularis and coracobrachialis. The *subscapularis* (/9) arises over much of the deep surface of the scapula and inserts on the medial tubercle of the humerus, distal to the axis of the shoulder joint. It braces the medial aspect of the joint. It is also a potential adductor of the arm and, like the infraspinatus, has an equivocal relationship to flexion and extension of the shoulder. It is supplied by the subscapular nerve from the brachial plexus. The *coracobrachialis* (/10) extends between the medial aspect of the supraglenoid tubercle and the proximal part of the shaft of the humerus. Too small to be of real significance, it is a fixator of the shoulder with the same equivocal relationship to shoulder flexion and extension. It is supplied by the proximal branch of the musculocutaneous nerve from the brachial plexus.

The *caudal* or flexor *group* comprises the deltoideus, teres major, and teres minor. The *deltoideus* has one head of origin in the horse and two in species possessing an acromion (/4,4′). The constant head arises from the caudal border and spine of the scapula; the inconstant second head arises from the acromion. Both insert on the deltoid tuberosity of the humerus. The *teres major* (/2) arises from the dorsal part of the caudal margin of the scapula and terminates on the teres tuberosity, midway down the humerus. The relatively insignificant *teres minor* lies over the caudolateral aspect of the joint between the deltoideus and infraspinatus. These three muscles are clearly primarily flexor; the deltoideus may also be an abductor and an outward rotator of the arm. The group is supplied by the axillary nerve from the brachial plexus.

In contrast to the well-defined group of flexors it seems that no muscles are clearly established as primarily extensors of the shoulder. The potential candidates—brachiocephalicus, biceps brachii, supraspinatus, and pectoralis ascendens—each have other, apparently more important, roles.

**Muscles Acting Primarily on the Elbow Joint.** There are extensor and flexor groups. The *extensor group,* which largely fills the angle between the scapula and humerus, consists of the triceps brachii, tensor fasciae antebrachii, and anconeus. The large and powerful *triceps brachii* (Fig. 2–54/6,6′,6″) possesses three heads of origin (but four in the dog). The long head, which arises from the caudal margin of the scapula, is potentially also a flexor of the shoulder. The lateral, medial, and (in the dog) accessory heads arise from the shaft of the humerus and have an action restricted to the elbow. The several heads combine to make a stout tendon that inserts on the summit of the olecranon where it is protected on its deep aspect—against the bone—by the tricipital bursa. A second, subcutaneous bursa often lies between the tendon and the skin.

The *tensor fasciae antebrachii* (/11) is a thin sheet, partly muscular, partly aponeurotic, that lies over the medial aspect of the long head of the triceps, extending from the scapula to the olecranon. The *anconeus* is much smaller and arises from the distal part of the humerus to insert on the lateral part of the olecranon; it is directly related to the elbow joint capsule and may have the additional function of tensing this so that it is not pinched between the humerus and ulna. All parts of the extensor group are supplied by the radial nerve from the brachial plexus.

The *flexor group* comprises the biceps brachii and brachialis. The biarticular *biceps brachii* (/12) arises from the supraglenoid tubercle of the scapula and runs through the intertubercular groove of the humerus before continuing distally to insert on the medial tuberosity of the proximal extremity of the radius, and on the adjacent part of the ulna. It is thus also a potential extensor of the shoulder. The *brachialis* (/8) arises from the proximocaudal part of the humerus and winds laterally in the spiral groove of this bone before inserting next to the biceps. Both are supplied by the musculocutaneous nerve.

**Pronator and Supinator Muscles of the Forearm.** Generalized mammals possess muscles that have supination or pronation as a prime function, but these muscles tend to become vestigial or to disappear when the capacity for the movements is reduced or lost. Among domestic species significant movement is possible only in the dog and cat in which there are two supinator muscles and two pronators. The *brachioradialis* or long supinator is a thin fleshy ribbon that extends from the lateral epicondyle of the humerus to the distal medial part of the forearm within the superficial fascia. It is quite prominent in the cat but is slight, often lost, in the dog. The short *supinator* muscle is more consistently developed. It is a small fusiform muscle, placed deep to the extensor muscles and passing obliquely over the flexor aspect of the elbow from the lateral humeral epicondyle to the upper quarter of the medial border of the radius. The supinator muscles are supplied by the radial nerve.

The *pronator teres* (Fig. 2–55/12) arises from the medial epicondyle of the humerus and converges on the insertion of the supinator on the radius. It is functional only in the dog and cat. The *pronator quadratus* is found only in carnivores. It

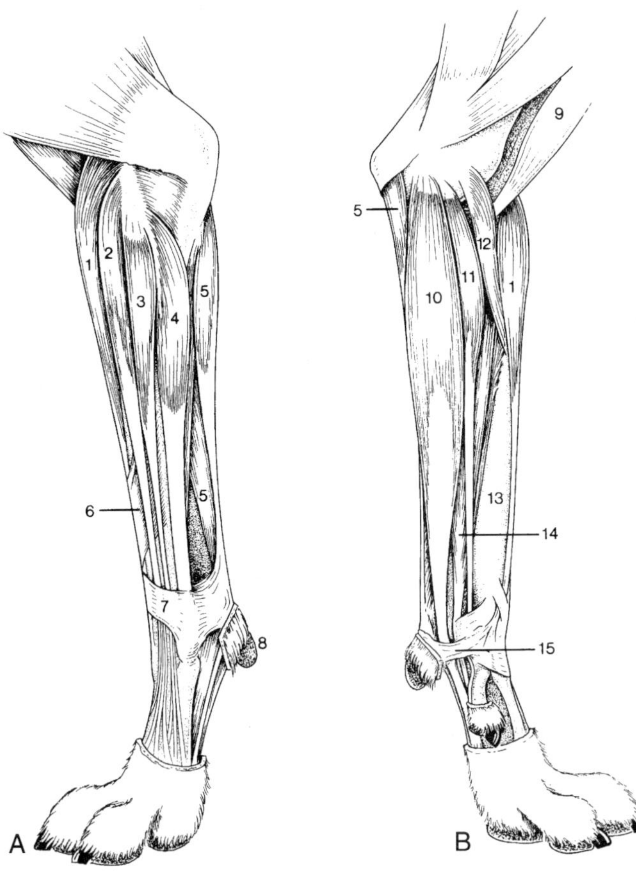


**Figure 2–55.** Muscles of the left forearm of the dog, lateral *(A)* and medial *(B)* views.

1, Extensor carpi radialis; 2, common digital extensor; 3, lateral digital extensor; 4, ulnaris lateralis; 5, flexor carpi ulnaris; 6, extensor carpi obliquus; 7, extensor retinaculum; 8, carpal pad; 9, biceps; 10, superficial digital flexor; 11, flexor carpi radialis; 12, pronator teres; 13, radius; 14, deep digital flexor; 15, flexor retinaculum.

passes from the shaft of the ulna to that of the radius, bridging the medial aspect of the interosseous space of the forearm. The pronator muscles are supplied by the median nerve.

The rotation from the neutral position that may be produced by these muscles is most free when the elbow is flexed. The movements are limited to about 40 degrees of pronation and about 45 degrees of supination in the dog, although the cat has a somewhat larger range.

**Muscles Acting Primarily on the Carpal and Digital Joints.** These are simply classified as flexor or extensor, although the action of one muscle is equivocal.

***The Extensor Muscles of the Carpus and Digits.*** These include digital extensor muscles in addition to those whose action is confined to the carpus. They have the following features in common: an extensor action at the carpus, a craniolateral position in the forearm, a radial nerve supply, and, with one exception, an origin from the cranial aspect of the lateral epicondyle of the humerus. The *extensor carpi radialis* (Fig. 2–55/1), the most medial member of the group, is situated directly cranial to the subcutaneous border of the radius. It inserts on the proximal extremity of the third (sometimes also second) metacarpal bone. The *ulnaris lateralis* (/4) [extensor carpi ulnaris] is the most lateral member and runs parallel to the ulnar flexor of the carpus on the outer aspect of the limb to insert on the accessory carpal and the upper end of the most lateral metacarpal bone. It may extend an already extended carpus but further flexes the joint that is in a flexed position. It may also deviate the paw laterally. Despite its equivocal character the ulnaris lateralis retains the extensor nerve supply. The *extensor carpi obliquus* (/6) (also known as the abductor pollicis longus) is distinguished by its origin from the cranial surface of the radius and by the oblique mediodistal course pursued by its tendon, which attaches to the most medial metacarpal bone present. It functions as an extensor of the carpus with, in dog and cat, a potential for medial deviation of the paw.

The long digital extensor muscles vary in arrangement, for although all species possess a common and a lateral muscle, the common one may be subdivided. The *common digital extensor*

(/2) inserts on the extensor process of the distal phalanx of each functional digit; the tendon is therefore unbranched in the horse; divides into two in the ruminants; and divides into four in the pig and dog (but into five in the cat). A subdivision of the common extensor, which is present in all species but the horse and cat, inserts on the most medial of the functional digits; it sends an oblique branch to the dewclaw in the dog. It is sometimes usefully termed medial digital extensor but this term is not official. The *lateral digital extensor* (/3) runs along the lateral edge of the common extensor; the undivided tendon inserts on the dorsal surface of the proximal phalanx in the horse. The muscle also has one insertion tendon in the ruminants, but two in the pig, three in the dog, and four in the cat; in these species the insertion is in common with the branch of the common extensor to the distal phalanx of the most lateral one, two, three, or four functional digits. In the smaller species separation of the digital divisions begins more proximally and is more complete.

*The Flexor Muscles of the Carpus and Digits.* The carpal flexor group includes digital flexor muscles in addition to muscles that act only at the carpus. They have certain common features: a flexor action at the carpus; a caudal position in the forearm; an origin, in part at least, from the caudal aspect of the medial epicondyle of the humerus; an innervation from the median or ulnar nerve, or from both these nerves. Some have additional—even principal—origins in the forearm and also act on the digital joints. The *flexor carpi radialis* (Fig. 2–55/11) is most medial and runs directly caudal to the subcutaneous border of the radius. It ends on the upper end of the second (sometimes third) metacarpal bone. The *flexor carpi ulnaris* (/5) is lateral and ends on the accessory carpal bone. Both muscles are solely carpal flexors.

The *superficial digital flexor* (/10) lies in the caudomedial part of the forearm and is not enclosed in a synovial sheath where it passes the carpus; later it divides into a branch for each functional digit that inserts in the region of the proximal interphalangeal joint. To reach these positions the branches of the tendon must first change position with those of the deep flexor that continue to more distal terminations. In principle (although the details vary), each branch of the superficial flexor tendon splits into two slips that diverge to the sides of the deep tendon, which then passes through the resulting arch. The *deep digital flexor* (/14) lies more deeply in the forearm and passes the carpus through the carpal canal before dividing into one to four digital branches; each perforates the corresponding branch of the superficial flexor tendon and then continues to its insertion on the palmar aspect of a distal phalanx.

**Short Digital Muscles.** *Interosseous muscles* support the metacarpophalangeal joints. They show marked species differences in number, structure (they are largely tendinous in the large species), and function. They arise from the palmar aspect of the proximal ends of the metacarpal bones and find initial insertion on the sesamoid bones at the metacarpophalangeal joints; from here they are continued by distal sesamoidean ligaments that attach to the phalanges, and by extensor branches that wind around to the dorsal aspect of the digit to join the extensor tendons. They are considered in detail later for the species in which they are important.

In the carnivores and pig a number of small digital muscles assist in the extension, flexion, abduction, or adduction of the abaxial digits—one, two, and five in dog and cat, two and five in pig. It is unnecessary to describe them.

## The Skeleton of the Hindlimb

### Pelvic Girdle

The pelvic girdle has been described with the trunk (p. 43) for the reason previously given.

### Skeleton of the Free Appendage

The *femur* (os femoris; Fig. 2–56), the skeleton of the thigh, is the strongest of the long bones. The proximal end curves medially so that the proximal articular surface, the head, is offset to the long axis of the shaft. The femoral head is hemispherical and is joined to the shaft by a neck, best defined in the smaller species. The articular surface is interrupted by a nonarticular area (fovea) to which the intracapsular ligament(s) attach(es); the fovea is round and central in the dog, wedge-shaped and extended to the medial periphery in the horse. A large process, the greater trochanter (/3), is placed lateral to the head; it rises level with the head in small animals but projects high above it in larger species (/3′,3″); it gives attachment to the bulk of the gluteal muscles, providing these extensors of the hip with a long lever arm. A plate of bone between the trochanter and the femoral neck helps bound the trochanteric fossa (/5), an excavation that is open caudally, and the site of insertion of the small rotator muscles of the hip.

The caudal aspect of the shaft is flattened, but the other aspects combine in a continuous smooth surface. The borders between the flat and rounded areas are emphasized by rough lines indicating

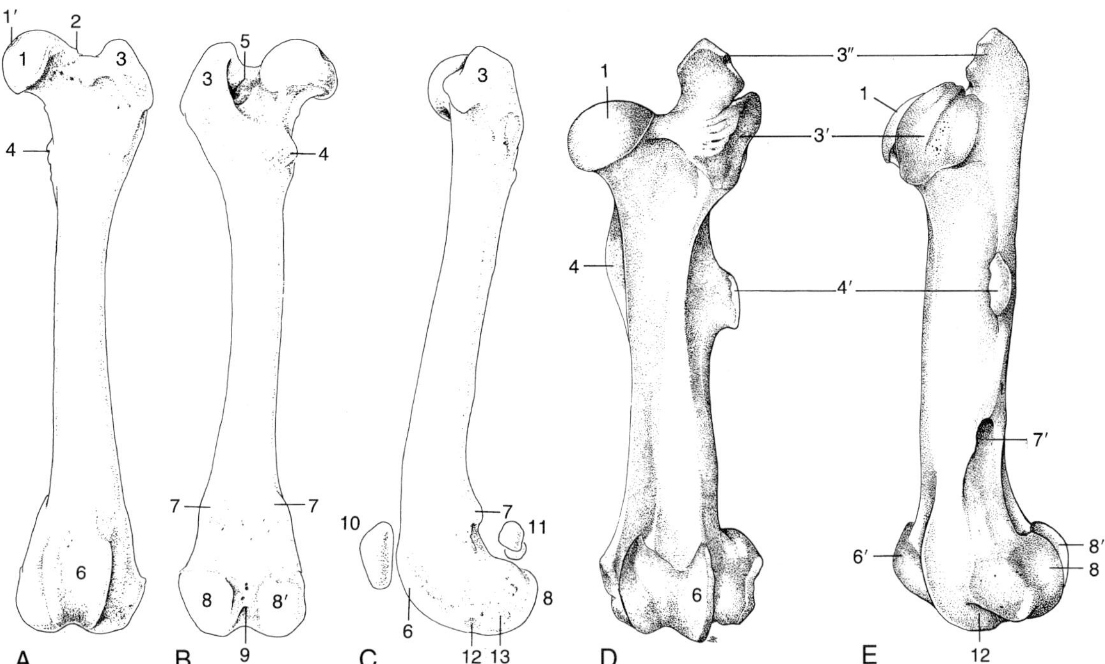


**Figure 2–56.** Left femur of the dog, cranial *(A)*, caudal *(B)*, and lateral *(C)* views. Cranial *(D)* and lateral *(E)* views of left equine femur.

1, Head; 1′, fovea; 2, neck; 3, greater trochanter; 3′, 3″, cranial and caudal parts of greater trochanter; 4, lesser trochanter; 4′, third trochanter; 5, trochanteric fossa; 6, trochlea; 6′, enlarged proximal end of medial trochlear ridge; 7, supracondylar tuberosities; 7′, supracondylar fossa; 8, 8′, lateral and medial condyles; 9, intercondylar fossa; 10, patella; 11, sesamoid bones (in gastrocnemius); 12, extensor fossa; 13, fossa for popliteus.

muscular attachment. Two processes mark the proximal half of the shaft. A low and rough lesser trochanter (/4) projects from the medial border and gives insertion to the iliopsoas muscle. An inconspicuous ridge at the base of the greater trochanter is known as the third trochanter (trochanter tertius). It is salient only in the horse and gives attachment to the gluteus superficialis (/4′). In the large animals the caudodistal part of the shaft exhibits a deep supracondylar fossa that increases the area of origin of the superficial digital flexor (/7′). The same function is fulfilled by tuberosities in the dog.

The distal extremity articulates with the tibia and the patella. The articulation with the tibia is accomplished by two condyles directed caudodistally and separated by a deep intercondylar fossa. The abaxial surfaces of the condyles are roughened and give attachment to the collateral ligaments of the stifle. The lateral condyle also carries two depressions close to the articular margin: the cranial one, the extensor fossa (/12), gives origin to the long digital extensor and peroneus tertius muscles; the caudal one (/13) gives origin to the popliteus. In the dog and cat the caudal aspect of each condyle is surmounted by a small flat facet for articulation with one of the small sesamoid bones (/11; formerly fabellae) in the origin of the gastrocnemius. A cranial trochlea (/6) articulates with the patella and extends proximally on the cranial surface. The bounding ridges are low and more or less equal in size in the dog and relatively larger and disparate in the horse and in cattle, in which the stouter medial ridge ends in a proximal enlargement (/6′).

The *patella,* the kneecap, is a sesamoid developed within the insertion of the quadriceps femoris, the main extensor of the stifle. It is ovoid in the dog but prismatic in the horse and in cattle. It is extended medially and laterally by parapatellar cartilages in the fresh state.

The *skeleton of the leg* consists of the tibia and fibula (Fig. 2–57), which, unlike the analogous elements of the forelimb, run side by side without any tendency to cross. The medial bone, the tibia, is always by far the larger of the two. The fibula is excluded from articulation with the femur and has only restricted contact with the hock skeleton.

The expanded proximal extremity of the *tibia* presents two condyles divided by a caudal popli-

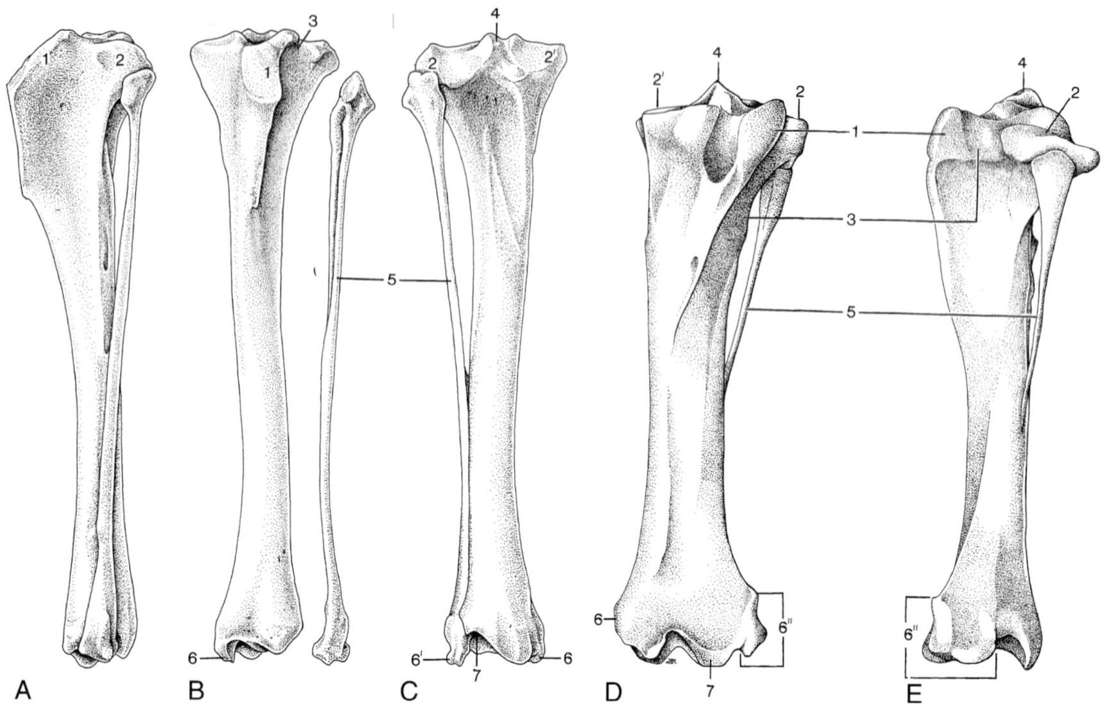


**Figure 2–57.** Left tibia and fibula of the dog, lateral *(A),* cranial *(B),* and caudal *(C)* views. Cranial *(D)* and lateral *(E)* views of left equine tibia and fibula.

1, Tibial tuberosity; 2, 2′, lateral and medial condyles; 3, extensor groove; 4, intercondylar eminence; 5, fibula; 6, 6′, medial and lateral malleoli; 6″, lateral malleolus in the horse (representing distal end of fibula); 7, cochlea.

teal notch that accommodates the like-named muscle. Each condyle has a gently undulating articular surface facing the corresponding condyle of the femur; a narrow intermediate nonarticular area carries a central eminence (/4) onto which the articular surfaces slope. A depression of the eminence, and less defined areas cranial and caudal to it, indicate ligamentous attachments. The very robust tibial tuberosity (/1) projecting from the cranial aspect of this extremity is a prominent landmark in life; it is continued by a gradually subsiding crest. A groove (/3) lodging the tendons of certain muscles of the leg (crus) separates the tuberosity from the cranial aspect of the lateral condyle. Caudal to this, the edge of the condyle carries a small facet for articulation with the fibula, although in some species the joint space is obliterated by fusion.

The proximal part of the tibial shaft is three-sided, but more distally the bone is craniocaudally compressed; the change is brought about by the smooth surface that faces craniolaterally in its proximal part but then twists to face directly forward. The entire medial surface (border distally) is subcutaneous and flat. The caudal surface is ridged for muscular attachment.

The distal extremity carries an articular area, known as the cochlea (/7), which is shaped to receive the trochlea of the talus. The central ridge and the flanking grooves of the cochlea have a craniolateral deflection, although the angle varies among species. A bony salience, the medial malleolus (/6), is present to the medial side of the cochlea. A similar lateral swelling is found only in the horse and represents the assimilated distal part of the fibula (/6″). In other species the corresponding feature (lateral malleolus) is provided by the fibula.

In carnivores and the pig the *fibula* is reduced in robustness but not in length. It is separated from the tibia by an interosseous space that runs the whole length of the leg in the pig but is limited to the proximal half in the dog. The shaft of the fibula regresses in ruminants; the proximal extremity persists as a tear-shaped process fused to the lateral condyle of the tibia; the distal extremity is isolated as a small compact malleolar bone that forms an interlocking joint with the tibia, completing the articular surface for the talus. The flattened proximal head of the fibula of the horse is closely applied to the tibia, and the slender shaft that leads from it converges on the tibia but fades toward the middle of the leg.

The *tarsal bones* are arranged in three tiers. The proximal tier consists of two relatively large bones, the talus medially and the calcaneus laterally; the middle tier comprises only a single central tarsal bone, while the distal tier comprises up to four bones, which are numbered in mediolateral sequence. The lateral fourth tarsal bone is constantly present and, being much deeper than the others, intrudes into the middle tier (Fig. 2–58).

The talus (Fig. 2–59) has a proximal trochlear surface shaped to fit the tibia. The distal surface, which articulates with the central bone, is flattened in the horse and more rounded in other species. The calcaneus lies mainly lateral to the talus but extends a shelflike process that overlaps the talus on its plantar surface; the process (sustentaculum tali; /3′) supports the deep digital flexor tendon. The larger part of the bone projects proximally behind the tibia as a free lever arm to which the common calcanean tendon attaches. It ends in a thickening that is the basis of the point of the hock (/3″) and corresponds to the human heel. The distal extremity of the calcaneus rests on the fourth tarsal bone (/6). The central tarsal bone is interposed between the talus proximally and the first, second, and third tarsal bones distally; its proximal surface conforms to the talus, being concave in most animals but flat in the horse; its distal articular surface is flattened. The central and fourth tarsal bones fuse in ruminants.

The distal tarsal bones are not always separate—the first and second are fused in the horse, the second and third in ruminants. Individually irregular, these bones together form a more or less flattened disc interposed between the central tarsal and the metatarsal bones. The much deeper fourth tarsal bone (/6) has a cuboidal form and is interposed between the calcaneus and the lateral metatarsal bones; in some species it also gives support to the talus.

The remaining bones of the hindlimb closely resemble those of the forelimb, although they tend to be less robust. The metatarsal bones are longer (by about 20%) than the metacarpals and are more rounded in cross section. The first metatarsal is rudimentary in the dog, in which only a few breeds consistently possess a dewclaw in the hindlimb.

## The Joints of the Hindlimb

The *hip joint* (Fig. 2–60) is a spheroidal joint formed between the lunate surface of the acetabulum and the head of the femur. The acetabular surface is enlarged by an articular labrum (/2′) continuous with the transverse acetabular ligament (/2″) that bridges the notch interrupting the medial wall of the socket. The walls of the articular cavity are completed by a synovial membrane supported externally by a fibrous covering. Although the fibrous capsule is not uniformly strong, there are no thickenings so definite that they need be recognized as specific ligaments. However, the head of the femur is joined to the depth of the acetabulum by the intracapsular ligament of the femoral head, which is covered by a reflection of the synovial membrane. In some species this ligament is known to convey blood vessels, but the importance of these to the nutrition of the head remains uncertain.

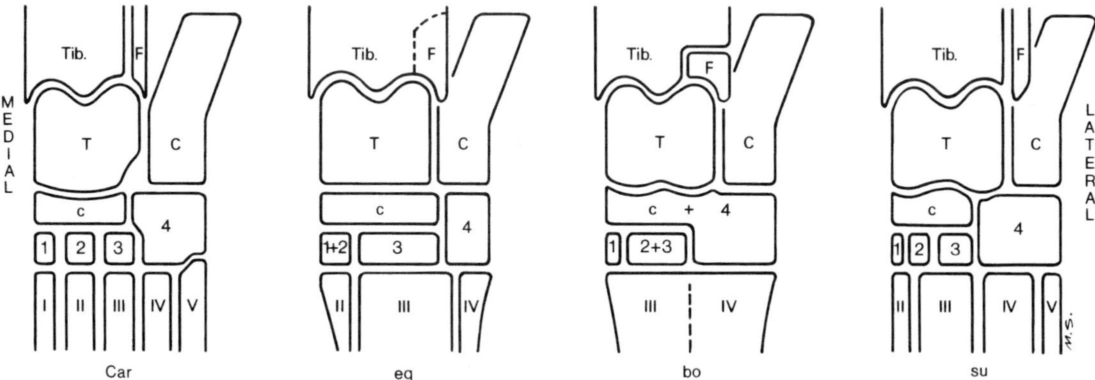


**Figure 2–58.** The bones of the tarsal skeleton in the carnivores (Car), horse (eq), cattle (bo), and pig (su), schematic. Roman numerals identify the metatarsal bones, Arabic numerals the distal tarsal bones.

Tib., Tibia; F, fibula; T, talus; C, calcaneus; c, central tarsal bone.

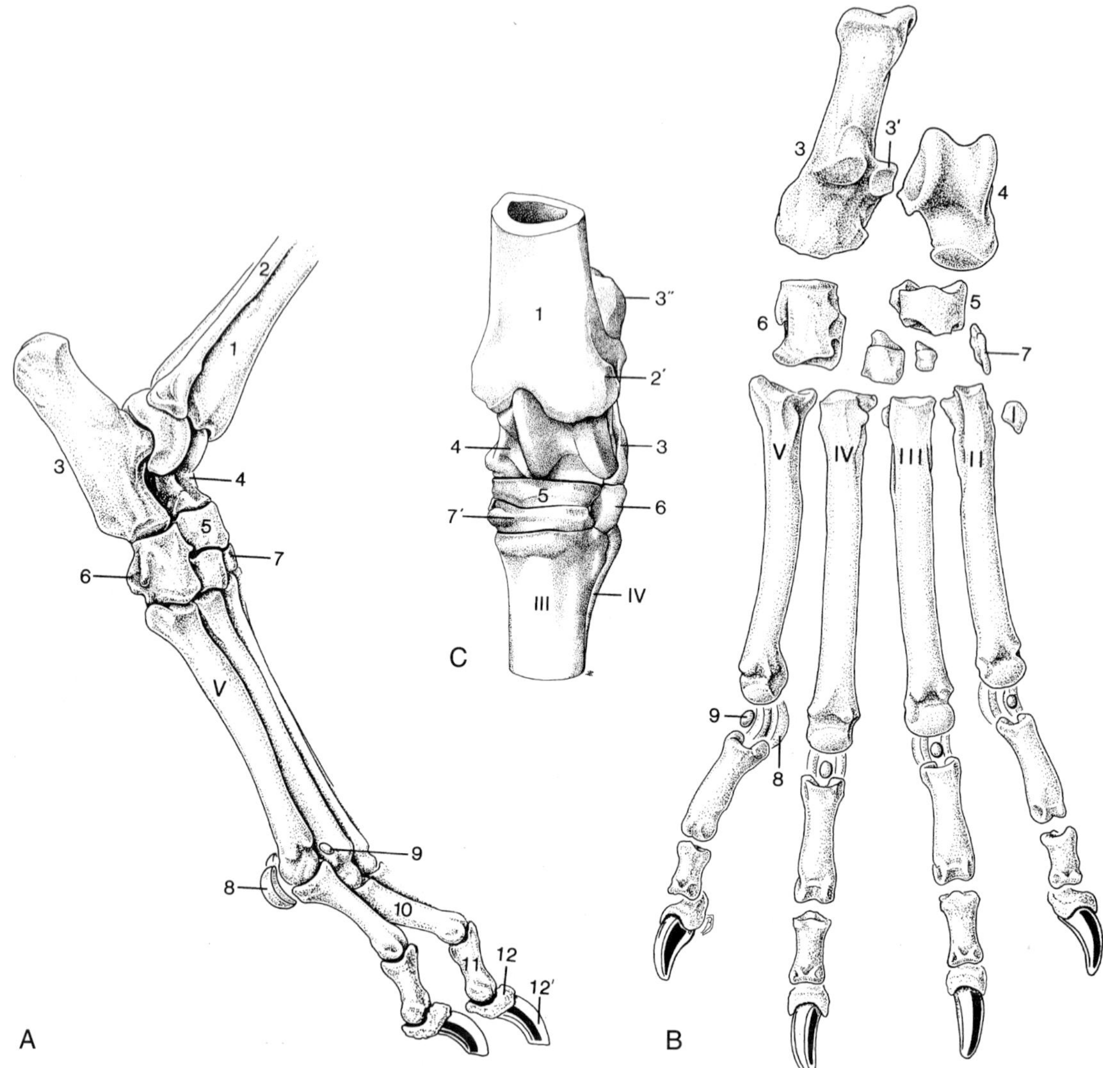


**Figure 2–59.** Skeleton of right pes of the dog; lateral *(A)* and dorsal *(B)* views. Dorsal *(C)* view of left equine tarsus. Roman numerals identify the metatarsal bones.

1, Tibia; 2, fibula; 2′, lateral malleolus; 3, calcaneus; 3′, sustentaculum tali; 3″, calcanean tuber (point of hock); 4, talus; 5, central tarsal; 6, fourth tarsal; 7, first, second, and third tarsal bones in distal row; 7′, third tarsal in the horse; 8, proximal sesamoid bones; 9, dorsal sesamoid bones; 10, 11, 12, proximal, middle, and distal phalanges; 12′, claw.

In the horse a second (accessory) ligament inserts on the nonarticular area of the head (p. 606).

Although a spheroidal joint, the hip does not enjoy the full range of movement expected of this class of joint. In the large animals movement is largely restricted to flexion and extension, with the capacity for rotation, abduction, and, especially, adduction being limited. In conformity with the dominance of sagittal movement, the articular area tends to extend onto the neck in ruminants. The restriction on movement owes much to the intra-articular ligament(s) but something to the massive medial muscles of the thigh. The joint has a more versatile employment in the dog.

The *stifle joint* (Fig. 2–61), corresponding to the human knee, comprises femorotibial, femoropatellar, and proximal tibiofibular joints; in the dog it also includes the joints between the femur and paired sesamoids in the origins of the gastrocnemius, and that between the tibia and the sesamoid in the popliteus tendon. In the dog, all these articulations share a common synovial cavity; in the large species the femoropatellar and the medial and lateral femorotibial compartments have more restricted communication with each other.

The femorotibial joint is unusual in having two fibrocartilaginous menisci (/10,17) interposed between the femoral and tibial condyles. The menisci, which compensate for the incongruence of the articular surfaces, are each semilunar in plan and wedge-shaped in section and have concave proximal and flattened distal surfaces. Each is secured by ligaments that extend between its cranial and caudal extremities and the central nonarticular area of the proximal extremity of the tibia; the lateral meniscus is also attached caudally to the intercondylar fossa of the femur.

Four ligaments join the femur to the bones of the leg. A medial collateral ligament passes between the femoral epicondyle and the proximal part of the tibia, toward the caudal part of the joint. The corresponding lateral ligament has a similar disposition but attaches to the fibular head. The cruciate ligaments are centrally placed. The cranial (lateral) cruciate ligament (/16) arises from the lateral condyle of the femur within the intercondylar fossa and runs craniodistally to attach on the tibia. The caudal (medial) cruciate ligament (/15) runs at right angles to the cranial one and attaches far back on the tibia near the popliteal notch.

The femoropatellar joint is formed between the femoral trochlea and the patella, extended by its parapatellar cartilages, of which the medial one is

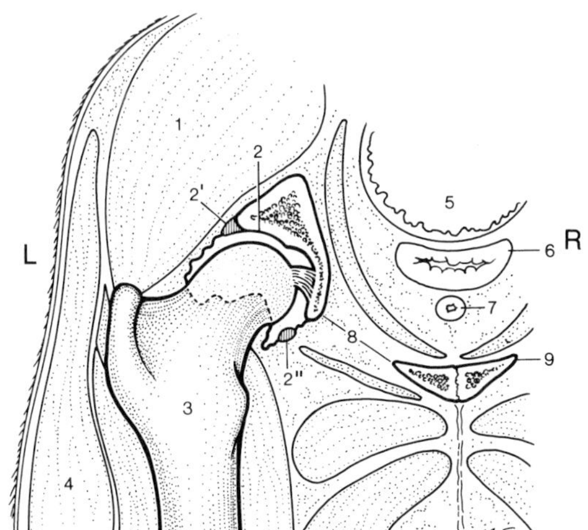


**Figure 2–60.** Schematic transverse section through the left hip joint of a dog. The femur has been drawn in relief.

1, Gluteus medius; 2, acetabulum, connected to the femoral head by the ligament of the head of the femur; 2′, fibrous rim (labrum) of acetabulum; 2″, transverse acetabular ligament; 3, femur; 4, biceps; 5, rectum; 6, vagina; 7, urethra; 8, obturator foramen; 9, pelvic floor.

especially well developed in the large animals. Relatively weak collateral femoropatellar ligaments (/12) run between the cartilages and the femur. Distally the patella is joined to the tibial tuberosity by a single patellar ligament, except in the horse and ox, in which three ligamentous thickenings are present—medial, intermediate, and lateral—connected by a fibrous sheet (see Fig. 24–4). The middle (or single) patellar ligament represents the insertion tendon of the quadriceps femoris; the others, when present, represent the continuation of other muscles inserting about the joint.

The synovial membrane attaches around the peripheries of the articular surfaces and the menisci. It covers the cruciate ligaments and here forms a partition, complete only in the horse, between the medial and lateral femorotibial joints. The femoropatellar portion of the cavity extends proximally between the femur and the quadriceps. In the horse it generally communicates only with the medial femorotibial compartment, but in other species it has free communication with both. Diverticula of the capsule embrace the lesser joints with the fibula and the sesamoid bones and extend along the tendons of origin of the long digital extensor and popliteus muscles.

Despite its complexity, the stifle functions as a hinge joint with free movement restricted to flexion and extension. The femoral condyles roll on the menisci, and these in turn slide over the tibial plateau—cranially on extension, caudally on flexion. The travel between the femur and menisci is about three times that between the menisci and the tibia. The spiral configuration of the femoral condyles—when viewed from the side—tightens the ligaments and slows the movement when the joint moves toward the extended position. The stability of the articulation depends much on the cruciate ligaments. Rupture of one of these—not an uncommon misfortune—allows the tibia unusual mobility; it may slip forward when the cranial ligament is torn and backward when the caudal ligament is torn. Rotation imposed on the joint, particularly when the joint is extended, places great strain upon the menisci and their attachments.

The *tarsal joint* of quadrupeds is usually known as the hock. It possesses four levels of articulation but in most species almost all movement occurs at the crurotarsal level. This is a hinge joint but not a typical one since the obliquity of the interlocking ridges and grooves of the tibia and talus imposes a lateral deviation of the foot when it is carried forward on flexion. In ruminants and carnivores limited flexion is also possible at the curved surfaces of the talocentral joint.

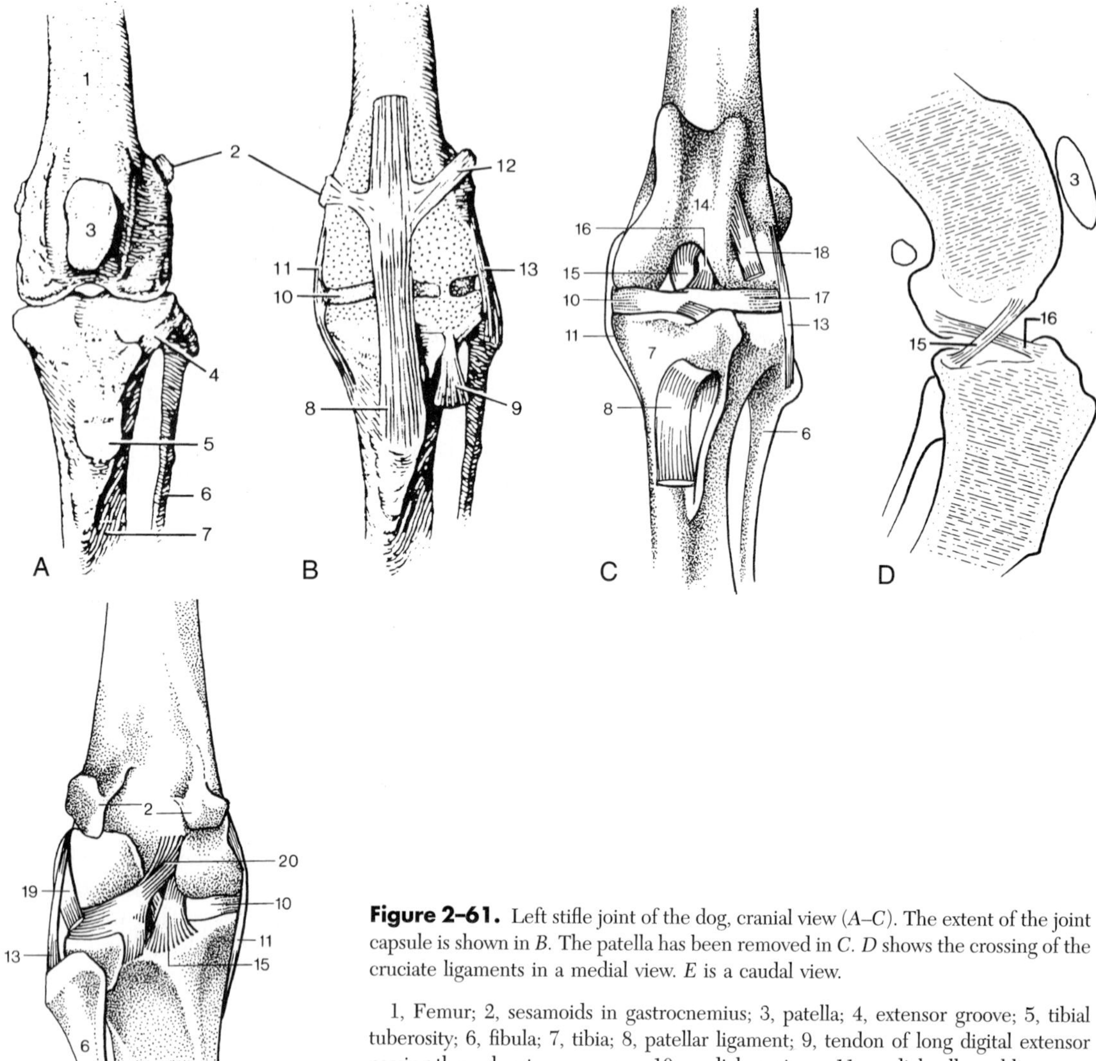


**Figure 2–61.** Left stifle joint of the dog, cranial view (*A–C*). The extent of the joint capsule is shown in *B*. The patella has been removed in *C*. *D* shows the crossing of the cruciate ligaments in a medial view. *E* is a caudal view.

1, Femur; 2, sesamoids in gastrocnemius; 3, patella; 4, extensor groove; 5, tibial tuberosity; 6, fibula; 7, tibia; 8, patellar ligament; 9, tendon of long digital extensor passing through extensor groove; 10, medial meniscus; 11, medial collateral ligament; 12, lateral femoropatellar ligament; 13, lateral collateral ligament; 14, trochlea; 15, caudal cruciate ligament; 16, cranial cruciate ligament; 17, lateral meniscus; 18, stump of 9; 19, popliteus tendon; 20, meniscofemoral ligament.

The ligaments are numerous. Those most important are the medial and lateral collateral ligaments, which extend, with intermediate attachments, from the tibia (and fibula) to the proximal extremity of the metatarsus. Each comprises a long superficial part of full extent and a shorter deeper part restricted to the proximal level of articulation. Another long ligament is found caudally, extending from the plantar surface of the calcaneus over the fourth tarsal bone to the metatarsus. The remaining smaller ligaments firmly hold the tarsal bones together.

There are several compartments to the joint. That between the tibia and talus is most capacious and may possess a number of local pouches, as the less supported parts of joint capsules are known. The other synovial sacs are much tighter and often communicate. The details are most important in the horse (p. 613).

The remaining joints of the hindlimb are considered in the regional chapters—insofar as they require to be differentiated from the corresponding forelimb joints.

## The Muscles of the Hindlimb

The girdle musculature has been described (p. 56).

## The Intrinsic Muscles of the Hindlimb

**Muscles Acting Primarily on the Hip Joint.** The muscles acting at the hip are arranged in gluteal, medial, deep, and caudal (hamstring) groups, a classification based primarily on topography.

The *gluteal group* comprises superficial, middle, and deep gluteal muscles and the tensor fasciae latae. The *gluteus superficialis* varies greatly. In the dog it is a relatively narrow muscle that covers the caudal part of the gluteus medius, extending from the gluteal and caudal fascia to the third trochanter of the femur (Fig. 2–62/4). In ungulates a part becomes incorporated within the biceps femoris, and sometimes also the semitendinosus, supplying these with vertebral heads of origin. It is an extensor of the hip and therefore a retractor of the limb. It is supplied by the caudal gluteal nerve.

The *gluteus medius* (/3) is by far the largest of the group. It arises from the outer surface of the ilium and the gluteal fascia and inserts on the greater trochanter. It is an exceptionally powerful extensor of the hip with some abduction potential. A deeper subdivision is known as gluteus accessorius. Neither it nor the small, more caudal piriformis need be considered separately; their actions are similar to those of the main mass. The muscle is principally supplied by the cranial gluteal nerve.

The much smaller *gluteus profundus* is completely covered by the gluteus medius. It arises from the ischial spine and adjacent region of the os coxae and inserts on the cranial part of the greater trochanter. It may also extend the hip, but because most fibers run more or less transversely, it is more advantageously placed to abduct the limb. It is also supplied by the cranial gluteal nerve.

The *tensor fasciae latae* (/2) is the most cranial muscle of the group. It arises from the coxal tuber (or equivalent) and from the adjacent part of the ilium and extends down the cranial border of the

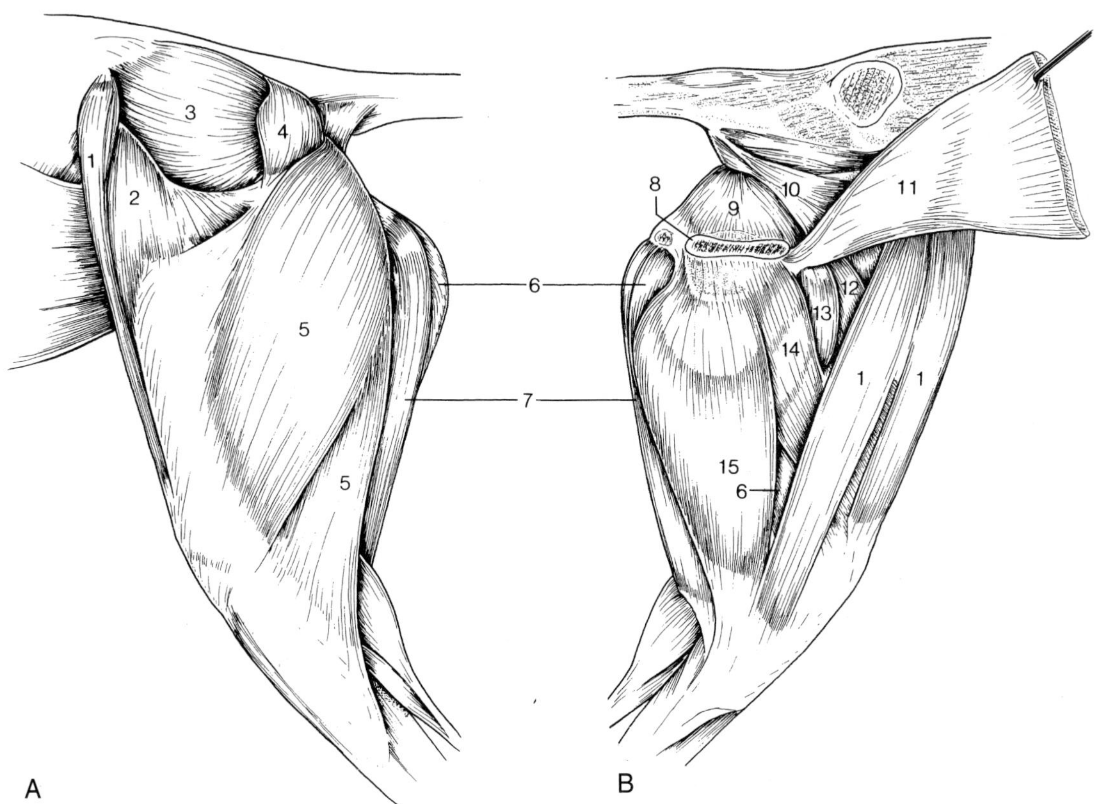


**Figure 2–62.** Muscles of the canine hindquarter and thigh, lateral *(A)* and medial *(B)* views.

1, Sartorius; 2, tensor fasciae latae; 3, gluteus medius; 4, gluteus superficialis; 5, biceps; 6, semimembranosus; 7, semitendinosus; 8, pelvic symphysis; 9, internal obturator; 10, levator ani; 11, rectus abdominis; 12, quadriceps; 13, pectineus; 14, adductor; 15, gracilis.

thigh before inserting into the heavy lateral femoral fascia, which serves as its insertion tendon and provides it with attachment to the patella and other structures of the stifle region. Supplied by the cranial gluteal nerve, it is primarily a flexor of the hip. In the horse its most caudal part extends toward and fuses with a cranial slip of the gluteus superficialis.

The *medial group* is principally employed to adduct the hindlimb, a term that of course also embraces the prevention of unwanted abduction. Most muscles of this group are supplied by the obturator nerve and these—gracilis, pectineus, adductor, and external obturator—are sometimes specifically termed "the adductors." The sartorius has a rather different origin and relationship.

The *gracilis,* a broad but thin muscle, takes an aponeurotic origin from the symphysial region of the pelvis (/15). Its insertion, also aponeurotic, merges with the crural fascia through which it finds attachment to the tibial crest and other medial structures of the stifle region.

The *pectineus* is a small fusiform muscle, which in the dog forms a prominent surface feature of the proximal part of the thigh (/13). It arises from the cranial branch of the pubis and from the prepubic tendon and inserts on the proximal part of the medial "rough line" of the femur. In the larger species, but not in the dog, a considerable part of the tendon of origin decussates with its fellow within the prepubic tendon.

The *adductor* is often divided into several individually named parts, but these distinctions are unnecessary. The muscle arises over an extensive area of the ventral aspect of the pelvic floor and inserts along the distal two thirds of the medial "rough line" of the femur and to the fascia and ligaments of the medial aspect of the stifle (/14).

The *obturator externus* is conveniently included here, although it has obvious affinities with the following deep group. It arises from the ventral surface of the pelvic floor, over and around the obturator foramen, and inserts within the ventral part of the trochanteric fossa. In addition to being an adductor, it is potentially an outward rotator of the thigh.

The *sartorius* is set apart from the other medial muscles by its innervation from the saphenous branch of the femoral nerve. It is superficial and follows the craniomedial aspect of the thigh; in the dog it consists of two parallel bellies, one of which forms the cranial contour of the thigh (/1). Except in the horse (in which it arises from the iliac fascia on the abdominal roof), it arises from the iliac crest and its insertion is to the medial structures of the stifle region. Flexion of the hip is probably its main action but it has some capacity for adduction of the thigh and extension of the stifle. The superficial space between the caudal margin of the sartorius and the pectineus is often designated the femoral canal.

The *deep muscles of the hip* form a rather heterogeneous community of small and essentially trivial muscles—the obturator internus, gemelli, quadratus femoris, and articularis coxae. Most are supplied by the sciatic nerve.

The *obturator internus* (/9) is a thin muscle that arises from the dorsal surface of the hip bone in the vicinity of the obturator foramen; in carnivores and in the horse its tendon leaves the pelvis by passing over the ischium, caudal to the acetabulum, to end in the trochanteric fossa. In other species the tendon passes through the obturator foramen; in this arrangement, the muscle may have its origin as a detachment from the external obturator. The muscle is an external rotator of the thigh.

The *gemelli* are two small "twin" bundles that pass from the ischial spine to the trochanteric fossa. They also are external rotators.

The *quadratus femoris* passes from the ventral aspect of the ischium to end on the femoral shaft close to the trochanteric fossa. It is described as an extensor but can be of no significance in this role.

The *articularis coxae* lies on the capsule over the cranial aspect of the hip and protects this from being nipped between the femoral and acetabular surfaces.

The *muscles of the caudal (hamstring) group*—biceps femoris, semitendinosus, and semimembranosus—flesh the caudal part of the thigh. They extend from the ischial tuber and adjacent part of the sacrotuberous ligament to a broad insertion both proximal and distal to the joint space of the stifle; certain components continue within the common calcanean tendon to the calcaneus. In ungulates one (or more) of these muscles is also extended proximally through the acquisition of an origin (vertebral head) from the sacrocaudal vertebrae. The vertebral heads are best developed in the horse and account for the full, rounded contour of the rump of this animal, which contrasts with the more angular appearance in the ox or dog. At least part of the vertebral extension is due to assimilation of a superficial gluteal component. The term *gluteobiceps* may be encountered for the combination.

The *biceps femoris* is most lateral (Fig. 2–62/5). In the horse and ruminants—but not in the dog—it has both vertebral and pelvic heads. In the lower part of the thigh the united muscle divides into insertions that attach, by way of the femoral and crural fascia, to the patella and ligaments of the stifle joint both proximal and distal to the joint space; an additional insertion to the point of the hock is achieved through a contribution (tarsal tendon) to the common calcanean tendon.

The *semitendinosus* (/7) forms the caudal contour of the thigh. It has a vertebral head only in the horse and pig. The insertion is to the medial aspect of the proximal extremity of the tibia and to the calcaneus. The insertions of the biceps and semitendinosus, one to each side of the depression (popliteal fossa) behind the stifle, can be palpated in life—they are the "strings of the ham" that give the group its name.

The *semimembranosus* (/6) is most medial and has a vertebral head only in the horse. The insertion is divided between a cranial part attaching to the medial femoral condyle and a caudal part attaching to the medial tibial condyle.

In the dog a ribbon-like *abductor cruris caudalis* lies on the deep face of the biceps and is probably derived from it. It has no great functional significance.

The vertebral heads of these muscles are generally supplied by the caudal gluteal nerve, and the pelvic heads by the sciatic nerve (or its tibial division).

Certain functions of these muscles are difficult to analyze, but their main role is undoubtedly the forceful extension of the hip joint that thrusts the trunk forward. In addition, the biceps has an abductor potential, the semimembranosus an adductor potential, at the hip.

When considering their action on the stifle it is probably more useful to divide the muscles into a cranial division inserting proximal to the joint axis and a caudal division inserting distal to this axis, rather than to consider the named units. The cranial division extends the stifle when the foot is planted on the ground. The caudal division has the same action when the foot is fixed but flexes the joint when the foot is free to move. The parts of the biceps and semitendinosus that insert on the calcaneus can obviously extend the hock. It is clear that not all these effects can be accomplished simultaneously; apart from the potential antagonism of the cranial and caudal divsions at the stifle it is unlikely that an animal would wish to flex the stifle while extending the hock. Indeed, in the horse in particular, this combination of actions is precluded by the reciprocal mechanism (p. 618). Different parts of these muscles must therefore be used at different times and in different combinations.

**Muscles Acting Primarily on the Stifle Joint.** There are extensor and flexor groups. The *quadriceps femoris,* the principal extensor of the stifle, forms the mass of muscle cranial to the femur (see Fig. 17–2/10). It consists of four parts, separate at their origins but joined distally. One, the rectus femoris, arises from the shaft of the ilium immediately cranial to the acetabulum. The others, vastus medialis, intermedius, and lateralis, arise from the medial, cranial, and lateral aspects of the femoral shaft. The common insertion appears to be on the patella but is actually on the tibial tuberosity since the muscle is continued distal to the patella by the patellar ligament(s). The rectus femoris has the potential secondary action of flexion of the hip, although it is ill placed for this purpose. The quadriceps is supplied by the femoral nerve.

The small *popliteus* muscle lies directly over the caudal aspect of the joint. It takes a tendinous and confined origin from the lateral condyle of the femur and fans out to a broad fleshy insertion on the proximal third of the caudal surface of the tibia (Fig. 2–63/15). Its tendon of origin contains a sesamoid in the dog and cat. In addition to being a flexor of the stifle, the popliteus rotates the distal part of the limb. It is supplied by the tibial nerve.

**Muscles Acting Primarily on the Tarsal and Digital Joints.** These comprise extensors and flexors of the hock and extensors and flexors of the digits. They are grouped in two masses, one craniolateral to the tibia, the other caudal to the tibia.

*Craniolateral Muscles of the Leg.* The craniolateral group comprises muscles with an action confined to flexion of the hock and others that have this action but continue to extend the digits. This arrangement contrasts with that of the corresponding muscles of the forelimb; here the longer units extend both carpal and distal joints. In addition to their position and action, the craniolateral crural muscles have their innervation—through the peroneal* nerve (/3)—in common.

A full set of the muscles that are pure flexors of the hock is not found in any domestic species; it would comprise the tibialis cranialis, peroneus tertius, peroneus longus, and peroneus brevis. The dog and cat lack the peroneus tertius, and ungulates lack the peroneus brevis; the horse also lacks the peroneus longus and has its peroneus tertius reduced to a tendinous cord.

The *tibialis cranialis,* always substantial, lies immediately cranial to the subcutaneous medial surface of the tibia (/5). It takes origin from the lateral condyle of the tibia and inserts on the mediodistal tarsal and adjacent metatarsal skele-

---

*The adjective *fibular* has equivalent meaning to peroneal and is substituted for it by many authors. At present peroneal (in its Latin form, *peroneus*) is official.

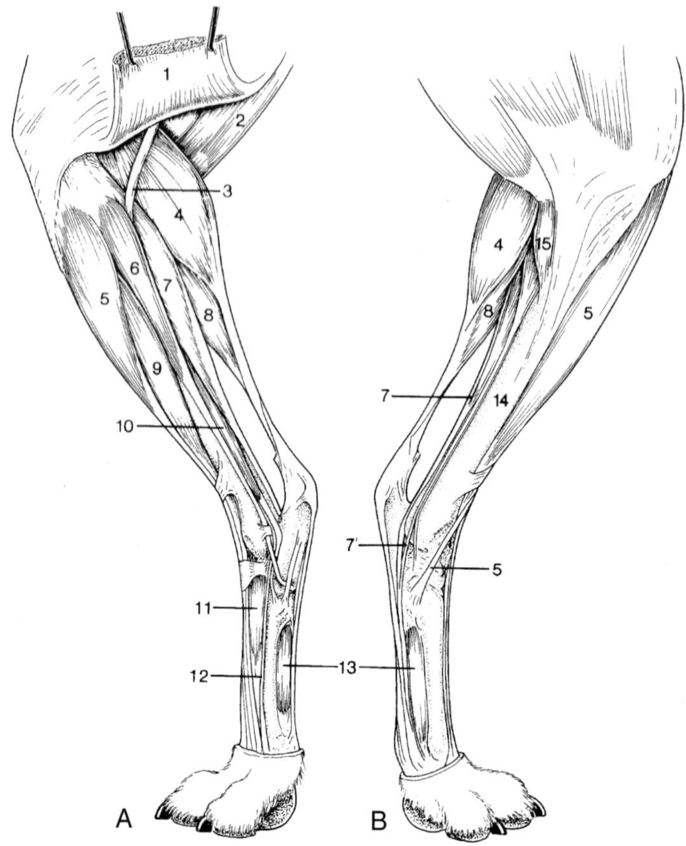


**Figure 2–63.** Muscles of the left canine leg, lateral *(A)* and medial *(B)* views.

1, Biceps; 2, semitendinosus; 3, peroneal nerve; 4, gastrocnemius; 5, tibialis cranialis; 6, peroneus longus; 7, lateral deep digital flexor, 7′, tendon of the smaller medial deep digital flexor; 8, superficial digital flexor; 9, long digital extensor; 10, peroneus brevis; 11, extensor brevis; 12, tendon of lateral digital extensor; 13, interossei; 14, tibia; 15, popliteus.

ton. It is a flexor of the hock with a secondary supinator role. The *peroneus tertius* is most important in the horse, in which it constitutes an essential component of the so-called reciprocal mechanism. It is described in that context on page 618.

The weak *peroneus longus* arises from and around the distal part of the lateral collateral ligament of the stifle joint (/6). It crosses the lateral aspect of the tarsus before turning medially, over the plantar aspect, to end on the proximal parts of the medial metatarsal bone. It is primarily a pronator of the foot but may also flex the hock. The *peroneus brevis* is of no practical importance.

The number and the arrangement of the extensor muscles of the digits are naturally correlated with the digital pattern. A *long digital extensor muscle* (/9) arises from the distal extremity of the femur and follows the lateral border of the tibialis cranialis. Its tendon crosses the dorsal surface of the hock, where it is held down by retinacula; later it splits into branches, one for each functional digit. Each branch inserts on the extensor process of a distal phalanx. In the dog, the tendons develop small sesamoid bones similar to those of the forelimb.

A *lateral digital extensor* (/12) arises from the head of the fibula, crosses the lateral aspect of the hock, and enters the most lateral functional digit, where it terminates either on the proximal phalanx (dog) or by joining the long extensor tendon (horse). In certain species, including the dog, a small discrete *extensor hallucis longus* is associated with the medial digit; it arises on the cranial border of the fibula and inserts on the proximal part of the digit.

*Caudal Muscles of the Leg.* The caudal group comprises the twin-bellied gastrocnemius, the soleus, and the superficial and deep digital flexors. All are supplied by the tibial nerve.

The gastrocnemius and the soleus, the latter insignificant (except in the cat) and absent in the dog, are sometimes collectively known as the triceps surae. The two heads of the *gastrocnemius* (Fig. 2–63/4) spring from the caudal aspect of the femur proximal to the condyles; two sesamoid bones are included in the origins in carnivores. The heads combine in the upper part of the crus and give rise to a single stout tendon that inserts on the point of the hock. It is the principal component of the common calcanean (Achilles) tendon. Despite its inclusion among the extensors of the hock, the role of the gastrocnemius is enigmatic, since its proximal attachment suggests that it is a potential flexor of the stifle; stifle and hock, however, normally move in unison. The apparent contradiction in these actions is not easily explained. It has been suggested that the prime function of the muscle is not to move either joint but to oppose bending of the tibia, ensuring that the strain is always directed aong its long axis.

The *superficial digital flexor* (/8) arises from a supracondylar fossa or tubercle on the caudal aspect of the femur, close to the origin of the gastrocnemius. It first runs deeply, between the two parts of the latter muscle; its tendon later winds around the medial border of the gastrocnemius tendon to gain the more superficial position. It forms a broad cap over the point of the hock, where part finds attachment through medial and lateral slips, before continuing over the plantar aspect of the calcaneus to enter the foot; it is then disposed like the corresponding tendon of the forelimb. The muscle is heavily infiltrated by connective tissue, especially in the horse, in which it becomes almost entirely tendinous and forms the caudal component of the reciprocal mechanism (p. 618).

There are three *deep digital flexor muscles* whose independence varies among species. The three—lateral and medial flexors and the tibialis caudalis—lie close together on the caudal surface of the tibia (and fibula) from which they take origin (/7). In the ungulates, the tendons of the lateral muscle and the tibialis caudalis unite above the tarsus and then run over the plantar aspect of the joint, medial to the calcaneus; this common tendon is then joined in the upper part of the metatarsus by that of the medial muscle which descends over the medial malleolus. The combined deep flexor tendon ends as the corresponding tendon of the forelimb. In the carnivores, only the lateral (/7) and medial (/7′) muscles unite; the rather small tibialis caudalis remains aloof and inserts separately upon the hock; this truncated course transforms it into an extensor of the hock and supinator of the foot.

The most important *short digital muscles* are the interossei (/13), which resemble those of the forelimb. A number of other small muscles that occur, especially in the dog, are of trivial significance.

CHAPTER 3

# The Digestive Apparatus

The digestive apparatus* comprises the organs concerned with the reception, mechanical reduction, chemical digestion, and absorption of food and drink and with the elimination of unabsorbed residues. It consists of the alimentary tract, extending from the mouth to the anus, and certain glands—the salivary glands, pancreas, and liver—that drain by ducts that open into the tract. The parts of the alimentary tract in proper sequence are the mouth, pharynx, esophagus, stomach, small intestine, and large intestine (Fig. 3–1). Some of the digestive organs have other, sometimes no less vital, functions quite distinct from the processing of the food intake.

These organs are primarily formed of endoderm, the germ layer that lines the yolk sac, although the muscle and connective tissues that support the epithelium are of mesodermal origin as elsewhere.

The separation of the digestive tube from the yolk sac is achieved in the folding process that converts the flat embryonic disc into a more or less cylindrical body. The folding is the result of the disc growing more rapidly than the extraembryonic tissue with which it is continuous; in consequence of the constraint exerted at the periphery, the disc buckles upward while its edges are folded or rolled under. Since growth is most rapid along the longitudinal axis, the folding is more pronounced at the head and tail extremities than along the lateral margins. This ensures that the part of the yolk sac taken into the body presents two horns extending cranially and caudally from a middle region that retains free communication with the larger part of the yolk sac remaining outside the embryo. The included part of the yolk sac is known as the *gut,* its three regions being the *foregut, midgut,* and *hindgut.* The midgut joins the other regions through tapering parts known as the *cranial* and *caudal intestinal portals* (Fig. 3–2).

The foregut and hindgut end blindly at the oral and cloacal membranes, circumscribed median areas where the endoderm and ectoderm are in direct contact, with no intervening mesoderm. These membranes form the floors of surface depressions known as the *stomadeum* and *proctodeum.* The depressions are deepened by the relatively rapid growth of the surrounding tissue; when the membranes break down the depressions become confluent with the gut, extending it at each end by a short passage lined with ectoderm. The cranial extension forms the larger part of the mouth, the caudal one the anal canal.

The foregut differentiates to form the pharynx, esophagus, stomach, and first part of the duodenum together with the structures formed by outgrowth from these parts. The midgut forms the remainder of the small intestine, the cecum, and the larger part of the colon. The hindgut forms the distal part of the colon, the rectum, and, after partitioning, part of the urogenital tract.

A more detailed account of the development of these organs must be deferred since it requires mention of parts and terms with which the reader is possibly not yet familiar.

## THE MOUTH

The term *mouth* (os, gen. oris) designates not only the cavity and its walls but also the accessory structures that project (teeth, tongue) and drain (salivary glands) into it. The mouth has as its main functions the prehension, mastication, and insalivation of food. It may also play a role in aggression and defense, while in ourselves it is important in the formulation of the sounds of speech. In most species it functions as an airway when flow through the nose is impaired.

The *mouth* (oral) *cavity* is entered between the lips and continues into the pharynx (Fig. 3–3) through a caudal narrowing at the level of the palatoglossal arches (see further on). It is divided by the teeth and margins of the jaws into an outer vestibule, bounded by the lips and cheeks externally, and the central mouth cavity proper. When the mouth is closed, these divisions communicate through gaps behind and between the teeth. The *vestibule* extends caudally toward the ramus of the mandible and the masseter muscle. The proportion

*The digestive, respiratory, urinary, and male and female reproductive organs constitute a series of systems or apparatuses whose study collectively is known as *splanchnology.* Most of the component parts are known as *viscera* (plural of viscus, Latin for organ).

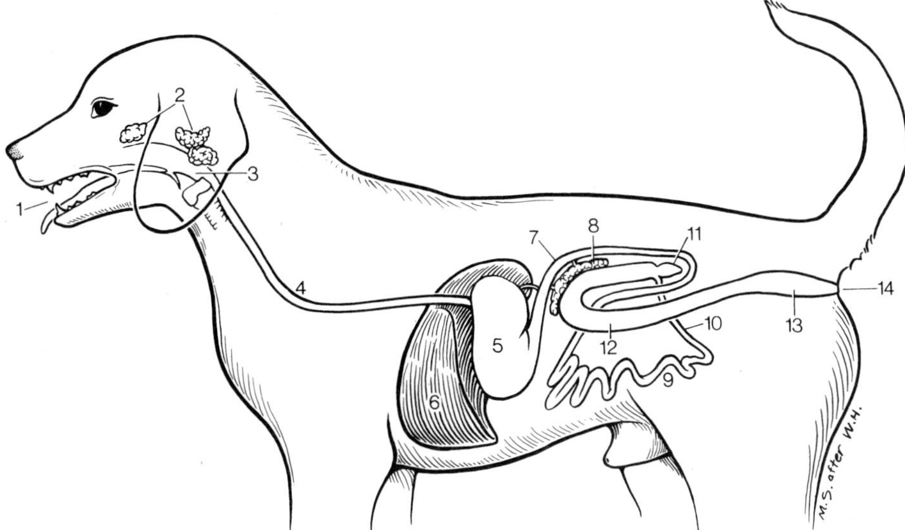


**Figure 3–1.** Schematic representation of the digestive apparatus in the dog.

1, Mouth; 2, salivary glands; 3, pharynx; 4, esophagus; 5, stomach; 6, liver; 7, duodenum; 8, pancreas; 9, jejunum; 10, ileum; 11, cecum; 12, colon; 13, rectum; 14, anus.

of its walls formed by the lips varies with feeding habits; a wide gape is necessary in species that feed greedily or use their teeth to seize prey or in fight, whereas a smaller opening suffices in most herbivores and rodents.

Diet and feeding habits also determine the form of the *lips* (labia oris). In some species, such as the horse, the lips are employed in collecting food and introducing it to the mouth; for this purpose they must be both sensitive and mobile. When other parts are more important in prehension the lips can be less mobile and reduced in size (e.g., cat) or thickened and insensitive (e.g., ox). The lips of the dog are extensive but thin, and although they can be drawn back from the teeth, they are not capable of other purposeful movements. Lip posture is an important factor in communication in this species and can signal aggressive intent or submission. In newborn animals the lips form the seal about the teat that is necessary for successful sucking.

The lips are composed of skin, an intermediate layer of muscle, tendon, and glands, and the oral mucosa. The skin and mucosa usually meet along the margin of the lips, though the boundary can be displaced in either direction. The muscles that make up the greater part of the lips belong to the mimetic musculature, the field of the facial nerve (p. 68). They include an orbicular muscle encircling the opening and, with some species variation, others that raise, depress, and retract the lips. Small salivary glands are scattered among the muscle bundles below the mucosa, especially toward the angles (commissures) where the two lips meet.

There is rarely anything remarkable in the arrangement of the lower lip. In the dog it is rather loose but fastened to the lower jaw at the level of the canine tooth and has a thin, serrated margin. Modifications of the upper lip are more frequent. Sometimes a median naked area is present continuous with the modified skin around the nostrils. The extensive moist and glandular nasolabial plate

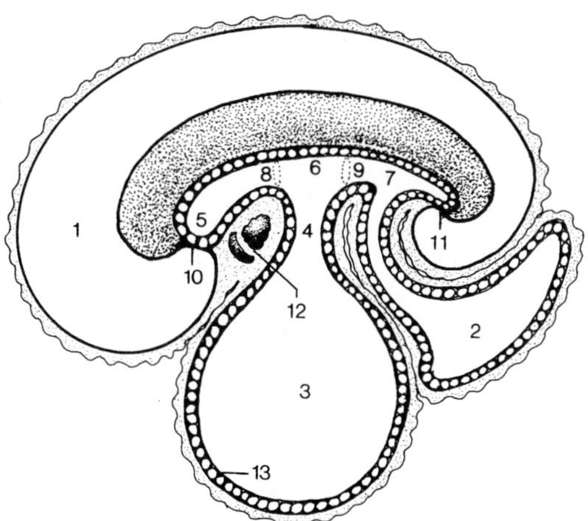


**Figure 3–2.** Sagittal section of an early embryo. Part of the yolk sac is taken into the body in the folding process.

1, Amniotic cavity; 2, allantoic cavity; 3, yolk sac; 4, stalk of yolk sac; 5, foregut; 6, midgut; 7, hindgut; 8, cranial intestinal portal; 9, caudal intestinal portal; 10, oral plate; 11, cloacal plate; 12, heart and pericardial cavity; 13, endoderm.

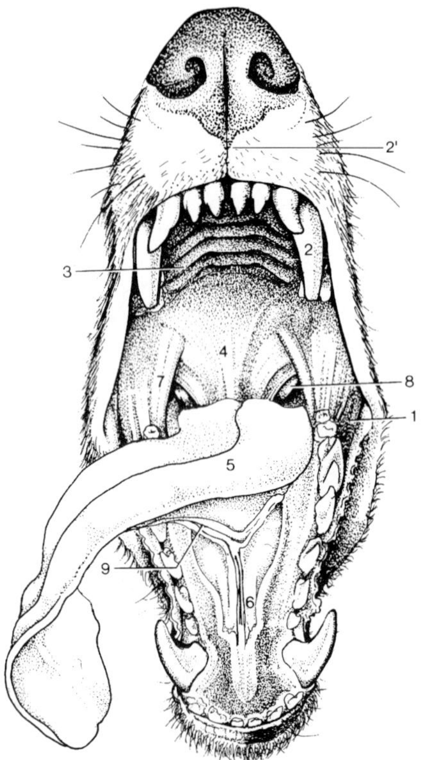


**Figure 3–3.** General view of the oral cavity of the dog.

1, Vestibule; 2, canine tooth; 2′, philtrum; 3, hard palate; 4, soft palate; 5, tongue; 6, sublingual caruncle; 7, palatoglossal arch; 8, palatine tonsil; 9, frenulum.

of the ox and the rostral disc of the pig are good examples of this. The area of modified skin is often much narrower and may be divided by a median groove (philtrum) as in the dog. Dog breeders refer to this modified region as the "nose leather" (Fig. 3–3). In man and in the horse a hairy integument extends across the entire upper lip.

The *cheeks* (buccae), which tend to be most capacious in herbivores, have a similar structure. The principal support is the buccinator muscle, which has the important function of returning to the central cavity any food that has escaped into the vestibule. There are additional salivary glands, sometimes aggregated in quite large masses—the zygomatic gland of the dog (Fig. 3–14/8), concealed below the zygomatic arch, has its origin in this way. The buccal mucosa must be sufficiently loose to allow the occasional maximal opening of the mouth while avoiding large folds that would at other times invite injury from the teeth (Fig. 3–4); it tends, therefore, to be tightly anchored here and there. In ruminants, whose food may be dry and rough, additional protection is required; since a very thick and much cornified epithelium would limit flexibility, protection is provided by large, closely spaced, pointed papillae (Fig. 3–7). A small papilla (in ourselves easily found with the tongue tip) carries the opening of the duct of the parotid gland.

Diverticula of the oral vestibule (cheek pouches) occur in certain rodents and monkeys. These pouches have a storage function and enable the animal to harvest its food rapidly, stowing it away for later mastication. They attain a considerable size in hamsters, reaching well onto the thorax; when developed to this degree, the pouches have their own supporting musculature.

The cavity within the dental arcades—the *mouth cavity proper*—is roofed by the palate; bounded laterally by the teeth, gums, and margins of the jaws; and floored by the tongue and the small area of mucosa left uncovered by the tongue. Most of the walls are rigid, and when the mouth is closed the size of the cavity can be altered only by raising or lowering the tongue and floor.

The larger, rostral part of the roof is based on a bony shelf formed of the palatine processes of the incisive, maxillary, and palatine bones and known as the *hard palate* (palatum durum). This is continued caudally, without external demarcation, by the soft palate, in which a connective tissue aponeurosis replaces the bone.

The hard palate is usually flat (though vaulted in ourselves) and is covered by a thick mucosa fashioned into a series of more or less transvere ridges (rugae), which may guide the food backward (Fig. 3–5). In general, they are most prominent, and their covering epithelium most heavily keratinized, in herbivores. A small median swelling, the incisive papilla, is commonly found behind the incisor

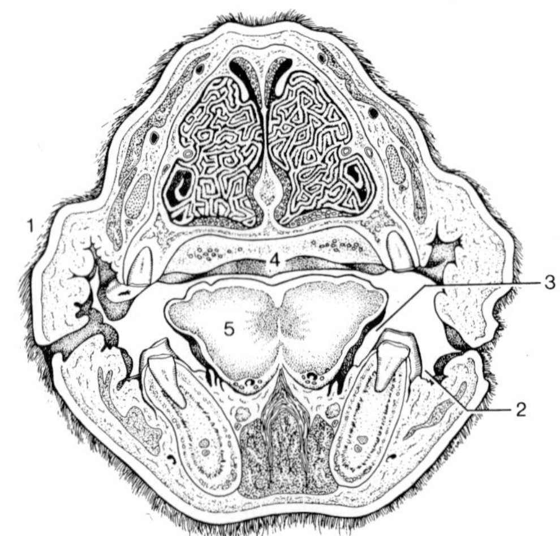


**Figure 3–4.** Transverse section of the head of the dog at the level of $P^2$.

1, Cheek (with buccal folds); 2, vestibule; 3, oral cavity proper; 4, hard palate (with venous plexus); 5, tongue.

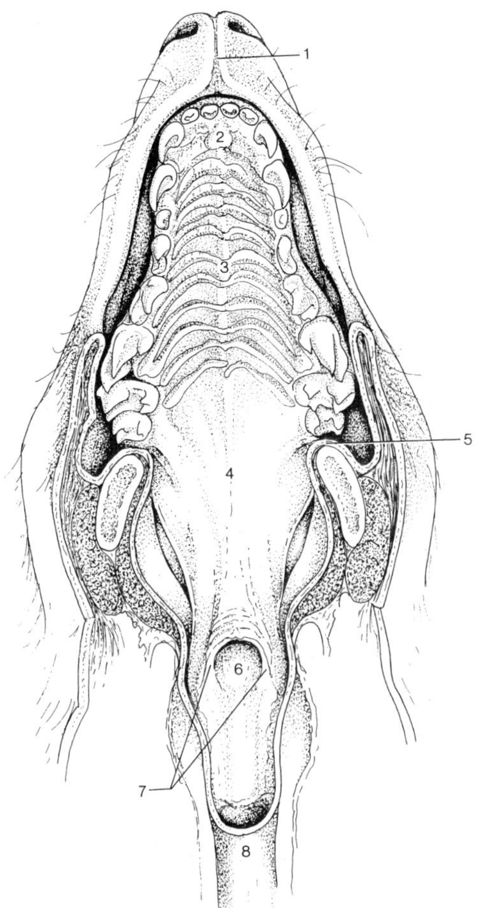


**Figure 3–5.** The hard and soft palate of the dog.

1, Philtrum; 2, incisive papilla; 3, hard palate with rugae; 4, soft palate; 5, palatoglossal arch; 6, intrapharyngeal ostium; 7, palatopharyngeal arches; 8, esophagus.

teeth, flanked by the orifices of small (incisive) ducts that perforate the palate. These ducts branch and lead to the nasal cavity and to the vomeronasal organ (Fig. 3–6). They convey small amounts of the fluid from the mouth for appraisal by the olfactory mucosa of the vomeronasal organ (p. 344).

A striking peculiarity in ruminants is the dental pad, a tough but yielding cushion in the position generally occupied by upper incisor teeth (lacking in these animals); the pad acts as a counterpart to the lower incisors in grazing (Fig. 3–7). A dense, richly vascularized tissue beneath the palatine epithelium functions both as the lamina propria of the mucosa and as the periosteum of the bone, attaching so tightly that not even the most vigorous mastication shifts it. Peripherally, the hard palate blends with the gums, the rather insensitive mucosa along the alveolar margins of the jaws.

The soft palate is described with the pharynx (p. 119).

## The Tongue

The tongue (lingua) occupies the greater part of the oral cavity but also extends into the oropharynx (Fig. 3–8). It has an attached root and body and a free apex and is a highly muscular organ capable of both vigorous and precise movements—as in

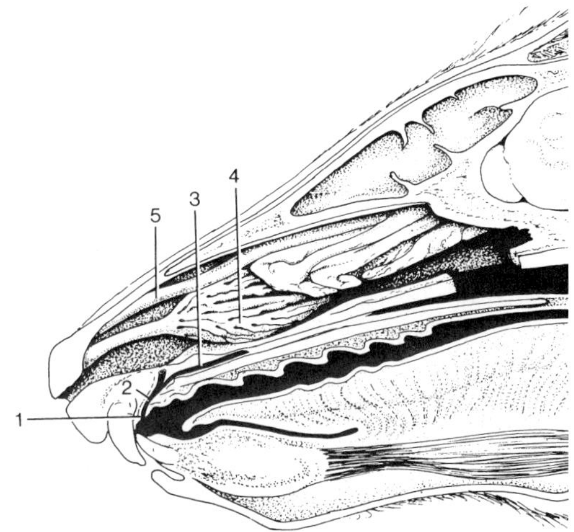


**Figure 3–6.** Paramedian section of the rostral part of the head of the dog. The plane of section fails to demonstrate the opening of the incisive duct into the nasal cavity.

1, Incisive papilla; 2, incisive duct; 3, vomeronasal organ; 4, ventral nasal concha; 5, dorsal nasal concha.

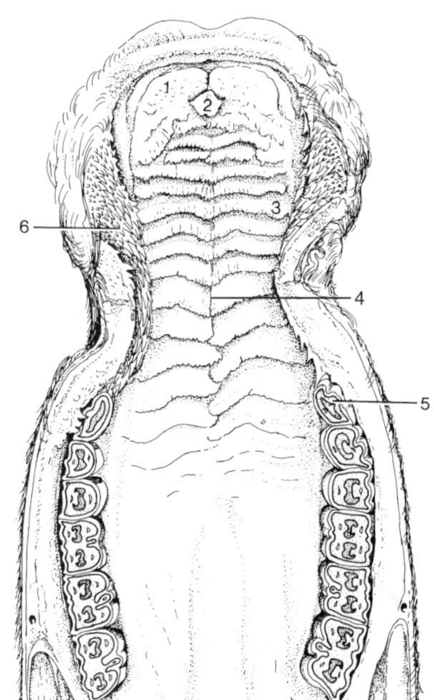


**Figure 3–7.** The hard palate of a cow.

1, Dental pad; 2, incisive papilla; 3, rugae of hard palate; 4, palatine raphe; 5, $P^3$; 6, buccal papillae.

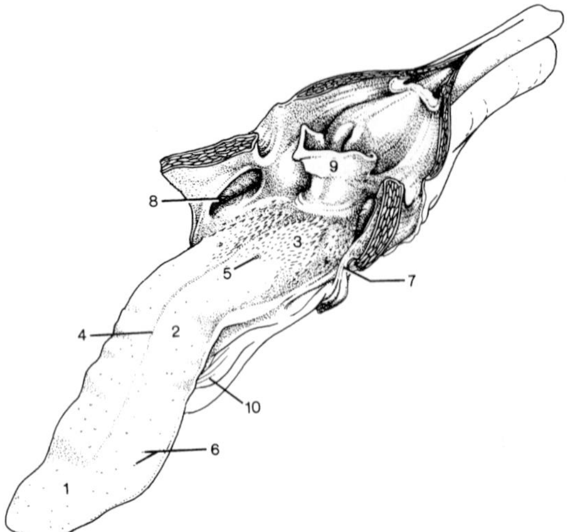


**Figure 3–8.** The tongue of the dog. The soft palate and the esophagus are sectioned in the median plane.

1, Apex; 2, body; 3, root, forming floor of oropharynx; 4, median groove; 5, vallate papilla; 6, fungiform papillae; 7, palatoglossal arch; 8, palatine tonsil in tonsillar fossa; 9, epiglottis; 10, frenulum.

prehension, lapping, grooming, and manipulating the food within the mouth on the one hand and speech articulation on the other. The mobility is achieved by restricting the attachments to the more caudal part, leaving the apex free to roam both within and beyond the mouth. The attachment of the root is to the hyoid bone, that of the body to the symphysial region of the mandible. The tongue is also supported by paired mylohyoideus muscles that sling it between the lower jaws. In the dog especially, the tongue is used to procure heat loss by panting, a process facilitated by the very generous supply of blood and the numerous arteriovenous anastomoses (p. 233).

In general shape, the tongue corresponds to the oral cavity. The apex is dorsoventrally compressed, the succeeding middle portion somewhat triangular in section (being joined to the oral floor by a mucosal fold or frenulum), while the root is uniformly wide to allow entry to the muscles passing forward from the hyoid bone. Mucosal reflections (palatoglossal arches; /7) also pass from each side of the root to join the soft palate; they demarcate the exit from the mouth.

The mucosa is tough and tightly adherent where repeated contact with abrasive food occurs but looser and less heavily keratinized where a softer diet or a more protected position allows. Much of the surface is covered by a variety of papillae. Some, like the soft threadlike (filiform) papillae that are scattered widely over the human tongue, provide additional protection; the harsh conical papillae that make the cat's tongue so efficient a rasp are a larger version of these. Other papillae carry taste buds and have a more restricted distribution, characteristic for each species (Fig. 3–9): their names—fungiform, foliate, and vallate papillae—give good indications of their shapes (Fig. 3–10). A few small salivary glands lie below the epithelium (/6).

The bulk of the tongue consists of muscle, usually divided into intrinsic and extrinsic groups. Four pairs of extrinsic muscles exist (Fig. 3–11). One, the geniohyoideus, lies somewhat apart and passes from the incisive part of the mandible to the

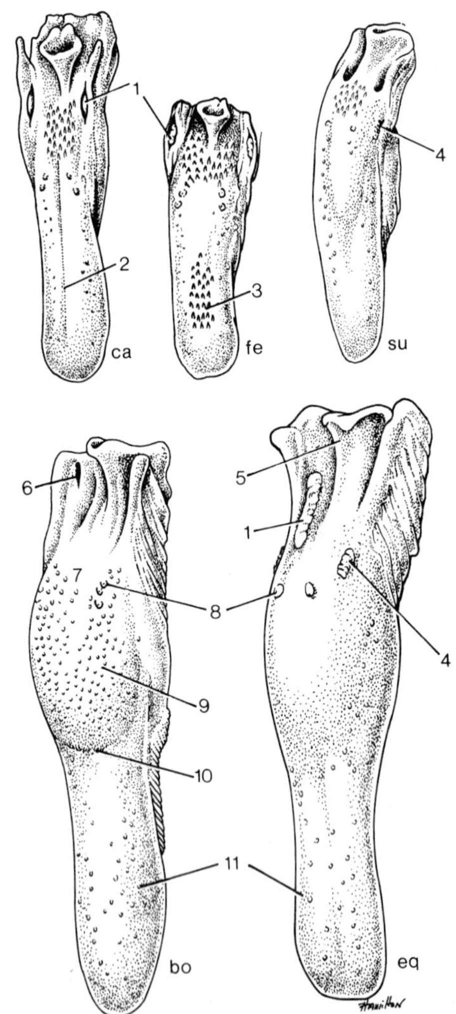


**Figure 3–9.** Dorsal view of the tongue and epiglottis of the dog (ca), cat (fe), pig (su), cattle (bo), and horse (eq).

1, Palatine tonsil; 2, median groove; 3, filiform papillae; 4, foliate papillae; 5, epiglottis; 6, tonsillar sinus; 7, root of tongue; 8, vallate papillae; 9, torus linguae; 10, fossa linguae; 11, fungiform papillae.

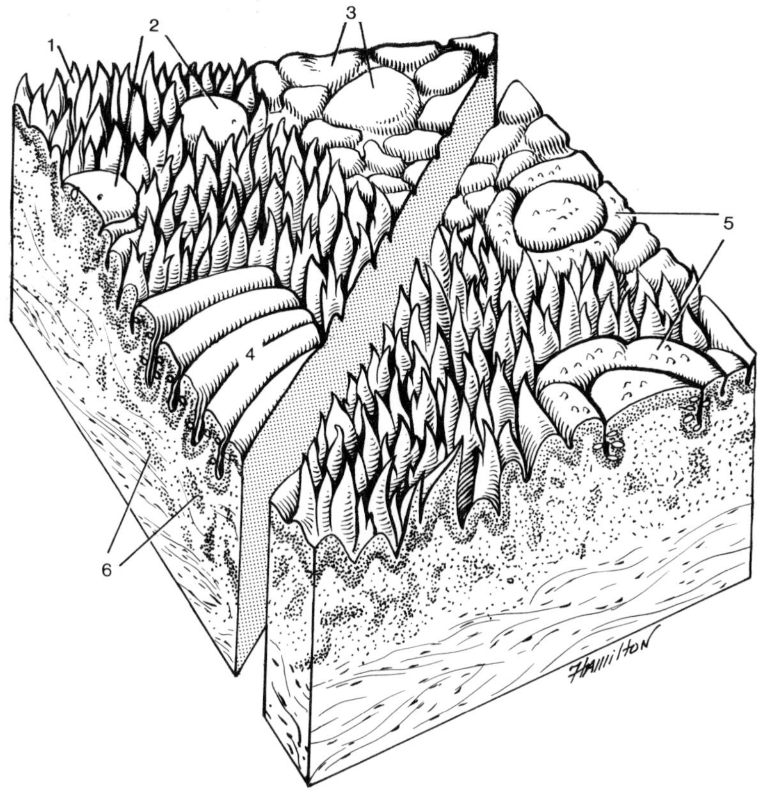


**Figure 3–10.** Blocks of tongue displaying the variety of lingual papillae.

1, Filiform papillae; 2, fungiform papillae; 3, lentiform papillae; 4, foliate papillae; 5, vallate papillae; 6, glands.

body of the hyoid bone; it therefore lies below the tongue rather than within it. It is able to draw the hyoid and thus the tongue forward. The genioglossus arises more dorsally than the geniohyoideus and first runs back below the floor of the mouth before dividing into bundles that fan upward in the sagittal plane. Those bundles that turn forward to the apex of the tongue retract this part; those that pass toward the root draw the whole tongue forward; the middle group passes toward the upper surface (dorsum), which it may depress. The other two muscles arise from the hyoid apparatus. The hyoglossus takes origin from the basihyoid and runs forward, lateral to the genioglossus; the styloglossus takes origin from the stylohyoid, yet farther to the side. Both draw the tongue back but in rather different fashions, the styloglossus tending to elevate it also. The intrinsic muscle is disposed in bundles that run longitudinally, transversely, and vertically (Fig. 4–2). Simultaneous contraction of the transverse and vertical bundles stiffens the tongue.

The muscle bundles are interspersed with considerable amounts of fat, an arrangement that

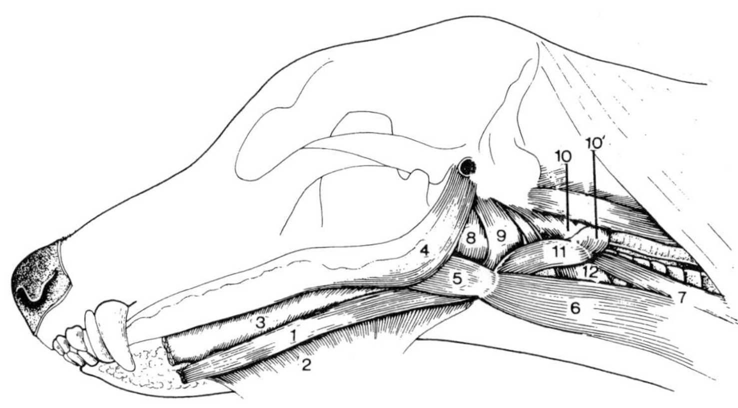


**Figure 3–11.** Muscles of the tongue and pharynx of the dog.

1, Gleniohyoideus; 2, mylohyoideus; 3, genioglossus; 4, styloglossus; 5, hyoglossus; 6, sternohyoideus; 7, sternothyroideus; 8,9, hyopharyngeus (two parts); 10, thyropharyngeus; 10′, cricopharyngeus; 11, thyrohyoideus; 12, cricothyroideus.

imparts a unique consistency and flavor to the cooked tongue. This fat is very resistant to mobilization in starvation.

In the dog, alone among the domestic species, the ventral part of the tongue contains a prominent fibrous condensation, the lyssa, easily recognized on palpation. A fibrous septum that extends from this is responsible for the conspicuous median groove on the upper surface.

The innervation accurately reflects the origin of the tongue as an unpaired swelling of the pharyngeal floor (Fig. 3–57) that is later extended by contributions from the ventral parts of the adjacent pharyngeal (branchial) arches (p. 141). The mucosa retains a sensory innervation from the corresponding arch nerves. The lingual branch of the mandibular nerve is responsible for general sensation over the rostral two thirds of the tongue; the chorda tympani, a branch of the facial nerve, for the special sensation of taste in the same area. Both general and special sensation of the root region are the responsibility of the glossopharyngeal and, to a small extent, the vagus nerves. The extrinsic and intrinsic muscles are all supplied by the hypoglossal nerve, although it is probable that the sensory fibers emanating from spindles and other receptors in these muscles travel mainly in the lingual nerve.

Relatively little of the *floor of the mouth* is left accessible rostral and lateral to the attachments of the tongue. The largest free area lies ventral to the apex, behind the incisor teeth. The mucosa here covers the incisive part of the mandible directly, but elsewhere it lies on muscle and the floor is yielding. The most prominent features are fleshy protuberances or caruncles behind the central incisors; these carry the common openings of the mandibular and major sublingual salivary ducts (Figs. 3–3 and 3–12). In some species, much smaller serial elevations to each side of the frenulum mark the openings of the lesser ducts of the sublingual gland. The mylohyoideus muscle passes below the mucosa and tongue from a linear attachment on the medial aspect of the mandible to meet its fellow of the other side in a median raphe; the two together suspend the tongue in a muscular hammock (Fig. 3–23/4). This muscle is supplied by the mandibular nerve and plays an important part in initiating swallowing (p. 121).

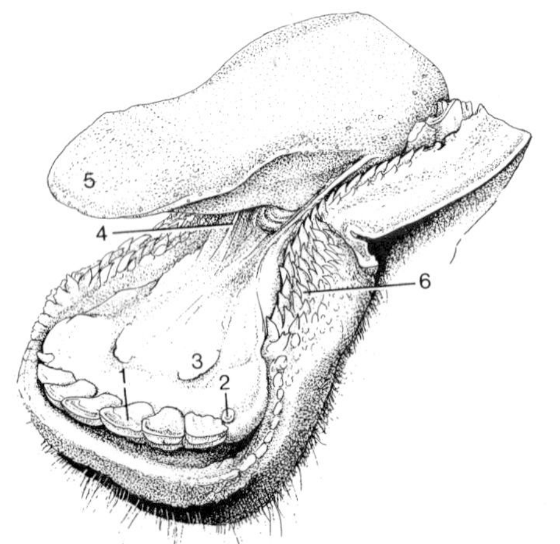


**Figure 3–12.** Floor of the bovine oral cavity and the apex of the tongue.

1, First incisor tooth; 2, fourth incisor (canine) tooth; 3, sublingual caruncle; 4, frenulum; 5, apex; 6, buccal papilla.

## The Salivary Glands

Numerous salivary glands drain into the oral cavity. Their secretion, the saliva, keeps the interior of the mouth moist, and when mixed with food, saliva facilitates mastication; when the food is eventually formed into a bolus for swallowing, the saliva lubricates its passage.

Small salivary glands have been mentioned as features of the lips, cheeks, and tongue; others are present in the soft palate, pharynx, and esophagus. Although individually unimportant, their collective contribution must be considerable. However, most saliva comes from certain larger glands situated at a greater distance from the mouth cavity into which they drain through longer ducts (Fig. 3–13). Unlike the minor glands, which mostly produce a mucous secretion, some of these major glands produce a more watery (serous) fluid containing the enzyme ptyalin, which plays a minor role in carbohydrate digestion.

The *parotid gland,* which is purely serous in most species (though not in the dog), obtains its name from its relationship to the ear, being molded around the ventral part of the auricular cartilage (Fig. 3–14). In the dog it is small and confined to the vicinity of the cartilage. Since the serous parotid secretion is important in moistening and softening food, the gland is larger and the flow more copious in herbivores. In these species the parotid gland extends rostrally onto the masseter muscle, ventrally toward the angle of the jaw, and caudally toward the atlantal fossa. In all species it is enclosed within a fascial covering that sends trabeculae inward to divide the gland into obvious lobules.

The major collecting ducts run within these trabeculae and eventually join to form a single duct that leaves the cranial aspect. In the dog this duct takes the short cut across the lateral surface of the masseter to open into the vestibule of the mouth opposite the fourth upper premolar tooth. In the

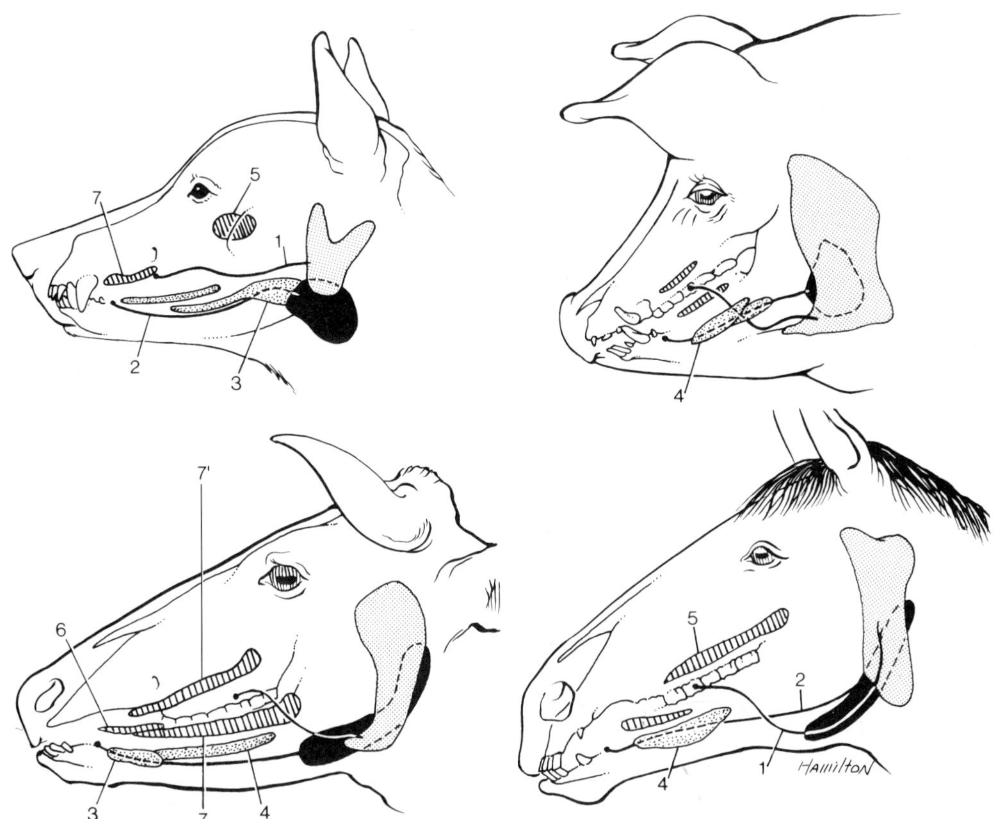


**Figure 3–13.** The major salivary glands of the dog, pig, cattle, and horse. *Gray:* parotid gland; *black:* mandibular gland; *stippled:* sublingual glands; *hatched:* buccal glands.

1, Parotid duct; 2, mandibular duct; 3, compact (monostomatic) part of sublingual gland; 4, diffuse (polystomatic) part of sublingual gland; 5, dorsal buccal glands (zygomatic gland in the dog); 6, middle buccal glands; 7, ventral buccal glands; 7′, dorsal buccal gland.

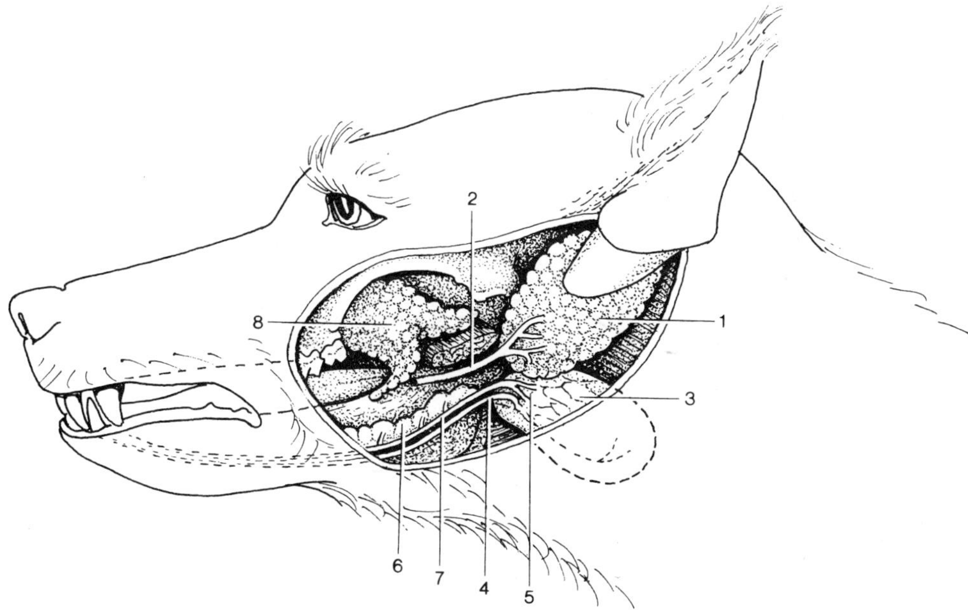


**Figure 3–14.** The salivary glands of the dog.

1, Parotid gland; 2, parotid duct; 3, mandibular gland; 4, mandibular duct; 5, caudal part of compact sublingual gland; 6, rostral part of compact sublingual gland; 7, major sublingual duct; 8, zygomatic gland.

large domestic animals the duct takes the longer but more protected route medial to the angle of the jaw and winds below the mandible to enter the face along the rostral margin of the masseter.

The *mandibular gland* produces a mixed mucous and serous secretion. Generally smaller than the parotid, it is more compact and is placed close to the angle of the jaw. It is a moderately large, very regular ovoid structure in the dog. It too is much larger in herbivores, in which it has a deeper position. This gland also drains by a single large duct that runs ventral to the mucous membrane of the floor of the mouth, close to the frenulum of the tongue, to open on the sublingual caruncle (Fig. 3–12).

The *sublingual gland* is also commonly mixed and sometimes consists of parts—one compact (monostomatic) and draining by a single duct, the other diffuse (polystomatic) and opening by several small ducts. In the dog the compact part fits over the rostral extremity of the mandibular gland, which it appears to continue. The duct that leaves this part runs close to the mandibular duct and discharges alongside this or through a common opening. The diffuse part, the only part present in the horse, is a thin strip lying below the mucosa of the oral floor; its many ducts open beside the frenulum.

The flow of saliva is normally continuous, although the rate is influenced by many factors. It is depressed by anxiety or fear and may be wholly suspended when the body is dehydrated, the resulting dryness of the mouth contributing to the sensation of thirst. It is increased when substances—even if inedible—are introduced into the mouth, although food is most effective, as was demonstrated by the classic experiments of Pavlov. Events indicating that feeding is imminent are also effective. The rate of secretion is controlled by the innervation. The salivary glands receive both sympathetic and parasympathetic supplies, the latter being vastly more important. The parasympathetic fibers come from the two salivatory nuclei of the brainstem and first travel in the facial and glossopharyngeal nerves; later the fibers pass into various branches of the trigeminal nerve that convey them to their destinations. The preganglionic fibers synapse close to the gland, and the postganglionic fibers terminate in direct contact with the secretory cells. Stimulation is followed by copious flow accompanied by vasodilation. Sympathetic stimulation produces vasoconstriction, which slows the rate of production and alters the composition of the saliva.

In addition to its cleansing, lubricant, and digestive functions, saliva serves as a route for the excretion of certain substances, some of which may accumulate as a deposit (tartar) on the teeth.

# THE MASTICATORY APPARATUS

The masticatory apparatus comprises the teeth and gums, the temporomandibular and symphysial joints of the jaws, and the masticatory muscles.

## Dentition

The mammalian *dentition** possesses certain characters that in combination, if not individually, are diagnostic of the class. The complement of teeth is limited to a fairly small number, rarely exceeding 44 in the permanent dentition, which is determined for each species—although minor variations may occur. Unlike those of most other vertebrates, the teeth are very differently developed in different regions of the mouth for better performance of special tasks; this character, known as *heterodonty,* allows the recognition of incisor, canine, premolar, and molar groups. A single replacement of the teeth first erupted is provided by a second, stronger set that is better adapted to the larger jaws and to the more vigorous mastication of the adult. The sequence is known as *diphyodonty* in contrast to the *polyphyodonty* (multiple succession) of most other vertebrates. Finally, the teeth are implanted in sockets set along the margins of the jaws, an arrangement described as *thecodont.*

The number and classification of the teeth in a particular species are conveniently represented by a formula. For the dog, the formula of the permanent dentition may be written

$$\frac{\text{I3-C1-P4-M2}}{\text{I3-C1-P4-M3}} = 42$$

or, more succinctly and no less clearly,

$$\frac{3\text{-}1\text{-}4\text{-}2}{3\text{-}1\text{-}4\text{-}3}$$

The temporary (milk or deciduous) dentition of the same animal may be represented

$$\frac{3\text{-}1\text{-}3}{3\text{-}1\text{-}3}$$

without risk of confusion, since molar teeth are always lacking in the milk set. There are various notations for the identification of individual teeth. According to the most convenient, $P^1$ may stand for the first permanent upper premolar, $i_2$ for the

*Terms relating to the teeth, for example dentine, periodontium, orthodontics, etc., are derived from the Latin *(dens)* or the Greek *(odous).*

secondary temporary lower incisor, and so forth, precision being achieved by the use of upper and lower case letters and superscript and subscript numerals.

The term *diastema* is used for a considerable gap between teeth in the one jaw, most usually for that between the incisors and premolars.

The *description of a simple tooth* may be considered before returning to the features of the different types of teeth. A tooth (dens) consists of crown and root, easily distinguished since the crown is encased in enamel, a very resistant, calcified, slightly opalescent, white material; and the root in cement, a softer, less shiny, yellowish tissue. The part of the tooth between root and crown is termed the *neck* (Fig. 3–15). Certain variations in structure may occur at the neck; the cement and enamel commonly abut, but the cement may overlie the enamel, while sometimes the two tissues fail to meet, exposing a narrow strip of dentine, the third calcified tissue of the tooth. The dentine, which is also known as ivory, provides the greater part of the substance of the tooth and contains a small central cavity that houses the connective tissue pulp. The pulp continues through a canal in the root of the tooth to merge with the connective tissue in the depth of the tooth socket (alveolus).

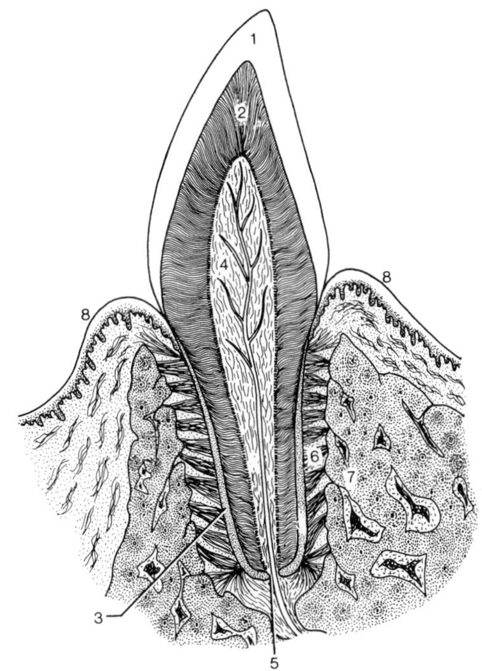


**Figure 3–15.** Schematic longitudinal section of a simple tooth.

1, Enamel; 2, dentine; 3, cement; 4, pulp; 5, apical foramen; 6, periodontal ligament; 7, socket (alveolus); 8, gum.

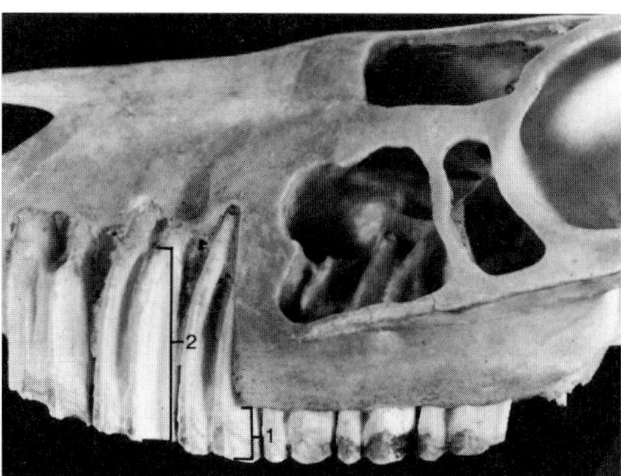


**Figure 3–16.** Premolar teeth exposed in the upper jaw of a horse. The part protruding above the gum is the clinical crown (1); the whole enamel-covered part is the anatomical crown or body (2) of the tooth.

Figure 3–15 depicts the idealized condition in which the gum (gingiva) embraces the neck and the crown corresponds to the exposed part of the tooth. The gums may recede with advancing age, exposing the cervical part of the root, a condition familiar in many older people who are said, on this account, to be "long in the tooth." The opposite condition, in which part of the enamel-covered crown is concealed below the gum line, occurs in many mammals; in some a large portion of the crown is initially held in reserve to be extruded gradually in compensation for the attrition at the masticatory surface. Such high-crowned teeth are said to be hypsodont (or hypseledont) and are characteristic of herbivores, which feed on abrasive food. Even in species such as primates or dogs with low-crowned (brachydont) teeth, suited to a softer diet producing less wear, it is common for part of the enamel-covered region to lie below the gum when the tooth first comes into use. For these reasons it is useful to distinguish the "clinical crown" from the anatomical crown, the first term specifyng the exposed part of the tooth regardless of its structure, and the second the enamel-covered part regardless of its location (Fig. 3–16).

The detailed description of the crown requires some system for indicating its various surfaces. The usual terms of relative position are inadequate for this purpose, since the curved line followed by the tooth row (arcade) alters the orientation of equivalent surfaces of successive teeth in the series. Less ambiguous terms are vestibular (labial, buccal) and lingual, and mesial and distal; their usage is indicated in Figure 3–20. Where adjacent teeth touch, the appropriate mesial and distal surfaces may both be termed contact surfaces. The working area, if extensive and not a mere cutting edge, is known as the occlusal or masticatory surface.

*Enamel* is a densely calcified tissue of ectodermal origin. It is acellular and therefore unable to react to injury—it cannot regenerate to patch a hole or repair a fracture. Since it is exposed to rough treatment, it is necessarily very hard, indeed uniquely so for a biological material. Despite this, the enamel casing may eventually be breached, exposing the softer dentine that wears away more rapidly. The thickness and the resistance of the enamel therefore largely determine the working life of the brachydont tooth. In species in which the tooth crown is high and only gradually passed above the gum line, the enamel may be folded in a very complicated fashion; this increases the efficiency of the masticatory surface, since the unequal resistance of the tissues exposed on opening the enamel casing results in an irregular ridged arrangement (Figs. 3–21 and 18–19).

*Cement* is the least hard of the calcified tissues of the tooth and resembles bone in structure, though lacking so regular an organization. The initial deposit over the root is thin but as deposition continues throughout life it may eventually form quite a thick crust. Collagen fibers extend from the cement into the periodontal ligament or membrane (periodontium), the specialized connective tissue that fastens the tooth in its socket. Although broadly comparable to bone in structure and development, cement differs in one important respect; it is relatively immune to pressure erosion. Orthodontists make use of this characteristic when they adjust the position of a tooth in the jaw by fitting an appliance that presses the tooth against the alveolar wall. If correctly adjusted, the pressure produces an erosion of the bone but leaves the tooth unaffected and free to shift into the space created. This lack of response to pressure is relative, not absolute, and excessive pressure causes resorption; indeed, the roots of the temporary teeth are resorbed under pressure from their permanent replacements thrusting against them.

*Dentine* is also similar to bone in having a calcified, collagen-rich matrix. In bone the osteoblasts become imprisoned in the matrix, but the dentine-producing cells (odontoblasts) recede from the newly formed dentine and remain as a continuous layer on the surface lining the dental (pulp) cavity. The odontoblasts retain their productive capacity throughout life, and a slow but continuous production of secondary dentine, with corresponding reduction of the dental cavity, continues into old age. This process may be accelerated when local damage or abrasion of the crown threatens to expose the pulp. Secondary dentine is easily recognized by its darker color. Although once disputed, it is generally believed that fine nerve processes enter a short distance into the dentine from the pulp.

The *dental cavity* reflects the external form of the tooth, sending a branch into each major elevation of the crown and through a narrow passage in the root where it opens at the apical foramen; when more than one root is present, each contains a channel that joins the central cavity.

The *pulp* that fills this space is a very delicate connective tissue margined by the odontoblast layer and richly vascularized. A lymphatic plexus also exists, although this is difficult to demonstrate. Numerous nerves run within the pulp; some are vasomotor, although most are sensory and possess endings that can be stimulated in various ways. Whatever the stimulus—thermal, mechanical, or chemical—the sensation perceived is pain; as the pulp is contained within unyielding walls, even a slight inflammatory swelling is quickly appreciated.

Each tooth is implanted in a separate socket in the margin of a jaw. The form of the socket corresponds to that of the root and is therefore often branched and irregular. Where the teeth lie close together the septa between adjacent sockets may be very delicate or even defective. Typically, the socket is lined by a thin lamina of compact bone perforated for the passage of the vessels and nerves that supply both the socket and the tooth. The outer surface of the lamina may be braced by trabeculae of spongy bone extending toward the surface of the jaw or radiating into surrounding parts; where the alveolar margin is narrow, however, the lamina merges with the external compacta of the jaw. The tooth is attached to the socket by means of the tough fibrous periodontal ligament. This is particularly rich in collagen fibers that attach to both the cement and the alveolar bone and are so oriented that the tooth is suspended in a sling; masticatory forces that tend to drive the tooth deeper into the socket are thus transformed into tension on the socket wall. The arrangement allows the tooth a certain though usually very limited mobility, and slight rotation and tilting are normal during mastication.

The vessels and nerves that supply the teeth are derived from the major trunks (superior and inferior alveolar arteries, veins, and nerves) that course through canals in the jaws.

Tooth *eruption* is a complicated and controversial process involving a number of factors—root growth, bone growth, pulpal proliferation, tissue pressure, and periodontal traction. Their relative importance is disputed but the last factor is probably the most significant. The temporary teeth rise in the jaws after the crown is completed but before the root is formed; this process carries the tooth closer to the surface and provides the space necessary for the formation of the root. The movement of the crown is facilitated by a loosening of the connective tissue of the dental follicle (p. 142) and gum and by the presence of remnants of the epithelium of the dental lamina, which define the line of passage. However, if these remnants are large and cystic, as sometimes happens, they may obstruct rather than facilitate the movement of the tooth and divert it from its true path, giving rise to troublesome anomalies of site and spacing. The retention of an epithelial covering over the unerupted crown ensures that no breach of continuity occurs when the tooth breaks through to the surface, as this remnant of the enamel organ fuses with the epithelium of the gums embracing the tooth (Fig. 3–17).

The eruption of the permanent teeth is more complicated. These develop in bony crypts deep to the roots of the equivalent teeth of the temporary set. To erupt they must escape from this confinement and displace their predecessors. The erosion of the roof and the continous adjustment of the walls of the embedded alveolus involve the usual processes of bone remodeling, and it is hardly too fanciful to say that the permanent tooth and its alveolus migrate as a unit through the jaw to enter the alveolus of the temporary tooth. The replacement tooth then presses on the root of the temporary tooth, causing its resorption. The attachment of the temporary tooth is loosened, allowing it to shift and become increasingly mobile during mastication; it is soon shed, and the permanent tooth then rises in its place. Proper eruption of the permanent tooth depends on the temporary teeth holding places ready for them; if the latter are prematurely lost, the filling of the alveoli by bone may make it difficult for the permanent teeth to establish their proper occlusal relationships.

The *dentition of the dog,* although relatively simple, is well adapted to the feeding habits of the animal (Fig. 3–18). The incisor teeth are small and peglike and are crowded together in the rostral part of each jaw. On eruption, each upper incisor presents a trilobed crown with a labial cutting edge. The lower incisors are bilobed. These features are lost as wear reduces the tooth to a simple prismatic peg. The name "incisor" suggests that these teeth are used for dividing food before it is taken into the mouth, but in this species a second and more efficient shear is provided by teeth farther back in the mouth, and the incisors are employed mainly in nibbling and grooming.

The *canine teeth* are particularly well developed, so much so that the generic name *(Canis)* for doglike animals provides the term by which these teeth are known in all mammals. Canines are large, curved, and laterally compressed teeth of simple form and are capable of inflicting a deep wound; they are used for aggressive and holding purposes. A large part of each canine tooth is implanted in the jaw; the extent and position of the embedded part of the upper canine are revealed by a bony ridge over the alveolus.

The premolar and molar teeth together constitute the "cheek teeth," a term more common and more useful in descriptions of the dentition of herbivorous species, in which the two groups have become assimilated to each other in form and function. In all mammals the first few (maximally four) cheek teeth are represented in both dentitions

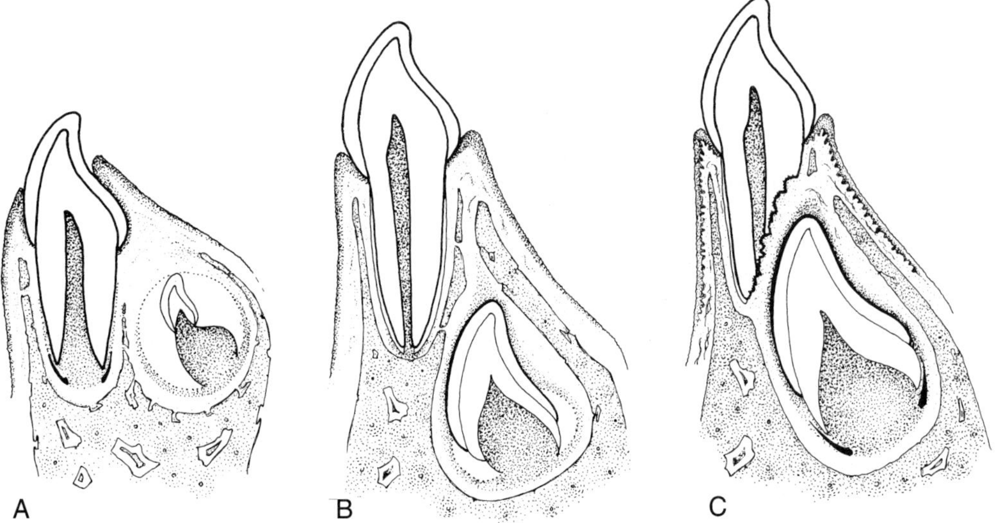


**Figure 3–17.** Schematic drawings representing tooth eruption and replacement. *A,* Eruption of a deciduous tooth. The primordium of the permanent tooth is located on the lingual side of the deciduous tooth. *B,* The fully developed deciduous tooth within a bony alveolus. The crown of the permanent tooth has already formed. *C,* The permanent tooth is ready to break through. The root of the deciduous tooth has been resorbed, formation of the root of the permanent tooth is in progress.

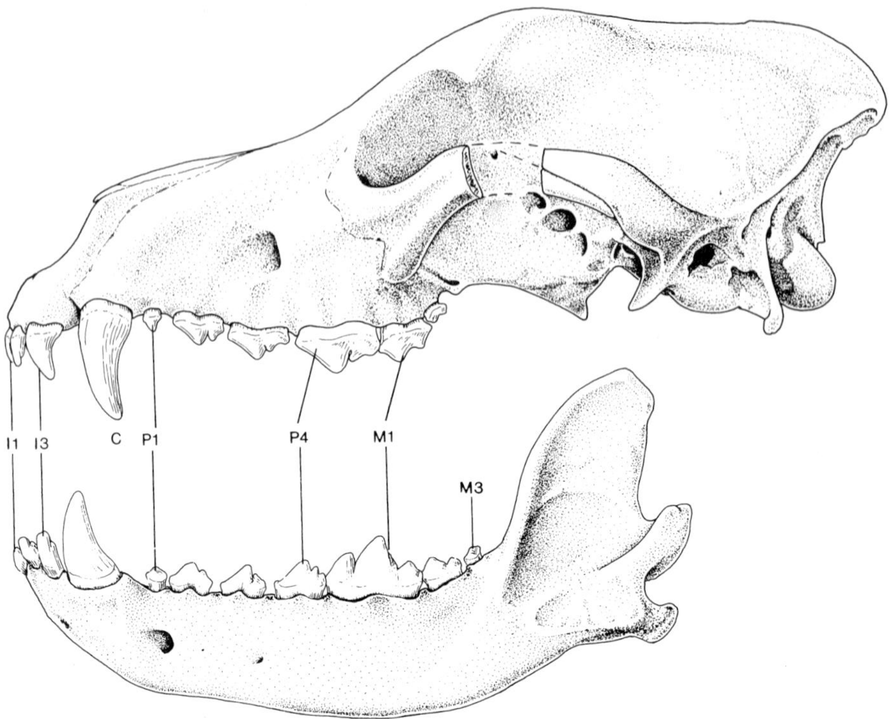


**Figure 3–18.** Lateral view of the permanent dentition of the dog.

and are assigned to the premolar group; the remainder (maximally three) are represented only in the permanent dentition and are known as molar teeth. The *premolars* of the dog form an irregular but fairly closely spaced series of increasing size and complexity. The cusps or projections of the individual crowns are aligned one behind the other to form a discontinuous serrated cutting edge rather resembling that of the pinking shears of a dressmaker and effective for the same reason—the elongation of the blade makes possible a more rapid and cleaner division while the notches help hold the food in place. The more caudal *molars* also possess a cutting potential but are principally developed for crushing and are distinguished by their broader and more extensive masticatory surfaces. The cusps or elevations that they carry are arranged in a pattern that is faithfully reproduced on the teeth of all members of the species; their homologues can be recognized, although sometimes only with great difficulty, in the teeth of other mammals.

Most of the cheek teeth, unlike the incisors and canines, have more than one root. Multiple roots, especially if divergent, provide firmer anchorage but make extraction difficult, if not impossible, without previous division of the crown into portions corersponding to the individual roots.

The *dentition of the cat* is reduced to

$$\frac{3\text{-}1\text{-}3\text{-}1}{3\text{-}1\text{-}2\text{-}1}$$

in the permanent set (Fig. 3–19). It is even more closely adapted to a fleshy diet, as the reduction of the molar series has largely eliminated the crushing potential presented by the dog's dentition. The cutting action of the cat's cheek teeth earns them the description *secodont;* the dual-purpose structure of the dog's molars is better described as tuberculosectorial. The incisors of cats are remarkably small and the canine teeth relatively large.

In other domestic species, the diet is much more abrasive and requires considerably more crushing and grinding. The dentition is modified accordingly. The details are presented in the later chapters, and here it is sufficient to note only the most conspicuous features.

In the *dentition of the pig* the broad crowns of the cheek teeth carry an elaborate formation of blunt cusps that make them very effective crushing instruments; teeth of this sort are said to be *bunodont* (Fig. 3–20). The canine teeth of this species remain open at the embedded end (root) so that accretion of dental tissues continues throughout the animal's life. This persistent growth, coupled with their curved form, allows them to assume very striking forms in older individuals, particularly in boars.

The other species are more restricted to a herbivorous diet than the omnivorous pig, and the *dentition of horses and ruminants* must allow for continuous and considerable wear at the masticatory surfaces. This requirement is met by the enlargement of these surfaces, by the increase in height of the crowns, which are only gradually extruded (the delayed development of the roots allows growth to continue for some years after the teeth have come into wear), and, above all, by complicated folding of the enamel. This folding has two important consequences. It increases the amount of the hardest and most durable component of the tooth that is exposed and so reduces the rate of attrition. It provides an alternation of harder and softer materials, which, wearing at different rates, produces an unevenness of the masticatory surface that gives it a rasplike quality (Figs. 3–21 and 3–22).

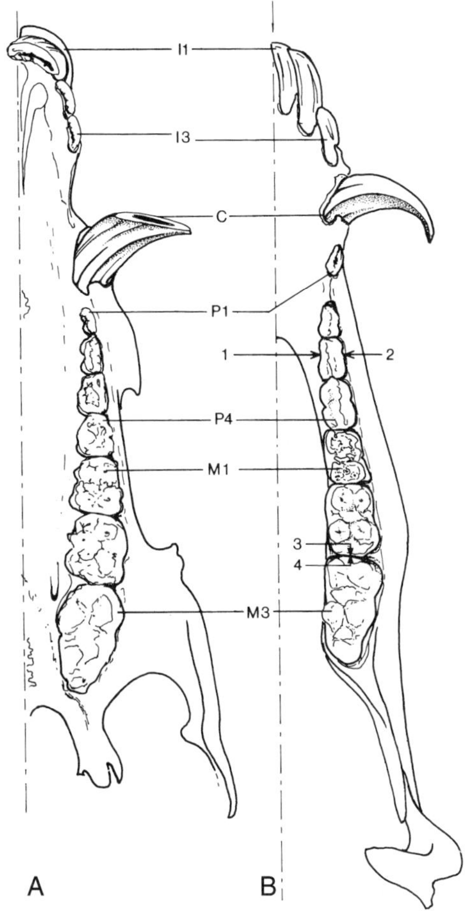


**Figure 3–20.** Permanent dentition of the pig; upper *(A)* and lower *(B)* jaws.

1, Lingual surface; 2, vestibular surface; 3, distal surface; 4, mesial surface.

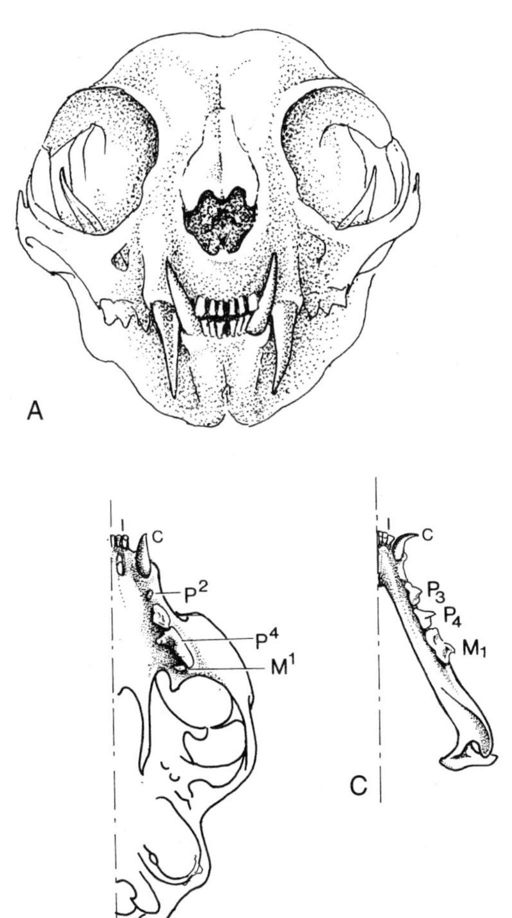


**Figure 3–19.** Permanent dentition of the cat. *A,* Rostral view. *B,* Upper jaw. *C,* Lower jaw.

## The Articulations of the Jaws

Although it is customary to describe two *temporomandibular joints,* these may be regarded as the widely separated halves of a single condylar joint (p. 21). Clearly, movement at one side must be accompanied by a movement, not necessarily identical, at the other side.

The articular surfaces are provided by the head, carried on a dorsal process of the ramus of the mandible, and the mandibular fossa of the skull, a facet mainly formed by the squamous temporal bone, though sometimes extending beyond it. The forms of the two surfaces reflect the feeding habits,

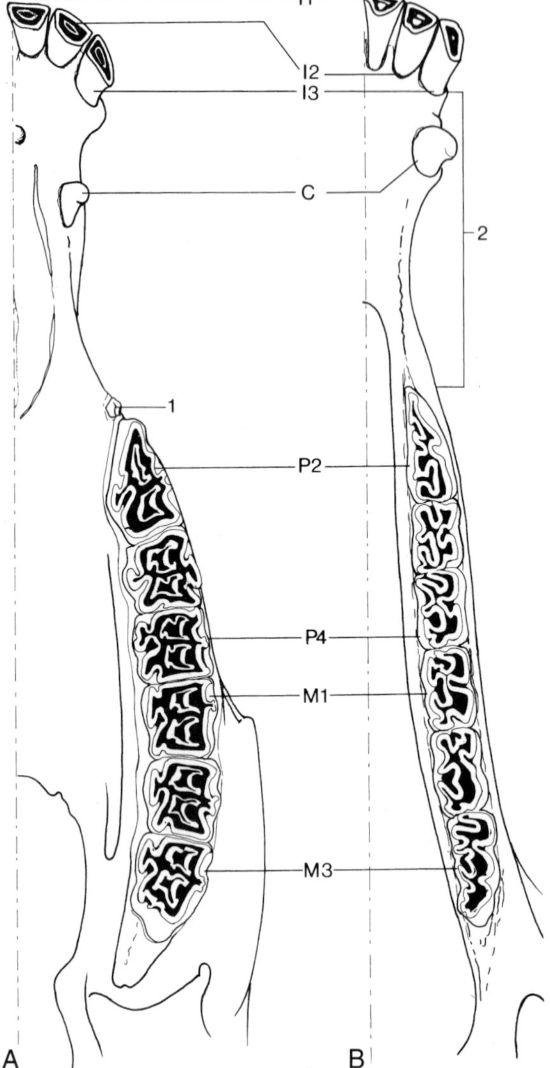


**Figure 3–21.** Permanent dentition of the horse; upper *(A)* and lower *(B)* jaws.

1, Wolf tooth ($P^1$); 2, diastema.

and in species such as the dog, in which hingelike movements of the lower jaw predominate, the head takes the form of a transverse condyle to which the fossa provides a corresponding gutter. Backward dislocation of the jaw is opposed by the prominent retroarticular process placed directly behind the mandibular fossa. A peculiarity of the joint is the presence of a fibrous or fibrocartilaginous articular disc that divides the cavity into upper and lower compartments. Although the phylogenetic origin of this structure is disputed, its functional significance may lie in its resolving the complex movements of the joint into simpler components; a hinge movement occurs between the mandible and the disc, while gross sliding movements (translations) of the mandible relative to the skull occur at the upper level. It is perhaps because the movements of the dog's jaw are so simple that the disc is rather thin and poorly developed in this species. In species in which lateral grinding movements predominate, the mandibular head is larger, the surface more plateau-like, and the disc thicker, although the details differ considerably.

In most species the two halves of the mandible are firmly fused together, but in the dog (and in ruminants) they articulate by means of a *symphysis,* providing a third joint. This much neglected joint allows small movements that may be important in securing more precise adjustment of the upper and lower tooth rows and therefore a more effective cutting or crushing mechanism. Two types of movement appear to be possible—a spreading movement, altering the angle between the two halves of the mandible, and one in which each half rotates about its own long axis so that the tooth cusps alter their inclination to the vertical. The dog appears to make use of these possibilities when adjusting the position of a bone between the teeth before attempting to crack it.

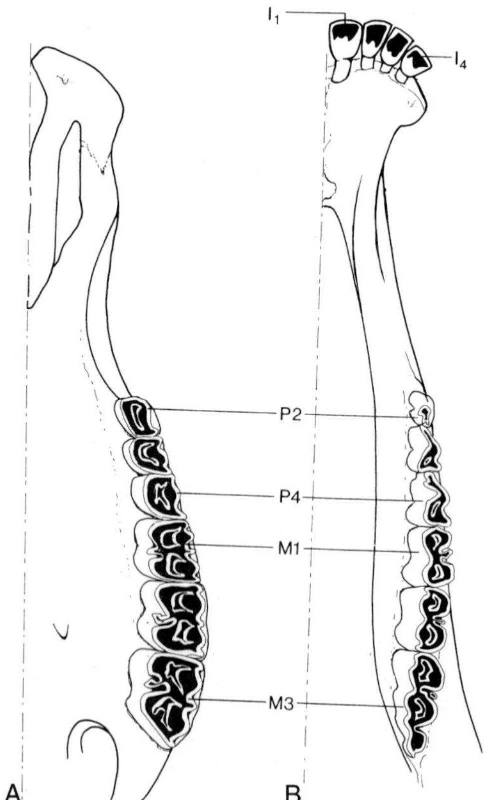


**Figure 3–22.** Permanent dentition of cattle; upper *(A)* and lower *(B)* jaws.

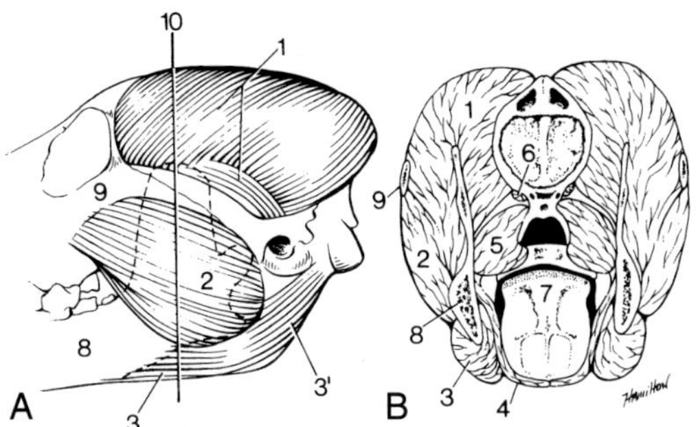


**Figure 3–23.** The muscles of mastication of the dog; left lateral aspect *(A)*, in section *(B)*.

1, Temporalis; 2, masseter; 3, 3′, rostral and caudal bellies of digastricus; 4, mylohyoideus; 5, medial pterygoid; 6, origin of lateral pterygoid; 7, tongue; 8, mandible; 9, zygomatic arch; 10, level of transection *(B)*.

## The Muscles of Mastication

The muscles that provide the masticatory forces are derived from the first pharyngeal arch, and in keeping with this, they are supplied by the mandibular nerve. They comprise the temporalis, masseter, pterygoideus medialis, and pterygoideus lateralis (Fig. 3–23). Other muscles that play some part in jaw movements, particularly in opening the mouth, are not normally included under the term "muscles of mastication."

The *temporalis* arises from an extensive area of the lateral surface of the cranium and converges to an insertion on the coronoid process of the mandible. On contraction the resultant force pulls the mandible upward, and the muscle is especially large in those species, such as the dog and cat, in which the chief jaw movement is scissor-like; a measure of its development is provided by the salience of the zygomatic arch—a well-sprung arch provides more room for this muscle. Although the main action is to raise the mandible, some fibers tend to draw it forward, others to pull the condyle against the retroarticular process.

The *masseter* lies lateral to the mandible. It takes its origin from the maxillary region of the skull and the zygomatic arch and has a wide insertion on the more caudal part of the mandible. It is frequently a multipennate muscle intersected by strong tendon plates. The fibers in the different strata do not all run parallel; different parts may have contrasting functions. Some may protrude the mandible, and others may retract it, but the general effect is to raise the mandible and draw it toward the active side, for mastication is restricted to one side at a time in domestic species. The masseter muscle is therefore rather small in the dog; it is proportionately better developed in herbivorous species that make lateral and rotational movements when chewing.

The *pterygoid* mass of muscle lies medial to the mandible and passes to this bone from the pterygopalatine region of the skull. Generally the mass is clearly divided into a small lateral and a larger medial muscle. Some fibers of the lateral pterygoid muscle attach to the articular disc and help to control its movements, but the principal function of the mass is to raise the mandible and draw it inward with some simultaneous protrusion. In species in which transverse movements are important the masseter and contralateral pterygoid muscles may form a functional pair.

Opening the mouth is assisted by gravity, but certain muscles are also available for the performance of this movement. The *digastricus* passes from the skull, caudal to the temporomandibular joint, to the ventral margin of the mandible and opens the mouth. The muscle consists of two parts arranged in tandem. The rostral portion is supplied by the mandibular nerve, the caudal portion by the facial, an indication that the muscle has a composite origin in the mesoderm of the first two pharyngeal arches. In species in which the sternocephalicus has a mandibular attachment it may open the mouth.

In most mammals the mouth is held closed at rest with the mandible supported by the tonic activity of the masticatory muscles, possibly assisted by the hermetic seal created by the application of the dorsum of the tongue to the palate. The jaws are symmetrically placed in relation to the median plane, and the upper and lower tooth rows are slightly separated or in gentle, interrupted contact. The arcade formed by the upper teeth is generally wider than its counterpart, and the tooth rows are superimposed for only part of their widths. In some species, such as the rat, simultaneous occlusion is impossible in both incisor and molar regions; in them, the lower jaw must be advanced and dropped to bring the incisor tips together, and withdrawn and raised for molar contact; such animals generally favor an intermediate position of the lower jaw at rest.

A slight increase in muscular activity brings the teeth into the more extensive contact known as centric occlusion. The relationships between the teeth in this position are variable, even in the same individual at different ages since the teeth come together in altered fashion as wear reduces the more salient projections (and in some species also by migration of teeth within the jaws). It is usual to find that each cheek tooth engages with two teeth of the opposite series, the lower teeth generally being a little mesial to their upper counterparts. In the dog, the largest teeth, the last upper premolar and the first lower molar, bite together and constitute the sectorial (or carnassial) teeth, the principal shear (Fig. 3–18). The teeth in front of the sectorials do not meet but leave open a carrying space, while the last cheek teeth make extensive contact. The lower canine engages in front of the upper canine, filling the space between this and the third incisor.

The relationship between the teeth is a dynamic one as is readily seen from the so frequently defective human dentition. A tooth deprived of normal support may drift under the influence of the masticatory forces; the pressures exerted by the lips, cheek, and tongue are also important in maintaining normal contact and alignment. It is evident from developmental studies that these associations are established before eruption and that common factors control the growth of the two jaws and the development of the teeth so that a harmonious relationship normally exists at all stages of development. But anomalies are not uncommon, and the "undershot" and "overshot" jaw are well illustrated by Bulldogs and by many Afghan Hounds.

The simplest activity that is common to all species, regardless of their masticatory habits, is the gaping that occurs on depression of the lower jaw. Gaping is achieved by slackening or cessation of activity in the masticatory muscles, by contraction of their antagonists, and by gravity. As the jaw is lowered the mandibular head rolls on the articular disc while the disc itself slides forward in the mandibular fossa, probably assisted by those lateral pterygoid fibers that attach to it. Closure of the mouth requires the reversal of these processes and must at times be vigorous enough to detach a morsel. Sometimes, the detachment is achieved by the incisors, and in certain species the hinge movement is complicated by a preliminary protrusion of the lower jaw to bring the incisor edges into alignment. When the cheek teeth are employed in biting, the action is unilateral. Herbivores employ the cheek teeth for grinding food already taken into the mouth, and the active (closing) movement is preceded by lateral displacement. The temporomandibular joint of these animals is situated high above the occlusal plane, and the lower teeth are drawn forward over their upper fellows as they approach. This contributes a grinding component that is absent when the joint and occlusal surfaces are more nearly level. The sheep and dog, typical examples of herbivore and carnivore, illustrate these differences in the position of the joint in relation to the teeth (Fig. 3–24).

## THE PHARYNX AND SOFT PALATE

The pharynx lies behind the mouth and continues into the esophagus. It is a funnel-shaped chamber contained between the base of the skull and first couple of cervical vertebrae dorsally, the larynx ventrally, and the pterygoid muscles, the mandible, and the dorsal part of the hyoid apparatus laterally. Since it communicates freely with other cavities in the head, it is rather difficult to form a clear conception of its boundaries and extent; a first impression may be obtained from Figures 3–25, 3–31, and 4–2. Figure 3–27 illustrates the crossing of the air and food pathways and is a reminder that the pharynx possesses a respiratory as well as an alimentary function.

The key to understanding the pharynx is provided by the soft palate, already encountered as the continuation of the hard palate beyond the choanal margin. In repose the soft palate lies on the tongue, but when the animal swallows, the soft palate is raised into a more horizontal position and then more obviously divides the pharynx into dorsal and ventral parts. Two pairs of arches connect the soft palate to adjacent structures. The caudal pair, the palatopharyngeal arches, pass onto the lateral wall of the pharynx and may be long enough to meet above the entrance to the esophagus (Fig. 3–25). Together with the free margin of the palate they circumscribe the constriction of the lumen—the intrapharyngeal ostium—that marks the separation of the pharynx into dorsal and ventral compartments. The dorsal compartment is known as the nasopharynx. The more rostral palatoglossal arches pass onto the sides of the tongue at its root; they demarcate the passage from the mouth to the oropharynx (Fig. 3–3). The oropharynx is somewhat arbitrarily divided from the

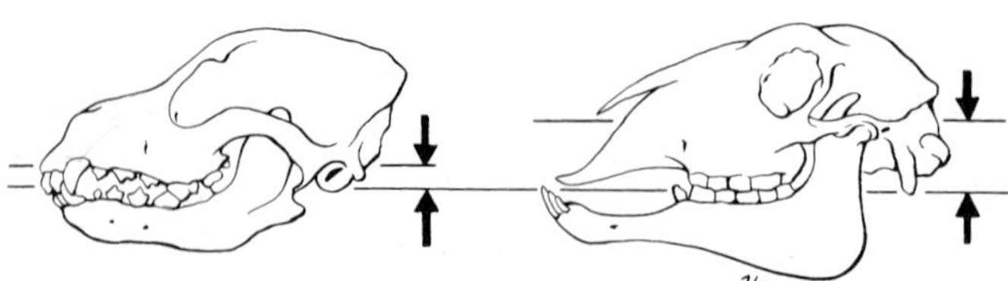


**Figure 3–24.** The relationships of the articular and occlusal surfaces in the dog and sheep (indicated by the upper and lower arrows, respectively).

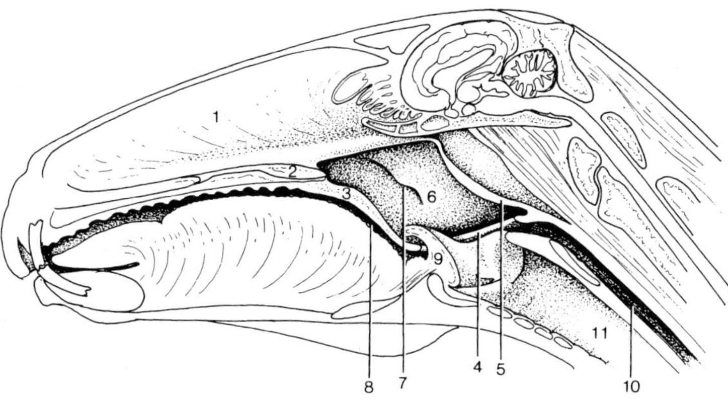


**Figure 3–25.** Paramedian section through the equine head.

1, Nasal septum; 2, hard palate; 3, soft palate; 4, palatopharyngeal arch; 5, roof of nasopharynx; 6, nasopharynx; 7, entrance to auditory tube; 8, oropharynx; 9, epiglottis; 10, esophagus; 11, trachea.

third subdivision, the laryngopharynx, at the level of the epiglottis. The laryngopharynx lies above the larynx and corresponds with this in extent.

Functional considerations suggest that the *nasopharynx* could well be regarded as a part of the nasal cavity. Food does not enter it, and it takes no part in the swallowing process but serves passively to convey air. The topography of the connection with the nasal cavity varies much among species; a single ductlike communication is present in the dog. In addition to the major connections, the nasopharynx communicates with the cavities of the middle ears through the auditory (Eustachian) tubes. The paired tubal openings are placed on the summits of small pimple-like elevations in the dog. Small muscle bundles radiate over the pharyngeal wall from the opening and provide a mechanism for dilating the orifice, thus allowing air to pass to or from the middle ear so that the pressure on the two sides of the eardrum may be equalized. Much of the wall of the nasopharynx is reduced to a thin mucosa that finds support by attaching to neighboring structures, mainly the base of the skull and the ventral straight muscles of the head. The mucosa possesses a typical respiratory epithelium and contains numerous mucous glands and much lymphoid tissue, some scattered, some in masses; the lymphoid masses that form elevations visible to the naked eye are known as the pharyngeal tonsils (adenoids in ourselves) and form part of the ring of lymphoid tissue that guards the passage from the nose and mouth to the pharynx and beyond (Fig. 3–26); like other lymphoid developments they are larger in infancy than later. Excessively enlarged tonsils impair the airflow.

The narrowness of the *oropharynx* limits the size of the morsels that can be swallowed. Its lateral walls are supported by a fascia and are the site of the palatine tonsils. These are very differently arranged in different species; in some (e.g., horse) they are diffuse (though raised slightly), whereas in others they constitute a compact mass that may project away from or toward the lumen, as in the ox and dog, respectively (Fig. 3–26). Tonsils that project into the lumen are overlain by flaps of mucosa that partly hide them from inspection through the open mouth (Fig. 3–8/8; Plate 16/*E*).

The *laryngopharynx* is the largest part of the pharynx. It is wide in front but narrows before joining the esophagus at a boundary that is well defined by a mucosal fold in the dog but more difficult to recognize in most other species. At rest, the lumen of the caudal part of the laryngopharynx is closed by the apposition of the lateral walls and roof to the floor. The floor is largely occupied by the entrance to the larynx, which presents the epiglottis, the arytenoid cartilages, and the aryepiglottic folds. The epiglottis serves as a breakwater to deflect fluids to the side, into gutters (piriform recesses) that run beside the projection of the larynx (Fig. 3–27).

Below an external fascia, the greater part of the pharyngeal wall is covered by a set of striated muscles. These fall into three groups—constrictor, dilator, and shortener—although no individual muscle has an action quite so simple as these terms suggest (Fig. 3–28). The constrictor muscles arise from certain fixed points conveniently placed to each side and run onto the roof of the pharynx; with their fellows they form a series of arches that enclose the lumen on its lateral and dorsal aspects. For most purposes it is sufficient to recognize rostral, middle, and caudal constrictor muscles, although each may be divided into lesser units. The rostral constrictor arises from the pterygoid region of the skull (pterygopharyngeus) and the aponeurosis of the soft palate (palatopharyngeus) and embraces the pharynx at the level of the palatopharyngeal arch; many fibers take an almost longitudinal course and thus also assist in shortening the pharynx, drawing it onto and over a bolus received

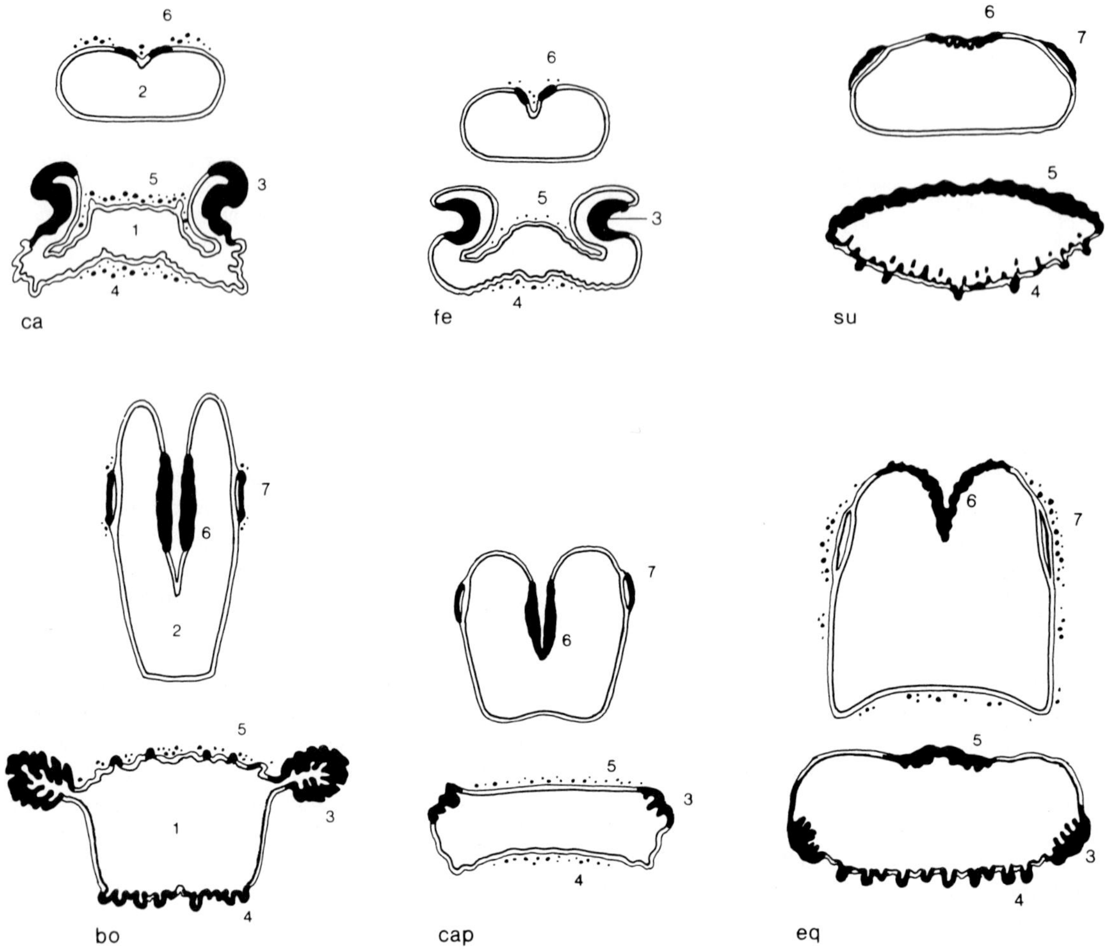

**Figure 3–26.** Tonsils in the wall of oro- and nasopharynx; ca, dog; fe, cat; su, pig; bo, cattle; cap, goat; eq, horse.

1, Oropharynx; 2, nasopharynx; 3, palatine tonsil; 4, lingual tonsil; 5, tonsil of the soft palate; 6, pharyngeal tonsil; 7, tubal tonsil.

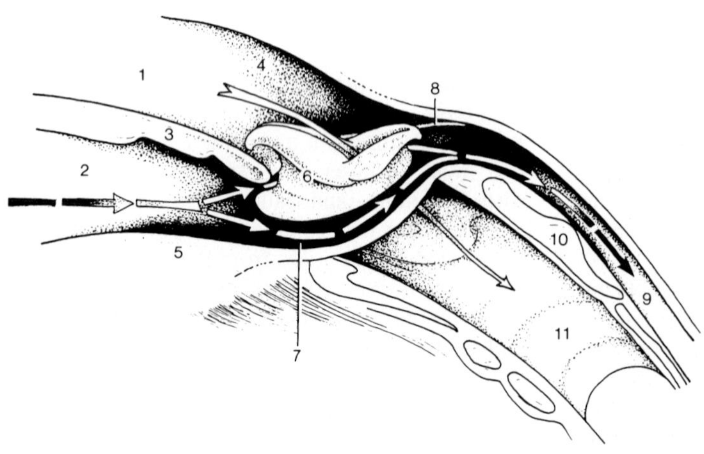


**Figure 3–27.** Schematic drawing of the pharynx showing its rostral connection with the nasal and oral cavities and caudal connection with the esophagus and larynx.

1, Nasal cavity; 2, oral cavity; 3, soft palate; 4, nasopharynx; 5, root of tongue; 6, larynx (protruding through pharyngeal floor); 7, laryngopharynx (piriform recess); 8, caudal end of palatopharyngeal arch; 9, esophagus; 10, lamina of cricoid cartilage; 11, trachea.

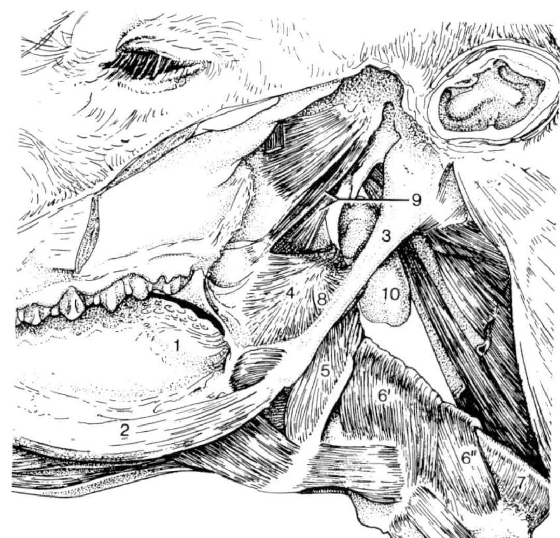


**Figure 3–28.** Lateral view of the connection of the pharynx with the base of the bovine skull.

1, Root of tongue; 2, styloglossus; 3, stylohyoid; 4, rostral pharyngeal constrictor; 5, middle pharyngeal constrictor; 6, caudal pharyngeal constrictor (6′, thyropharyngeus, 6″, cricopharyngeus); 7, esophagus; 8, pharyngeal dilator (stylopharyngeus caudalis); 9, tensor and levator veli palatini; 10, medial retropharyngeal lymph node.

from the mouth. The middle constrictor (hyopharyngeus) arises from neighboring parts of the hyoid bone. The caudal constrictor arises in two parts, from the thyroid (thyropharyngeus) and cricoid (cricopharyngeus) cartilages. When the three constrictors contract in succession they hurry the bolus distally into the esophagus. The dilator muscle (stylopharyngeus caudalis) also arises from the hyoid apparatus but runs more transversely to fan out in the pharyngeal wall; when active it widens the rostral part of the pharynx, enabling it to accept the bolus more easily.

A fibroelastic aponeurosis internal to the muscles supports the mucosa. It also provides a median raphe to which many fibers of the paired muscles insert and which, continuing to the skull, serves to fix the whole organ in position. The mucous membrane of the oral and laryngeal parts of the pharynx is covered by a stratified squamous epithelium and possesses many small salivary glands that provide additional lubrication to the passage of food.

The *soft palate* (velum palatinum) is bounded by a respiratory mucosa on its dorsal surface and an oral mucosa ventrally. It is braced by a stout aponeurosis below the dorsal mucosa; the part ventral to the aponeurosis mainly consists of close-packed salivary glands, interrupted toward the midline by the longitudinally disposed palatinus muscle, which shortens the palate. Two small muscles that arise from the muscular process of the temporal bone insert into the lateral part of the aponeurosis after following slightly different courses. As their names indicate, one muscle (tensor veli palatini) tenses the soft palate by exerting lateral traction; the other (levator veli palatini) raises the soft palate. The mucous membrane of the pharynx and soft palate and the muscles, except the tensor, which is supplied by the mandibular nerve, obtain their innervation from a plexus to which the vagus makes the chief, the glossopharyngeal nerve a minor, contribution.

## THE ESOPHAGUS

The esophagus (or gullet) conveys food from the pharynx to the stomach. This relatively narrow tube begins dorsal to the cricoid cartilage of the larynx and follows the trachea down the neck, at first inclining to the left but regaining a median position above the trachea before or shortly after entering the thorax (Fig. 3–29). Within the thorax it runs in the mediastinum (p. 158) and, continuing beyond the tracheal bifurcation, it passes over the heart before penetrating the esophageal hiatus of the diaphragm. It then makes its way over the dorsal border of the liver to join the stomach at the

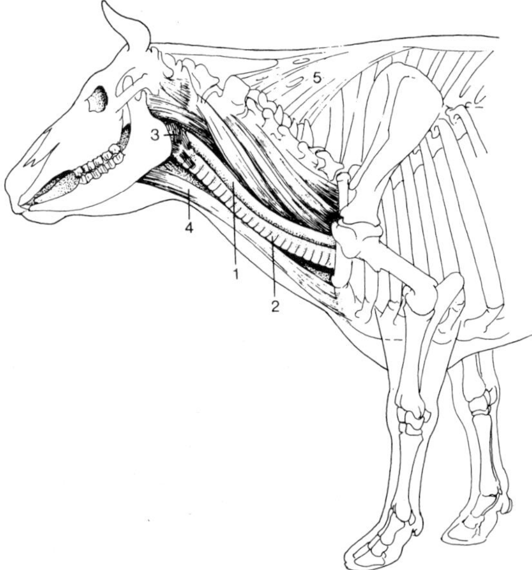


**Figure 3–29.** Lateral view of the bovine neck. In midneck the esophagus lies on the left dorsolateral aspect of the trachea.

1, Esophagus; 2, trachea; 3, pharyngeal musculature; 4, sternocephalicus muscle; 5, nuchal ligament.

cardia. It thus consists of cervical, thoracic, and abdominal portions, although the last is very short.

Only a few of the more important features of its topography are mentioned here. The cervical part runs within the visceral space of the neck, related to the subvertebral muscles dorsally and the left side of the trachea medioventrally (Fig. 3–29). For much of its length it is accompanied by the left common carotid artery and vagosympathetic and recurrent laryngeal nerves.

The thoracic part crosses to the right of the aortic arch, which may deflect it from its sagittal course; more caudally its dorsal and ventral borders are followed by the trunks into which the fibers of the right and left vagus nerves are regrouped.

The structure of the esophagus conforms to a pattern that is common to the remainder of the alimentary canal. The outer coat is a loose connective tissue (adventitia) in the neck, but this is largely replaced by serosa* in the thorax and abdomen. The muscle is striated at the origin of the esophagus, but in some species (e.g., cat, pig, and horse) the striated muscle is replaced by smooth muscle at some point within the thorax (Plate 1/*F,G*). It is usual to describe two muscle strata; both are spiral and they wind in opposite directions in the first part of the esophagus; closer to the stomach the outer coat becomes more longitudinal and the inner one more circular (Fig. 3–30). The arrangement is quite complicated in detail and reveals considerable interlacing of muscle bundles that exchange between the two layers. Although morphological evidence for their existence is unconvincing, a number of sphincters are suggested by functional studies. They include a cranial sphincter, probably provided by fibers of the cricopharyngeus muscle, and possibly others within the thorax, where the passage of food tends to be delayed. A thickening suggestive of a sphincter occurs at the junction of the esophagus with the stomach, although the flow of food is more obviously impeded at a slightly more cranial level, immediately in front of the diaphragm. However, no anatomical evidence exists for a prediaphragmatic sphincter.

The inner part of the wall is divided between submucosa and mucosa by a fenestrated muscularis mucosae, usually more prominent in the thoracic esophagus (Plate 1/*G*); it helps throw the lining of the empty organ into longitudinal folds.

*Most organs contained within the body cavities (divisions of the embryonic celom) are protected by "serous membranes" (serosae). These coverings, which extend to line the walls of the body cavities, consist of a layer of flat mesothelial cells supported by a delicate connective tissue. A small amount of watery (serous) fluid keeps the membranes moist and minimizes friction when opposing surfaces move against each other.

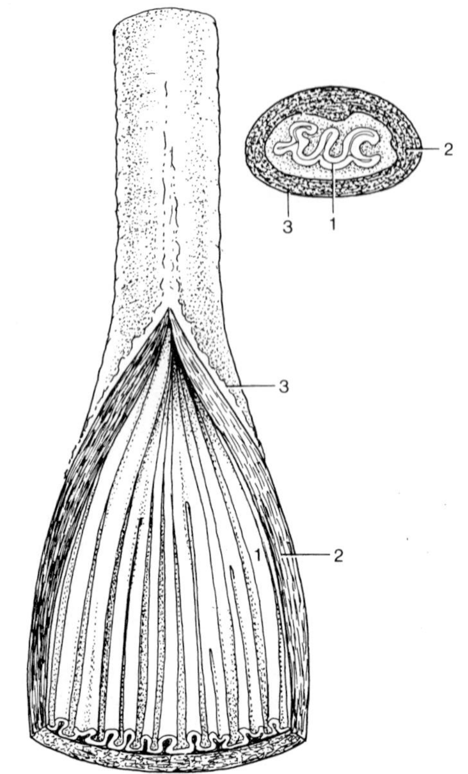


**Figure 3–30.** Semischematic drawing of the structure of the esophagus, sectioned longitudinally and transversely.

1, Mucosa; 2, muscular layer (longitudinal and circular); 3, adventitia.

The surface epithelium is generally stratified squamous, with the degree of keratinization reflecting the relative harshness of a species' habitual diet. This is nicely illustrated by comparing the esophageal epithelium of the dog (Plate 1/*F*) with the thicker epithelium of the goat, which has a much rougher diet (Plate 1/*G*). Another striking difference between these species is provided by the many mucus-secreting tubuloacinar glands present in the submucosa of the canine esophagus. The boundary between esophageal and gastric epithelia is sharp and may be displaced to either side of the cardia. In humans, prolonged or repeated exposure to gastric juice (e.g., heartburn) may provoke transformation of the stratified epithelium of the lower esophagus into the columnar gastric variety.

The esophagus receives its innervation from the sympathetic and vagus nerves, including the recurrent laryngeal branches. The vagal supply is the more important. The striated muscle arises from the mesoderm of the pharyngeal arches and is under control of the general visceral motor neurons of the vagus, whereas the smooth muscle portions are under direct control of the intrinsic nervous system and indirect control of the autonomic nervous system. A myenteric plexus extends the length of the esophagus.

The blood supply from various local arteries presents no features of special interest.

## DEGLUTITION

The first stage of deglutition (swallowing; Fig. 3–31/*B*) is a voluntary act, but once the food has left the mouth its progress is not under control of the will.

Food that has been sufficiently prepared by mastication and insalivation is collected in a recess formed by cupping the dorsal surface of the tongue and then isolated by pressing the apex of the tongue against the palate. The jaws are closed and brisk contraction of the mylohyoid, hyoglossal, and styloglossal muscles raises the tongue and impels the bolus into the oropharynx. Inevitably the food touches the pharyngeal mucosa, and this contact initiates the reflex that completes the act. The afferent nerves include branches of the mandibular, glossopharyngeal, and vagal trunks. As the food passes caudally, the soft palate is raised and its free margin drawn toward the dorsocaudal pharyngeal wall. Closure of the intrapharyngeal ostium prevents dissipation of the pressure generated in the mouth and ensures that the food is carried toward the esophagus by denying escape into the nasopharynx. This stage is accompanied by brief inhibition of breathing, with the glottis closed. The hyoid apparatus and the larynx are simultaneously drawn forward, and the epiglottis, meeting the tongue, is tilted back to provide some cover to the laryngeal entrance; however, no question of it fitting into the opening (as often assumed) exists, and it is known that surgical resection of most of the human epiglottis does not seriously impair swallowing efficiency. The food passes over the epiglottis, or to the side of this, with the impetus maintained by the coordinated successive and rapid contraction of the constrictor muscles. The pharynx, which was dilated for reception of the bolus by the caudal stylopharyngeus muscle, is then shortened and in effect drawn onto and over the bolus by the longitudinal fibers of the constrictor muscles. The caudal end of the pharynx relaxes to receive the food, which is then hastened through the esophagus by a wave of peristalsis that commences just distal to the cricopharyngeal fibers. This last movement is probably coordinated by a local reflex, unlike the preceding events which are controlled by a deglutition center in the brainstem.

Fluid is swallowed in essentially the same way. It passes mainly through the piriform recesses, and the initial impetus may be sufficient to project it well into the esophagus.

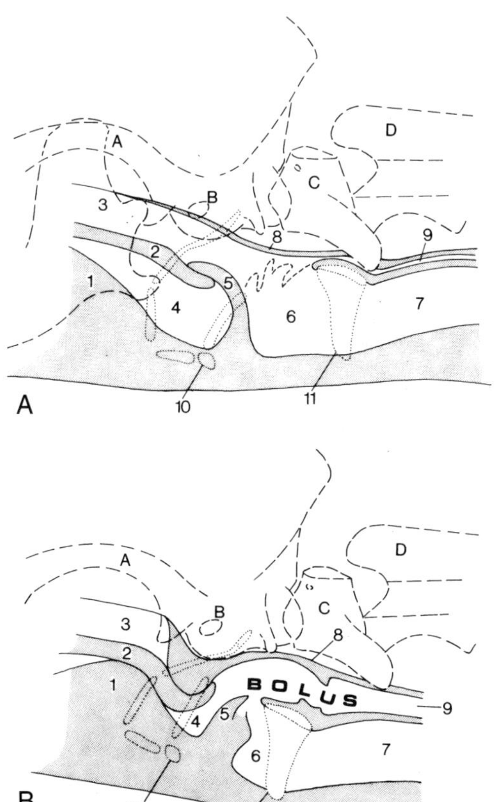


**Figure 3-31.** Pharynx of the dog. *A*, Nose breathing. *B*, Swallowing. (Drawn from radiographs.)

A, Zygomatic arch; B, external acoustic meatus; C, atlas; D, axis. 1, Tongue; 2, soft palate; 3, nasopharynx; 4, oropharynx; 5, epiglottis; 6, larynx; 7, trachea; 8, roof of nasopharynx; 9, esophagus; 10, basihyoid; 11, cricoid cartilage.

## THE ABDOMINAL CAVITY

Some general observations concerning the abdominal cavity are necessary before continuing the description of the digestive system.

The abdomen is the portion of the trunk that lies caudal to the diaphragm (p. 32). It contains the largest of the body cavities, which is continuous at a plane passing through the sacral promontory and the pubic brim with the more caudal and very much smaller pelvic cavity (see Fig. 2–2). The more cranial (intrathoracic) part of the abdominal cavity is protected by the hindmost ribs and costal cartilages and is rather restricted in the variations in size that it may experience; the more caudal part is supported by the skeleton only on its dorsal aspect and is therefore more variable. The pelvic cavity has the most extensive bony support and the most constant size, although even here a certain latitude is allowed by changes in the soft tissue components of its walls (p. 208).

The structure of the abdominal and pelvic walls has been described with the locomotor apparatus. Comparative features, including conformation and the factors that influence this in different species are considered in later chapters. The abdominal and pelvic cavities contain the peritoneal sac; the stomach, small and large intestine, and associated liver and pancreas; the spleen; the kidneys, ureters, bladder, and urethra (in part); the ovaries and most of the reproductive system in the female, a smaller part of the reproductive tract in the male; the adrenal glands; and many nerves, blood vessels, and lymph nodes and vessels.

## Peritoneal Structures

An incision through the whole thickness of the abdominal wall enters the peritoneal cavity, a division of the celom that is bounded by a delicate serous membrane, the peritoneum. The *peritoneal cavity* is completely enclosed in the male, but in the female a potential communication with the exterior exists at the abdominal opening of each uterine tube. The peritoneal cavity contains only a small amount of serous fluid, since the abdominal organs are excluded from the space by their peritoneal covering. Nonetheless, it is common to designate as intraperitoneal those organs that are suspended from the abdominal roof within the peritoneal reflections. Although misleading, the term is useful in emphasizing the difference between this and the alternative retroperitoneal arrangement of other organs that are directly joined to the abdominal wall. A diagram (Fig. 3–32) may make the distinction plain. The same diagram illustrates the division of the peritoneum into a parietal part lining the walls (parietes), a visceral part directly enshrouding the organs (viscera), and a series of double folds connecting the parietal to the visceral parts. These folds are often collectively known as mesenteries, but properly this term is restricted to the fold suspending the small intestine (and more specifically only the jejunum and ileum); certain similar folds are conveniently named mesocolon, mesovarium, and so on, according to the organ that they support; others, for example, the greater omentum, have names less immediately revealing.

A small outpouching (infracardiac bursa) of the parietal peritoneum extends a little way into the mediastinum within the thorax along the right face of the esophagus where this penetrates the diaphragm.

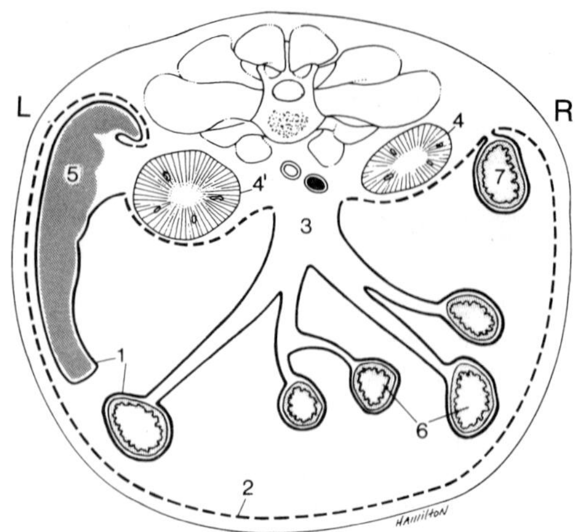


**Figure 3–32.** Schematic transverse section through the abdomen of the dog.

1, Visceral peritoneum *(continuous line)*; 2, parietal peritoneum *(broken line)*; 3, root of mesentery; 4, 4′, right and left kidneys (retroperitoneal); 5, spleen; 6, jejunum; 7, descending duodenum.

The *peritoneum* consists of a single layer of flattened mesothelial cells supported by a fibroelastic tissue that attaches, more or less firmly according to position, to the underlying structures. A considerable amount of fat is often stored below the peritoneum, with some locations especially favored. In the healthy animal the peritoneal cavity is reduced to a series of clefts between the closely packed abdominal organs. Most clefts are of capillary dimensions, and the total volume of the peritoneal fluid is therefore small—a few milliliters in a dog. The fluid is nonetheless of vital importance, for it lubricates the viscera, allowing them to slip freely over each other or against the abdominal wall in the performance of their own functions or when displaced by other activities. The fluid is constantly turned over, although the mechanism of resorption is disputed. Whatever its nature, the large surface area (2 $m^2$ in humans) of the peritoneum aids rapid removal, and drugs are sometimes administered by intraperitoneal injection. Toxins are also readily absorbed and, since the warm and moist peritoneal cavity affords ideal conditions for bacterial growth, inflammation of the peritoneum is never regarded lightly.

Inflamed serous sheets have a tendency to stick together, and in the course of time these adhesions may become organized and permanent. For this reason the surgeon often turns in the edges of the wound, bringing serosal surfaces together, when closing an incision. Adhesion between organs that are normally free to move over each other is a possible and undesirable sequel to infection or trauma of the peritoneum. Clearly, any attachment that limits mobility may interfere with normal function. However, it must also be noted that adhesion of apposed serosal surfaces (with the obliteration of the intervening space) is commonplace in development and explains the definitive position and arrangement of many organs and mesenteries.

In early development the gastrointestinal tract pursues a sagittal course through the body cavity. It is attached along its whole length to the roof of the embryonic trunk by a primitive dorsal "mesentery," but only a portion of the foregut (that which becomes the stomach and first part of the duodenum) and a short caudal portion of the hindgut have similar ventral attachments. The parts of the dorsal mesentery associated with the differentiating organs are assigned appropriate names and may be listed in succession—(dorsal) mesogastrium, mesoduodenum, mesojejunum, mesoileum, mesocolon, and mesorectum. The ventral connection to the stomach is known as the ventral mesogastrium. The mesojejunum and mesoileum together constitute the (great) mesentery of adult anatomy. Most portions of the dorsal mesentery persist in more or less unmodified form (at least in the dog) but the mesogastria have a more complicated fate dictated by the later development of the stomach.

The dorsal mesogastrium becomes drawn out and folded on itself during development and is then known as the greater omentum. The folding creates a pouch, the omental bursa, enclosing a portion of the peritoneal cavity. However, the pouch is flattened and its walls brought into close contact so that the cavity is potential, not actual. The greater omentum of the dog is turned caudally between the viscera and the abdominal floor, and its walls are described as parietal (ventral) and visceral (dorsal) because of their relationship to abdominal wall and viscera. It is the first structure to appear when the abdominal floor is opened. The later growth of the liver reduces access to the interior of the bursa to a narrow opening, the epiploic (omental) foramen, through which the cavity of the omental bursa remains in open, if restricted, communication with the major part of the peritoneal cavity. The main features of the arrangement are shown in Figures 3–33 and 3–60. The differential growth and the secondary attachments that determine the adult arrangement vary considerably between species, and those details that possess a practical importance are mentioned in context. In most species the greater omentum is lacelike, an effect produced by the deposition of fat in strands along the course of the blood vessels; in ruminants so much fat may be present that the omentum appears to consist entirely of this tissue. The omentum has no intrinsic capacity for movement but is liable to be shifted about the abdomen by the movements of other structures. Since it possesses the common tendency of serous membranes to adhere when inflamed, it is often found attached in regions of infection and helps to wall these off. The surgeon may stitch the greater omentum over a closed incision of a viscus as an extra insurance against leakage.

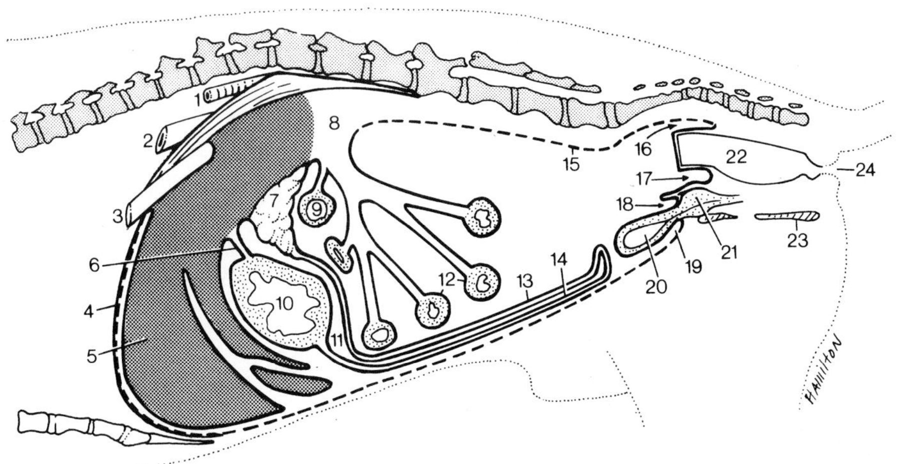


**Figure 3–33.** Paramedian section of the abdominal cavity of a dog to show the dispostion of the peritoneum (schematic).

1, Aorta; 2, esophagus; 3, caudal vena cava; 4, diaphragm; 5, liver; 6, lesser omentum; 7, pancreas; 8, root of mesentery; 9, transverse colon; 10, stomach; 11, omental bursa; 12, small intestine; 13, deep wall of greater omentum; 14, superficial wall of greater omentum; 15, parietal peritoneum; 16, pararectal fossa; 17, rectogenital pouch; 18, vesicogenital pouch; 19, pubovesical pouch; 20, bladder; 21, prostate; 22, rectum; 23, ischium; 24, anus.

The no less complicated arrangement of peritoneal folds that develop—mainly in the pelvic cavity—in association with the urogenital organs is best described with these organs (p. 181).

## Visceral Topography

The general disposition of the viscera is determined by the form of the cavity in which they are retained; their detailed arrangement is influenced by individual features of attachment, motility, and distention. Since the peritoneal cavity is hermetically sealed and most abdominal contents are incompressible, it follows that any change in the position or contours of one organ must be followed by adjustment of the abdominal wall or by a reciprocal change in a neighboring organ. In this way a quite trivial change in one organ may set in motion a chain reaction extending into all parts of the abdomen. The weight of the abdominal contents is considerable, especially in the larger herbivores. They "float" within the serous fluid, and the gravitational forces are opposed by the tension actively and passively developed by the structures of the abdominal wall, by the cranial pull on the diaphragm exerted by the negative pressure within the thorax and, to a lesser and uncertain extent, by the mesenteries and vessels that support particular organs.

The essence of the situation can be conveyed schematically (Fig. 3–34). It is seen that the internal pressure varies at different heights within the abdomen; it is less than the ambient pressure in the most dorsal part, equal to this at one particular level, and increasingly greater than this toward the abdominal floor. This explains the concavity of the upper part of the flank and also the tendency for air to rush into the rectum when exploration of this part is clumsily performed. Clearly, the local internal pressures also vary with respiratory changes in intrathoracic pressure and with posture.

The significance of the mesenteries and other attachments in determining visceral topography is disputed. Some of the more robust attachments—for example, those between the liver and the diaphragm—anchor organs quite firmly; others are too frail to play a significant role, and the organs to which they attach must be held in place by mutual contact and by the "lift" of the diaphragm. Certainly, they drop as soon as air is introduced into the peritoneal cavity. The potbellied appearance familiar in many older people is alleged to be in part a consequence of the loss of elasticity in the lungs with resulting reduction of the diaphragmatic "pull." Some of the arteries that branch from the aorta to supply abdominal organs possess an unusually thick adventitia, and this may allow them to bear some weight when the enclosing mesenteries are fully stretched.

In the dead animal the viscera commonly conform to a fixed pattern; if allowance is made for such obvious factors as the recent consumption of a meal, a tolerably accurate forecast of their disposition can be made before the abdomen is opened, although this introduces air and hence some sagging is inevitable. Therefore, good reason once existed for believing that each of the hollow organs possessed a fairly constant "normal" form. The introduction of radiography in the early years of last century threw doubt on, and broadening use destroyed, this comfortable illusion—though not before many patients had their organs "tailored"to fit the preconceptions of surgeons reared on traditional anatomy. Unfortunately, the awareness among veterinary students of the incessant alterations in size and conformation, and therefore also in position and relation, of the abdominal organs is still insufficient. It can hardly be stressed too strongly that detailed assertions of "normal" form and position have no place in the description of the hollow organs.

When describing the positions of the abdominal organs it is often sufficient to relate them to

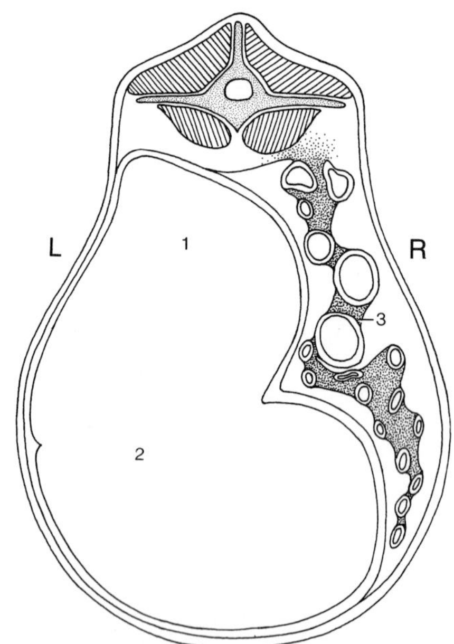


**Figure 3–34.** Section through the abdomen of a goat. The greater pressure in the lower part of the abdomen causes the convex form of the lower part of the abdominal wall. The pressure within the upper part of the abdomen is below that of the atmosphere, and the flank is sunken.

1, Gas in upper part of rumen; 2, ingesta in the lower part of rumen; 3, intestines.

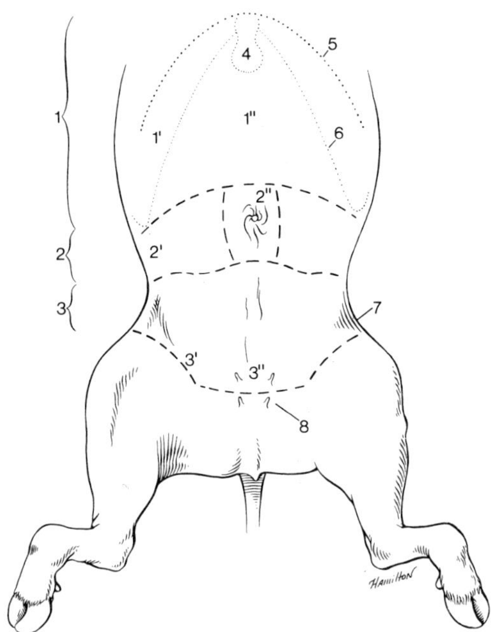


**Figure 3–35.** Abdominal regions shown on a heifer.

1, Cranial abdominal region; 1′, hypochondriac region; 1″, xiphoid region; 2, middle abdominal region; 2′, flank; 2″, umbilical region; 3, caudal abdominal region; 3′, inguinal region; 3″, pubic region; 4, xiphoid cartilage; 5, cranial extent of diaphragm; 6, costal arch; 7, fold of the flank; 8, juvenile udder.

the abdominal wall by means of everyday expressions; if greater precision is required, recourse may be had to the conventional terms illustrated in Figure 3–35.

## THE STOMACH

The stomach, interposed between the esophagus and small intestine, is the dilated part of the digestive tract in which the processes of digestion are initiated. It is succeeded by the intestine, which consists of a proximal small intestine (in most species the principal organ of digestion and absorption) and a distal large intestine (generally much shorter and especially concerned with the dehydration of the food residue).

However, among mammals there exists very considerable diversity in the form and structure of these two parts of the digestive system, which are closely associated in function and which are collectively known as the gastrointestinal tract. Much of this diversity is clearly adaptive and reflects the habitual diet of the various groups. The concentrated diet of carnivores is most easily digested, and these animals have a small and simple stomach (Plate 1/A) and a relatively short and uncomplicated intestine. The fodder of herbivores is less easily managed; it has a lower nutritive value and must be consumed in large amounts. Moreover, a major part consists of celluloses and other complex carbohydrates that are not susceptible to the action of mammalian digestive enzymes. These substances can be utilized only if they are first broken down by symbiotic microorganisms; this is a relatively slow process that requires the provision of a large fermentation chamber where food may be held in an environment favorable to the multiplication and activity of the microorganisms. In some herbivorous species such a chamber is supplied by a greatly enlarged and subdivided stomach, in others by a voluminous and complicated large intestine. Ruminants illustrate the first alternative, the horse the second. Some indication of the range of variation of gastrointestinal anatomy among domestic species is provided by Figure 3–36. Detailed accounts are found in the chapters concerned with individual species; the description that follows is largely confined to the simple organs of the dog and cat.

The *stomach* (ventriculus)* receives food from the esophagus and retains it for a time before discharging it into the duodenum, the first part of the small intestine. The stomach of the dog has a relatively modest capacity—ranging from 0.5 to 6.0 liters according to breed—and conforms to a pattern that is common to most carnivores and indeed to many other mammals, including ourselves. It consists of two distinct parts that converge and join at a ventral angle (Fig. 3–37). The larger part, into which the esophagus opens at the cardia, lies mainly to the left of the median plane, well forward under cover of the ribs and in direct contact with the liver and the diaphragm; it is relatively distensible and rapidly expands to accommodate a meal. The second part is narrower, has thicker walls, and is more constant in appearance since it is less affected by the presence of a meal; it passes to the right to continue into the duodenum at the pylorus (Plate 1/*B*). The cranial (parietal) aspect of both parts is mainly in contact with the liver, while the more numerous relations of the caudal (visceral) surface include the intestinal mass, left kidney, pancreas, and greater omentum. The left part of the margin is applied to the hilar region of the spleen.

Other terms are available when it is necessary to refer to particular regions of the stomach more precisely. The large left sac is divided between a

*The alternative term *gaster,* derived from the Greek, is the root of most clinical terms: gastritis, gastrectomy.

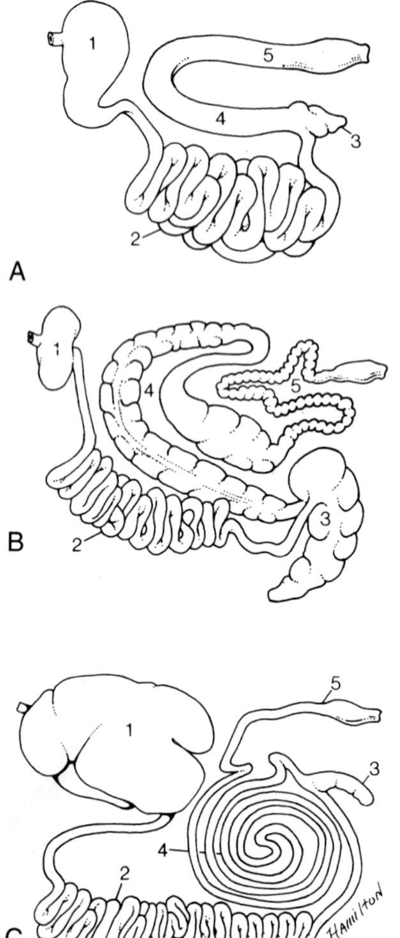


**Figure 3–36.** Gastrointestinal tracts of the dog *(A)*, of the horse *(B)*, and of cattle *(C)* laid out in one plane.

1, Stomach; 2, small intestine; 3, cecum; 4, ascending colon; 5, descending colon.

blind dome (fundus) rising above the cardia and a body (corpus) extending from the cardia to the ventral angle. The more tubular right or pyloric part is divided between a more proximal pyloric antrum and a more distal pyloric canal, the distinction being based on the terminal muscular thickening (Plate 1/*B*). The margin separating the two surfaces is divided between greater and lesser curvatures, each of which runs between the cardiac and pyloric openings. The convex greater curvature gives attachment to the greater omentum, of which a part (gastrosplenic ligament) connects the spleen with the stomach. The shorter, concave lesser curvature is connected with the liver by the lesser omentum. This curvature is marked by a sharp change in direction known as the angular notch (incisura).

The *stomach wall* is composed of layers corresponding to those of the esophagus and intestine. The external peritoneum or serosa covers the entire organ, adhering to the underlying muscle, except along the curvatures where it is reflected to continue into the omenta; its absence from the curvatures makes them the parts most likely to burst when the organ is excessively distended.

The next coat is of smooth muscle and is arranged in three layers, each incomplete but with its deficiencies compensated by the others. The external layer is more or less longitudinal and continues the outer muscle of the esophagus; it is concentrated along the curvatures, although it spreads more widely over the pyloric part. The middle layer is disposed in hoops, with those most proximal forming a weak sphincter around the cardia; beyond this the pattern is interrupted by the projection of the fundus but it is resumed at a lower level. It then continues to the pyloric canal where the hoops are bunched together on the lesser

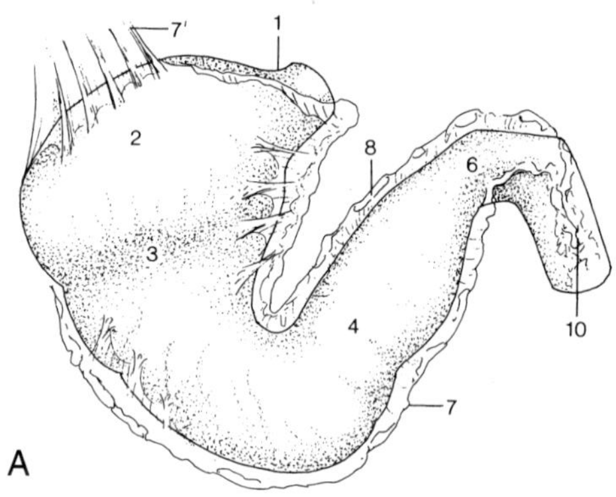


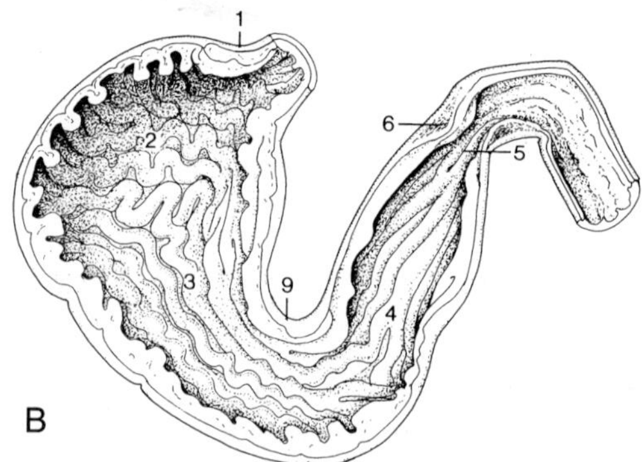


**Figure 3–37.** Caudal view of the canine stomach. *A*, Exterior. *B*, Interior.

1. Cardia; 2, fundus; 3, body; 4–6, pyloric part; 4, pyloric antrum; 5, pyloric canal; 6, pylorus; 7, greater omentum; 7′, gastrosplenic ligament; 8, lesser omentum; 9, angular notch; 10, mergence of attachment of greater and lesser omenta.

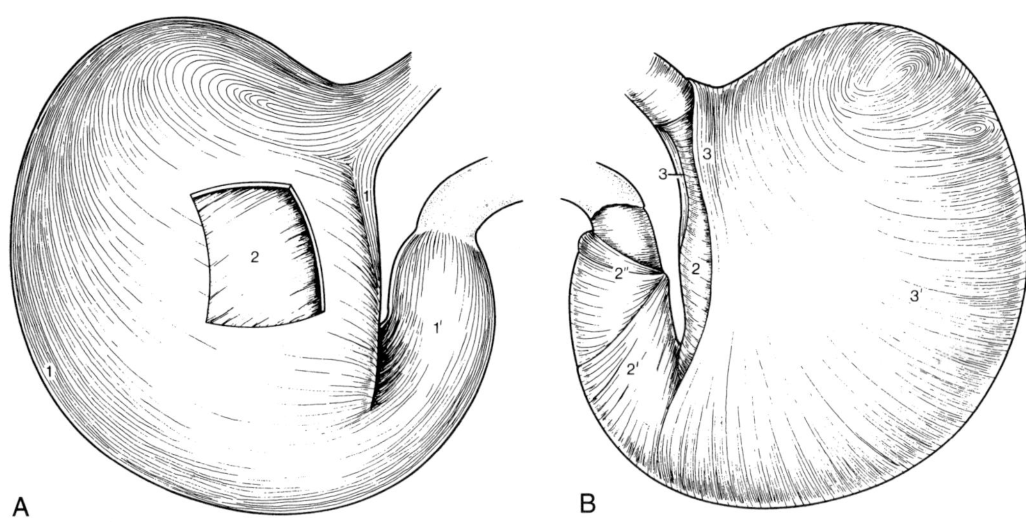


**Figure 3–38.** The tunica muscularis of the canine stomach. *A*, Visceral surface after removal of the serosa. *B*, Stomach turned inside out with the mucosa removed.

The tunica muscularis comprises outer longitudinal, middle circular, and inner oblique layers. The *longitudinal layer* clothes the curvatures (1) and the pyloric part (1′) but is thin over the body. The *circular layer* surrounds the body (2) and is especially prominent on the pyloric part (2′), where it furnishes the pyloric sphincters (2″). The *oblique layer* is thickest along the lesser curvature where it forms two lips that fuse over the cardia (cardiac loop); it is thin where it lines the fundus and body (3′).

curvature, forming a muscular knot (that in some species produces an obvious projection into the lumen), and fanning out on the greater curvature; the edges of this "fan" are sometimes held to constitute proximal and distal pyloric sphincters. The innermost layer is very incomplete but compensates for the deficiencies in the circular muscle; particularly stout fascicles arch above the cardia before continuing distally to each side of the lesser curvature extending toward, but not beyond, the angular notch (Fig. 3–38).

The thin submucosa internal to the muscle is separated from the mucosa proper by a plexiform muscularis mucosae. It contains major arterial and venous plexuses and also a wealth of elastic fibers that help the muscularis mucosae throw the mucosa of the empty organ into the folds (rugae) that provide the characteristic surface relief (Fig. 3–37; Plate 1/*C*). These folds are predominantly longitudinal in orientation, although individually tortuous; they are completely effaced only when the stomach is grossly distended.

The entire gastric mucosa is densely pockmarked by innumerable tiny depressions. These so-called gastric pits—many would be better described as crevices—are invisible to the naked eye but account for the surface folding seen in histological sections (Plate 1/*E*). The surface epithelium of columnar, mucus-secreting cells continues into the pits and even extends into the uppermost parts of the gastric glands that deliver their products into the depth of the pits. This epithelium is largely responsible for the protective coat that makes gastric mucosa slimy to the touch. The gastric glands are of three varieties, which are termed cardiac, proper gastric (fundic), and pyloric, although it must be stressed that in many species, including the dog, their distribution does not exactly coincide with the gross regions that bear the same names. The cardiac and pyloric glands produce additional mucus whereas the proper gastric glands are alone responsible for the gastric juice active in digestion by virtue of its pepsin and hydrochloric acid content. The enzyme is the product of its most numerous (chief) cell type, the acid of the fewer parietal cells; there is also a further contingent of mucus-secreting cells. It is claimed that the proper gastric glandular region has a somewhat darker hue than the remainder of the mucosa.

The *blood supply* to the stomach comes from all three chief branches of the celiac artery and is particularly generous along the two curvatures (Fig. 3–39). The arteries anastomose quite freely externally and also within the stomach wall. For the most part, the arteries that penetrate the wall pass to the submucosa before branching to form an elaborate plexus from which both the muscular and the mucosal coats are fed. The mucosal branches supply unusually wide-bored capillaries below the epithelium and about the glands.

The veins are similarly arranged and ultimately

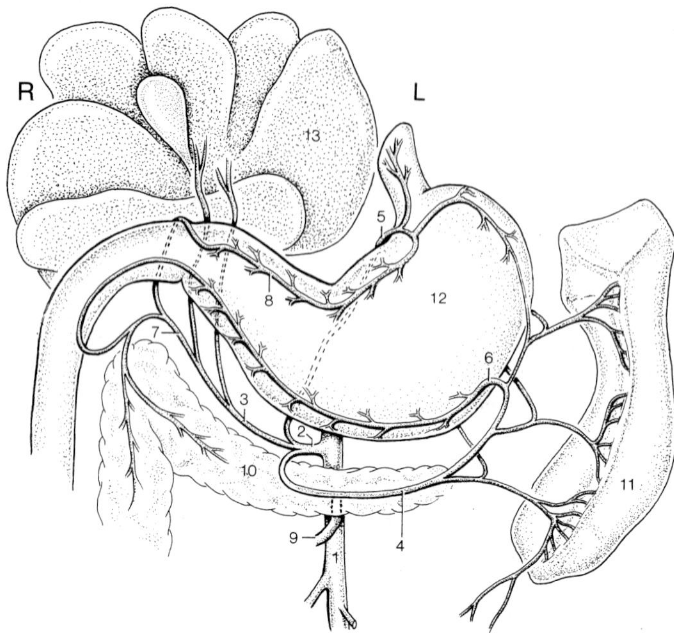


**Figure 3–39.** Distribution of the celiac artery of the dog (ventral view).

1, Aorta; 2, celiac artery; 3, hepatic artery; 4, splenic artery; 5, left gastric artery; 6, left gastroepiploic artery; 7, gastroduodenal artery; 8, right gastric artery; 9, cranial mesenteric artery; 10, pancreas; 11, spleen; 12, stomach; 13, liver.

combine to form trunks that join the portal vein. Numerous arteriovenous anastomoses provide a means of regulating mucosal blood supply, with much blood being diverted from the capillary bed of the fasting organ.

Lymph vessels are present in profusion, particularly in the submucosa. They lead to several gastric nodes, each charged with the drainage of a particular territory.

The stomach is innervated by parasympathetic fibers within the two vagal trunks and by sympathetic fibers that reach the organ with the arteries. The efferent fibers of both sets are accompanied by more numerous afferent fibers. Parasympathetic fibers of the vagus synapse on ganglion cells in intramural plexuses within the submucosa and between the muscle coats and exert a high measure of control over gastric motility. The effects of vagal stimulation on the proximal and distal regions of the stomach are dissimilar: In the proximal stomach vagal activity suppresses muscular contraction and leads to adaptive relaxation, whereas in the distal stomach vagal stimulation causes intense peristaltic activity. Vagal stimulation of distal antral motility is mediated by acetylcholine, but the identity of the inhibitory mediator is not well established; it may be vasoactive intestinal peptide. The intramural plexuses are involved in the local reflexes in which the stomach wall reacts to direct stimulation. Sympathetic and parasympathetic fibers also innervate the surface epithelium and glands, but only parasympathetic fibers end on the intragastric endocrine cells.* Division of the vagal nerves—either the main trunks or selected branches—reduces gastric activity and secretion.

The *topography* and the form of the living stomach of the dog are much influenced by functional changes. The empty stomach is small and contracted toward the fixed point of the esophageal entrance. It lies entirely within the rib cage and fails to reach the abdominal floor. The wall is generally inert except for occasional weak peristaltic contractions, and little secretion from the glands occurs. Any residual peristaltic activity ceases as soon as food is offered (or anticipated). Secretion increases as a reflex response to the taste of food or the effort of mastication; it appears to be independent of food actually reaching the stomach. When food does arrive, it first collects in layers—since as yet no mixing movements are present—and largely occupies the body, which expands in all directions but principally ventrally and caudally. A motor response is delayed, and when it begins it is relatively slow in building to a peak. Peristaltic contractions commence near the cardia and course distally, accelerating and becoming more vigorous when they reach the muscular

*There are several varieties of these, the most important being the gastrin-secreting cells scattered singly within the epithelium of gastric glands, especially those of the antral region. The release of gastrin is stimulated by the vagal nerves and also, more directly, by distention of the stomach by a meal. Gastrin is passed into the portal circulation, returning within the arterial blood to promote increased activity, both glandular and muscular, of the stomach wall.

pyloric antrum. The terminal segment contracts en masse, and the injection of ingesta into the duodenum therefore occurs when the wave is still some distance from the pylorus. Radiographic studies suggest that the pylorus is open for about one third of the time; it is probable that emptying is more dependent on intermittent increase of the intragastric pressure than on the regular peristaltic activity.

The effects of feeding on topography and relations are considerable, especially in animals kept under regimens that allow them to feed seldom but to repletion. The fully distended stomach may extend almost to the umbilicus—or even beyond this in the puppy—pushing the intestinal mass dorsally and caudally. The liver is pushed to the right while the spleen, tethered to the left part of the greater curvature, follows the expansion of that side of the stomach.

# THE INTESTINE

The intestine* commences at the pylorus and continues to the anus. It is divided between the proximal small intestine (intestinum tenue) and the distal large intestine (intestinum crassum), parts that do not always differ as much in caliber as their names suggest. However, the boundary is made obvious by the outgrowth of a blind diverticulum, the cecum, at the origin of the large intestine (Fig. 3–40). The small intestine consists of three parts: an initial duodenum, which is short and rather closely fixed in position, and the jejunum and ileum, which are carried by the great mesentery. The large intestine also comprises three parts; recognition of the blind-ending cecum presents no problem, but the separation of colon from rectum is arbitrarily put at the pelvic inlet. The rectum joins the short anal canal that leads to the exterior, but this canal is not part of the intestine in the strict sense.

The length of the intestine may be given in absolute terms or, more usefully, in measures of body length. Unfortunately, the figures commonly quoted cannot be taken too seriously, since formidable difficulties to measurement are present in life and uncertainty is introduced by relaxation of the gut after death. The dog, in keeping with its diet, has a relatively short gut—perhaps some three or four times its body length in life. Intestinal length in herbivores varies with the nature of the gastrointestinal adaptation but may be as much as 25 times the body length in sheep.

*The Greek word *enteron* provides the stem for many terms: enteritis, mesentery, and so forth.

## The Small Intestine

The *duodenum* is short and closely attached to the abdominal roof by a short mesoduodenum. The initial portion continues from the pyloric part of the stomach and passes toward the right body wall before being deflected caudally to descend to a point between the right kidney and the pelvic inlet. It then passes medially, behind the root of the mesentery, before ascending a short distance; it ends by bending ventrally to enter the mesentery, where it is continued as the jejunum. The more constant relations of the dog's duodenum are to the liver at its origin, thereafter to the right body wall laterally, the pancreas and later the right kidney medially, and, overall, to other parts of the intestinal mass. Although the first part of the duodenum is not expanded to form a distinct "duodenal bulb" or "cap," so commonly the site of ulcers in people, its functional independence is retained.

The *jejunum* and *ileum* are less closely fixed in position, but, although the arrangement of individual coils continually adjusts, this gut as a whole occupies a more or less constant position in the ventral part of the abdominal cavity (Fig. 3–41; Plate 19/*D*). The coils are carried by the mesentery, which conveys the vessels and nerves; the mesentery is bunched at its root around the origin of the cranial mesenteric artery from the aorta and widens to the length of the gut at its other margin. The initial and final portions of the mesentery are shortest and ease the transitions with the relatively

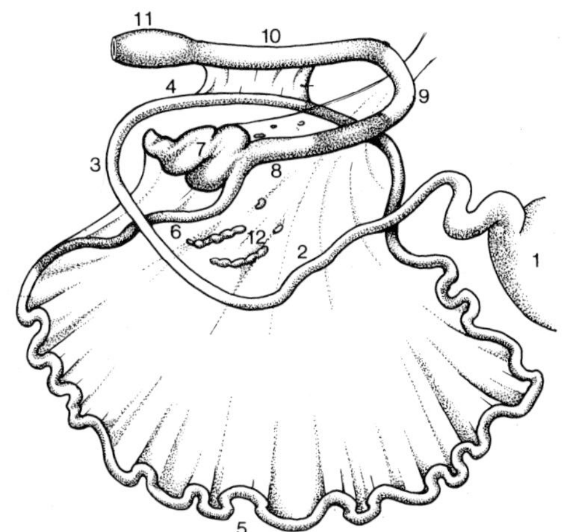


**Figure 3–40.** Intestinal tract of the dog (schematic).

1, Stomach; 2, descending duodenum; 3, caudal flexure; 4, ascending duodenum; 5, jejunum; 6, ileum; 7, cecum; 8, ascending colon; 9, transverse colon; 10, descending colon; 11, rectal ampulla; 12, jejunal lymph nodes.

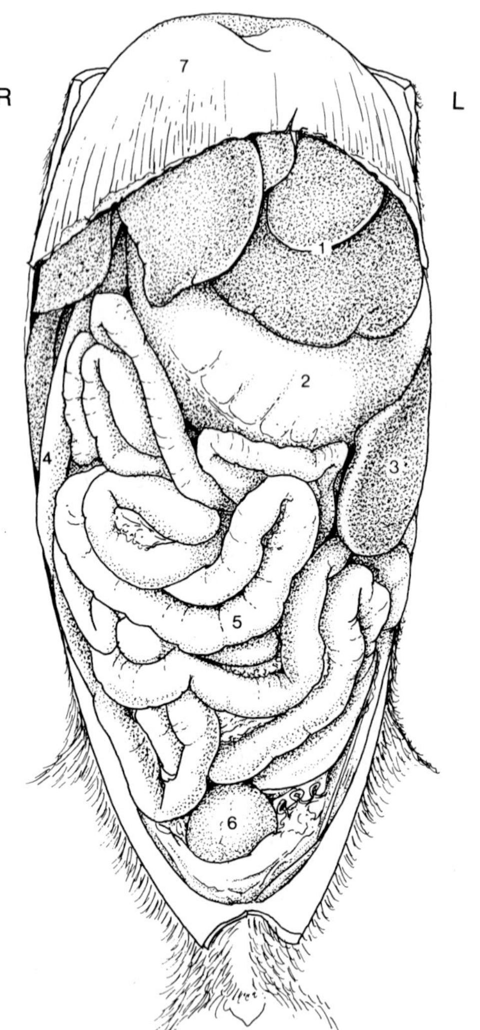


**Figure 3–41.** Ventral view of the abdominal organs of the dog after removal of the greater omentum.

1, Liver; 2, stomach; 3, spleen; 4, descending duodenum; 5, jejunum; 6, bladder; 7, diaphragm.

fixed duodenum at one end and with the ascending colon at the other (Fig. 3–40). The distinction betwen jejunum and ileum is arbitrary and perhaps unnecessary, for although certain progressive structural changes occur, these do not allow recognition of a sharp boundary. The convention that we follow limits the ileum to a short, relatively more muscular (and hence firmer) final portion with a direct peritoneal connection with the cecum. Many Anglo-Saxon anatomists assume a more or less equal division between the two parts.

The jejunum fills those parts of the abdomen that are not preempted by other viscera. In the dog, in which the large intestine is relatively small, it lies more or less symmetrically about the midline, between the liver and stomach cranially and the urinary bladder caudally. It lies on the abdominal floor, though separated from the parietal peritoneum by the intervention of the greater omentum. The coils are quite mobile, and at first sight their disposition appears to be haphazard; closer inspection shows that there is some pattern to the arrangement. The mainly sagittal coils of the proximal part lie largely cranial to the more transverse coils of the distal part (Fig. 3–41). The ileum pursues a rather direct cranial, dorsal, and dextral course toward its junction with the large intestine. In life the intestine is not uniformly full, and at any moment most parts are flattened and molded by the pressures of adjacent viscera. The lumen may be locally obliterated and, when a passage is retained, it is more often than not reduced to a narrow channel along one margin—a "keyhole" form when viewed in section. This explains the narrow streaks that are the common representation of the small intestine in radiographs obtained after the administration of a barium suspension. Segmental and peristaltic movements continually alter the configuration in life.

The intestine is composed of the usual four tunics (Fig. 3–42). The luminal surface has a velvety appearance since it presents innumerable tiny but densely packed projections, the intestinal

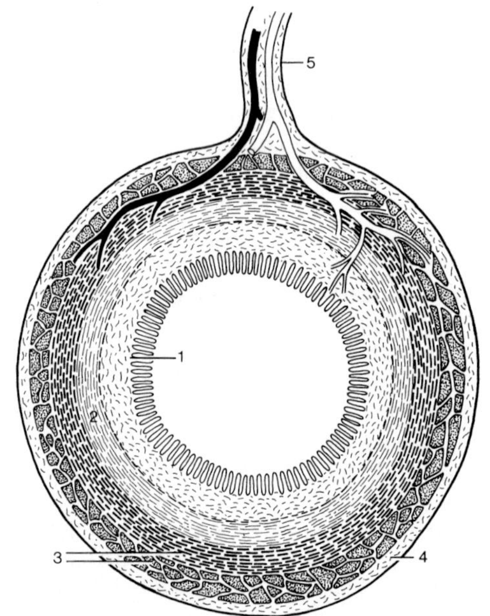


**Figure 3–42.** Transverse section through the gut. The artery and vein reach the gut via the mesentery; the larger branches fail to reach the antimesenteric border.

1, Mucosa; 2, submucosa; 3, muscle layer; 4, serosa; 5, mesentery.

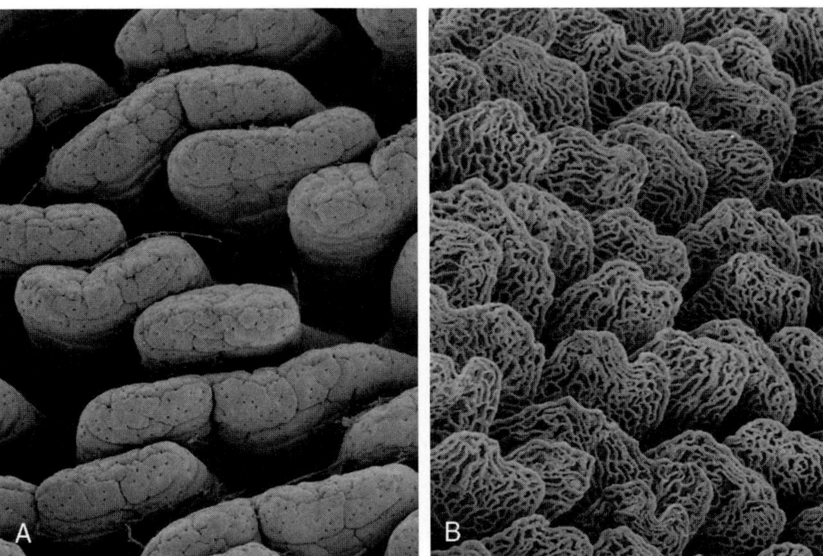


**Figure 3–43.** Scanning electron micrographs of rat duodenal villi *(A)* and of a vascular cast of the same tissue demonstrating subepithelial capillary plexuses *(B)*.

villi. These are finger-like in the dog and horse but broader and leaflike in many species (Fig. 3–43). In addition to the interspecific differences, variations in form and dimension may be present at different locations along the length of the small intestine. The appearance, and the detailed morphology, may be profoundly influenced by changes in diet (early weaning) or disease (microbial infections). The villi greatly increase the area of epithelium available for absorption; the efficiency of the process is enhanced by very generous subepithelial capillary plexuses (/*B*). Microscopic intestinal glands (crypts) open to the surface between the bases of the villi. The crypts produce a mucous secretion that coats the surface of the bowel and various enzymes that contribute to the further digestion of carbohydrate and protein breakdown products.

Larger (Brunner's) glands confined to the submucosa of the duodenum, especially its initial part, also secrete a protective mucus. A proportion of the cells lining the crypts—perhaps 1% of the total population—belong to the enteroendocrine (enterochromaffin) system (p. 216). Of several varieties, these cells form a series, commencing with the gastrin-producing cells of the stomach and extending through the small into the large intestine, that produces a number of hormones that influence various aspects of gastrointestinal activity. The intestinal components of the series, unlike that of the stomach, are under regulation by intrinsic nerves of the organ wall and largely outweigh the influence of the extrinsic nerve supply to the gut. Cholecystokinin, which provokes contraction of the gallbladder, is an important member of the set.

The great length and the villous surface of the small intestine combine to increase the absorptive area. In some species the absorptive area is also increased by permanent longitudinal and spiral folds; these are not pronounced in the dog, and the mucosal relief sometimes visible in radiographs is produced by temporary ridges.

The mucosa is rich in nodules of lymphoid tissue, both solitary and clumped; the larger aggregations (Peyer's patches*; [Plate 23/*H*]) cause visible depressions and elevations of the mucosa that may become more obvious by the absence of a covering pile of villi. These aggregations tend to be more numerous and individually larger toward the junction with the large intestine.

Attention must be directed, however briefly, to the remarkable cycle of epithelial renewal exhibited by the lining of the small intestine throughout life. The epithelium is renewed by the mitotic division of cells in the depths of the crypts. The cells lining the crypts, continuously recruited in this way, gradually ascend to the surface, spread to embrace the bases of the villi, and continue up

*These patches may be initial sites for the accumulation, after ingestion, of the infective agents responsible for the transmissable spongiform encephalopathies ("new variant" Creutzfeldt Jacob disease, bovine spongiform encephalopathy [BSE], scrapie) that have claimed so much attention in recent years.

these to the summits where they are finally shed into the gut lumen. The passage from the bottom of a crypt to the summit of a villus takes about 3 days and involves a prodigious wastage—one calculation suggests a loss of about 1 g of epithelial cells for every centimeter stretch of the human small intestine every day. The process has the fortunate consequence of permitting rapid renewal of the integrity of the gut lining following extensive damage, such as the necrosis and loss by sloughing of the surface layer that occurs in certain infections in various domestic species. While repair is in train, the villi are reduced in size; they are not fully restored until a sufficiency of epithelial cells has again become available to clothe villi of normal height and proportions.

Both the liver and the pancreas discharge into the duodenum. The arrangement in the dog is for the bile duct and one pancreatic duct to discharge by separate openings on a (major duodenal) papilla a few centimeters beyond the pylorus, while the second larger pancreatic duct discharges on a smaller papilla a little farther on. Neither papilla is conspicuous.

## The Large Intestine

In its most elementary form the mammalian large intestine is a short tube, little wider than the small intestine from which it arises to pursue a direct course to the anus. The canine large intestine is somewhat more complicated, though still simple if compared with that of herbivores (Fig. 3–44). As in most species, it is clearly divided into cecum, colon, and rectum, while the colon is itself differentiated into ascending, transverse, and descending parts (/3,4,5). The cecum is a blind-ending piece of gut that arises at the junction of the ileum and colon. The division of the colon follows from the

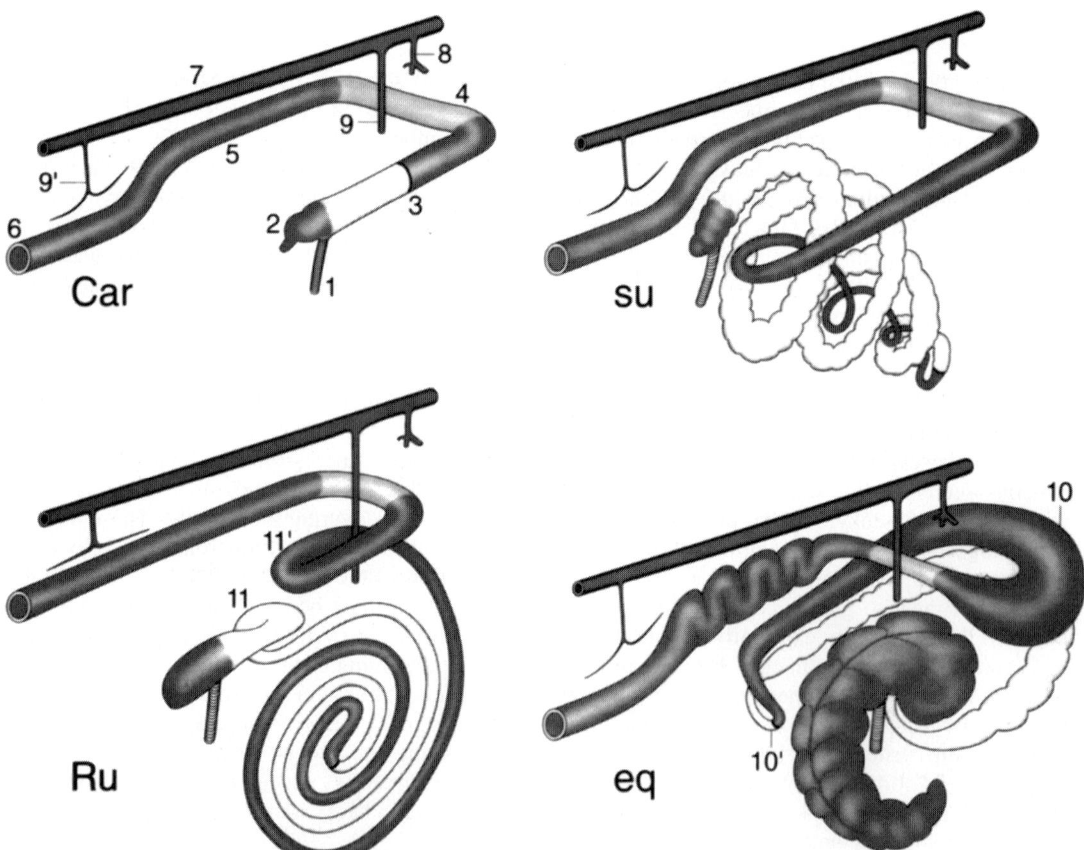


**Figure 3–44.** Schematic drawing of the large intestine of the domestic mammals: carnivores (Car), the pig (su), ruminants (Ru), and the horse (eq). Cranial is to the upper right.

1, Ileum; 2, cecum; 3, ascending colon; 4, transverse colon; 5, descending colon; 6, rectum and anus; 7, aorta; 8, celiac artery; 9, 9′, cranial and caudal mesenteric arteries; 10, 10′, dorsal diaphragmatic and pelvic flexures of ascending colon; 11, 11′, proximal and distal loops of ascending colon.

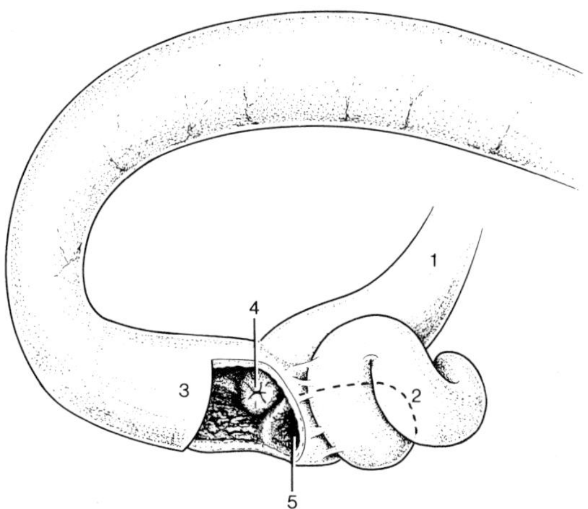


**Figure 3–45.** The ileocolic junction and its relation to the cecum in the dog.

1, Ileum; 2, cecum; 3, ascending colon; 4, ileal orifice surrounded by annular fold; 5, cecocolic orifice.

rotation of the embryonic gut imposing on the adult organ a conformation that resembles a question mark (when viewed from below; Fig. 3–61).

The canine *cecum* is unusual in having no direct connection with the ileum, but since it is conventional to regard the cecum as the first part of the large intestine, the description commences with it. The cecum of the dog is short and at first sight appears even shorter, since it is drawn into a spiral and held against the ileum by folds of peritoneum. It is only slightly wider than the small intestine and tapers slightly toward its rounded blind extremity. The lumen communicates with the interior of the colon, immediately beyond the ileocolic junction, through an opening that is guarded by an inner circular muscular ring (the cecocolic sphincter) (Fig. 3–45).

The smooth, externally featureless *colon* has a caliber that is uniformly and significantly, though not remarkably, greater than that of the small bowel. It is suspended throughout its length by a moderately long mesocolon, which allows it some mobility, and its position and relations vary within certain limits; the flexures that divide it into ascending, transverse, and descending parts are not precisely fixed. The short ascending part continues the axis of the ileum from a junction defined internally by an ileocolic opening of similar appearance and construction to that at the origin of the cecum. The transverse part runs across the abdomen from right to left, between the stomach cranially and the mass of small intestine and cranial mesenteric artery caudally. The descending part is the longest; it follows the left flank before edging medially to enter the pelvic cavity where it is continued as the rectum without other visible demarcation than the passage across the abdominopelvic boundary. The term rectum implies a straight course, but often this part of the bowel is deflected to one side by pressure from other viscera, most usually a distended bladder. The *rectum* is the most dorsal of the pelvic viscera and lies above the reproductive organs, bladder, and urethra. Its cranial part has the same relationship to the peritoneum as the colon, but this changes as the mesorectum shortens and the serosal covering is reflected laterally to continue into the parietal peritoneum of the pelvic cavity and ventrally to continue over the urogenital organs. The terminal part is wholly retroperitoneal and is directly attached to the vagina in the female, to the urethra in the male, and to the pelvic diaphragm in both sexes.

The mucosa of the large intestine is generally smooth since villi are lacking. No permanent mucosal folds are present, but there are numerous scattered lymph nodules, especially in the rectum where they tend to be conspicuous; this is because the summits of the swellings are here depressed, leading to tiny pits. In many species, including the horse and pig among domestic animals, the outer muscle coat of the large intestine is mainly concentrated in a number of bands (teniae), which, on shortening, pucker the gut so that a linear series of sacculations (haustra) is produced (see Fig. 21–11). Such bands are not present on the intestine of the dog and cat.

The *anal canal* joins the bowel to the exterior. It is a short passage that is derived from the proctodeum, the invagination of the surface ectoderm. The lumen is constricted at the rectoanal junction where the mucosa is thrown into longitudinal folds, normally pressed together to occlude the orifice (Fig. 3–46). Anal continence, however, depends primarily on the presence of two sphincters; the internal anal sphincter is merely a thickening of the circular smooth muscle of the gut, but

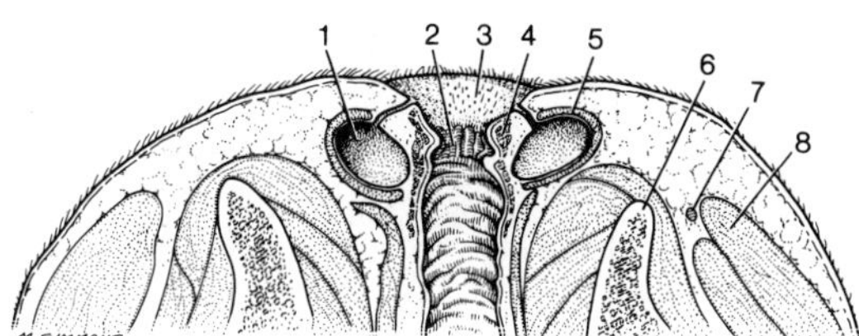


**Figure 3–46.** Dorsal (horizontal) section through the canine anal canal.

1, Anal sac; 2, columnar zone of the anal canal; 3, cutaneous zone; 4, internal and sphincter; 5, external anal sphincter; 6, ischium; 7, sacrotuberous ligament; 8, gluteus superficialis.

the external sphincter is striated, of somatic origin, and under voluntary control (Fig. 3–47).

Many glands are always present in the anal region, both in the mucosa and in the surrounding skin. Most are small but the dog and cat also possess two so-called *anal sacs* (sinus paranales). Each is roughly the size of a hazelnut (in the dog) and is located ventrolateral to the anus betwen the internal and external sphincters (see Fig. 10–28. The fundus of the sac secretes an evil-smelling fluid that drains through a single duct to an opening near the anocutaneous junction. The sac is compressed at defecation, expelling the secretion, which probably serves as a territorial marker. Such sacs are found in most carnivores and are most notorious in the skunk.

The *blood supply* to the intestinal tract is mainly provided by the cranial and caudal mesenteric arteries; however, the initial part of the duodenum is supplied through the hepatic branch of the celiac artery and the caudal part of the rectum by rectal branches of the internal pudendal artery. The cranial mesenteric artery supplies the bulk of the small intestine, the ileocecocolic junctional region, and the midpart of the colon through its three primary divisions; the details of branching vary among species and also, though to a lesser extent, among individuals. The smaller caudal mesenteric artery has a distribution restricted to the descending colon and cranial part of the rectum. The arrangement in the dog is illustrated (Figs. 3–42 and 3–48); although its relevance in surgery suggests that the pattern of arterial branching should be known, the richness of the anastomoses is of even greater importance. These ensure that the intestine can normally survive the complete obstruction of a major supplying vessel. The chain of anastomoses continues beyond the territories of the mesenteric arteries to connect with those of the celiac and internal pudendal arteries.

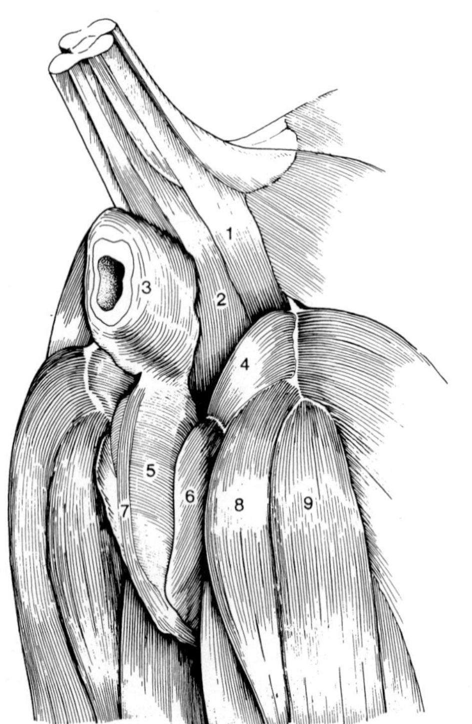


**Figure 3–47.** The muscles of the perineal region of the male dog.

1, Coccygeus; 2, levator ani; 3, external anal sphincter; 4, internal obturator; 5, bulbospongiosus; 6, ischiocavernosus; 7, retractor penis; 8, semimembranosus; 9, semitendinosus.

The veins are broadly comparable and join to form the cranial and caudal mesenteric veins, two of the main radicles—the splenic vein is the third—of the portal vein (Fig. 3–49). Certain tributary veins connect with systemic veins at the extremities of their territories—the thoracic esophagus and anal canal, parts that normally drain by systemic routes. Congestion within the portal circulation (p. 137) may lead to enlargement of submucosal veins in both these (and other) parts but is much more important in human than in veterinary medicine. The gut wall contains a considerable proportion of the lymphocyte population and represents an important component of the body's defense mechanism, one capable of barring entry to a variety of antigens.

The lymphatic drainage, of the small intestine in particular, is copious since some of the products of digestion are absorbed by this route. When these products include fat, the lymph is milky and the intestinal lymphatic vessels ("lacteals") are unusually conspicuous. The flow is directed toward certain nodes through which the lymph percolates before joining the cisterna chyli, the dilated origin of the thoracic duct, the most important lymphatic vessel (p. 254). In the dog these nodes are large but few and are centralized toward the root of the mesentery (Fig. 3–40); in other species they may be more numerous and more widely scattered and may include many that are peripheral, close to the gut itself.

The intestine receives both sympathetic and parasympathetic nerves. The sympathetic pathways lead through the celiac, cranial mesenteric, and caudal mesenteric ganglia, with the postganglionic fibers enmeshing the relevant arteries (see Fig. 8–77). The parasympathetic pathways involve both vagal and pelvic nerves. The former supply the intestine to the junction of the transverse and descending parts of the colon; the latter supply the descending colon and rectum. The parasympa-

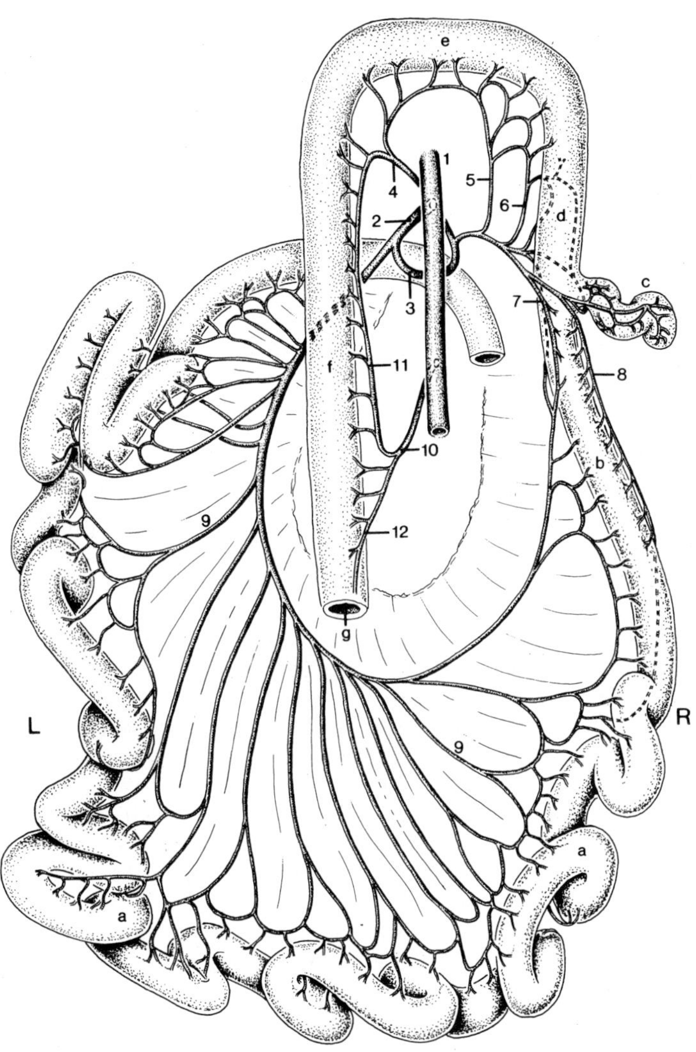


**Figure 3–48.** Distribution of the cranial and caudal mesenteric arteries to the intestines of the dog (dorsal view).

a, Jejunum; b, ileum; c, cecum; d, ascending colon; e, transverse colon; f, descending colon; g, rectum.

1, Aorta; 2, cranial mesenteric artery; 3, ileocolic artery; 4, middle colic artery; 5, right colic artery; 6, colic branch of ileocolic artery; 7, mesenteric ileal branch; 8, antimesenteric ileal branch; 9, jejunal arteries; 10, caudal mesenteric artery; 11, left colic artery; 12, cranial rectal artery.

thetic nerves augment peristalsis, but the effects of intestinal denervation are far less striking than those of gastric denervation.

Under stress, vasoconstriction may close the capillary bed of the intestinal wall, leading to abnormal permeability that allows large molecules to overcome the gut barrier, with septic shock being an eventual possibility.

## THE LIVER

The liver (hepar) is located in the most cranial part of the abdomen, immediately behind the diaphragm. It is by far the largest gland in the body and performs many functions essential for life. The most obvious is the production of bile, but the parts it plays in protein, carbohydrate, and fat metabolism are even more important and depend on the liver's situation astride the blood stream draining the gastrointestinal tract. This ensures that the products of digestion, which are conveyed in the blood stream after absorption, are presented to the hepatic cells before entering the general circulation.

The metabolic functions of the liver explain the wide interspecific variation in size, average values being about 3% to 5% of body weight in carnivores, 2% to 3% in omnivores, and as little as 1% to 1.5% in herbivores. The liver is substantially heavier in the young animal than in the adult; it often shows considerable atrophy in old age. Usually brownish-red, the fresh liver is soft with a characteristic friable consistency.

The adult liver intervenes between the diaphragm cranially and the stomach and intestinal mass caudally. Although extended across the median plane, the bulk lies to the right in all

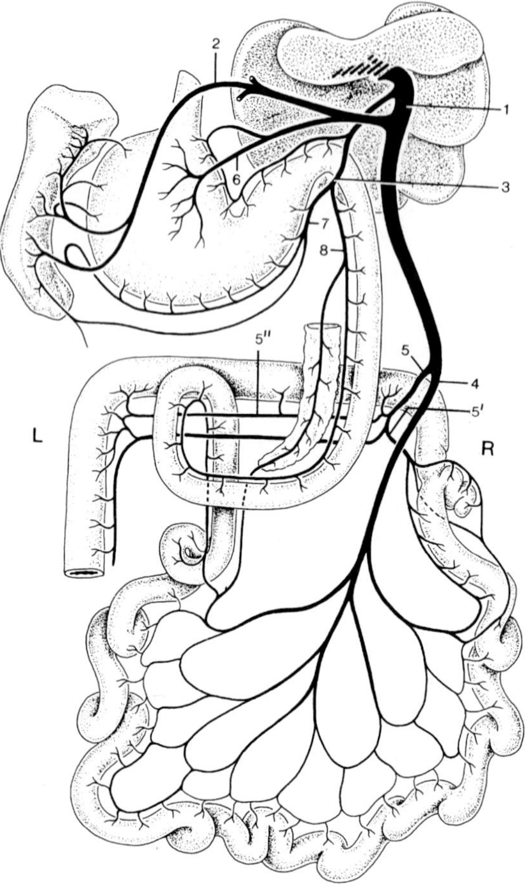


**Figure 3–49.** Semischematic dorsal view of the formation of the portal vein (dog).

1, Portal vein; 2, splenic vein; 3, gastroduodenal vein; 4, cranial mesenteric vein; 5, caudal mesenteric vein; 5′, ileocolic vein; 5″, middle colic vein; 6, left gastric vein; 7, right gastroepiploic vein; 8, cranial pancreaticoduodenal vein.

species (Fig. 3–50). It is not so very asymmetrical in the dog, the proportions to the right and left of the median plane being about 3:2. In most species, including the dog, the liver is grossly divided into lobes by a series of fissures that extend inward from the ventral margin (Plate 2/*A*,*C*). The lobation pattern shows many features of resemblance among different mammals, and considerable effort has been given to determining the homologies of individual lobes and fissures. The theoretical pattern—which accords the dog's liver left lateral, left medial, right lateral, right medial, quadrate, and caudate lobes, the last enlarged by papillary and caudate processes—is illustrated (Fig. 3–51). It should not be regarded as more than a convenient fiction that facilitates description. Recent studies minimize the significance of the external fissuration and rely more on the internal ramifications of the vessels to establish homologies. Such studies have had the useful byproduct of providing the surgeon with the detailed knowledge of the vascular architecture necessary for the safe removal of diseased parts of the human liver.

In life the liver adapts to the form of neighboring organs, and when fixed in situ it retains the conformation and impressions these impose. The rather large liver of the dog is therefore bluntly conical, with its cranial surface matching the curvature of the diaphragm against which it is pressed. The caudal surface is concave; to the left it exhibits a large excavation for the stomach, which is then extended over the median plane into a narrow duodenal groove. The dorsal border extends more caudally and reaches farther dorsally on the right side, where it is further extended by the caudate process which carries a deep impression for the cranial pole of the right kidney. Toward the median plane, this border carries a groove for the passage of the caudal vena cava and, to the left of this, a notch for the esophagus. The gallbladder lies between the quadrate and right medial lobes; it is partly attached, partly free, and in some dogs is so deeply embedded that it reaches the parietal surface and so makes contact with the diaphragm (Fig. 3–51).

The liver is clothed in peritoneum except for relatively small areas at the porta (hilus), in the fossa for the gallbladder, and at the origin of certain peritoneal reflections. The right and left triangular, the coronary, and the falciform ligaments that pass to the diaphragm from the parietal surface have fibrous cores and attach the liver firmly; the lesser omentum, which passes from the visceral surface to the stomach and duodenum, is more fragile. A tunica fibrosa encloses the parenchyma beneath the serosa; it enters the substance at the porta and detaches extensions that convey the blood vessels inward, dividing where the vessels divide and thinning at each division. The finer trabeculae pervade the entire organ and divide the liver into innumerable small units, the hepatic lobules of the classic description. Though particularly marked in the pig's liver (Plate 2/*D*), the lobular pattern is also quite obtrusive in that of the dog, in which the lobules appear as hexagonal areas (about 1 mm across) on the intact surface and in gross and histological sections.

The liver receives a very generous *blood supply* through the hepatic artery, a branch of the celiac artery, and the portal vein. The relative importance of these two supplies varies among species. The proportions are not known with certainty for the dog; the artery supplies the human liver with only one fifth of the blood but about three fifths of the oxygen. The branches of the hepatic artery that actually enter the liver are effectively end-arteries. However, provision exists for a collateral circulation outside the liver, between the hepatic artery and the other branches of the celiac artery that supply the stomach and duodenum (Fig. 3–39). The intrahepatic arteries divide in company with branches of the portal vein and tributaries of the hepatic duct. They supply the connective tissue structures en route to the hepatic sinusoids into which both they and the branches of the portal vein eventually discharge.

The portal vein is formed by the union of tributaries draining the digestive tract, pancreas, and spleen (Fig. 3–49). It is connected to systemic veins in the cardioesophageal and rectoanal regions at the extremities of its territory. These connections provide alternative outlets for portal blood when the flow through the liver is obstructed or impaired. The effects of obstruction vary between species and reflect the varying effectiveness of the hepatic artery in supplying oxygen. In the dog complete obstruction is rapidly fatal.

All blood delivered to the liver is collected by a single set of veins of which the central veins of the hepatic lobules are the smallest radicles. These eventually form the few large hepatic veins that open into the caudal vena cava as this tunnels through the liver substance. The circulation through the liver possesses numerous anastomoses—interarterial, intervenous, and arteriovenous; it is also controlled by various sphincter mechanisms, and together these features make it capable of very subtle regulation. A relatively rare congenital defect allows portal blood to pass directly to the caudal caval vein.

The liver receives sympathetic and parasympathetic nerves by way of periarterial plexuses and the vagal trunks, respectively.

The *hepatic duct system* begins with microscopic canaliculi within the lobules. These open into larger ductules that by successive unions within the connective tissue between the lobules ultimately form a few large hepatic ducts. Before, or shortly after, leaving the liver at the porta these

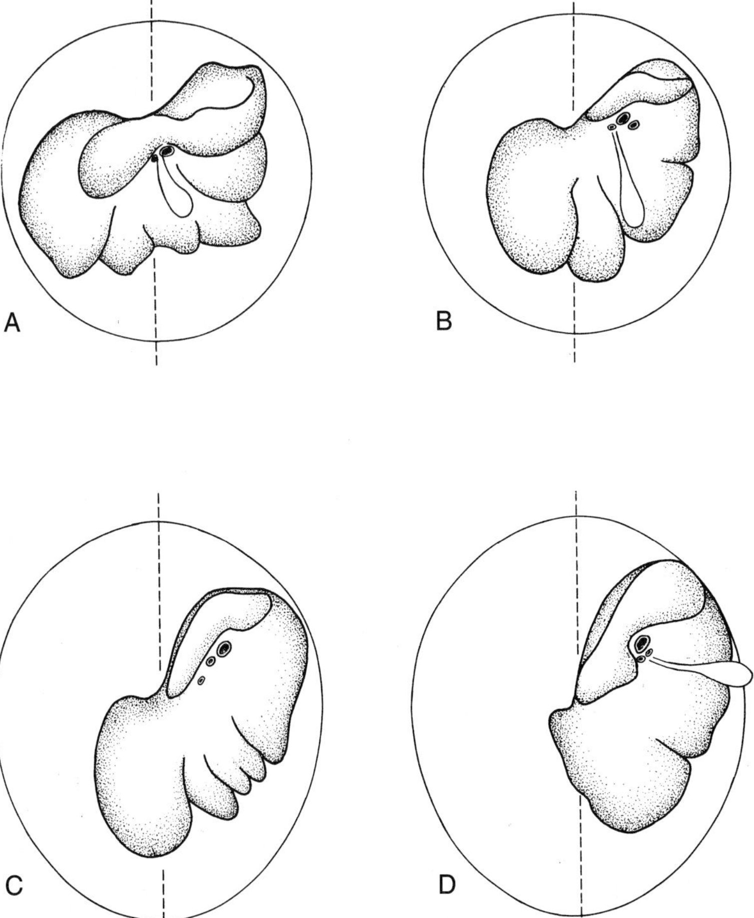


**Figure 3–50.** Caudal surface of the liver of the dog *(A)*, pig *(B)*, horse *(C)*, and cattle *(D)*. The median planes are indicated. The liver is asymmetrical, less so in the dog, more so in the pig and horse, and most in cattle, in which the bulk of the organ is displaced to the right. Note the absence of a gallbladder from the horse liver.

combine in a single trunk that runs to the duodenum (Fig. 3–52). A tortuous side branch (cystic duct) that arises from the common trunk leads to the pear-shaped gallbladder (Plate 2/*B*). The part of the common trunk that is distal to the origin of the cystic duct is known as the bile duct (ductus choledochus). Variation in the duct system is frequent; some hepatic ducts may enter the gallbladder directly, others may join the main outlet distal to the cystic duct. The gallbladder not only stores the bile but also concentrates it by absorption through the folded mucosa. As is well known, a gallbladder is not essential; it is lacking in the horse, the rat, and certain other species, which compensate by enlargement of the duct system (Fig. 3–50).

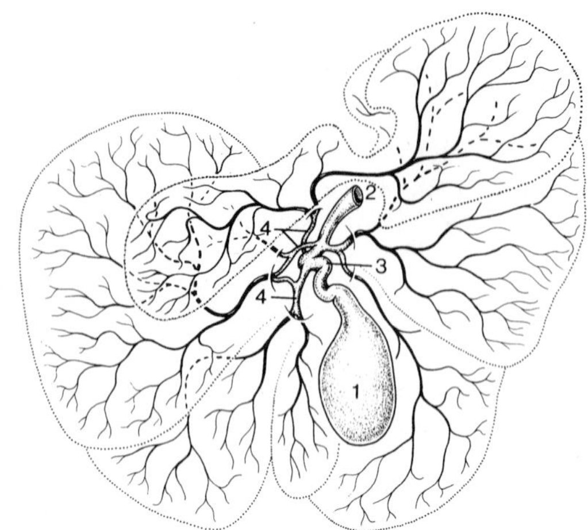


**Figure 3–52.** The bile drainage system of the dog.

1, Gallbladder; 2, bile duct; 3, cystic duct; 4, hepatic ducts.

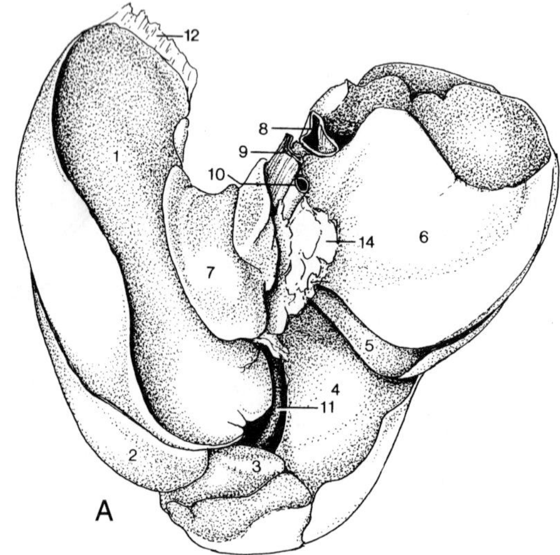


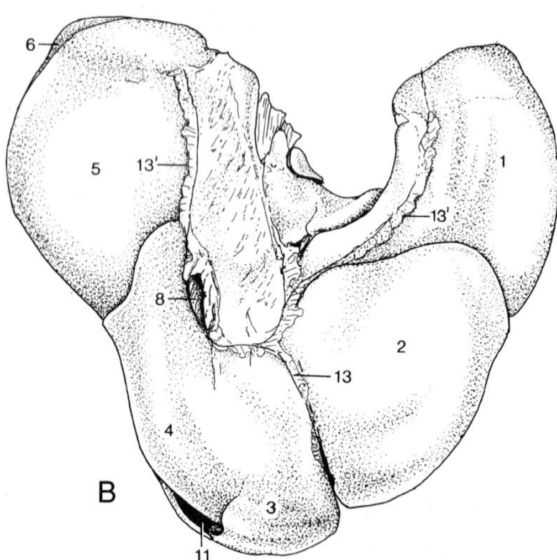


**Figure 3–51.** Visceral *(A)* and diaphragmatic *(B)* surfaces of the canine liver.

1, Left lateral lobe; 2, left medial lobe; 3, quadrate lobe; 4, right medial lobe; 5, right lateral lobe; 6, caudate process (of caudate lobe); 7, papillary process (of caudate lobe); 8, caudal vena cava; 9, portal vein; 10, hepatic artery; 11, gallbladder; 12, left triangular ligament; 13, falciform ligament; 13′, coronary ligaments; 14, lesser omentum.

The muscle of the bladder wall and duct, including the sphincter at the entrance to the duodenum, is supplied by parasympathetic nerves. Pain arising from the duct system, common in human patients, is abolished by section of the (sympathetic) splanchnic nerves.

## THE PANCREAS

The pancreas is a much smaller gland closely related to the duodenum in the dorsal part of the abdominal cavity. It is yellowish and bears some resemblance to a salivary gland, although it is softer and more loosely knit than most of these. It combines exocrine and endocrine functions.

The exocrine component is by far the larger; it produces a digestive juice that is discharged into the proximal part of the duodenum through one or two ducts. The juice contains enzymes that break down protein, carbohydrates, and fats. The endocrine component comprises the pancreatic islets, cell clumps that are scattered between the exocrine acini and are the source of insulin, glucagon, and gastrin; the islets are therefore of prime importance in carbohydrate metabolism (p. 216).

The pancreas is conventionally regarded as consisting of a body and two lobes, a description that suits the canine pancreas but is less apt for those of some other species (Fig. 3–53). When hardened in situ, the canine pancreas is acutely flexed with the apex of the V nestling close to the cranial flexure of the duodenum. The slender right lobe runs within the mesoduodenum; the thicker but shorter left lobe extends over the caudal surface of the stomach toward the spleen, within the greater omentum (Fig. 3–33/7).

The pancreas arises from two primordia that bud from the proximal part of the duodenum. The buds later merge, but in many species evidence of the dual origin of the pancreas is provided by its duct system. A greater pancreatic duct commonly drains the part of the pancreas that arises from the ventral primordium and opens into the duodenum together with, or just beside, the bile duct. A lesser (accessory) duct emerges from the part of the pancreas formed by the dorsal primordium and opens on the opposite aspect of the gut. This is the arrangement usually found in the dog, although the terminal part of one duct sometimes regresses; since the duct systems of the two lobes communicate within the gland, the absence of one or the other outlet is of no significance. In some species only one duct commonly survives.

The generous blood supply is from the cranial and caudal pancreaticoduodenal arteries, the former branching from the celiac, the latter from the cranial mesenteric artery. The veins drain to the portal vein. The gland is supplied by both sympathetic and parasympathetic nerves.

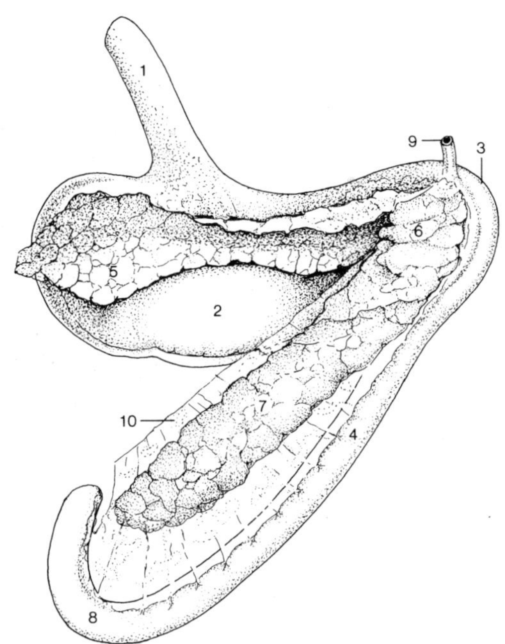


**Figure 3–53.** The pancreas of the dog (caudal view).

1, Esophagus; 2, stomach; 3, cranial flexure of duodenum; 4, descending duodenum; 5, left lobe of pancreas; 6, body; 7, right lobe; 8, caudal flexure of duodenum; 9, bile duct; 10, mesoduodenum.

# THE DEVELOPMENT OF THE DIGESTIVE APPARATUS

It is now necessary to amplify the very brief account given at the beginning of this chapter. The illustration (Fig. 3–2) that accompanied this should be consulted again.

## The Mouth

The stomodeum or depression that revealed the position of the future mouth is carried ventrally in the folding process and comes to lie between the swelling of the forebrain dorsally and that over the developing heart ventrally. The depression is still separated from the blind rostral extremity of the foregut by the oral membrane, but this shortly breaks down; with its disappearance it is no longer possible to recognize the extent of the ectodermal contribution to the lining of the mouth. A small dorsal diverticulum of the ectoderm grows out immediately in front of the plate and extends toward the undersurface of the brain. This diverticulum (saccus hypophysialis) becomes associated with a downgrowth from the forebrain; it loses its connection with the oral ectoderm and is later transformed into the anterior lobe of the hypophysis (pituitary gland) (p. 211).

The mouth is built up by the forward growth of certain processes that appear around the margins of the oral plate; dorsally, a frontal process appears as the result of a spurt in growth of the paraxial mesoderm around the forebrain; laterally and ventrally, the margin is formed by the mandibular arch, the first of the thickenings (see further on) that develop in the mesoderm lateral to the presumptive pharynx, the most rostral part of the foregut.

The frontal process is initially a simple prominence (Fig. 3–54/1). Soon bilateral thickenings, olfactory placodes, appear in the covering ectoderm immediately bounding the oral depression. These placodes sink below the surface when growth of the surrounding mesoderm throws up a rim around each. The rim has the form of a horseshoe with a ventral interruption leading to a groove extending to the mouth. The interruption divides the lateral and medial parts of the rim, which are known hereafter as the lateral and

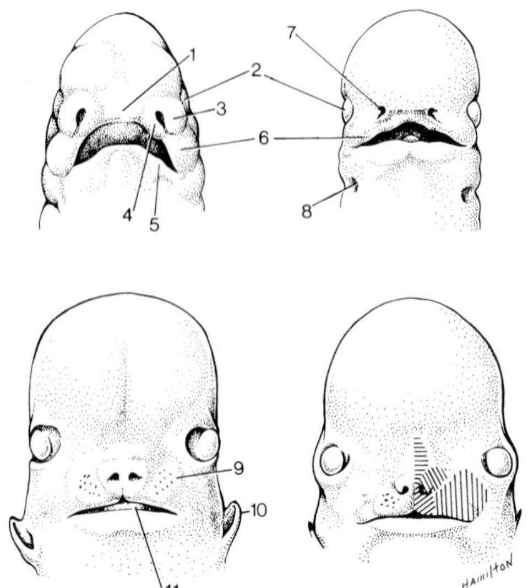


**Figure 3–54.** Development of the face (dog).

1, Frontal process; 2, eye; 3, lateral nasal process; 4, medial nasal process; 5, mandibular arch; 6, maxillary process; 7, nostril; 8, external acoustic meatus; 9, papillae of tactile hairs; 10, ear; 11, tongue.

Origin of the upper jaw and nose: *horizontal hatching,* frontal process; *vertical hatching,* maxillary process; *oblique hatching above nostril,* lateral nasal process; *oblique hatching below nostril,* medial nasal process.

medial nasal processes. The mandibular arches also expand and grow toward each other at this time; they soon fuse ventral to the oral depression, forming the continuous shelf of the lower jaw and mouth floor. In addition, the upper end of each mandibular arch detaches a maxillary process which extends forward between the frontal and mandibular processes to enclose the mouth laterally. The various swellings gradually merge.

Fusion of the mandibular and maxillary processes at the corner of the mouth builds up the cheek. The details of the conjunction of the maxillary and nasal processes are quite complicated and may vary between species. It is claimed that in some species the two maxillary processes approach and join directly, excluding the nasal processes from the dorsal margin of the mouth; that in other species the maxillary processes grow across and submerge the medial nasal processes; and that in a third group they fail to meet, allowing the medial nasal processes to form the entire central region of the upper lip. It is sometimes asserted that the modified skin around the nostrils reveals an origin from the ectoderm over the nasal processes, whereas ordinary hairy skin reveals an origin from that over the maxillary processes. One interpretation of the various contributions to the final pattern of the face is shown in Figure 3–54.

The depressions in which the olfactory placodes are contained originally communicate with the oral cavity, but these connections are lost when the placodes sink more deeply within blind pits, the nasal fossae, that now excavate the upper jaw. The tissue that remains between these pits and the mouth constitutes the primary palate. Communication between nose and mouth is regained when the pits eventually break through into the mouth cavity at two openings known as the primitive choanae (Fig. 3–55). The disruption is considerable, and only the most rostral part of the original roof to the mouth, the primary palate, survives.

The definitive nasal cavities arise from a fresh subdivision of the temporarily combined nasal and oral spaces. The inner aspect of each maxillary process sends out a flange, the palatine process, which first hangs ventrally to the side of the developing tongue. At a certain stage it undergoes a very rapid reorientation in which it is swung inward and upward to meet its fellow of the other side (Fig. 3–56). It fuses with this, with the residue of the primary palate, and with the lower edge of the septum between the nasal fossae; a horizontal shelf is thus formed between the nasal fossae and the mouth. Fusion of the residual primary palate (the region of the incisive papilla) with the palatine processes is almost complete but leaves open the small passages that become the incisive ducts. The shelf that now divides the nasal and oral cavities constitutes the secondary (definitive) palate, which later differentiates into rostral hard and caudal soft parts. The mechanism of its formation is complicated and not wholly understood; the timing is

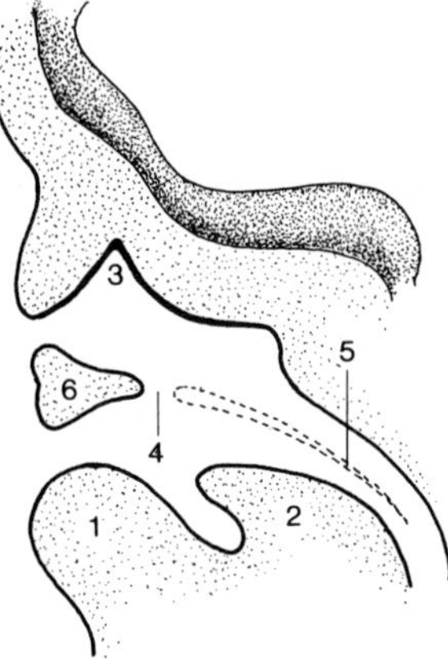


**Figure 3–55.** Sagittal section through the nasal and oral cavity of a young embryo.

1, Lower lip; 2, tongue; 3, nasal cavity; 4, primitive choana (future incisive duct); 5, position of future secondary palate; 6, primary palate.

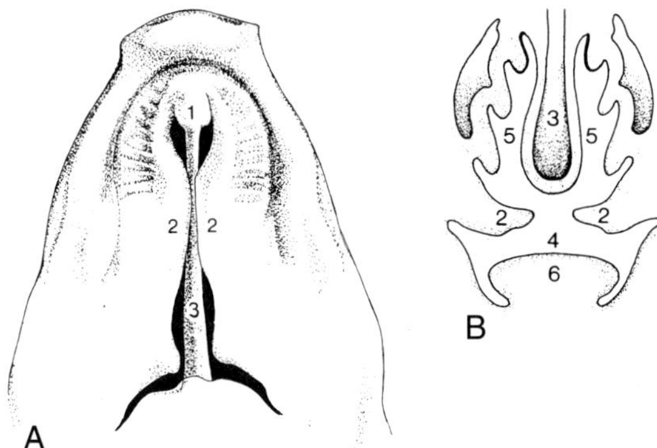


**Figure 3–56.** *A*, Ventral view of the development of the palate (pig). *B*, Transverse section through oral and nasal cavity before closure of the secondary palate.

1, Primary palate; 2, palatine processes (secondary palate); 3, nasal septum; 4, oral cavity; 5, nasal cavity; 6, tongue.

critical, since the stage at which the secondary palate forms is normally soon followed by a marked widening of the head. If reorientation of the palatine processes is delayed, they are too short to bridge the gap and fail to fuse with each other and with the ventral edge of the nasal septum, leaving the secondary palate divided by a median fissure through which the nasal and oral cavities communicate. The consequences of this anomaly (cleft palate) can be severe, not least because of resulting difficulties in feeding from the teat.

The skeleton of the face and jaws is formed by intramembranous ossification within the mesoderm. The mandible is preceded by a cartilage bar, but this is soon overlain and enveloped by bone of membranous origin; the bar thus makes no significant contribution to the definitive lower jaw.

The division of the mouth cavity into its vestibular and central parts is foreshadowed by the appearance of ectodermal thickenings that run parallel to the margins of both the maxillary and the mandibular processes. These thickenings are soon transformed into grooves, known as labiogingival grooves, since they mark the division of the lips from the outer aspect of the gums; deepening of the grooves creates and then enlarges the vestibular space. Second, similar formation internal to the labiogingival groove of the mandibular process separates the internal aspect of the gum from the lateral margin of the tongue, which is developing in the floor of the mouth. Continuing fusion of the maxillary and mandibular processes at the angle of the mouth enlarges the part of the vestibular wall that is formed by the cheek at the expense of that formed by the lips.

The salivary glands, both major and minor, are formed from solid outgrowths of epithelium that push into the underlying mesenchyme. These branch repeatedly and are later canalized to form both gland acini and ducts. It is tempting to suppose that their sites of origin correspond with the points of entry of the adult ducts; however, some evidence suggests that the openings may be relocated when grooves in the oral epithelium are bridged over, extending the ducts.

The *tongue* develops in the floor of the mouth. It has a complicated origin, being formed by the mergence of several swellings (Fig. 3–57). One, a median (distal) tongue swelling, appears on the pharyngeal floor between the lower ends of the mandibular arches and later fuses with more lateral swellings that appear over the adjacent parts of these arches. A more caudal (proximal) swelling extends from the floor onto the ventral parts of the second, third, and, possibly, fourth pharyngeal arches. The caudal swelling divides, the caudal part becoming the epiglottis, the rostral part blending with the other contributions to the tongue. The thyroid gland develops from the pharyngeal floor between the median and proximal swellings. It initially has a connection (thyroglossal duct) with the pharyngeal epithelium; although this is later lost, a pit (foramen cecum) may occasionally mark the boundary of the rostral and caudal contributions to the adult tongue in humans, although never in domestic species. The substance of the tongue is supposed to derive mainly from myotomes of occipital somites. It is alleged that material from these myotomes migrates forward under the floor of the mouth, and although the evidence is not wholly convincing, the theory satisfactorily accounts for the innervation of the lingual muscles by the hypoglossal nerve—the nerve specific to the

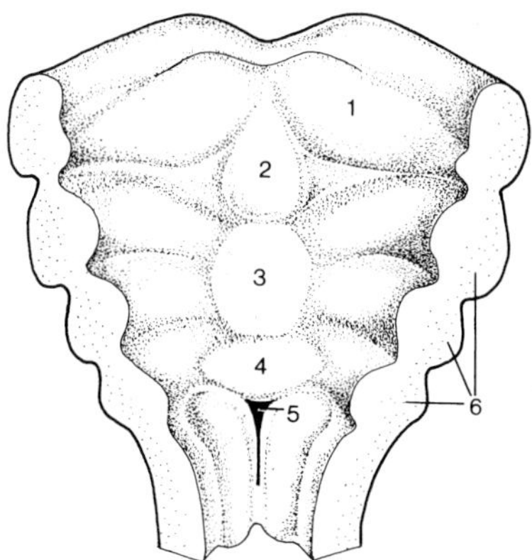


**Figure 3–57.** Development of the tongue in the floor of the oral cavity.

1, Distal (lateral) tongue swelling; 2, median tongue swelling; 3, proximal tongue swelling; 4, primordium of epiglottis; 5, laryngeal entrance; 6, pharyngeal arches.

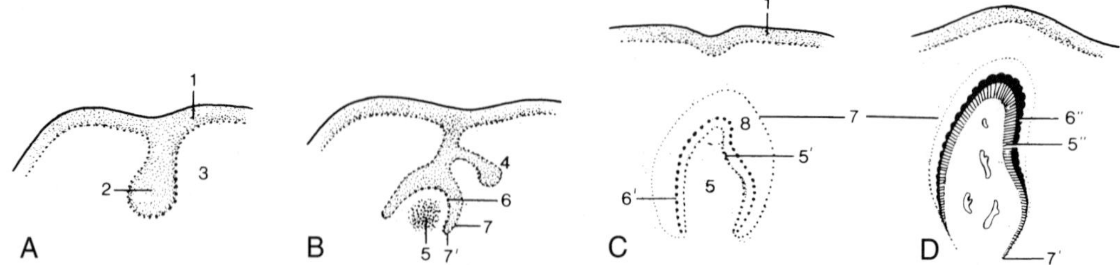


**Figure 3–58.** *A,* Development of dental plate. *B,* Development of an enamel organ. *C,* Enamel organ. *D,* Deciduous tooth before eruption.

1, Epithelium of oral cavity; 2, dental plate; 3, mesenchyme; 4, bud of a permanent tooth; 5, dental papilla; 5′, odontoblasts (differentiated from the outer cell layer of the papilla); 5″, dentine; 6, inner dental epithelium (future ameloblasts); 6′, ameloblasts; 6″, enamel; 7, outer dental epithelium; 7′, transition of inner and outer dental epithelia (where root formation occurs); 8, enamel reticulum.

occipital somites. The sensory supply to the lingual epithelium involves the mandibular, fascial, glossopharyngeal, and vagus nerves, the nerves associated with the first, second, third, and fourth arches.

The separation of the tongue from the floor is gradual; it is more complete for the part that derives from the median swelling and first arches (apex and body) than for that which derives from the proximal swelling (root).

The first indications of the *teeth* are ribbon-like thickenings of the epithelium parallel but internal to the labiogingival thickenings previously described. The thickenings extend as plates, dental laminae, into the subjacent mesenchyme (Fig. 3–58); quite soon a linear series of knoblike swellings buds from the deep margin of each. The swellings represent the enamel organs of the temporary teeth, and their number corresponds to the dental formula of the species. Occasionally it is greater; the disparity occurs when primordia appear—and possibly develop quite far—for teeth that later regress without erupting. The upper incisors of ruminants are examples of teeth whose development is aborted in this way.

The mesenchyme condenses against the free surfaces of each bud; when the bud shortly invaginates, the dense mesoderm, which is now known as the dental papilla, fills the resulting cup. The whole tooth germ—the enamel organ together with the dental papilla—is enclosed by a mesenchymal thickening that merges with the papilla at its base, forming the dental sac or follicle that later gives rise to the periodontal membrane and the root cement.

The enamel organ consists of an inner dental epithelium (over the concave surface applied to the dental papilla), an outer dental epithelium (over the convex surface facing the dental follicle), and an intervening loose and sparsely cellular tissue (enamel reticulum) resembling the Wharton's jelly of the umbilical cord (Fig. 3–58). The cells of the inner dental epithelium are known as ameloblasts, since they produce enamel. Enamel formation begins over the center of the crown but soon spreads outward from this focus. As the layer thickens, the ameloblasts retreat in a centrifugal direction until finally they meet and fuse with the outer dental epithelium to form an epithelial cuticle or membrane. This covers the completed crown and remains until worn away after eruption.

Meanwhile, certain cells of the mesodermal papilla have become arranged in a sheet facing the ameloblasts. Since they produce dentine, they are known as odontoblasts. The first dentine also appears toward the center of the crown, a little later than the first deposition of enamel. Thereafter dentine deposition also spreads out in all directions. As the layer thickens the odontoblasts withdraw in a centripetal direction, and when a dentine production has ceased they remain as a covering to the pulp, the surviving less differentiated portion of the original papilla.

The root of the tooth develops somewhat later than the crown. It is ensheathed by a prolongation of the enamel organ, simplified by the omission of the intermediate reticulum and not productive of enamel. The sheath later breaks down when the follicular tissue produces cement to encase the dentine of the root.

After the enamel organs of the temporary teeth have appeared the dental lamina undergoes extensive destruction. However, its free edge remains to produce a second crop of buds, the enamel organs of the replacement teeth; these remain dormant for a time, but when activated the sequence of events replicates that seen in the development of the temporary teeth.

## The Pharynx

Many details of the development of the pharyngeal region are more appropriately considered in Chapters 2 and 6. The pharynx is initially dorsoventrally flattened and widest immediately behind the oral plate, but the simple initial form is altered by the unequal growth of the mesoderm flanking the endodermal tube (Fig. 3–59). This mesoderm forms serial thickenings—the pharyngeal (branchial) arches—which protrude into the pharyngeal lumen and bulge on the surface of the neck. The internal modeling of the lumen defines a series of pharyngeal pouches with which corresponding grooves coincide externally (Fig. 3–59). The number of arches (and therefore of pouches) is disputed and many well vary among mammalian species. It is most commonly assumed that five arches exist and that these represent the first four and the sixth of the somewhat longer series that develops in other vertebrates; apparently the fifth is always suppressed. Each arch develops an internal skeleton and musculature with which a particular cranial nerve is associated; the fates of these have been tabulated elsewhere (p. 58). Each pouch of the pharyngeal lumen has also its specific fate (see Fig. 6–5). The features of immediate interest include the contribution of the first, and possibly the second, pouch to the cavity of the middle ear—a fate revealed in the adult by the site of entry of the auditory tube into the nasopharynx. The ventral part of the second pouch forms the tonsillar sinus, a landmark that in the adult provides some clue to the position of the boundary between the ectodermal and endodermal parts of the oral lining.

The outgrowth of the lower respiratory tract at the caudal limit of the pharynx is considered in the following chapter.

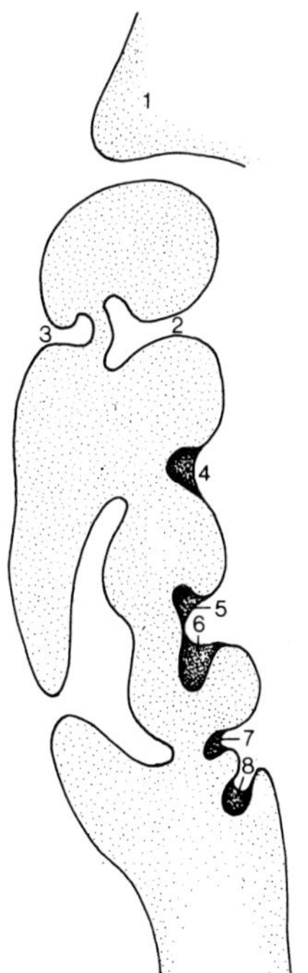


**Figure 3–59.** Dorsal section of the left side of the pharynx showing the development of the pharyngeal arches and pouches.

1, Maxillary process; 2, pharyngotympanic tube (future auditory tube); 3, external auditory meatus; 4, palatine tonsil (in tonsillar sinus); 5, parathyroid gland III; 6, thymus; 7, parathyroid gland IV; 8, ultimobranchial body.

## The Caudal Part of the Foregut

A fusiform enlargement identifies the stomach at an early stage. The portion of the foregut between this and the caudal limit of the pharynx becomes the esophagus, which is initially very short but elongates as the heart descends from the neck into the thorax. The esophagus is involved in the origin of the lower respiratory tract (pp. 164–165) but, this apart, presents little of interest in its development. At one stage, the rapid proliferation of the endodermal lining completely obstructs the lumen, but the passage is later restored.

The development of the stomach involves displacement, reorientation, and differential enlargement. The displacement carries the stomach from a position in the neck to one ventral to the caudal thoracic segments. Although reorientation appears to involve rotations about two axes, it is possibly the result of unequal growth of the stomach wall. However, it is usual and simpler to assume that the rotations do occur. Rotation about the long axis of the stomach spindle carries the originally dorsal aspect to the left, where it is later distinguished as the convex greater curvature. The dorsal megogastrium, which becomes the greater omentum, shares in the process. The second rotation, about a dorsoventral axis, swings the cranial (cardiac) extremity to the left, the caudal (pyloric) one to the right (Fig. 3–60). In the dog the most conspicuous change in shape is an asymmetrical enlargement to the left of the cardia that produces the fundus; a much more radical reshaping is required in ruminants to produce the four compartments of their stomachs. The various tunics of the stomach wall differentiate quite early; in the human fetus the gastric glands are established and capable of secretion by midterm.

The short portion of foregut between the gastric spindle and the midgut forms the initial part of the

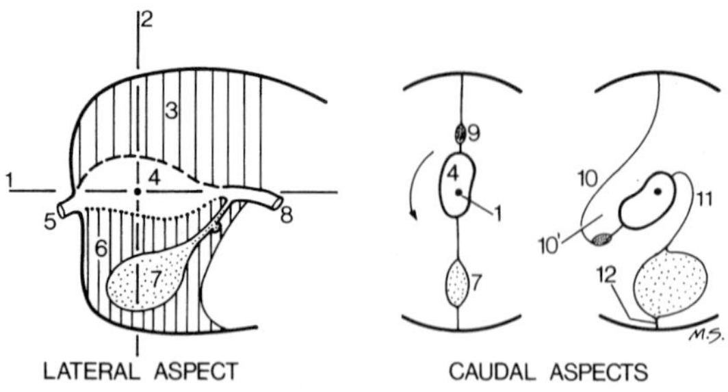


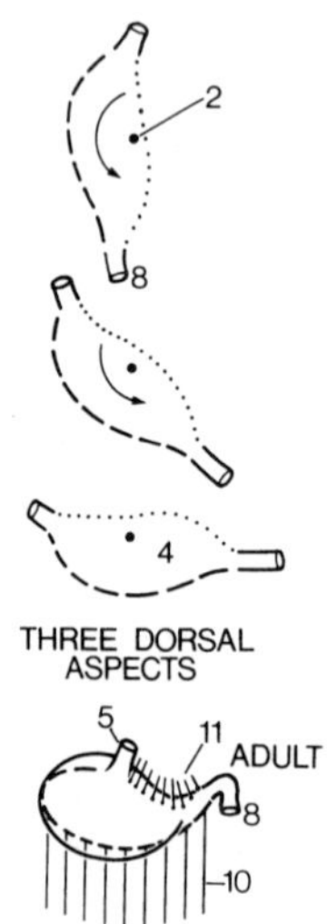


**Figure 3–60.** The reorientation of the developing simple stomach. It rotates counterclockwise (as seen from behind) around a longitudinal axis (caudal aspects [1]) and continues counterclockwise (as seen from above) around a dorsoventral axis (three dorsal aspects [2]).

1, Longitudinal axis; 2, dorsoventral (vertical) axis; 3, dorsal mesogastrium; 4, stomach primordium; 5, esophagus; 6, ventral mesogastrium; 7, developing liver; 8, duodenum; 9, developing spleen; 10, greater omentum; 10′, omental bursa; 11, lesser omentum; 12, developing ligaments of the liver.

duodenum that terminates at the entrance of the bile and pancreatic ducts. The sites of origin of the primordia of the liver and pancreas are the relevant landmarks in the young embryo. This part of the duodenum is transported to the right in the rotation of the stomach.

## The Liver and Pancreas

The liver appears as an endodermal diverticulum at the junction of the fore- and midguts. It quickly divides into a cranial branch, which forms the gland tissue and hepatic ducts, and a caudal branch, which forms the gallbladder and cystic duct (Fig. 3–61).

The cranial branch extends finger-like processes into the splanchnic mesoderm of the adjacent septum transversum, carried here with the formation of the head fold. As the processes penetrate the mesoderm they engage with the vitelloumbilical system of veins, which follows this route from the extraembryonic membranes. Very soon a three-dimensional spongework of hepatic cell-cords and plates is formed, surrounded on all sides by thin-walled blood vessels—a precocious realization of the adult arrangement. The developing liver is confined to the dorsal part of the septum transversum, since its rapid growth causes it to draw away from the ventral part (which gives rise to much of the substance of the diaphragm). The connection between the dorsal and ventral parts of the septum survives in modified form as the parietal ligaments of the liver. A similar attenuation of the connection between the liver and the gut becomes the lesser omentum.

Canalization of the caudal branch of the primordium creates the gallbladder and distal duct system, whose entrance to the gut is shifted dorsally by differential growth of the duodenal wall.

The growth of the liver, extremely rapid in younger embryos, is a major factor in the caudal shift of the stomach and the temporary herniation of the midgut (see further on). Although it slows later, the liver remains disproportionately large (by comparison with that of the adult) until well after birth. One relevant factor is the exercise before birth of an erythropoietic activity that is later

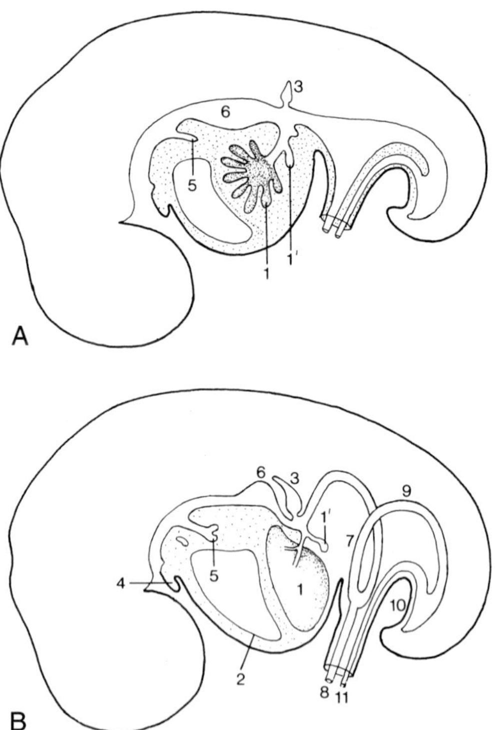


**Figure 3–61.** Development of the liver. *A,* Early development: a cranial branch (1) of the endodermal diverticulum invades the septum transversum; a caudal branch (1′) forms the gallbladder and cystic duct. *B,* A later stage, in which the developing liver expands caudally into the abdominal cavity.

1, Liver; 1′, gallbladder; 2, pericardium and heart; 3, dorsal primordium of pancreas; 4, tongue; 5, tracheobronchial diverticulum; 6, stomach; 7, loop of midgut; 8, vitelline duct; 9, hindgut; 10, cloacal membrane; 11, allantoic stalk.

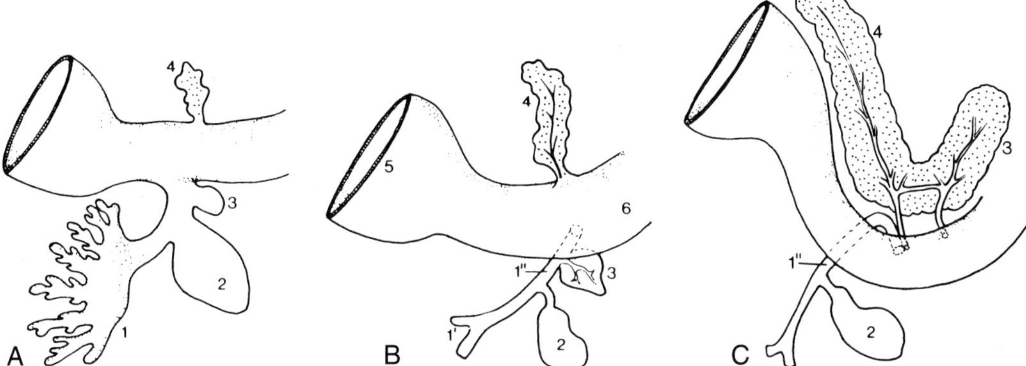


**Figure 3–62.** Development of the pancreas. *A,* Early stage. *B,* A later stage showing separate duct systems in the two primordia. *C,* The two primordia have fused after the migration of the ventral pancreas. The dorsal pancreas now drains mainly via the ventral duct system.

1, Liver premordium; 1′, hepatic ducts; 1″, bile duct; 2, gallbladder; 3, ventral primordium of pancreas; 4, dorsal primordium of pancreas; 5, stomach; 6, duodenum.

relinquished. The secretory and metabolic functions are established by midterm in the human fetus.

The pancreas arises from the same portion of the foregut as the liver. The initial development takes the form of two primordia, one dorsal, the second ventral and associated with the hepatic outgrowth (Fig. 3–62). The enlargement of the ventral outgrowth brings it into contact and later fusion with the dorsal bud. This usually involves combination of the two duct systems, following which one or the other may lose its connection with the gut. The islet tissue develops by budding from the ducts. Both endocrine and exocrine components are competent well before birth.

The celiac artery is associated with the postpharyngeal part of the foregut.

## The Midgut

The midgut forms the bulk of the intestine, from the entry of the bile duct to the junction of the transverse and descending parts of the colon. Its initial wide connection with the yolk sac is quickly reduced to a narrow (vitelline) duct midway along its length. Ultimately even this connection is lost, although a small (Meckel's) diverticulum of the adult jejunum occasionally marks the site.

The early growth of the midgut is very rapid, causing it to hang in a loop from an elongated mesentery in which the midgut (cranial mesenteric) artery runs. The liver, also expanding fast, soon claims so large a part of the abdominal cavity that insufficient room remains for the intestine. The long mesentery permits the midgut to slip out of the abdominal cavity into the umbilical cord—a process known as physiological herniation—where growth continues. The cranial limb of the herniated loop (which has the attachment of the vitelline duct at its apex) becomes the small intestine; the appearance of a diverticulum, the future cecum, indicates the division of the caudal limb into the terminal part of the small intestine and the initial part of the colon. The cranial limb grows more rapidly and soon becomes much coiled. The key event is the rotation of the loop about the arterial axis (Fig. 3–63), a rotation that carries the originally caudal limb forward on the left, then across the abdomen before it passes caudally on the right side, completing a rotation through 270 degrees or so—three quarters of a full turn. This rotation, which is clockwise when viewed from above, brings the intestines more or less into their adult disposition when they are returned to the abdomen (Fig. 3–64). The return is possible because the rate of liver increase slows and falls behind the general growth of the embryo. The final species-specific arrangement may depend on local shortenings of the mesentery and fusions of apposed peritoneum-clad surfaces.

## The Hindgut

The hindgut develops into the descending colon and the rectum, parts supplied by the caudal mesenteric artery in the adult. Initially this part of the gut ends blindly against the cloacal plate, the membrane that forms the floor of the proctodeum, the pit analogous to the stomodeum. Except in the horse, in which the descending colon shows a

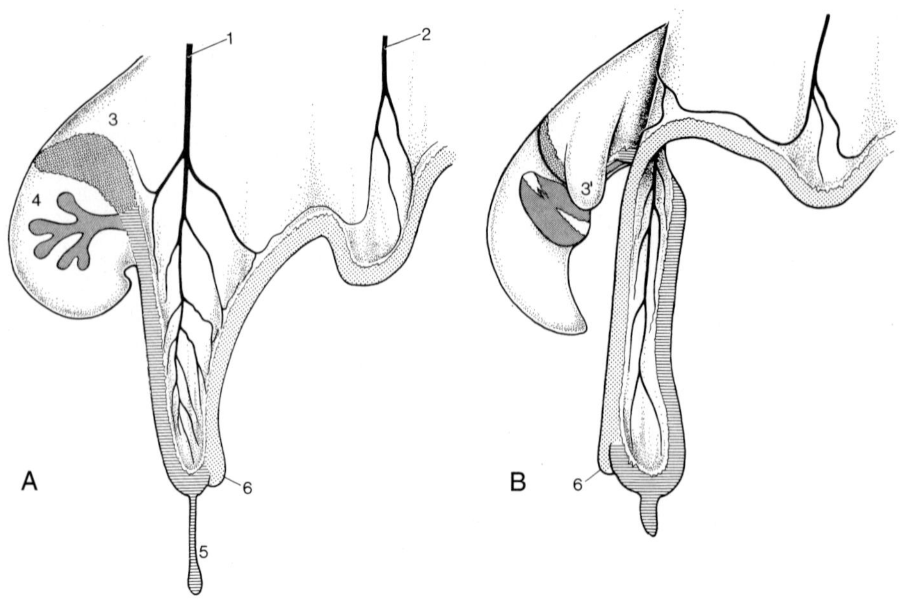

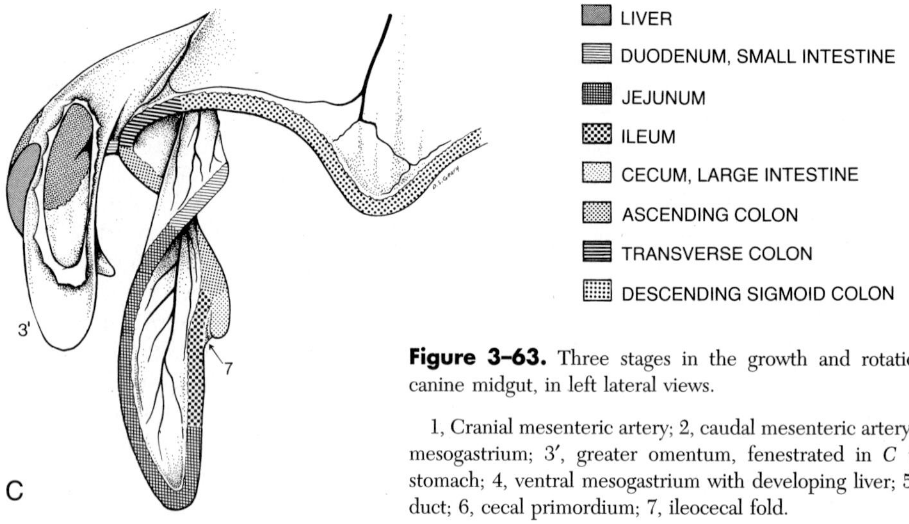

1
2
3
4
3'
5
6
A
B

3'
7
C
STOMACH
LIVER
DUODENUM, SMALL INTESTINE
JEJUNUM
ILEUM
CECUM, LARGE INTESTINE
ASCENDING COLON
TRANSVERSE COLON
DESCENDING SIGMOID COLON

**Figure 3–63.** Three stages in the growth and rotation of the canine midgut, in left lateral views.

1, Cranial mesenteric artery; 2, caudal mesenteric artery; 3, dorsal mesogastrium; 3′, greater omentum, fenestrated in *C* to expose stomach; 4, ventral mesogastrium with developing liver; 5, vitelline duct; 6, cecal primordium; 7, ileocecal fold.

6 1
2
3
4
5
10
9
8
7
11

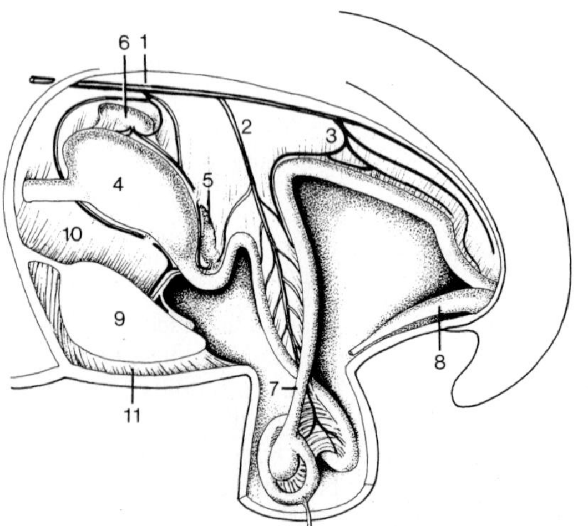

**Figure 3–64.** Development of the intestinal tract during the rotation process. The midgut loop is herniated into the extraembryonic celom.

1, Celiac artery; 2, cranial mesenteric artery; 3, caudal mesenteric artery; 4, stomach; 5, pancreas; 6, spleen; 7, loop of midgut; 8, bladder expansion of the urogenital sinus; 9, liver; 10, lesser omentum; 11, falciform ligament.

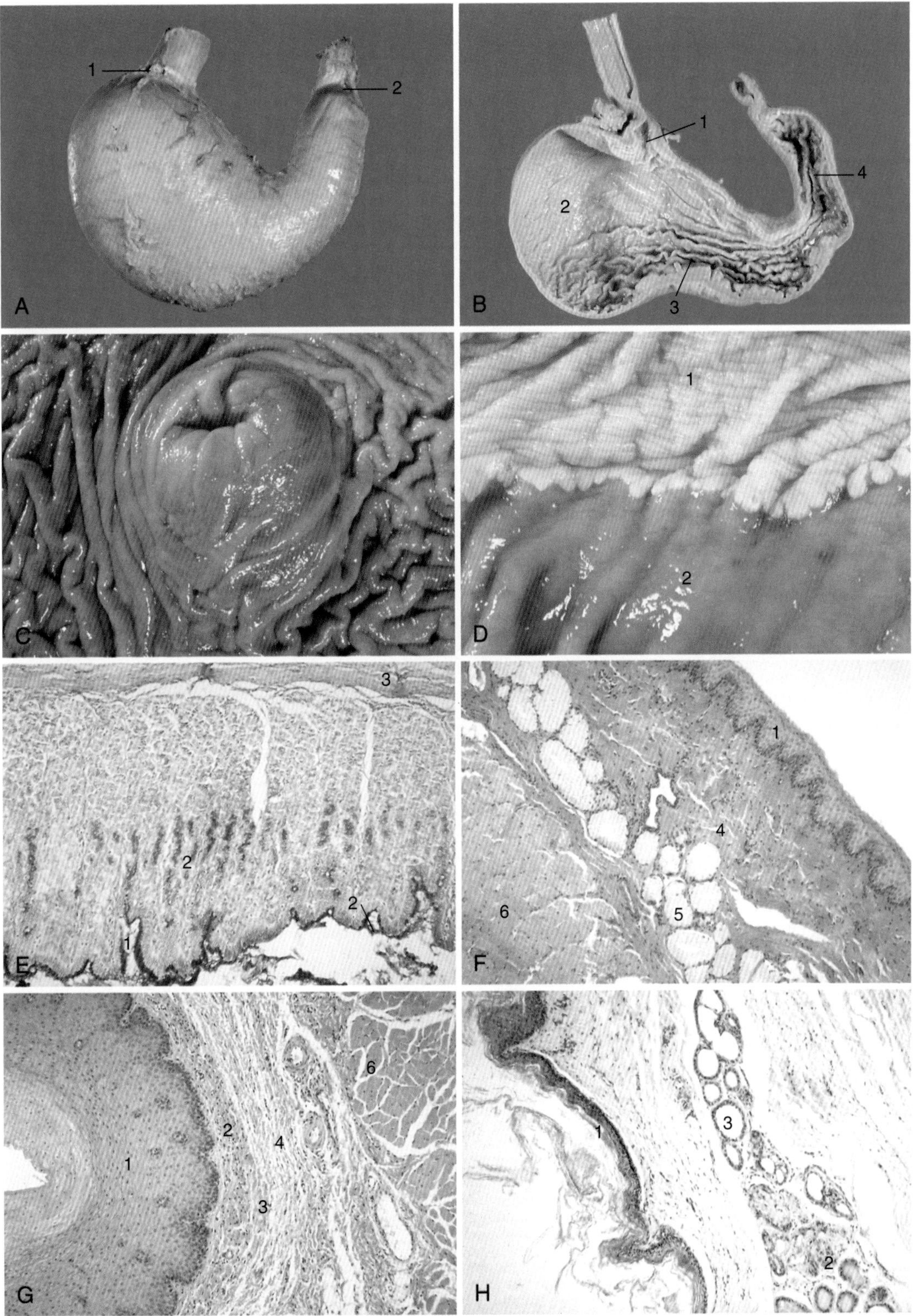

**Plate 1.** *A,* Visceral surface of stomach (dog): 1, cardia; 2, pylorus. *B,* Interior of stomach (dog): 1, cardiac opening; 2, fundus; 3 pyloric antrum; 4, pyloric canal. *C,* Protruding cardia (dog). *D,* Demarcation between nonglandular (1) and glandular (2) (cardiac) regions of the stomach (pig). *E,* Mucosa of the stomach (PAS-H; 70×) (dog): 1, gastric pit; 2, mucopolysaccharide secreting cells; 3, lam. muscularis mucosae. *F* and *G,* Esophagus (dog) and (goat), respectively (70×): 1, stratif. squam. epithelium; 2, lam. propria; 3, lam. muscularis mucosae; 4, submucosa; 5, mucus-secreting tubuoacinar glands; 6, muscularis interna. *H,* Anal sac and associated glands (dog) (70×): 1, cutaneous epithelium; 2, tubuloalveolar glands; 3, ducts.

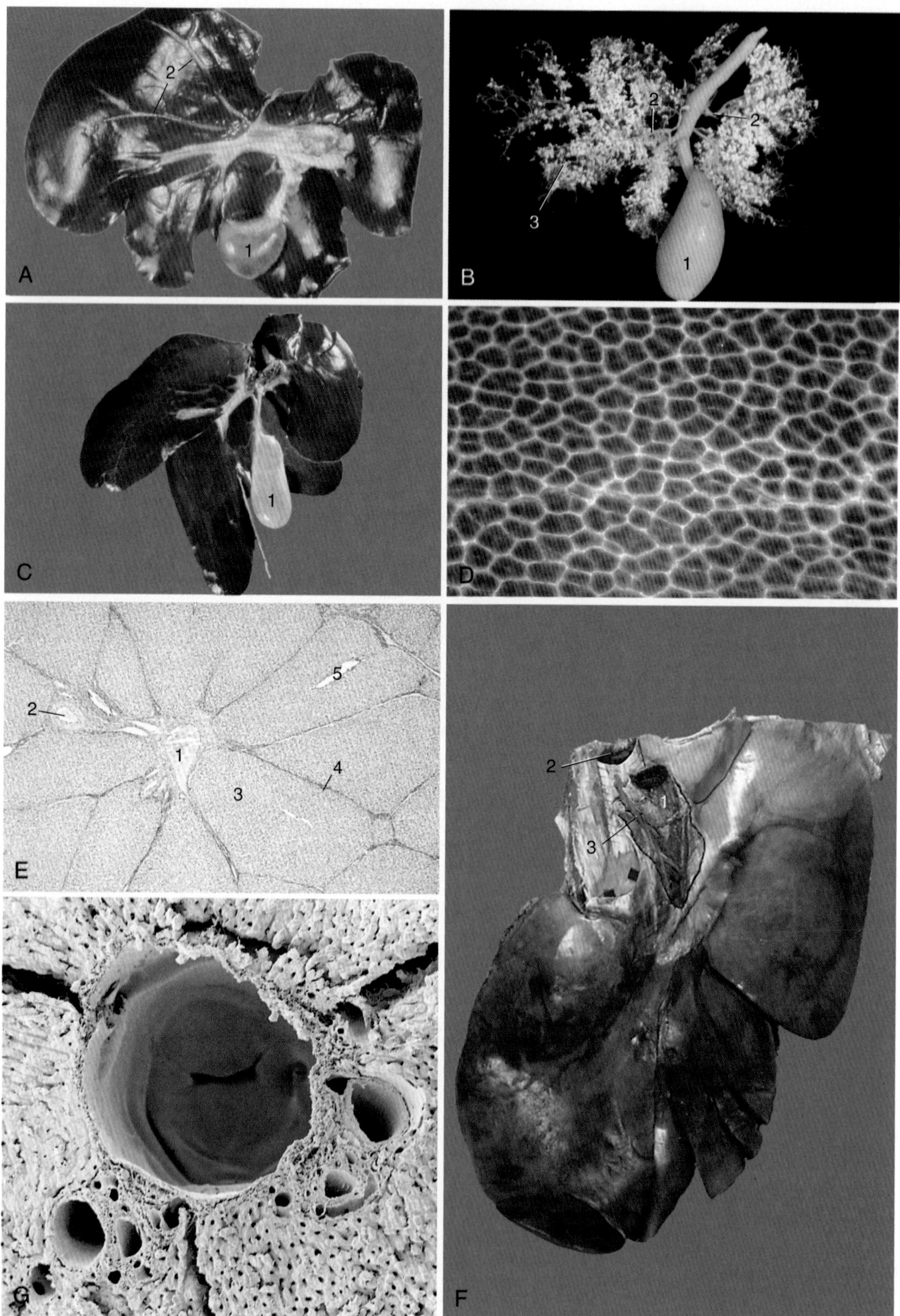


**Plate 2.** *A,* Visceral surface of liver (dog): 1, gallbladder; 2, hapetic ducts. *B,* Corrosion cast of hepatic duct system (dog): 1, gallbladder; 2, major hepatic ducts; 3, ductules. *C,* Visceral surface of liver (pig): 1, distended gallbladder. *D,* Surface of liver (enlarged) with clearly defined hepatic lobules (pig). *E,* Liver (pig) (28×): 1, central v.; 2, interlobular a.; 3, hepatic lobule; 4, interlobular connective tissue; 5, centrolobular venule. *F,* Visceral surface of liver (horse): 1, portal v.; 2, caudal caval v.; 3, hepatic a. *G,* S.E.M. of corrosion cast of hepatic vessels (rat); note valve within central v.

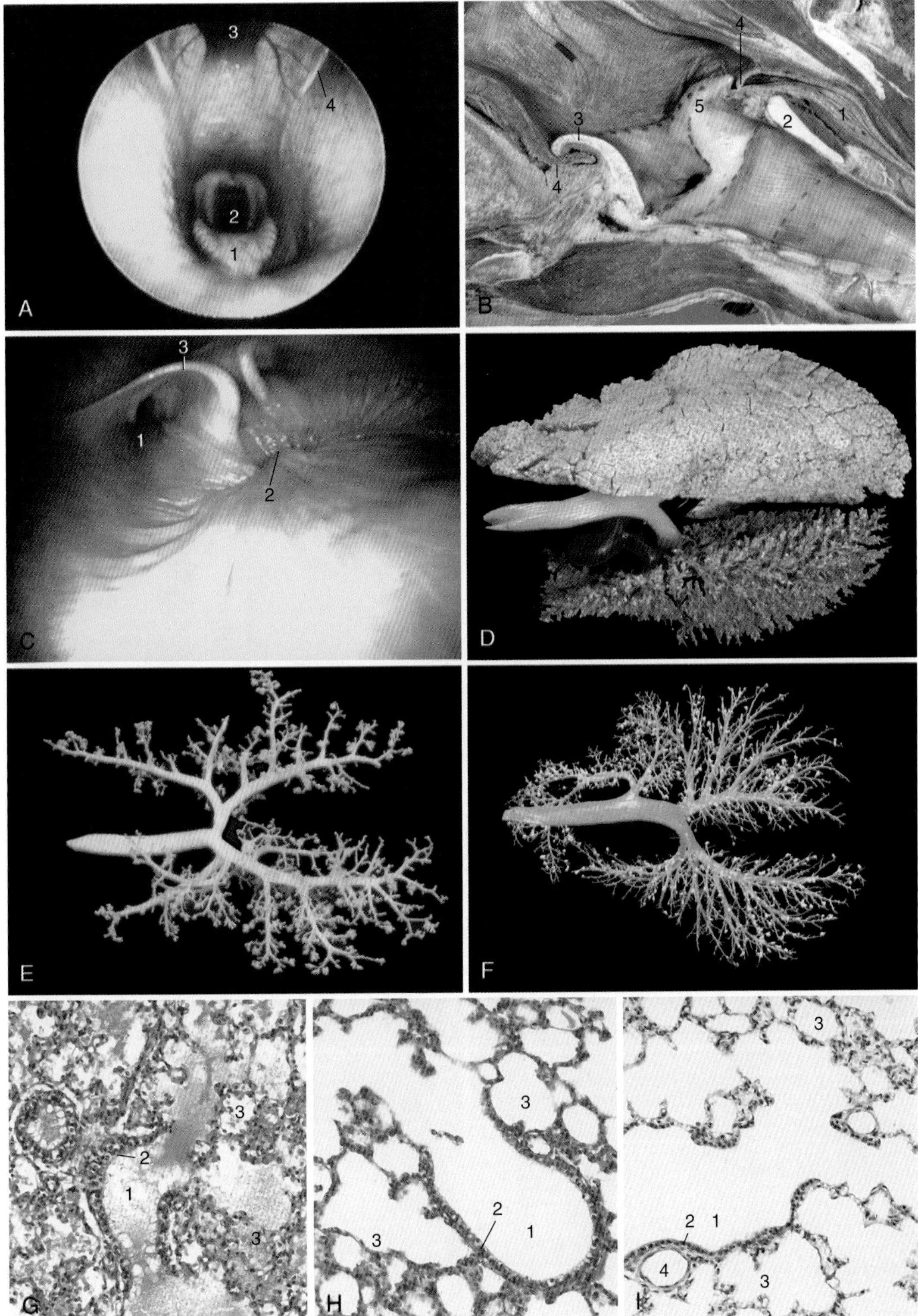


**Plate 3.** *A,* Endoscopic view of equine nasopharynx: 1, epiglottis; 2, laryngeal entrance; 3, pharyngeal recess; 4, entrance to auditory tube. *B,* Sagittal section of junction of pharynx with larynx (horse): 1, esophagus; 2, cricoid lamina; 3, epiglottis; 4, palatropharyngeal arch; 5, corniculate process of arytenoid cartilage. *C,* Caudal part of nasopharynx during swallowing (horse): 1, entrance to auditory tube; 2, closure between the rostral and caudal parts of the nasopharynx (during swallowing); 3, cartilage flange supporting the auditory tube. *D,* Corrosion cast of bronchial tree of pig (yellow), pulmonary a. (red) and pulmonary vv. (blue). *E,* Corrosion cast of bronchial tree (cat). *F,* Corrosion cast of bronchial tree (calf). *G,* Lung of pig fetus (140×); note presence of fluid in bronchioles and alveoli; 1, terminal bronchioles; 2, bronchiolar exocrinocyte (clara) cells; 3, alveoli; 4, venule. *H,* Lung of 1-day-old piglet (140×). *I,* Lung of an adult pig (140×).

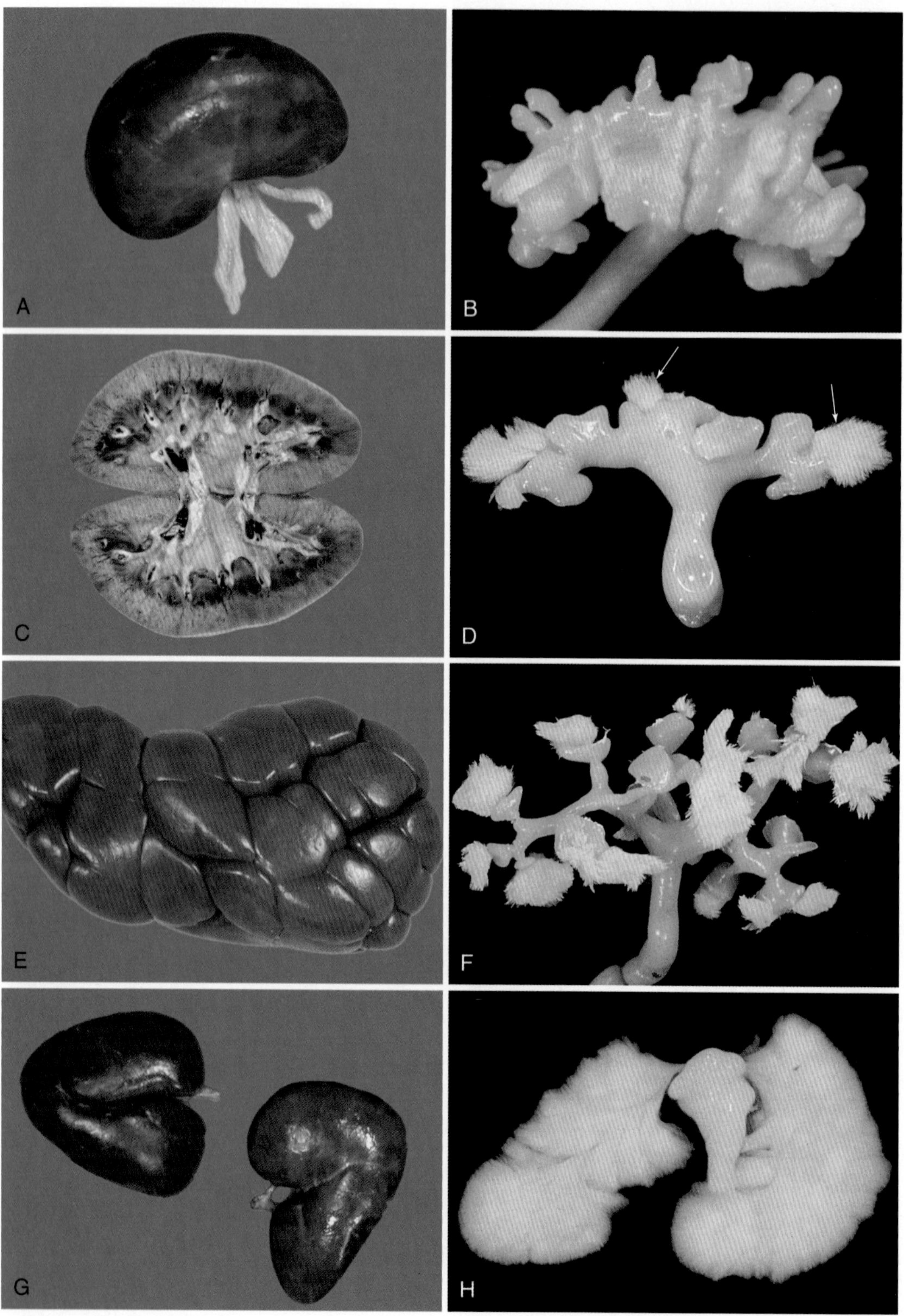


**Plate 4.** *A,* Kidney (dog). *B,* Corrosion cast of renal pelvis (dog). *C,* Sectioned kidney (pig). *D,* Corrosion cast of renal pelvis (pig); note papillary ducts *(arrows)*. *E,* Kidney (cow). *F,* Corrosion cast of renal pelvis (cow); note papillary ducts. *G,* Right (heart-shaped) and left kidneys (horse). *H,* Corrosion cast of renal pelvis (horse): note papillary ducts.

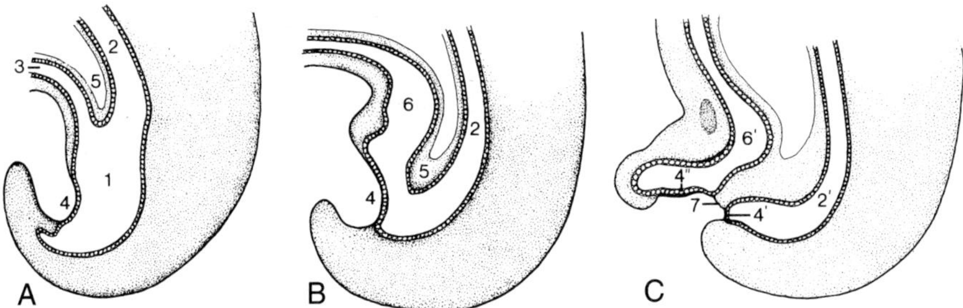


**Figure 3–65.** Division of the distal part of the hindgut into rectum and urogenital sinus. *A*, Formation of the allantois and beginning of the caudal extension of the urorectal septum (5). *B*, The urorectal septum now approaches the cloacal membrane. *C*, Complete division of urogenital sinus and anorectal canal.

1, Cloaca; 2, hindgut; 2′, anorectal canal; 3, allantois; 4, cloacal membrane; 4′, anal membrane; 4″, urogenital membrane; 5, urorectal septum; 6, primitive urogenital sinus; 6′, urogenital sinus; 7, tissue bridge ventral to future anus.

considerable secondary increase in length, significant changes affect only the terminal part of the hindgut. A bud, the allantois, grows from its ventral aspect toward and through the umbilical opening in the abdominal wall; once outside the embryo it enlarges to form the capacious allantoic sac, an important component of the fetal membranes. A wedge of tissue (urorectal septum) enlarging in the angle between the gut and this diverticulum thrusts toward the cloacal membrane (Fig. 3–65). When it meets this, it divides the gut into two completely separate tubes; the dorsal one is continuous with the descending colon; the ventral one is continuous with the allantois and is destined to form the lower urogenital tract (p. 167). Meantime, proliferation of mesoderm beneath the ectoderm around the proctodeum has deepened the pit; when the dorsal part (anal membrane) of the cloacal membrane breaks down, this deepening is added to the gut, providing it with the anal canal that leads to the exterior.

# CHAPTER 4

# The Respiratory Apparatus

The essential organs of respiration are the lungs, in which gaseous exchange takes place between the inspired air and the blood stream. The ancillary organs comprise the passages through which air is led to and from the lungs. The nose is included, although it may alternatively be considered among the organs of special sense since it evolved as the organ of olfaction. The pharynx, in which the air and food streams cross, is more conveniently considered among the digestive organs, although its upper part (nasopharynx) is purely an airway. A short account of the development follows the description of the adult anatomy.

## THE NOSE

The nose* (nasus) in the broad sense comprises the external nose, the paired nasal cavities, and the paranasal sinuses. A case may be argued for also including the nasopharynx.

An *external nose* such as forms so conspicuous a feature of the human face is hardly to be recognized in the domestic species, in which it is merged within the general contours of the muzzle (Fig. 4–1). Its extent is more easily determined on palpation since it more or less corresponds with the part of the muzzle skeleton that is cartilaginous and therefore flexible. It is divided internally into two cavities, the nasal vestibules, each entered through a nostril and leading through a region of constriction to the much larger nasal cavity placed beyond. The form and size of the nostrils, their orientation, and the nature of the surrounding integument all show considerable species differences. The integument around the nostrils is naked and sharply demarcated from the unmodified skin in all domestic species other than the horse. According to its extent, the modified region is variously known as the nasal (carnivores, small ruminants), nasolabial (cattle), or rostral (pigs) plate. The nasal plate may be divided by a median groove or philtrum (/2). The plate is kept moist in cattle, pigs, and dogs; in the first two species the moisture is derived from closely packed underlying glands, whereas in the dog it is an overflow of the secretion of glands of the nasal mucosa, principally the lateral nasal glands.

The cartilages that support the external nose are variable in form, relative size, and even number. The rostral end of the nasal septum forms the median partition between the right and left vestibules and includes a small bone (os rostrale) in the pig. The free edge of the septum gives attachment to other cartilages that support the dorsal and lateral margins of the nostril and determine the form of the opening. One, the alar cartilage, is especially large in the horse and accounts for the curious comma form of the nostril, which is divided in this species into a ventral part, the so-called true nostril leading to the nasal cavity, and a dorsal part, the false nostril leading to a skin-lined diverticulum occupying the nasoincisive notch (see Fig. 18–3). The nostril is round in the pig, but in most other species it is prolonged laterally by a slitlike extension. The form of the nostril may be altered, principally by raising the lateral "wing" (ala) actively by certain facial muscles or passively when the air flow is increased in strenuous breathing or when sniffing. These changes can be very pronounced in the horse, leading to compression and almost complete obliteration of the diverticulum.

The integument is carried some distance into the vestibule, where it meets the nasal mucosa at a sharply defined line near which several ducts may open. In the horse these include the nasolacrimal (tear) duct, whose opening is very evident on inspection of the vestibular floor of the live animal; the opening is less easily found in other species, either because the tissues are less pliant (cattle) or because it is placed more deeply (dog). The much smaller openings of the long ducts of the serous lateral nasal glands also discharge in this area. This arrangement aids humidification of the incoming air since the acceleration of flow at the constriction favors vaporization of tears and other watery discharge.

The two *nasal cavities* occupy a large part of the face since they extend caudally to the transverse bony septum at the rostral end of the cranial cavity

*The Greek word for nose, *rhin,* provides the stem for many medical terms, for example, rhinitis.

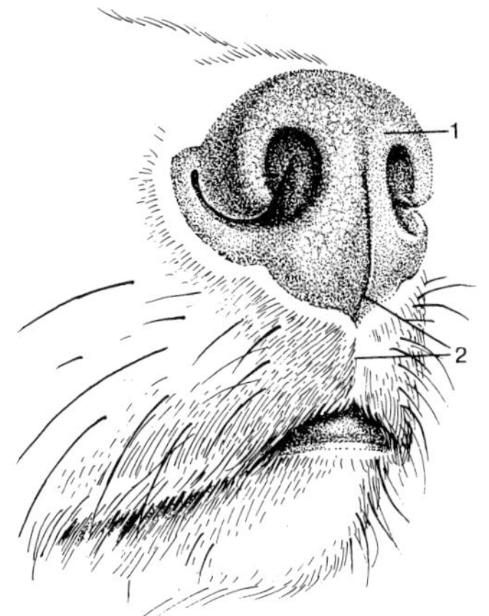


**Figure 4–1.** The canine muzzle.

1, Nasal plate; 2, philtrum.

(Fig. 4–2). Their size may be gauged from the conformation of the head, but the first impression is apt to be grossly misleading. Several features greatly reduce the extent of the cavities below expectation. In the first place, certain bones bounding the cavity are thickened by air spaces (paranasal sinuses) that communicate with the cavity but do not form part of it. Secondly, the embedded portions of the upper cheek teeth occupy a surprising amount of space, especially in the horse. The potential space is also much reduced by certain very delicate mucosa-covered turbinate bones (conchae) that project into the interior from the dorsal and lateral walls. Finally, the walls are covered by a mucosa locally thickened by vascular plexuses (Figs. 4–3, 4–4, and 4–5).

The right and left cavities are divided by the nasal septum, which is largely cartilaginous but ossified in its most caudal part (the perpendicular plate of the ethmoid bone). The septum meets the upper surface of the hard palate, which separates the nasal and mouth cavities, but the details vary greatly between species (Fig. 4–5). In the horse the septum meets the whole length of the hard palate so that each nasal cavity communicates with the pharynx through a separate opening (choana) (see Fig. 18–10). In other species (e.g., ox, dog) the caudal part of the septum fails to meet the palate and a single opening is shared by the two sides (Figs. 4–4/7 and 25–10).

The conchae, which intrude on the cavity, have a complicated and variable pattern. Classified by topography (and not by morphology), they comprise a caudal system (of ethmoidal conchae) constituting the lateral mass or labyrinth of the ethmoid bone and a rostral (nasal) system in which

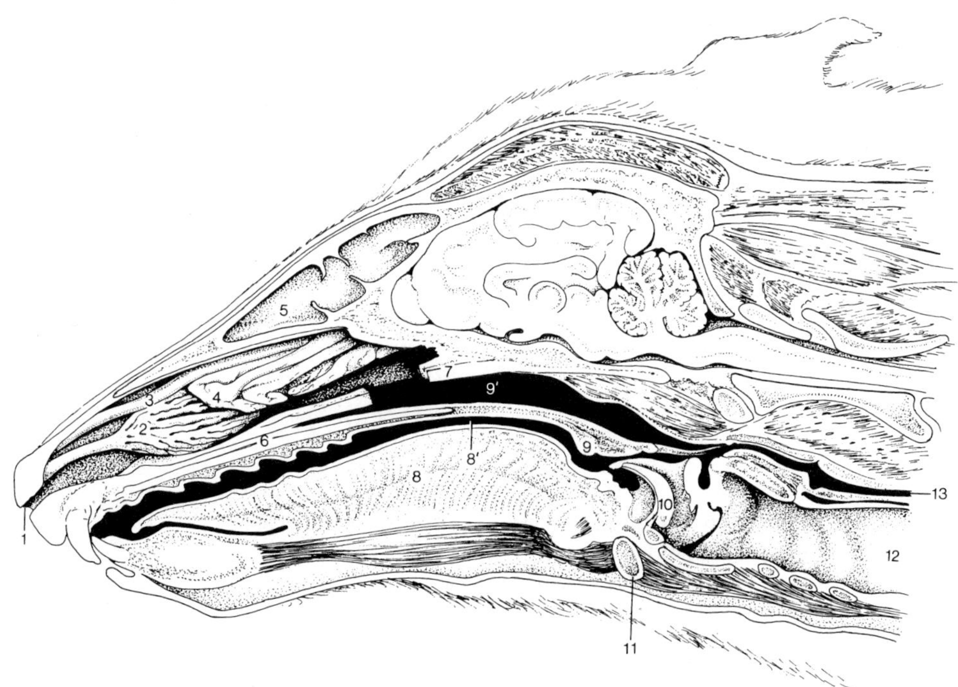


**Figure 4–2.** Paramedian section of the canine head; the nasal septum has been removed.

1, Right nostril; 2, ventral nasal concha; 3, dorsal nasal concha; 4, ethmoidal conchae; 5, frontal sinus; 6, hard palate; 7, vomer, resected; 8, tongue; 8′, oropharynx; 9, soft palate; 9′, nasopharynx; 10, epiglottis; 11, basihyoid; 12, trachea; 13, esophagus.

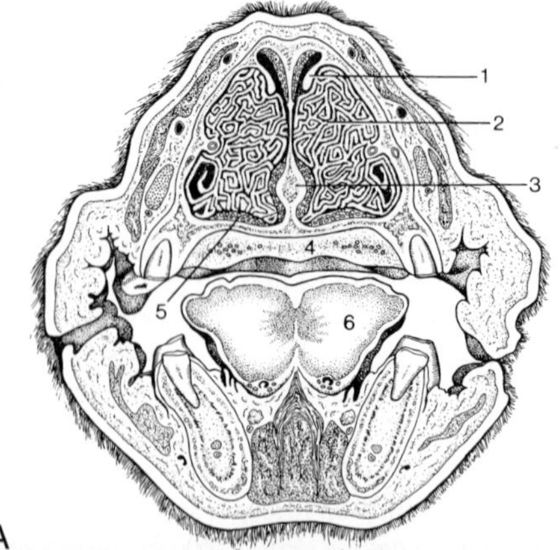


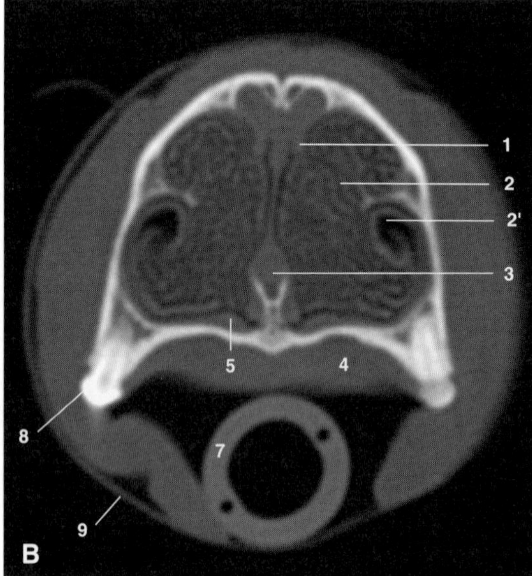


**Figure 4–3.** *(A)*, Transverse section of the canine head at the level of $P^2$. *(B)* CT image taken at the same level but without tongue and structures of the lower jaw.

1, Dorsal concha; 2, ventral concha; 2′, recess of ventral concha; 3, nasal septum; 4, hard palate; 5, venous plexus in nasal mucosa; 6, tongue; 7, endotracheal tube; 8, $P^2$; 9, tape to keep endotracheal tube against hard palate during CT procedure.

large dorsal and ventral—and a much smaller middle—conchae predominate (Figs. 4–2 and 25–10). The numerous ethmoidal conchae are separated by narrow clefts (ethmoidal meatuses), and their pattern is most complicated in species that place much reliance on the sense of smell (Fig. 4–4/5,6). The dorsal and ventral nasal conchae impose the meatal pattern of the middle and more rostral parts of the cavity. They are formed of fragile laminae coiled on themselves in a manner that varies with the species and the location. Rostrally, the lamina does not recurve to meet itself and thus bounds a recess of the nasal cavity; more caudally the coil meets itself or the lateral nasal wall to enclose a space that is part of the paranasal sinus system. The conchae reduce the cavity to a series of clefts or meatuses in an arrangement that may be likened to the letter E in transverse section (Fig. 4–5); in other words, the major conchae define dorsal, middle, and ventral meatuses branching from a common meatus against the septum. The dorsal meatus leads directly to the fundus of the nasal cavity and presents air to the olfactory mucosa. The middle meatus usually gives access to the sinus system. The ventral and common meatuses provide the principal airway leading to the pharynx. The relatively wide space at their junction is the route chosen for passage of an instrument such as a stomach tube.

The nasal mucosa blends with the underlying periosteum and varies in thickness. In some parts it is thin, but elsewhere, and especially ventrally, it is much thickened by the inclusion of cavernous blood spaces that make it a semierectile tissue (/8). The thickness of the mucosa varies with the degree of vascular congestion; when the vessels are most congested they greatly impede the air flow, causing the stuffiness associated with a head cold.

Apart from olfaction, the nasal cavity has the important function of modifying the incoming air before it is presented to the lower respiratory passages. The air is warmed by passing over the very vascular mucosa, humidified by the vaporiza-

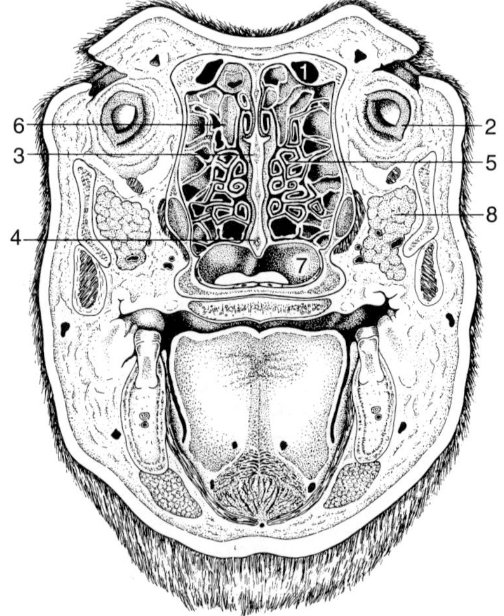


**Figure 4–4.** Transverse section of the canine head at the level of the eyeball.

1, Frontal sinus; 2, eyeball; 3, ethmoid bone; 4, vomer; 5, 6, ethmoidal conchae; 7, choana; 8, zygomatic gland.

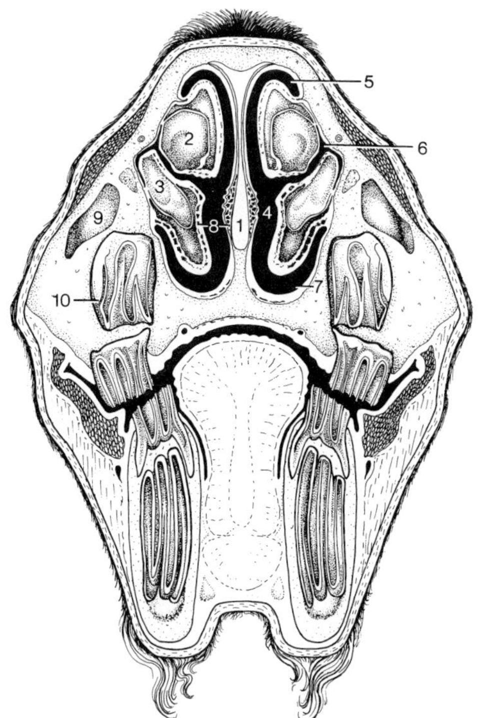


**Figure 4–5.** Transverse section of the equine head at the level of $P^4$.

1, Nasal septum; 2, dorsal concha; 3, ventral concha; 4, common meatus; 5, dorsal meatus; 6, middle meatus; 7, ventral meatus; 8, venous plexus in nasal mucosa; 9, rostral maxillary sinus; 10, $P^4$.

tion of the tears and serous nasal secretion, and cleansed by contact with the secretion of numerous scattered mucous glands. These glands spread a carpet of mucus over the nasal mucosa that entraps particles and droplets that come into contact with it. The carpet is moved toward the pharynx by the ciliary action of the lining epithelium and is then swallowed. It is said that in the human species as much as half a liter of mucus is swallowed unconsciously each day.

The *paranasal sinuses* are diverticula of the nasal cavity that excavate the skull bones (Fig. 4–6), largely after birth. The separation of the inner and outer tables of the bones alters the conformation of the head and is especially striking in pigs and cattle (Figs. 4–7 and 25–12), in which certain sinuses eventually extend dorsal and even caudal to the cranial cavity. The sinuses retain their connections with the nasal cavity, but since the openings are generally narrow a relatively slow exchange of air occurs. The narrowness and locations of the openings make them prone to blockage when the mucosa is thickened by inflammation or congestion. Not all the sinuses are of equal clinical importance; the surface projections of those commonly involved in disease are considered in the topographical chapters.

All species have frontal and maxillary systems, neither communicating with its contralateral counterpart. The frontal system consists of one or more spaces within the bones at the border between the nasal and cranial cavities. In most species the various frontal compartments open separately into the ethmoidal meatuses in the nasal fundus, but in the horse the frontal sinus communicates with the nasal cavity indirectly via the caudal maxillary sinus.

The maxillary sinus system occupies the caudolateral part of the upper jaw, above the caudal cheek teeth; in some species it sends extensions, variously described as separate sinuses or as diverticula, into the hard palate, the sphenoid bones, the medial aspect of the orbit, and the ventral concha. In the horse the maxillary sinus is divided into caudal and rostral parts, both connected to the middle nasal meatus. In the dog the

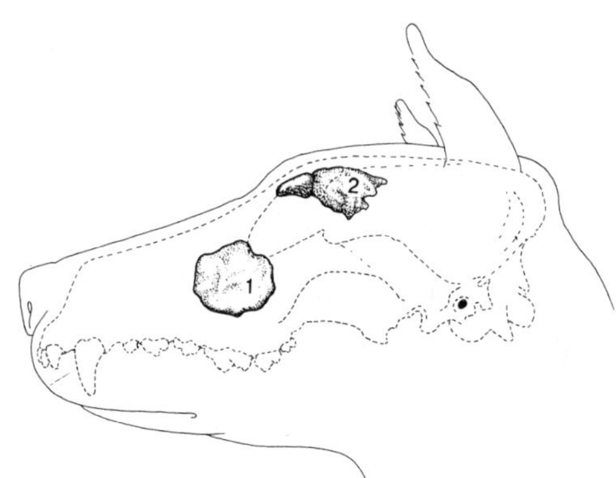


**Figure 4–6.** Paranasal sinuses in the dog.

1, Maxillary recess; 2, frontal sinus.

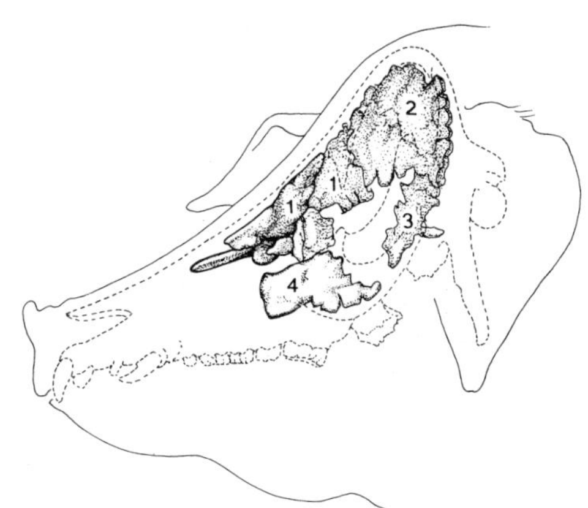


**Figure 4–7.** Paranasal sinuses in the pig.

1, Rostral frontal sinus; 2, caudal frontal sinus; 3, sphenoidal sinus; 4, maxillary sinus.

cavity communicates freely with that of the nose and is known as the maxillary recess.

The function of the sinuses is obscure; they offer some thermal and mechanical protection to the orbit and nasal and cranial cavities, enlarge the skull areas available for muscular attachment without unduly increasing weight, and affect the resonance of the voice.

# THE LARYNX

The larynx forms the connection between the pharynx and the tracheobronchial tree. It lies below the pharynx and behind the mouth, suspended from the cranial base by the hyoid apparatus; in most species it is partly contained between the rami of the mandible and partly extended into the neck, where its cartilaginous skeleton is easily recognized on palpation of the living animal (Fig. 4–8). Because of its connection with the tongue and hyoid apparatus, the larynx shifts its position when the animal swallows.

## The Cartilages

The forms of the laryngeal cartilages, and even the number of the minor elements, vary from species to species, but few differences are of great practical significance. The major consistently present cartilages comprise the median epiglottic, thyroid, and cricoid cartilages, and the paired arytenoid cartilages (Figs. 4–9 and 4–10).

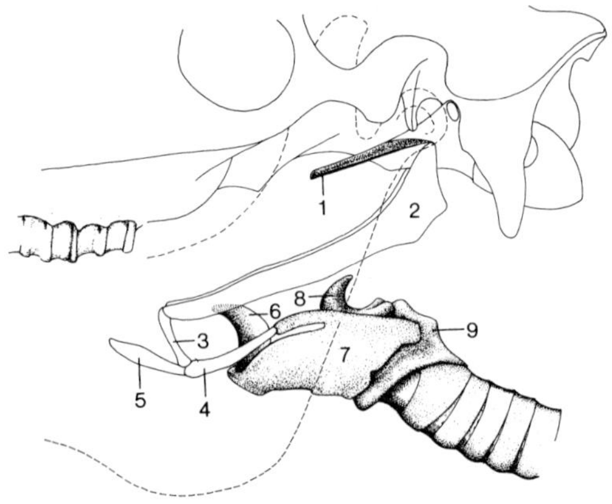


**Figure 4–8.** Hyoid apparatus suspending the larynx from the base of the skull (horse). The broken line indicates the mandible.

1, Cartilage of auditory tube; 2, stylohyoid; 3, keratohyoid; 4, thyrohyoid; 5, lingual process of basihyoid; 6, epiglottic cartilage; 7, thyroid cartilage; 8, arytenoid cartilage; 9, cricoid cartilage.

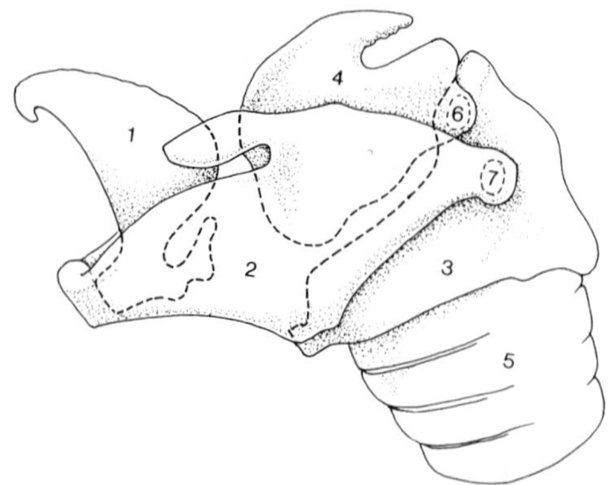


**Figure 4–9.** Lateral view of the equine laryngeal skeleton. The outlines of those parts of the cartilages that are covered by others are indicated by broken lines.

1, Epiglottic cartilage; 2, thyroid cartilage; 3, cricoid cartilage; 4, arytenoid cartilage; 5, trachea; 6, cricoarytenoid joint; 7, cricothyroid joint.

The *epiglottic cartilage* is most rostral. It consists of a small stalk and a large leaflike blade. The stalk is embedded between the root of the tongue, the basihyoid, and the body of the thyroid cartilage and is attached to all of these structures. At rest, the blade inclines dorsorostrally behind the soft palate (the retrovelar position), but it may be tilted backward to partially cover the entrance to the larynx when the animal swallows. It is composed of elastic cartilage and is flexible.

The *thyroid cartilage* is the largest of the series. It consists of two lateral plates that meet ventrally, where they fuse to a varying degree, forming a major part of the laryngeal floor (Fig. 4–10/3). The body formed by this ventral fusion is least extensive in the horse, in which a large, forward-pointing notch provides a convenient route of entry for laryngeal surgery. The most rostral part of the body is generally thickened and corresponds to the "Adam's apple," which is more salient in the human than in domestic species. The rostral and caudal extremities of the dorsal edge of each lamina articulate with the thyrohyoid and arch of the cricoid cartilage, respectively. The thyroid cartilage is hyaline and susceptible to the age changes that affect this tissue; islands of calcification and even ossification make it more brittle with advancing age.

The *cricoid cartilage* is fashioned like a signet ring and consists of an expanded dorsal "seal" (lamina) and a narrower ventral arch (/4). The dorsal part carries a median crest and, on its rostral rim, two facets for the arytenoid cartilages. The arch carries on each side a facet for articulation with the thyroid cartilage. The cricoid cartilage is also hyaline and subject to the aging process.

The *arytenoid cartilages* have a very irregular form best described as pyramidal (/2). However, the details are of little importance, and for most purposes it is sufficient to recognize only a few features. A caudal facet articulates with the rostral margin of the cricoid lamina and from this radiates a vocal process that projects ventrally into the laryngeal lumen, and to which the vocal fold attaches; a muscular process that extends laterally; and a corniculate process that extends dorsomedially, forming the caudal margin of the laryngeal entrance with its fellow of the other side. The arytenoid cartilage is mainly hyaline, but the *corniculate process* is elastic.

Among the smaller and less prominent cartilages are the elastic *cuneiform processes* that support mucosal folds passing from the epiglottis to the arytenoids. These processes do not occur in all species and, when present, they may be free or fused with the epiglottis or with the arytenoid cartilages. A discrete nodule of hyaline cartilage—the *interarytenoid cartilage*—may be found between the arytenoid cartilages dorsally.

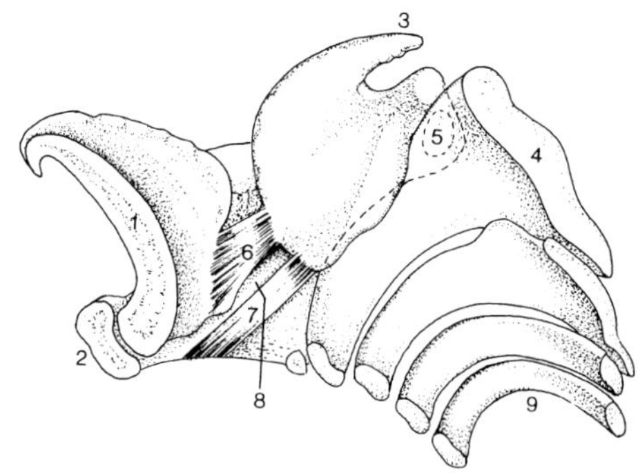


**Figure 4–11.** Median section of the equine larynx after removal of the mucosa.

1, Epiglottic cartilage; 2, sectioned body of thyroid cartilage; 3, corniculate process of arytenoid cartilage; 4, sectioned lamina of cricoid cartilage; 5, cricoarytenoid joint; 6, ventricularis; 7, vocalis; 8, laryngeal ventricle; 9, tracheal rings.

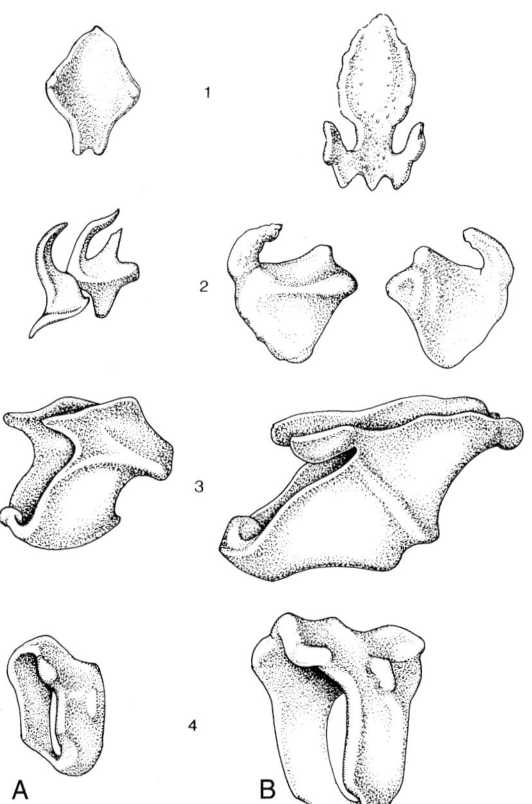


**Figure 4–10.** Laryngeal cartilages of the dog *(A)* and the horse *(B)*.

1, Epiglottic cartilage; 2, arytenoid cartilage; 3, thyroid cartilage; 4, cricoid cartilage.

## The Articulations, Ligaments, and Membranes

In most mammals a synovial articulation is present between the thyrohyoid and the dorsorostral angle of the thyroid cartilage. Rotation occurs about a transverse axis common to the right and left joints. The joints between the dorsocaudal angles of the thyroid cartilage and the lateral facets of the cricoid cartilage also allow rotation about a common transverse axis. The third pair of synovial joints is formed between the arytenoid and cricoid cartilages (Figs. 4–9 and 4–11). They are more complex and allow rotation about both sagittal and transverse axes as well as sliding movements that bring the two arytenoid cartilages closer together or carry them farther apart. Movement at the cricoarytenoid joints is the most important factor in regulating the size of the glottic opening, the narrow stretch of the lumen of the larynx. All of these joints possess the usual attributes of synovial joints.

The cartilages are additionally joined by various membranes and ligaments that balance the laryngeal musculature and determine the resting posture of the larynx when the latter is inactive.

Elastic membranes join the epiglottis to the thyroid and arytenoid cartilages, the thyroid to the cricoid cartilage, and the cricoid to the first tracheal ring. Other less elastic ligaments form the basis of the vocal folds (and the vestibular folds when these are present) that pass between the arytenoid cartilages and the laryngeal floor.

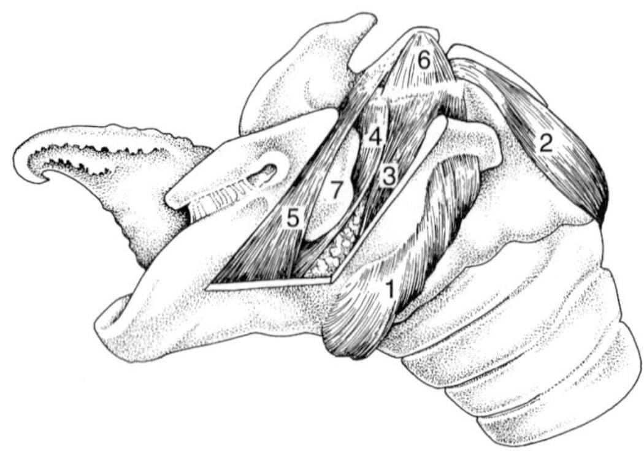


**Figure 4–12.** Intrinsic muscles of the equine larynx.

1, Cricothyroideus; 2, cricoarytenoideus dorsalis; 3, cricoarytenoideus lateralis; 4, vocalis; 5, ventricularis (4 + 5 = thyroarytenoideus); 6, arytenoideus transversus; 7, laryngeal ventricle.

## The Musculature

In addition to the extrinsic laryngeal muscles that pass between this organ and the pharynx, tongue, hyoid bone, and sternum, a suite of small paired intrinsic muscles connects the laryngeal cartilages and influences their mutual relations (Fig. 4–12).

One of these muscles, the *cricothyroideus* (/1), is somewhat set apart from the rest through its superficial position and its innervation by the cranial laryngeal nerve, a branch of the vagus. It runs between the lateral surfaces of the thyroid lamina and cricoid arch ventral to the cricothyroid joint; on contraction it approximates these attachments and thus carries the dorsal part of the cricoid (and the attached arytenoid cartilages) caudally and so tenses the vocal folds.

The other muscles lie more deeply, attach to the arytenoid cartilage, and are innervated by the caudal (recurrent) laryngeal branch of the vagus nerve. The *cricoarytenoideus dorsalis* (/2) arises from the dorsal surface of the cricoid lamina, and its fibers converge rostrolaterally to insert on the muscular process of the arytenoid cartilage. On contraction it abducts the vocal process and thereby the vocal fold and so widens the glottis. The *cricoarytenoideus lateralis* (/3) takes origin from the rostroventral part of the cricoid arch and passes dorsally to an insertion on the muscular process. It is, therefore, an adductor of the vocal processes and thus narrows the glottis. The *thyroarytenoideus* arises from the cranial part of the laryngeal floor (chiefly the thyroid cartilage) and runs dorsocaudally to insert on the muscular process and adjacent part of the arytenoid cartilage. In certain species (horse and dog included) it is divided into two units, a rostral ventricularis (/5) and a caudal vocalis (/4), which occupy the vestibular and vocal folds. This muscle adjusts the tension of the fold(s) and forms part of the sphincter arrangement. The *arytenoideus transversus* (/6) runs from the muscular process of the arytenoid cartilage to a median raphe (sometimes containing the interarytenoid nodule); some fibers may cross the midline to reach the arytenoid cartilage of the other side. It approximates the arytenoid cartilages and completes the sphincter.

## The Cavity of the Larynx

The cavity of the larynx may be divided into three sections, arranged in series (Figs. 4–13 and 18–31). The vestibule extends from the laryngeal entrance to the rostral margin of the arytenoid cartilages and vocal folds; the glottic cleft is bounded by the arytenoid cartilages dorsally and the vocal folds ventrolaterally and can be varied in size; the third, infraglottic, cavity is of fixed dimensions and leads smoothly to the lumen of the trachea (Plate 3/*B*).

The structures bounding the *entrance to the larynx* (aditus laryngis) project into the lumen of the pharynx; they may protrude through the intrapharyngeal ostium into the nasopharynx where they may be grasped by the free margin of the soft palate and its continuation by the palatopharyngeal arches. The rostral part of the wall of the entrance is provided by the epiglottis, the lateral parts by the (aryepiglottic) folds extending between the epiglottis and the arytenoid cartilages, and the caudal part by the corniculate processes of the arytenoid cartilages. The interior of the *vestibule* may present a number of important features, but none of these is found in every species. In some animals a vestibu-

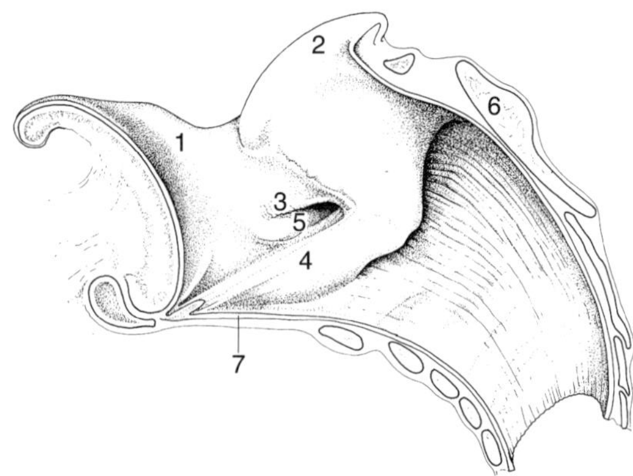


**Figure 4–13.** Median section of the equine larynx.

1, Epiglottis; 2, corniculate process of arytenoid cartilage; 3, vestibular fold; 4, vocal fold; 5, laryngeal ventricle; 6, lamina of cricoid cartilage; 7, cricothyroid ligament.

lar fold runs roughly parallel to the vocal fold but at a more rostral level (Fig. 4–13/3). This fold goes paired with an outpouching of the mucosa to form a ventricle or diverticulum that is entered between the vestibular and vocal folds. These features are especially prominent in the horse and receive more attention later. The mucous membrane bounding the vestibule is tightly adherent to the epiglottic and arytenoid cartilages, looser elsewhere where it rests on fat.

The *glottic cleft* (rima glottidis) is narrower than the vestibule; the dorsal part is bounded by the vocal processes and adjacent parts of the arytenoid cartilages, the ventral part by the vocal folds (the folds and the arytenoid cartilages constitute the glottis). The cleft, laterally compressed and diamond-shaped, varies in dimensions and disappears when the glottis is closed. The vocal folds run caudodorsally from the rostral part of the laryngeal floor to their attachments on the arytenoid cartilages. Each fold contains a ligament in its free margin and, lateral to this, the vocalis muscle, which is surrounded on most sides by fat. The vestibular folds, when present, have a similar construction but form no part of the glottis in the strict sense. The mucosa is tightly adherent to the arytenoid cartilages and along the free margin of the folds; it is much looser elsewhere.

The *infraglottic cavity* has few features of interest, its form reflecting that of the cricoid cartilage. It may be slightly reduced in size where it continues into the trachea. The mucosa is relatively firmly attached.

The *laryngeal mucous membrane* contains numerous mucous glands (especially massed within the ventricles when these are present) and also lymphoid aggregations (especially in the infraglottic region). It is surfaced by an epithelium whose character varies from region to region according to its use. This epithelium is stratified squamous about the entrance, where it risks abrasion from the passage of food, and also on the free edges of the folds, which at times are abruptly brought together; elsewhere it is pseudostratified and ciliated like the epithelium lining most respiratory passages. The sensory innervation is from the cranial and caudal (recurrent) laryngeal nerves, the boundary between the territories coinciding with the glottis.

## The Mechanism of the Larynx

The larynx originally develops as a device to protect the lower respiratory passages against inundation. Protection remains its primary role, although phonation—the production of voice—is the function that most often comes to mind.

Protection of the lower passages against the entrance of food and drink is achieved in two ways. On swallowing, the larynx is drawn forward, and the epiglottis, tilted somewhat backward by coming against the root of the tongue, forms a partial cover to the laryngeal entrance (see Fig. 3–31/5). The resemblance between the outlines of the epiglottis and the aditus suggests a much closer fit than actually occurs. Solid foods are swiftly carried over the laryngeal entrance by the pharyngeal muscles, whereas fluids are deflected by the epiglottis through the piriform recesses of the pharyngeal floor. It is known that removal of the larger part of the human epiglottis does not interfere with normal swallowing. A second, active protection is provided at a deeper level by the glottis, which is closed by the adduction of the vocal folds (see Fig. 18–31). Inhibition of inspiration at this time further reduces the risk of food being drawn into the larynx. In fact, food comparatively rarely "goes down the wrong way," but, when it does, contact with the vestibular mucosa initiates reflex coughing.

On inspiration, abduction of the vocal folds may widen the rima glottidis, but the effect is pronounced only when breathing is unusually vigorous. Abduction is the task of the dorsal cricoarytenoideus, subsequent adduction the task of the lateral cricoarytenoideus muscle (Fig. 4–14/5,6 and *arrows*), and it will be noticed that these antagonistic muscles are supplied by the same nerve, contrary to the common arrangement.

Closure of the glottis also occurs in a number of other functional contexts in which free passage of air to or from the lungs must be prevented. A build-up of expiratory forces against a closed glottis allows for a forceful expulsion when the air is eventually released; this is the mechanism used when coughing to clear the lower passages of mucus accumulations or foreign matter. Sustained closure with elevation of the intrathoracic pressure is also used in activities involving straining—defecation, micturition, and parturition; the blockage of the escape route for air helps maintain the intrathoracic pressure and by so stabilizing the diaphragm aids the action of the muscles of the abdominal wall.

The skeleton of the thorax can also be more effectively fixed to provide a firm base for muscles attaching to the ribs when the glottis is closed. This combination of activities is well illustrated in ourselves when we attempt to lift a heavy weight or to draw the trunk toward a handhold above the head.

The production of voice is a further important function of the larynx. The sounds of human speech are more complex than those produced by

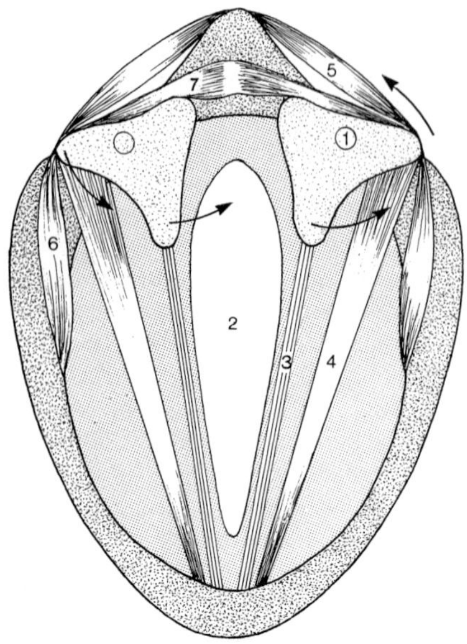


**Figure 4–14.** Schematic transverse section of the larynx. Arrows on the left: action of cricoarytenoideus lateralis (6) on arytenoid cartilage; arrows on the right: action of cricoarytenoideus dorsalis (5) on arytenoid cartilage.

1, Location of the cricoarytenoid joint; 2, glottic cleft; 3, vocal ligament in vocal fold; 4, thyroarytenoideus; 5, cricoarytenoideus dorsalis; 6, cricoarytenoideus lateralis; 7, arytenoideus transversus.

other species, although no greater complexity of laryngeal structure is present. Indeed the complex laryngeal mechanism is not indispensable to this task; the human patient can learn to use the expulsion of air from the esophagus to produce voice, though sadly unnatural, after the surgical removal of the larynx, an operation sometimes required by malignant disease. Even in normal circumstances the voice does not issue from the larynx in its final form but is much modified and "colored" by the resonance chambers provided by other cavities of the head. Some controversy exists over the manner in which the basic sound is produced in the larynx. The air stream is made to vibrate as it passes through the glottis. The pitch is controlled by the thickness, the length, and the tension of the vocal folds and is thus to some extent variable, to some extent determined by permanent (or semipermanent, since a boy's voice breaks with growth) and individual features of laryngeal anatomy. The tension of the folds, or of part of them, is varied by the cricothyroideus muscle acting as the coarse, the vocalis muscle as the fine, adjustment. Most workers believe the folds are made to vibrate passively by the flow of air passing between them. An alternative theory suggested that the muscles contract and relax at the appropriate rate, but as some tones of the human voice exceed 200 cycles per second, and tonic contraction of the vocalis muscle occurs with stimuli repeated 67 times per second, this theory is untenable.

Electromyographic studies show that purring in cats is produced by fast twitching of laryngeal muscles and of the diaphragm. The laryngeal muscles rapidly narrow and widen the glottis, which causes the respiratory air to vibrate and make the sound.

## THE TRACHEA

The trachea and bronchi form a continuous system of tubes conducting air between the larynx and the smaller passages (bronchioli) in the lungs. They

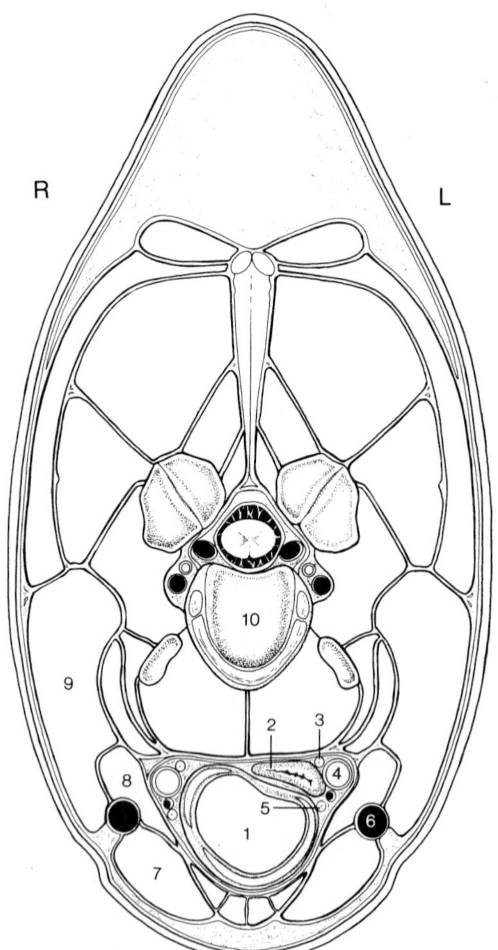


**Figure 4–15.** Transverse section of the neck (horse) at the level of the fourth cervical vertebra.

1, Trachea; 2, esophagus; 3, vagosympathetic trunk; 4, common carotid artery; 5, caudal (recurrent) laryngeal nerve; 6, external jugular vein; 7, sternocephalicus; 8, omohyoideus; 9, brachiocephalicus; 10, body of the fourth cervical vertebra.

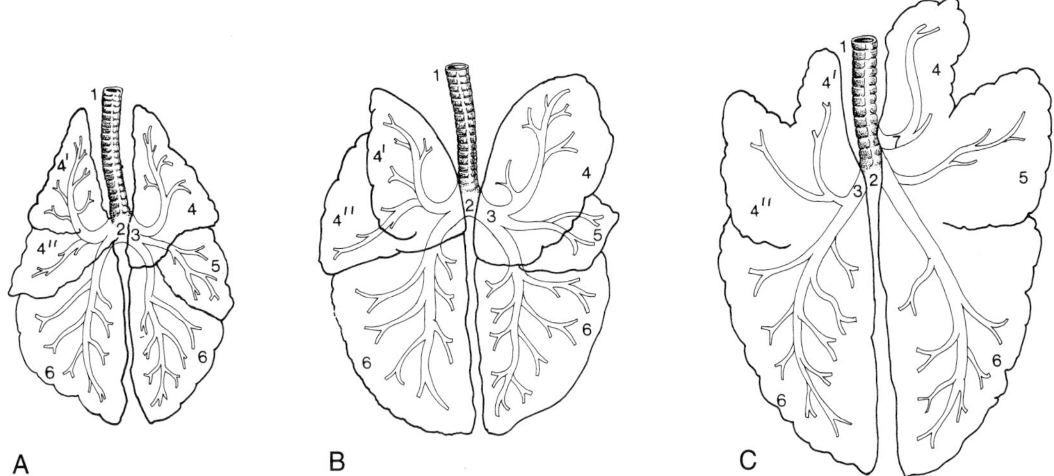


**Figure 4–16.** Dorsal views of the bronchial tree and lungs of the cat *(A),* dog *(B),* and pig *(C),* schematic.

1, Trachea; 2, bifurcation of trachea; 3, chief bronchus; 4, right cranial lobe; 4′, 4″, cranial and caudal parts of left cranial lobe; 5, middle lobe; 6, caudal lobe; 7, tracheal bronchus.

have a very similar construction and together are sometimes termed the tracheobronchial tree.

The trachea leads from the larynx through the visceral space of the neck, enters the mediastinum at the thoracic inlet, and continues to its terminal bifurcation above the heart. The two chief bronchi diverge from the line of the trachea to enter the corresponding lungs at their roots. In ruminants and pigs a separate tracheal bronchus arises proximal to the tracheal bifurcation and separately aerates the cranial lobe of the right lung. The cervical part of the trachea maintains a more or less median position, although its relationship to the esophagus alters at different levels and in different postures of the head and neck (see Figs. 3–29 and 4–15/1). Other relations in the neck include the ventral strap muscles of the neck and the carotid sheath and its contents; the common carotid artery commences ventrolaterally but gradually climbs to a dorsolateral position where the trachea originates from the larynx.

The thoracic part of the trachea is deflected slightly to the right where it crosses the aortic arch. It is related ventrally to the cranial vena cava, to the arteries arising from the aortic arch, and to various tributaries and branches of these vessels; it is related dorsally to the esophagus and related variously to mediastinal lymph nodes and, in young subjects, to the thymus. The bifurcation lies in the region of the fourth to sixth intercostal spaces but varies with the species and with the respiratory phase.

The chief *bronchi* very quickly enter the lungs (Fig. 4–16; Plate 3/*E,F*) in which they ramify according to a pattern described later (p. 161).

The wall of the trachea is composed of an inner mucosa, a fibrocartilaginous middle layer, and an adventitia (in the neck) or serosa (in the thorax) (Fig. 4–17). The mucosa continues that lining the infraglottic part of the larynx and may show slight longitudinal folding when the lumen is narrowed. It contains both uni- and multicellular mucous glands that produce a protective covering of mucus that is continuously moved toward the larynx by the ciliary action of the epithelium. This mucus eventually reaches the pharynx and is swallowed without being noticed. Excessive mucus accumulations may irritate the mucosa, stimulating coughing to clear the airway. The fibrocartilaginous coat is composed of numerous strips of cartilage that are bent to form "rings" that are incomplete dorsally where the ends may fail to meet or may overlap. The edges of the strips are connected to each other by sheets of rather elastic connective tissue continuous with the perichondrium. The ends are joined by the smooth tracheal muscle (/4), which bridges the gap within the "ring" in most species but is placed externally in the dog and cat.

The construction of the trachea prevents it from collapsing and allows it to make the necessary adjustment in length when the neck is extended and also when the diaphragm contracts. It is attached to the diaphragm indirectly by the pulmonary ligaments and mediastinal connective tissue and also, more effectively, by the negative intrapleural pressure that couples the lungs to the chest wall, including the diaphragm. Variations in diameter are regulated by the tracheal muscle. In addition to these functional changes, there are

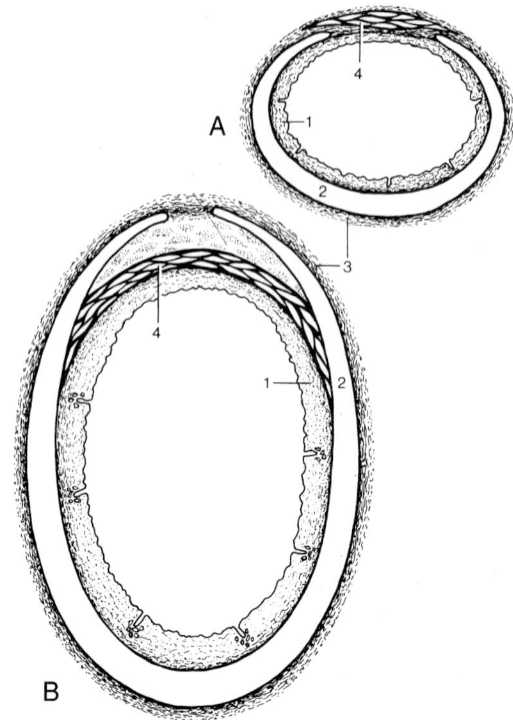


**Figure 4–17.** Transverse sections of the canine *(A)* and bovine *(B)* trachea.

1, Mucous membrane; 2, tracheal cartilage; 3, adventitia; 4, tracheal muscle (external in dogs, internal in cattle).

permanent species and regional variations in the cross-sectional form and area of the trachea.

The structure of the larger bronchi is identical to that of the trachea if allowance is made for the mergence of their outer surfaces with the peribronchial connective tissue (and through this with the stroma of the lung). On the smaller bronchi the cartilage rings are gradually replaced by irregular plaques, and it is the shedding of the last of these that defines the bronchobronchiolar transition.

Variations in the diameter of the bronchi and bronchioli are relatively greater and more significant than those of the trachea.

Before proceeding it may be advisable to reread the section on the shape and function of the thoracic cavity (p. 52).

## THE PLEURA

Each lung is invested by a serous membrane, the pleura, which also lines the corresponding "half" of the thoracic cavity. Thus, two pleural membranes exist, each arranged as a closed invaginated sac. The space between the right and left sacs forms the mediastinum, a more or less median partition in the thorax within which the heart and other thoracic organs are situated (Fig. 4–18/7).

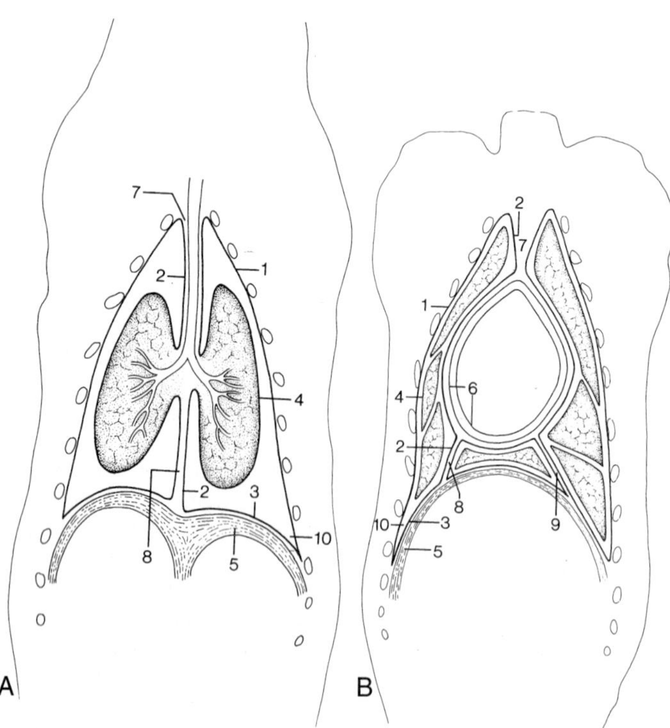


**Figure 4–18.** Schematic dorsal sections of the pleural cavities (dog); at the level of the tracheal bifurcation *(A)* and at the level of the heart *(B)*.

1–3, Parietal pleura, later subdivided; 1, costal pleura; 2, mediastinal pleura; 3, diaphragmatic pleura; 4, visceral pleura; 5, diaphragm; 6, parietal and visceral pericardium; 7, cranial mediastinum; 8, caudal mediastinum; 9, plica venae cavae; 10, costodiaphragmatic recess.

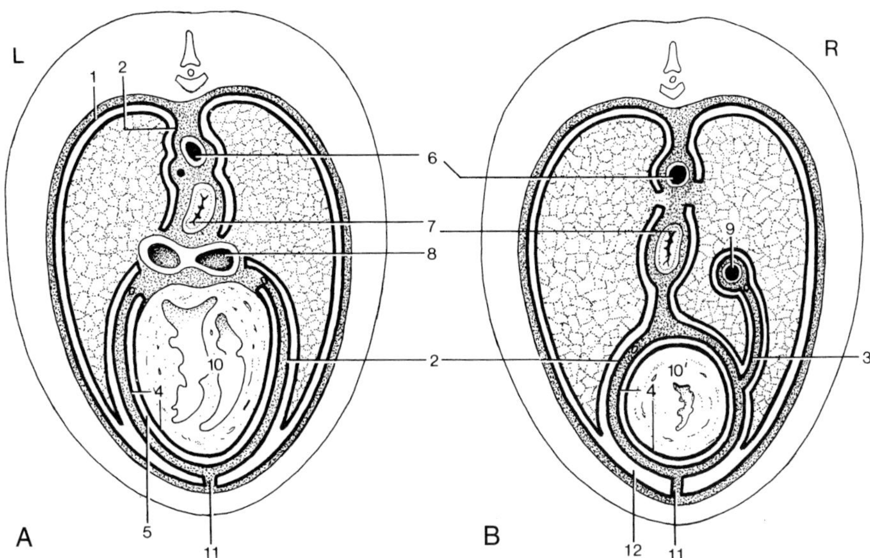


**Figure 4–19.** Schematic transverse section of the thorax at the level of the heart *(A)* and at the transition of heart to caudal mediastinum *(B)*.

1, Costal pleura; 2, mediastinal pleura; 3, plica venae cavae; 4, parietal and visceral pericardium; 5, pericardial space; 6, aorta; 7, esophagus; 8, tracheal bifurcation; 9, caudal vena cava; 10, heart; 10′, apex of heart; 11, sternopericardial ligament; 12, costomediastinal recess.

The part of the pleura that clothes the lung directly is known as the visceral or pulmonary pleura (/4). It is reflected around, and also behind, the root of the lung to become continuous with the mediastinal pleura which, in turn, is continuous with the costal and diaphragmatic pleura; these last three parts are together termed the parietal pleura.

In the healthy animal the pleural cavity is a potential rather than an actual space, and it contains only a small amount (a few milliliters) of serous fluid, which is thinly spread over the pleural surface and facilitates the smooth movement of the lung against the chest wall and of one lung lobe against another. The pressure within the pleural cavity, which is about −5 cm $H_2O$ in the neutral resting position of the chest, represents the difference between the forces that tend to recoil the lung and those that tend to expand the chest. The pressure is not uniform throughout the pleural cavity, and in addition to the expected dorsoventral gradient, local and partly unexplained differences exist; these variations in intrapleural pressure account for regional differences in the expansion and aeration of the lungs. The prevailing negative pressure explains why a surgical or traumatic opening in the chest wall causes an inrush of air into the pleural cavity, collapsing the lung and producing the condition known as pneumothorax.

The pleural sac is always more extensive than the lung, and in certain regions facing surfaces of parietal pleura are directly applied to each other. The most important example of such an arrangement is found caudal to the basal border of the lung where the peripheral part of the diaphragmatic pleura rests against the costal pleura lining the chest wall (the costodiaphragmatic recess; /10); although the extent of the recess varies with the phase of respiration, it remains considerable even in full inspiration, and the potential of this portion of the pleural sac is therefore never realized (Fig. 4–21/6). A similar but smaller costomediastinal recess is present ventral to the lung (Fig. 4–19/12).

Cranially, the costal and mediastinal portions of the pleura come together to form a dome, the cupula pleurae, which may extend in front of the first rib where it is obviously vulnerable to injury (Fig. 4–20/8′). The mediastinum is not symmetrical but is deflected to the left at certain levels. The important deflection of the caudal mediastinum is produced by the greater size of the base of the right lung (/9).

A special fold (plica venae cavae) of the pleura of the right sac extends between the diaphragm and pericardium and carries the caudal vena cava in its free dorsal border (Fig. 4–19/3,9). This triangular partition helps define a recess into which the accessory lobe of the right lung fits (Fig. 4–20).

Considerable practical significance attaches to the strength of the mediastinum, which varies much between species. In some, for example, the ruminants, the mediastinum is thick and able to

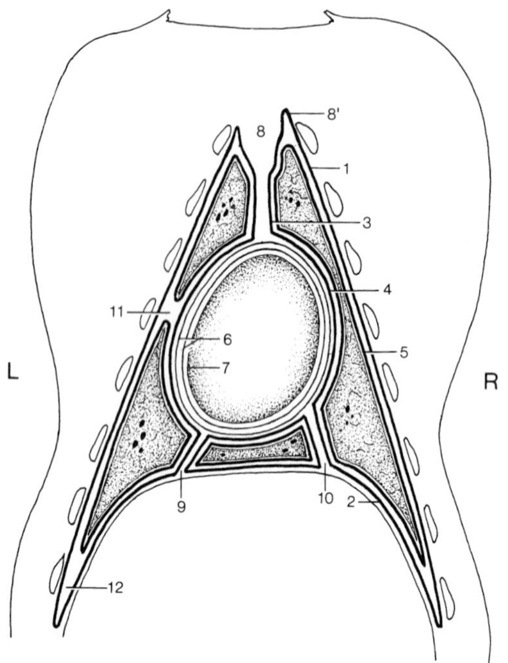


**Figure 4–20.** The distribution of the pleura and pericardium, schematic. The heavy lines indicate the pleura.

1–4, Parietal pleura, later subdivided; 1, costal pleura; 2, diaphragmatic pleura; 3, mediastinal pleura; 4, pericardial pleura; 5, visceral (pulmonary) pleura; 6, parietal pericardium; its outer fibrous layer tightly adheres to its inner serous layer; 7, visceral pericardium, adherent to heart (epicardium); 8, cranial mediastinum; 8′, cupula pleurae; 9, caudal mediastinum; 10, plica venae cavae; 11, left cardiac notch; 12, costodiaphragmatic recess.

withstand a considerable pressure difference between the two pleural cavities; consequently, collapse of one lung may be tolerated. In others, for example, the dog, cat, and horse, it is very delicate and ruptures readily. Indeed, the horse is among those species in which the mediastinum of the dead specimen always presents numerous small openings that place the right and left pleural cavities in communication.

## THE LUNGS

The right and left lungs (pulmones,* pl.) are each invaginated into the corresponding pleural sac and are free, except at the roots where they are attached to the mediastinum. They have no fixed size or shape since they comply with respiratory changes in the dimensions of the thorax. The lungs are normally kept expanded by the air pressure within the respiratory tree and, being elastic, they recoil and collapse as soon as air is admitted into the pleural cavities by trauma, surgery, or dissection. They have a soft, spongy texture, and the residual air they contain, even when collapsed, causes them to crepitate when squeezed and to float when placed in water. In contrast, the unexpanded lungs of the fetus or stillborn animal feel solid; they sink when immersed, and this provides the pathologist with an easy means of determining that the animal from which they came had not breathed. The color of healthy lungs varies in intensity with the blood content and therefore with the manner of death; it is a fresh pink in many slaughterhouse specimens but a much deeper red in lungs obtained from animals that were not bled. The frequently patchy coloration is produced by uneven distribution of blood, often the result of gravitation after death. The lungs of animals that spent their lives in heavily polluted atmospheres acquire a grayish tinge from deposition of soot or other inhaled particles.

Anatomical descriptions are generally based on specimens hardened in situ before the thorax was opened; at death such lungs retain their size, which is intermediate between those adopted in full inspiration and full expiration (Fig. 4–21). The two lungs are grossly alike and mirror each other in shape, although the right one is always larger; this asymmetry, partly due to the skewed position of the heart, is most obvious in the lungs of cattle. Each has some resemblance to the half of a cone, making it possible to recognize the following features: an apex presented toward the thoracic inlet; a wide, concave base related to the face of the diaphragm; a convex costal surface fitted against the lateral chest wall; an irregular medial surface modeled on the contents of the mediastinum; a thick dorsal border occupying the gutter between the vertebrae and ribs; and a thin border that comprises a ventral part bordering the costomediastinal recess, and a basal (caudoventral) part bordering the costodiaphragmatic recess (Figs. 4–19 and 4–21). The ventral part is indented over the heart (cardiac notch; incisura cardiaca).

Certain features of the mediastinal surface and base require further attention. The many indentations carried by the mediastinal surface include the large and deep cardiac impression, created by the heart and naturally larger on the left lung, since the heart itself is biased to this side. The impression extends to the ventral border, which is deeply notched at this level in most species, allowing the heart (or more accurately, the peri-

*Both the Latin term, *pulmo,* and its Greek equivalent, *pneumon,* are used as stems in the production of medical terms; pulmonitis and pneumonia both describe inflammation of the lungs.

cardium) direct contact with the thoracic wall (Fig. 4–21). The root of the lung, situated dorsal to the cardiac impression, is formed by the bunching together of the chief bronchus and the pulmonary artery, veins, lymphatics, and nerves within a covering of pleura provided by the reflection of the mediastinal pleura onto the lung. The reflection extends caudal to the root in a tapering fashion that leaves bare an area of lung that is directly joined by mediastinal connective tissue to the corresponding part of its partner. In some species, including the dog and cat, the empty part of the reflection,

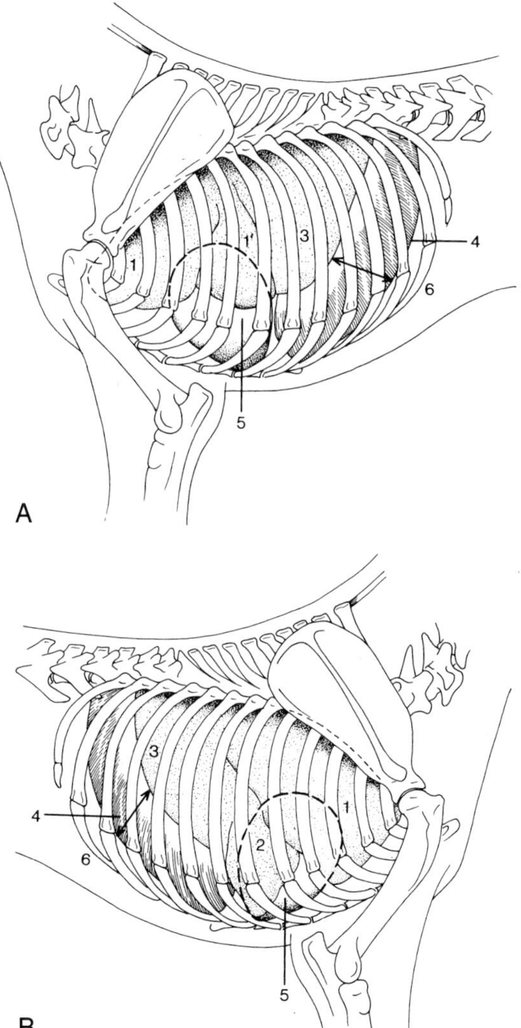


**Figure 4–21.** Semischematic drawings of the thoracic organs of the dog on the left *(A)* and right *(B)* sides. The outline of the heart is indicated by a broken line.

1, Cranial lobe; 1′, caudal part of left cranial lobe; 2, middle lobe; 3, caudal lobe; 4, diaphragm; 5, heart; 6, costodiaphragmatic recess *(arrow)*.

which is known as the pulmonary ligament, extends onto the base of the lung, which thus finds additional attachment to the diaphragm (Fig. 4–22/10). In ruminants and pigs the bronchus that arises from the trachea prior to its bifurcation, and the associated vessels, create a smaller second root of the right lung (Plate 3/*F*).

The base of the right lung reveals the small accessory lobe, which is separated from the medial surface of the caudal lobe by a fissure that widens at its dorsal limit to accommodate the caudal vena cava in its passage between the caval foramen of the diaphragm and the right atrium. The accessory lobe sits, as it were, astride the vein (/5,6).

In most species one or more fissures extend into the substance toward the root, dividing each lung into parts that are commonly equated with lobes. The lobes are properly defined by the ramification of the bronchial tree, and scope for confusion exists since many older texts employed the external demarcations for this purpose. According to the current practice, the left lung consists of cranial and caudal lobes, the right one of cranial, middle, caudal, and accessory lobes; however, the cranial lobe is commonly subdivided by an external fissure, whereas the right lung of the horse lacks a middle lobe. The fissures are much deeper in the lungs of the dog and cat than in those of other species, but it is difficult to find convincing functional significance in such differences; the deeper fissures may allow the parts to slip over each other more easily and facilitate the adaptation of the lungs to the pronounced changes in thoracic form that occur in animals that employ a bounding gallop.

The bulk of the lung substance is provided by the bronchi, pulmonary vessels, and peribronchial and perivascular connective tissue. The right and left chief bronchi arise at the tracheal bifurcation above the heart, and after entering the lung at its root each detaches a bronchus to the cranial lobe before continuing caudally (Figs. 4–16 and 4–25; Plate 3/*E,F*). The two generations of subdivisions that follow next have a fairly consistent pattern of origin, but subsequent ramifications are less predictable. The number of bronchial generations before the smaller bronchi are succeeded by bronchioles varies among species and also among parts of the one lung; in mice and other small animals only four or five generations of bronchi are present, whereas more than a dozen may be necessary in large animals. The consistency in the pattern of the first branchings allows the recognition of the so-called bronchopulmonary segments, specific portions of the lung supplied by identifiable bronchi and partly defined by connective tissue septa that extend from the peribronchial and

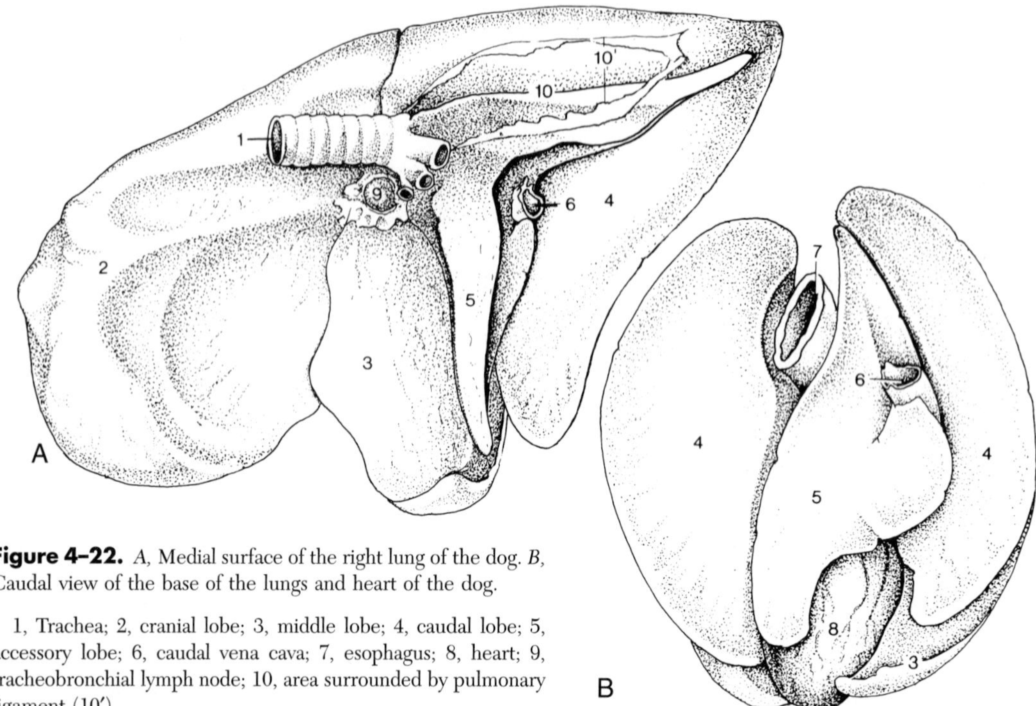


**Figure 4–22.** *A,* Medial surface of the right lung of the dog. *B,* Caudal view of the base of the lungs and heart of the dog.

1, Trachea; 2, cranial lobe; 3, middle lobe; 4, caudal lobe; 5, accessory lobe; 6, caudal vena cava; 7, esophagus; 8, heart; 9, tracheobronchial lymph node; 10, area surrounded by pulmonary ligament (10′).

perivascular tissue (and are responsible for the surface marbling where they impinge upon the visceral pleura). Although bronchopulmonary segmentation has been studied in domestic species, it has yet to find important application; it is not yet common veterinary practice to resect portions of diseased lungs. It is the elasticity of the connective tissue stroma that allows the lungs to expand on inspiration and collapse on subsequent expiration. Loss of this elasticity, which occurs naturally with aging (but also in certain pathological conditions), reduces respiratory efficiency.

The structure of the major bronchi resembles that of the trachea, but with each successive division the supporting cartilages become smaller and more irregular, while the muscle expands to enclose the lumen on all sides. The lumen is lined by a pseudostratified epithelium comprising tall ciliated columnar cells interspersed with goblet and serous-secreting cells, and with stem cells that proliferate to repair depletions of the other types. Larger glands are included within the submucosa of the major bronchi. The transition from bronchus to bronchiole is defined by the disappearance of the last cartilage plate and of the submucosal glands. Bronchioles are narrow—less than 1 mm in diameter—and also pass through several generations. The last of these is characterized by the loss of goblet cells and their replacement by the exocrinocytes (Clara cells) thought to secrete a component of lung surfactant. The terminal bronchioles present scattered alveolar outpouchings of

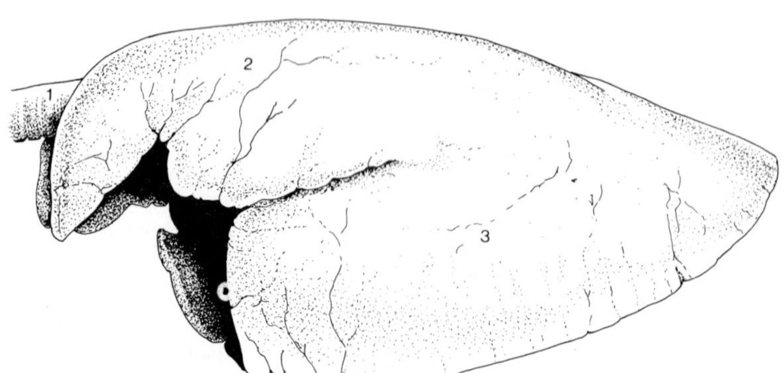


**Figure 4–23.** Left lateral view of the equine lungs. Note the poor lobation and lobulation.

1, Trachea; 2, cranial lobe; 3, caudal lobe.

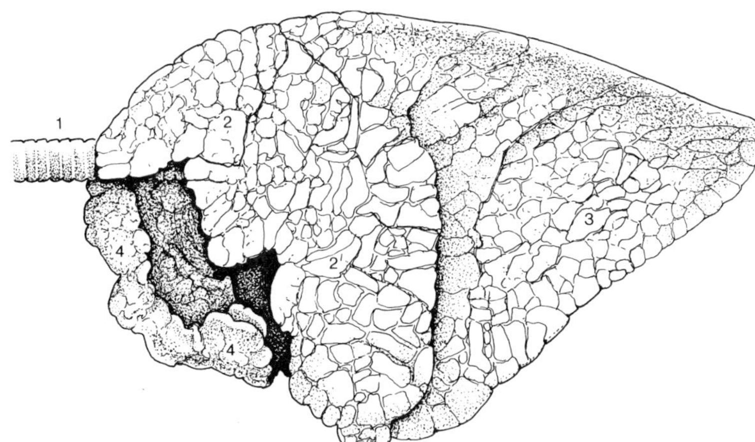


**Figure 4–24.** Left lateral view of the bovine lungs. Note the definite lobation and lobulation.

1, Trachea; 2, 2′, cranial and caudal parts of left cranial lobe; 3, caudal lobe; 4, right cranial lobe.

their walls, and are continued by alveolar ducts, thence alveolar sacs, and ultimately by the saclike alveoli—the spaces where gaseous exchange takes place through a flattened epithelium closely related to the pulmonary capillaries. Patency of the finer passages, which are unsupported by cartilage, is ensured by elastic fibers which anchor them to the pulmonary stroma. At the first breath, the alveoli fill with air and dilate (Plate 3/*G,H*), although for a time they remain significantly smaller than those of the adult (Plate 3/*H,I*).

The identification of the lungs of individual species is most conveniently based on the degrees of lobation and lobulation. The lungs of horses show almost no lobation and very inconspicuous lobulation externally (Fig. 4–23); those of ruminants (Fig. 4–24) and pigs are conspicuously lobated and lobulated (though not uniformly in sheep and goats), whereas those of carnivores are very deeply fissured into lobes but show little external evidence of lobulation (Fig. 4–22).

The *pulmonary arteries* generally follow the bronchi (Fig. 4–25), while the pulmonary veins sometimes run separately, alternating in position with the bronchoarterial associations. The pattern not only varies with the species but also with location in the one lung. These differences may find clinical significance if lung surgery becomes more common. Then it will be important to know the vascular arrangements and to be aware that both interarterial and intervenous anastomoses are to be found crossing the connective tissue partitions. A set of bronchial arteries arises from the aorta to supply the bronchi and associated connective tissue wholly independently of the pulmonary arteries (Fig. 4–26). A corresponding set of bronchial veins may return this blood to the right atrium via the azygous vein, but often the bronchial flow is entirely returned to the left atrium. Arteriovenous anastomoses appear to be absent, and this makes the lung an effective filter preventing the further spread of emboli and tumor cells. This accounts for the frequent occurrence of abscesses and tumor metastases in lung tissue, secondary to disease of other organs.

Lymph drains to the tracheobronchial and mediastinal lymph nodes, directly or after initial passage through small pulmonary nodes set on the bronchial tree within the lung substance; the details are

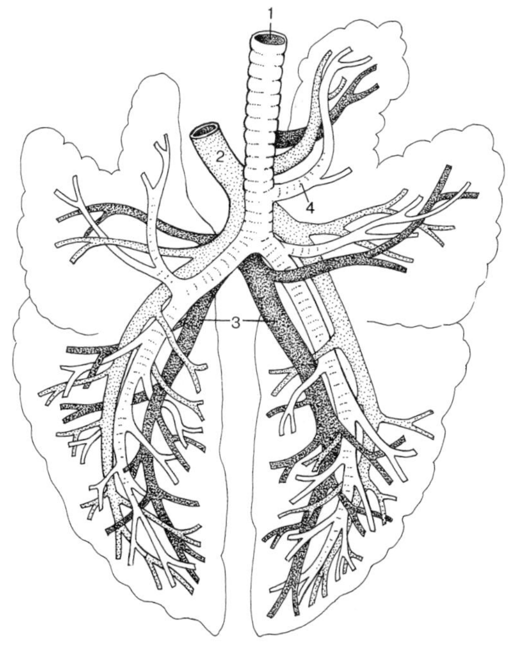


**4–25.** Dorsal view of the bronchial tree and accompanying blood vessels of the pig (corrosion cast).

1, Trachea; 2, pulmonary trunk; 3, pulmonary veins; 4, tracheal bronchus.

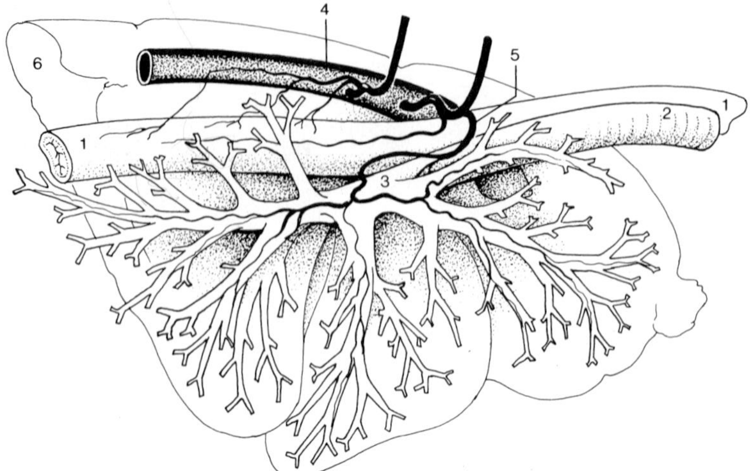


**Figure 4–26.** Corrosion specimen of the lungs and part of the aorta of a dog. On the right side the resin in the bronchioli and smaller bronchi has been removed to expose the main tracheobronchial tree.

1, Esophagus; 2, trachea; 3, tracheal bifurcation; 4, aorta; 5, bronchial artery; 6, caudal lobe of left lung.

complicated, vary among species, and receive later notice when of pathological relevance.

The nerves to the lungs are delivered through a pulmonary plexus within the mediastinum to which both sympathetic and parasympathetic (vagal) fibers contribute. The efferent fibers pass to the bronchial glands and musculature and to the blood vessels. Afferent fibers come from the bronchial mucosa (cough reflex), from vessels, and from stretch receptors. Vagal section has been found to relieve pain in inoperable bronchial carcinoma of human patients.

The features of the lungs of greatest clinical significance are their projection on the surface of the body and their radiographic appearance. The projections vary among species and are described later; meanwhile it may be stressed that they obviously vary with the phase of respiration. Moreover, the areas over which auscultation and percussion can usefully be employed are more limited than might initially be supposed; this is partly because intervention of the upper part of the forelimb denies access to part of the lung field and partly because the lower border of the lung is too thin to provide much useful information.

Since radiography of the lungs is done mainly in small animals (dogs and cats), the relevant observations on their appearance on radiographs and figures will be found in Chapter 13.

## THE DEVELOPMENT OF THE RESPIRATORY APPARATUS

The development of the nose was considered in the previous chapter in relation to the development of the mouth and face (p. 140). The larynx, trachea, and lungs find a common origin in a ventral outgrowth from the foregut, directly caudal to the second of the two swellings that form the tongue (Fig. 4–27). The primordium extends caudally as a (tracheobronchial) groove in the pharyngoesophageal floor; the groove is later converted into a tube by infolding and fusion of its lips; fusion commences caudally and extends forward until the esophagus and pharynx are divided from the

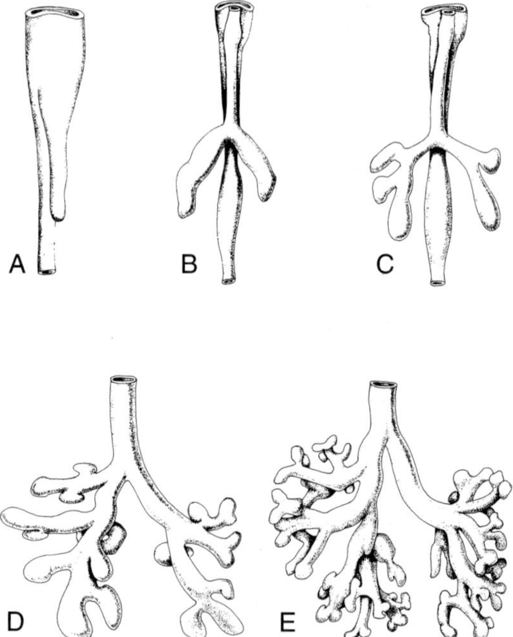


**Figure 4–27.** Five stages in the development of the trachea and lungs (ventral view). *A,* Caudal growth of the tracheobronchial tube. *B,* Its division into two lung buds. *C,* Further division into three bronchi on the right and two on the left. *D, E,* Further development of the bronchial tree.

respiratory tract, except for a small cranial opening that persists as the entrance to the larynx. The fact that the initial development has the form of a groove, rather than a tube, is important since it explains the wide variety of communications between the esophagus and trachea that may occur as congenital anomalies when the process of division has been locally unsuccessful.

The further differentiation of the larynx includes the appearance of the separate cartilages and muscles by condensation and differentiation of the mesoderm of the neighboring pharyngeal arches. The epiglottis has a somewhat different origin, developing as a caudal division of the second of the two median swellings that give rise to the tongue.

After separation from the esophagus, the caudal end of the respiratory tract grows down the neck and comes to lie in the median mesoderm that intervenes between the two forward-pointing extensions of the celom that become the pleural cavities. The apex of the tract splits into two lung buds *(/B),* whose further splitting first reproduces the pattern of the bronchial tree and then creates the smaller respiratory passages that succeed the bronchi. In babies about 18 divisions succeed the stem bronchi by the time of birth; however, the process is not yet complete, and further divisions are added during infancy. The branches of the lung buds become invested by the splanchnic mesoderm into which they thrust, and it is this mesoderm that forms the tissues of the respiratory organs other than the lining epithelium (which is, of course, supplied by the foregut endoderm). The histological development of the lungs encompasses three phases named after the dominant microscopic characters: the first (glandular) phase establishes the bronchial pattern; the second (canalicular) phase establishes the respiratory portion of the lung; the third and final (alveolar) phase is concerned with the development of the alveoli.

The production of surfactant, a substance secreted by certain alveolar cells and necessary to reduce the surface tension to allow alveolar expansion when breathing commences, is of rather late occurrence. The respiratory distress syndrome of the newborn is associated with immaturity of this feature of development.

CHAPTER 5

# The Urogenital Apparatus

The official nomenclature brings the urinary and reproductive organs together under one heading, apparatus urogenitalis. The chief justification for this convention lies in the common origin of certain elements of both organ complexes in the intermediate mesoderm and adjacent part of the celomic epithelium. In addition, the urinary and reproductive systems of the adult share the final portions of the tracts that deliver their products to the exterior; the part used in common is limited to the urethra in the male and the vestibule in the female.

Because of the close developmental associations of the urinary and reproductive systems, we have chosen in this chapter to precede the account of the adult anatomy by a review of the development. The uninitiated reader is therefore advised to consult Figures 5–1 and 5–2, which show the general layout of the urogenital apparatus in each sex, before reading further.

## THE DEVELOPMENT OF THE UROGENITAL APPARATUS

### Development of the Urinary Organs

The intermediate mesoderm reflects in muted fashion the segmentation that is so evident in the adjoining somites. It soon forms in its caudal domain a continuous solid longitudinal (nephrogenic) thickening from which arise, in craniocaudal and temporal sequence, three attempts at the formation of an excretory organ. The first attempt constitutes the pronephros, which forms in the presumptive neck region; this has a transient existence and is not functional in mammals. The second attempt, the mesonephros, forms in the thoracic and lumbar regions and is more successful; it is functional through a large part of embryonic life. The third attempt, the metanephros, forms in the lumbar region; it becomes the adult kidney (Fig. 5–3).

All three structures have as their essential histological feature a series of excretory tubules. In the *pronephros* one end of each tubule turns caudally to meet its neighbor, and in this way a continuous pronephric duct is formed (/4), which at its caudal end grows toward and opens into the cloaca. The duct survives the regression of the pronephric tubules and is adopted as the means of drainage of the mesonephric tubules that now appear. Since the pronephric tubules are nonfunctional their peculiarities of construction need not be noted.

The mesonephric tubules are much more numerous. Each resembles in structure and function a rather simple version of the nephron of the adult kidney. The blind end is invaginated by a capillary tuft to form a filtration mechanism while the connection of the other end with the pronephric duct, now more appropriately termed the *mesonephric duct,* provides an outlet for the urine that is formed. The *mesonephros* may be a very prominent organ at its apogee, when it projects from the roof of the abdomen. Its size varies among species and is in inverse proportion to the permeability (and thus the excretory efficiency) of the placenta. The mesonephros is supplanted by the metanephros when it begins to regress, a process that occurs in a craniocaudal direction. Parts, however, survive to be given fresh use by the male reproductive system (Fig. 5–5).

The *metanephros* has two primordia. One is provided by an outgrowth, the ureteric bud, from the lower end of the mesonephric duct close to its opening into the cloaca. This bud grows cranially into the metanephric blastema constituted by the caudal part of the nephrogenic cord (Fig. 5–3/5). The extremity of the bud undergoes a dozen or so dichotomous divisions. Branches of the later orders become the collecting tubules of the kidney, while those of the first few orders are later reabsorbed into the terminal expansion of the duct in a variable fashion that accounts for the specific forms of the renal pelvis and calices. The outer part of the metanephric mass forms the capsule and interstitium of the kidney, while cellular condensation in the inner part creates the cell cords that are transformed into nephrons. One end of each cell cord makes contact with a connecting duct,

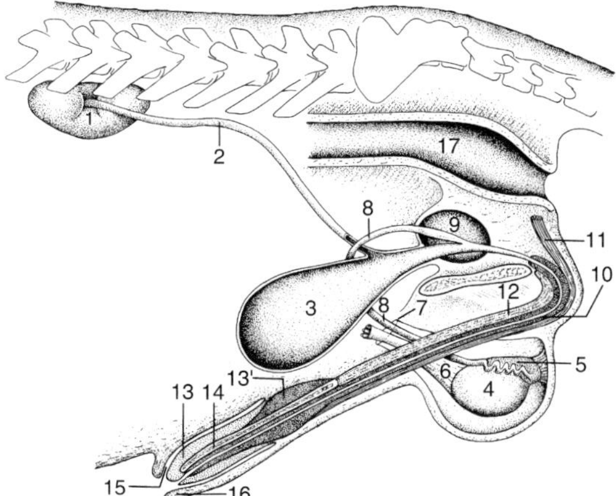


**Figure 5–1.** The urinary and male reproductive organs (dog).

1, Right kidney; 2, ureter; 3, bladder; 4, testis; 5, epididymis; 6, spermatic cord; 7, vaginal ring; 8, deferent duct; 9, prostate; 10, corpus spongiosum (spongy body); 11, retractor penis; 12, corpus cavernosum (cavernous body); 13, glans penis; 13′, bulb of glans; 14, os penis; 15, preputial cavity; 16, prepuce; 17, rectum.

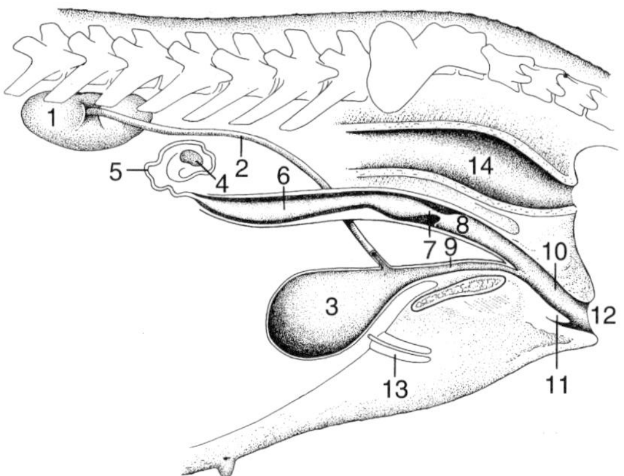


**Figure 5–2.** The urinary and female reproductive organs (bitch).

1, Right kidney; 2, ureter; 3, bladder; 4, ovary; 5, uterine tube; 6, uterine horn; 7, cervix; 8, vagina; 9, urethra; 10, vestibule; 11, clitoris; 12, vulva; 13, vaginal process; 14, rectum.

and once canalization has occurred a continuous passage is established (Fig. 5–6). The other extremity of the nephron becomes invaginated by a vascular tuft supplied from a local branch of the aorta; this forms the glomerulus.

The lower urinary passages are formed by the horizontal division of the cloacal region of the hindgut. The division is effected by the caudal growth of a wedge of mesoderm present within the angle between the hindgut and the allantoic bud (Fig. 5–5/9). This wedge, the urorectal septum, eventually reaches the cloacal membrane, which is thus divided into dorsal (anal) and ventral (urogenital) parts. The fusion site corresponds to the perineal body. When the anal membrane breaks down, the dorsal passage becomes a continuous rectoanal canal. A similar rupture of the urogenital membrane provides the ventral passage with a separate opening to the surface of the body. This urogenital passage differentiates into a cranial part, the future bladder and allantois, and a caudal part from which the urethra is formed.

The bladder then appears as a widening that is continued cranially by the allantoic duct and caudally by an undilated urethra. The allantoic duct or *urachus* (Fig. 5–3/6) can be followed

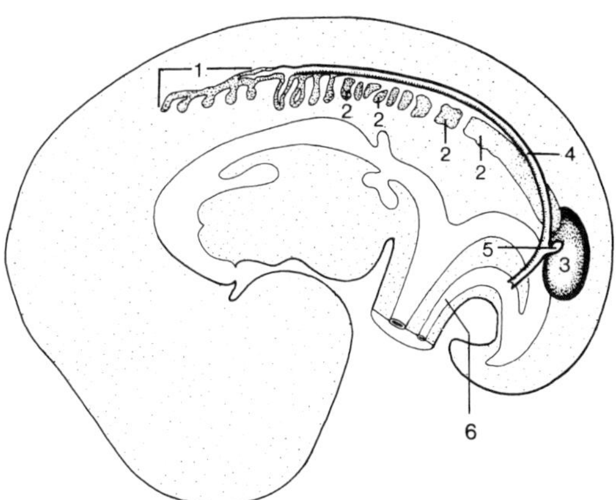


**Figure 5–3.** Differentiation of the intermediate mesoderm.

1, Pronephros; 2, mesonephros, segmented cranially but continuous caudally; 3, metanephros; 4, pronephric (later mesonephric) duct; 5, ureteric bud; 6, urachus.

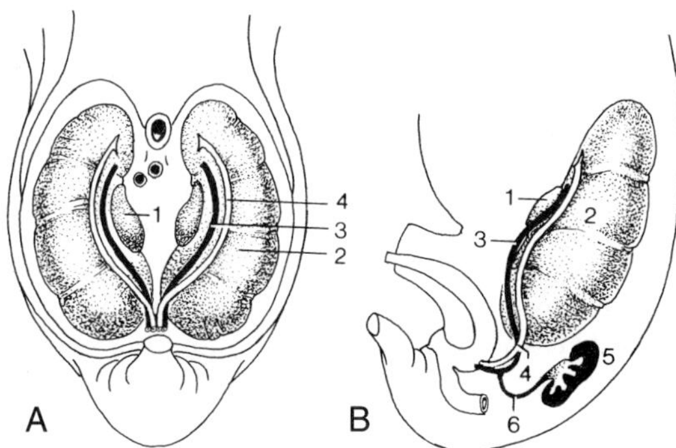


**Figure 5–4.** Ventral *(A)* and lateral *(B)* views of the abdominal roof in a pig embryo of 2.5 cm. The pronephric duct drains the mesonephros and is now more aptly termed the *mesonephric duct.*

1, Developing gonad; 2, mesonephros; 3, mesonephric duct; 4, paramesonephric duct; 5, metanephros; 6, ureter.

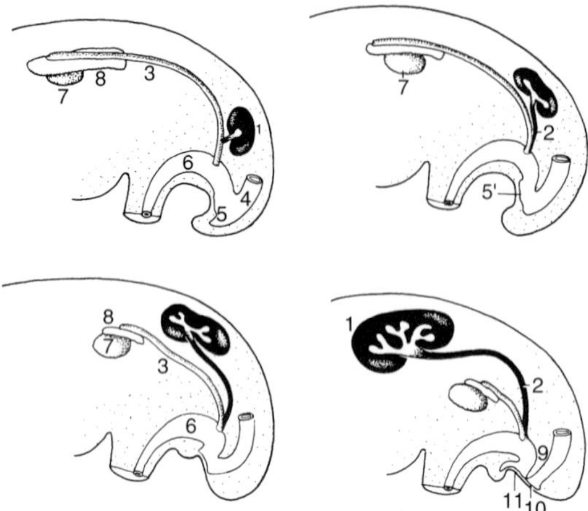


**Figure 5–5.** The development of the metanephros from two primordia (metanephric cord and ureteric bud). Note the gradual regression of the mesonephros.

1, Metanephros; 2, ureteric bud (future ureter); 3, mesonephric (deferent) duct; 4, rectum; 5, cloaca; 5′, cloacal membrane; 6, urogenital sinus; 7, gonad; 8, remnant of mesonephros (future epididymis); 9, urorectal septum; 10, anal membrane; 11, urogenital membrane.

through the umbilical opening to an extraembryonic expansion (the allantois) in which urine accumulates and which is discarded at birth. The part of the duct within the fetus then shrivels and is finally represented only by the cicatrix or scar on the apex of the bladder. The caudal part of the primordium is transformed into the urethra—the entire urethra in the female but only the short pelvic urethra in the male (in which the penile urethra develops with the genital system). The definitive positions of the openings of the mesonephric and metanephric ducts result from the incorporation of their lower ends within the larger passage. The rearrangement brings the opening of the metanephric duct (ureter) into the bladder, while that of the mesonephric duct (deferent duct) becomes situated more caudally within the urogenital sinus (Fig. 5–5). In this process the mesoderm of the mesonephric duct provides the epithelium of the dorsal trigonal region (p. 181) of the bladder, while the epithelium of the remaining part is provided by hindgut endoderm. The outer layers of the bladder wall differentiate from local mesoderm.

## Development of the Male Reproductive Organs

Although the genetic sex of the embryo is decided when the male and female gametes combine, the early stages of morphological differentiation of the reproductive organs follow an indifferent pattern that is common to the two sexes. In both, the gonadal primordium appears as a thickening of the celomic epithelium on the medial aspect of the mesonephros. It projects as a swelling when the underlying mesenchyme proliferates (Fig. 5–7/*A*,5). Cords of cells that develop from the covering epithelium penetrate the interior of the swelling (*B*,5). These cords shortly incorporate the primordial germ cells, which, rather surprisingly, have a distant origin in the endoderm of a restricted portion of the yolk sac where they are identifiable by their large size. They reach the gonad by migration over the gut and its mesentery, but carriage in the blood stream also seems possible.

An early indication that the gonad will become a testis is provided by a marked mesenchymal condensation (tunica albuginea) below the celomic epithelium. Now isolated from the surface epithelium, the cords increase in size and in complexity of arrangement (Fig. 5–8/3). They connect to a plexus or network (rete) within the testis. On the other side the plexus makes contact with the blind ends of the few tubules that have survived the general regression of the mesonephros (/*B*, 3–5). Differentiation within the cell cords permits recognition of two cell lineages. One provides the sustentacular (Sertoli) cells of the seminiferous tubules; the second, contributed by the primordial germ cells, provides the germinal epithelium.

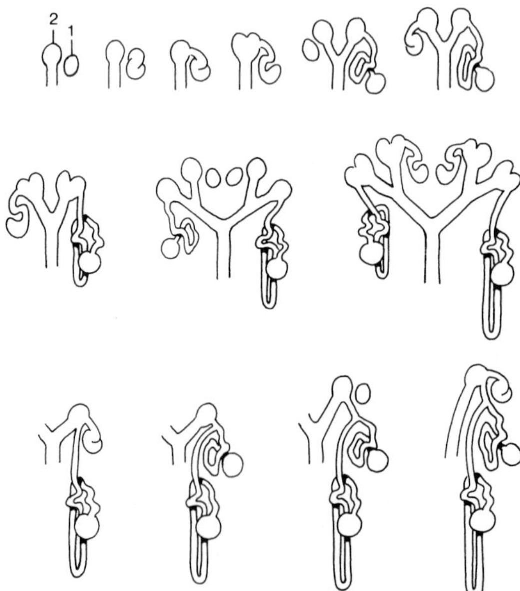


**Figure 5–6.** This series of schematic drawings depicts the connections between developing nephrons (1) and branches (2) of the ureteric bud. Note the dichotomous division of the drainage system (ureteric bud).

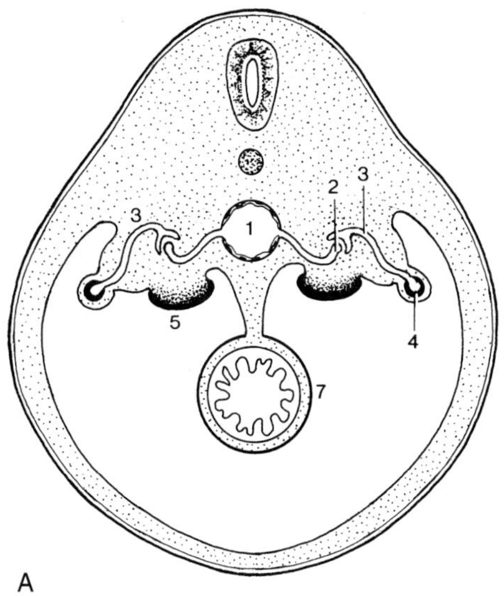


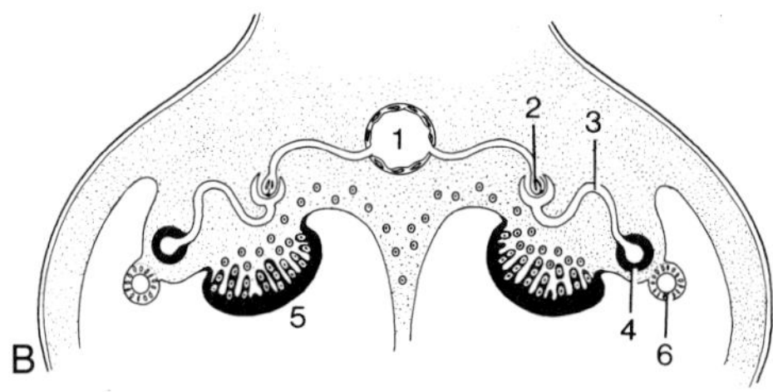


**Figure 5–7.** *A,* Early development of the indifferent gonad. *B,* Invasion of the gonad by epithelial cords, which then incorporate primordial germ cells.

1, Aorta; 2, capillary tuft (in nephron); 3, nephron (tubule); 4, mesonephric duct; 5, gonad; 6, paramesonephric duct; 7, gut.

During fetal development the primordial germ cells differentiate into gonocytes, which after birth give rise to spermatogonia. At puberty, the spermatogonia proliferate, and differentiate to supply cells which undergo meiosis and spermiogenesis to form male gametes (Plate 6/*F*). Sections through the adult testis show seminiferous tubules cut in various planes. The walls of the highly convoluted tubules are lined by a stratified germinal epithelium consisting of cells in various stages of differentiation. Supporting Sertoli cells nourish the germ cells. Cells of an additional type can be identified. These, the Leydig cells, produce the steroid testosterone that is essential if spermatogenesis is to continue. Their progenitors, like those of Sertoli and primordial germ cells, presumably migrate from the mesonephros during fetal development to become embedded in a mesenchymal interstitium, while around puberty, when the process of spermatogenesis is initiated, a second generation of Leydig cells develops. The initial formation of the seminiferous cords is followed in later fetal life by canalization of the cords, to create a series of passages leading to the mesonephric duct which thus becomes the outlet for the gamete products of the testis. The peripheral parts of the cords become seminiferous tubules, the central parts become the rete testis, and the mesonephric tubules become the efferent ductules (Fig. 5–8/*C*). The first part of the mesonephric duct convolutes and forms the duct of the epididymis within the dense connective tissue of that organ; the remaining part retains a straighter course, and as the deferent duct (Fig. 5–5/3) it opens into that part of the cloaca that becomes the urogenital sinus (/6). Glandular proliferation of the lining of the duct toward its termination produces the ampullary thickening, while in most species, but not in carnivores, a subterminal budding enlarges as the vesicular gland (Fig. 5–9/5). In some species a final short passage, the ejaculatory duct, persists, but in others later adjustments cause the deferent and vesicular ducts to open separately. Gonadal enlargement causes the testis to hang within a fold (mesorchium) arising from the regressing mesonephros. The duct is carried within this supporting fold, which in its caudal stretch inclines medially to form with its neighbor the genital fold of peritoneum that helps subdivide the peritoneal cavity of the pelvis. The testis later migrates outside the abdomen (p. 173) before the initiation of spermatogenesis (Plate 6/*F*).

The division of the cloaca has been described (p. 147). The caudal part of the sinus constitutes the pelvic part of the urethra. Outgrowths from its lining differentiate into the prostate and bulbourethral glands in a species-characteristic fashion (Fig. 5–9). The greater part of the male urethra lies within the penis and has a different origin. Thickenings appear around the margin of the urogenital membrane in the indifferent stage (Fig. 5–10). One, ventral and median, constitutes the *genital (phallic) tubercle* or swelling (/1), which gives rise to the greater part of the penis; other thickenings that are more lateral in position contribute the scrotum. A further *urogenital fold* that appears medial to each scrotal swelling makes an additional contribution to the penis. A groove extends along the (initially) dorsal surface of the genital tubercle; it is gradually closed by the approach and mergence of these urogenital folds. This process is rather complex since the lining of the penile urethra is provided by an extension of the endoderm of the urogenital sinus, although the initial swellings have ectodermal coverings. The corpus spongiosum (spongy body) of the penile

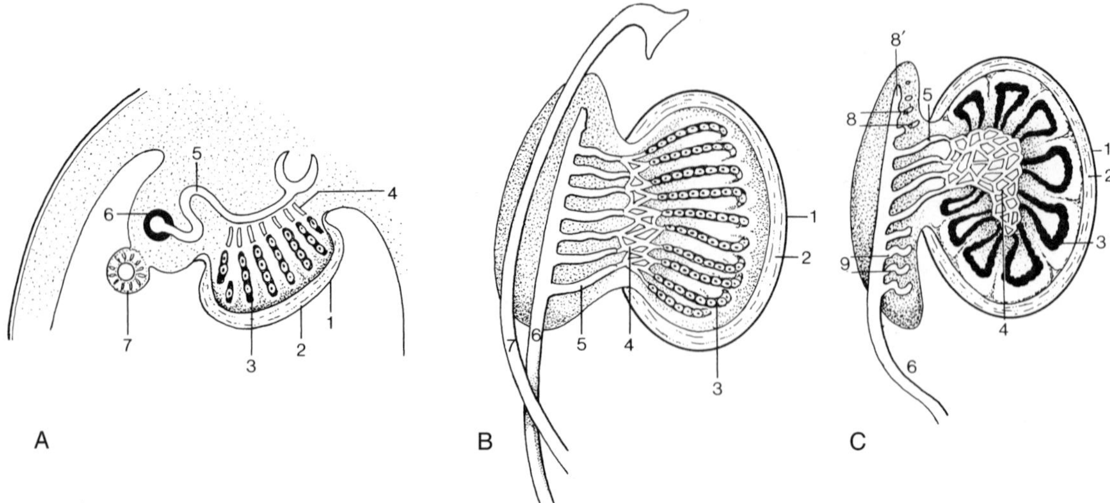


**Figure 5–8.** Three stages in the development of the testis. *A,* The epithelial cords are isolated from the surface epithelium by the formation of the tunica albuginea. *B,* The epithelial cords, rete, and mesonephric tubules have interconnected. *C,* The epithelial cords become seminiferous tubules, and the mesonephros is gradually transformed into part of the epididymis.

1, Celom epithelium; 2, tunica albuginea; 3, epithelial cords, seminiferous tubules; 4, rete testis; 5, mesonephric tubules, efferent ductules; 6, mesonephric (later deferent) duct; 7, paramesonephric duct; 8, cranial remnant of mesonephric tubules (aberrant ductules); 8′, remnant of 6 (appendix of epididymis); 9, caudal remnant (paradidymis).

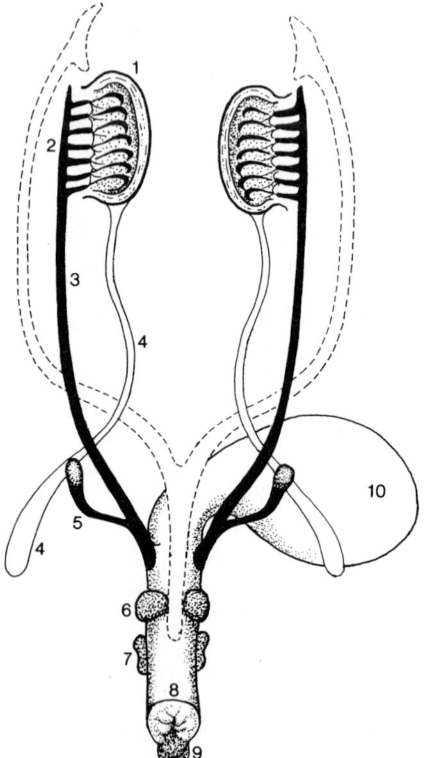


**Figure 5–9.** Differentiation of the urogenital sinus. Note the budding of the prostate and bulbourethral glands and the enlargement of the genital tubercle. The regressed paramesonephric ducts are indicated by the broken lines.

1, Testis; 2, epididymis; 3, deferent duct; 4, gubernaculum; 5, vesicular gland; 6, prostate; 7, bulbourethral gland; 8, urogenital sinus (urethra); 9, genital tubercle; 10, bladder.

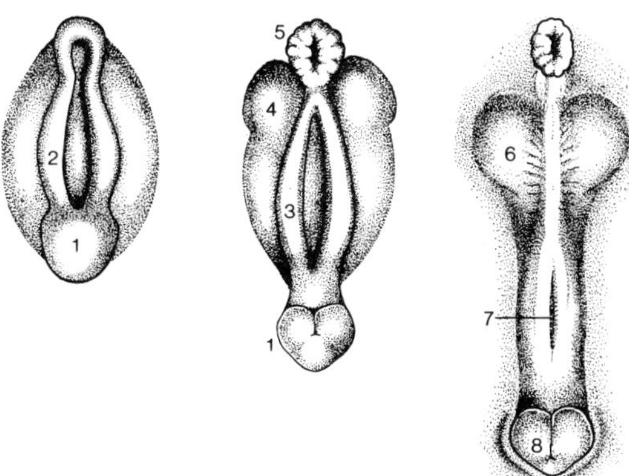


**Figure 5–10.** Development of the male external genitalia.

1, Genital tubercle; 2, cloacal fold; 3, urogenital fold; 4, lateral (scrotal) swelling; 5, anus; 6, scrotum; 7, groove closing to form the penile urethra; 8 glans penis.

urethra directly continues the bulbar tissue of the pelvic urethra, while the corpus cavernosum penis forms within the genital swelling. The lateral swellings grow and join together to form the scrotum, which retains evidence of its bilateral origin in a median raphe and septum.

Differentiation of the male efferent duct system, accessory glands, and external genitalia depends on the presence of testosterone, the male sex hormone produced by the developing testes. The testes also produce several other hormones, for example, the antimüllerian hormone (AMH) and insulin-like factor 3 (descendine), respectively responsible for the disappearance of the müllerian duct and the outgrowth of the gubernaculum. Without exposure to these three hormones the genital tract would develop in the female direction.

## Development of the Female Reproductive Organs

The initial stages of gonadal development resemble those described for the male. Later the cell cords fragment into cell clusters, each enclosing an immigrant germ cell. The cords penetrate less deeply into the interior of the gonad than in the male. The primordial follicles are formed here. Rete formation is less pronounced in the ovary and since no connection is established with mesonephric tubules, no uninterrupted tubular outlet for the escape of gametes is created (Fig. 5–11).

Consequently, follicular rupture releases the female gametes at the surface of the ovary by tissue breakdown, a process made easier by the absence of a thick tunica albuginea. The same feature allows for the formation of further sex cords, with the establishment of additional follicles, during a large part of prenatal life; indeed in certain species this process may continue for a time after birth. Even so, it ceases eventually and the number of female gametes is then at its maximum; it is afterward depleted by loss through atresia and, to a much smaller extent, through ovulation. Ovarian descent is very limited in most species, being greatest in the ruminants in which the ovaries shift caudally to the abdominopelvic boundary.

The duct system of the female is largely provided by the *paramesonephric ducts* (Fig. 5–11/7), which have only vestigial importance in the male. These ducts first develop by invagination of the celomic epithelium lateral to the mesonephric ducts, and secondly by active growth in the

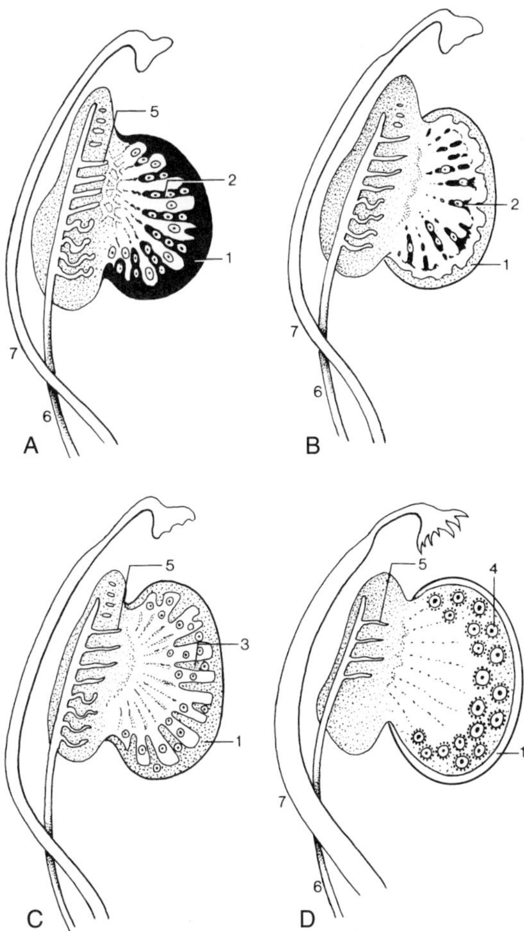


**Figure 5–11.** Successive stages in the development of the ovary.

1, Celomic epithelium; 2, epithelial cords, penetrating *(A)* and regressing *(B)*; 3, second formation of sex cords *(C)*; 4, primitive follicles; 5, remnants of mesonephric tubules; 6, mesonephric duct; 7, paramesonephric duct *(D)*.

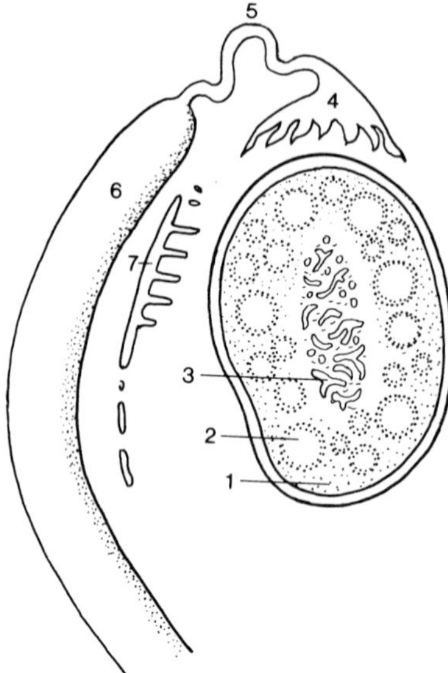


**Figure 5–12.** Differentiation of paramesonephric duct and regression of mesonephric duct.

1, Interstitial tissue of the ovary; 2, primitive follicles; 3, ovarian rete; 4, infundibulum; 5, uterine tube; 6, uterine horn (4, 5, and 6 differentiate from paramesonephric duct); 7, remnants of the mesonephric tubules and duct (epoöphoron and paroöphoron).

direction of the urogenital sinus within the genital folds. In contrast, the mesonephric ducts regress in craniocaudal sequence (Fig. 5–12), and only remnants survive within the broad ligaments and in the vaginal wall (ducts of Gartner, ductus epöophori longitudinales) where they are occasionally the seat of anomalous processes. The cranial part of each paramesonephric duct runs lateral to the mesonephric duct, but it crosses this more caudally where it inclines to meet and fuse with its fellow (Fig. 5–13/6). The cranial end of each paramesonephric duct remains open to the peritoneal cavity (abdominal ostium of the uterine tube), while the caudal end of the united duct initially ends blindly against a solid outgrowth from the dorsal wall of the urogenital sinus (Fig. 5–14). The uterine tubes and the horns, body, and cervix of the uterus form from the paramesonephric ducts; their caudal parts fuse to an extent that varies with the species and accounts for the very different form and proportions of the uterus of adult animals (p. 195) (Fig. 5–15). The supporting genital fold becomes the broad ligament with its various parts. The vaginal lumen appears within the solid outgrowth from the sinus, although a tissue partition, the hymen, may persist near the junction with the fused paramesonephric ducts. A hymen is present only in virgin animals and is rarely well formed in domestic species. Some dispute exists over the contribution of the urogenital and paramesonephric epithelia to the lining of the vagina in the adult, with a suggestion that the boundary may divide regions with the different responses to hormonal influences that are observed in some species.

The urogenital sinus becomes the vestibule with relatively little further change. Epithelial outgrowths form the vestibular glands in species-variable fashion. The external genital parts are formed from the same structures as in the male,

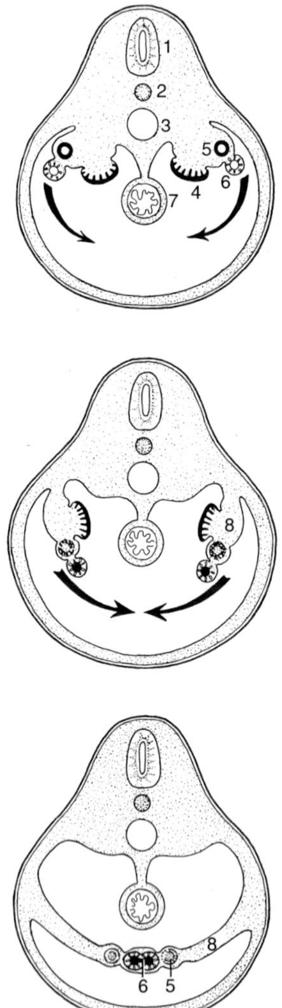


**Figure 5–13.** Transverse sections (from cranial to caudal) through the caudal part of the abdomen, illustrating the creation of the genital fold in the female embryo.

1, Neural tube; 2, notochord; 3, aorta; 4, gonad; 5, mesonephric duct (regressing); 6, paramesonephric duct (merged in the caudal section); 7, gut; 8, genital fold.

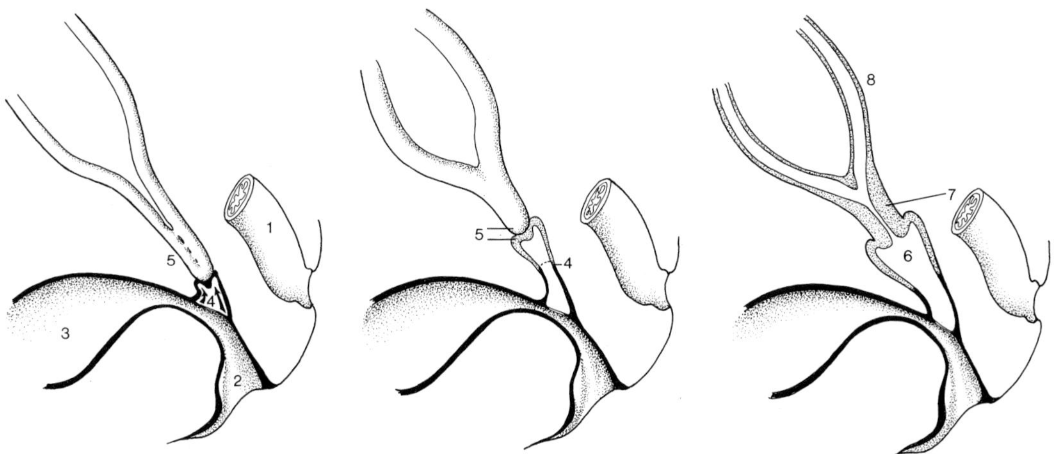


**Figure 5–14.** The fusion of the combined paramesonephric ducts with a bud from the urogenital sinus forms the vagina.

1, Rectum; 2, caudal part of urogenital sinus (vestibule); 3, cranial part of urogenital sinus (bladder, urethra); 4, bud from urogenital sinus; 5, fused paramesonephric ducts; 6, vagina; 7, cervix uteri; 8, uterine horn.

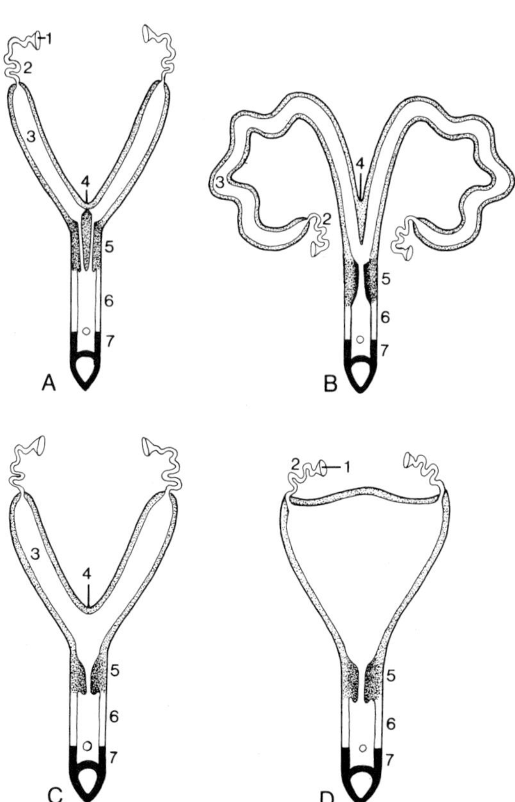


**Figure 5–15.** Different degrees of fusion of the paramesonephric ducts *(gray)*. *A,* Uterus duplex (rabbit). *B,* Uterus bicornis (small body: sow, cow). *C,* Uterus bicornis (large body: mare). *D,* Uterus simplex (woman).

1, Infundibulum; 2, uterine tube; 3, uterine horn; 4, fusion site of the two ducts; 5, cervix; 6, vagina; 7, vestibule.

genital tubercle and lateral folds (swellings) appearing first (Fig. 5–16). The former produces the clitoris, while the lateral folds, which form the labia majora of human anatomy, regress—with a possible reservation for the bitch (p. 442). The labia of the vulva of the domestic species are provided by the *urogenital folds* (/3) that appear medial to the lateral swellings and correspond to the labia minora of women.

## The Process of Testicular Descent

The descent of the testis into a scrotal position is necessary in most mammals to obtain normal fertility. The process depends on the existence of a mesenchymal condensation, the *gubernaculum*

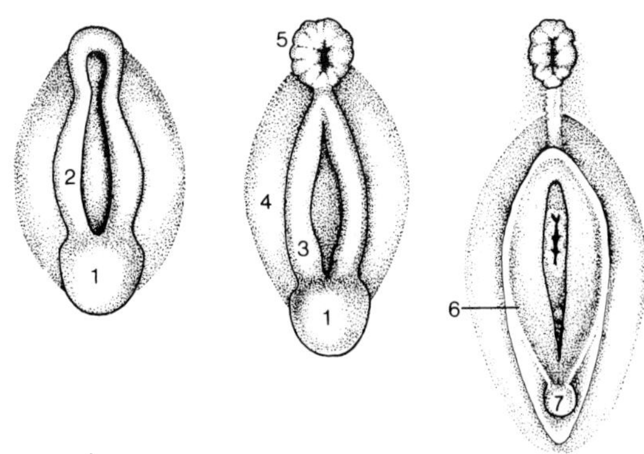

**Figure 5–16.** Development of the female external genitalia.

1, Genital tubercle; 2, cloacal fold; 3, urogenital fold; 4, lateral swelling; 5, anus; 6, labia of vulva; 7, clitoris.

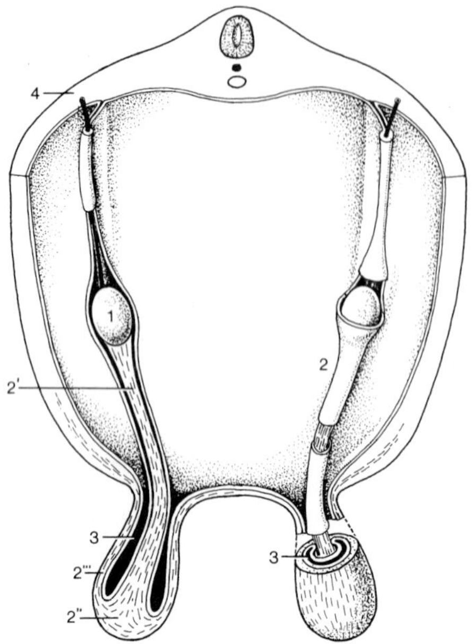


**Figure 5–17.** Schematic representation of the testis and gubernaculum within the peritoneal fold in which descent takes place.

1, Testis; 2, gubernaculum; 2′, pars propria; 2″, pars infravaginalis; 2‴, pars vaginalis; 3, vaginal process; 4, testicular artery.

*testis,* within a detachment from the genital fold that leads from the testis toward and through the inguinal canal (Fig. 5–17 and Plate 5/*A,B*). At a certain critical period of development (which varies in timing among different species) the distal part of the gubernaculum, which extends through the inguinal canal to the groin, enlarges very rapidly and considerably. The gubernaculum is invaded by an extension of the peritoneal lining of the abdomen (Fig. 5–17/3). In this way the vaginal process, which provides the space into which the testis will be drawn, is formed. The invasion by the vaginal process divides the gubernaculum into three parts: the proximal part (pars propria) is enclosed by the inner (future visceral) peritoneal lining of the process; the second part (pars vaginalis) surrounds the outer (future parietal) peritoneal lining of the process; and the third part (pars infravaginalis) lies distal to the invagination and is thus continuous with the other parts. The swelling of the gubernaculum commences distally, causing it to exert pressure on the body wall about the superficial ring of the inguinal canal. This displaces the testis distally, toward the abdominal entrance of the canal. The swelling then gradually extends proximally, and when at its peak the part adjacent to the testis (and within the inguinal canal) is as thick as the testis itself (Plate 5/*A,B*). At this stage any slight increase in intra-abdominal pressure may be sufficient to expel the testis from the abdomen into the inguinal canal, although for a time its return to the abdomen is still possible. The descent is complete and irreversible once the core of the gubernaculum has regressed (Fig. 5–18). A well-timed gubernacular regression is therefore as indispensable to normal descent as is the earlier swelling. Since the timing is critical and the process subject to various disturbances, it is not surprising that abdominal retention and abnormal descent are both relatively frequent. Failure of the testis to appear in the groin is known as cryptorchidism (hidden testis). It takes various forms; it may be unilateral or bilateral, and may present the testis held within the abdomen or trapped within the inguinal canal. As a result of the higher temperature to which an undescended testis is exposed, spermatogenesis is not initiated at puberty. The condition is clearly undesirable and although unilaterally cryptorchid animals may be

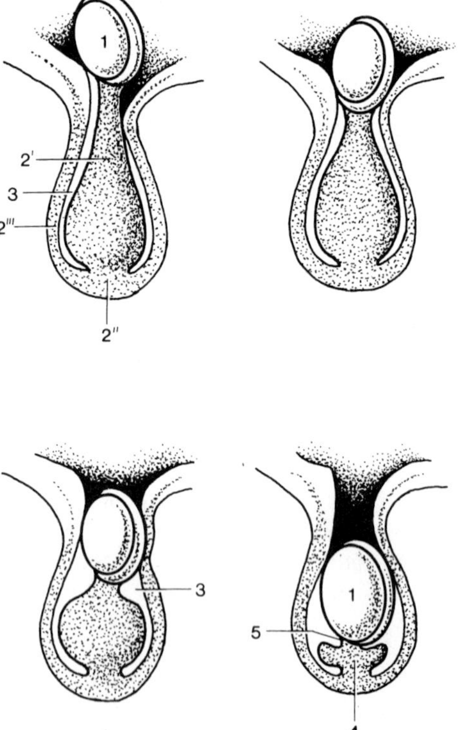


**Figure 5–18.** Successive stages in gubernacular regression in the pig fetus. Observe the migration of the testis caused by this regression.

1, Testis and epididymis; 2, gubernaculum; 2′, pars propria; 2″, pars infravaginalis; 2‴, pars vaginalis; 3, vaginal process; 4, ligament of the tail of the epididymis; 5, proper ligament of the testis.

fertile, they should be excluded from breeding since the condition is often hereditary.

Similar structures are formed in the female sex but do not develop significantly, except in the bitch among domestic mammals, in which the existence of the vaginal process is occasionally troublesome (p. 440).

## THE URINARY ORGANS

The urinary system comprises paired kidneys that form the urine from the blood; ureters that convey the urine from the kidneys; the bladder, where urine is stored until it can be discharged conveniently; and the urethra, through which it finally passes to the exterior. Since almost the entire male urethra also conveys the reproductive products, it is usual to describe it with the reproductive organs.

### The Kidneys

The kidneys have as their prime task the maintenance of the milieu intérieur. They do this by filtering the plasma, initially extracting an enormous volume of fluid before subjecting this ultrafiltrate to further processing in which useful substances are selectively reabsorbed, waste substances concentrated for elimination, and the volume adjusted by the conservation of sufficient water to maintain the composition of the plasma within the appropriate range. Some figures may give an impression of the dimensions of this task. In large dogs (and animals of similar size), 1000 to 2000 L of blood perfuse the kidneys daily; the 200 to 300 L of fluid that are filtered from this volume are later reduced by reabsorption until only 1 or 2 L of urine remain to be discharged.

The endocrine function of the kidneys consists of the production and release of two hormones: renin, which plays a vital role in the regulation of systemic blood pressure, and erythropoietin, which influences erythropoiesis. Both are produced within the juxtoglomerular complexes, localized regions of intimate association between arterioles, formed by the union of afferent glomerular capillaries, with adjacent portions of the distal convoluted tubules (p. 216).

The kidneys are firm, reddish-brown glands whose appearance varies considerably among mammals (Fig. 5–19). The most familiar form, that which has introduced the term "kidney-shaped" to the common vocabulary, is encountered in the dog, cat, and small ruminants. The kidneys of the pig are a much flattened version, whereas those of the horse are more heart-shaped (*/C*). In contrast, the bovine kidneys are very unlike and have a surface deeply fissured to outline many lobes (*/D*). Even greater subdivision is shown by the kidneys of certain marine species (*/E*), which resemble trusses of grapes with the lobes only slightly fused and mainly held together by the branching "stalk."

The kidneys are usually found pressed against the abdominal roof, one to each side of the vertebral column, and predominantly in the lumbar region, although often extending forward under the last ribs. Their positions change with the excursions of the diaphragm and they move, perhaps by half the length of a vertebra, with each breath. They are rarely symmetrical; in domestic animals, other than pigs, the right one is about half a kidney-length in advance of its fellow. The cranial extremity of the right kidney commonly fits into a fossa of the liver, which helps fix its position. The left one, lacking this lodgment, is more mobile and is more likely to sag within the abdomen. The pendulous left kidney of ruminants is thrust into the right half of the abdomen by the enormous development of the stomach. In general, kidneys pressed against the abdominal roof are largely retroperitoneal, whereas those suspended at a lower level have a more extensive peritoneal covering (Fig. 5–20).

Each kidney lies within a splitting of the sublumbar fascia, which also holds considerable fat, sometimes enough to hide the kidney completely. The fat protects against distorting pressures from neighboring organs. The surface of a kidney is generally smoothly convex except for an indentation of the medial border. This indentation leads to a concealed space (renal sinus; Fig. 5–21/6) occupied by the dilated origin (renal pelvis) of the ureter, the vessels and nerves passing to and from the renal hilus, and more fat.

The general organization of the kidney is most conveniently shown in a section that divides the organ into dorsal and ventral "halves" (Fig. 5–21). Such a section shows that the parenchyma is enclosed within a tough fibrous capsule (see Plate 4/*C;* and Fig. 36–11). The capsule restricts the kidney's ability to expand; the swelling that occurs in certain disease conditions therefore tends to compress the tissue and narrow the internal passages. The capsule strips readily from the healthy kidney but adheres where the underlying substance has been scarred by former lesions.

The parenchyma is visibly divided into an outer cortex and an inner medulla. The cortex (/1) is distinguished by its reddish-brown color and finely granular appearance. The medulla (/2) consists of a dark, purplish outer zone, from which stripes (medullary rays) extend into the cortex, and a paler, grayish-red, and radially striated inner zone

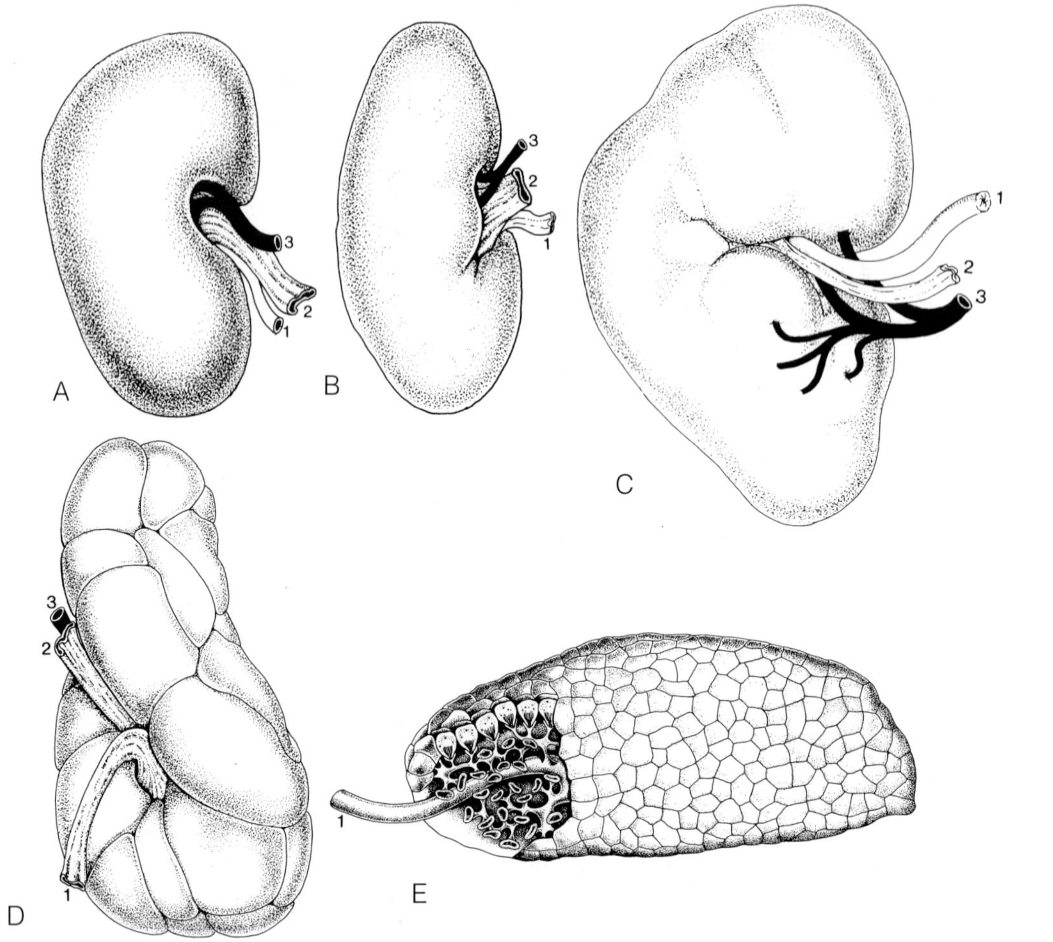

**Figure 5–19.** Left kidney of the dog *(A)*, pig *(B)*, horse *(C)*, cattle *(D)*, and dolphin *(E)*.

1, Ureter; 2, renal vein; 3, renal artery.

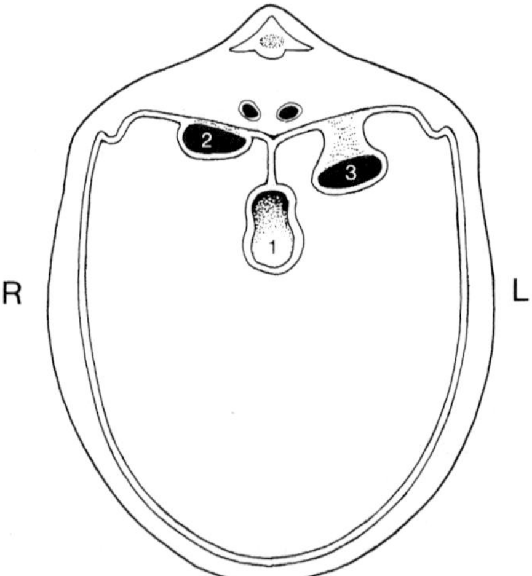


**Figure 5–20.** Schematic representation of the position of the kidneys in relation to the peritoneal cavity.

1, Gut; 2, right kidney (retroperitoneal); 3, left kidney (intraperitoneal—pendulous or "floating").

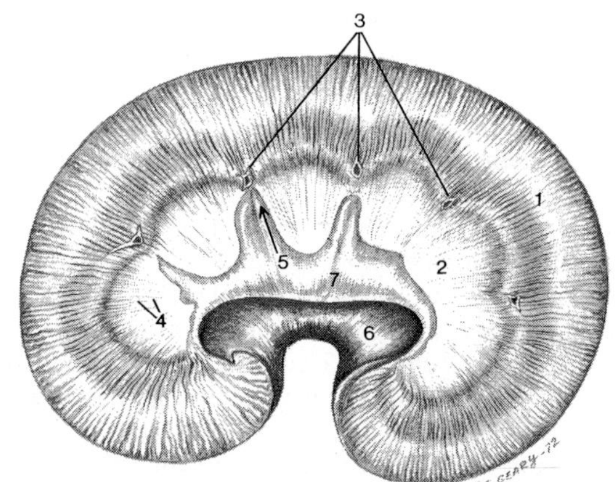


**Figure 5–21.** Dorsal section of a unipyramidal kidney (dog).

1, Cortex; 2, medulla; 3, arcuate arteries; 4, collecting tubules; 5, recess of renal pelvis; 6, renal sinus; 7, renal crest.

that extends toward the renal sinus. The gross arrangement of the medulla shows very marked species differences. In many species the medulla is arranged as several (or even many) discrete masses, each roughly pyramidal in form. In kidneys of this type a portion of the cortex is associated with each pyramid and caps its base, the aspect directed toward the outer surface. The apex of the pyramid points toward the renal sinus and forms a *papilla* (/3) that fits into a cuplike expansion (calix) of the renal pelvis. Each medullary pyramid with its associated cortex constitutes a *renal lobe.* Kidneys that retain this organization are said to be *multipyramidal* or multilobar. In some multipyramidal kidneys, such as those of cattle (Fig. 28–28; and Plate 4/*E*), the boundaries between the lobes are revealed by the fissures that penetrate from the surface; in others, including those of pigs, no external evidence of lobation is present (Fig. 5–19/*B*).

All mammalian kidneys pass through a multipyramidal phase in their development, although in most species the number of lobes is later drastically reduced. In some species, including the dog, horse, and sheep, all the pyramids finally fuse to form a single medullary mass that confines the cortex to the periphery where it forms a continuous shell. Even this *unipyramidal* or unilobar type of kidney retains some evidence of its complex ontogeny; a slight scalloping of the corticomedullary junction, punctuated by the arteries that mark the interlobar boundaries, shows where the pyramids fused. The fusion joins the papillae in a common crest (Figs. 5–21/7 and 5–22) that may be modeled to reveal its composite origin; it is so modeled in the dog but not in the horse.

The functional units within the kidney are known as renal tubules or *nephrons.* These epithelial tubules are supported by a connective tissue interstitium and are estimated to number several hundred thousand or even a million in canine kidneys. The structure and the functions of the nephron are more appropriately described in texts of microscopic anatomy and physiology; only a few points, mainly those discernible to the naked eye, are mentioned here.

Each nephron begins with a blind expansion that is invaginated by a cluster of capillaries known as a *glomerulus* (Figs. 5–23/1 and 5–24). The glomerulus and its epithelial covering together constitute a *renal corpuscle* (Fig. 5–23/1′), a structure just large enough to be visible to the unaided eye, especially if the capillaries are congested. The corpuscles are scattered throughout the cortex and give it a finely granular appearance.

The remaining part of the nephron forms a long tubule differentiated into several successive segments. The first, the proximal convoluted tubule, is very tortuous and is located close to the corpuscle from which it arises (/2). This part gradually straightens and enters one of the narrow rays that penetrate the cortex from the medulla. The tubule then forms a long hairpin loop (formerly known as the loop of Henle) within the medulla. The first part of the loop, the descending limb, is relatively narrow and runs through the medulla to approach the papilla before turning back. The ascending limb is generally thicker—although the change in caliber need not coincide with the change in direction—and runs back to regain the medullary ray. On leaving this, the tubule forms a second or distal convoluted part that is also placed close to the corpuscle of origin (/4). A short junctional section then runs to join a collecting tubule within the medullary ray. Each *collecting tubule* (/5), which serves many nephrons, runs through the medulla before opening into a larger vessel, a *papillary duct,* close to the apex (/6). Several score of papillary ducts drain into the renal pelvis. The papillary ducts can be clearly demonstrated in resin injection specimens (Plate 4/*D,F,H*). The

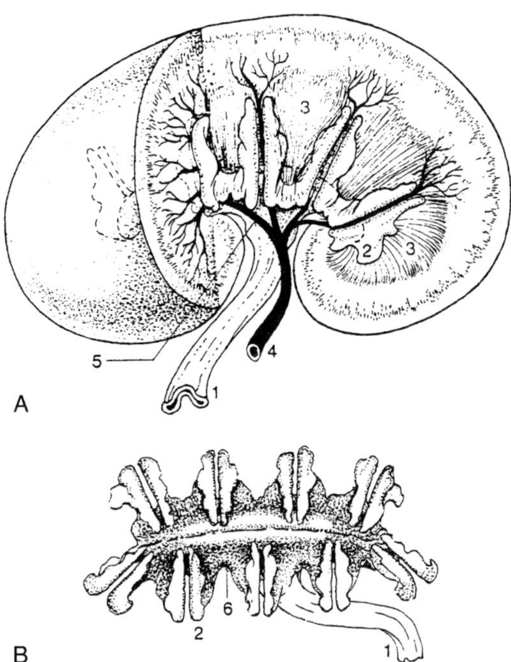


**Figure 5–22.** Semischematic drawing of the canine kidney *(A).* The papillae have joined in an irregular common crest; the thickenings of the crest alternate with recesses of the renal pelvis as shown by the corrosion cast of the pelvis *(B).*

1, Ureter; 2, pelvis recess; 3, medulla with papillary ducts; 4, renal artery; 5, interlobar arteries at the pyramidal boundaries; 6, impression of renal crest.

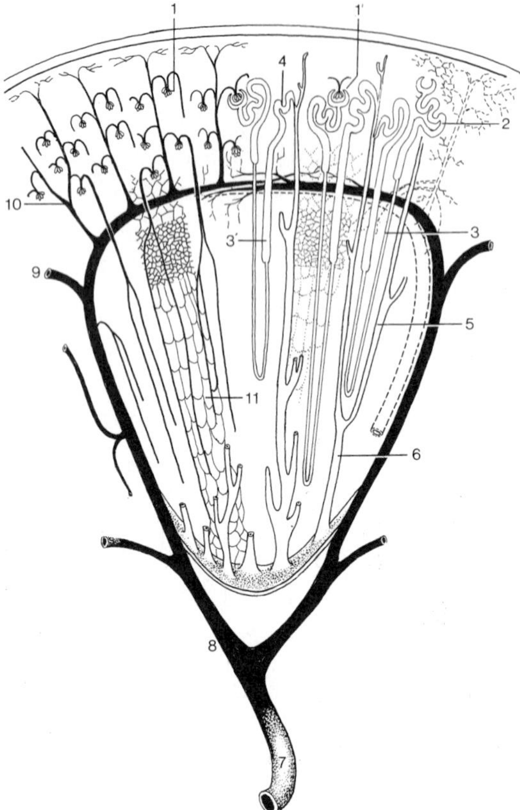


**Figure 5–23.** Schematic drawing of a kidney lobe.

1, Glomerulus; 1′, renal corpuscle; 2, proximal convoluted tubule; 3, descending limb of nephron; 3′, ascending limb; 4, distal convoluted tubule; 5, collecting tubule; 6, papillary duct; 7, renal artery; 8, interlobar artery; 9, arcuate artery; 10, interlobular artery; 11, capillary plexus.

perforated (cribriform) areas where they discharge are confined to the apices of independent papillae or to specific regions of a common crest.

Variations in the location of the corpuscles and in the overall length and proportions of the tubules have functional importances that cannot be discussed here.

Each kidney is supplied by a *renal artery,* a branch of the abdominal aorta, which may carry rather more than a tenth of the total output of the left ventricle! The renal artery divides into several *interlobar arteries* (/8) that follow the divisions, former or extant, between the renal pyramids at the corticomedullary junction. These vessels are prominent in gross sections of the kidney. They give rise to branches known as *arcuate arteries* that curve over the bases of the pyramids (/9). These in turn give origin to numerous *interlobular arteries* that supply the units or lobules into which the cortex is divided by the medullary rays. Each interlobular artery gives rise to many branches that supply individual glomeruli. The glomerular capillaries rejoin in one emissary vessel at the distal pole of the glomerulus, and this then supplies a further capillary plexus around the tubules (/11). The flow of blood through this second capillary bed is countercurrent to the direction of the urine flow. The vessels that issue from the juxtomedullary corpuscles (those in the innermost layer of the cortex) have a particular importance in the supply of the medulla. The renal circulation is actually more complicated than is described here and provides opportunities for collateral circulation. However, the interlobular arteries are certainly, the interlobar arteries possibly, functional end-arteries.

The veins, which lead ultimately to the caudal vena cava, are broadly satellite. Lymphatic vessels drain to nodes of the lumbar series that accompanies the aorta. The sympathetic nerves to the kidneys are routed through the celiacomesenteric plexus and thence along the renal arteries. The synapses may be located within the major ganglia or within smaller (aorticorenal) ganglia within peripheral parts of the plexus. The vagus contributes the parasympathetic supply.

## The Renal Pelvis and Ureter

In cattle the ureter is formed by the coming together of the short passages that lead from the calices that enclose individual renal papillae (see

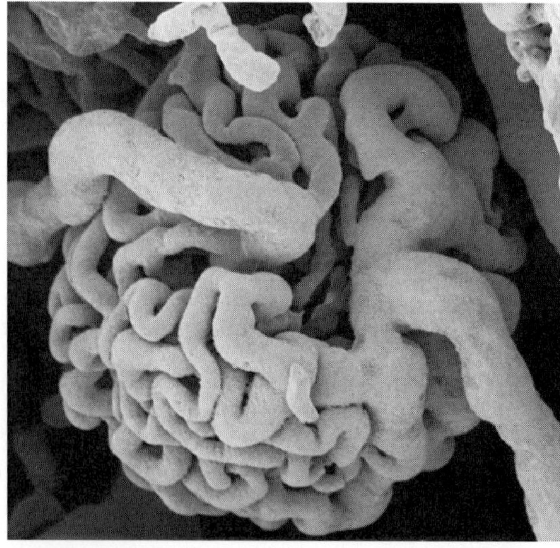

**Figure 5–24.** Scanning electron micrograph of a corrosion cast of a rat renal glomerulus.

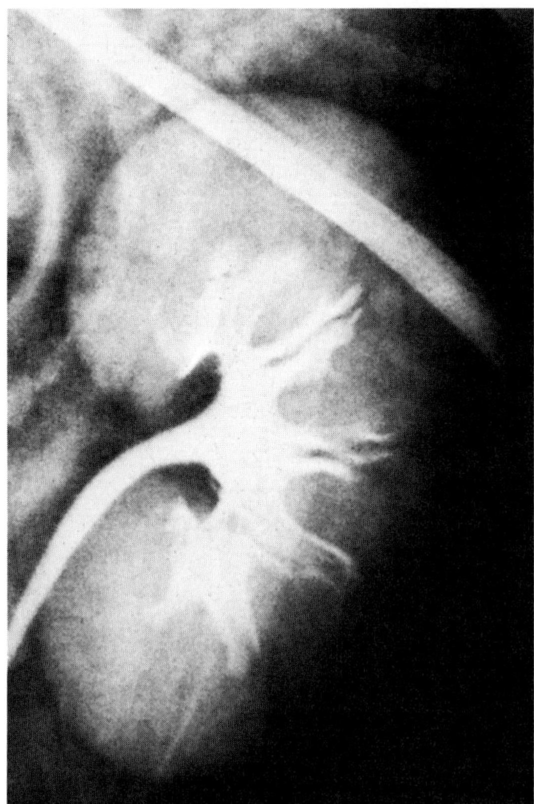

**Figure 5–25.** Radiograph of renal pelvis of the dog. Note the pelvic recesses.

Fig. 28–28). In most domestic species the ureter begins in a common expansion, the renal pelvis, into which all the papillary ducts open—although in different ways in different species (Figs. 5–22 and 21–23). Few differences in pelvic anatomy are of practical significance. However, in the dog and cat the form of the renal pelvis obtains an importance lacking in the other species from its ready depiction in radiographs. The renal pelvis of these animals is molded on the renal crest and extends flanges dorsal and ventral to this. Each flange shows a number of local expansions or recesses that are divided from each other by projections of renal tissue (Figs. 5–22 and 5–25). Neighboring recesses are also separated by the interlobar vessels.

The remaining tubular part of each ureter has a fairly even caliber. It follows a broadly sagittal course against the abdominal roof, although it may exhibit occasional sharp changes in direction. On reaching the pelvic cavity the ureter bends medially to enter the genital fold in the male, the broad ligament in the female; this carries the ureter over the dorsal surface of the bladder, into which it opens near the neck (Fig. 5–26). In the male the ureter passes dorsal to the corresponding deferent duct.

The ureter penetrates the bladder wall very obliquely. The length of the intramural course guards against reflux of urine into the ureter when the pressure is raised within the bladder (Fig. 5–27). It does not prevent further filling of the bladder since the resistance is overcome by peristaltic contractions of the ureteric wall. The wall of the renal pelvis and ureter possesses an external adventitia, a middle muscularis, and an internal mucosa. The muscle coat is well developed, and although its peristalsis helps move urine to the bladder, it can enter spasm when provoked by local irritation such as is provided by a urinary calculus.

## The Urinary Bladder

The bladder is a distensible storage organ and thus can have no constant size, position, or relationships. It is small and globular when fully contracted and is then remarkable for the great thickness of its walls and the negligible extent of its lumen. The contracted bladder rests on the pubic bones; it is confined to the pelvic cavity in the larger species but extends into the abdomen in carnivores. When the bladder enlarges it becomes pear-shaped, presenting a cranial vertex (apex), an intermediate body, and a caudal neck that narrows to the internal urethral orifice at the junction with the urethra. Although continuing distention carries an ever-increasing portion of the bladder into the abdomen, the neck remains fixed within the pelvis through its continuity with the urethra (Fig. 5–28/11).

No immediate increase in internal pressure occurs when the bladder begins to fill. But once a certain, quite considerable, volume has been attained, the pressure rises sharply; this creates the urge to void urine, an urge that is obeyed without hesitation in many species. In house-trained animals the urge may temporarily disappear if resisted, although discomfort, and later pain, may be experienced if the bladder becomes overfull. In the well-trained dog the distention may be very great, carrying the apex cranial to the umbilicus and stretching the walls to paper thinness with risk of rupture. Though the outline of the grossly distended bladder is smooth, that of the more modestly distended organ is irregular since the low internal pressure allows it to be indented by its firmer neighbors (Fig. 5–26).

In the larger species the contracted bladder is largely retroperitoneal, but most of the surface becomes intraperitoneal when the organ is even

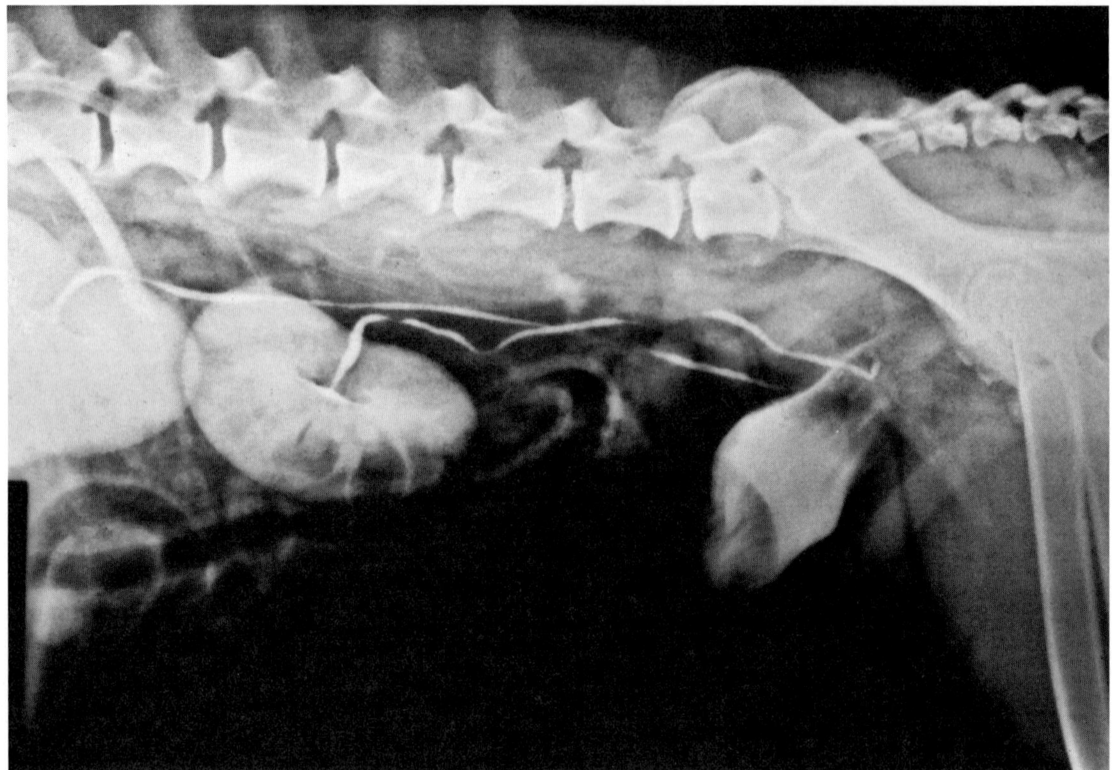

**Figure 5–26.** Radiograph of renal pelves, ureters, and bladder of the dog.

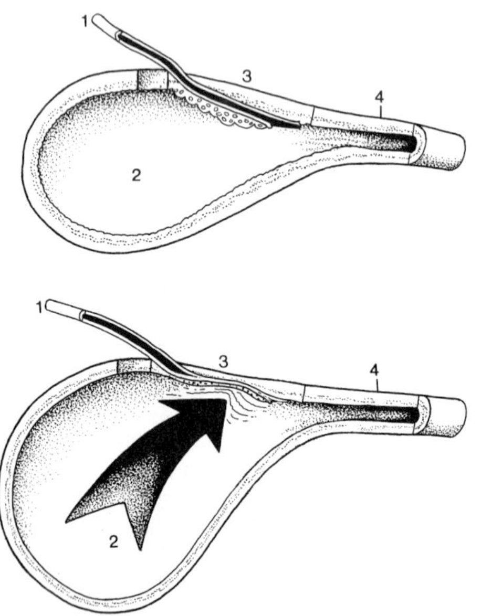


**Figure 5–27.** The ureterovesical junction. Because of its oblique passage through the wall, the ureter is compressed as the intravesical pressure rises.

1, Ureter; 2, bladder lumen; 3, bladder wall; 4, bladder neck.

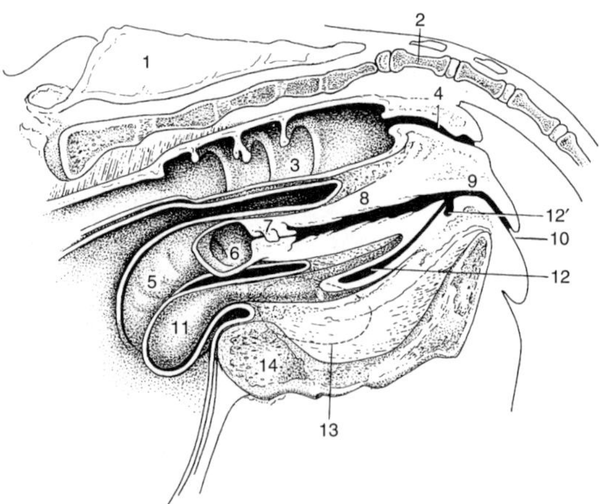


**Figure 5–28.** Median section of the bovine pelvis.

1, Sacrum; 2, first caudal vertebra; 3, interior of rectum; 4, anal canal; 5, exterior of right uterine horn; 6, interior of stump of left uterine horn; 7, cervix; 8, vagina; 9, vestibule; 10, vulva; 11, exterior of bladder; 12, urethra; 12′, suburethral diverticulum; 13, obturator foramen; 14, pelvis symphysis.

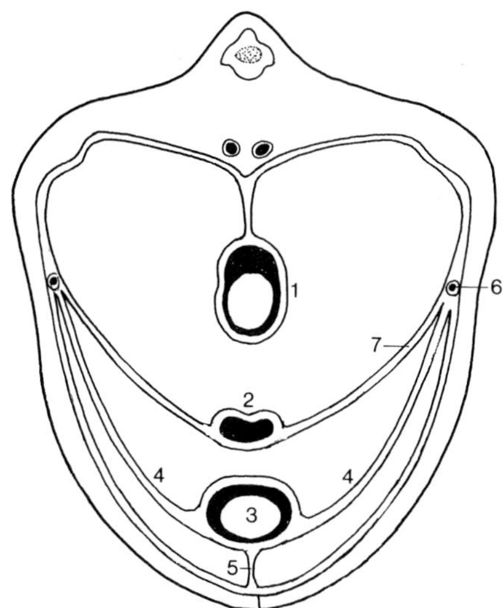


**Figure 5–29.** Peritoneal disposition in the caudal part of the abdomen.

1, Colon; 2, uterus; 3, bladder; 4, lateral vesical ligaments; 5, median vesical ligament; 6, ureter; 7, broad ligament of uterus (mesometrium).

moderately expanded. Three folds continue this serosal covering onto the abdominal and pelvic walls (Fig. 5–29). Paired *lateral vesical folds* convey the round ligaments of the bladder; these vestiges of the umbilical arteries retain narrow lumina through which some blood reaches the cranial part of the bladder. The third, *median vesical fold,* is empty in the adult, but in the fetus it supports the urachus, the constricted cranial continuation of the bladder that passes forward to leave the abdomen through the umbilical foramen before expanding externally into the allantoic sac. Urachus and umbilical arteries rupture at birth; the urachus survives as a scar on the bladder vertex, while the umbilical arteries are transformed into the round ligaments. The folds in the adult bound the ventral pair of the several excavations into which the pelvic peritoneal cavity is divided (Fig. 5–29).

The constant dorsal relations of the bladder are to the reproductive organs and their supporting folds—the uterus and vagina within the broad ligament in the female, the deferent duct (and perhaps the vesicular glands) within the genital fold in the male. The bladder may also make indirect contact with the rectum through these folds. The ventral surface touches the pelvic and abdominal floor. Other relations of the intra-abdominal part of the bladder are less predictable and may be numerous when the bladder is greatly enlarged.

The loose attachment of the bladder mucosa and its ability to stretch allow marked change in the appearance of the interior with altered physiological status. The surface, much folded when the lumen is small, becomes generally smooth when the bladder fills. However, two particular folds resist effacement. These run from the slitlike orifices of the ureters, converge at the exit from the bladder, and fuse to form a median *urethral crest* that continues into the pelvic urethra (Fig. 5–30/5). The triangle bounded by the ureteric and urethral openings is termed the trigone; it appears to have a different origin from the remainder of bladder wall (p. 168) and is believed to have an enhanced sensitivity (/4). The bladder epithelium is of the transitional kind.

The *bladder muscle* is arranged in three sheets that exchange fascicles. The muscle is probably entirely detrusor—available to squeeze and empty the bladder—and fails to form an internal sphincter, although one is often described. Many now believe that, in place of this, some muscle bundles form a series of arcades whose summits are directed toward the orifice; they therefore dilate rather than occlude the exit when they contract. If this is so, continence depends on the tension

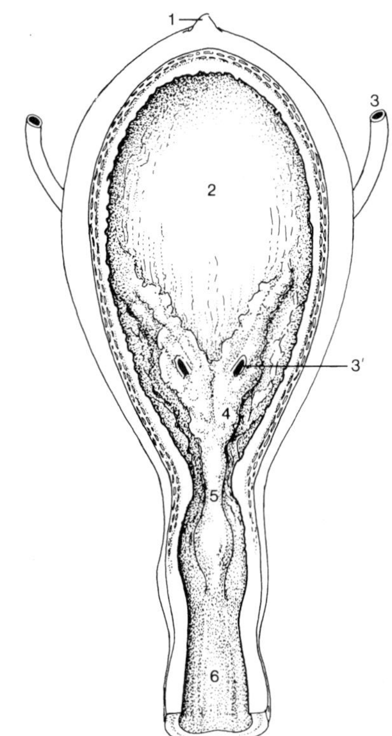


**Figure 5–30.** The interior of the urinary bladder.

1, Scar of urachus; 2, bladder; 3, ureter; 3′, ureteric orifice; 4, trigone of bladder; 5, urethral crest; 6, urethra.

passively exerted by the elastic elements within the mucosa and on the action of the external sphincter, the striated urethralis. This interpretation is consistent with the recent demonstration that in certain species (dog, goat) the proximal part of the urethra forms part of the urine reservoir, expanding as the bladder fills. The functional boundary between bladder and urethra would thus appear to be represented by the cranial limit of the urethralis in these species.

Autonomic fibers reach the bladder through the sympathetic hypogastric and parasympathetic pelvic nerves; the latter innervate the detrusor muscle. Sensory fibers are routed through the pudendal nerve. The main blood supply is from the vaginal (or prostatic) artery, but, as has been mentioned, it is supplemented by the reduced umbilical arteries.

## The Female Urethra

The female urethra runs caudally on the pelvic floor below the reproductive tract. It passes obliquely through the vaginal wall to open ventrally at the junction of vagina and vestibule (Fig. 5–31). Its length and breadth vary considerably among species; it is conspicuously short and wide in mares. In some animals, such as the cow and sow, it opens together with a suburethral diverticulum (Fig. 5–28/12′), in others, such as the bitch, on a hummock. Both arrangements create difficulties when catheterization of the bladder is attempted.

When a *diverticulum* is present it is enclosed within the urethralis, which surrounds the urethra along most of its length. The cranial fascicles of this muscle encircle the urethra, while the caudal ones support it within U-shaped loops that arise and end on the vaginal wall. Contraction of this part of the muscle closes the urethra by pressing the two organs together; it also narrows the vagina. The urethralis obtains a somatic innervation through the pudendal nerve, but sympathetic and parasympathetic involvement is also described.

The urethral submucosa contains many veins that constitute a form of erectile tissue that may contribute to continence by assisting mucosal apposition. These features apart, the structure of the urethra continues that of the bladder.

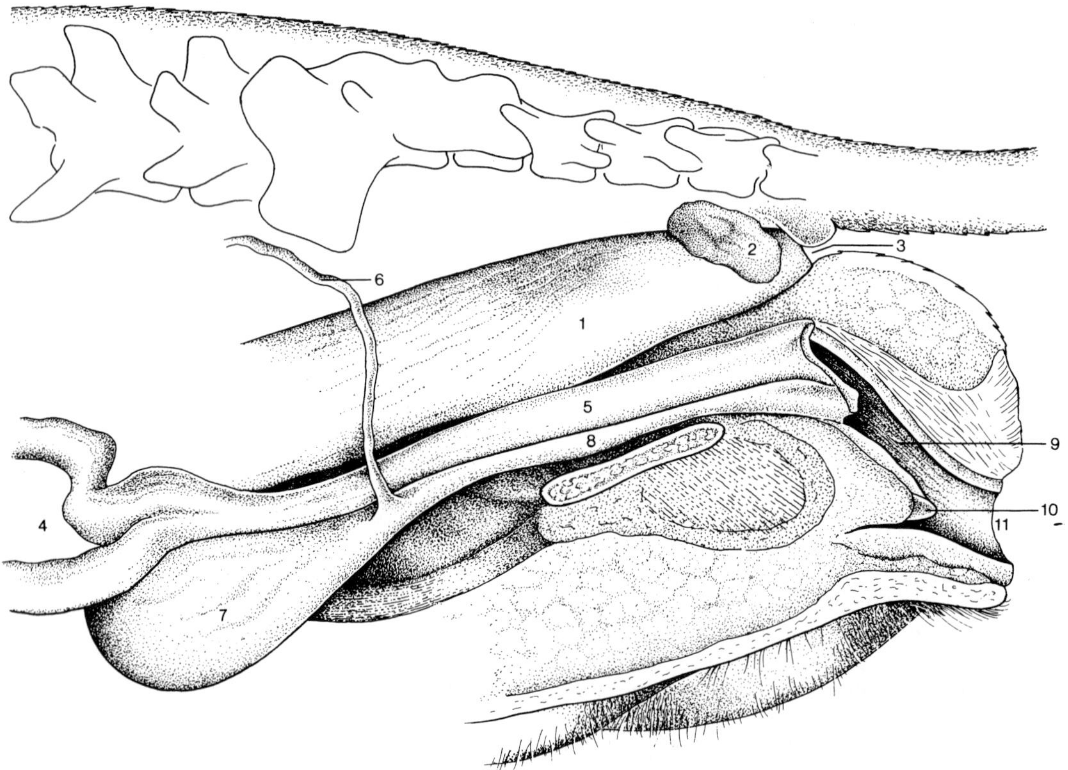


**Figure 5–31.** Pelvic organs of the bitch. The lateral pelvic wall and the lateral wall of the vestibule have been removed. 1, Rectum; 2, anal sac; 3, anus; 4, uterus; 5, vagina; 6, ureter; 7, bladder; 8, urethra; 9, vestibule; 10, clitoris; 11, vulva.

# THE MALE REPRODUCTIVE ORGANS

The male reproductive organs include paired gonads, the testes, which produce both male gametes (sperm) and hormones; paired gonadal duct systems, each consisting of an epididymis and deferent duct (ductus deferens), which convey the exocrine products of the testes to the urethra; a suite of accessory glands, which contributes the bulk of the semen; the male urethra, which extends from the bladder to the free extremity of the penis and serves for the passage of both urine and semen; the penis, the male copulatory organ, which deposits the semen within the reproductive tract of the female; and skin adaptations, the scrotum and the prepuce, developed in relation to the testes and the penis.

## The Testes and Their Adnexa

### *The Testis*

The testis combines endocrine and exocrine components within a common capsule. The endocrine component functions normally at the core temperature of the body, but in most mammals the successful production of the male gametes requires a temperature a few degrees lower than that within the abdomen. Hence, though the testes develop within the abdomen, they later migrate, descending through the inguinal canals to come to lie within the scrotum (see p. 174), a pouch of skin and underlying fasciae variously placed between the groin and perineum. That plausible though rather facile explanation of the descent fails to account for the ability of spermatogenesis to occur normally at the core temperature in a few mammals (known as testiconda: e.g., elephants, hyraxes) in which the testes remain within the abdomen throughout life. It is consistent with the periodic changes exhibited in many small mammals (chiefly found among rodents, insectivores, and bats) in which the testes descend into the scrotum for the breeding season, after which they return to the abdomen. This is brought about by contraction of the cremaster muscle sac found in these species.

The testes are solid ellipsoidal organs whose bulk bears no fixed proportion to the body size. Among domestic species they are conspicuously small in cats and impressively large in sheep and goats. Their orientation also varies. They are carried with their long axes vertical in ruminants (necessitating a deep and pendulous scrotum), horizontal in horses and dogs, and tilted toward the anus in pigs and cats. These differences are broadly correlated with the position of the scrotum, which is below the caudal part of the abdomen in ruminants, perineal in pigs and cats, and intermediate in position in horses and dogs (Fig. 5–32). Each testis is separately suspended within the scrotum by a spermatic cord, a bundle

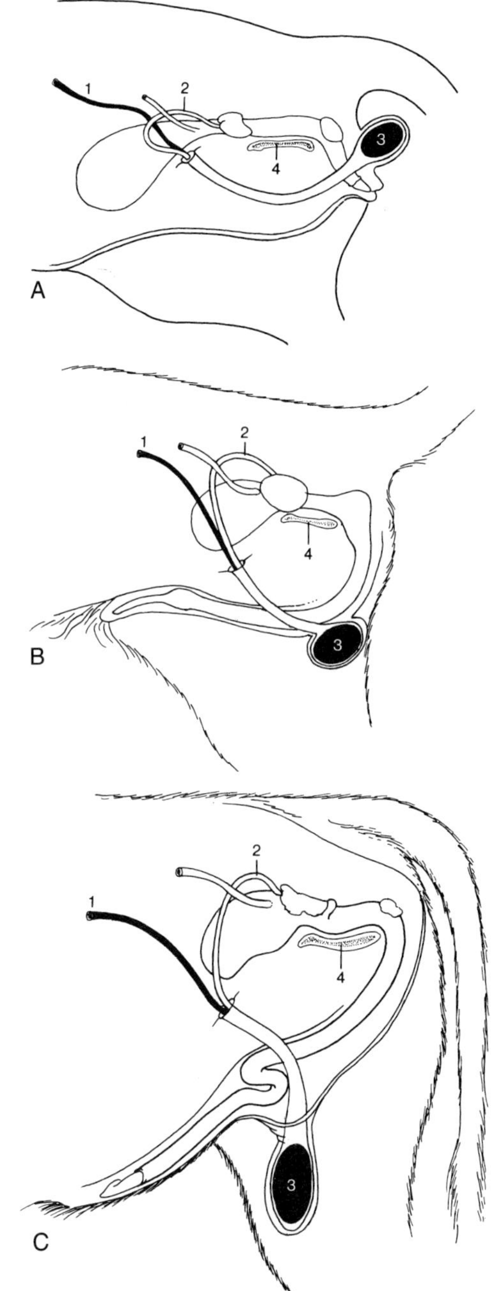


**Figure 5–32.** The perineal, intermediate, and inguinal positions of the scrotum exhibited by the tomcat *(A)*, dog *(B)*, and bull *(C)*.

1, Testicular artery; 2, deferent duct; 3, testis; 4, pelvic symphysis.

of structures that includes the deferent duct and the supplying vessels and nerves enclosed within a double covering of peritoneum.

The outer surface of the testis is made smooth by the direct peritoneal investment, except at the poles and along one margin where the testis is attached to the epididymis, a structure formed by the coiled initial portion of the external duct system. The peritoneum covers a thickish capsule *(tunica albuginea)* mainly composed of dense connective tissue but sometimes including smooth muscle. The larger branches of the testicular artery and vein run within the capsule, where they are visible in a pattern that is species-characteristic. The parenchyma is contained under moderate pressure, which accounts for its pouting through any incision of the capsule. It is probable that slight swelling of the parenchyma can be accommodated by the testis assuming a more globular form, but any significant expansion raises the intratesticular pressure and produces pain, which may be severe when the testis is inflamed (orchitis).* The capsule detaches septa and trabeculae that divide the parenchyma into lobules. The septa are not always conspicuous, but in those species in which they are well developed they may be seen to converge on a substantial thickening (mediastinum testis); this may be axial or displaced toward the side bordering the epididymis.

The soft, yellowish or brownish parenchyma consists of intermingled seminiferous tubules and interstitial tissue. The latter consists of massed interstitial (Leydig) cells supported by a delicate connective tissue framework in which run small blood and lymphatic vessels (Plate 6/*F*). The interstitial cells are the principal producers of the steroid androgenic hormones. The greater part (60% in boars and stallions, 90% in rams and bulls) of the parenchyma is formed by the tubules in which the process of spermatogenesis is conducted.

Each *seminiferous tubule* (Fig. 5–33) is much contorted, and also looped so that both ends open into the rete testis (/5), a plexus of spaces within the mediastinum. Within the seminiferous tubules two cell types can be discerned: the Sertoli cells which support and nourish the germ cells by the production of hormones and growth factors, and the seminiferous epithelium (Plate 6/*F*). The rete drains by a dozen or so efferent ductules (/6) that pierce the capsule to join the head of the epididymis.

The endocrine functions of the testis are performed by the interstitial (Leydig) cells, responsible for androgen production, and the sustentacular (Sertoli) cells, responsible for inhibin production. Both types are normally under the pulsatile but more or less tonic control of gonadotropins (luteinizing hormone [LH] and follicle-stimulating hormone [FSH], respectively) produced in the pituitary (p. 212). The sustentacular cell hormone (inhibin) seems to regulate secretion of FSH via a negative feedback mechanism either directly or indirectly via a hypothalamic site of action. Androgens clearly have distinct local function but are also responsible for secondary sex characteristics such as the maturation of the accessory sex glands, male skeletomuscular development, skin characteristics, and even the prenatal differentiation of certain brain and spinal cord nuclei. They are also partly responsible for the behavior typical of the male. They also exert a negative feedback on pituitary gonadotropin secretion; part of this feedback is effected at the level of the hypothalamus. In the fetal period, active production of androgens may take place without pituitary con-

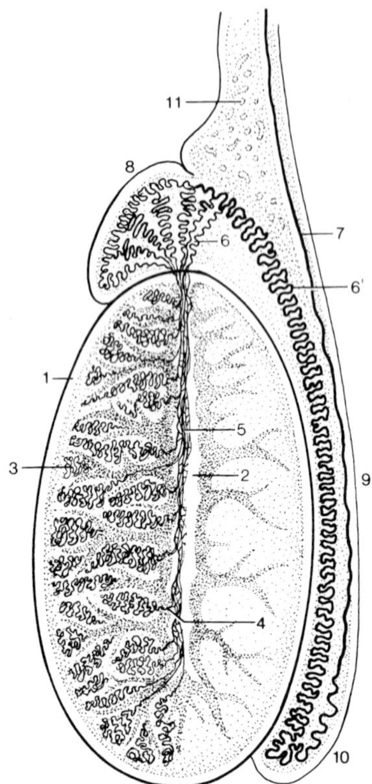


**Figure 5–33.** Longitudinal section of a testis and epididymis, schematic.

1, Tunica albuginea; 2, mediastinum; 3, seminiferous tubules; 4, straight tubules; 5, rete testis; 6, efferent ductules; 6′, epididymal duct; 7, deferent duct; 8, head of epididymis; 9, body of epididymis; 10, tail of epididymis; 11, pampiniform plexus.

*Many derivative terms are based on the alternative name, *orchis,* derived from the Greek.

trol. The interstitial cells in this period are also responsible for the production of the insulin-like factor 3 that recently was associated with gubernacular outgrowth and thus with testicular descent. In the fetal period the sustentacular cells produce the AMH that exerts an inhibitory effect on the paramesonephric ducts (p. 171) causing the disappearance of most of the female duct system.

## The Epididymis

The epididymis is a firm organ that is largely formed by the numerous convolutions of the single epididymal duct within a connective tissue matrix. It is attached along one of the longer borders—dorsal in the dog, caudomedial in the bull—of the testis and usually spreads some distance over both poles (Plate 6/*A*). It is conventionally divided into three parts—head, body, and tail—but these rather arbitrary divisions do not always correspond to functional distinctions.

The head (Fig. 5–33/8) is firmly attached to the testicular capsule. It receives the efferent ductules, which immediately or after some coiling join to form the wider *epididymal duct* (/6′). The body may be less completely attached to the surface of the testis, and in that case an intervening space (testicular bursa, homologous with the ovarian bursa) is created (Fig. 5–34/2′,3). The tail is firmly attached to the testis by a ligament (proper ligament of the testis) and also to the parietal layer of the enveloping peritoneal sac by the ligament of the tail of the epididymis (/7,8). The tail finally tapers and the duct emerges to continue as the deferent duct (/4). The epididymis appears spongy in section since the coiled duct is inevitably cut across many times.

## The Deferent Duct

The deferent duct is undulating where it emerges but gradually straightens when followed toward the abdomen (Plate 6/*E*). It first runs medial to the epididymis as it heads toward the testicular vessels that form the bulkier components of the spermatic cord. The constituents of the cord remain together as they pass through the inguinal canal but disperse at the vaginal ring (Plate 24/*C*). The duct here turns caudomedially to pass under the ureter before gaining the dorsal surface of the bladder (Fig. 5–32); it penetrates the prostate before finally entering the urethra a little way beyond the urethra's origin from the bladder. The abdominal part continues to be supported by a peritoneal fold (mesoductus), which joins its contralateral partner to produce a horizontal genital fold above the bladder. The greater part of the duct is of uniform appearance and structure; its lumen is rather narrow in relation to the thick muscular wall. In most species the subterminal stretch lying on the bladder exhibits a fusiform enlargement, the *ampulla of the deferent duct* or ampullary gland (Fig. 5–40/4). Although the term suggests a widening of the lumen, the thickening is mainly due to glandular proliferation in the wall of the duct, largely in the locally folded mucosa.

In most domestic mammals a second accessory gland grows from the duct close to its termination. This, the vesicular gland, is described in a later section, but it may be noted in the meantime that the short, shared passage is known as the *ejaculatory duct*.

## The Vaginal Tunic and Spermatic Cord

The peritoneal process (vaginal tunic) that encloses the testis is an evagination of the lining of

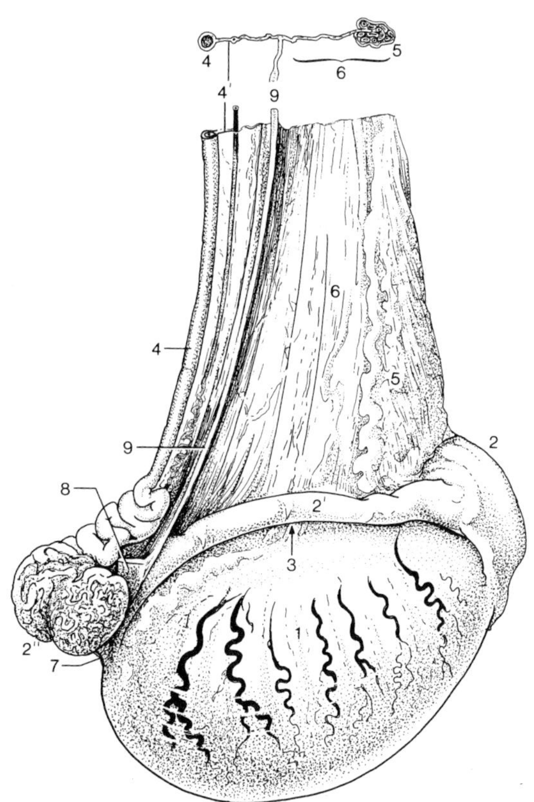


**Figure 5–34.** Lateral view of the right testis of a stallion.

1, Testis; 2, head of epididymis; 2′, body of epididymis; 2″, tail of epididymis; 3, testicular bursa; 4, deferent duct; 4′, mesoductus deferens; 5, pampiniform plexus; 6, mesorchium; 7, proper ligament of testis; 8, ligament of tail of epididymis; 9, cut edge of fold connecting visceral and parietal layers of the vaginal tunic.

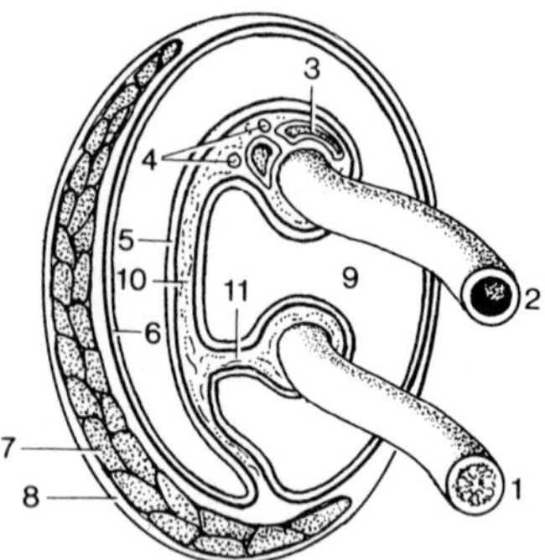


**Figure 5–35.** Transverse section of the spermatic cord and its immediate investments, schematic.

1, Deferent duct; 2, testicular artery (coiled); 3, pampiniform plexus; 4, testicular nerves and lymph vessels; 5, visceral layer of vaginal tunic; 6, parietal layer of vaginal tunic; 7, cremaster muscle; 8, external spermatic fascia; 9, vaginal cavity; 10, mesorchium; 11, mesoductus.

the abdomen through the inguinal canal. The narrow proximal part that surrounds the spermatic cord widens distally to form within the scrotum a flasklike expansion that encloses the testis and epididymis. The parietal and visceral layers of the tunic are connected by a fold that extends from the vaginal ring to the tail of the epididymis (Fig. 5–34/9).* The cavity between the parietal and visceral layers (Fig. 5–35/9) normally contains only a minute amount of serous fluid. It communicates with the peritoneal cavity of the abdomen through the vaginal ring, a narrow slitlike opening placed within the internal opening of the inguinal canal. Sometimes a loop of small intestine or another abdominal organ herniates into the peritoneal process through the vaginal ring; this complication is often encountered at castration. It is worth mentioning that in human infants the neck of the peritoneal process usually becomes obliterated shortly after birth, isolating the cavity about the testis.

The spermatic cord varies in length and shape according to the position and orientation of the testis. It is shortest and most compact in those species in which the testis hangs vertically in the inguinal region. The bulk of the cord is provided by the *testicular artery* and veins, both remarkably modified. The artery branches from the abdominal aorta and first pursues a fairly direct course toward the vaginal ring where the constituents of the spermatic cord are assembled. The more distal part is extraordinarily convoluted—one account describes no less than 7 m of artery packed within a 10-cm stretch of cord (Fig. 5–36 and Plate 6/*C*). These particular figures perhaps exaggerate the usual arrangement but serve to emphasize its extravagance. The testicular veins constitute a very elaborate close-meshed *pampiniform plexus* in which the contortions of the artery are embedded (Fig. 5–37); the plexus ultimately reduces to a single vein that runs to the caudal vena cava. Arteriovenous anastomoses are present between

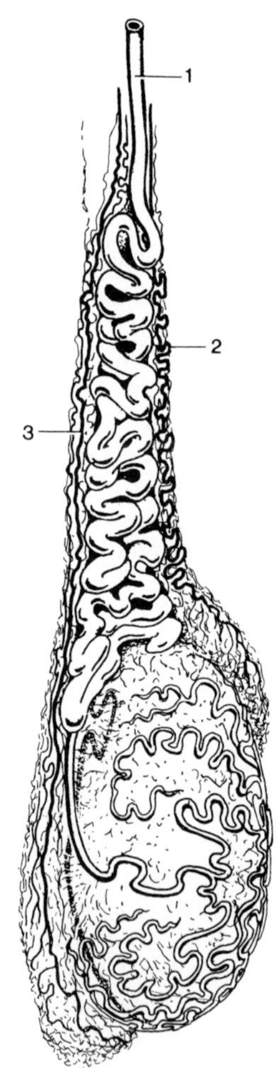


**Figure 5–36.** The arterial blood supply to the bovine testis and epididymis. Observe the course of arterial branches on the testicular surface.

1, Testicular artery (becoming very tortuous as it approaches the testis); 2, cranial epididymal branch; 3, caudal epididymal branch.

*The mesorchium is the visceral tunic between the fold (Fig. 5–34/9) and the epididymal border of the testis but also includes the long peritoneal fold (/6) that conveys the testicular vessels and nerves from their origin at the abdominal roof to the testis; it thus forms a considerable portion of the spermatic cord. The narrow fold that attaches the deferent duct to the pelvic and abdominal walls and (more distally) to the mesorchium is the mesoductus deferens (/4′).

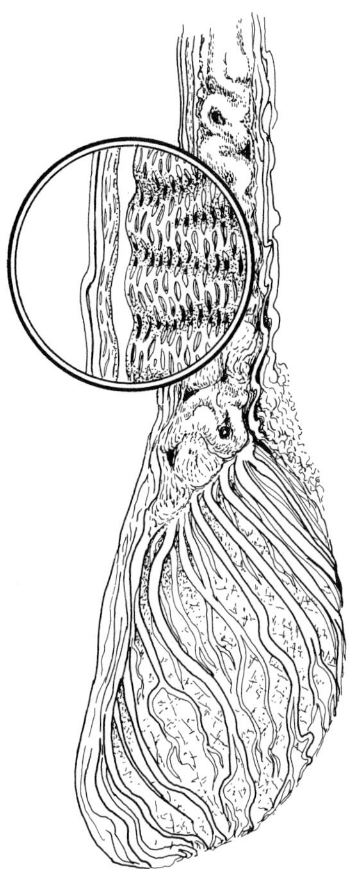

**Figure 5–37.** Testicular veins on the surface of the bovine testis, and the pampiniform plexus *(magnified in inset)*.

the coiled testicular artery and its epididymal branches and the veins of the pampiniform plexus. A generous lymphatic drainage passes to lymph nodes placed about the bifurcation of the aorta. In some species a small lymph node is present near the inguinal canal. The lymph conveys a substantial fraction of the hormone production of the testis. The inconspicuous testicular nerves are of sympathetic origin.

## The Scrotum

Variations in the location and form of the scrotum have been noted (Fig. 5–32). Externally, a median groove marks the division into right and left compartments; it often betrays a striking asymmetry of the testes. The lower part of the scrotum is molded on the testes and adjusts as their position varies with the ambient temperature (see p. 188).

The relatively thin scrotal skin is well provided with both sweat and sebaceous glands. It is sometimes rather bare, but this is not a constant feature—indeed, the scrotum is hidden by hair in the cat and densely covered by fleece in sheep of certain breeds. When bare, it is often pigmented. The scrotal skin adheres to a tough fibromuscular layer *(tunica dartos),* which also extends as a septum between the compartments that separately lodge the testes. Internal to the dartos, a (spermatic) fascia is present that may be resolved into several layers, which are believed to correspond to the layers of the abdominal wall. The predominant layer is the *external spermatic fascia,* which can be clearly separated from the dartos (Fig. 5–38). The loose intermediate stratum allows the vaginal tunic independent movement within the scrotal sac; in addition to its functional significance (see further on), this facilitates castration by the closed method (in which the testis is brought to the exterior within the vaginal tunic before the cord is severed proximally). The dense external spermatic fascia that supports the vaginal tunic also invests the *cremaster,* a slip of muscle that passes onto the cord on detachment from the caudal margin of the internal oblique muscle of the abdomen.

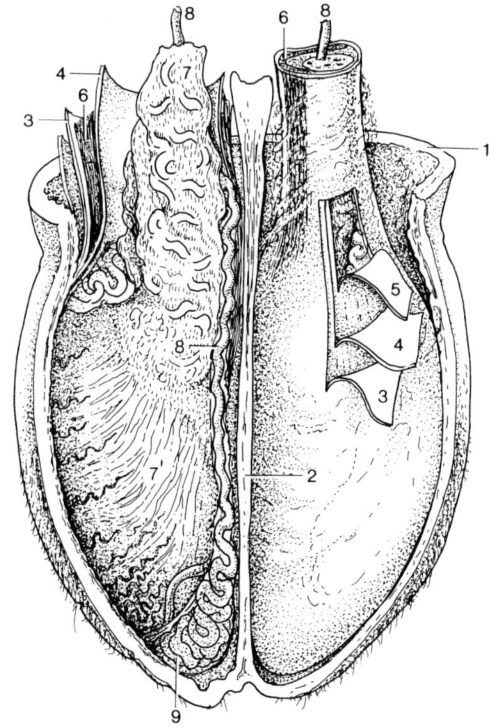


**Figure 5–38.** Cranial view of the opened scrotum of a bull; the investments of the testis have been partly dissected.

1, Scrotal skin and dartos; 2, scrotal septum; 3, external spermatic fascia; 4, parietal layer of vaginal tunic; 5, visceral layer (dissected from surface of testis); 6, cremaster muscle; 7, visceral layer of vaginal tunic covering structures in spermatic cord; 7′, visceral layer on testis; 8, deferent duct; 9, tail of epididymis.

### *Testicular Function*

In most wild mammals the breeding period is seasonal, and this is reflected by changes in the morphology and activity of the reproductive organs of both sexes. Little of this seasonality remains among male domestic animals, in which the seminiferous epithelium is active throughout the year with, at most, only slight variation in sperm output. Although the process of spermatogenesis is not described, the reader is reminded that the serial cell divisions and maturation processes that constitute the cycle are not synchronous in every part of the seminiferous epithelium. Instead, adjacent segments show successive stages so that a "lucky" longitudinal section of a tubule displays the different stages of the process occurring as a wave spreading along its length (Plate 6/*F*).

The process of spermatogenesis is influenced by temperature and, as already stated, it cannot proceed normally at the core temperature of the body. The seminiferous epithelium is damaged in testes that fail to descend into the scrotum (the "cryptorchid condition"), and these do not produce sperm. Similar changes are evident in testes that, having descended successfully, are later returned to the abdomen—and indeed, in scrotal testes that are overheated by an unusually thick covering of hair or fleece. Since the interstitial tissue is less susceptible to temperature, it follows that libido and potency may be normal in cryptorchid animals that are infertile.

Many factors help maintain the appropriate endotesticular temperature. The exposed position of the scrotum, the absence of fat within the scrotal fascia, and the intracapsular situation of large testicular vessels all favor heat loss by radiation; the generous supply of sweat glands allows additional loss through evaporation from the skin surface. Perhaps more importantly, the extensive contact between the vessels within the cord precools the blood within the artery as this follows its winding course in relation to the venous plexus (Plate 6/*C,E*). The opportunities for heat loss are such that the testicular temperature could be lowered excessively in colder climates. Countermeasures are available. Contraction of the tunica dartos, directly sensitive to temperature change, tightens and bunches the scrotum, thereby reducing the exposed surface and also drawing the testes toward the warmer trunk. The testes may also be separately raised within the scrotum by contraction of the cremaster muscles which pull on the vaginal tunics; being striated, these muscles react briskly to pull the testes away from potentially harmful stimuli.

Castration of surplus male animals has long been practiced to make them more manageable or to promote particular carcass qualities. Modern husbandry, the effects of selective breeding, and changes in consumer requirements now make it possible to bring food animals to slaughter at earlier ages than before, and the necessity for, and economic advantage of, routine castration are beginning to be questioned. The direct influence of castration on the reproductive organs is considered in some detail for cattle, the species about which most is known, on page 720.

## The Pelvic Reproductive Organs

### *The Male Urethra*

The male urethra extends from an internal orifice at the bladder neck to an external orifice at the free extremity of the penis. It is thus divisible into an internal or pelvic part and an external or spongy part, the last adjective referring to the very vascular tissue that surrounds the urethra on its leaving the pelvic cavity. The spongy part is largely incorporated within the penis and is appropriately considered as a component of that organ. The pelvic part is joined by the deferent and vesicular (or combined ejaculatory) duct(s) a short distance from its origin from the bladder; by far the greater part of the urethra thus serves to discharge both urine and semen.

Although the pelvic urethra shows regional and specific variations, it consists essentially of a mucosal tube successively invested by a vascular submucosa and a muscular tunic. The mucous membrane is thrown into longitudinal folds in the inactive state. The initial part also carries a dorsal crest that continues from the urethral orifice to end in a thickening *(colliculus seminalis)*. The colliculus displays on its sides the slitlike orifices of the deferent ducts and the much smaller openings through which the many prostatic ducts discharge (Fig. 5–39/7). Similar but more distal openings mark the entry of the ducts of other accessory glands (/8). The submucosa contains a rather inconspicuous system of connecting blood spaces that is continuous with the vastly more generous spongy investment of the second part of the urethra. The major component of the muscle coat is the striated *urethralis* that encircles the tube.

The urethra is embedded in fat and other connective tissues where it lies on the pelvic floor. The dorsal surface is related to the rectum and, with species differences, to various accessory reproductive glands; usually only a narrow median strip that faces directly into the rectogenital pouch

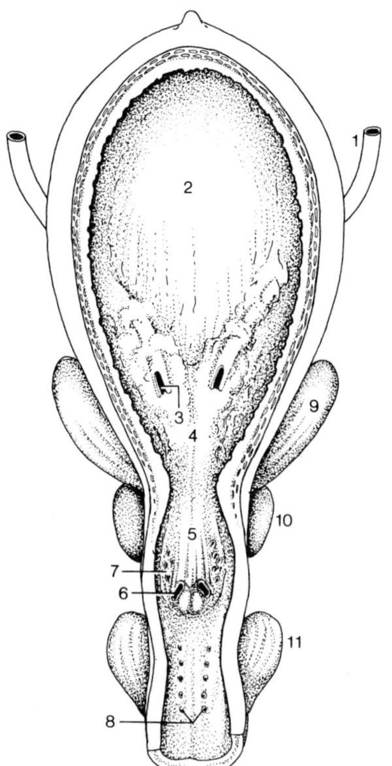


**Figure 5–39.** Ventral view of the opened bladder and urethra of a stallion.

1, Ureter; 2, bladder; 3, ureteric orifice; 4, trigone of bladder; 5, urethral crest and seminal colliculus; 6, opening of ejaculatory duct; 7, multiple openings of prostatic ducts; 8, multiple openings of bulbourethral ducts; 9, vesicular gland; 10, prostate; 11, bulbourethral gland.

is covered by peritoneum. The urethra is easily palpated per rectum, a procedure that may stimulate rhythmic activity of its muscle.

## The Accessory Reproductive Glands

The full set comprises ampullary, vesicular, prostate, and bulbourethral glands, although not all of these are present in every species (Fig. 5–40). The *ampullary glands* have been sufficiently described (p. 185).

Paired *vesicular glands* (/5) are present in all domestic species except the dog and cat. Each buds from the distal part of the deferent duct in the embryo and this relationship commonly persists; in the pig the later absorption of the ejaculatory duct into the urethra causes the vesicular gland to open separately. These glands vary greatly in appearance; in the horse they are large, externally smooth, and bladder-like, resembling the human organs that were formerly known as seminal "vesicles." This term is inappropriate since in most species the glands are knobby and thick-walled with rather narrow branched lumina. The vesicular glands lie wholly or partly within the genital fold, each lateral to the corresponding deferent duct.

A *prostate* (/6) is present in all domestic species. In some it consists of two parts, one diffusely spread within the wall of the pelvic urethra, the other a compact body placed external to the urethralis. Both parts drain by many small ducts. The small ruminants have only the diffuse or disseminate part, the horse only the compact part. The disseminate part is vestigial in the dog and cat, but the compact part is very large and globular and

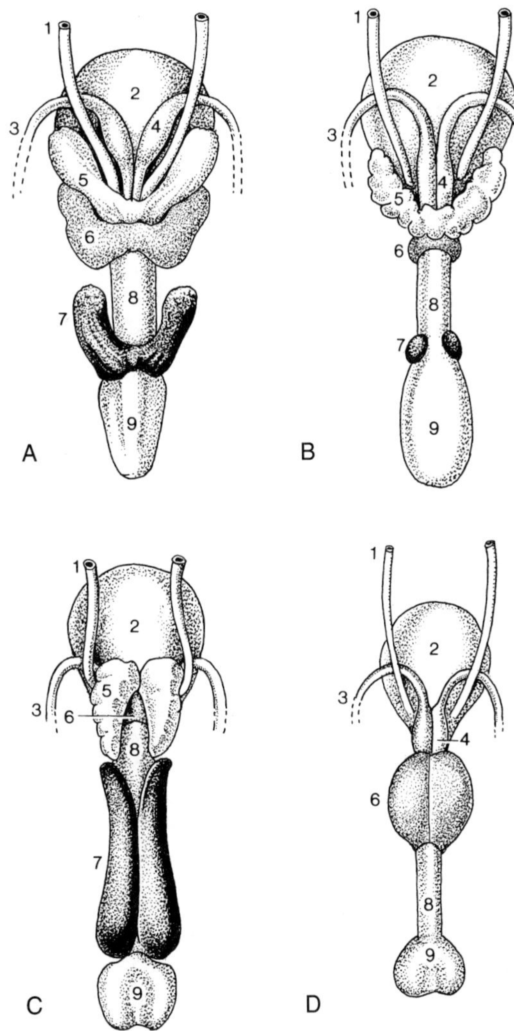


**Figure 5–40.** Accessory reproductive glands of the stallion *(A)*, bull *(B)*, boar *(C)*, and dog *(D)*; dorsal view.

1, Ureter; 2, bladder; 3, deferent duct; 4, ampullary gland; 5, vesicular gland; 6, body of prostate; 7, bulbourethral gland; 8, urethra, 9, bulb of penis.

so well developed that it surrounds the urethra entirely (dog) or almost so (cat).

Paired *bulbourethral glands* (/7; Plate 29/*F*), compound tubular glands with a secretory epithelium, lie on the dorsal aspect of the urethra close to the pelvic exit. They are found in all species other than the dog (although they are vestigial in the cat). They are of moderate size in horses and ruminants but are very substantial in the pig, in which they appear as rather irregular elongated cylinders placed to each side of the urethra. They may drain by one or by several ducts.

All the larger glands possess well-developed capsules and internal septa in which much smooth muscle is present that expels the secretion at the appropriate time.

## The Penis and Prepuce

The penis is suspended below the trunk and is partly contained between the thighs, where it is anchored to the floor of the pelvis by a suspensory ligament in the large species (see Fig. 22–20/21). In the quiescent state, the free extremity is concealed within an invagination of the abdominal skin, the prepuce, which opens at a variable site behind the umbilicus. The organ is mainly constructed of three columns of erectile tissue (Fig. 5–41). These are independent caudally where they constitute the root of the penis, but their major parts are combined in the body of the penis.

The paired dorsal columns are known as the *crura of the penis* (/1) at their widely separated origins from the ischial arch. They converge, bend forward, and run below the pelvic floor before joining. Each consists of a core of cavernous tissue enclosed within a thick connective tissue casing (tunica albuginea), the complex being known as a *corpus cavernosum* (/4). A septum exists between the two corpora cavernosa in the proximal part of the body, but in most species this will be found to weaken and ultimately disappear when traced distally toward the apex of the penis. In carnivores the septum is complete. The combined structure is grooved ventrally to accommodate the third component, the urethra within its enveloping vascular sleeve, the *corpus spongiosum* (/3). The blood spaces within the crura and corpus cavernosum communicate freely.

The corpus cavernosum does not extend to the apex of the penis, which is formed by an expansion of the corpus spongiosum. The corpus spongiosum commences at the pelvic outlet with the sudden enlargement of the meager spongy tissue of the pelvic urethra. The expansion constitutes the *bulb of the penis* (/2), a bilobed structure that tapers to continue as a more uniform sleeve. The corpus spongiosum is more delicate than the corpus cavernosum, having larger blood spaces separated by thinner septa. Its cranial expansion over the distal end of the corpus cavernosum, usually known as the *glans* (/9), forms the apex of the whole organ. Since the corpus spongiosum surrounds the urethra, the urethral orifice is brought to the very extremity of the penis; indeed, in small ruminants a free urethral process prolongs the urethra well beyond this.

Other pronounced species differences in penis structure exist. In the dog and cat the distal part of the corpus cavernosum is transformed into bone, the *os penis*. The glans has very different forms. It is minimally developed in the pig, insubstantial in the ruminants, but large and mushroom-shaped in the horse. It is most specialized in the dog, in which it presents bulbar proximal and long cylindrical distal parts. The penis of the cat is unique (among domestic species) in pointing caudoventrally from the ischial arch; this retention of the embryonic posture affects the manner of copulation.

The construction of the corpus cavernosum also exhibits major differences. In some species it contains small blood spaces enclosed within and divided by substantial amounts of tough fibroelastic tissue. Relatively little additional blood need be retained to make this *fibroelastic type* of penis become erect (Fig. 5–42/*A*); this construction is found in the penis of the boar and ruminant species in which the quiescent organ exhibits a sigmoid flexure of that part of its body carried between the

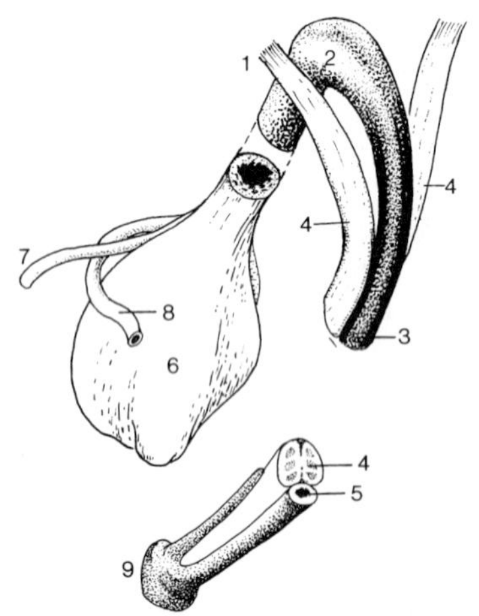


**Figure 5–41.** Schematic drawing of the components that constitute the equine penis at its root, and at its apex.

1, Crus penis; 2, bulb; 3, corpus spongiosum; 4, corpus cavernosum; 5, urethra; 6, bladder; 7, ureter; 8, deferent duct; 9, glans.

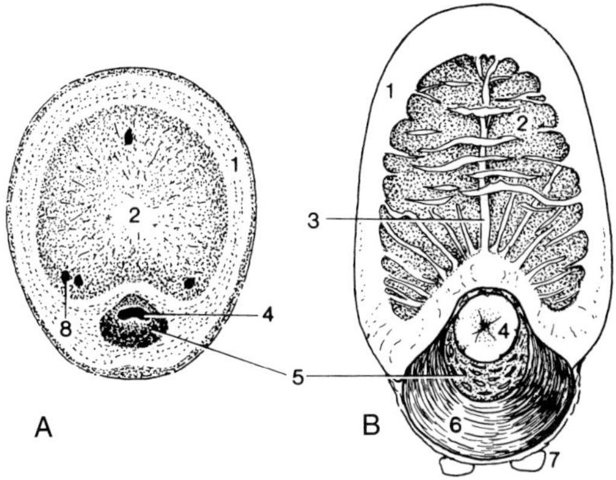


**Figure 5–42.** Transverse sections of the fibroelastic penis of a bull (*A*) and the musculocavernous penis of a stallion (*B*).

1, Tunica albuginea; 2, corpus cavernosum; 3, septum; 4, urethra; 5, corpus spongiosum; 6, bulbospongiosus; 7, retractor penis; 8, large thick-walled veins.

thighs. In the other type, the blood spaces are relatively larger, and the enclosure and intervening septa more delicate and more muscular (/*B*); a relatively much greater quantity of blood is required to achieve erection, which involves significant increases in both length and girth. This *musculocavernous type* of penis is found in the stallion and, in atypical form, in the dog.

The prepuce or sheath is a tubular fold consisting of an external layer (lamina externa), continuous with the general integument, and an internal layer (lamina interna) that faces the free end of the penis; the internal layer continues as the covering of the free part of the penis after reflection in the depth of the preputial cavity. Both the internal layer and the penile covering are hairless but often well provided with smegma-secreting glands and lymphoid tissue. In the newborn male the penis and sheath are fused, and separation is gradually achieved during the period before puberty (p. 720). The attachments of the adult prepuce are sufficiently loose to allow the internal lamina to be reflected onto the erect penis when this is protruded through the preputial orifice.

Certain muscles are associated with the penis. The *bulbospongiosus* is the thick extrapelvic continuation of the urethralis. It begins abruptly and extends distally to end on the surface of the corpus spongiosum at a variable distance beyond the point at which this is incorporated within the penis.

The powerful paired *ischiocavernosi* arise from the ischial arch, almost enclose the crura, and follow them to their fusion.

The *retractor penis* is also paired. It arises from the caudal vertebrae and descends through the perineum, bending laterally to pass around the anal canal, to reach the penis. Unlike the other muscles associated with the penis, the retractor is mainly composed of smooth muscle fibers.

Narrow slips of striated muscle (*cranial* and *caudal preputial*) may pass onto the prepuce and attach near its opening. The caudal muscles are less frequently encountered and retract the prepuce, so uncovering the extremity of the penis. The cranial muscles protract the prepuce. Both caudal and cranial muscles must be regarded as detachments of the cutaneous trunci; they are best developed in the bull but lacking in the stallion.

The penis obtains its exclusive (in the horse, principal) *blood supply* from the artery of the penis, a terminal branch of the internal pudendal. The artery of the penis has a very short course and at the ischial arch it quickly divides to form an artery of the bulb, which enters the bulb of the penis and supplies the corpus spongiosum; a deep artery, which pierces the tunica albuginea to supply the corpus cavernosum; and the dorsal artery, which passes apically on the dorsal border of the organ to supply the free end. The dorsal artery may be reinforced by anastomosis with the obturator artery (horse) and generally by anastomosis with the external pudendal artery for the supply of the prepuce. The veins are broadly satellite. Interspecific details are considered in the later chapters when they are significant.

The nerves to the penis accompany the vessels. The motor fibers are predominantly parasympathetic, from the pelvic nerves.

## Sperm Transport in the Male Tract; Erection of the Penis

The sperm are immotile when released into the lumen of the seminiferous tubules, where they float in fluid secreted by the sustentacular (Sertoli) cells of the epithelial lining. Their passage through the rete testis into the head of the epididymis is effected by the current generated by the combination of the testicular secretory pressure and the resorption of fluid by the lining of the efferent ductules. Onward progress through the epididymis appears to depend on several factors, among which spontaneous peristalsis of the muscular epididymal duct is probably most important. Hydrostatic pressure may continue to play a part, and in many species the sperm have themselves acquired the capacity for coordinated movement by the time they reach the tail of the epididymis. Many aspects of the process remain obscure, and it is not clear whether the physiological maturation of the sperm—which require to spend some days in their passage through the epididymis—is merely the result of aging or whether it is due to specific features of the milieu. Fertilization with epididymal sperm has been achieved under experimental conditions, most readily when utilizing sperm removed from the tail. Secretory activity of the lining of the epididymal duct is maintained by androgens, and it is possible that these also have a direct influence on sperm. The deferent duct also exhibits peristalsis, which gradually moves the sperm toward the ampullary region. In sexually inactive animals, sperm are lost from here by seepage into the urethra whence they are flushed away by urine. A few may be resorbed by the lining of the duct system.

This regular but slow emission of sperm contrasts with the vigorous ejaculation that occurs during coitus. Erection of the penis is a necessary preliminary to this and is brought about by the engorgement of the cavernous and spongy spaces. This engorgement both stiffens and enlarges the penis, causing its free extremity to protrude from the prepuce, so making possible intromission, the introduction of the penis into the vagina. The details of the process, which differs significantly among species, are largely dependent on the structure of the penis. In species in which the penis is "fibroelastic," little additional blood need be retained in order to distend the cavernous spaces fully; the penis therefore does not increase greatly in size and its protrusion is largely due to effacement of the preexisting sigmoid flexure. Moreover, because relatively little additional blood is required, full erection may be achieved rapidly. The cavernous spaces are much larger and more dilatable in the "musculocavernous" penis possessed by horses and dogs. In these species a much greater increase in both length and girth occurs. The process requires more time for its completion.

Two distinct phases of erection are recognized. In the first stages of sexual excitement, blood flow into the penis increases as the walls of the supplying arteries relax; at the same time the venous outflow is obstructed. The pressure within the cavernous spaces rises rapidly and soon equals that within the arteries that deliver blood to the corpus cavernosum via the crura and to the corpus spongiosum via the bulb.

The venous outflow is restricted at the proximal extremity of the organ where the veins are compressed against the ischial arch; this has more effect on the drainage of the crura and corpus cavernosum than on that of the corpus spongiosum whose more distal outlet is as yet unaffected (see Fig. 15–17).

The process continues and intensifies after intromission. Rhythmic contractions of the ischiocavernosus and bulbospongiosus muscles now begin, impelling blood forward through the corpus cavernosum and corpus spongiosum. The internal pressures fluctuate in time with this activity. The additional blood pumped distally within the corpus cavernosum cannot escape since the emissary veins are compressed; the pressure therefore rises further. In contrast, the contractions of the bulbospongiosus produce only intermittent rises in pressure since some blood continues to escape at the free extremity of the penis; the effect of this flow is to massage the urethra, supplying a further impulse to the forward movement of semen when ejaculation takes place.

In most species the pressures drop rapidly after ejaculation, first reaching that within the arteries and then dropping to the resting pressure (a mere 15 to 20 mm Hg). As the blood escapes the penis shrinks, becomes more flaccid, and is returned to the prepuce. The return is brought about by the active involvement of the retractor penis muscles.

The volume and composition of the ejaculate vary with species and also with recent sexual activity. Only a small part of the semen is provided by the sperm-rich fraction emanating from the testes and epididymides, most coming from the accessory reproductive glands. Since semen volume is dependent on the bulk of these glands it could be anticipated that the ejaculate would be greatest in the boar. The various contributions to the semen are very imperfectly mixed when expelled into the urethra, but information on the sequence of discharge and on the specific proportions and function of the different glandular secretions must be sought elsewhere. The semen is moved through the urethra by the activity of striated muscles (urethralis, bulbospongiosus), and its ejaculation into the vagina or cervix (according to species) is therefore forceful.

## THE FEMALE REPRODUCTIVE ORGANS

The female reproductive organs include paired female gonads, or ovaries, which produce both female gametes (ova) and hormones; paired uterine tubes, which capture the ova on their release from the ovaries and convey them to the uterus; the uterus, in which the fertilized ova are retained and nourished until prenatal development is complete; the vagina, which serves both as copulatory organ and as birth canal; and the vestibule, which continues the vagina to open externally at the vulva but which also doubles as a urinary passage (Fig. 5–2).

Age and functional changes are particularly obtrusive where these organs are concerned. Age changes include the rapid growth and maturation associated with puberty and also the regression that occurs as the capacity for reproduction wanes with increasing age. Functional changes include those that are relatively transient and recur with each reproductive cycle as well as others, more lasting, that are associated with pregnancy and giving birth. To avoid unnecessary complications, the initial account concentrates on the description of the organs of the mature nonpregnant animal; growth and functional changes are left for later comment. Even so, it may be helpful to introduce a few general terms at this point.

Female mammals generally accept the male only close to the time of ovulation, a period characterized by various structural changes and by general excitability as well as specific behavioral features; the period is known as "heat" or "season" in lay language and as "estrus" more technically. Estrus recurs with varying frequency according to a program that is characteristic for each species although subject to environmental modification. In certain wild mammals the breeding season is confined to a certain part of the year, and sexual receptivity, with the concomitant structural and behavioral changes, occurs only once (monestrous species) or perhaps several times (seasonally polyestrous species) within this period. In other (truly polyestrous) species the cycle is repeated throughout the year; the adoption of the polyestrous mode often distinguishes domestic and laboratory species from their wild progenitors. The condition in which female receptivity is continuous and not linked to ovulation occurs only in women and some higher primate species (e.g., bonobo, the pygmy chimpanzee); in most of the latter it appears to be more common among, if not confined to, menagerie specimens.

The estrous cycle is divided into several phases. Estrus, the climax, is prefaced by proestrus, a period of follicular development; it is followed by a period of luteal activity divided between metestrus and diestrus. In monestrous species a lengthy period (anestrus) of sexual inactivity occurs before the cycle is renewed with a preparatory period of proestrus. In polyestrous species, proestrus follows directly on diestrus.

Proestrus and estrus together represent the follicular phase, when the reproductive condition is predominantly determined by the rising levels of estrogen produced in the batch of ovarian follicles then rapidly developing to maturity and rupture. Metestrus and diestrus represent the luteal phase, when the dominant hormonal influence is exerted by progesterone, the hormone produced by the corpora lutea, the transient endocrine glands that replace the ruptured follicles.

Other helpful terms tell whether a female animal has or has not borne young. Animals that have are said to be parous; those that have not are nulliparous; uniparous and multiparous extend this terminology in obvious fashion. These terms are sometimes confused with others that refer to the number of young habitually carried by the gravid female. A mare with its (generally) single foal is monotocous; a sow with its litter of piglets is polytocous.*

## The Ovaries

The ovaries possess both gametogenic and endocrine functions. Each ovary is a solid, basically ellipsoidal body, though commonly made irregular by the projection from the surface of large follicles and corpora lutea (Plate 7/*B–G*). The irregularity is naturally greatest in polytocous species, in which follicles ripen in batches. The ovaries, though much smaller than the testes of conspecific males, like these bear no constant proportion to body size. Those of the mare are relatively large and also peculiar in being kidney-shaped (Fig. 5–43/4). Ovaries are usually found in the dorsal part of the abdomen, close to the tips of the horns of the uterus since they do not shift far from their place of development. This migration, generally modest, occurs in the absence of any apparent endocrine influence: it is most considerable in ruminants in which the ovaries come to lie close by the pelvic inlet. Each ovary is suspended within the cranial part (mesovarium) of the broad ligament, the common suspension of the female reproductive tract.

A section through the ovary of a mature animal shows it to consist of a central looser and more vascular part contained within a denser shell. The *parenchymatous zone* (cortex) is bounded by a tunica albuginea directly below the peritoneum and is strewn with follicles in various stages of development and regression. Each *follicle* contains a single ovum; the stages through which it passes are shown in schematic fashion in Figure 5–44. The rapid enlargement undergone by those follicles selected to come to maturity in the current cycle is mainly due to the accumulation of the fluid by which the ova are swept out on ovulation. The cavity within the ruptured follicle, though it may initially fill with blood, is soon occupied by hypertrophy of the granulosa and theca cells that

*Unfortunately, there is some conflict in the use of these terms, many authors reserving uniparous and multiparous for the senses in which we employ monotocous and polytocous.

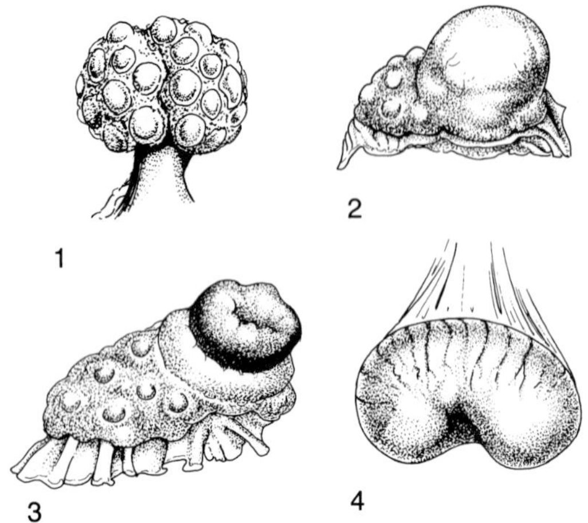


**Figure 5–43.** Specific and functional variations in ovarian morphology.

1, Ovary of a polytocous animal (sow); 2, ovary of a monotocous animal (cow) with ripening follicle; 3, ovary of a monotocous animal (cow) with a fully developed corpus luteum; 4, kidney-shaped ovary of mare.

originally lined the space (Plate 7/*H*). This produces a solid body, known as the corpus luteum (yellow body) on account of its color. *Corpora lutea* are transient structures that wax and wane between one estrous period and the next (assuming pregnancy does not ensue) (Fig. 5–43/3). Degeneration of the corpora lutea is characterized by vacuolization of the cytoplasm of the luteal cells, due to lipid accumulation and nuclear shrinkage (Plate 7/*J*). Though transient, they are important as the source of progesterone, just as the ripening follicles are the source of estrogen. Corpora lutea finally regress and are replaced by connective tissue scars, corpora albicantes (white bodies). The alternation in the levels of estrogen and progesterone determines the changes in the behavior pattern and in the morphology and activity of the reproductive tract.

## The Uterine Tubes

The uterine tubes* are narrow and generally very flexuous. They capture the ova released from the ovaries and convey them toward the uterus; since they also convey the sperm in their ascent, fertilization normally occurs within the tubes.

The free cranial extremity takes the form of a thin-walled funnel (*infundibulum;* Fig. 5–45/2) placed close to the cranial pole of the ovary. The free edge of the funnel is ragged, and the tags (fimbriae) come into contact with and sometimes adhere to the surface of the ovary. A small (abdominal) orifice in the depth of the funnel leads to the longer tubular part that is divided into two more or less equal segments. The proximal one, known as the *ampulla,* is followed by the more convoluted and narrower *isthmus,* but it must be admitted that the distinction between these segments is not equally obvious in all species or at all phases of the cycle (/3,4). The isthmus joins the apex of the horn of the uterus at the uterotubal (salpingouterine) junction, a region of very variable appearance. The junction is gradual in ruminants and pigs, abrupt in horses and carnivores; indeed, in the mare, and to a lesser extent also in the bitch and cat, the terminal part of the tube is thrust into the apex of the horn to raise a small papilla perforated by the (uterine) orifice of

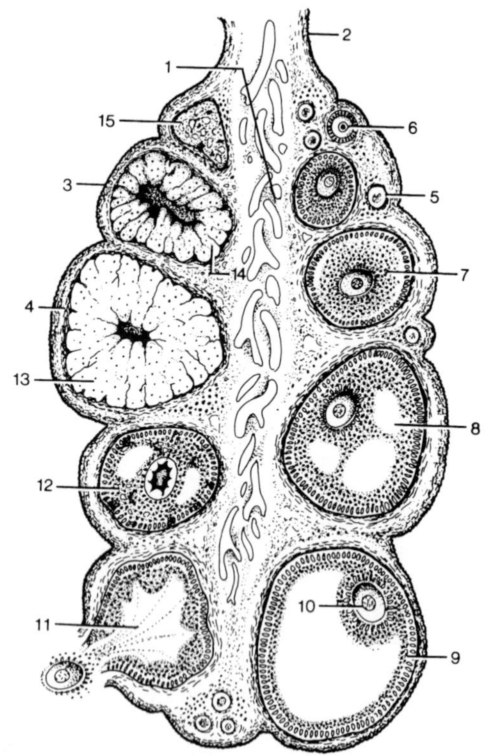


**Figure 5–44.** Schematic representation of the different functional stages in ovarian activity.

1, Medulla; 2, mesovarium; 3, surface epithelium; 4, tunica albuginea (poorly developed); 5, primordial follicle; 6, primary follicle; 7, secondary follicle; 8, early tertiary follicle; 9, mature follicle; 10, oocyte; 11, ruptured follicle; 12, atretic follicle; 13, corpus luteum; 14, atretic corpus luteum; 15, corpus albicans.

*The obsolete terms *fallopian tubes* and *oviducts* are still encountered, perhaps most commonly in medical writing. Another term, *salpinx,* receives official recognition; though less frequently encountered, it is the stem of such derivatives as mesosalpinx and salpingitis (inflammation of the uterine tube).

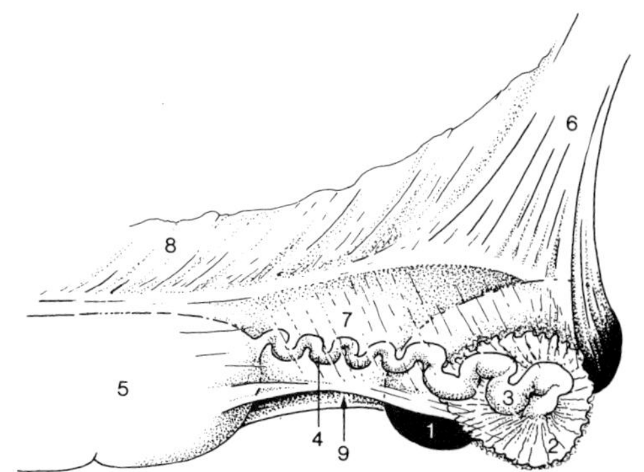


**Figure 5–45.** Lateral view of the suspension of the right ovary, uterine tube, and uterine horn of a mare.

1, Ovary; 2, infundibulum of tube; 3, ampulla of tube; 4, isthmus of tube; 5, uterine horn; 6, mesovarium; 7, mesosalpinx; 8, mesometrium; 9, arrow indicates entrance to ovarian bursa.

the tube. Too much should not be made of these differences since, regardless of its appearance, the junction always represents a real barrier, impeding both the ascent of sperm and the descent of ova. The tube wall consists of external serosal, middle muscular, and internal mucosal tunics. The mucosa is folded longitudinally along its whole length from infundibulum to isthmus; secondary and even tertiary folds reduce the lumen of the ampulla to a series of narrow branching clefts. The tube is carried in a side-fold (mesosalpinx) of the part of the broad ligament that supports the ovary.

## The Uterus

The uterus,* the womb in popular speech, is the enlarged part of the tract in which embryos come to rest, where they establish a means of physiological exchange with the mother's blood stream, and where they are protected and nourished until ready to be delivered to the outside world. It is the part of the tract that displays the most striking specific differences (although the most extreme forms do not occur among domestic species). These differences find a ready explanation in the manner of formation of the reproductive tract (p. 172) from two paramesonephric ducts that grow caudally to meet and fuse with each other and with the median urogenital sinus, the ventral division of the cloaca (Figs. 5–14 and 5–15). In some species, including many rodents, fusion of the ducts is limited to the most caudal portions, which contribute to the vagina; the more cranial parts remain distinct, and the uterus thus consists of paired tubes that open separately into the vagina (double uterus—uterus duplex). In contrast, in women and most other primates, fusion is much more extensive and only the uterine tubes remain paired; a median uterus with a simple undivided lumen is present. In the intermediate variety (bicornuate uterus) found in all major domestic species the uterus comprises a caudal median part from which paired horns diverge cranially to continue as the uterine tubes.

In all domestic mammals the median part of the uterus has two segments. The caudal, very thick-walled segment, the *cervix* (Fig. 5–46/8), provides

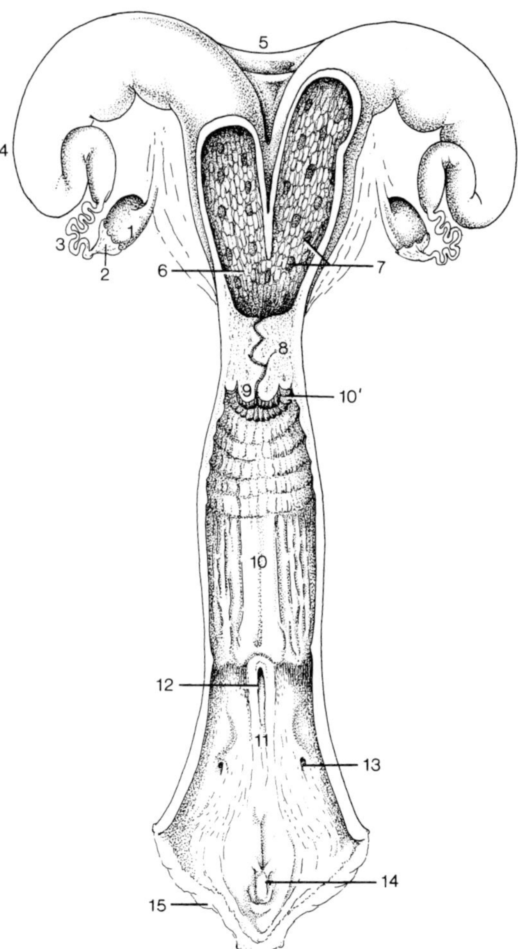


**Figure 5–46.** The reproductive tract of a cow, opened dorsally.

1, Ovary; 2, infundibulum; 3, uterine tube; 4, horn of uterus; 5, intercornual ligaments; 6, body of uterus; 7, caruncles; 8, cervix; 9, vaginal part of cervix; 10, vagina; 10′, fornix; 11, vestibule; 12, external urethral opening; 13, opening of major vestibular gland; 14, clitoris; 15, vulva.

*Compound terms are generally derived from the alternative name, metrium—for example, mesometrium and metritis; surgical removal of the uterus, however, is termed hysterectomy (Greek, *hystera,* uterus).

a sphincter controlling access to and from the vagina. A part of the cervix (/9) (portio vaginalis) usually projects into the vaginal lumen with which it communicates at the external ostium. The lumen of the cervix (cervical canal) is constricted and often almost occluded by mucosal folds; it opens into the *body of the uterus* (/6) at the internal ostium. The body is generally a rather small segment in domestic species, although the proportions vary (Fig. 5–15); it is largest in the mare. The division of the interior is not always obvious externally since an internal septum may partially divide an apparently single space. Although visual inspection generally fails to reveal the extent of the cervix, this is easily discovered on palpation since it is much firmer than the adjacent parts.

The *horns* (cornua) vary greatly in length, and it is hardly surprising that they are longest in polytocous species. Their disposition also varies; they are characteristically wound in ruminants, straight and divergent in mares and bitches, and cast into intestine-like loops in sows. The cervix generally lies within the pelvic cavity, interposed between the rectum and the bladder (Fig. 5–28/7), but the body and horns of the uterus typically lie within the abdomen above the mass of intestines.

The uterus possesses serosal, muscular, and mucosal coats that are known as the *perimetrium, myometrium,* and *endometrium,* respectively. The serosal covering reaches the uterus by extension from the supporting broad ligament (mesometrium; Fig. 5–29/7). The muscle is arranged as weak external longitudinal and thicker internal circular layers that are separated by a very vascular stratum of connective tissue. The tissues, especially the external muscle layer, extend (as parametrium) into the supporting broad ligaments. Dense connective tissue intermingles with the muscle of the cervix and makes this a very indistensible part of the tract at most times.

The endometrium is thick. Its surface relief varies among species and is most remarkable in ruminants, in which numerous permanent elevations (caruncles) mark the sites where the embryonic membranes firmly attach during pregnancy (Fig. 5–46/7). Numerous tubular glands open on the surface, which is generally lined by a simple columnar epithelium. The mucosa within the cervix is prominently modeled by both longitudinal and circular folds whose interdigitation helps close the passage (/8). Mucus secreted by cervical glands plugs the canal at most times and so helps seal the uterus from the vagina. The passage is open only at estrus and immediately before, during, and, for a short time, following parturition.

## The Vagina

The remainder of the female tract, though sometimes loosely termed the vagina, consists of two parts. The cranial part, the vagina in the strict sense (Fig. 5–46/10), is a purely reproductive passage that runs from the cervix to the entrance of the urethra. The caudal part, the vestibule (/11), extends from the urethral orifice to the external vulva and combines reproductive and urinary functions. The two parts together constitute the female copulatory organ and birth canal.

The *vagina* is a relatively long, thin-walled tube that is distensible in length and width. It occupies a median position within the pelvic cavity, related to the rectum dorsally and the bladder and urethra ventrally (Fig. 5–28/8). It is mostly retroperitoneal, although peritoneum does cover the cranial parts of both the dorsal and the ventral surfaces to a variable extent. Incision of this part of the dorsal wall, a relatively easy procedure to perform from within the vagina in larger species, provides a convenient access to the peritoneal cavity (see Fig. 22–7/2,8). The corresponding ventral approach is prohibited by the presence of a plexus of veins draining the uterus and vagina.

The vaginal muscle, although weaker, has a similar disposition to that of the uterus. The mucosa is lined by a stratified squamous epithelium that reacts—more emphatically in some species than in others—to changes in hormone levels throughout the estrous cycle. Glands are confined to the cranial part of the vagina, although the moisture may diffuse more widely. The surface is smooth, but circular, and longitudinal folds may form when the walls of the inactive organ collapse inward. The intrusion of the cervix into the cranial part of the vagina reduces the lumen of this part to a (generally) ringlike space known as the *fornix* (Fig. 5–46/10′).

The junction of vagina and vestibule is supposedly marked in virgin animals by a transverse mucosal fold (hymen). This is best developed in the filly and the gilt, but even in these it is rarely very prominent. It does not survive coitus. The junctional region is less distensible than the parts of the tract cranial and caudal to it.

## The Vestibule and Vulva

The vestibule, much shorter than the vagina, lies mainly if not entirely caudal to the ischial arch, a circumstance that permits it to slope ventrally to its opening at the vulva. The amount of "drop" is variable, both among species and individuals

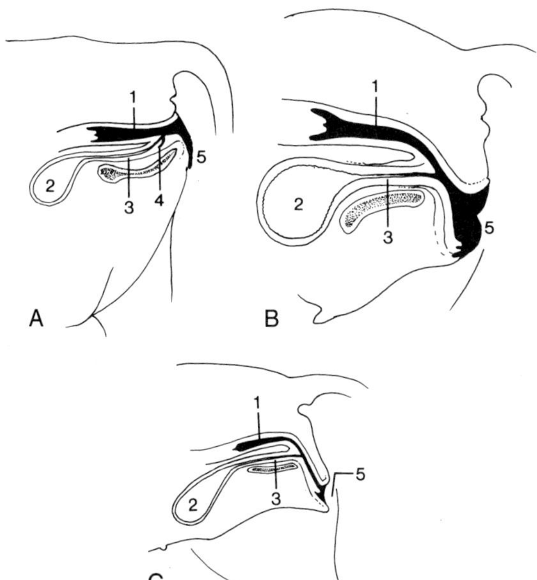


**Figure 5–47.** Variation in the position of the vestibule in relation to the ischial arch (*A,* cow; *B,* mare; *C,* bitch).

1, Vagina; 2, bladder; 3, urethra; 4, suburethral diverticulum; 5, vulva.

(Fig. 5–47). The resulting inflection of the axis of the genital passage must be borne in mind when introducing a vaginal speculum or other instrument.

The walls of the vestibule are less elastic than those of the vagina and come together at rest, reducing the lumen to a vertical cleft. The urethra opens on the floor, directly caudal to whatever indication of a hymen may exist. In some animals, for example the bitch, the urethral opening is raised above the general level of the vestibular floor (Fig. 5–31); in others, such as the cow, it is associated with a *suburethral diverticulum* (Fig. 5–28/12′). More caudally, the vestibular walls are marked by the entrances of the ducts of *vestibular glands.* In certain species (e.g., bitch) the glands are small but numerous and the duct orifices form linear series; in others (e.g., cow) a large glandular mass to each side drains by a single duct (Fig. 5–46/13). In a few species (e.g., ewe) both minor and major vestibular glands are present. These glands produce a mucous secretion that lubricates the passage at coitus and at parturition. At estrus the odor of the secretion has a sexually stimulating effect on the male. The vestibular wall is exceptionally well vascularized with a concentration of veins forming a lateral patch of erectile tissue known as the vestibular bulb and regarded as the homologue of the bulb of the penis.

The vestibule opens to the exterior at the vulva. The vertical vulvar opening is bounded by labia that meet at dorsal and ventral commissures. Except in the mare, the dorsal commissure is rounded, the ventral one pointed and raised above the level of the surrounding skin. The labia correspond to the (inner) labia minora of human anatomy; the (outer) labia majora are suppressed in domestic species.

The *clitoris,* the female homologue of the penis, lies just within the ventral commissure (/14). It is formed of two crura, a body and a glans, in the same fashion as its much larger male homologue. Without dissection, only the glans is visible where it projects within a fossa on the vestibular floor, partly enveloped by a mucosal fold constituting a prepuce.

## The Adnexa

The *broad ligaments,* the principal attachments of the female reproductive tract, are bilateral sheets that take extended origin from the abdominal roof and pelvic walls. The cranial part of each hangs vertically and suspends the ovary, uterine tube, and horn of the uterus (see Fig. 22–9/17). The caudal part passes more horizontally to attach to the side of the body of the uterus, cervix, and cranial part of the vagina; the right and left caudal parts with their visceral inclusion thus divide the pelvic cavity into dorsal and ventral spaces (Figs. 5–29/7, 22–7, and 29–8). Different parts of the broad ligaments obtain the specific designations already mentioned (e.g., mesovarium). These ligaments are unlike most peritoneal folds since the serosal membranes are held apart by considerable amounts of tissue, mainly smooth muscle; this sometimes makes it difficult to point to the exact boundary between the uterus and its adnexa. The muscle enables the ligaments to take an active part in the support and disposition of the reproductive organs in addition to conveying vessels and nerves.

When followed distally from its attachment to the abdominal roof, the *mesovarium,* which supports the ovary, releases a lateral fold (mesosalpinx) that passes onto the uterine tube (Figs. 5–45/7 and 5–48/2). Mesosalpinx and mesovarium enclose a pouch, the *ovarian bursa,* into which the ovary projects. The bursa may be shallow and unable to hold the ovary (mare; Fig. 5–45/9) or deep and so enclosed by the fusion of apposed serosal surfaces that the ovary is permanently trapped (bitch; Fig. 5–49/*B*). In certain nondomestic species (e.g., mouse) fusion is so complete that the space within the bursa no longer communicates

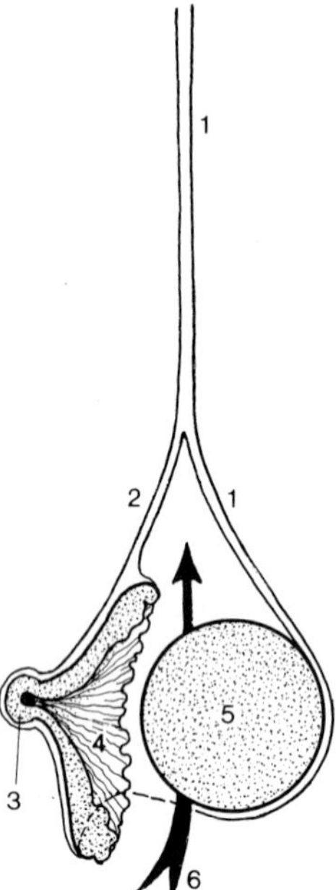


**Figure 5–48.** Schematic section of the ovary and its suspensory system.

1, Mesovarium; 2, mesosalpinx; 3, abdominal opening of uterine tube; 4, infundibulum; 5, ovary; 6, the arrow is in the ovarian bursa.

with the peritoneal cavity. The walls of the bursa may contain so much fat that the ovary is quite hidden. The mesovarium also supports a fibromuscular band, the proper ligament of the ovary, which extends from the caudal pole of the ovary to the adjacent tip of the horn of the uterus.

The large part of the broad ligament that passes onto the horn and body of the uterus helps to give the organ the shape characteristic of the species. The two serosal membranes are very widely separated by fat where they attach to the cervix and especially to the vagina; the lateral part of the vagina is therefore retroperitoneal (see Fig. 29–9). A cord of fibrous tissue and smooth muscle, the *round ligament of the uterus,* passes from the tip of the horn of the uterus toward (and in the bitch, through) the inguinal canal, supported by a special fold of peritoneum detached from the lateral surface of the broad ligament.

The muscles and fasciae associated with the female reproductive organs are best considered in topographical contexts for those animals in which they have special importance (p. 703). It will be recalled that the pelvic outlet is closed by a musculofascial partition of complicated form and structure. The dorsal part, the *pelvic diaphragm,* closes the outlet about the anus. The ventral part, the *urogenital diaphragm* (membrana perinei), closes the outlet about the vestibule. Muscle forms the principal component of the pelvic diaphragm, while the fasciae predominate in the urogenital diaphragm.

The blood supply to the female reproductive organs is obtained from several sources. The *ovarian artery,* a direct branch of the aorta, supplies the ovary and branches to the uterine tube and cranial part of the horn of the uterus; the pattern of branching varies in detail. The ovarian artery assumes an extraordinarily convoluted course and, depending on species, is more or less closely related to the ovarian vein. The uterine branch anastomoses with the uterine artery within the broad ligament (Fig. 5–50/1′,2).

The *uterine artery* arises as an indirect branch of the internal iliac artery (except in the mare) and runs forward within the broad ligament. It detaches a series of anastomosing branches to the body and horn of the uterus; the most cranial anastomoses with the ovarian artery, the most caudal with the vaginal artery. Thus, an arterial arcade is established, running the length of the uterus and supplied from both ends (Fig. 5–51). Much rather inconclusive discussion has occurred on the significance of this arrangement in determining the generosity of the blood supply to different parts of the uterus—and therefore to particular implantation sites in the pregnant animal. Some believe that differences in arterial pressure disfavor certain sites and that this explains the location of the runts that are so common in polytocous species.

The more caudal parts of the tract are variously supplied by branches of the *internal pudendal* and *vaginal arteries;* some more important species differences are mentioned elsewhere.

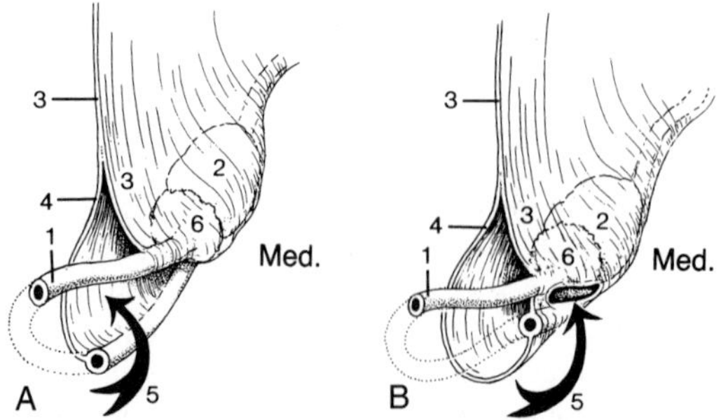


**Figure 5–49.** Schematic representations of the suspensory system of the ovary and uterine tube and of the varying form of the ovarian bursa. *A,* Spacious bursa with large entrance (cow, mare). *B,* Bursa with constricted entrance and entrapped ovary (bitch).

1, Uterine tube; 2, ovary; 3, mesovarium; 4, mesosalpinx; 5, arrow entering the ovarian bursa; 6, infundibulum.

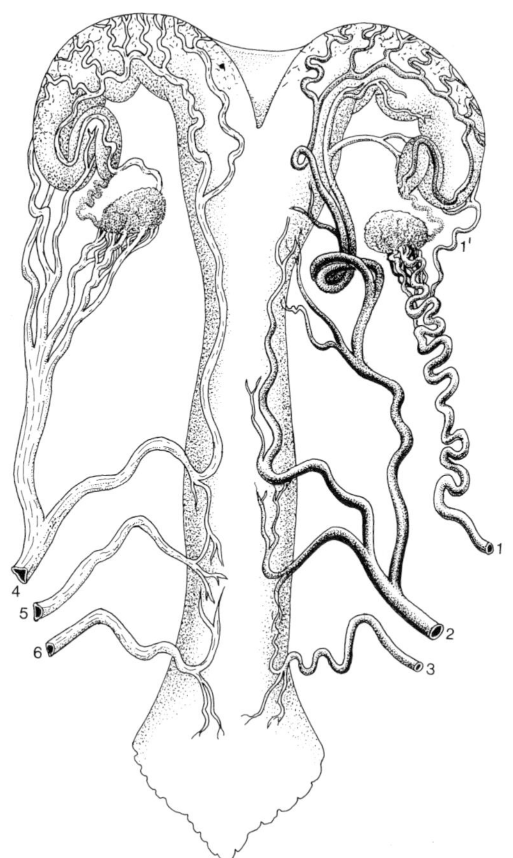


**Figure 5–50.** Semischematic ventral view of the blood supply to the reproductive tract of the cow. The arteries are depicted on the right side, the veins on the left.

1, Ovarian artery; 1′, uterine branch; 2, uterine artery; 3, vaginal artery; 4, ovarian vein; 5, accessory vaginal vein; 6, vaginal vein.

The veins, broadly satellite to the arteries, do not correspond to their companions in relative importance. The plexiform *ovarian vein* is relatively much larger, the uterine vein relatively much smaller, than the accompanying artery (Fig. 5–50). A prominent and elaborate venous plexus present on the ventral aspect of the uterus and vagina drains both organs; it allows blood to escape by any of the paired ovarian, uterine, and vaginal veins. The close relation between the artery and ovarian vein, best seen in ruminants and sows, provides a means for the countercurrent transfer of the luteolytic hormone (prostaglandin) from venous to arterial blood (p. 207).

The lymphatics from the ovaries and more cranial parts of the tract pass to the aortic and medial iliac nodes, those from more caudal parts to the medial iliac and other nodes within the pelvis.

*Innervation* of the female reproductive organs is provided by both sympathetic and parasympathetic fibers, by routes that have yet to be fully clarified. Sympathetic fibers run to the ovary together with the ovarian artery, but although they reach ripening follicles, their significance is unclear since denervation hardly disturbs ovarian function. The fibers to the uterine tube, uterus, and vagina mainly follow the other arteries to form plexuses within the broad ligaments and the genital organs themselves. In the caudal part of the broad ligaments these fibers are augmented by other sympathetic fibers that travel by way of the plexus located in the retroperitoneal pelvic tissue.

The parasympathetic fibers branch from the pelvic nerves and reach the genital organs via the pelvic plexus. A large proportion goes to erectile tissue.

Both sympathetic and parasympathetic fibers seem to be concerned with uterine activity, although their precise roles in stimulation and inhibition are still controversial. The uterus is able to coordinate contractions and accomplish a normal birth even after denervation.

## Age and Functional Changes in the Female Tract

Only a general account of the important age and functional changes is presented in this chapter, which glosses over the many species differences that affect all aspects but particularly the timing and duration of events.

### Age and Cyclic Changes

The *juvenile* reproductive organs are disproportionately small. At birth the ovaries provide no evidence of their future endocrine role, which is not established until shortly before puberty when ripening follicles, and the corpora lutea that replace them, produce the hormones that stimulate the growth, tissue differentiation, and activity of the reproductive tract, and the manifestation of female behavior. In contrast, the gametogenic or exocrine function was established in the young fetus with the migration into the ovary of premordial germ cells (p. 168). These immigrant cells proliferate rapidly to produce a population of perhaps 3 million at its maximum, but this number soon begins to be progressively reduced in a process that continues to puberty and beyond. Only a few hundred thousand generally survive at birth and, since no later accession to their number is possible, this determines the later much more niggardly release of female than of male gametes. Each surviving oocyte is initially surrounded by a

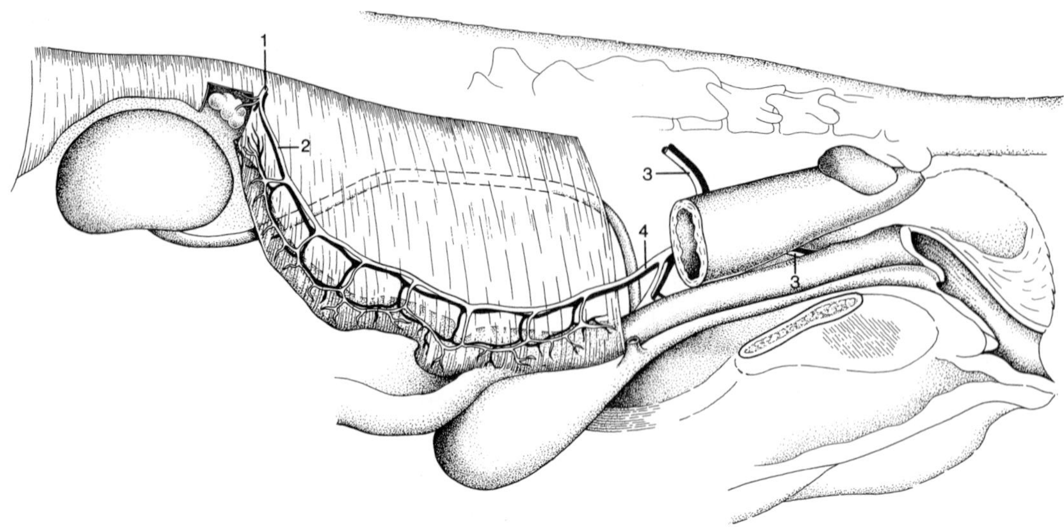


**Figure 5–51.** Semischematic drawing of the blood supply of the female reproductive tract (bitch).

1, Ovarian artery; 2, uterine branch of the ovarian artery; 3, vaginal artery; 4, uterine artery.

single layer of flattened epithelial (granulosa) cells to form the structure known as the primordial follicle. Most primordial follicles remain in arrested development, or undergo atresia, but some transform into primary follicles that are distinguished by the enlargement of the oocyte and its enclosure within a covering of granulosa cells that have assumed a cuboidal confirmation.

The neonatal and juvenile tubular reproductive organs are delicate, thin-walled, and slack; they are rather poorly vascularized and the arteries are unobtrusive and relatively straight. The uterus is symmetrical, the layers of its wall poorly differentiated, and the cervix soft, distensible, and free from the distortions common in parous animals. The broad ligaments are thin and translucent since they contain little parametrial tissue. A hymen may be present, but, this apart, the vagina, vestibule, and vulva present no features of special interest. *Growth* of these organs is initially isometric, keeping pace with general somatic growth. After puberty the actions of ovarian hormones, cumulative over the first few cycles, bring about a rapid enlargement and a better differentiation of the component tissues. Follicles in all stages of development may now be found within the ovaries together with corpora lutea and replacing scars (Fig. 5–44 ).

There is a continuous slow growth of many follicles within the adult ovaries. In the ovary of anestrous animals the follicles grow to the early antral stage (Plate 7/*H*) but then degenerate. The onset of the breeding season is heralded by a more rapid development of a few, chosen from this larger population according to obscure criteria. These favored follicles enlarge at an exponential rate under the influence of FSH of the pituitary. Their growth is explained by the proliferation of granulosa and theca cells and the accumulation of follicular fluid. This fluid increasingly distends a central vesicle (antrum) into which the ovum projects, raised on a mound of cells (cumulus oophorus) and enclosed within a cellular covering (corona radiata). The follicle is bounded by a two-layered capsule (theca interna and externa) differentiated from the surrounding stroma (Fig. 5–44/9). As each follicle grows it shifts toward the surface of the ovary, where it forms an increasingly salient projection. The granulosa cells of the ripening follicle produce estrogen, and it is the peak level of production of this hormone that induces both the behavioral pattern and the structural changes that characterize the animal in heat.

Estrogen has an epitheliotropic effect most evident in promoting proliferation of the vaginal epithelium and simple lengthening of the uterine glands. It also produces edema and hyperemia of the tissues of the reproductive tract; edema may produce a visible swelling of the vulva, while congestion of the endometrium may lead in some species (notably the bitch) to the appearance of blood in the external discharge. It also enhances the irritability of the myometrium that is detectable through the uterus, including the cervix, becoming more responsive to manipulation.

*Ovulation* occurs late in estrus or shortly after its termination and is stimulated by LH, also of pituitary origin. Ovulation is spontaneous in most species, but in some, including the cat, the mechanical stimulus of coitus is necessary to set in train the events that culminate in follicular rupture (Table 5–1). Once shed into the peritoneal cavity, an ovum is soon gathered into the expanded end of the uterine tube. How this is effected is uncertain, although it is clear that the nonmotile ovum can play no active part. The most likely mechanisms are the production of a current in the suspending fluid by the ciliary beat of the tubal epithelium, and grasping movements of the muscular fimbriae which are closely applied to the surface of the ovary at this time. Both mechanisms would be assisted by the surface irregularity provided by adherent corona cells. However, none of this convincingly explains how ova may be captured after transperitoneal migration; that this is possible is shown by animals sometimes becoming pregnant after removal of one ovary and the contralateral tube.

The space within the vacated follicle fills with blood when rupture has been attended by considerable hemorrhage, but any clot is soon replaced by proliferation of the surviving granulosa and internal theca cells to form a solid body, the corpus luteum (Plate 7/*I*). This structure grows rapidly and may soon equal the follicle that it replaces. It produces progesterone, the hormone that continues the preparation of the uterus for the reception of the embryo and for the maintenance of pregnancy. In animals that become pregnant it survives well into or throughout pregnancy (according to species), but it regresses quite rapidly in cycles that are infertile (Plate 7/*J*). Responsibility for its regression rests with a luteolytic hormone (prostaglandin) produced by the "empty" uterus. The effects of progesterone reinforce those produced by previous exposure to estrogen and stimulate further growth of the uterine glands, which now become branched, tortuous, and more active, secreting the so-called uterine milk that nourishes the embryo before implantation. Progesterone also dampens the activity of the myometrium.

The transport of ova within the tube is achieved by the combination of ciliary and muscular activity. If mating has occurred the ova rendezvous with the sperm within the ampulla. Although sperm may reach this site within a few minutes of coitus, a longer sojourn within the female tract is required before they become capable of fertilization. According to species, semen is initially deposited within the vagina or the cervix, where it forms a coagulum from which some sperm soon emerge. Even when the semen is deposited in the vagina, churning movements soon bring some sperm into contact with the cervical mucus, which provides a more hospitable environment than the acid secretion of the vagina. The physicochemical properties of the cervical mucus at this time help align the sperm, directing them on their upward path. Even so, the movement of sperm would be slow if they depended on their own puny efforts; transport is mainly effected by muscular contractions, evoked by prostaglandin within the semen, and by oxytocin reflexly released into the blood stream at coitus. Though sperm are produced with great prodigality, only a small propertion, say 1% or 2% of the many millions within an ejaculate deposited within the vagina, succeed in passing the cervical barrier. The uterotubal junction, the next major impediment, is successively negotiated by even fewer sperm (and those necessarily of normal motility). In species in which intrauterine deposition of sperm takes place, the uterotubal junction is the first barrier. Movement within the tube is more

**Table 5–1.** Some Specific Parameters in Reproduction

| Species | Puberty (mo) | Cycle Length (days) | Duration of Estrus | Ovulation | Pregnancy Duration (days) |
|---|---|---|---|---|---|
| Dog | 6–9 | ≥90 | 9 days | 3 days after the beginning of estrus | 62 |
| Cat | 6–9 | Variable | 7–10 days | 24 hr after coitus | 63–65 |
| Horse | 20 | 21 (19–22) | 5–6 days | 1–2 days before the end of estrus | 330 |
| Cattle | 6–18 | 21 (18–24) | 18 hr | 10–12 hr after the end of estrus | 280 |
| Sheep | 6–12 | 17 (16–18) | 24–36 hr | 30–36 hr after the beginning of estrus | 150 |
| Goat | 4–8 | 21 | 24–36 hr | 30–36 hr after the beginning of estrus | 150 |
| Pig | 5–10 | 21 (19–21) | 48–72 hr | 35–45 hr after the beginning of estrus | 114 |

erratic since the muscular contractions on which it depends are ill-coordinated. In most species sperm remain fertile for a day or two following coitus, and many apparently find temporary refuge in cervical glands and other niches.

*Fertilization* activates the ovum, and cleavage begins within a short time. Its later fate is considered in the following section.

## The Course of Pregnancy

The evolution of the gravid uterus affects its size, position, form, and relations, changes that naturally become increasingly evident as pregnancy advances. Even so, it will be convenient to take brief note of certain of them now, before resuming the history of the fertilized ovum. The principles effecting change in size are more or less the same in all animals, but the other aspects vary among species and are best considered separately for each (see the appropriate later chapters). The increase in size may ultimately be as much as 100-fold (as in the cow) but the greater part of this is represented by the contents of the uterus which comprise the fetal membranes and fluids in addition to the conceptus(es). The more modest growth of the organ involves all its components. The endometrium remains hyperemic and edematous, and the myometrium enlarges owing to a vast increase in the size of individual muscle cells (although the possibility of addition to their number cannot always be excluded). Despite this hypertrophy, the uterine wall is unable to keep pace with the growth of the contents and it stretches markedly, so much so that in rats and other species of similar size it becomes transparent. The broad ligaments share in the increase and come to contain large amounts of muscle. The arteries enlarge greatly as it becomes necessary to satisfy an ever-increasing demand for blood. Activity of the cervical glands continually renews the mucous plug that seals the cervical canal.

Resuming the history of the fertilized ovum, we remind the reader that cleavage continues as the ovum is transported through the uterine tube. This transport takes several days, spent mainly within the isthmus section, and when the conceptus, as the fertilized ovum is now conveniently known, is passed into the uterus it is in the morula or early blastocyst stage of development. The timing of its arrival may be critical since if it loiters, or makes overhasty passage, it may encounter an inhospitable, even hostile reception. The appropriate welcome is obtained from an endometrium that has been progesterone-primed and then additionally prepared by a suitably timed stimulus of estrogen. The conceptus must shortly establish a fixed relationship to the endometrium if it is to survive; meanwhile it lies free to shift within the lumen and relies on the secretion of uterine glands for sustenance. This delay before attachment (implantation) provides multiple conceptuses opportunity to find favorable locations in which to settle, and they are later found to be spaced at more or less equal intervals within the uterine horns, an arrangement that allows for the most extensive and equitable use of the endometrium by the placentas that will shortly develop. The spacing is achieved by peristaltic contractions that spread from the extremities of the horns and in both directions from the locus of each conceptus; each conceptus is repulsed by the contractions emanating from its neighbors and therefore moves until it is stabilized by encountering forces of comparable magnitude from both sides. Even single conceptuses show consistent preference for certain locations within the uterus; the equine conceptus, for example, always comes to rest in the part of the horn adjacent to the body.

*Implantation* involves reaction from the apposed epithelial layers of the blastocyst and endometrium and in some species considerable erosion of maternal tissue takes place as the attachment develops (see later). This erosion occurs mainly in species in which the blastocyst remains small before implantation and either seeks out a nidus (nest) in a cleft of the endometrium or burrows into its substance. The blastocysts of domestic species grow considerably before implantation and remain centrally within the lumen and thus related to the whole circumference of the endometrium. In some species it is not always easy to decide when the closeness of association amounts to implantation, and in domestic ungulates the event is probably significantly longer delayed than the 2 weeks after coitus suggested for many other mammals. Two circumstances exist in which implantation is unusually delayed. In some species, including rats and mice, suckling prolongs the preimplantation stage, a (facultative) delay that ensures that a later litter does not find itself in competition for milk with its predecessor. A much longer prolongation (obligatory delay or diapause) occurs regularly in certain wild species (e.g., roe deer and badger) in which both pairing and birth are seasonal; the suspension of development for several months, and the timing of its resumption, ensure that birth will occur when conditions are most favorable for rearing young.

Implantation and the initial development of the fetal membranes may be regarded as concluding the preembryonic period, the first of the three periods into which development is conventionally divided. Its principal features may be summarized:

the intrauterine migration and eventual settlement of the blastocyst; its rapid transformation from a spherical to a threadlike form in many species (which include the ruminants and pig, but not the horse); the demarcation of the inner cell mass (the future embryonic body) from the embryonic adnexa (fetal membranes); the establishment of the three primary germ layers (ecto-, meso-, and endoderm); and the apposition of embryonic and maternal tissue in anticipation of the formation of the placenta and the transition from histiotrophic to hemotrophic nutrition and exchange.

The second or embryonic period is occupied by the establishment of a fully functional placenta, the differentiation of the various tissues and organ systems (for which see the relevant systematic chapters), and the initiation of various functions, most notably an embryonic circulation. Overall growth is still relatively modest but by the end of this period the external conformation is sufficiently developed to identify the major taxon—order, perhaps family—to which the embryo belongs, though not yet the particular species.

The remaining part of the intrauterine development is assigned to a third or fetal period although the determination of the boundary is necessarily somewhat arbitrary and imprecise.* Organogenesis continues throughout the fetal period, and for many organs well into postnatal life, but the changes that now bring the different systems into the degree of structural and functional competence necessary for survival after birth are less dramatic than those that took place earlier. The rapid growth, which is the foremost characteristic of the fetal period, continues into postnatal life without significant interruption about the time of birth, in the sheep (chosen for illustration) and many other species, and lends itself to graphical representation in a variety of complementary ways in Figure 5–52. Taken together, these show that growth, from conception through the first months of postnatal life, follows an S-curve; that the onset of

*Since many processes continue uninterrupted from one period to the next, there is unavoidable overlap and inconsistency in the use of the terms "embryo" and "fetus."

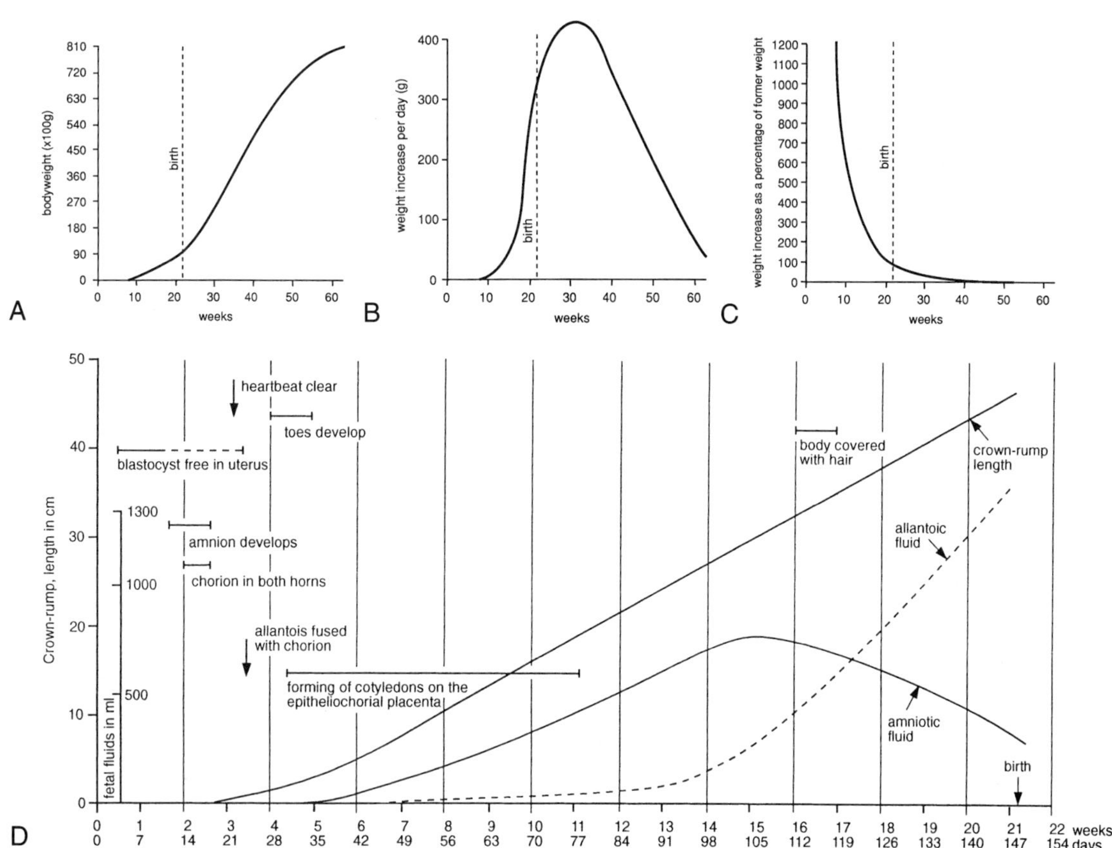


**Figure 5–52.** The growth of lambs. *A, B,* and *C* record the growth in weight of lambs during fetal and early postnatal life. *D,* Schematic summary of metrical and other features of the development of the fetal lamb and its adnexa.

rapid growth is delayed until some way into fetal life; that weight increase accelerates week on week through most of the rapid growth period; but that the weekly accession diminishes when expressed as a percentage of the former weight. Although weight is commonly regarded as the more revealing parameter, it is often more convenient to use linear measurements, especially crown-rump length; however, it will be appreciated that there must be a tolerably close fit between linear measurements and the cube root of weight. The last part *(D)* of the figure correlates crown-rump length with other salient features of the development of the sheep fetus and its adnexa.

The slopes of the curves, the timing of the onset of rapid growth, and other features are subject to both species and individual variation. Individual variation is in part determined by the fetal genome but is also influenced by intrauterine conditions which, for many species, include litter size and the relative advantage or disadvantage provided by different locations within the uterus (Fig. 5–53). A normal rate of growth presumes adequate supplies of nutrients and oxygen, and the rate will be depressed if the uterine circulation is impaired, if there is insufficient healthy placental tissue, or if the mother is severely malnourished. Although it is widely accepted that an inverse correlation exists between litter size and individual fetal and neonatal weight, the effect, which generally only becomes apparent toward full term, is usually modest when other conditions are favorable and litter size is not extreme. Fetuses exposed to any circumstance that deflects them from the expected growth curve are generally able to recover if exposure was neither too severe nor too prolonged, although "catching-up" may be deferred until after birth.

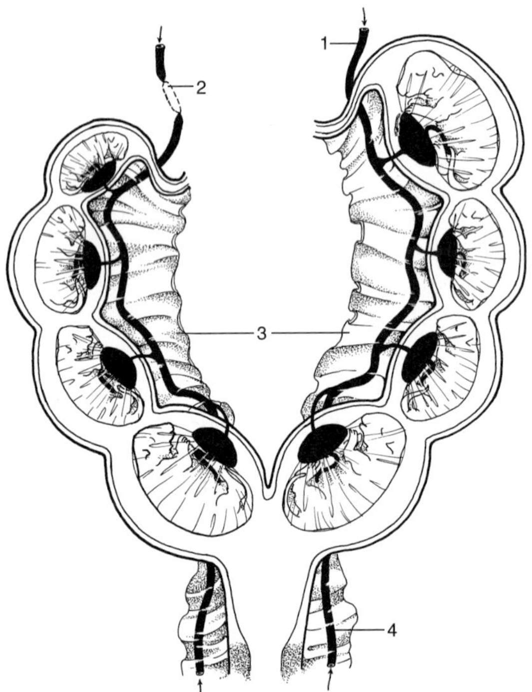


**Figure 5–53.** Schematic drawing of uterus of sow with arterial blood supply partly interrupted. Fetal size depends on position in uterus and the relation between blood supply and position.

1, Uterine branch of ovarian artery; 2, ligated artery; 3, broad ligaments; 4, uterine artery.

The early transformations and the complexities of organogenesis provide ample opportunity for development to go awry, and death or malformation is common in the first two periods. This is probably true for all mammals although data are most reliably available for the human and the pig. Some losses and abnormalities are due to intrinsic defects of the conceptus, some to an unreceptive state of the uterus, and some to exposure of the mother to any of a variety of environmental insults. It is known, for example, that chromosomal abnormality, of structure or number, is demonstrable in about 10% of clinically detectable human pregnancies, including spontaneous early abortions, and it is believed to be even more common in conceptuses lost at earlier stages before awareness of pregnancy exists. In contrast, chromosomal abnormality is identified in a much smaller proportion, perhaps 0.5%, of human infants delivered at term. Although the fertilization rate in pigs is high—possibly exceeding 95% in some herds—it has been estimated that only 60% or so of conceptuses come to term. Most deaths occur within the first 40 days (of a gestation period of 114 days) but, since conceptuses lost at an early stage are generally resorbed and leave no trace, the figure must be interpreted with caution. The rates for fertilization and delivery at term for other species vary too much from herd to herd, and stud to stud, to be susceptible to convenient or safe summary.

Considerable attention has recently been given to the recognition of mixoploidy in the blastocysts of a variety of mammalian species. The term describes the existence of polyploid cells—those with more than the usual complement of chromosomal sets—admixed with the normal population of diploid cells. Some investigations have revealed a considerable proportion, upward of 25% in one study, of the total cell population exhibiting this aberrant feature. Many affected conceptuses are destined to die at a very early stage but some may survive. There are indications that the deviant cells tend to be segregated to the trophoblast. It has been postulated that the greater frequency of certain reproductive failures in cattle—stillbirths, reduced postnatal viability, the "large calf" syndrome—encountered following manipulation of blastocysts in vitro may have this causation. These defects may therefore be due to disturbance of placental function rather than to a direct effect upon the calf itself.

The environmental insults that may affect development adversely cannot be comprehensively listed, far less adequately considered here. They include ionizing radiation, viral infections, inorganic and organic chemicals, including some that are constituents of plants (e.g., clover, soya and certain other legumes, *Veratrum californicum*) potentially present in pasture or other feedstuffs. Many of these agents are better known from their effects in the laboratory than in the field and, while some are lethal, others are more likely to produce abnormalities that are survivable, if sometimes only for a time. Such agents (teratogens) are most likely to produce abnormality when exposure occurs during the embryonic period when so many complicated and critically timed procedures are under way; earlier exposure is more likely to result in death.

Familiar examples of indictable infective agents are provided by bovine viral diarrhea (BVD), hog cholera (swine fever) (HCV), border disease virus (BDV), and human rubella and cytomegalovirus. These viruses are notorious for causing fetal death resulting in abortion or stillbirth, and for producing defects, of brain and eye especially, or growth retardation, in young born to mothers infected in early pregnancy. Fetuses infected at a later stage with BVD or HCV become immunotolerant to these viruses and may be born apparently healthy. Since they are persistently infected they represent a real danger to other livestock on the farm.

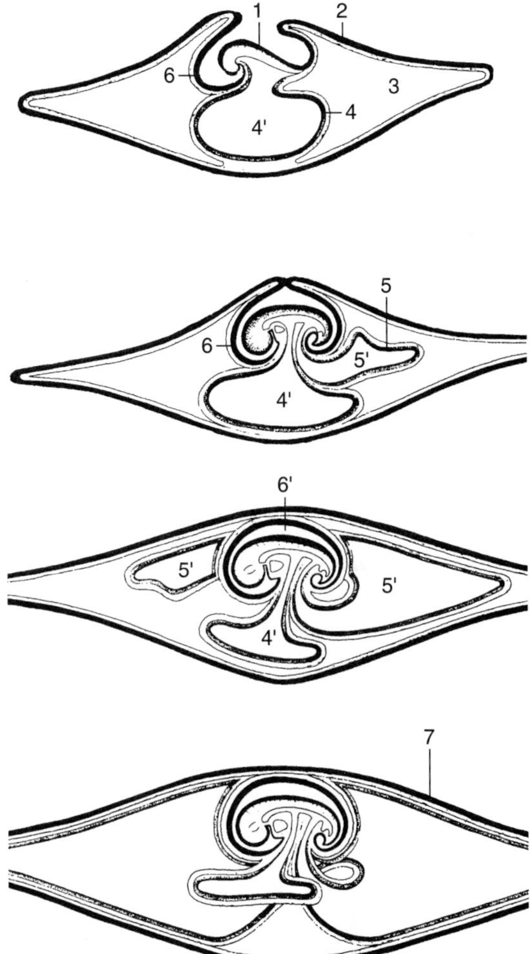


**Figure 5–54.** Schematic representation of the formation of extraembryonic membranes.

1, Embryo; 2, chorion; 3, extraembryonic celom; 4, yolk sac; 4′, yolk sac cavity; 5, allantois; 5′, allantoic cavity; 6, amnion; 6′, amniotic cavity; 7, chorioallantois.

## *Fetal Membranes and Placentation*

We have insufficient space to describe the formation of the embryonic or fetal membranes but include diagrams (Fig. 5–54) as reminders of the principal points. The definitive gross arrangement is shown for the dog (Plate 8/*G*), horse (Plate 8/*E*), and ruminant (Plate 8/*C,D*) conceptuses. These membranes concur with the endometrium in the formation of the placenta, an organ that may be defined as an apposition or fusion of fetal and maternal tissue for the purposes of physiological exchange and hormone production. A provisional placenta, furnished by a vascularized yolk sac, may provide a useful organ of exchange in early pregnancy. This omphaloplacenta is important in the first third or so of equine pregnancy, but in most species the chorioallantoic placenta, the definitive placenta of eutherian mammals, becomes competent at a relatively earlier stage. In the definitive arrangement, the chorion, intimately associated with the endometrium, is vascularized by vessels that reach it by following the allantoic outgrowth from the hindgut. The stalk of the allantois (urachus), the accompanying vessels which become the umbilical arteries and veins, and the ensheathing connective tissue (the fetal variety known as Wharton's jelly), constitute the umbilical cord, which persists as the communication between fetus and placenta until ruptured in the course of birth or shortly thereafter.

**Table 5–2.** Placental Classification

| | Carnivores | Horse | Ruminants | Pig |
|---|---|---|---|---|
| Gross form | Zonary and labyrinthine | Diffuse | Cotyledonary | Diffuse and folded |
| Histological type | Endotheliochorial | Epitheliochorial | Epitheliochorial | Epitheliochorial |
| Separation | Semideciduate | Nondeciduate | Semideciduate | Nondeciduate |

The *chorioallantoic placenta* takes many forms that may be classified in several complementary ways. The first system refers to the gross distribution of the chorionic villi, minute outgrowths of the chorionic surface that engage with depressions of the endometrial surface to provide the areas of exchange. In horse and pig these villi are spread in small clumps (microcotyledons) over virtually the entire surface of the chorion; such placentas are *diffuse* (Plate 9/*A,B*). In ruminants the villi develop in scattered patches or cotyledons opposite the endometrial caruncles; each cotyledon and associated caruncle forms a separate unit or placentome and these collectively constitute a *cotyledonary placenta* (/*C,D*). In dog and cat the villi develop in a band of chorion that encircles the trunk of the embryo, forming a *zonary placenta** (/*E,H*). The fourth and last type does not occur in domestic species; in this, the common pattern in primates and rodents, the villi are concentrated in one large patch, forming a *discoidal placenta.*

The second system refers to the tissue layers that separate the fetal and maternal blood streams. Initially, six layers are present: chorionic capillary endothelium, connective tissue, and epithelium; endometrial epithelium, connective tissue, and capillary endothelium. The tissue barrier at the areas of exchange is always later reduced, sometimes only by the closer approach of the two sets of capillaries but often by tissue loss. In theory, the six layers persist in the epitheliochorial placenta seen in the mare and sow; they are reduced to four, by the loss of the endometrial epithelium and connective tissue, in the endotheliochorial placenta seen in dogs and cats (/*F,H*); they suffer the ultimate reduction to one layer, embryonic endothelium, in the hemoendothelial placenta of bats. Ruminants were long described as having a syndesmochorial placenta, in which only the uterine epithelium had been lost; modern studies discount this loss, and it is now believed that these animals also have epitheliochorial placentas. Indeed, the syndesmochorial "slot" in the classification is currently empty since no example of this arrangement has been confirmed by electron microscopy.

The third system refers to the loss of maternal tissue that occurs at birth. In some species the fetal and maternal layers part cleanly, no maternal tissue is shed, and the description "nondeciduate" is appropriate. When implantation is interstitial, considerable maternal loss may be expected; the human placenta is of this "deciduate" type. Minor loss of uterine tissue occurs in an intermediate semideciduate type found in ruminants (Table 5–2).

The histological system appears to define different degrees of placental permeability. While this is broadly true, histological differences provide an incomplete explanation of variations in permeability. It must be borne in mind that the barrier may not be exactly as implied by the description; moreover, the placenta evolves and changes in structure during pregnancy and significant regional differences may exist side by side. Freely diffusible molecules cross from one circulation to the other according to their relative concentrations, and in this respect the human hemochorial placenta certainly allows more rapid passage than the "thicker" epitheliochorial placenta of the larger domestic species. The transport of larger molecules depends on other factors, including specialized unidirectional mechanisms.

Differences in the barrier to the passage of immunoglobulin G (IgG) are of particular veterinary significance. In some species a mechanism exists for the transfer to the fetus of maternal antibodies produced in response to infection; these may confer some immediate protection upon the newborn, possibly delivered into an environment contaminated by the same infective agent. This prenatally acquired immunity is denied to offspring of species (including horses and farm animals) with epitheliochorial placentas; their neonates rely upon colostrum, the milk first produced as the source of antibodies that may provide temporary protection.

Fetal antigens, present in plasma or borne by blood cells, may leak into the maternal blood stream with potentially damaging consequences. The classic illustration is furnished by the hemolytic disease (erythroblastosis fetalis) of human infants; this condition develops in a second or later

*In the dog a permanent zone of leaking blood creates marginal hematomas (Plate 8/*G*). In the cat this zone is diffuse and temporary and therefore not as striking as that of the dog.

child confronted by antibody produced by a Rhesus-negative mother in reaction to the incompatibility of her Rhesus factor with that of a previous Rhesus-positive child. Antibody production by the mother develops so slowly that the child (usually the first) provoking the response generally escapes serious harm. Similar conditions occur in other species, including horses and pigs, but damage to their offspring can be prevented by denying them access to colostrum, which contains the relevant antibody.

The endocrine functions of the placenta are both complex and lacking in uniformity among species, even between those that are closely related. The topic will therefore be treated concisely with the interested reader referred to specialized works for fuller information. In certain respects the placenta or, for some species, the fetoplacental unit, assumes functions that are undertaken by the ovary and pituitary of the nonpregnant animal. Thus, the placenta produces progesterone in amounts that vary among species and at different stages, often showing a gradual increase as gestation proceeds. This production supports, and in some species eventually supplants, that of the corpus luteum within the ovary; in species of the latter grouping the ovary may be removed in later gestation without jeopardizing the continuation of pregnancy. Although sheep tolerate this intervention, goats do not—a good example of the risk contained in applying results obtained from one species to another, even to one of especially close kinship. Progesterone promotes the growth of the uterus, among other effects stimulating activity of the endometrial glands; but it depresses the excitability of the uterine muscle. The effects are obtained in collaboration with estrogen which is also, in part, of placental origin. The fetal component of the placenta is also responsible, again to varying degree and with unequal significance, for the production of chorionic gonadotropin. The horse is of unusual interest in this context since equine chorionic gonadotropin is produced from structures unique to Equidae, the endometrial cups (Plate 8/*F;* and p. 558).

Elevated levels of steroid hormones in blood and urine provide the basis for diagnostic tests for pregnancy in women; even the DIY tests now widely marketed are generally reliable, if not infallible. Tests of comparable reliability, simplicity, and economy are not yet available for domestic species for which reliance is still largely placed upon clinical procedures, including ultrasonography.

The placenta is one, though not the only, source of other hormones relevant to pregnancy. Lactogen, a hormone related to growth hormone, acts with other hormones to develop the mammary glands for the approaching lactation, while relaxin, which is also secreted by the corpus luteum, helps prepare the reproductive tract and pelvic parietes for parturition (p. 208); later, acting in synergy with oxytocin, it stimulates the expulsive activity of the myometrium.

Although prostaglandin is not a product of the placenta it may be convenient to take notice of it here. This hormone is manufactured by the endometrium of the "empty" uterus, with production delayed for 2 weeks (or so) after the corpus luteum first forms. It leaves the uterus in the uterine vein and in some species, including ruminants, it reaches the ipsilateral ovary after countercurrent transfer to the ovarian artery (Fig. 29–20); in others, for example, horse, in which contact between artery and vein is less close, it reaches the ovaries only after diffusion through the general circulation. Within the ovary, prostaglandin promotes luteolysis (regression of the corpus luteum) with consequent decline and eventual cessation of progesterone secretion and release. The production of prostaglandin is stimulated by oxytocin, but in pregnancy the conceptus produces a factor that blocks endometrial receptivity to oxytocin, and thus indirectly protects the corpus luteum whose integrity is now required.

Before concluding the account of the fetal membranes and placenta, brief attention may be given to the fluids contained within the amniotic and allantoic cavities. These fluids, whose main claim to notice sometimes appears to be their rather dramatic release at the time of birth—the "breaking of the waters"—actually have rather important functions to perform throughout gestation and at certain stages they account for a very considerable fraction of the total content of the gravid uterus. The fluid within the amniotic cavity immediately surrounds and supports the embryo or fetus, cushioning it against compression and protecting it against chance blows to the mother's abdomen. This protection is most required by the young embryo whose skeleton is still largely unformed and whose external covering—hardly yet to be called skin—is delicate and vulnerable to trauma. Later, when these structures are better developed, the amniotic fluid tends to be reduced in amount (Fig. 5–52), relative to the size of the fetus in large species, in absolute terms in small mammals, though the precise amount is always rather variable. At its maximum, it measures about 3 to 5 L in cattle, perhaps a little more in horses; in pigs it varies around 100 mL and it is about 10 to 30 mL in dogs and cats. It is often assumed that amniotic fluid is more or less stagnant but there is a brisk turnover with production and resorption roughly matched in the short term. In early stages, the fluid is a dialysate from vessels of the embryonic skin and amnion; later, once rupture of the urogenital membrane has opened a passage from the bladder, it consists largely of urine and as more is added the fluid already present is reduced by being swallowed. Deficient and excessive amounts of this fluid (oligohydramnios and polyhydramnios, respectively) are possible complications of pregnancy, the former often indicating anomalous development of the kidneys, the latter potentially open to correction by the addition of a "sweetener" to encourage deglutition. This fluid is not normally a significant contributor to that present in the respiratory passages of the fetus and newborn, although this is sometimes suggested. Being slightly mucoid, amniotic fluid has additional value as a lubricant of the birth canal at parturition.

The allantoic cavity is large in all domestic species but the human allantois fails to expand and is soon reduced to a negligible vestige. It is possibly the consequent lack of medical interest that explains the relative paucity of information concerning the formation, turnover, and role of allantoic fluid. The allantoic cavity does, of course, receive urine through the urachus before the urethral route is established and this helps maintain the osmotic pressure of the fetal plasma at a level that prevents fluid loss to the maternal blood stream. A second function may be to maintain sufficient radial pressure to hold the chorion firmly against the endometrium in those species in which the placental attachment is less firm. There is rather more allantoic than amniotic fluid in the large species, about the same amount in dogs and cats; although there is about 100 mL in the pig at midterm, the quantity is reduced to very little at full term. But the quantities are rather variable in all species.

## *Parturition and the Puerperal Period: The Neonate**

Parturition is chiefly initiated by the fetus although the mother is not without all influence. Mares, for example, tend to postpone giving birth when conditions in the stable are disturbed; most foals—approaching 90% in some surveys—are born in the quieter night hours. At the risk of oversimplification, the sequence of fetal events may be summarized: enhanced activity along the adrenocorticotropic hormone (ACTH)–adrenal cortex axis boosts the output of cortical hormones, which, on reaching the placenta, alter the estrogen-to-progesterone ratio in the former's favor; this stimulates the production and release of certain gonadotropins, which are the decisive agents in determining both the preparatory soft tissue changes and the later expulsive activity of the myometrium. They are assisted in the first task by relaxin, and in the second by oxytocin.

Changes in the soft tissues take some time for their achievement. They affect many structures, increasing their water content and loosening the larger collagen accumulations. In the cow, the effect is revealed externally by insinking beside the tail head, a sign of impending parturition long appreciated by stockmen and caused by slackening of the sacrotuberous ligaments, and by swelling of the vulva, most apparent in heifers calving for the first time (Plate 30/*H,I*). Parallel but concealed changes soften the caudal reproductive tract, including, most significantly, the cervix; cervical "ripening," to use the midwife's term, relaxes and allows dilation of this sphincter, which has, till now, guarded the exit from the uterus. Despite these preparations, soft tissue structures may still impede birth, resistance to passage of the fetus being offered by the cervix, the relatively tight vaginovestibular junction, and the vulva. In some species there is significant weakening of the pelvic symphysis, proceeding to complete dissolution in the guinea pig; articular changes in the domestic animals are not pronounced and are limited to some loosening of the sacroiliac joints. Comparable changes in the pelvic joints of women are responsible for the pelvic instability encountered as a frequent complication of late pregnancy, and of the period following childbirth. The skeletal obstructions to fetal passage, most important in species carrying a single offspring that is large in relation to the birth canal, are considered in appropriate later chapters.

The posture and orientation adopted by the fetus in the final phase of pregnancy are of crucial importance to the achievement of an easy delivery. In early pregnancy, when the embryo is small and the amniotic cavity disproportionately large, the posture is a matter of indifference and is probably subject to frequent change. As the fetus enlarges, it becomes constrained by the conformation of the uterus and its long axis aligns with that of the containing horn; since its body flexes most freely in the ventral direction, it generally presents its convex back toward the greater curvature of the uterus. This attitude is not immediately fixed and in calves, the animal for which most is known, the number presenting the head rather than the rump toward the cervix fluctuates, reaching a minimum (ca. 45%) about the seventh month, and then rising steadily to reach 95% at term. The change is

*The period immediately following parturition is known as the puerperium (Latin for childbirth).

brought about by the more rapid growth and weight increase of the hindquarters, which therefore sink, and by the restriction upon further change imposed by progressive reduction of the volume of amniotic fluid. The final posture of foals is even more strongly biased (99%) in favor of a head presentation. The advantages of this presentation are obvious. When labor begins, the contractions of the uterus tend to impel the extended forelimbs, and then the head and slender neck, into a birth canal already widened by a wedge of fluid-distended fetal membranes; the bulkier trunk and hindquarters eventually follow. In its final passage to the exterior, the fetus rotates about its own long axis so that its back, previously directed toward its mother's belly, comes to lie uppermost. This is not the result of a fetal initiative but is the passive consequence of the curvature and dimensions of the birth canal.

In polytocous species the fore- and hindquarters are more nearly equal and the advantage of a head presentation is less. The proportion of fetuses delivered "headfirst" varies among these species, and according to different reports, but is of the order of 60% to 80%. As each fetus is delivered from a uterine horn the emptied part contracts, bringing those left behind closer to the exit.

In the dog and cat, the fetal membranes are delivered with the neonate, to which they remain joined by the intact umbilical cord. Detachment is achieved by the mother biting through the cord, following, or in cats often preceding, her consumption of the membranes. In the larger species the cord tends to be ruptured in the course of parturition and the membranes remain in place for a time before they are expelled as the "afterbirth." In cows, their expulsion sometimes does not occur spontaneously and the decomposing fetal component of the placenta must then be separated from the uterine caruncles and removed by human intervention.

Following parturition, the organs tend to return to their former state, although the first pregnancy generally leaves a permanent legacy in increased size and thickening of the entire tract, loss of virgin symmetry, and, frequently, damage to the cervix and vulva. The stretched uterine wall contracts directly after delivery. The organ loses much of the weight gain of pregnancy within a few days of birth. Although involution then slows, it may continue until the uterus is temporarily smaller than its usual size while lactation continues (superinvolution).

It is difficult to separate aging changes from those of repeated pregnancy in animals that have led active reproductive lives. The tract of older animals is often marked by its larger size, greater toughness, asymmetry, endometrial staining (due to diapedesis of blood when hyperemic), more coiled and more prominent arteries, and evidence of cervical and vulvar trauma. Although ovaries do not sustain injury in pregnancy, they are often distorted in age, and many older animals have adventitious adhesions between the ovaries and their peritoneal supports.

Before concluding this section and chapter, a few sentences may be devoted to the status of the newborn, which exhibits interspecific differences that are both striking and important. Neonates of so-called precocial species possess a remarkable ability to fend for themselves more or less at once (Plate 10/*A,B*), while those of altricial species are initially much more reliant upon maternal care and the warmth and protection of a nest (/*C,D*). The young of the ungulate orders—both perissodactyls and artiodactyls—are generally precocial, those of carnivores and primates, including human infants, are predominately less developed. Young rodents are divided between the two categories; those like rats (myomorphs) are born naked, unable to maintain body temperature independently, barely capable of struggling to reach the dam's teats, and have their eyelids joined and external ear canals closed by epithelial fusion; in contrast, guinea pigs and their close relatives (caviomorphs) are born fully haired, mobile, equipped with vision and hearing, and have the ability to seek and ingest solid food within hours of being born (although they may take milk during the first 2 or 3 weeks) (/*B,D*). The differences among domestic species are significant if less extreme. Foals, like most newborn ungulates, are able to stand and attend their mothers almost at once; their skeletons are well developed with most secondary ossification centers not only present but well advanced in modeling toward their adult form; relatively efficient locomotor coordination allows them to follow the herd or flock within a short time (/*A*). Kittens and puppies, on the other hand, have skeletons that are less mature, with many ossification centers yet to make their appearance (Plate 10/*E–G*); the forelimb musculature is sufficiently developed and controlled to enable them to scramble toward the teats, but that of the hindlimbs is less competent and contributes little to this progress; the development of the sense organs is somewhat retarded and the eyelids do not part until the 10th day or shortly thereafter (/*C*). These differences in neonatal status are gradually "ironed out" and most mammals—ourselves excluded—show comparable maturity by the end of the usual lactation period.

CHAPTER 6

# The Endocrine Glands

The endocrine or ductless glands are those that deliver their secretory products (hormones) into the blood, lymph, or tissue fluid, which transports them to the target organs susceptible to the instructions these products represent. Each gland has its particular and distinctive function; collectively, they collaborate with the nervous system in maintaining the internal environment and securing the appropriate general and specific responses to stimuli from both external and internal sources. Unlike the actions of the nervous system, those of the hormones tend to be slower in taking effect but of longer duration.

The study of the anatomy of the glands, the production and the chemistry of the hormones, the responses of the target organs, and the complicated interplay of the various endocrine tissues with each other and with the nervous system is entitled endocrinology. Endocrinology is one of the most important and currently most active branches of biology and, since derangements are common in clinical medicine, its significance is not to be measured by the brevity of this chapter, which is essentially concerned with the gross anatomy of the glands.

Some writers regard these organs as together constituting an "endocrine system." Though there is no serious objection to this practice, it must be appreciated that the components, unlike those of other body systems, are scattered, achieve no physical continuity, and have very diverse embryological origins. They are united only by their general subservience to the central nervous system (hypothalamus) and by the similar patterns of their government of other organs and by some common features of structure; these comprise the epithelioid character of the secretory cells, the absence of drainage ducts, the sparse supporting frameworks, the generous vascularity, and the intimate association with blood vascular or other transport media (Fig. 6–1).

Three types of endocrine organ may be recognized pragmatically. The first comprises the few discrete organs of a primary endocrine nature: the hypophysis, the epiphysis, and the thyroid, parathyroid, and adrenal glands. The second comprises those organs that combine major endocrine with other important related functions: the pancreas, testes, ovaries, and placenta. The last comprises organs with a quite different primary function but which include an unobtrusive endocrine component; the kidneys, liver, thymus, heart, and the gastrointestinal tract are the best examples.

The existing knowledge of endocrine functions has been obtained in part from observation of human and animal patients with derangements of these glands, in part from experimental studies. Although much remains to be discovered, it is already clear that notable species differences exist.

## THE HYPOPHYSIS

The hypophysis or pituitary gland is sometimes described as the master endocrine organ since it produces certain hormones that directly influence the activities of other endocrine glands. Its location as an appendage of the brain also points to its significance as the relay between the nervous and humoral mechanisms that jointly control certain functions.

The hypophysis is a dark ellipsoidal body measuring about $1 \times 0.75 \times 0.5$ cm in the medium-sized dog. It is suspended below the hypothalamus by a narrow, fragile stalk and is received into a depression (hypophysial fossa) of the cranial floor that is defined by rostral and caudal crests of bone. A covering of dura directly invests the gland and also roofs the depression, extending from its margins to embrace and confine the hypophysial stalk from all sides; this arrangement (diaphragma sellae) makes it exceedingly difficult to remove the brain at autopsy with the hypophysis attached.

Certain other features of topography have a clinical or experimental interest. A large venous channel (cavernous sinus) to each side of the hypophysis provides a longitudinal connection between the ophthalmic plexus (and thus the veins of the face) rostrally, and the external jugular vein and vertebral venous plexus caudally (p. 304); transverse (intercavernous) sinuses rostral and caudal to the gland complete an encircling venous ring. The internal carotid artery (or the emissary vessel from the rete mirabile that replaces this in the cat, ruminants, and pig [p. 302]) runs through the cavernous sinus to join the arterial circle below

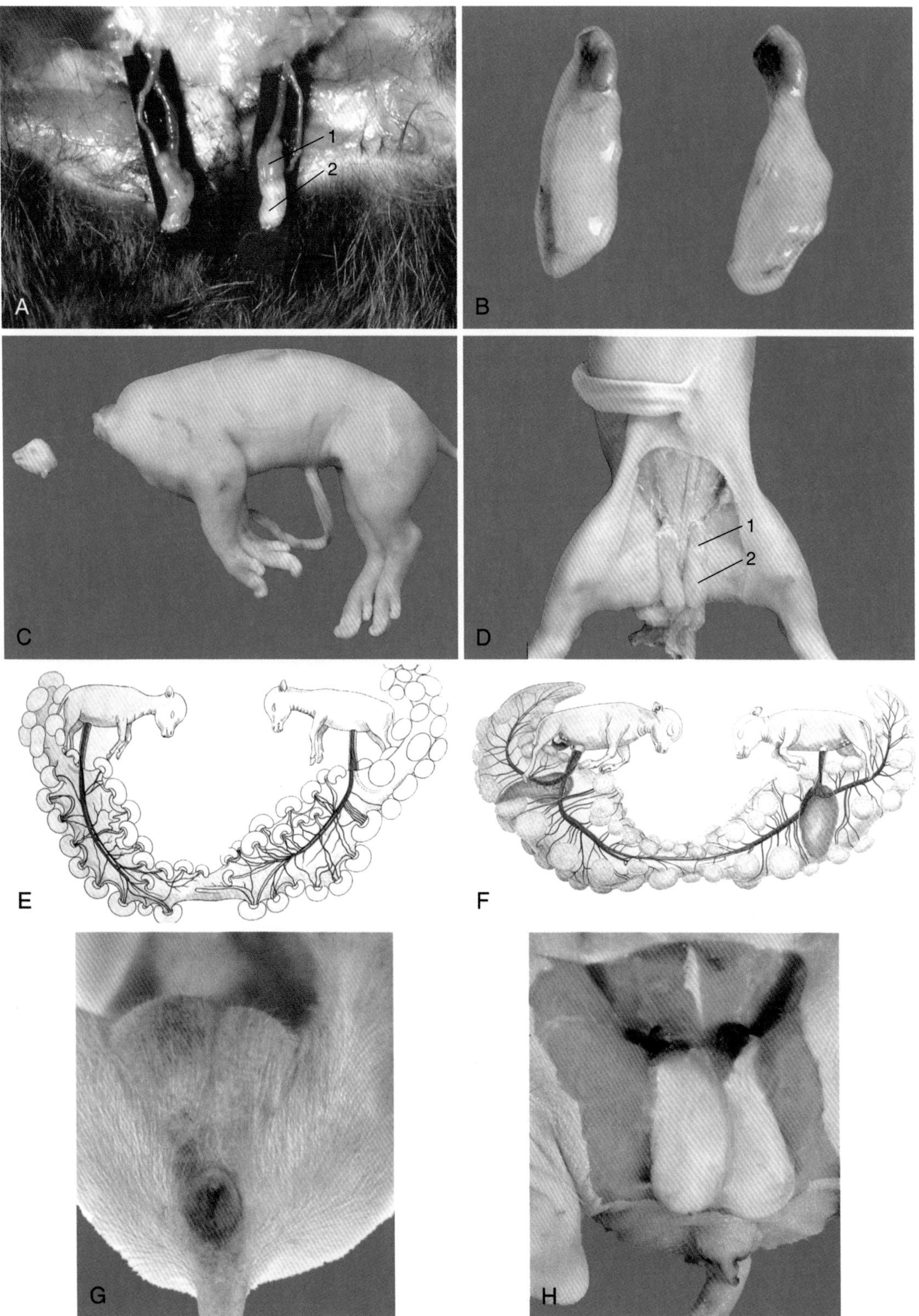


**Plate 5.** *A,* Inguinal area of newborn pup: 1, testis; 2, exposed gubernaculum. *B,* Testes and gubernacula of pig fetus (110 days). *C,* Pig fetus (near term), decapitated in utero at 42 days. *D,* Fetus shown in *C* with inguinal area dissected to show gubernacula unaffected by removal of pituitary gland: 1, testis; 2, gubernaculum. *E,* Twin ovine pregnancy showing separate circulations. *F,* Twin bovine pregnancy showing conjoined circulations (freemartin development possible). *G,* Freemartin (genetically female) piglet at day 0: gubernacular outgrowth. *H,* Gubernacula of *G* exposed.

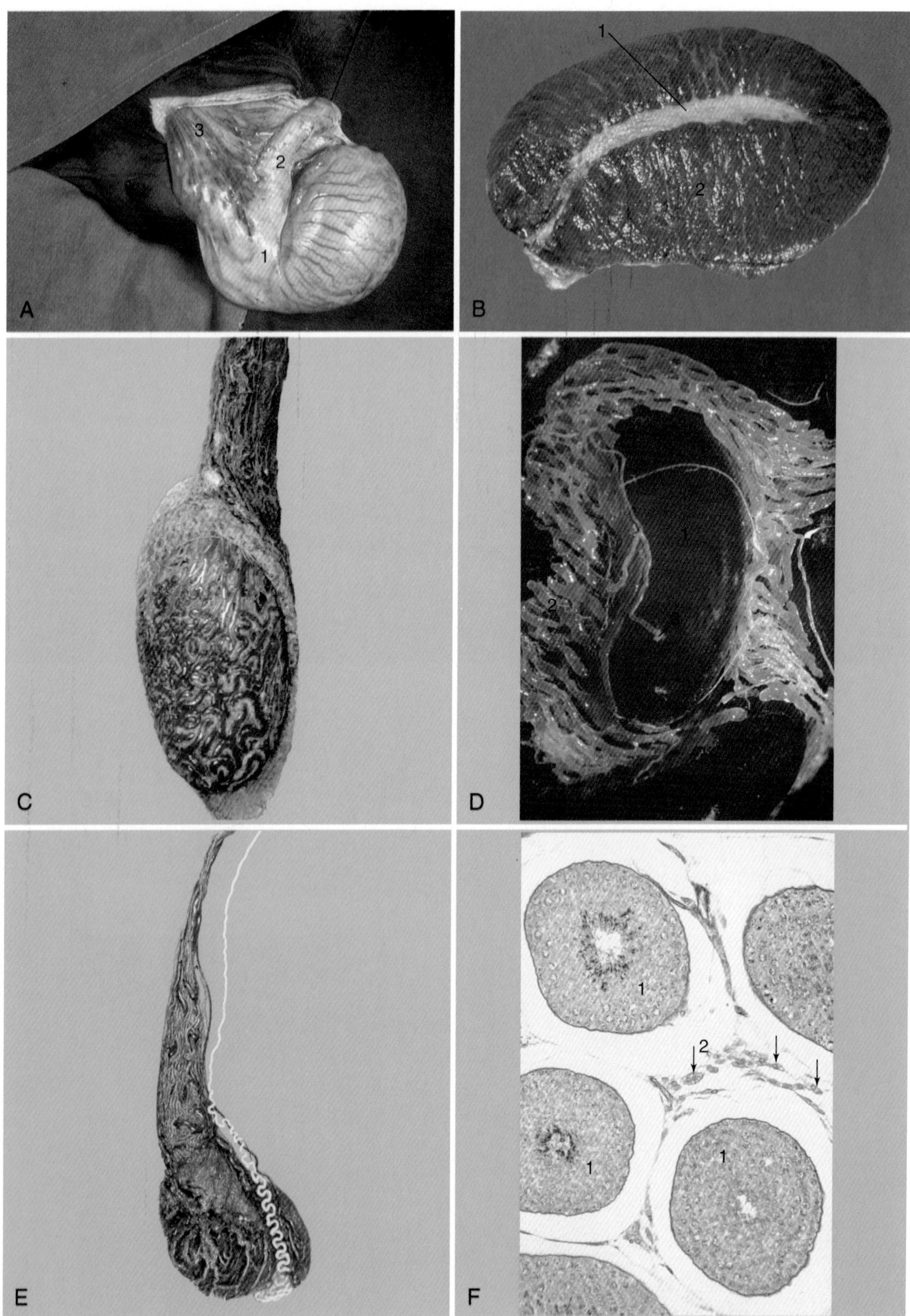


**Plate 6.** *A*, Testis (horse): 1, head of epididymis; 2, body of epididymis; 3, pampiniform plexus. *B*, Median section of testis (bull): 1, rete testis; 2, testicular parenchyma. *C*, Corrosion of cast of vessels within testis and of pampiniform plexus (bull). *D*, Corrosion cast of testicular a.: 1, coil of artery; 2, pampiniform plexus; 3, a-v anastomosis (plexus filled via this anastomosis). *E*, Corrosion cast (dog) of testicular a. (red), pampiniform plexus (blue), and deferent duct (yellow). *F*, Testis (dog) (140×): 1, seminiferous tubules (showing spermatogenesis); 2, interstitial tissue with androgen-producing (Leydig) cells *(arrows)*.

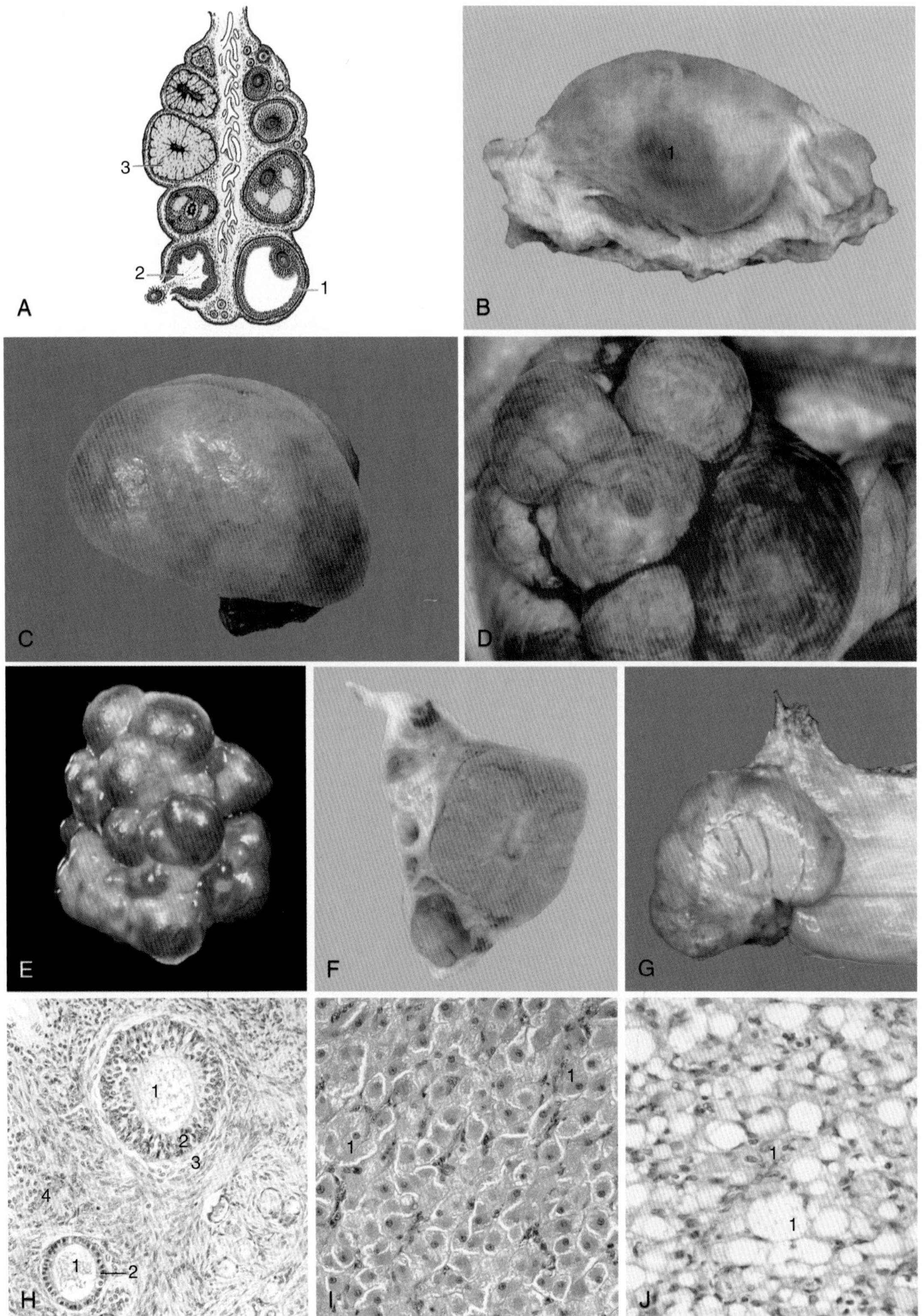


**Plate 7.** *A,* Schematic representation of ovarian activity: 1, mature follicle; 2, ruptured follicle; 3, corpus luteum (see text Fig. 5–44). *B,* Ovary (cow): 1, mature follicle. *C,* Ovary (bitch). *D,* Ovary (bitch) exhibiting several mature follicles. *E,* Ovary (sow) exhibiting mature follicles. *F,* Section of ovary (cow) containing a large corpus luteum. *G,* Ovary (mare), with ovulation fossa. *H,* Ovary (bitch) in anestrus with preantral follicles (140×): 1, oocyte; 2, granulosa cells; 3, theca cells; 4, stroma. *I,* Active corpus luteum (queen) (140×): 1, luteal cells. *J,* Inactive corpus luteum (queen) (140×): 1, luteal cells.

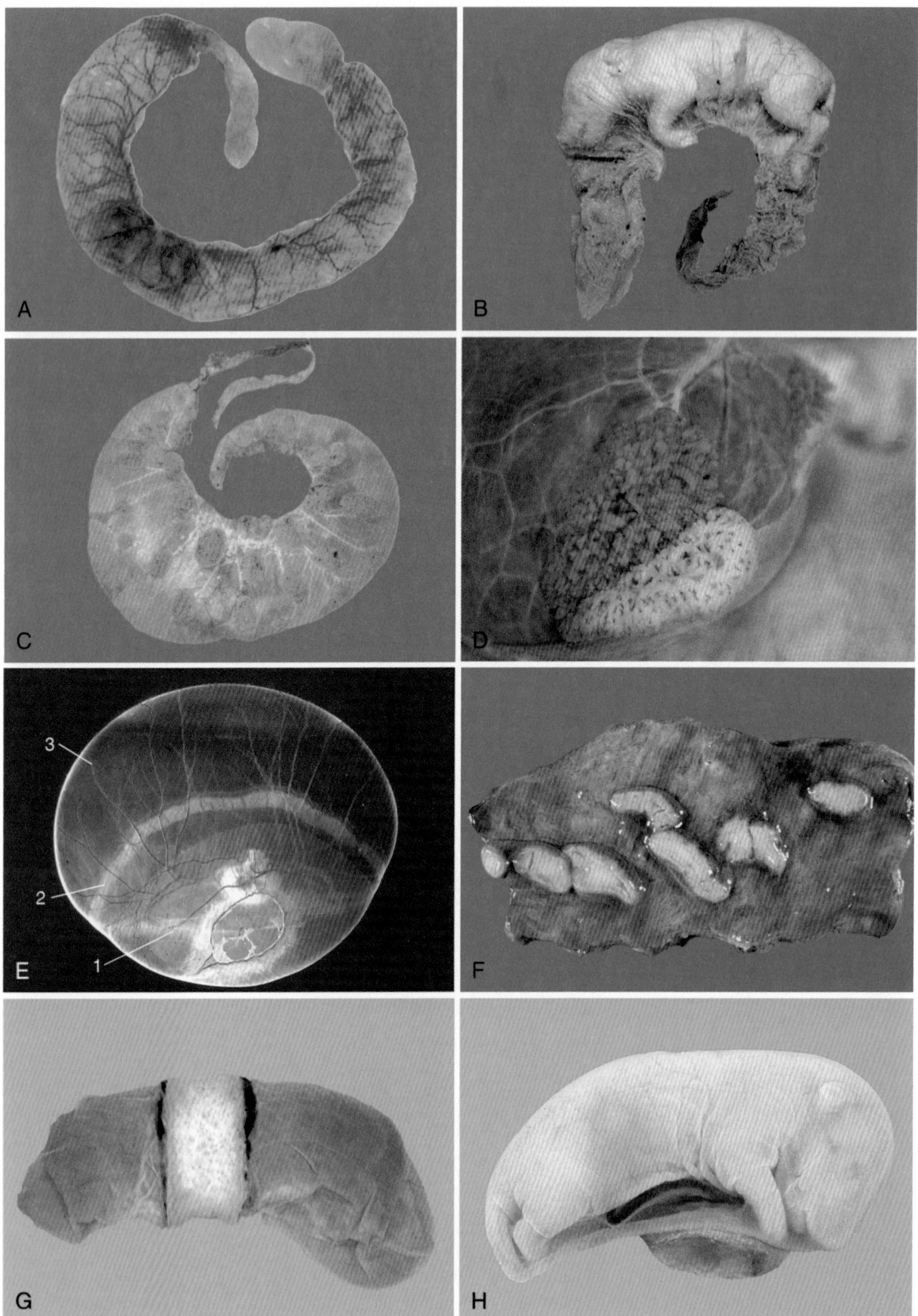


**Plate 8.** *A,* Chorionic sac (pig), with nonvascularized tips; the embryo is within the amniotic sac (blue injected). *B,* Pig fetus near term, surrounded by fetal membranes. *C,* Cotyledonary placenta (ruminant). *D,* Partial separation of maternal and fetal parts of placentome (cow). *E,* Young conceptus (horse): 1, yolk sac; 2, chorionic girdle; 3, allantochorion. *F,* Endometrial cups (mare) during early pregnancy. *G,* Zonary placenta (carnivores). *H,* Discoidal placenta (rat).

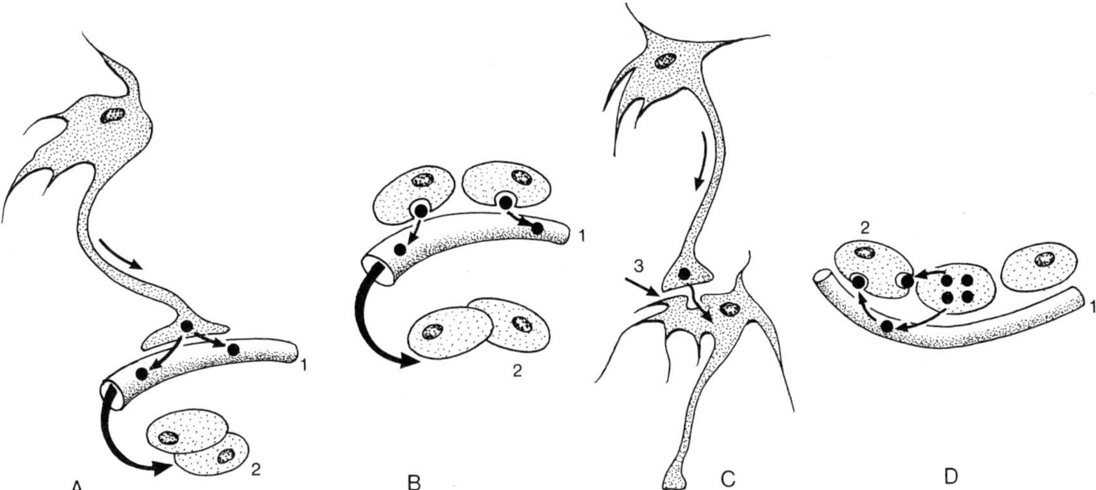


**Figure 6–1.** Illustrates and names the various ways in which hormones reach their targets. *A,* Neuroendocrine; *B,* endocrine; *C,* neurotransmitter, neuromodulator (action on postsynaptic membrane); *D,* paracrine (localized hormone action).

1, Blood stream; 2, target cell; 3, synapse.

the brain. The optic chiasm is directly rostral to the hypophysis (see Fig. 8–22/24, 21) while laterally, flanking the cavernous sinus, are the cranial nerves that supply the adnexa of the eye (the oculomotor, trochlear, ophthalmic, and abducent nerves). Physiological increase in the size of the hypophysis, which occurs in pregnancy, or pathological growth may exert pressure on these structures—especially on the optic nerves. Specific features in topography affect both the manner of expansion and the most convenient surgical approach. This is made via the nose and the sphenoidal sinus (within the cranial base, rostroventral to the hypophysial fossa) in human patients but more directly from below, via mouth, pharynx, and sphenoid in the dog. A temporal approach has been used in the pig.

Although the hypophysis appears to be a solid unitary organ, it comprises parts of very different origin and function and includes certain spaces. One part, the neurohypophysis (posterior lobe), is formed by a downgrowth of the hypothalamus; the stalk that persists as the connection with the brain includes an extension of the third ventricle. The other part, the adenohypophysis (anterior lobe), is formed by an epithelial outgrowth of the roof of the developing mouth. It contains a flattened vestigial space, the hypophysial cleft; the tissue caudal to the cleft is directly applied to the neurohypophysis and is distinguished as the pars intermedia (intermediate lobe). The topographical relationships of the three "lobes" show some interspecific differences, but these need concern few readers (Fig. 6–2).

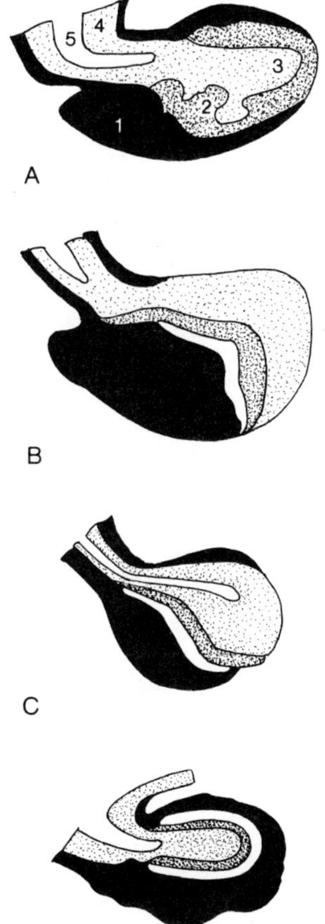


**Figure 6–2.** Median sections of the hypophysis of the horse *(A)*, ox *(B)*, pig *(C)*, and dog *(D)*. The rostral extremity of the gland is to the left.

1, Adenohypophysis; 2, intermediate part; 3, neurohypophysis; 4, hypophysial stalk; 5, recess of third ventricle.

The adenohypophysis produces several hormones commonly designated by acronyms: growth (somatotropic) hormone (STH); gonadotropic hormones—follicle-stimulating (FSH) and luteinizing (LH); adrenocorticotropic hormone (ACTH); thyroid-stimulating hormone (TSH); and prolactin. The intermediate part produces α-melanocyte–stimulating hormone (MSH). The production of all these is controlled by regulating, hypophysiotropic hormones, releasing or inhibitory factors such as gonadotropin-releasing hormone (GnRH), somatostatin (SS), growth hormone–releasing hormone (GRH), and corticotropin-releasing hormone (CRH), to name the most important. They are produced by neurosecretory cells in several hypothalamic nuclei, particularly the paraventricular nucleus, preoptic area, arcuate nucleus, and periventricular nucleus. These hormones are secreted from their axon terminals and are discharged into fenestrated capillaries within the median eminence (Fig. 8–66/6); these releasing and inhibitory hormones are conveyed to a sinusoidal network within the adenohypophysis (Fig. 6–3).

The hormones stored and later released into the circulation by the neurohypophysis include certain peptides, oxytocin and vasopressin. Oxytocin stimulates contraction of the smooth muscle of the uterus and of the myoepithelial cells of the udder. Vasopressin stimulates vasoconstriction and promotes fluid reabsorption by the kidneys. These substances are produced by magnocellular neurosecretory neurons within the supraoptic and paraventricular nuclei of the hypothalamus and are conveyed along the axons for direct release into the neurohypophysial capillary bed.

The adenohypophysis and neurohypophysis are separately vascularized. The latter is supplied by small branches from the internal carotid artery (or substitute vessel) and the arterial circle of the brain. The former is supplied indirectly; rostral hypophysial arteries, also from the internal carotid, expend themselves within the floor of the hypo-

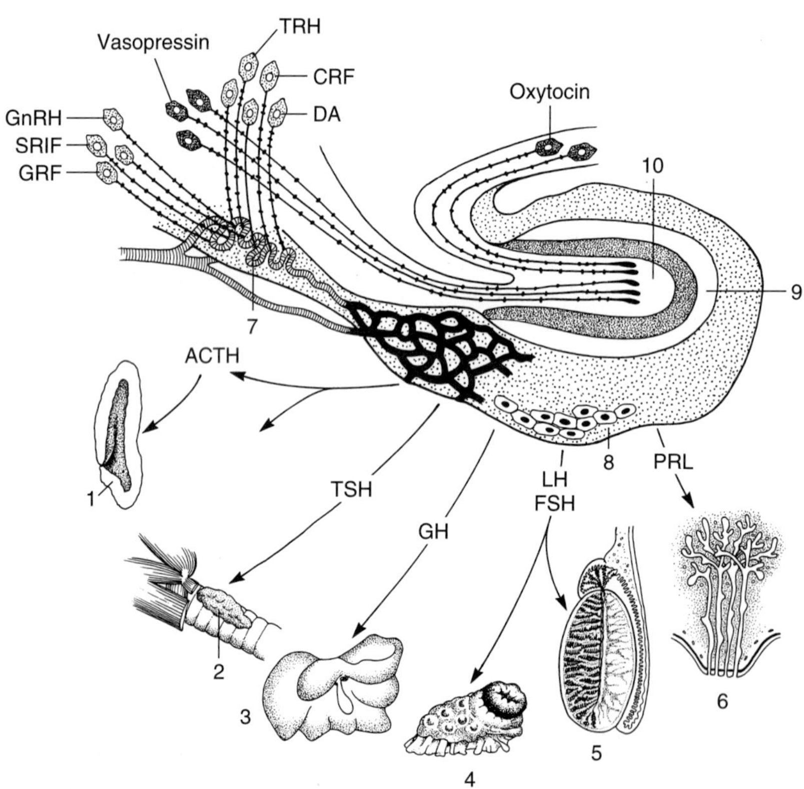


**Figure 6–3.** Organization of the brain-pituitary–peripheral organ axis.

1, Adrenal cortex; 2, thyroid; 3, liver; 4, ovary; 5, testis; 6, mammary gland; 7, median eminence; 8, anterior lobe of pituitary; 9, intermediate lobe of pituitary; 10, neural lobe of pituitary. TRH, thyroid-releasing hormone; CRF, corticotropin-releasing factor; DA, dopamine; GnRH, gonadotropin-releasing hormone; SRIF, somatotropin-release inhibiting factor; GRF, gonadotropin-releasing factor; ACTH, adrenocorticotropic hormone; TSH, thyroid-stimulating hormone; GH, growth hormone; LH, luteinizing hormone; FSH, follicle-stimulating hormone; PRL, prolactin.

thalamus whence the blood is conveyed through the stalk by a portal system of veins. The capillary network of the adenohypophysis subsequently drains into the cavernous sinus.

Certain regions of the brain, collectively known as the circumventricular organs (CVOs), are distinguished from other parts by their susceptibility to direct chemosensory stimulation by substances carried within the blood stream. They owe this distinction to the fenestration of perfusing capillaries which allows large molecules to exchange between the plasma and the extracellular milieu of the CVO, a possibility elsewhere excluded by the existence of the blood-brain barrier. The name given to the assembly emphasizes the proximity of the component regions to the system of ventricles within the brain, which suggests a role for the cerebrospinal fluid in the diffusion of the chemical messengers. The neurons within the different regions are of course able to communicate through synaptic connections in the usual way, but also allow CVOs to use neurohormonal mechanisms to influence peripheral function. The CVOs comprise the subfornical organ, the pineal body, the subcommissural organ, the area postrema, the posterior and intermediate lobes of the pituitary, the median eminence, and the vascular organ of the lamina terminalis (Fig. 8–66). It is difficult, if not impossible, to assign specific functions to different regions and it is perhaps sufficient to say that they are broadly concerned with homeostatic and autonomic function (feedback regulation), and with the provision of neuroendocrine mechanisms of peripheral effect dependent on the entry of substances, produced by neurons in certain circumventricular regions, into the fenestrated capillaries for diffusion within the general circulation.

## THE EPIPHYSIS

The epiphysis or pineal gland, named from the fancied resemblance of the human structure to a pine cone, is a small, darkly pigmented outgrowth from the dorsal aspect of the brain at the caudal end of the roof of the third ventricle and directly before the rostral colliculi (see Fig. 8–22/11). In certain species it is related to a large outpouching (epiphysial recess) of the pia-ependyma that roofs the ventricle. It is concealed between the cerebral hemispheres and cerebellum in the intact brain.

The epiphysis is solid but is not always homogeneous since foci of calcification ("brain sand") often develop with advancing age. Its functions were long obscure. It produces melatonin, an indolamine related to serotonin, which possesses an antigonadotropic circadian effect. The existence of this hormone was first postulated from the observation that tumors that destroy the secretory tissue are frequently associated with precocious puberty.

The driving endogenous circadian clock is located in the suprachiasmatic nucleus and its rhythm controls the rhythm of melatonin secretion by the pineal gland. Fine-tuning of this clock can be achieved by gradual changes in daylight, regulating both long-term (seasonal) and short-term (diurnal) variation in gonadal activity.

## THE THYROID GLAND

The thyroid gland lies on the trachea directly behind, and sometimes overlapping, the larynx. Its form varies greatly; in the dog and cat the gland consists of separate masses that are occasionally connected by an isthmus (Fig. 6–4/*A*); in the horse paired lobes are widely dissociated but connected by an insubstantial isthmus (/*B*); in cattle the lobes are connected by a wide isthmus of parenchymal tissue (/*C*); in small ruminants the isthmus is inconstant and when present is a mere connective tissue strand. In yet other species the thyroid has a more compact form and exhibits a relatively large median (pyramidal) lobe in addition to the lateral lobes. This arrangement, found in pigs and human subjects, provides a cover on the trachea that extends toward the thoracic inlet (/*D*); it explains the name given to the gland.*

The gland has its origin in a median outgrowth from the part of the pharyngeal floor that contributes to the tongue (p. 141). The primordium extends caudally on the ventral surface of the trachea before dividing at its apex into divergent processes that extend dorsolaterally to reach the boundary between the trachea and the esophagus (Fig. 6–5/2). In most mammals the connection with the developing tongue (thyroglossal duct) is never patent and it later regresses in its entirety.

The mature gland is enclosed within a connective tissue capsule that is loosely attached to neighboring organs. Its substance, generally brick-red, obtains a rather granular texture from the many enclosed follicles of which it is composed. In some species (e.g., cattle) these give the intact organ an irregular appearance, but in others (e.g., dog) the surface is quite smooth. The tissue is relatively firm, and this consistency, allied to the form, size, and location, enables the lobes to be identified in larger species by palpation caudal to the larynx. They are not palpable in the healthy dog.

*Greek, *thyreos,* a shield.

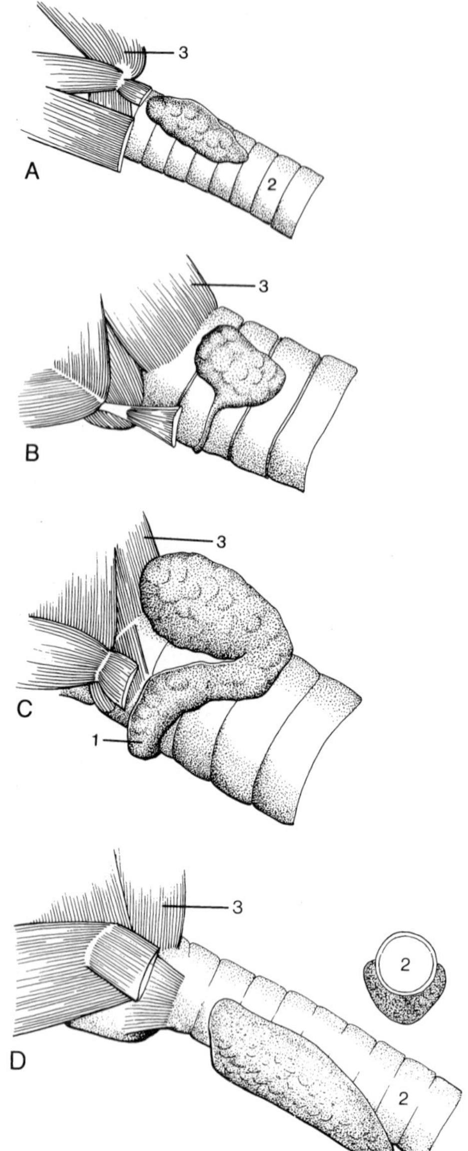


**Figure 6–4.** The thyroid gland of the dog *(A)*, horse *(B)*, cattle *(C)*, and pig *(D)*. The inset to *D* illustrates the subtracheal connection in transverse section in the pig.

1, Isthmus; 2, trachea; 3, cricopharyngeus.

The size of the thyroid gland varies greatly, depending to a great extent on the iodine content of the diet; when this content is deficient, enlargement (goiter) may develop, and in some parts of the world it is customary to add iodine to table salt as a preventive measure. In dogs the relative weight of the thyroid may vary by a factor of as much as six, although the increasing use of commercial foods (of uniform composition) now tends to reduce this variation. Average dimensions in medium-sized dogs are of the order of $6 \times 1.5 \times 0.5$ cm. Accessory masses of thyroid tissue are sometimes located along the cervical trachea and are occasionally carried into the thorax by the descending heart.

The gland is mainly supplied by the cranial thyroid artery, which arises from the common carotid artery and arches around the cranial pole. A subsidiary supply is occasionally provided by a caudal thyroid artery, which takes a more proximal origin. In the dog the two vessels are connected by a substantial anastomosis along the dorsal margin. The venous drainage is to the internal jugular vein. The glandular tissue receives both sympathetic and parasympathetic fibers, the former routed through the cranial cervical ganglia, the latter through the laryngeal branches of the vagus nerves. The fibers are predominantly vasomotor, and denervation has little effect on secretory activity.

The main lymph drainage of the thyroid in the dog proceeds to the cranial deep cervical nodes.

The thyroid hormones, concerned with metabolism and growth, are produced by the follicular cells that compose the bulk of the parenchyma. They are stored in the follicular fluid and later broken down to yield the final products, which are released into the blood stream.

A small portion of the parenchyma is provided by parafollicular (or C) cells. These appear to have their origin in the ultimobranchial bodies that derive from epithelial clusters of the fourth pharyngeal pouches that are invaded by neural crest cells (Fig. 6–5/8). C cells produce calcitonin, a hormone antagonistic to parathormone in some species. It also seems to play a role in fetal bone

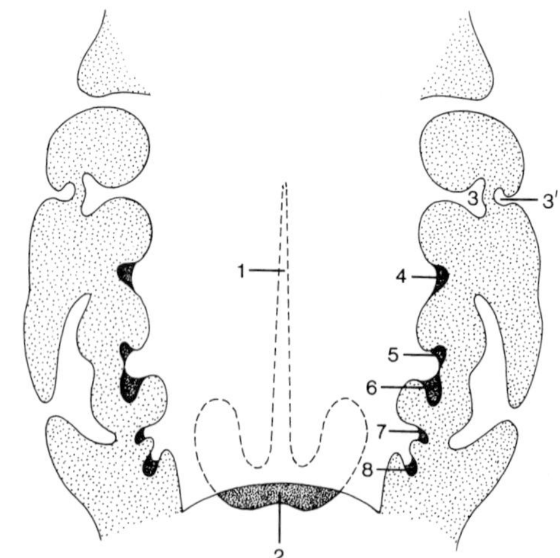


**Figure 6–5.** The pharyngeal primordia of certain endocrine structures; dorsal view, schematic.

1, Thyroglossal duct; 2, thyroid gland; 3, first pharyngeal pouch; 3′ external acoustic meatus; 4, palatine tonsil (second pouch); 5, parathyroid III; 6, thymus; 7, parathyroid IV; 8, ultimobranchial body.

growth and it protects the maternal skeleton against excessive demineralization.

## THE PARATHYROID GLANDS

Usually four parathyroid glands, small epithelial bodies located close to, or embedded within, the much larger thyroid, are present. The parathyroid glands also develop from the pharyngeal lining; one pair (parathyroids III or external parathyroid glands) comes from the third pharyngeal pouches, and the other (parathyroids IV or internal parathyroid glands) from the fourth pouches (/5,7). In the dog, cat, and small ruminants the parathyroid glands generally become recessed or embedded within the substance of the thyroid gland and frequently escape notice in routine dissections. Once exposed, they can be identified by their pale color, which contrasts with the thyroid tissue. In cattle and the horse they are usually located close to the thyroid gland.

The parathyroids III are carried down the neck by the developing thymus and come to rest at various levels, generally near the carotid bifurcations but much farther caudally in the horse (in which they may approach the thoracic inlet). They are also not always easily recognizable since they resemble small lymph nodes; however, they are paler and lack the smooth, glistening exterior of these. In the dog these glands are usually located at the rostral, in the cat at the caudal, end of the thyroid gland.

The parathyroid hormone (parathormone) plays a vital role in the regulation of various aspects of calcium metabolism: absorption from the gut, mobilization from the skeleton, and excretion in the urine. The production of the hormone is largely regulated by the calcium plasma concentration. The close relationship of the parathyroid glands to the thyroid points to the need for caution in thyroid surgery.

## THE ADRENAL GLANDS

The paired adrenal glands lie against the roof of the abdomen near the thoracolumbar junction. They are retroperitoneal and usually located craniomedial to the corresponding kidney (more directly medial in the horse). Although they obtain their name from this relationship, they are in fact more closely connected with the major vessels in the abdomen—the aorta on the left, caudal vena cava on the right—and they adhere to these when the kidneys shift from the accustomed positions (e.g., the left kidney of the ruminant; see p. 687).

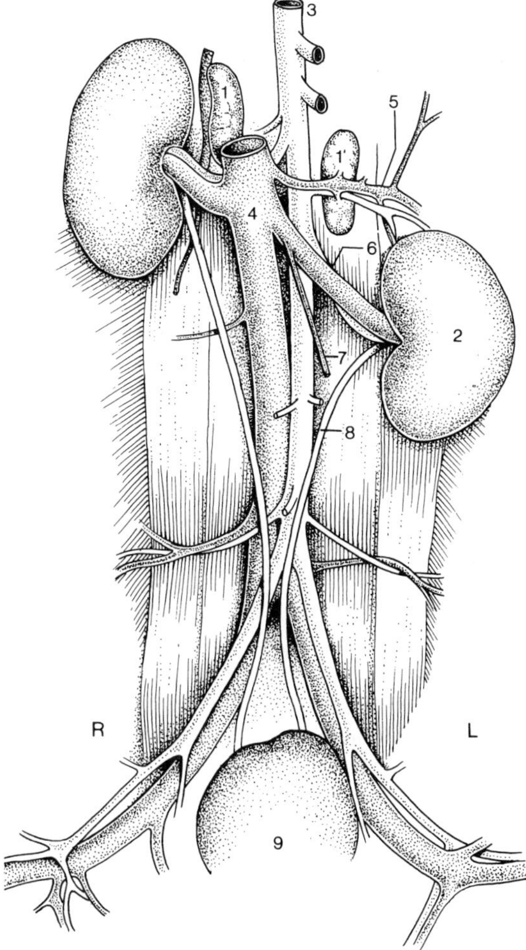


**Figure 6–6.** The topography of the canine adrenal glands.

1, 1′, Right and left adrenal glands; 2, left kidney; 3, aorta; 4, caudal vena cava; 5, phrenicoabdominal vessels; 6, renal vessels; 7, ovarian vein; 8, ureter; 9, bladder.

Although generally elongated, the glands are often asymmetrical and quite irregular, being molded upon neighboring vessels (Fig. 6–6/1). It is difficult to specify their size since this appears to be influenced by several factors; they are relatively larger in wild than in related domestic forms, in juvenile than in adult individuals, and in pregnant and lactating females than in those reproductively inactive. Those of a medium-sized dog commonly measure about 2.5 × 1 × 0.5 cm.

Adrenal glands are firm, solid bodies that fracture readily when flexed. The fractured (or sectioned) surface exposes the division of the interior into an outer cortex and an inner medulla. The cortex, covered by a fibrous capsule, is yellowish and radially striated; the much darker medulla has a more uniform appearance. The two parts also contrast in origin, in microscopic structure, and in function.

The cortex is mesodermal and derived from a patch of celomic epithelium close to the gonadal fold. On gross inspection, certain color changes vaguely suggest a subdivision into several concentric shells (zones) but these distinctions become clear only in microscopic preparations. The outer zone produces the mineralocorticoid hormone. The subjacent zones produce glucocorticoids and certain sex steroids.

The medulla is of ectodermal origin, being contributed by a parcel of the cells that migrate from the neural crest to provide the neurons of the peripheral sympathetic ganglia. The medullary cells produce the transmitter substances norepinephrine and epinephrine and thus share with the sympathetic nervous system in the control of the body's response ("flight or fight") to acute stress situations. These cells obtain the additional designation chromaffin from their marked affinity for the salts of chromium and other heavy metals.

The adrenal glands are variously but always generously vascularized by small branches from several neighboring trunks—the aorta and the renal, lumbar, phrenicoabdominal, and cranial mesenteric arteries. After perfusing the gland, the blood pools within a central vein from which emissary vessels lead through a hilus to join the caudal vena cava or a tributary. Though not easily found, fine nerves within the cortex subject the tissue to hypothalamic control. Nerve bundles are more readily demonstrated within the medulla; appropriately, these are predominantly sympathetic preganglionic fibers passing to the medullary cells, which are equivalent to sympathetic postganglionic neurons elsewhere.

Accessory masses of cortical and medullary tissue both occur. Those of cortical tissue may be incorporated within any of several organs but are most commonly found attached to the capsule of the adrenal gland itself. Accessory chromaffin cells form the bodies known as paraganglia, endocrine cell clusters particularly associated with sympathetic nerves; a prominent example is found within the plexus on the aorta, close to the origin of the cranial mesenteric artery. Similar clumps of nonchromaffin cells, usually assigned to the parasympathetic system, are best known from the carotid and aortic bodies (described in Chapter 7, p. 234).

## OTHER ENDOCRINE TISSUES

The other endocrine tissues are incorporated within organs of composite function. The most familiar example is provided by the endocrine component of the pancreas, the pancreatic islets, also known as the islets of Langerhans. The general anatomy of the pancreas has already been described (p. 138). The endocrine component comprises many hundred (or thousand) islets of varying size unevenly distributed among the predominant exocrine tissue. The islets are not normally visible to the naked eye, but the larger ones—of pinhead size—can be made apparent by the use of intravital dyes. The islet tissue has the same origin as the exocrine pancreas and buds from the epithelial cords at an early stage; it remains solid when the remainder of the "tree" canalizes.

The islet cells are of several types (the exact number is disputed); the two most numerous are the alpha and beta types, which produce glucagon and insulin, respectively. These hormones affect carbohydrate metabolism, their role being best known from the diabetes that develops when insufficient insulin is produced by the islet tissue. The pancreas is also the source of certain other hormones, including somatostatin and pancreatic polypeptide. Other less numerous cells manufacture gastrin; the distinction and functions of yet other types are in dispute. The relative frequencies of the different types are not the same in all parts of the pancreas, and some evidence exists that different ratios occur in the parts that originate from the dorsal and ventral primordia.

The endocrine components and functions of the testes (p. 184), ovaries (p. 200), and placenta (p. 207) were sufficiently mentioned in Chapter 5.

The endocrine components of other organs are even more discrete, and since they make no gross representation are not described. The most important examples are the renin-producing juxtaglomerular complexes within the kidney and the variety of enteroendocrine cells scattered within the gastric and intestinal epithelia (p. 131). The number, distinctions, and functions of the enteroendocrine cell types are inadequately known. Although mainly scattered singly, these cells are so numerous that they would constitute a considerable gland if massed together. They are considered to belong to the so-called APUD* cell system (now shown to be of endodermal origin, not neuroectodermal as formerly supposed) and are believed to produce gastrin, secretin, glucagon, vasoactive intestinal peptide, gastric inhibitory peptide, and several other hormones.

---

*An acronym for *a*mine *p*recursor *u*ptake and *d*ecarboxylation.

# CHAPTER 7

# The Cardiovascular System

The blood vascular and lymphatic systems are combined under a single heading, angiologia, in the official terminology. Angiology strictly means the study of vessels, but its scope is conveniently enlarged to include the heart, spleen, and various lymphatic organs in addition to the arteries, veins, and other vessels.

A circulatory system is essential to any organism that exceeds that relatively trivial size in which diffusion can deliver the metabolic fuel and other substances required by the tissues and convey away their products, whether waste for excretion or materials that are utilized elsewhere. Obviously, the critical mass must vary with the level of metabolic activity. It is soon reached in the rapidly growing mammalian embryo, in which the circulatory system, though not the first to be laid down, is the first body system to reach a "working state."

The circulatory organs and the blood cells have a common origin in clusters of mesenchymal cells that first appear in the wall of the yolk sac. The outermost cells of these "blood islets" flatten and become arranged as an endothelium that lines spaces in which the remaining cells, hemocytoblasts or stem blood cells, float within a fluid plasma. The islets first formed are soon supplemented by others that appear in the mesoderm of the chorioallantois and within the body of the embryo; as the various patches spread and link up they form a diffuse system of connecting vessels that is then extended further by branching from existing channels. The principal vessels thus form independently of each other and in relation to the appearance and growth of the regions and organs of the embryo.

Since no proper circulation through this system can occur until a means of pumping blood is created, the heart necessarily makes a very early appearance. It is formed by differentiation of channels within a part of the mesoderm appropriately known as the cardiogenic area. This area lies in front of the oral membrane of the discoidal embryo, and the heart rudiments are related from the outset to the most rostral of the tissue spaces that later coalesce to form the celomic cavity, which divides the somatopleure from the splanchnopleure. The cardiogenic area, including both heart and pericardial rudiments, becomes folded ventrally and carried caudally in the process that converts the embryonic disc into a cylindrical body (p. 100). At this stage the heart consists of paired endothelial (endocardial) tubes placed ventral to the foregut, but these shortly fuse to form a single median organ that gradually shifts caudally to the level of the thoracic somites (Fig. 7–1/5,7).

The heart is from the beginning connected at one extremity with the vessels that become the aorta and at the other with those that form three sets of veins: the vitelline (omphalomesenteric) veins that drain the yolk sac, the umbilical veins that drain the chorioallantoic placenta, and the cardinal veins that drain the body. The ventral aorta, continuous with the heart, is soon joined to an independently formed dorsal aorta by a system of aortic loops contained within the pharyngeal (branchial) arches lateral to the pharynx (Fig. 7–2). It is possible to trace the origin of certain arteries of adult anatomy from the six pairs of aortic arches that develop (although not all persist), but the reader must refer to textbooks of embryology for details of this process and for a description of the even more complicated evolution of the veins. The reader is reminded that a hallmark of the developing circulatory system is its ability to respond to changing functional requirements by refashioning the pattern of vessels, always retaining obsolescent parts until their replacements have become operative.

Descriptions of the development of the heart itself (p. 228), and of the particularly dramatic changes that occur in the circulation at birth (p. 249) are found later in this chapter.

## THE HEART

The heart (cor) is the central organ that by rhythmic contraction pumps blood continuously through the blood vessels. In the adult it consists of four chambers: right atrium, left atrium, right ventricle, and left ventricle (Fig. 7–3). The two atria are separated by an internal septum as are the

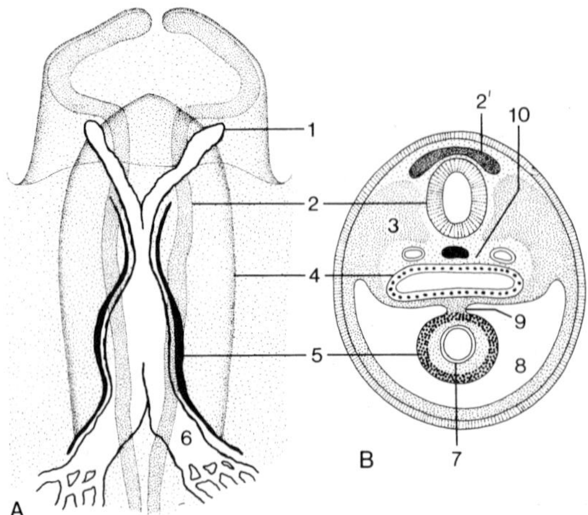


**Figure 7–1.** *A,* Ventral view of the cranial part of a 15-day-old pig embryo after fusion of the endocardial tube. *B,* Transverse section of a seven- to eight-somite embryo taken at the level of 5.

1, First aortic arch; 2, neural tube; 2′, neural crest; 3, somite; 4, foregut; 5, epimyocardial wall of the fused endocardial tubes; 6, vitelline vein; 7, endocardial tube; 8, pericardial cavity; 9, dorsal mesocardium; 10, notochord and dorsal aortae.

two ventricles, but the atrium and ventricle of each side communicate through a large opening. The heart thus consists of two pumps that are arranged in series but combined within a single organ. The right pump receives deoxygenated ("venous") blood from the body and ejects it into the pulmonary trunk, which carries it to the lungs for reoxygenation; the left pump receives the oxygenated ("arterial") blood from the lungs and ejects it into the aorta, which distributes it once more to the body (Fig. 7–4).

The size of the heart varies considerably among species and also among individuals; as a rule it is relatively larger in smaller species and in smaller individuals, but it may become markedly hypertrophied by hard training. As a rough guide it may be said to provide about 0.75% of the body weight, less in lethargic animals, considerably more in those renowned athletes—the Thoroughbred horse and racing Greyhound.

The construction, the form, and the general position of the heart are similar in all mammals and, as most differences in the first two have only theoretical implications, they receive little attention. Differences in topography do have practical importance since they modify the methods used for clinical examination and the interpretation of the evidence that this examination provides; these points are mentioned in later chapters.

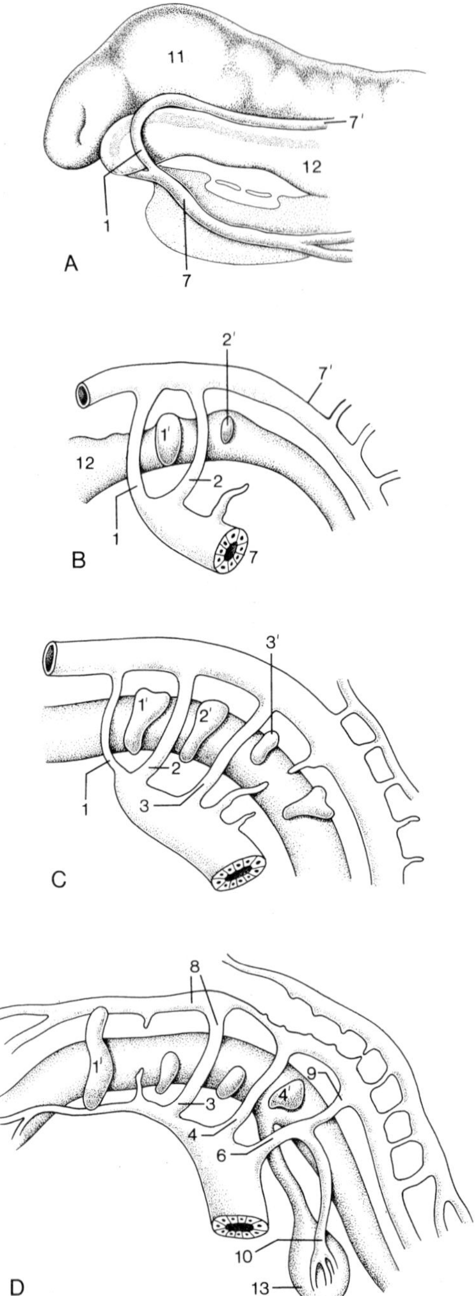


**Figure 7–2.** Left lateral view of the aortic arches and their transformation. *A,* Dorsal and ventral aortae are connected by the first aortic arches. *B,* First and second aortic arches are present. *C,* The first arch begins to disappear, the third is complete, and the fourth and sixth develop. *D,* The third arch and the cranial part of the dorsal aorta are now transformed into the internal carotid artery, while the sixth gives rise to the pulmonary trunk and ductus arteriosus.

1–4, 6, Aortic arches; 1′–4′, pharyngeal pouches; 7, 7′, ventral and dorsal aortae; 8, internal carotid artery; 9, ductus arteriosus; 10, left pulmonary artery; 11, brain vesicle; 12, foregut; 13, lung bud.

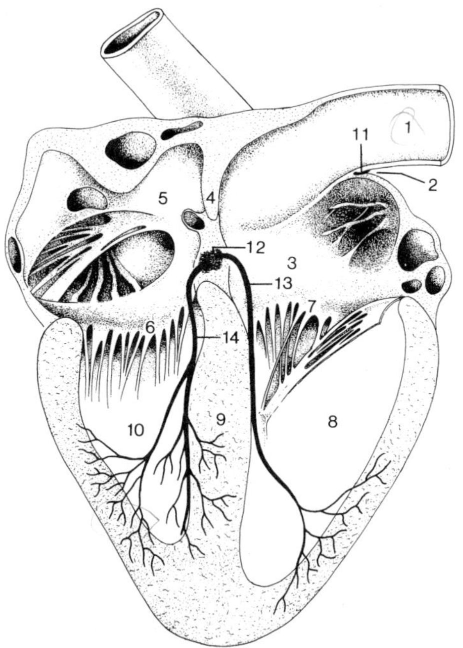


**Figure 7–3.** Section of the heart exposing the four chambers.

1, Cranial vena cava; 2, terminal sulcus; 3, right atrium; 4, interatrial septum; 5, left atrium; 6, left atrioventricular valve; 7, right atrioventricular valve; 8, right ventricle; 9, interventricular septum; 10, left ventricle; 11, sinuatrial node; 12, atrioventricular node; 13, 14, right and left limbs of atrioventricular bundle.

## The Pericardium and the Topography of the Heart

The heart is almost completely invested by the pericardium, which fits snugly about it (Fig. 7–5). The pericardium is essentially a closed serous sac that is so deeply invaginated by the heart that its lumen is reduced to a mere capillary cleft (/4). The space contains serous fluid, normally just sufficient in amount to allow easy movement of the heart wall against its covering. The visceral and parietal layers of the pericardium continue into each other at a complicated reflection that runs over the atria and the roots of the great vessels. The visceral layer is so closely adherent to the heart wall that it may be described as a component of this, the epicardium. The parietal layer obtains a thick external fibrous covering (/6) that blends with the adventitia of the great vessels dorsally and continues into a ligament at the ventral apex of the sac. This usually attaches to the sternum (*sternopericardial ligament;* /8) but attaches to the diaphragm *(phrenicopericardial ligament)* in species in which the heart axis is more oblique. These attachments place a severe restraint on the mobility of the heart, although slight movement does occur with each respiratory excursion.

Although the pericardium distorts to accommodate the changing form of the heart during the cardiac cycle, its fibrous component prevents any significant distention in the short term. It may stretch over longer periods should the heart become enlarged by exercise or disease or should effusion or pus collect within the pericardial cavity.

The heart (within the pericardium)* is included within the mediastinum, the partition that separates the right and left pleural cavities (see Fig. 4–19/*A*). It is conical and is placed asymmetrically within the thorax with the larger part (say 60%) lying to the left of the median plane (see Figs. 13–8 and 20–9). The base is dorsal and reaches approxi-

*This qualification, necessary for strict accuracy, may be assumed in later references to the relations of the heart.

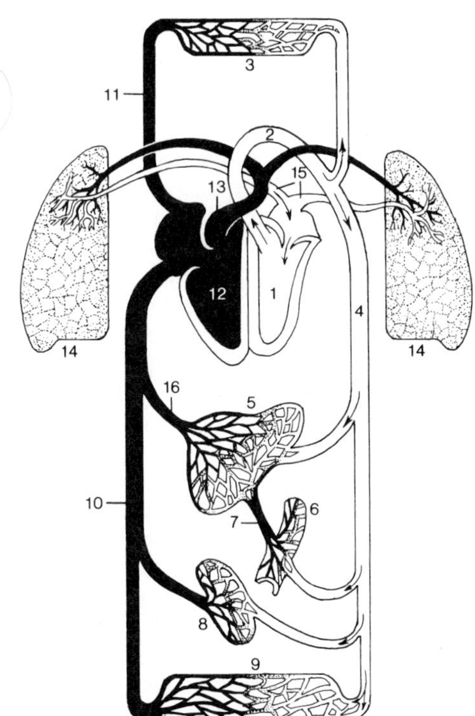


**Figure 7–4.** Schematic drawing of the systemic and pulmonary circulation.

1, Left ventricle; 2, aorta; 3, capillary bed of head, neck, and forelimb; 4, abdominal aorta; 5, liver; 6, capillary bed of intestines; 7, portal vein; 8, capillary bed of kidneys; 9, capillary bed of caudal part of the body; 10, caudal vena cava; 11, cranial vena cava; 12, right ventricle; 13, pulmonary trunk; 14, capillary bed of lungs; 15, pulmonary vein; 16, hepatic veins.

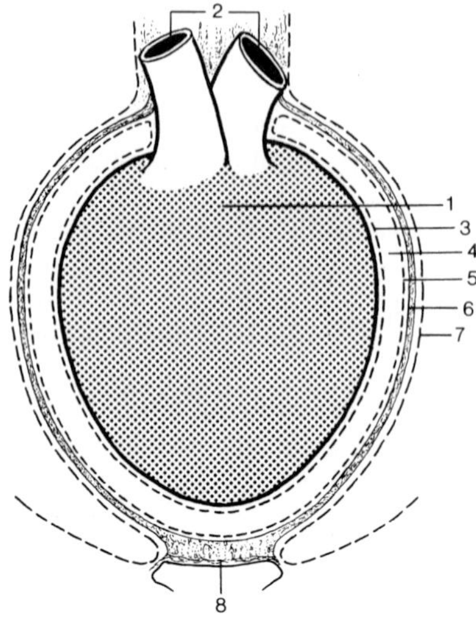


**Figure 7–5.** Schematic illustration of the pericardium.

1, Heart; 2, great vessels; 3, visceral pericardium (epicardium); 4, pericardial cavity (exaggerated in size); 5, parietal pericardium; 6, connective tissue layer of the parietal pericardium; 7, mediastinal pleura; 8, sternopericardial ligament.

mately to the horizontal (dorsal) plane that bisects the first rib; in some species (e.g., dog) it is tilted in varying degree to face craniodorsally. The apex is placed close to the sternum, opposite the sixth costal cartilage. The long axis that joins the center of the base to the apex thus slopes caudoventrally, with some deviation to the left imposed by the skewed orientation (Fig. 7–6). The projection of the heart on the chest wall extends between the third and sixth ribs (or thereabouts); it follows that much of the heart is under cover of the forelimbs, a considerable handicap to clinical examination, especially in larger species (see Figs. 20–2 and 27–1).

Although generally conical, the heart displays some lateral compression to conform to the similar compression of the thorax of most quadrupeds. This better defines right and left surfaces that face toward the corresponding lungs, which are shaped to fit. The cardiac notch in the ventral border of each lung allows the heart a restricted contact with the chest wall, which is normally greater on the left side because of the asymmetrical position (see Fig. 13–4). Each lateral surface is also crossed by the corresponding phrenic nerve. The cranial aspect is extensively related to the thymus (in the young animal) while the caudal surface faces toward the diaphragm and may be indirectly related through this to cranial abdominal organs (see Plate 29/*B*)—a point of importance in certain species (p. 662).

## General Anatomy of the Heart

The base of the heart is formed by the thin-walled atria, which are clearly separated from the ventricles by an encircling *coronary groove* that contains the main trunks of the coronary vessels within a concealment of fat. The right and left atria combine in a continuous U-shaped formation that embraces the origin of the aorta; the formation is interrupted craniosinistrally where each atrium ends in a free blind appendage, the auricle (Fig. 7–7/*A*,6,3), which overlaps the origin of the

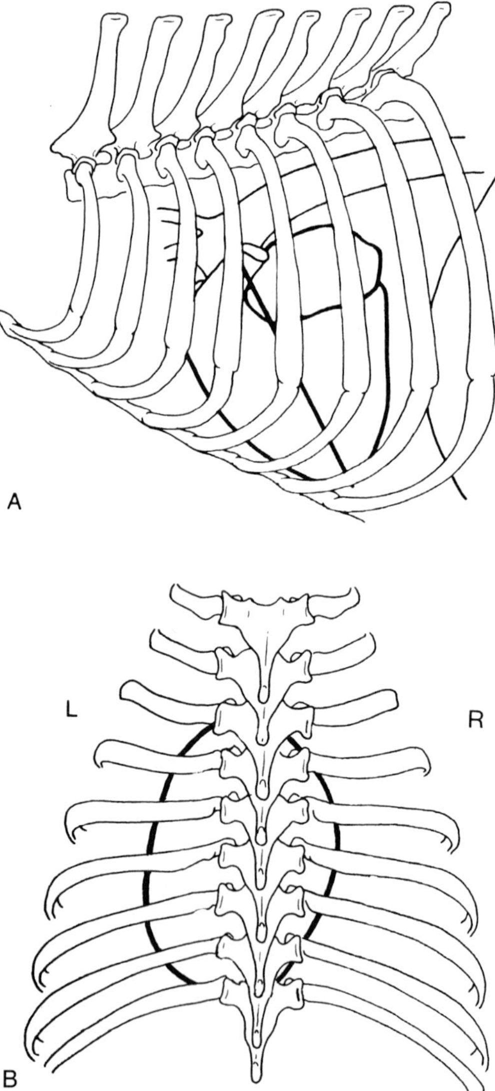


**Figure 7–6.** Schematic drawings to show the position of the canine heart, based on radiographs. *A*, Left lateral view; the caudoventrally sloping long axis *(straight line)* of the heart is indicated. *B*, Dorsoventral view showing the asymmetrical position of the heart.

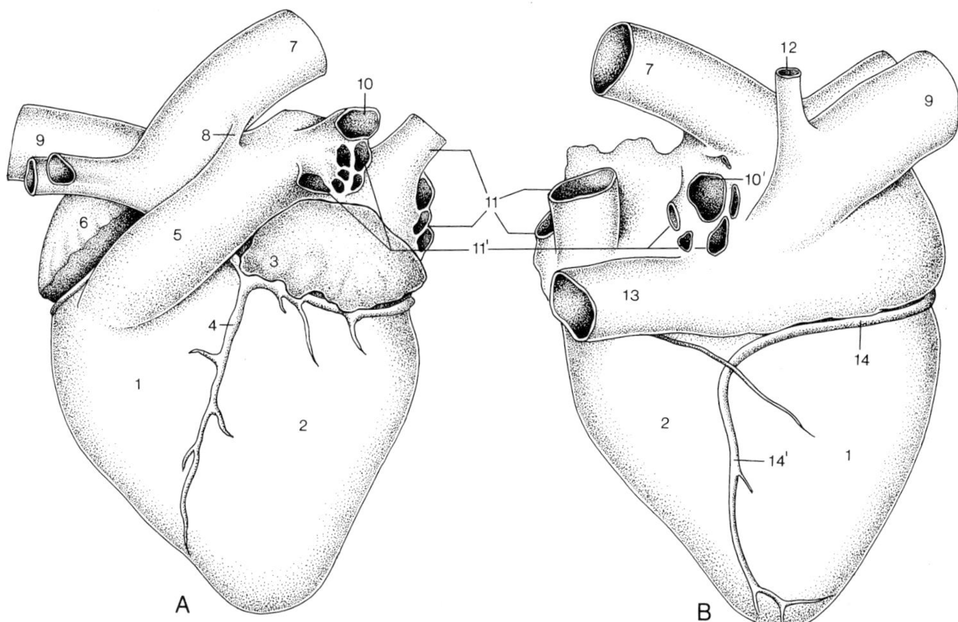


**Figure 7–7.** Left *(A)* and right *(B)* views of the equine heart.

1, Right ventricle; 2, left ventricle; 3, left auricle; 4, paraconal interventricular branch of left coronary artery; 5, pulmonary trunk; 6, right auricle; 7, aorta; 8, ligamentum arteriosum; 9, cranial vena cava; 10, 10′, left and right pulmonary arteries; 11, 11′, left and right pulmonary veins; 12, right azygous vein; 13, caudal vena cava; 14, right coronary artery; 14′, subsinuosal interventricular branch of right coronary artery.

pulmonary trunk. The margins of the atria are often crenated.

The ventricles provide a much larger part of the heart that is also much firmer because of the greater thickness of the walls. Although the ventricles merge externally, their separate extents are defined by shallow grooves that descend toward the apex. The *paraconal (left) groove* runs close to the cranial aspect of the heart (/*A*,4); the *subsinuosal (right) groove* runs close to the caudal aspect (/*B*,14′); both convey substantial vessels that follow the edges of the interventricular septum and together they reveal the asymmetrical disposition of the ventricles. The right chamber lies as much cranially as to the right of the left one (Fig. 7–10). Additional branches of the coronary vessels extend some distance over the ventricular surface in a less constant pattern but, these apart, the external surface is smooth and featureless. Although it is not apparent externally, a fibrous skeleton separates the atrial from the ventricular muscle mass.

## The Right Atrium

This chamber lies mainly on the right although the auricular cul-de-sac extends to the cranial face of the pulmonary trunk to appear on the left side. The greater part forms a chamber (sinus venarum) into which the principal systemic veins discharge (Fig. 7–8/1). The caudal vena cava enters the caudodorsal part of this chamber, above the opening of the much smaller vein (*coronary sinus;* /7) that drains the heart itself. The cranial vena cava opens craniodorsally at the *terminal crest* (/8). An azygous vein enters variously; when a *right azygous* is present (as in the horse, dog, and ruminants) it enters dorsally, either by joining the cranial vena cava (6′) or discharging between the caval openings; when a *left azygous* is present (as in ruminants and the pig), it joins the coronary sinus close to its termination after winding around the caudal aspect of the base from the left side (Fig. 7–9/*A*,12).

The interior of the atrium is smooth between the vein entrances, which are unobstructed by valves. Its roof dips between the caval openings, being indented by the passage of pulmonary veins returning across the right atrium to enter the left atrium. The ridge (*intervenous tubercle;* Fig. 7–8/5) produced by the indentation prevents confrontation between the caval streams by deflecting both ventrally, toward the atrioventricular ostium (/3) that occupies much of the floor. A depressed membranous area (*fossa ovalis;* /9) of the septal wall is present caudal to the tubercle; it corresponds to the foramen ovale of fetal life. In sharp contrast, the interior of the auricle (/1′) is made irregular by a series of ridges (musculi pectinati) that branch from the terminal crest that marks the boundary between the auricle and the main compartment.

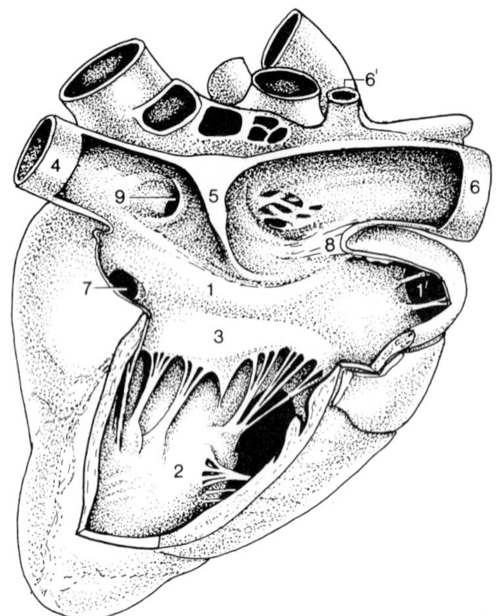


**Figure 7–8.** Overview of the interior of the right atrium and right ventricle of the equine heart.

1, Right atrium; 1′, right auricle; 2, right ventricle; 3, right atrioventricular valve; 4, caudal vena cava; 5, intervenous tubercle; 6, cranial vena cava; 6′, right azygous vein; 7, coronary sinus; 8, terminal crest; 9, fossa ovalis.

## The Left Atrium

This has a generally similar form. It receives the pulmonary veins, which enter, separately or in groups, at two or three sites: craniosinistral, craniodextral, and in some species, caudal (Figs. 7–7/11,11′ and 7–9/11,11′). The septal wall may present a scar marking the position of the valve of the fetal foramen ovale. The auricle resembles that of the right side.

## The Right Ventricle

This chamber, crescentic in transverse section, is wrapped around the right and cranial aspects of the left ventricle (Fig. 7–10). It is incompletely divided by a stout muscular beam (supraventricular crest) that projects from the roof cranial to the atrioventricular ostium (Fig. 7–11/7). The main part of the chamber lies below this large elongated

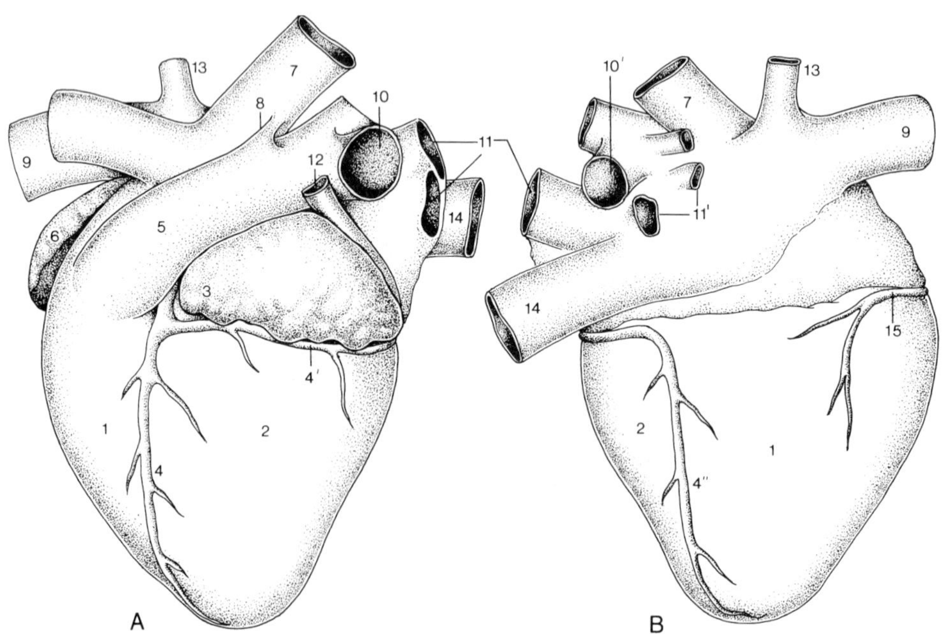


**Figure 7–9.** Left *(A)* and right *(B)* views of the bovine heart.

1, Right ventricle; 2, left ventricle; 3, left auricle; 4, paraconal interventricular branch of left coronary artery; 4′, circumflex branch of left coronary artery; 4″, subsinuosal interventricular branch of left coronary artery; 5, pulmonary trunk; 6, right auricle; 7, aorta; 8, ligamentum arteriosum; 9, cranial vena cava; 10, 10′, left and right pulmonary arteries; 11, 11′, left and right pulmonary veins; 12, left azygous vein; 13, right azygous vein; 14, caudal vena cava; 15, right coronary artery.

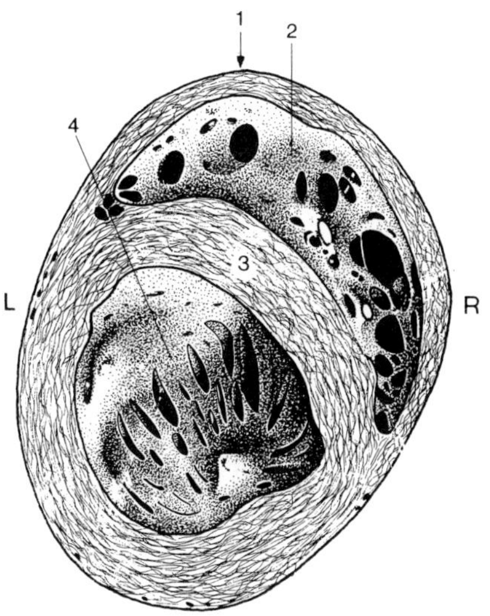


**Figure 7–10.** Transverse section through the ventricles. Note the different thicknesses of the walls of the right and left ventricles.

1, Most cranial point; 2, right ventricle; 3, interventricular septum; 4, left ventricle.

opening while the extension to the left, the *conus arteriosus* (/6), leads directly to the much smaller circular exit into the pulmonary trunk.

The *right atrioventricular (tricuspid) valve* is composed of three flaps or cusps that attach to a fibrous ring that encircles the opening. The cusps are fused at their attachment but part toward the center of the opening where their free margins are thick and irregular, especially in later life. Each cusp is joined by fibrous strands (chordae tendineae) that descend into the ventricular cavity to insert on projections from the walls *(papillary muscles)*. Generally, three of these muscles are present, and the chordae tendineae are so arranged that they connect each cusp to two muscles, each muscle to two cusps (Fig. 7–12/2,3). The arrangement prevents eversion of the cusps into the atrium during ventricular contraction (systole). The lumen of the ventricle is crossed by a thin band of muscle *(trabecula septomarginalis)* that passes from the septal to the outer wall (Fig. 7–11/8). It provides a shortcut for a bundle of the conducting tissue, so ensuring a more nearly simultaneous contraction of all parts of the ventricle (Fig. 7–3). A further modification of the muscle is provided by the many irregular ridges (trabeculae carneae) that give the lower part of the wall a spongy appearance. These are confined to the "inflow" part of the cavity and are thought to reduce blood turbulence.

The opening into the pulmonary trunk lies at a more dorsal level than the atrioventricular ostium and is craniosinistral to the origin of the aorta (Figs. 7–13/4). It is closed during ventricular relaxation (diastole) by the backflow of blood forcing together the three cusps that arise around its margin and constitute the *pulmonary valve*. The cusps are semilunar and deeply hollowed on the arterial side, fitting together tightly when the valve is closed; thickenings of the contact areas, sometimes pronounced in older animals, improve the seal.

## The Left Ventricle

This chamber is circular in section (Fig. 7–10) and forms the apex of the heart as a whole. Except toward the apex, its wall is much thicker than that of the right ventricle in conformity with the greater work it must perform; however, the impression that the chamber is also much smaller is illusory. The *left atrioventricular* (*bicuspid* or *mitral*) *valve* that closes the atrioventricular ostium generally has only two major cusps but is otherwise comparable to that of the right side. It lies largely to the left of the median plane (Fig. 7–13/2 and

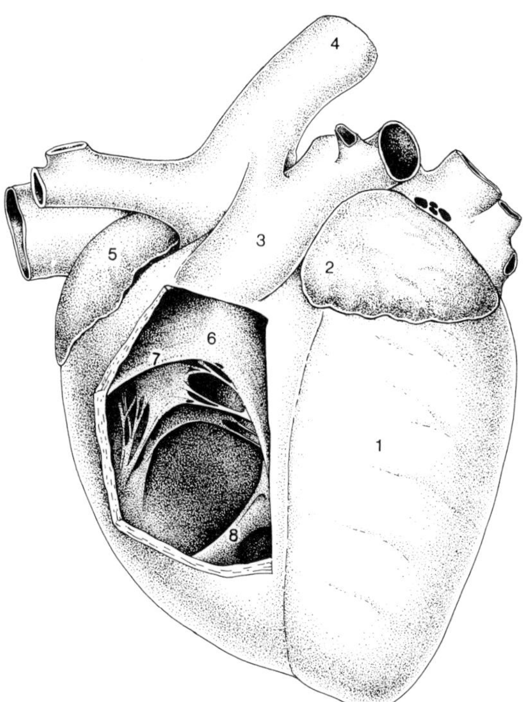


**Figure 7–11.** Craniosinistral view of the heart after removal of part of the wall of the right ventricle.

1, Left ventricle; 2, left auricle; 3, pulmonary trunk; 4, aorta; 5, right auricle; 6, conus arteriosus; 7, supraventricular crest; 8, trabecula septomarginalis.

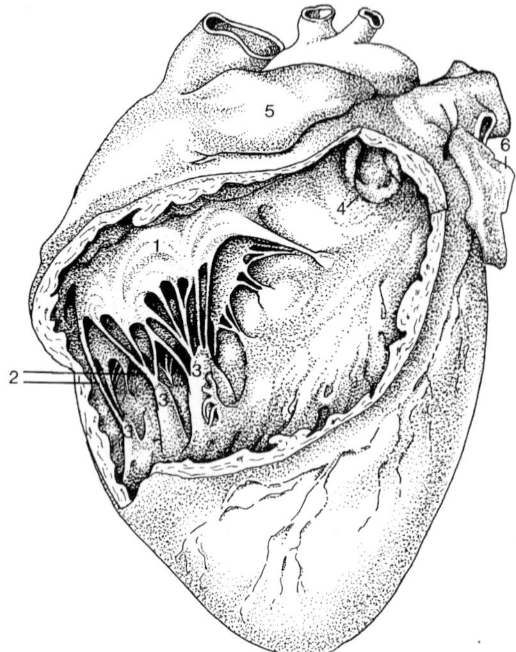


**Figure 7–12.** Cranioventral view of the interior of the right ventricle.

1, Cusp of right atrioventricular valve; 2, chordae tendineae; 3, papillary muscles; 4, pulmonary valve; 5, right auricle; 6, left auricle.

Plate 11/*E*). The exit to the aorta takes a more central position within the heart (/3).

The *aortic valve,* generally resembling the pulmonary valve, shows a different orientation of its cusps. The nodular thickenings in the free margins of the aortic cusps are conspicuous.

## The Structure of the Heart

The thick middle layer of the wall *(myocardium)* is composed of cardiac muscle, a variety of striated muscle peculiar to this organ. It is covered externally by the visceral pericardium *(epicardium)* and internally by the *endocardium,* a thin smooth-surfaced layer continuous with the lining of the blood vessels.

The atrial and ventricular parts of the muscle are separated by a fibrous skeleton that is mainly formed by the conjunction of the rings that encircle the four heart orifices. The skeleton contains islands of fibrocartilage in which nodules of bone *(ossa cordis)* may develop (Fig. 7–13/5). Although these bones appear precociously in the hearts of cattle, they are not confined to this species as is sometimes suggested. The fibrous skeleton is perforated in one place (near the entrance of the coronary sinus) to allow passage to the *atrioventricular bundle* of specialized tissue that conducts the impulse to contract and constitutes the only direct connection between the atrial and ventricular muscles. Delicate extensions of the fibrous tissue also provide the cores of the cusps of the various valves.

The atrial muscle is thin—indeed, the auricular wall may be translucent between the pectinate ridges. It is arranged in superficial and deep bundles; some of the former are common to both atria, but the remainder, and all of the deep bundles, are confined to one. It has been postulated that the fascicles that surround the various venous inlets, both systemic and pulmonary, act as throttles to oppose reflux of blood into the veins during atrial systole.

The much thicker ventricular muscle is also arranged in superficial and deep bundles. Some superficial bundles coil around both chambers, utilizing the septum to complete a figure-of-eight course. Others, like the deeper bundles, encircle only the one chamber. The arrangement of the muscle is actually very complicated, and analyses

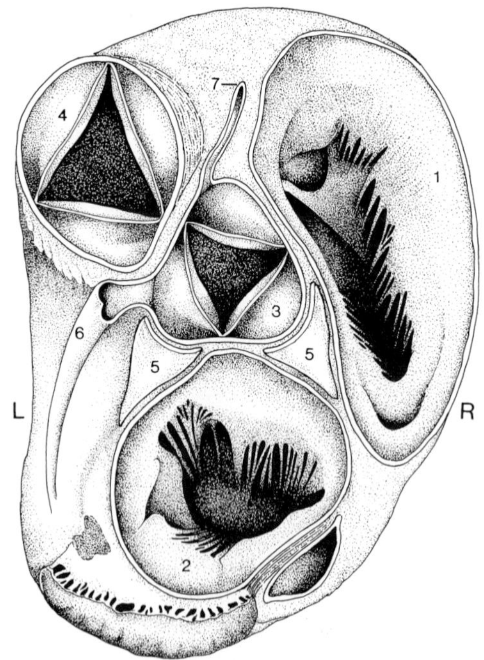


**Figure 7–13.** Dorsal view of the base of the bovine heart after removal of the atria. The ossa cordis on both sides of the aortic valve have been exposed.

1, Right atrioventricular valve; 2, left atrioventricular valve; 3, aortic valve; 4, pulmonary valve; 5, ossa cordis; 6, left coronary artery; 7, right coronary artery.

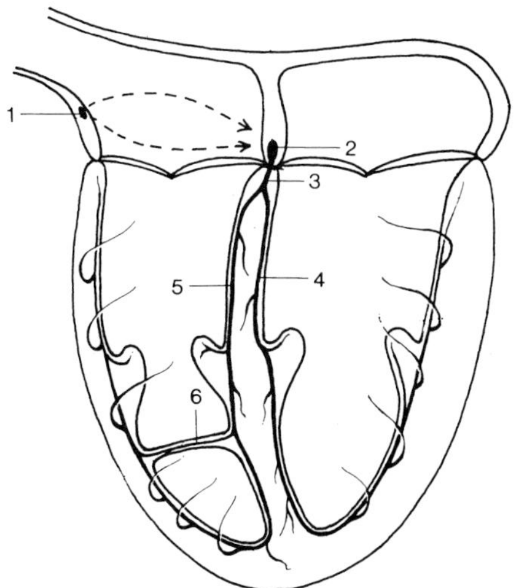


**Figure 7–14.** Schematic drawing of the conducting system of the heart. The broken lines suggest the passage of the excitation wave through the atrial wall.

1, Sinuatrial node; 2, atrioventricular node; 3, atrioventricular bundle; 4, left limb; 5, right limb; 6, branch of right limb traversing the septomarginal band.

of the contraction mechanism still leave much obscure.

The inherent rhythm of the heart is controlled by a pacemaker, a small, richly innervated *sinuatrial node* of modified cardiac fibers (nodal myofibers) that provide the conducting tissue (Plate 12/*A*). This node, which is not apparent to the naked eye, lies below the epicardium of the right atrial wall ventral to the cranial caval opening (Fig. 7–3/11). With each heart cycle, a wave of excitation, which arises in the sinuatrial node and spreads throughout the atrial muscle, reaches the atrioventricular node (Fig. 7–14; Plate 12/*B,C*). In ungulates, specialized conductive tissue is present subendocardially in the atrium, mainly on the pectinate muscle. From the *atrioventricular node* an excitatory stimulus passes rapidly throughout the whole ventricular myocardium via the *atrioventricular bundle,* largely composed of Purkinje fibers, modified cardiac muscle fibers which conduct impulses much more rapidly than those of the common sort (Fig. 7–14). The atrioventricular node consists of modified nodal and Purkinje fibers and is found within the interatrial septum, cranial to the opening of the coronary sinus; it is richly innervated. This node gives origin to the *atrioventricular bundle,* which penetrates the fibrous skeleton before dividing into right and left limbs (crura) that straddle the interventricular septum (Fig. 7–14). Each limb continues ventrally close to the endocardium and branches to reach all parts of the heart muscle; part of the right bundle travels to the outer wall by way of the septomarginal band. The main conducting structures are not difficult to display by dissection of the beef heart.

## Cardiac Vessels and Nerves

The heart is lavishly supplied with blood, receiving about 15% of the output of the left ventricle. The supply is led through the coronary arteries that spring from two of the three sinuses above the semilunar cusps at the beginning of the aorta (Fig. 7–15).

The *left coronary artery* is usually the larger. It arises above the caudosinistral cusp and reaches the coronary groove by passing between the left auricle and the pulmonary trunk; it divides almost at once. The left (paraconal) interventricular branch follows the like-named groove toward the apex of the heart (Fig. 7–16/2′). The trunk continues as a circumflex branch (/2″) that follows the coronary groove toward the caudal aspect of the heart where it may terminate close to the origin of the right (subsinuosal) interventricular groove (horse and pig) or continue into this (carnivores and ruminants) (Fig. 7–17/*A,B* and Plate 11/*C*).

The *right coronary artery* arises above the cranial cusp (Fig. 7–15/6) and reaches the coronary groove after passage between the right auricle

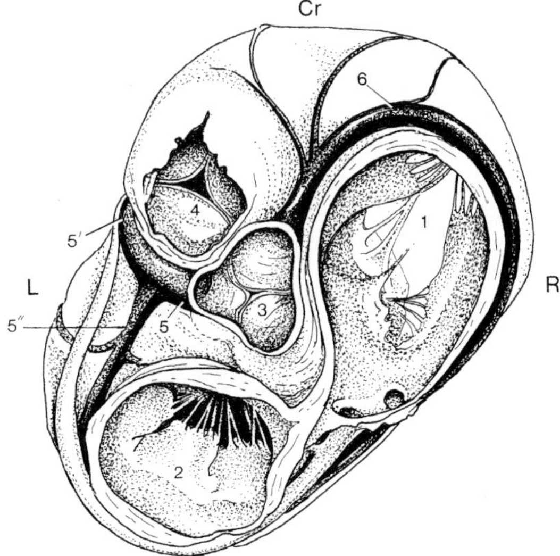


**Figure 7–15.** Dorsal view of the base of the heart after removal of the atria. The coronary arteries are exposed.

1, Right atrioventricular valve; 2, left atrioventricular valve; 3, aortic valve; 4, pulmonary valve; 5, left coronary artery; 5′, paraconal interventricular branch; 5″, circumflex branch; 6, right coronary artery. Cr, cranial.

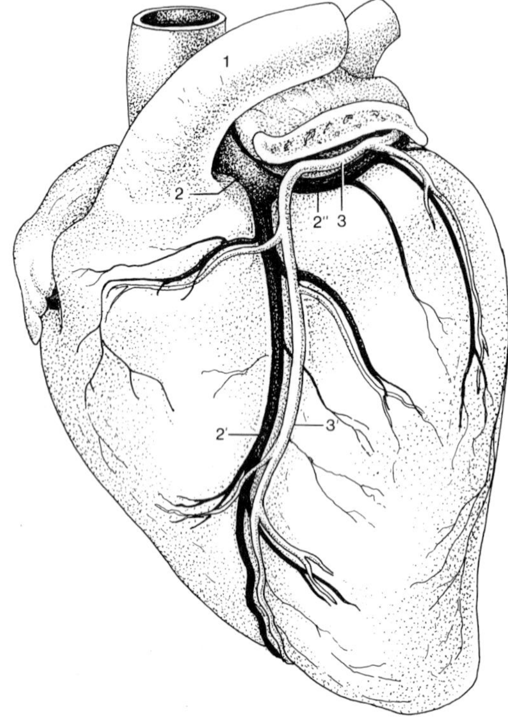


**Figure 7–16.** Branching of the left coronary artery of the heart, viewed from the left. The left auricle has been shortened.

1, Pulmonary trunk; 2, left coronary artery; 2′, paraconal interventricular branch; 2″, circumflex branch; 3, great cardiac vein (continued by the coronary sinus on the right side of the heart); 3′, paraconal interventricular tributary of 3.

and pulmonary trunk. It pursues a circumflex course that either fades toward the origin of the subsinuosal groove or turns into it in those species in which the left artery has the restricted distribution. Both coronary arteries send other branches, of varying size and constancy of position, to neighboring parts of the atrial and ventricular walls. Very small twigs extend some distance into the cores of the valve cusps (Plate 11/*D*).

Anastomoses are not formed between the main branches of the coronary arteries but are numerous between the lesser branches. Even so, sudden closure of one of these small vessels cannot usually be compensated; it leads to local infarction of the cardiac muscle.

Blood is principally returned to the heart through the *great cardiac vein* that opens separately into the right atrium via the coronary sinus (Fig. 7–17/4,3). Rather surprisingly, many very much lesser (Thebesian) veins open directly into all four heart chambers.

The innervation of the heart is complicated topographically, but happily the details mainly concern physiologists. A sympathetic contribution is routed through the caudal cervical and first few thoracic ganglia of the sympathetic trunk. The postganglionic fibers form cardiac plexuses within the cranial mediastinum before extending to the heart wall (Fig. 7–18). Parasympathetic fibers branch from the vagus nerves, either directly or after short passage within the recurrent laryngeal nerves. They end on nerve cells in the heart wall, especially within and about the sinuatrial and atrioventricular nodes; many of the postganglionic fibers pass to the nodes, others reach the periphery of the heart by following the atrioventricular bundle and its branches.

## Functional Anatomy

An indication of the exacting task required of the heart is provided by the following figures, culled from various sources: 60% of the total volume of blood within the human body passes through the heart each minute while the corresponding figures for dogs and horses are 80% and 100%, respectively.

Coordinated contraction is essential for efficient pumping; asynchronous contraction of muscle fascicles (fibrillation) is ineffectual and is rapidly fatal when it involves the ventricular muscle. The sinuatrial node is the pacemaker from which the wave of excitation normally spreads to all parts of the muscle; it has the highest rate of spontaneous activity when relieved from external stimuli, but in normal circumstances its discharge is determined by the fine balance of accelerating sympathetic and retarding vagal inputs. The wave of excitation that spreads from the sinuatrial node through the atrial muscle soon reaches the atrioventricular node (Fig. 7–14/2 and Plate 11/*G,H*). This does not respond at once, the short delay permitting completion of atrial contraction. The impulse then spreads to the ventricular muscle through the atrioventricular conducting tissue. Although ventricular contraction is almost synchronous, the subendocardial layer, which includes the papillary muscles, gains a slight lead.

The flow of blood is related to these activities. Blood enters the atria for as long as the pressure within the veins exceeds that within the heart. Several factors of uncertain and varying magnitude contribute to the venous pressure. The force exerted upstream (vis a tergo) is the summation of the residual pressure imparted to the blood by ventricular contraction; the forces exerted by muscles, visceral activity, and arterial pulsation; and the so-called abdominal pump in which contraction of the diaphragm expels blood from the caudal vena cava and its large tributaries within the abdomen. The downstream force (vis a fronte) oscillates between a negative aspirating effect (provided by thoracic expansion and atrial relaxation) and a positive pressure developed on atrial systole. A lateral pressure may be exerted by contraction of the muscular coat of the great veins. Gravity also plays a part, sometimes assisting, sometimes impeding flow according to posture. Much blood flows directly into the ventricles through open atrioventricular ostia and only a "topping-up" effect is exerted by the atrial contraction, which coincides with the last stage of ventricular relaxation. When the atria do contract, some blood may reflux into veins (despite the conjectured throttle mechanism already mentioned); a jugular pulse may be visible evidence of this.

The pulmonary and aortic (arterial) valves are closed during ventricular relaxation when the arterial pressure exceeds that within these chambers. Ventricular contraction closes the atrioventricular valves, eversion of the cusps into the atria being prevented by the timely contraction of the papillary muscles. As the contraction develops, blood forces the arterial valves open and the conducting arteries are expanded by this sudden input. The two ventricles do not contract identically. The right ventricular lumen is squeezed in a "bellows" action in which the outer wall is drawn toward the septum (Fig. 7–19). The more cylindrical left ventricle contracts radially and in length; radial contraction is believed to have the greater effect.

Closure of the heart valves produces distinctive sounds that are audible on auscultation. Their character provides valuable information on the condition of the valves. Because of the vagaries of sound conduction through tissues of different densities, the projections of the heart valves on the chest wall are not necessarily the spots (puncta maxima) where the sounds are most clearly heard. As a rough guide, leaving aside species and breed variations and other factors, it may be said that the

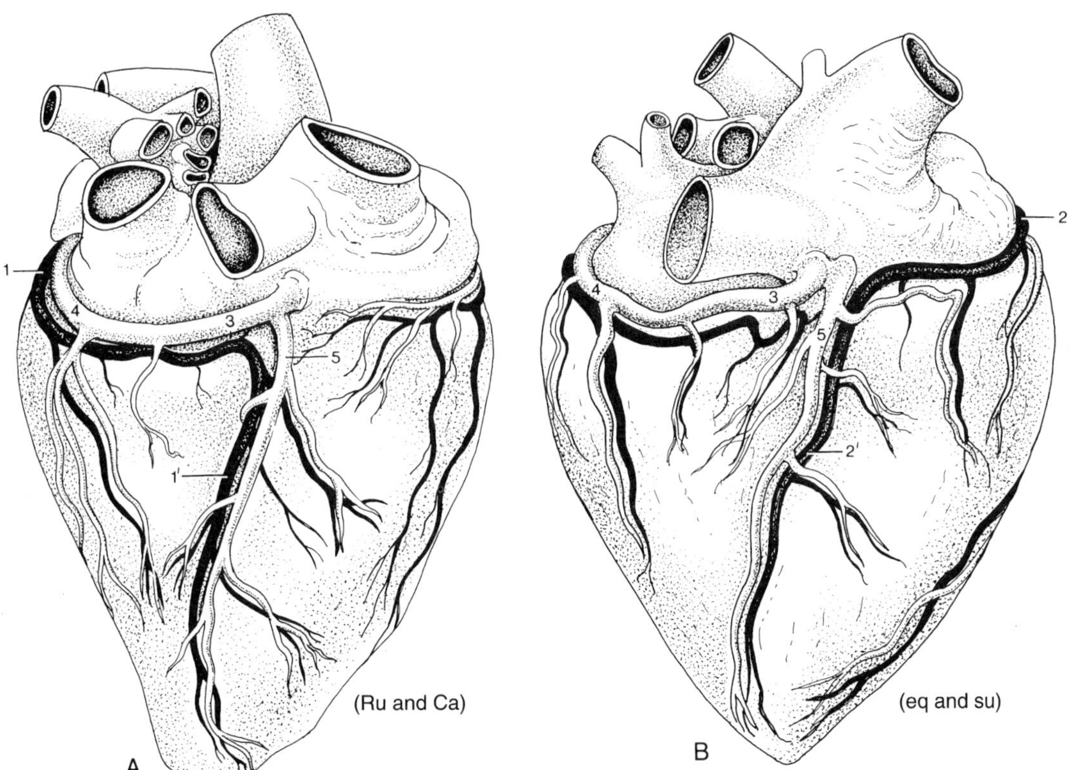


**Figure 7–17.** Patterns of coronary circulation of the heart viewed from the right. *A,* Situation in ruminants and carnivores; the right (subsinuosal) interventricular branch (1′) is a continuation of the left coronary artery. *B,* Situation in the horse and pig; the right (subsinuosal) interventricular branch (2′) is a continuation of the right coronary artery. Ru (ruminants), Ca (cat), su (pig), eq (horse).

1, Circumflex branch of left coronary artery; 1′, right (subsinuosal) interventricular branch; 2, right coronary artery; 2′, right (subsinuosal) interventricular branch; 3, coronary sinus; 4, great cardiac vein; 5, middle cardiac vein.

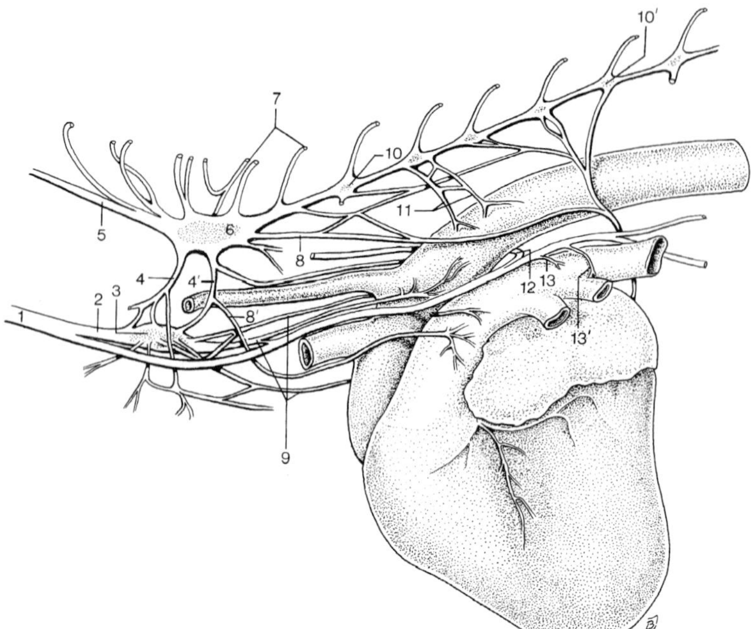


**Figure 7–18.** Cardiac nerves and related ganglia of the dog; left lateral view.

1, Vagosympathetic trunk; 2, sympathetic trunk; 3, middle cervical ganglion; 4, 4′, cranial and caudal limbs of ansa subclavia; 5, vertebral n.; 6, cervicothoracic ganglion; 7, communicating branches; 8, 8′, caudodorsal and caudoventral cervicothoracic cardiac nn.; 9, vertebral cardiac nn.; 10, 10′, third and seventh thoracic ganglia; 11, thoracic cardiac nn.; 12, left recurrent laryngeal n.; 13, 13′, cranial and caudal vagal cardiac nn.

pulmonary, aortic, and left atrioventricular valves are best auscultated over the third, fourth, and fifth ribs of the left side, and the right atrioventricular valve over the fourth rib on the right. The arterial valves are somewhat dorsal to the atrioventricular valves, although the slope of the heart is clearly relevant to this detail. Percussion is also used as a means of evaluating the size of the heart. The quality of cardiac dullness contrasts with the high pitch obtained on percussing over the lungs. The boundary of the cardiac area is not sharply defined since the lung tissue covering the heart grades in thickness about the cardiac notch.

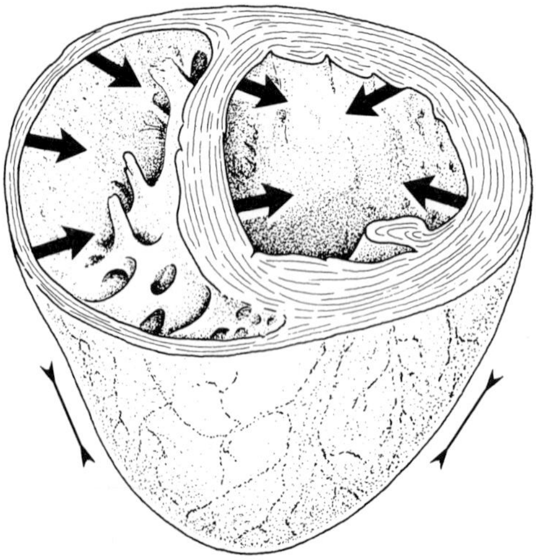

**Figure 7–19.** Schematic drawing of the mode of contraction of the left and right ventricles. The wall of the left ventricle contracts radially, while the right ventricular lumen is squeezed in a "bellows" action.

## The Development of the Heart

The primitive heart, the single median structure formed by the fusion of paired rudiments, is carried ventral to the foregut by the reversal process reshaping the head end of the embryo (p. 100). Though initially consisting of a simple endothelial tube, the heart soon acquires an investment of mesoderm that forms the myocardial and epicardial components of its wall. The cranial part of the tube, which will later form the truncus arteriosus and ventricles, is at this stage contained within the pericardial cavity and suspended by a fold (dorsal mesocardium) extending between the myoepicardium and the pericardial wall (Fig. 7–1/*B*,9). The caudal part, which forms the atria and sinus venosus, first lies caudal to the pericardial cavity embedded within the septum transversum. The enclosed (truncoventricular) part of the heart grows more rapidly than the pericardial space and is forced into a flexure whose apex is directed ventrocaudally and somewhat to the right. The atrial expansions of the initially paired endothelial tubes have now fused in a single common atrium continuous with the sinus venosus; this presents an unpaired transverse part that receives the paired

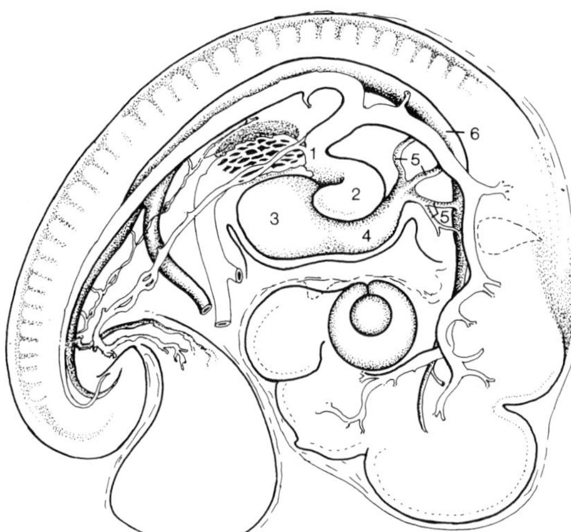


**Figure 7–20.** The developing heart after the fusion of the initially bilateral tubes. The truncus arteriosus is connected by several aortic arches to the single dorsal aorta.

1, Sinus venosus; 2, atrium; 3, ventricle; 4, truncus arteriosus; 5, aortic arches; 6, dorsal aorta.

horns created by the entry of the veins (Figs. 7–20 and 7–21).

Four heart chambers are apparent at this stage—sinus venosus, atrium, ventricle, and truncus arteriosus in caudocranial sequence. The last three are separated by regions of constriction; that between the atrium and ventricle is known as the atrioventricular canal while the transition from ventricle to truncus forms the arterial conus (bulb of the heart). The truncus continues rostrally into the aortic arches, which now appear in the mesoderm to each side of the pharynx (Figs. 7–2/*B* and 7–20). The sinus venosus receives the cardinal, vitelline, and umbilical systems of veins that extend from the body of the embryo, the yolk sac, and the chorioallantois, respectively (Fig. 7–21). The bifid character of the sinus venosus persists for a time, but its wide communication with the atrium gradually shifts toward the right as the amount of blood entering the left horn is diminished after the obliteration of the left umbilical and left vitelline veins. When the sinus is eventually incorporated within the atrium it is the undivided part and the right horn that contribute the sinus venarum, the smooth-walled portion of the adult right atrium; the left horn is reduced to the coronary sinus. By this stage the sinus venosus and common atrium have also become included within the pericardial cavity where they lie dorsal to the ventricle.

Division of the common atrium into right and left chambers is first achieved by the appearance and subsequent growth of a crescentic ridge (Fig. 7–22/2). This projects ventrally into the lumen, and at its ends it grows toward thickenings of the wall of the atrioventricular canal known as the endocardial cushions (/6). The ridge is known as the septum primum; the opening between its free margin and the cushions is known as the *ostium primum* (/4). The ostium primum is gradually occluded by the further enlargement of the cushions, but before closure is complete a number of perforations appear within the septum and coalesce to form a fresh communication, the *ostium secundum* (/5), between the two atria. The definitive division of the atria is achieved by a second crest (/3) that now appears to the right of the primary partition. The concave free ventral margin of this second crest overlaps the ostium secundum; the passage between the atria is reduced to a narrow space between the second septum and the remains of the first (/*C*). The passage is known as the *foramen ovale;* the covering provided by the remnant of the septum primum forms the valve of the foramen ovale. The final closure of the opening is accomplished after birth by the apposition and subsequent fusion of the valve to the septum secundum (p. 250).

Further growth and eventual mergence of the endocardial cushions divide the canal into the two openings that become the right and left atrioventricular ostia (Figs. 7–23 and 7–24/*B*).

The septation of the truncus arteriosus and bulbus is achieved by the appearance, growth, and

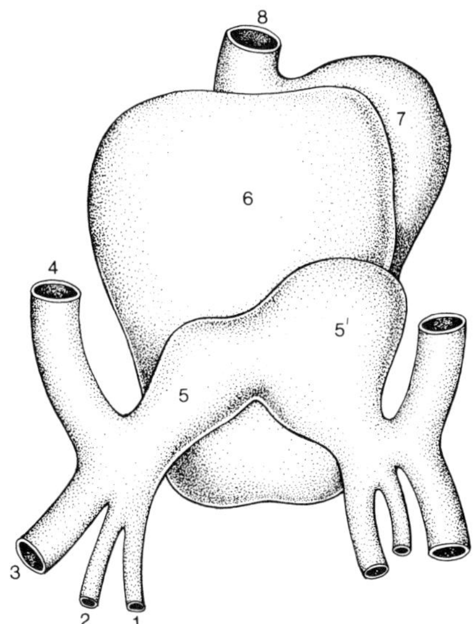


**Figure 7–21.** Dorsal view of the developing heart.

1, Vitelline vein; 2, umbilical vein; 3, caudal cardinal vein; 4, cranial cardinal vein; 5, 5′, left and right horns of sinus venosus; 6, atrium, 7, ventricle; 8, truncus arteriosus.

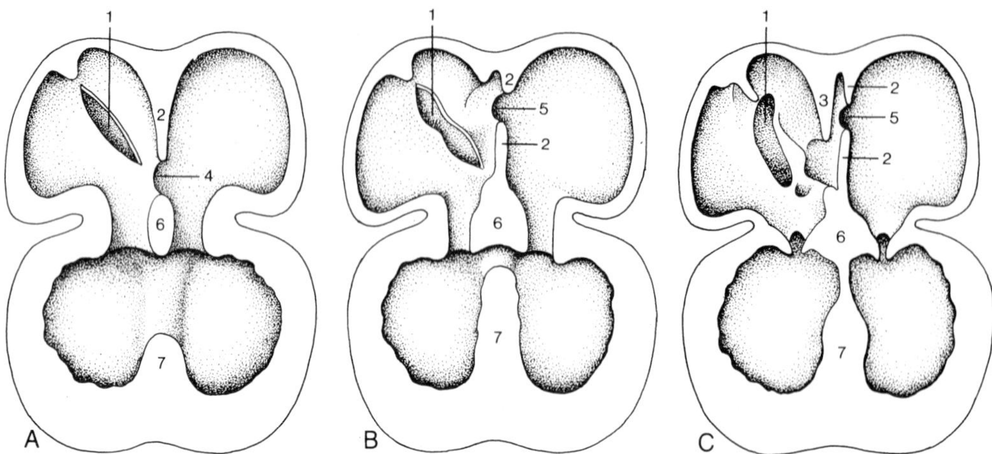


**Figure 7–22.** The partitioning of the atrium and ventricle, schematic. *A,* The primary atrial septum has formed, and development of the interventricular septum has begun. *B,* The primary atrial septum has fused with the endocardial cushions, and a secondary foramen (5) has been formed. *C,* The secondary atrial septum has formed, and a passage (foramen ovale) between primary and secondary septa connects the right and left atria. Note the fusion of the interventricular septum with the endocardial cushions.

1, Sinuatrial opening; 2, primary atrial septum; 3, secondary atrial septum; 4, ostium primum; 5, ostium secundum; 6, fused endocardial cushions; 7, interventricular septum.

fusion of two endocardial ridges that run along the length of the truncus. The left one is known as the septal, the right one as the parietal or dorsal ridge. Fusion of the ridges commences at the distal extremity of the truncus and gradually extends proximally, producing a partition that ends in a free edge arched over the common ventricle (Fig. 7–24/*B*,2,3). The lower end of the parietal ridge expands within the ventricle and contributes to the closure of the atrioventricular ostium (Fig. 7–25/4). The septal ridge fuses with the most cranial part of the interventricular septum that has been developing in the meantime.

This interventricular septum first appears as a falciform crest formed by local thickening of the myocardium at the apex of the ventricle; as it extends it divides the common cavity into right and left chambers (Fig. 7–22/7). Although the external conformation of the heart at this stage already approximates to its final form, the truncus arteriosus (although now divided internally) appears to arise solely from the right ventricle (Fig. 7–24/*A*). The two ventricles still communicate with each other over the free edge of the interventricular septum but are in separate communication with the atria through the paired slitlike openings created by the subdivision of the atrioventricular canal. The right atrioventricular opening is substantially bounded by the right part of the caudal endocardial cushion, less extensively by the cranial cushion, and partly, as already mentioned, by the parietal ridge of the truncus (Fig. 7–25). These three contributions each form a separate cusp of the valve, the truncus ridge contributing the parietal cusp.

The left atrioventricular valve has a similar origin, mainly from the cranial and caudal endocardial cushions but with a small additional (lateral) cushion forming the parietal cusp. The division of the ventricles is largely completed by fusion of the interventricular septum with the caudal cushion; it is finally achieved by fusion of the lower edge of the truncus septum with the right part of the caudal cushion and with the interventricular septum (Fig. 7–25). Since the same process completes the aortic part of the truncus the output of the heart is now divided into a stream from the

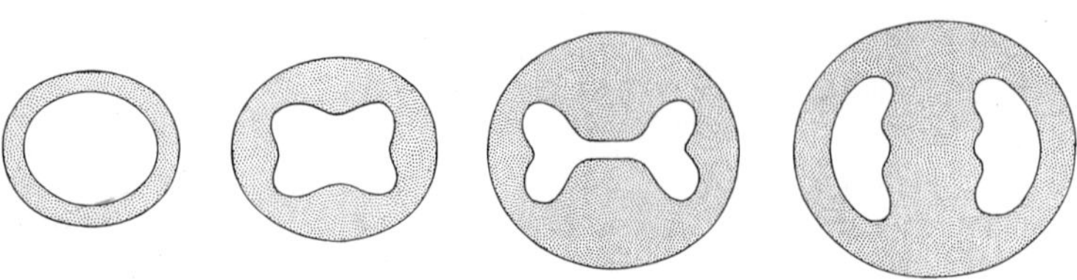

**Figure 7–23.** Partitioning of the atrioventricular canal by the endocardial cushions. The single atrioventricular canal is gradually divided into right and left atrioventricular openings.

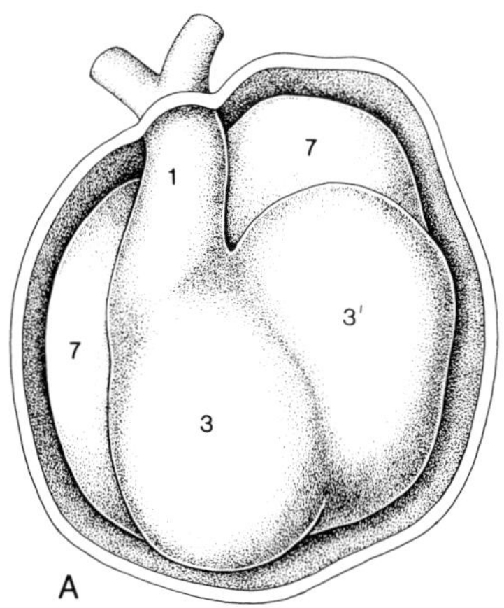


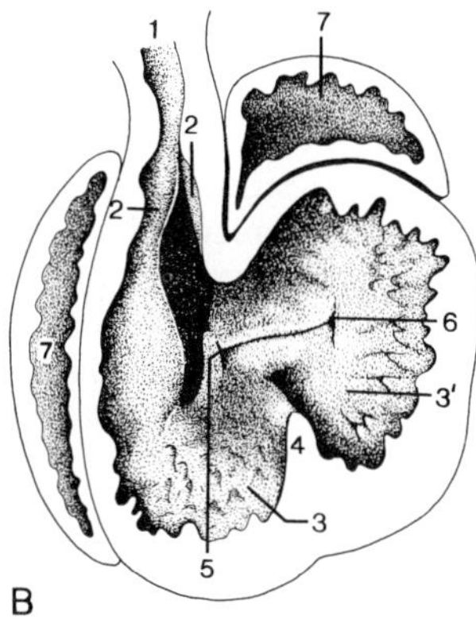


**Figure 7–24.** The partitioning of the truncus arteriosus. *A*, Ventral view of the developing heart. *B*, The ventral part of the heart has been removed to expose the developing ridges (2) in the truncus arteriosus.

1, Truncus arteriosus; 2, ridges in truncus; 3, right ventricle; 3′, left ventricle; 4, interventricular septum; 5, right atrioventricular canal; 6, left atrioventricular canal; 7, atrium.

left ventricle into the aorta and one from the right ventricle into the pulmonary trunk (/1,2).

So complicated a process, requiring the meeting and fusion of various elements in precisely the right place at precisely the right time, is clearly open to mishap; it is therefore unsurprising that heart malformations are among the most common congenital abnormalities. Various surveys suggest that their incidence approaches 1% of all human births; although reliable figures are not available, heart malformations are also frequent in domestic animals. The more common malformations are defects of the cardiac septa, atresia or stenosis of the pulmonary or aortic trunks, or some combination of these anomalies (e.g., the tetralogy of Fallot: pulmonary stenosis, enlarged overriding aorta, ventricular septal defect, and hypertrophy of the right ventricle). Failure of closure of the oval foramen is generally without functional significance, but most other malformations are incompatible with normal life after birth. Surgical correction is neither practicable nor advisable in those affected animals that do not die spontaneously.

## THE BLOOD VESSELS

The arteries, capillaries, and veins form a continuous system lined by an unbroken low-friction endothelium. The other layers of their walls vary greatly in construction, thickness, and even presence, in evident or presumed adaptation to different functional requirements.

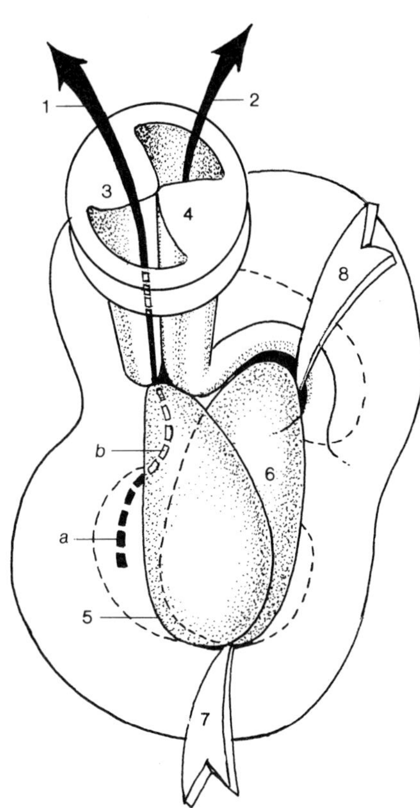


**Figure 7–25.** Caudodorsal view of the developing heart. Arrow 1 illustrates the connection between the left ventricle and the aorta, arrow 2 the connection between the right ventricle and the pulmonary trunk. Part *a* of arrow 1 is located in the left ventricle, part *b* in the aortic orifice of the left ventricle (between the interventricular septum and the cranial endocardial cushion).

1, Outflow of aorta; 2, outflow of pulmonary trunk; 3, septal ridge; 4, parietal ridge; 5, cranial endocardial cushion; 6, caudal endocardial cushion; 7, arrow leading to left atrioventricular canal; 8, arrow leading to right atrioventricular canal.

## The Arteries

The arterial wall is composed of three concentric tunics (Fig. 7–26). The endothelium of the inner one *(tunica interna)* is supported by a thin layer of specialized connective tissue that is bounded externally by a well-developed, fenestrated elastic sheet, the inner elastic membrane (/2). The subendothelial connective tissue is frequently affected by arteriosclerotic changes ("hardening of the arteries"), particularly, though not exclusively, in human subjects. The middle tunic *(tunica media)* is the thickest and most variable layer. It is composed of an elaborately organized admixture of elastic tissue and smooth muscle in varying proportions (/3). The outer tunic *(tunica adventitia)* is predominantly fibrous and grades into the fibroareolar tissue within which many arteries are embedded (/4). Its importance in limiting expansion of the artery, safeguarding against spontaneous rupture, is not always sufficiently recognized.

Differences in the structure of the media allow the convenient recognition of three major classes of arteries, although it should not be assumed that these are sharply distinguished. A few very large arteries—those that are required to expand considerably when they receive the systolic output of the ventricles—have a media predominantly composed of concentric, fenestrated elastic membranes with relatively little muscle interspersed. The elastic tissue stretches to absorb and store the energy contained in the moving blood stream; later, on recoil, it releases this energy to forward the flow of blood toward the periphery. These elastic or conducting arteries comprise the first part of the aorta, certain of its major branches, and the pulmonary trunk.

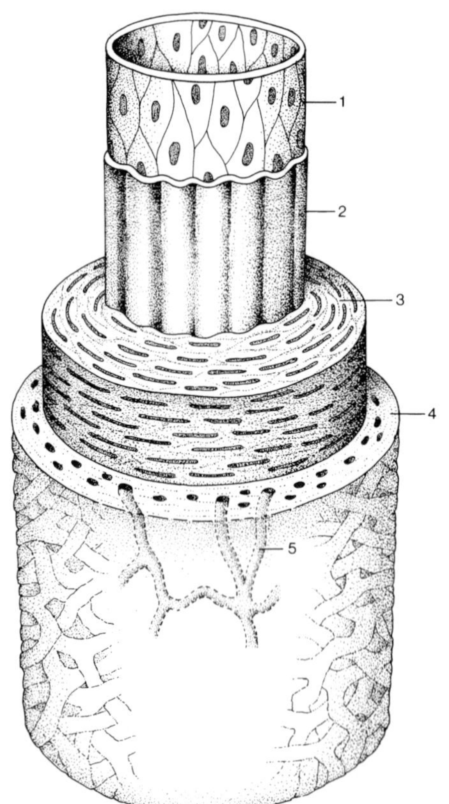


**Figure 7–26.** The components of the arterial wall.

1, 2, Tunica interna; 1, endothelium; 2, inner elastic membrane; 3, tunica media; 4, tunica adventitia; 5, vasa vasorum.

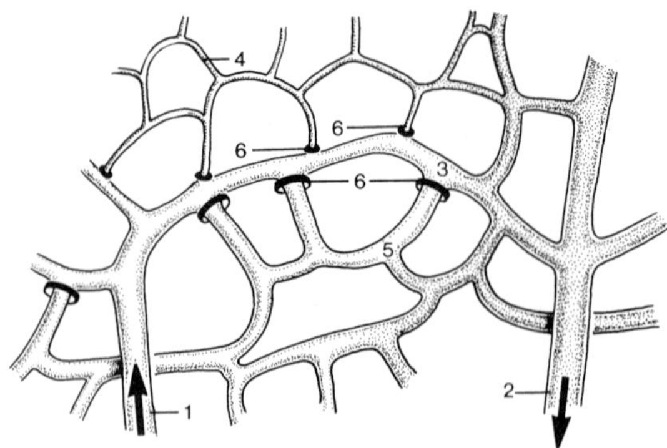


**Figure 7–27.** Schematic drawing of a capillary plexus.

1, Arteriole; 2, venule; 3, communicating (low-resistance) channel; 4, closed capillaries; 5, open capillaries; 6, precapillary sphincters.

Most named arteries and others of smaller size have a media that consists largely of smooth muscle arranged in many closely spiraled layers. The caliber of these muscular or distributing arteries is closely controlled by an autonomic innervation.

The smallest arteries, known as *arterioles,* principally regulate the resistance to the flow of blood and hence the peripheral blood pressure. The muscle is reduced to a few layers that are progressively shed. Although arterioles may be little wider than the capillaries into which they open, they are distinguished from these by the retention of some muscle in their walls. The sphincters about the openings to the capillaries are the means of determining the fraction of the capillary bed that is open to perfusion at any time (Fig. 7–27).

## The Capillaries and Sinusoids

The capillaries are reduced to narrow endothelial tubes supported by a very delicate connective tissue investment. They are the exchange vessels from which fluid passes from the blood into the tissue interstitium at the arterial end of the loop and into which some fluid is resorbed toward the venous end (Fig. 7–27). They permeate almost every tissue, although the density of the network varies very considerably. The endothelium is described as complete, but minute pores are present in the (fenestrated) capillaries that are typical of some situations—intestinal villi and renal glomeruli are two examples.

Sinusoids constitute a special type of capillary found in certain organs, including the liver, spleen, and bone marrow. They are wider, less regular, and more commonly fenestrated than the ordinary capillary, and their endothelial cells are able to extract colloidal substances from the blood.

## The Veins

Though thinner-walled, the larger veins have a construction similar to that of arteries. The smallest ones, the venules, do not possess muscle and may pass through several successive confluences before acquiring this component of the wall. The tunica interna is always thin and lacks an elastic membrane; its chief distinction is its involvement in the formation of the valves whose form, disposition, and function have already been noted (p. 28). The media is relatively weak and is mainly muscular with little admixture of elastic elements. Elastic fibers are more plentiful in the adventitia.

The structure of veins is much less uniform than that of arteries but, although many specializations have been described, it has not yet been possible to assign specific adaptive significance to all. However, longitudinal bundles of smooth muscle within the adventitia of some veins can be correlated with a capacity to alter in length with changes in circumstance. Clear indications exist that the muscular layer can increase in thickness in response to elevated venous pressure (e.g., the digital veins of horses).

## Arteriovenous Anastomoses

Direct connections between small arteries and veins exist in many parts of the body where they are used to short-circuit the capillary bed (Fig. 7–28). One purpose is to shunt blood away from tissues of intermittent activity when they are resting; good examples are supplied by the thyroid gland and the gastric mucosa (Plate 6/*D*). Arteriovenous anastomoses are also concerned with temperature regulation. To this end, they are plentiful in the exposed appendages of the body—the digits, external ears, and nose. Paradoxically, they appear to be used in two ways. They open in a cold environment to prevent local overchilling of the appendages; they also open when the animal is overheated and then promote heat loss by increasing the throughput of blood close to the body's surface. A special example of the last use is provided by the panting dog; the circulation of blood through the many arteriovenous anastomoses within the tongue promotes the evaporation of saliva from the surface, compensating to some degree for the restricted distribution of sweat glands in canine skin.

The use of radioactive-labeled microspheres has made it possible to estimate the amount of blood that can circumvent the capillary bed. In the pig, up to 30% of the total cardiac output sometimes passes through arteriovenous anastomoses.

The structure of these interconnecting channels is not uniform. Some are distinguished by having very muscular walls, others by the muscle cells taking on a peculiar epithelioid character; these epithelioid cells are believed to swell on response to specific chemical stimuli, thereby closing the channel.

## Erectile Tissue

Erectile or cavernous tissue is a vascular specialization in which many close-packed, endothelium-lined spaces are set in continuity with the blood stream. The spaces are usually closed, but as they are directly fed by arterioles they rapidly engorge under appropriate nervous stimulation. Erectile

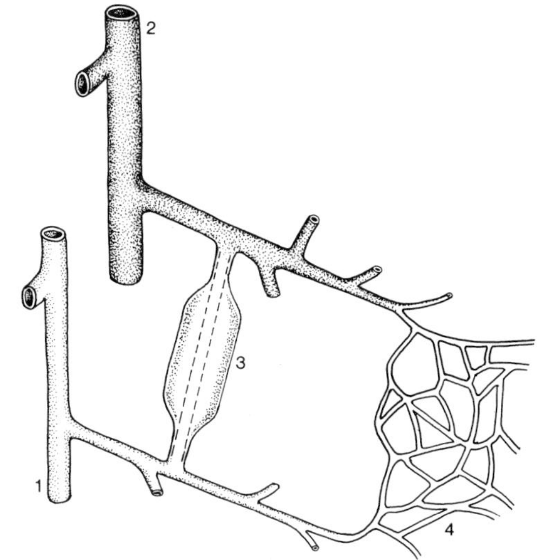


**Figure 7–28.** A precapillary arteriovenous anastomosis.

1, Artery; 2, vein; 3, arteriovenous anastomosis; 4, capillary plexus.

tissue is best known in connection with the genital system; it provides a large part of the structure of the penis (p. 190) and of the smaller but comparable female equivalent. In modified form it is also found in the teat wall, the nasal mucosa, the vomeronasal organ, and a few other sites. A simultaneous response of the genital and nasal erectile tissue is common and has provoked curious speculation; the association is less surprising than it may seem at first, since the perception of odors plays a significant part in the sexual behavior of many animals.

"Blood-cushions" formed by a concentration of veins, although not strictly comparable, may be mentioned here. Several of these arrangements are associated with the gastrointestinal tract. One of veterinary interest is provided by the ileal papilla of the horse (p. 536), which has a considerable capacity for engorgement. Another, less relevant, example is supplied by the human anal mucosa; pads formed by the underlying veins are believed to contribute to closure of the orifice, and it has been claimed that the postnatal elaboration of these veins is correlated with the development of continence by the infant.

## Vascularization and Innervation of the Vessel Wall

Like other tissues, blood vessel walls require nutrition. Diffusion from the lumen is sufficient to supply the needs of smaller vessels but requires supplementation by an intramural circulation in those of larger size. The supplying arteries (vasa vasorum) most often arise at some distance from the stretch of wall they feed, frequently coming from collateral branches. They penetrate the adventitia from outside and ramify within this layer and the adjoining part of the media (Fig. 7–29/1). They do not penetrate beyond the middle of the media in arteries, probably because capillaries in

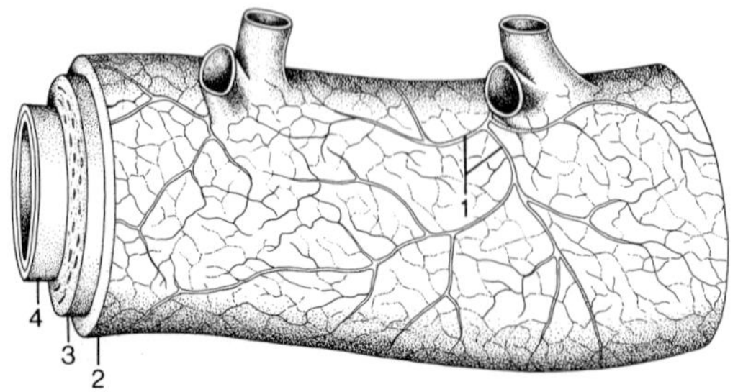


**Figure 7–29.** Vasa vasorum in the wall of a large artery.

1, Vasa vasorum; 2, tunica adventitia; 3, tunica media; 4, tunica interna.

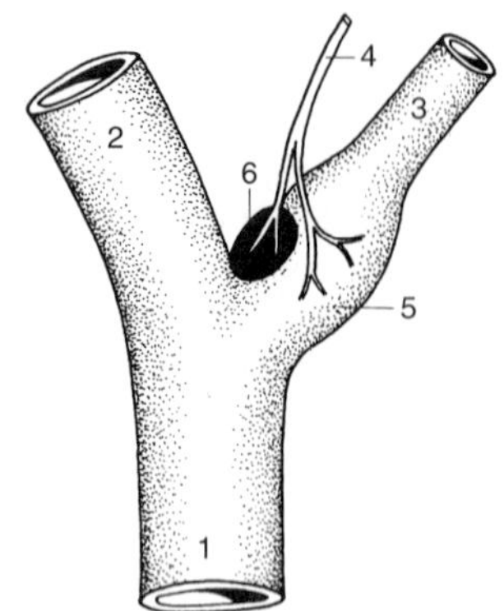


**Figure 7–30.** Baro- and chemoreceptors at the origin of the internal carotid artery.

1, Common carotid artery; 2, external carotid artery; 3, internal carotid artery; 4, carotid sinus branch of the glossopharyngeal nerve; 5, carotid sinus (baroreceptor); 6, carotid body (chemoreceptor).

the inner part of the wall would be closed by the radial pressure generated by the blood stream within the lumen. The tunica intima is never vascularized unless diseased.

Arteries and veins receive both a motor and a sensory innervation. The vasomotor nerves to the arteries are particularly important since they control the diameters of the lumina and hence the peripheral resistance. Most are vasoconstrictor fibers of sympathetic origin. Some pass directly to the great arteries from sympathetic plexuses within the mediastinum, but most first travel within local nerve trunks from which they later emerge to enmesh the peripheral arteries. The afferent supply is concerned in local and general vascular reflexes; some fibers mediate the sensation of pain perceived from arterial lesions.

In addition, certain specific sites are much more richly supplied with nerves whose endings respond to pressure or chemical stimuli. These baroreceptor and chemoreceptor concentrations, of great importance in the regulation of the circulation, are confined to arteries originating in the pharyngeal (branchial) arches—the internal carotid arteries, the aortic arch, the right subclavian artery, and the pulmonary trunk. The best-known examples of each type, the carotid sinus and carotid body (glomus caroticum), are found in close association at the origin of the internal carotid artery (Fig. 7–30).

The carotid sinus may be recognized in the cadaver as a slightly expanded and especially distensible stretch at the origin of the internal carotid. Its receptors are stimulated by pressure changes that alter the mechanical tension in its wall. The carotid body is a neighboring nodule (sometimes palpable) that is composed of a richly vascularized mass of epithelioid cells. The chemoreceptors respond to changes in oxygen and carbon dioxide tension and hydrogen ion concentration in the perfusing blood. The afferent fibers from both receptor types travel in the carotid sinus branch (known to physiologists as the nerve of Hering) of the glossopharyngeal nerve to project upon centers within the brainstem.

The less familiar receptor areas in the other arteries named are similar but less important. Specific differences exist, and in some animals they appear to decline in importance with the attainment of maturity.

## Patterns of Arterial Distribution

We have already mentioned certain more obvious features of arterial distribution—the increase in total cross-sectional area at each branching, the variation in the angle of branching, the preference for protected courses within the limbs, and the generosity of interarterial anastomoses (p. 28). Amplification of the description of certain features is required.

### Collateral Circulation

Few arteries of any size proceed to their terminations in capillary beds without first detaching side or collateral branches. Most collateral branches, whether large or small, connect with their neighbors, although the profusion of anastomoses may not be apparent on dissection since so many are concealed within muscles and other organs (Fig. 7–31). The anastomoses enlarge when the blood stream is diverted from its normal route by occlusion of a principal trunk; initially the widening is due to relaxation and stretching of the wall, later to reconstruction of the anastomotic links. Thus, provided that sufficient blood can pass in the meantime, tissues deprived of their usual sources of supply generally survive, though possibly with temporary loss of function of the ischemic parts. Experiments have shown that in healthy dogs even the aorta can be ligated (caudal to the origin of the renal arteries) with fair, perhaps 50%, expectation of survival. This does not mean that any artery can be ligated with impunity. The ability to develop an adequate collateral circulation is increased when the obstruction develops slowly; it is lessened by sudden onset and by aging or frankly pathological changes in the vessel wall.

Some arteries have a patency that is essential, with interruption to flow producing an infarct, the death of a block of tissue (typically shaped like a cone about the vascular axis). These arteries, known as end-arteries, are paradoxically more numerous among smaller arteries than their parent trunks which generally have more extensive collateral connections. By strict definition, the end-artery is a rarity, but "functional" end-arteries—in which the collateral connections are of insufficient caliber—are more common (Fig. 7–32). It is impossible to assess the adequacy of collateral circulation from purely morphological evidence; for example, although intramuscular arteries appear to anastomose freely, occlusion of one frequently leads to local necrosis. Other good examples of arteries in which anastomoses are poor are the central artery of the retina and many small vessels within the brain; the consequence of their obstruction may be immediate and catastrophic—destruction of the retina or the death of a nucleus or tract with permanent sensory or motor disability. This may be contrasted with the freedom of anastomoses between the major arteries that conjoin to form the arterial circle on the ventral

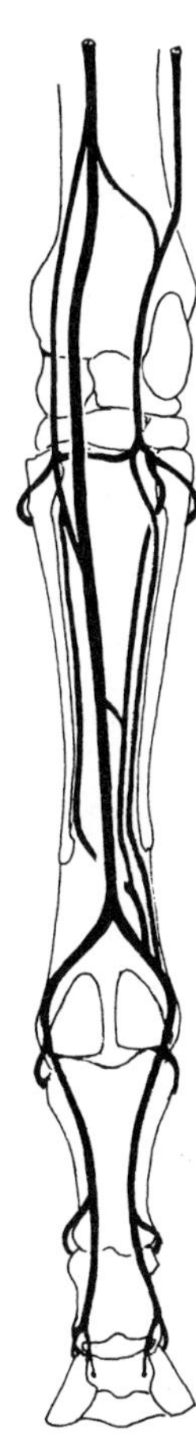

**Figure 7–31.** This illustration of the arterial pattern of the equine limb shows the generosity of interarterial anastomoses.

surface of the brain. Anastomoses between finer branches of the coronary arteries are also poor and usually incapable of maintaining an adequate collateral circulation; even so, not all coronary embolisms are fatal; much may depend on the size and specific site of the infarct and on the immediate medical care.

Anastomoses between small arteries within the limbs are especially numerous in the regions of the joints and sometimes form visible networks or retia; a prominent example exists over the dorsal aspect of the carpus of the horse (rete carpi dorsale).

The retia just described are not to be confused with the so-called retia mirabilia of more restricted occurrence. Retia mirabilia are found where a main trunk splits more or less at once into a leash of parallel vessels. In one variety the parallel trunks later reunite, a "bipolar" arrangement found on the arteries to the brain (in certain species) (Fig. 7–33/7) and, on a diminished scale, in the renal glomeruli (see Fig. 5–23/1). Other examples are "unipolar"—the branches remain separate. Examples are found within the limbs of slow-moving arboreal creatures (sloths, lemurs) and in the thoracic cavity of whales and other diving mammals. No convincing explanations exist of the adaptive value of most of these, the renal glomeruli being the obvious exception (p. 178).

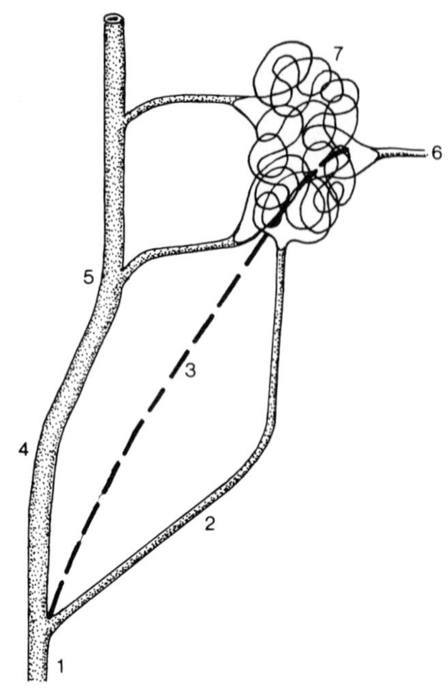


**Figure 7–33.** A rete mirabile interposed on the blood supply to the bovine brain.

1, Common carotid artery; 2, occipital artery; 3, internal carotid artery (regresses after birth); 4, external carotid artery; 5, maxillary artery; 6, branch from rete to arterial circle of the brain; 7, rostral epidural rete mirabile.

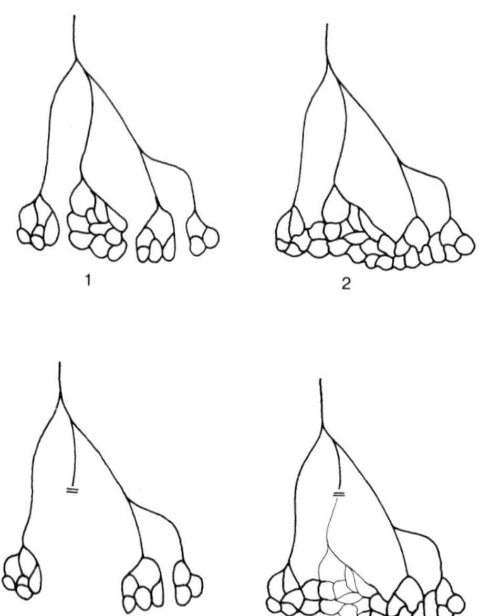


**Figure 7–32.** True (1) and functional (2) end-arteries. Closure of an end-artery leads to necrosis of the tissue it supplies (1′). In the case of a functional end-artery (2), a potential but inadequate alternative route exists (2′).

# SYSTEMATIC ANGIOLOGY

It is not our intention to provide in one place a comprehensive description of all the blood vessels. Few things would be more tedious and there seems to be a pragmatic advantage in fragmenting the account, dealing with the vascularization of particular organs and regions in other chapters where it is easier to emphasize those features that have a special functional importance or clinical interest. Even so, it is advisable to have somewhere an outline of the arterial and venous trees. Since species differences are numerous and would, if given attention, require many qualifications of the description, the dog is used as model; only a few most salient comparative features are noted.

## The Pulmonary Circulation

### *The Pulmonary Arteries*

The *pulmonary trunk* arises from the pulmonary orifice of the right ventricle on the craniosinistral aspect of the heart. It is slightly expanded at its origin where it presents a small sinus above each cusp of the pulmonary valve. The trunk

(Fig. 7–9/*A*,5) passes between the two auricles, then bends caudally over the base of the heart where it is joined on its right face by the ligamentum arteriosum, the fibrosed remnant of the ductus arteriosus (p. 250). After penetrating the pericardium it divides into right and left *pulmonary arteries,* each directed to the hilus of the corresponding lung in company with the principal bronchus and pulmonary veins (/10,10′). The course of the right artery carries it ventral to the trachea.

The pulmonary arteries make their initial branching before entering the lung (Fig. 4–22); their further ramifications have already been briefly noted (p. 163).

### The Pulmonary Veins

The pulmonary veins open variously into the roof of the left atrium. They form two clusters in the dog, one for the veins draining each lung; in some other species the veins draining the caudal lobes of both lungs form a separate third cluster. Valves are absent from these veins.

## The Systemic Circulation

### The Systemic Arteries

**The Aortic Arch.** The origin of the aorta is similar to that of the pulmonary trunk but is from the left ventricle. The initial portion, the aortic bulb, is concealed between the atria and forms sinuses above the three cusps of the aortic valve; the right coronary artery arises from the cranial sinus, the left artery from the caudosinistral sinus (Fig. 7–15/6,5). Beyond this, the aorta arches cranially, dorsally, and caudally, penetrating the pericardium to ascend within the mediastinum to reach the sinistroventral aspect of the vertebral column about the level of the seventh thoracic vertebra (Fig. 7–34). In addition to the *coronary arteries* (p. 225) the first part of the aorta gives origin to the paired subclavian and paired common carotid arteries. These vessels amalgamate at their origins to form a short, cranially directed *brachiocephalic trunk* in the larger species (Fig. 7–35); in the dog and pig the left subclavian artery remains distinct and takes a separate, more distal origin (Fig. 7–34/4). The common carotid arteries supply structures of the head (p. 240).

The *subclavian artery* (/4) supplies blood to the forelimb and to structures of the neck and cervicothoracic junction. It winds around the cranial border of the first rib to enter the limb through the axilla; it changes its name to axillary at this point. The subclavian detaches four branches in its intrathoracic course. The first, the *vertebral artery* (/6), runs craniodorsally, dives between the scalenus and longus colli muscles, and then passes through the successive transverse foramina of the sixth to first cervical vertebrae. After receiving

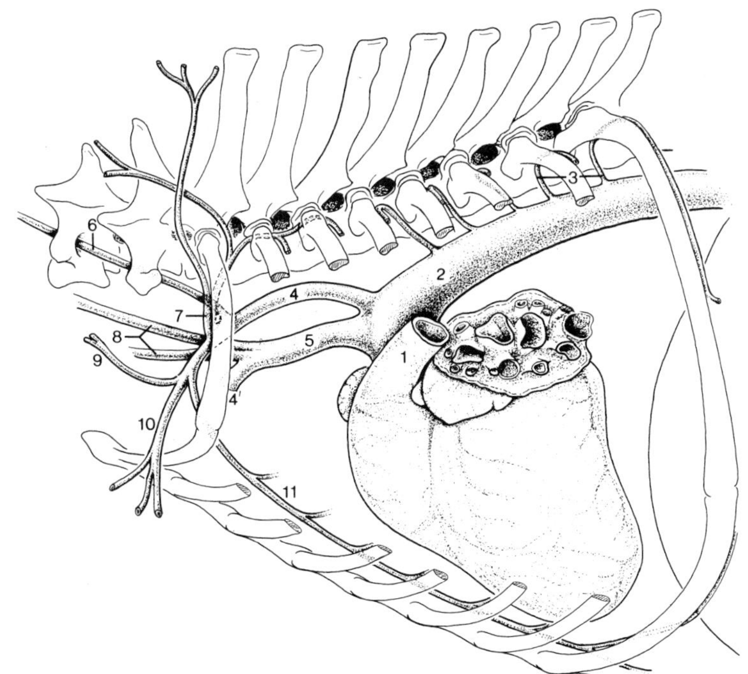


**Figure 7–34.** Branching of the aortic arch in the dog. (In this series of figures, not all arteries depicted are named.)

1, Pulmonary trunk; 2, aorta; 3, intercostal aa.; 4, left subclavian a.; 4′, right subclavian a.; 5, brachiocephalic trunk; 6, vertebral a.; 7, costocervical trunk; 8, left and right common carotid aa.; 9, superficial cervical a.; 10, axillary a.; 11, internal thoracic a.

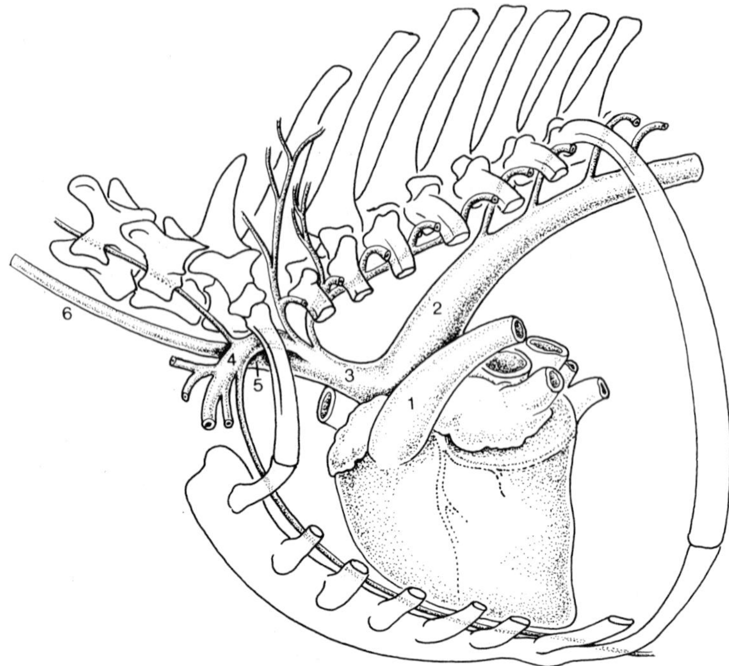


**Figure 7–35.** Branching of the aortic arch in the horse. The arteries to the head and neck and to the forelimbs originate from a short brachiocephalic trunk (3).

1, Pulmonary trunk; 2, aortic arch; 3, brachiocephalic trunk; 4, left subclavian a.; 5, bicarotid trunk; 6, left common carotid a.

the termination of the occipital artery it enters the vertebral canal within the atlas and there divides into a basilar artery to the brain and the ventral artery of the spinal cord (p. 302). Twigs are detached en route to the vertebral column, covering muscles, and contents of the vertebral canal.

The larger second branch, the *costocervical trunk* (/7), provides the first few dorsal intercostal intercostal arteries and the *deep cervical artery,* which ascends the neck within the dorsal cervical musculature that it supplies.

The *internal thoracic artery* (/11), the third branch, curves ventrally within the mediastinum to pass between the transversus thoracis and the sternum. It follows the sternum and tunnels below the diaphragm to continue as the cranial epigastric artery of the abdominal floor. Collateral branches include twigs to the pleura, thymus, and pericardium, perforating branches to the pectoral muscles and thoracic mammary glands, and ventral intercostal arteries; the more caudal ventral intercostal branches arise from a common trunk, the musculophrenic artery, which follows the lateral attachment of the diaphragm. The *cranial epigastric artery* divides into superficial and deep branches; the latter follows the deep face of the rectus abdominis to an anastomosis with the caudal epigastric artery within the substance of this muscle. The superficial branch passes to the superficial fascia where it assists in the supply of the abdominal mammary glands.

The *superficial cervical artery* (/9), the fourth branch, arises from the subclavian opposite the origin of the internal thoracic. It supplies muscles of the ventral part of the neck, the cranial part of the shoulder, and the upper arm.

- Aortic arch
  - Coronary aa.
  - Brachiocephalic trunk
    - Right subclavian a.
      - Vertebral a.
      - Costocervical trunk
        - Deep cervical a.
      - Internal thoracic a.
        - Ventral intercostal aa.
        - Cranial epigastric a.
        - Musculophrenic a.
      - Superficial cervical a.
    - Common carotid aa.
  - Left subclavian a. (its branches correspond to those of the right subclavian a.)

**The Axillary Artery.** The *axillary artery* (Fig. 7–36/1), the magistral trunk of the forelimb, crosses the axilla to continue distally over the medial surface of the arm, caudal to the humerus. It changes its name again when level with the teres major tuberosity where it becomes the brachial artery (/6). The axillary gives *external* and *lateral thoracic arteries* to the chest wall and one important collateral branch to the limb, the *subscapular artery* (/3). This runs dorsally along the caudal border of the scapula between the subscapularis and teres major. It supplies branches to the muscles of the shoulder.

The *brachial artery* (/6) passes obliquely over the medial surface of the humerus to reach the craniomedial aspect of the elbow; it continues into the forearm where it shortly changes its name yet again, becoming the median artery. Its collateral branches include several to the muscles of the arm, principally the *deep brachial* (/7) to the tricipital mass; toward the elbow it detaches *collateral ulnar* and *superficial brachial arteries* (/8,9) that pass to the caudal and cranial aspects of the forearm, respectively. Branches of the superficial brachial run subcutaneously beside the cephalic vein and superficial branch of the radial nerve to reach the dorsum of the paw. The *transverse cubital artery* (/10) is detached just proximal to the elbow joint. A substantial branch, the *common interosseous artery,* originates from the main artery distal to the elbow.

The *common interosseous artery* (/11) detaches the *ulnar artery* (/13) for the digital and carpal flexors and the caudal interosseous artery, which runs between the radius and ulna to reach the palmar arches of the proximal metacarpus. A cranial interosseous penetrates the interosseous space to supply the dorsal muscles of the forearm.

The *median artery* (/12) runs down the caudomedial aspect of the forearm in company with the median nerve and under protection of the flexor carpi radialis. It passes through the carpal canal to end by concurring with branches of the common interosseous in forming palmar arterial arches (/15,16) from which the palmar aspect of the forepaw is supplied.

The paw receives its principal blood supply on its palmar aspect where (deep) palmer metacarpal and (more superficial) palmar common digital arteries run at the boundaries of the metacarpal bones before dividing at their distal ends into proper palmar digital arteries that follow the axial borders of the digits. The corresponding but narrower dorsal common and proper digital arteries follow a similar pattern. The arrangements are more easily illustrated than described, and the details are in truth of very limited practical importance (Fig. 7–37).

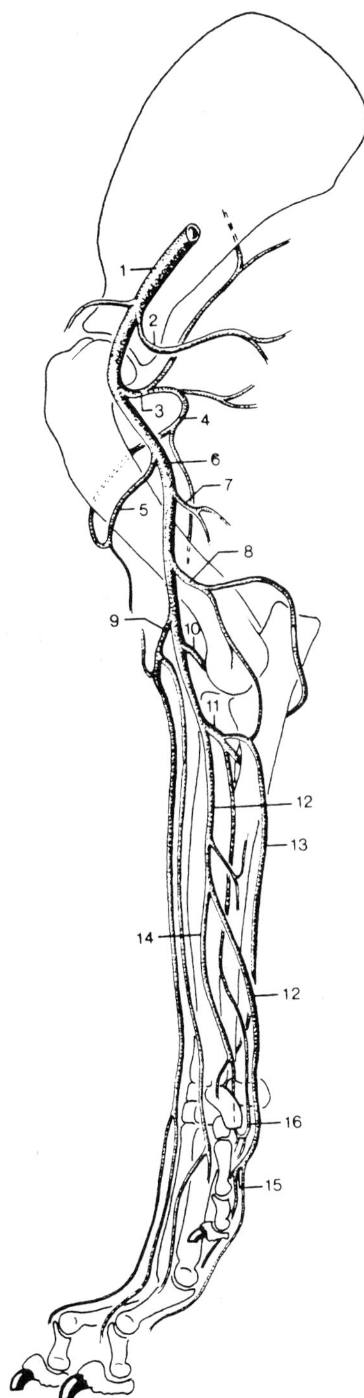


**Figure 7–36.** Arteries of the canine forelimb.

1, Axillary a.; 2, lateral thoracic a.; 3, subscapular a.; 4, caudal circumflex humeral a.; 5, cranial circumflex humeral a.; 6, brachial a.; 7, deep brachial a.; 8, collateral ulnar a.; 9, superficial brachial a.; 10, transverse cubital a.; 11, common interosseous a.; 12, median a.; 13, ulnar a.; 14, radial a.; 15, superficial palmar arch; 16, deep palmar arch.

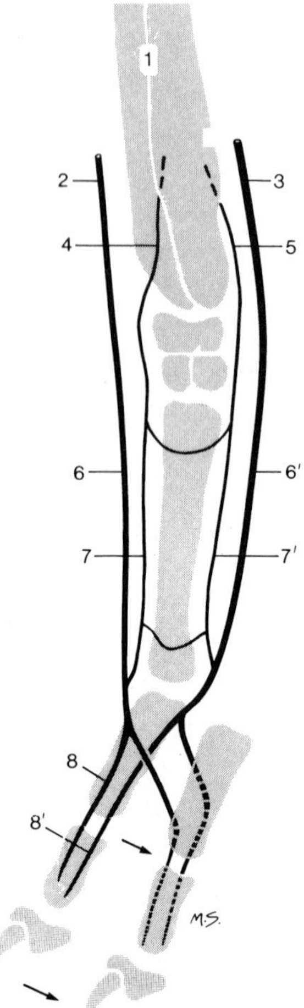


**Figure 7–37.** Schema for the naming of the arteries of the metacarpus and digit, lateral view; based on the dog. The common digital and the metacarpal (-tarsal) vessels (and nerves) are numbered according to the ray (digit) medial to them.

1, Radius and ulna; 2, 3, superficial aa. entering the paw, continuations of the superficial brachial a. and median a., respectively; 4, 5, deep aa. entering the paw, continuations of the cranial and caudal interosseous (or other deep) aa., respectively; 6, 6′, dorsal and palmar common digital arteries—common to neighboring digits *(arrows);* 7, 7′, dorsal and palmar metacarpal aa., connected by proximal and distal perforating branches; 8, 8′, dorsal and palmar proper digital aa.

Axillary a.
- External thoracic a.
- Lateral thoracic a.
- Subscapular a.

Brachial a.
- Deep brachial a.
- Collateral ulnar a.
- Superficial brachial a.
    - Cranial superficial antebrachial a.
        - Dorsal common digital aa.
- Transverse cubital a.
- Common interosseous a.
    - Ulnar a.
    - Cranial interosseous a.
    - Caudal interosseous a.
        - Superficial palmar arch
            - Palmar common digital aa.
        - Deep palmar arch
            - Palmar metacarpal aa.

Median a.
- Radial a.

(The small arteries of the forepaw arise from anastomoses not listed.)

**The Common Carotid Artery.** The common carotid arteries arise separately in the dog (Fig. 7–34/8) and by a short common (bicarotid) trunk in ungulates (Fig. 7–35/5). Each crosses the ventrolateral face of the trachea (or esophagus on the left) in its ascent of the neck where it is accompanied by the vagosympathetic trunk. The artery ends by dividing above the larynx into external and internal carotid arteries. The only significant collateral branches of the common carotid are detached close to its termination; they are the *caudal* and *cranial thyroid arteries,* the latter being the origin of laryngeal and pharyngeal branches.

The *external carotid artery* is the larger of the terminal branches and appears as the direct continuation of the parent trunk (Fig. 7–38/1,2). In the dog it shortly detaches the occipital artery, which branches from the internal carotid in some other species. The external carotid is continued as the maxillary artery (/11), the distinction being rather arbitrarily determined by the origin of the superficial temporal artery.

The external carotid in this narrow sense forms a short dorsally convex arch resting on the pharynx and covered by the mandibular gland and digastricus. Its branches are the occipital, cranial laryngeal, ascending pharyngeal, lingual, facial, caudal auricular, parotid, and superficial temporal arteries.

The *occipital artery* (/4) runs to the condyloid fossa where it divides into several branches that supply, among other structures, the middle and internal ear and the caudal meninges. The largest branch, effectively the continuation of the stem, passes to the atlantal fossa to an anastomosis with the vertebral; it thus takes part in the supply to the brain (p. 303).

The *cranial laryngeal* and *ascending pharyngeal arteries* (/5,6) are the principal supplies to these organs (larynx, pharynx). The large *lingual artery* (/7) pursues a rostroventral course over the pharynx to enter the tongue between the genioglossus and hyoglossus muscles. It principally supplies the tongue, but collateral branches detached en route include one to the palatine tonsil that is of potential importance to the surgeon (p. 376).

The *facial artery* (/8) arises near the angle of the jaw and runs within the intermandibular space before winding around the ventral border of the mandible where it is conveniently located for pulse-taking in larger species; it then divides into various branches for the lips, lateral nose, and angle of the mouth. The relatively large *caudal auricular artery* (/9) generously supplies the external ear and associated muscles. The *parotid artery* supplies the parotid gland.

The *superficial temporal artery* (/10) winds onto the face and runs forward to supply the masseter. In the dog it branches to the upper and lower eyelids and dorsum of the nose. The position and firm support of one of the branches (transverse facial artery) suit it to pulse-taking in larger species.

The *maxillary artery* (/11) heads in the direction of the alar canal through which it passes to enter the pterygopalatine fossa. Before reaching the canal its main branch is the *inferior alveolar* (/12), which enters the mandible to supply the alveoli and teeth and, through mental branches that emerge from the bone, the lower lip and the chin region. Other maxillary branches pass to the tympanic cavity, muscles of mastication, and cranial meninges (the last passing through the oval foramen). No branches are detached from the stretch of artery within the canal but a sheaf of diverging vessels comes off directly it reaches the pterygopalatine fossa. The most important is the *external ophthalmic artery* (/13) going to the contents of the orbit (p. 335). Others include the *ethmoidal artery* to the nasal cavity, the *major* and *minor palatine arteries* to the hard and soft palates, respectively, and the continuation *(infraorbital artery)* of the main trunk into the superior alveolar canal (/14).

The *internal carotid artery* (/3) enters the cranial cavity through the jugular foramen and carotid canal, taking a rather indirect course in the dog (p. 302). It divides within the cavity into divergent caudal and rostral branches that concur with their contralateral counterparts and with the basilar artery in forming the arterial circle from which the brain is supplied (p. 302).

Common carotid a.
- Caudal thyroid a.
- Cranial thyroid a.
- External carotid a.
  - Occipital a.
  - Cranial laryngeal a.
  - Ascending pharyngeal a.
  - Lingual a.
  - Facial a.
  - Caudal auricular a.
  - Parotid a.
  - Superficial temporal a.
  - Maxillary a.
    - Inferior alveolar a.
    - External ophthalmic a.
    - Ethmoidal a.
    - Palatine aa.
    - Infraorbital a.
- Internal carotid a.

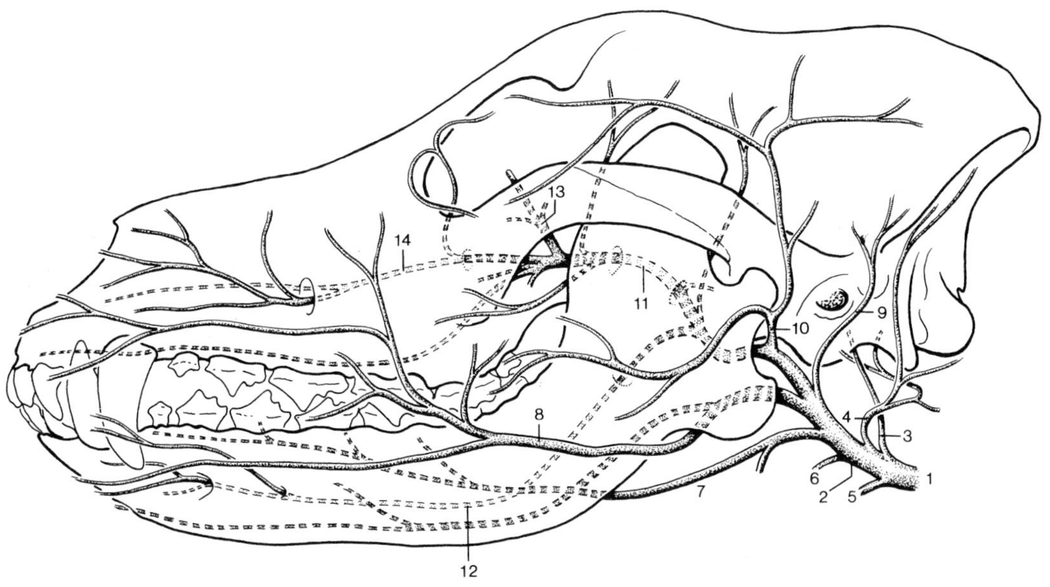


**Figure 7–38.** Arteries of the canine head.

1, Common carotid a.; 2, external carotid a.; 3, internal carotid a.; 4, occipital a.; 5, cranial laryngeal a.; 6, ascending pharyngeal a.; 7, lingual a.; 8, facial a.; 9, caudal auricular a.; 10, superficial temporal a.; 11, maxillary a.; 12, inferior alveolar a.; 13, external ophthalmic a.; 14, infraorbital a.

**The Thoracic Aorta.** The thoracic aorta runs caudally below the roof of the thorax to enter the abdomen by the aortic hiatus of the diaphragm. It continues as the abdominal aorta in company with the azygous vein and thoracic duct. The branches of the thoracic aorta are dorsal intercostal arteries (excepting those to the first few spaces), which arise variously, and often by common trunks for the right and left vessels, and a bronchoesophageal artery, which is rather erratic in its origin (Figs. 7–34 and 7–35).

Despite their names, which suggest rather restricted distribution within the intercostal spaces, the *dorsal intercostal arteries* detach substantial branches to the vertebral column and associated structures. They end by anastomosing with ventral intercostal arteries from the internal thoracic artery and its musculophrenic branch, thereby completing arterial loops within the spaces. The corresponding artery behind the last rib is known as the dorsal costoabdominal. The bronchoesophageal artery descends to the root of the lungs where it gives rise to bronchial branches for the tissues of the lungs and esophageal branches for much of the thoracic esophagus.

Thoracic aorta
- Dorsal intercostal aa.
- Bronchoesophageal a.
  - Bronchial branches
  - Esophageal branches
- Dorsal costoabdominal a.

**The Abdominal Aorta.** The abdominal aorta follows the roof of the abdomen, related to the caudal vena cava on its right and the psoas muscles on its left. Shortly after releasing the paired external iliac artery, the abdominal aorta terminates in the dog below the last lumbar vertebra by branching off the internal iliac arteries and continues as the very much smaller *median sacral artery* that extends into the tail (Fig. 7–39/2,3,4). Along its course the abdominal aorta detaches both visceral and parietal branches.

The visceral arteries have been considered with the organs they supply. They comprise the unpaired celiac (p. 127), cranial mesenteric (p. 134), and caudal mesenteric (p. 134) arteries and the paired renal (p. 178) and testicular (p. 186; or ovarian [p. 198]) arteries. The unpaired vessels represent the arteries of the caudal foregut, midgut, and hindgut of the embryo (see Fig. 3–64).

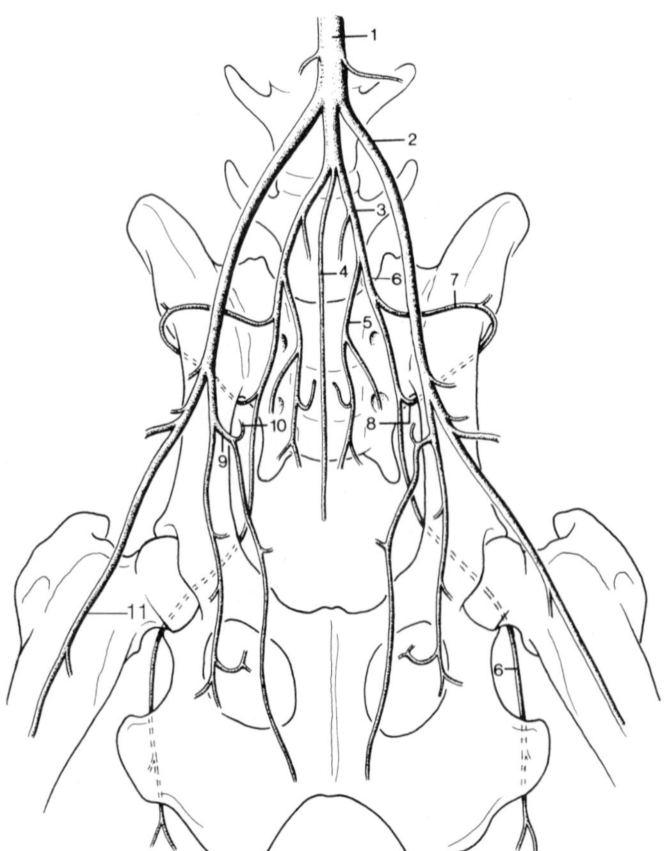


**Figure 7–39.** Termination of the canine abdominal aorta (ventral view).

1, Aorta; 2, external iliac a.; 3, internal iliac a.; 4, median sacral a.; 5, internal pudendal a.; 6, caudal gluteal a.; 7, iliolumbar a.; 8, cranial gluteal a.; 9, deep femoral a.; 10, pudendoepigastric trunk; 11, femoral a.

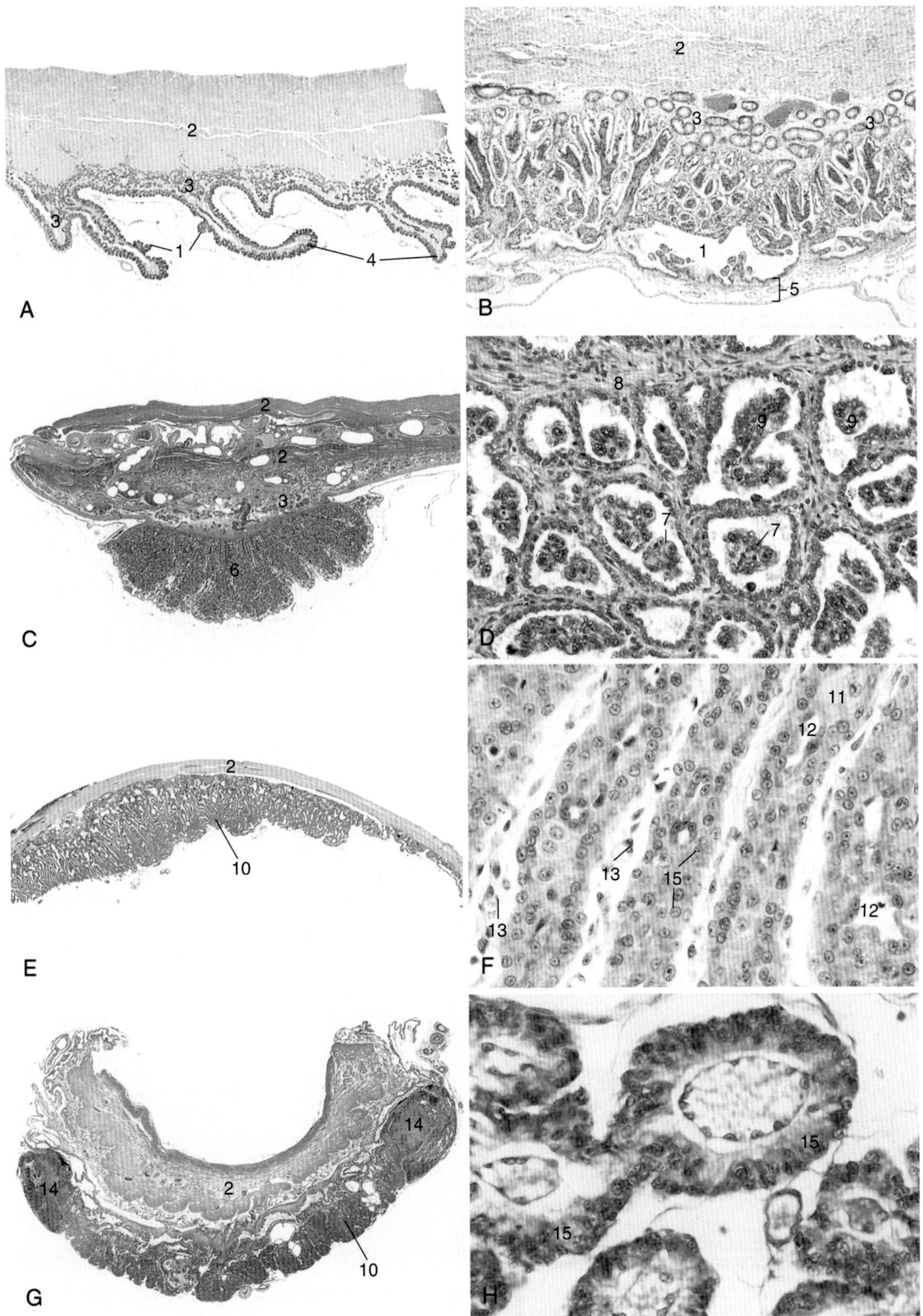


**Plate 9.** *A* to *H*, Placental histology (see *H* for label descriptions). *A*, Diffuse folded villous placenta (pig) (4×). *B*, Diffuse villous placenta (horse) (28×). *C* and *D*, Cotyledonary villous placenta (cow) (4×/140×). *E* and *F*, Zonary labyrinthine placenta (cat) (4×/279×). *G* and *H*, Zonary labyrinthine placenta (dog) (4×/279×): 1, areola; 2, myometrium; 3, endometrial glands; 4, primary fold; 5, allantochorion; 6, placentome; 7, trophoblastic giant cells; 8, uterine septum; 9, chorionic villi; 10, placental labyrinth; 11, decidual cell; 12, maternal capillaries; 13, fetal capillaries; 14, marginal hematomas; 15, trophoblast cells.

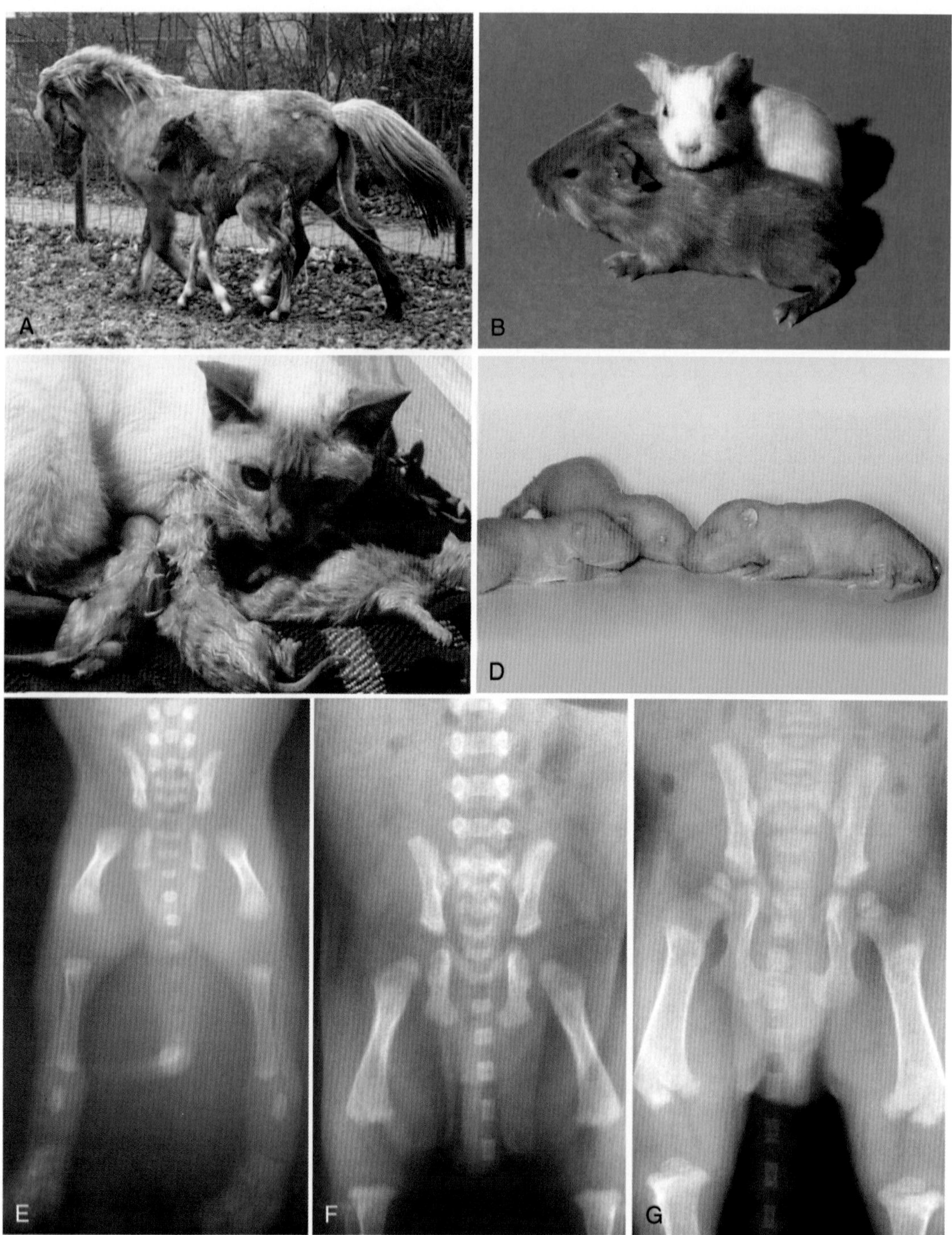

**Plate 10.** Developmental status shortly after birth. *A,* Newborn foal with mother (the mare has yet to discharge the fetal membranes (afterbirth). *B,* Newborn guinea pigs. *C,* Newborn kittens. *D,* Newborn and two-day-old rats. *E, F,* and *G,* Progress of skeletal ossification in puppy: 1, 14, and 28 days after birth, respectively.

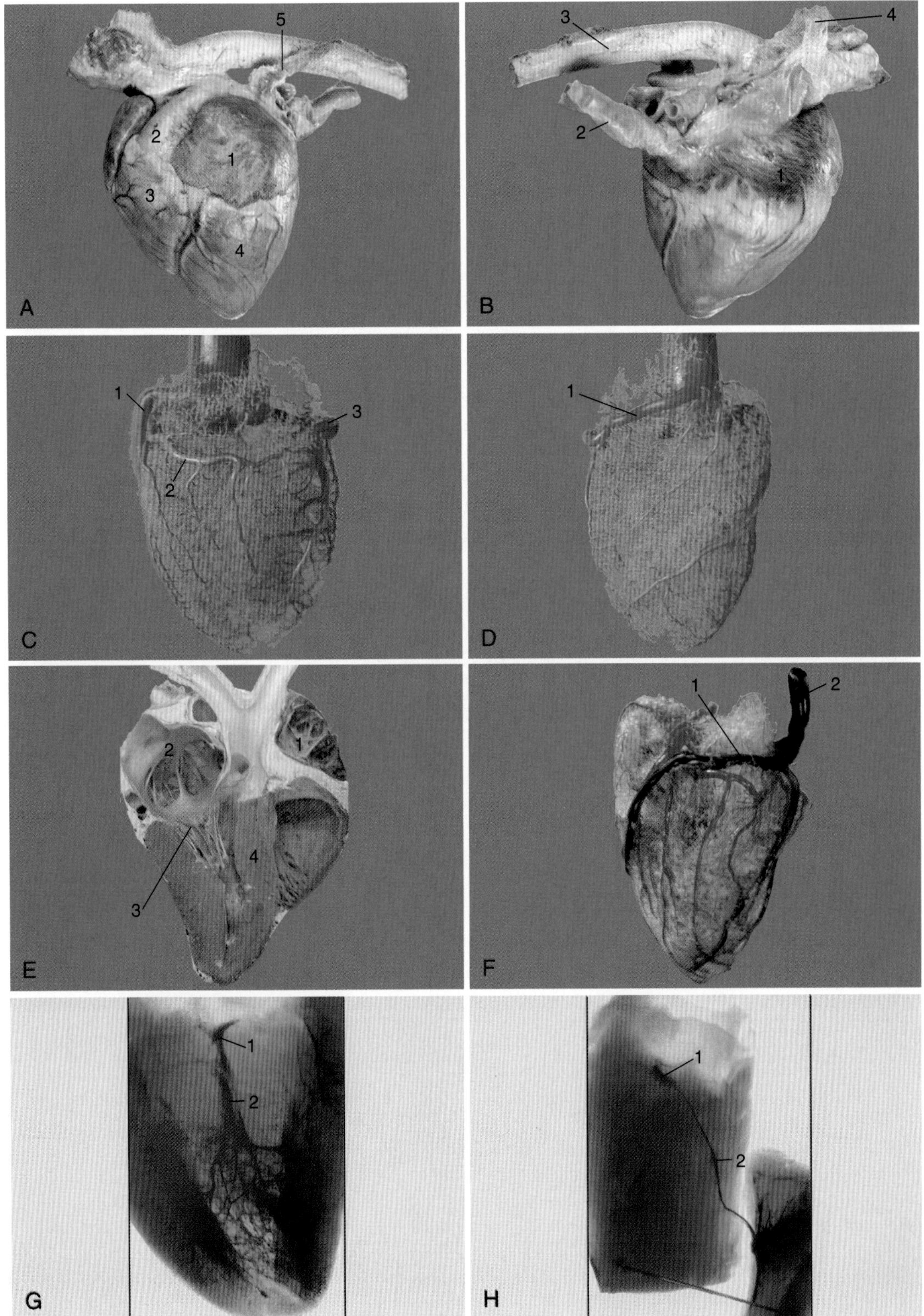


**Plate 11.** *A,* Left surface of the heart (pig): 1, left auricle; 2, pulmonary trunk; 3, right ventricle; 4, left ventricle; 5, left azygous v. *B,* Right surface of the heart (pig): 1, right atrium; 2, caudal v. cava; 3, aorta; 4, right azygous v. (opening into cranial v. cava). *C,* Corrosion cast of aorta and coronary circulation (pig): 1, left coronary a.; 2, ramus circumflexus; 3, right coronary a. *D,* Corrosion cast of aorta and coronary circulation (pig): 1, right coronary a. *E,* Section of heart (cow): 1, right auricle; 2, left atrium; 3, left atrioventricular valve; 4, interventricular septum. *F,* Corrosion cast of coronary aa. and v. (cow): 1, v. cordis magna; 2, left azygous v. *G,* Cleared specimen of left ventricle: 1, atrioventricular node; 2, left crus of atrioventricular trunk (injected blue). *H,* Cleared specimen of right ventricle: 1, atrioventricular node; 2, right crus of the atrioventricular trunk, continuing into the moderator band.

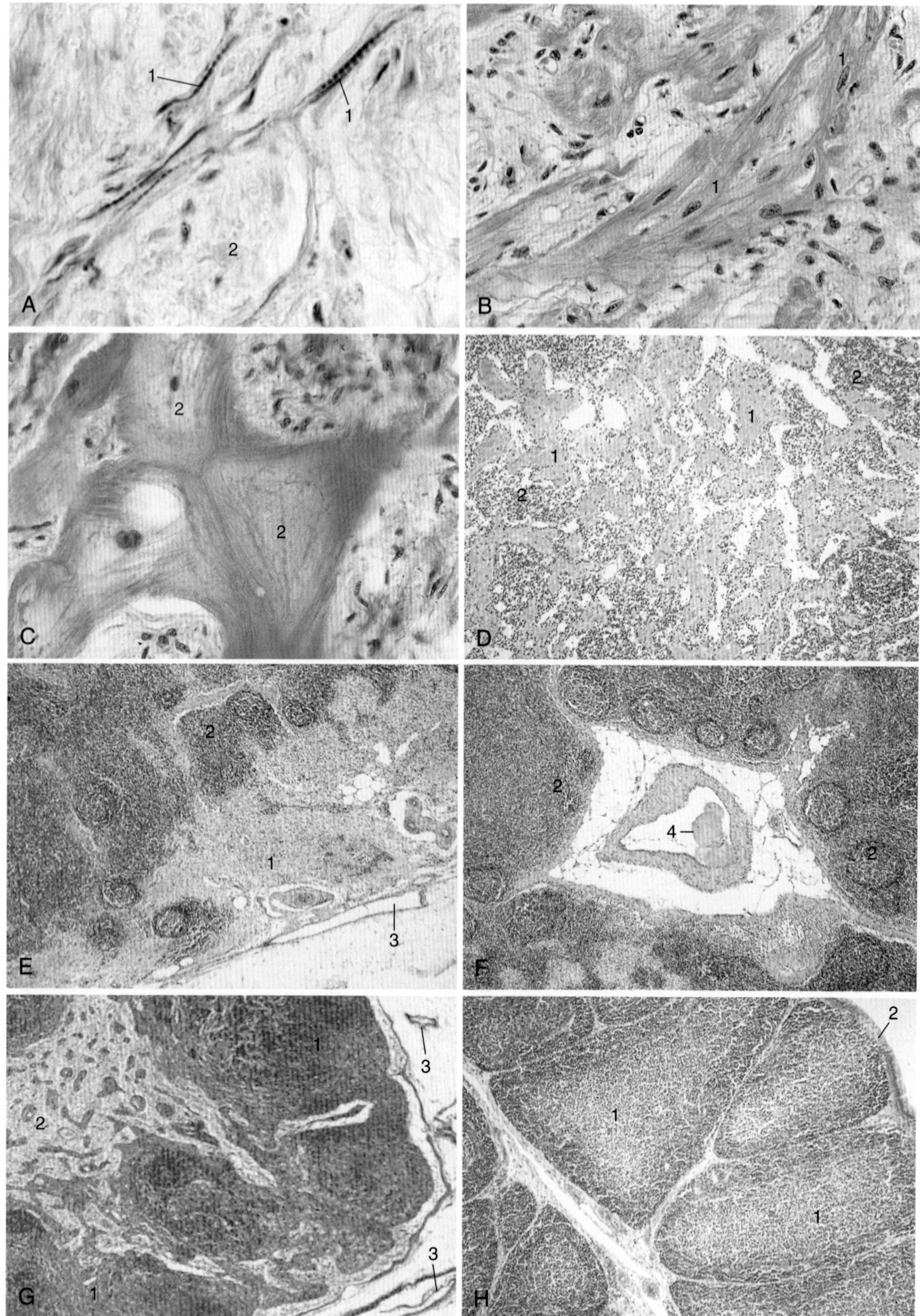


**Plate 12.** *A,* Sinuatrial node of equine heart (I-HE) (279×): 1, nodal myofibers; 2, bundle of nerve fibers. *B* and *C,* Atrioventricular node of equine heart (HE) (279×): 1, nodal myofibers; 2, purkinje cells with abundant glycogen. *D,* Hemal node of sheep (HE) (70×): 1, erythrocytes; 2, lymphocytes. *E* and *F,* Lymph node (pig) (28×): 1, loose lymphoreticular tissue; 2, lymph nodules in centrally located "cortex"; 3, efferent lymph vessels; 4, centrally located afferent lymph vessel, with valve. *G,* Lymph node (dog) (28×): 1, cortex with lymph nodules; 2, medulla; 3, afferent lymph vessels. *H,* Thymus of calf (HE) (70×): 1, thymic lobules; 2, capsule.

The collateral parietal branches begin with the caudal phrenic and cranial abdominal arteries which share a common *phrenicoabdominal* origin in the dog. They also include the paired *lumbar arteries* to the tissues and structures of the back, the *deep circumflex iliac* to the flank, the *external iliac artery* to the hindlimb, and the *internal iliac artery* which serves both pelvic viscera and pelvic walls.

Abdominal aorta
- Phrenicoabdominal aa.
- Lumbar aa.
- Celiac a.
  - L. gastric a.
  - Hepatic a.
    - Hepatic branches
    - R. gastric a.
    - Gastroduodenal a.
    - Cranial pancreaticoduodenal a.
    - R. gastroepiploic a.
  - Splenic a.
    - Pancreatic branches
    - Short gastric aa.
    - L. gastroepiploic a.
- Cranial mesenteric a.
  - Caudal pancreaticoduodenal a.
  - Jejunal aa.
  - Ileal aa.
  - Ileocolic a.
    - Middle colic a.
    - R. colic a.
    - Cecal aa.
- Renal aa.
- Testicular (ovarian) aa.
- Caudal mesenteric a.
  - L. colic a.
  - Cranial rectal a.
- Deep circumflex iliac aa.
- External iliac aa.
- Internal iliac aa.
- Median sacral a.
  - Lumbar a. VI
- Median caudal a.

It is worth drawing attention at this point to the existence of several pathways, established by anastamosis, that mitigate the effects of constriction or blockage of the aorta (e.g., by thrombosis, especially common in the cat). The collateral pathways include those formed along the spinal cord by anastomoses between successive lumbar arteries, those along the gut formed by connections between the principal visceral arteries, and those within the abdominal floor formed by the cranial and caudal epigastric arteries.

**The External Iliac Artery.** This is the principal artery of the hindlimb. It arises close to the termination of the aorta and runs obliquely over the abdominal roof to leave the abdomen by the vascular lacuna above the caudodorsal corner of the flank (Fig. 7–40/3). It detaches one branch within the abdomen, the *deep femoral artery* (/12), which is the common origin of the pudendoepigastric trunk and an important branch to the adductor

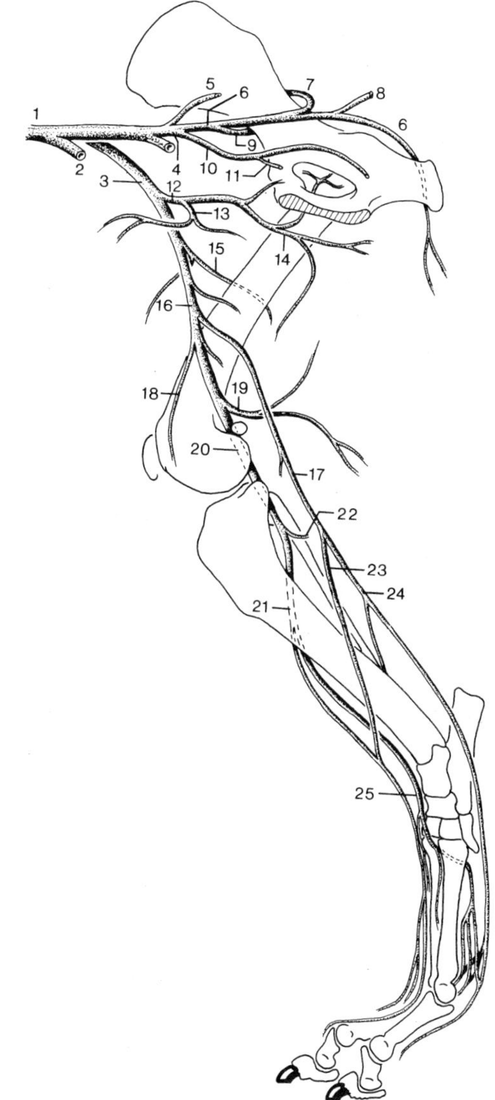


**Figure 7–40.** Arteries of the canine hindlimb.

1, Abdominal aorta; 2, left external iliac a.; 3, right external iliac a.; 4, left and right internal iliac aa.; 5, median sacral a.; 6, caudal gluteal a.; 7, cranial gluteal a.; 8, lateral caudal a.; 9, iliolumbar a.; 10, internal pudendal a.; 11, vaginal (prostatic) a.; 12, deep femoral a.; 13, pudendoepigastric trunk; 14, medial circumflex femoral a.; 15, lateral circumflex femoral a.; 16, femoral a.; 17, saphenous a.; 18, descending genicular a.; 19, distal caudal femoral a.; 20, popliteal a.; 21, cranial tibial a.; 22, caudal tibial a.; 23, cranial branch of the saphenous a.; 24, caudal branch of the saphenous a.; 25, dorsal pedal a.

muscles of the thigh. The short *pudendoepigastric trunk* (/13) ends by giving rise to the *caudal epigastric* and the *external pudendal arteries.* The former divides in similar fashion to the cranial epigastric; the latter passes through the inguinal canal to supply structures in the groin, including the prepuce in the male and the caudal mammary glands (via the caudal superficial epigastric artery) in the bitch (see Fig. 14–1).

The external iliac continues as the *femoral artery* (Fig. 7–40/16) on leaving the abdomen. Its first part has a superficial position in the femoral triangle—between the sartorius and pectineus where it raises a visible ridge and is ideally located for pulse-taking. It then burrows more deeply among the muscles to cross the medial surface of the femur to gain the caudal aspect of the thigh; it continues directly over the capsule of the stifle joint as the popliteal artery. The femoral artery has many branches, named and unnamed, to the muscles of the thigh, but most do not require individual notice. One branch that does merit attention is the *saphenous artery* (/17), which is detached in midthigh. This is a more important vessel in carnivores than in the larger species; it descends over the medial aspect of the limb before dividing into cranial and caudal branches. The cranial branch (/23) supplies the dorsal crural muscles before crossing the dorsal aspect of the hock to continue as the *dorsal common digital arteries.* The caudal branch (/24) takes a deep course between the muscles of the caudal aspect of the leg (crus), which it supplies, crosses the caudal face of the hock, and terminates as the plantar common digital arteries, which are comparable to the corresponding forelimb arteries.

The *popliteal* (/20) divides into cranial and caudal tibial arteries. The *cranial tibial artery* (/21) passes through the interosseous space between the tibia and fibula to run distally with the deep peroneal nerve. It crosses the dorsal aspect of the hock (as the dorsal pedal artery; /25) and gives rise to the dorsal metatarsal arteries among other branches. One of these metatarsal arteries reinforces the caudal branch of the saphenous on the plantar aspect of the limb after passing between the second and third metatarsal bones. The *caudal tibial artery* (/22) is of little account in carnivores. The following list includes various muscular branches not mentioned in the text.

- External iliac a.
  - Deep femoral a.
    - Pudendoepigastric trunk
      - Caudal epigastric a.
      - External pudendal a.
  - Femoral a.
    - Lateral circumflex femoral a.
    - Proximal, middle, and distal caudal femoral aa.
    - Saphenous a.
      - Cranial branch
        - Dorsal common digital aa.
      - Caudal branch
        - Plantar common digital aa.
  - Popliteal a.
    - Cranial tibial a.
      - Dorsal pedal a.
        - Dorsal metatarsal aa.
        - Plantar metatarsal aa.
    - Caudal tibial a.

**The Internal Iliac Artery.** This is the supply of the pelvic viscera and walls, including the overlying muscles of the gluteal region and those of the proximocaudal part of the thigh. The internal iliac artery continues caudoventrally from its origin, and in the dog it has a single branch, the *umbilical artery* (Fig. 7–41/5), a rather unimportant vestige of the placental supply of the fetus (p. 249). The proximal part of the umbilical artery carries a little blood to the cranial part of the bladder; the distal part is transformed into the round ligament of the bladder within the lateral vesical fold.

The internal iliac artery terminates by dividing into the caudal gluteal and internal pudendal arteries. The parietal branch, the *caudal gluteal artery* (/6), turns out of the pelvis with the sciatic nerve. This trunk, with its *iliolumbar* and *cranial gluteal* (/7) branches, supplies the muscles about the lumbosacral junction and those of the gluteal and proximocaudal femoral regions; the structures of the last-named region include the proximal parts of the hamstring muscles in which the caudal gluteal terminates.

The second terminal branch is the *internal pudendal artery* (/8) to the pelvic viscera (see also pp. 554 and 693). Its branches are differently named and disposed in the two sexes. The first branch is the prostatic artery in the male dog, the vaginal artery (/9) in the female. The *prostatic artery* supplies the middle rectal artery to the penultimate part of the rectum and various branches to the caudal parts of the ureter and bladder, the prostate, and the first part of the urethra. The *vaginal artery* also supplies the rectum and urinary organs in addition to the uterus and vagina. Its cranial branch, the uterine artery, forms the caudal part of the arterial arcade within the broad ligament (p. 198).

The next artery, the *urethral artery* (/10), is the same in both sexes. It supplies the caudal part of the pelvic urethra. The terminal branches of the

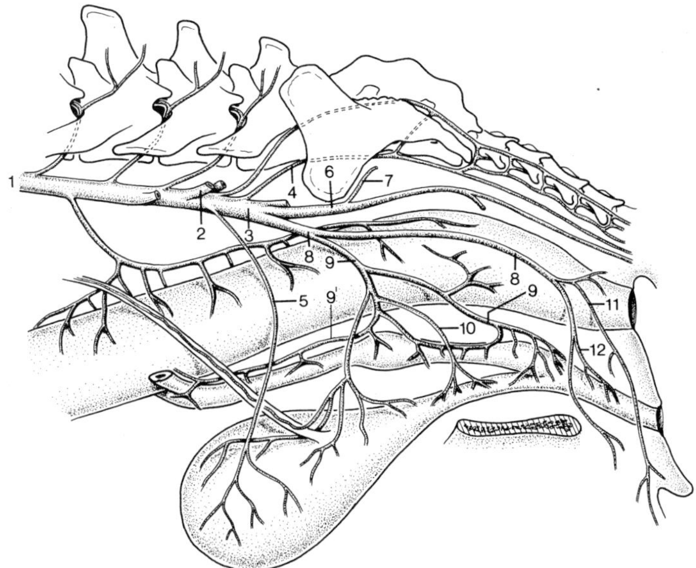


**Figure 7–41.** Arteries of the female pelvis, left lateral view (bitch).

1, Abdominal aorta; 2, external iliac a.; 3, internal iliac a.; 4, median sacral a.; 5, umbilical a.; 6, caudal gluteal a.; 7, cranial gluteal a.; 8, internal pudendal a.; 9, vaginal a.; 9′, uterine a.; 10, urethral a. (frequently a branch of the vaginal a.); 11, ventral perineal a.; 12, a. of the clitoris.

internal pudendal are the ventral perineal artery and the artery of the penis or clitoris. The *ventral perineal artery* (/11) supplies a caudal rectal artery to the last part of the rectum and branches to the scrotum (or labia of the vulva). The *artery of the penis* runs the length of the upper border of this organ to the region of the bulbus glandis; it becomes known as the dorsal artery of the penis after detachment of a branch to the penis bulb, which also supplies the corpus spongiosum and pars longa glandis, and a deep branch to the corpus cavernosum (p. 448 and Fig. 15–17). The *artery of the clitoris* (Fig. 7–41/12) is similar but on a less substantial scale.

Internal iliac a.
- Umbilical a.
- Caudal gluteal a.
  - Iliolumbar a.
  - Cranial gluteal a.
- Internal pudendal a.
  - Prostatic (vaginal) a.
    - A. of deferent duct (uterine a.)
    - Caudal vesicle a.
    - Middle rectal a.
  - Urethral artery
  - Ventral perineal a.
    - Caudal rectal a.
  - Artery of penis (clitoris)
    - Artery of bulb
    - Deep artery
    - Dorsal artery

## *The Systemic Veins*

The systemic veins return blood to the heart through the cranial vena cava, caudal vena cava, and coronary sinus.* The *coronary sinus* returns the bulk of the blood from the heart wall (p. 226); in ruminants and pigs it is joined by the left azygous vein. In the horse and the dog the equivalent (azygous) territory is drained by the right azygous (Figs. 7–9/12 and 7–7/12).

**The Cranial Vena Cava.** The cranial vena cava is formed close to the entrance to the chest by the union of the external jugular and subclavian veins, which drain the head and neck and the forelimb, respectively. In the dog the subclavian and jugular veins of each side join in a common trunk (brachiocephalic vein; Fig. 7–42/2), which then combines with its fellow; another arrangement is the union of the two jugulars in a single bijugular trunk (/4), which is then joined by the subclavian veins. The cranial vena cava runs through the cranial mediastinum, ventral and to the right of the trachea and related to the brachiocephalic trunk (dorsally at its origin, later at its left face). It is joined by various tributaries broadly corresponding to branches of the subclavian artery and by the larger right azygous vein toward its

*Because we do not give a full systematic account of the veins, it is convenient to depart from common practice and describe them according to the direction of the flow of blood.

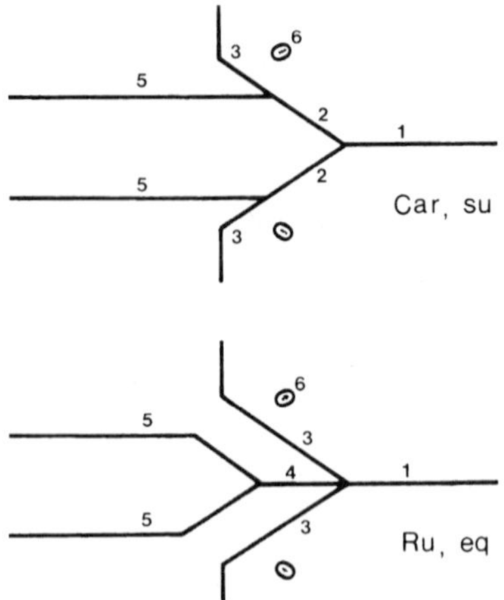


**Figure 7–42.** Formation of the cranial vena cava (1) at the thoracic inlet, schematic; dorsal view, cranial is to the left. Car (dog and cat), su (pig), Ru (ruminants), eq (horse).

1, Cranial vena cava; 2, brachiocephalic v.; 3, subclavian v.; 4, bijugular trunk; 5, external jugular v.; 6, position of first pair of ribs.

termination (Fig. 7–43/3)—unless this makes separate entry to the right atrium as in the horse.

The *azygous vein* (/3) is formed by the union of the first lumbar veins and passes through the aortic hiatus into the chest where it is reinforced by intercostal veins from the caudal and middle intercostal spaces. Right and left veins are present in the embryo, but the pattern is later commonly simplified: in horses and dogs the right azygous vein persists as the main trunk, in ruminants and pigs the left one—unless, as is usual in ruminants, both remain of some size. The right azygous vein arches ventrally, passing in front of the root of the right lung to reach the terminal part of the cranial vena cava or the adjacent part of the right atrium (horse). The left vein arches in front of the root of the left lung and must then run caudally, over the left atrium, to reach its confluence with the coronary sinus (Fig. 7–9/*A*,12). The cranial intercostal veins that do not drain into this system join various tributaries of the subclavian or go

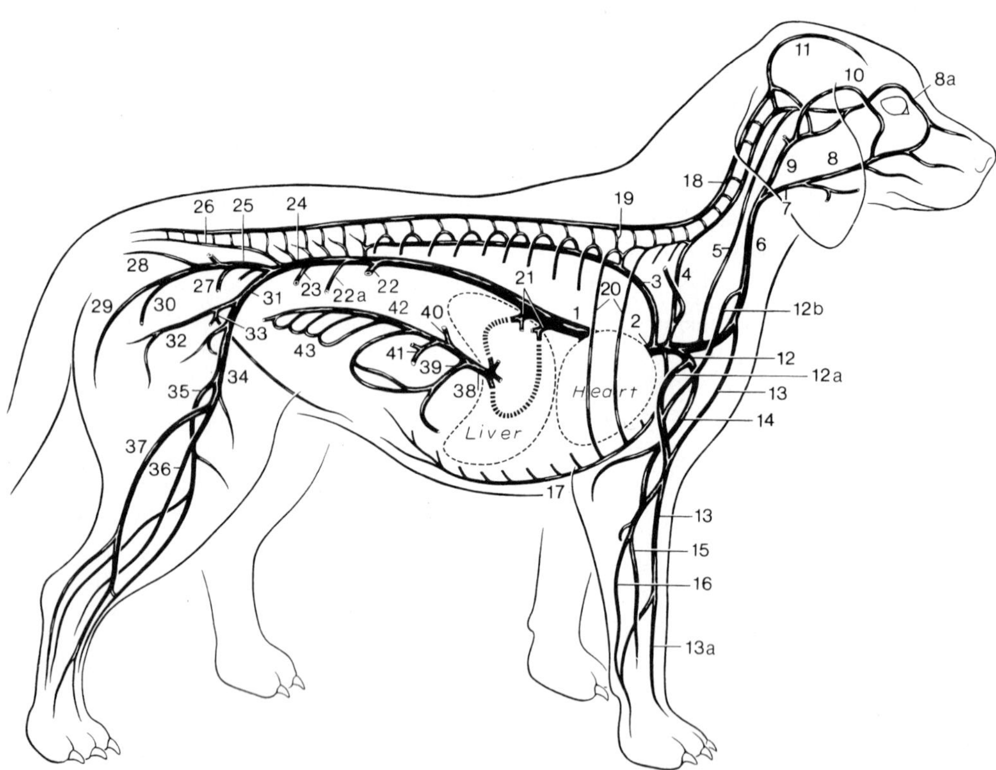


**Figure 7–43.** Schematic representation of the venous system (dog).

1, Caudal vena cava; 2, cranial vena cava; 3, azygous v.; 4, vertebral v.; 5, internal jugular v.; 6, external jugular v.; 7, linguofacial v.; 8, facial v.; 8a, angularis oculi v.; 9, maxillary v.; 10, superficial temporal v.; 11, dorsal sagittal sinus; 12, subclavian v.; 12a, axillobrachial v.; 12b, omobrachial v.; 13, cephalic v.; 13a, accessory cephalic v.; 14, brachial v.; 15, radial v.; 16, ulnar v.; 17, internal thoracic v.; 18, vertebral venous plexus; 19, intervertebral v.; 20, intercostal vv.; 21, hepatic vv.; 22, renal v.; 22a, testicular or ovarian v.; 23, deep circumflex iliac v.; 24, common iliac v.; 25, right internal iliac v.; 26, median sacral v.; 27, prostatic or vaginal v.; 28, lateral caudal v.; 29, caudal gluteal v.; 30, internal pudendal v.; 31, right external iliac v.; 32, deep femoral v.; 33, pudendoepigastric trunk; 34, femoral v.; 35, medial saphenous v.; 36, cranial tibial v.; 37, lateral saphenous v.; 38, portal v.; 39, gastroduodenal v.; 40, splenic v.; 41, caudal mesenteric v.; 42, cranial mesenteric v.; 43, jejunal vv.

directly to the cranial vena cava. The special importance of the azygous system in draining the plexus within the vertebral canal is considered elsewhere (p. 305).

The *subclavian vein* generally corresponds to the subclavian artery and most tributaries in the upper part of the limb are satellite to arterial branches. The pattern is different in the distal part of the limb where important unaccompanied superficial veins are present. Although these are connected with the deeper veins at various levels they also continue into the *cephalic vein* (Fig. 7–43/13), which in the arm runs between the pectoral and brachiocephalic muscles to join the external jugular vein in the lower part of the neck.

Two pairs of jugular veins exist within the neck. The deep *internal jugular* (/5) runs with the common carotid artery within the visceral space of the neck; however, except in the dog and cat, it is very much reduced in size or even absent in postnatal animals; even in the dog and cat it is of minor importance. The *external jugular vein* (/6) is formed near the angle of the jaw by the union of linguofacial and maxillary veins. Its course through the neck occupies a (jugular) groove between the brachiocephalicus dorsally, the sternocephalicus ventrally in the larger species, while in the dog it lies on the sternocephalicus. It is easily raised for intravenous injection and blood sampling, and in the larger species it is the first choice for these procedures. The territories of its linguofacial and maxillary tributaries show considerable overlap and some species variation; the former vein is in general the principal drainage of the more superficial and more rostral structures of the head, the latter of those deeper and more caudal, including the contents of the cranial cavity (see Fig. 11–28).

**The Caudal Vena Cava.** The caudal vena cava is formed on the roof of the abdomen, near the pelvic inlet, by the union of right and left common iliac veins, each formed in its turn by the union of an *internal iliac vein,* which drains the pelvic walls and much of the contents of the pelvic cavity, and an *external iliac vein,* which drains the hindlimb (Fig. 7–43/25,31). The external iliac vein and the bulk of its tributaries are satellite to arteries. The independent medial and lateral saphenous veins of the leg (/35,37) drain the superficial veins of the foot.

In its intra-abdominal course the caudal vena cava is joined by additional tributaries draining the abdominal roof, including large *renal veins,* before it dips ventrally to tunnel through the liver and subsequently the diaphragm at the caval foramen. It enters the thoracic cavity at a relatively ventral level and pursues a course within the free edge of the plica venae cavae between the caudal and accessory lobes of the right lung (see Fig. 4–19/*B*,9). It joins the right atrium dorsal to the inlet of the coronary sinus.

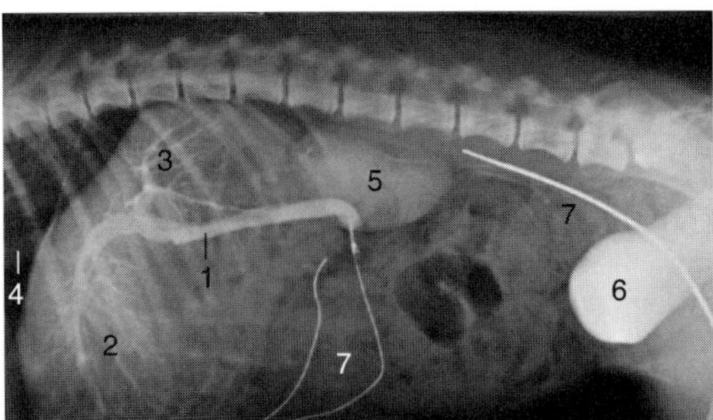


**Figure 7–44.** Cannulation of the portal vein of a dog.

1, Portal vein; 2, branches to the quadrate, left medial and lateral liver lobes; 3, branches to the remaining liver lobes; 4, caudal vena cava; 5, kidney; 6, bladder, filled with opaque medium; 7, catheters.

In its intrahepatic course the caudal vena cava receives the *hepatic veins,* which drain the liver (Fig. 7–43/21).

The *portal vein* drains the spleen, the intra-abdominal digestive organs, the caudal part of the thoracic esophagus, and the bulk of the rectum (/38 and Fig. 7–44). It is formed variously from three main tributaries (see Fig. 3–49/2,4,5). The splenic tributary corresponds to the celiac artery (excluding its hepatic branches) and therefore drains the last part of the esophagus, the stomach, parts of the duodenum and pancreas, and the spleen. The cranial and caudal mesenteric veins drain the territories of the like-named arteries and usually join in a common trunk before combining with the splenic.

The last part of the rectum and the anal region differ from the remainder of the gut in draining toward the internal iliac vein. The veins of this part form one of the portosystemic connections that provide alternative (although not very capacious) outlets from the portal drainage territory that are used when the intrahepatic circulation is impaired, as, for example, by cirrhosis (hepatic fibrosis).

## THE CIRCULATION IN THE FETUS AND THE CHANGES AFTER BIRTH

During fetal life the placenta combines the roles that are later performed by the lungs, the digestive tract, and the kidneys. The blood is therefore replenished with oxygen, provided with nutrients, and cleansed of waste in its circulation through the placenta. It is returned to the fetus by two large umbilical veins that wind within the umbilical cord and join as one where they enter the body at the navel (Fig. 7–45/11). The single intra-abdominal umbilical vein runs forward to penetrate the liver at the umbilical fissure before it divides. It detaches collateral branches that vascularize the left portions (umbilical moiety) of the liver while a further branch bends toward the right to make a wide connection with the portal vein (/12), which vascularizes the right portions (portal moiety). A direct continuation of the umbilical trunk, the ductus venosus (/9), tunnels through the substance of the liver, bypassing the hepatic circulation, to join the caudal vena cava. The ductus venosus, present in all young embryos, soon becomes vestigial in those of the horse and pig. It persists in other species but varies in caliber and importance and tends to become reduced toward term. The division of the liver into umbilical and portal moieties has obvious functional and possibly also clinical importance. The portal moiety is less generously supplied with oxygen, and this stimulates more active hemopoiesis; the umbilical moiety is more likely to suffer from infections acquired in utero.

The caudal vena cava (/8) receives the umbilical blood after its passage through the liver and adds it to the deoxygenated blood returned from the hindpart of the body. The oxygen content of the caudal caval stream is therefore already reduced below that of the placental return before it reaches the heart where the stream impinges on the cranial margin of the foramen ovale (Fig. 7–46/2,4). This divides it into two: one part continues into the right atrium (/3), the other passes through the foramen ovale into the left atrium (/8). The relative sizes of the two streams change as gestation advances, a continuing shift of the margin of the foramen to the left increasing the flow into the right atrium. The right stream mixes with the return from other systemic veins (/1), and the oxygen content of the blood passed to the right ventricle is thus further diminished. This blood is ejected into the pulmonary trunk (/6), which in the fetus communicates with the aorta through a wide channel, the ductus arteriosus (/7′). The ductus enters the aorta beyond the origin of the brachiocephalic trunk and is as wide as the pulmonary trunk (it is in fact its direct continuation—the right and left pulmonary arteries [/7] are the side branches). The ductus arteriosus receives most of the output of the right ventricle since the vascular bed of the unexpanded lungs offers a more considerable resistance to blood flow.

The small flow that is returned to the left atrium

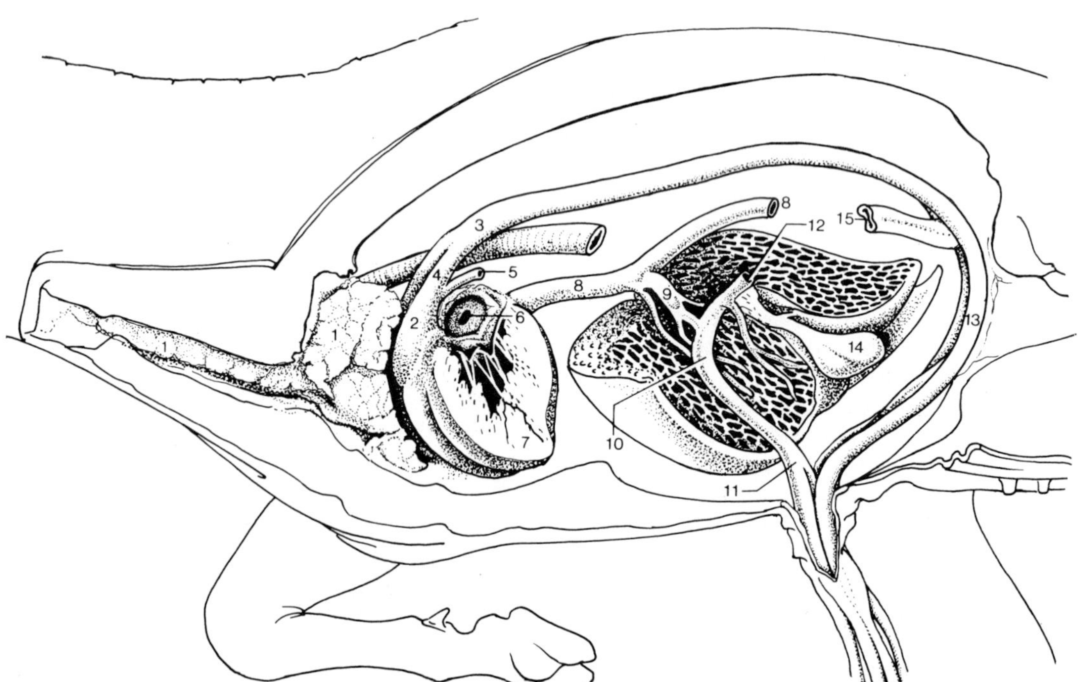


**Figure 7–45.** Semischematic drawing of fetal circulation (calf).

1, Thymus; 2, pulmonary trunk; 3, aortic arch; 4, ductus arteriosus; 5, pulmonary artery; 6, foramen ovale; 7, wall of left ventricle; 8, caudal vena cava; 9, ductus venosus; 10, junction of umbilical and portal branches within the liver; 11, umbilical vein; 12, stump of portal vein; 13, left umbilical artery; 14, gallbladder; 15, descending colon.

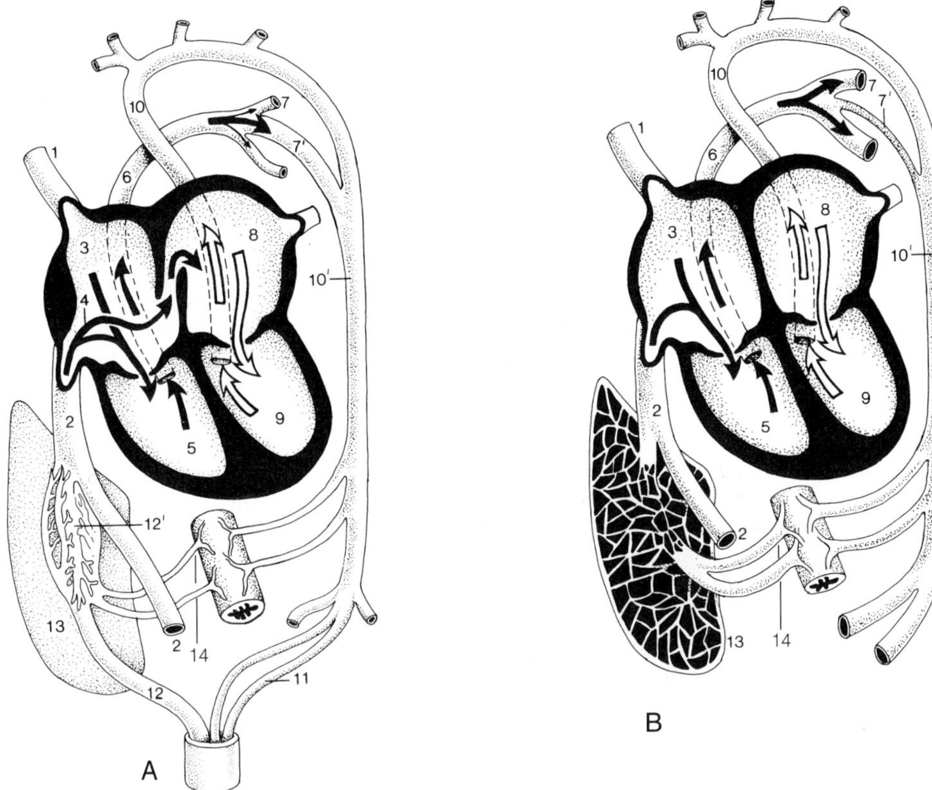


**Figure 7–46.** Diagrams of the fetal *(A)* and postnatal *(B)* circulatory systems.

1, Cranial vena cava; 2, caudal vena cava; 3, right atrium; 4, arrow entering oval foramen; 5, right ventricle; 6, pulmonary trunk; 7, pulmonary artery; 7′, ductus arteriosus (in *B*, vestige); 8, left atrium; 9, left ventricle; 10, aortic arch; 10′, descending aorta; 11, umbilical artery; 12, umbilical vein; 12′, ductus venosus; 13, liver; 14, portal vein.

from the lungs mixes there with the greater volume of blood that passed through the foramen ovale. The blood that enters the aorta (/10) is therefore relatively well oxygenated; part of this stream enters the coronary and carotid arteries. The head and brain are therefore favored by receiving a richer supply of oxygen than is given to organs supplied from those branches of the aorta that arise distal to the entry of the ductus arteriosus; these later branches receive the mixed output of both ventricles. The placenta receives the greater share of the flow through the descending aorta (/10′) by way of the umbilical arteries (/11); these branch from the internal iliac arteries and leave the fetus at the umbilicus, together with the allantoic duct (Fig. 7–45/13). The fetal blood stream is brought into close apposition with the maternal blood stream within the placenta, although the intervening tissue barrier varies in thickness and permeability among species (p. 206).

The changes in the circulation that follow birth are not completed as promptly as many believe, and some hours, or even days, may be necessary before a stable circulation of adult pattern is established. The permanent closure of the redundant fetal channels requires a much longer time. The arrest of the placental circulation may precede or follow the initiation of pulmonary ventilation according to the circumstances of parturition. The umbilical vessels are either bitten across by the mother (e.g., puppy) or are ruptured, being unable to support the weight of the offspring (e.g., calf); in species in which the latter fate is usual they divide at predetermined levels. In both circumstances little hemorrhaging occurs since the rough treatment stimulates contraction of the muscle in the vessel wall. The arterial stumps are slowly transformed into the round ligaments of the bladder. The stump of the umbilical vein outside the abdomen shrivels, the intra-abdominal part is in time transformed into the round ligament of the liver (p. 419). The raw umbilical surfaces provide potential entry to infection ("navel ill"), the allantoic duct and thrombosed vein being convenient routes for its spread.

The ductus venosus closes within a short time,

but how this is achieved and whether closure is to be measured within hours or days are controversial points. Its elimination from the circulation allows the portal vein to perfuse all parts of the liver.

The loss of the umbilical return reduces both the volume and the pressure of the caudal caval stream. This, combined with the concurrent increase in left atrial pressure, halts the shunt through the foramen ovale. Contraction of the muscular wall of the ductus arteriosus is stimulated by the raised oxygen tension of the perfusing blood; it is not effected at once, and for some hours or days blood may shunt in either direction according to the relative pressures in the aorta and pulmonary artery. Expansion of the lungs reduces the resistance of their vascular bed and the drop in pulmonary arterial pressure results in the flow through the ductus normally being from the aorta. The passage of blood through the constricted tube causes vibration of its wall, which may be detected on auscultation as a continuous murmur during the first day or two of postnatal life in calves and foals. Permanent structural changes eventually obliterate the lumen, converting the duct into the fibrous structure (ligamentum arteriosum); but for some time after birth the ductus dilates in circumstances that produce hypoxia, and it is often found widely open in the neonatal postmortem specimen.

The increased venous return from the lungs raises the pressure within the left atrium, and this forces the valve of the foramen ovale against the atrial septum, closing the foramen (Figs. 7–22 and 7–46). The valve is a simple flap in carnivores, more elaborate and tubular in ungulates, in which muscle causes it to crumple, improving closure. Although fibrosis eventually seals the valve in place, this takes some time, and it is not uncommon for the opening to be patent to a probe for months or even years; such patency is rarely of significance.

Hypertrophy of the left ventricular wall occurs as a response to the increased workload that is now placed on that chamber. Although little exact information is available on this point for most species, significant relative thickening of the left ventricular wall is already apparent by the end of the first postnatal week in puppies.

## THE ORGANIZATION OF THE LYMPHATIC SYSTEM

The lymphatic system is responsible for the immunological defense of the body. It protects the body from exogenous (foreign) and abnormal endogenous macromolecules and from viruses, bacteria, and other invasive microorganisms. It includes all the lymphatic organs: thymus, tonsils, spleen, lymph nodes and hemal nodes, and the diffuse lymphatic tissue and lymphatic nodules present in many mucous membranes. The circulating lymphocytes, and the lymphocytes and plasma cells that are widely disseminated throughout the organism, also participate in this protective system.

Two types of functionally distinct lymphocytes are recognized: T-lymphocytes and B-lymphocytes. Both result from antigen-independent proliferation and differentiation of stem cells in the primary lymphatic organs (T-cells from the thymus, and B-cells from the bursa of Fabricius in birds, the bone marrow in mammals); from the primary organs both types of lymphocytes seed the secondary lymphatic organs and within these, B- and T-lymphocytes undergo antigen-dependent proliferation and differentiation into effector cells which either attend to the disposal of particular antigens or provide the memory cells which become temporarily inactive. There is, in addition, a reserve population of undifferentiated lymphocytes.

The brief introduction to the system presented in Chapter 1 emphasizes the role of the lymphatic capillaries and larger vessels in returning an important fraction of the tissue fluid to the circulating blood. This role justifies the inclusion of these vessels, and of the nodes through which the lymph is passed, within the broad concept of a circulatory system (see Fig. 1–34). The framework that supports the lymphatic nodules (germinal centers) contains phagocytic cells that remove particulate matter, including microorganisms on occasion, from the percolating lymph; this element must be included within the widely diffused macrophage or reticuloendothelial system that also includes the tissue macrophages and the endothelium of the hepatic, splenic, and bone marrow sinusoids. The vital uniting theme is defense, both humoral and cellular, against foreign invasion of the body. Since some of these functions do not intrude on the scope of gross anatomy, the present account concentrates on the lymphatic vessels and nodes as drainage and filtration mechanisms.

Before considering the topographical layout of the lymphatic system, mention must be made of the so-called lymphoepithelial structures comprising aggregations of unencapsulated lymph nodules within various mucosae. These are conveniently generically termed *tonsils,* although the name is most often used specifically for those in the pharyngeal region where they guard against the passage of infection to deeper parts of the respiratory and digestive systems (Fig. 7–47/2). Pharyngeal and palatine tonsils are mentioned on page 117. Other tonsils are found in the mucosae

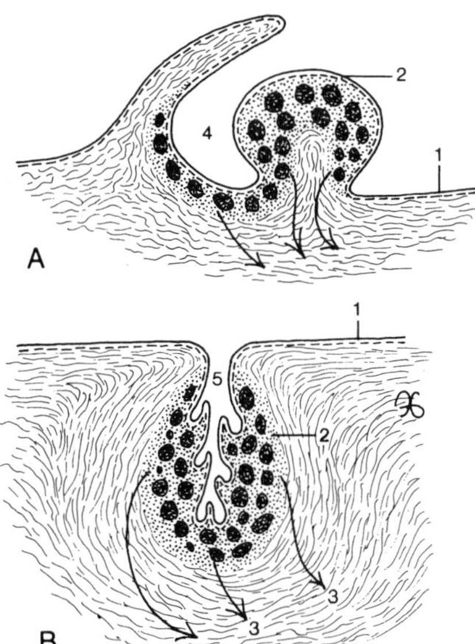


**Figure 7–47.** Schematic drawing of the palatine tonsils of the dog *(A)* and cattle *(B)*. The tonsils of the dog develop around a fossa but protrude into the oropharynx. Those of cattle surround the tonsillar sinus within the oropharyngeal wall.

1, Epithelium; 2, palatine tonsil; 3, efferent vessels *(arrows)*; 4, tonsillar fossa; 5, tonsillar sinus.

of the larynx, intestine, prepuce, and vagina and other parts of the female tract. The common features that distinguish tonsils from lymph nodes are the absence of a capsule, the close relationship to a moist epithelial surface, and the position at the origin of a lymphatic drainage pathway.

In addition to the ordinary lymph node, a second variety of similar structure exists but is positioned athwart the blood stream. These *hemal nodes* (Plate 12/*D*) are not found in all species and are most familiar in sheep in which their dark color (due to the contained blood) contrasts them with the white fat in which they are commonly embedded. They are mainly found below the roof of the abdomen and thorax. A so-called third variety, the hemolymph node, is probably only a lymph node that contains red blood cells in its sinuses as a result of hemorrhage in its tributary field.

It is uncertain whether lymph vessels develop independently and later make secondary entry to veins, bud from existing veins, or arise by a combination of these methods. Both methods account for the existence of the lymphaticovenous connections between the major lymphatic trunks and the great veins at the entrance to the chest. In some (nondomestic) mammals additional connections are described, often with renal veins. Such additional openings into the venous system can develop in later life when the normal flow is obstructed.

Lymph nodes initially form as mesenchymal condensations placed along the lymphatic capillary plexus. They are later populated by lymphocytes that emigrate from the central lymphoid organ, the thymus. All lymphoid structures are especially well developed in juveniles.

As already mentioned (p. 29) there are important species differences in the disposition of the components of the lymph nodes. In most animals, the lymph nodules are located in the peripheral cortex close to where the afferent lymph vessels penetrate the capsule (Fig. 7–48; Plate 12/*G*). The central medulla consists of loose lymphoreticular tissue where the efferent vessels take origin to

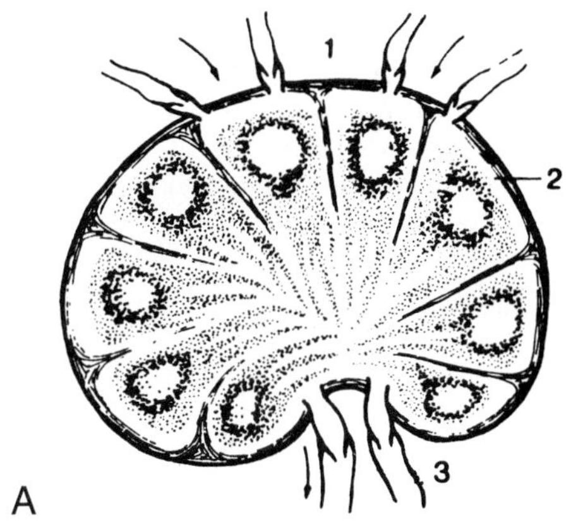


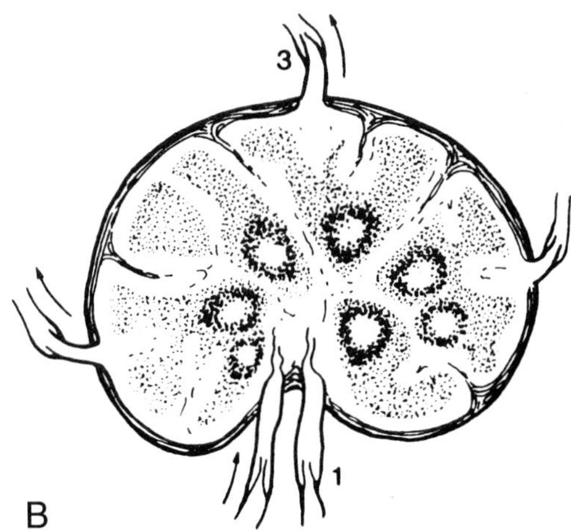


**Figure 7–48.** Structure of a lymph node *(A)* in which the germinal centers (lymph nodules) occupy the cortical region. In the pig *(B)* the germinal centers lie centrally. The arrows indicate the direction of lymph flow.

1, Afferent lymphatics; 2, subcapsular sinus; 3, efferent lymphatics.

leave the node in the indented hilar region. In contrast, in porcine nodes, the "cortical" tissue is central where most nodules lie alongside the trabecular sinuses. The afferent vessels penetrate the capsule at one or more sites and follow the trabeculae to reach the centrally located nodules. The periphery of the node is largely occupied by loose lymphoreticular tissue (Plate 12/*E,F*), and it is from here that the efferent lymph vessels emerge.

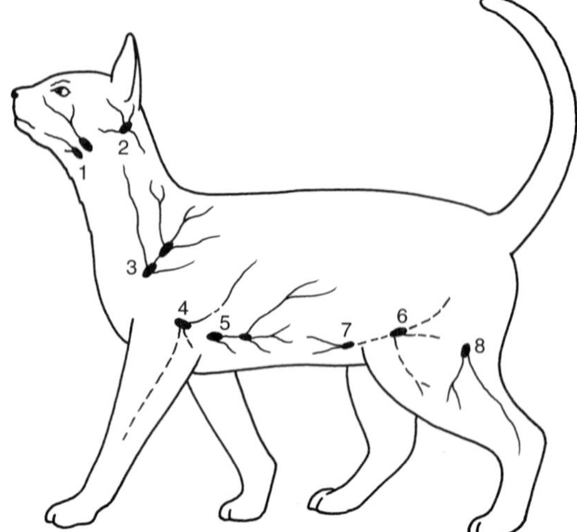


**Figure 7–50.** Palpable lymph nodes of the cat.

1, Mandibular; 2, lateral retropharyngeal; 3, dorsal superficial cervical; 4, axillary; 5, accessory axillary; 6, superficial inguinal; 7, caudal epigastric; 8, popliteal.

## The Topography of Lymphatic Drainage

The applied importance of the lymphatic drainage has been stressed, and accounts of its organization in different species are presented later. Since these accounts are necessarily fragmented by the regional character of the later chapters, it may be useful to give here a short general account in which species variations and clinical significance are subordinated to the presentation of a view of the system as a whole. We begin with Figures 7–49 and 7–50 which show the palpable lymph nodes of the dog and cat.

### The Lymph Nodes of the Head

Three lymphocenters are present in the head. The *parotid center* consists of one or more nodes placed on the masseter close to the temporomandibular joint and commonly covered by the parotid gland (Fig. 7–51/2). These nodes receive lymph from dorsal structures of the head, including skin, the dorsal bones of the skull, the contents of the orbit, and the masticatory muscles (in part).

The *mandibular center* (/1) comprises a group of nodes placed within the intermandibular space or more caudally by the angle of the jaw. They drain structures of the muzzle, the salivary glands, the intermandibular space (including the tongue), and a further part of the masticatory muscles.

The *retropharyngeal center* comprises two groups of nodes, medial and lateral; the former (/4) lie against the roof of the pharynx, the latter (/3) are contained within the atlantal fossa. Together, they drain deeper structures of the head and adjacent parts of the neck, including the pharynx and larynx; one or the other also receives lymph that has already passed through the more peripheral centers. In most species the medial group serves as the collecting center for the head, receiving the output from the lateral retropharyngeal, parotid, and mandibular nodes; in cattle this role is taken by the lateral group (see Fig. 25–28).

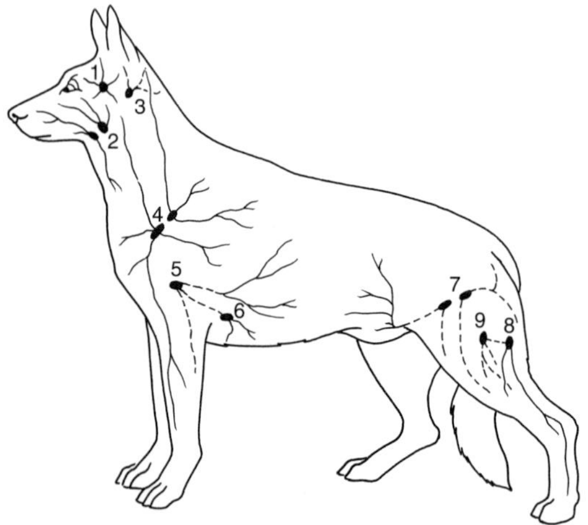


**Figure 7–49.** Palpable lymph nodes of the dog.

1, Parotid; 2, mandibular; 3, lateral retropharyngeal (inconstant); 4, superficial cervical; 5, axillary; 6, accessory axillary (inconstant); 7, superficial inguinal; 8, popliteal; 9, femoral (inconstant).

### The Lymph Nodes of the Neck

The *superficial cervical center* (Fig. 7–51/6) lies in front of the shoulder joint, under cover of the lateral superficial muscles of the neck; it consists of one or more nodes that drain a very wide but predominantly superficial territory. This extends from the nape to the middle of the trunk and includes the proximal part of the forelimb. The outflow is usually to the lymphatics at the thoracic inlet (/12).

The *deep cervical center* (/5) comprises a chain of nodes, usually described as packeted in cranial, middle, and caudal groups but often irregular in disposition. The nodes are placed along the trachea within the visceral space of the neck and mainly drain deeper and more ventral structures; much of this lymph percolates through successive nodes of the chain before entering one of the major lymphatic channels at the entrance to the chest.

## The Tracheal Duct

In most species the tracheal duct (/12) is a large paired vessel that follows the course of the trachea within the neck. Except in the horse, it takes origin in the retropharyngeal nodes that serve as the collecting center of the head; it may be augmented by tributaries from deep cervical nodes before it joins the thoracic (on the left side) or right lymphatic duct. Alternatively, one or both tracheal ducts may enter the corresponding jugular or other vein at the venous confluence at the entrance to the thorax (see Fig. 1–34). In the horse the flow may be interrupted by serial passage through deep cervical nodes (see Fig. 18–38/7).

## The Lymph Nodes of the Forelimb

One *axillary center* exists. The principal nodes are contained within the axilla where they lie on the medial muscles of the shoulder; additional nodes may be found in relation to the first rib or more caudally on the chest wall. In the horse alone, a more distal group of cubital nodes is placed over the medial aspect of the elbow. The center drains the deeper structures of the entire limb and the more superficial structures of the distal segments. The efferent vessels pass directly, or after serial passage through several nodes, to one of the major lymphatic or venous channels at the entrance to the chest.

## The Lymph Nodes of the Thorax

Four lymphocenters attend to the drainage of the thoracic walls and contents. The nodes within certain groups are rather diffusely spread, and it is not always easy to decide their correct designation (see Fig. 35–6).

The *dorsal thoracic center* comprises two groups of small, inconstant nodes; the intercostal set (Fig. 7–52/6) is found within the upper parts of a few intercostal spaces; the thoracic aortic set is dispersed along the course of the vessel. The center drains the back and deeper tissues of the thoracic wall and sends its outflow, possibly after serial passage through several nodes, to the thoracic duct or the mediastinal nodes (/8).

The *ventral thoracic center* comprises cranial sternal nodes (/10) by the manubrium of the sternum and, but only in ruminants, caudal sternal nodes placed against both surfaces of the transversus thoracis muscle. The center drains the deeper structures of the ventral part of the thoracic wall and sends its efferent flow either to mediastinal nodes or to one of the larger collecting vessels.

The *mediastinal center* is divided into a group of nodes within the cranial mediastinum (/8), a middle group about the base of the heart, and a caudal group (absent in carnivores) near the esophagus as it approaches the diaphragm (see Fig. 27–8/5,6). The various nodes drain structures of the thoracic wall, mainly after first passage of the lymph through other primary nodes, and thoracic

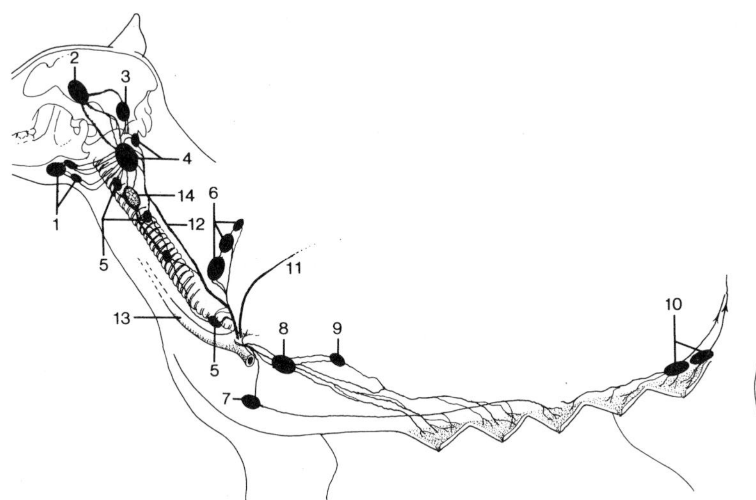


**Figure 7–51.** Lymph drainage of the head, neck, and mammary glands of the dog.

1, Mandibular nodes; 2, parotid node; 3, lateral retropharyngeal node; 4, medial retropharyngeal nodes; 5, cranial and caudal deep cervical nodes; 6, superficial cervical nodes; 7, sternal node; 8, axillary node; 9, accessory axillary node; 10, superficial inguinal nodes; 11, thoracic duct; 12, tracheal duct; 13, external jugular vein; 14, thyroid gland.

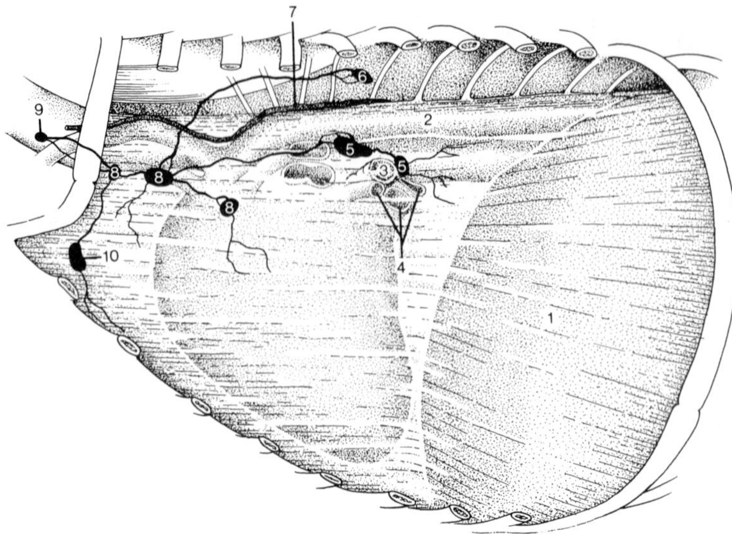


**Figure 7–52.** Thoracic lymph nodes in the dog. Left lung removed; the outline of the heart is visible within the mediastinum.

1, Diaphragm; 2, thoracic aorta; 3, left bronchus; 4, pulmonary vessels; 5, tracheobronchial nodes; 6, intercostal node; 7, thoracic duct; 8, cranial mediastinal nodes; 9, caudal deep cervical node; 10, sternal node.

viscera; they provide a secondary station for lymph from the lungs that has already passed through tracheobronchial nodes. The outflow goes to the large collecting vessels at the entrance to the chest, in part after serial passage through several nodes.

The *bronchial center* consists of groups of tracheobronchial nodes placed about the tracheal bifurcation, and, in many animals, small pulmonary nodes embedded within the substance of the lung (Figs. 7–52/5 and 7–53). The former groups are individually named (left, middle, right, and [in ruminants and pigs] cranial tracheobronchial nodes)

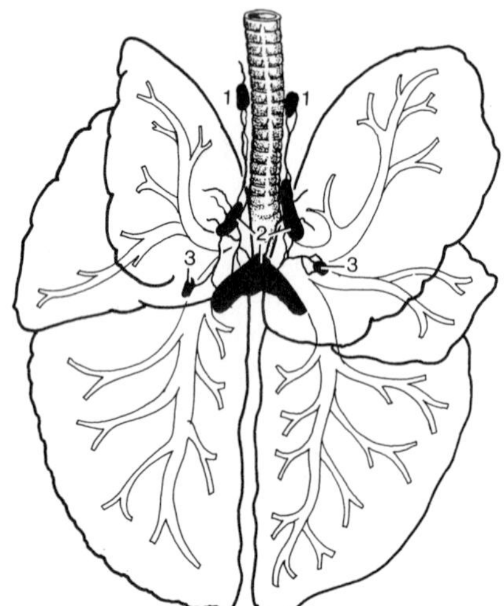


**Figure 7–53.** Lymph nodes associated with trachea and lungs of the dog.

1, Cranial mediastinal nodes; 2, tracheobronchial nodes; 3, pulmonary nodes.

according to their relationships to the major bronchi. They collect lymph from the lungs and send it in inconstant fashion to middle and caudal mediastinal nodes, sometimes directly to the thoracic duct.

## The Thoracic Duct

The thoracic duct is the major lymph-collecting channel. It arises from the cisterna chyli, which receives lymph from the abdomen, pelvis, and hindlimbs (see Fig. 1–34/5,7). The cisterna has a very irregular, even plexiform, shape, and although it is mainly contained between the aorta and the vertebrae at the thoracolumbar junction, it may also extend ventrally around the vena cava and the origin of the celiac artery. The thoracic duct passes through the aortic hiatus into the mediastinum. Its further course takes it cranially and ventrally, over the left face of the trachea, to a termination within one or other vein of the confluence that forms the cranial vena cava; it most often enters the left jugular vein or the vena cava itself (Fig. 7–54). The duct receives additional lymph from the structures and nodes of the left side of the chest. A separate right lymphatic duct provides similar drainage for cranial thoracic structures of the right side and proceeds to a similar termination. One or both commonly receive the corresponding tracheal duct(s).

## The Lymph Nodes of the Abdominal Viscera and Loins

The roof of the abdomen is drained by a *lumbar center* comprising various nodes spread along the abdominal aorta and possibly also within the spaces between the lumbar transverse processes

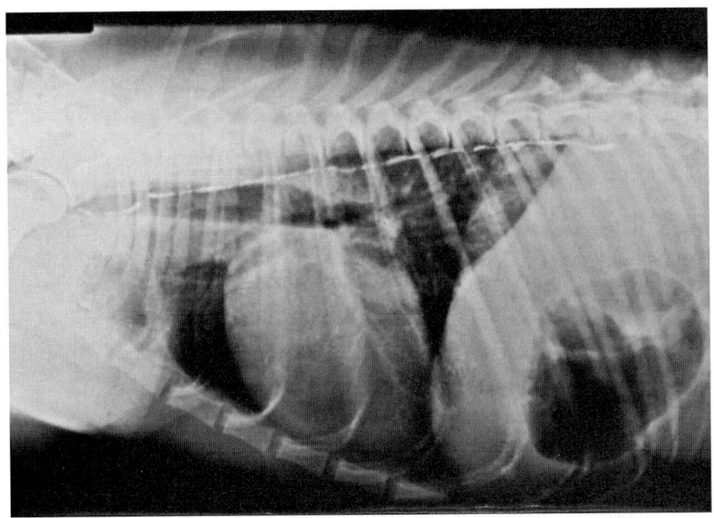

**Figure 7–54.** Lymphangiogram of the canine thoracic duct.

(Fig. 7–55). Usually those (renal) nodes (/7) that are associated with the kidneys are larger than others in the series. In addition to draining the structures of the loins, kidneys, and adrenal glands, these nodes may receive some lymph from reproductive organs. The flow is to the cisterna chyli (/5) directly or after serial passage.

Three centers associated with the drainage of the abdominal viscera have territories broadly corresponding to those of the celiac, cranial mesenteric, and caudal mesenteric arteries. They show very considerable interspecific distinctions, and bare mention of the nodes assigned to each center must be sufficient in this general account (Fig. 7–56). The *celiac center* comprises splenic, gastric (subdivided in ruminants), hepatic, and pancreaticoduodenal nodes (/3,2,1,4). The *cranial mesenteric center* comprises cranial mesenteric nodes toward the root of the mesentery and more peripheral jejunal, cecal, and colic nodes (/5,6,7). The *caudal mesenteric center* comprises caudal mesenteric nodes associated with the descending colon (/8). The three centers give rise to various visceral trunks that converge on the cisterna chyli.

## The Lymph Nodes of the Hindlimb, Pelvis, and Abdominal Wall

Though an inconveniently large territory to consider together, this cannot be subdivided since the responsibilities of certain nodes do not coincide with the usual division of the body. The description is most suitably begun with the most peripheral *popliteal center,* which consists of a node (or nodes) placed within the popliteal fossa caudal to the stifle (Figs. 7–49/8 and 7–57/5). The nodes

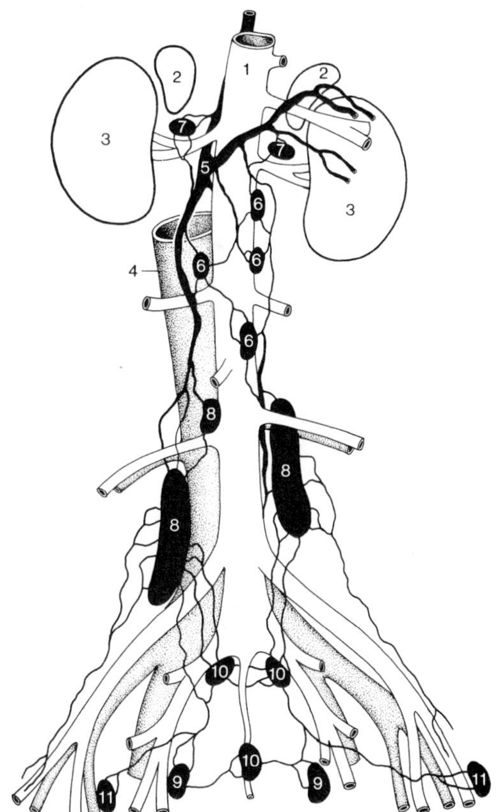


**Figure 7–55.** Lymph drainage of the canine lumbosacral area; ventral view.

1, Aorta; 2, adrenals; 3, kidneys; 4, caudal vena cava; 5, cisterna chyli; 6, lumbar aortic nodes; 7, renal nodes; 8, medial iliac nodes; 9, hypogastric nodes; 10, sacral nodes; 11, deep inguinal (iliofemoral) nodes.

drain the distal part of the limb and direct their efferent flow to the medial iliac center (except in the horse, in which it passes to deep inguinal nodes).

The *ischial center* has one element, the ischial node placed on the lateral aspect of the sacrosciatic ligament (of ungulates [see Fig. 33–11/6]—no comparable node exists in carnivores). It collects from the muscles and skin of the rump and proximal thigh and sends its outflow to various nodes of the iliosacral center.

The *deep inguinal* (iliofemoral) *center* comprises nodes placed along the course of the external iliac artery or its femoral continuation (Fig. 7–55/11). They primarily drain part of the thigh but also accept lymph from the popliteal nodes for onward passage to the iliosacral center.

The *superficial inguinal center* is more peripheral. It includes the superficial inguinal nodes of the groin, the subiliac nodes of the flank fold (except in the dog), the coxal node, and those of the paralumbar fossa of cattle (Figs. 7–51/10 and 33–9/10,2). The superficial inguinal nodes are also named scrotal or mammary since they drain the external male reproductive organs or the udder (in dogs, caudal mammary glands) in addition to the groin region. The subiliac node drains skin and deeper structures extending from the midflank to the thigh. The efferent lymph passes to the iliosacral center, directly or after passage through the deep inguinal nodes.

The *iliosacral center* is a very large, widely spread collection of nodes placed against the roof of the caudal part of the abdomen and within the pelvic cavity (Fig. 7–55). The main components are the medial iliac nodes (/8), near the origin of the external and internal iliac arteries, and, though not in the dog, the lateral iliac about the breakup of the deep circumflex iliac vessels. Other nodes are found within the pelvic cavity, both on the walls (sacral nodes) and about the viscera (hypogastric and anorectal nodes). These various small nodes are the primary filtration centers for adjacent structures and secondary stages on the drainage of the hindlimb and reproductive and other pelvic organs; the flow is funneled toward the medial iliac nodes that give origin to the lumbar trunks.

## The Lumbar Trunks

These are mainly formed by efferent vessels from the medial iliac nodes. They form a plexus on the

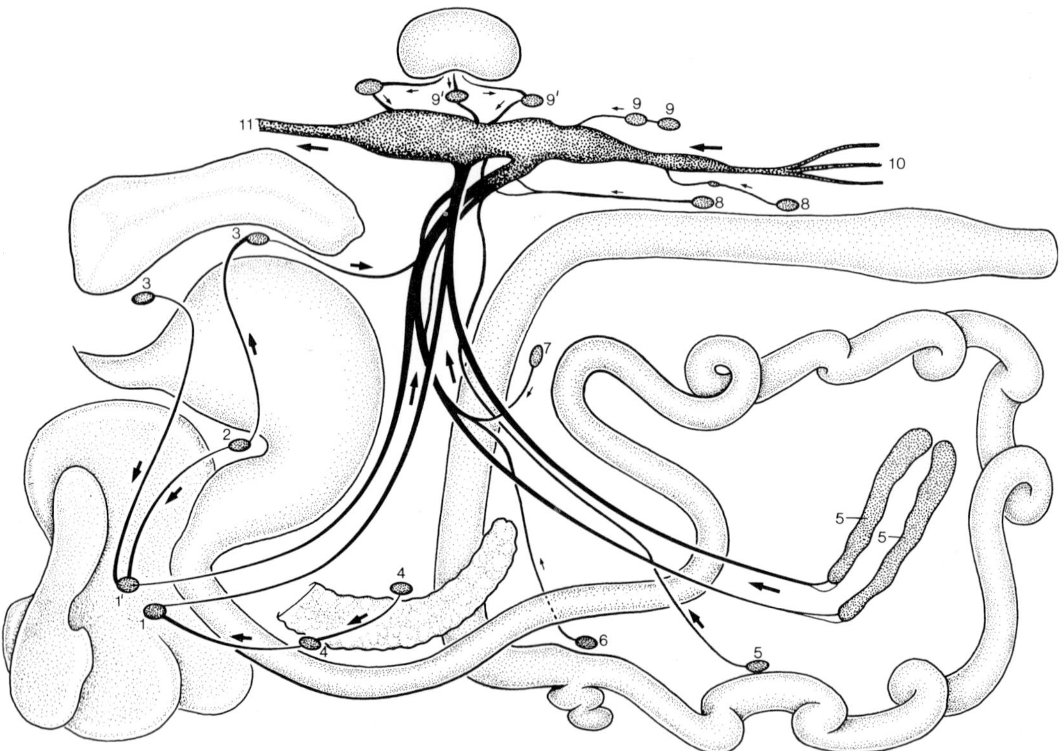


**Figure 7–56.** Lymph drainage from the organs in the canine abdominal and pelvic cavities (schematized).

1, 1′, Right and left hepatic nodes; 2, gastric node; 3, splenic nodes; 4, pancreaticoduodenal nodes; 5, jejunal nodes; 6, right colic node; 7, middle colic node; 8, caudal mesenteric nodes; 9, lumbar aortic nodes; 9′, renal nodes; 10, efferents from the iliosacral region; 11, continuation of cisterna chyli as thoracic duct.

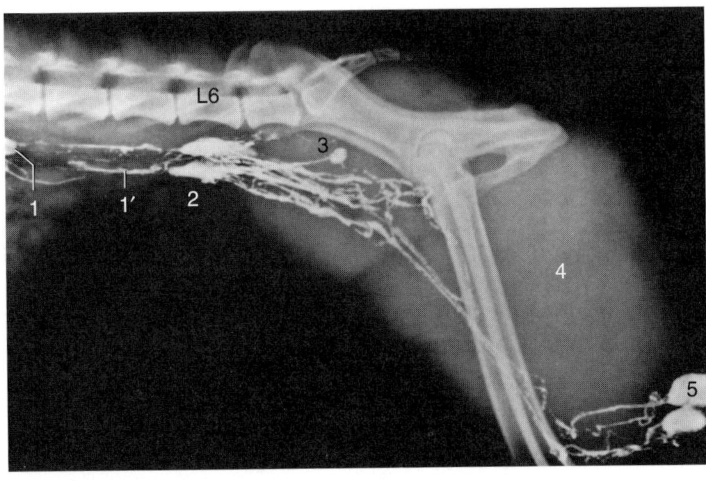


**Figure 7–57.** Lymphangiogram of the canine lumbar area, pelvis, and thigh.

1, Lumbar aortic lymph node; 1′, lumbar trunks; 2, medial iliac nodes; 3, hypogastric node; 4, thigh muscles; 5, popliteal nodes; L6, sixth lumbar vertebra.

roof of the abdomen where they are augmented by part of the lumbar outflow before they expand as the cisterna chyli (/5 and Fig. 7–57/1′). This also receives visceral trunks from the digestive organs.

## THE SPLEEN

The spleen* is contained within the left cranial part of the abdomen where it is joined to the greater curvature of the stomach by inclusion within the greater omentum. This helps fix its position, which cannot be defined with great precision since it is dependent on the degree of filling of the stomach and on its own blood content. The basic form is very dissimilar in the various domestic species, being dumbbell-shaped in the dog and cat, strap-like in the pig, a broader oblong shape in cattle, and falciform in the horse (Fig. 7–58). Its capsule extends trabeculae into the interior. In some species (carnivores) the capsule and trabeculae are very muscular, in others (ruminants) much less so; these differences determine the extent of the physiological variation in size that may occur. When relaxed, the spleen of the dog and cat

*The official name, lien, is the stem for many descriptive terms, for example, a. lienalis, the splenic artery.

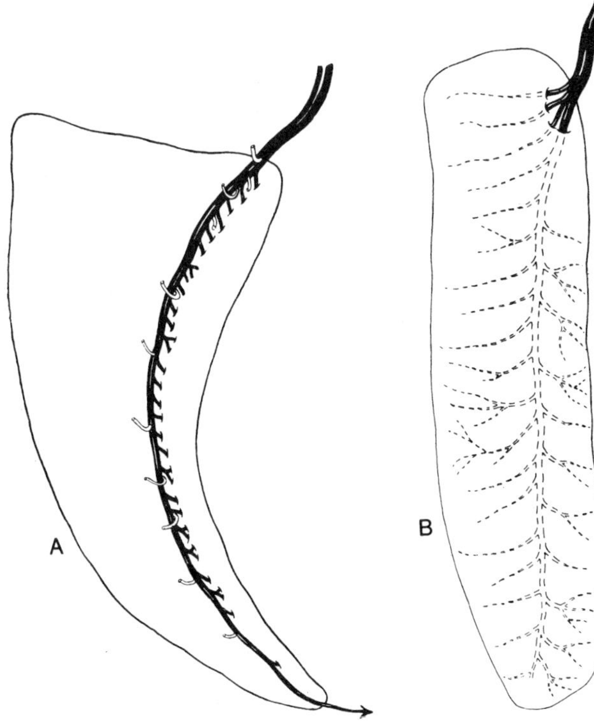


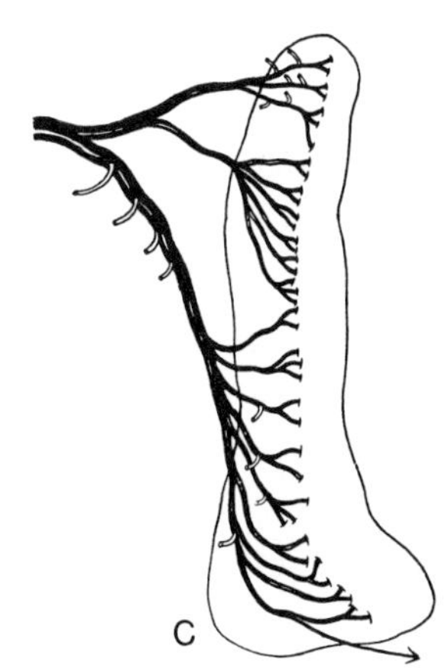


**Figure 7–58.** Visceral surface of the spleens of horse *(A)*, cattle *(B)*, and dog *(C)* to show the distribution of the splenic arteries. Branches to other structures are shown in white.

increases severalfold from its contracted state and it is therefore particularly effective as a reservoir from which the cell content of the circulation may be recruited in times of stress.

The soft tissue contained within the supporting framework is divided between red and white pulp; the former consists of spaces in series with the blood vessels and occupied by a concentration of the cellular elements of the blood. The white pulp, which is divided into foci that are usually just visible to the naked eye, is formed of lymph nodules within a supporting reticuloendothelial framework. This tissue has the usual lymphogenic and phagocytic properties.

The functions of the spleen are blood storage, the removal of particulate matter from the circulation, the destruction of worn-out erythrocytes, and the production of lymphocytes. The first role is familiar to all who have experienced a "stitch," the pain that sometimes accompanies physical stress and is associated with contraction of the splenic capsule.

The spleen is supplied by the splenic artery, a branch of the celiac artery that is generously sized in relation to the organ (see Fig. 3–39/4). The venous drainage through the splenic vein leads to the portal vein (see Fig. 3–49/2,1). Important specific features in the arrangement of these vessels exist. The artery and vein may pass undivided through a confined hilus (ruminants; Fig. 7–58/*B*); run the length of the organ detaching branches at intervals (horse, pig; *A*); or divide as they approach the spleen into branches that vascularize splenic compartments that are normally independent, although they do communicate (dog, cat; /*C*). The lymph vessels found in the capsule and trabeculae do not extend into the pulp. The sympathetic and parasympathetic nerves approach with the artery.

The spleen develops from a mesodermal condensation within the dorsal mesogastrium (which becomes the greater omentum) (see Fig. 3–64/6). The part of the sheet intervening between the stomach and the spleen may be specifically distinguished as the gastrosplenic ligament.

## THE THYMUS

The thymus is an organ whose importance is greatest in the young animal. It begins to regress about the time of puberty and may eventually almost disappear; even when a more sizable vestige persists, this will be found to consist largely of fat and fibrous elements, with suppression of the thymic tissue.

The thymus has a paired origin from the third pharyngeal pouch (see Fig. 6–5/6), although some uncertainty exists about the precise contribution made by the endoderm and subjacent mesoderm and even a conjectured ectodermal contribution in some species. The buds grow down the neck beside the trachea and invade the mediastinum in which they extend to the pericardium. The cervical part regresses prematurely in many species (including the dog) and the thymus then appears as a single, median organ whose bilateral nature is anything but obvious. At its apogee it is a lobulated structure (with some resemblance to a salivary gland) that fills the ventral part of the cranial mediastinum, fitting about the other contents of this space.

The thymus is divisible in microscopic preparations into a cortex and medulla. The cortex produces the immunocompetent T-lymphocytes, which enter the blood stream for distribution to the peripheral lymphoid organs (nodes and scattered lymph nodules) where they settle and multiply. The medulla is formed of epithelioid cells of more speculative significance (Plate 12/*H*). Because of its relevance to the postnatal development and maintenance of immunological competence, the thymus is of vital importance.

# CHAPTER 8

# The Nervous System

*In collaboration with Dr. G. J. Molenaar*

## INTRODUCTORY CONCEPTS

Every living organism must be able to react appropriately to changes in its environment if it is to survive, and by surviving to increase the chance of survival of the species. The regulation of these reactions is the responsibility of the nervous system, incomparably the most complicated of the body systems.

A purely descriptive account, of the brain in particular, has a very limited value or appeal; an account that attempts an adequate explanation of function encounters certain problems. Many of the structures and pathways of which the central nervous system is composed are neither discrete nor identifiable by the usual methods of anatomy; the majority of the "functional units" that it is convenient to recognize have multifarious and complex connections with other such units; there are parts to which it is impossible to pin specific functional labels, some because their significance is unknown, others because of a multiplicity of associations.

The compromise adopted in this chapter is the presentation of an initial formal description followed by short and rather elementary digressions upon the functional significance of a few selected "units." These digressions have as their prime purpose the attachment of some "meaning" to the structures previously described. We do so knowing that more complete functional analyses will be provided by concurrent or later courses of physiology or neurology.

### The Structural Elements

An appropriate environmental change provides a stimulus that is recognized by a receptor organ; the reaction or response that may be provoked in answer to the stimulus is performed by an effector organ (Fig. 8–1). In multicellular organisms the receptor and effector organs are separate and are connected by a chain of neurons, highly specialized cells in which the general cytoplasmic properties of irritability and conductivity are developed to extreme degrees. Whatever the stimulus, the receptor neuron translates it into an electrical potential, and the message is transmitted in this coded form. The impulse travels the length of the neuron before transmission to the next cell in the chain; this may be another neuron or interneuron, but ultimately, at the end of the chain, the motor neuron will end on an effector muscle or gland cell. Neurons thus provide the basic units from which the nervous system is constructed.

The typical *neuron* is an elongated cell that consists of a cell body, containing the nucleus and therefore known as the perikaryon, and various processes (Fig. 8–2). The processes, which vary considerably in number, length, and form, are of two varieties most obviously and usefully distinguished by the direction in which they transmit impulses. One variety, the dendrite, is usually multiple and transmits impulses toward the perikaryon; the other, the axon, is always single at its origin (although it may divide at some distance from the perikaryon) and conveys impulses away. The nerve cell is thus clearly polarized. The arrangement of the processes permits a simple morphological classification of neurons. Most are *multipolar* and possess a number, often a very large number, of branching dendrites that join the perikaryon at scattered points (Fig. 8–2). In a second type, *bipolar,* the dendrites join in a common trunk before reaching the perikaryon at a site remote from the origin of the axon. In the third type, *unipolar,* the dendrite tree and axon first combine in a single extension of the perikaryon that later branches; such neurons are sometimes described as pseudo-unipolar since they initially develop as bipolar cells. Dendrites and axons are superficially alike, and both are commonly described as nerve fibers. As a general rule to which there are many exceptions, dendrites are relatively short and axons relatively long.

The different varieties of neuron have specific distributions that are related to their particular functions. Clearly, a much-branched dendritic tree enables a neuron to receive impulses from many sources. Conversely, a much-branched axon makes

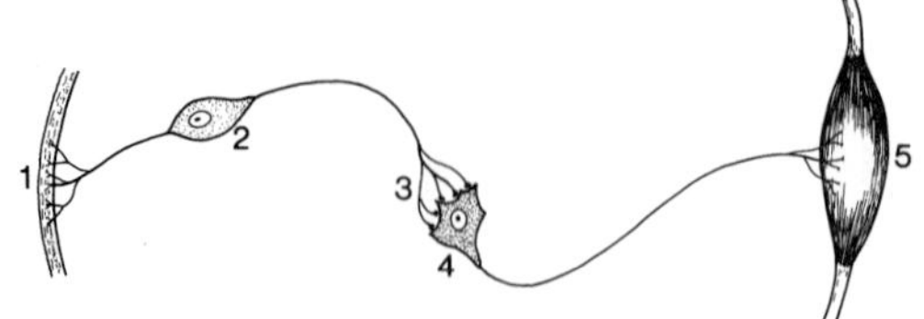


**Figure 8–1.** A simplified receptor-effector system.

1, Skin receptor; 2, afferent neuron; 3, synapse; 4, efferent neuron; 5, striated muscle (effector organ).

connection with and stimulates many cells. The first arrangement allows a convergence of impulses from various origins; the second provides for a divergence or diffusion of a message.

Interneuronal connections are known as *synapses,* a term usually broadened to include neuromuscular connections also. An axon may establish synaptic connections with the bodies, dendrites, or axons of other neurons—varieties of synapses distinguished as axosomatic, axodendritic, and axoaxonic. Most neurons establish many synapses—some have many thousands of synaptic sites, though not in relation to so many other cells. Synapses have a variable but always complicated morphology, but only an elementary description is required here. The participating cells are neither continuous nor in direct contact but are always separated by a very narrow gap. A nerve impulse (action potential) arriving at the presynaptic part of an axon does not jump from cell to cell; instead, it prompts the release of a specific chemical transmitter substance that diffuses across the gap. When this substance arrives at the postsynaptic plasma membrane (of the following cell) it produces one of two effects: it either depolarizes the membrane, initiating a fresh impulse, which is then propagated the length of the postsynaptic cell, or it hyperpolarizes the membrane, producing a blocking or inhibitory effect. The existence of both excitatory and inhibitory synapses, sometimes upon the same cell, provides a means for a great diversity of response. Many transmitter substances are known; the most common include acetylcholine, glycine, noradrenaline, and serotonin.

Neurons are supported by other specialized cells. The supporting tissue of the brain and spinal cord is known as *neuroglia* and comprises several cell types that we shall not distinguish. Neuroglial cells not only support the neurons but also assist in their nutrition; additionally, neuroglial cells provide nerve fibers within the brain and cord with cytoplasmic investments that insulate them from their surroundings, preventing leakage of the impulses they convey. The insulating material, myelin, incidentally imparts a white color to nerve fibers seen en masse. Nerve fibers within peripheral trunks (outside the brain and spinal cord) receive similar insulation—of very variable thickness—from another type of supporting cell, the *Schwann cell* (neurolemmocytus; Fig. 8–3). Peripheral nerve trunks are further protected, supported, and subdivided by connective tissue sheaths and septa, but the brain and cord, although included within a series of connective tissue investments (meninges), are not penetrated by connective tissue in this way.

Groups of perikarya are distinguished by their darker color, especially when set off by the whiteness of adjacent fiber bundles; this permits the ready distinction of the gray and white substance of the brain and cord. Isolated neuronal aggregations within the brain are generally known as *nuclei;* many are too small to be distinguished by the naked eye.

Fiber bundles of common origin, destination, and function tend to be aggregated within the brain and cord into *fasciculi* or *tracts,* although the limits of these are not normally evident and can be made so only by experimental means. Most such tracts are named by the combination of their origin, employed as prefix, with their destination, employed as suffix; the significance of such names as the spinocerebellar and cerebellospinal tracts is thus revealed directly.

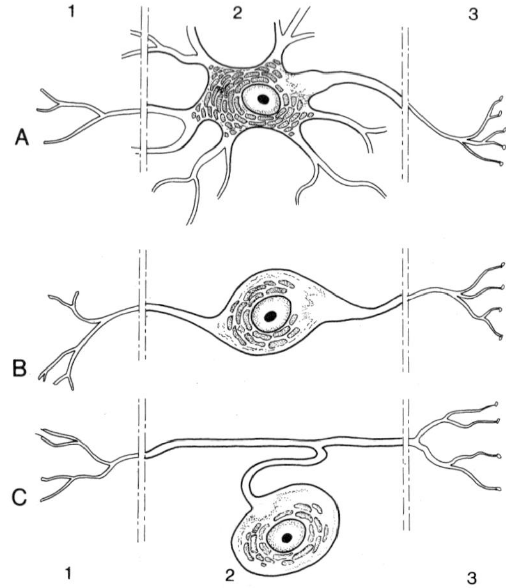


**Figure 8–2.** Multipolar *(A),* bipolar *(B),* and pseudounipolar *(C)* neurons.

1, Receptor side (dendrites); 2, cell body (perikaryon); 3, effector side (axon).

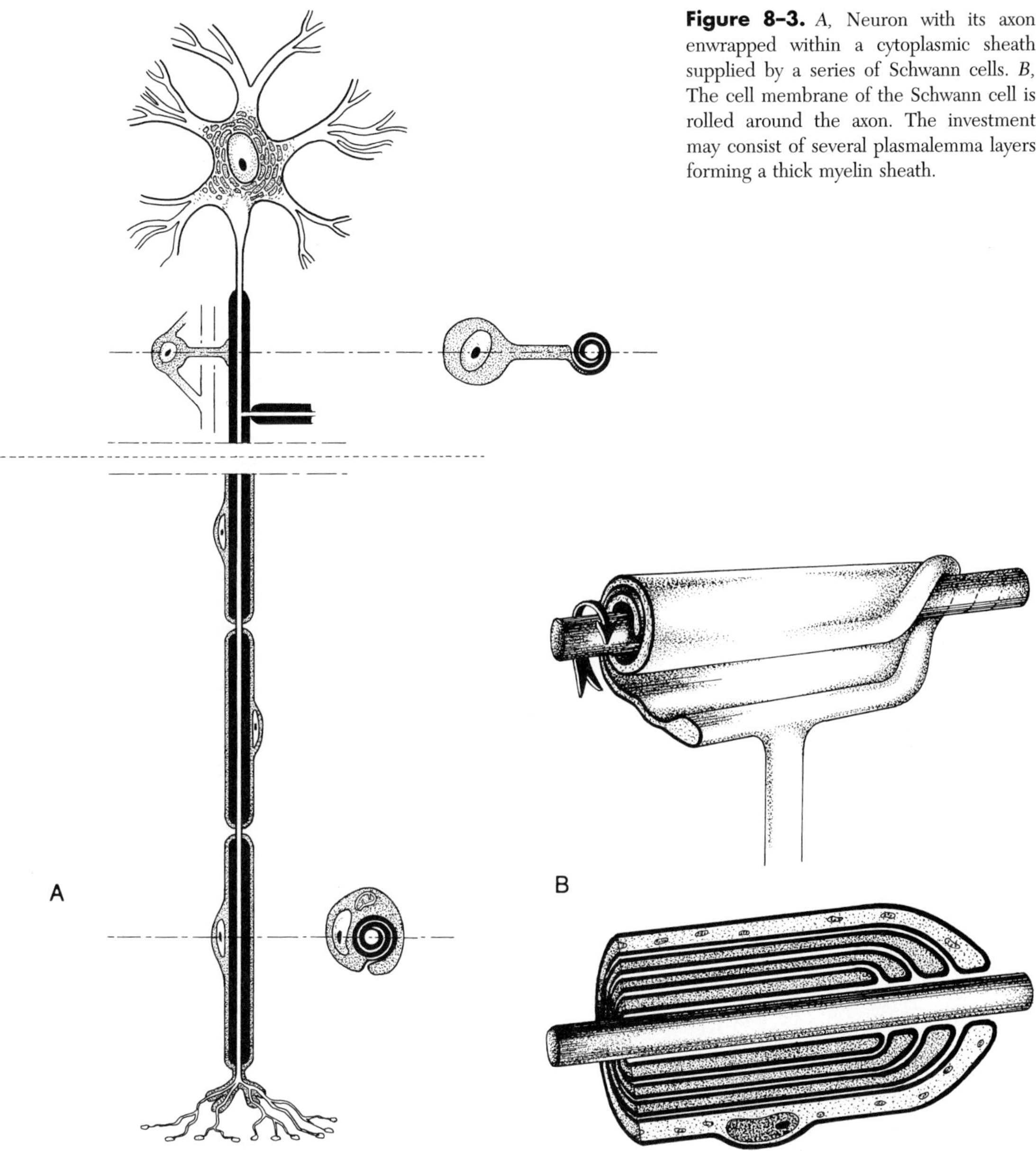


**Figure 8–3.** *A,* Neuron with its axon enwrapped within a cytoplasmic sheath supplied by a series of Schwann cells. *B,* The cell membrane of the Schwann cell is rolled around the axon. The investment may consist of several plasmalemma layers forming a thick myelin sheath.

Neuronal aggregations upon peripheral nerves may form visible swellings; they may also be distinguished by their color and texture, which are darker and firmer than those of the related nerve trunks. They are universally known as *ganglia.*

## Stimulus-Response Apparatus

Having established these fundamental points, we may now return to consider the stimulus-response apparatus. In the simplest form found in mammals, this apparatus comprises five elements arranged in series: a receptor region adapted to respond to a stimulus of a particular modality* (sound, touch, and so forth); an afferent neuron that conveys an impulse centrally, toward the brain or cord; a synapse; the remainder of the efferent neuron that conveys an impulse from the center to the periphery; and an effector, which may be a muscle,

*In fact, stimuli to certain neurons may be perceived in different ways, depending on their intensity, duration, and frequency of delivery.

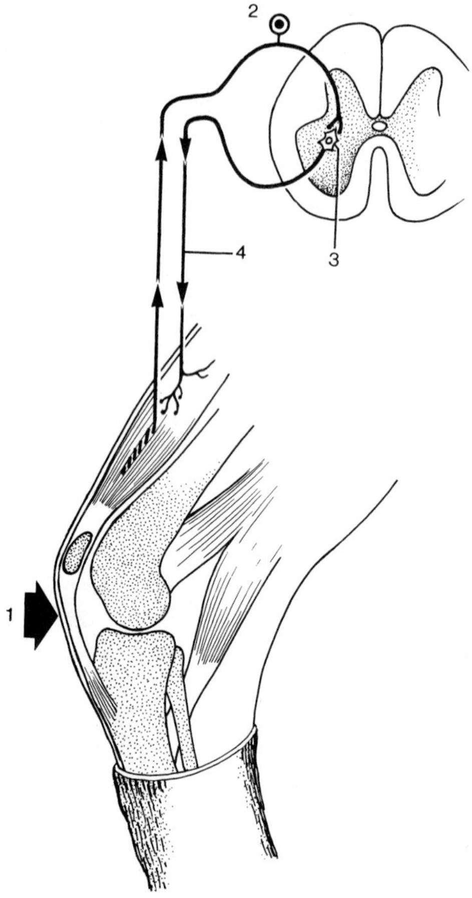


**Figure 8–4.** The monosynaptic patellar reflex. The stretch stimulus on the tendon (1) travels via the afferent neuron (2) to the spinal cord. The impulse is then transmitted to the efferent neuron (3), which stimulates the quadriceps muscle (4).

gland, or neurosecretory cell (Fig. 8–1). This sequence constitutes a primary, elementary, or monosynaptic reflex arc.

The *monosynaptic reflex arc* is actually a most uncommon arrangement, although it does provide the basis of one familiar example—the patellar or knee-jerk reflex (Fig. 8–4). This is a stretch (myotactic) reflex that, as many readers will know, can be elicited by an appropriate tap upon the patellar ligament, the functional continuation of the quadriceps femoris muscle. The tap stretches the muscle and thus stimulates muscle spindles and other receptors within its belly and tendon; an impulse travels along afferent fibers within the femoral nerve to reach the spinal cord, where it is projected upon efferent (lower motor) neurons; the axons of these neurons return within the femoral nerve and the impulse is then projected upon the constituent fibers of the muscle, stimulating their contraction to effect the abrupt extension of the joint.

In most reflexes one or more additional neurons are interposed in the chain between the afferent and efferent neurons (Fig. 8–5). These are conveniently known as *interneurons,* although several synonyms exist. The system may still be described as simple if only an unbranched neuronal chain is involved. However, most reflexes involve more complicated circuitry in which additional neurons are stimulated (or inhibited). Collateral branching enables the exercise of a more refined control and possibly the intrusion of the activity upon consciousness.

A good example of an integrated response is given by the limb of a standing animal subjected to a prick or other noxious stimulus. The limb is withdrawn by the coordinated action of the flexor muscles of several joints, movements that are facilitated by the relaxation of the previously active and antagonistic extensor muscles. The branching pathways involved in securing this response extend through several segments of the cord in order to reach and excite, or inhibit, the efferent neurons that supply the various muscles. At the same time, the animal has to adjust to the removal of one of its supporting props by redistributing its weight over the other limbs; the pathways necessary for this wider adjustment extend through considerable stretches of the cord, some crossing to the contralateral side (Fig. 8–6).

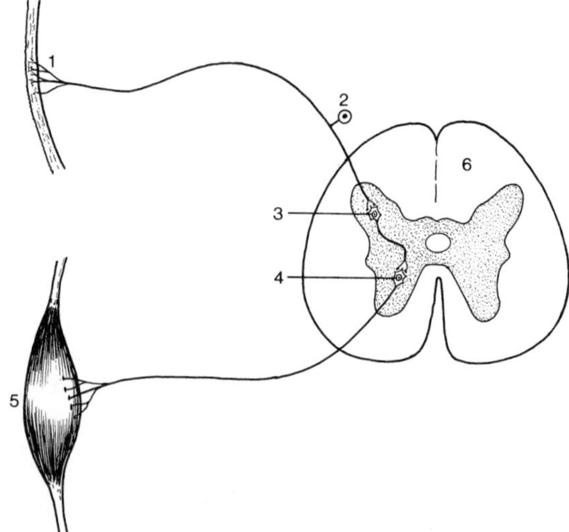


**Figure 8–5.** Schematic representation of a reflex chain in which an interneuron is interposed.

1, Skin receptor; 2, afferent neuron; 3, synapse at interneuron; 4, synapse at efferent neuron; 5, muscle; 6, spinal cord.

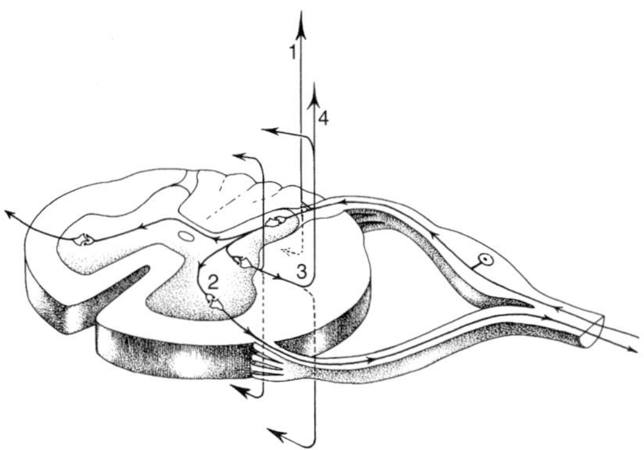


**Figure 8–6.** The course of fibers within the spinal cord. Some afferent fibers in the dorsal funiculus travel directly toward the brain (1); others end on interneurons in the dorsal horn. From here impulses can be transmitted directly to efferent neurons (2) or to other interneurons that transmit impulses caudally or cranially within the spinal cord (3), some extending to the brain (4).

Coordination of the changes so that balance may be maintained involves higher centers within the brain, to which the message must ascend, in addition to integration within the cord. The process is unlikely to go unnoticed; the cortex is involved and the animal assesses the situation and considers whether a more general response, such as flight or retaliation against the aggressor, would be appropriate. This considered response is a far cry from the simple, monosynaptic, and monosegmental response of the knee jerk and involves integrative apparatuses of various degrees of complexity, spread through the cord and brain, and drawing upon those higher centers that are concerned with memory and judgment.

## The Subdivisions of the Nervous System

Although the nervous system in reality forms a single, integrated whole, it is convenient—indeed necessary for many purposes—to divide it into parts. The most fundamental division can be made on topographical grounds, distinguishing the *central nervous system* (brain and spinal cord, or neuraxis) from the *peripheral nervous system* (the cranial, spinal, and autonomic nerve trunks with their associated ganglia). The division facilitates description but at the cost of making an artificial distinction that even assigns different parts of the same neurons to the two divisions—as, for example, the perikarya and axons of the efferent neurons of the patellar reflex arc.

An alternative division that would purport to have more regard to function is based on the direction in which impulses travel and on the nature of the information these impulses convey. It distinguishes *afferent* from *efferent* systems. The former conduct impulses toward the spinal cord and particular brain parts; the latter convey impulses away from these structures. Afferent pathways withn the peripheral nerves are frequently termed sensory; the impulses travel from the periphery toward the brain or spinal cord. Within the cord they are more often described as ascending; the impulses travel from "lower" (more caudal) toward "higher" (more cranial) parts. Efferent pathways usually conduct impulses from "higher" to "lower" levels within the brain and cord, and from these to the periphery; the alternative names to describe these systems are descending and motor. The equivalence of certain of these terms does not withstand close scrutiny, particularly when applied to integrative systems within the cord; many descending fiber bundles are not motor and many ascending bundles are not sensory.

The nature of the information that is conveyed, and of the activities that are directed, permits the further distinction of somatic and visceral nervous systems. The *somatic system* is concerned with those functions, like locomotion and so forth, that determine the relationship of the organism to the outside world. The *visceral system* is concerned with functions that relate to the internal environment—the regulation of the vascular system and heart rate, the control of glandular activity and digestive processes, and so forth. As a general but not invariable rule, there is a greater awareness and greater voluntary control of somatic than visceral functions. The somatic and autonomic and enteric systems, of course, work in close collaboration.

A more elaborate classification is possible. Afferent systems are initially divisible into somatic and visceral divisions, and these in turn into general and special subdivisions.

*Somatic afferent* pathways originate in receptors within the skin and deeper somatic tissues of the body wall and limbs. The pathways that arise from skin receptors are concerned with the *exteroceptive* sensations, such as touch, temperature, and pain, that respond to stimuli delivered from outside the organism; receptors within the deeper tissues include the additional *proprioceptive* category concerned with such "deep" sensations as those that inform on the present angulation of the joints and tension within muscles and tendons, and on changes in these conditions. Somatic afferent fibers are carried by all spinal nerves and by the fifth cranial (trigeminal) nerve (see Table 8–2, p. 276).

*Special somatic afferent* pathways have a more restricted origin within certain special sense organs—the retina of the eye and the cochlear and vestibular components of the inner ear—which are concerned with vision, hearing, and balance, respectively. The fibers concerned with vision and hearing are exteroceptive, those concerned with balance proprioceptive. Special somatic afferent fibers are thus found only within two cranial nerves, the optic and vestibulocochlear nerves.

*Visceral afferent* pathways originate in the (enteroceptive) receptors of vessels and glands and the viscera of the head and trunk that mostly respond to stretch and chemical stimuli. The fibers of this division are found in the cranial nerves III, V, VII, IX, and X, certain sympathetic and parasympathetic nerves, and all spinal nerves.

*Special visceral afferent* pathways arise from the special sense organs of smell and taste. Fibers conveying olfactory information are confined to the olfactory nerve, those conveying gustatory (taste) information to a small group of cranial nerves.

Efferent systems are divided more simply.

*Somatic efferent* pathways lead to striated muscles of somitic and branchiomeric* origin.

*Visceral efferent* pathways lead to the smooth muscle of the viscera and vessels, to heart muscle, and to glands. Most of these organs receive a double innervation through the sympathetic and parasympathetic divisions of the autonomic nervous system (p. 317), which are often described as antagonistic, although "balancing" might better suggest their cooperative role. Visceral efferent fibers of the *sympathetic division* leave the central nervous system via the spinal nerves in the thoracolumbar regions of the cord; those of the *parasympathetic division* are limited to a small group of cranial nerves and to the sacral contingent of spinal nerves. However, many visceral efferent fibers later join other nerves so that they finally obtain a very widespread peripheral distribution.

## Somatotopy

The fibers and cell bodies within many tracts and relaying nuclei, and within areas of the cerebral and cerebellar cortices upon which these may project, preserve very orderly point-to-point arrangements that reflect the topography of the parts of the body from which afferent impulses arise or to which efferent impulses are delivered. These do not always, or even usually, reproduce the true proportions but represent the parts of the body in relation to the densities of their innervation. The representations take the form of grotesque caricatures, sometimes known as homunculi—although animalcula would better fit veterinary anatomy—in which very sensitive parts, such as the lips and muzzle of the horse, or those capable of very refined and accurate movements, such as the fingers of a human or the prehensile tail of a monkey, are of exaggerated size. The concept of somatotopy is of great importance when considering the significance of pathological lesions, in the conduct of neurosurgery, and in experimental stimulation.

*This term identifies structures originating in the serial pharyngeal (branchial) arches.

# GENERAL MORPHOLOGY AND EMBRYOLOGY OF THE CENTRAL NERVOUS SYSTEM

## Introductory Survey

The brain† and spinal cord‡ are continuous without any clear demarcation. The brain is a very irregular organ whose shape conforms very approximately to the cranial cavity in which it is lodged, whereas the slender elongated cord has a more regular and uniform appearance.

The size of the brain bears no constant relationship to that of the animal from which it came but is relatively smaller in large species and is certainly proportionately greater in more advanced mammals. The weights of the brains of the human, dog, and horse are of the order of 1200 to 1500 g, 70 to 150 g, and 400 to 700 g, respectively; these figures yield ratios of brain weight to body weight of the order of 1:48 (human), 1:100 to 400 (dog), and 1:800 (horse). The large variation in the relative weight of the canine brain, although it might be expected from the variety of breeds, does provide some indication of the difficulties of interpretation of such figures. A more obvious significance attaches to the relative development of particular parts of the brain; there is a relative preponderance of "newer" parts (in the phylogenetic sense) and particularly of the cerebrum in mammals generally, and in "higher" mammals in particular, when comparison is made with lower forms. The great size and complexity of the human cerebral hemispheres provide the extreme example of this evolutionary trend (Fig. 8–7).

†The official term, *encephalon,* is rarely met but provides a much-used stem, e.g., encephalitis and electroencephalography.

‡The official term is *medulla spinalis.* Unfortunately, medulla (marrow) is used in several contexts. The term *medulla tout court* generally signifies medulla oblongata, the hindmost part of the brainstem.

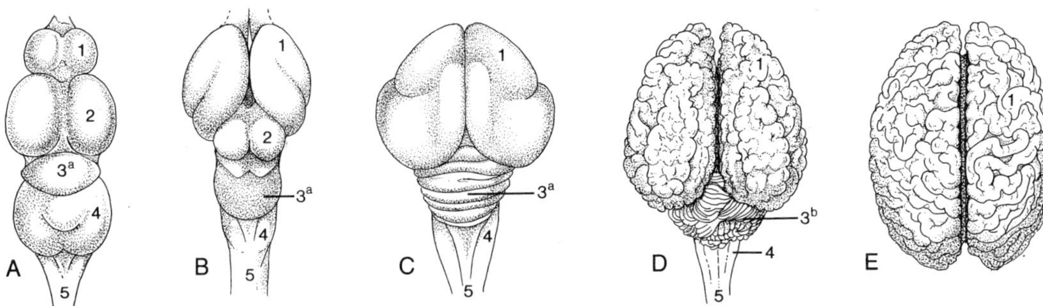


**Figure 8–7.** Vertebrate brains illustrating the phylogenetic development. The increase in volume and complexity of the telencephalon and cerebellum is most striking. *A,* fish (carp); *B,* reptile (python); *C,* bird (duck); *D,* mammal (cattle); *E,* mammal (human).

1, Telencephalon; 2, mesencephalon; $3^a$, $3^b$, metencephalon; $3^a$, archicerebellum; $3^b$, neocerebellum; 4, myelencephalon; 5, spinal cord.

More detailed descriptions of the parts of the central nervous system are given shortly, but a first appreciation of these will be facilitated by an initial survey of the brain as a whole followed by an account of its development. Repeated references should be made to the figures in order to locate and identify the structures named.

When viewed from the dorsal direction the dominant features of the brain are the cerebral hemispheres and cerebellum; only a small part of the medulla oblongata is visible in continuity with the spinal cord (Fig. 8–17). The semi-ovoid cerebral hemispheres are divided from each other by a deep longitudinal fissure and from the cerebellum by a transverse fissure; when the brain is in situ both fissures are occupied by folds of the tough dural membrane that lines the cranial cavity. Each hemisphere is molded to display a pattern of ridges (gyri) and grooves (sulci) in patterns that differ significantly among the various species. The cerebellum has an even more pronounced surface marking.

The ventral aspect of the brain is flatter overall and reveals the subdivisions of the brain more clearly. The caudal part is provided by the medulla oblongata, which expands when followed forward until it terminates behind a prominent transverse ridge, the pons, which can be traced over the lateral aspect to join the cerebellum (Fig. 8–18). The midbrain in front of this, hidden in dorsal view, appears as two divergent columns, the crura cerebri (/12), which continue rostrally to disappear into the depths of the hemispheres. They are separated by the interpeduncular fossa (/13). The forebrain lies in front of this; its most prominent ventral median features are the hypothalamus (to which the hypophysis [pituitary gland] is attached by a stalk) and the crossing or chiasm formed by the optic nerves. The larger part of the forebrain is provided by the paired cerebral hemispheres, which have as their most prominent ventral features the rounded piriform lobes (/3), flanking the crura cerebri, and the olfactory tracts (/2), which originate in the olfactory bulbs that project at the rostral extremity. The superficial origins of the cranial nerves—all except the trochlear (IV) pair—are also visible on the ventral surface.

The cerebral hemispheres and cerebellum develop dorsal to the other parts, and when they are removed all that remains is referred to as the brainstem (Fig. 8–23). This is a direct, though highly modified, continuation of the spinal cord.

## Development

Since the anatomy of the brain is most easily understood by reference to its development, it may be useful to give a general account of this before proceeding further; additional details will be mentioned later.

The nervous system makes a very early appearance, becoming evident at the embryonic disc stage as an elongated thickening (neural plate) of the ectoderm that overlies the notochord and paraxial mesoderm. The lateral parts of this thickening, the neural plate, are soon raised above the surrounding surface by growth of the underlying mesoderm and form bilateral neural folds that slope toward an axial crease, the neural groove. As the process continues, the edges of the folds become increasingly prominent and then bend inward toward each other; eventually they meet and fuse, converting the neural groove into a neural tube (Fig. 8–8). The tube, which is the primordium of the brain and spinal cord, then sinks below the surface, which is simultaneously closed above it by the fusion of the non-neural ectoderm

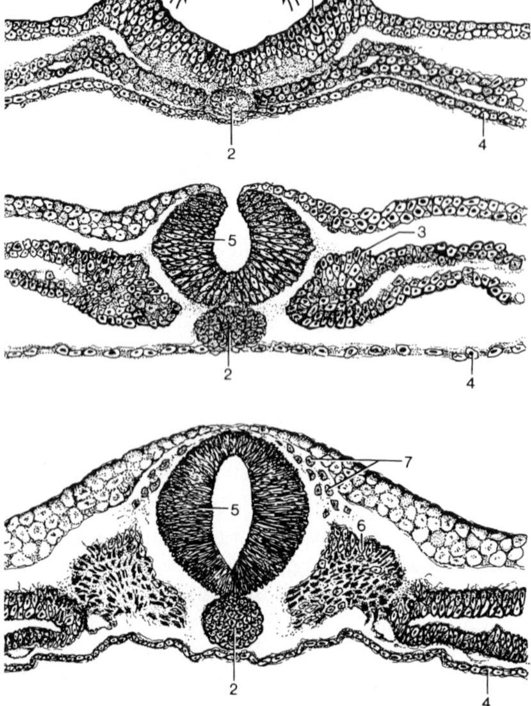


**Figure 8–8.** Three stages in the closure of the neural plate.

1, Neural plate; 2, notochord; 3, paraxial mesoderm; 4, endoderm; 5, neural tube; 6, somite; 7, neural crest.

to each side. At the same time, cells within the margins of the folds break away to form continuous cords, the neural crests, that run almost the whole length of the tube at its dorsolateral aspects. The neural crests contribute to peripheral ganglia, both somatic (dorsal root) and visceral, to the enteric nervous system, to the medullary parts of the adrenal glands, to glia, to skin melanocytes, and to a variety of craniofacial connective tissues. The sympathetic ganglia develop in the mid trunk of the embryo while neural crest cells from more cranial and more caudal regions migrate into the gut to form the enteric nervous system.

Closure of the neural tube is initially limited to the presumptive occipital region but soon spreads rostrally and caudally until only two small openings (neuropores; Fig. 8–9/3,5) remain to provide communication at the surface of the embryo between the lumen of the tube and the amniotic cavity. These openings do not persist long; the rostral neuropore closes first; the caudal one remains open for another day or two while the tube continues to lengthen at its caudal extremity by extension and subsequent infolding of the neural plate. The abnormal persistence of these openings produces relatively common defects of the brain and spinal cord in which nervous tissue may be exposed on the surface of the body. Failure at the rostral extremity leads to malformation of the fore- and midbrain with accompanying anomalies of the skull; it is known as anencephaly and, though the term implies complete failure of brain development, it can show considerable variation in severity; most forms are incompatible with life after birth. Failure at the caudal extremity is more common and is known as spina bifida. It is associated with defective closure of the vertebral arches. Children and young animals with this malformation may live after birth, though with

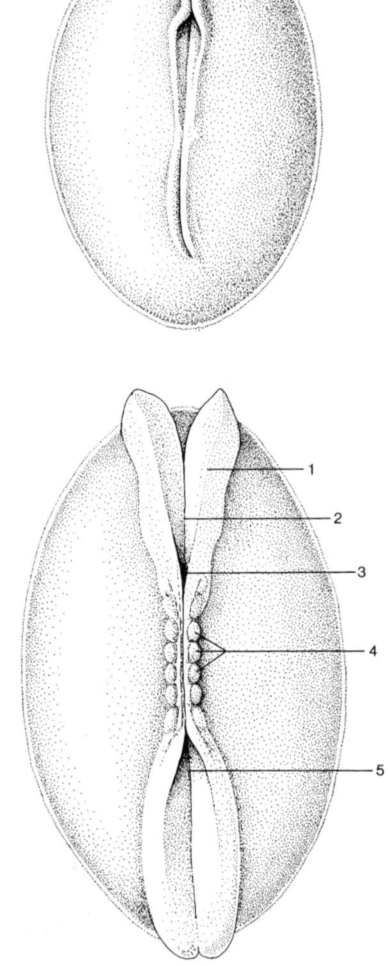


**Figure 8–9.** Dorsal views of developing embryos. Two stages in the formation and fusion of the neural folds are illustrated.

1, Neural fold; 2, neural groove; 3, rostral neuropore; 4, somites; 5, caudal neuropore.

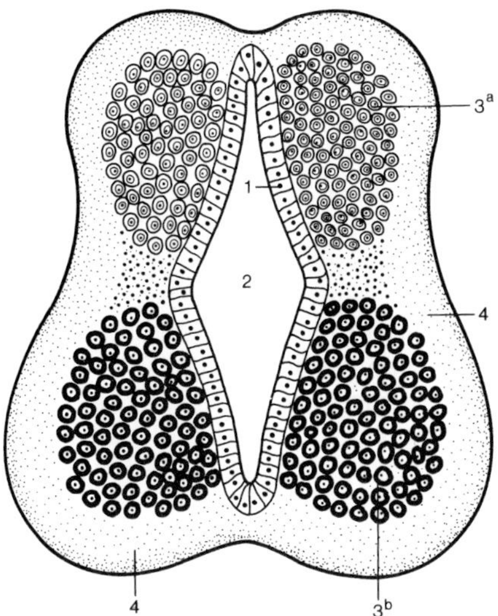


**Figure 8–10.** Differentiation of the neural tube.

1, Neuroepithelial (ependymal) layer; 2, central canal; 3[a], 3[b], mantle layer; 3[a], dorsal column (alar lamina); 3[b], ventral column (basal lamina); 4, marginal layer.

severe functional disturbance; affected animals are not usually permitted to survive.

The part of the neural tube that forms the brain is wider from the outset and shows localized expansions even before the tube is completely closed. These define three primary brain vesicles; prosencephalon (forebrain), mesencephalon (midbrain), and rhombencephalon (hindbrain). The remaining, more uniform part of the tube becomes the spinal cord. The differentiation of the wall is initially similar along the length of the tube but becomes modified later in the part that becomes the brain, and increasingly so toward its rostral extremity. It is convenient to consider first the differentiation of the spinal cord.

A transverse section of the tube at its formation reveals three concentric layers in its structure (Fig. 8–10). These are unequally developed around the circumference, which is divisible into thick lateral parts connected by thinner roof and floor plates. The innermost layer bounding the lumen is provided by a sheet of neuroepithelial cells that persists as the ependyma lining the central canal and ventricular system of the adult cord and brain. These cells proliferate rapidly and, although some daughter cells remain as a surface lining, most migrate outward, into the middle (mantle) layer of the lateral wall. These immigrant cells are neuroblasts, precursors of neurons and glia. The mantle layer itself becomes the gray substance to which the bodies of the neurons are confined. The processes from the cells within the mantle layer extend outward and form the outer (marginal) layer consisting of dendrites and axons. The marginal layer becomes the white substance of the cord in which fibers descend or ascend for various distances.

The cells of the mantle layer now become arranged in dorsal and ventral columns that bulge into the lumen of the tube, where they are separated by a longitudinal limiting groove (Fig. 8–11/4). The dorsal bulge (alar plate) provides the dorsal horn or column of the gray substance of the cord; its constituent neurons are those of the afferent systems. The ventral bulge (basal plate) becomes the ventral horn or column, the location of the efferent neurons; both horns also contain many interneurons. Neurons with somatic functions segregate from those with visceral functions, and four groups of neurons are then arranged in dorsoventral sequence; somatic afferent, visceral afferent, visceral efferent, and somatic efferent (Fig. 8–12). The roof and floor plates provide commissures through which nerve fibers pass from one side of the cord to the other.

Further growth of the alar and basal plates causes the lateral parts of the tube wall to expand outward in all directions, submerging the roof and floor plates and creating the dorsal sulcus and the ventral fissure that divide the adult cord into its right and left halves. A serial segmentation is created by the appearance of the roots of the spinal nerves. The dorsal roots are provided by neurons within the dorsal root ganglia, local condensations of neural crest cells. The axon processes of these cells extend medially to reach and penetrate the

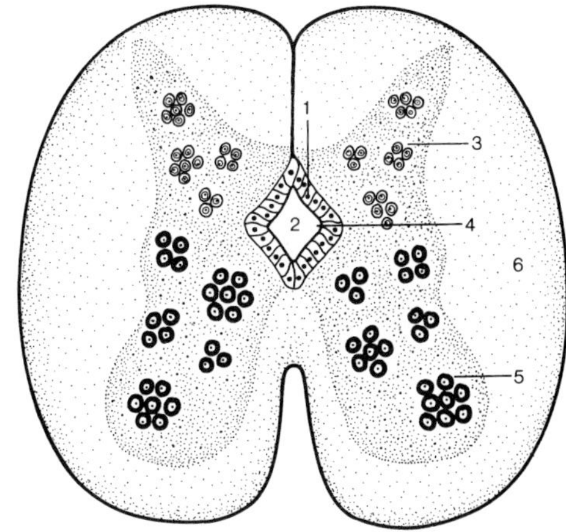


**Figure 8–11.** Further differentiation of the neural tube (spinal cord).

1, Neuroepithelial layer, 2, central canal; 3, dorsal column of mantle layer; 4, longitudinal limiting groove; 5, ventral column of mantle layer; 6, marginal layer.

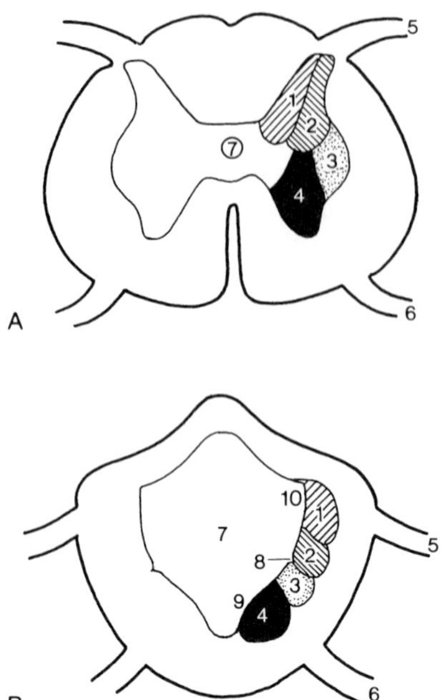


**Figure 8–12.** Organization of the gray substance of the spinal cord *(A)* and medulla oblongata *(B)*.

1, Somatic afferent column; 2, visceral afferent column; 3, visceral efferent column; 4, somatic efferent column (lower motor neurons); 5, dorsal root; 6, ventral root; 7, central canal or fourth ventricle; 8, sulcus limitans; 9, basal lamina (plate); 10, alar lamina (plate).

marginal layer, where they divide. Branches of these axons diffuse over several segments before entering the mantle layer to terminate on dorsal column cells; some of greater length extend to reach higher levels within the central nervous system (Fig. 8–6). The ventral roots are formed by axons of efferent neurons within the ventral column, which grow through the marginal layer to emerge on the surface of the cord, where they converge. The appearance of the roots divides the white substance into the dorsal, lateral, and ventral funiculi (Fig. 8–13/7,8,9).

Although the histogenesis of the nervous system will not be described, two points must be made. In most parts of the brain the full complement of neurons is established shortly after, if not before, birth. However, and contrary to former beliefs, in some regions there is a significant, more protracted postnatal recruitment, in some areas continuing into later life. Adult life is marked by a gradual depletion of their number in a process that accelerates with advancing age. Different authors provide very different estimates of neuronal loss in the human brain, in which the phenomenon is of the most obvious interest. One commonly quoted assertion is that some 20% of the juvenile complement is lost by the age of 65 or 70. The second point relates to the process of myelinization of the fibers within the central nervous system. Different tracts within the brain and cord acquire adequate insulation (essential to their function) at different stages of development. There are important species differences in this process.

The three primary brain vesicles are evident before closure of the neural tube. At this time the prosencephalon has already extended the evaginations that become the optic cups (p. 333). The brain grows more rapidly than the tissues that enclose it, and the constraint that this exercises enforces a remodeling of its form. Flexures appear at three locations. The most caudal flexure is more marked in ourselves than in quadrupeds. It bends the brain ventrally at its junction with the cord. A second flexure at midbrain level is almost simultaneous and is sufficiently pronounced to bring the ventral surfaces of the fore- and hindbrains close together; this relationship is later reversed by the third flexure, which folds the hindbrain dorsally upon itself (Fig. 8–14). The plan of the chief parts is completed by the appearance of paired lateral evaginations from the alar plates of the prosencephalon, directly behind the rostral limit of this part. These outgrowths, the future cerebral hemispheres, constitute the telencephalon; the unpaired median portion of the prosencephalon, hereafter known as the diencephalon, differentiates as the thalamus and related structures. The telencephalic vesicles expand in all directions but chiefly in a curve that extends dorsally and caudally to overlap the diencephalon, to which they make secondary fusions at the apposed surfaces (Fig. 8–33).

The development of the cerebellum is initially by bilateral formations in the alar plates of the metencephalon; these later extend to a median fusion.

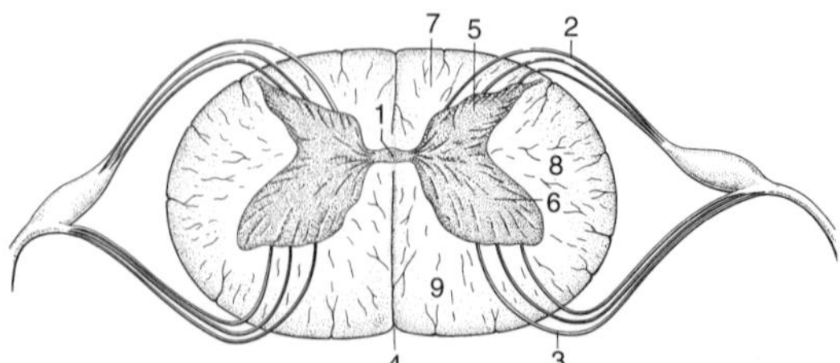


**Figure 8–13.** Transverse section of spinal cord showing the subdivision of the white substance by the dorsal and ventral roots of the spinal nerves.

1, Central canal; 2, fibers of dorsal root; 3, fibers of ventral root; 4, ventral median fissure; 5, dorsal horn; 6, ventral horn; 7, dorsal funiculus; 8, lateral funiculus; 9, ventral funiculus.

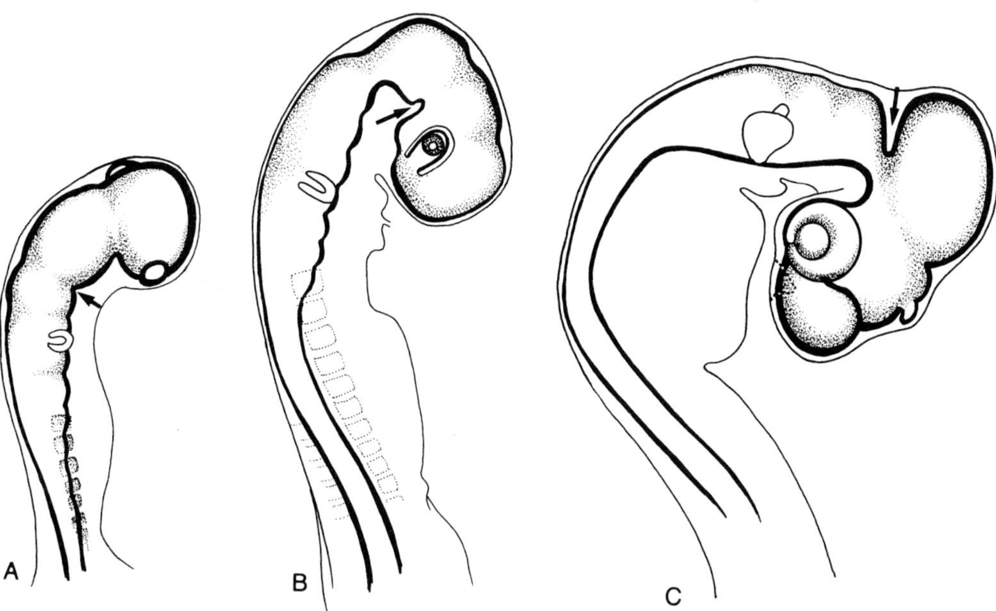


**Figure 8–14.** Formation of the caudal ventral *(A)*, rostral ventral *(B)*, and dorsal *(C)* flexures *(arrows)*.

The origin of the major components and cavities of the brain may be conveniently summarized in tabular form (Table 8–1).

The neural tube receives an early direct investment provided by mesodermal cells, with some supplementation in the forebrain region from cells that migrate from the neural crests; they form two sheets (pia mater and arachnoid; p. 298) that are separated by a space. An outer covering (dura mater) is provided by condensation from the surrounding mesoderm; it is separated from the arachnoid by a much narrower space.

**Table 8–1.** Derivatives of the Neural Tube

| Primary Division | Subdivisions | Major Derivates | Lumen |
|---|---|---|---|
| Prosencephalon | Telencephalon | Cerebral cortex<br>Basal nuclei<br>Limbic system | Lateral ventricle |
| | Diencephalon | Epithalamus<br>Thalamus<br>Hypothalamus | Third ventricle |
| Mesencephalon | | Tectum (corpora quadrigemina)<br>Tegmentum<br>Cerebral peduncles | Cerebral aqueduct |
| Rhombencephalon | Metencephalon | Pons<br>Cerebellum | Rostral part of fourth ventricle |
| | Myelencephalon | Medulla oblongata | Caudal part of fourth ventricle |
| Remainder of neural tube | | Spinal cord | Central canal |

# DESCRIPTIVE ANATOMY OF THE CENTRAL NERVOUS SYSTEM

## The Spinal Cord

The spinal cord (medulla spinalis) is an elongated structure, more or less cylindrical but with some dorsoventral flattening and certain regional variations in form and dimensions. The most important of these are the thickenings *(intumescentiae*; Fig. 8–15*)* of the parts that give origin to the nerves supplying the fore- and hindlimbs, and the final caudal tapering *(conus medullaris)* (see Fig. 19–5). The cord is divided into segments corresponding to the somites by the serial origins of the roots of the paired spinal nerves; the formation of these nerves has been described (p. 30); the relation of the segments to the vertebrae are considered in later chapters.

A simple transverse section shows a central mass of gray substance perforated in the midline by a small central canal, the residue of the lumen of the embryonic neural tube (Fig. 8–13). The gray substance, which has a crude resemblance to a butterfly or an H, is commonly described as exhibiting dorsal and ventral horns or columns, the former a rather misleading term since the "horns" extend the length of the cord (Fig. 8–16). The grayness is of course produced by the restriction of the perikarya to this part. The dorsal horn corresponds to the alar plate. It contains somatic afferent neurons dorsomedially and visceral afferent neurons ventrolaterally (Fig. 8–19). The ventral horn corresponds to the basal plate; it is composed of somatic efferent neurons, which are located ventrally, and visceral efferent neurons, which form an additional lateral horn confined to the thoracolumbar and sacral regions of the cord.

The neurons within each horn are more specifically grouped according to their functional and topical associations, but this is not grossly discernible.

The white substance that envelops the gray is divided into three funiculi on each side (Fig. 8–20/I,II,III). The dorsal funiculus is contained between a shallow dorsal sulcus, extended deeply by a median glial septum, and the line of origin of the dorsal roots of the spinal nerves (Fig. 8–13); the lateral funiculus is contained between the lines of the dorsal and ventral roots; the ventral funiculus is contained between the line of the ventral roots and a ventral fissure that penetrates far into the white substance, although leaving a considerable commissure connecting the right and left halves. This ventral fissure is occupied by a

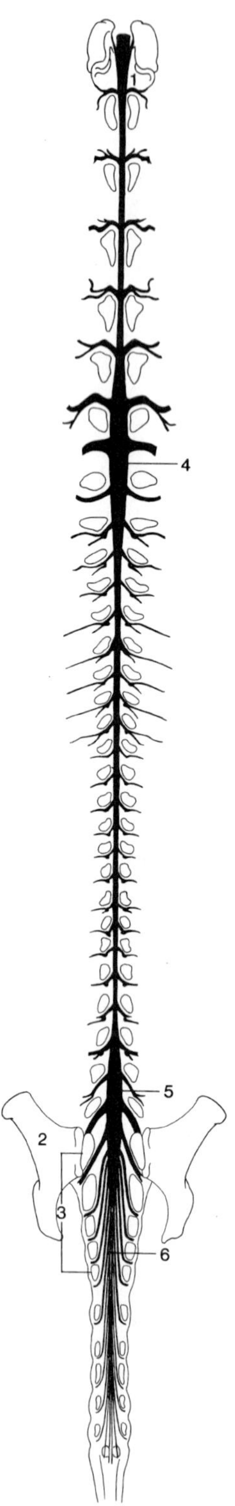


**Figure 8–15.** Dorsal view of the spinal cord and the vertebral pedicles of the horse. The spinal cord is shorter than the vertebral canal (ascensus medullae spinalis).

1, Atlas; 2, ilium; 3, sacrum; 4, cervical intumescence; 5, lumbar intumescence; 6, cauda equina.

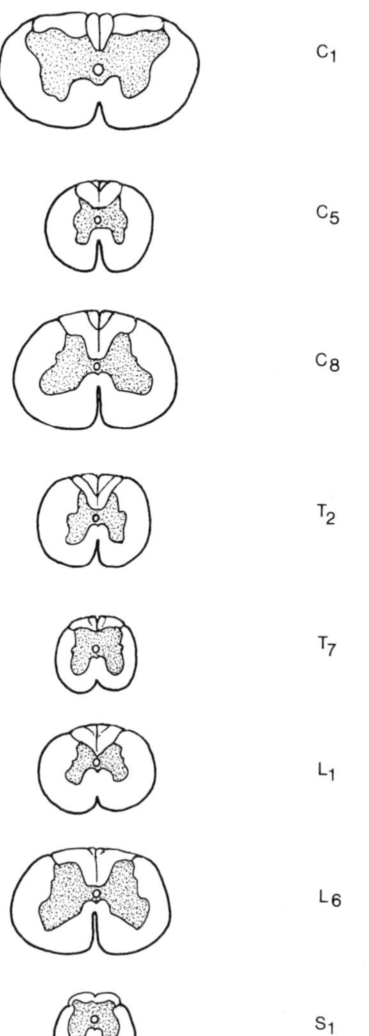


**Figure 8–16.** Transverse sections of the canine spinal cord (the levels are indicated). Note the changes in diameter of the cord and in the relative proportions of gray and white substance.

mass of pia that appears as a glistening streak on the surface of the cord.

The funiculi are composed of ascending and descending nerve fibers, many grouped within bundles (fasciculi or tracts) of common origin, destination, and function (Fig. 8–20). Certain of these are mentioned later.

## The Hindbrain

The hindbrain (rhombencephalon) comprises the medulla oblongata, pons, and cerebellum. These parts differentiate from the caudal brain vesicle shortly after closure of the neural tube. Attenuation of the roofplate weakens the structure and causes the vesicle to flatten as the pontine flexure develops. The flattening splays the side walls outward so that the luminal surfaces come to face dorsomedially, the alar plates now lying lateral to the basal plates (Fig. 8–24). The part caudal to the flexure (myelencephalon) becomes the medulla oblongata of adult anatomy. The rostral part develops to become metencephalon, externally marked by the pons and cerebellum. The parts of the roofplate caudal and rostral to the cerebellum remain thin and constitute the medullary vela that complete the enclosure of the lumen, now known as the fourth ventricle (Fig. 8–23).

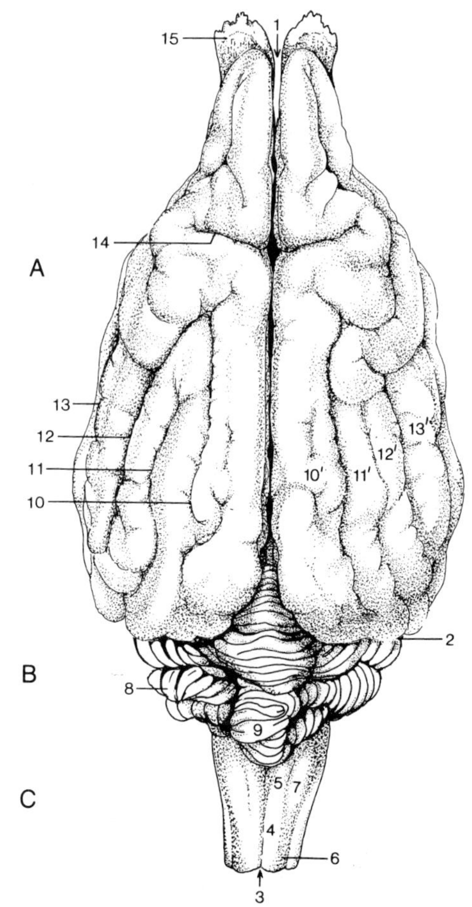


**Figure 8–17.** Dorsal view of the canine brain. *A*, Cerebral hemispheres; *B*, cerebellum; *C*, medulla oblongata.

1, Longitudinal fissure; 2, transverse fissure; 3, dorsal median sulcus; 4, tractus gracilis; 5, nucleus gracilis; 6, tractus cuneatus; 7, nucleus cuneatus; 8, cerebellar hemisphere; 9, cerebellar vermis; 10, marginal sulcus; 10′, marginal gyrus; 11, ectomarginal sulcus; 11′, ectomarginal gyrus; 12, suprasylvian sulcus; 12′, suprasylvian gyrus; 13, ectosylvian sulcus; 13′, ectosylvian gyrus; 14, cruciate sulcus; 15, olfactory bulb.

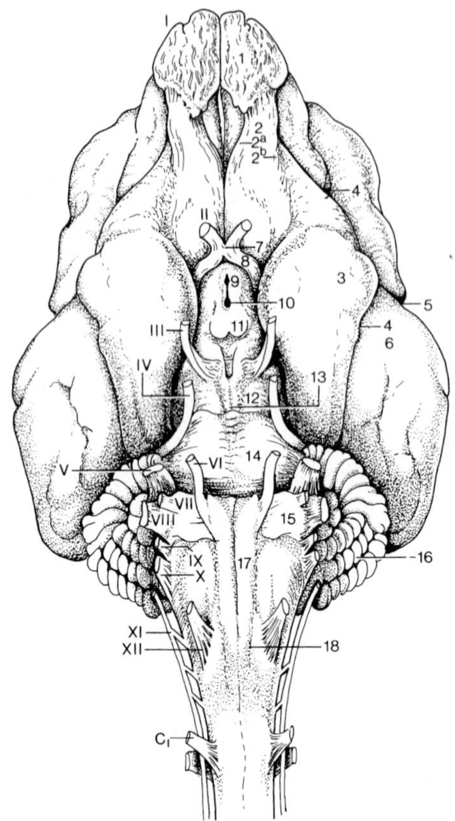


**Figure 8–18.** Ventral view of the canine brain.

1, Olfactory bulb; 2, olfactory tract; $2^a$, medial olfactory tract; $2^b$, lateral olfactory tract; 3, piriform lobe; 4, rhinal sulcus; 5, sylvian sulcus; 6, ectosylvian gyrus; 7, optic chiasm; 8, optic tract; 9, tuber cinereum; 10, infundibulum (the hypophysis has been detached); 11, mamillary body; 12, crus cerebri; 13, interpeduncular fossa; 14, pons; 15, trapezoid body; 16, cerebellar hemisphere; 17, pyramidal tract; 18, crossing of pyramidal tracts. I–XII designate the appropriate cranial nerves.

## The Medulla Oblongata and Pons

The medulla oblongata and pons form successive portions of the brainstem, the pons corresponding in extent to the large transverse bar that encloses the ventral and lateral aspects and continues into the cerebellum as the *middle cerebellar peduncles* (/9). Despite the clear external distinction, continuity of the internal organization makes the division of pons from medulla a rather artificial concept.

Although the medulla oblongata continues the spinal cord directly, it widens toward its rostral end as the result of the developmental flattening. Its ventral surface is marked by a median fissure continuous with that of the cord and flanked by longitudinal ridges, the *pyramids* (Fig. 8–18/17; Plate 13/E). Many of the constituent fibers of the pyramids decussate at the transition of spinal cord and medulla, forming interlacing bundles within the fissure (/18). A lesser transverse ridge, the *trapezoid body* (/15), crosses the ventral surface of the medulla oblongata directly caudal to the larger pontine bar. The other noteworthy features on this surface are the superficial origins of many of the cranial nerves. The trigeminal nerve (V) appears at the lateral aspect of the transverse pontine bar; the

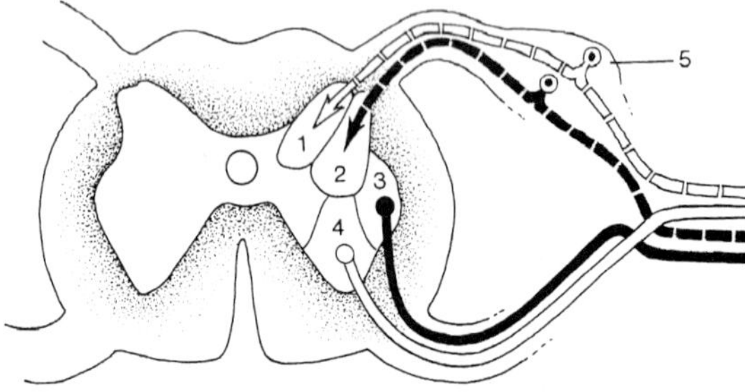


**Figure 8–19.** Schematized subdivision of the gray substances in the spinal cord.

1, Somatic afferent neurons; 2, visceral afferent neurons (1 and 2 form the dorsal horn); 3, visceral efferent neurons; 4, somatic efferent neurons (3 and 4 form the ventral horn); 5, dorsal root ganglion.

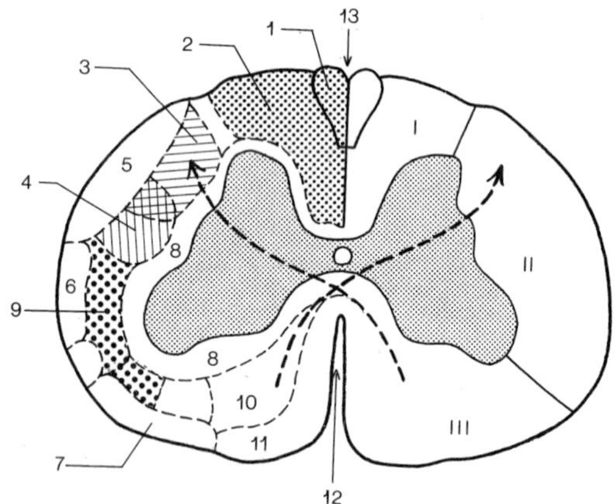


**Figure 8–20.** Hypothetical transverse section of the canine spinal cord showing the location of some principal tracts. The curved arrows indicate the crossing of the pyramidal tracts. (The drawing has been simplified for the sake of clarity.)

I, Dorsal funiculus; II, lateral funiculus; III, ventral funiculus. 1, Fasciculus gracilis; 2, fasciculus cuneatus; 3, lateral corticospinal tract; 4, rubrospinal tract; 5, dorsal spinocerebellar tract; 6, ventral spinocerebellar tract; 7, spino-olivary and olivospinal tracts; 8, propriospinal system (fasciculi proprii); 9, spinothalamic tract; 10, ventral corticospinal tract; 11, vestibulospinal tract; 12, ventral median fissure; 13, dorsal median sulcus.

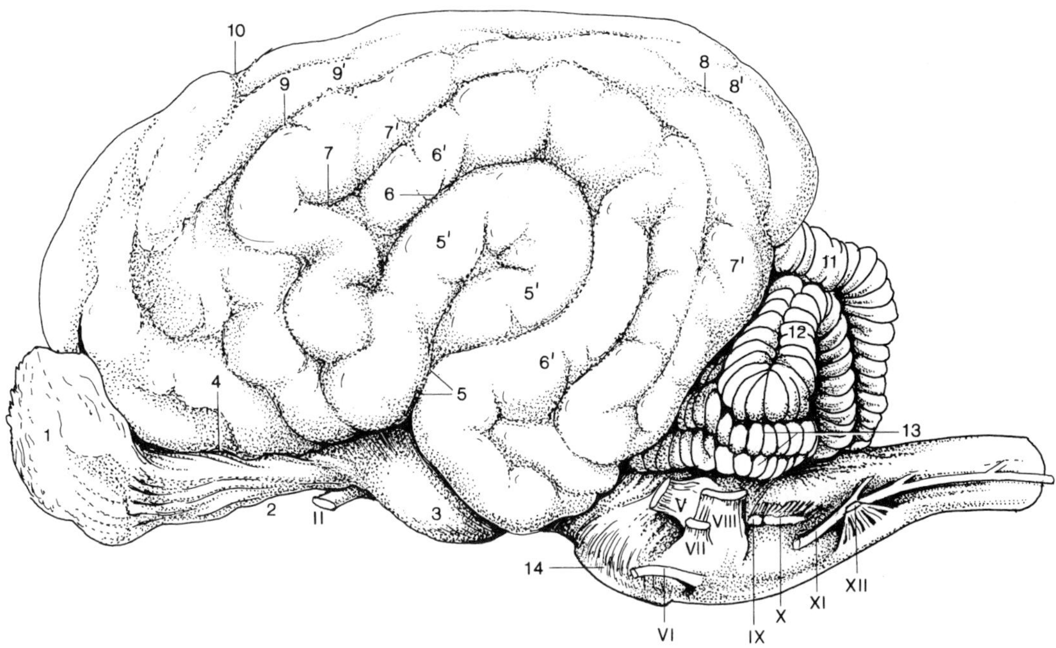


**Figure 8–21.** Lateral view of the canine brain.

1, Olfactory bulb; 2, olfactory tract; 3, piriform lobe; 4, rhinal sulcus; 5, sylvian sulcus; 5′, sylvian gyrus; 6, ectosylvian sulcus; 6′, ectosylvian gyrus; 7, suprasylvian sulcus; 7′, suprasylvian gyrus; 8, ectomarginal sulcus; 8′, ectomarginal gyrus; 9, coronal sulcus; 9′, coronal gyrus; 10, cruciate sulcus; 11, cerebellar vermis; 12, cerebellar hemisphere; 13, paraflocculus; 14, pons.

abducent nerve (VI) emerges caudal to this and more medially, through the trapezoid body lateral to the pyramid; the facial (VII) and vestibulocochlear (VIII) nerves appear to continue the trapezoid body laterally; the glossopharyngeal (IX), vagus (X), and accessory (XI) nerves arise from the lateral aspect of the medulla oblongata in close succession; the hypoglossal nerve (XII) takes a more ventral origin in line with that of the abducent nerve and the ventral roots of the spinal nerves (Fig. 8–18 and 8–21; Plate 13/*A,C*).

It may be helpful to study a median section (Fig. 8–22) of the brain before examining the dorsal aspect of the medulla oblongata and pons. This section shows that the fourth ventricle (/27‴) is brought close to the upper surface of the brainstem by a dorsal inclination of the central canal within the short caudal part of the medulla. The ventricle is covered by a tented roof formed by the cerebellum and the *caudal* and *rostral medullary vela* (/15′,15), which extend from the cerebellum to the closed caudal part of the medulla oblongata and to the midbrain, respectively. Exposure of the dorsal surface of the medulla and pons requires the removal of the cerebellum by transection of its peduncles, an operation that almost inevitably destroys the fragile vela (Fig. 8–23).

The *fourth ventricle* is diamond-shaped and is aptly named the rhomboidal fossa; it has its widest part at the pontinomedullary junction. The margins of the fossa are provided by the three pairs of cerebellar peduncles. The floor is rather irregular and is marked by a median sulcus and paired *lateral (limiting) sulci.* The most rostral part of the rostral velum, a part that commonly survives removal of the cerebellum, shows the superficial origins of the trochlear nerves (IV), the only nerves to emerge from the dorsal aspect of the brain.

The dorsal surface of the medulla oblongata flanking the caudal part of the fourth ventricle presents inconspicuous eminences, the *gracile* and *cuneate nuclei* (Fig. 8–17/5,7), at the termination of the like-named fasciculi within the dorsal funiculus of the spinal cord.

The principal features of the *internal anatomy* of the medulla oblongata and pons are as follows: the nuclei of the cranial nerves, the olivary and pontine nuclei, and the reticular formation and certain ascending and descending fiber tracts that connect the spinal cord with higher levels within the brain. The various categories of structure are described seriatim but without excessive attention to establishing their topographical relationships.

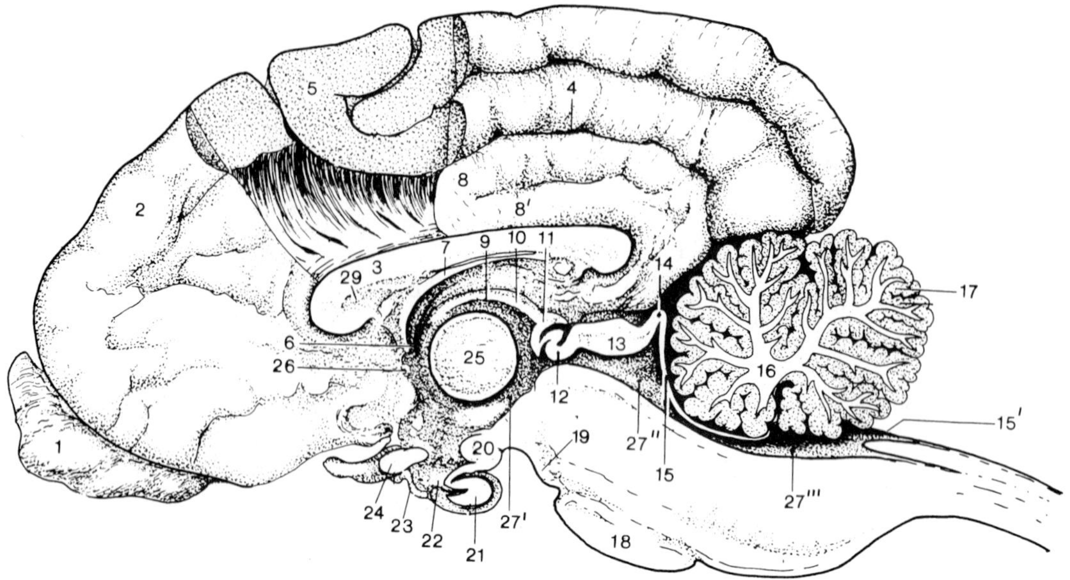


**Figure 8–22.** Median section of the canine brain. Part of the medial wall of the hemisphere has been removed.

1, Olfactory bulb; 2, hemisphere; 3, corpus callosum; 4, splenial sulcus; 5, cerebral cortex; 6, interventricular foramen; 7, fornix; 8, cingulate gyrus; 8′, supracallosal gyrus; 9, thalamus; 10, epithalamus; 11, epiphysis; 12, posterior commissure; 13, 14, commissures of rostral and caudal colliculi; 15, rostral medullary velum; 15′, caudal medullary velum; 16, corpus medullare; 17, cerebellar cortex; 18, pons; 19, crus cerebri; 20, mamillary body; 21, hypophysis; 22, infundibulum; 23, tuber cinereum; 24, optic chiasm; 25, interthalamic adhesion; 26, anterior commissure; 27′, third ventricle; 27″, mesencephalic aqueduct; 27‴, fourth ventricle; 29, septum telencephali (pellucidum).

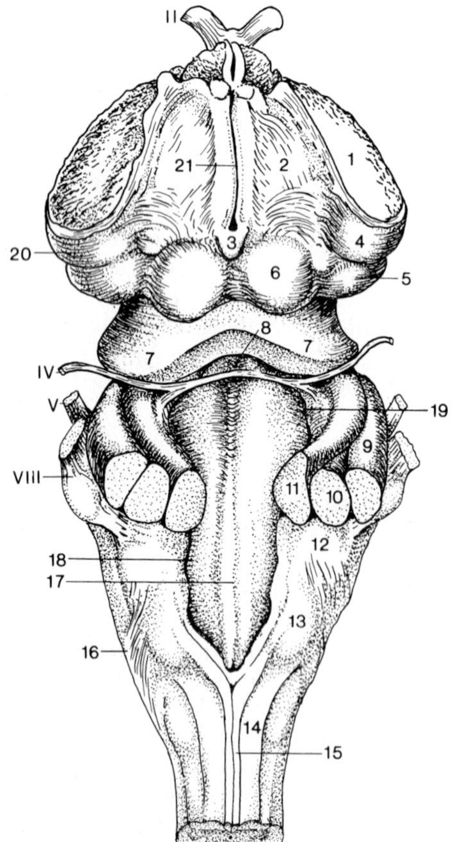


**Figure 8–23.** Dorsal view of the canine brainstem with the cerebellum removed and the fourth ventricle opened.

1, Cut fibers of internal capsule; 2, dorsal part of thalamus; 3, epiphysis; 4, lateral geniculate body; 5, medial geniculate body; 6, rostral colliculus; 7, caudal colliculus; 8, decussating fibers of trochlear nerves in the rostral velum; 9, middle cerebellar peduncle; 10, caudal cerebellar peduncle; 11, rostral cerebellar peduncle; 12, dorsal cochlear nucleus; 13, cuneate tubercle; 14, fasciculus cuneatus; 15, fasciculus gracilis; 16, superficial arcuate fibers; 17; median sulcus; 18, medial eminence; 19, sulcus limitans; 20, optic tract; 21, margin of roof of third ventricle.

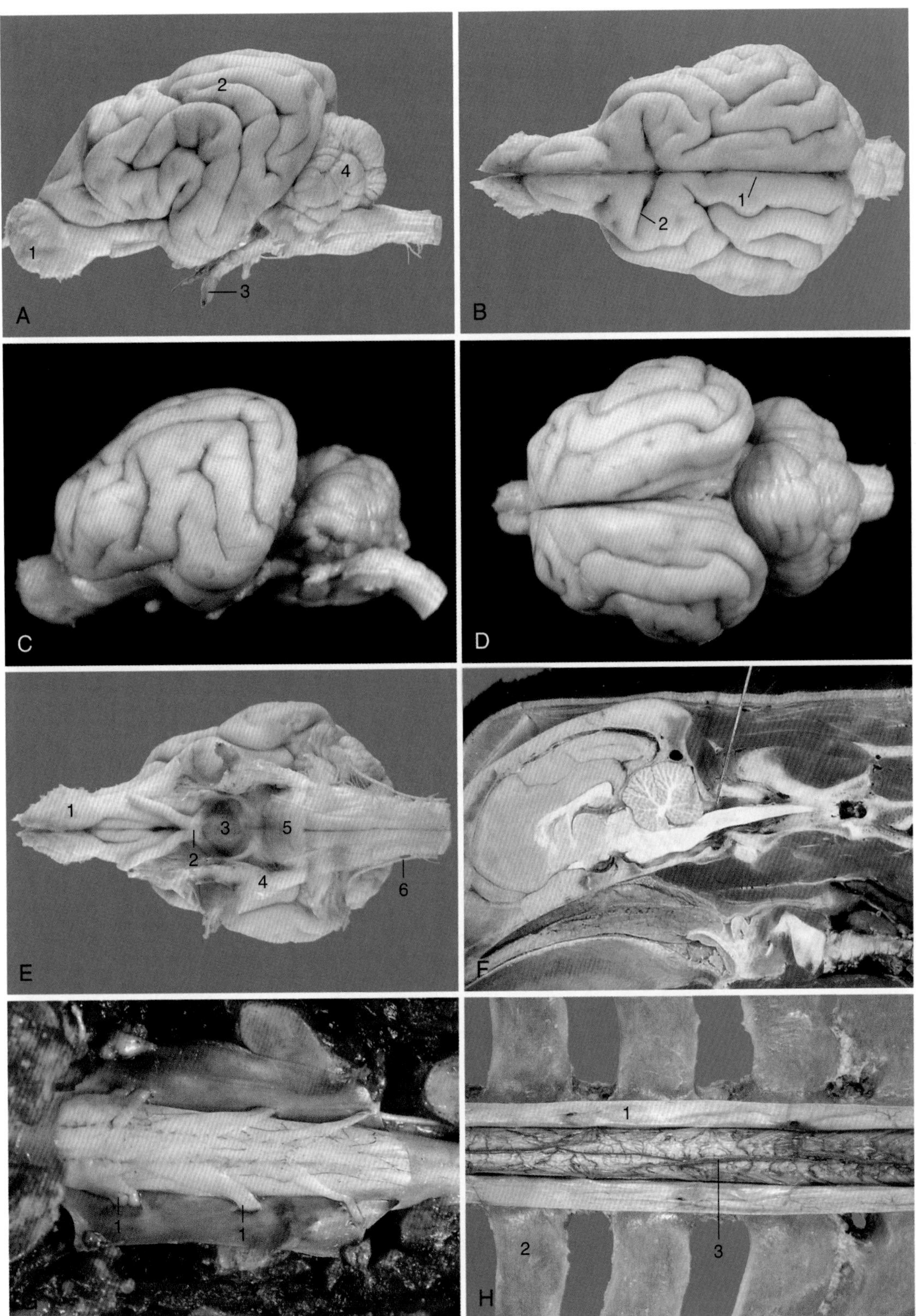


**Plate 13.** *A,* Lateral view of canine brain: 1, olfactory bulb; 2, ectosylvian gyrus; 3, optic n.; 4, cerebellar hemisphere. *B,* Dorsal view of canine brain: 1, marginal gyrus; 2, cruciate sulcus. *C,* Lateral view of feline brain. *D,* Dorsal view of feline brain. *E,* Ventral view of canine brain: 1, olfactory bulb; 2, optic chiasm; 3, pituitary gland; 4, trigeminal n.; 5, pons; 6, accessory n. *F,* Median section of head and neck (dog); the needle penetrates the atlantooccipital space to enter the subarachnoid cerebellomedullary cistern. *G,* Dorsal view of opened vertebral canal (cat): 1, spinal nn. penetrating arachnoid and dura mater. *H,* Dorsal view of opened vertebral canal (horse): 1, dura; 2, 3rd lumbar vertebra; 3, dorsal spinal v.

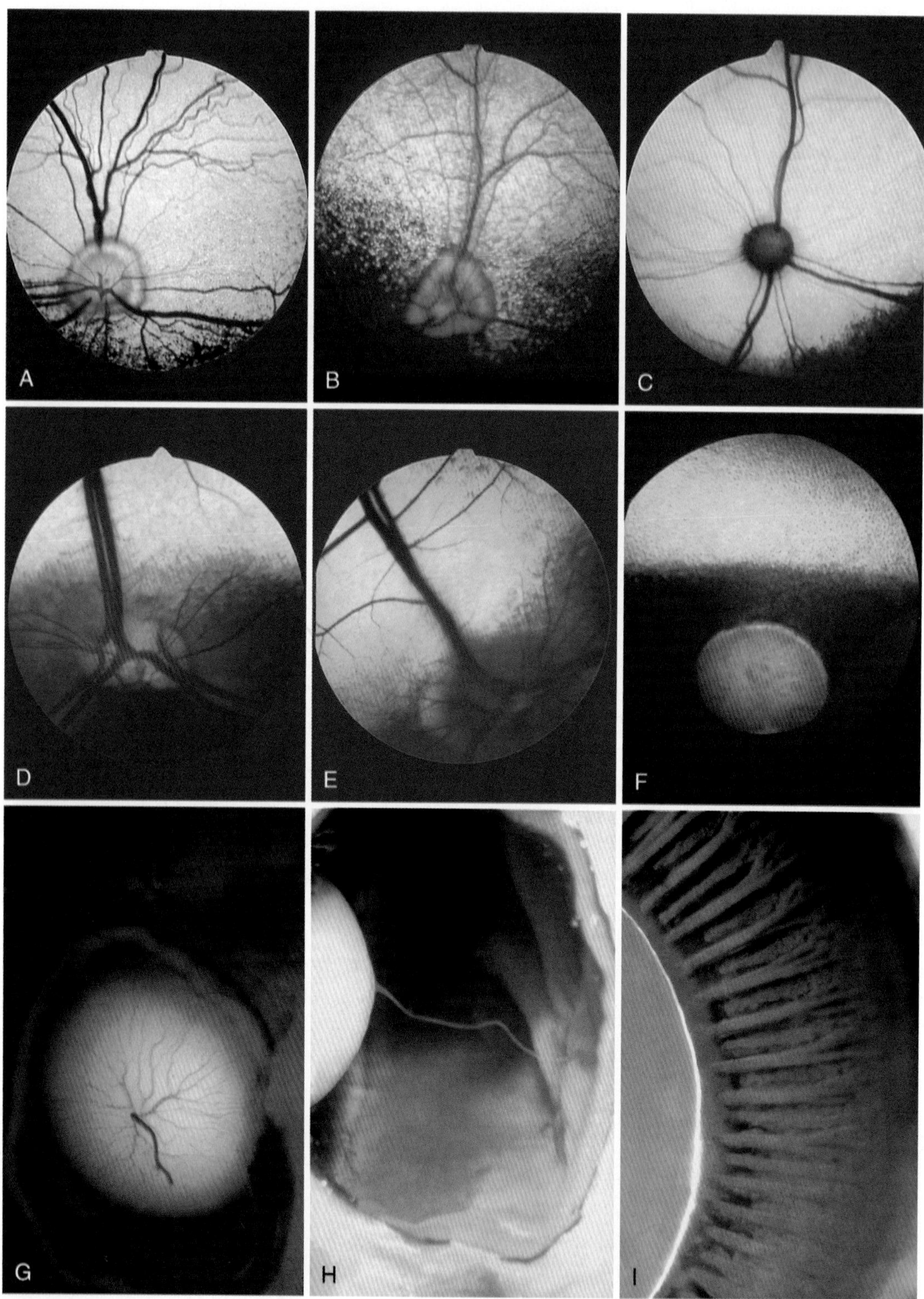


**Plate 14.** *A* to *F*, Fundus of eye. *A*, Dutch sheepdog. *B*, Old English sheepdog. *C*, Cat. *D*, Cow. *E*, Goat. *F*, Horse. *G*, Posterior surface of lens (newborn puppy) showing remnant of hyaloid a. *H*, Persistent hyaloid a. (dog). *I*, Posterior view of ciliary body with ciliary processes (horse).

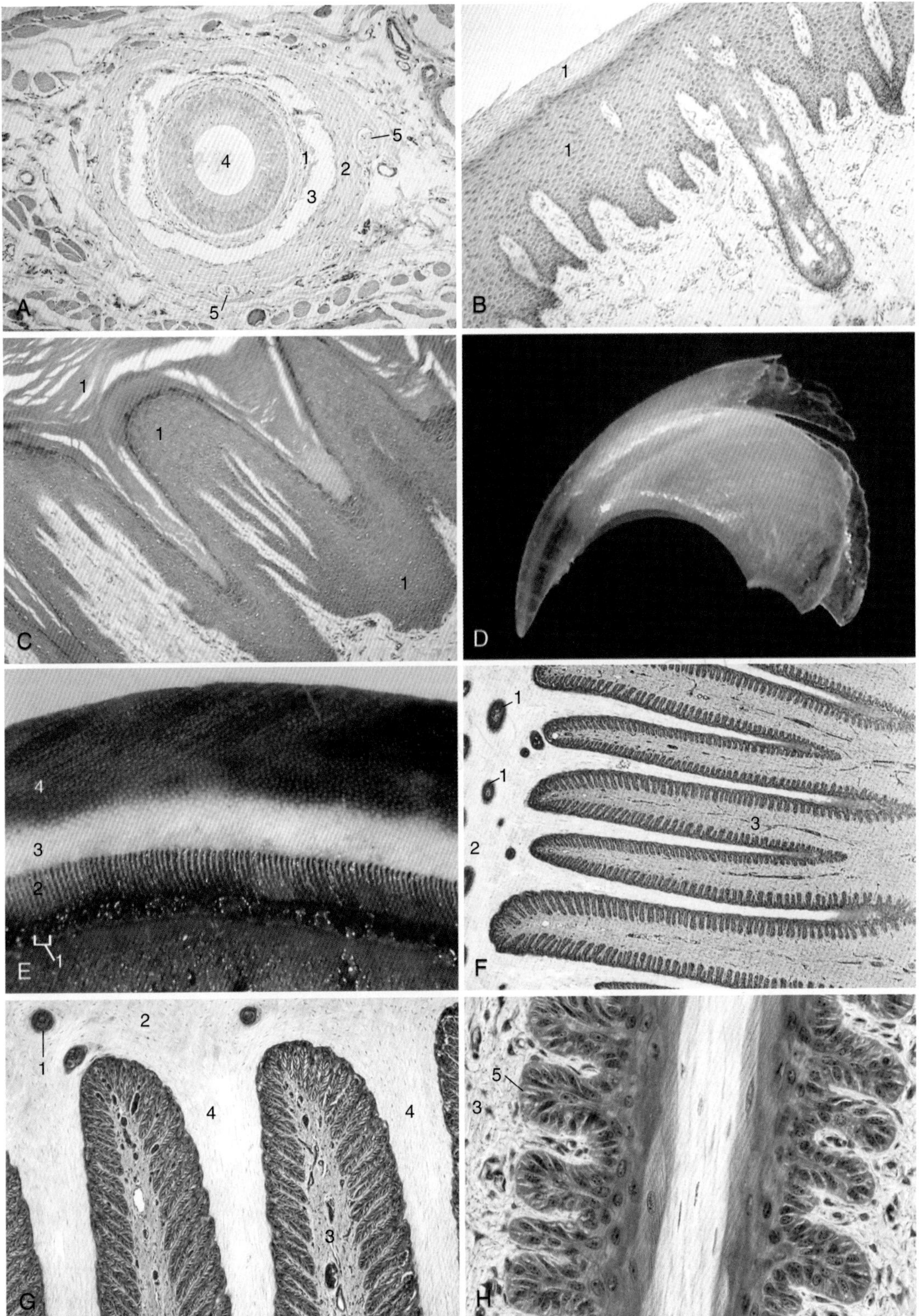


**Plate 15.** *A,* Tactile hair follicle of pig (HE) (70×): 1,2, inner and outer layers of dermal sheath; 3, trabeculated blood sinus; 4, medulla and cortex of hair; 5, nerve ending. *B,* Stratif. squam. epithelium of nasal plate of calf (HE) (70×). *C,* Stratif. squam. epithelium of footpad of dog (HE) (70×): 1, very thick stratum corneum. *D,* Outer layer of horn shed from cat claw. *E,* Cross section of hoofwall and third phalanx: 1, laminar corium; 2, horny lamellae; 3, horn tubules; 4, stratum medium. *F, G,* and *H,* Cross sections of equine hoof wall (modified analine blue stain) (28×/70×/279×): 1, horn tubules growing from epidermis over coronary dermal papillae; 2, intertubular horn; 3, primary dermal lamellae; 4, primary horny lamellae; 5, secondary dermal lamellae.

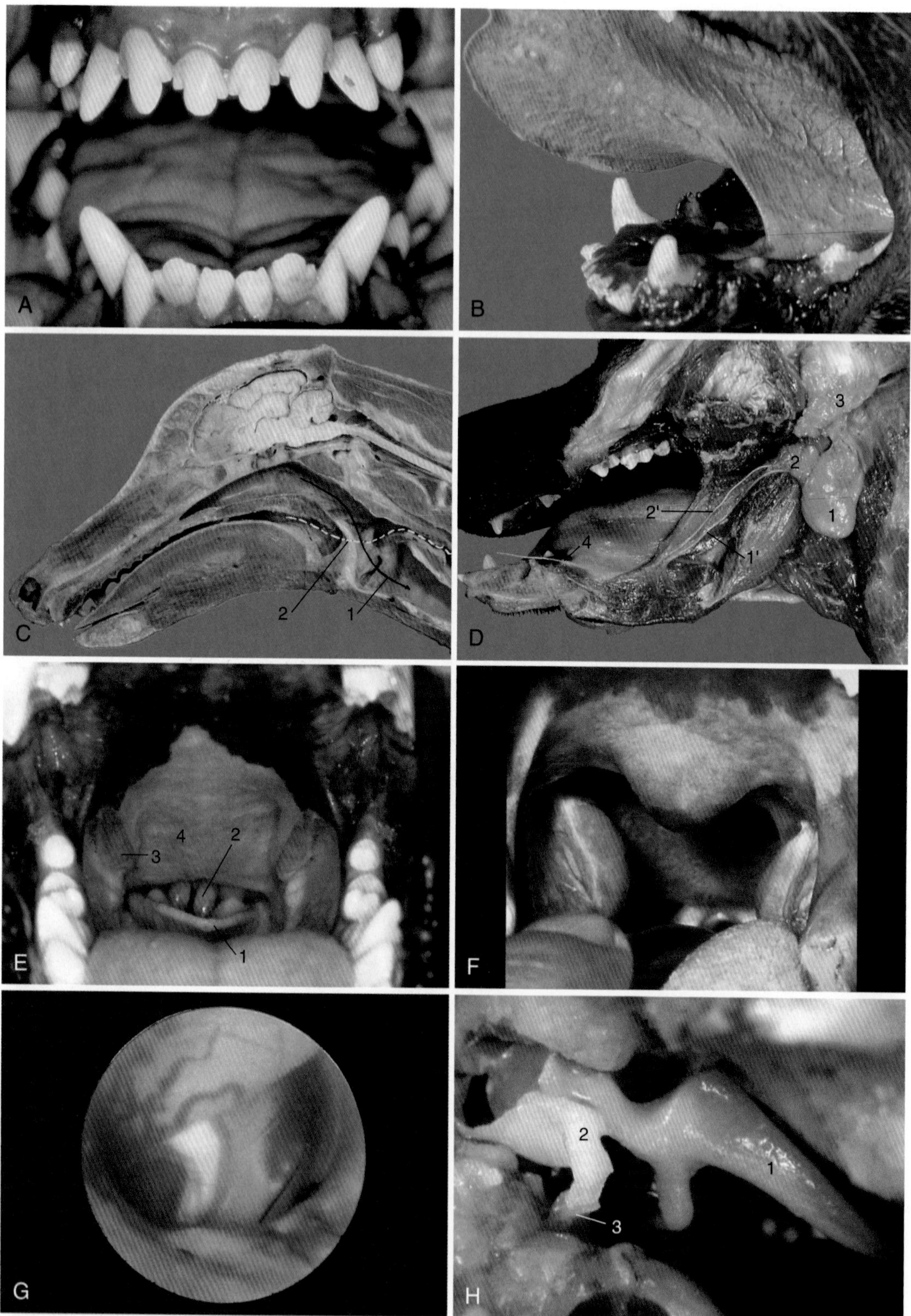


**Plate 16.** *A* to *H,* Dog parts. *A,* Trilobular form of upper incisors. *B,* Tongue with frenulum. *C,* Median section of head and neck: 1, route from nasopharynx to trachea *(solid line);* 2, route of food from mouth to esophagus *(broken line). D,* Salivary glands: 1, mandibular gland; 1′, mandibular duct; 2, sublingual gland, monostomatic part; 2′, its duct; 3, parotid gland; 4, sublingual caruncle. *E,* Oropharynx: 1, epiglottis; 2, cuneiform processes of arytenoid cartilages; 3, palatine tonsils; 4, soft palate. *F,* Palatine tonsils; the caudal part of the soft palate is missing. *G,* Otoscopic view of eardrum showing handle of malleus. *H,* Dissection of middle ear: 1, malleus; 2, incus; 3, stapes.

## The Nuclei of the Cranial Nerves

The nuclei of the cranial nerves represent the continuation of the four functional components—somatic afferent, visceral afferent, visceral efferent, and somatic efferent—that compose the gray matter of the spinal cord (Fig. 8–12), supplemented by two additional components—special somatic afferent and special visceral afferent—that appear in the medulla oblongata in connection with the innervation of structures of the head that have no counterparts in the trunk or limbs (Fig. 8–24). The four components are massed together within the gray matter of the cord but separate into parallel columns within the medulla (Fig. 8–12). In part, this is the consequence of the flattening of the medulla and the widening, and dorsal shift in the position of its lumen.

These components now exhibit a lateromedial rather than dorsoventral sequence with the somatic afferent column laterally, the somatic efferent column medially. Certain of the columns also fragment into discrete parts (nuclei), while at some levels the relationships are further adjusted to allow the intrusion of the additional components. The consequences of all this are that those cranial nerves that contain more than one functional component arise from more than one nucleus, and that certain nuclei give rise to similar components of more than one nerve. The general arrangement of the six components is illustrated in Figure 8–25, in schematic fashion but sufficiently exact for many needs.

The *somatic efferent column* serves muscles that have originated from somites and branchiomeres of the head. Its medial part is fragmented into a long *hypoglossal* and a smaller *abducent nucleus* within the floor of the fourth ventricle (and *trochlear* and *oculomotor nuclei* within the tegmentum of the midbrain). The fibers from the oculomotor, abducent, and hypoglossal nuclei take the expected courses to emerge on the ventral aspect of the brain, close to the midline and in line with each other and the ventral roots of the spinal nerves (Fig. 8–18). Those that compose the trochlear nerve emerge from the dorsal aspect of the brain after decussation within the rostral medullary velum (Fig. 8–23/IV), an aberrant course for which there is no satisfactory explanation.

The lateral (branchiomeric) portion of the somatic efferent column (Fig. 8–25) supplies the striated masticatory, mimetic, laryngeal, and pharyngeal muscles through the trigeminal, facial, glossopharyngeal, vagus, and accessory nerves. This portion is divided into the motor *nuclei* of the *trigeminal* and *facial nerves* (Fig. 8–25/17,16) and the *nucleus ambiguus* (/14) shared by the glossopharyngeal and vagus nerves. The fibers emerge from the ventrolateral surface of the brainstem but do not always take the most direct internal course to do so.

The *visceral efferent column* supplies the autonomic (parasympathetic) motor component of certain cranial nerves. It is the lateral of the efferent columns (Fig. 8–24/4) and is divided into the *parasympathetic nucleus of the vagus* (Fig. 8–25/13), the *caudal salivatory nucleus* of the glossopharyngeal, and the *rostral salivatory nucleus* of the facial nerve (/15) (and the parasympathetic nucleus of the oculomotor nerve [/18] in the midbrain). The distribution of the vagal fibers of this category is to the cervical, thoracic, and abdominal (but not pelvic) viscera, of those within

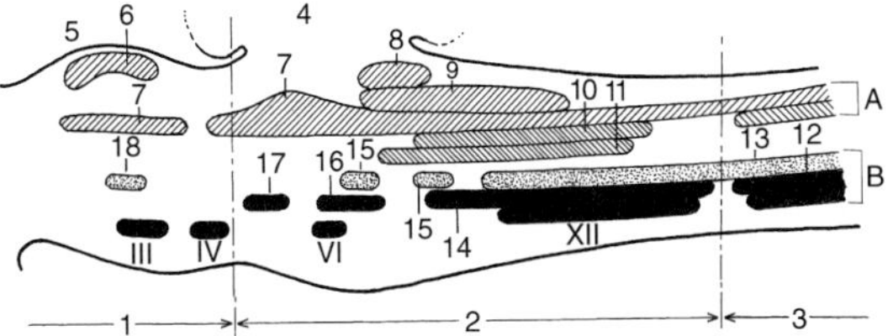


**Figure 8–25.** Schematic representation of the brainstem showing the nuclei in an adult mammal. Roman numerals are used for nuclei of some cranial nerves. A = afferent nuclei; B = efferent nuclei.

1, Mesencephalon; 2, rhombencephalon; 3, spinal cord; 4, cerebellum; 5, tectum mesencephali; 6, rostral colliculus (SSA); 7, trigeminal nuclei (SA); 8, cochlear nuclei (SSA); 9, vestibular nuclei (SSA); 10, solitary nucleus of VII, IX, X (VA); 11, gustatory nuclei of VII, IX (SVA); 12, motor nucleus of XI (SE); 13, motor nucleus of X (VE); 14, nucleus ambiguus of IX, X (SE); 15, salivatory nuclei of VII, IX (VE); 16, motor nucleus of VII (SE); 17, motor nucleus of V (SE); 18, parasympathetic nucleus of III (VE).

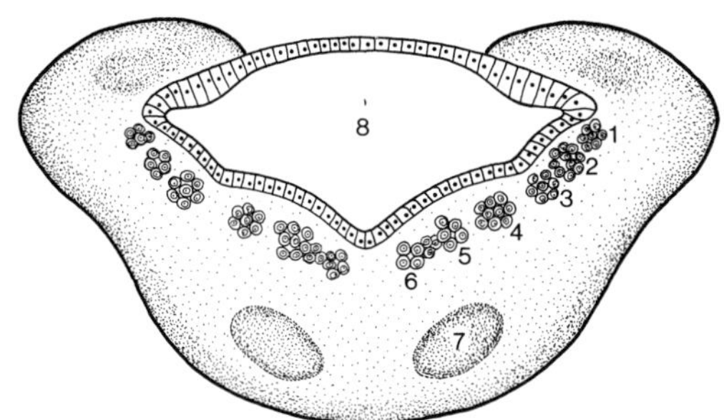


**Figure 8–24.** Schematic transverse section of the metencephalon. The special somatic afferent nuclei are not shown.

1, Somatic afferent column; 2, visceral afferent column; 3, special visceral afferent column; 4, visceral efferent column; 5, 6, somatic efferent column; 7, nuclei of pons; 8, fourth ventricle.

the glossopharyngeal and facial nerves to glands of the head (and of those within the oculomotor nerve to intrinsic muscles of the eyeball).

The *visceral afferent column* (Fig. 8–24/3,2) is in fact double and is shared by visceral and special visceral afferent neurons. It forms a single very long nucleus (*of the solitary tract* [Fig. 8–25/10]) that is subdivided in relation to the associated facial, glossopharyngeal, and vagus nerves. Many neurons are concerned with visceral sensation in the caudal part of the mouth and the cervical, thoracic, and abdominal viscera; the special component, which is concerned with taste, is spread between all three named nerves.

The *somatic afferent column* (Fig. 8–24/1) extends from the cervical part of the spinal cord through the medulla and pons into the mesencephalon. It is broken into several nuclei. One—the *mesencephalic nucleus of the trigeminal nerve* (Fig. 8–25/7)—is concerned with proprioception; it presents a unique feature, the inclusion of the primary afferent neuron cell bodies within the central nervous system (the one exception to an otherwise inviolable rule that the cell bodies of primary afferent neurons are located within peripheral ganglia). The two exteroceptive nuclei (/7) are the *nucleus of the descending (spinal) tract of the trigeminal nerve,* which extends from the level of the nerve's entrance into the cervical part of the spinal cord, and the *principal sensory nucleus of the trigeminal nerve* within the pons.

The *special somatic afferent column* is associated with the optic and vestibulocochlear nerves and therefore with the special somatic senses of vision (II), balance (vestibular division of VIII), and hearing (cochlear division of VIII) (Fig. 8–25/6,9,8). The afferent pathways of these important senses are considered elsewhere; our present purpose is to locate the relevant nuclei within the brainstem. The four closely related *vestibular nuclei* are spread through part of the medulla oblongata and pons, medial to the caudal cerebellar peduncle. The two (dorsal and ventral) *cochlear nuclei* are located within the most rostral part of the medulla oblongata close to the entry of the eighth nerve.

The fiber composition of the nerves can be summarized conveniently within Table 8–2.

## Other Internal Features

The *olivary nuclear complex* occupies a position in the caudal part of the medulla oblongata, dorsolateral to the pyramidal tract, where it sometimes raises a gentle surface swelling (Fig. 8–26/10). It is composed of several parts and varies considerably in form among species, generally taking the form of a nuclear lamina folded onto itself to form a bag. It is an important feature of the motor feedback regulatory mechanism (p. 293). Several other nuclei within the pons (Fig. 8–27) are also concerned with motor control (p. 292).

The *reticular formation* is a diffuse system of nuclei and fiber tracts (Figs. 8–26/8 and 8–28/13) that extends from the spinal cord to the forebrain and occupies a large part of the core of the medulla oblongata and pons. It is discussed on p. 289.

The principal fiber tracts that pass through this part of the brainstem also receive attention later. The large descending tract that produces the *pyramid* externally (Fig. 8–26/11) and the ascending tract known as the *medial lemniscus* (Fig. 8–28/9) are prominent in transverse sections. The medial lemniscus is formed of fibers that issue

**Table 8–2.** Cranial Nerve Components*

| | Nerve | Components | | | | | |
|---|---|---|---|---|---|---|---|
| | | *SE* | *VE* | *SA* | *SSA* | *VA* | *SVA* |
| I | Olfactory | – | – | – | – | – | + |
| II | Optic | – | – | – | + | – | – |
| III | Oculomotor | + | + | – | – | – | – |
| IV | Trochlear | + | – | – | – | – | – |
| V | Trigeminal | + | – | + | – | – | – |
| VI | Abducent | + | – | – | – | – | – |
| VII | Facial | + | + | – | – | + | + |
| VIII | Vestibulocochlear | – | – | – | + | – | – |
| IX | Glossopharyngeal | + | + | – | – | + | + |
| X | Vagus | + | + | – | – | + | + |
| XI | Accessory | + | + | – | – | + | – |
| XII | Hypoglossal | + | – | – | – | – | – |

*Certain points are controversial, notably the nerve trunks followed by fibers conveying proprioceptive information from various muscles of the head, and the precise distribution of the medullary component of the accessory nerve.

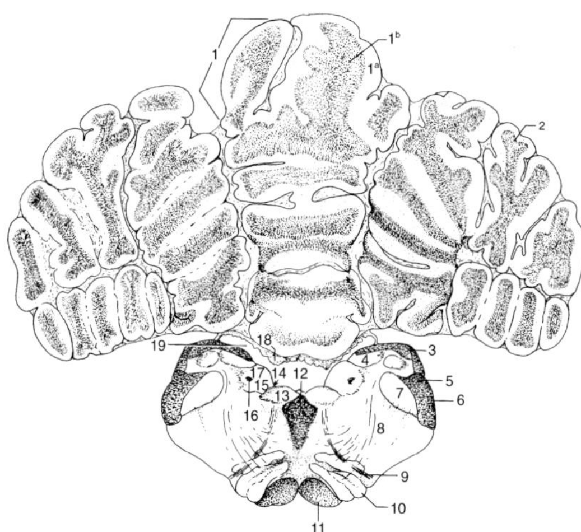


**Figure 8–26.** Transverse section of the canine brain at the level of the hypoglossal nerve (XII).

1, Cerebellar vermis; $1^{a}$, cortex; $1^{b}$, medulla; 2, cerebellar hemisphere; 3, fasciculi gracilis and cuneatus; 4, gracile and cuneate nuclei; 5, caudal cerebellar peduncle; 6, spinal tract of the trigeminal nerve; 7, nucleus of the spinal tract of the trigeminal nerve; 8, reticular formation; 9, root of hypoglossal nerve; 10, caudal olivary nucleus; 11, pyramidal tract; 12, medial longitudinal fasciculus; 13, motor nucleus of XII; 14, sulcus limitans; 15, motor nucleus of X; 16, solitary tract (special visceral afferents of VII, IX, and X); 17, solitary nucleus; 18, choroid plexus; 19, fourth ventricle.

from the gracile and cuneate nuclei, run ventrally (as the deep [internal] arcuate fibers), and cross the midline in the ventral part of the caudal medulla before turning rostrally as a large medial lemniscal bundle. This area also includes fibers of the trigeminothalamic and cervicothalamic tracts, which emanate from the principal sensory nucleus of the trigeminal nerve and the lateral cervical nucleus, respectively. Other conspicuous fiber aggregations compose the three cerebellar peduncles whose composition, origin, and destination are given later.

## The Cerebellum

The cerebellum is a roughly globular, much-fissured mass located above the pons and medulla oblongata and connected to the brainstem by three peduncles on each side (Fig. 8–23/9,10,11). It is separated from the cerebral hemispheres by the transverse fissure occupied by the membranous tentorium cerebelli (p. 299) when the brain is in situ.

The cerebellum consists of large lateral hemispheres and a narrow median ridge named the *vermis* from its fancied resemblance to an earthworm. A division of greater functional and phylogenetic significance is created by a series of transverse fissures. The deepest divide a small caudal *flocculonodular lobe* from the larger mass, which is itself divided into *caudal* and *rostral lobes* (Fig. 8–21). Smaller fissures divide the lobes into lobules and these into yet smaller units known as folia. The caudal lobe is particularly well developed in higher forms and most so in primates. The lobules are individually named, but neither their names nor their exact forms are important.

The arrangement of the gray and white substance sharply contrasts that found in the spinal cord and medulla oblongata. In the cerebellum the bulk of the gray substance is arranged as an external cortex that encloses the white substance or "medulla" (Fig. 8–22). The medulla arises from the peduncles and radiates through the various lobes, lobules, and folia, forming a branching structure with some resemblance to a tree. Because of this appearance, and because of an ancient belief that it is the seat of the soul, it is sometimes known as the *arbor vitae*—the tree of life. Some additional gray substance forms a series of nuclei

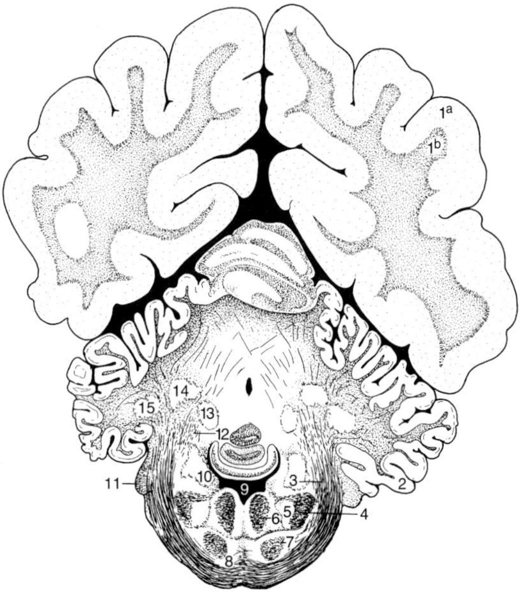


**Figure 8–27.** Transverse section of the canine brain at the level of the middle cerebellar peduncle.

$1^{a}$, $1^{b}$, cerebral hemisphere; $1^{a}$, neocortex; $1^{b}$, fibers; 2, paraflocculus lateralis; 3, middle cerebellar peduncle; 4, spinal tract of the trigeminal nerve; 5, nucleus of the spinal tract of the trigeminal nerve; 6, medial longitudinal fasciculus; 7, pyramidal tract; 8, pontine nuclei; 9, fourth ventricle; 10, nuclei of the vestibulocochlear nerve (VIII); 11, root of VIII; 12, rostral cerebellar peduncle; 13, fastigial nucleus; 14, nucleus interpositus; 15, lateral cerebellar nucleus.

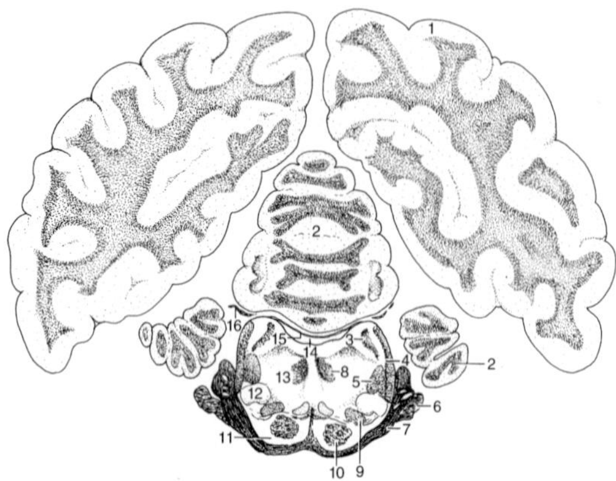


**Figure 8–28.** Transverse section of the canine brain at the level of the trigeminal nerve.

1, Cerebral hemisphere; 2, cerebellum; 3, rostral cerebellar peduncle; 4, lateral lemniscus; 5, rubrospinal tract; 6, root of V; 7, middle cerebellar peduncle; 8, medial longitudinal fasciculus; 9, medial lemniscus; 10, pyramidal tract; 11, pontine nuclei; 12, nucleus of lateral lemniscus; 13, reticular formation; 14, fourth ventricle; 15, rostral medullary velum; 16, root of IV.

embedded within the medulla; the most important of these are the *fastigial nuclei* (Fig. 8–27/13) close to the midline, the *lateral cerebellar (dentate) nucleus* (/15) laterally, and the *nuclei interpositi* (/14).

The cerebellum is attached to the brainstem by the three *cerebellar peduncles* on each side and by the caudal and rostral medullary vela (Fig. 8–23). The caudal peduncle (/10) connects with the medulla oblongata and is largely composed of afferent fibers, some running from origins within the spinal cord, others from the vestibular nuclei, the olivary nucleus, and the reticular formation. The middle peduncle (brachium pontis; /9) is also composed of afferent fibers; these arise from pontine nuclei. The rostral peduncle (brachium conjunctivum; /11) is attached to the midbrain; it is largely composed of efferent fibers dispatched toward the red nucleus, reticular formation, and thalamus but also includes a considerable afferent component that continues the ventral spinocerebellar tract. The three peduncles are closely compressed together at their attachments to the cerebellum.

The functions of the cerebellum are concerned with the control of balance and the coordination of postural and locomotor activities. Balance is located in the flocculonodular node. The caudal lobe is concerned with the feedback regulation of motor function, and to this end it receives a direct input from pontine and olivary nuclei and an indirect input from the other parts of the cerebellum. The rostral lobe receives an input of proprioceptive information. There is a somatotopic representation of the body in the cerebellar cortex.

## The Midbrain

The midbrain (mesencephalon) is a short, rather constricted portion that better preserves the basic organization of the neural tube than do other parts of the brainstem.

The midbrain is exposed on the ventral surface of the intact brain, to which it contributes the crura cerebri, the interpeduncular fossa, and the superficial origin of the oculomotor nerves (III). It is concealed dorsally by the overhanging cerebral hemispheres and cerebellum. Its lumen, the aqueduct, is a simple passage joining the much larger cavities of the third and fourth ventricles. The mesencephalon has a stratified structure, comprising tectum, tegmentum, and cerebral peduncle in dorsoventral sequence (Fig. 8–29). Formally, all parts except the tectum are included within the cerebral peduncles, but in practice the latter term is frequently equated with the crus cerebri, the part ventral to the tegmentum.

The *tectum* lies dorsal to the aqueduct. Its major features are four rounded surface swellings (Fig. 8–23). The paired caudal swellings, the *caudal colliculi,* are widely spaced and are joined by a substantial commissure. They are integration centers upon auditory pathways (p. 291). There is a connection with the ipsilateral medial geniculate body (a swelling of the thalamus) via a distinct ridge (brachium). The *rostral colliculi* are placed closer together and are joined to the lateral geniculate bodies by similar but less obtrusive brachia. The rostral colliculi are staging posts upon

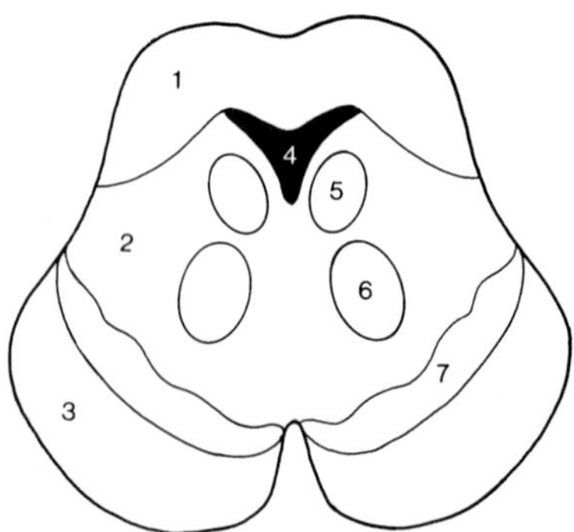


**Figure 8–29.** Schematic transverse section of the mesencephalon.

1, Tectum; 2, tegmentum; 3, crus cerebri; 4, mesencephalic aqueduct; 5, oculomotor nucleus (III); 6, red nucleus; 7, substantia nigra.

the visual pathways and are involved in somatic reflexes resulting from visual input, such as the response to being startled by a flash of intense light. They are also spatial integration centers.

The *tegmentum* comprises the core of the midbrain and is directly continuous with the corresponding stratum of the metencephalon. Much of it is formed by the reticular formation. The principal mesencephalic nuclei are the *mesencephalic nuclei of the trigeminal nerves* (V), the *trochlear nuclei* (IV), the *principal and parasympathetic oculomotor nuclei* (III), the *red nuclei* (named for their pronounced vascularity), and the *periaqueductal gray,* a core of gray substance about the aqueduct. The *substantia nigra* is a prominent lamina that can be identified in transverse sections by its darker color, which is due to the gradual accumulation of pigment within the constituent neurons. Like the red nucleus, it is associated with the basal nuclei (p. 282) in the control of voluntary movement.

The *crura cerebri* are visible on the ventral surface of the brain. They comprise fiber tracts that are in passage between the telencephalon and caudal brainstem. On emerging from the telencephalon they converge, although separated by the interpeduncular fossa (Fig. 8–18). The oculomotor nerves (III) emerge in this region, directly rostral to the pons.

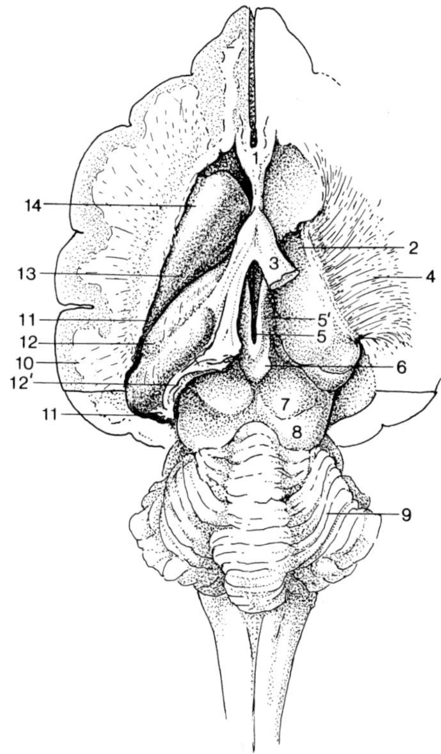


**Figure 8–30.** Dorsal view of the canine brain. Part of the left hemisphere has been removed, opening the lateral ventricle. On the right, the hippocampus and basal nuclei have also been removed, exposing the thalamus and the internal capsule.

1, Septal nuclei; 2, dorsal surface of thalamus; 3, fornix (cut); 4, internal capsule; 5, dorsal part of third ventricle; 5′, habenular nuclei (in roof of third ventricle); 6, epiphysis; 7, rostral colliculus; 8, caudal colliculus; 9, cerebellum; 10, cut lateral wall of hemisphere; 11, lumen of lateral ventricle; 12, hippocampus; 12′, cut-edge of denticulate gyrus; 13, tail of caudate nucleus; 14, head of caudate nucleus.

## The Forebrain

The forebrain comprises the median diencephalon and the paired cerebral hemispheres (telencephalon). The hemispheres overlap the dorsolateral aspects of the diencephalon to which they have become fused by the growth of fiber tracts across the gaps.

### The Diencephalon

The diencephalon (there is no convenient alternative name) forms the most rostral part of the brainstem. Only its most ventral part, the hypothalamus, is visible on the external surface of the intact brain (Fig. 8–18), but it is more extensively revealed in median section (Fig. 8–22). It comprises three parts: epithalamus, thalamus (including subthalamus), and hypothalamus, which develop in relation to the roof, walls, and floor of the third ventricle, respectively.

The *epithalamus,* the most dorsal part, comprises the pineal gland (epiphysis cerebri), habenular striae, habenulae, and habenular commissure (Fig. 8–30). The *pineal gland* (/6) is a small, median body projecting dorsally from the brainstem behind an evagination of the roof of the third ventricle that is composed only of pia and ependyma. Although the pineal gland has long been suspected to play some part in sexual development and behavior, its functions are only now becoming clear; it is believed to be particularly concerned in the seasonal regulation of ovarian activity in response to changing day length. The pineal gland produces melatonin, the pineal antigonadotropin that is also important in circadian rhythms (p. 213). The *habenular stria* is a fiber bundle that among others connects the septal area with the habenular nuclei (/5′). It is an important pathway in the limbic system. The *habenulae* are nuclear complexes of enigmatic function that develop within the most dorsal parts of the ventricular walls. They receive fibers (habenular stria) from the hippocampus and other parts of the telencephalon and send fibers to mesencephalic nuclei. The left and right habenular nuclei are interconnected via the *habenular commissure.*

The *thalamus* is the largest component of the diencephalon. It develops within the lateral walls of the third ventricle but in many, including the domestic, species it later bulges into the ventricle to form a bridge with its fellow. This, the intermediate mass or *interthalamic adhesion,* reduces the ventricle to an encircling annular space (Fig. 8–31/3). The relations of the thalamus are difficult to envisage because of its deep position and lack of separation from the neighboring structures. It extends to the *lamina terminalis grisea* rostrally and to the midbrain caudally; its dorsal surface faces toward the fornix and floor of the lateral ventricle; its ventral surface rests upon the hypothalamus; and its lateral face is covered by the internal capsule of fibers ascending to and descending from the cerebral cortex (Fig. 8–30).

The thalamus is composed of a very large number of nuclei named according to their topographical relationships to each other. These nuclei have various specific functions and collectively form one of the most important relay and integration centers of the brainstem. The ventral group receives most afferent systems (but excluding the pathways concerned with olfaction) and also provides relays on feedback control systems of motor pathways (Fig. 8–33).

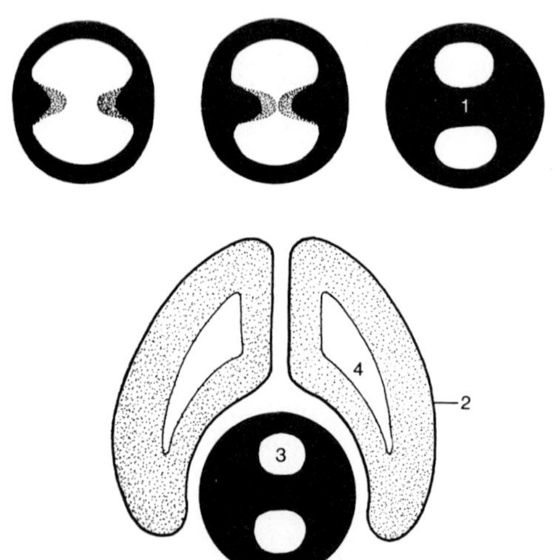


**Figure 8–31.** The formation of the interthalamic adhesion by median fusion of outgrowths of the lateral walls of the diencephalon.

1, Interthalamic adhesion; 2, telencephalon; 3, third ventricle; 4, lateral ventricle.

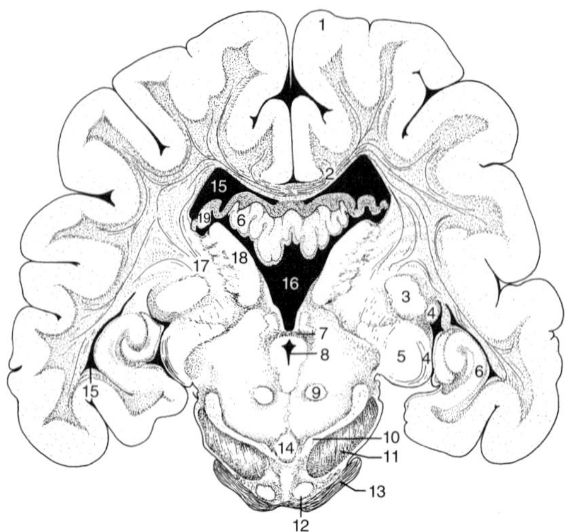


**Figure 8–32.** Transverse section of the canine brain at the boundary between the mesencephalon and diencephalon.

1, Cerebral hemisphere; 2, corpus callosum; 3, lateral geniculate nucleus; 4, optic tract; 5, medial geniculate nucleus; 6, hippocampus; 7, caudal commissure; 8, mesencephalic aqueduct; 9, red nucleus; 10, substantia nigra; 11, crus cerebri; 12, rostral extension of pontine nuclei; 13, middle cerebellar peduncle; 14, interpeduncular nucleus; 15, lateral ventricle; 16, third ventricle; 17, internal capsule; 18, thalamic nuclei; 19, fornix.

The *subthalamus* contains the subthalamic and endopeduncular nuclei and the zona incerta. The subthalamic nucleus acts as a relay station on the extrapyramidal motor pathway, whereas the other nuclei serve as links between the limbic system and the somatic and visceral motor systems.

The *metathalamus,* the caudolateral part of the thalamus, comprises the *medial* and *lateral geniculate bodies* (Fig. 8–32/5,3), whose presence and position were noted in the description of the midbrain. The lateral geniculate body, although not conspicuous in itself, is joined by the optic tract, which sweeps caudodorsally toward it, over the surface of the thalamus. The medial geniculate body lies ventromedial to the lateral one and receives acoustic fibers via the caudal colliculus (p. 291). The nuclei within these swellings relay visual and acoustic information to the cerebral cortex.

The *hypothalamus* forms the lower parts of the lateral walls of the third ventricle. It appears on the external surface of the brain between the *preoptic region* (rostral to the optic chiasm) and the cerebral peduncles and interpeduncular fossa (Fig. 8–18). Its salient surface features are the region known as the *tuber cinereum,* which extends the stalk or infundibulum that suspends the hypophysis below the brain, and the rounded *mamillary body* (Fig. 8–22). Internally it contains a number of nuclei associated with the visceral nervous system and hormonal regulation.

The gonadotropin-releasing hormone (Gn-RH)–producing neurons (see p. 294) have a curious history. They originate from outside the brain in the olfactory placode and migrate along the route taken by the developing olfactory, vomeronasal, and terminal nerves to enter the forebrain. Pheromone stimuli can directly influence the Gn-RH cells.

The *hypophysis* is a dark, solid body. It is located within a recess of the floor of the cranial cavity and is usually left behind when the brain is removed since the infundibulum, hollowed by a recess of the third ventricle, is easily torn across. The hypophysis is also held in place by a fold of dura mater (p. 299). The functions of the hypophysis are described elsewhere (p. 212).

## The Telencephalon (Cerebrum)

The telencephalon consists of the paired hemispheres and the *lamina terminalis grisea,* the thin plate forming the rostral wall of the third ventricle. Since the hemispheres develop as outgrowths of the diencephalon their walls and lumina (lateral ventricles) remain in direct continuity with the corresponding features of that part. The adult hemispheres are semi-ovoid structures that form the largest part of the brain, their growth causing them to extend caudally over the brainstem to reach to within a short distance of the cerebellum. This growth brings them close together, and their flattened medial surfaces face toward each other across the narrow *longitudinal fissure* into which the falx cerebri fits when the brain is in situ. The remainder of the outer wall is divided between convex dorsolateral and flattish ventral (basal) surfaces (Figs. 8–32 and 8–33; Plate 13/*B,D*).

The walls of the hemispheres thicken unequally. Much of the medial wall of each hemisphere remains particularly thin and in fetal life a part rolls inward, invaginating the pia mater and the ependymal lining into the ventricle, where it develops into the *choroid plexus* (p. 300) associated with this cavity. The ventrolateral (striatal) part of the wall becomes much thickened when a number of large nuclei—the basal nuclei—develop within it. The alternation of these nuclei with the fiber aggregations in which they are embedded lends this region a striated appearance when exposed by section (Fig. 8–33); it is therefore appropriately known as the *corpus striatum.* The remainder of the wall is initially known as the *pallium* but when it acquires an external covering of gray substance, again by migration from the ependyma, it is more frequently termed the *cortex,* although this term strictly designates only the outer gray substance.

Three regions of the pallium (or cortex) are distinguished on the basis of evolutionary history, structure, and function. The paleopallium initially served a purely olfactory function; it has retained this association in the highly developed mammals. The archipallium was also initially concerned with olfaction but, unlike the paleopallium, it has largely lost this association. The youngest part, the neopallium, made a very modest initial appearance in vertebrate history but has undergone a spectacular enlargement in mammals in which it is both the largest and functionally dominant part of the telencephalon. These parts are now described separately, but in a different order for convenience. First, it may be helpful to dispose of the concept of a *rhinencephalon* ("smell-brain") of primary olfactory function. Although it is true that the telencephalon of lower vertebrates developed specifically in relation to this sense, many parts have since discarded their original function and acquired new roles. The term rhinencephalon therefore no longer describes the functions of these parts at all adequately and since it is now used in many conflicting ways, there is little in favor of its retention.

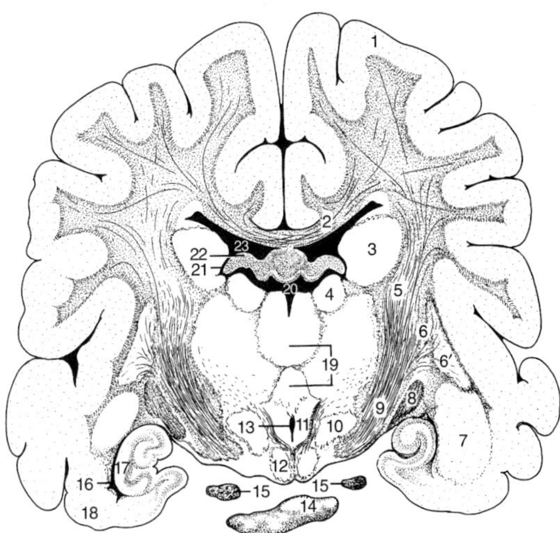


**Figure 8–33.** Transverse section of the canine brain at the transition between crus cerebri and internal capsule.

1, Cerebral hemisphere; 2, corpus callosum; 3, caudate nucleus; 4, thalamic nuclei; 5, internal capsule; 6, 6′, lentiform nucleus; 6, globus pallidus; 6′, putamen; 7, amygdala; 8, optic tract; 9, crus cerebri; 10, hypothalamic nuclei; 11, mamillothalamic tract; 12, mamillary body; 13, ventral part of third ventricle; 14, hypophysis; 15, oculomotor nerve; 16, ventral part of lateral ventricle; 17, hippocampus; 18, piriform lobe; 19, interthalamic adhesion; 20, dorsal part of third ventricle; 21, interventricular foramen; 22, fornix; 23, lateral ventricle.

## The Paleopallium

The paleopallium is confined to the basal part of the brain; it is separated from the neopallium by the *rhinal sulcus* (Fig. 8–34/4) on the lateral surface and, although less clearly, from the archipallium medially. Its rostral extremity is provided by an appendage, the *olfactory bulb* (/1), that fits into a recess of the ethmoid bone. The surface apposed to the bone is made shaggy by the entrance of the numerous filaments that together form the olfactory nerve (I); these arise from receptors within the nasal mucosa and pass through the many perforations in the cribriform plate of the ethmoid bone. In the bulb the olfactory stimuli are conveyed to second-stage neurons. The bulb is continued caudally by the *common olfactory tract* (Fig. 8–18/2), which soon divides into medial and lateral divisions separated by a triangular area. The *medial tract* runs toward the medial aspect of the hemisphere (precommissural area), where the information is conveyed to third-stage neurons. Some of the continuing fibers terminate within certain cortical gyri; others pass through the narrow *anterior commissure* in the rostral wall of the third ventricle to reach the corresponding region of the opposite hemisphere. The *lateral tract* continues caudally to join the large *piriform lobe* (/3), the most salient feature of the basal surface of the hemisphere; not all the fibers in this tract reach the piriform lobe, some being precociously detached en route, mainly to the amygdaloid body.

## The Basal Nuclei

The large nuclei known by this title lie dorsal to the paleopallium, where a number of them combine with the white substance to form the *corpus striatum.* The complex may have had its original importance in relation to olfaction but has now acquired additional functions in relation to other sensory input and to the regulation of motor function.

The nuclei composing the striatal complex are listed variously but most commonly as follows: the caudate nucleus, lentiform nucleus, amygdala, and claustrum. The *caudate nucleus* (Fig. 8–33/3) has the general form of a comma with a large head bulging into the floor of the main part of the lateral ventricle, a body following the caudal bend of the cavity, and a tail related to the roof of its ventral extension (Fig. 8–30/13,14). The *lentiform nucleus* is more lateral and is divided by a fiber intersection into two parts—the medial globus pallidus and the lateral putamen (Fig. 8–33/6,6′). The lentiform nucleus is separated from the caudate nucleus by

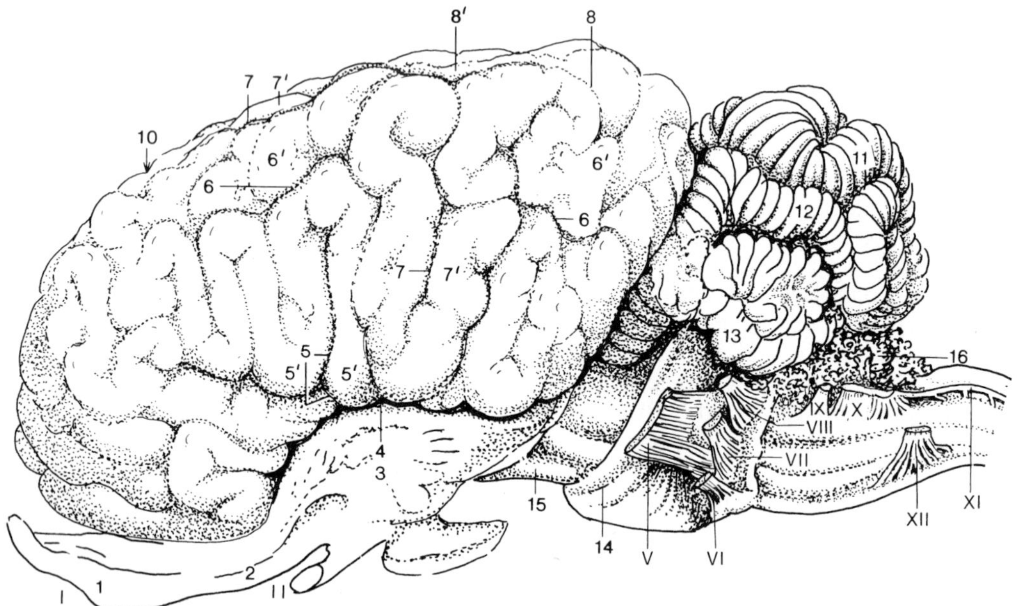


**Figure 8–34.** Lateral view of the equine brain.

1, Olfactory bulb; 2, olfactory tract; 3, piriform lobe; 4, rhinal sulcus; 5, sylvian sulcus; 5′, sylvian gyrus; 6, ectosylvian sulcus; 6′, ectosylvian gyrus; 7, suprasylvian sulcus; 7′, suprasylvian gyrus; 8, ectomarginal sulcus; 8′, ectomarginal gyrus; 10, cruciate sulcus; 11, cerebellar vermis; 12, cerebellar hemisphere; 13, paraflocculus; 14, pons; 15, crus cerebri; 16, caudal medullary velum.

the rostral limb of the fiber mass known as the internal capsule (/5), and from the thalamus by the caudal limb of the same formation.

The other basal nuclei are the smaller *amygdala* (/7), located near the tail of the caudate nucleus, and the *claustrum,* which is interposed between the lentiform nucleus and neopallium; it is separated from these by other fiber laminae, that on its lateral face being known as the *external capsule.*

## The Neopallium

The neopallium constitutes the major part of the telencephalon—all that is visible in dorsal view and the bulk of that visible in lateral and medial views. References to the "cortex," or even to the cerebrum without further qualification, usually have the neopallium specifically in mind. It is divided from the paleopallium by the rhinal sulcus on the lateral side of the hemisphere (Fig. 8–21/4) and from the archipallium by the *splenial sulcus* medially (Fig. 8–22/4). In some mammals, generally those that are of smaller size, its outer surface is smooth but in larger mammals, including domestic species, it displays a complicated arrangement of alternating ridges (gyri) and grooves (sulci) (Fig. 8–17). Though it is tempting to regard the more intricate modeling as evidence of greater intelligence and increased capacity for complex responses, the underlying cause appears to be physical. The ridges, which are mainly longitudinal, are produced by restraints imposed upon the expanding telencephalic vesicle by the rigid corpus striatum and corpus callosum, while additional folding is necessary to maintain the relationship between volume (which increases by the cube) and cortical area (which increases by the square) in large brains.

The pattern of the gyri is reasonably constant within one species but differs among species. The features of greatest consistency include the *cruciate sulcus,* running transversely on the rostrodorsal aspect, a few sulci and gyri that follow the dorsomedial border, and the *sylvian sulcus* on the lateral side. Although other features provide useful landmarks for the investigator seeking to establish the functional significance of particular cortical areas, the names of most are of little consequence to the student. A simpler, rather arbitrary, division of more general utility distinguishes four regions or lobes named from their proximity to overlying bones; this division recognizes *frontal, parietal,* and *occipital* lobes in rostrocaudal sequence, and a *temporal lobe* lying lateral to the last two; only the frontal lobe is clearly demarcated since it is bounded caudally by the cruciate sulcus (Figs. 8–17/14 and 8–35).

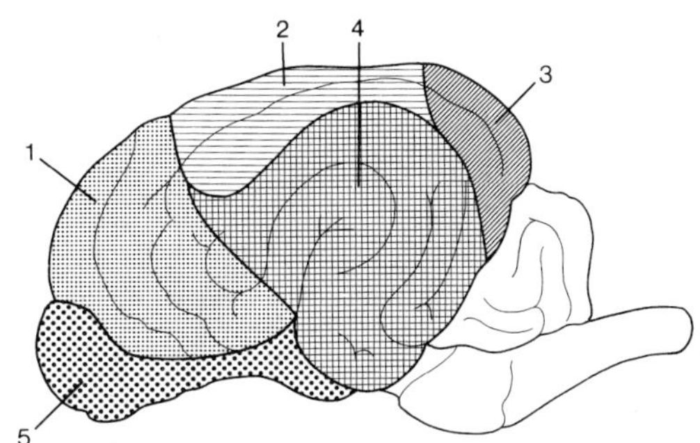


**Figure 8–35.** Cortical lobes of the canine brain. Lateral view.

1, Frontal lobe; 2, parietal lobe; 3, occipital lobe; 4, temporal lobe; 5, olfactory lobe.

The structure of the neopallium is more elaborate than that of other cortical areas and is remarkably uniform. It exhibits six superimposed strata that are densely populated by neurons and are separated by cell-free divisions. The neurons are broadly of two types: some more or less spherical (granular) neurons are provided with processes of very limited extent, other (pyramidal) neurons have processes that range more distantly within the underlying white substance. The pyramidal neurons can be classified by their connections. Association fibers connect parts of the neopallium of the same hemisphere after passage directly below the cortex. Commissural fibers connect the two hemispheres, generally linking equivalent contralateral parts. They run over the roof of the lateral ventricle and mainly cross within the *corpus callosum,* the major telencephalic commissure that is shaped to form a rostral genu, middle trunk, and caudal splenium (Fig. 8–22/3). Descending projection fibers from the cortex connect with lower parts of the central nervous system; most converge upon the internal capsule squeezed between the basal nuclei and thalamus (Figs. 8–36/7 and 8–37/1). In their courses to, from, and within the capsule the projection fibers are ordered according to their functional associations and somatotopic relationships.

## The Archipallium

This part of the cortex was once concerned with the correlation of olfactory with other sensory information but has acquired new functions in modern mammals. It is included in the limbic system, which comprises the cingulate, supracallosal and geniculate gyri, the hippocampal formation, and the dentate gyrus.

The archipallium is no longer a conspicuous feature of the telencephalon. The relatively reduced

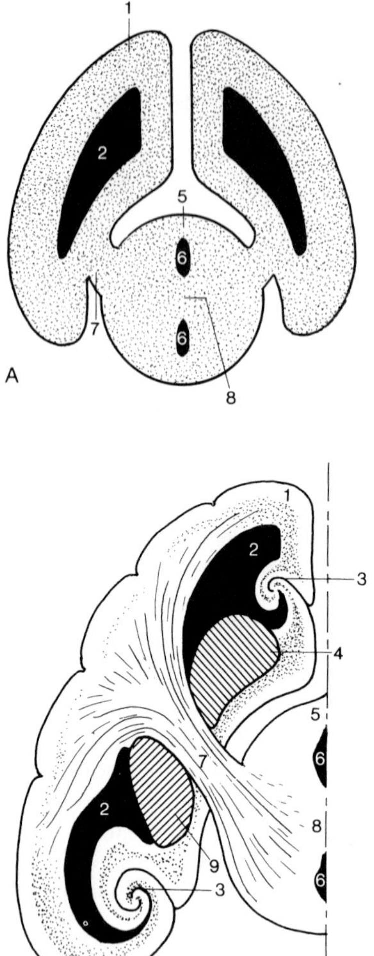


**Figure 8–36.** *A*, The connection between the cerebral hemisphere and diencephalon via the internal capsule (7). *B*, The lateral ventricle, basal nuclei, and hippocampus form concentric arches over the internal capsule.

1, Cerebral hemisphere; 2, lateral ventricle; 3, hippocampus; 4, caudate nucleus; 5, diencephalon; 6, third ventricle; 7, internal capsule; 8, interthalamic adhesion; 9, globus pallidus and putamen.

importance of the olfactory sense and the enormous development of the neopallium have caused the archipallium to be displaced to the medial wall of the hemisphere; it is further reduced in prominence by a large part being rolled inward to lie upon the floor of the lateral ventricle. The archipallium is topographically divided by the corpus callosum into a dorsal part that remains on the surface of the hemisphere (forming the *cingulate* and *supracallosal gyri* between the splenial sulcus and the corpus callosum; Fig. 8–22/8,8′) and a ventral part composed of the inflected portion usually known as the *hippocampus* (Fig. 8–38/2). The archipallium is curved in conformity with the shape assumed by the expanding telencephalic vesicle and fits around the dorsal, caudal, and ventral aspects of the thalamus. This arrangement is difficult to envisage, and it is helpful to remember that the archipallium is interposed between the olfactory bulb and the hypothalamus. The pathway is thus bent into a hairpin loop by the expansion of the hemisphere (Fig. 8–39); the proximal limb extends, with a ventral concavity, caudally toward the apex of the loop, where a spiral twist sets the distal limb upon a parallel returning course.

The proximal limb is provided by the surface gyri; beneath that run the longitudinal association fibers *(cingulum)* from the septal area. The fibers of this multisynaptic pathway enter the caudal extremity of the hippocampus and form a covering to it. The fibers leaving the hippocampus run rostrally over its surface, gradually consolidating into a thick bundle, the fornix. The *fornix* lies directly below the corpus callosum at its commencement but deviates ventrally as it passes forward; it curves around the rostral extremity of the thalamus to enter the hypothalamus, where it terminates within the mamillary body (Figs. 8–38 and 8–40). The right and left hippocampi are joined by the *commissure of the fornix.* There are thus three telencephalic commissures: the neopallial corpus callosum, the paleopallial anterior commissure, and the archipallial fornical commissure (also known as the commissure of the hippocampus).

When the fornix parts company with the corpus callosum it remains connected to it by a thin septum that increases in depth toward its rostral end. This *septum telencephali (pellucidum)* forms part of the medial wall of the lateral ventricle (Fig. 8–22/29). It is a bilateral structure that is separated

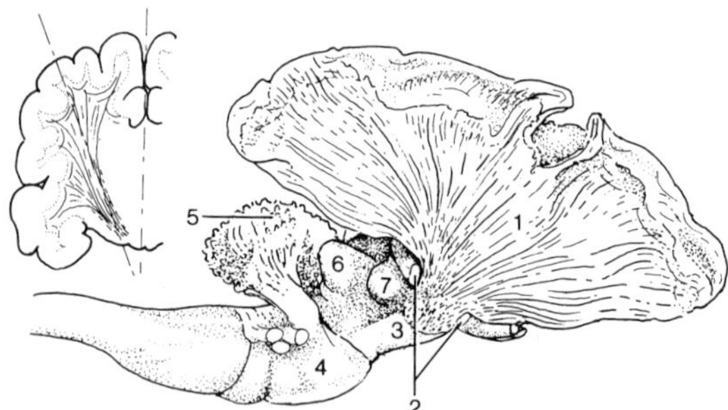


**Figure 8–37.** The internal capsule in the canine brain. A part of the cerebral cortex and the cortex of the cerebellum have been removed. The resected part of the telencephalon is indicated in the inset.

1, Fibers of the internal capsule; 2, optic tract, partly removed; 3, crus cerebri; 4, pons; 5, corpus medullare of cerebellum; 6, caudal colliculus; 7, medial geniculate body.

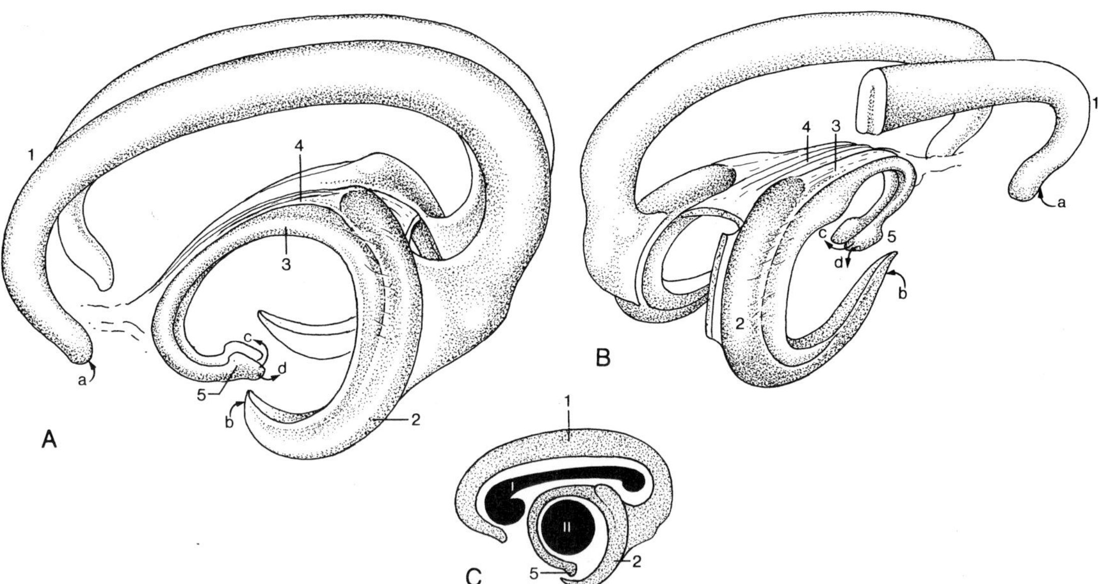


**Figure 8–38.** A three-dimensional representation of the archipallium. *A,* Left lateral view. *B,* Right caudolateral view. *C,* The positions of the corpus callosum (I) and the thalamus (II) are shown in lateral projection.

1, Supracallosal and cingulate gyri; 2, hippocampus; 3, fornix; 4, commissure of fornix; 5, hypothalamus with mamillary body.
a, Input from the medial olfactory tract; b, input from the piriform lobe; c, output to the mamillothalamic tract; d, output to the brainstem.

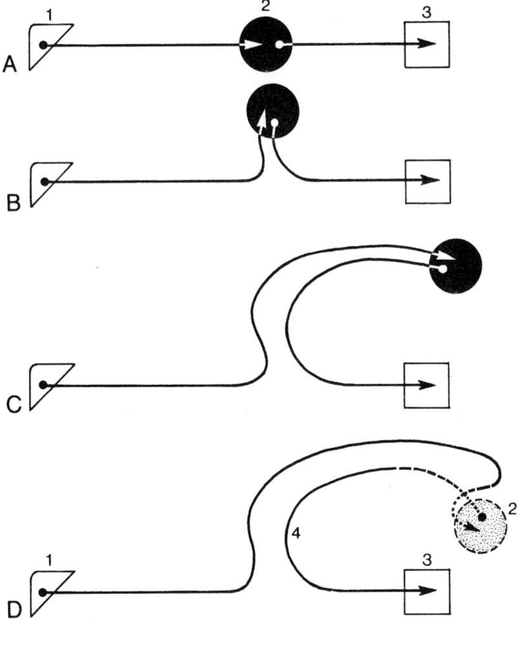


**Figure 8–39.** Diagram illustrating conjectured course of fibers running to and from the hippocampus. Because of differential growth of various parts of the brain, the hippocampus extends first dorsally *(B),* then caudally *(C),* and finally laterally *(D).*

1, Olfactory bulb; 2, hippocampus; 3, hypothalamus; 4, fornix.

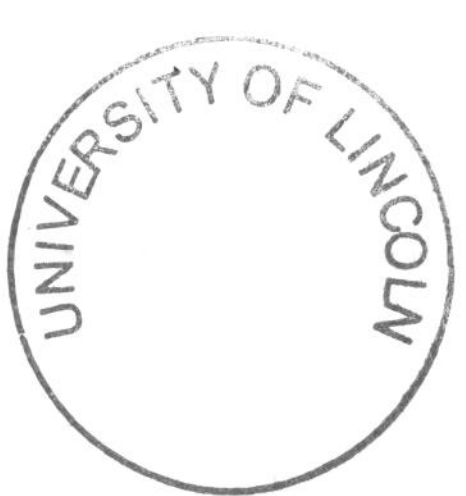
UNIVERSITY OF LINCOLN

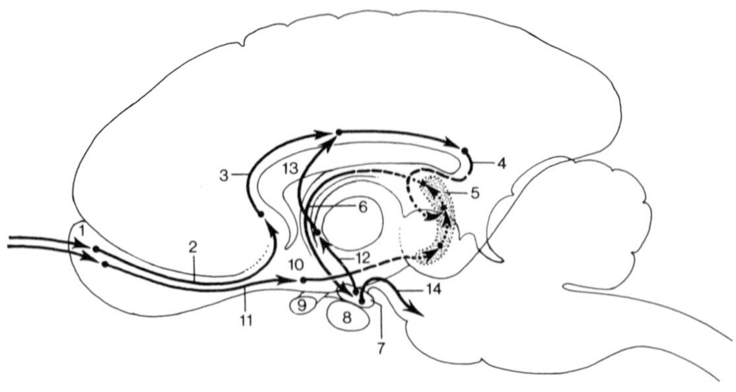


**Figure 8–40.** A simplified conjectured diagram of the relay scheme of the limbic system. The fiber tracts indicated by dotted lines are bent laterally out of the plane of the drawing.

1, Olfactory bulb; 2, medial olfactory tract; 3, cingulum (in gyri supracallosus and cinguli); 4, gyrus dentatus; 5, hippocampus; 6, fornix; 7, mamillary body; 8, hypophysis; 9, optic chiasm; 10, piriform lobe; 11, lateral olfactory tract; 12, mamillothalamic tract; 13, projection fibers entering the cingulum; 14, projection fibers to reticular formation.

from its neighbor by a narrow, completely enclosed cleft and in its ventrorostral part contains septal nuclei in which fibers from the medial olfactory tract terminate.

## THE FUNCTIONAL MORPHOLOGY OF THE CENTRAL NERVOUS SYSTEM

Despite the pretensions of the heading this section will deal only with certain rather fundamental topics involving, for the most part, relatively discrete structured pathways.

### Somatic Afferent Pathways

The designation "somatic afferent" is applied to those pathways of fiber tracts and intercalated nuclei that convey information from the wide array of receptors of various types that are scattered throughout the skin and the deeper somatic tissues. It excludes the special somatic afferent pathways from the eye and inner ear and, obviously, the pathways from visceral receptors.

The somatic afferent system is concerned with a variety of sensory modalities: touch, pressure, vibratory sensation, thermal sensation, pain, and the kinesthetic sensations relating to joint angulation and muscle tension. The primary neurons concerned with all these senses are located within the dorsal root ganglia of the spinal nerves (and corresponding ganglion of the trigeminal nerve where structures of the head are concerned), and their axons enter the central nervous system by way of the dorsal roots of the spinal nerves (and afferent root of the trigeminal nerve). The axons branch on entering the central nervous system. Some branches end on interneurons within the gray substance of the segment of entry or of an adjacent segment; these neurons in turn project upon ventral horn cells of the same or neighboring segment, so completing the short neuron chain that provides the anatomical basis for local reflex responses. (The interneuron is omitted from the simplest reflex arc of all—that of the tendon jerk; Fig. 8–4.) The ventral horn neuron whose axon ends directly on the effector is called the lower motor neuron.

Other branches of the primary axons connect directly, or through interneurons, with higher centers and so provide pathways that initiate more complex integrated responses. The ascending pathways concerned with most sensory modalities (even including a fraction of those concerned with registering joint position) ultimately reach the somatosensory area of the cerebral cortex, providing the mechanism for conscious perception. None of these ascending pathways is entirely isolated from other parts of the brain—all are variously connected to other centers by collateral branches at different levels.

#### *The Lemniscal System*

There are two large ascending pathways that enter consciousness. One, termed here the *lemniscal system* though other names are used, is followed by impulses that provide for a high degree of spatial discrimination of touch, for accurate assessment of the intensity of pressure, for repetitive vibratory sensation, and for a part of joint proprioception. The initial link in this pathway is provided by the chief branches of the axons of the primary sensory neurons that enter the cord (Fig. 8–6). These pass at once to the dorsal funiculus of the cord, where they adopt a very orderly arrangement (Fig. 8–20); those that enter through sacral nerves occupy the most medial positions, while those that enter at more cranial levels assume progressively more lateral positions. A glial septum that appears within the dorsal funiculus at midthoracic level divides it into two parts: the medial division, which constitutes the *gracile fasciculus,* contains fibers from the hindlimb and caudal trunk; the lateral division, the *cuneate fasciculus,* contains fibers from the forelimb, the cranial part of the trunk, and neck. Both tracts end within like-named nuclei of the dorsal part of the medulla oblongata, where they raise slight surface elevations, the gracile and cuneate tubercles (Fig. 8–23/13). The axons of the second-stage neurons leave the ventral aspects of the *gracile* and *medial cuneate nuclei* and at once decussate to the opposite side and turn rostrally as the large fiber tract known as the medial lemniscus. The *medial lemniscus* runs forward within the ventral part of the medulla, dorsal to the pyramid and close to the median plane, to reach a specific part of the *caudoventral nuclear complex of the thalamus* (Fig. 8–41). After synapses within the thalamus, axons of third-stage neurons project through the thalamic radiation to the somatosensory area of the cerebral cortex (neopallium), chiefly to a region directly caudal to the cruciate sulcus. In its course through the brainstem the medial lemniscus is joined by equivalent fibers from the lateral cervical nucleus, the nucleus of the descending tract of the trigeminal nerve, and the rostral (principal) sensory nucleus of the trigeminal nerve following a decussation within the metencephalon (Figs. 8–41 and 8–42).

The somatotopic organization of this pathway is preserved throughout its length, including the thalamic nucleus and the cortex. The cortical representation is of contralateral parts of the body and reflects the generosity of their sensory innervation, not their absolute sizes. There is also some segregation by modality.

## The Extralemniscal System

The extralemniscal system conveys a second group of somatic afferent modalities, characterized by slower propagation and less precise localization of the originating stimuli. The information conveyed relates to the cruder varieties of touch and pressure, to temperature, and to pain. The primary axons of this system end on neurons of the dorsal horns within a segment or two of entry. The information is processed via several interneurons before leaving the dorsal horn (Fig. 8–6). The axons of the second-stage neuron then pass into the white substance of the cord and ascend to higher brain centers. The projection of pain signals from the spinal cord to the brain occurs via multiple ascending systems, which can be divided into medial and lateral groups by their projections.

The tracts of the medial group tend to project into the core of the neuraxis to the level of the limbic system. The group comprises the spinothalamic tract (Fig. 8–42) that projects into the medial and intralaminar thalamic nuclei, the spinoreticular tract composed of fiber bundles located bilaterally within the ventral and ventrolateral zones of the spinal white substance and ending in the reticular formation of the brainstem as far rostrally as the diencephalon, and a loosely organized group of propriospinal pathways that originates and ends in the spinal gray substance and forms a multisynaptic ascending fiber system. The medial group, in contrast to the lateral, shows little variation among vertebrates.

The lateral group also comprises tracts projecting onto the medial caudoventral nuclear complex of the thalamus (MCV) and thence to the neocortex: the spinothalamic tract, the spinocervicothalamic system, and the second-order dorsal column pathway (Figs. 8–42 and 8–43).

The (neo)spinothalamic tract constitutes the classical pain tract of primates, including humans. It is entirely crossed and ascends on the ventrolateral aspect of the ventral horn toward the MCV.

The spinocervicothalamic system is well developed in subprimate mammals, particularly carnivores. Second-order axons ascend ipsilaterally as the spinocervical tract, which occupies the dorsolateral quadrant of the white substance and ends in

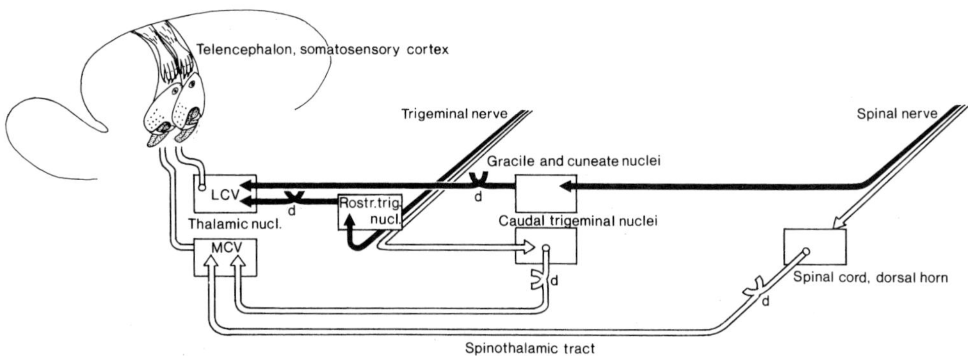


**Figure 8–41.** The lemniscal *(black)* and extralemniscal *(white)* projections from the trunk and head to the telencephalon. d, Decussation; LCV, lateral part; MCV, medial part of the caudoventral thalamic nucleus.

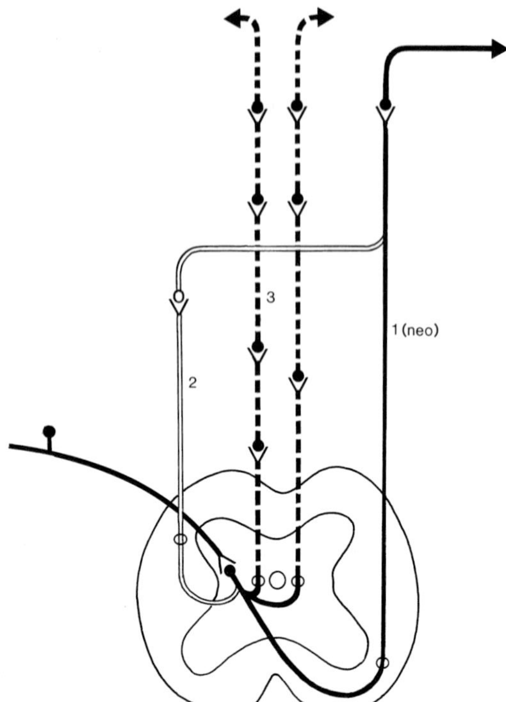


**Figure 8–42.** A simplified scheme of the extralemniscal projections ascending from the spinal cord to the telencephalon. The *uninterrupted black and white lines* represent the projections within the lateral system; the *interrupted black lines* represent the bilateral and multisynaptic projections within the medial system. The (paleo)spinothalamic tract is not represented in this scheme.

1, Spinothalamic tract; 2, spinocervicothalamic tract; 3, spinoreticulothalamic tract.

Models have been proposed to explain the respective roles of the lateral and medial pain-signaling systems in the generation of pain sensation and behavior. It has been proposed that the lateral and medial systems contribute differentially to the psychological dimensions of pain experience, with the suggestion that the lateral system conveys information regarding the sensory-discriminative dimensions of pain, whereas the medial is mainly involved in the motivational-affective dimension via the reticular formation, medial thalamus, and limbic system. Another model suggests that the lateral system is tuned preferentially to the sudden onset of noxious stimuli and thus may be related to the threat modality of pain. In contrast, the medial system is tuned to persistent components of pain and is thus better suited to mediate signals relating to existing tissue damage.

## Other Ascending Pathways

Ascending pathways transmit information—from muscle and tendon receptors—of which there is no conscious appreciation. The pathways commence in the usual way with primary axons that terminate on dorsal horn cells within the initial and adjacent segments. The axons of the second-stage neurons associate in *dorsal* and *ventral spinocerebellar tracts* (Fig. 8–20/5,6), which follow separate routes to their projections on the cerebellar cortex. The dorsal tract takes a direct ipsilateral pathway that enters the cerebellum through the caudal

the lateral cervical nucleus, located at the junction of spinal cord and brainstem. The axons that emanate from this nucleus cross the midline and follow the medial lemniscus to end in the MCV, where they overlap the projection site of the (neo)spinothalamic tract.

The third system has been found in cats. It is composed of second-order axons that, surprisingly, ascend through the dorsal columns; in addition to non-nociceptive these are mainly composed of primary afferents. The postsynaptic, pain-conveying axons end in ipsilateral dorsal column nuclei. The third-order axons that cross the midline also run to the MCV. Second-order trigeminal axons arise from the caudal part of the descending trigeminal nucleus. Axons either join the lateral system and ascend to the MCV or join the medial system into the thalamic reticular formation. The third-stage axons project upon an area of the somatosensory cortex rostral to the area allocated to the lemniscal system.

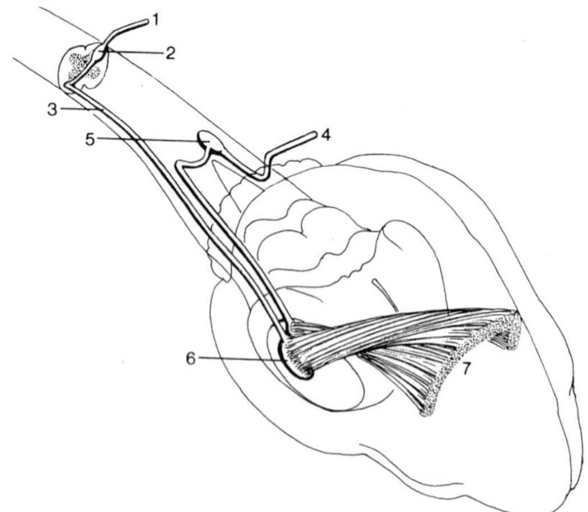


**Figure 8–43.** Three-dimensional representation of the extralemniscal projection in the dog.

1, Spinal nerve; 2, dorsal horn of spinal cord; 3, spinothalamic tract; 4, trigeminal nerve; 5, nucleus of the spinal tract of the trigeminal nerve; 6, medial part of the caudoventral thalamic nucleus; 7, somatosensory cortex.

peduncle; the information it conveys is obtained from stimulation of muscle spindles. In contrast, the ventral spinocerebellar tract is mainly concerned with transmitting information provided by tendon receptors. The fibers of this tract decussate within the cord close to their origins; they then ascend to midbrain level before they turn back to enter the cerebellum through the rostral peduncle. A second decussation within the cerebellar medulla restores the fibers to the side of the origin of the stimulus before they terminate within the cerebellar cortex. These two tracts are concerned only with information from the trunk and hindlimb; the equivalent representation of the forelimb follows a different pathway that will not be described.

A further diffuse ascending pathway is provided within the reticular formation, the subject of the following section. It provides a means for integrating information conveyed by the pathways previously described with information from other afferent systems, somatic and visceral, general and special.

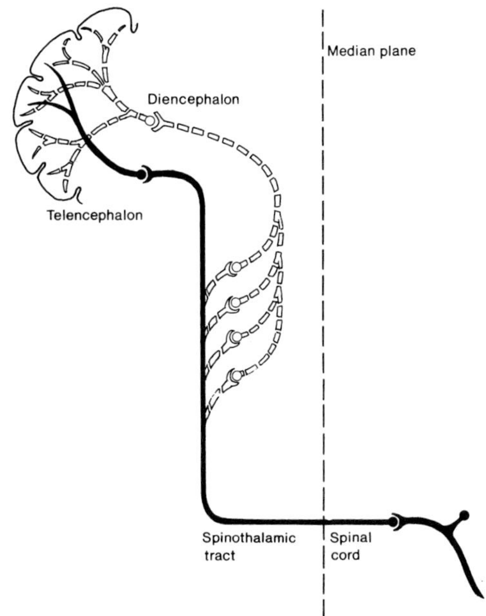


**Figure 8–44.** A multisynaptic ascending tract *(white dotted line)* to the telencephalon via the reticular formation. The collateral tract in this example represents the extralemniscal projection *(black)*.

## *The Reticular Formation*

The reticular formation extends from the spinal cord throughout the brainstem as a diffuse arrangement of neurons interspersed with fiber tracts. In the evolutionary sense it is an old system.

Despite the impression of diffusion and lack of organization it initially creates, closer analysis permits the recognition of numerous nuclear aggregations of varying size and architectonic character; some are sufficiently distinctive for their homologues to be recognizable in different species.

The reticular formation is connected to all projection systems within the central nervous system, whether afferent or efferent, and has reciprocal connections with the major integration centers within the brain. Thus, among its many ascending, descending, and transverse connections there are such tracts as reticulocerebellar and cerebelloreticular, reticulothalamocortical and corticoreticular tracts. The inescapable inference is that the reticular formation plays an important role in modulating the activities of these integration centers.

The reticular formation occupies a large part of the brainstem; it is spread within the core, and when it reaches the thalamus it contributes some of the nuclear groups of this complex structure; it also extends into the cervical part of the spinal cord.

The formation may be divided into parts distinguished by their morphology. The medial part, the *periventricular gray,* is arranged mainly in relation to the ventricular system of the brain. It has proved impossible to analyze in detail but appears to provide multisynaptic pathways composed of an indeterminable number of neurons with short and much-branched processes.

The *second component* exhibits a more obvious organization with more readily identifiable nuclei and tracts. It is restricted to the brainstem, extending from the floor of the medulla oblongata through the midbrain to the "reticular" nuclei of the thalamus. The reticular nuclei of the thalamus receive an input from lower parts of the formation and project diffusely upon the entire neopallium. The *spinoreticulothalamic tract,* an important component of the system, may provide an alternative or complementary route to the spinothalamic system. The spinoreticulothalamic tract commences with the projection of primary afferent neurons on neurons within the dorsal horn. It contains axons that project for long distances and conduct more rapidly than those found in the spinothalamic tract.

One extensive ascending pathway that ultimately projects beyond the thalamus to the cortex is known as the *ascending reticular activating system.* It receives an input through collateral branches from all sensory systems—whether exteroceptive or enteroceptive (Fig. 8–44). Its activation arouses the animal, making it more conscious of its circumstances and surroundings;

diminution of activity induces lethargy or sleep. The reticular activating system has been regarded as the seat of consciousness, but most neurologists would assert that "there is no room or place where consciousness dwells."

The reticular system also plays an essential role in motor control by means of a descending pathway that extends from the telencephalon to ultimate destinations on lower motor neurons of the brainstem and cord (p. 291).

## Special Somatic Afferent Pathways

### *The Visual Pathways*

Visual information is conveyed from the retina by the optic nerve. After entering the cranial cavity by the optic foramen the nerve converges to meet its fellow in the optic chiasm on the ventral surface of the brain. There is here a partial decussation of fibers, and the proportion crossing has been correlated with the degree of binocular vision enjoyed by the species. In birds all fibers cross and vision was considered to be monocular; recent information indicates, however, that some birds have an even larger binocular vision than humans. In ungulates, the binocular field of vision is much restricted, a very large percentage (85% to 90%) of fibers cross. A smaller proportion (75%) cross in carnivores and about 50% in primates, in which binocular vision is best developed.

This reassortment brings fibers from both retinae into each optic tract, which arches over the lateral surface of the thalamus (Fig. 8–23/20). The larger proportion terminates within the lateral geniculate nucleus, which raises a swelling on the upper end of the tract, or within the pulvinar nucleus medial to it. The primary optic pathway ends here. The fibers of the second-stage neurons project, via the optic radiation within the internal capsule, on the visual cortex, which is located within the occipital lobe of the cerebrum and is the seat of conscious visual perception (Fig. 8–45/6).

A smaller number of the fibers project upon various mesencephalic nuclei, some after preliminary relay in the lateral geniculate nucleus. The foremost of these mesencephalic visual integration centers and nuclei are the rostral colliculi. From the mesencephalic nuclei there are relays through various neuronal chains by which the various visual and optic reflexes—concerned with direction of gaze, accommodation, pupillary diameter—are effected. Fibers from the rostral colliculi also end on lower motor neurons in the cervical spinal cord and constitute the tectospinal tract, part of the so-called extrapyramidal system.

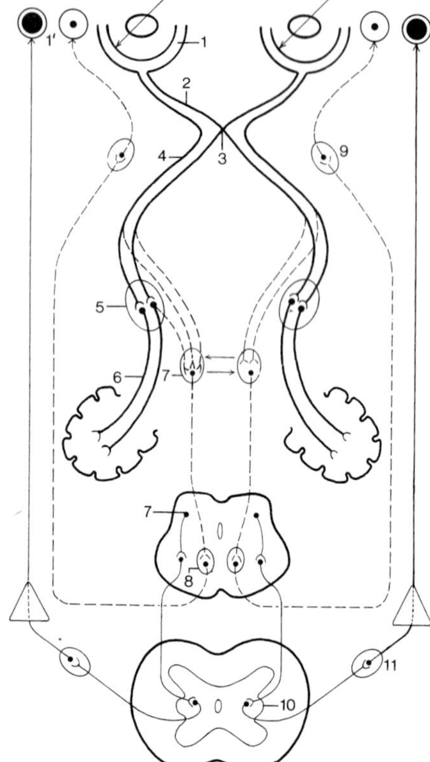


**Figure 8–45.** A simplified schema of the visual and pupillary reflex pathways. *Thick lines,* special somatic visual fibers; *thin lines,* sympathetic fibers; *broken lines,* parasympathetic fibers.

1, Retina; 1′, dilated and constricted pupils; 2, optic nerve; 3, optic chiasm; 4, optic tract; 5, lateral geniculate nucleus; 6, optic radiation; 7, rostral colliculus and pretectal nuclei; 8, oculomotor nucleus (parasympathetic part); 9, ciliary ganglion; 10, lateral visceral efferent column; 11, cranial cervical ganglion.

### *Vestibular Pathways*

The vestibular fibers enter the brainstem within the common vestibulocochlear trunk that penetrates the trapezoid body. They then terminate on, or detach collateral branches to, neurons of the vestibular nuclei (Fig. 8–46/2). Those that continue unbroken reach the cerebellum by way of the caudal peduncle. The secondary fibers from the vestibular nuclei are divided between those that also pass to the cerebellum and the remainder, which run to the spinal cord via the vestibulospinal tract and medial longitudinal fasciculus. Within the cord they project via a series of interneurons on lower motor neurons of the ventral column. Other fibers proceed to the nuclei of the cranial nerves supplying the external ocular muscles; they follow the medial longitudinal fasciculus (/4) and the reticular formation. These tracts are part of the extrapyramidal system.

The fibers that lead to conscious perception of vestibular stimuli proceed via the lateral lemniscus and thalamic nuclei to a particular region of the cerebral cortex of the temporal lobe.

## Auditory Pathways

The fibers of the cochlear component of the vestibulocochlear nerve relay within the dorsal and ventral cochlear nuclei located on the surface of the brainstem (Fig. 8–47/1,2). The second-stage fibers from the ventral nucleus then proceed to a further synapse within an ipsi- or contralateral nucleus of the trapezoid body (/3). The pathway is then continued by fibers of third-stage neurons carried within the lateral lemniscus. A proportion of these synapse within the nucleus of this tract, a second contingent proceeds to the caudal colliculus (/6), while a third, concerned with the conscious perception of sound, synapses in the medial geniculate nucleus before going to the auditory cortex, which is located within the temporal lobe.

The fibers that emerge from the dorsal cochlear nuclei join the ipsi- or contralateral lateral lemniscus and thereafter follow the same courses as those that proceed from the ventral cochlear nuclei.

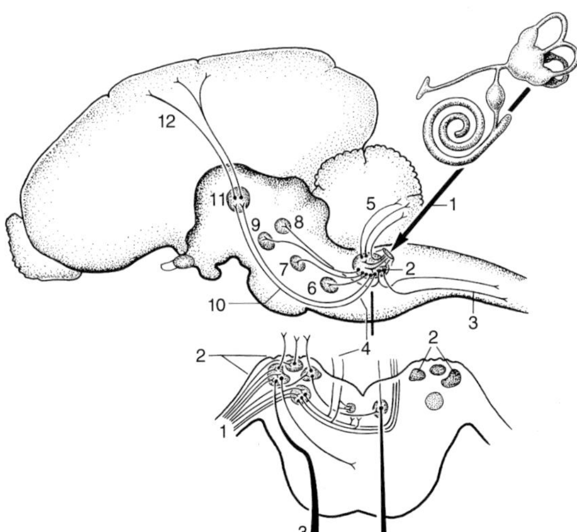


**Figure 8–46.** A simplified scheme of the vestibular pathways.

1, Vestibular fibers in vestibulocochlear nerve; 2, vestibular nuclei; 3, vestibulospinal tract; 4, medial longitudinal fasciculus; 5, vestibulocerebellar tract; 6, abducent nucleus; 7, trochlear nucleus; 8, oculomotor nucleus; 9, red nucleus; 10, vestibulothalamic tract (in lateral lemniscus); 11, thalamic nuclei; 12, thalamocortical projection fibers.

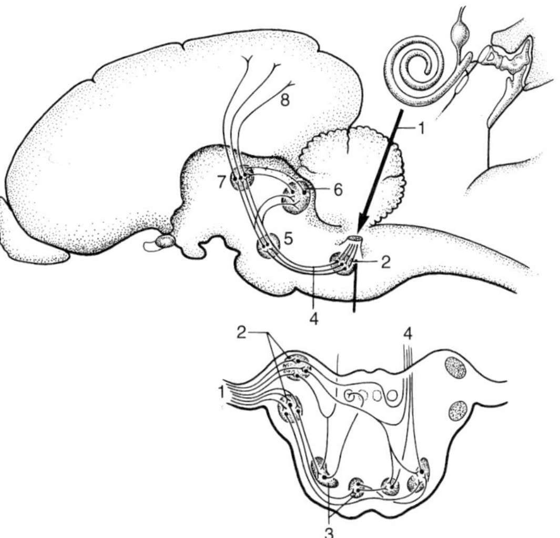


**Figure 8–47.** A simplified scheme of the auditory pathways.

1, Cochlear fibers in the vestibulocochlear nerve; 2, cochlear nuclei (dorsal and ventral); 3, nuclei in trapezoid body; 4, lateral lemniscus; 5, nucleus in lateral lemniscus; 6, caudal colliculus; 7, medial geniculate nucleus; 8, projection fibers for conscious perception.

## Somatic Motor Pathways

Somatic motor activity is regulated at two levels within the central nervous system by separate groups of nerve cells conveniently designated the lower and upper motor neurons.

The *lower motor neurons* are located within the ventral column of the gray substance of the spinal cord (Fig. 8–12/4) and within the somatic motor nuclei of those cranial nerves that contain somatic efferent components. Their axons are conveyed within the spinal and relevant cranial nerves to the skeletal muscles, where each terminates on a group of muscle fibers (Fig. 8–48), the size of the group varying with the precision of performance required of the particular muscle (p. 25). Lower motor neurons provide the efferent limbs of simple reflexes but are in most other circumstances directed by upper motor neurons.

The *upper motor neurons* are involved in more complicated reflexes and also initiate voluntary movements. They are mainly located within the motor area of the neopallium but also in other regions of the brain, including the reticular formation and red nucleus. The cortical areas allocated to neurons controlling the muscles of different parts of the body vary in extent with the importance and complexity of the movements of these parts in the habitual activities of the species; thus the hand occupies a relatively much larger

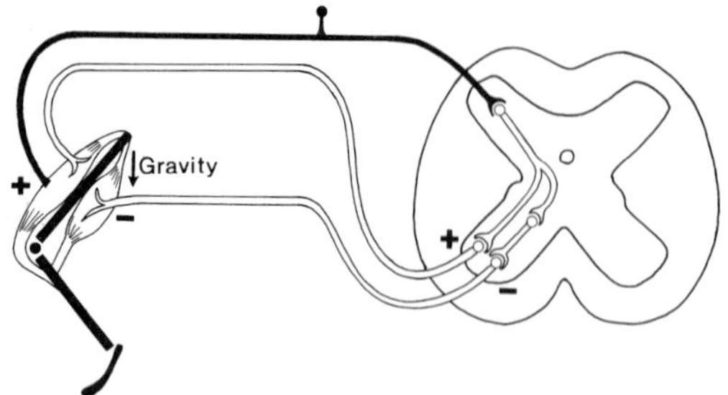


**Figure 8–48.** A myotactic reflex arc. Gravity *(arrow)* stretches the extensor muscle, stimulating its contraction via the reflex arc. The flexor muscle is inhibited by a collateral fiber and an inhibiting interneuron.

area of the human cortex than that allocated to the whole limb in ungulates. Upper motor neurons do not project directly upon muscle fibers but exert their control by excitation or inhibition of lower motor neurons.

The connections of the upper with lower motor neurons follow various pathways that vary considerably among species in their relative development and details of organization. The primary distinction is made between so-called pyramidal and extrapyramidal systems, although the two are coordinated and work in close collaboration. The pyramidal system is mostly concerned with the exercise of finely adjusted movements, while the extrapyramidal system is employed in the control of coarser movements, particularly in stereotyped locomotor patterns. It follows that the pyramidal system must be better developed in primates than in domestic species, a distinction that explains the different consequences of lesions to the pyramidal pathway. Severe damage to the pyramidal pathway produces a complete and permanent paralysis of the contralateral voluntary musculature in ourselves, while the effects in domestic species are mainly confined to disturbance of contralateral postural reactions from which partial recovery occurs after a few days. Both pyramidal and extrapyramidal systems are provided with elaborate feedback mechanisms that allow for the continuous monitoring and adjustment of motor activity.

## The Pyramidal System

The *pyramidal system* takes origin from neurons within various regions of the neopallium, particularly the primary motor area. The axons of these neurons converge toward their exit from the telencephalon and form an important fraction of the internal capsule; in their passage they preserve the orderly point-to-point arrangement of the cortical representation. They then continue over the lateral aspect of the thalamus to enter the crus cerebri on the ventral surface of the brain (Fig. 8–33/9); after traversing the ventral portion of the pons, they reappear on the surface as the pyramids of the medulla oblongata (Fig. 8–18/17). Three fiber groups may be distinguished within the system: *corticospinal fibers* continue through the medulla oblongata into the spinal cord; *corticobulbar fibers* peel off at appropriate levels of the brainstem to reach various nuclei of contralateral cranial nerves; and *corticopontine fibers* pass to various nuclei in the pons (Fig. 8–49/a,b,c).

Certain of the corticospinal fibers decussate within the medulla oblongata, while the others continue directly into the cord and decussate only when close to their terminations. The fibers with a medullary decussation form a *lateral corticospinal tract* within the lateral funiculus; those that continue uncrossed constitute a *ventral corticospinal tract* within the ventral funiculus (Fig. 8–20/3,10). The fibers of both tracts finally project upon ventral column cells of the side contralateral to their origin. In domestic species, as in the generality of mammals, a short interneuron is always interposed; this interneuron is omitted from certain connections of the primate system.

There are other differences among species. In primates and carnivores, pyramidal fibers reach all levels of the cord; in the dog about 50% terminate in cervical segments, 20% in thoracic segments, and 30% in lumbosacrocaudal segments. In contrast, the pyramidal system of ungulates appears to have terminated by the level of origin of the brachial plexus (Fig. 8–50), although there are hints of a diffuse continuation to lower levels within the dorsal funiculus—the route, inciden-

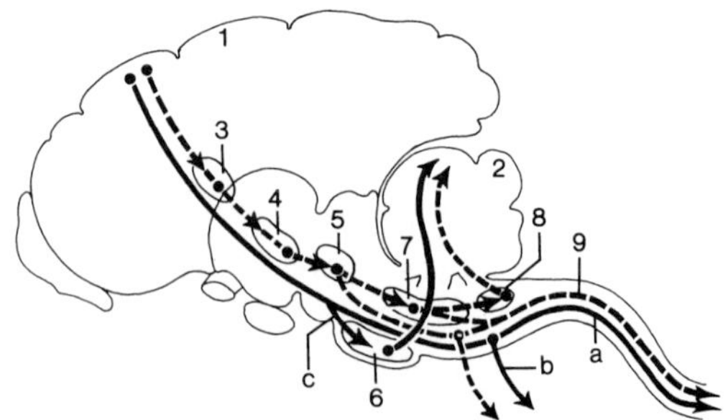


**Figure 8–49.** Relay diagram of the pyramidal (continuous line) and the extrapyramidal (interrupted line) systems.

1, Motor cortex; 2, cerebellum; 3, basal nuclei; 4, substantia nigra (mesencephalon); 5, red nucleus (mesencephalon); 6, pontine nuclei (metencephalon); 7, reticular formation; 8, olivary nucleus; 9, rubrospinal tract.

a, Corticospinal fibers; b, corticobulbar fibers; c, corticopontine fibers.

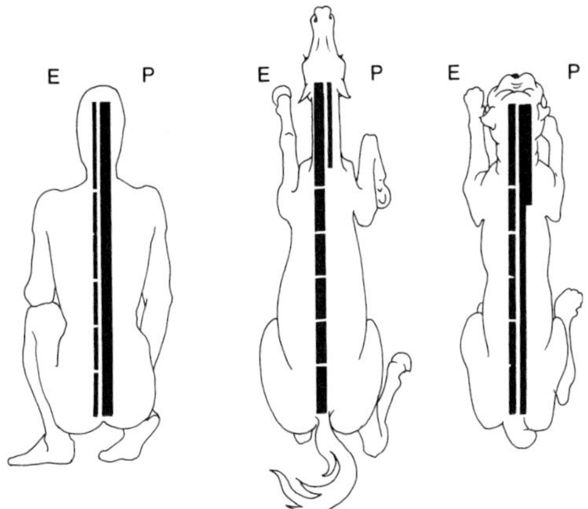


**Figure 8–50.** Comparison of the pyramidal (P) and extrapyramidal (E) systems of human, horse, and dog. The multisynaptic composition of the extrapyramidal system is indicated by the interruptions in this column; the width of the columns is an indication of their importance.

tally, that is favored by the entire system in rodents. The proportion of fibers that decussate within the medulla oblongata also varies; about 50% do so in ungulates, 75% in primates, while all, or almost all, do so in the dog and cat.

The corticopontine fibers end within nuclei of the ventral pons; the axons of the neurons of the second order then decussate and pass within the transverse lamina of the pons to enter the cerebellum through its middle peduncle. Further successive synapses occur within the cerebellar cortex, and then within the nuclei of the cerebellum whence the return to the cerebral cortex is completed by relay through ventral thalamic nuclei (Fig. 8–51). This arrangement constitutes the pyramidal feedback system.

## *The Extrapyramidal System*

The extrapyramidal motor system includes all brain areas involved in regulating motor functions that are not included within the pyramidal system. It is more complicated and involves various multisynaptic pathways that relay within a series of nuclei dispersed through the brain from the telencephalon to the medulla oblongata. Some of these nuclei are large, grossly visible structures; others are small or diffuse, constituting a descending reticular system within the reticular formation of the brainstem. Tracts originating in the tectum and in the lateral vestibular nucleus are dealt with under visual and vestibular pathways (p. 290).

The extrapyramidal system also takes origin from various parts of the cortex, including the primary motor area. The relay stations include the caudate nucleus among the basal nuclei, small subthalamic nuclei, the substantia nigra and red nucleus of the mesencephalon, the reticular formation, and the olive in the medulla oblongata (Fig. 8–49). Only the reticular formation and the red nucleus contain neurons that project directly (via interneurons) upon the lower motor neurons of the brainstem and spinal cord; the other nuclei, and also some neurons within the red nucleus, project only upon cells within nuclei lower in the series.

The fibers from the red nucleus decussate at once before descending through the ventrolateral part of the medulla oblongata to constitute a discrete (rubrospinal) tract bordering on the lateral corticospinal tract within the lateral funiculus of the cord (Fig. 8–20/4). This tract reaches to the most caudal part of the cord, projecting en route on ventral column cells (lower motor neurons) via short interneurons. This is an important tract in carnivores and is the best developed of all motor pathways in ungulates (Fig. 8–50). It serves as a modulator of pattern generators that are located in the spinal cord itself.

The reticulospinal system is divided between well-defined dorsal and ventral tracts located within the lateral funiculus and a third (pontine reticulospinal) tract within the ventral funiculus.

The activities of the various nuclei and connecting tracts of the extrapyramidal system are closely coordinated and so finely balanced that damage to any part may seriously impair the ability to maintain posture or to execute intended movements. Different parts of the system play different roles, some being facilitatory, others inhibitory,

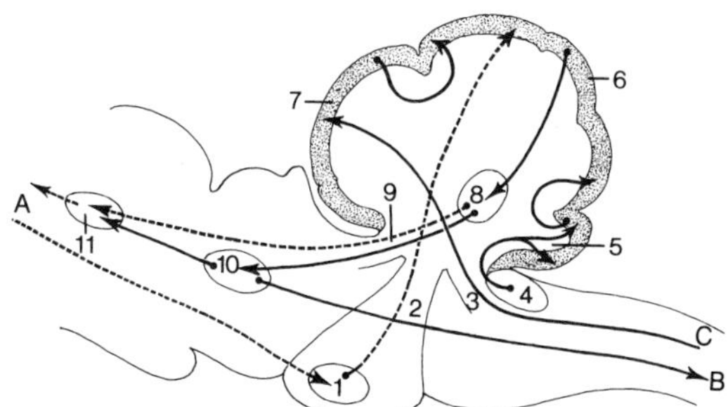


**Figure 8–51.** Some important fiber connections of the cerebellum. The connections with the neocortex are represented by *broken lines. A,* Tracts to and from the neocortex; *B,* tracts to the motor column of the spinal cord (extrapyramidal); *C,* proprioceptive tracts.

1, Pontine nuclei; 2, middle cerebellar peduncle; 3, caudal cerebellar peduncle; 4, cochlear nuclei; 5, flocculonodular lobe of the cerebellum; 6, neocerebellum; 7, rostral cerebellar lobe; 8, cerebellar nuclei; 9, rostral cerebellar peduncle; 10, red nucleus; 11, thalamic nuclei.

and yet others facilitatory through removal of other inhibitory influences.

The numerous feedback circuits associated with the extrapyramidal system maintain the necessary balance between these facilitatory and inhibitory influences. The various circuits are, however, all subordinated to the overall control of the cerebellum to which all nuclei of the system project via relays within the olivary nuclear complex (Fig. 8–49). This complex projects, by way of the caudal cerebellar peduncle, to the contralateral cerebellar cortex before returning from the cerebellum to the various nuclei. The most important return limb runs from the cerebellum to the thalamic nuclei and thence to the motor cortex and basal nuclei; other pathways take shorter courses to project upon the red nucleus and reticular formation.

### *Cerebellar Function*

Although the cerebellum does not itself initiate movement, it ensures that movements are executed as intended by controlling both pyramidal and extrapyramidal systems. To this end, it receives a continuous stream of information that flows from the pyramidal and extrapyramidal feedbacks to the caudal lobe, from the vestibular apparatus via the vestibular nuclei to the flocculonodular lobe, and from proprioceptors that feed into the rostral lobe.

The directions that are based on the integration of these various inputs within the cerebellar cortex are relayed through the cerebellar nuclei before issuing through the various peduncles to the contralateral red and thalamic nuclei, the reticular formation, and the vestibular nuclei (for the coordination of vestibular reflexes).

## THE VISCERAL NERVOUS SYSTEM

The visceral nervous system governs the visceral functions. It has many particular responsibilities, which in summation may be defined as the maintenance of the internal environment within the permissible limits. The common concentration upon the peripheral (sympathetic and parasympathetic) motor pathways distracts attention from the central controlling structures and the afferent pathways that supply the information necessary for appropriate responses.

### The Hypothalamus

An important integration center is the hypothalamus of which the rostral part is concealed and the caudal part—exemplified by the tuber cinereum and mamillary bodies—exposed on the surface of the brain (Figs. 8–18/9,11 and 8–22). The hypothalamus includes many areas of specialized function and responsibility. A brief summation of its functions must include the control of appetite, water balance, body temperature, cardiovascular performance, sexual behavior and activity, and emotion. Several hypothalamic cell groups implicated in reproductive function are sexually dimorphic. Since almost every body function has visceral implications the hypothalamus must receive (and coordinate) information from most other parts of the nervous system, including those of ostensibly somatic function. Information on the somatic activities is projected via the basal nuclei, relays upon the extrapyramidal motor pathways, and via the thalamic nuclei to which the somatic afferent pathways lead. Information concerning visceral function is received from mesencephalic nuclei and the reticular formation. The nucleus of the solitary tract is the principal visceral sensory nucleus that receives topographically organized input from major organ systems by way of the glossopharyngeus (IX) and vagus (X) nerves. As such it is the region of initial processing of visceral, cardiovascular and respiratory, and gustatory information. A further very important contribution comes from the telencephalon, especially the hippocampus, via the fornix. This enables emotional inputs to be related to and coordinated with the rest. Hypothalamic input from peripheral organ systems is also possible by way of bloodborne signals.

The hypothalamus regulates activity through both nervous and humoral mechanisms, sometimes in combination. The nervous pathways extend to the brainstem and spinal cord, by direct routes or by multisynaptic pathways within the reticular formation, in which final integration takes place. Other projections provide a feedback to the forebrain routed through rostral thalamic nuclei.

The humoral pathway operates through neurosecretory cells whose products may enter the blood stream directly for general distribution or may be conveyed specifically to the hypophysis by means of a system of portal vessels (see Fig. 6–3).

### The Hypophysis

The hypophysis (pituitary gland; Fig. 8–52) suspended below the hypothalamus by the infundibulum, consists of two parts. One, the neurohypophysis (posterior lobe), is an outgrowth of the brain itself; the other, the adenohypophysis, is developed from oral ectoderm (p. 140) and comprises anterior and intermediate lobes; interspecific differences in

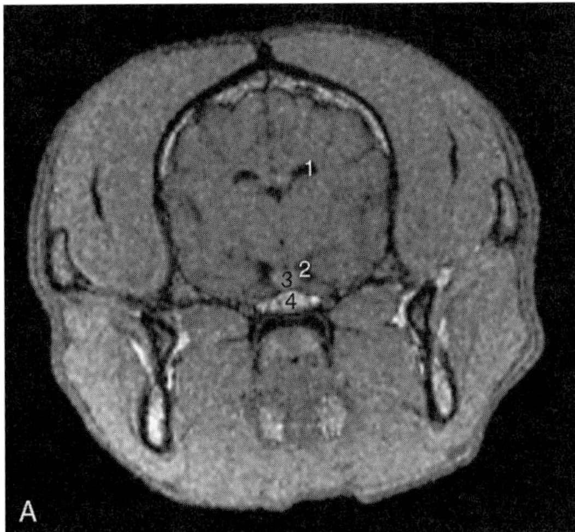


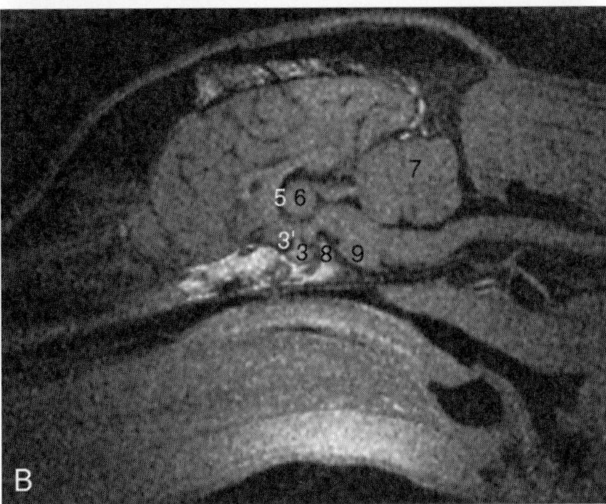


**Figure 8–52.** Transverse image at the level of the pituitary fossa *(A)*, and median image *(B)*, of 1-mm-thick T1-weighted gradient-echo magnetic resonance slices of the canine head.

1, Lateral ventricle; 2, basal cistern; 3, pituitary gland; 3′, infundibulum; 4, fat in sphenoid bone; 5, third ventricle; 6, interthalamic adhesion; 7, cerebellum; 8, dorsum sellae; 9, pons.

the topographical interrelationship of the lobes are not of present concern (see Fig. 6–2).

The three lobes produce or store several hormones (p. 212). The posterior lobe hormones are produced by neurosecretory cells within the supraoptic and paraventricular nuclei of the hypothalamus and are conveyed along the axons for direct release into the neurohypophysial capillary bed (see Fig. 6–3).

## Visceral Afferent Pathways

There are both "general" and special visceral afferent pathways, the latter concerned with taste and smell. The receptors of the general visceral afferent pathway are found within viscera and blood vessels; most are mechanoreceptors responsive to pressure, stretch, and, less commonly, flow, while a minority are chemoreceptors responsive to such stimuli as the carbon dioxide content of the blood. The fibers that convey impulses from these receptors travel within any conveniently located nerve trunk, utilizing those of mainly somatic composition as well as those whose other components are visceral efferent. The bodies of the primary neurons are located within the dorsal root ganglia of all spinal nerves (and the equivalent ganglia of certain cranial nerves); the axons project upon interneurons and projection neurons within the visceral afferent column of the spinal cord and brainstem (Fig. 8–12/2).

Short chains of interneurons provide for simple visceral reflexes that have their last two relays within the visceral efferent column and the peripheral autonomic ganglia. The projection neurons form ascending pathways that follow somatic systems, both lemniscal and extralemniscal, to end (like these) within nuclei of the ventrocaudal thalamus. A final projection to the cortex may give rise to conscious perception, although most visceral activity goes unnoticed. (The sense of fullness arising from digestive organs or the bladder is among the visceral activities of which awareness is most common.) Pronounced contraction and serious overdistention of visceral organs may be perceived as pain. Pain of visceral origin may be "referred" to the surface of the body, presumably in consequence of the convergence of the cutaneous somatic and visceral afferent pathways on the same neurons at some point along their course.

The special visceral afferent pathway concerned with taste follows a similar route to that taken by the general visceral sensory modalities. The course from the taste buds within the facial, glossopharyngeal, and vagus nerves terminates in the nucleus of the solitary tract.

The more complicated olfactory pathways are described elsewhere (Fig. 8–40).

## Visceral Efferent Pathways

Unlike the afferent component, the efferent component of the visceral nervous system is arranged in two divisions, sympathetic and parasympathetic, distinguished by morphology, pharmacology, and physiology. The final conducting pathway of both divisions, unlike that of the somatic system, includes two motor neurons in succession; the first has its perikaryon within the central nervous system, the second is stationed within a peripheral ganglion (Fig. 8–53). The two are most frequently distinguished as preganglionic and postganglionic neurons and together are equivalent to the lower motor neuron of the somatic system.

The preganglionic neurons of the sympathetic division are located within the lateral (visceral efferent) column of the spinal cord between the first thoracic and middle lumbar segments (with some interspecific variation) (Fig. 8–75). The postganglionic neurons are found in paravertebral ganglia of the sympathetic chain or subvertebral ganglia on the aorta; both groups are relatively close to the cord.

The parasympathetic preganglionic neurons are restricted to nuclei of origin of the oculomotor, facial, glossopharyngeal, and vagus nerves within the brainstem, and the lateral columns of certain sacral segments of the cord (Fig. 8–74). The postganglionic neurons are stationed within small ganglia in close proximity to or actually incorporated within the walls of the organs they supply.

The transmitter substance at the last sympathetic relay is norepinephrine, that of the parasympathetic division, acetylcholine. The two divisions therefore react differently to autonomic stimulant and depressant drugs.

The two systems have broadly similar distributions and are frequently described as antagonist, one inhibiting while the other stimulates a particular activity. This rule is less absolute than was once supposed, and their roles are better regarded as collaborative. The more diffuse anatomy of the peripheral sympathetic nerves (which are described later) and the use of norepinephrine as a transmitter point to the more general effects produced by sympathetic activity, in contrast to those of parasympathetic activity, which are often local, effecting single specific functions.

The central control is exerted by neurons within the hypothalamus; those that influence the sympathetic division are generally caudal to those controlling the parasympathetic division. The pathways from both sets follow various routes, some direct, others by multisynaptic chains within the reticular formation.

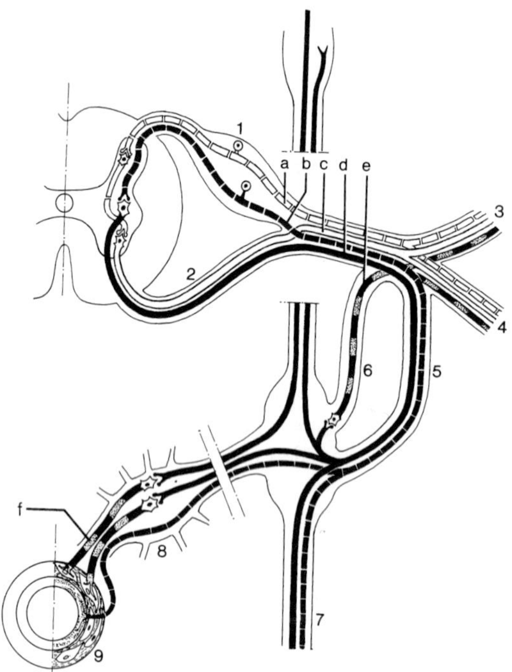


**Figure 8–53.** Comparison of the organization of the visceral *(black)* and the somatic *(open)* nervous system at the thoracolumbar level of the spinal cord. Afferent fibers are indicated by *interrupted lines,* efferent fibers by *solid lines.* The postganglionic sympathetic fibers are indicated by alternating *black* and *stippled lines.*

1, Dorsal root ganglion; 2, ventral root; 3, dorsal branch of spinal nerve; 4, ventral branch of spinal nerve; 5, 6, white (preganglionic) and gray (postganglionic) communicating branches, often fused; 7, sympathetic trunk with ganglia; 8, prevertebral ganglion; 9, gut.

a, Somatic afferent fibers; b, visceral afferent fibers; c, somatic efferent fibers; d, visceral efferent fibers (preganglionic sympathetic); e, postganglionic sympathetic (to peripheral structures); f, postganglionic sympathetic (to abdominal organs).

## The Limbic System

The limbic system has a complex organization and is composed of the limbic cortex and many subcortical nuclei. The cortical part forms a ring at the medial surface of the cerebral hemisphere, including, among other structures, the cingulate and supracallosal gyri, the piriform lobe, and the hippocampus. The subcortical part is composed of the hypothalamus, septal area, anterior thalamic nuclei, intrathalamic nuclei, caudate nucleus, putamen, amygdala, habenular nuclei, and dorsal part of the mesencephalic tegmentum. There are numerous associations between these structures and other regions of the brain. The limbic system is often considered to be primarily a "visceral brain," because its major functions are expressed by visceral motor activity.

Olfactory impulses passing by way of the piriform lobes may influence many structures of the system. Of all the sensory inputs, olfaction exhibits the most profound effects on visceral motor activities that are associated with emotional behavior such as eating, rage, sexual activity, fear, and drinking. The system also receives optic, auditory, extroceptive, and introceptive stimuli.

The efferent pathways from the cortical regions involve nearly all the subcortical nuclei of the system. A major portion of the influences of the limbic cortex is mediated through the efferent systems of the amygdaloid nuclei. Electrical stimulation of the amygdala produces a wide variety of visceral, somatic, and many behavioral reactions. The types of behavior most influenced by the amygdala are those essential for the preservation of the individual or the species.

The hippocampus probably plays the predominant part in the limbic system's control of emotional expression and behavior through regulation of autonomic, endocrine, and somatic functions. It is also concerned with memory functions, in the processing of recently acquired memory and in its more permanent consolidation. In its activities the limbic system is closely associated with the reticular formation of the brainstem.

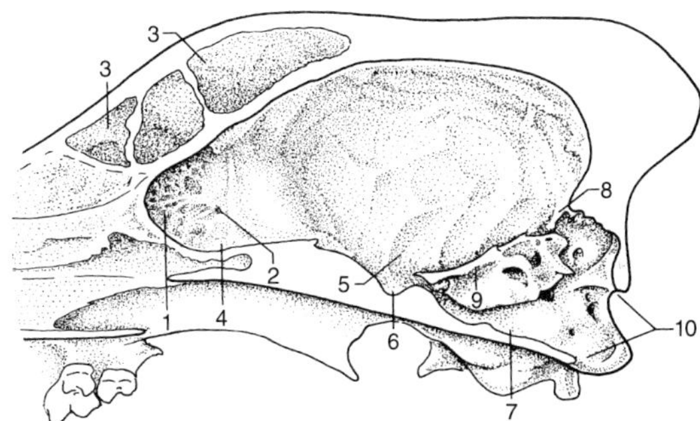


**Figure 8–54.** Sagittal section of the cranium of the dog.

1, Cribriform plate; 2, ethmoid foramen; 3, frontal sinus; 4, rostral fossa; 5, middle fossa; 6, hypophysial fossa; 7, caudal fossa; 8, tentorium cerebelli osseum; 9, petrosal crest; 10, foramen magnum.

# THE TOPOGRAPHY, ENVIRONMENT, AND VASCULARIZATION OF THE BRAIN AND SPINAL CORD

## Topography

The brain and spinal cord are contained within a continuous space provided by the cranial cavity of the skull and the canal formed by successive bony rings and connecting ligaments and discs of the vertebral column.

The *cranial cavity* lies directly behind the nasal cavities. Smaller than is commonly supposed, its form and extent are not easily predicted from external inspection since the paranasal sinuses, horns, muscular ridges and other projections of the skull, and the temporal muscles all contribute significantly to the conformation of this part of the head. The closest agreement between the external contours and the cavity within the cranium is found in the newborn of all species; among adults this agreement is best retained in cats and in dogs of brachycephalic breeds. Fortunately, the exact location of the brain is rarely of practical significance except in the humane slaughter techniques mentioned in later chapters. It is probably sufficient to state meanwhile that the caudal limit of the cavity extends to the caudal wall of the skull—thickened by the frontal sinus in cattle—while the rostral limit shows considerable variation; it ends level with the caudal margin of the zygomatic processes of the frontal bones in dogs and cats, with the rostral level of these processes in horses and cattle, but extends to the middle of the orbit in pigs and small ruminants.

The interior of the cranial cavity shows a fairly close correspondence with the contours of the brain, although significant intracranial space is required for the meninges and intermeningeal spaces that surround the brain and for the capacious intracranial venous sinuses. While the roof (calvaria) of the cavity remains largely undivided, the base is divided into three fossae; these need not be described in detail since the main features are depicted in Figure 8–54. The rostral fossa is formed by the sphenoid and ethmoid bones, and extends to the level of the optic canals, the passages of exit of the optic nerves. It contains the olfactory bulbs, within recesses of the cribriform plate (/1), and the rostral parts of the cerebral hemispheres. The middle fossa extends from the optic canals to the sharp petrosal crests (/9) that project inward from the petrous temporal bones of the lateral walls. The floor is formed by the sphenoid bone, which carries the median hypophysial fossa (sella turcica) into which the hypophysis fits; it also presents various foramina of exit—the orbital fissure and the round and oval foramina—that were encountered in the previous description of the skull (p. 62). This, the widest part of the cranial cavity, contains the temporal and parietal lobes of the cerebral hemispheres. The caudal fossa extends from the caudal limit of the hypophysial fossa to the foramen magnum in the caudal wall. Its principal features are the contributions to its lateral walls made by the petrous parts of the temporal bones (each perforated by an internal acoustic meatus) and the jugular and hypoglossal foramina in the floor. The caudal fossa lodges the midbrain, pons, and medulla ventrally, and the cerebellum dorsally.

The caudal, dorsal, and lateral walls of the entire cranial cavity blend together. Their most prominent internal feature is the tentorium cerebelli osseum (/8), a large projection at the junction of the dorsal and caudal walls forming the middle portion of the tentorium cerebelli within the

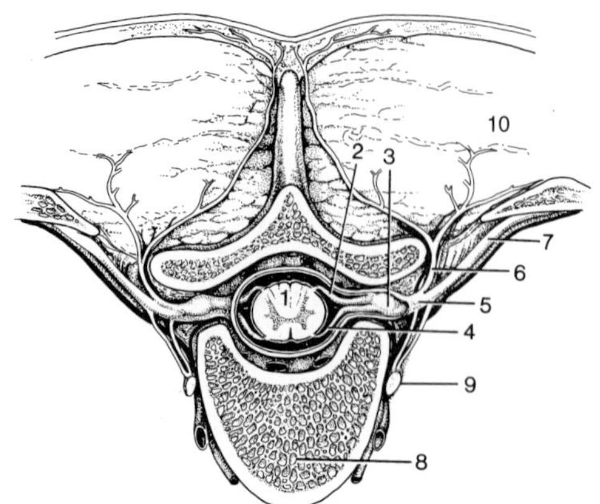


**Figure 8–55.** Transection of the vertebral column to show the formation of a spinal nerve.

1, Spinal cord; 2, dorsal root; 3, spinal ganglion; 4, ventral root; 5, spinal nerve; 6, dorsal branch of spinal nerve; 7, ventral branch of spinal nerve; 8, body of vertebra; 9, sympathetic trunk; 10, epaxial muscles.

transverse fissure of the brain. It presents passages through which emerge emissary branches of the dorsal intracranial venous sinuses.

The *vertebral canal* is widest within the atlas and tapers rapidly within the sacrum; in between, it is most expanded where it contains the cervical and lumbar swellings of the spinal cord from which arise the nerves that form the limb plexuses (Fig. 8–55). The topography of the spinal cord is of considerable importance in veterinary practice since injections into the canal are frequently made, particularly of local anesthetic solution with the intention of blocking specific spinal nerves; in addition, there is sometimes a need to locate central nervous lesions to specific vertebral levels, a procedure made possible by association of specific sensory and motor deficits with particular spinal segments.

Even with the inclusion of its meningeal wrappings, the spinal cord is considerably smaller than the vertebral canal (Fig. 8–55). It is also considerably shorter. This is due to the unequal later growth of the spinal cord and vertebral column, an inequality that begins well before birth and continues after it. The relative shift in position (ascensus medullae) carries the segments of the cord cranially from their original positions within vertebrae of the same numerical designations. The shift of the more caudal segments is most pronounced and explains the peculiar arrangement of the associated spinal nerves. These take progressively longer courses within the canal to reach their fixed foramina of exit, forming a leash (known as the cauda equina from a superficial resemblance to a horse's tail) to each side of the conus medullaris (see Fig. 12–8/9). The level at which the cord ends varies among species (and, in early life, with age); it is within L5 or L6 in the pig, L6 in ruminants, L6 or L7 in the dog, S2 in the horse, and rather variably between L6 and S3 in the cat (Fig. 8–56).

## The Meninges and Fluid Environment

The brain and spinal cord are surrounded by three continuous membranes or meninges that exhibit certain topographical differences of importance in their cranial and vertebral parts.

The tough outermost membrane, the *dura mater,* is fused with the inner periosteum of the skull bones; it splits from this within the margin of the foramen magnum to form a free tube separated

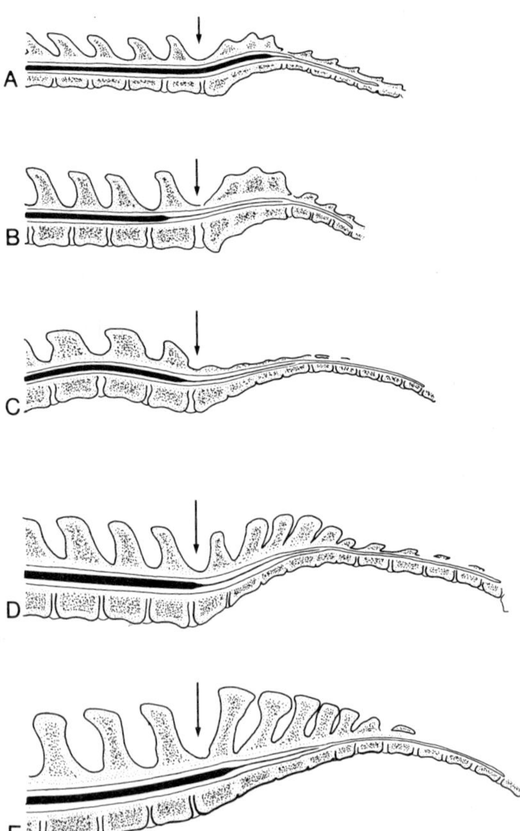


**Figure 8–56.** Median section of the vertebral canal and spinal cord of cat *(A)*, dog *(B)*, pig *(C)*, cattle *(D)*, and horse *(E)*. The lumbosacral interarcuate space is indicated by an arrow. Notice the difference in caudal extent of the spinal cord in the different species. The thin extension of the spinal cord is the filum terminale that ends on the caudal vertebrae (not shown).

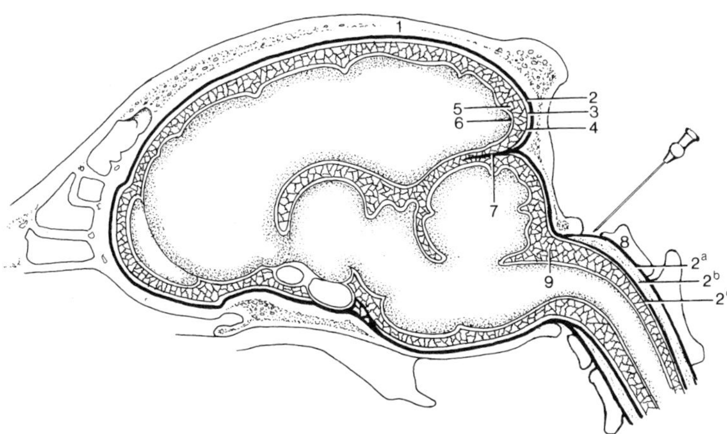


**Figure 8–57.** Schematic representation of the meninges of the brain. The needle points to the atlanto-occipital space and the cerebellomedullary cistern.

1, Calvaria; 2, dura mater (also connected to the bone as periosteum); $2^a$, periosteum of vertebral canal; $2^b$, epidural space (with fat); $2^c$, dura mater of spinal cord; 3, subdural space; 4, arachnoid; 5, subarachnoid space; 6, pia mater; 7, membranous tentorium cerebelli; 8, atlas; 9, cerebellomedullary cistern.

from the wall of the vertebral canal by a wide though varying epidural space. The *epidural space* is occupied by fat, more fluid in life than in the post-mortem specimen, and by the internal vertebral venous plexus; the fat and vessels together cushion the spinal cord and allow it to adjust to the movements of the neck and back (Fig. 8–55). The dural tube is attached at its caudal end, where the several meninges finally combine in a fibrous strand (filum terminale) that fuses with the upper surface of the caudal vertebrae.

The fusion of the cranial dura with the periosteum obliterates the epidural space within the skull, and the cranial venous sinuses thus come to be enclosed within the thickness of the combined membrane. In addition to lining the cavity, the cranial dura forms certain folds that project inward and limit shuddering movements of the brain; these are a considerable hindrance to the removal of the intact brain at autopsy. One, the *falx cerebri,* extends from the dorsal and rostral cranial walls between the two cerebral hemispheres; caudally it joins a second, transverse fold, the *membranous tentorium cerebelli,* which separates the cerebellum from the cerebrum (Fig. 8–57/7). The tentorium is ossified in its median part. A third specialization of the dura roofs the hypophysial fossa in which the hypophysis is seated, forming a diaphragm around the infundibular stalk.

A capillary space divides the dura from the *arachnoid* (/4), the first of the two more delicate inner membranes. This subdural space normally contains only a minute amount of a clear lymph-like fluid but may be enlarged by effusion of blood following injury. The spinal part of the subdural space is crossed by a bilateral series of triangular (denticulate) ligaments that alternates with the origins of the spinal nerves; they attach the inner meninges to the dural tube and thus indirectly sling the cord (Fig. 8–58/6; Plate 13/*G,H*). The outer part of the arachnoid forms a continuous membrane molded against the dural envelope. Its inner surface is joined to the pia mater by numerous trabeculae and filaments, imaginatively compared to a spider's web (the origin of the name "arachnoid"). The *pia mater* is directly attached to the brain and cord, and follows every change in their contours. The subarachnoid space, which

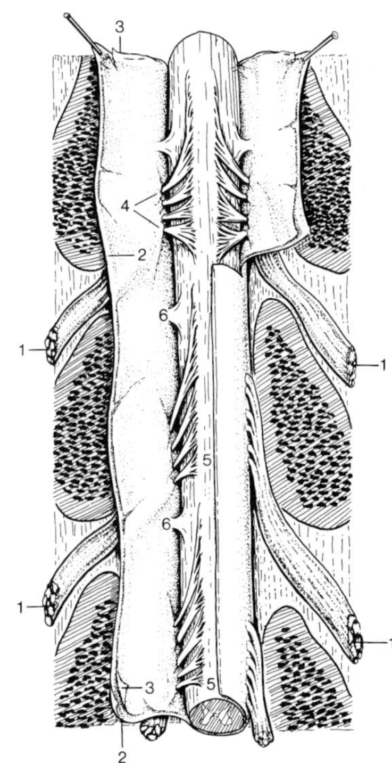


**Figure 8–58.** Dorsal view of the opened vertebral canal. The dura mater has been dissected and is partly reflected.

1, Spinal nerves; 2, dura mater; 3, outer layer of arachnoid; 4, dorsal rootlets of a spinal nerve; 5, spinal cord (covered by pia mater); 6, denticulate ligament.

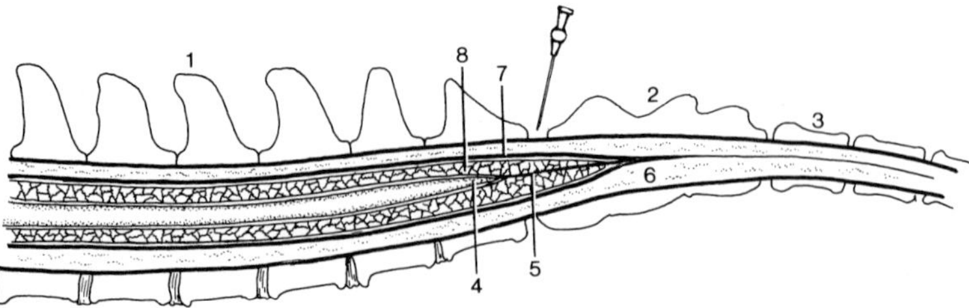


**Figure 8–59.** Schematic median section of the vertebral canal and its contents. The needle points to the lumbosacral interarcuate space.

1, Lumbar vertebra; 2, sacrum; 3, caudal vertebra; 4, conus medullaris; 5, filum terminale; 6, epidural space; 7, dura mater; 8, subarachnoid space with cerebrospinal fluid.

contains the clear, watery cerebrospinal fluid, is much wider than the subdural space but less uniform, particularly in its cranial part (Fig. 8–57).

The widest parts ("cisterns") of the cranial *subarachnoid space* are located between the more salient parts of the ventral surface of the brain and in the angle between the cerebellum and the dorsal aspect of the medulla. The dorsal widening, the *cerebellomedullary cistern,* is especially large and may be reached in the living animal by passing a needle between the atlas and the skull (Fig. 8–57; Plate 13/*F*). Cisternal puncture is employed in both clinical and experimental work for obtaining samples of cerebrospinal fluid. The spinal subarachnoid space is more uniform but widens around the conus medullaris, a fortunate circumstance since access to the vertebral canal is easiest through the lumbosacral interarcuate space (Fig. 8–59).

The pia mater is firmly attached to the outer surface of the brain and cord, and many branches from arteries within the pia penetrate the brain and cord substance. These vessels are initially enclosed by pial sleeves but these soon merge with the vascular walls. A thickening of the pia fills the ventral fissure of the spinal cord, where it appears as a glittering silver line.

All three meninges form cuffs around the roots of origin of the cranial and spinal nerves.

The cerebrospinal fluid within the subarachnoid space forms a water jacket that buoys up and protects the soft brain and cord. It is largely a product of the ependymal lining of the ventricular system within the brain, the overwhelmingly larger part being produced where this covers the choroid plexuses, vascular tufts that invaginate the ventricles (Fig. 8–60/6,9). An additional contribution to the fluid is made by the pial vessels.

The ventricles are local modifications of the lumen of the neural tube; they have complicated shapes, but since these are illustrated (Fig. 8–61) and since the details have little veterinary significance, they need not be described. It is more important to understand their relationship to the choroid plexuses. The plexuses of the lateral and third ventricles, which merge within the interventricular foramen, develop within a duplicature of the pia that becomes entrapped between the expanding telencephalic vesicles and the roof of the diencephalon (Fig. 8–62). The plexuses of the fourth ventricle develop separately within the pia over the caudal medullary velum. In the course of development these plexuses thrust themselves into the lumen of the fourth ventricle; parts later reemerge into the subarachnoid space by herniating through paired lateral openings in the roof (Fig. 8–63).

The clear colorless cerebrospinal fluid is largely formed from the blood plasma by ultrafiltration through the "blood-cerebospinal fluid barrier" (blood-brain barrier) composed of vascular endo-

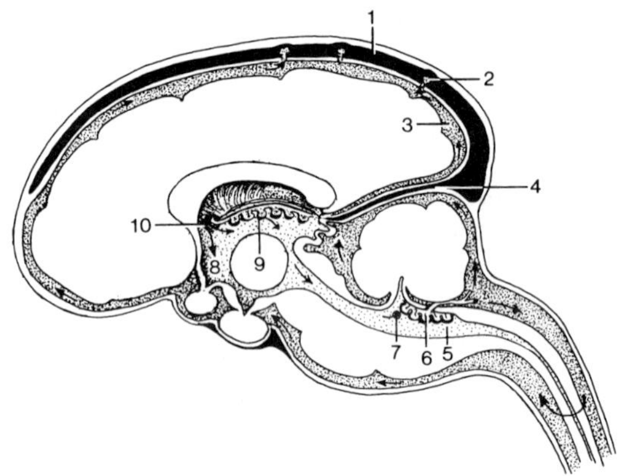


**Figure 8–60.** The production and circulation of cerebrospinal fluid (sagittal section). The blood vessels are in *black,* the subarachnoid spaces are *heavily shaded,* the ventricles are *lightly shaded,* and the nervous tissue is *white.* The direction of the flow of the cerebrospinal fluid is indicated by *arrows.* The cerebrospinal fluid is secreted by the choroid plexus (6, 9) of the lateral, third, and fourth ventricles. It escapes into the subarachnoid space via the aperture of the fourth ventricle (7). The cerebrospinal fluid is transferred to the systemic circulation (1) at the arachnoid villi (2).

1, Dorsal sagittal sinus; 2, arachnoid villus; 3, subarachnoid space; 4, membranous tentorium cerebelli; 5, fourth ventricle; 6, choroid plexus of fourth ventricle; 7, aperture of fourth ventricle; 8, third ventricle; 9, choroid plexus of third ventricle; 10, interventricular foramen, connecting the lateral and third ventricles.

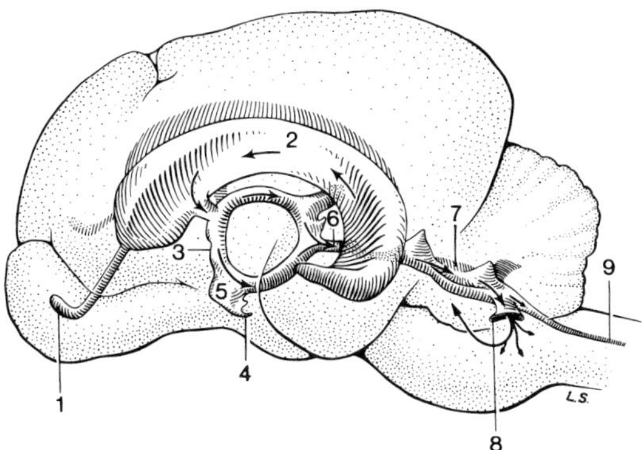


**Figure 8–61.** Lateral view of a cast of the ventricles of the brain of the dog.

1, Cavity of olfactory bulb; 2, lateral ventricle; 3, third ventricle; 4, infundibular recess; 5, optic recess; 6, mesencephalic aqueduct; 7, fourth ventricle; 8, lateral recess; 9, central canal.

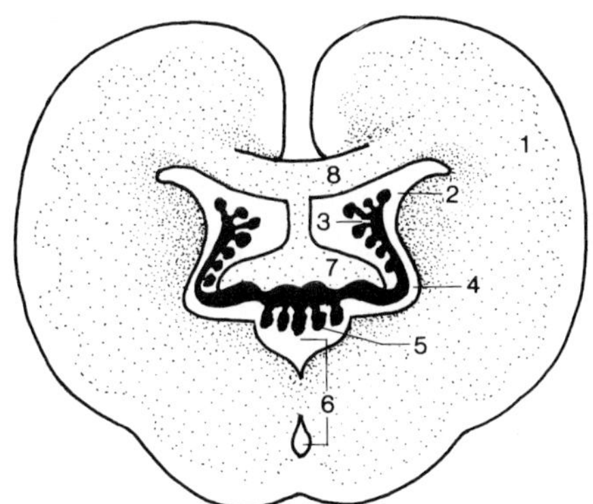


**Figure 8–62.** Schematic section of the brain illustrating the interrelations of the third and lateral ventricles and of their choroid plexuses.

1, Cerebral hemisphere; 2, lateral ventricle; 3, choroid plexus of lateral ventricle; 4, interventricular foramen; 5, choroid plexus of third ventricle; 6, third ventricle; 7, fornix; 8, corpus callosum.

thelial cells. The fluid has a higher concentration of potassium and calcium ions and a lower concentration of sodium, magnesium, and chloride ions than the plasma; it is also rather deficient in glucose and, most importantly, contains little protein since the barrier is impermeable to larger molecules, which of course include those of many antibiotic and other drugs.

In addition to its mechanical role, the cerebrospinal fluid protects the brain through its chemical buffering capacity, which provides a rather stable milieu. It also transports nutrients, flushes away waste products, and serves as a medium for the diffusion of neuroendocrine and neurotransmitter substances.

The fluid is produced continuously, at a rate of some 30 mL per hour in the dog, and first circulates through the ventricular system, moved onward by the filtration pressure and ciliary activity of the ependymal lining. It then escapes from the interior of the brain through the lateral apertures of the fourth ventricle (Fig. 8–60/7; in some species there is a third median opening unrelated to the plexus). The fluid bathes the brain and cord before returning to the blood, mostly through the arachnoid granulations (villi), projections of the arachnoid and subarachnoid space that pierce the dura to enter the dorsal sagittal venous sinus of the brain (Fig. 8–64/10); these formations

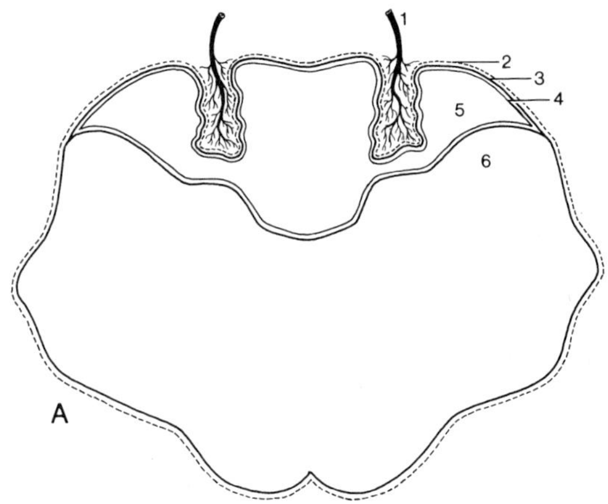


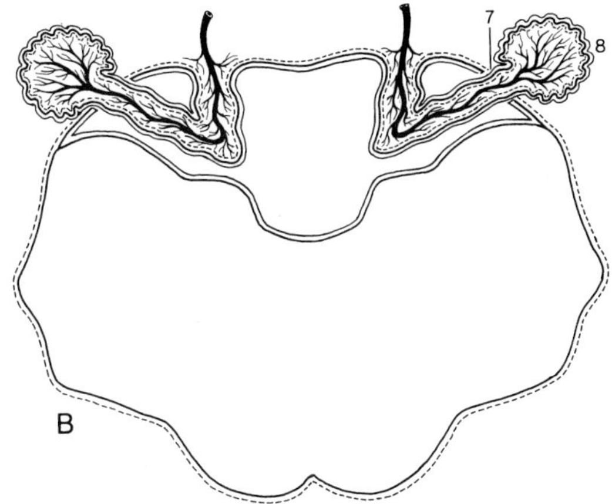


**Figure 8–63.** The formation of the choroid plexus in the roof of the fourth ventricle *(A)* and of its later extension into the subarachnoid space *(B)*.

1, Blood vessel invagination; 2, pia mater; 3, caudal medullary velum; 4, ependyma; 5, fourth ventricle; 6, myelencephalon; 7, aperture of fourth ventricle; 8, choroid plexus extending into subarachnoid space.

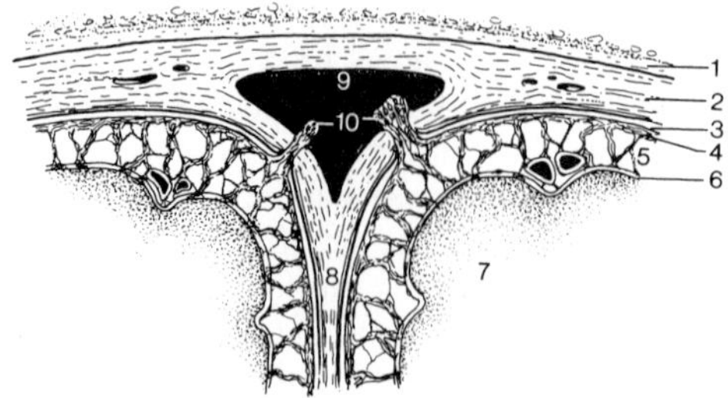


**Figure 8–64.** Transverse section of the dorsal sagittal sinus and adjacent meninges. Cerebrospinal fluid is transferred from the subarachnoid space to the sinus via the arachnoid granulations (villi).

1, Roof of cranial cavity; 2, fused dura mater and periosteum; 3, subdural space; 4, arachnoid; 5, subarachnoid space; 6, pia mater; 7, cerebral hemisphere; 8, falx cerebri; 9, dorsal sagittal sinus; 10, arachnoid granulations (villi).

become increasingly prominent with age. (Obliteration of the villi results in hydrocephalus since drainage of the fluid is hampered while its production continues and is not influenced by a feedback mechanism.) A smaller part of the fluid percolates along the meningeal cuffs that surround the cranial and spinal nerves at their origins and is eventually absorbed by perineural lymphatics; these connections are believed to provide potential routes for the retrograde (i.e., toward the meninges and nervous tissue) spread of infection.

## The Arterial Blood Supply

The blood supply to the brain comes mainly from the *circulus arteriosus cerebri* (formerly known as the circle of Willis), which lies ventral to the hypothalamus where it forms a ring around—but at some distance from—the infundibular stalk. The appearance of the circle and the pattern of its major branches are remarkably constant among mammals, although the sources from which the circle is supplied, and the directions in which blood flows in certain vessels, vary. For this reason, the initial account is based on the arrangements in the dog, an animal in which the arrangement is not only relatively simple but of the most common pattern.

The arterial circle of the dog is supplied from three sources, paired internal carotid arteries laterally and the basilar artery caudally (Fig. 8–65). The *internal carotid artery* (/5) is a terminal branch of the common carotid from which it springs opposite the pharynx. It then runs toward the base of the skull. In many species the artery makes immediate entry to the cranial cavity through a carotid foramen in the cranial floor, but in the dog it must first traverse a tunnel (carotid canal) in the bone medial to the tympanic bulla. The artery is released at the rostral end of the tunnel and describes a loop that first carries it ventrally, then dorsally, before it finally gains the cranial cavity. It then penetrates the outer meninges, which involves passage through the cavernous venous sinus enclosed within a splitting of the drua, before dividing into divergent branches. The rostral branch unites with its fellow to complete the rostral half of the circle, the half from which the large rostral and middle cerebral arteries arise. The caudal branch anastomoses with a branch of the *basilar artery* (which reaches the circle along the midventral surface of the brainstem) to complete the circle (/11). The caudal cerebral and rostral cerebellar arteries leave the caudal half of the circle; the fifth major artery to the brain, the caudal cerebellar, leaves the basilar artery directly.

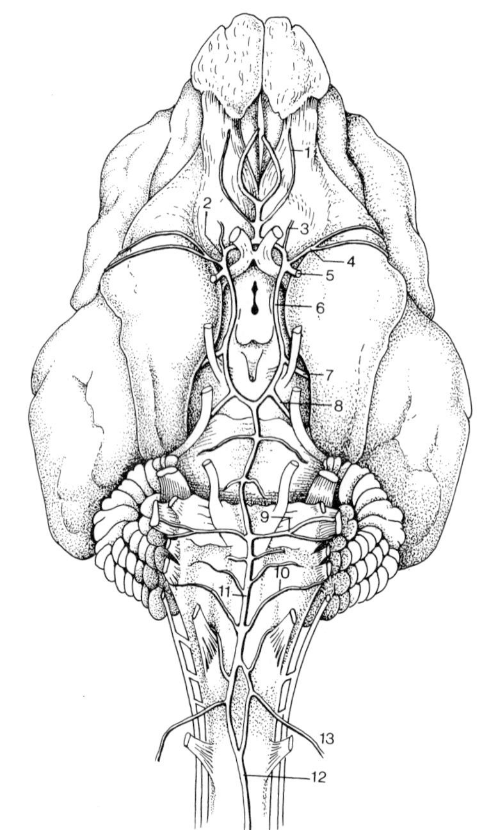


**Figure 8–65.** Arteries on the ventral surface of the canine brain.

1, Internal ethmoidal a.; 2, rostral cerebral a.; 3, internal ophthalmic a., 4, middle cerebral a.; 5, internal carotid a.; 6, caudal communicating a.; 7, caudal cerebral a.; 8, rostral cerebellar a.; 9, labyrinthine a.; 10, caudal cerebellar a; 11, basilar a.; 12, ventral spinal a.; 13, vertebral a.

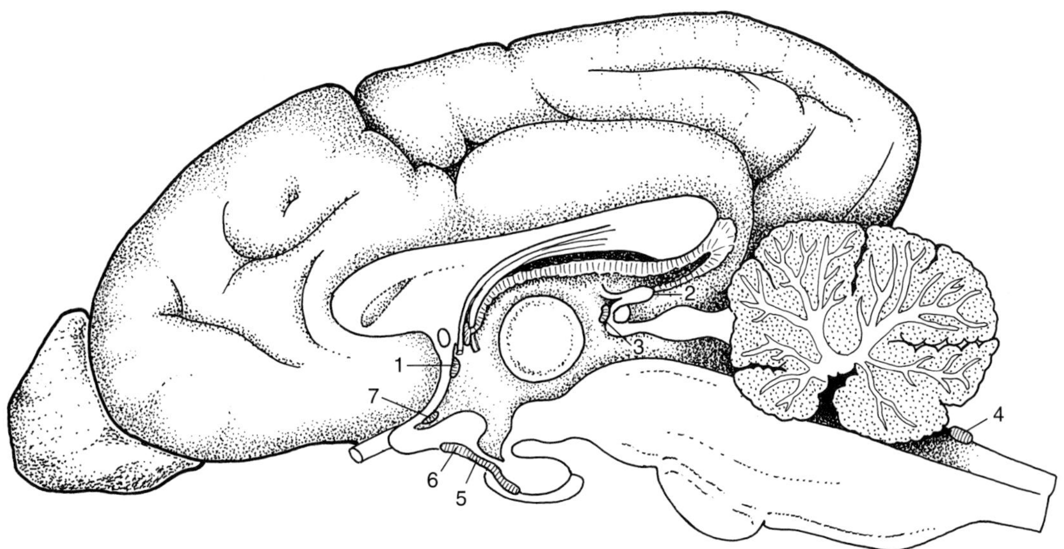


**Figure 8–66.** Schematic median section of the canine brain with an indication of the locations of the circumventricular organs (CVO).

1, Subfornical organ; 2, pineal body; 3, subcommisular organ; 4, area postrema; 5, posterior and intermediate lobes of pituitary; 6, median eminence; 7, vascular organ of lamina terminalis.

The blood within the basilar artery has a composite origin. The artery appears to be the direct continuation of the small ventral spinal artery but is greatly reinforced by anastomosis with the vertebral artery (/13), which passes into the vertebral canal through the atlas. The *vertebral artery* itself receives anastomotic branches (dog and horse) from the occipital artery (another branch of the common carotid) before entering the canal, and it would thus appear that this vessel (occipital artery) also contributes to the supply of the brain. However, the vertebral artery is the main, if not sole, supply to the occipital lobes of the cerebral hemispheres and other caudal parts of the brain.

The arrangement is more complicated in many other species. In these the internal carotid connects with other arteries of the head, especially the maxillary, before discharging into the arterial circle. The anastomosis may be small initially, but in many species it later enlarges and detaches many tortuous branches, which together substitute for the original single channel. This arrangement, which may present a rather tangled appearance, is known as a rete mirabile and has a rather enigmatic significance; the arrangement enhances the efficiency of the blood-cooling mechanism that is discussed shortly. In some species the lumen of the part of the internal carotid artery proximal to the rete becomes obliterated, sometimes only a considerable time after birth; when this happens the emissary artery from the rete delivers blood that is wholly of external carotid origin (see Fig. 7–33). This arrangement is found in both sheep and cattle, although these species differ in other features of the arterial supply to the brain (p. 645).

The brain, particularly its gray substance, has very high metabolic requirements and the arterial supply is commensurate with this, amounting to some 15% or 20% of the cardiac output. Despite this, the vessels that actually penetrate the brain are uniformly small, a feature that may be related to the need to avoid large, pulsating trunks within the delicate brain tissue. Moreover, in sharp contrast to the wide anastomoses between the feeding vessels, any intracerebral anastomoses are narrow and mostly connect functional end-arteries. This fact, coupled with the very limited regeneration capacity of brain tissue, explains why the most serious consequences may attend occlusion or rupture of a small vessel that may be the sole effective supply to some vital nucleus or tract. Notorious examples are provided by the small arteries within the human corpus striatum, where hemorrhage is so often the cause of a "stroke."

The permeability of the blood capillaries of the nervous tissue is reduced, resulting in the "blood-brain barrier." The main structural components of this barrier are provided by the continuity between the endothelial cells of these capillaries and pericytes, astrocytes, and the basement membrane surrounding these capillaries (see p. 213; Fig. 8–66).

The spinal cord is supplied by three arteries that run its length. The largest, the *ventral spinal artery,* follows the surface of the ventral fissure of the cord; paired *dorsolateral spinal arteries* run close to the furrow from which the dorsal roots of the spinal nerves arise. All three are periodically reinforced by branches from regional arteries—vertebral in the neck and intercostal, lumbar, and sacral in the trunk. These enter at the intervertebral foramina, often in the form of narrow vessels that accompany the roots of the spinal nerves; they form plexuses on the surface of the cord with which the major longitudinal arteries connect. This theoretically regular pattern is subject to much variation, both specific and individual, in which many expected reinforcing arteries are lacking, the plexus is unevenly developed, and stretches of the longitudinal trunks are attenuated.

Branches of the ventral spinal artery supply the "core" of the cord, the gray substance, and the adjacent layer of white substance by an approach through the ventral fissure (see Fig. 19–6). The greater part of the white substance is supplied by radial twigs from the dorsolateral arteries and surface plexus. Internal anastomoses between the two sets of vessels, although common, are of questionable efficiency.

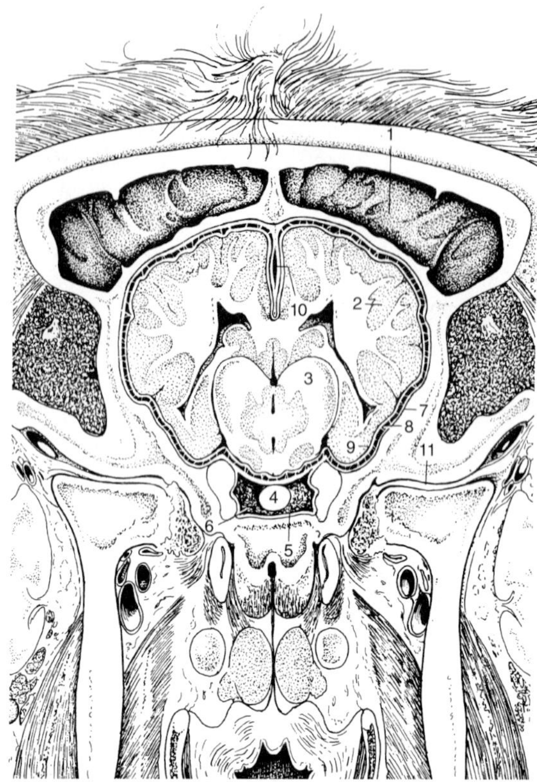


**Figure 8–67.** Position of the brain in relation to the roof of the bovine skull. Some features of the meninges are also shown.

1, Frontal sinus; 2, cerebral cortex; 3, diencephalon; 4, hypophysis; 5, sella turcica; 6, cavernous sinus; 7, dura mater; 8, arachnoid; 9, pia mater; 10, falx cerebri with dorsal sagittal sinus; 11, temporomandibular joint.

## The Venous Drainage

A complicated system of venous sinuses within the cranial cavity and vertebral canal is connected at intervals to the exposed regional veins. The cranial sinuses enclosed within the dura mater are divided into dorsal and ventral systems between which there is only limited communication (Fig. 8–67). The dorsal system collects blood from the dorsal parts of the brain and the diplöe of the bones of the cranial vault. It includes a *dorsal sagittal sinus* within the falx cerebri. The dorsal sagittal sinus receives numerous tributary veins directly from the cerebral hemispheres, and it is joined toward its caudal end by the *straight sinus,* which runs within the ventral part of the falx and collects blood from a major vein draining deeper parts of the brain. The dorsal sinus splits (in a variable manner) into bilateral *transverse sinuses* within the tentorium cerebelli; each later divides—one branch leaving the skull through a foramen, the other connecting with the ventral system.

The ventral or *basilar system* drains the ventral part of the brain (and other cranial contents and walls) and also receives a major inflow from a vein that enters the cranial cavity from the orbit after draining much of the face, including the nasal cavity. The rostral part of the longitudinal trunk of the ventral system, the *cavernous sinus* (/6), is connected with its fellow both before and behind the hypophysis. It divides caudally into the *basilar sinus,* which continues through the foramen magnum as the main component of the internal vertebral plexus, and a branch that receives a connection from the dorsal system before emerging through a ventral foramen to contribute to the maxillary vein.

The flow of blood into the cranial cavity from the face is noteworthy for two reasons. First, it provides a potential pathway for the spread of infection from the face to the cranial contents. Secondly, it provides for cooling the arterial supply to the hypothalamus, the part of the brain responsive to, and concerned with the regulation of, body temperature. The cooling is due to the passage of the internal carotid artery (or rete substitute) through the cavernous sinus, where bathing by venous blood at a somewhat lower temperature (since drained from the nose and superficial structures of the head) promotes heat exchange. (An additional mechanism for protecting the brain from damaging hyperthermia is provided by the course of the common carotid artery, which is extensively related to the trachea at no great depth below the skin. These relationships promote heat loss, especially because any physical exertion that tends to raise body temperature also increases the flow of air within the upper respiratory tract.)

The *vertebral venous plexus* is probably more important clinically. It runs the whole length of the vertebral column and drains blood from the vertebrae, the adjacent musculature, and the structures within the vertebral canal. It gives rise to segmental veins that leave the canal through the intervertebral foramina to join the principal venous channels of the neck and trunk—the vertebral, cranial caval, azygous, and caudal caval veins (see Fig. 7–43/18). The major part of the plexus consists of paired channels within the epidural space ventral to the cord. They are composed of crescentic segments that extend between successive intervertebral foramina (see Fig. 26–5/1). The enlarged midpart of each segment swings toward and is generally joined to its neighbor over the middle of the vertebra, producing a ladder-like pattern of vessels. The connections with segmental veins through the intervertebral foramina form a plexus around the emerging spinal nerves, protecting them from injury.

The veins composing the plexus are thin walled and, being without valves, may pass blood in either direction. They are capacious and adjust in size to compensate for variations in venous return to the heart induced by the intrathoracic pressure changes that accompany respiration. Since the system provides alternative channels to the major systemic veins it may mitigate the effects of jugular obstruction (when the neck is compressed) or of caudal caval obstruction (when pressure within the abdomen is raised). The intermittency of flow caused by these several factors facilitates the spread of septic or neoplastic disease to the vertebral column when the lungs would be the expected destination; blood diverted into the vertebral plexus when the flow through other channels is impeded may be temporarily held stagnant, allowing tumor seeds or microorganisms to settle within the tributaries that issue from the bones.

A further point of clinical importance lies in the risk of hemorrhage when epidural or subarachnoid puncture is performed. The risk is greatest at the atlanto-occipital space, where tributaries of the plexus most often encircle the dural tube.

There are no lymphatics in the central nervous tissue.

# THE CRANIAL NERVES

The names and sequence of the cranial nerves should now be familiar. Though these nerves lack the relative uniformity of make-up and distribution pattern that is found with the spinal nerves, it is possible to arrange them in three groupings: those exclusively concerned with special senses (the olfactory, optic, and vestibulocochlear nerves); those that supply head muscles of somitic origin (the oculomotor, trochlear, abducent, and hypoglossal nerves); and those primarily concerned with structures of pharyngeal arch origin (the trigeminal, facial, glossopharyngeal, vagus, and accessory nerves). However, it is probably more convenient to deal with them in numerical, that is in rostrocaudal, sequence.

## The Olfactory Nerve (I)

The fibers that compose the olfactory nerve arise as the central processes of the olfactory cells of the nasal mucosa. They are collected into a number of filaments that separately traverse the cribriform plate to join the adjacent surface of the olfactory bulb (Fig. 8–18/1). The further course of the olfactory pathways has been described (p. 282).

The short course and deep location protect these nerves against casual injury, and though they may be involved in infectious or neoplastic disease, interference with the sense of smell is more often due to blockage of the air passages leading to the olfactory mucosa. The filaments are surrounded by meningeal sheaths enclosing extensions of the subarachnoid space, which provide potential routes for the spread of infection from the nose to the cranial cavity.

## The Optic Nerve (II)

The optic nerve mediates the visual sense and is more accurately regarded as a brain tract connecting the retina with the diencephalon (from which it originated). The intracranial part of the nerve extends from the optic chiasm (/7), where varying proportions of the fibers decussate (p. 290), to the optic foramen at the apex of the orbital cone; the intraorbital course is described elsewhere (p. 336) (see Fig. 9–11/9). The optic nerve is also enclosed within extensions of the meninges, the dura blending with the sclera where the nerve joins the eyeball. Section of the nerve obviously results in blindness of that eye.

## The Oculomotor Nerve (III)

The oculomotor nerve consists of somatic efferent fibers from the principal (motor) nucleus and visceral efferent fibers from the parasympathetic nucleus (of Edinger-Westphal), both within the tegmentum of the midbrain (Fig. 8–25). Fibers of the two categories emerge together at the superficial origin from the ventral aspect of the midbrain, close to the midline and in series with other cranial nerves of predominantly somatic efferent composition, and with the ventral roots of spinal nerves (Fig. 8–18). In its intracranial course the oculomotor is related to the trochlear, abducent and ophthalmic nerves, and to the cavernous sinus, and it passes through the orbital fissure in their company. It divides within the orbit to supply the dorsal, medial, and ventral recti, the ventral oblique, and the levator muscle of the upper eyelid (some authors also include part of the retractor bulbi). The preganglionic parasympathetic fibers synapse within the small ciliary ganglion placed upon one of the branches (Fig. 8–45/9 and 8–70/1,6). From here, postganglionic fibers pass within the short ciliary nerves to supply the intraocular ciliary and constrictor pupillae muscles. Isolated injury or involvement in disease is not common; the effects can be deduced from consideration of the actions of the muscles it supplies (p. 336).

## The Trochlear Nerve (IV)

The trochlear nerve, which is small, is motor to the dorsal oblique muscle. The nucleus of origin within the tegmentum of the midbrain gives rise to a fiber bundle that decussates internally before emerging from the rostral medullary velum (Fig. 8–23/8). The nerve then follows the edge of the tentorium cerebelli to the floor of the cranial cavity. In some species it makes a separate entrance to the orbit but usually it passes through the orbital fissure. The effects of section are those of paralysis of the dorsal oblique (p. 330).

## The Trigeminal Nerve (V)

The trigeminal nerve, the largest of the cranial nerves, is sensory to the skin and deeper tissues of the face and motor to the muscles of first pharyngeal (mandibular) arch origin. The proprioceptive fibers (which include many from muscles that receive their motor innervation from other cranial nerves) pass to the rostral sensory mesencephalic nucleus; the other afferent fibers pass to the pontine and spinal nuclei; the efferent fibers originate in the motor nucleus (Fig. 8–25/7,17). The peripheral nerve is formed by the fusion of sensory and motor roots that attach to the ventrolateral aspect of the pons. The larger sensory root carries the massive trigeminal ganglion and, just beyond this, divides into the trio of primary branches that give the trunk its name. The mandibular branch unites with the motor root to constitute the mixed mandibular nerve; the ophthalmic and maxillary divisions remain purely sensory at this level, although peripheral connections with other cranial nerves introduce somatic and visceral efferent fibers into certain branches. The mandibular nerve emerges through the oval foramen in the floor of the cranial cavity. The ophthalmic and maxillary nerves run rostrally to emerge through the orbital fissure and round foramen, respectively (in ruminants the two openings are combined).

The three primary divisions are initially each restricted to a different process of the embryonic face, which explains the crisply defined adult territories (cf. the dermatomes of the trunk). The ophthalmic nerve supplies the frontonasal process, the primordium of the forehead and nose regions; the maxillary nerve supplies the maxillary process, the primordium of the upper jaw and associated parts; the mandibular nerve supplies the mandibular process, the primordium of the lower jaw and associated parts, which include the masticatory and other first pharyngeal arch muscles (Fig. 8–68).

The **ophthalmic nerve** (/1), for which the convenient notation is **V-1,** divides into three divergent branches soon after entering the orbit. The *lacrimal nerve* (/3) passes to the lateral part of the orbital perimeter and, after detaching branches to the lacrimal gland and other deeper structures, emerges to supply the skin about the lateral angle of the eye. The more considerable territory of the *frontal nerve* (/2) includes much of the upper eyelid, the forehead, and, through branches that penetrate the bone, the mucosa of the frontal sinus.

The *nasociliary nerve* (/4) runs toward the medial wall of the orbit. One branch, the *infratrochlear nerve* (/4′), emerges on the face after supplying structures at the medial angle; it supplies another portion of the mucosa of the frontal sinus and in small ruminants detaches the principal nerve to the horn. Other branches of the nasociliary nerve include long ciliary and ethmoidal nerves. The *long ciliary nerves* (/4″) penetrate the posterior aspect of the eyeball to supply sensitive tissues, including the cornea; the *ethmoidal nerve* first re-enters the cranial cavity through the ethmoidal foramen and subsequently passes to the

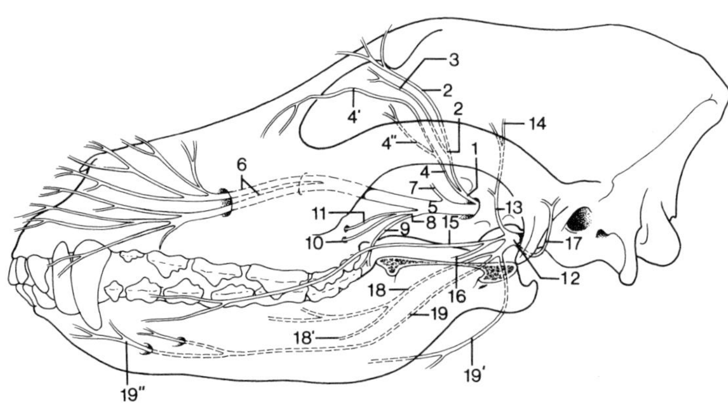


**Figure 8–68.** Distribution pattern of the trigeminal nerve of the dog.

1, Ophthalmic n.; 2, frontal n.; 3, lacrimal n.; 4, nasociliary n.; 4′, infratrochlear n.; 4″, long ciliary n.; 5, maxillary n; 6, infraorbital n.; 7, zygomatic n.; 8, pterygopalatine n.; 9, lesser palatine n.; 10, greater palatine n.; 11, caudal nasal n.; 12, mandibular n.; 13, masticatory n.; 14, deep temporal n.; 15, buccal n.; 16, pterygoid n.; 17, auriculotemporal n.; 18, lingual n.; 18′, sublingual n.; 19, inferior alveolar n.; 19′, mylohyoid n.; 19″, mental n.

nasal cavity via the cribriform plate before dividing into medial and lateral branches to the mucosa.

The **maxillary nerve (V-2)** runs across the wall of the pterygopalatine fossa ventral to the orbit (/5). It bears, or lies close to, the pterygopalatine ganglion but the relationship is purely topographical. It then enters the infraorbital canal at the maxillary foramen, where it becomes known as the infraorbital nerve in anticipation of its reappearance on the face at the infraorbital foramen (/6).

Collateral branches detached within the pterygopalatine fossa include the *zygomatic nerve* (/7) which supplies the lower eyelid and adjacent skin and is the origin of the principal nerve of the horn in cattle.

The second branch, the *pterygopalatine nerve* (/8), detaches; the *lesser palatine nerve* (/9) to the soft palate; the *greater palatine nerve* (/10), which reaches the hard palate after traversing the palatine canal and supplies both the palatine mucosa and the floor of the nasal vestibule; and the *caudal nasal nerve* (/11), which passes through the pterygopalatine foramen to supply mucosa of the ventral part of the nasal cavity, maxillary sinus, and palate.

Within the infraorbital canal the *infraorbital nerve* (/6) detaches short twigs to the alveoli of the cheek teeth and nasal mucosa, and longer rostral alveolar branches that continue within the bone, beyond the infraorbital foramen, to the alveoli of the canine and incisor teeth. After emerging at the infraorbital foramen the infraorbital nerve supplies various labial and nasal branches to the structures of the muzzle, including some branches that run back over the nose to the edge of the infratrochlear territory. Although covered by muscle at its emergence, the infraorbital nerve may usually be palpated, stimulated by pressure, or blocked by injection of local anesthetic solution.

On leaving the cranium, the **mandibular nerve (V-3)** detaches in close succession several nerves that pass to the masseter, temporalis, medial and lateral pterygoid, tensor veli palatini, and tensor tympani muscles (/12). There are minor variations in their pattern, and those to the masseter and temporalis are often initially conjoined in a short masticatory nerve (/13). The *masseteric nerve* passes to that muscle between the coronoid and condylar processes of the mandible. The *deep temporal nerves* (/14) run dorsomedially to the temporalis. The otic ganglion lies close to the origin of the *pterygoid nerves* (/16).

The next branch, the *buccal nerve* (/15), is sensory to the tissues of the cheek, which it reaches after first passing between the pterygoideus and temporalis, and then between the maxillary tuber and mandible. Its origin is followed by that of the *auriculotemporal nerve* (/17), which bends around the caudal border of the mandible to enter the face a little ventral to the temporomandibular joint. It is sensory to the skin of the temporal region and over much of the external ear, including the lining of the canal leading to the eardrum. The continuation onto the face, the *transverse facial branch,* supplies a strip of skin extending to the corner of the mouth.

The mandibular nerve continues between the medial and lateral pterygoid muscles before dividing into its end-branches, the lingual and inferior alveolar nerves.

The *lingual nerve* (/18) detaches twigs to the oropharyngeal mucosa before dividing into a deep branch that enters the tongue and a superficial branch, the *sublingual nerve* (/18′), that runs medial to the mylohyoideus below the mucosa of the oral floor that it supplies. The branch to the tongue is joined by the *chorda tympani,* a branch of the facial, which introduces visceral efferent fibers to salivary glands that synapse in the adjacent mandibular ganglion, and gustatory fibers (special visceral afferent) from the taste buds of the rostral two thirds of the tongue. Other sensory fibers supply general sensation in the same area of the lingual mucosa.

The *inferior alveolar nerve* (/19) detaches the *mylohyoid nerve* (/19′) for the mylohyoideus and rostral belly of the digastricus before entering the mandibular canal at the mandibular foramen. The inferior alveolar nerve supplies the lower cheek teeth before a large part reappears at the mental foramen as the *mental nerve* (/19″), which supplies tissues of the lower lip and chin. In some species several mental branches exit through as many foramina. Though also covered by muscle, the mental nerve(s) can be palpated, compressed, and blocked at emergence.

Injuries to, or disease of, the branches of the trigeminal nerve produce sensory deficiencies in their territories and sometimes manifest themselves by chronic facial irritation; some branches are frequently blocked for minor surgery of the head. Destructive lesions of the mandibular nerve produce paralysis of the muscles that raise the jaw; when the lesion is unilateral the resulting atrophy may be more obvious than any motor disability. A temporary idiopathic bilateral paralysis of the trigeminal musculature, characterized by a dropped jaw, has been reported in dogs.

## The Abducent Nerve (VI)

The fibers of the abducent nerve originate within the caudal brainstem and make the expected appearance (for general somatic efferent fibers) close to the midline (Fig. 8–18). The intracranial course leads to the orbital fissure (or the foramen orbitorotundum); within the orbit the nerve branches to go to the lateral rectus and the retractor, although the exact innervation of the latter muscle is still controversial. Injury produces inability to deviate the eyeball laterally (p. 330).

## The Facial Nerve (VII)

The facial nerve is sometimes known as the intermediofacial nerve, a term that indicates its composite nature. The intermediate component is a visceral nerve with sensory, including gustatory, and motor (parasympathetic) functions; the facial component is the nerve of the second pharyngeal arch whose main distribution is to the mimetic musculature.

The facial and vestibulocochlear nerves arise close together at the lateral extremity of the trapezoid body (Fig. 8–21/VII,VIII) and run within common meningeal investments to the internal acoustic meatus of the petrous temporal bone. They part here and the facial nerve enters a passage (facial canal) within the bone that leads, via a sharp caudal convexity ("genu"), to the stylomastoid foramen, where the nerve appears at the surface of the skull. The facial nerve carries the appropriately named *geniculate ganglion* at the summit of the bend. With the exception of the small branch to the stapedius muscle, the branches detached within the bone represent the intermediate component, those detached after leaving the bone represent the facial component (Fig. 8–69/1).

The *greater petrosal nerve* is detached at the level of the ganglion and emerges through an independent foramen. It is initially parasympathetic but is shortly joined by sympathetic fibers to form a composite autonomic nerve; this, the nerve of the pterygoid canal, runs through that fine passage to reach the pterygopalatine ganglion within the pterygopalatine fossa (Fig. 8–70/12,7). The nerve of the pterygoid canal is discussed more fully later (p. 319). The *stapedial nerve,* which arises next, is motor to the stapedius muscle of the middle ear (p. 339). The next branch, the *chorda tympani* (/14), crosses the tympanic cavity to emerge at the petrotympanic fissure, after which

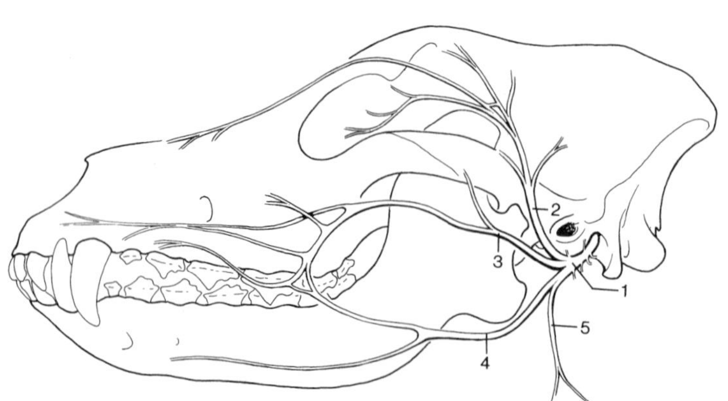


**Figure 8–69.** Distribution pattern of the facial nerve of the dog.

1, Facial n.; 2, auriculopalpebral n.; 3, dorsal buccal branch; 4, ventral buccal branch; 5, cervical branch.

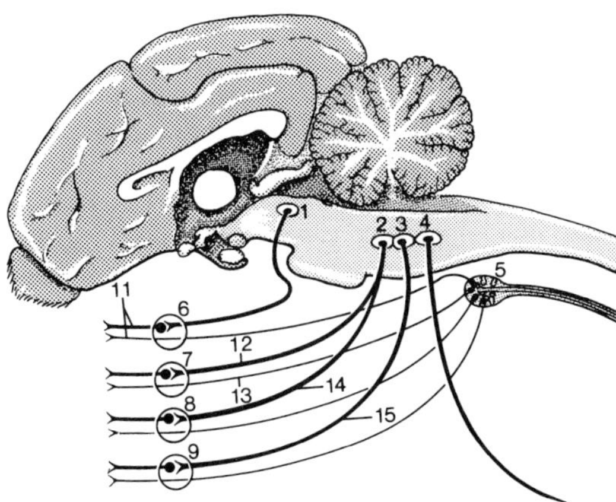


**Figure 8–70.** Schematic representation of the autonomic innervation of structures of the head.

1, Parasympathetic oculomotor nucleus (III); 2, parasympathetic facial nucleus (VII); 3, parasympathetic glossopharyngeal nucleus; 4, parasympathetic vagus nucleus; 5, cranial cervical ganglion; 6, ciliary ganglion; 7, pterygopalatine ganglion; 8, mandibular ganglion; 9, otic ganglion; 11, short ciliary nerves; 12, greater petrosal nerve; 13, deep petrosal nerve; 14, chorda tympani; 15, tympanic plexus, short petrosal nerve.

it converges upon, and becomes incorporated within, the lingual branch of the mandibular nerve (p. 342).

The first branches of the free portion of the facial nerve are the *internal* and *caudal auricular nerves,* which supply muscles of the external ear and other branches to some hyoid muscles, including the caudal belly of the digastricus. The main trunk enters the face by turning around the mandible, where it is first contained between the masseter and the parotid gland. It divides at about this level—there are species differences—into three terminal branches.

In some species the *auriculopalpebral nerve* (Fig. 8–69/2) is detached before the main trunk reaches the face, and it is then less vulnerable to injury from superficial trauma to the side of the head. It crosses the zygomatic arch, heading for the space between the upper eyelid and external ear, before dividing into branches that supply the muscles of the eyelids (excluding levator palpebrae superioris) and the auricular muscles in front of the external ear.

The *dorsal buccal branch* (/3), which may take the form of a leash of divergent branches, crosses the masseter en route to the muzzle.

In some species the *ventral buccal branch* (/4) may take a similar path at a slightly more ventral level, but in others it takes a divergent course, first running within the intermandibular space before entering the face with the parotid duct and facial vessels, where they cross the mandible in front of the masseter. Together, the buccal branches supply the muscles of the cheek, lips, and nostrils. Their peripheral branches join with those of the trigeminal nerve at various levels, and many of the smaller trunks combine motor (facial) and sensory (trigeminal) fibers.

The effects of injury or disease clearly depend on the site of the lesion. Lesions that are situated more centrally, which tend to have more sinister origins, affect the whole facial field and lead to loss of secretory activity by the lacrimal and salivary (except the parotid) glands in addition to muscular paralysis. Lesions involving the main trunk near its exit from the bone paralyze the entire mimetic musculature, while more peripheral lesions may spare some groups, depending on their site, and specific and individual variations in the branching pattern. Those confined to the auriculopalpebral nerve produce drooping of the external ear and narrowing of the palpebral fissure with inability to close the eye. Damage to the buccal branches may paralyze the muscles of the lips and cheeks, allowing a quid of food to collect in the oral vestibule. It may also lead to deformation of the muzzle, which is drawn out of symmetry by the unopposed activity of the muscles on the sound side. The alteration in appearance is not always very striking, and the uninjured side, to which the muzzle is drawn, may sometimes appear to have the more distorted aspect. The distortion tends to be more pronounced in the horse and sheep than in other domestic species. (It is important to be aware that in unilateral facial spasm, seen occasionally in the dog, the nose may be drawn toward the affected side.)

The auriculopalpebral nerve is sometimes blocked to facilitate examination of the eye.

## The Vestibulocochlear Nerve (VIII)

The vestibulocochlear nerve divides at the internal acoustic meatus into its vestibular and cochlear parts, which make their separate ways through the petrous temporal bone to the vestibular and cochlear components of the membranous labyrinth of the inner ear. They are discussed further with the special sense organs of balance and hearing (p. 342).

## The Glossopharyngeal Nerve (IX)

The glossopharyngeal nerve combines fibers concerned with the innervation of structures of third pharyngeal arch origin with important visceral efferent (parasympathetic) and afferent components. It is motor to part of the palatopharyngeal musculature and to certain salivary glands, and sensory to mucosa of the root of the tongue, palate, and pharynx. In addition, there is an important branch to the carotid sinus and body.

The glossopharyngeal nerve arises from the ventrolateral aspect of the medulla oblongata, from the most rostral rootlets of the linear series that also gives origin to the vagus and the medullary part of the accessory nerve (Figs. 8–18 and 8-21). It runs with these nerves to the jugular foramen and at about this level bears two small and rather indistinct ganglia. The first branch, the *tympanic nerve,* enters the tympanic cavity, where it participates with branches of the facial and internal carotid (sympathetic) nerves in forming a plexus from which a nerve leads to the otic ganglion for the supply of the parotid gland (Fig. 8–70/3,15).

The main trunk cleaves for a spell to the vagus and accessory nerves, and at this level detaches the *carotid sinus branch,* which proceeds to the carotid sinus, where it terminates in baroreceptors within the sinus wall and chemoreceptors of the carotid body. The glossopharyngeal nerve then turns rostroventrally, parallel to the stylohyoid, before dividing into pharyngeal and lingual branches. The *pharyngeal branches* include one to the stylopharyngeus caudalis; the others become diffused within the pharyngeal plexus to which the vagus also contributes. Although most fibers are sensory to the mucosa, the possibility of a further contribution to the pharyngeal musculature seems likely.

The larger *lingual branch* enters the tongue parallel to the lingual artery, the lingual branch of the mandibular nerve and the hypoglossal nerve. It is sensory to the mucosa of the root of the tongue (including the taste buds in this area) and motor to the levator palatini muscle and the glands of the soft palate. Damage to the nerve—most common in horses as the result of inflammation of the guttural pouch—may lead to difficulties in swallowing. Since the vagus may also be affected it is difficult to know the extent to which the paresis of palate and pharynx is due to glossopharyngeal involvement. Experimental studies suggest that the role of the glossopharyngeal nerve is more important than most authors have claimed.

## The Vagus Nerve (X)

The vagus nerve is the nerve of the fourth and subsequent pharyngeal arches. It also contains the parasympathetic fibers that innervate the cervical, thoracic, and abdominal viscera. The second component gives it by far the most widespread distribution of any cranial nerve (Fig. 8–74/5).

The vagus forms part of the bundle of nerves that passes through the jugular foramen. It bears two small ganglia on the stretch that lies within and immediately external to the foramen, and beyond this runs in close association with the glossopharyngeal and accessory nerves. After the glossopharyngeal nerve turns rostrally, the vagus continues with the accessory and later acquires a relationship with the cranial cervical ganglion. It then continues down the neck in close contact with the sympathetic trunk, with which it is bound within a common fascial sheath, on the dorsal margin of the common carotid artery and related to the trachea. The left vagosympathetic trunk has an additional contact with the esophagus (Fig. 8–76/5). The vagus and sympathetic nerves part at the entrance to the chest, after which the vagus continues more or less horizontally through the mediastinum until it divides over the pericardium into dorsal and ventral branches. These combine with the corresponding contralateral branches to form the dorsal and ventral vagal trunks that enter the abdomen along the corresponding borders of the esophagus. Within the abdomen the two nerves branch freely, participating with the sympathetic fibers in forming the plexuses from which the abdominal viscera are supplied (p. 319).

The first significant detachment after the nerve leaves the skull is an *auricular branch* that takes part in the innervation of the skin of the external ear. This is followed by *pharyngeal branches* that combine with those of the glossopharyngeal, cranial laryngeal, and sympathetic nerves in forming the pharyngeal plexus. An extension of the plexus supplies the cervical esophagus. The *cranial laryngeal nerve* goes to the larynx, where it divides into an external branch for the cricothyroid muscle and an internal branch for the laryngeal mucosa from the aditus to the glottis. This branch makes connections with the recurrent laryngeal nerve. The *depressor nerve* to the heart is partly formed of fibers from the cranial laryngeal nerve, partly of fibers from the main vagal nerve; it is difficult to follow since in most animals it rejoins the main trunk for its further progress through the neck and thorax to the heart.

The thoracic portion of the vagus detaches *cardiac branches* that form a mediastinal plexus with sympathetic fibers with the same destination. A large *caudal (recurrent) laryngeal nerve* is also detached within the thorax. That of the right side changes direction by winding around a branch of the subclavian artery, while the left one winds around the aorta. The recurrent laryngeal nerve reascends the neck ventral to the common carotid artery in a course that leads it back to the larynx, where it supplies the bulk of the intrinsic laryngeal musculature (all but the cricothyroideus) and the mucosa caudal to the glottis. Small twigs detached en route pass to the cardiac plexus and to the trachea and esophagus. The distribution of the main trunk is completed by pulmonary branches that combine in a common plexus with sympathetic nerves.

Damage to the vagus nerve and its branches may be manifested in a variety of ways, including difficulties in swallowing and altered functioning of the heart and the other viscera. Degeneration of the recurrent laryngeal nerve is especially common in horses, producing the condition known as roaring (p. 502); it also occurs in dogs.

### The Accessory Nerve (XI)

The accessory nerve is curiously formed of two roots. The spinal root is provided by filaments that emerge midway between the dorsal and ventral roots of the first five (or so) spinal nerves (Figs. 8–18 and 8-21). These combine in a trunk that runs within the spinal subarachnoid space to enter the skull through the foramen magnum; it then approaches the cranial root, which is formed by the most caudal rootlets of the glossopharyngeal-vagus series. There is only brief contact between the two roots, and although some fibers may be exchanged, the cranial root then amalgamates with the vagus to which it probably furnishes the fibers that reach the laryngeal musculature via the recurrent laryngeal nerve. It is the spinal root that forms the accessory nerve of descriptive anatomy. This passes through the jugular foramen to divide within the atlantal fossa into dorsal and ventral branches.

The *dorsal branch* runs caudally over the splenius and serratus ventralis before it supplies the covering brachiocephalicus, omotransversarius, and trapezius. The *ventral branch* supplies only one muscle, the sternocephalicus, which it enters close to its cranial attachment.

There is no convincing explanation of the curious detour made by the spinal fibers of this nerve.

### The Hypoglossal Nerve (XII)

The hypoglossal nerve is motor to the intrinsic and extrinsic muscles of the tongue, which originate in the myotomes of occipital somites. After leaving the ventral aspect of the medulla oblongata (Fig. 8–18), the nerve passes through the hypoglossal canal before crossing the nerves of the vagus group to continue toward the tongue, which it enters ventral to the glossopharyngeal nerve. It ramifies within the tongue substance to reach the various muscles.

A destructive lesion of this nerve paralyzes the ipsilateral muscles, allowing a deviation of the tongue toward the normal side. A marked atrophy eventually develops.

## THE SPINAL NERVES

A general account of the formation and distribution of the spinal nerves has been given (see p. 30). That account described the formation of each nerve by the union of dorsal and ventral roots and its later division into dorsal and ventral primary rami, which diverge on passing through the intervertebral foramen (see Fig. 1–36). The rather consistent pattern of distribution of the dorsal rami may be represented by a single description; important regional features of the ventral rami require separate attention.

### The Dorsal Rami

As a rule, the dorsal rami are considerably smaller than the ventral and have simpler distributions. Each divides into a medial branch that supplies the local part of the epaxial musculature of the neck, trunk, or tail and a lateral branch that is distributed to the dorsal part of the skin segment (dermatome) served by the particular spinal nerve (see Fig. 1–37). These areas extend from the dorsal midline for a variable distance over the side of the animal. The territories of the first few cervical nerves extend onto the poll region of the head in addition to supplying skin over the neck; those of the nerves to each side of the cervicothoracic junction supply skin over the upper part of the shoulder; those of the middle and caudal thoracic and lumbar regions serve increasingly larger areas of the skin of the chest wall and flank; but those of the sacral nerves are again restricted. Inconspicuous connections between neighboring nerves form a continuous plexus through which exchange of fibers blurs the boundaries between the areas supplied by individual nerves; indeed, it is probable that every part of the skin receives sensory fibers from two, if not three, spinal nerves (Fig. 8–71).

### The Ventral Rami

The larger ventral rami supply the hypaxial muscles, including those of the limbs (excepting the thoracic girdle muscles supplied by the eleventh cranial nerve, and the rhomboideus supplied in some species by dorsal rami) and the remaining skin of the neck, trunk, and limbs. Except in the thoracic region, where a more precise segmental

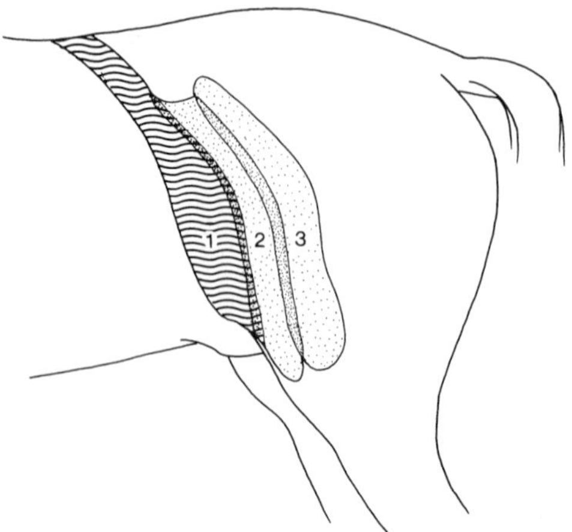


**Figure 8–71.** Cutaneous innervation of the flank. Note the overlap of the three zones.

1, Innervation by T18; 2, innervation by ventral branch of L1 (iliohypogastric nerve); 3, innervation by ventral branch of L2 (ilioinguinal nerve).

distribution is retained, the ventral rami are also joined with their neighbors by connecting branches. These connections are greatly exaggerated at the levels of origin of the nerves to the fore- and hindlimb, where they constitute the brachial and lumbosacral plexuses, respectively (Fig. 1–38).

## The Cervical Ventral Rami

The cutaneous distribution of the first two cervical ventral rami extends to the external ear and the masseteric and throat regions. The more caudal members of the series contribute to the phrenic nerve and brachial plexus while retaining local responsibilities.

In domestic species the *phrenic nerve* is generally formed by the fifth, sixth, and seventh cervical nerves. The contributions run ventrally over the scalenus muscle to join in a trunk (see Fig. 1–38) that winds below the muscle to enter the mediastinum between the two first ribs. The phrenic nerve runs caudally within the mediastinum, crossing the lateral face of the pericardium, to reach the diaphragm; the right nerve utilizes the plica venae cavae in the last part of its course (see Fig. 13–10/7). The phrenic nerves ramify within the diaphragm to which they are the sole motor innervation; their sensory fibers are supplemented by others channeled through intercostal nerves. It is worth emphasizing that the phrenic nerves are typical muscle nerves; it must not be inferred from the normally involuntary nature of breathing that they are autonomic. Experiments (in several species) have shown that bilateral section of the phrenic nerves has little effect, although respiratory embarrassment may become evident when the animal is severely stressed.

## The Brachial Plexus

The brachial plexus supplies almost all structures of the forelimb, the exceptions being the trapezius, omotransversarius, brachiocephalicus, and rhomboideus, and the skin over the upper shoulder region.

The plexus is usually formed by contributions from the last three cervical and first two thoracic nerves; the fifth cervical nerve sometimes participates, and the contribution of the second thoracic nerve is then reduced or lacking. The plexus reaches the axilla by passing between the parts of the scalenus and quickly splits into peripheral branches that diverge toward their separate destinations (Fig. 8–72). Several branches have very restricted local distributions and bare mention of their names and destinations is all that is required; they comprise the *long thoracic nerve* (/9) to the serratus ventralis, the *thoracodorsal nerve* (/9′) to the latissimus dorsi, *cranial* and *caudal pectoral nerves* (/3,9‴) to the pectoral muscles (including the subclavius), the *subscapular nerve* (/2) to the subscapularis, and the *lateral thoracic nerve* (9″) to the cutaneous trunci and to skin over the ventral part of the thorax and abdomen. The other branches require fuller description. Though some exhibit interspecies differences, these are rarely of importance except in the manus, and even these will be largely disregarded in the meantime.

The *suprascapular nerve* (/1) leaves the cranial part of the brachial plexus (C6–C7). It passes between the supraspinatus and subscapularis to reach the cranial margin of the neck of the scapula, around which it winds to the lateral aspect of the bone, where it is expended within the supra- and infraspinatus muscles. Like other nerves directly related to bone, it is vulnerable to injury—in this case usually by being stretched against the scapula when the limb is overabducted or violently retracted. The resulting paralysis of the lateral shoulder muscles does not affect the standing posture but may result in an obvious lateral movement of the shoulder joint (“shoulder slip”) during the stride. The condition occurs most frequently in horses, in which it is also known as “sweeny”; it manifests itself after a time by obvious wasting of the muscles beside the scapular spine.

The *musculocutaneous nerve* (/4) is also of cervical origin (C7–C8). After a short course within the axilla the nerve branches off the proximal muscular branch (/4′), which supplies the coracobrachialis and biceps in the upper part of the arm. In the dog the continuation beyond the proximal muscular branch remains separate from the median nerve until in the distal third of the arm a communicating branch passes distocaudally to the median nerve. The continuing nerve passes under the terminal part of the biceps brachii, where it divides into the distal muscular branch (/4″), which supplies the brachialis, and the medial cutaneous nerve of the forearm (/4‴), which crosses the flexor aspect of the elbow before ramifying in skin.

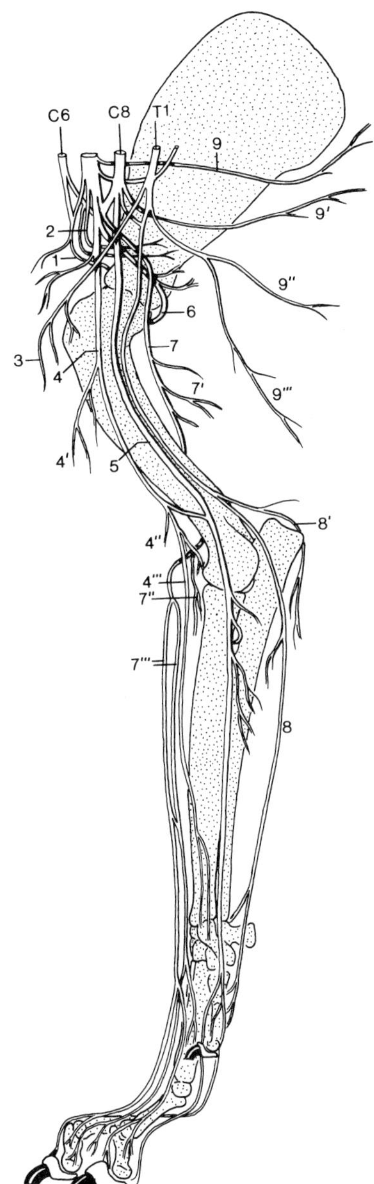


**Figure 8–72.** The nerves of the right forelimb of the dog; medial view.

1, Suprascapular n.; 2, subscapular nn.; 3, cranial pectoral nn.; 4, musculocutaneous n.; 4′, proximal muscular branch; 4″, distal muscular branch; 4‴, medial cutaneous antebrachial n.; 5, median n.; 6, axillary n.; 7, radial n.; 7′, muscular branches to triceps; 7″, muscular branches to extensors; 7‴, cranial cutaneous antebrachial n.; 8, ulnar n.; 8′, caudal cutaneous antebrachial n.; 9, long thoracic n.; 9′, thoracodorsal n.; 9″, lateral thoracic n.; 9‴, caudal pectoral n.

In ungulates generally, the musculocutaneous nerve loops around the axillary artery to join the median nerve in which its identity is for a time submerged; the musculocutaneous fibers again separate from the median nerve in the upper and lower parts of the arm, where they form the proximal and distal muscular branches of the musculocutaneous nerve. In the horse alone the cutaneous branch extends beyond the carpus to the fetlock.

Section of the main musculocutaneous trunk is an unlikely injury; it would paralyze the main flexors of the elbow, although compensation would probably be found from activity of the carpal and digital extensors.

The *axillary nerve* (C8) (/6) passes behind the shoulder jont to reach the lateral aspect of the limb. En route it supplies the teres major, teres minor, capsularis, and deltoideus—the true flexors of the shoulder joint. It also supplies twigs to the distal part of the brachiocephalicus, which, it will be recalled, is of deltoid origin. A cutaneous branch supplies skin over the cranial aspect of the arm and forearm.

The three remaining branches of the plexus have the most complicated courses and the most extensive distributions. The *radial nerve* (Fig. 8–72/7) arises from the last two cervical and first thoracic nerves (C7–T1). It first runs distally within the arm, caudal to the brachial artery, before diving between the long and medial heads of the triceps to follow the spiral groove of the humerus, which leads it to the craniolateral aspect of the limb. While buried by the triceps it supplies branches to the various heads of this muscle (/7′), and to tensor fasciae antebrachii and anconeus. In the lower part of the arm the radial nerve supplies a further set of muscular branches (/7″) to all carpal and digital extensor muscles, including the anomalous ulnaris lateralis. A cutaneous branch (/7‴), often replicated, descends over the craniolateral aspect of the forearm and carpus to reach the dorsal surface of the digits—except in the horse, in which it fades about the level of the carpus, part of the more distal duty being assumed by the musculocutaneous nerve.

Damage to the radial nerve can have three obvious consequences: paralysis of the elbow extensors, paralysis of the carpal and digital extensors, and anesthesia of the skin territory. The combination of all three disabilities points to injury proximal to the middle of the arm; the combination of the second and third points to injury in the distal part of the arm; a purely sensory deficit suggests injury beyond the origin of the distal motor branches. Injury in the arm is quite common since in places only a thin layer of muscle separates the nerve from the humerus and it may be involved in fracture or tumor of this bone. Extensive damage to the radial nerve proximal to the origin of the tricipital branches is serious since it prevents fixation of the elbow, prohibiting the limb from bearing weight; the foot is dragged with its dorsal surface on the ground. More distal lesions are less serious since the elbow can be fixed and most animals learn to compensate for paralysis of the forearm muscles by flicking the limb forward and planting the foot before the impetus is lost.

The *median nerve* (/5) comes mainly from the last cervical and first thoracic nerves (C8–T1). It runs down the medial surface of the arm caudal to the main artery and enters the forearm over the medial collateral ligament of the elbow joint. It then inclines caudally, passes under the flexor carpi radialis, and maintains this protected situation until it reaches the carpus. It divides in the distal part of the forearm, or within the carpal canal, into two or more divisions that descend through the carpal canal to supply most structures of the palmar part of the foot. The median nerve supplies most of the flexor muscles of the carpus and digit in a pattern that overlaps (but does not quite coincide) with the distribution of the ulnar. Because of this, damage confined to the median nerve does not usually manifest itself through any abnormality of posture or gait.

The *ulnar nerve* (Fig. 8–72/8) leaves the caudal part of the plexus (C8–T2). It runs down the arm beside, and possibly (as in the dog) for a stretch united to, the median nerve before deviating in the direction of the olecranon to cross the caudal aspect of the elbow joint. Within the arm it detaches the caudal cutaneous antebrachial nerve. The main trunk is severely depleted by detachment of the branches to the carpal and digital flexor muscles in the upper part of the forearm, and the narrow continuation runs down the caudal aspect of the forearm. It finally divides a short distance above the accessory carpal bone. The dorsal branch emerges between the tendons of the ulnar carpal flexor and ulnaris lateralis, and descends over the lateral face of the accessory bone to supply the skin on the lateral aspect of the forefoot. The palmar branch continues through the carpal canal and later supplies the interosseous and other small muscles of the foot. It also supplies sensory branches to skin and deeper structures. The distribution within the foot is in close collaboration with the median nerve, partly through combined trunks. The innervation of the forefoot, a topic of considerable practical importance in horses and cattle, is later considered separately for the different species.

Damage confined to this nerve is unlikely to impair locomotion; the sensory deficits show considerable interspecies variation.

## The Thoracic Ventral Rami

These show a more strictly segmental distribution than is found in other regions. The first two contribute to the brachial plexus, but generally the thoracic ventral rami provide the intercostal nerves that run ventrally within the intercostal spaces, either directly below the pleura or between the two intercostal muscle layers—the relation varies according to location and species. Apart from supplying the intercostal muscles, the intercostal nerves detach lateral cutaneous branches that supply a band of skin over the lateral aspect, and ventral cutaneous branches that supply the ventral aspect of the chest wall; the more caudal members of the series are also concerned in the supply of the abdominal floor. There are a few minor connections with nerves of the brachial plexus. In the sow, bitch, and cat the lateral cutaneous branches detach twigs to thoracic mammary glands.

The last thoracic ventral branch (costoabdominal nerve) is slightly different in its course and distribution since it runs behind the last rib. It collaborates with lumbar ventral branches in the supply of the flank.

## The Lumbar Ventral Rami

The lumbar and sacral ventral rami form a continuous plexus, best developed where the last three or four lumbar and first two sacral nerves form the lumbosacral plexus that supplies the hindlimb. The more cranial lumbar ventral rami have a considerable importance in cattle since they are frequently blocked for abdominal surgery. They are given individual names; in species (including cattle) in which there are six lumbar nerves the first ventral ramus is known as the *iliohypogastric,* the second as the *ilioinguinal,* and the third and fourth combine to form the *genitofemoral nerve.* In species with seven lumbar nerves the first two ventral rami are distinguished as the *cranial and caudal iliohypogastric;* the third supplies the ilioinguinal and also makes a contribution to the genitofemoral nerve. The genitofemoral nerve divides into a femoral branch that supplies the skin over the medial aspect of the thigh and a genital branch that supplies the spermatic fasciae, the scrotum, and the prepuce.

The caudoventral inclination of the ventral rami that becomes increasingly apparent with the caudal intercostal nerves is further accentuated with the lumbar rami; the locations where the nerves can most easily be reached by injection of local anesthetic solution, and the positions of their dermatomes, are both considerably more caudal than would naturally be supposed (see Fig. 28–2). The nerves pass through the transversus close to the tip of the transverse processes and then run deep to the internal oblique toward the abdominal floor (see Fig. 1–37). In addition to supplying the flank and rectus muscles, they detach lateral and ventral cutaneous branches; the former appear subcutaneously at increasingly dorsal levels as the series is followed caudally.

## *The Lumbosacral Plexus*

The lumbosacral plexus that gives origin to the nerves of the hindlimb (with the minor exceptions of those to certain proximal skin areas) is an enhancement of the continuous plexus. It usually begins with the ventral ramus of the fourth lumbar nerve and ends with that of the second sacral (L4–S2); it thus has an additional root in species possessing seven lumbar nerves (Fig. 8–73).

The *femoral nerve* (/1) arises from the cranial part (L4–L6) of the plexus and pursues a course through the psoas muscles to reach the gap between the dorsocaudal corner of the flank and the iliopsoas muscle. It is accompanied by the external iliac artery and vein, and on entering the thigh it runs in a protected position between the sartorius and pectineus. It soon detaches the saphenous nerve and after a very short further course it dives between the rectus femoris and vastus medialis to be expended within the quadriceps mass (/1′). Severe damage to this nerve, though relatively infrequent, has serious consequences since paralysis of the quadriceps precludes fixation of the stifle joint, rendering the whole limb incapable of supporting weight. No compensation for this defect is possible.

The *saphenous nerve* (/1″) gives a branch to the sartorius before continuing to supply skin over the medial aspect of the limb from the stifle to the metatarsus.

The *obturator nerve* (/2) has broadly the same origin (L4–L6) as the femoral nerve. It follows the medial aspect of the shaft of the ilium to reach the obturator foramen through which it passes to the adductor muscles of the thigh; the group

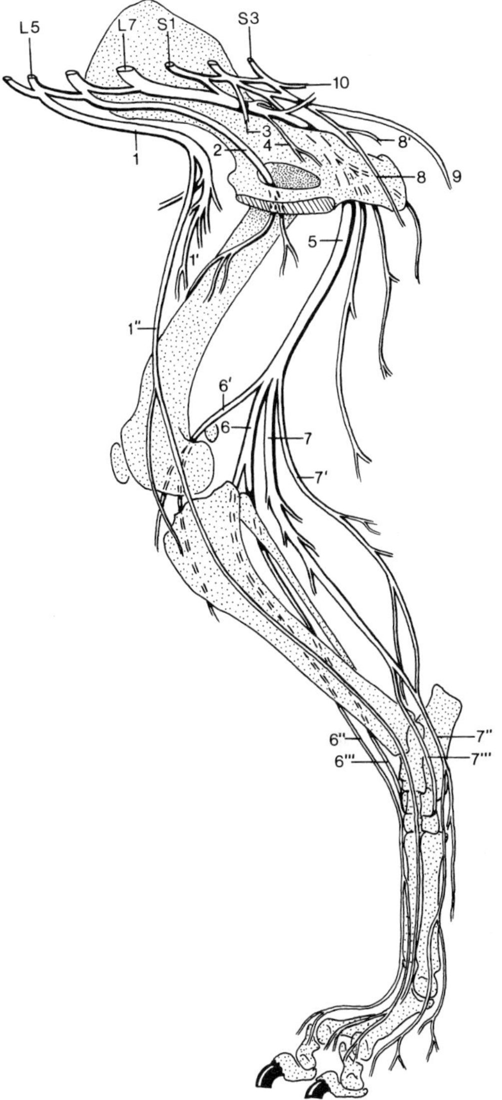


**Figure 8–73.** The lumbar and sacral nerves of the dog; medial view.

1, Femoral n.; 1′, branches to quadriceps; 1″, saphenous n.; 2, obturator n.; 3, pelvic n.; 4, branch to obturator internus, gemelli, and quadratus femoris; 5, sciatic n.; 6, peroneal n.; 6′, lateral cutaneous sural n.; 6″, superficial peroneal n.; 6‴, deep peroneal n.; 7, tibial n.; 7′, caudal cutaneous sural n.; 7″, medial plantar n.; 7‴, lateral plantar n.; 8, pudendal n.; 8′, deep perineal n.; 9, caudal cutaneous femoral n.; 10, caudal rectal n.

comprises gracilis, pectineus, adductor, and obturator externus—and obturator internus in ruminants and pig.* The relationship to bone is potentially dangerous, exposing the nerve to risk

*The variation may be more apparent than real; it has been suggested that the internal obturator of Artiodactyla is actually an intrapelvic part of the external obturator.

of laceration in fractures and of compression during calving and foaling (the risk is less in species in which the young are small relative to the pelvic cavity). The effects of injury vary with its extent but are greater in heavier animals and are exaggerated by a requirement to walk on smooth ground when the limb tends to slip sideways.

The remaining branches of the plexus arise from a common *lumbosacral trunk* that is largely formed by the last lumbar and first two sacral nerves with a smaller contribution from the penultimate lumbar nerve. The trunk leaves the pelvis through the greater sciatic foramen and almost at once detaches three branches.

The *short cranial gluteal nerve* supplies the tensor fasciae latae and the middle and deep, and in some species part of the superficial, gluteal muscles, a group that—contrary to the usual expectation—includes both flexor and extensor muscles of the hip.

The *caudal gluteal nerve* supplies the superficial gluteal muscle and the vertebral heads of origin of the hamstring muscles (biceps femoris, semitendinosus, and semimembranosus), parts supposed to represent assimilation of elements of the superficial gluteal. It thus supplies extensor muscles of the hip.

The *caudal cutaneous femoral nerve* (/9) supplies skin over the caudal aspect of the thigh.

The *sciatic nerve* (/5) continues the lumbosacral trunk distally, passing between the middle and deep gluteal muscles before turning into the thigh caudal to the hip joint, where it is protected by the greater trochanter of the femur. It then runs between the biceps femoris laterally, the semitendinosus medially, before dividing into its terminal branches, the common peroneal and tibial nerves, at a level that varies among species. In the proximal part of its course it detaches twigs to the unimportant internal obturator (except in ruminants and pigs), gemelli, and quadratus femoris (/4); other muscular branches that may appear to arise directly from the sciatic nerve are usually referred to its common peroneal and tibial divisions.

The *common peroneal nerve* (Fig. 8–73/6), the lesser of the terminal branches, arises from the lumbar roots of the lumbosacral trunk. It runs first with the tibial nerve but separates from this in order to pass over the lateral head of the gastrocnemius to enter the leg. It detaches a branch, the lateral sural nerve (/6′), to the skin over the lateral aspect of the leg before dividing into superficial and deep branches when close to the head of the fibula. The *superficial peroneal nerve* (/6″) supplies skin over the dorsal aspect of the leg and entire foot—except in the horse, in which it fades about the level of the fetlock joint. The *deep peroneal nerve* (/6‴) supplies the dorsolateral muscles of the leg (flexors of the hock and extensors of the digits) and is also sensory to the structures of the foot. Since the sensory innervation of pedal structures varies considerably, the details are deferred until the accounts of individual species.

Paralysis of the common peroneal nerve produces overextension of the hock and flexion of the digits, which may be rested upon their dorsal surfaces. The foot may be passively placed to support weight and in time compensation may be possible (cf. radial paralysis, p. 314). There is also a considerable sensory deficit.

The *tibial nerve* (/7) arises from the sacral roots of the lumbosacral trunk. It detaches important proximal muscular branches to the pelvic heads of the hamstring muscles before freeing itself from the parent trunk to enter the leg by passing between the two heads of the gastrocnemius. About this level it detaches, first, a caudal sural nerve (/7′) to the skin of this aspect of the leg, and later, distal muscular branches to the gastrocnemius, soleus, popliteus, and caudal crural muscles. The nerve continues as an almost exclusively sensory trunk (although it will supply short digital muscles) within the fascial plate between the common calcanean tendon and the caudal crural muscles; it ends by dividing into medial and lateral plantar nerves when level with the point of the hock. The *plantar nerves* (/7″,7‴) continue into the plantar aspect of the foot to supply sensation to plantar structures chiefly, but with some dorsal penetration that varies among species.

Section or severe damage to the tibial nerve is manifested by overflexion of the hock and overextension of the digits. Similar damage to the parent trunk combines the effects of common peroneal and tibial nerve injuries, rendering the limb largely incapable, although fixation of the stifle joint by the unaffected quadriceps may allow it to support some weight.

## The Sacral and Caudal Ventral Rami

The sacral ventral rami caudal to and overlapping the roots of the lumbosacral plexus give rise to other important individual nerves. The *pelvic nerves* (/3) composed of the parasympathetic outflow are considered in the following section.

The *pudendal nerve* (/8) arises variously (S1–S3 in the dog, S2–S4 in ruminants, S[2]3–S4 in the horse). It is sensory to the rectum, internal and external reproductive organs, and perineal skin, and motor to much of the striated perineal musculature. It has both physiological and applied importance but since it is very variable it must for the present suffice to say that its course takes it obliquely through the pelvis toward the ventral part of the outlet (see Fig. 29–5/7,7‴). It provides deep and superficial perineal nerves in addition to various cutaneous branches, and finally continues as the dorsal nerve of the penis (or clitoris). The *superficial perineal branch* supplies the skin of the anus, vulva, and ventral perineal region, the strict perineal location.

The *deep perineal nerve* supplies the ventral part of the striated musculature of the perineum, particularly that of the reproductive organs. The main trunk also supplies branches to the skin of the prepuce and scrotum in the male, and of the caudal part of the udder in the female.

The *caudal rectal nerves* (Fig. 8–73/10) arise from the most caudal sacral nerves, sometimes overlapping the origin of the pudendal nerve. They supply sensory fibers to the rectum, anus, and perianal skin, and motor fibers to the dorsal perineal striated musculature, including the levator ani. The division of territory between these nerves and the pudendal is rather variable.

The ventral rami of the caudal nerves supply the ventral or depressor muscles of the tail.

## THE PERIPHERAL AUTONOMIC NERVOUS SYSTEM

Although the appropriate regulation of "visceral" activities clearly presumes the existence of receptors in the viscera and vessels, the autonomic nervous system was originally defined as wholly efferent. This offers a certain convenience since visceral afferent pathways are in general indistinguishable in structure and arrangement from their somatic counterparts. The visceral efferent pathways, on the other hand, are clearly distinguished, particularly by the location of the last neuron in the chain within a peripheral ganglion and by the restriction of the neurons that drive these ganglion cells to specific nuclei of the brainstem and particular regions of the cord (Figs. 8–74 and 8–75). The peripheral efferent pathway thus consists of a preganglionic (myelinated, and therefore white) fiber and a postganglionic (little myelinated, and therefore gray) fiber. Moreover, certain anatomical, physiological, and pharmacological features distinguish two contrasting—sympathetic and parasympathetic—efferent systems, whereas no similar distinction is possible for the visceral afferent fibers presumed to be included in all cranial and spinal nerves (if only because of the ubiquitous distribution of blood vessels). It has been shown (p. 295) that cerebrospinal (somatic) and autonomic (visceral) mechanisms cannot be

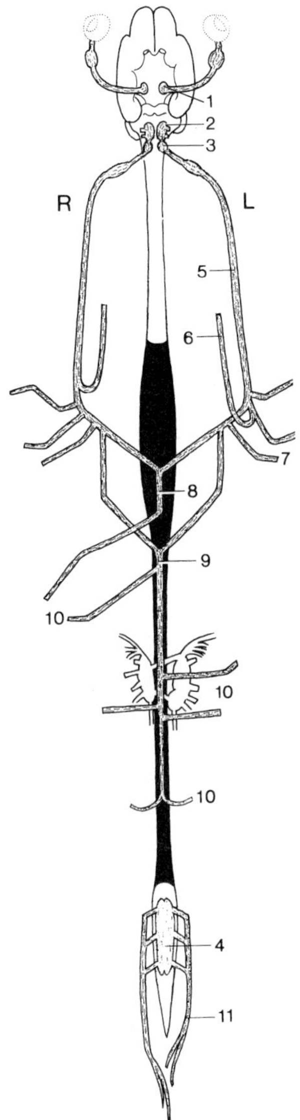


**Figure 8–74.** Origin and distribution of the parasympathetic nervous system. Ventral view, schematic.

1, Parasympathetic oculomotor nucleus; 2, rostral and middle parasympathetic nuclei of the medulla oblongata; 3, dorsal vagal nucleus; 4, sacral outflow; 5, vagus nerve; 6, recurrent laryngeal nerve; 7, parasympathetic fibers to heart and lungs; 8, ventral vagal trunk; 9, dorsal vagal trunk; 10, parasympathetic fibers to the abdominal organs; 11, pelvic nerves.

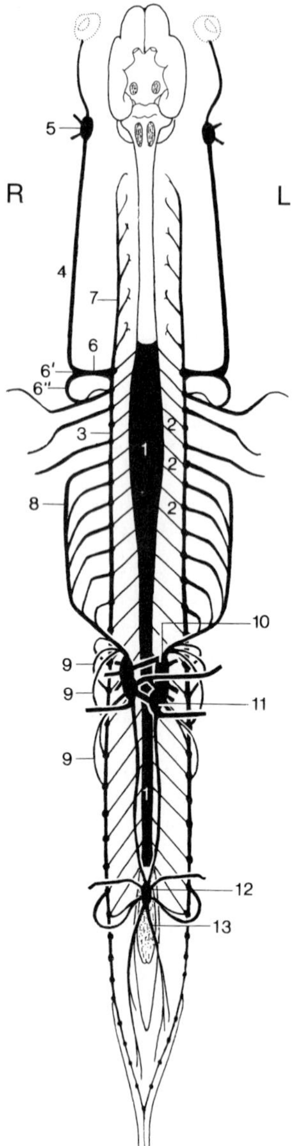


**Figure 8–75.** Origin and distribution of the sympathetic nervous system. Ventral view, schematic. The parasympathetic nuclei in brain and spinal cord are indicated in gray.

1, Sympathetic outflow from T1 to L3; 2, communicating branches; 3, 4, sympathetic trunk; 5, cranial cervical ganglion; 6, cervicothoracic ganglion; 6′, middle cervical ganglion; 6″, ansa subclavia; 7, vertebral n.; 8, greater splanchnic n.; 9, lesser splanchnic nn.; 10, celiac ganglion; 11, cranial mesenteric ganglion; 12, caudal mesenteric ganglion; 13, hypogastric n.

entirely separated since the cerebral cortex directs both types.

Some contrasting physiological actions of the two systems are summarized later (p. 322), but it may be said now that they partly rest upon the use of norepinephrine as the mediating substance at the last synapse of the sympathetic pathway, while acetylcholine is used at the corresponding parasympathetic synapse. Epinephrine is produced by the adrenal medulla and when generally diffused by the blood stream it evokes a mass sympathetic response. Acetylcholine is liberated and destroyed locally. The activities of the parasympathetic system therefore tend to be more specific and discrete than those of the sympathetic system. The narrower localization of parasympathetic responses is further assisted by the location of parasympathetic ganglia close by or even within the target organ, whereas the sympathetic ganglia are close to the central nervous system and the postganglionic fibers radiate more widely.

## The Parasympathetic System

The preganglionic cells of the parasympathetic system are restricted to a number of discrete nuclei within the brainstem and to the lateral column of a short stretch of the spinal cord, generally the second, third, and possibly fourth sacral segments (Fig. 8–74). The aptly designated craniosacral outflow is confined to the oculomotor, facial, glossopharyngeal, vagus, and pelvic nerves.

The cranial parasympathetic pathways have rather limited anatomical independence. Varying parts of their courses are incorporated within nerves of predominantly somatic composition. Exclusively parasympathetic bundles are found only close to the target organs. The chief grossly visible features of the cranial parasympathetic outflow have been described with the relevant nerves, and it now remains to draw these threads together.

The most rostral parasympathetic nucleus, the parasympathetic oculomotor nucleus, lies within the midbrain in association with the motor nucleus of the third cranial nerve. The parasympathetic preganglionic fibers emerge from the main trunk within the orbit to constitute the oculomotor (short) root of the ciliary ganglion. Beyond the ganglion, the postganglionic fibers proceed as the short ciliary nerves, which also incorporate sympathetic and sensory fibers; these nerves penetrate the sclera to form the ciliary plexus from which the parasympathetic fibers extend to the ciliary and pupillary sphincter muscles (Fig. 8–70/6,11).

The parasympathetic component of the facial nerve originates in the rostral parasympathetic (salivatory) nucleus of the medulla oblongata (/2). The preganglionic fibers are incorporated within the main facial trunk, run through the somatic geniculate ganglion without interruption, and later leave in the chorda tympani and the greater petrosal nerve (/14,12). The chorda tympani introduces its complement to the lingual nerve from which the parasympathetic fibers later emerge to synapse within the mandibular ganglion; the postganglionic fibers supply the mandibular and sublingual salivary glands.

The greater petrosal nerve is joined by the deep petrosal (sympathetic) nerve (/13) to constitute the nerve of the pterygoid canal, which leads to the pterygopalatine ganglion (/7). The postganglionic fibers join the lacrimal nerve (after passage through the zygomatic nerve) en route to the lacrimal gland, and various other branches of the maxillary nerve en route to glands within the nasal and palatine mucosae.

The parasympathetic component of the glossopharyngeal nerve originates from the middle parasympathetic nucleus in the medulla oblongata (/3). The preganglionic fibers pass through the somatic ganglion of this nerve before joining the tympanic plexus; from this they proceed to the otic ganglion (/9). The postganglionic fibers are carried via the pterygoid nerve and a communicating branch with the auriculotemporal nerve to the parotid gland.

The parasympathetic component supplies the bulk of the vagus nerve, indeed the whole complement distal to the origin of the recurrent laryngeal nerve (Fig. 8–74/5,6). The preganglionic fibers proceed to numerous small ganglia scattered along the nerve plexuses that supply, and are often located within, the tissues of the target organs. The plexuses include the cardiac and pulmonary plexuses within the chest (/7), and the gastric, hepatic, mesenteric, gonadal, and renal plexuses formed by the confluence of branches of the vagal trunks with sympathetic nerves within the abdomen (/10). Broadly, the dorsal vagal trunk supplies hepatic and gastric plexuses, the larger ventral vagal trunk supplying celiac, mesenteric, renal, and gonadal plexuses. Particular features of the distribution in ruminants are mentioned elsewhere (p. 681).

The sacral part of the parasympathetic outflow constitutes the pelvic nerves (/11). The fibers of the parasympathetic outflow are initially incorporated within the relevant ventral sacral rami from which they emerge to constitute the pelvic nerves. These form a retroperitoneal plexus that is joined by sympathetic fibers delivered by the hypogastric nerves that descend from the caudal mesenteric ganglion. Numerous minute ganglia are found scattered in the plexus while other (terminal) ganglia are embedded within the walls of predominantly pelvic viscera: the descending colon, and rectum, bladder, uterus, and vagina (in the female); accessory reproductive glands (in the male); and the genital erectile tissue. The parasympathetic pathways have their peripheral synapses exclusively in the terminal ganglia while some sympathetic peripheral synapses are divided among the plexus and terminal ganglia.

## The Sympathetic System

The preganglionic fibers of the sympathetic system take their origin from the lateral column of the thoracolumbar part of the spinal cord (Fig. 8–75/1) and pass into the ventral roots of the thoracic and first several lumbar nerves. They continue into the spinal nerves and then issue from the ventral rami, constituting the white communicating branches, which join the ganglia of the sympathetic trunks (Fig. 8–53/5,7). The bilateral trunks run the length of the neck and back. Each has a basically segmental arrangement, although strict correspondence of the ganglia with spinal nerves is evident only in the thoracic and cranial lumbar regions.

The cervical part of the trunk begins at the large, spindle-shaped, cranial cervical ganglion placed close to the base of the skull (Fig. 8–75/5). The trunk is associated with the vagus within the carotid sheath, forming the vagosympathetic trunk that proceeds down the neck. The two components part company at the entrance to the chest, where the sympathetic trunk often bears a middle cervical ganglion by the first rib (Fig. 8–76/7′). The trunk then continues subpleurally, over the line of the costovertebral articulations, before passing dorsal to the diaphragm to gain admission to the abdomen. Its thoracic part shows a regular arrangement of ganglia, although the first one or two are fused with a caudal cervical element to form the large cervicothoracic ganglion deep to the head of the first rib (/7). The lumbar part of the trunk, which lies between the psoas musculature and vertebral bodies, at first also carries a regular complement of ganglia, but the arrangement later becomes more erratic, with some caudal lumbar ganglia splitting into two or, less commonly, fusing with their neighbors. The sacral part is even less regular and may fuse, temporarily or finally, with its fellow before extending into the tail, where it rapidly fades (Fig. 8–75/3).

Since the sympathetic outflow is restricted it follows that only the thoracic and cranial lumbar ganglia are joined by white communicating branches. But all spinal and many cranial nerves are joined by bundles (gray communicating branches) of postganglionic fibers destined for

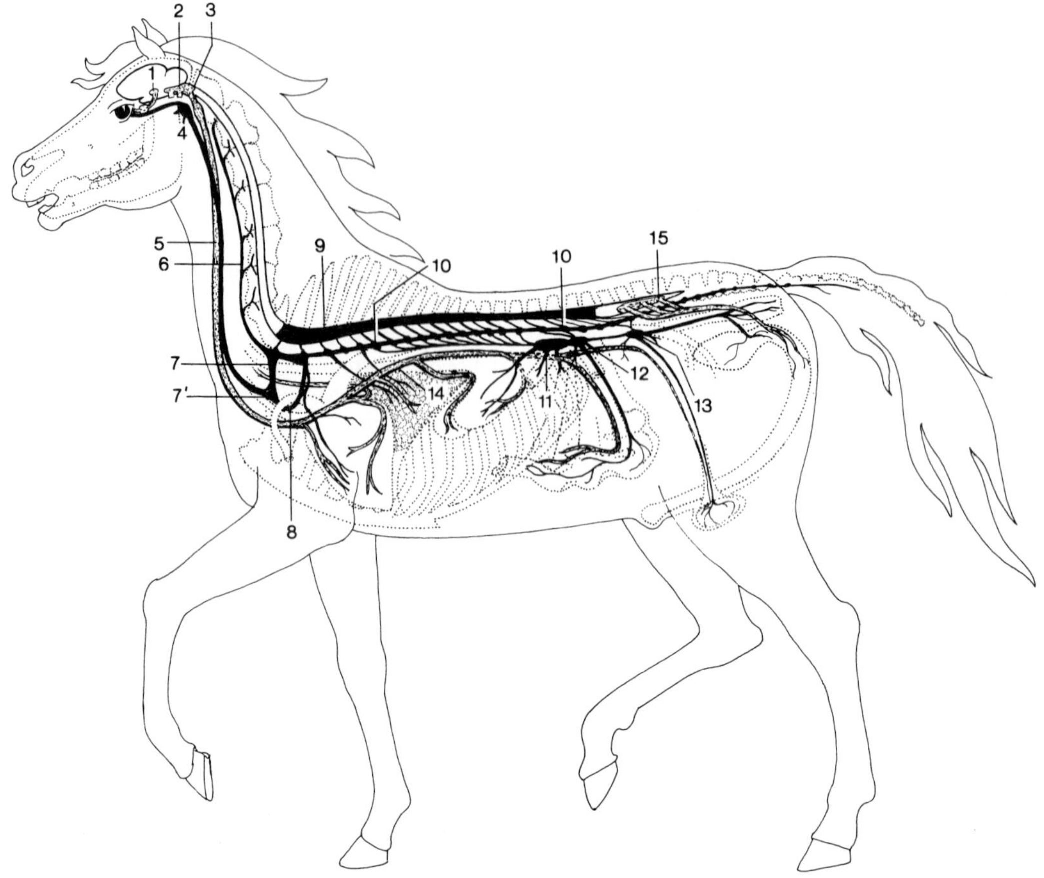


**Figure 8–76.** Distribution of sympathetic *(black)* and parasympathetic *(gray)* nervous systems, semischematic.

1, Parasympathetic oculomotor nucleus; 2, salivatory nuclei (rostral and middle parasympathetic nuclei); 3, dorsal vagal nucleus; 4, cranial cervical ganglion; 5, vagosympathetic trunk; 6, vertebral nerve; 7, cervicothoracic ganglion; 7′, middle cervical ganglion; 8, ansa subclavia; 9, sympathetic outflow from spinal cord; 10, sympathetic trunk with paravertebral ganglia; 11, celiac ganglion; 12, cranial mesenteric ganglion; 13, caudal mesenteric ganglion; 14, vagus nerve with distribution to thoracic and abdominal organs; 15, sacral outflow of parasympathetic nervous system.

vessels, skin glands, and so forth. It should be stressed that the body wall and limbs are innervated only by these postganglionic sympathetic fibers. Those to most cervical nerves join within a single trunk, the vertebral nerve, which runs from the cervicothoracic ganglion through the foramina of successive cervical transverse processes (/7). The postganglionic sympathetic fibers to the first two cervical nerves, and to cranial nerves, extend from the cranial cervical ganglion; many form the internal carotid nerve that follows the like-named artery.

Several alternative fates are open to the preganglionic fibers that enter the sympathetic chain, each to project on many ganglion cells. Some fibers synapse immediately within the local ganglion, others run cranially or caudally within the trunk to synapse within ganglia that are more cranial or caudal in the series, while yet others pass uninterruptedly through the trunk to proceed to a second set of (prevertebral) ganglia placed about the origin of the visceral branches of the abdominal aorta (Figs. 8–75/10,11 and 8–76/11,12). This last group constitutes the splanchnic nerves, which are rather variable in arrangement; usually one *greater splanchnic nerve* is formed by preganglionic fibers that leave the trunk from about the sixth to the penultimate thoracic ganglia with *lesser thoracic and lumbar splanchnic nerves* arising at more caudal levels (Fig. 8–75/8,9).

The viscera and vessels of the head receive their sympathetic innervation via the cranial cervical ganglion. The postganglionic fibers that emerge from this ganglion radiate in a number of directions that carry them into the territories of the cranial and first two cervical nerves. Though many pass through parasympathetic ganglia, they of course do so without interruption. The details are of rather limited clinical importance (although relevant to experimental work), and only a few points are presented here (Fig. 8–70).

One large group of fibers follows the internal carotid artery into the cranial cavity and there provides twigs to the intracranial vessels and fiber bundles that join various nerves, especially the trigeminal and those to the extraocular muscles. Another group of fibers passes through the ciliary ganglion to the eyeball for ultimate distribution to the dilator pupillae. At a more proximal level, the *internal carotid nerve* gives off the deep petrosal nerve, which combines with the greater petrosal nerve (/12) in its passage through the pterygoid canal to the pterygopalatine ganglion (/7). These fibers are ultimately dispersed with the various nerves that supply structures within the orbit, nasal cavity, sinuses, and palate.

Other branches concur with parasympathetic fibers in forming a plexus within the tympanic cavity from which the parotid gland is supplied after passage beyond the otic ganglion. Yet other bundles of fibers entwine the external carotid artery and its branches.

The thoracic organs—heart, trachea, and lungs—are supplied by postganglionic fibers that form cardiac and pulmonary plexuses within the mediastinum after leaving the thoracic portion of the sympathetic trunk. These plexuses combine with the corresponding parasympathetic component (Fig. 8–76).

The abdominal and pelvic organs receive their sympathetic innervation through the various splanchnic nerves that lead to the celiac, cranial mesenteric, renal, aorticorenal, gonadal, and caudal mesenteric ganglia placed on the ventral face of the aorta by the origins of the visceral arteries. The preganglionic fibers synapse in these ganglia and the postganglionic fibers that emerge from intricate plexuses (combining vagal contributions) that enmesh, and run parallel to, the visceral arteries from which they obtain their names (Fig. 8–77).

The pelvic organs are supplied with postganglionic fibers that leave the caudal mesenteric ganglion within the paired hypogastric nerves (/8). These enter the pelvic cavity below the peritoneum to form a common pelvic plexus with the parasympathetic pelvic nerves (Fig. 8–76). As already mentioned, the sympathetic contribution to the pelvic plexus includes preganglionic fibers that have deferred their synapses to peripheral locations within the pelvis.

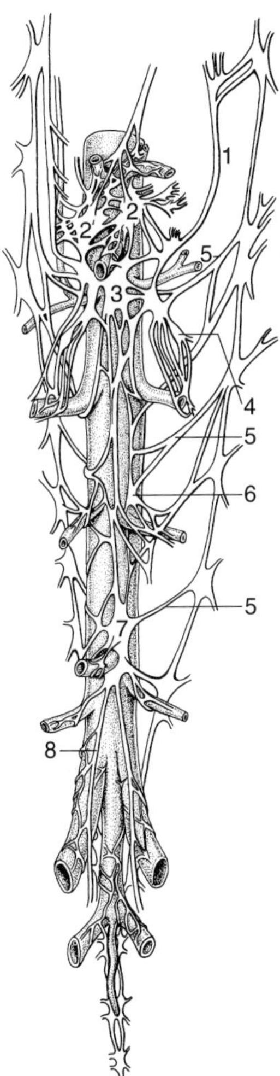


**Figure 8–77.** Ganglia and plexuses of the abdominal cavity. Ventral view.

1, Greater splanchnic n.; 2, left celiac ganglion; 2′, right celiac ganglion; 3, cranial mesenteric ganglion; 4, renal ganglion; 5, lumbar splanchnic nn.; 6, gonadal ganglion; 7, caudal mesenteric ganglion; 8, right hypogastric n.

## Summary of Autonomic Innervation

Certain effects of the autonomic nervous system are tabulated (Table 8–3) by way of illustration, but for more controversial points, such as the innervation of the bladder and urethra, or those requiring more detailed description, the reader is referred to modern works of physiology.

**Table 8–3.** Actions Controlled by the Autonomic Nervous System

| Sympathetic Innervation | | | Parasympathetic Innervation | |
|---|---|---|---|---|
| *Source* | *Effect* | **Target Organ** | *Effect* | *Source* |
| Cranial thoracic segment via cranial cervical ganglion | Dilation of pupil | Iris | Contraction of pupil | Oculomotor n. via ciliary ganglion |
| Cranial thoracic segment via cranial cervical ganglion | Relaxation: Accommodation for distant vision | Ciliary muscle | Contraction: Accommodation for near vision | Oculomotor n. via ciliary ganglion |
| Cranial thoracic segment via cranial cervical ganglion | Vasoconstriction and contraction of myoepithelial cells | Salivary glands | Vasodilation and secretion | Facial n. via mandibular ganglion<br>Glossopharyngeal n. via otic ganglion |
| Cranial thoracic segment via cranial cervical ganglion | Vasoconstriction | Lacrimal gland | Secretion | Facial n. via pterygopalatine ganglion |
| Cranial thoracic segments | Increased activity | Heart | Reduced activity | Vagus n. via cardiac ganglia |
| Thoracic and lumbar segments | Vasoconstriction in some tissues, e.g., skin; vasodilation in others, e.g., skeletal muscle | Blood vessels | Vasodilation, and possibly vasoconstriction in some vessels | |
| Cranial thoracic segments | Relaxation | Bronchi | Constriction | Vagus n. |
| Caudal thoracic segments | Secretion | Adrenal medulla | | |
| Caudal thoracic and lumbar segments via abdominal ganglia | Decreased activity | Gastrointestinal tract | Increased motility and secretion | Vagus n. and pelvic nn. |
| Lumbar segments via abdominal ganglia | Relaxation | Bladder wall | Contraction | Pelvic nn. |
| | | Erectile tissue | Vasodilation | Pelvic nn. |

# CHAPTER 9

# The Sense Organs

A stabled animal, for example a dairy cow tied to a stanchion, experiences few environmental changes—and these by and large are routine. It is quite different with a wild animal, which, if it is to survive, must constantly check its environment. It must see obstacles, hear predators, smell other animals to distinguish outsiders from members of its own group, taste in order to discard harmful substances in its food, and, in a more general way, be in touch with its surroundings "through its skin" by perceiving touch, pressure, and temperature. This is made possible by those organs that represent the special senses (eye, ear, olfactory organ, and organ of taste) and those others that are widely diffused, especially in the skin, where they mediate a cutaneous sense. The former are concentrations of highly specialized sensory cells; the latter are composed of numerous peripheral specialized endings of centrally located sensory cell bodies. Associated with the ear are sensory cells that respond to gravity and to movements of the head and so give the animal its sense of balance.

All these senses are conscious, that is to say, the animal is aware of what it has registered. But there are other systems concerned with muscle and visceral sense of which the animal is less aware and by which it is in touch with the "internal environment" of its own body.

The organs of special sense are described first.

## THE EYE

The eye, the organ of vision, consists of the eyeball and various adnexa—accessory structures such as the ocular muscles that move the eyeball, the lids that protect it, and the lacrimal apparatus that keeps its exposed parts moist. Most of these are housed in the orbit, where the eyeball is embedded in generous quantities of fat. The eyelids arise from the bony margins of the orbit and, like curtains, are intermittently drawn over the exposed part of the eye (blinking) to distribute the tears or lacrimal fluid for protection; they are kept across the eye during sleep when vision is not required.

The eyes of the domestic mammals protrude more from the surface of the face than do those of primates, ourselves included. Their position in the head is related to the animal's environment, habits, and method of feeding. In general, predatory species (cat, dog) have eyes set well forward, whereas those that are the hunted (herbivores: horse, ruminants, rabbits) carry their eyes more laterally (Fig. 9–1). The former position of the eyes provides a large field of binocular vision that allows for concentration on near objects and for the perception of depth. In the latter, the right and left fields of vision hardly overlap; consequently, though these animals are constantly aware of a large segment of their surroundings, they have little capacity for binocular vision.

When an animal is emaciated the orbital fat is reduced and the eyes sink within the orbits, giving the face a gaunt, suffering appearance.

### The Eyeball

The eyeball (bulbus oculi) of the domestic mammals is nearly spherical but with some anteroposterior* compression in horses and cattle. In addition, the cornea, the transparent part of the eyeball, bulges from the anterior surface by virtue of its smaller radius of curvature (Fig. 9–2).

The highest point on the cornea is the *anterior pole,* the highest point on the posterior surface, the *posterior pole* of the eyeball; the straight line passing through both poles is the *optic axis.* The *equator* is an imaginary line about the eyeball, which, like that of the Earth, is equidistant from the poles. A *meridian* is one of the many lines passing from pole to pole that intersect the equator at right angles. The optic nerve (/6) leaves the eyeball slightly ventral to the posterior pole.

The eyeball has three thin tunics that, being in close apposition, form a laminated sheet that surrounds the partly liquid, partly gelatinous center. The three tunics are (1) an external fibrous tunic that gives form to and protects the eyeball—it is the only complete tunic; (2) a middle vascular tunic that consists largely of blood vessels

*Anterior and posterior, in front of and behind, are used instead of rostral and caudal when referring to the eye.

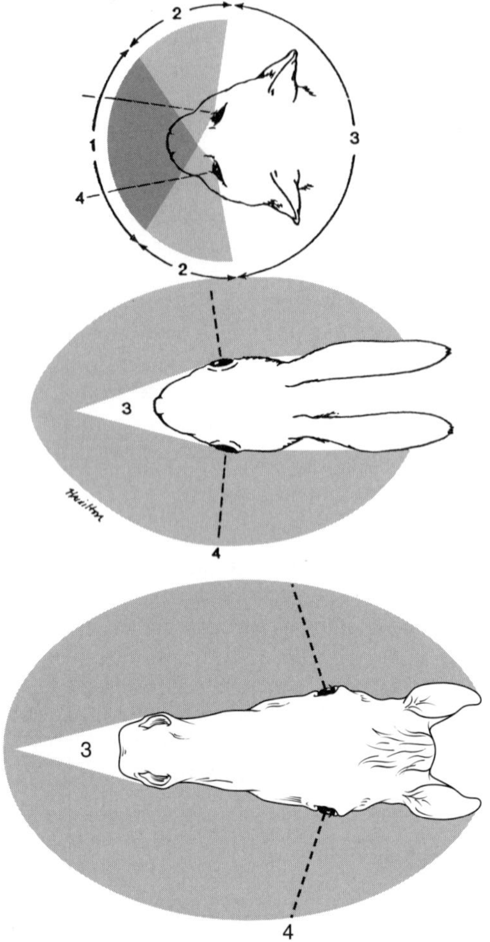


**Figure 9–1.** Visual fields of cat, rabbit, and horse.

1, Binocular vision; 2, monocular vision; 3, blind area; 4, visual axis of eye in central position.

and smooth muscle and is concerned with the nutrition of the eyeball and the regulation of the shape of the lens and size of the pupil; and (3) an internal nervous tunic that consists largely of nervous tissue and is the layer most directly concerned with vision, that is, the translation of visual stimuli into nerve impulses for interpretation by the brain.

## The Fibrous Tunic

The fibrous tunic of the eyeball is made up of very dense collagenous tissue, which, by resisting the internal pressure, gives the eye shape and stiffness. It consists of the sclera and cornea, which meet at the *limbus* (Fig. 9–2/7).

The *sclera* is the opaque posterior part of the fibrous tunic. It consists of a dense feltwork of collagenous and elastic fibers and is generally white ("the white of the eye"), though with a bluish tinge; in some species it contains pigmented cells that render it gray. Ventral to the posterior pole it presents a small cribriform area (Fig. 9–3/13) through which pass the fibers of the optic nerve. The nerve is surrounded by a connective tissue sheath that continues the dura mater to the sclera. The sclera is also pierced by several small ciliary arteries and nerves, and by larger vorticose veins. It gives attachment to the tendons of the ocular muscles anterior to the equator. Posteriorly, except for the areas taken up by the retractor bulbi muscle, it is covered by a thin membrane (vagina bulbi; /5) that separates it from the retrobulbar fat, providing a socket in which the eyeball can play.

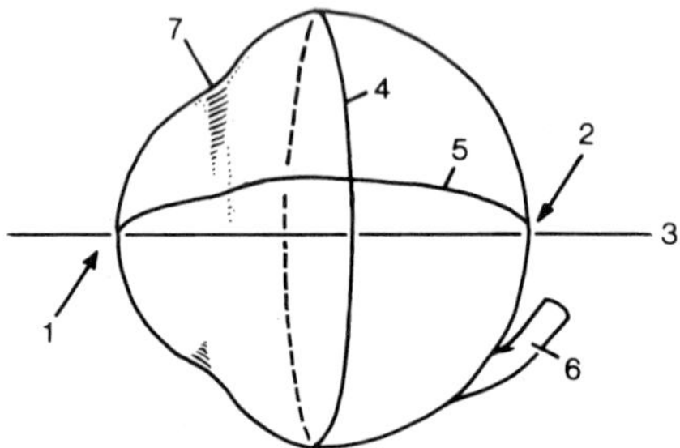


**Figure 9–2.** Medial view of right eyeball.

1, Anterior pole; 2, posterior pole; 3, optic axis; 4, equator; 5, a meridian; 6, optic nerve; 7, limbus.

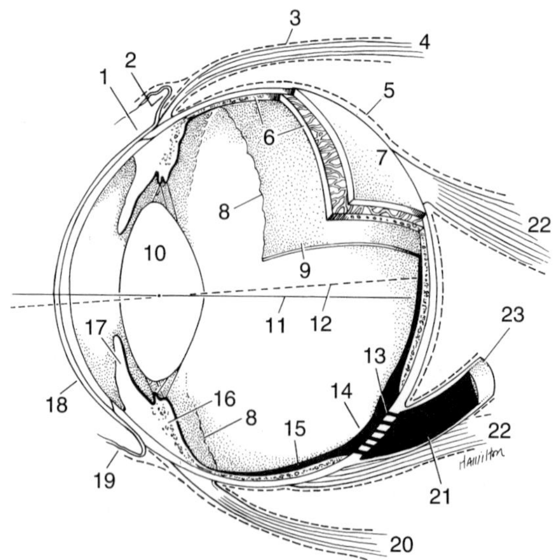


**Figure 9–3.** Eye opened to show the three tunics, which have been drawn thicker than they actually are.

1, Limbus; 2, upper fornix; 3, deep muscular fascia; 4, dorsal rectus muscle; 5, vagina bulbi; 6, choroid; 7, sclera; 8, ora serrata; 9, retina; 10, lens; 11, optic axis; 12, visual axis; 13, area cribrosa; 14, optic disc; 15, retina; 16, ciliary body; 17, iris; 18, cornea; 19, conjunctiva; 20, ventral rectus muscle; 21, optic nerve; 22, retractor bulbi; 23, sheath of optic nerve.

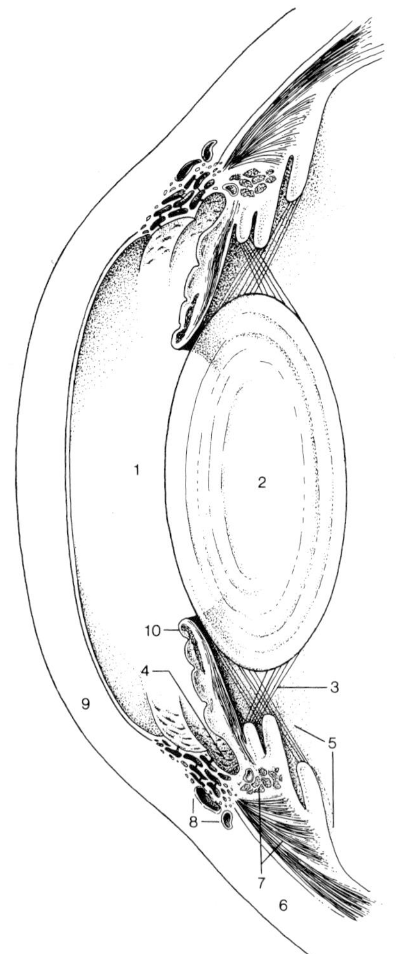


**Figure 9–4.** Anterior part of the eye in section.

1, Anterior chamber; 2, lens; 3, zonular fibers; 4, iridocorneal angle; 5, ciliary body; 6, sclera; 7, ciliary muscles; 8, venous plexus of sclera; 9, cornea; 10, iris with the sphincter and dilator muscles shown.

Near the limbus the sclera is covered by conjunctiva (see further on), which furnishes connection to the inside of the lids (/19).

The *cornea* forms about one quarter of the fibrous tunic and bulges forward (Plate 18/*E*). It is composed of a special kind of dense connective tissue arranged in lamellar form. It is generally recognized that, despite the careful arrangement of its fibers, transparency is not only a structural but also a physiological phenomenon and depends on the continuous pumping out of interstitial fluids, a process that has been localized in the posterior epithelium. Its main bulk (substantia propria) is continuous with the sclera (Fig. 9–4/9,6) and encased by anterior and posterior limiting membranes and epithelial layers. The anterior epithelial layer is continuous with the epithelium of the conjunctiva, while the posterior epithelial layer unites with the anterior surface of the iris across the iridocorneal angle (/4). The cornea does not contain blood vessels; nutrients for its cells permeate the substantia propria from vessels in the limbus or are carried to its surfaces in the lacrimal fluid and aqueous humor. The surface of the cornea is very sensitive owing to the presence of free nerve endings near the anterior epithelium. These arise from the long ciliary nerves, branches of the ophthalmic nerve (see further on). Their axons form the afferent limb of the *corneal reflex,* which closes the lids when the cornea is touched. This reflex is employed when monitoring deep anesthesia.

## The Vascular Tunic

The vascular tunic of the eye (also known as the uvea) lies deep to the sclera to which it is applied. It consists of three zones: choroid, ciliary body, and iris, given in posteroanterior sequence (Fig. 9–3). The choroid lines the sclera from the optic nerve almost to the limbus, the ciliary body follows as a thickened zone opposite the limbus, and the iris projects into the cavity of the eyeball posterior to the cornea; the iris is the only internal structure readily seen through the cornea without recourse to instruments (ophthalmoscope). Although blood supply is its principal function, the vascular tunic suspends the lens, regulates its curvature, and adjusts the size of the pupil by means of the smooth muscle in the ciliary body and iris (Fig. 9–4).

The *choroid* contains a dense network of blood vessels embedded in heavily pigmented connective tissue. The network is supplied by the posterior ciliary arteries and is drained by the vorticose veins. A flat sheet of capillaries on the internal surface is responsible for the nutrition of the external layers of the nervous tunic (retina), which lies deep (internal) to it. The blood in these capillaries produces the redness of the fundus (interior surface of the posterior hemisphere) seen when the eye is examined with an ophthalmoscope. In the dorsal part of the fundus the choroid forms a variously colored, light-reflecting area known as the *tapetum lucidum* (Plate 14/*A–F*). This is an avascular layer (cellular in carnivores, fibrous in ruminants and horses) between the capillaries and the network of larger vessels. The tapetal cells contain crystalline rods arranged in such a way that light striking them is split into its components, resulting in the characteristic iridescence. The packaging of the collagen in the fibrous tapetum has the same effect. The tapetum makes the eyes of animals "shine" when they look toward a light, such as the headlights of an oncoming car. Our eyes, and those of the pig, do not have a tapetum and therefore do not give this effect. It is believed that the tapetum is a nocturnal adaptation since by reflecting incident light it increases the stimulation of the light-sensitive receptor cells in the overlying retina and thus aids vision in dark places. The choroid adheres so closely to the pigmented external layer of the retina that the latter remains when the bulk of the retina is removed during dissection. The retina is without pigment where it overlies the tapetum lucidum.

Toward the limbus the choroid thickens to form the *ciliary body* (Fig. 9–4/5). This is a raised ring with ridges converging toward the lens in the center; anteriorly the ring is continued by the iris. The ciliary body is best comprehended when seen in its entirety by looking into the anterior part of the eye from behind (Fig. 9–5/2; Plate 14/*I*). The radial ridges, known as the *ciliary processes,* extend *zonular fibers* (Fig. 9–4/3) to the equator of the lens, suspending it around its periphery. Between the ciliary body and the sclera is the smooth *ciliary muscle* (/7), which functions in accommodation (the ability of the eye to focus on near or distant objects by changing the shape of the lens) (see further on).

The third and smallest part of the vascular tunic is the *iris* (/10), which is suspended between the cornea and lens. It is a flat ring of tissue attached at its periphery to the sclera (by the pectinate ligament; Fig. 9–8/7) and to the ciliary body; the opening in the center is the *pupil* (Fig. 9–6) through which light enters the posterior part of the eye. The size of the pupil and therefore the amount of light reaching the retina are regulated by smooth sphincter and dilator muscles in the iris. The sphincter lies near the pupillary margin, while the fibers of the dilator are arranged radially and upon contraction enlarge the pupil. Irregular outgrowths (iridic granules; /3; Plate 18/*H*) containing coils of capillaries are often seen on the upper and lower pupillary margins of ungulates; their significance is not known, though there are suggestions that they act as "shades."

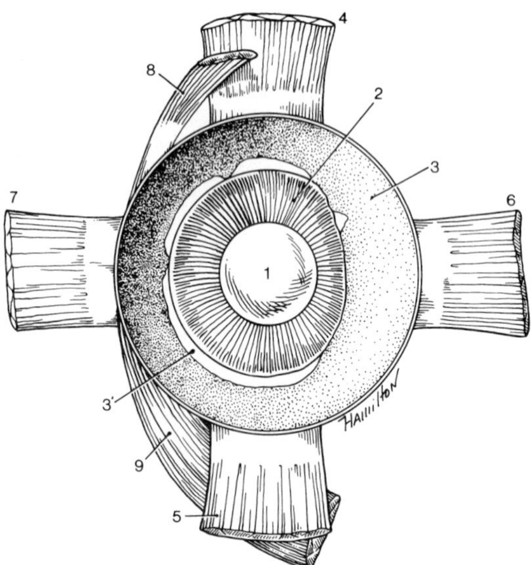


**Figure 9–5.** Anterior half of the left equine eye, viewed from behind.

1, Lens; 2, cililary body; 3, choroid covered by pigmented outer layer of retina; 3′, remnants of inner nervous layer of retina, which has been removed; 4–7, dorsal, ventral, medial, and lateral rectus muscles; 8, 9, dorsal and ventral oblique muscles.

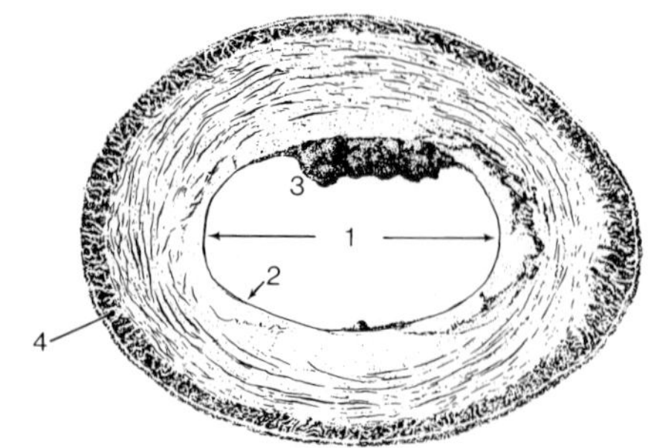


**Figure 9–6.** Anterior surface of the equine iris.

1, Pupil; 2, pupillary margin; 3, iridic granule; 4, pectinate ligament connecting iris to sclera in the iridocorneal angle.

The iris divides the space between the lens and cornea into anterior and posterior chambers that communicate through the pupil (Fig. 9–8). Both are filled with *aqueous humor,* a clear watery fluid (see further on).

The iris consists of three layers: an anterior epithelial layer continues across the iridocorneal angle and blends with the posterior epithelium of the cornea, a middle layer of connective tissue stroma contains the two smooth muscles, and the posterior layer of pigmented epithelium is the forward extension of the pigmented layer of the retina mentioned when we described the choroid; it is known as the iridic part of the retina and is closely related to the dilator pupillae (Fig. 9–4/10).

The color of the iris determines the "color of the eye" and depends on the number of pigmented cells present in its stroma and on the type of pigment in the cells. If the pigmented (melanin) cells are tightly packed the iris is dark brown; with fewer cells the iris is lighter and yellowish (Plate 18/*C,G*); and with a minimum of pigmented cells the iris appears bluish. In albinos pigment is also absent from the iridic part of the retina, that is to say, the iris is totally devoid of pigment; their eyes appear red because the blood in the capillaries is not obscured.

## The Internal Tunic

The internal or nervous tunic of the eyeball contains the light-sensitive receptor cells and is known as the *retina* (Fig. 9–3/9,15). It is an extension of the brain to which it remains connected by the optic nerve. The retina begins where the nerve penetrates the choroid; shaped like a hollow cup, it lines this and ends at the pupillary margin. Only the posterior two thirds or so of the retina can be reached by light entering the pupil. Consequently, only that part (pars optica retinae) is provided with receptor cells; it is relatively thick. The remaining third is "blind" (pars ceca retinae) and is mainly represented by the thin pigmented layer that continues on to the ciliary body and the back of the iris. The edge caused by the abrupt decrease in thickness at the junction of optic and blind parts is the *ora serrata* (/8); it also demarcates the choroid from the ciliary body. The two layers of the retina develop from the inner and outer layers of the optic cup with which the eye makes its appearance in the embryo (Fig. 9–17/4). The gap between the layers of the optic cup, though obliterated postnatally, remains a weakness where delamination produces "detachment of the retina."

The presence of so much retinal and choroidal pigment makes the interior of the posterior part of the eye dark like the inside of a camera so that the pupil appears black. The black walls absorb scattered and reflected light and prevent it from striking the retina a second time, which would contribute to blurred vision.

The layers in the pars optica retinae are as follows, beginning at the choroid: a single layer of pigmented cells; a neuroepithelial layer containing the receptor cells, rods and cones and their nuclei, the rods, so far as we know, being concerned with black and white (night) and the cones with color (day) vision; a layer of bipolar ganglion cells; and a layer of multipolar ganglion cells whose nonmyelinated axons, lying internal (deep) to the cells, pass to the optic disc where they aggregate to form the optic nerve. It will be clear from this arrangement that light passes through all layers except the first before reaching and stimulating the rods and cones (Fig. 9–7).

The area where the axons of the fourth layer concentrate to leave the eye, the *optic disc,* can easily be seen when examining the fundus with an ophthalmoscope (Plate 14/*A,F*). Because the axons here turn in toward the cribriform area of the sclera there is no room for receptor cells; the optic disc, therefore, is a blind spot. In contrast, an area of maximum optical resolution (macula) is located a short distance dorsolateral to the optic disc. It is believed that when we examine objects intently we focus them on the macula. It is not known whether animals do the same. In some species the macula is faintly visible with the ophthalmoscope. The *visual axis* is the line connecting the macula, the center of the lens, and the object viewed. It does not quite coincide with the optic axis because the macula is slightly dorsal to the posterior pole of the eyeball (Fig. 9–3).

Arterioles and venules emerging from the optic disc spread out in various species-specific patterns to nourish and drain the retina (Plate 14/*A,F*). The arterioles are branches of the central artery of the retina, which arrives at the optic disc in the center of the optic nerve.

The anteroposterior compression of the equine eyeball has led to the assumption that the horse has a ramp retina. A ramp retina is one in which all parts are not equidistant from the posterior pole of the lens; the distance from the lens becomes progressively greater as the retina is followed dorsally. Presumably, as increasingly closer objects are viewed they are focused on the more dorsal parts of the retina; focal length is automatically increased and little accommodation of the lens is required (p. 504).

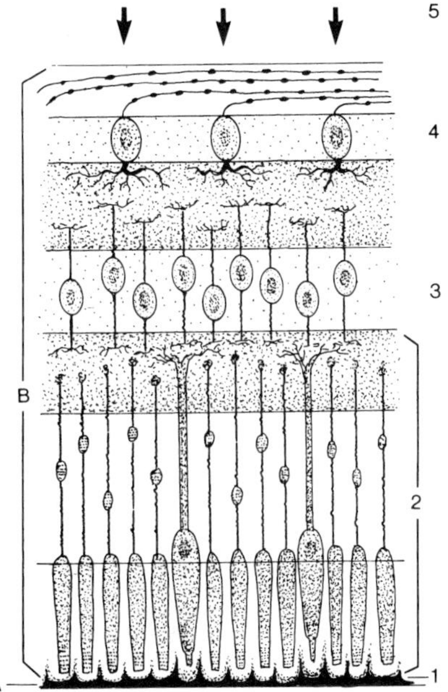


**Figure 9–7.** Outer pigmented layer (*A*) and inner neuroepithelial layer (*B*) of retina.

1, Pigmented cells; 2, receptor cells (rods and cones); 3, bipolar ganglion cells; 4, multipolar ganglion cells; 5, incoming light (*arrows*).

## *The Refractive Media of the Eyeball*

Now that the laminated wall has been described, it remains to say something of the interior of the eyeball, which is concerned with the manipulation of the light rays that enter it. It is best to do this by following the path taken by the light. Several interior structures have already been mentioned and require little further description.

The *cornea* is an integral part of the supporting fibrous tunic. Although dense and tough, it has the quality of being transparent and thus enables light to enter the eye. The cornea plays a major role in refraction, that is to say, it is capable, as is the lens, of bending light so that what is seen by the animal is miniaturized sufficiently to be focused on the retina.

The rays next encounter the *aqueous humor* filling the space between cornea and lens. The aqueous humor is a clear watery fluid that, apart from its refractive properties, plays an important role in the maintenance of intraocular pressure. It is continuously produced by cells of the ciliary processes and enters the system in the posterior chamber. From here it passes through the pupil into the anterior chamber and thence through the spaces in the trabecular tissue (pectinate ligament) at the iridocorneal angle. These spaces convey it to venous sinuses in the sclera and thus into the blood stream (Fig. 9–8). In the healthy eye the rate of production balances the rate of drainage, maintaining a constant pressure. Interference with drainage allows excess fluid to accumulate, causing the intraocular pressure to rise (glaucoma). This serious condition, common in humans, is rarely seen in animals.

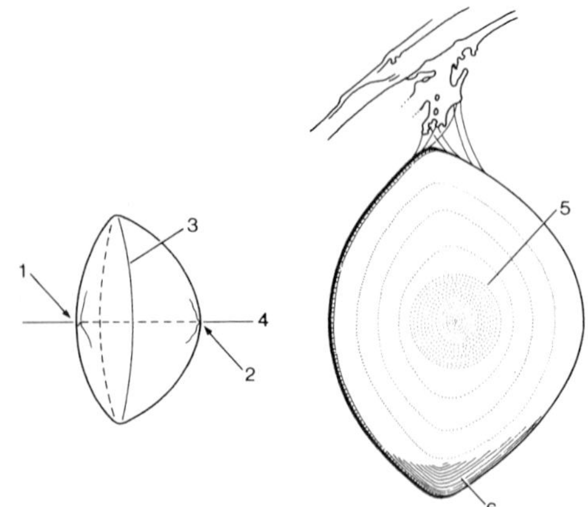


**Figure 9–9.** Bovine lens; on the right, a meridional section.

1, Anterior pole with lens star; 2, posterior pole with lens star; 3, equator; 4, optic axis; 5, nucleus; 6, layers of lens fibers, shown only in part.

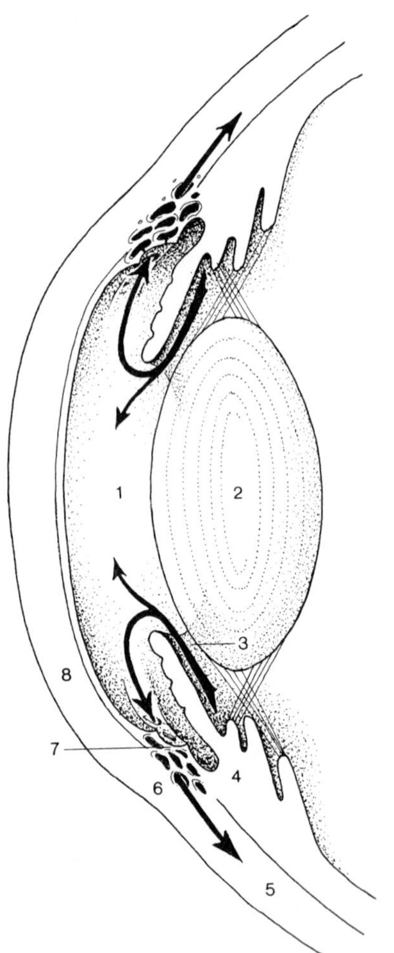


**Figure 9–8.** The flow *(arrows)* of aqueous humor.

1, Anterior chamber; 2, lens; 3, posterior chamber; 4, ciliary body; 5, sclera; 6, venous plexus; 7, pectinate ligament; 8, cornea.

The *lens* (Fig. 9–9), in contrast to its liquid neighbors, is a solid structure, though sufficiently elastic to be able to change in shape. It is biconvex and has anterior and posterior poles, an equator, and a central axis that coincides with the optic axis of the eye. The posterior surface is usually more convex than the anterior. The lens has an outer capsule that is thicker anteriorly and thickest at the equator, where the zonular fibers of the ciliary body are secured. The capsule of the lens is elastic and is permanently under tension, which, if unopposed by the pull exerted at the periphery, would cause the lens to assume a more spherical shape. The substance of the lens consists of very regularly arranged fibers. These form concentric sheets that can be peeled off like the layers of an onion. Within each sheet the fibers are so arranged that they loop from a point on the anterior surface to one on the posterior surface. Their ends are cemented to the ends of other fibers, forming visible sutures shaped like little three-pointed stars (radii lentis; /1,2). In the peripheral, or cortical, part of the lens the fibers are relatively soft; they are firmer and thinner toward the center where they form a harder nucleus. Owing to its elastic properties the cortex can be molded so that the lens changes shape during accommodation. In many older animals the lens becomes cloudy, impairing vision; the condition is known as cataract (Plate 18/*C,D*).

**Accommodation.** As we have said, the elastic capsule of the lens would squeeze the relatively soft cortex into a rounder shape unless opposed by the zonular fibers that arise from the ciliary processes and exert a constant radial pull on the equator. This pull flattens the lens into the shape described; this is the resting shape of the lens adapted for far vision and is present during sleep. When the animal wants to focus on a near object the muscle on the surface of the ciliary body contracts, thickening the ciliary body. This displaces the processes toward the lens and thus relaxes the zonular fibers. The lens, released from the tension at its equator, rounds out and brings the object into focus. Compared with the human condition, the ciliary muscle and, therefore, the ability to accommodate are poorly developed in domestic animals.

After passing through the lens the light rays enter the *vitreous body.* This is a gel-like mass consisting mainly of water (vitreous humor) but with a stroma of fine transparent fibers that condenses into a membrane at the surface. The vitreous body occupies the space between lens and retina and holds the latter against the choroid. In the embryo the lens is nourished by the hyaloid artery, a branch of the central retinal artery that passes through the vitreous body. The artery usually degenerates after birth and the lens is then nourished by diffusion. Unlike the aqueous humor, the vitreous humor is not continuously replaced; it is therefore constant in volume.

## The Adnexa of the Eye

The structures that protect and move the eyeball include the orbital fasciae, the ocular muscles, the eyelids and tunica conjunctiva, and the lacrimal apparatus; most are contained within the *orbit.* This is a cone-shaped cavity on the lateral surface of the skull that is delimited externally by a bony margin (base of cone). In the carnivores and pig the bone is deficient laterally but the ring is completed by the *orbital ligament* (see Fig. 2–31/1). The wall of the human orbit is entirely osseous, but in the domestic mammals the lateral and ventral parts are formed by the fibrous periorbita, one of the orbital fasciae (see further on).

### The Orbital Fasciae

The eyeball is surrounded by three roughly conical fascial layers. The most external of these is the periorbita, which has just been mentioned; internal to the periorbita are superficial and deep muscular fasciae (Fig. 9–10).

The *periorbita* is attached near the optic foramen at the apex of the cone. It blends with the periosteum at the orbital margin and on the medial and dorsal walls of the orbit. Elsewhere (mainly laterally and ventrally) it is free and forms a substantial fibrous partition between orbital and extraorbital structures (Fig. 9–11/11). The periorbita splits at the orbital margin. One part is continued as the periosteum of the facial bones; the other, the *orbital septum* (/2), forms two semilunar folds with thickened free margins (tarsi) that stiffen the edges of the upper and lower eyelids. The *trochlea* (/6), a flat piece of cartilage embedded in the dorsomedial wall close to the orbital margin, provides a pulley around which the dorsal oblique muscle winds to change direction by nearly 90 degrees.

The *superficial muscular fascia* lies within the periorbita; it is loose and fatty, and envelops the levator palpebrae superioris and the lacrimal gland (Fig. 9–10/3). The *deep muscular fascia* is more fibrous; it arises from the eyelids and from the limbus of the eyeball, which it closely invests. It is reflected around the muscles attaching to the eyeball, providing each (and also the optic nerve), with a fascial envelope. It is known as the vagina

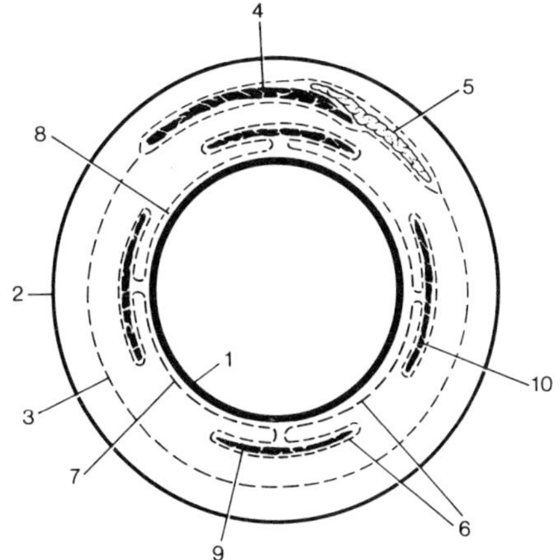


**Figure 9–10.** Schematic representation of the orbital fasciae: transection of orbital structures at the level of the eyeball. Part of the deep fascia (6) forms the vagina bulbi (7).

1, Eyeball; 2, periorbita; 3, superficial muscular fascia; 4, levator palpebrae; 5, lacrimal gland; 6, deep muscular fascia; 7, vagina bulbi; 8, episcleral space; 9, ventral rectus muscle; 10, lateral rectus muscle.

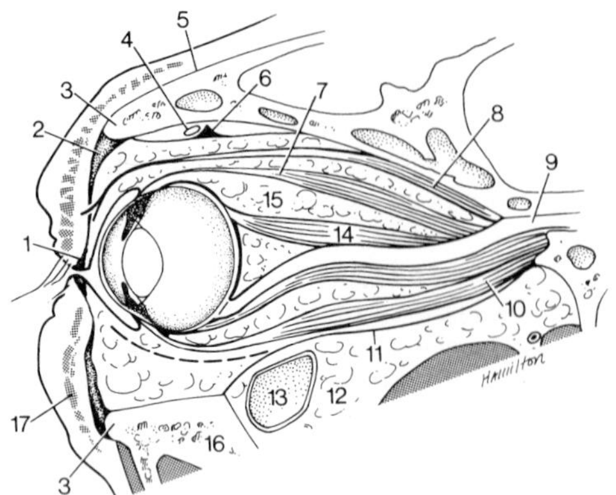


**Figure 9–11.** Right bovine eye cut along orbital axis, rostromedial surface.

1, Tarsus; 2, orbital septum; 3, orbital margin; 4, dorsal oblique muscle; 5, periosteum of face; 6, trochlea; 7, dorsal rectus muscle; 8, levator palpebrae superioris; 9, optic nerve in optic foramen; 10, ventral rectus muscle; 11, periorbita; 12, extraperiorbital fat; 13, lacrimal bulla, a caudal recess of the maxillary sinus; 14, retractor bulbi; 15, intraperiorbital fat; 16, zygomatic arch; 17, orbicularis.

bulbi (/7), where it is applied to the eyeball, though separated by a narrow episcleral space. The presence of this space facilitates the movement of the eyeball against the retrobulbar fat. In enucleation (removal of the eye), advantage is usually taken of this arrangement; the eyeball is freed and the vagina bulbi and the retrobulbar structures it covers are left in place.

## The Muscles of the Eyeball

The muscles that move the eye are located behind the eyeball. All except one originate in the vicinity of the optic foramen at the apex of the orbital cone. There are four rectus muscles, two oblique muscles, and a retractor.

The four *rectus muscles*—dorsal, ventral, medial, and lateral—are inserted anterior to the equator by wide but very thin tendons (Fig. 9–5). The *dorsal* and *ventral oblique muscles* attach to the eyeball near the equator and on contraction tend to rotate the eyeball around the visual axis (Fig. 9–12/1,7). The dorsal oblique muscle also arises close to the optic foramen and passes forward on the dorsomedial wall of the orbit before it is deflected around the trochlea to end on the dorsolateral surface of the eyeball beneath the tendon of the dorsal rectus muscle. A small synovial sheath protects the muscle as it passes around the trochlea, which in fact is its functional origin. If this muscle were to contract by itself, it would pull the dorsal part of the eyeball medially.

The ventral oblique muscle, uniquely, does not arise from the vicinity of the optic foramen. Instead, it takes its origin from a depression in the ventromedial wall of the orbit, passing laterally below the eyeball and the tendon of the ventral rectus muscle before inserting on the ventrolateral part of the eyeball. Its contraction, if isolated from the action of the other muscles, would rotate the eyeball around the visual axis so that the dorsal portion of the eyeball would move laterally. The *retractor bulbi* (Fig. 9–11/14) arises from the vicinity of the optic foramen but is inserted on the eyeball posterior to the equator. It forms a nearly complete muscular cone about the optic nerve (Fig. 9–13/7). The retractor is not present in ourselves, and it is still a matter of conjecture why we do not possess the ability to retract our eyes; perhaps we do not need the additional protection provided to the more protruding eyes of animals.

The movements of the eyes are much more complex than the origins and insertions of the individual muscles suggest. As far as we know, none ever acts singly. It seems that the tonus is increased or decreased in opposing groups for smooth transition from one eye position to another. The most difficult actions to explain are those of the oblique muscles, since there is no significant rotation around the visual axis in any usual movement. Their participation is required for the following reason. The rectus muscles arise slightly medioventral to the point where the visual axis, if extended caudally, would strike the skull. That is to say, the visual axis does not coincide with the axis of the orbital cone. As a result, the dorsal rectus muscle, to take one example, would not simply elevate the cranial pole of the eyeball but would also rotate the eyeball so that its dorsal part

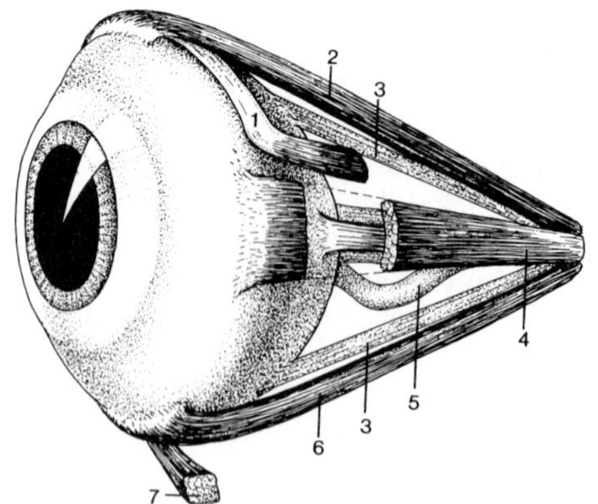


**Figure 9–12.** Ocular muscles.

1, Dorsal oblique m.; 2, dorsal rectus m.; 3, retractor bulbi; 4, medial rectus m.; 5, optic nerve; 6, ventral rectus m.; 7, ventral oblique m.

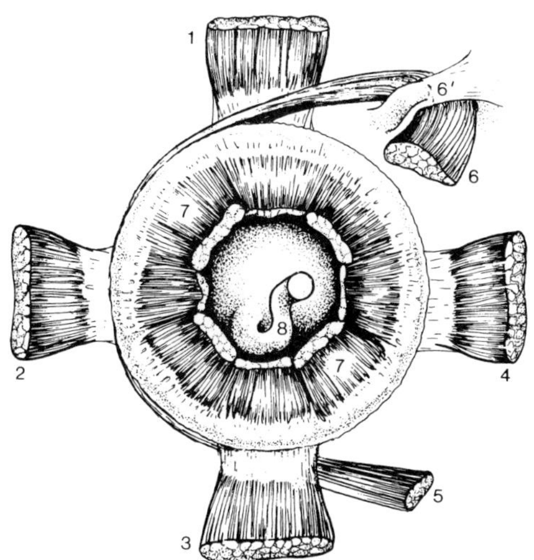


**Figure 9–13.** Stumps of ocular muscles viewed from behind the left eyeball.

1, Dorsal rectus m.; 2, lateral rectus m.; 3, ventral rectus m.; 4, medial rectus m.; 5, ventral oblique m.; 6, dorsal oblique m.; 6′, trochlea; 7, retractor bulbi; 8, optic nerve.

moved slightly medially. This slight intorsion is reflexively resisted by the ventral oblique, and the result is a smooth elevation of the anterior pole. The reverse happens in depression of the eyeball when the ventral rectus and the dorsal oblique muscles are involved.

An additional striated muscle within the orbit is conveniently considered here. This is the *levator palpebrae superioris* (Fig. 9–11/8). It does not attach to the eyeball but passes over it to enter and elevate the upper eyelid.

In addition to these striated muscles there are three sheets of smooth muscle, although they are rarely observed during routine dissection. One (m. orbitalis) consists of a sheet of circular (with regard to visual axis) fibers applied to the internal surface of the periorbita. A ventral longitudinal sheet extends from the sheath of the ventral rectus muscle into the lower lid (as the m. tarsalis inferior) and into the third eyelid (see further on). A medial longitudinal sheet extends from the sheath of the medial rectus muscle and from the trochlea into the upper eyelid (as the m. tarsalis superior) and into the third eyelid. Tonus in these sheets maintains the normal protruded position of the eye and retracted position of the eyelids.

## The Eyelids and Conjunctiva

The eyelids (palpebrae) are two musculofibrous folds of which the upper is the more extensive and more mobile. The free margins of the lids meet at the medial and lateral *angles of the eye* and bound an opening known as the *palpebral fissure.*

The eyelids consist of three layers: skin, a middle musculofibrous layer, and a mucous membrane, known as the palpebral conjunctiva, facing the eye (Fig. 9–14).

The *skin* of the lids is thin and delicate, and is covered with short hairs; it may also carry a few prominent tactile hairs.

The *musculofibrous layer* is formed by the orbicularis oculi, the orbital septum, the aponeurosis of the levator muscle, and the smooth tarsal muscle. The orbital septum arises from the margin of the orbit; the aponeurosis of the levator and the tarsal muscle originate in the orbit. Except for the orbicularis oculi, which lies directly under the skin and can be dissected away, the components of this layer intermingle inseparably. Toward the free margin these components are succeeded by the *tarsus* (/2′), a platelike fibrous condensation that stabilizes the edge of the lid. The ends of the two

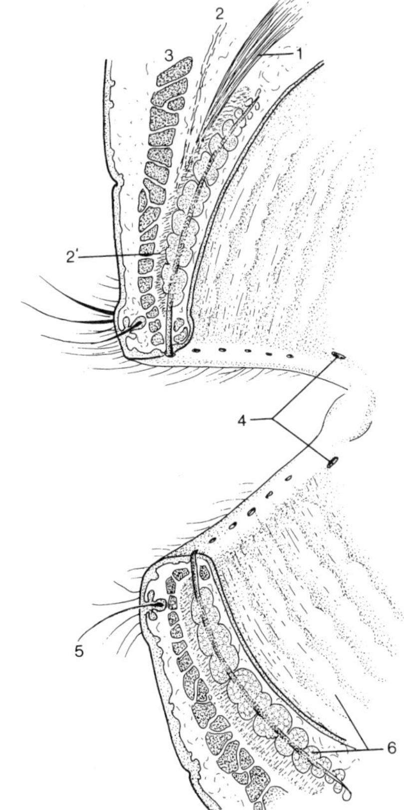


**Figure 9–14.** Eyelids, sectioned and viewed obliquely from behind.

1, Levator palpebrae superioris; 2, orbital septum; 2′, tarsus; 3, orbicularis oculi; 4, puncta lacrimalia; 5, cilium with associated ciliary and sebaceous glands; 6, tarsal glands.

tarsi are anchored to the orbital margin by medial and lateral *palpebral ligaments* that assure an elongated palpebral fissure when the eye is closed (by the orbicularis oculi). Deep to the tarsus, and opening onto the edge of the lid by a row of tiny openings, is a series of *tarsal glands* (/6) that secrete a fatty material. Just in front of these glandular openings are the *cilia* (eyelashes), which are usually more prominent and numerous on the upper than on the lower lid; conspicuous cilia are absent from the lower lid of carnivores. Small ciliary and sebaceous glands are associated with the roots of the cilia; the common stye (hordeolum) is an inflammation of one of these glands.

The posterior surface of the lid is lined with conjunctiva, a thin, transparent mucous membrane. The *palpebral conjunctiva* is reflected at the base of the lids to continue on the sclera as the *bulbar conjunctiva,* which ends at the limbus although the epithelium continues as the anterior epithelium of the cornea. The potential space between the lids and the eyeball is known as the *conjunctival sac* whose dorsal and ventral extremities are the *fornices* (Fig. 9–3/2). The transparency of the conjunctiva renders the smaller blood vessels visible, especially when they are congested in infections. Those in the bulbar conjunctiva move with this loosely attached layer; the deeper scleral vessels do not. Advantage is taken of this arrangement to distinguish inflammation of the conjunctiva from that of deeper structures. A pale conjunctiva suggests anemia, shock, or internal hemorrhage.

A slight mucosal elevation, the *lacrimal caruncle,* is present in the medial angle of the eye; it bears a few fine hairs in the large species (Fig. 9–15/2).

Between the lacrimal caruncle and the eyeball is a dorsoventrally oriented conjunctival fold known as the *third eyelid* (/6). Unlike a true lid, it is covered with conjunctiva on both sides and is invisible when the eye is closed. The third eyelid is supported by a T-shaped piece of cartilage (/6′) whose bar lies in the free edge of the fold and whose stem points backward into the orbit medial to the eyeball. The stem of the cartilage is surrounded by an additional lacrimal gland, the *gland of the third eyelid;* pigs and cattle also have a second, deeper gland. The secretion of these glands enters the conjunctival sac on the bulbar surface of the third eyelid. The third eyelid is kept retracted by smooth muscle (m. orbitalis) under sympathetic influence. It slides over the eyeball when the latter is retracted or pushed into the orbit. The lid, in conjunction with the retractor bulbi muscle, is thought to provide added protection to the protruding eyes of animals.

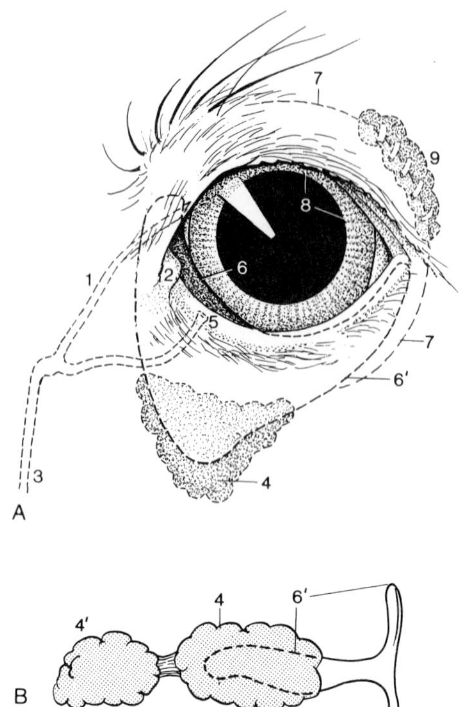


**Figure 9–15.** *A,* Left eye of dog showing third eyelid and lacrimal apparatus. *B,* Isolated cartilage of the third eyelid and associated glands of a pig.

1, Upper canaliculus; 2, lacrimal caruncle; 3, nasolacrimal duct; 4, gland of third eyelid; 4′, deep gland of third eyelid; 5, punctum lacrimale; 6, third eyelid; 6′, cartilage of third eyelid; 7, position of conjunctival fornix; 8, pupil; 9, lacrimal gland.

## The Lacrimal Apparatus

This consists of the lacrimal gland proper, the gland(s) associated with the third eyelid, several small accessory glands, and a duct system that conveys the lacrimal fluid (tears), after it has washed over the eye, into the nasal cavity for evaporation. The *lacrimal gland* is flat and lies between the eyeball and the dorsolateral wall of the orbit (/9). Its secretion is drained by many minute ducts into the dorsal fornix of the conjunctival sac where it mixes with the secretions of the lesser glands. Blinking movements distribute the lacrimal fluid over the exposed part of the eye, which is thus kept moist; the tears carry away foreign material and supply the cornea with some nutriment. The fluid, being repelled by the fatty secretion of the tarsal glands along the edge of the lids, is normally pooled at the medial angle of the eye in the so-called *lacrimal lake,* a shallow depression surrounding the lacrimal caruncle, before being drawn by capillary action into the duct system through the puncta lacrimalia (Fig. 9–14/4). Lacrimal fluid escapes onto the face only when produced in excessive amounts or when normal drainage is impaired.

The *puncta lacrimalia* are minute slits, one on the edge of each lid next to the caruncle. Each punctum leads to a short, narrow *canaliculus* through which the fluid flows to the much longer *nasolacrimal duct* (Fig. 9–15/3). The beginning of the nasolacrimal duct is slightly enlarged, forming the *lacrimal sac,* which occupies a funnel-shaped fossa near the bony margin of the orbit. The nasolacrimal duct runs rostrally, at first within the thickness of the maxilla, then on its internal surface where it is covered by nasal mucosa. In some species it ends at the nostril, in others more deeply in the nasal cavity.

The tear film washing the eye consists of three layers. The outermost lipid layer is derived from the secretion of the tarsal glands; it helps spread the tears evenly and retards the breakup of the film. The thick middle aqueous layer is derived from the lacrimal glands; it moistens and nourishes the cornea. The innermost mucinous layer is produced by goblet cells in the conjunctiva and holds the tear film intimately to the cornea. Tear flow can be increased by drugs or reflexively after stimulation of the conjunctiva, cornea, or nasal mucosa. Weeping as an expression of emotion is a purely human phenomenon.

## The Development of the Eye

A brief account of the development of the eye will aid in understanding this complex organ. The eye develops from neuroectoderm of the neural tube and from the mesoderm and surface ectoderm that surround and cover this. The neuroectoderm contributes the retina and optic nerve; the mesoderm forms the remaining structures except the lens, the lacrimal glands, and the epithelia of the conjunctival sac and lids, which are supplied by the surface ectoderm. The three layers of the eyeball—the retina, choroid, and sclera—reflect the eyeball's origin as an outgrowth of the embryonic brain; the retina corresponds to and is continuous with the brain tissue, the choroid corresponds to the pia-arachnoid, and the sclera corresponds to the dura mater.

Development begins with a lateral evagination (optic vesicle) from the rostral end of the neural tube. This makes contact with the overlying ectoderm and stimulates it to thicken (Fig. 9–16/1). Soon thereafter, the distal (anterior) part of the vesicle invaginates to form a double-walled (optic) cup (/6). The invagination is incomplete ventrally, leaving a fissure (/8) that extends proximally along the stalk of the cup that has been drawn out in the meantime. The thickened ectoderm (lens placode) overlying the cup invaginates, becomes detached, and rounds off into a smaller (lens) vesicle, which occupies the mouth of the optic cup.

The two walls of the optic cup give rise to the pigmented and sensory layers of the retina (Fig. 9–17/4). The space that at first separates them disappears, though the layers will easily separate postnatally. The outer layer remains thin and soon acquires pigment granules. The inner layer thickens, especially in its posterior two thirds (pars optica retinae). Its cells form layers reminiscent of those in the developing forebrain from which the cup arose. The outermost cells, those closest to the pigment layer, differentiate into the rods and cones. The cells internal to this form the ganglion and glia cells. The processes growing from the ganglion cells occupy the innermost layer, where they converge on the optic fissure that conducts them to the brain. The anterior third of the inner cup wall (pars ceca retinae) remains thin and, together with the pigment layer, lines the posterior surface of the ciliary body and iris, which have yet

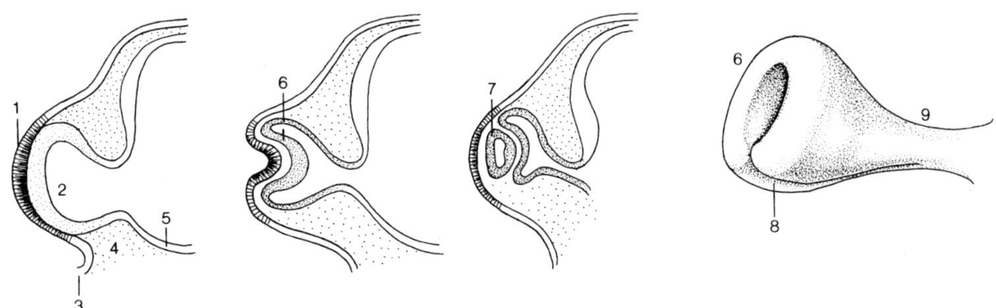


**Figure 9–16.** Early development of the eye.

1, Lens placode; 2, optic vesicle; 3, ectoderm; 4, mesoderm; 5, neuroectoderm of neural tube; 6, optic cup; 7, lens vesicle; 8, optic fissure; 9, optic stalk.

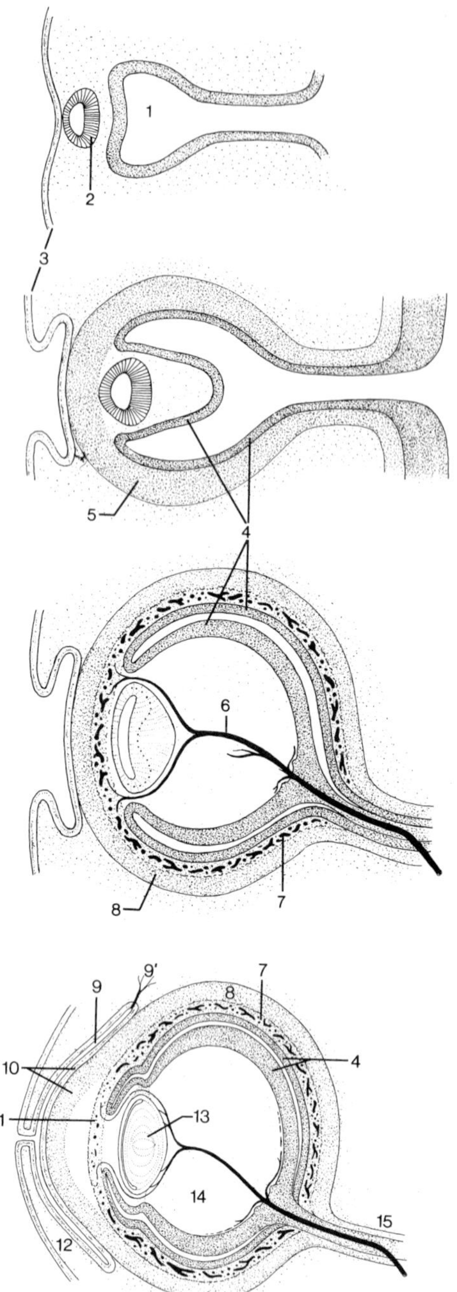


**Figure 9–17.** Development of the eye.

1, Optic cup; 2, lens vesicle; 3, ectoderm; 4, inner and outer layers of optic cup, forming retina; 5, condensed mesoderm; 6, hyaloid artery; 7, choroid; 8, sclera; 9, conjunctival sac; 9′, sprouts of lacrimal gland; 10, cornea; 11, iridopupillary membrane; 12, lower eyelid; 13, lens; 14, vitreous body; 15, optic nerve.

to be established. The cup enlarges while these cellular changes are taking place. Its edges creep over the anterior surface of the lens vesicle and eventually bound the pupil.

The mesenchyme (primary vitreous body) occupying the optic cup is invaded through the optic fissure by (hyaloid) blood vessels (/6; Plate 14/*G,H*) that spread over the inner layer of the cup and the posterior surface of the lens vesicle. It is not clear whether the inner layer of the cup or the mesenchyme lying against it elaborates the secondary (definitive) vitreous body that gradually surrounds the primary substance and restricts it to a central (hyaloid) canal running from the optic disc to the lens. The edges of the optic fissure close over the hyaloid artery and nerve fibers, incorporating them into the optic stalk. The artery eventually regresses but the nerve fibers increase and transform the stalk into the optic nerve.

The anterior wall of the lens vesicle remains thin; it develops into the single layer of epithelial cells present on the anterior surface of the functional lens. The posterior wall thickens in an anterior direction, reducing and finally eliminating the lumen of the vesicle (/13). Its cells grow into long fibers that form a sphere destined to become the nucleus of the lens. More fibers are added to the equator; these form the softer substance that surrounds the nucleus.

The mesenchyme that surrounds the optic cup and stalk, and is present between the surface ectoderm and the lens vesicle, condenses and completely encloses cup and lens (/5). The tissue adjacent to the cup remains loosely arranged and gives rise to the vascular tunic (choroid, ciliary body, and iris). The mesenchyme outside this continues to condense into the sclera and the bulk of the cornea, the anterior epithelial layer of the latter being supplied by the surface ectoderm. The mesenchyme between the developing cornea and lens splits into a thin layer destined to become the posterior epithelial layer of the cornea and a thicker layer that gives rise to the iris. The latter, however, is continuous across the anterior surface of the lens as the iridopupillary membrane, which eventually disappears (/11). The space created by the split is the beginning of the anterior eye chamber. It communicates with a similar excavation between the lens and developing iris once the iridopupillary membrane has broken down, leaving free pupillary margins.

The lids begin to form when the anterior eye chamber appears. They grow over the developing cornea and fuse, creating and temporarily closing the conjunctival sac. The third eyelid develops much later as a vertical fold pushing into the medial part of the conjunctival sac. Sprouts (/9′) of conjunctival sac epithelium grow into the mesenchyme surrounding the eyeball and give rise to the lacrimal gland and the accessory glands, including those of the third eyelid. The lids of ungulates separate again close to birth. Puppies, like kittens (and most rodents), are born with their eyes still closed; their lids separate about 10 days after birth. The nasolacrimal duct develops from the surface ectoderm of the groove running rostrally from the eye between the maxillary and lateral nasal processes. The floor of the groove becomes separated from the surface and is later canalized to connect the conjunctival sac with the nasal cavity (see Fig. 3–52).

## The Blood Supply of the Eye

The blood supply to the eyeball and its adnexa is complex (Fig. 9–18). The blood supply to the human eye enters the orbit with the optic nerve. This route is represented in the domestic mammals by the rudimentary internal ophthalmic artery (/2), which loses its identity when joined by a sizable anastomosis (/4) from the external ophthalmic. The principal supply is carried by the *external ophthalmic artery* (/3), a branch detached from the maxillary as this passes ventral to the orbit to supply more rostral structures of the face. The arteries arising from the external ophthalmic and malar arteries (a further, smaller branch of the maxillary) can be divided into three groups: (1) those supplying the eyeball, (2) those supplying ocular muscles, and (3) those leaving the orbit to supply adjacent structures whether or not these are associated with the eye.

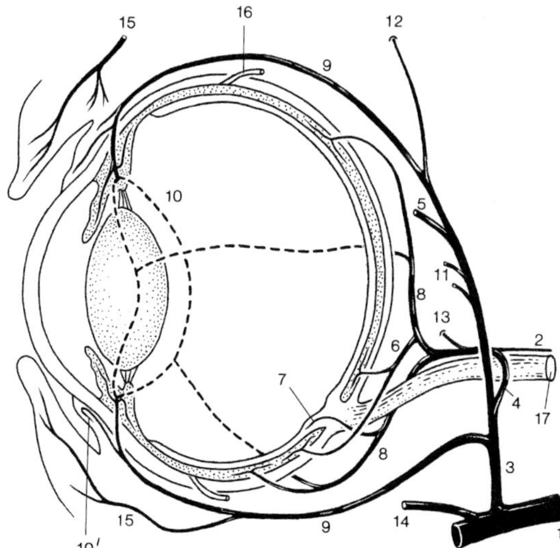


**Figure 9–18.** The principal arteries supplying the eye.

1, Maxillary a.; 2, rudimentary internal ophthalmic a.; 3, external ophthalmic a.; 4, anastomosis between external and internal ophthalmic aa.; 5, lacrimal a. to lacrimal gland and upper lid; 6, short posterior ciliary aa.; 7, retinal aa.; 8, long posterior ciliary aa.; 9, anterior ciliary aa., substantial branches to 10 in horse, lesser branches in the other domestic species; 10, greater arterial circle of the iris; 10′, annular pericorneal network; 11, muscular branches; 12 supraorbital a. and foramen; 13, external ethmoidal a. and foramen; 14, malar a.; 15, palpebral branches; 16, vorticose veins; 17, optic nerve.

1. The branches of the external ophthalmic artery for the eyeball penetrate the sclera to reach the vascular tunic and the retina. *Short posterior ciliary arteries* (/6) penetrate near the optic nerve and supply the adjacent choroid in addition to branches to the optic nerve. The latter form the *central artery of the retina,* the parent vessel for the retinal arteries (/7; Plate 14/*A–F*). *Long posterior ciliary arteries* (/8) pass through the sclera somewhat closer to the equator. The *anterior ciliary arteries* (/9) penetrate near the limbus and supply the anterior portion of the choroid, the ciliary body, and the iris. These arteries anastomose to form the *greater arterial circle of the iris* (/10) from which numerous fine branches pass toward the pupil and into the ciliary body. Capillaries near the limbus nourish the cornea by diffusion. The anterior ciliary arteries also send branches to the conjunctiva (Plate 18/*F*). The principal venous return is by several *vorticose veins* (/16) that emerge from the sclera near the equator. The extraocular veins of carnivores and ruminants form substantial venous plexuses within the periorbita. Venous blood returning from the retina leaves at the optic disc through small veins satellite to the short posterior ciliary arteries.

2. No more need be said about the arteries supplying the ocular muscles except that most enter the muscles proximally. The absence of larger vessels in the distal ends reduces bleeding when the muscles are cut during enucleation.

3. Only four of the arteries that leave the orbit require mention. The *lacrimal artery* (/5) passes forward in the lateral part of the orbital cone and, after supplying the lacrimal gland en route, crosses the dorsolateral part of the orbital margin to supply lateral parts of the eyelids and conjunctiva. The *supraorbital artery* (/12) passes dorsally and leaves the orbit by the supraorbital foramen. It ramifies subcutaneously medial to the orbit and may send branches into the upper eyelid. (Carnivores have no supraorbital foramen and artery; the blood supply to their eyelids comes from long branches of the superficial temporal artery.) The *malar artery* (/14) arises directly from the maxillary and passes over the ventral wall of the orbit to the medial angle of the eye, where it supplies the eyelids and also the adjacent area of the face. The *external ethmoidal artery* (/13) has the shortest intraorbital course of the four. It leaves the orbit through the ethmoidal foramen and supplies the ethmoid labyrinth of the nasal cavity.

Most of the arteries described also take part in supplying the fat, fascia, and nerves within the orbit. There is some interspecific variation but this is rarely of practical concern. However, it may be noted that the external ophthalmic artery of the ruminants breaks up and forms a small arterial network (rete mirabile ophthalmicum) on entering the orbit. The various arteries, except the malar, arise from this.

### The Nerve Supply of the Eye

The nerve supply to the eye and its accessory structures is derived from no fewer than six cranial nerves. Most of these enter the orbital cone but some reach accessory structures directly.

The *optic nerve* (II) enters the orbit through the optic foramen and passes to the light receptor cells in the retina. It is rather slack in order to allow for the movements of the eye and is covered by meninges that it acquired during its development as the stalk of the optic cup.

Though the name of the *oculomotor nerve* (III) implies that it controls movement of the eyeball, it does not innervate all the ocular muscles. It enters the orbit through the orbital foramen (fissure; foramen orbitorotundum in ruminants and pig) and sends branches to the levator palpebrae, the dorsal, medial, and ventral recti, the ventral oblique, and part of the retractor muscles.

The *trochlear nerve* (IV) accompanies the third nerve and innervates the dorsal oblique muscle.

The ophthalmic and maxillary divisions of the *trigeminal nerve* (V) send branches to the eye. The *ophthalmic nerve* passes through the orbital foramen and supplies the following sensory branches: long ciliary nerves to the eyeball, especially the cornea; a lacrimal nerve to the eyelids and conjunctiva of the lateral angle; a supraorbital nerve that accompanies the like-named artery through the supraorbital foramen to supply the upper eyelid and skin medial to the orbit; an infratrochlear nerve (not present in all species) sensory to structures near the medial angle of the eye; and an ethmoidal nerve that follows the ethmoidal artery to innervate the caudal part of the nasal cavity. The *maxillary nerve* has only one relevant branch; this, the zygomatic nerve, supplies the lateroventral segment of the eyelids and conjunctiva by a zygomaticofacial branch, and skin caudal to the orbit by a zygomaticotemporal branch. In horned cattle the zygomaticotemporal branch furnishes the clinically important cornual nerve to the horn. These sensory nerves to the orbit provide the afferent limbs of the palpebral and corneal reflexes that stimulate the orbicularis oculi to close the eye when the lids or cornea are touched.

The *abducent nerve* (VI) enters through the orbital foramen. It innervates most of the retractor bulbi and the lateral rectus muscles.

The auriculopalpebral branch of the *facial nerve* (VII) passes between the eye and ear, and thus approaches the eyelids from behind. It innervates the orbicularis oculi. It may be blocked in order to immobilize the lids or to relieve the "pressure" on a painful globe that the tonus of the muscle may exert. (The levator palpebrae is not immobilized by this block.)

*Sympathetic nerve fibers* arising from the cranial cervical ganglion follow arteries or the ophthalmic nerve to the orbit, where they innervate the orbital muscle and dilator of the pupil. Tonus in the orbital muscle keeps the eyeball protruded, the third eyelid retracted, and the palpebral fissure open. Loss of sympathetic innervation results in a sunken eye, protrusion of the third eyelid, and constriction of the pupil (Horner's syndrome). Dilation of the pupil (mydriasis) is initiated by fear, excitement, or pain.

*Parasympathetic* presynaptic *nerve fibers* enter the orbit within the oculomotor nerve. They synapse in the ciliary ganglion and the postsynaptic fibers (which form the short ciliary nerves) innervate the ciliary muscle and the constrictor of the pupil. They control both the accommodation of the lens and the pupillary contraction (miosis) response to light.

## THE EAR

The ear is appropriately called the *vestibulocochlear organ* since it not only enables the animal to hear but also provides it with a sense of balance. The mechanical stimuli produced by sound waves are transformed into nerve impulses in the *cochlea;* and the action of small amounts of fluid and microscopic crystals on neuroreceptors within the *vestibule* provides the animal with a perception of the attitude and movement of its head with respect to gravity. Both functions are performed in the internal ear, the most medial of the three subdivisions of the ear as a whole. The other subdivisions are the middle ear and the external ear. Only the external ear is visible in the intact animal, the other two being housed in the temporal bone (Fig. 9–19/24).

### The External Ear

The external ear consists of two parts, the auricle and the external acoustic meatus (/1,2). The auricle, or pinna, is the "ear" as it is understood by the layperson, the part that sticks out from the

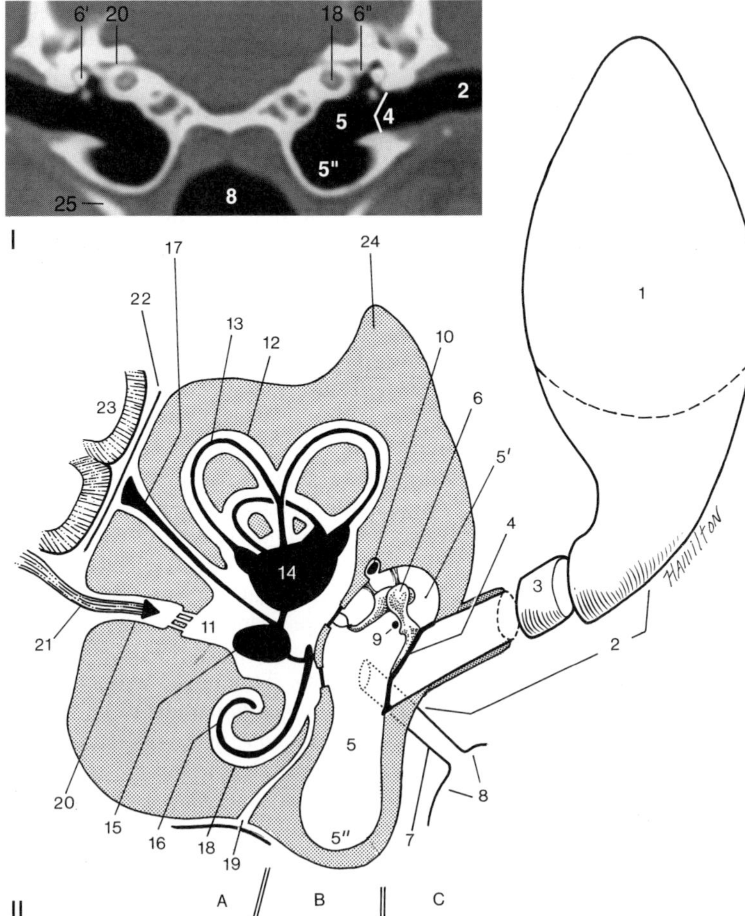


**Figure 9–19.** *I,* Transverse image of a 2-mm-thick computed tomographic slice of the canine tympanic bullae and petrous temporal bones. (Bone settings were used.) *II,* Schema of the right ear, caudal view. Note that the sizes of the structures shown are out of proportion to each other. *A,* Internal ear. *B,* Middle ear. *C,* External ear.

1, Auricle; 2, external acoustic meatus; 3, annular cartilage; 4, tympanic membrane; 5, tympanic cavity; 5′, epitympanic recess; 5″, tympanic bulla; 6, auditory ossicles; 6′, malleus; 6″, base of stapes in vestibular window; 7, auditory tube; 8, nasopharynx; 9, chorda tympani; 10, facial nerve; 11, vestibule; 12, semicircular canals; 13, semicircular ducts; 14, utricle; 15, saccule; 16, cochlear duct; 17, endolymphatic duct; 18, cochlea; 19, perilymphatic duct; 20, internal acoustic meatus; 21, vestibulocochlear nerve in internal acoustic meatus; 22, meninges; 23, brain; 24, petrous temporal bone; 25, stylohyoid bone.

head. The external acoustic meatus is the canal that leads from the base of the auricle to the eardrum (tympanic membrane) stretched across an opening in the temporal bone.

The auricle is shaped like a funnel; distally it is wide open to receive the sound, and more proximally it is rolled up to form a tube that bends medially for connection with the external acoustic meatus. The auricle can be turned toward the source of sound; right and left auricles can move independently so that each can focus on separate sounds. The animal does not have to turn its head as we with our immobile "ears" are obliged to do.

The shape of the auricle is determined by the supporting *auricular cartilage.* In most domestic mammals this is sufficiently stiff to keep the auricle erect at all times. In many breeds of dogs and in certain other animals, the cartilage is relatively soft, allowing the auricle to collapse; even so, most dogs can prick their ears and make them turn when attention to sound requires it. The parts of the auricular cartilage and the separate annular cartilage, which supports part of the external acoustic meatus, are shown in Figure 9–20.

A complex set of *auricular muscles,* all voluntary, is responsible for the movement of the ear. These muscles arise from various points on the skull and adjacent fasciae and attach to the base of the auricle. A flat, palpable (scutiform) cartilage rostral to the ear redirects the pull of some. The auricular muscles are innervated by branches of the facial nerve.

The *external acoustic meatus* begins where the rolled-up part of the auricular cartilage narrows and ends at the eardrum (Fig. 9–19/2). The meatus therefore has cartilaginous and osseous parts. It is lined with skin that contains sebaceous and tubular ceruminous glands. The latter secrete the earwax (cerumen), which is thought to prevent dust from reaching the delicate tympanic membrane. The ear of the dog is of the most clinical interest. Unfortunately, its external acoustic meatus is curved, making the passage of the straight otoscope for the examination of the proximal part of the meatus and eardrum difficult.

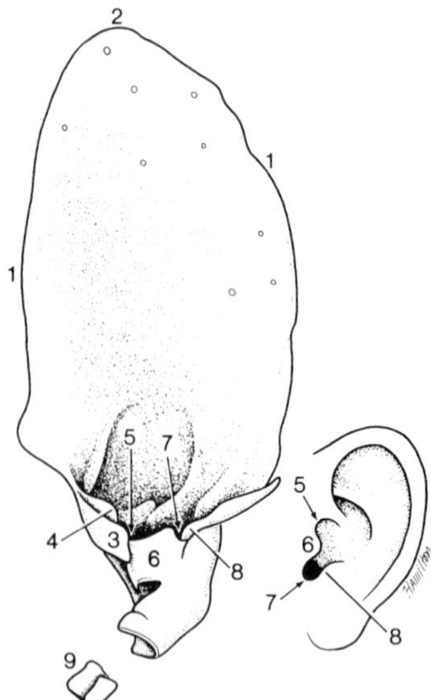


**Figure 9–20.** Left auricular cartilage of dog compared with human ear.

1, Helix; 2, apex; 3, medial crus of helix; 4, lateral crus of helix; 5, pretragic notch; 6, tragus; 7, intertragic notch; 8, antitragus; 9, annular cartilage.

## The Middle Ear

The middle ear is housed in the temporal bone and is essentially the small air-filled space known as the *tympanic cavity* (Fig. 9–19/5). It is lined with a thin mucous membrane and communicates with the nasopharynx by the auditory tube (/7). The upper part of the tympanic cavity is compressed from side to side and slanted outward. The lateral wall of the cavity incorporates the *tympanic membrane* (/4). The medial wall is formed by the petrous part of the temporal bone, which houses the internal ear. It contains two windows (fenestrae), closed in the natural state, through which the mechanical stimuli produced by sound waves enter the internal ear for translation into nerve impulses. The more dorsal *vestibular window* connects the tympanic cavity with the vestibule of the internal ear. In the live animal it is occupied by the stapes, the most medial of the auditory ossicles (/6). The other, the *cochlear window,* leads to the cavity of the cochlea (/18). It is closed by the thin secondary tympanic membrane. Ventral to the two windows the medial wall bulges over the cochlea, forming the promontory.

The tympanic cavity may be divided into dorsal, middle, and ventral parts. The dorsal part (epitympanic recess) is situated above the level of the tympanic membrane. It contains the chain of auditory ossicles and the two associated muscles. The middle part includes the tympanic membrane in its lateral wall and opens rostrally into the nasopharynx via the auditory tube. The ventral part is an enlarged bulbous extension of the temporal bone known as the *tympanic bulla* (/5″). The bulla varies in prominence among species; in some it is subdivided into numerous bony cells. The function is not known with certainty but it has been suggested that it may improve the perception of sounds of very low and very high frequencies.

The *tympanic membrane* (Fig. 9–21) is a thin partition separating the lumen of the external acoustic meatus from that of the tympanic cavity. Like the tympanic cavity, it is slanted so that its dorsal part is more lateral than its ventral part, and its surface area is thus considerably larger than that of the transected external acoustic meatus; the dog's eardrum on average measures 10 × 15 mm; its long axis is oriented rostrocaudally. Its lateral surface is covered with an epidermis continuous with that of the meatus, its medial surface by the mucosa lining the tympanic cavity. A layer of fibrous tissue between epidermis and mucosa firmly attaches the membrane to the osseous tympanic ring of the temporal bone. The tympanic ring is interrupted dorsally by a notch that extends onto the roof of the external acoustic meatus. The part of the tympanic membrane attached to the tympanic ring is tense; the part that closes the notch is flaccid.

The handle of the malleus (/4), the most lateral of the ear ossicles, is embedded in the medial

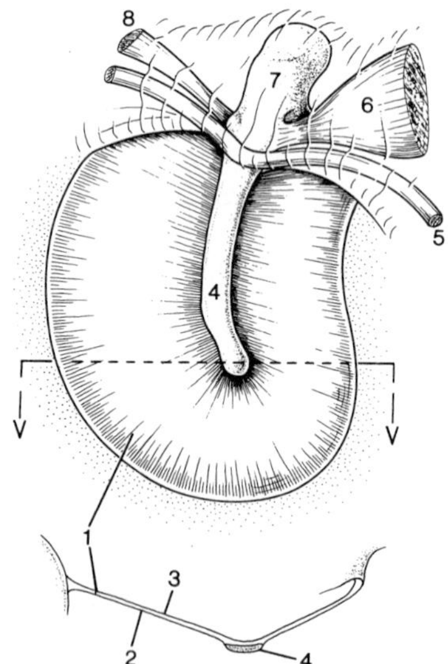


**Figure 9–21.** Medial surface and transverse section *(below)* of canine tympanic membrane.

1, Tense part of tympanic membrane; 2, medial surface; 3, lateral surface; 4, handle of malleus; 5, chorda tympani; 6, tensor tympani; 7, head of malleus; 8, one of the ligaments associated with the malleus.

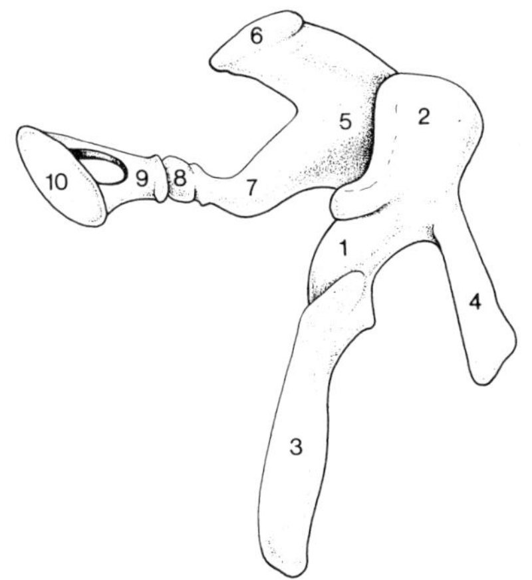


**Figure 9–22.** Left auditory ossicles of the horse, craniomedial view.

1, Malleus; 2, head of malleus; 3, handle of malleus; 4, rostral process; 5, incus; 6, short crus; 7, long crus; 8, os lenticulare; 9, head of stapes; 10, base (footplate) of stapes.

surface of the tympanic membrane. Tension in the chain of ossicles pulls the tympanic membrane medially, hollowing its lateral surface. The handle shines through the thin membrane and is visible as a light band (stria mallearis) when the eardrum is examined with an otoscope (see Fig. 11–25/2; Plate 16/*G*).

## Auditory Ossicles

The transmission of sound waves across the tympanic cavity is mediated by the three auditory ossicles (Fig. 9–19/6) known, in lateromedial sequence, as malleus, incus, and stapes (Latin names for hammer, anvil, and stirrup, from their rather fanciful resemblance to these objects; Plate 16/*H*).

The handle (manubrium) of the *malleus* (Fig. 9–22/3) is embedded in the tympanic membrane so that the head of the malleus protrudes above the membrane by a few millimeters. The head articulates with the body of the *incus* and the latter articulates with the head of the stapes by means of its long crus. The base (footplate) of the *stapes* sits in the vestibular window in the medial wall of the tympanic cavity.

The oscillations of the tympanic membrane perceived by the handle of the malleus are magnified and transmitted to the vestibular window by lever action through the chain of ossicles. The base of the stapes is set in motion, which causes the fluid in the internal ear to vibrate. This stimulates the neuroreceptor cells in the membranous labyrinth and sound is perceived.

The mechanism of sound transmission from the outside to the internal ear may not, in fact, be quite so simple. There is evidence that sound waves are also transmitted to the fluid through the walls of the tympanic cavity and directly through the cochlear window.

The auditory ossicles are attached to the wall of the epitympanic recess by several ligaments, and their relationships can be altered by two small muscles (tensor tympani and stapedius). These are believed to tense the tympanic membrane and the chain of ossicles in an effort to decrease the amplitude of their vibrations in the lower frequencies and to protect the system from damage caused by sudden overload (see p. 221 for their innervation).

## Auditory Tube

This structure, often called the Eustachian tube, connects the tympanic cavity with the nasopharynx (Fig. 9–19/8). It is short with a narrow lumen that is laterally compressed and usually collapsed. The tube is confined by an inverted cartilaginous trough except along its ventral border. The membranous wall of the horse's auditory tube evaginates through this ventral defect in the cartilaginous support to form the large, thin-walled *guttural pouch* dorsolateral to the nasopharynx (see p. 497).

The *pharyngeal openings of the auditory tubes* are located in the lateral walls of the nasopharynx and are marked by accumulations of lymphoid tissue (tubal tonsils) (see Fig. 18–10/8). The cartilage of the auditory tube extends into the medial wall of the pharyngeal opening and stiffens it. The auditory tubes allow equalization of the pressures on the two sides of the delicate eardrums. The pressure sometimes becomes unbalanced, for example, during a ride in an express elevator, and its sudden restoration causes our ears to pop. The auditory tubes temporarily open each time we swallow or yawn. This permits the slight secretion from the goblet cells and the glands in the lining of the tympanic cavity to escape.

# The Internal Ear

The mechanical stimuli produced by sound and by the positional changes of the head are transformed into nerve impulses in the internal ear. This is a delicate mechanism, no larger than about 12 mm across in the dog, and is completely enclosed in the very hard petrous temporal bone for protection and proper functioning (Fig. 9–19/*A*). It is exposed to sound vibrations on the lateral surface and the impulses into which these are converted leave the bone in nerve fibers that pass through the internal acoustic meatus on the medial surface.

The internal ear consists of a closed system of tiny membranous ducts and cavities known, because of its complexity, as the *membranous labyrinth* (Fig. 9–23/*A*). This contains endolymph whose movement inside the system stimulates sensory cells in the membranous wall. Two enlargements in the center of the membranous labyrinth are known as the utriculus and sacculus. From the *utriculus* arise three semicircular ducts concerned with balance, and from the *sacculus,* the spiral cochlear duct, which is concerned with hearing.

The *semicircular ducts* stand roughly at right angles to each other and are designated anterior, posterior, and lateral; one end of each duct is ampullated close to the utriculus. The endolymph within them is set in motion by movements of the head, and this results in pressure on minute barriers (cristae ampullares) present in each ampulla (/9,10). These pressures deflect sensory hairs projecting from the receptor cells of the cristae, stimulating the individual cells to send impulses to the central nervous system.

Two further receptor areas called *maculae* (/6,7) are present in the walls of the utriculus and sacculus. They monitor the position of the head with respect to gravity. Although the maculae are bathed in endolymph, they react to a layer of crystals (statoconia) adhering to a gelatinous layer that surrounds the sensory hairs of the receptor cells. When the gelatinous layer of the maculae faces toward the ground the cells are maximally stimulated by the gravitational pull. The maculae thus record the *position* of the head, whereas the cristae record the *movements* of the head.

The sacculus gives origin to the endolymphatic duct which ends blindly in the epidural space (Fig. 9–19/17). It is thought to function in the resorption of the endolymph secreted by the epithelial lining of the membranous labyrinth.

The membranous labyrinth is housed in a similar but slightly larger *osseous labyrinth,* a complex excavation in the temporal bone (Fig. 9–24/4). The central chamber of the osseous labyrinth, the vestibule, houses the utriculus and the sacculus. The semicircular ducts lie within the osseous semicircular canals. The cochlear duct passes up the spiral canal of the cochlea, which is an excavation very similar to the inside of a snail's shell (/6). The center of the cochlea is an osseous pyramid known as the modiolus (Fig. 9–25/2). Running around the modiolus is the spiral canal—the actual lumen of the cochlea—which ends blindly at the apex of the modiolus. Projecting into the spiral canal from the modiolus is an osseous

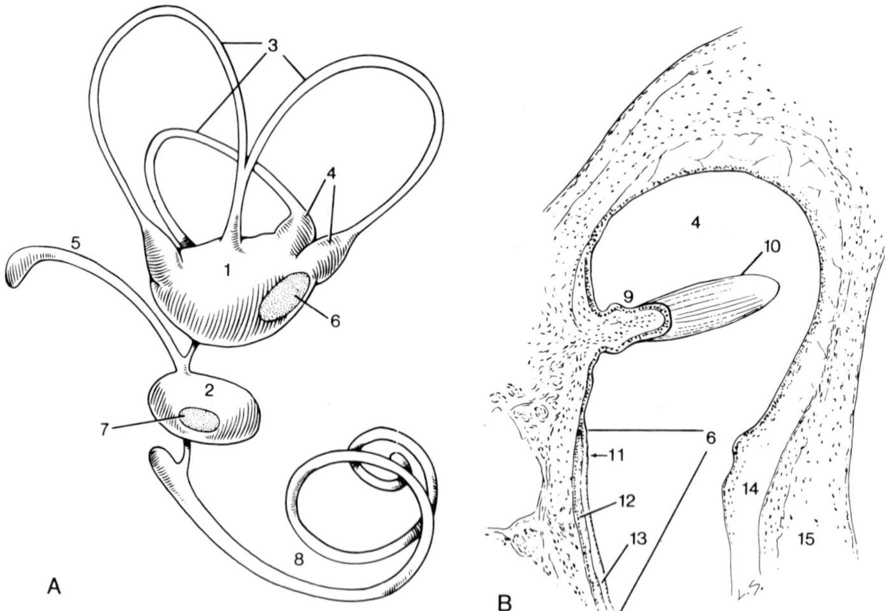


**Figure 9–23.** *A,* Membranous labyrinth. *B,* Section of ampulla.

1, Utriculus; 2, sacculus; 3, semicircular ducts; 4, ampullae containing ampullary crests; 5, endolymphatic duct; 6, 7, maculae; 8, cochlear duct; 9, ampullary crest; 10, cupula containing sensory hairs; 11, layer of neuroepithelial hair cells; 12, statoconia; 13, gelatinous layer of macula; 14, perilymphatic space; 15, wall of osseous labyrinth.

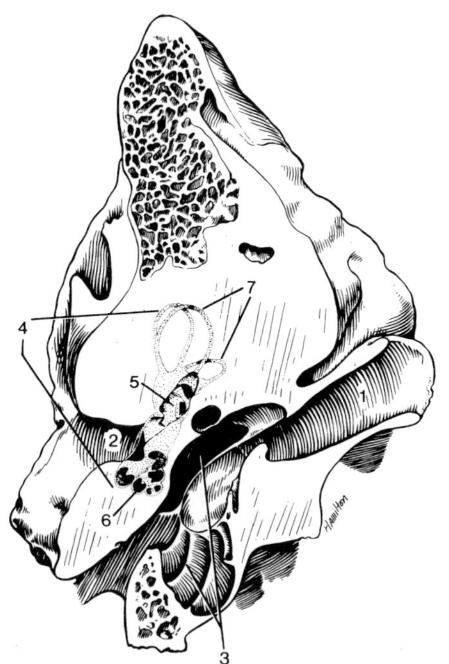


**Figure 9–24.** Left petrous temporal bone of a horse, sectioned through both external and internal acoustic meatuses.

1, External acoustic meatus; 2, internal acoustic meatus; 3, tympanic cavity; 4, osseous labyrinth; 5, vestibule; 6, cochlea; 7, semicircular canals.

shelf, the spiral lamina (/5), which terminates in the blind end of the spiral canal of the cochlea. The spiral lamina itself is hollow, forming the spiral canal of the modiolus.

Since the osseous labyrinth is slightly larger than the membranous labyrinth it encloses, there is between the two a minute space containing perilymph. Only the two perilymphatic spaces (scala tympani and scala vestibuli) accompanymg the cochlear duct into the cochlea need be considered further.

The spiral canal of the cochlea is divided by a split longitudinal membrane into three channels (/6,7,8), all running around the modiolus to the apex of the cochlea. The membrane arises centrally from the spiral lamina and, after splitting, attaches to the outside wall of the spiral canal. The uppermost channel is the scala vestibuli, the middle one the cochlear duct, and the lowest is the scala tympani. The two scalae communicate at the apex of the cochlea around the blind end of the cochlear duct. At the base of the cochlea, the scala vestibuli communicates with the perilymphatic space in the vestibule, and the scala tympani ends at the secondary tympanic membrane (Fig. 9–19).

An enlarged transverse section of the spiral canal of the cochlea shows the composition of the split membrane, particularly the part that forms the walls of the triangular cochlear duct (Fig. 9–25/7).

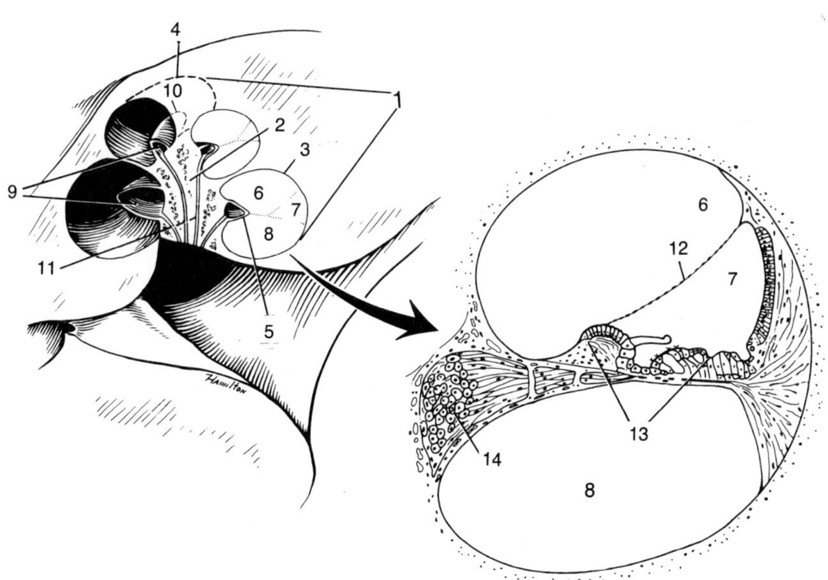


**Figure 9–25.** Cochlea and enlarged cochlear duct.

1, Cochlea; 2, modiolus; 3, 4, spiral canal of cochlea; 5, osseous spiral lamina; 6, scala vestibuli; 7, cochlear duct; 8, scala tympani; 9, 10, spiral canal of modiolus; 11, longitudinal canals; 12, spiral membrane; 13, spiral organ; 14, spiral ganglion.

The simplest of these walls separates the cochlear duct from the scala vestibuli; it consists of a single layer of cells and is known as the spiral membrane. The wall of the cochlear duct facing the scala tympani is complex by virtue of the large neuroreceptor and other cells found in it. Its connective tissue component is the basilar lamina, which plays an important role in the perception of sound. The cells form the *spiral organ* (/13) in which originate the nerve impulses that are produced by the sounds received by the external ear.

The impulses travel toward the modiolus to ganglion cells housed in the spiral canal. The aggregate of these cells forms the *spiral ganglion* (/14), which also winds around the modiolus. From the spiral ganglion the impulses travel along nerve fibers within canals to the base of the modiolus where the fibers join to form the cochlear part of the vestibulocochlear nerve.

As the base of the stapes rocks in the vestibular window in unison with the vibrations of the tympanic membrane, it compresses the perilymph in the closed system of perilymphatic spaces. Since fluids are incompressible the required "give" is found in similar vibrations of the secondary tympanic membrane closing the cochlear window. The way in which the mechanical stimuli in the vibrating columns of fluid within the cochlea act on the receptor cells in the spiral organ is complex and beyond the scope of this book. The width and structure of the basilar lamina suggests that, at least in humans, lower-pitched sound is "read" by a relatively short stretch of the spiral organ near the apex of the cochlea. The remaining much longer stretch of the spiral organ responds to sounds of higher frequency, including those of speech.

The anatomy of the internal and middle ear is complicated by the passage of the facial nerve through this area (Fig. 9–19/10). The facial nerve enters the internal acoustic meatus together with the vestibulocochlear nerve and, within an osseous facial canal, traverses the temporal bone to emerge at the stylomastoid foramen. The facial canal makes a sharp kneelike bend within the temporal bone and at this point the nerve is enlarged by the geniculate ganglion. From this arises the major petrosal nerve, which regulates secretion of the lacrimal and nasal glands. The chorda tympani, regulating the sublingual and mandibular glands but also relaying taste from the rostral two thirds of the tongue, leaves the facial nerve a little more distally. The chorda tympani is so named because, for a short segment of its course, it lies on the upper part of the tympanic membrane (Fig. 9–21/5). Both major petrosal and chorda tympani nerves leave the temporal bone through foramina on the rostroventral aspect of the bone. The facial nerve also supplies the stapedius muscle. (The tensor tympani is activated through the mandibular division of the trigeminal nerve [V3].)

The vestibulocochlear nerve (VIII) divides into vestibular and cochlear parts as it enters the internal acoustic meatus. The branches of the vestibular part pass to the neuroreceptor areas in the utriculus and sacculus, conveying impulses concerned with balance; the cochlear part passes into the base of the cochlea to mediate the impulses concerned with hearing.

## The Development of the Ear

The external ear develops from ectoderm of the first branchial groove, the middle ear from endoderm of the first pharyngeal pouch, and the inner ear from a patch of ectoderm lateral to the developing hindbrain—there is no outgrowth from the neural tube as described for the nervous component of the eye.

The formation of the external acoustic meatus precedes that of the auricle. It begins with a deepening and thinning of the first branchial groove, as a result of which a blind tube is formed (Fig. 9–26/3). The medial end of the tube comes to lie lateroventral to the dorsal part of the first pharyngeal pouch (/4), which gives rise to the tympanic cavity. The slanted mesenchymal partition between the tube and the pouch foreshadows the tilted orientation of the eardrum. As the meatus lengthens, it is supported by cartilage derived from the surrounding mesenchyme. The dorsal wall of

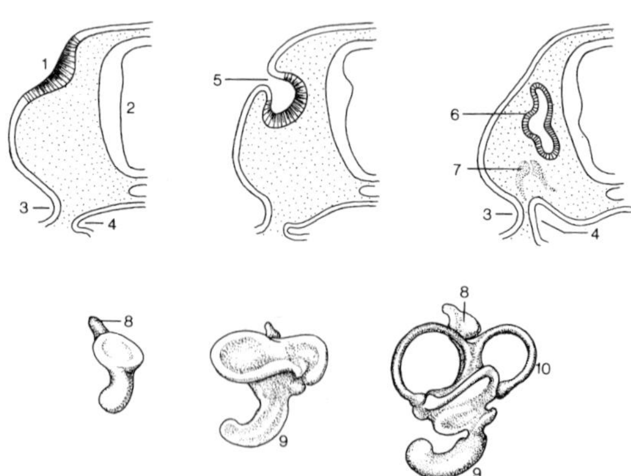


**Figure 9–26.** Early development of the ear. Transverse sections at the level of the hindbrain, and the formation of the membranous labyrinth *(below)*.

1, Otic placode; 2, hindbrain; 3, first branchial groove; 4, first pharyngeal pouch; 5, otic pit; 6, otic vesicle; 7, ossicles; 8, endolymphatic duct; 9, cochlear duct; 10, semicircular canals.

its most medial part becomes the eardrum to which the branchial groove ectoderm supplies the outer epithelial layer. The auricle arises from a number of elevations bordering the branchial groove. Those caudal to the groove grow more rapidly and furnish the pinna, which grows rostrally, covering the ear canal. The rostral elevations remain small; they become the saliences rostral and ventral to the definitive ear opening. The primitive ear canal is gradually occluded by epithelial overgrowth of its walls so that in most species it is functionally closed at birth. In the dog it is said to be patent again about 10 days after birth.

The middle ear develops from the endoderm of the first pharyngeal pouch, the tympanic cavity from the dorsal part, and the auditory tube from the proximal part, or neck, of the pouch. The neck remains patent and is drawn out to furnish the permanent connection (auditory tube) between the definitive tympanic cavity and the nasopharynx.

The dorsal part of the pouch expands upward and makes contact lateroventrally with the developing external acoustic meatus and dorsomedially with the otic vesicle, the primordium of the inner ear (see further on). It is surrounded by loosely arranged mesenchyme in which the ear ossicles (/7) and associated muscles take shape. Malleus, incus, and tensor tympani are derived from the dorsal end of the first (mandibular) pharyngeal arch; the muscle is thus innervated by the mandibular branch of the trigeminal nerve. The stapes and the stapedius muscle originate in the dorsal end of the second pharyngeal arch and the muscle is supplied by the facial nerve. The dorsal part of the pharyngeal pouch now enlarges and gradually engulfs the ossicles and muscles so that they receive an epithelial covering and come to lie within the developing cavity. Small amounts of mesenchyme trapped in the process form the ligaments (and joints) that attach the ossicles to each other and to the wall of the definitive tympanic cavity.

The development of the inner ear begins with the formation of an ectodermal (otic) placode overlying the lateral surface of the future hindbrain (/1). The placode sinks below the surface (otic pit) and closes over to form the otic vesicle. As the distance between the vesicle and the surface ectoderm increases, the upward-growing first pharyngeal pouch takes up a position lateral to the vesicle and medial to the developing external acoustic meatus, thus establishing the lateral-to-medial sequence of the external, middle, and inner ear. The otic vesicle gives rise to the membranous labyrinth. Its dorsomedial wall is drawn out early to form the endolymphatic duct (/8). The ventral part of the vesicle enlarges to form the saccule, and this in turn gives rise to the cochlear duct, which spirals away rostroventrally. The middle and dorsolateral parts of the vesicle form the utriculus and the semicircular canals, respectively. The medial surface detaches neuroblasts that proliferate into the bipolar cells forming the vestibular and spiral ganglia; lateral processes connect with the sensory cells of the ampullae, maculae, and spiral organ, while proximal processes go to the brain, forming the vestibulocochlear nerve.

The mesenchyme that surrounds the developing membranous labyrinth differentiates to form a cartilaginous capsule. The interior of the capsule mimics the shape of the labyrinth but leaves between the two an irregular space filled with gel-like tissue. The capsule is continuous with the other parts of the chondrocranium. During the last third of gestation (in the dog) it is transformed into the osseous labyrinth. The malleus and the tympanic ring (to which the eardrum attaches) ossify earlier than that, the incus and stapes later. The gel-filled spaces between osseous and membranous labyrinths become more and more vacuolated and form the areolar tissue of the perilymphatic spaces; in the cochlea, substantial partitions remain and divide the perilymphatic space into the scala vestibuli and scala tympani that accompany the cochlear duct.

## THE OLFACTORY ORGAN

The sense of smell is much better developed in the domestic mammals than in ourselves; this is particularly true of the dog, which can detect airborne substances in incredibly low concentrations. Much of the "contact" with the environment and with other animals is made through this sense, and the examples given here underscore the importance of olfaction in animal life. This capability is exploited when dogs are used to "point" at game, to follow a scent in tracking fugitives (or detect drugs and explosives), and when dogs and pigs are trained to find buried truffles. Dams recognize their offspring largely by the sense of smell; wild animals identify the extent of their territory by odorants on the ground; wild herbivores test the air for the scent of predators.

The olfactory organ is of course situated in the nose. In animals with a well-developed sense of smell it consists of a relatively large area of *olfactory mucosa* covering the lateral wall and the ethmoidal conchae in the caudal part of the nasal cavity. Although claimed to be a little more yellowish than the respiratory mucosa rostral to it, the olfactory mucosa cannot convincingly be identified by gross inspection. Histological sections show the presence of olfactory cells that, like the light-receptor cells in the retina, are bipolar neurons. Their dendrites reach the surface of the epithelium, presenting several minute olfactory hairs (cilia) to the air in the nasal cavity. The axons of the cells combine to form the fascicles of the olfactory nerve (cranial nerve I) that pass through the cribriform plate to the nearby olfactory bulb. Serous *olfactory glands* below the olfactory epithelium moisten the surface of the epithelium, presumably to wash away previously perceived odorants no longer present in the air.

The *vomeronasal organ** found in the nasal cavity is also concerned with olfaction. It consists of two narrow parallel ducts that are embedded in the hard palate, one to each side of its junction with the nasal septum. The ducts, which are supported laterally, ventrally, and medially by thin cartilages, are lined in part with olfactory mucosa (Plate 17/*F,I*). Caudally they end blindly, but rostrally they open into the incisive ducts which in most mammals connect the nasal and oral cavities through openings in the hard palate. The communication with the oral cavity is lacking in horses and donkeys. This organ has received considerable attention from animal behaviorists and reproductive physiologists because of its involvement in sexual activity, particularly in the lip-curl (Flehmen) reaction demonstrated by male animals aroused by the odor of vaginal secretion or urine from estrous females (Plate 24/*D*; Fig. 9–27). Whether the Flehmen reaction, and the accompanying extension of the head, helps the odorants reach the vomeronasal organ is still a matter of speculation. Experimental blockage of the incisive ducts modifies, but does not eliminate, the Flehmen and other responses of bulls exposed to the pheromones contained within the vaginal secretion of cows in heat.

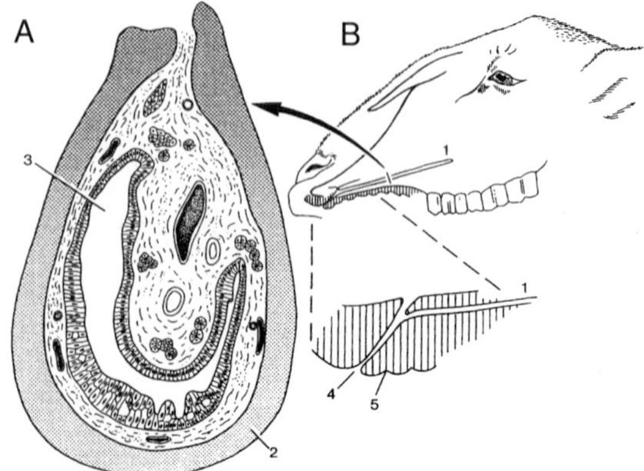


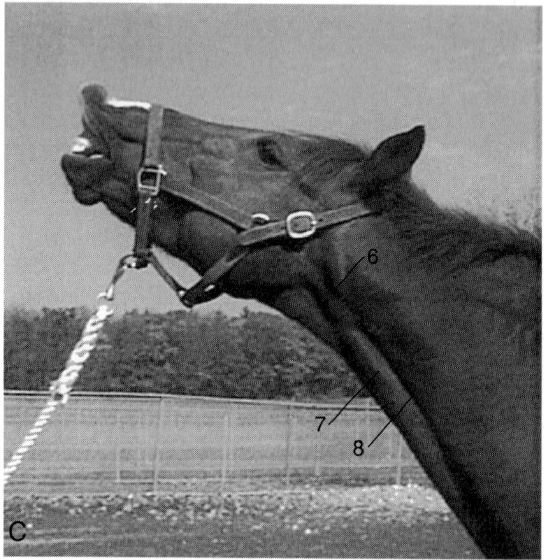


**Figure 9–27.** *A,* Transverse section of vomeronasal organ of sheep. *B,* Vomeronasal organ of sheep in situ. *C,* During the Flehmen reaction the head is fully extended, accentuating several features of the neck.

1, Vomeronasal organ; 2, vomeronasal cartilage; 3, vomeronasal duct; 4, incisive duct; 5, palate; 6, wing of atlas; 7, sternocephalicus; 8, jugular groove.

## THE GUSTATORY ORGAN

The receptors for the sense of taste are the *taste buds* (Fig. 9–28), microscopic nests of cells mainly associated with the papillae of the tongue, although small numbers are also found in the soft palate and in the vicinity of the epiglottis. Taste buds are about as tall as the epithelium in which they lie and communicate with the oral cavity by taste pores through which solutions enter in order to stimulate the receptor cells. Taste pores cannot be seen with the naked eye.

The taste buds consist of sustentacular or supporting cells in addition to the receptor or *gustatory cells.* The latter have elongated nuclei and at their free tips bear microvilli (taste hairs) that project into the taste pore. Glands deep to the papillae discharge a serous secretion on the surface of the epithelium. It is believed that the secretion cleanses the taste pores and enhances perception by the gustatory cells.

In order to be discerned, food substances have to be in solution. One of the reasons food is

*A vomeronasal organ is not found in human adults; it makes an appearance during development but later regresses, although vestiges occasionally survive within the nasal septum.

Since stimulation of the vomeronasal organ is known to affect the activity of gonadotropin-releasing hormone (GnRH) neurons, it is interesting to learn that these neurons have an unusual origin in the olfactory placodes. Their definitive locations are diffusely and variously spread (according to species) within the hypothalamic region of the brain.

insalivated is to dissolve parts for sampling by the taste buds. The principal taste sensations are sweetness, sourness, and saltiness. It appears that, in the dog, sweetness and saltiness are perceived in the rostral two thirds of the tongue where taste buds are present on the fungiform papillae. Sour substances are perceived over the entire tongue. The caudal third of the tongue, which incorporates the vallate and foliate papillae, therefore seems to respond only to what tastes sour.

The afferent pathways mediating these sensations are similarly divided. In the rostral two thirds of the tongue the pathways travel at first in the lingual nerve and then in the chorda tympani—which we encountered in the description of the ear. After passing through the geniculate ganglion of the seventh cranial nerve they enter the medulla oblongata. The afferent fibers from the caudal third of the tongue travel in the glossopharyngeal nerve (and to a small extent in the vagus) to the medulla oblongata.

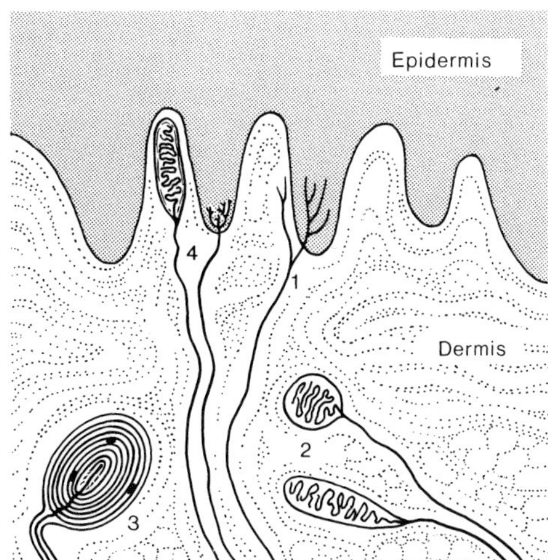


**Figure 9–29.** Sensory nerve endings of the skin, schematic.

1, Free nerve endings (pain); 2, bulbous corpuscles (heat or cold); 3, lamellar corpuscles (vibration); 4, meniscoid nerve endings (touch).

## THE CUTANEOUS SENSE

As mentioned at the beginning of the chapter, much of the more immediate environment is experienced by the animal through its skin. The sensations are touch, pressure, pain, heat, and cold—touch being a light stimulus such as is produced by a fly on the haircoat, and pressure a stronger and deeper stimulus such as a horse feels from a saddle or girth. The receptors responsible for the detection of these stimuli vary considerably in structure. Unfortunately, many intermediate forms exist so that it is difficult to classify them and to assign clear-cut functions to each kind. The simple classification given here is probably adequate for the purpose of this book.

The sensory receptors of the skin can be divided into free nerve endings and those that bear terminal corpuscles. The *free nerve endings* are tufts formed by the branches of nerve fibers that terminate either in fine points or in button-like swellings; they are found principally in the epidermis and are thought to be pain receptors (Fig. 9–29/1). The *corpuscular endings* fall into three kinds: bulbous, lamellar, and meniscoid. The bulbous corpuscles, which are encapsulated terminal tufts of nerve fibers found in the dermis, are thought to respond to heat or cold (/2). The lamellar corpuscles are large (2 to 3 mm) and consist of many concentric lamellae (flattened cells) in the center of which is the nerve fiber; they are found in the subcutis and are thought to be pressure receptors (/3). Meniscoid corpuscles consist of small cup-shaped discs (menisci) at the ends of nerve fibers with which they contact "tactile" cells; they are found, usually encapsulated, both in the papillary layer of the dermis and free in the adjacent epidermis and are thought to be touch receptors (/4).

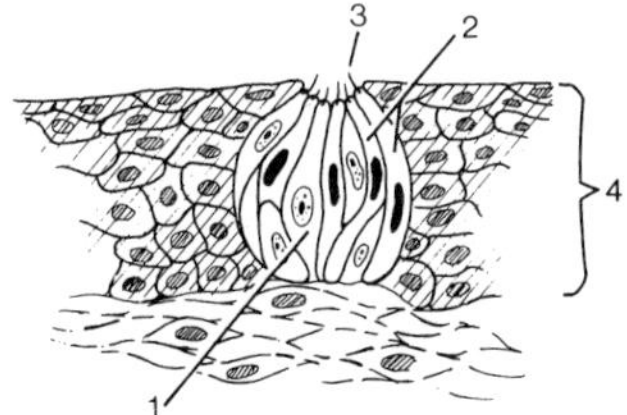


**Figure 9–28.** Histological section of a taste bud.

1, Sustentacular cell; 2, gustatory cells; 3, taste pore; 4, epithelium.

A special sort of cutaneous sense is mediated by the *tactile hairs.* These are long, protrude from the head, and are substantially thicker than the hairs forming the haircoat. The cat's whiskers are good examples but all domestic mammals have them, principally about their muzzle and eyes. The walls of blood spaces (sinuses) surrounding the roots of these hairs contain numerous nerve endings. When the tips of the sinus hairs are touched, these nerve endings are stimulated and an impulse is sent to the central nervous system (see also p. 352).

## PROPRIOCEPTION

This depends on the action of numerous nerve endings (proprioceptors) embedded in skeletal muscle, tendons, joint capsules, and ligaments.

These specialized nerve endings are not unlike some of the skin receptors. They respond to stretching or compression and inform the animal not only of the degree to which a muscle is contracted, a tendon tensed, or a joint flexed but also of the rate at which these changes occur. This information travels centrally through sensory cell bodies in the dorsal root ganglia near the spinal cord and activates reflexes indispensable for the coordination of muscle groups in maintaining posture and effecting movement. (It is proprioception that enables us to describe the exact position and attitude, of our lower limbs, i.e., without having to look at them.) If for some reason proprioception is disturbed, movements become ataxic, that is, muscular coordination is lost. Receptors that mediate pain, particularly of joints, are closely associated with the proprioceptors; the impulses from these travel in pathways that accompany those of proprioception to the spinal cord and thence to higher centers.

## ENTEROCEPTION

Receptors present in the hollow viscera respond to extreme dilation, to contraction or spasm (colic), and to chemical irritation. These sensations are translated as pain and, when the affected organ is in the abdominal cavity, are often accompanied by reflex contraction of the abdominal muscles and cessation of abdominal breathing. A rigid abdomen is an important accompanying diagnostic sign.

*Referred pain,* although important in human medicine, is of doubtful significance in animals. Pain impulses from the viscera share spinal cord pathways with sensory impulses arising from cutaneous zones that do not necessarily overlie these viscera but develop at the same embryological level. Since these pathways are much more often used by impulses from the cutaneous zones, it is not surprising that the brain misinterprets the origin of the much less frequent pain impulses from the viscera. The most widely known example is the pain referred to the presternal region, neck, shoulders, and inner aspect of the left arm in human sufferers from angina pectoris—a lack of oxygen to the heart tissue due to an inadequate blood supply.

Small cutaneous zones have been identified in the cow as being related through the nervous system with certain abdominal organs. These zones become hypersensitive when the corresponding organs are diseased. It is interesting that these zones broadly coincide with the acupuncture points specified in the animal "maps" from China that have become known to the Western world in recent years.

# CHAPTER 10

# The Common Integument

The term *common integument* comprehends ordinary skin with its covering of hair and variety of skin glands as well as more specialized parts such as claws, hoofs, and horns. The skin completely encloses the body and blends with the mucous membranes at the various natural openings. In its common form it protects against surface wear and tear, and invasion by microorganisms, plays an important part in thermoregulation (p. 349), and, being practically impermeable to water, prevents the body from drying out (with the accompanying loss of electrolytes and other vital substances); conversely, it prevents excessive water uptake in aquatic mammals. Certain lipid substances can penetrate skin and are used (in the form of ointments) as vehicles for administration of medication.

The color of skin (and hair) depends partly on the presence of pigment granules in certain component cells. These protect against ultraviolet radiation and are related to the ability to reflect solar heat which may raise body temperature; their effects partly explain why skin and coat color affects the adaptability of animals to life in sunny climates. The color of naked and nonpigmented areas is also affected in various ways by the blood in the vessels that perfuse its deeper layers; blushing in humans provides the most obvious example of such effects but the pallor of anemia or shock, the blue tint (cyanosis) that indicates oxygen lack, and the yellow (icterus) of jaundice are of greater veterinary relevance. Very spectacular color changes, such as that for which the chameleon is famous, do not occur in mammals, although mention may be made of the garish coloration of the skin of the mask and perineum of male mandrills and related monkeys.

## THE STRUCTURE OF SKIN

Some recapitulation and amplification of the earlier account (p. 9) of basic skin structure is now required. It will be recalled that skin is composed of two parts: a superficial epithelium (epidermis) and a tough fibrous layer (dermis) that rests on a stratum of loose connective tissue (subcutis) (see Fig 1–7).

The *epidermis* is continuously renewed. The surface cells are sloughed in flakes (e.g., dandruff) or as smaller particles (those of human skin accounting for much household dust), and this loss is made good by cell division in the deepest layer followed by migration of daughter cells toward the surface. As the epidermal cells drift superficially, they undergo a series of internal changes that gradually brings about their deaths, and when presented to the environment they are incapable of reacting to the various influences to which they are then exposed. The sequence of changes, shown schematically in Figure 10–1, imposes an obvious stratification. The deepest layer (stratum basale) is closely molded on the irregularities of the underlying dermis and has a considerably greater area than the surface of the body (/2). As the cells move into the stratum spinosum they shrink and draw apart, though remaining connected by intercellular bridges (desmosomes). The process of keratinization (cornification) now begins, and in the next layer (stratum granulosum) the cells contain scattered keratohyalin granules (/4). In some regions this layer is followed by a narrow stratum lucidum (not represented in Fig. 10–1) in which the flattened cells, which have already lost their nuclei and distinct outlines, obtain a homogeneous appearance from the even dispersal of the granules. Finally, the outermost layer (stratum corneum; /5) consists of squames densely packed with the fibrous protein keratin, the true horny substance, into which keratohyalin has been transformed. It is keratin that gives epidermal specializations (e.g., hair, hoof, and horn) their hardness and their strength.

The epidermal layers are thickest and most clearly differentiated where the skin is exposed to hard usage, as on the footpads of a dog (Plate 15/*C*). Where abrasion is less severe, as in haired regions, the epidermis is much thinner and neither the stratum granulosum nor the stratum lucidum may be clearly represented. The thickness of the epidermis depends on the mitotic rate within the stratum basale, which is adjusted by a substance (epidermal chalone) that inhibits cell division.

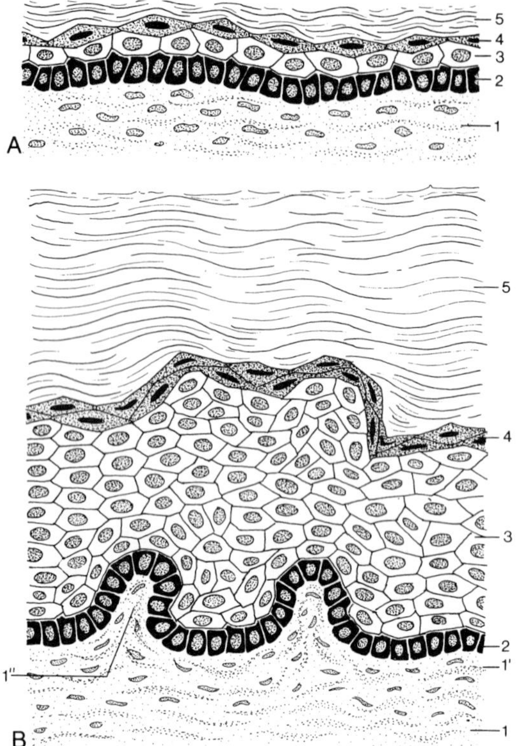


**Figure 10–1.** Structure of adult skin, schematic, *A,* Skin from the flank of a dog (hair not shown). *B,* Skin from a region exposed to wear. Note the increased keratinization and the formation of dermal papillae.

1, Dermis; 1′, papillary layer; 1″, dermal papilla; 2, stratum basale; 3, stratum spinosum; 4, stratum granulosum; 5, stratum corneum.

Although cell production and loss normally match to maintain an even epidermal thickness, this balance may be disturbed in certain circumstances.

There are no blood or lymphatic vessels in the epidermis, which is nourished by diffusion from the subjacent dermis.

The *dermis* is largely composed of collagen bundles, thickly felted together, as can be demonstrated by teasing leather (tanned dermis). Elastic fibers, which are also present, make the skin pliable and are able to restore its shape after being wrinkled or deformed. It is these fibers that draw apart the edges of a wound, making it gape (Fig. 10–2). Chronic tension damages the structure of the dermis, rupturing the connective tissue bundles; subsequent repair is usually by lighter scar tissue. A physiological example of this process is provided by the white lines (striae) of abdominal skin that appear following the completion of a pregnancy, especially in women.

The dermis is generously vascularized and innervated. It is also invaded by hair follicles and sweat, sebaceous, and other glands growing from the epidermis (see Fig. 1–7).

The interface across which nutrients and waste substances diffuse between the epidermis and the dermis is enlarged by the complicated molding of these components. The finger- and ridgelike projections (papillae; Fig. 10–1/1″) of the dermis fit closely into reciprocal depressions of the epidermis, and under normal conditions adhesion between the two structures is not easily disturbed. Trauma, such as that caused by the rubbing of an ill-fitting boot or shoe, sometimes separates them forcibly, allowing interstitial fluid to collect in a blister. Rupture of the blister exposes the raw surface of the dermis; normally this is quickly covered by epithelium growing inward from the margin of the sore.

The larger dermal ridges and papillae, generally developed where the covering epithelium is thickest, are reflected by corresponding epidermal contours. These are permanent and individually distinct and provide a means of identification, widely used in ourselves (fingerprinting), less commonly in other species (noseprinting of dogs and cattle; Figs. 10–3, 25–4, and Plate 15/*B*).

The *subcutis* consists of loose connective tissue interspersed with fat. It varies in amount according to situation and is thin or even absent where movement is undesirable (e.g., over the lips, eyelids, and teats). It is particularly ample in dogs and cats, whose easily shifted skin can be grasped in large folds over much of the body (Fig. 10–3). In the pig and ourselves, the subcutis contains more substantial accumulations of fat, even in relatively ill-nourished individuals; this constitutes the panniculus adiposus familiar in sliced bacon (see Fig. 1–10/2).

The clinical significance of the effects of dehydration or edema of the subcutis has been mentioned (p. 9).

The cutaneous blood vessels come from those that supply the fasciae and superficial muscles. The arteries form a series of networks within the

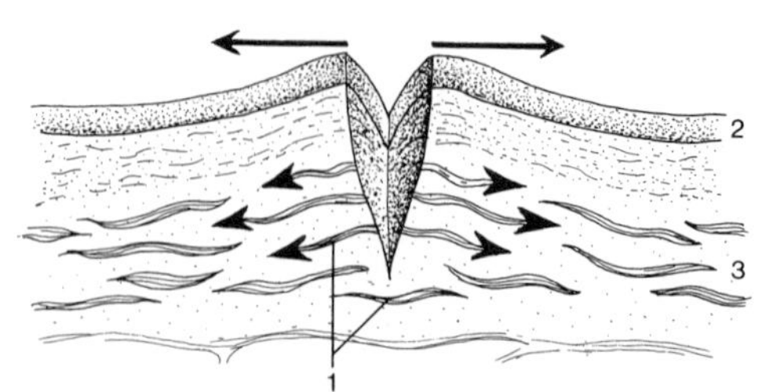


**Figure 10–2.** Skin incision. Elastic fibers in the dermis cause the wound to gape.

1, Elastic fibers; 2, epidermis; 3, dermis.

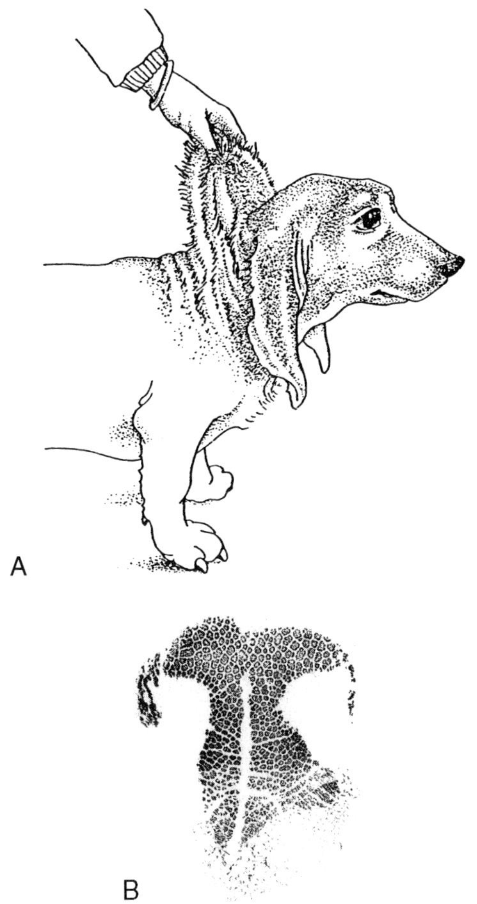


**Figure 10–3.** *A,* Loose skin on the neck of a Basset Hound. Ample subcutis permis shifting of the skin. *B,* Noseprint of a dog.

dermis. The most superficial network lies at the bases of the papillae and provides end-arteries that enter the papillae to release numerous capillaries from which fluid passes to nourish the basal epidermal cells. Other capillary plexuses surround the hair follicles and associated glands (see Fig. 1–7). Variation in flow through the superficial vessels plays an important role in temperature regulation. When the body temperature is raised, vasodilation promotes heat loss—directly by surface radiation and indirectly by favoring the activity of the glands that produce sweat, which then evaporates. Conversely, the surface vessels constrict in cold environments or when the internal temperature drops. The regulation of flow is in part achieved by opening or closing numerous anastomoses connecting the cutaneous arteries with veins. The skin vessels normally contain a considerable volume of blood but much can be recalled to the musculature and internal organs after hemorrhage or shock.

Skin has a rich sensory innervation. The nerves accompany the vessels through the fasciae and form networks within the dermis. From these, fibers disperse to a variety of sensory receptors, some even penetrating a little way into the epidermis (see Fig. 9–29). Other (autonomic) fibers regulate the caliber of the smaller vessels, control the activity of skin glands, and excite the arrector pili muscles that attach to the hair follicles.

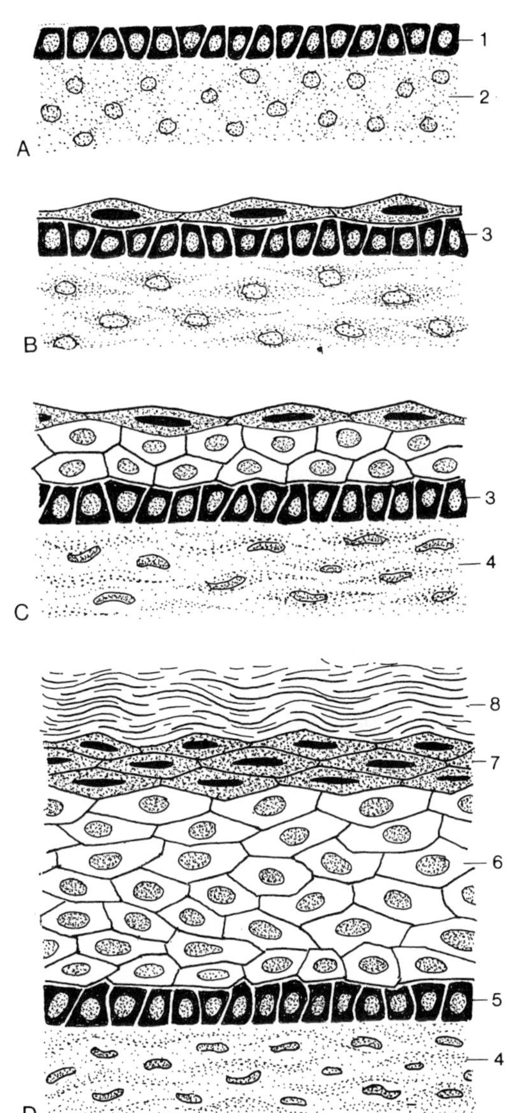


**Figure 10–4.** Development of skin, schematic. *A,* Skin of an early embryo. *B,* Differentiation of epidermis and dermis. *C,* Further differentiation of the epidermis. *D,* Complete differentiation of the epidermis and dermis.

1, Ectoderm; 2, mesoderm (mesenchyme); 3, primitive stratum basale; 4, dermis; 5, stratum basale; 6, stratum spinosum; 7, stratum granulosum; 8, stratum corneum.

The epidermis develops from the embryonic ectoderm. This is initially a single layer of cells lying on a bed of mesenchyme that in time gives rise to the dermis (Fig. 10–4/*A*). Long before birth the ectodermal cells begin to proliferate, pushing new cells toward the surface to produce a multilayered epithelium, while local condensations grow into the mesenchyme as the epithelial buds from which hair and glands differentiate. By the time of birth the skin of domestic mammals has a basically adult character, unlike that of many rodents and other small mammals that are born naked.

## HAIR

Hair is a mammalian feature, diagnostic of the class. In most species a thick haircoat is spread over the body, except about the mouth and other openings and on the surfaces of the feet; in a few, including the domestic pig (though not its ancestors), the covering is sparse (Fig. 10–8/*E*). The individual hairs take a variety of intergrading forms, but only three need be distinguished here: straight, rather stiff guard hairs provide a "topcoat"; fine, wavy wool hairs provide an "undercoat"; stout tactile hairs of restricted distribution are associated with touch receptors.

*Guard hairs* mostly lie close against the skin and sweep uniformly in broad tracts, giving the coat a smooth appearance disturbed only by the whorls, crests, and partings formed where different streams converge and combine, or diverge from one another. The regularity of the arrangement is significant since it promotes the runoff of rain, preventing the chilling that would occur if water were allowed to penetrate the pile to reach the skin. Occasionally, animals are born with a disturbed coat pattern, which may seriously impair their ability to withstand severe weather. However, as with so many other features, breeders have chosen to promote deviant mutant arrangements as attributes of particular breeds, particularly of dogs, cats, and rabbits.

Each hair grows from a tiny pit or follicle from which it protrudes above the surface of the skin. The follicle develops from an ectodermal bud that grows into the underlying mesenchyme in the embryonic stage of life. In addition to forming the hair, the bud branches give rise to skin glands (Fig. 10–5). The distal end of the bud forms a bulbous enlargement, which is then indented by a mesenchymal (dermal) papilla to form a primitive hair follicle. The epithelial cells lying against the papilla multiply, forming a hair matrix; the cells produced here keratinize and combine to form a primitive hair that grows through the center of the bud until it rises above the epidermis on the surface of the skin. Its passage takes it past the sebaceous glands that develop to the side of the

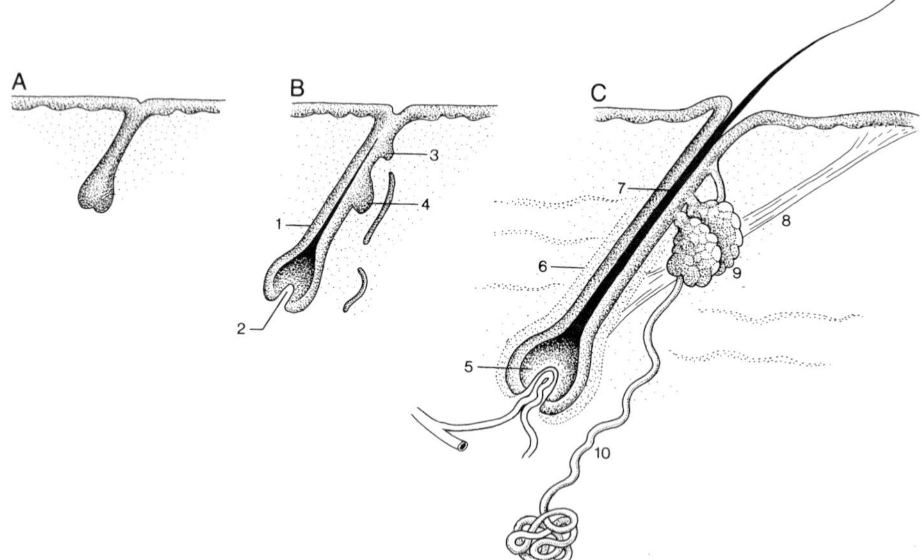


**Figure 10–5.** Development of hair and associated sebaceous and sweat glands, schematic. *A,* Ectodermal bud growing into mesenchyme. *B,* Differentiation of the bud; indications of glands appear. *C,* Hair follicle with accessory structures.

1, Primitive hair follicle; 2, dermal papilla; 3, bud of sweat gland; 4, bud of sebaceous gland; 5, bulb (hair matrix) of hair; 6, hair follicle; 7, root of hair; 8, arrector pili muscle; 9, sebaceous gland; 10, sweat gland. In the adult, many glands open independently, not into hair follicles.

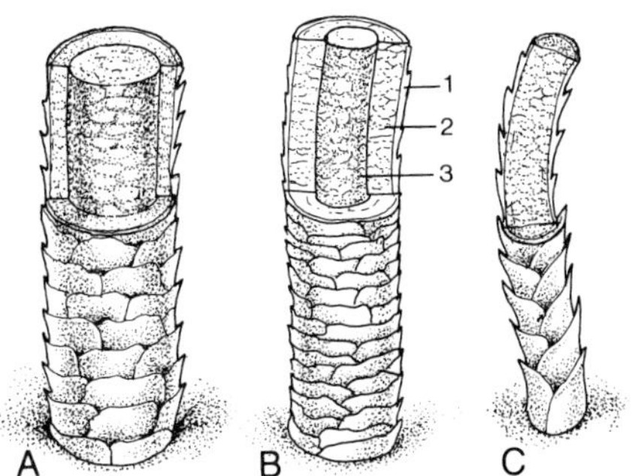


**Figure 10–6.** Schematic representation of three kinds of hair. *A*, Guard hair with thick medulla. *B*, Guard hair with thick cortex and thin medulla. *C*, Wool hair; the medulla is absent.

1, Cuticle; 2, cortex; 3, medulla.

follicle, and this arrangement allows the hair to obtain the oily coating so important for its health. While the ectoderm differentiates in this way, the mesoderm also condenses so that the tiny sheath around the embedded part of the hair acquires an outer mesodermal component.

Figure 10–6 shows the essential features; other texts must be consulted for the histological details. It must suffice here to say that, in essence, a hair consists of a flexible column of closely consolidated and heavily keratinized, and hence dead, epithelial cells. Their arrangement permits the distinction of a medulla or core, a cortex, and an outer "scaly" cuticle. The proportions of the parts and the details of their arrangement vary and permit the microscopic determination of the origin of a hair sample. In general, hairs with a thick medulla are straight and rather brittle, whereas those in which the cortex predominates are stronger and more pliable.

The proximal end of the follicle is joined by a tiny arrector pili muscle passing from an attachment near the dermal papillae (Fig. 10–5/8). Contraction of this muscle is involuntary and may be stimulated by a low ambient temperature. It results in erection of the hair from its normally oblique posture; when this happens to hairs en masse, the thickened pile traps more air and so improves the insulation of the body. Though functionally unimportant in the human species, the effect is very obvious in our relatively naked skin when little mounds ("goose pimples") appear over the courses of the arrector muscles. A similar effect occurs in the "fight-or-flight" reaction mediated by the sympathetic nervous system; the pronounced response by the hairs of the neck and back raises the "hackles" that give an animal a threatening appearance.

There are many local variations in the form and development of guard hairs. Familiar examples are the stiff, sparsely scattered bristles of pigs (Fig. 10–8/*E*); the coarse hair of the mane and tail of horses; the long tail hairs of cattle; the fetlock tufts of horses; and the feathering of the tail and limbs of certain breeds of dogs. Local variations that are hormone dependent are particularly evident in the human species; they include the male beard and the sexually dimorphic distribution of body hair. Baldness as an accompaniment of advancing age is especially a problem of the human male. Its causation is complicated and in part obscure; testosterone, which is responsible for the growth of the beard and coarse body hair, paradoxically seems to trigger early baldness in genetically predisposed individuals; a reduced blood level of thyroxine, which initiates and controls hair growth, also plays some part.

Hairs have restricted lives and are discarded sooner or later. In humans this shedding is a continuous process that involves only a few hairs at a time; in most other species it is intermittent, related to the season, and affects many hairs together (though never so many that the animal is denuded). Seasonal shedding is most pronounced in wild species, but even domesticated animals protected from the more extreme climatic changes show a recurrent pattern with peaks in the spring and fall. Shedding is obviously most noticeable in animals that are not regularly groomed to remove dead hair. Information on these matters is not abundant, and most accounts rely heavily on casual observation. This is particularly so where companion animals are concerned, and veterinarians are frequently embarrassed by too-penetrating inquiry from owners. Although there seems to be much variation, most dogs molt most heavily in the spring and fall; the spring shedding is more pronounced and lasts about 5 weeks. Cats also molt most heavily in spring but this is followed by a less substantial loss that continues through the summer and fall; it is not until winter that shedding ceases and the coat attains its prime condition. For the same reason, the pelts of furbearing species are harvested in winter, although in reduced numbers as the trade in furs is regarded with increasing disfavor.

The seasonal replacement begins with a slowing of the growth of existing hair; although this appears to be mainly conditioned by a rise in temperature, other factors, including nutrition and day length, play their parts. As growth slows (in the so-called catagen phase) the hair matrix and covering papilla both atrophy (Fig. 10–7/*B*). No growth occurs in the ensuing (telogen) phase when the follicle, including the papilla, shortens, causing

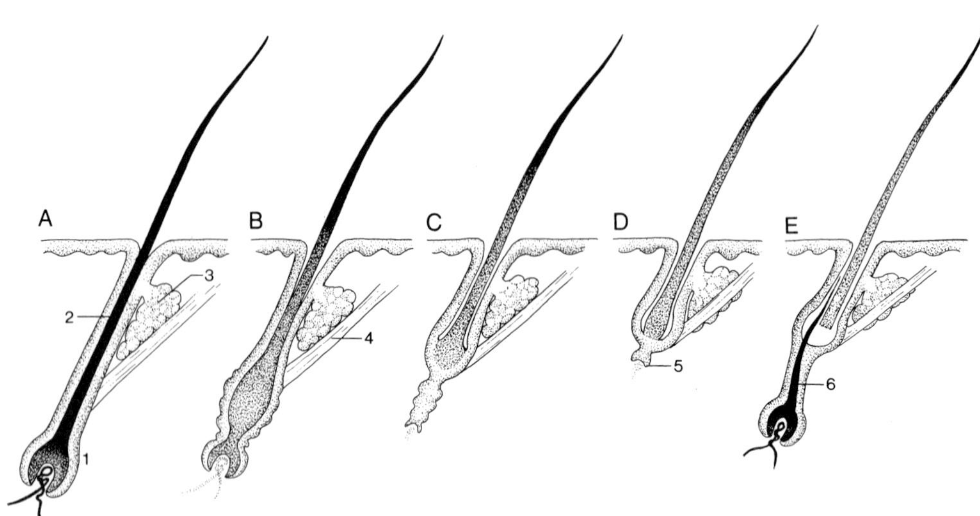


**Figure 10–7.** Phases of the hair cycle. *A,* Fully functional hair follicle, anagen phase. *B,* Follicle begins to atrophy, early catagen phase. *C,* Further atrophy of follicle, late catagen phase. *D,* Atrophied follicle. Hair is displaced distally and new hair matrix begins to form, telogen phase. *E,* New hair matrix established and new hair begins to grow, early anagen phase.

1, Hair follicle; 2, root of hair; 3, sebaceous gland; 4, arrector pili muscle; 5, new hair matrix; 6, new hair.

a larger part of the hair to project above the skin in simulation of growth (/*D*). When growth resumes, the follicle, with its matrix now reactivated, lengthens, and as it again extends away from the surface it loses its grip upon the old hair, which falls out. A replacement hair then forms in the active growth (anagen) phase that follows; this new hair gradually grows from the depth of the follicle until it emerges on the surface of the skin.

*Wool hairs* provide the soft undercoat. They are thin, wavy, and in most species, shorter and more numerous than the guard hairs by which they are concealed. The distinction between hair fiber types is not always clear-cut and intermediate forms exist to complicate description. The sheep fleece presents particular problems as well as obvious interest.* Wool is not, of course, confined to sheep among domestic animals. Cashmere and Angora goats, Angora rabbits, and alpacas all produce wools of distinctive quality that are utilized in the production of luxury yarns and textiles.

In many species, including mature dogs and cats, several hairs share a single follicle opening (Fig. 10–8/*B,C,D*). The central (primary) hair is longest and of the guard type, while the surrounding (secondary) hairs are shorter and softer; they provide the undercoat and may be designated wool hairs since they have little medulla.

The grouping of the hair follicles shows considerable inter- and intraspecific variation. This may be revealed in products prepared from animal skin. The study of vellum of different periods has been used to trace the evolution of the fleece of modern breeds of sheep from the haircoat of their wild

*The coat of wild sheep and of extant primitive breeds exhibits an outer coat of very coarse, hollow-cored guard hairs, known as kemp, which conceals and protects, by facilitating the runoff of rain, a short undercoat of much finer wool fibers. The growth of both fiber types is seasonally restricted and is succeeded by a spring molt when the shed wool forms tangled mats that are eventually cast. The wool is harvested by being gathered from the pasture and plucked directly from the animals. Evolution of the fleece under domestication has been characterized by loss of pigmentation, and by reduction in the amount of kemp, partly by depletion of the number of kemp hairs, partly by the transformation of a proportion of these into finer and more typical forms of hair. The wool now grows continuously and at a more rapid rate, though showing seasonal variation, and elimination of the spring molt introduces the necessity for shearing. The more rapid growth results in increased fiber length in the annual wool clip; other changes affect fiber waviness (crimp) and introduce greater diversity in the relative incidences of fibers of different diameters. The variations in these acquired features account for the characters, and therefore the values, of the fleeces of different breeds. The coarse, hairy fleece of some is most appropriate for the less valuable carpet trade; the improved fleece of others is suited to the production of finer yarns and fabrics. The weight of wool produced annually also varies widely with breed, ranging from as little as 3 to as much as 20 pounds (1.4 to 9 kg).

ancestors. Fragments of the Dead Sea Scrolls are among the materials utilized.

*Tactile hairs* are substantially thicker and generally protrude beyond the neighboring guard hairs. Most are found on the face, principally on the upper lip and about the eyes, although others are scattered (in species-variable fashion) on the lower lip, the chin, and elsewhere on the head. The cat, whose whiskers are particularly good examples (Fig. 10–9), also possesses a cluster of similar hairs at the carpus. Tactile hair follicles reach deeply into the subcutis, or even the superficial muscles. They are characterized by the presence of a venous sinus filled with blood and located between inner and outer layers of the dermal sheath (Plate 15/*A*). The nerve endings responsive to mechanical stimulation are also contained within the dermal sheath (Fig. 10–10/*B*,6). The stimulus provided by disturbance of the hair is amplified by wave motion in the blood. The follicles of tactile hairs appear early in development, before those of the coat hairs, and their staged appearances provide useful criteria for aging embryos.

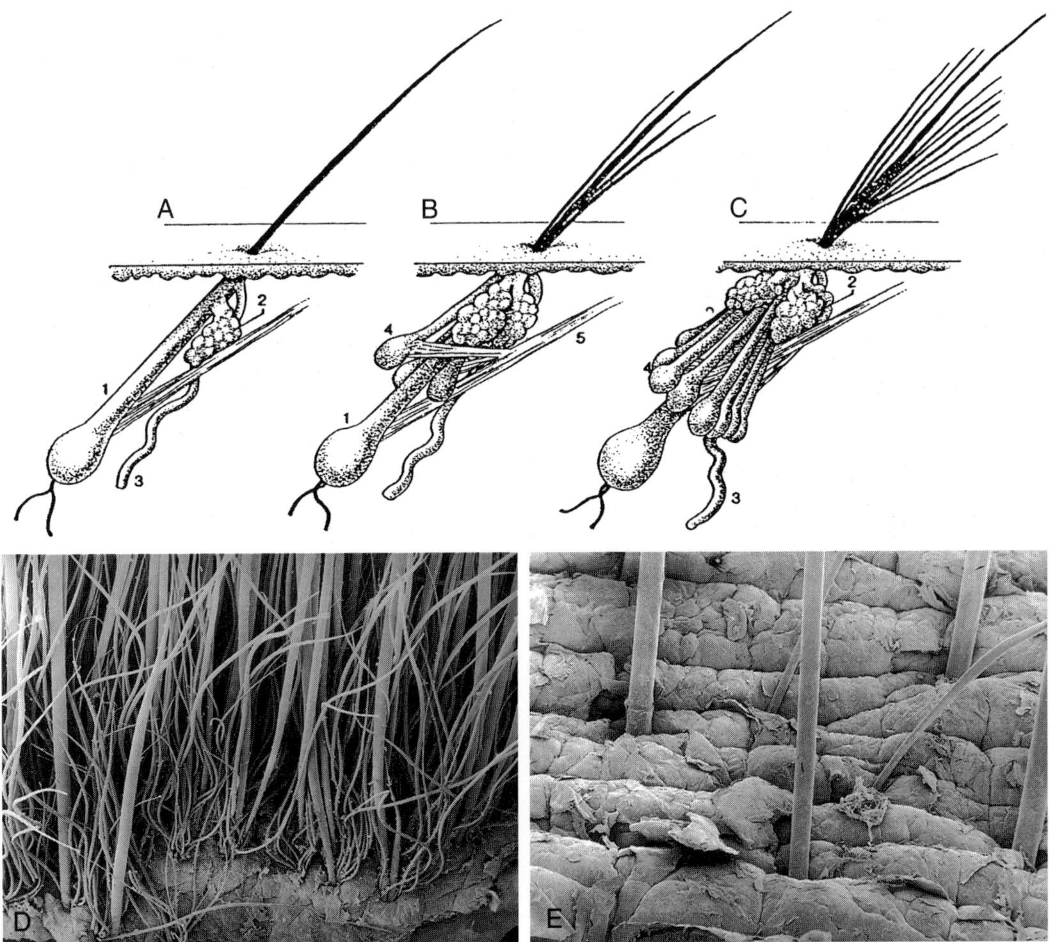


**Figure 10–8.** *A–C,* Hair follicles of the dog. *A,* Simple follicle present shortly after birth. *B,* Follicle present during the first few months following birth. *C,* Complex adult follicle; the primary hair is surrounded by several secondary hairs. *D,* Scanning electron micrograph of adult canine skin; note one or two follicles without primary (guard) hairs. *E,* "Naked" skin of a pig with sparse primary hairs (bristles) and surface debris.

1, Primary hair follicle; 2, sebaceous gland; 3, duct of sweat gland; 4, secondary hair follicle; 5, arrector pili muscle.

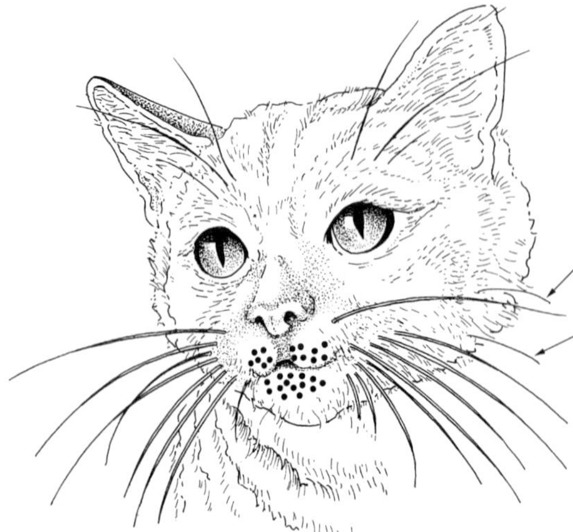

**Figure 10–9.** Tactile hairs on the head of the cat. The dots on the lips show the position of the circumoral glands. The arrows point to the buccal (tactile) hairs.

The skin of dogs and cats presents minute scattered tactile elevations (toruli tactiles) usually associated with special (tylotrich) guard hairs; the roots of these are surrounded by venous sinuses similar to, though smaller than, those of true tactile hairs. These elevations are also sensitive to touch (Fig. 10–11).

Many breeds of domestic animals, such as Holstein cattle and Dalmatian dogs, are immediately recognizable from the distinctive patterns of their coats. These patterns are created by the restricted distribution of various pigments, polymers of melanin ranging from black, through brown and red, to lighter shades, that are present in granule form* within cells of the epidermis, hair follicles, and hair. The pigments protect the skin from potentially harmful ultraviolet radiation and are unnecessary within those epidermal regions that are covered by a dense coat of hair. In most mammals, unlike humankind, skin pigmentation is therefore restricted to a few exposed parts that include the modified area associated with the external nose. It may be lacking here in white-coated individuals that obtain equivalent protection from a thickened stratum corneum.

*The pigment granules are produced within melanocytes, specialized cells of neural crest origin that are confined to the basal layer of the epidermis and hair follicles. The granules move to the tips of the dendritic processes of the melanocytes and are pinched off and subsequently phagocytized by neighboring cells (keratinocytes), in a process that continues until widespread. Melanin production is influenced by many factors; it is dependent upon the presence of a sufficiency of copper, with a deficiency of this mineral resulting in reduced pigmentation (among other abnormalities of hair), and its regulation is one function of the melanocyte-stimulating hormone (MSH). Changes in productivity may be intermittent, resulting in hair of banded (agouti) appearance, confined to a portion of the melanocyte population, or general, and then perhaps of seasonal occurrence, as in those lagomorphs and mustelids that adopt a white pelage in anticipation of winter snow. Local depression of melanogenesis is also a sign of aging, familiar in the white hair of the muzzle of older dogs and in that on our own heads.

## FOOTPADS

The footpads (tori) are the cushions on which animals walk. They are covered by a naked, densely cornified epidermis (Plate 15/*C*). The dermis is unremarkable, and the bulk of their substance is provided by a thick, resilient subcutis, an admixture of collagenous and elastic fibers interspersed with adipose tissue.

Footpads are best developed in plantigrade mammals (e.g., bears), in which digital, metacarpal (-tarsal), and carpal (tarsal) pads are all present (Fig. 10–12). In the digitigrade dog and cat, only digital and metacarpal (-tarsal) pads make ground contact; there is a carpal pad of no obvious use but no corresponding tarsal pad (Fig. 10–13).

Only digital pads are functional and in contact with the ground in ungulates, in which they are (generally) incorporated in the hoof, providing the features known as the bulb in ruminants and pigs, and the more complex frog in horses. The bulbs of the pig are soft and well set off from the sole (see further on); in ruminants they are harder, though less so than other parts of the hoof (Fig. 10–14/1).

The digital cushion (pulvinus digitalis) deep to the frog of the horse consists of an apex and a base. The apex lies deep to the horny frog on the ground surface of the hoof (Fig. 10–15/4), while the base helps shape the palmar (plantar) surface, forming the swellings at the heels. These, the bulbs of the heels (/3), do not make contact with the ground and are covered by periople, the softer horn produced at the junction of the skin with the wall of the hoof. The horse, unlike the other domestic ungulates, also has rudimentary metacarpal (-tarsal) pads ("ergots"; /2) embedded in a tuft of hair behind the fetlock joint and vestigial carpal (tarsal) pads (chestnuts; /1,1′).

The subcutis of the canine footpads, porcine bulbs, and equine frog contains sweat glands whose ducts channel through the thick, cornified epidermis. The secretions function as territorial or trail markers.

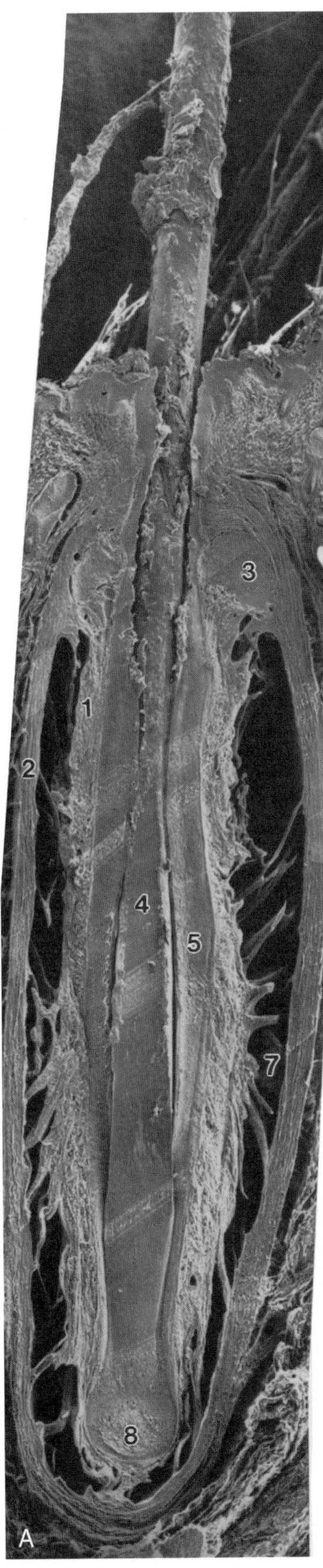


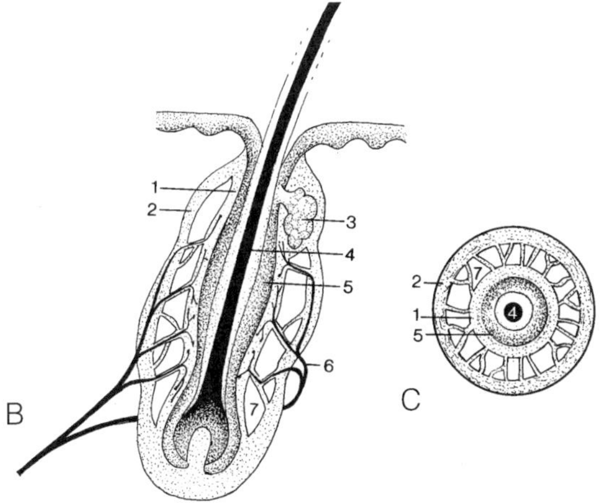


**Figure 10–10.** *A,* Scanning electron micrograph of an equine tactile hair follicle in longitudinal section. *B* and *C,* Schematic longitudinal and transverse sections of a tactile hair follicle.

1, 2, Internal and external walls of blood sinus; 3, sebaceous gland; 4, root of hair; 5, epidermal wall of hair follicle; 6, nerve ending in wall of blood sinus; 7, blood sinus; 8, dermal papilla.

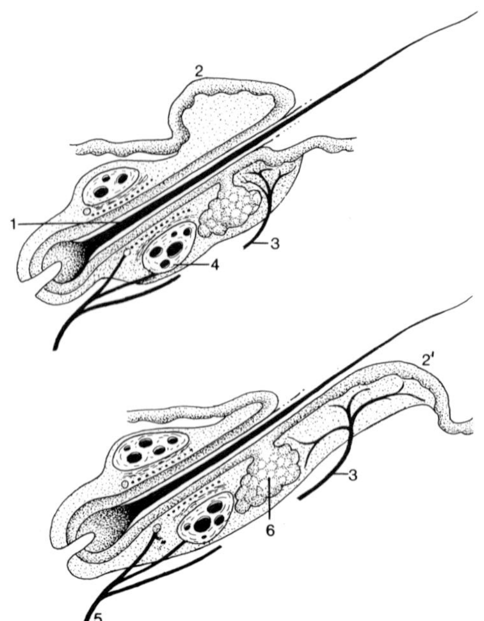


**Figure 10–11.** Tylotrich hairs below *(top)* and above *(bottom)* tactile elevations (2,2′).

1, Root of hair; 2, 2′, tactile elevations; 3, nerve endings associated with tactile elevations; 4, blood sinus; 5, nerve endings associated with blood sinus; 6, sebaceous gland.

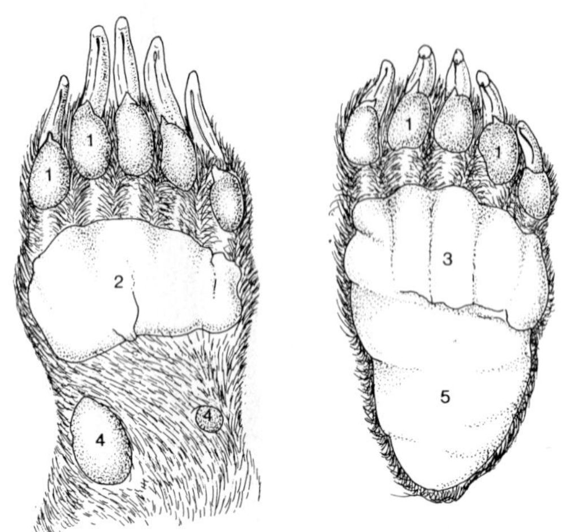


**Figure 10–12.** Footpads of a bear: forelimb *(left)*, hindlimb *(right)*.

1, Digital pads; 2, metacarpal pad; 3, metatarsal pad; 4, carpal pads; 5, tarsal pad, fused with the metatarsal pad.

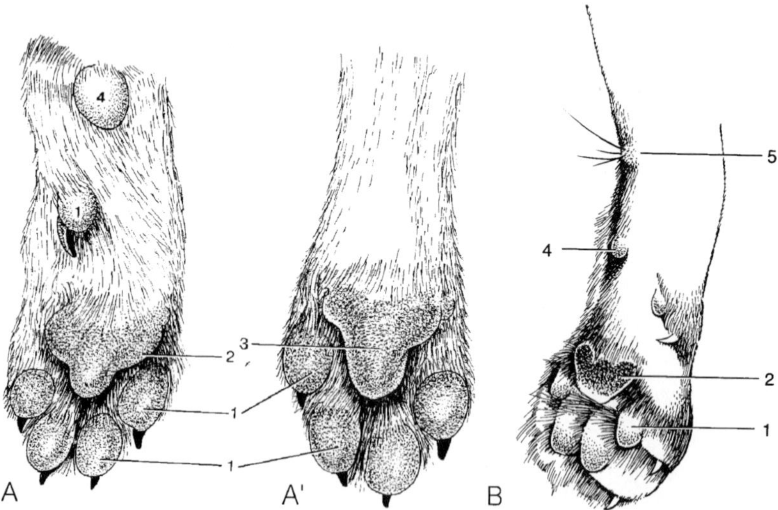


**Figure 10–13.** Footpads of canine fore- and hindlimbs *(A, A′)* and of feline forelimb *(B)*.

1, Digital pads; 2, metacarpal pad; 3, metatarsal pad; 4, carpal pad; 5, carpal gland and associated tactile hairs.

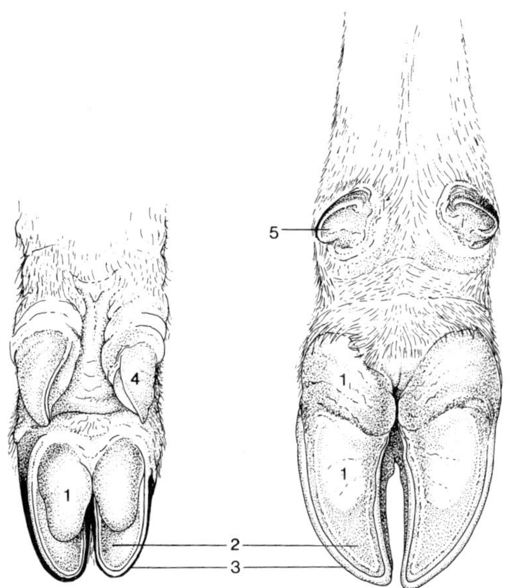


**Figure 10–14.** Palmar surface of foot of the pig *(left)* and of cattle *(right)*.

1, Bulb (digital pad) of hoof; 2, sole of hoof; 3, wall of hoof; 4, hoof of accessory digit; 5, rudimentary hoof of dewclaw.

## NAILS, CLAWS, AND HOOFS

Although these structures enclosing the distal phalanx appear strikingly different at first glance, they are in fact basically similar. Their origins as local modifications of skin are reflected in their retention of epidermal, dermal, and subcutis layers (though perhaps in greatly altered form). Nails, claws, and hoofs serve primarily to protect the underlying tissues, but each is also used for other purposes, such as scratching or digging or as a weapon. The equine hoof, the most complex, reduces concussion on foot impact, when its elastic nature also aids the return of blood to the heart. Figure 10–16 shows the correspondences between these appendages, each of which presents three parts: wall, sole, and associated pad. It is only in ungulates that the last forms part of the horny structure; it corresponds with the digital bulb of primates and the digital pad of carnivores.

The *nail* (wall) of primates grows from the epidermis covering a curved fold of dermis at its base. The epidermis under most of the nail produces a little horn that helps maintain adhesion as the nail gradually slides distally. The dermis under this rather unproductive portion of the epidermis is gathered into a few low, longitudinal folds (laminae) that interdigitate with corresponding epidermal laminae; increased dermoepidermal contact strengthens the bond between the nail and the deeper tissues. The epidermis underlying the free border of the nail produces small amounts of soft "sole horn" (/2).

The wall of the *claw* of carnivores can be likened to a nail that has been laterally compressed and so has obtained a sharp dorsal border. Its proximal part, and the germinal layer from which it is derived, are similarly shaped and are lodged with the associated dermis within the unguicular crest of the distinctively shaped distal phalanx (/*D*). The epidermis deep to the wall is minimally productive. The dermis that covers the unguicular process fuses with the periosteum and, as with the primate nail, longitudinal interdigitations between dermal and epidermal laminae strongly bond the

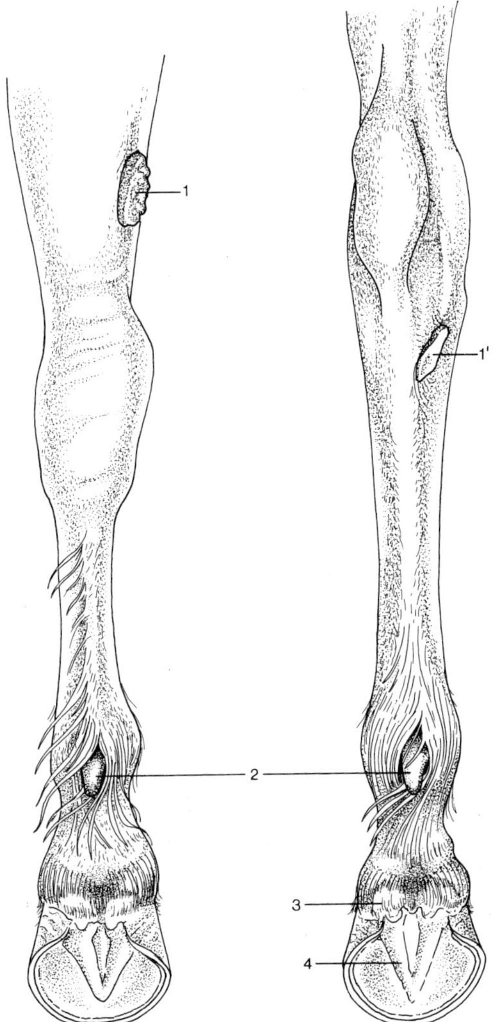


**Figure 10–15.** Left forelimb *(on the left)* and left hindlimb *(on the right)* of the horse, caudal view.

1, 1′, Chestnuts above carpus and below hock, respectively; 2, ergots; 3, bulbs of the heels; 4, frog.

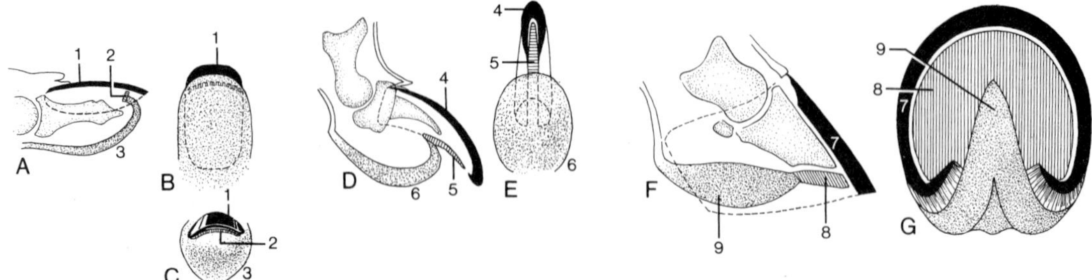


**Figure 10–16.** Schematic representation of nail, claw, and hoof. *A–C,* Longitudinal section, palmar surface, and head-on view of human fingertip. *D, E,* Longitudinal section and palmar surface of canine claw. *F, G,* Longitudinal section and ground surface of equine hoof.

1, Nail (wall); 2, "sole horn" of nail; 3, bulb of finger; 4, wall of claw; 5, "sole" of claw; 6, digital pad; 7, wall of hoof; 8, sole of hoof; 9, frog.

claw to the dorsal border of the bone. The space between the free margins of the wall on the undersurface of the unguicular process is filled with flaky "sole horn" (/5).

The wall of the *horse's hoof* is also strongly curved with the sides sharply inflected to form the so-called bars (Fig. 10–17/2″). The space between the bars is occupied by the frog, the part of the footpad that makes contact with the ground. The sole horn that fills the ground surface between wall and frog meets the wall at a junction known as the white line (zona alba; /5). The wall grows distally from the epidermis over a bulging (coronary) dermis* studded with numerous papillae directed toward the ground. The epidermis covering these papillae produces horn tubules that run distally, toward the weight-bearing margin of the wall. The tubules are embedded in less structured intertubular horn formed by the epidermis over the interpapillary regions of the dermis; the combination of horn types gives the tissue a finely striated appearance. The (laminar) epidermis deep to the wall is again only minimally productive. It is arranged as several hundred well-formed laminae that tightly interdigitate with an equal number of dermal laminae (p. 593), bonding the wall to the underlying distal phalanx. It is well to remember that this is a living bond that allows the wall to slide gradually toward the ground where its distal border is worn away. A band of soft horn (periople) lies over the external surface of the wall near its junction with the skin (Fig. 10–18/1). It descends with the wall and dries to a protective glossy layer. The band widens at the back of the hoof, where it covers the bulbs of the heels and part of the frog.

The *hoofs of ruminants and pig,* though resembling those of the horse in principle, differ in several respects: the wall is sharply bent to form a dorsal border (like that of the claw); the footpad (bulb) is relatively large and furnishes the entire caudal part of the hoof (Fig. 10–17/*B*,4); the sole between the bulb and wall is small; and the interdigitating laminae are less developed (Fig. 10–19/2).

*Formerly, and still commonly, termed *corium.*

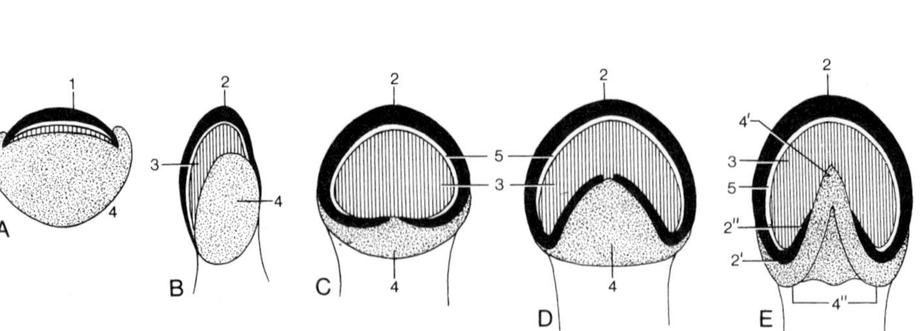


**Figure 10–17.** An "interpretation" of the phylogenetic "development" of the horn structures associated with the distal phalanx. *A,* A human fingertip. *B,* Pig. *C,* Rhinoceros. *D,* Tapir. *E,* Horse.

1, Nail; 2, wall of hoof; 2′, 2″, heel and bar (of horse); 3, sole; 4, footpad (bulb in human finger and pig); 4′, 4″, frog and bulbs of the heels (of horse); 5, white line.

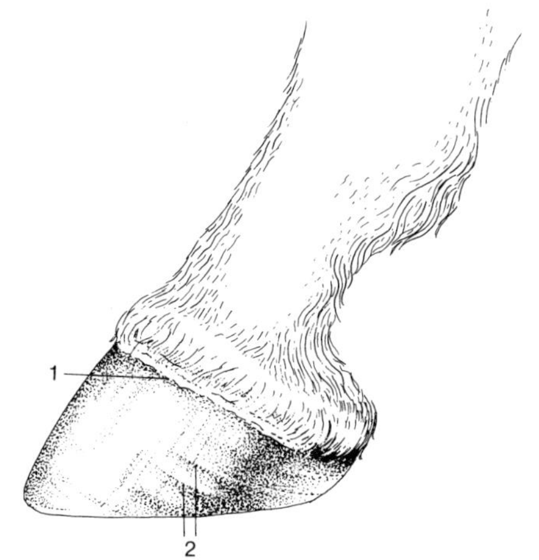


**Figure 10–18.** Equine hoof.

1, Periople; 2, rings indicating uneven horn growth.

In all species, periods of disturbed or lessened horn production create ridges on the wall parallel to the formative region at the junction with the skin (Fig. 10–18/2).

Fuller accounts of these specializations are found in the appropriate later chapters.

## HORNS

The horns of domestic ruminants have osseous bases provided by the cornual processes of the frontal bones. Unlike antlers, which are shed and replaced yearly, horns are permanent* and grow continuously following their first appearance soon after birth.

The dermis is tightly adherent to the cornual process and bears numerous short papillae that are slanted apically, ensuring that the horn elongates as well as thickens as it grows (Fig. 10–20). The horn substance resembles that of the hoof in being an admixture of tubules and intertubular horn. The horn (epiceras) produced by the epidermis at the base is soft and somewhat transparent, resembling the periople of the hoof. It gives the horn its glossy sheen.

In general, horns are found in both sexes—though obviously not in naturally polled breeds—but those of males are usually more massive. Their shape is strongly characteristic of the breed and reflects the shape and size of the cornual process. In cattle, these processes are invaded by the frontal sinuses (/1), which are therefore opened when an adult animal is dehorned.

The horny shell separates from the bony core on maceration, and this explains the (obsolete) zoological designation Cavicornia (hollow-horned animals) sometimes given to ruminants with permanent horns. Ruminants of the deer family (Cervidae) have antlers and are specifically excluded from this grouping. Antlers are sturdy outgrowths of the skull that are initially covered with skin but become exposed when the skin dies. The dead skin, "velvet," is removed by rubbing against trees and other objects. The osseous processes lose their blood supply when exposed, die, and are shed, leaving the animal relatively defenseless until a new set of antlers grows next season.

*Uniquely, the horns of the American Pronghorn are shed annually.

## SKIN GLANDS

The glands of the skin develop as epidermal sprouts that invade the underlying mesoderm. They generally develop from primitive hair follicles and retain these connections; the ducts deliver the secretion into the adult follicles from which it oozes onto the skin surface beside the projecting hairs (Fig. 10–5/9,10). Two basic types—sweat and sebaceous glands—are distinguished, but each occurs in various subvarieties and in more definitely specialized forms.

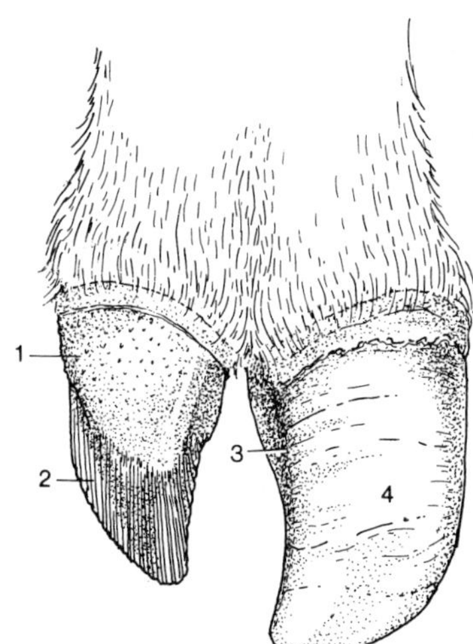


**Figure 10–19.** Bovine foot, dorsal view. The horn shoe (epidermis) has been pulled off one digit, exposing the dermis.

1, Coronary dermis—the wall of the hoof grows distally from the epidermis over this wide band; 2, dermal laminae; 3, dorsal border of hoof; 4, wall of hoof.

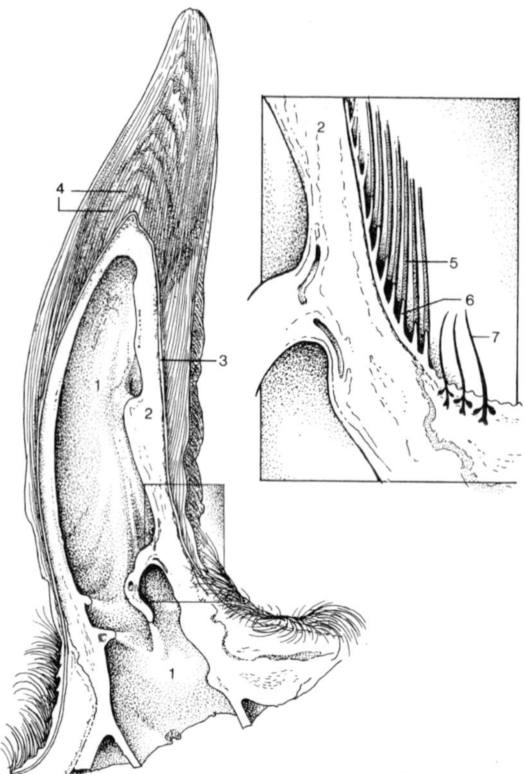


**Figure 10–20.** Longitudinal section of bovine horn.

1, Caudal frontal sinus extending into horn; 2, cornual process of frontal bone; 3, combined periosteum, dermis, and noncornified stratum of epidermis; 4, horn tubules separated by intertubular horn; 5, horn tubules *(inset)*; 6, dermal papilla; 7, hair.

## The Sebaceous Glands

These produce a fatty secretion (sebum) that lubricates and waterproofs the skin and coat. It also promotes the spread of sweat, retards bacterial growth, and, in certain instances, serves as a territorial marker that is recognized by other members of the species. The odor of the wet dog is due to these glands. Certain substances (pheromones) present in sebum are known to be sexually attractive; the rate of production is controlled by steroid hormones, androgens generally promoting and estrogens retarding secretion. A good illustration of a selective effect of androgens is found in the reaction of the so-called acne region of the human adolescent.

The sebum of the fleece of sheep is collected and processed; known as lanolin commercially, it is used as a base for ointments, in cosmetics, and as a cleansing agent in soaps. The secretions of certain specialized glands (e.g., the preputial glands of musk deer and the anal glands of the civet) have long been collected for use by the perfume industry.

The major localized accumulations of sebaceous glands of domestic animals, those of a size visible to the naked eye, are listed; several are associated with skin pouches.

### *Circumoral Glands* (Fig. 10–9)

These large glands are found in the lips of cats, which use them to mark their territories. The secretion is deposited directly by the animal's rubbing its head against an object or ingratiatingly against its owner, and indirectly after transference to the body during grooming.

### *Horn Glands* (Fig. 10–21)

These musk or scent glands are present in goats of both sexes, caudomedial to the horn base (or at the corresponding site in polled animals). They are larger and more productive in the breeding season; those of males, stimulated by testosterone, produce a secretion with an odor so pungent that some owners insist on their surgical removal.

### *Glands of the Infraorbital Pouch* (Fig. 10–22)

These glands are contained in a cutaneous pouch rostral to the eye and opening ventrolaterally upon

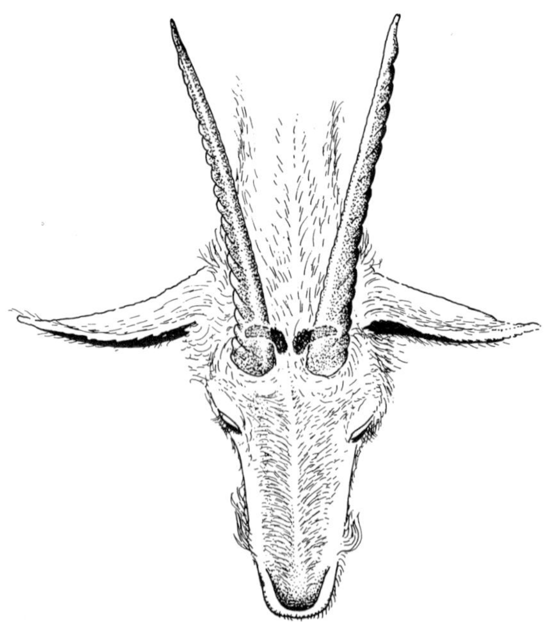

**Figure 10–21.** Horn glands caudomedial to the base of the horns in the goat.

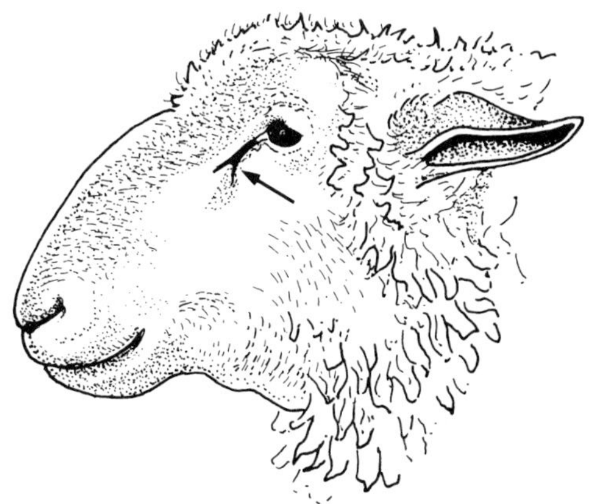

**Figure 10–22.** Infraorbital pouch *(arrow)* of the sheep.

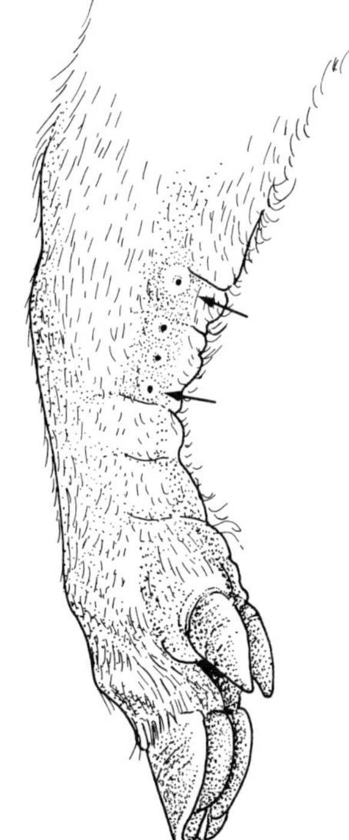

**Figure 10–23.** Carpal glands *(arrows)* of the pig, medial view.

the face of sheep. The pouch wall contains both sebaceous and tubular serous glands whose mixed secretion stains the skin when it escapes from the pouch. The glands, which serve as territorial markers, are larger in rams.

## *Carpal Glands* (Fig. 10–23)

These are present in pigs and cats. In pigs they surround several cutaneous invaginations on the mediopalmar aspect of the carpus. They are found in both sexes and serve to indicate territorial claims; boars are said to make particular use of them when "marking" sows during copulation.

The location of the glands in cats is marked by a tuft of a few tactile hairs proximal to the carpal pad. The site is betrayed by a palpable thickening of the skin (Fig. 10–13/*B*,5).

## *Glands of the Interdigital Pouch* (Fig. 10–24)

Interdigital pouches are found on the fore- and hindlimbs of sheep of both sexes. The pouches are tubular invaginations of the skin whose walls contain branched sebaceous and serous glands. The waxy secretion is discharged through a single opening above the hoofs and serves as a "trail marker." Many gregarious wild species have similar glands.

## *Glands of the Inguinal Pouch* (Fig. 10–25)

Inguinal pouches, found near the base of the udder or scrotum of sheep, contain both sebaceous and sweat glands. The secretion escapes as a brown waxy substance whose odor may assist the lamb to find the udder.

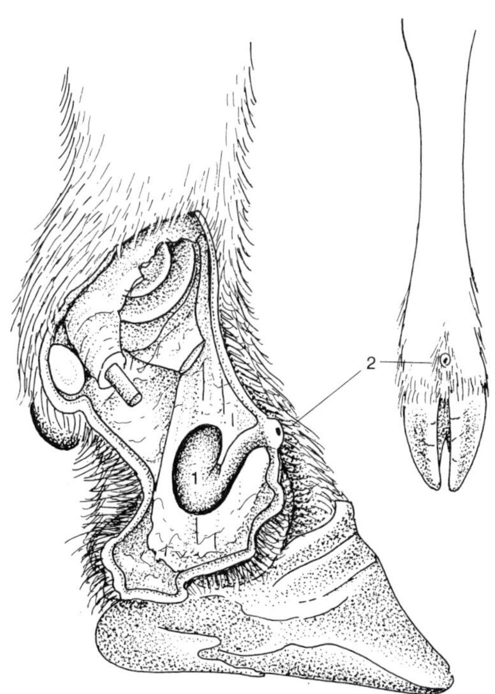


**Figure 10–24.** Interdigital pouch (1), and its opening (2), of the sheep.

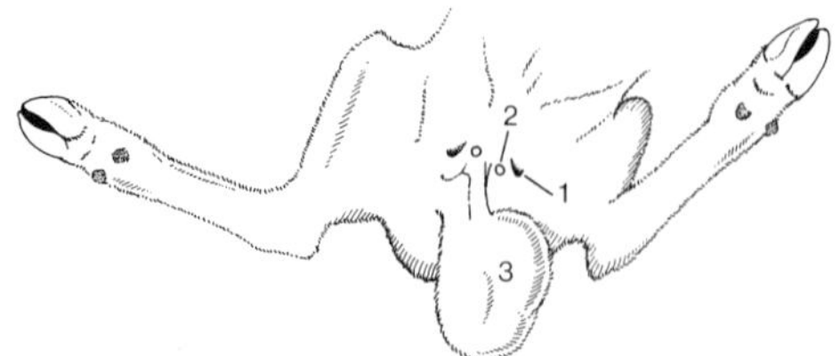


**Figure 10–25.** Inguinal region of the ram.

1, Inguinal pouch; 2, rudimentary teat; 3, scrotum.

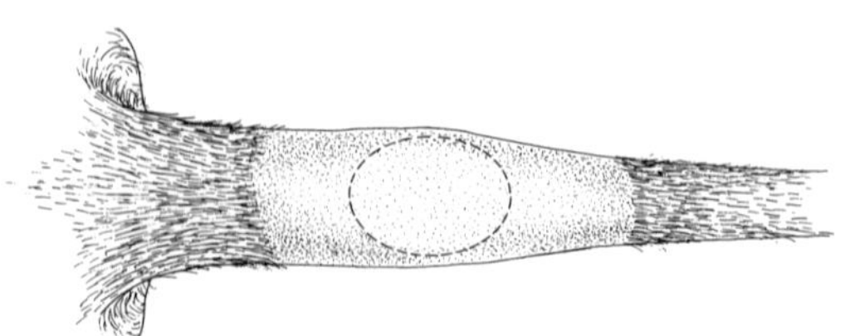

**Figure 10–26.** Location of the tail glands of the dog.

### *Preputial Glands*

Sebaceous and apocrine sweat glands within the prepuce produce secretions that combine with desquamated cells to form the crumbly substance known as smegma. They are best developed in the boar, in which they are massed within a dorsal diverticulum of the preputial cavity (see Fig. 37–10/5). Their secretion gives the boar its characteristic odor. They are present but less offensive in other species (which lack the diverticulum).

### *Tail Glands*

Collections of large sebaceous and serous glands are found in an oval patch on the dorsal surface of the tail of certain carnivores. The skin over these glands is often defined by its sparser hair and yellowish color. Activity is greatest during the breeding season. The patch is situated more proximally in cats, toward the root of the tail, than in dogs (Fig. 10–26).

### *Circumanal Glands* (Fig. 10–27)

These sebaceous glands are restricted to the perianal skin of certain carnivores, including dogs, where they drain into (and are believed to influence) special sweat glands. It is probably their secretion that excites the particular attention paid to the anal region when dogs confer. It has been suggested that some of these glands have an endocrine function.

### *Glands of the Anal Sacs* (Fig. 10–28)

Sebaceous and serous glands are found in the walls of the anal sacs, cutaneous pouches that open beside the anus of carnivores (Fig. 10–27/2). The secretion, which is particularly foul-smelling, is expressed during defecation and apparently serves as a marker. It is well-known that skunks can forcefully expel the contents of the sacs to fend off aggressors.

## The Sweat Glands

Sweat glands are scattered over the entire body, though somewhat sparsely in carnivores and pigs. Two types are distinguished by (a probably erroneous interpretation of) the histology of the secretory process. Apocrine sweat glands discharge an albuminous sweat into hair follicles over most of the body.* Eccrine glands secrete a more watery sweat directly onto certain naked, or nearly naked, regions of the skin (e.g., the nasolabial plate of cattle and the footpads of dogs). The apocrine variety predominates, and its secretion and subsequent evaporation are important in salt metabolism and temperature regulation. The secretion is degraded by bacteria, forming substances that provide the characteristic body odor. The product of the eccrine variety is thought to play a lesser role in temperature regulation.

*There are important species differences. The distribution and other features of human (and other primate) sweat glands differ significantly.

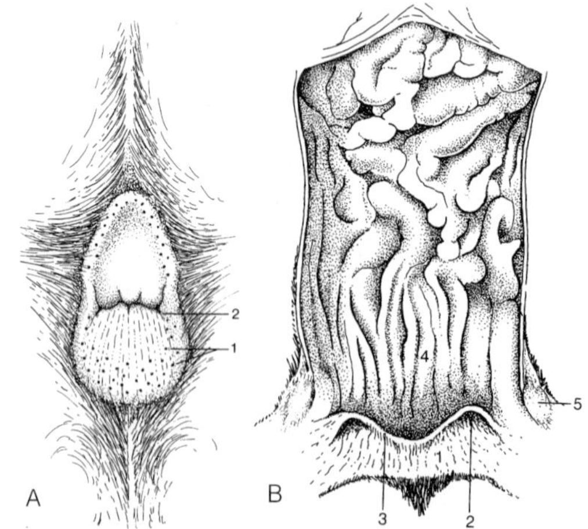


**Figure 10–27.** *A*, Cutaneous zone of the canine anal canal. *B*, Feline anal canal opened dorsally.

1, Cutaneous zone with circumanal glands forming a ring around the anus of the dog; 2, opening of the right anal sac; 3, anocutaneous line; 4, columnar zone; 5, right anal sac.

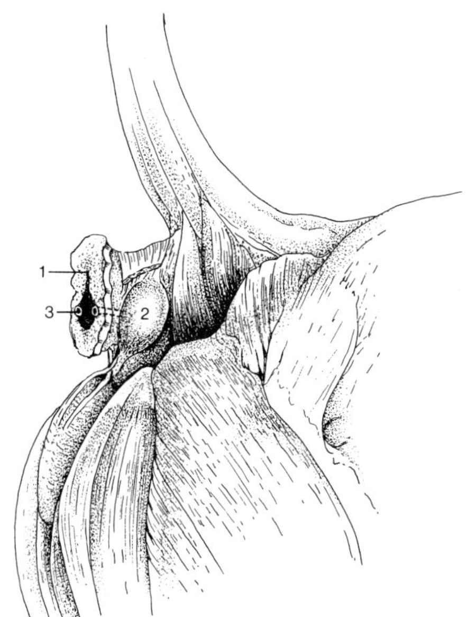


**Figure 10–28.** Exposed right anal sac of a dog.

1, Anus; 2, anal sac; 3, opening of excretory duct of anal sac (emphasized; see Fig. 10–27/*A*,2).

Most mammals possess fewer glands and sweat less profusely than humans. However, impressions can be misleading since the sweating that does occur tends to be masked by the more generous coat. The horse is an obvious exception to the general statement since it not only sweats abundantly but also produces an especially albuminous sweat that froths when worked by movement of the skin and coat ("lathering up"). Certain breeds of cattle also sweat visibly along the neck and over the flanks; in this species there are well-established differences between temperate and tropical breeds in the number, size, and distribution of the glands. Surprisingly, the Asiatic buffalo has fewer sweat glands than cattle and resorts to wallowing in water in compensation. Among domestic species, dogs and cats sweat least, although the skin of short-haired individuals sometimes feels moist.

## The Mammary Glands

Mammary glands (mammae) are greatly modified, much enlarged sweat glands whose secretion nourishes the young. The modified milk (colostrum) produced immediately after parturition has an additional role in the passive transfer of immunity to the newborn. Its importance varies among species, there being some correlation with the nature of the placental barrier. Each mammary gland is a compound tubuloalveolar gland that consists of secretory units grouped into lobules defined by intervening connective tissue septa (Plate 30/*G*). The mammary glands develop as epithelial buds that grow into the underlying mesenchyme from linear ectodermal thickenings (mammary ridges). These ridges may extend from the axilla to the groin (as in carnivores and pigs) or may be of more limited extent, restricted to the axilla (as in elephants), the thorax (as in women), or the groin (as in ruminants and horses). Usually more buds appear than survive in the adult, and while most extra buds soon regress, some persist to give rise to *supernumerary* teats. These may be independent or attached to other, better developed glands (see Fig. 31–2). They are unsightly and since they may interfere with milking they are often removed from the udders of cows and goats.

Proliferation of the mesenchyme surrounding the bud raises a teat (papilla) upon the surface of the body. One or more epidermal sprouts grow from the mammary bud into the connective tissue of the teat and begin to canalize at about the time of birth. Each sprout is destined to form a separate duct system with associated glandular tissue. When there is only one sprout, the mammary gland arising from it has a single duct system leading to a single orifice on the tip of the teat (Fig. 10–29/*A*).

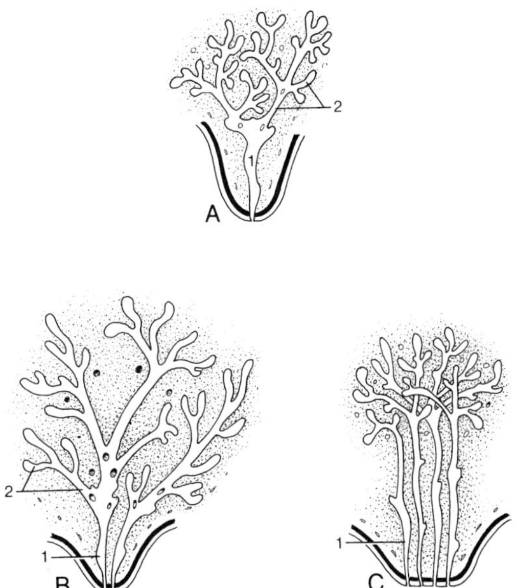


**Figure 10–29.** Developing duct systems growing proximally from the tip of the fetal teat. *A*, Cow, ewe, and goat. *B*, Mare and sow. *C*, Bitch and cat (only four primary sprouts are shown).

1, Primary sprout, which gives rise to the lactiferous sinus; 2, secondary and tertiary sprouts, which give rise to the lactiferous ducts.

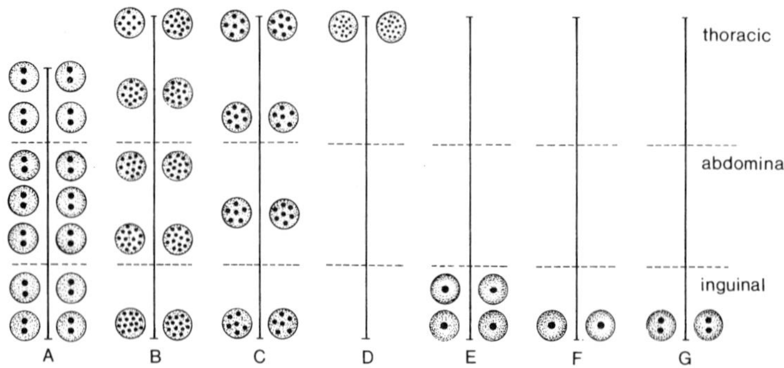


**Figure 10–30.** Distribution of mammary glands in certain mammals. The dots indicate the number of orifices on the teat. *A,* Sow. *B,* Bitch. *C,* Cat. *D,* Woman. *E,* Cow. *F,* Ewe and she-goat. *G,* Mare.

When there are more, say two or four as in our illustration, there will be that number of separate duct systems, each with an associated glandular mass and separate orifice. The growth of the ducts and gland tissue is continued after puberty and especially during the first pregnancy, forming the swelling that pushes the teat away from the body wall. The process is controlled by the intricate interplay of several hormones from the hypophysis, ovaries, and other endocrine glands.

Examination of one of the several units formed along the trunk of a lactating sow (see Fig. 35–1) reveals that it is composed of glandular tissue supported and enclosed by a fibrous tissue framework in which run the mammary vessels and nerves. The whole formation is pervaded with fat and covered by skin. Sometimes, as in ruminants and horses, the mammary glands are so closely placed that they appear to merge in a single consolidated complex—the udder. Though the glands of the pig, like those of the dog and cat, remain more distinctly separated, this collective term is sometimes used also in the sow. The number of mammary glands (as well as their duct systems) in the domestic species is shown schematically in Figure 10–30.

The more detailed organization is illustrated by reference to the cow. The glandular tissue is arranged in lobules (Fig. 10–31/1 and Plate 30/*G*), each 1 mm or perhaps a little more in diameter and consisting of about 200 alveoli. The milk drains to an intralobular duct that joins others to form a larger interlobular duct (/2′). Interlobular ducts lead in their turn to a system of lactiferous (milk-carrying) ducts that ultimately convey the milk to the relatively large cavity known as the lactiferous sinus (/4). The lactiferous ducts of successive orders increase in diameter but diminish in number so that only 10 or so enter the sinus. Unlike most ducts, they have alternating narrow and dilated portions; contraction of the muscular wall of the narrow portions holds the milk in the expansions before it is "let down" when the cow suckles or is milked. The lactiferous sinus extends into the teat and is incompletely divided into gland and teat sinuses by a constriction. The teat sinus is continued by the papillary duct, which opens at the tip of the teat where the orifice is surrounded by a smooth muscle sphincter (/8).

Corresponding parts can be identified in other species, including those in which each gland contains several small lactiferous sinuses, each

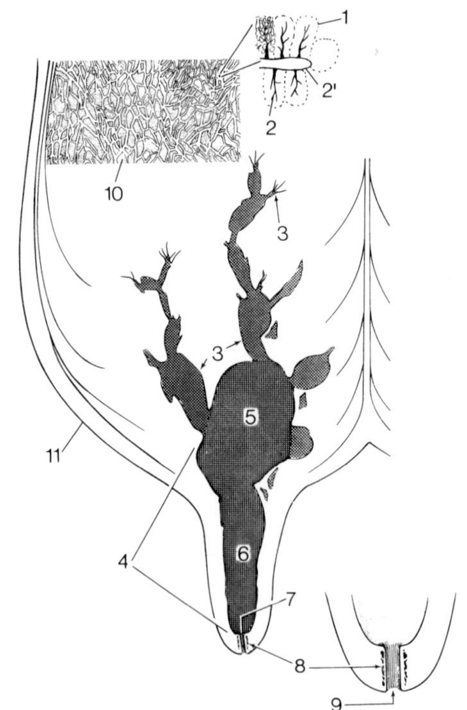


**Figure 10–31.** Duct system of the bovine mammary gland.

1, Lobule; 2, intralobular duct; 2′, interlobular duct; 3, lactiferous ducts of various diameters; 4, lactiferous sinus; 5, gland sinus; 6, teat sinus; 7, papillary duct; 8, teat sphincter; 9, teat orifice; 10, parenchyma of gland; 11, skin.

served by a separate duct system and each opening independently.

It must be stressed that mammary glands are fully developed and fully functional only at the height of lactation. They are then large and show a predominance of yellow glandular tissue over the paler fibrous stroma. When the dam weans her young, involution sets in and the parenchyma regresses (Plate 30/*F*); the connective tissues now form the bulk of the organ. However, the gland never quite reverts to its prelactation size and it grows a little more with each pregnancy.

Mammary buds also form in male embryos and persist to give rise to the rudimentary teats found on the ventral surface of the trunk (carnivores and pig) or on the cranial surface of the scrotum (ruminants) (Fig. 10–25/2). They are less common in horses but occasionally appear beside the prepuce. On the other hand, in certain species, such as rats, the male glands regress completely.

# CHAPTER 11

# The Head and Ventral Neck of the Carnivores



The series of chapters (11–17 inclusive) that begins here is concerned with the anatomy of the two companion species, the dog and cat. Although both are included within the one order, Carnivora, the dichotomy between Canoidea and Feloidea, the suborders to which the two species respectively belong, was of ancient occurrence. Despite this, and despite the existence of certain differentiating specializations, the general anatomies of the two domestic species are sufficiently alike for it to be possible to consider them together. Though cats rival, and in many countries now surpass, dogs in popularity, it is both conventional and convenient (because of the greater wealth of literature) to base the initial accounts upon the dog and follow these with mention of the clinically significant differences in the cat. Distinctions that are essentially matters of dimension and proportion are more usefully covered by illustration than description.

Dogs of course differ very considerably among themselves, and where no specific breed features are mentioned it may be assumed that the description, as well as any measurements that are given, refers to animals of moderate size and generalized conformation such as are represented by the Beagle.

The reader is also reminded that the systematic chapters (1–10 inclusive) are largely based on the anatomy of the dog, which supplies the bulk of their illustrations. In order to facilitate review, page references to earlier material will be found under many subheadings in the chapters that now follow.

## CONFORMATION AND EXTERNAL FEATURES

Conformation varies more in dogs than in other domesticated species. The preferences, frequently ill-conceived, of fanciers have produced a variety of breeds that are not only strikingly different from each other, and from their common wolf ancestor, but are also sometimes incapable of leading a full existence without human cosseting. This variation is nowhere better expressed than in the head.

The appearance of the dog's head is largely determined by the shape of the skull, the position and size of the eyes, and the form and carriage of the ears. The ears may be held erect, hang from the side, or have an intermediate carriage that is erect at the base and pendulous toward the tip. Certain differences are permanent attributes of breed, others no more than temporary expressions of mood.

The bare skin around the nostrils, the *nasal plate,* is divided by a median philtrum that continues ventrally to groove the upper lip (see Fig. 4–1). It is very pronounced in some breeds. The surface of the plate is irregularly divided, creating a pattern believed to be individual and therefore available as a means of identification (noseprinting; Fig. 10–3/*B*).

The adult *skull* has been described (p. 58). It is characterized by a well-developed facial part, large orbits and temporal fossae, incomplete postorbital bars, the absence of supraorbital foramina, and prominent tympanic bullae. It is widest behind the eyes, where the zygomatic arches are widely spread. Breed differences in the skull relate largely to the relative length of the facial part. Dolichocephalic, brachycephalic, and mesaticephalic (long, short, and intermediate head length) breeds are recognized. A good example of the first is the Greyhound, whose head is long and narrow (Fig. 11–1/*A*). The dorsal surfaces of nose and cranium form two nearly parallel planes that are divided at the level of the eyes by a break (nasofrontal angle or stop) where the cranium descends to the level of the nose. The long facial part is often accompanied by an underbite jaw (brachygnathism). The well-muscled head of a dolichocephalic dog has a prominent external sagittal crest for expanded attachment of the temporalis muscles. Examples of the brachycephalic types are the English Bulldog and the Pekingese. In these the facial part is extremely short and the cranium exceptionally wide and globular; the stop is pronounced and the dorsal surface of the cranium is convex with a much reduced external sagittal crest; numerous skin folds mark the face; and the eyes are widely spaced. Certain brachycephalic breeds are prognathic, the lower jaw not sharing fully in the foreshortening of the face. Difficulties with nasal breathing and with the occlusion of the teeth are not uncommon. Most breeds, however, belong to the mesaticephalic type, in which the length of the skull is more harmoniously proportional to its width.

An impression of the general shape of a skull is conveyed by the cephalic index, obtained from the formula:

$$\frac{100 \times \text{breadth of skull}}{\text{length of skull}}.$$

In the dog this index varies from below 50 in long-headed breeds to almost 100 in those with the shortest heads. The craniofacial index is possibly more revealing; this is obtained from the formula:

$$\frac{\text{length of cranium}}{\text{length of face}},$$

taking the frontonasal suture as the boundary. The index may considerably exceed 3 in the most distorted short-headed breeds with "pushed-in" faces and prominent stops. It is about 2 in the mesaticephalic beagle.

The face of the dog is more expressive of emotion than that of other species, and everyone is familiar with the signs that indicate aggressive intent, submission, or pain, even if unable to particularize them. Owners frequently assert, and with some reason, that they can interpret other more subtle changes. Age is also clearly revealed in dogs of pigmented coat by a "graying" that begins at the upper lip and later spreads, reaching the area about the eyes by about the eighth year or a little later.

Redundancy of facial skin is a feature of several breeds, Bulldogs and Bloodhounds among others, and in extreme form may result in frontal folds that obscure the vision and, by turning the upper eyelid inward (entropion), irritate the cornea through contact with hairy skin. The problem is encountered in grotesque form in Shar-Peis, a consequence of ill-considered breeding policy. Mitigation may be obtained by carefully adjusted surgery.

The cat's head also exhibits features distinctive of breed, or rather type. In most cats the face is relatively short but in certain Oriental breeds, especially the Siamese, it is proportionately longer and the whole head is more wedge-shaped with a less pronounced stop (Fig. 11–2/*A*). In contrast, Persian cats have very short "pushed-in" faces; when exaggerated, this trait may be associated with blockage of the tear ducts, leading to persistent weeping. The eyes and orbits are relatively large and they face more directly forward than in dogs, providing a wider field of binocular vision (Fig. 10–9). The infraorbital foramen is small and not easily found on palpation; it lies very close to the orbit. The ears are wide at the base and are carried erect, except in the Scottish Fold in which the distal part of the pinna flops. The contrast between the rather short, rounded ears of most European breeds and the larger, pointed ears of the Oriental has little practical importance but contributes much to breed "character." The tactile hairs (whiskers) are prominent.

In cats, in contrast to the breeds of dog recently mentioned, the bare sufficiency of the skin of the scalp creates problems when it is necessary to close large wounds.

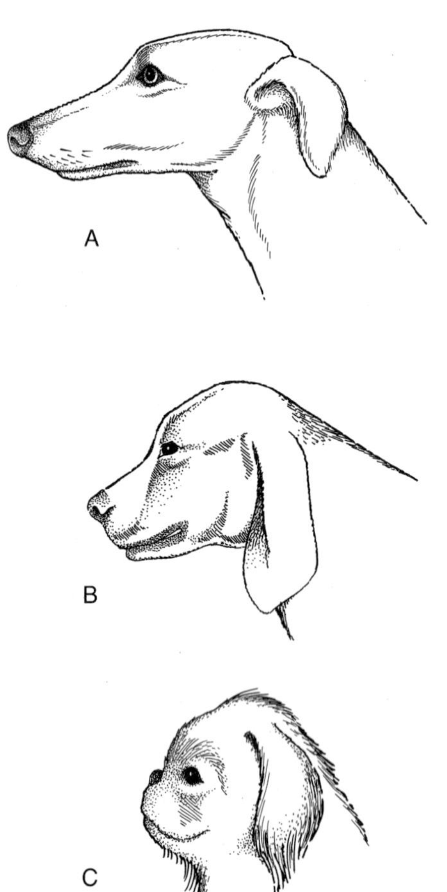


**Figure 11–1.** Representatives of dolichocephalic (*A*), mesaticephalic (*B*), and brachycephalic (*C*) breeds.

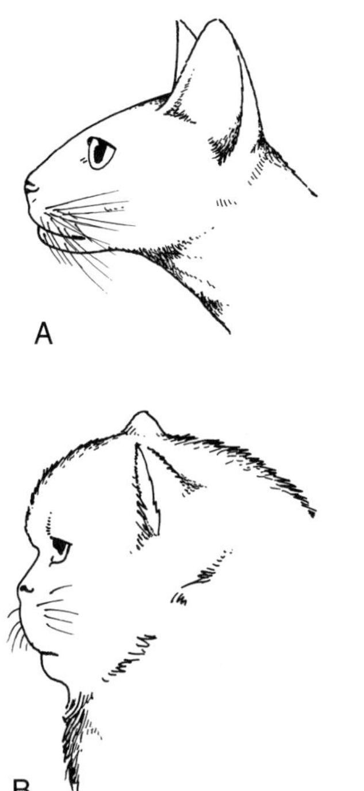


**Figure 11–2.** Representatives of long-headed Oriental *(A)* and short-headed Persian *(B)* types of cat.

## SUPERFICIAL STRUCTURES

Much of the surface of the skull can be palpated since it is either directly subcutaneous or covered only by a thin layer of muscle. Palpable features of the face include the infraorbital and mental foramina, and the ridge over the long root of the upper canine tooth. The masticatory muscles are massive, and the temporalis and masseter remove the lateral plate of the frontal and parietal bones, and the ramus of the mandible, from direct reach. The boundary between these muscles is provided by the zygomatic arch, a relatively vulnerable region of the skull prone to traumatic separation at the oblique suture between the zygomatic and temporal bones (see Fig. 2–34). The fontanelle, characteristic of the neonatal skull, may persist into adult life in certain toy breeds in which it remains a palpable feature. The brain case is surmounted by the sagittal crest and by the nuchal crest, which connects the caudal end of the sagittal crest with the base of the ear, providing the dorsal boundary of the triangular caudal (nuchal) surface of the skull. Both crests are palpable, although little of the nuchal surface can be appreciated. In the puppy's skull the cranial exceeds the facial part in size, being relatively much wider than it becomes in the adult (see Fig. 1–18); the sagittal crest has yet to form and the nuchal crest, although visible on the skull, is not palpable.

Other superficial structures, some palpable, may be identified with the aid of Figure 11–3/*A*, which omits certain of the smaller cutaneous muscles. The dorsal buccal branch (/7) of the facial nerve runs across the dorsal half of the masseter; the ventral branch takes the more protected course along the ventral edge; they are joined by communicating branches at the cranial border of the muscle. The auriculopalpebral branch of the facial nerve (/*A*6) passes across the zygomatic arch, where it can be blocked to eliminate blinking (m. orbicularis oculi) during examination of the eye. The *parotid duct* (/*A*8) also crosses the masseter, midway between the two branches of the facial nerve; it can sometimes be palpated before it passes deep to the communicating nerves and the facial vessels to open into the cheek cavity opposite the upper fourth cheek tooth. Accessory lobules of the parotid gland may accompany the duct. The end of this duct is occasionally transplanted into the conjunctival sac when the flow of tears is insufficient to keep the conjunctiva moist.

The ventral border of the mandible and the prominent angular process at its caudal end are easily palpated. The halves of the mandible meet in a cartilaginous joint that persists throughout life. Separation at this synchondrosis and fractures of the mandible are both common injuries, especially from traffic accidents. The parotid and mandibular glands and the mandibular lymph nodes can be palpated caudal to the mandible (Plate 16/*D*). The *mandibular gland* (/*A*12) is embraced by the maxillary and linguofacial veins, which join to form the external jugular vein. The linguofacial vein is short since the lingual tributary, which is joined to its fellow by a subcutaneous anastomosis level with the (palpable) basihyoid, enters close by the gland. The *facial vein,* when followed rostrally, first passes over the mandibular lymph nodes and then along the ventral border of the masseter before crossing the face obliquely. It arises from the fusion of prominent dorsal nasal and angularis oculi veins rostral to the eye. These run the risk of injury when surgical access is made to the nasal cavity and frontal sinuses. The angularis oculi vein, which emerges from the orbit, is also vulnerable during enucleation (removal) of the eye. The facial artery and accompanying vein serve the lips, cheek, and muzzle; the side of the nose is supplied by an artery that emerges from the infraorbital foramen.

The distribution of the cutaneous nerves follows the general pattern (see Fig. 8–68).

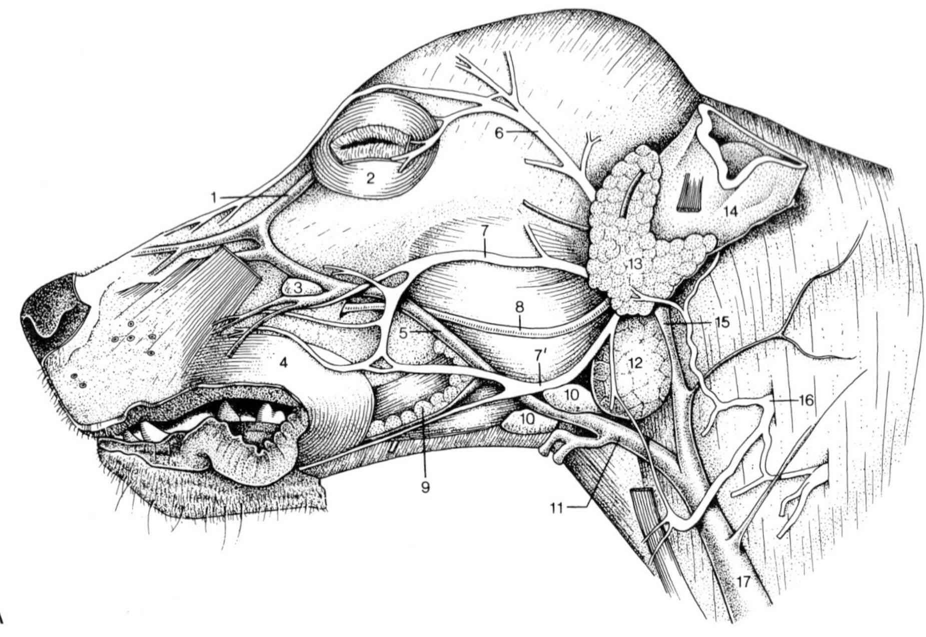


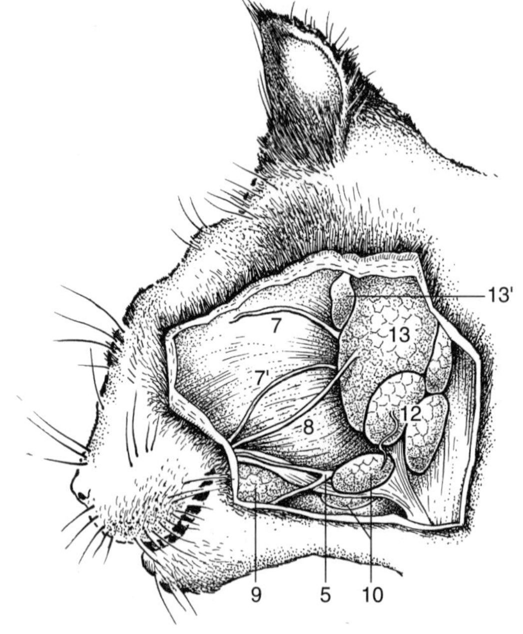


**Figure 11–3.** Superficial dissection of the canine *(A)* and feline *(B)* heads.

1, Angularis oculi vein; 2, orbicularis oculi; 3, facial lymph node; 4, orbicularis oris; 5, facial vein; 6, auriculopalpebral nerve; 7,7′, dorsal and ventral buccal branches of facial nerve; 8, parotid duct; 9, buccal salivary glands; 10, mandibular lymph nodes; 11, linguofacial vein; 12, mandibular gland; 13, parotid gland; 13′, parotid lymph node; 14, base of ear; 15, maxillary vein; 16, second cervical nerve; 17, external jugular vein.

## THE NASAL CAVITY AND PARANASAL SINUSES

*(See also pp. 148–152.)*

The nasal cavity extends to the level of the eyes. Its rostral part is roughly tubular, while caudal to the level of the infraorbital foramen it widens and gains in height (Fig. 11–4). Only the caudal and dorsal parts of the nasal septum ossify. The rostral extremity, which projects beyond the skull, remains cartilaginous, and this accounts for the passive mobility of the tip of the nose. The cavity is more tightly filled with nasal and ethmoidal *conchae* than in other species, and the intervening meatuses are narrow. The rostral half lodges the

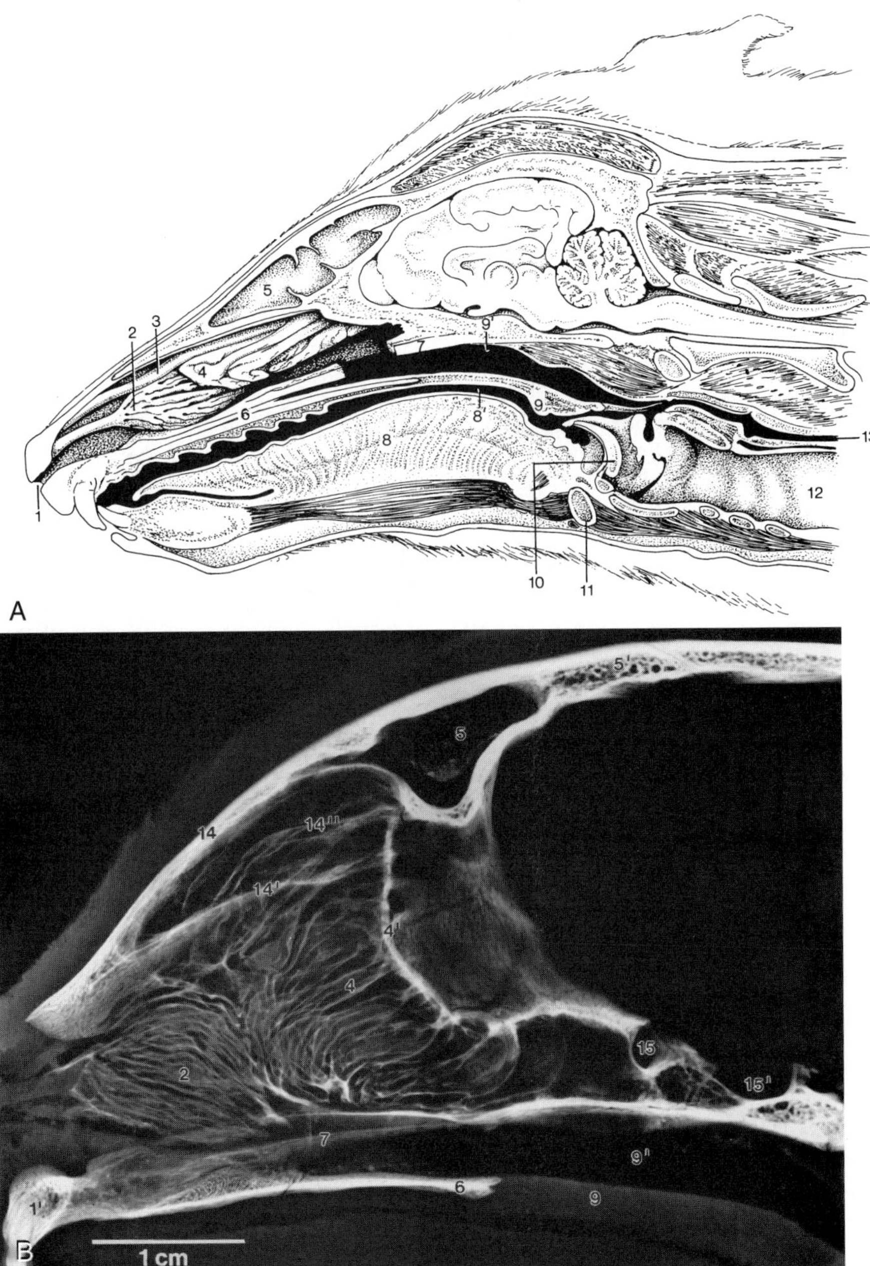


**Figure 11–4.** Paramedian section of the canine head *(A)* and tomogram of the feline nasal cavity *(B)*.

1, Right nostril; 1′, incisive bone with incisor; 2, ventral nasal concha; 3, dorsal nasal concha; 4, ethmoidal conchae; 4′, cribriform plate; 5, frontal sinus; 5′, frontal bone; 6, hard palate; 7, vomer (resected in A); 8, tongue; 8′, oropharynx; 9, soft palate; 9′, nasopharynx; 10, epiglottis; 11, basihyoid; 12, trachea; 13, esophagus; 14, nasal bone; 14′, horizontal crest of nasal bone; 14″, dorsal part of nasal cavity invaded by ethmoidal conchae; 15, optic canal; 15′, hypophysial fossa.

dorsal and ventral nasal conchae. The dorsal one (/A3) is a simple plate where it arises from the nasal bone, but it widens caudally where it attaches to the ethmoid. The ventral concha, which is thick but short, arises from the maxilla and breaks up to form many scrolls that greatly enlarge the area of richly vascularized mucosa (see Fig. 4–3). It is continued rostrally by the alar fold, which ends in a bulbous swelling, visible through the nostril, on the lateral wall of the vestibule. In some brachycephalic dogs the swelling is large enough to hamper breathing and must be resected.

The *nasolacrimal duct* (Fig. 11–5) opens where the floor of the vestibule meets the alar fold and is visible when the nostril is spread. As often as not, there is a second, more caudal, opening level with the canine tooth. The duct of the *lateral nasal gland* opens directly caudal to the vestibular orifice of the nasolacrimal duct, on the lateral wall above the alar fold. The gland lies in the lateral nasal wall close by the entrance to the maxillary recess (see further on). The watery secretions of the lacrimal, lateral nasal, and scattered minor nasal glands moisten the nasal plate, which has no intrinsic glands. As is well-known, a moist nose is generally regarded as a sign of health. The secretion of the lateral nasal gland may have a social significance that accounts for the nose-to-nose sniffing common when dogs meet.

The caudal half of the nasal cavity is almost filled by ethmoidal conchae covered with olfactory mucosa; they are so extensive that they also invade the lower part of the frontal sinuses. Collectively, the ethmoidal conchae are larger than the nasal conchae—an indication of the dog's keen sense of smell (Fig. 11–6/11).

The *sinus system* of the dog is poorly developed. The three frontal compartments, which drain separately into the nasal cavity through ethmoidal meatuses, may be invaded by ethmoidal conchae. The lateral compartment is the largest and occupies much of the frontal bone, including its zygomatic process; it may extend to the level of the temporomandibular joints in larger animals (especially if they are long-headed) (Fig. 11–7).

The maxillary sinus communicates so freely with the nasal cavity that the term *maxillary recess* is preferred. The communication faces forward and is at the level of the sectorial tooth ($P^4$). The recess occupies the face immediately rostral to the orbit above the roots of the last three cheek teeth. Root abscesses may break into the recess and later onto the surface of the skull. Surgical drainage is most conveniently achieved by the extraction of the sectorial tooth to open a passage to the mouth since the presence of the infraorbital canal makes the direct lateral approach unwise (see Fig. 4–6).

The sinus system of the cat comprises frontal, sphenoidal, and maxillary compartments, among which the frontal is the most important (Figs. 11–4/*B*, 5 and 11–8/1). It occupies the same general position as the corresponding sinus of the dog but is undivided and extends rather far ventrally within the medial wall of the orbit. The communication with the nasal cavity is in the rostral part of the sinus and may provide ineffective drainage in the bacterial sinusitis that commonly complicates viral infections of the upper

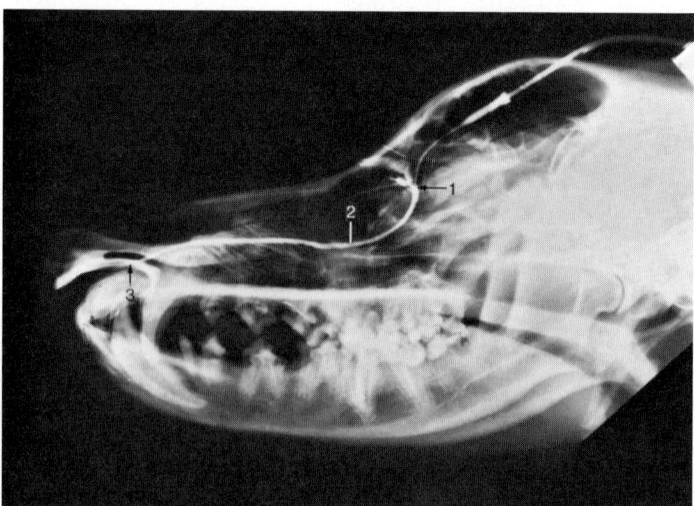


**Figure 11–5.** Contrast medium outlining the canine nasolacrimal duct in a radiograph.

1, Position of ventral punctum; 2, nasolacrimal duct; 3, opening of duct at the nostril.

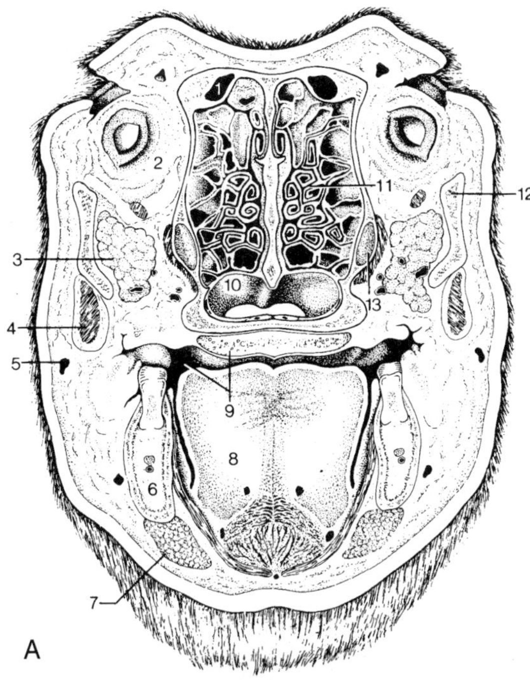


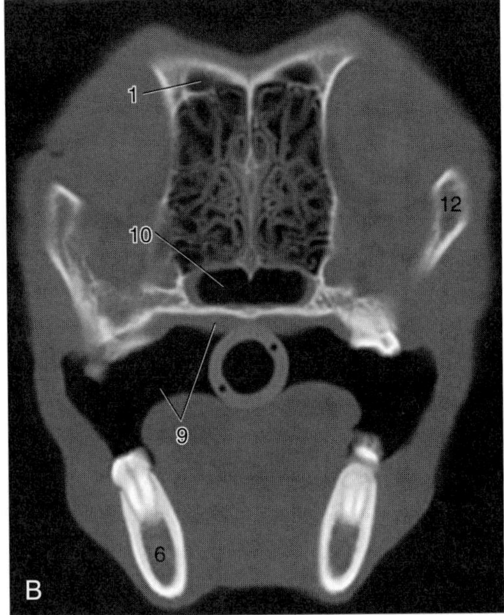


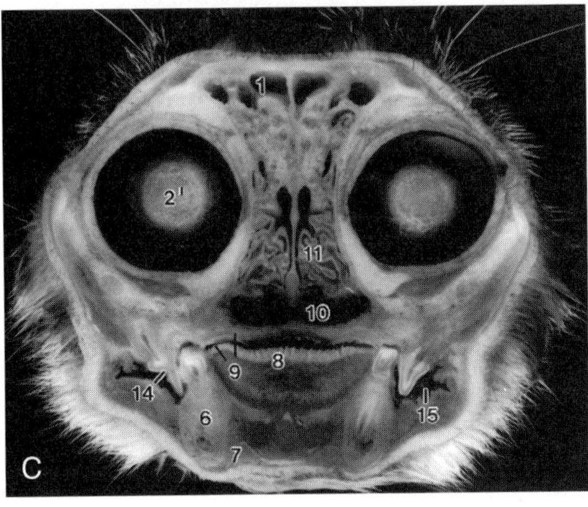


**Figure 11–6.** Transverse section of the canine *(A)* and feline *(C)* heads through the rostral part of the orbit, rostral surface. *(B)* CT scan (bone window) of canine head at the level of A.

1, Frontal sinus; 2, orbital structures; 2′, eye; 3, zygomatic gland; 4, masseter; 5, facial vein; 6, mandible; 7, digastricus; 8, tongue; 9, oral cavity and hard palate; 10, choana; 11, ethmoidal conchae; 12, zygomatic arch; 13, maxillary recess; 14, sectorial teeth, $P^4$ engaging $M_1$; 15, oral vestibule.

respiratory tract. Surgical drainage may then be required.

## THE MOUTH AND OROPHARYNX

*(See also pp. 100–106 and 116–119.)*

The wide gape of carnivores is made possible by the caudal situation of the angles of the mouth and the correspondingly short length of the cheeks. The interior of the mouth, including the oropharynx, is therefore easily examined.

The edge of the lower lip carries blunt papillae. The upper lip is pendulous and presses on the lower one, which is everted near the commissure in certain breeds, such as Spaniels, with ample head skin (Fig. 11–3 and Plate 16/*B*). The resulting creases predispose to infection. The general looseness of the lips creates a large vestibule—an advantage when administering liquid medicines, which then escape behind the cheek teeth into the central cavity (Fig. 11–6/*C*, 15). The ducts of the parotid and zygomatic salivary glands open into the vestibule, the former by a single orifice on a small papilla opposite the upper fourth premolar, the latter by a row of four or five orifices on a mucosal ridge a little farther caudally. The ducts of the mandibular and compact (monostomatic) sublingual glands open on the floor of the mouth at the sublingual caruncle. They run below the mucous membrane that connects the side of the tongue

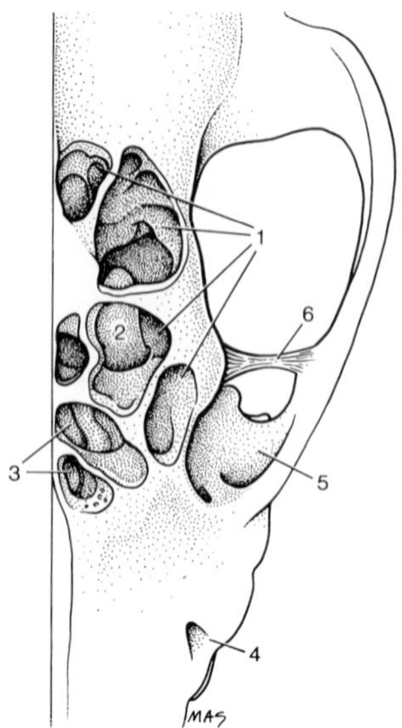


**Figure 11–7.** The canine frontal sinuses, dorsal view.

1, Lateral frontal sinus; 2, ethmoidal concha invading the sinus; 3, medial and rostral frontal sinuses; 4, infraorbital foramen; 5, orbit; 6, orbital ligament.

with the gums; when a duct is damaged, saliva may escape to form a large submucosal swelling (ranula) lateral to the tongue. The larger salivary ducts are occasionally cannulated to remove obstructions or to inject a contrast medium for radiographic examination (sialography; Plate 16/*D* and Fig. 11–9).

The oral cavity proper, like the nasal cavity above it, widens from front to back until it contracts at the level of the palatoglossal arches, beyond which it is continued by the oropharynx.

The hard palate presents transverse ridges and a prominent incisive papilla (see Fig. 3–5). The narrow incisive ducts that open beside the papilla furnish communication with the vomeronasal organs and nasal cavity. The oral mucosa, generally pink, may be pigmented locally. The wide and flat apex of the *tongue* is depressed centrally (like a spoon) when liquids are lapped. A short median rod (lyssa) of connective, muscular, and cartilaginous tissue is embedded close to the ventral surface of the tongue. Its significance is not known, though a fanciful connection with rabies was postulated in former times. The (sublingual) veins that can be raised on the smooth undersurface of the apex may be used, as a last resort, for intravenous injection during anesthesia (Plate 16/*B*). The dorsal surface of the tongue is roughened by *papillae.* Filiform papillae predominate but are replaced by stouter conical papillae toward the root; both have protective and mechanical functions. Other papillae are concerned with the perception of taste; round fungiform papillae are dotted among the filiform papillae; foliate papillae—represented by a few shallow grooves—are present on the lateral border, near the palatoglossal arch; and four to six vallate papillae form a rostrally open V on the root (see Fig. 3–8).

The tongue of the newborn is fringed with lacelike (marginal) papillae that persist for the first 2 weeks and are thought to assist in fitting the tongue to the dam's teat.

The notoriously abrasive nature of the cat's tongue is due to the strong keratinization of the epithelium of the large conical papillae that replace the more delicate filiform papillae of most species.

The *oropharynx* is dorsoventrally flattened; it extends from the palatoglossal arches, which are not easily detected unless made to stand out by pulling the tongue forward. During normal breathing the soft palate lies on the tongue with its free edge rostral to the epiglottis (Plate 16/*C*). In many brachycephalic dogs, the soft palate is disproportionately long and rests over the entrance to the larynx, causing respiratory difficulties.

The fusiform *palatine tonsil* occupies a fossa in the lateral wall of the oropharynx and is covered medially by a semilunar fold hanging from the lateral part of the soft palate (see Figs. 3–8/8 and 3–26/3 and Plate 16/*E,F*). The tonsils are relatively large in young dogs and often protrude from the fossae; similar protrusion in grown dogs usually

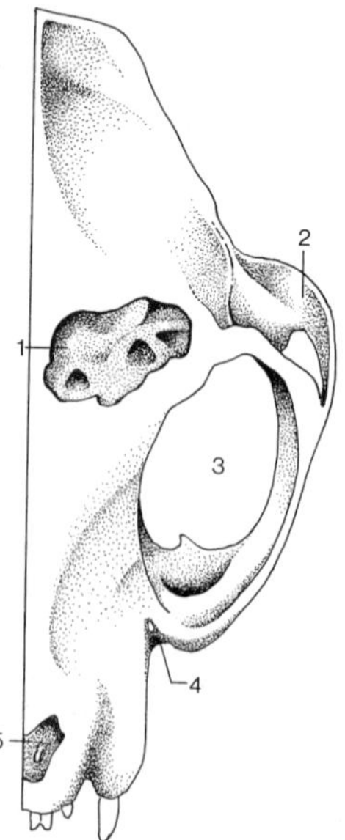


**Figure 11–8.** The feline frontal sinus, dorsal view.

1, Frontal sinus, opened; 2, zygomatic arch; 3, orbit; 4, position of infraorbital foramen; 5, nasal aperture.

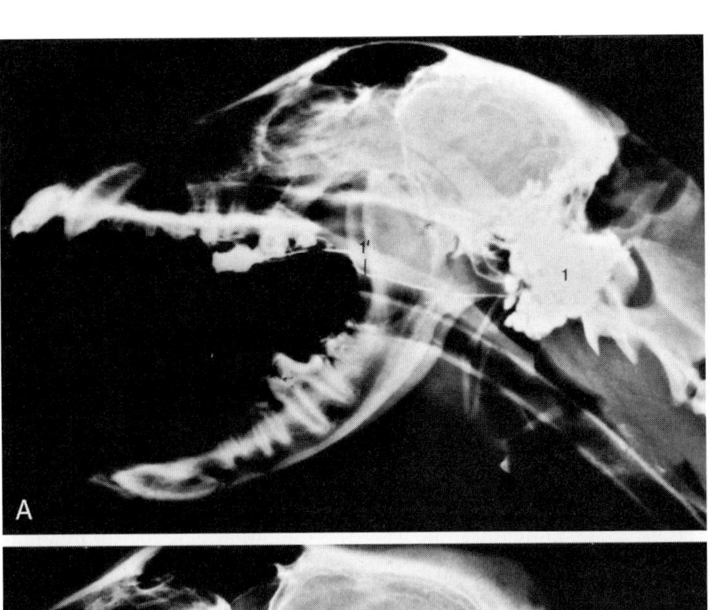


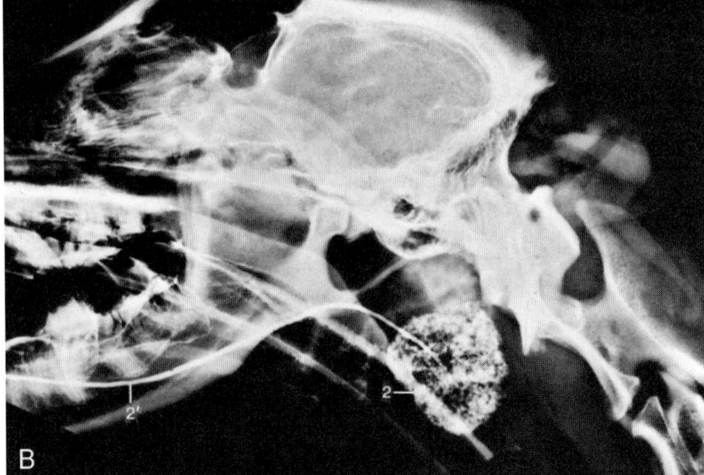


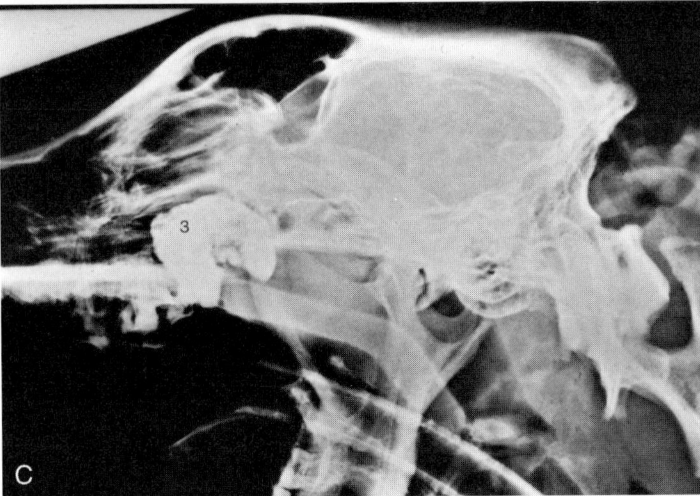


**Figure 11–9.** Contrast medium outlining the canine parotid *(A)*, mandibular *(B)*, and zygomatic *(C)* glands.

1, Parotid gland; 1′, duct; 2, mandibular gland; 2′, duct; 3, zygomatic gland.

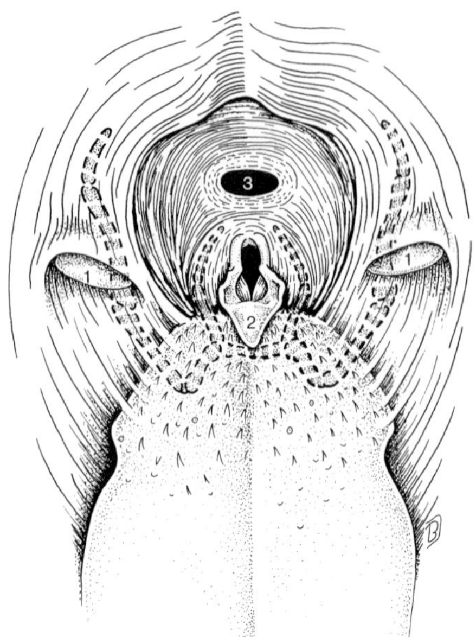


**Figure 11–10.** The canine oropharynx. Note the palatine tonsils (1), the epiglottis (2), and the entrance to the esophagus (3). The position of the hyoid apparatus is outlined by the broken lines.

indicates pathological swelling. The reddish lymphoid tissue lines the fossa dorsal to the tonsil and must also be removed if tonsillectomy is to be complete. The lingual nerve and the mandibular and major sublingual ducts lie lateral to the tonsil and are at some risk in this operation. The palatine tonsil is supplied by tonsillar and hyoid vessels, branches of the lingual artery, which courses ventrolateral to the tonsil.

Contact with the oropharyngeal wall during examination of the mouth normally causes dogs to retch; the absence of this (gag) reflex suggests damage to the glossopharyngeal and vagus nerves. The epihyoid crosses the lateral wall of the oropharynx and provides a useful landmark. It is related laterally to the lingual artery and the hypoglossal nerve, which here pursue rostroventral courses to the root of the tongue.

The *oral cavity of the cat* is short and wide and is easily examined in cooperative subjects (Plate 17/*C*). The filiform papillae on the dorsum of the tongue are caudally directed and hooked; this assists in grooming but makes it more difficult for cats to eject threadlike objects that have been taken into the mouth (Plate 17/*A,B*). Hairs removed from the coat during grooming therefore accumulate in the stomach ("hairballs"); they mingle with the ingesta and may be expelled with the feces or ejected through the mouth. The labial skin glands, present in large numbers, are thought to add a conditioning substance to the coat in the grooming activity in which cats indulge with such relish. The secretion has a more certain social role.

## DENTITION

*(See also pp. 108–113.)*

Much of the general description of the teeth was based on the dentition of the dog, in which the most remarkable features are the prominence of the canine teeth and the marked regional specialization of the others (see Fig. 3–18). The upper dental arch, despite having fewer teeth, is slightly longer than the lower one; the upper teeth therefore bite on the buccal side of the lower ones in a shearing action. This feature precludes lateral movement of the lower jaw, making grinding impossible. There is little occlusal contact between upper and lower teeth except caudally, where some crushing of food is possible. The first few premolars do not touch at all, creating the so-called carrying space. Dogs and cats bolt rather than chew their food.

The formula for the temporary dentition is $\frac{3\text{–}1\text{–}3}{3\text{–}1\text{–}3}$, and for the permanent set, $\frac{3\text{–}1\text{–}4\text{–}2}{3\text{–}1\text{–}4\text{–}3}$. Brachygnathic breeds often have a lesser number, upper and lower P1 and M3 being the teeth most often missing. The cheek teeth of these breeds may be more obliquely placed than normal to fit within the foreshortened jaws.

Though a pup is toothless at birth, the first teeth appear within a few weeks and the deciduous set is complete and functional by the end of the second month. The first replacement tooth erupts after a further month, or little more, and the permanent set is complete by the sixth or seventh month, a remarkably early age (Table 11–1). The

**Table 11–1.** Eruption Dates of the Dog's Teeth

| | Eruption of Temporary Tooth (wk) | Eruption of Permanent Tooth (mo)* |
|---|---|---|
| Incisor 1 | 4–6 | 3–5 |
| Incisor 2 | 4–6 | 3–5 |
| Incisor 3 | 4–6 | 4–5 |
| Canine | 3–5 | 5–7 |
| Premolar 1 | | 4–5 |
| Premolar 2 | 5–6 | 5–6 |
| Premolar 3 | 5–6 | 5–6 |
| Premolar 4 | 5–6 | 4–5 |
| Molar 1 | | 5–6 |
| Molar 2 | | 5–6 |
| Molar 3 | | 6–7 |

*Permanent teeth erupt slightly earlier in large breeds.
Based in part on Schummer et al., 1979, and Evans, 1993.

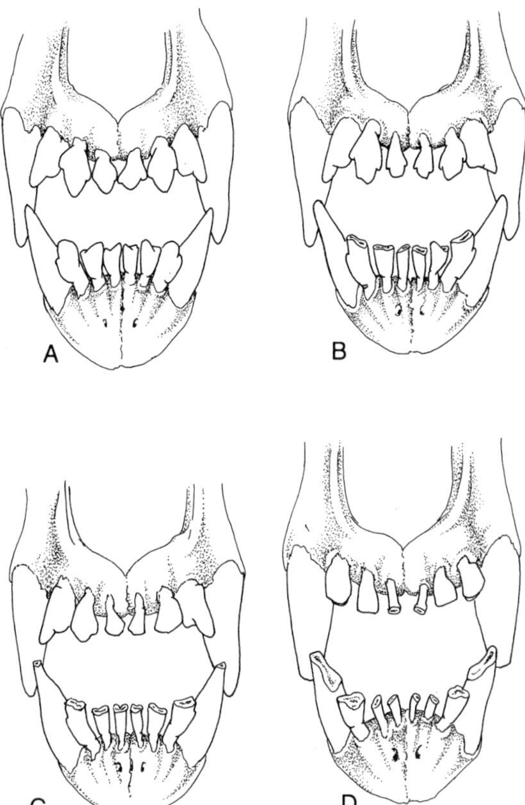


**Figure 11–11.** Changes in the canine incisors with increasing age. *A*, Six months. *B*, About 2½ years. *C*, About 6 years. *D*, About 10 years.

corresponding dates for cats are little different. However, there is much individual and breed variation in eruption and replacement dates, which are unreliable guides to age.

The small permanent *incisors* are rather loosely embedded and are mainly used for nibbling, both in grooming and when detaching small morsels. The upper incisor crowns present a central cusp that is flanked by two smaller ones but the mesial cusp is lacking on the lower incisors (Plate 16/*A,B*). These features are lost as wear reduces the incisors to simple prismatic pegs. The wear of the incisors gives some indication of a dog's age but is not very reliable because of differences in skull size, frequency of malocclusion, and variations in the diet and habits of individuals (Fig. 11–11).

The root of the *canine* is especially massive—larger, indeed, than the crown—and curves caudally to lie dorsal (or ventral) to the first premolar (Fig. 11–12). These teeth are occasionally removed in aggressive dogs. Simple extraction is made impossible by the size and firm implantation of the root; attempts to draw one free risk fracture of the jaw, and it is necessary to resect the bone over the lateral surface of the root before it can be elevated from its socket. Abscesses of the upper canine teeth may fistulate into the nasal cavity.

The four *premolars* increase in size and complexity from first to last in both jaws. The laterally compressed crowns are triangular in profile, presenting small mesial and distal cusps to each side of the principal one. The last upper premolar, $P^4$, is massive and has a small medial part, with its own root, which encroaches upon the hard palate.

The *molars* decrease in size from first to last. The two upper molars, though still tuberculate, have flatter crowns than the premolars. They have three roots and are oriented transversely rather than rostrocaudally as are the premolars (Fig. 11–13/*A*). The first of the lower molars, $M_1$, the sectorial tooth, is the largest in the lower series. It is flattened from side to side and has two thick, divergent roots that occupy most of the width of the jaw. Extractions must be performed carefully to avoid fracture of the mandible. $M_2$ and $M_3$ are much smaller; they engage the last upper molar and, like it, have flat tuberculate crowns.

Most of the cheek teeth have more than one root. It is important to know the pattern of the sockets to ensure that no part is left behind when extracting a tooth (Figs. 11–12 and 11–13). Multiple roots always diverge and it is frequently necessary to divide a tooth before it can be extracted to avoid causing excessive trauma.

The *temporary teeth* in general resemble the definitive set but are smaller and sharper. They have long slender roots. A temporary canine is sometimes retained after the replacement tooth has erupted since the latter appears alongside its predecessor, producing an asymmetrical and sometimes insufficient resorption pressure. In such cases the temporary canine is found caudal to its replacement in the upper jaw and lateral to it in the lower jaw. Retained teeth should be removed to allow their replacements to attain normal position. The three temporary premolars are properly designated $p^2$, $p^3$, and $p^4$; the tooth known as the first premolar erupts several weeks later than these and as a part of the permanent dentition (Table 11–1).

The upper teeth are innervated by the infraorbital nerve, and the rostral members of the series can be desensitized by blocking the nerve within the infraorbital foramen. The lower teeth are supplied by the inferior alveolar nerve, which can be blocked at a site a centimeter or so caudal to the last tooth, before it enters the mandible. The rostral members of this series can be desensitized by blocking the appropriate nerve branches within the mandibular canal.

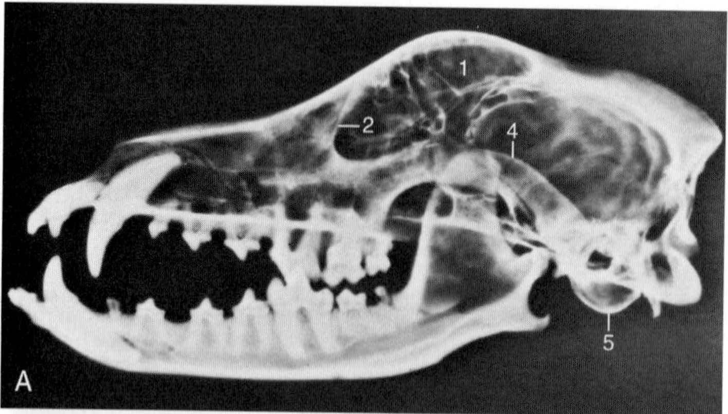


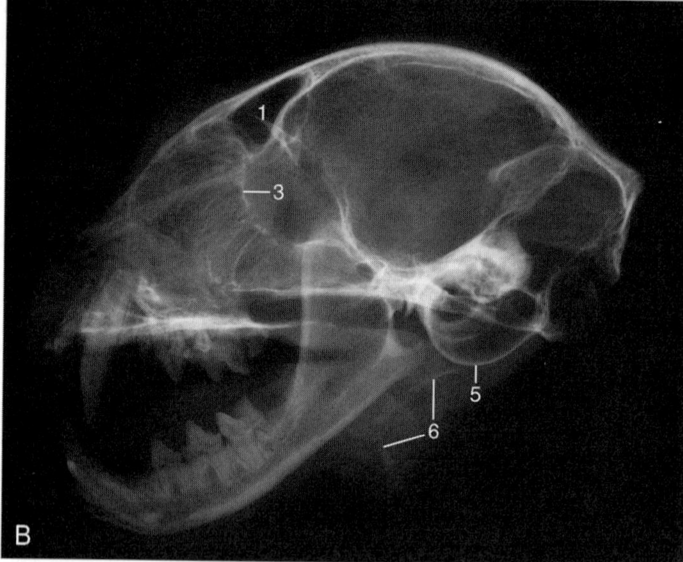


**Figure 11–12.** *A,* Radiograph of half of a canine skull showing the permanent teeth and their roots. *B,* Radiograph of half of a feline head.

1, Frontal sinus; 2, orbital rim; 3, cribriform plate; 4, zygomatic arch; 5, tympanic bulla; 6, hyoid apparatus.

The formula for the temporary *dentition of the cat* reads $\frac{3\text{–}1\text{–}3}{3\text{–}1\text{–}2}$, and for the permanent dentition, $\frac{3\text{–}1\text{–}3\text{–}1}{3\text{–}1\text{–}2\text{–}1}$. The reduction in the cheek teeth is due to the absence of $P^1$ and $M^2$ in the upper jaw and of $P_1$, $P_2$, $M_2$, and $M_3$ in the lower (see Fig. 3–19). The molar loss deprives the cat of flat-crowned crushing teeth, leaving an exclusively shearing bite (Fig. 11–14). $P^4$, the upper sectorial, alone has three roots, which are implanted only a few millimeters from the ventral wall of the orbit. Its lower counterpart is $M_1$. The eruption dates of the cat's teeth are given in Table 11–2.

It is not uncommon to find that one or more of the smaller incisor teeth have been shed by the time cats settle into middle age, and without obvious cause. Plaque deposition, and consequent periodontal disease, are common in both companion species.

## THE TEMPOROMANDIBULAR JOINT

*(See also pp. 113–114.)*

The articular surfaces of the temporomandibular joint are nearly congruent. The transversely oriented cylinder provided by the mandible fits within a trough-shaped fossa on the undersurface of the zygomatic process of the temporal bone (Figs. 11–15 and 11–19/4′). The trough is enlarged caudally by a prominent retroarticular process that securely cups the cylinder and prevents its luxation in a caudal direction. In keeping with the congruence of the joint, the articular disc is thin. The joint capsule is strengthened by a lateral ligament.

Movement of the mandible is almost exclusively of a hinge nature with only slight protrusion possible when the mouth is fully open. Some lateral movement may be produced by trauma and occasionally is so severe that the coronoid process engages the zygomatic arch, locking the jaws in the depressed position.

The joint lies under cover of the caudal part of the masseter, where the dorsal buccal branch of the facial nerve crosses the border of the muscle. It is cranial to the parotid salivary gland.

The masticatory muscles have been sufficiently described (p. 115).

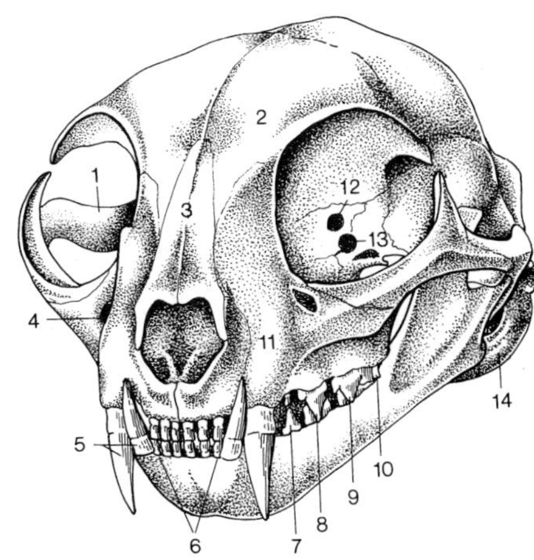


**Figure 11–14.** Feline skull, left craniolateral view.

1, Zygomatic arch; 2, frontal bone; 3, nasal bones; 4, infraorbital foramen; 5, upper and lower canine teeth; 6, upper and lower incisors, in incisive bones and mandible, respectively; 7, $P_3$ opposite small $P^2$; 8, $P^3$ covering $P_4$; 9, $P^4$ covering $M_1$; 10, $M^1$; 11, maxilla; 12, optic canal; 13, orbital fissure; 14, tympanic bulla.

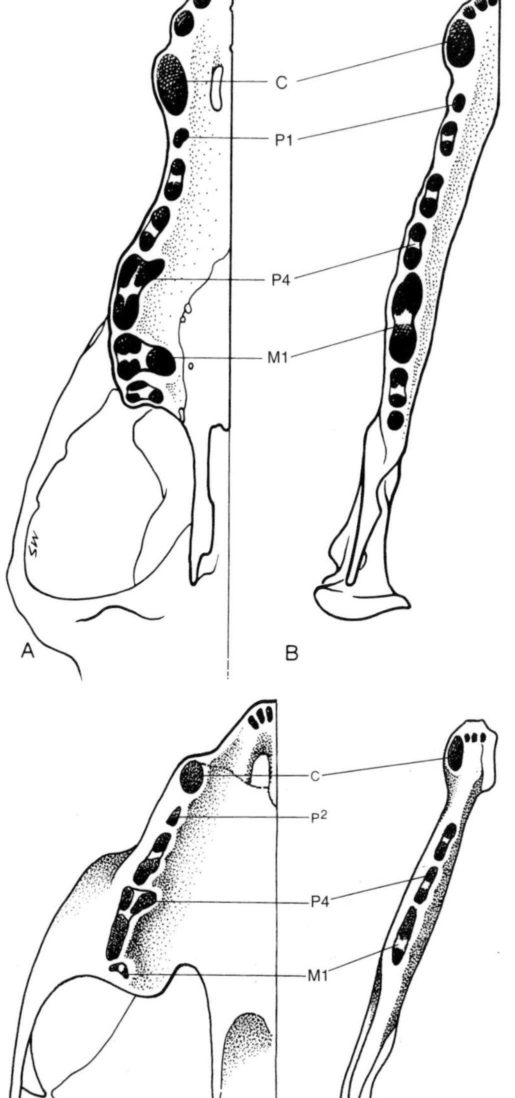


**Figure 11–13.** The tooth sockets in canine *(top)* and feline *(bottom)* upper *(A)* and lower *(B)* jaws to show the number and disposition of the roots.

**Table 11–2.** Eruption Dates of the Cat's Teeth

| | Eruption of Temporary Tooth (wk) | Eruption of Permanent Tooth (mo) |
|---|---|---|
| Incisor 1 | 3–4 | 3½–5½ |
| Incisor 2 | 3–4 | 3½–5½ |
| Incisor 3 | 3–4 | 3½–5½ |
| Canine | 3–4 | 5½–6½ |
| Premolar 2 | 5–6 | 4–5 |
| Premolar 3 | 5–6 | 4–5 |
| Premolar 4 | 5–6 | 4–5 |
| Molar 1 | | 5–6 |

From Schummer et al., 1979.

## THE SALIVARY GLANDS

*(See also pp. 106–108.)*

The *parotid gland* (Fig. 11–3/*A*13 and Plate 16/*D*) is roughly triangular, relatively thin, and molded around the proximal portion of the auricular cartilage, against which it can be rolled on palpation. It occupies a depression between the masseter, the wing of the atlas, and the auricular cartilage. Ventral to the cartilage it is related medially to the facial nerve and maxillary vein, and more cranially to the parotid lymph node and temporomandibular joint.

The *mandibular gland* (/12) is large, ovoid, and contained within a strong fibrous capsule that gives it definite form. This, with its firm attachment, makes it easily palpable, in contrast to the adjacent mandibular lymph nodes that "float" under exploring fingers (/10). The gland has these relations: cranially, the mandibular nodes, sublingual gland, and masseter and digastricus muscles; medially, the digastricus, external carotid artery, and medial retropharyngeal lymph node; and caudally, the muscles of the neck. Its capsule continues cranially onto the compact part of the sublingual gland to which it is firmly fused (see Fig. 3–14).

The narrow *compact sublingual gland* continues forward from the mandibular gland. It follows the mandibular duct between the digastricus ventrally and the medial pterygoideus dorsally, and soon gains a position lateral to the root of the tongue, ending variously at the level of the cheek teeth. Its duct follows that of the mandibular gland forward to the sublingual caruncle. The *diffuse sublingual gland* comprises a chain of lobules spread along the two ducts. The lobules open separately on the floor of the mouth, next to the tongue.

There are also dorsal and ventral buccal glands. The latter constitute a short chain lateral to the mandible; the former are consolidated in a mass generally known as the *zygomatic gland* because of its position medial to the rostral end of the zygomatic arch (Figs. 11–6/*A* and 11–9/*C*). This large gland is related medially to the maxillary artery and nerve, and medial pterygoideus, and dorsally to the periorbita. Its swelling may cause protrusion of the eyeball or bulging of the oral mucosa near the last upper cheek tooth where the ducts open into the vestibule.

The *cat's salivary glands* are shown in Figures 11–3/*B* and 11–16.

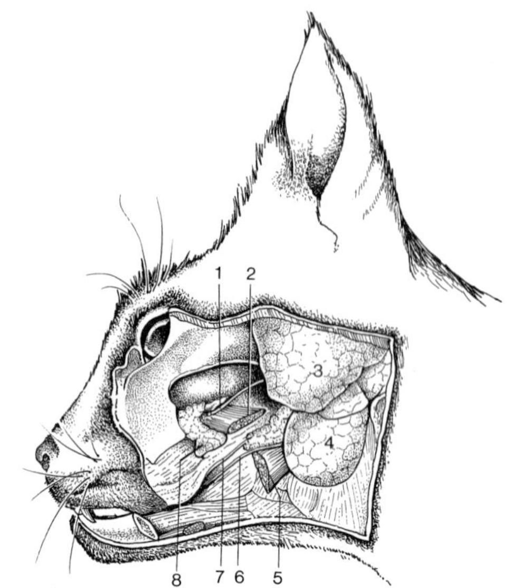


**Figure 11–16.** Deep dissection of the feline head to expose the zygomatic salivary gland (8).

1, Parotid duct, cut; 2, medial pterygoid muscle; 3, parotid gland; 4, mandibular gland; 5, digastricus muscle; 6, mandibular duct; 7, sublingual duct emerging from the rostral end of the monostomatic sublingual salivary gland; 8, zygomatic salivary gland.

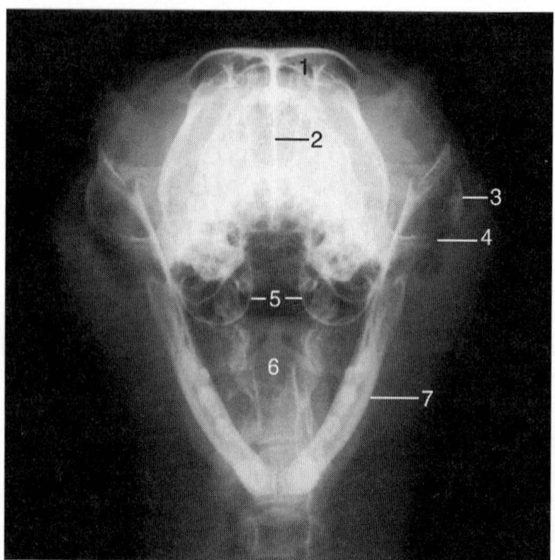


**Figure 11–15.** Rostrocaudal open-mouth radiograph of a feline head.

1, Frontal sinus; 2, nasal septum; 3, zygomatic arch; 4, temporomandibular joint; 5, tympanic bullae; 6, axis with dens; 7, mandible.

## THE LARYNX

*(See also pp. 152–156.)*

The larynx lies caudal to the intermandibular space and ventral to the first two or three cervical vertebrae. Its cranial parts can be examined through the mouth in the sedated dog when the soft palate is raised with a spatula (Plate 16/*E*). Palpation through the skin reveals, in caudorostral succession, the cricoid cartilage (especially its arch), the rounded ventral surface of the thyroid cartilage, and the prominent thyrohyoids that connect the rostral horns of the thyroid cartilage with the basihyoid. The remaining bones of the hyoid apparatus, except for the stylohyoids, are also palpable (see Figs. 2–34 and 11–17/*B*).

The epiglottis is pointed. Its sides are continued caudally to the arytenoid cartilages by the aryepiglottic folds that form the lateral boundaries of the entrance to the laryngeal cavity. The folds contain the remarkably large cuneiform processes of the arytenoid cartilages, which define and stiffen the free edges (Fig. 11–10). The caudal end of the laryngeal entrance is formed by the corniculate processes of the arytenoid cartilages, which take the form of paramedian tubercles (see Fig. 3–8). The vocal folds can be seen through the laryngeal entrance. They are separated from the more rostral vestibular folds by the laryngeal ventricles, lateral evaginations of the mucosa that extend to the thyroid cartilage. Solitary lymph nodules are found in the wall of the ventricles and sometimes on the laryngeal surface of the epiglottis.

The parts of the larynx surrounding the entrance project into the pharynx. Except during swallowing or breathing through the mouth, the free border of the soft palate is wedged below the epiglottis, aligning the laryngeal lumen with that of the nasopharynx (see Fig. 11–17).

The larynx is covered ventrally by the subcutaneous sternohyoideus muscles (Fig. 11–25). It is related laterally to the medial retropharyngeal lymph node, the common carotid artery and vagosympathetic trunk (/6), the linguofacial vein, and the mandibular lymph nodes. It is related dorsally to the caudal end of the laryngopharynx leading to the esophagus (/10).

The larynx is innervated by the cranial and caudal (recurrent) laryngeal nerves. Idiopathic paralysis, comparable to roaring in the horse (p. 502), occurs in certain breeds, notably the Bouvier.

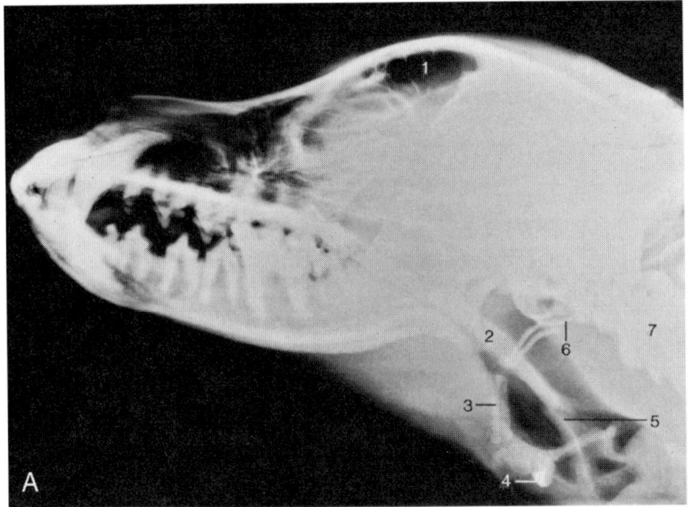


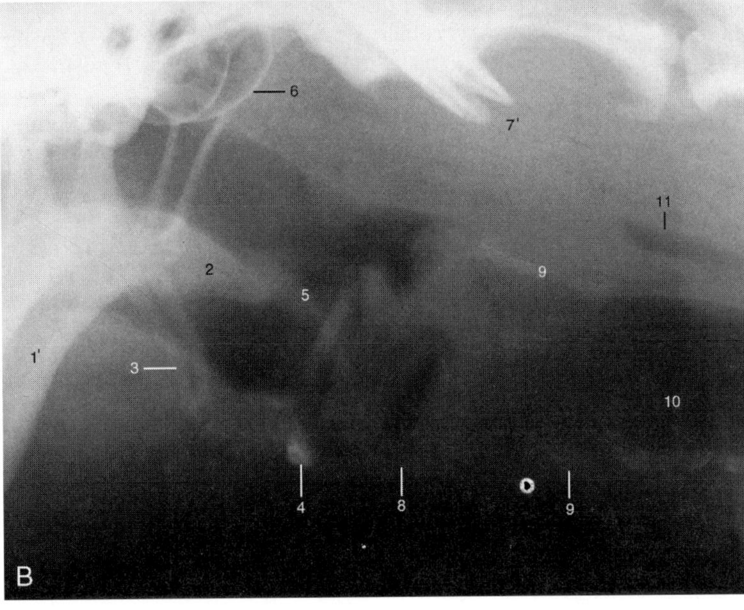


**Figure 11–17.** *A*, Radiograph of the canine head to show the relation of the hyoid apparatus to the skull and atlas. *B*, Enlargement of the laryngeal region of another dog.

1, Frontal sinus; 1′, mandible; 2, soft palate; 3, hyoid apparatus (epihyoid); 4, basihyoid; 5, epiglottis; 6, tympanic bulla; 7, atlas; 7′, wings of atlas; 8, thyroid cartilage; 9, cricoid cartilage; 10, trachea; 11, air in esophagus.

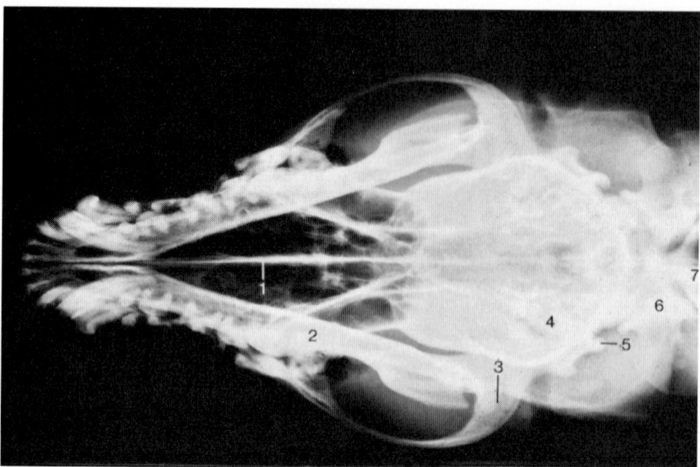


**Figure 11–18.** Ventrodorsal radiograph of the canine head. Note the position and size of the brain case.

1, Nasal septum; 2, mandible; 3, temporomandibular joint; 4, petrous temporal bone; 5, paracondylar process; 6, atlas; 7, axis.

The *cat's larynx* may be depicted in radiographs (Fig. 11–19) and is shown in median section (Fig. 11–21). Its arytenoid cartilages lack both cuneiform and corniculate processes. The aryepiglottic folds bypass the arytenoid cartilages and connect the sides of the epiglottis directly to the cricoid lamina. The vocal folds are thick and rounded; in contrast, the vestibular folds are thin and present sharp margins. There are no ventricles, but pouches of the vestibule extend lateral to the vestibular folds to reach the vocal processes of the arytenoid cartilages. Solitary lymph nodules are present on the laryngeal surface of the epiglottis, while aggregated nodules (paraepiglottic tonsils) thicken the aryepiglottic folds.

Electromyographic studies show that purring in cats is produced by fast twitching of muscles in the larynx and of the diaphragm. The laryngeal muscles rapidly narrow and widen the glottis, which causes the respiratory air to vibrate and make the sound.

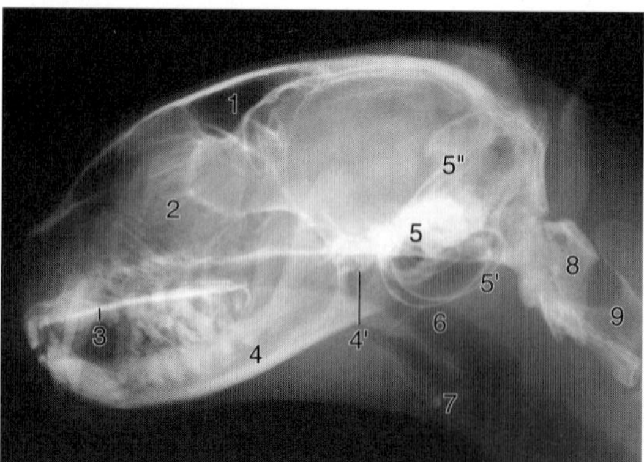


**Figure 11–19.** Radiograph of the feline head.

1, Frontal sinus; 2, cribriform plate and ethmoidal conchae; 3, hard palate; 4, mandible; 4′, temporomandibular joint; 5, petrous temporal bone; 5′, tympanic bullae; 5″, tentorium cerebelli; 6, nasopharynx; 7, basihyoid; 8, atlas; 9, axis.

## THE EYE AND ORBIT

*(See also pp. 323–333.)*

The margins of the *orbits* are easily palpable. They are largely formed by the frontal, lacrimal, and zygomatic bones with the gap in the dorsolateral segment closed by the orbital ligament (Fig. 11–7/6). Only the medial third of the orbital wall is osseous, the remainder being provided by the periorbita. The orbital axis takes a dorsal, lateral, and anterior direction from the apex of the cone. In brachycephalic dogs, particularly those with wide skulls, the axes point more laterally, restricting binocular vision.

The openings into the orbit comprise the optic canal, orbital fissure, duplicated ethmoidal foramina, and fossa of the lacrimal sac. The optic canal transmits the optic nerve and internal ophthalmic artery; the orbital fissure transmits the oculomotor, trochlear, abducent, and ophthalmic nerves; the ethmoidal foramina transmit divisions of the like-named nerve and artery; the fossa contains the slight enlargement at the origin of the nasolacrimal duct.

The osseous wall of the orbit is related dorsomedially to the frontal sinus and rostromedially to the maxillary recess; infection in either of these cavities can easily spread to orbital structures. The periorbita is related as follows: medioventrally, to the medial pterygoid muscle; ventrally, to a pad of

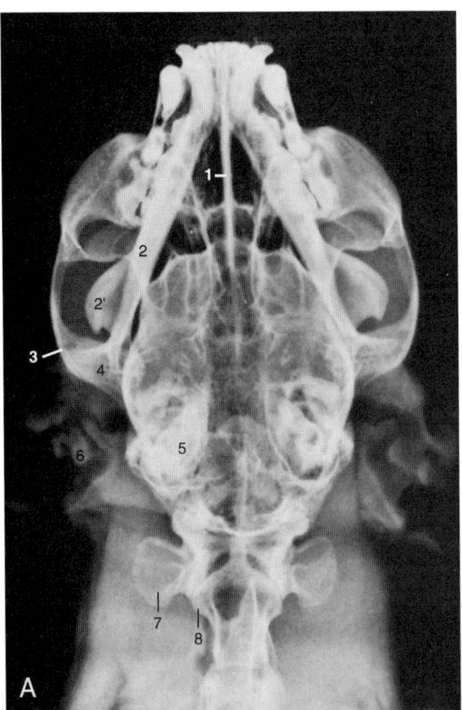


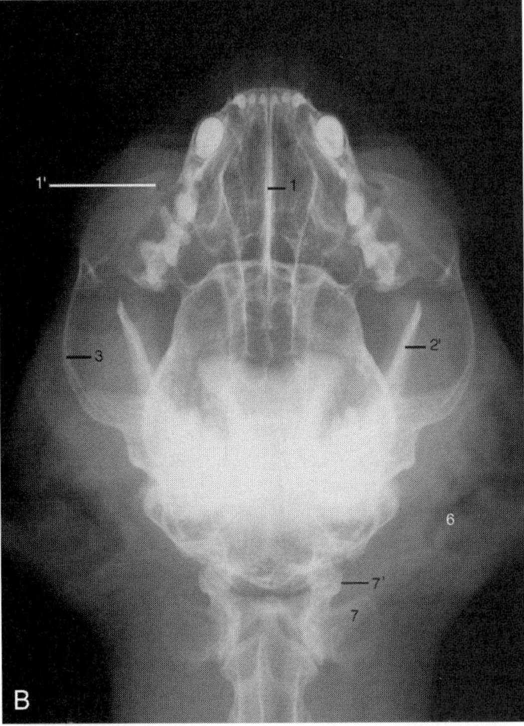


**Figure 11–20.** Radiographs of the feline head. *A,* Ventrodorsal view. *B,* Ventrodorsal view with mouth fully opened.

1, Nasal septum; 1′, infraorbital foramen; 2, mandible; 2′, coronoid process; 3, zygomatic arch; 4, temporomandibular joint; 5, petrous temporal bone; 6, external ear; 7, wing of atlas; 7′, atlanto-occipital joint; 8, axis.

fat caudal to the orbital margin, the zygomatic gland, and the large deep facial vein; laterally, to the zygomatic arch; and caudodorsally, to the orbital ligament and temporalis muscle. The dorsolateral aspect of the orbit is accessible to surgery without resection of bone.

The important maxillary artery and nerve, and their branches to the face and palate, course ventral to the orbit between the medial pterygoid and the zygomatic gland (Fig. 11–22). The maxillary artery gives off the external ophthalmic artery, which pierces the periorbita near its apex to supply the structures within the cone. The temporalis, which surrounds the coronoid process of the mandible, impinges on the periorbita when the mouth is opened. This may cause pain when the orbital contents are diseased, as, for example, by a retrobulbar abscess. The proximity to the oral cavity permits drainage of such abscesses into the mouth, behind the last cheek tooth.

The dimensions of the orbital rim of large and small dogs differ less than might be expected; since the diameter of the eyeball varies even less, the surgical "working" space is generally narrower in larger dogs. However, the position of the eyeball within the orbit differs markedly. In dolichocephalic dogs, the eyeball is deeply placed and the palpebral fissure is small. The eyes of brachycephalic dogs protrude and are more susceptible to injury to the cornea.

The *lacrimal gland* is flat, lobulated, and about 12 to 15 mm in diameter. It lies between the eyeball and the orbital ligament, dorsal to the lateral angle of the eye (/7). The gland must be identified and removed in enucleation (removal) of the eye. The thin edge of the third eyelid is visible in the medial angle of the eye in the "resting state." More is seen when the upper and lower lids are retracted with the fingers while full protrusion is obtained by gentle pressure on the eyeball through the upper lid (see Fig. 9–15/6). Although the superficial gland that surrounds the cartilage of the third lid is not normally visible, it appears when the eyeball is retracted, the increased retrobulbar pressure pushing it to the fore. Active protrusion of the third eyelid, effected by a specific muscular arrangement, is common in cats and may have an emotional or physical origin. The bizarre appearance frequently evokes an exaggerated response from the animal's owner. Abnormal retrobulbar pressure may cause this gland to be everted into the medial angle of the eye, where it appears as a round swelling below a covering of conjunctiva. The subepithelial lymph nodules present on the bulbar surface of the third eyelid may become inflamed.

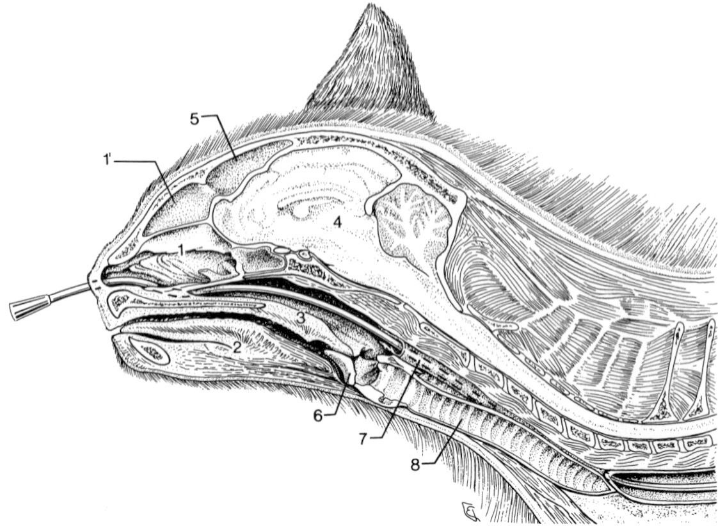


**Figure 11–21.** Paramedian section of the feline head and neck. A nasogastric tube is in place.

1, Nasal cavity; 1′, dorsal part of nasal cavity; 2, tongue; 3, soft palate; 4, brain; 5, frontal sinus; 6, epiglottis; 7, esophagus; 8, trachea.

The puncta lacrimalia (/5) are 2 to 4 mm from the medial angle of the eye, often located at the junction of pigmented and nonpigmented epithelia. Though they are often difficult to find, and accepting that the lower one may be absent or displaced to the bulbar surface of the lid, it is possible to cannulate them for the purpose of irrigation of the lacrimal passages (Fig. 11–5). Eyelashes are sparse (Plate 18/*C,D*). Occasionally, aberrant hairs protrude from the openings of the tarsal glands and these may irritate the cornea.

The *eyeball* is nearly spherical and relatively large. The cornea is slightly oval, its larger diameter being mediolateral in keeping with the shape of the globe itself (Plate 18/*C–E*). It is slightly thicker at the anterior pole than at the periphery. The canine iris is brown, golden yellow, or bluish. Whether dilated or contracted, the pupil remains round, like ours. It is said to be smaller in older dogs under standard light conditions. Remnants of the pupillary membrane may be seen on its upper margin in young puppies (up to the age of 5 weeks). The fundus is illustrated in Plate 14/*A,B*. The triangular tapetum lucidum, which nearly fills the dorsal half, includes the optic disc in large dogs. The retinal vessels emerge from the disc;

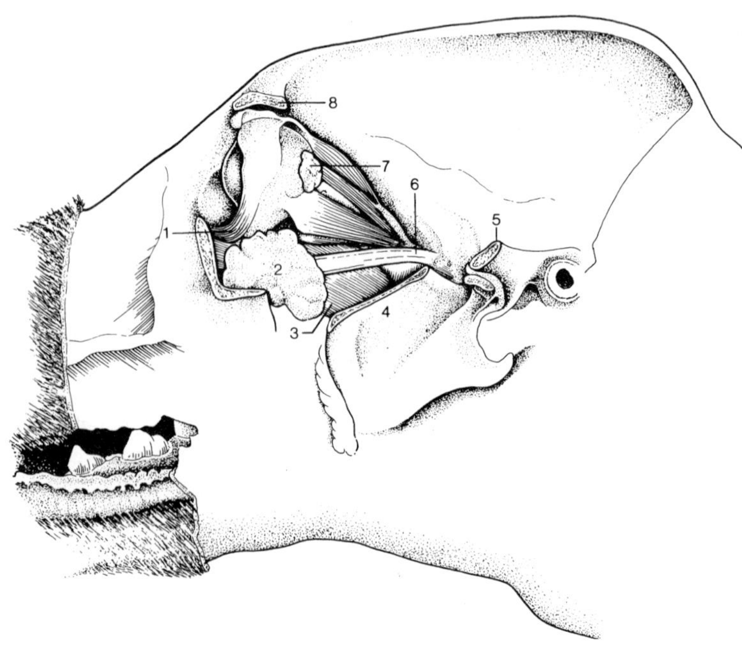


**Figure 11–22.** Dissection of the canine orbit and pterygopalatine fossa, lateral view.

1, Ventral oblique muscle; 2, zygomatic gland; 3, medial pterygoid muscle; 4, coronoid process of mandible, cut; 5, caudal stump of zygomatic arch; 6, maxillary nerve; 7, lacrimal gland; 8, zygomatic process of frontal bone.

prominent venules may form a partial circle from which tributaries usually spread dorsally, medio- and lateroventrally, and ventrally; thinner arterioles radiate in all directions, many in company with the venules.

In the *cat* there is little surgical "working" space between the eye and the orbital margin. The third eyelid is large and in certain circumstances it may be drawn completely over the cornea. As in the dog, it responds to retraction of the eyeball. The cornea is relatively large and permits a wide visual field. The color of the iris ranges from blue through green to golden, the last color said to be due to pigment cells containing phenomelanin, a modified melanin. In certain breeds iris color is strictly prescribed to meet show standards. Kittens are usually born with blue eyes that later change color. The pupils of domestic cats are round when dilated, vertical slits when constricted (Plate 18/*B,A*). (Those of the large wild "cats" remain round at all times.) The vertical form is due to the dorsoventral orientation of the muscle fibers that extend from the periphery of the iris and decussate at the extremities of the constricted pupil. The fundus is dominated by a large tapetum lucidum that surrounds the optic disc. The tapetum is yellowish- or bluish-green and because of its brilliance is thought to be more effective in reflecting light than that of the dog, a convenience in nocturnal wandering (Plate 14/*C*).

## THE EAR

*(See also pp. 336–342.)*

The auricle, known as the ear leather to dog fanciers, is shaped like a lopsided funnel. The part above the ear opening is supported by relatively soft cartilage that allows the ear to flop. However, many dogs can make their ears stand erect. There is a small cutaneous pouch on the caudal border (helix) a short distance above the ear opening (Fig. 11–23/5). The skin adheres more firmly to the cartilage on its concave surface. The large blood vessels that lie on the convex outer surface of the cartilage are branches of the caudal auricular artery, a branch of the external carotid; they send finer branches to the skin over the concave surface through small holes in the cartilage. Vigorous and repeated headshaking or scratching, in most instances elicited by parasites or infection of the ear canal, may injure the vessels and cause hematomas, especially in pendulous ears.

The rostral border of the auricle divides into two crura as it approaches the ear opening; the medial crus forms a prominent ridge on the inside of the ear cavity, and the lateral one ends at the pretragic notch (/1) near the rostral end of the opening. Two named parts of the rolled-up auricular cartilage, the tragus and antitragus, are found caudal to the pretragic notch. The tragus is rectangular and is separated from the antitragus by the intertragic notch (/3). Pretragic and intertragic notches are useful surgical landmarks. The antitragus forms the caudal part of the ear opening and sweeps up toward the end of the lateral helix.

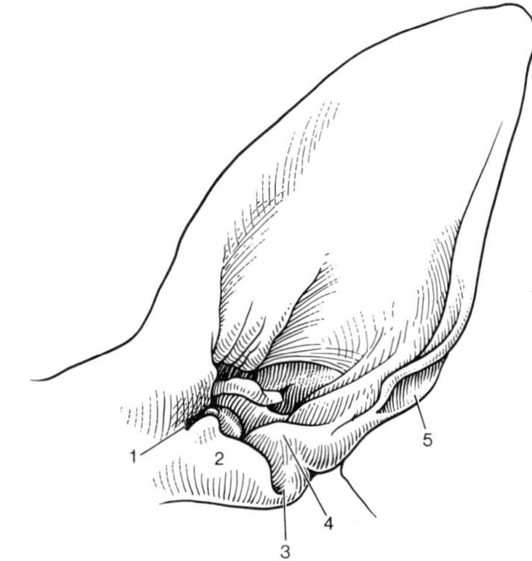


**Figure 11–23.** Left canine ear, shaved.

1, Pretragic notch; 2, tragus; 3, intertragic notch; 4, antitragus; 5, cutaneous pouch.

The ear opening is the beginning of the external acoustic meatus, or ear canal, where it is supported by the rolled-up part of the auricular cartilage. The auricular cartilage bends toward the skull and is succeeded by a small annular cartilage through which the auricle is attached to the skull. The ear canal is first directed ventrally and then rostromedially, the change in direction hampering passage of the straight otoscope for examination of the proximal part of the canal and of the eardrum. The canal may be straightened by pulling the ear first caudally, then ventrally as the otoscope is advanced (Fig. 11–24). The ear canal is about 7 cm long. It generally contains only a few fine hairs but in some breeds, Poodles for example, hair is abundant and may require plucking. The appearance of the eardrum through an otoscope is shown in Figure 11–25 and Plates 16/*G* and 17/*D*.

One surgical procedure to correct infection of the ear canal (otitis externa) removes the lateral wall of the funnel-shaped cavity at the base of the ear, so taking the curve out of the canal; pus can then drain to the outside through the proximal, more medially directed part that is left intact.

The base of the auricle and the ear canal are related laterally and ventrally to the parotid gland.

The facial nerve crosses the ventral surface of the canal deep to the gland before breaking into the auriculopalpebral nerve and the two buccal branches. The former passes dorsally in front of the ear in company with the superficial temporal vessels. The facial nerve here also detaches a caudal auricular nerve and a branch to the interior of the ear canal. The veins of the area join the maxillary, which descends toward the mandibular gland from its formation by substantial caudal and cranial auricular, and superficial temporal veins, that may pass through the parotid gland (Fig. 11–28). The arteries lies more deeply. The external carotid, having detached the caudal auricular artery to the convex surface of the auricle, ends rostroventral to the ear canal by dividing into maxillary and superficial temporal arteries. The latter, with the like-named vein, lies deep to the parotid gland close to the rostral surface of the ear canal.

The middle and inner ears show few special features of importance. The auditory tubes are narrow and open on the dorsolateral wall of the nasopharynx, level with the landmark provided by the hamulus of the pterygoid bone, which is palpable through the mouth caudomedial to the last cheek tooth. The tympanic bullae are relatively large, convex ventrally, and, except for a serrated septum in their rostral half, undivided (Fig. 11–12/5).

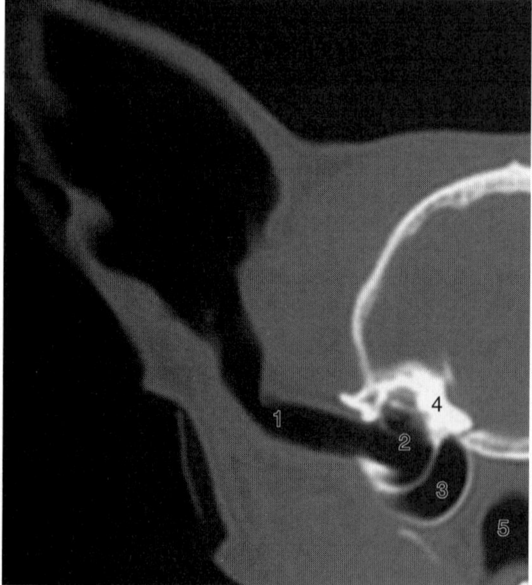


**Figure 11–24.** Transverse CT scan (bone window) of half of a feline head showing ear canal and middle ear.

1, Ear canal; 2, tympanic cavity; 3, tympanic bulla; 4, petrous temporal bone; 5, nasopharynx.

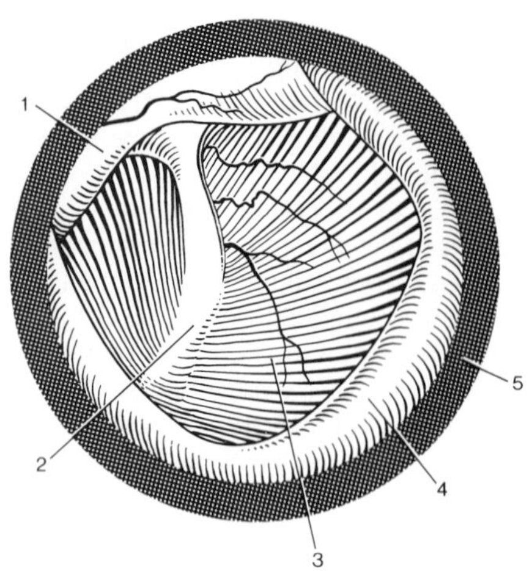


**Figure 11–25.** Lateral surface of the canine tympanic membrane as seen through an otoscope.

1, Flaccid part of tympanic membrane; 2, handle of malleus, shining through tympanic membrane; 3, tense part of tympanic membrane; 4, skin of external acoustic meatus raised by tube of otoscope; 5, tube of otoscope.

Middle ear infections (otitis media) may be drained into the nasopharynx through the bulla, which can be palpated through the oropharynx and soft palate, caudal to the hamulus. The inflated, hemispherical tympanic bulla of the cat is easily found on palpation through the skin, between the wing of the atlas and the zygomatic arch.

The radiographic appearance of the skull of dog and cat is shown in Figures 11–17 to 11–20.

## THE VENTRAL PART OF THE NECK

*(See also pp. 70–71.)*

It is convenient to describe with the head the part of the neck that lies ventral to the vertebrae. The dorsal part of the neck will be dealt with in the next chapter (p. 398). The skin on the ventral surface of the neck is loose and in some breeds forms longitudinal folds. When fat is present subcutaneously it is concentrated caudally, especially in the depression dorsolateral to the manubrium.

The *external jugular vein* sinks into this depression after following a course along the lateral surface of the sternocephalicus (Fig. 11–27/*A,B,* 12). It does not lie in a distinct jugular groove as in the larger species. Although the external jugular is the principal vein draining the head, it is assisted by smaller vessels associated with the vertebrae (vertebral vein, internal vertebral plexus) and accompanying the common carotid artery (internal jugular vein; Fig. 11–28/2′); these mainly drain deeper structures. The external jugular vein is formed by tributaries embracing the mandibular gland; these are easily raised by pressure on the jugular and provide an additional means for the positive distinction of the gland from the mandibular lymph nodes (Fig. 11–3). The large diameter of the jugular vein makes it a convenient alternative to the cephalic when considerable amounts of blood have to be collected. It is especially useful in the cat, in which the limb veins are naturally rather small.

The visceral space ventral to the cervical vertebrae is enclosed by four superficial and two deep muscles. The *sternohyoideus* ventral to the trachea extends from the manubrium to the basihyoid; it is loosely connected to its fellow in the midline. The *sternothyroideus,* also thin and straplike, lies lateral to the trachea, ending on the lateral surface of the thyroid cartilage. These are the only structures that intervene between the trachea and the skin in the cranial half of the neck (Fig. 11–26). They are covered by the *sternocephalicus* in the caudal half. This muscle consists of two parts, sternomastoideus and sterno-occipitalis, which diverge toward the head. The dorsal sterno-occipitalis ends on the back of the skull. The *brachiocephalicus* also has two parts in the neck, the cleidomastoideus and cleidocervicalis. The former passes deep to the sterno-occipitalis to a common insertion with the sternomastoideus on the mastoid process of the temporal bone. The latter sweeps over the lateral surface of the neck to meet its fellow in the dorsal midline (see Fig. 2–53/2). Sternocephalicus and brachiocephalicus are fused except caudally, where their separation allows the external jugular vein to become subcutaneous (Fig. 11–27).

The deep muscles comprise the *longus capitis,* ventrolateral to the cervical vertebrae, and the *longus colli* more medially (Fig. 11–26/5,4). The fascia that covers these muscles ventrally detaches a superficial leaf that encloses the structures in the visceral space.

These structures are the esophagus, trachea, thyroid and parathyroid glands, common carotid arteries, vagosympathetic trunks, internal jugular veins, recurrent nerves, and tracheal lymph trunks (Fig. 11–27/*A*). There is no cervical component of the thymus.

The *esophagus* continues form the laryngopharynx. It first lies dorsal to the trachea but it deviates to the left in the middle of the neck and maintains this position through the thoracic inlet. Esophagus and trachea are thus both in contact with the longus colli in the caudal half of the neck. The esophagus

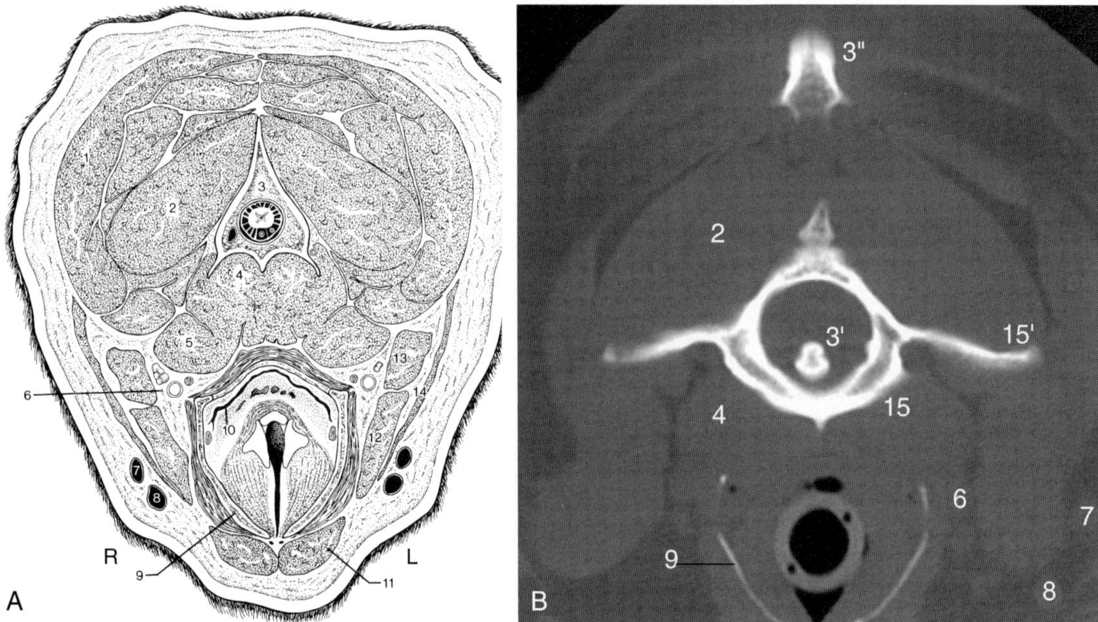


**Figure 11–26.** *A,* Transverse section of the canine neck at the level of the axis. *B,* Corresponding CT scan (bone window), slightly more cranial than *A.*

1, Splenius; 2, obliquus capitis caudalis; 3, axis; 3′, dens of axis; 3″, cranial tip of spine of axis; 4, longus colli; 5, longus capitis; 6, common carotid artery, vagosympathetic trunk, and medial retropharyngeal lymph node; 7, maxillary vein; 8, linguofacial vein; 9, thyroid cartilage (calcified); 10, laryngopharynx, leading into esophagus; 11, sternohyoideus; 12, sternomastoideus; 13, cleidomastoideus; 14, sterno-occipitalis; 15, atlas; 15′, wing of atlas.

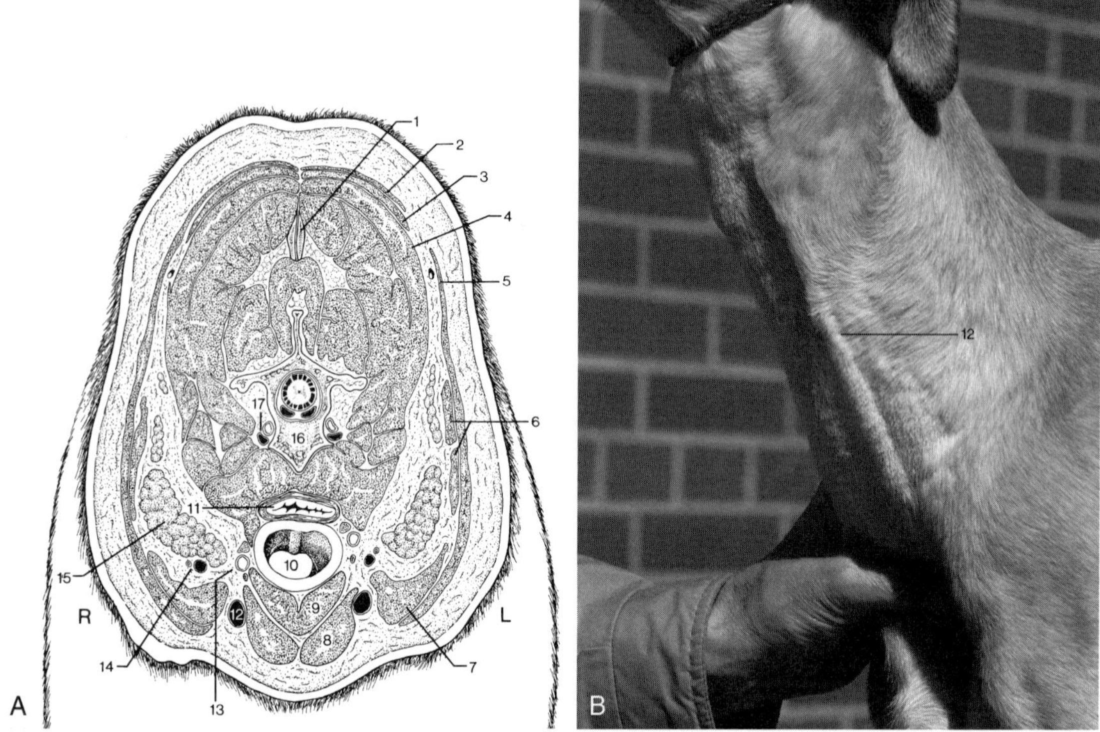


**Figure 11–27.** *A,* Transverse section of the canine neck at the level of the fifth cervical vertebra. *B,* Left external jugular vein raised by thumb pressure at the base of the neck.

1, Nuchal ligament; 2, trapezius; 3, rhomboideus; 4, splenius; 5, cleidocervicalis; 6, omotransversarius; 7, cleidomastoideus; 8, sternocephalicus; 9, sternothyrohyoideus; 10, trachea; 11, esophagus; 12, external jugular vein; 13, common carotid artery, vagosympathetic trunk, and recurrent laryngeal nerve; 14, superficial cervical vessels; 15, superficial cervical lymph nodes; 16, fifth cervical vertebra; 17, vertebral vessels.

may be felt with the finger tips as a pliable tube sinistrodorsal to the trachea. The habit of dogs of bolting their food often leads to obstructions. Large pieces of meat, gristle, or bone—and not infrequently, stones—tend to lodge at the thoracic inlet where the esophagus is prevented from expanding fully.

The *trachea* continues from the larynx and because of its firmness is easily palpated. Unlike the esophagus, it can be grasped so that the flat dorsal surface between the ends of the tracheal rings can be appreciated.*

*In normal dogs it may be possible to demonstrate modest changes in tracheal diameter in synchrony with the phases of respiration. The cervical trachea, especially its caudal part, narrows slightly during inspiration only to recover during expiration. The changes in the thoracic trachea are reciprocal. This physiological variation is not to be confused with the more severe narrowing of the tracheal lumen, possibly amounting to collapse, that sometimes occurs consequential to congenital or acquired degeneration of the supporting cartilages. In this pathological condition the cervicothoracic transitional portion of the trachea is most often affected.

The *thyroid gland* consists of two elongated, rather flattened lobes placed against and loosely attached to the lateral aspects of the first few tracheal cartilages under cover of the sternothyroid muscles (see Fig. 6–4/A). Their caudal poles are sometimes connected across the ventral surface of the trachea by a vestigial isthmus. The lobes in medium-sized dogs are about 5 cm long.

The major blood supply to each lobe is provided by a cranial thyroid artery, a vessel with a larger distribution than its name suggests. Its thyroid branches include one that follows the dorsal margin caudally to an anastomosis with the much smaller caudal thyroid artery (if present); one that follows the ventral margin partway before fading; and others that pass directly to the cranial pole (and to the external parathyroid gland). Twigs from all these result in the thyroid being supplied at scattered points around most of its periphery. Blood leaving the gland enters the nearby internal jugular veins, while some is conveyed to the large veins at the thoracic inlet by an unpaired (caudal thyroid) vein lying on the ventral surface of the trachea.

Each lobe is closely associated with two *parathyroid glands* (discounting the possible existence of accessory parathyroid tissue) in a relationship of obvious relevance to the performance of thyroid surgery. The external (III) parathyroid is generally found close to or against the cranial pole of the thyroid, to which it is loosely joined; in cats more often than in dogs, this gland descends unusually far from its site of origin (p. 215) and comes to rest near the caudal pole. The internal (IV) parathyroid is located within the connective tissue capsule of the thyroid and may be difficult to discover, especially when completely submerged within thyroid glandular tissue as sometimes happens. Recognition is assisted by its pale color which contrasts with the brownish-red thyroid tissue; it can, however, be identified on or within the thyroid gland by ultrasonography. The size of the parathyroid glands is rather variable but, on average, they are about 3 mm in diameter in dogs. Partial or complete thyroidectomy may be performed in the treatment of thyroid hyperplasia and neoplasia, the former condition now recognized as occurring with great frequency in cats. Certain surgical procedures (intracapsular thyroidectomy) make the concomitant removal of a considerable fraction of the total parathyroid tissue more or less inevitable;this loss is generally tolerated provided the integrity of the blood supply to the remaining part is preserved. Caution is obviously most necessary when surgery is bilateral.

The *common carotid artery* runs dorsolateral to the trachea (though the left one is commonly displaced to the side by the esophagus in the caudal half of the neck). It arises from the brachiocephalic trunk within the thorax and crosses the lateral surface of the trachea (esophagus on the left) obliquely to gain a dorsolateral position in the neck. The cranial thyroid artery, which arises level with the larynx, is the only cervical branch of consequence. The common carotid artery ends at the level of the atlanto-occipital joint by dividing into internal and external carotid arteries. The former enters the skull by the jugular foramen, and the latter continues as the principal supply to structures of the head (Figs. 11–28/1,5,6 and 7–38/3,2).

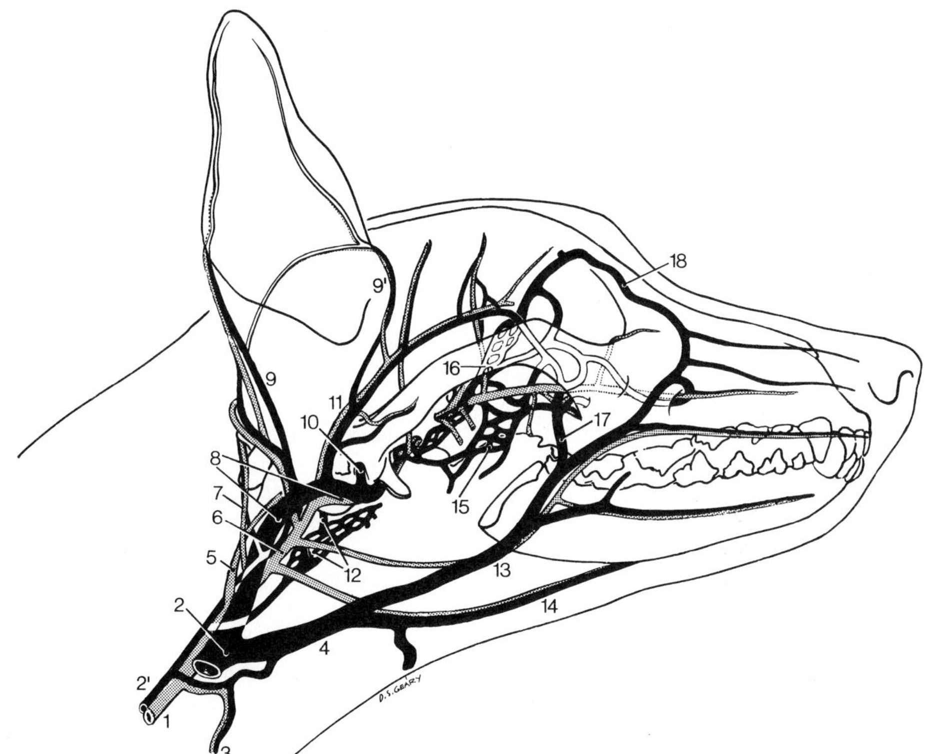


**Figure 11–28.** The major arteries *(gray)* and veins *(black)* of the canine head. The ramus of the mandible has been removed.

1, Common carotid; 2, external jugular; 2′, internal jugular; 3, cranial thyroid; 4, linguofacial; 5, internal carotid; 6, external carotid; 7, occipital; 8, maxillary; 9, 9′, caudal and rostral auricular; 10, dorsal emissary; 11, superficial temporal; 12, ventral emissary and pharyngeal plexus; 13, facial; 14, lingual; 15, pterygoid plexus; 16, ophthalmic plexus; 17, deep facial; 18, angularis oculi.

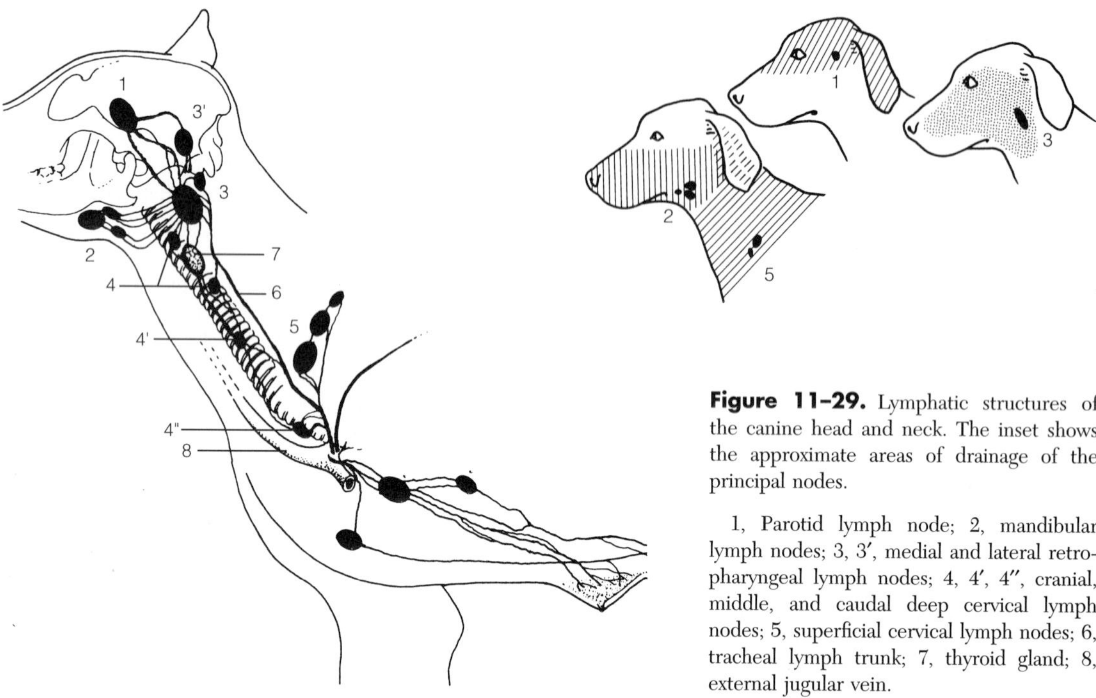


**Figure 11–29.** Lymphatic structures of the canine head and neck. The inset shows the approximate areas of drainage of the principal nodes.

1, Parotid lymph node; 2, mandibular lymph nodes; 3, 3′, medial and lateral retropharyngeal lymph nodes; 4, 4′, 4″, cranial, middle, and caudal deep cervical lymph nodes; 5, superficial cervical lymph nodes; 6, tracheal lymph trunk; 7, thyroid gland; 8, external jugular vein.

The *vagosympathetic trunk* adheres to the dorsal surface of the common carotid artery; the recurrent nerve and internal jugular vein accompany the artery ventrally. The *tracheal lymph trunk* is formed by efferents of the medial retropharyngeal lymph nodes and drains to a larger collecting duct, or directly to a vein, at the thoracic inlet.

The mobility of the structures in the visceral space (and of the ventral muscles) facilitates their exposure in midneck by a median skin incision followed by blunt dissection. Cervical intervertebral discs are occasionally approached (for fenestration to relieve pressure on the spinal cord) by this route.

## THE LYMPH NODES OF THE HEAD AND NECK

Except for the unimportant facial node, the lymph nodes of the head are concentrated in an area caudal to the mandible; those of the neck are found at shoulder level and, inconstantly, scattered along the trachea (Fig. 11–29).

The *parotid lymph node* lies on the caudal border of the masseter cranial to the base of the ear. It drains superficial structures, broadly, those dorsal to the palate and ear. It is not always palpable (/1).

The *mandibular lymph nodes* are grouped around the facial vein near the angle of the mandible. They drain superficial structures of the face and also the intermandibular space. They are always palpable (Fig. 11–3/10).

The large *medial retropharyngeal lymph node* lies medial to the mandibular gland and sternomastoideus, between the wing of the atlas and the larynx. It drains the deep structures, including the palatine tonsil, and receives lymph from other nodes of the head. Its efferents form the tracheal lymph trunk. It cannot be palpated (Fig. 11–29/3).

The inconstant *lateral retropharyngeal lymph node* may be palpated at the caudal border of the parotid and mandibular glands. It drains deep structures dorsal to it.

The *superficial cervical lymph nodes* (/5), which are sometimes rather large, lie on the cranial border of the supraspinatus under cover of the omotransversarius. They drain the skin of the neck, the shoulder region, and the forelimb. They can be palpated. (Small deep cervical lymph nodes are occasionally found in the vicinity of the thyroid gland and trachea.)

### Selected Bibliography

Abood, S.K., and C.A. Buffington: Improved nasogastric intubation technique for administration of nutritional support in dogs. JAVMA 199:577–579, 1991.

Adams, D.R., D.W. Deyoung, and R. Griffith: The lateral nasal gland of dog: Its structure and secretory content. J. Anat. 132:29–37, 1981.

Alsup, J.C., C.L. Greenfield, L.L. Hungerford, et al: Comparison of unilateral arytenoid lateralization and ventral ventriculocordectomy for the treatment of experimentally induced laryngeal paralysis in dogs. Can. Vet. J. 38:287–293, 1997.

Barnett, K.C.: The canine ocular fundus: Normal variations. Compend. Small Anim. 16:348–356, 1994.

Barrie, K.P., G.G. Glenwood, D.A. Samuelson, and K.N. Gelatt: Morphologic studies of uveoscleral outflow in normotensive and glaucomatous Beagles with fluorescein-labeled dextran. Am. J. Vet. Res. 46:89–97, 1985.

Beckman, S.L., W.B. Henry, Jr, and P. Cechner: Total ear canal ablation combining bulla osteotomy and curettage in dogs with chronic otitis externa and media. JAVMA 196:84–90, 1990.

Bellenger, C.R., and D.J. Simpson: Canine sialocoeles—60 clinical cases. J. Small Anim. Clin. Sci. 33:376–380, 1992.

Belz G.T., and T.J. Heath: Lymph pathways of the medial retropharyngeal lymph node in dogs. J. Anat. 186:517–526, 1995.

Belz, G.T., and T.J. Heath: Pathways of blood flow to and through superficial lymph nodes in the dog. J. Anat. 187:413–421, 1995.

Belz, G.T., and T.J. Heath: Lymphatic drainage from the tonsil of the soft palate in pigs. J. Anat. 187:491–495, 1995.

Biknevicius, A.R., and B. van Valkenburgh: Design for killing: Craniodental adaptations of predators. In Gittleman, J.L. (ed): Carnivore Behavior, Ecology and Evolution. vol. 2, Ithaca, N.Y., Cornell University Press, 1996.

Boothe, H.W., Jr.: Surgical management of otitis media and otitis interna. Vet. Clin. North Am. Small Anim. Pract. 18:855–899, 901–911, 1988.

Boyd, J.S.: Color Atlas of Clinical Anatomy of the Dog and Cat. St. Louis, Mosby–Year Book, 1991.

Brooks, D.E.: Glaucoma in the dog and cat. Vet. Clin. North Am. Small Anim. Pract. 20:775–797, 1990.

Burbidge, H.M., B.E. Goulden, and B.R. Jones: Laryngeal paralysis in dogs: An evaluation of the bilateral arytenoid lateralisation procedure. J. Small Anim. Pract. 34:515–519, 1993.

Burk, R.L.: Computed tomographic anatomy of the canine nasal passages. Vet. Radiol. Ultrasound 33:170–176, 1992.

Constantinescu, G.H., and R.C. McClure: Anatomy of the orbital fasciae and the third eyelid in dogs. Am. J. Vet. Res. 51:260–263, 1990.

Cook, C.S.: Surgery for glaucoma. Vet. Clin. North Am. Small Anim. Pract. 27:1109–1129, 1997.

Coyne, B.E., and R.B. Fingland: Hypoplasia of the trachea in dogs: 103 cases (1974–1990). JAVMA 201:768–772, 1992.

deLahunta, A., and R.E. Habel: Applied Veterinary Anatomy. Philadelphia, W.B. Saunders Company, 1986.

De Schaepdrijver, L., P. Simoens, H. Lauwers, and J.P. De Geest: Retinal vascular patterns in domestic animals. Vet. Sci. 47:34–42, 1989.

Dole, R.S., and T.L. Spurgeon. Frequency of supernumerary teeth in a dolichocephalic canine breed, the Greyhound. Am. J. Vet. Res. 59:16–17, 1998.

Dubielzig, R.R., J.W. Wilson, and A.A. Seireg: Pathogenesis of canine aural hematomas. JAVMA 185:873–875, 1984.

Evans, H.E.: Miller's Anatomy of the Dog, 3rd ed. Philadelphia, W.B. Saunders, 1993.

Fahie, M.A., B.J. Smith, J.B. Ballard, et al.: Regional peripheral vascular supply based on the superficial temporal artery in dogs and cats. Anat. Histol. Embryol. 27:205–208, 1998.

Flanders, J.A., H.J. Harvey, and H.N. Erb: Feline thyroidectomy—a comparison of postoperative hypocalcemia associated with three different surgical techniques. Vet. Surg. 16:362–366, 1987.

Gamm, D.J., P.E. Howard, H. Walia, and D.J. Nencka: Prevalence and morphologic features of apical deltas in the canine teeth of dogs. JAVMA 202:63–70, 1993.

George II, T.F., and J.E. Smallwood: Anatomic atlas for computed tomography in the mesaticephalic dog: Head and neck. Vet. Radiol. Ultrasound 33:217–240, 1992.

Greenfield, C.L.: Canine laryngeal paralysis. Compend. Contin. Educ. Pract. Vet. 9:1011–1017, 1987.

Gross, M.E., E.R. Pope, D. O'Brien, et al.: Regional anesthesia of the infraorbital and inferior alveolar nerves during noninvasive tooth pulp stimulation in halothane-anesthetized dogs. JAVMA 211:1403–1405, 1997.

Harvey, C.E.: Tooth extraction in dogs and cats. Compend. Contin. Educ. Pract. Vet. 10:175–186, 1988.

Hennet, P.R., and C.E. Harvey: Apical root canal anatomy of canine teeth in cats. Am. J. Vet. Res. 57:1545–1548, 1996.

Holmberg, D.L., C. Fries, J. Cockshutt, and D. Van Pelt: Ventral rhinotomy in the dog and cat. Vet. Surg. 18:446–449, 1989.

Horowitz, A.: The Fundamental Principles of Anatomy: Dissection of the Dog. Saskatoon, University of Saskatchewan, 1970. Published by the author.

Hudson, L.C., and W.P. Hamilton: Atlas of Feline Anatomy for Veterinarians. Philadelphia, W.B. Saunders Company, 1993.

Janssens, L.A.A.: Devocalization of dogs—a new technique. Vet. Surg. 15:375–377, 1986.

Johnson, L.R., and W.H. Fales: Clinical and microbiologic findings in dogs with bronchoscopically diagnosed tracheal collapse: 37 cases (1990–1995). JAVMA 219:1247–1250, 2001.

Kern, T.J., M.C. Aromando, and H.N. Erb: Horner's syndrome in dogs and cats: 100 cases (1975–1985). JAVMA 195:369–373, 1989.

Koblik, P.D., and C.R. Berry. Dorsal plane computed tomographic imaging of the ethmoid region to evaluate chronic nasal disease in the dog. Vet. Radiol. Ultrasound 31:92–97, 1990.

Lantz, G.C.: Intermittent open-mouth locking of the temporomandibular joint in a cat. JAVMA 190:1574, 1987.

Lantz, G.C., and H.D. Cantwell: Intermittent open-mouth jaw locking in five dogs. JAVMA 188:1403–1405, 1986.

Little, C.J.L., and J.G. Lane: The surgical anatomy of the feline bulla tympanica. J Small Anim. Pract. 27:371–378, 1986.

Little, C.J.L., and J.G. Lane: An evaluation of tympanometry, otoscopy and palpation for assessment of the canine tympanic membrane. Vet. Rec. 124:5–8, 1989.

Lorinson, D., R.M. Bright, and R.A.S. White: Brachycephalic airway obstruction syndrome—a review of 118 cases. Canine Pract. 22(5–6):18–21, 1997.

Mason, L.K., C.E. Harvey, and R.J. Orsher: Total ear canal ablation combined with lateral bulla osteotomy for end-stage otitis in dogs—results in thirty dogs. Vet. Surg. 17:263–268, 1988.

Matthiesen, D.T., and T. Scavelli: Total ear canal ablation and lateral bulla osteotomy in 38 dogs. J. Am. Anim. Hosp. Assoc. 26:257–267, 1990.

Morgan, J.P., and T. Miyabayashi: Dental radiology: Aging changes in permanent teeth of beagle dogs. J. Small Anim. Pract. 32:11–18, 1991.

Morgan, R.V.: Ultrasonography of retrobulbar diseases of the dog and cat. J. Am. Anim. Hosp. Assoc. 25:393–399, 1989.

Morgan, R.V., J.M. Duddy, and K. McClurg: Prolapse of the gland of the third eyelid in dogs: A retrospecitve study of 89 cases (1980–1990). J. Am. Anim. Hosp. Assoc. 29:56–60, 1993.

Niebauer, G.W., J.E. Eigenmann, and T.J. Van Winkle: Study of long-term survival after transsphenoidal hypophysectomy in clinically normal dogs. Am. J. Vet. Res. 51:677–681, 1990.

Orsini, P., and P. Hennet: Anatomy of the mouth and teeth of the cat. Vet. Clin. North Am. Small. Anim. Pract. 22:1265–1277, 1992.

Ramsey, D.T., S.M. Marretta, R.E. Hamor, et al.: Ophthalmic manifestations and complications of dental disease in dogs and cats. J. Am. Anim. Hosp. Assoc. 32:215–224, 1996.

Reusch, C.E., K. Tomsa, C. Zimmer, et al.: Ultrasonography of the parathyroid gland as an aid in differentiation of acute and chronic renal failure in dogs. JAVMA 217:1849–1852, 2000.

Roush, J.K., P.E. Howard, and J.W. Wilson: Normal blood supply to the canine mandible and mandibular teeth. Am. J. Vet. Res. 50:904–907, 1989.

Saidla, J.: Veterinary dentistry '89. J. Vet. Dent. 7:16–20, 1990.

Schebitz, H., and H. Wilkens: Atlas of Radiographic Anatomy of the Dog and Cat, 4th ed. Berlin, Paul Parey Verlag, 1986.

Schramm, U., K. Unger, and C. Keeler: Functional morphology of the nictitating membrane in the domestic cat. Ann. Anat. 176:101–108, 1994.

Schummer, A., R. Nickel, and W.O. Sack: The Viscera of the Domestic Mammals, 2nd ed. New York, Springer-Verlag, 1979.

Sharp, N.J.H.: Chronic otitis externa and otitis media treated by total ear canal ablation and ventral bulla osteotomy in thirteen dogs. Vet. Surg. 19:162–166, 1990.

Simoens, P., P. Poels, and H. Lauwers: Morphometric analysis of the foramen magnum in Pekingese dogs. Am. J. Vet. Res. 55:34–39, 1994.

Skrabalak, D.S., and A.L. Looney: Supernumerary tooth associated with facial swelling in a dog. JAVMA 203:266, 1993.

Smeak, D.D., and W.D. deHoff: Total ear canal ablation. Clinical results in the dog and cat. Vet. Surg. 15:161–170, 1986.

Smith, M.M.: The clinical significance of root morphology in periodontal disease in dogs. Compend. Contin. Pract. Vet. Educ. 17:625–635, 1995.

Spodnick, G.J., L.C. Hudson, G.N. Clark, and M.M. Pavletic: Use of a caudal auricular axial pattern flap in cats. JAVMA 208:1679–1682, 1996.

Stogdale, L., and J.B. Delack: Feline purring. Compend. Contin. Vet. Pract. Educ. 7:551–553, 1985.

Trevor, P.B., and R.A. Martin: Tympanic bulla osteotomy for treatment of middle-ear disease in cats: 19 cases (1984–1991). JAVMA 202:123–128, 1993.

Vázquez, J.M., A. Arencibia, F. Gil, et al.: Magnetic resonance imaging of the normal canine larynx. Anat. Histol. Embryol. 27:263–270, 1998.

Venker-van Haagen, A.J., W. Hartman, and W. Th. C. Wolvekamp: Contributions of the glossopharyngeal nerve and the pharyngeal branch of the vagus nerve to the swallowing process in dogs. Am. J. Vet. Res. 47:1300–1307, 1986.

Voorhout, G.: Cisternography combined with linear tomography for visualization of the pituitary gland in healthy dogs. Vet. Radiol. Ultrasound 31:68–73, 1990.

Watson, A.G., A. de Lahunta, and H.E. Evans: Dorsal notch of foramen magnum due to incomplete ossification of supraoccipital bone in dogs. J. Small Anim. Pract. 30:666–673, 1989.

Willis, A.M., C.L. Martin, J. Stiles, and S.E. Kirschner: Brow suspension for treatment of ptosis and entropion in dogs with redundant facial skin folds. JAVMA 214:660–662, 1999.

Wisner, E.R., J.S. Mattoon, T.G. Nyland, et al.: Normal ultrasonographic anatomy of the canine neck. Vet. Radiol. Ultrasound 32:185–190, 1991.

CHAPTER 12

# The Neck, Back, and Vertebral Column of the Carnivores*

## CONFORMATION AND SURFACE ANATOMY

The length and proportions of the neck vary with the breed; its transverse section, generally circular in smaller dogs, is somewhat compressed from side to side in larger breeds but widens toward the trunk with which it blends smoothly. Only a few dogs show a significant elevation at the withers. In most breeds the back slopes slightly downward toward the tail, in some others it is level, and in a few (including the Greyhound) it rises toward the loins after dipping over the thorax. The carriage of the tail is very variable. Some conformations are characteristic of certain breeds, the tightly coiled tail of the Spitz breeds being a good example, while others express temporary mood, such as the stiffened tail, held level or upright that may denote aggressive intent, and the tail depressed to cover the anus in the cringing submissive attitude. The back of the sitting dog is almost straight, that of the cat strongly arched.

Surprisingly little of the vertebral column is palpable, even in moderately lean subjects. The external occipital protuberance (of the skull) is a distinct landmark at the cranial limit of the neck, and behind this the wings of the atlas and the spinous process of the axis are easily appreciated, confirming the position of these two vertebrae close to the dorsal surface. The remaining cervical vertebrae are more deeply placed, and it is sometimes only with difficulty—if at all—that their transverse and spinous processes can be appreciated. Only the tips of the spinous processes can be palpated with certainty in the remainder of the column until the tail is reached. The dorsal parts of the scapulae and iliac crests provide other certain landmarks in the regions of the withers and hindquarters.

In cats the dorsal borders of the scapulae are very prominent and bound a hollow over the adjacent part of the vertebral column. The hollow deepens and the scapular ridges become very pronounced when the trunk is lowered between their forelimbs in the posture cats assume when stalking.

Cats also vary in the conformation of the neck, trunk, and tail.† Many European Shorthairs can be described as "cobby," the adjective suggesting a short, thick neck and a thick, deep, and fairly short trunk that is carried rather close to the ground. Cats of Oriental breeds are more slender with a longer, narrower trunk, raised from the ground on limbs that are proportionately longer, especially behind. The slinky, svelte appearance is accentuated by the longer tail and smooth, flat coat.

## THE VERTEBRAL COLUMN

(See also pp. 35–39).

The dog has 7 cervical, 13 thoracic, 7 lumbar, and 3 sacral vertebrae as a rule; the most common variation is the reduction to six of the lumbar vertebrae (see Fig. 2–1). The precaudal vertebral formula is the same in cats, in which the individual

*See introductory remarks on page 367.

†The neutral carriage of the tail is slightly drooping but changes from this posture are frequent and revealing to observers of cat behavior. All felids, large and small, commonly spray urine upon objects in their environment, presumably to mark their territory. They back toward the chosen object with the tail upright and, usually quivering, eject urine from the standing position, a posture in marked contrast to the squatting adopted for routine elimination. Domestic cats, uniquely and as a behavioral trait acquired in domestication, often carry the tail upright in other circumstances, when they are apparently content and at ease—as when greeting an attentive owner or meeting a conspecific from which they anticipate a friendly reception. The tucked-under position of the tail of the fearful cat, crouching in submission, and the side-to-side lashing of the cat in pugnacious mood, or merely irritated by unwanted attention, will be universally familiar.

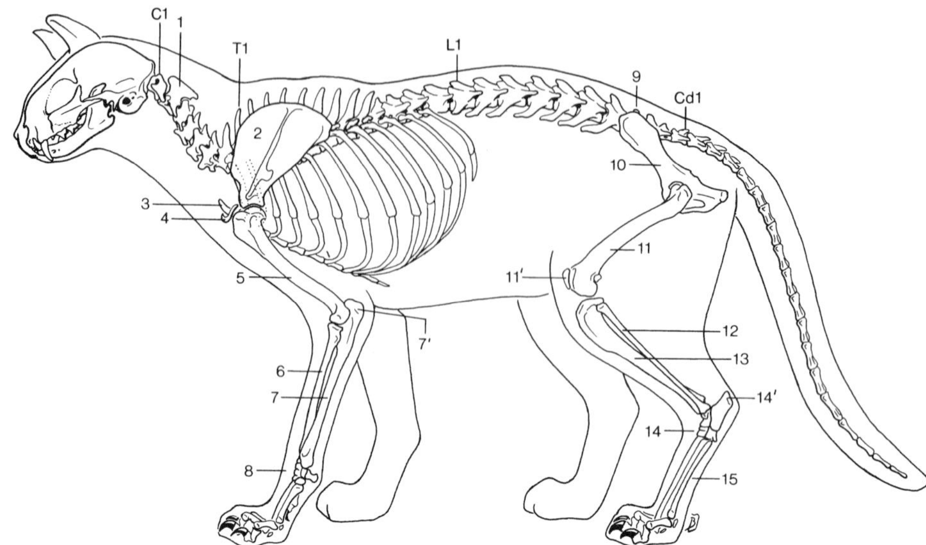


**Figure 12–1.** The feline skeleton.

1, Axis (C2); 2, scapula; 3, manubrium of sternum; 4, clavicle; 5, humerus; 6, radius; 7, ulna; 7′, olecranon; 8, carpal bones; 9, sacrum; 10, hip bone (os coxae); 11, femur; 11′, patella; 12, fibula; 13, tibia; 14, tarsal bones; 14′, calcaneus; 15, metatarsal bones; C1, T1, L1, and Cd1, first cervical, thoracic, lumbar, and caudal (tail) vertebrae.

bones are generally more slender and differ from those of the dog in subtle ways that are easy to recognize but difficult to define (Figs. 12–1, 12–2, 12–4, and 12–5).

The intervertebral discs of both dog and cat are relatively longer than in most species and contribute some 15% and 17% to 20%, respectively, of the total length of the column. Longitudinal growth of the column continues until the 12th month or so, when the epiphyses fuse with bodies of the vertebrae—except in the sacral region where there is some delay. The contours of the vertebral column do not reproduce the dorsal profile of the standing animal. The convex nape is followed by a relatively straight cervical section (Fig. 12–1). A pronounced but concealed change in direction of the vertebrae at the cervicothoracic junction redirects the column on an ascending course in relation to the contour of the back. The caudal thoracic and lumbar segments are fairly straight (depending on the breed), but over the pelvis the column curves ventrally into the tail.

The caudal end of the cervical segment is the most flexible part, and this enables the dog to reach almost every part of its trunk and limbs with its mouth. Ventral flexion to lower the head to the ground is mainly the result of movement in the cranial thoracic joints, and the cervical vertebrae

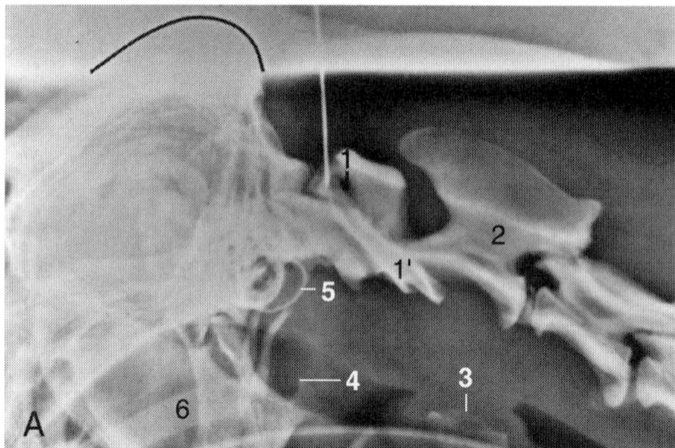


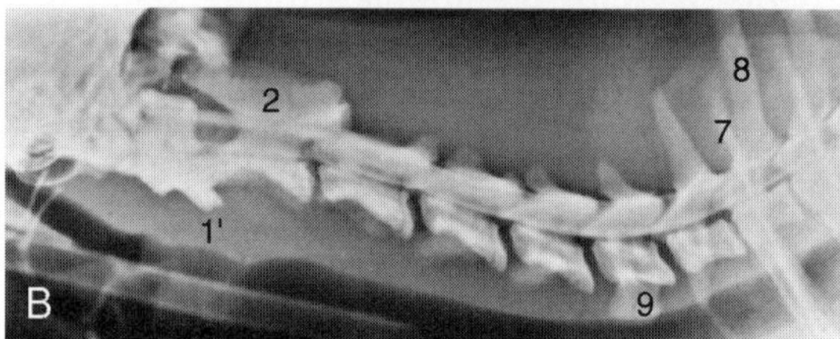


**Figure 12–2.** *A*, Lateral radiograph of the head-neck junction of an intubated dog. Note the needle in the atlanto-occipital space for a cerebrospinal fluid tap. The dorsal contour of the skull is marked. *B*, Myelogram of an intubated dog.

1, Lateral vertebral foramen of atlas; 1′, wing of atlas; 2, axis; 3, cricoid cartilage; 4, angular process of mandible; 5, tympanic bulla; 6, soft palate; 7, spine of scapula; 8, spinous process of T1; 9, ventral tubercle of C6.

**Table 12–1.** Development and Maturation of the Canine* Vertebral Column

| Ossification Centers Present at Birth (after Birth) | Approximate Age at Growth Plate Closure Observed on Radiographs |
|---|---|
| Vertebrae, except C1 and C2 | |
| Cranial epiphysis (2–8 wk) | 7–14 mo† |
| Body | |
| Caudal epiphysis (2–8 wk) | 7–14 mo† |
| Two sides of arch | |
| Atlas | |
| Ventral arch | |
| Two sides of dorsal arch | 4 mo‡ |
| Axis | |
| Apex of dens (3–4 mo) | 3–4 mo‡ |
| Dens and cran. articular surface | 7–9 mo‡ |
| Intercentrum (3 wk) | 4 mo‡ |
| Body | |
| Caudal epiphysis (3 wk) | 7–9 mo‡ |
| Two sides of arch | 3 mo‡ |

*Similar information for the cat appears to be lacking.
†Based on Hare, W. C. D.: Zur Ossifikation und Vereinigung der Wirbelepiphysen beim Hund. Wien. Tierärztl. Monatsschr. 48:210–215, 1961.
‡Based on Hare, W. C. D.: Radiographic anatomy of the cervical region of the canine vertebral column. JAVMA 139:209–220, 1961.
From deLahunta, A., and R. E. Habel, 1986.

are merely brought into line. Considerable mobility of the caudal thoracic and lumbar joints is necessary for the alternating sagittal flexion and extension of the back in the bounding gallop used by both dogs and cats when moving at speed. This enables the hindlimbs to be placed alongside (if not ahead of) the forelimbs after which the hindlimb joints, and those of the column, extend to hurl the body forward. Lateral flexion of the joints of the thoracic and lumbar segments is surprisingly free and enables dogs to curl up when sleeping. The spine of the cat is even more supple.

From the clinical point of view it is important to be familiar with the appearance of the vertebral column in radiographs of both juvenile and mature animals. The atlanto-occipital, atlantoaxial, and lumbosacral junctions merit particular attention. Table 12–1 records the ages at which the secondary ossification centers of the vertebrae appear and those at which they later fuse.

The ventral arch of the *atlas* is considerably narrower (craniocaudally) than the dorsal. The lateral vertebral foramen for the first cervical nerve is close to the cranial border of the dorsal arch; a notch in the cranial border of the wing replaces the alar foramen of other species and transmits the ventral branch of the same nerve. The wing slants caudally and overlaps the atlantoaxial junction. Its base is perforated by the transverse foramen. Both arches participate in the deep cranial articular foveae, which receive the occipital condyles. The joint capsules are widely spaced dorsally but communicate ventrally. The dorsal deficiency is bridged by the atlanto-occipital membrane, which extends from the dorsal border of the foramen magnum to the dorsal arch of the atlas. By attaching laterally to the joint capsules it closes the atlanto-occipital aperture. This membrane is punctured in the collection of cerebrospinal fluid and in the injection of radiopaque contrast agent into the subarachnoid space to outline the spinal cord (contrast myelography) (Fig. 12–2/*A,B* and Plate 13/*F*).

The *axis* is characterized by its length and its enormous spinous process, which overhangs both the dorsal arch of the atlas and the laminae of the following vertebra. The cranial extent of the spinous process matches that of the dens, which rests on the dorsal surface of the ventral arch of the atlas (Fig. 12–3/4′,2′). Between the two is a large (cranial vertebral) notch, which transmits the second cervical nerve. A thin transverse process projects caudolaterally, overlapping the junction with the next vertebra; it carries the transverse foramen in its base. The atlantoaxial joint is enclosed by a single capsule. The two bones are held in apposition by a thin median ligament (lig. apicis dentis), which connects the tip of the dens with the ventral border of the foramen magnum (see Fig. 2–13), and paired (alar) ligaments, which pass obliquely from the dens to the ventrolateral borders of the foramen. The dens is further secured by a transverse ligament connecting the inner walls of the ventral arch of the atlas across its dorsal

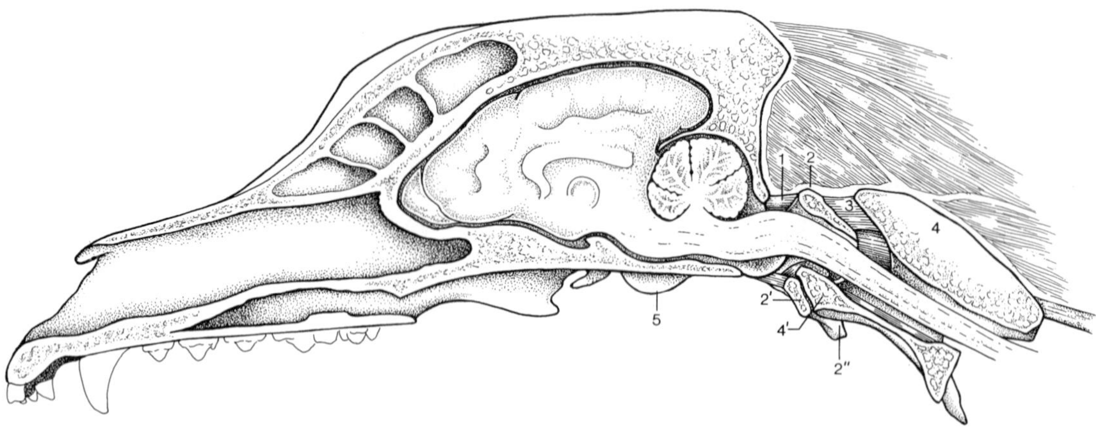


**Figure 12–3.** Paramedian section of the canine head-neck junction.

1, Dorsal atlanto-occipital membrane; 2, dorsal arch of atlas; 2′, ventral arch of atlas; 2″, wing of atlas; 3, dorsal atlantoaxial ligament; 4, spinous process of axis; 4′, dens; 5, tympanic bulla.

surface. An atlantoaxial membrane closes the interarcuate space; its median part is thickened by elastic fibers that connect the cranial tip of the spine of the axis with the tubercle on the dorsal arch of the atlas (dorsal atlantoaxial lig.; Fig. 12–3/3).

The spinous processes of the remaining *cervical vertebrae* increase in height and in cranial inclination. The ventral crests are most prominent at the caudal ends of the bodies, marking the positions of the intervertebral discs directly caudal to them. The transverse processes have distinct cranial and caudal extensions (ventral and dorsal tubercles). The ventral tubercle of the sixth vertebra is a nearly sagittal plate that projects considerably below the contour of the body (Fig. 12–2/9). The transverse process of the seventh is a rodlike lateral projection that does not overlap the body ventrally. The flat articular surfaces of the synovial joints are nearly horizontal. The cranial articular processes, which provide the ventral component of these joints, narrow the large intervertebral foramina from above.

The bodies of the *thoracic vertebrae* are relatively short but increase in length from the 10th caudally (Fig. 12–4). This increase continues in the lumbar region, where the bodies are each about twice as long as those of the first few thoracic vertebrae. The long spinous processes of the first half of the thoracic region are of about equal length. Those of the second half gradually decrease in height; their caudal inclination changes at the 11th thoracic, the anticlinal vertebra (/3). A more noteworthy change occurs in the orientation of the

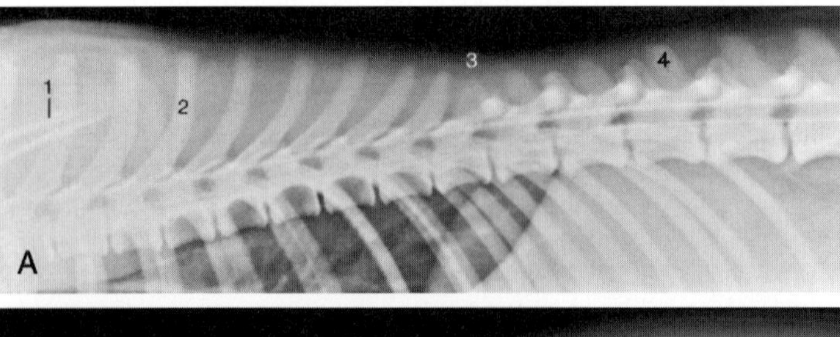


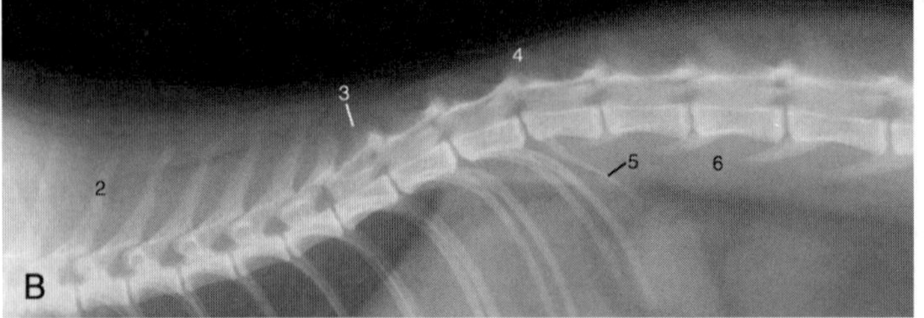


**Figure 12–4.** Lateral radiographs of canine *(A)* and feline *(B)* thoracic and lumbar vertebrae. Radiograph *A* was obtained after the injection of a contrast agent into the subarachnoid space.

1, Scapular spines; 2, spinous process of T5; 3, anticlinal vertebra (T11); 4, spinous process of L1; 5, rudimentary rib; 6, sublumbar muscles.

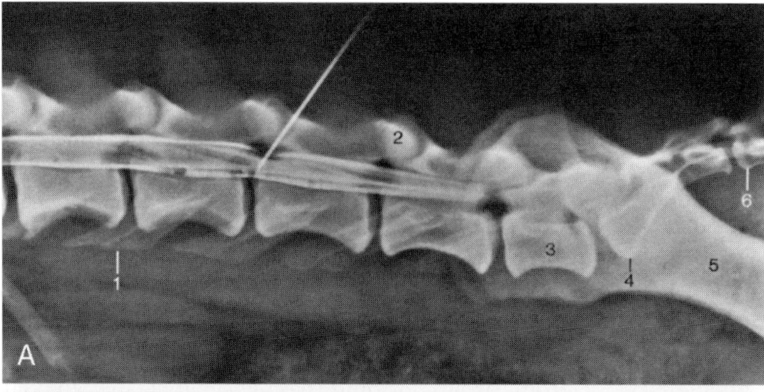


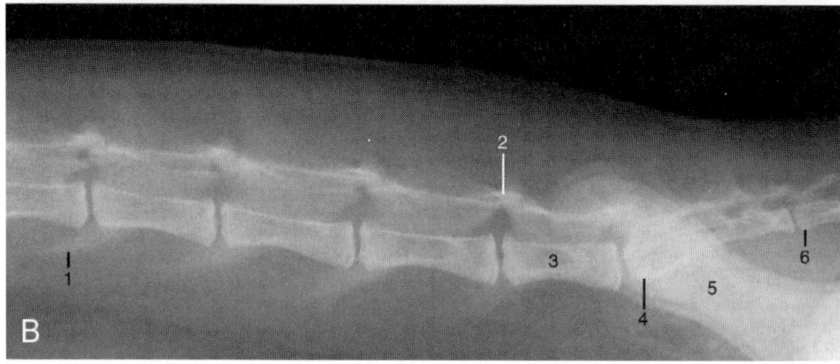


**Figure 12–5.** *A*, Lateral radiograph of the lumbar area of a dog with a myelogram. A needle is in the interarcual space between L4 and L5. *B*, Same structures and view of a cat.

1, Transverse processes of L4; 2, articular processes; 3, last lumbar vertebra (L7); 4, promontory (of sacrum); 5, shaft of ilium; 6, first tail vertebra (Cd1).

articular surfaces. On the first 10 (or so) thoracic vertebrae these surfaces lie roughly in a dorsal plane (like those of the cervical vertebrae); caudal to this they are nearly sagittal, with the cranial articular processes enclosing the caudal ones (see Fig. 2–10). The articular spaces of the former joints are best depicted in lateral, those of the latter in ventrodorsal radiographs. The more cranial thoracic vertebrae favor lateral movement of the column, while the more caudal bones favor sagittal flexion and extension. Further features of the canine and feline vertebrae are the mamillary and accessory processes. The mamillary processes are short dorsal projections of the transverse processes that begin at the third thoracic vertebra and later, from the 11th, migrate dorsally to surmount the cranial articular processes. The accessory processes arise from the caudal border of the pedicle and are present from the midthoracic to midlumbar regions; they are confined to the last three thoracic vertebrae in cats (see Fig. 2–11/1,2).

The *lumbar vertebrae* continue several features of the thoracic vertebrae but are characterized by long transverse processes that sweep cranioventrally, overlapping the preceding vertebra (Fig. 12–5/1). The ventral deflection of these processes is even more pronounced in the cat. The interarcuate spaces of both lumbar and thoracic segments are very small, making access with a needle to this part of the vertebral canal difficult. The space at the lumbosacral junction is much better suited for this purpose. It is about 1 cm in diameter (in a medium-sized dog) and lies in the transverse plane of the highest palpable points on the wings of the ilia but about 2 cm deeper.

Fusion of the three segments that constitute the sacrum may not be completed until 1½ years after birth. The sacrum is deeply embedded between the wings of the ilia so that only the spinous processes (sacral crest) are palpable through the skin; however, its caudoventral part and the first few (of the score or more) *caudal vertebrae* can be palpated digitally per rectum. A feature of certain caudal vertebrae (usually the fourth to sixth) are hemal arches, small V-shaped bones attached to the caudal ends of the ventral surfaces (see Fig. 2–12/9). Short (hemal) processes are found in similar positions on several more segments.

Congenital anomalies of the cat tail include the distinctive Manx "bob" and the kinking formerly common in Siamese though largely bred out of the modern breed.

Most vertebrae are joined by the intervertebral discs, paired synovial joints, and short and long ligaments (p. 40). The functional importance of the intervertebral discs lies in the contributions they make to the flexibility of the spine and to the distribution of pressure over the extremities of the vertebrae. Their clinical significance lies in the frequency with which degenerative changes occur. When not too profound, these changes may almost be regarded as part of the normal aging process.

They include the replacement of fibrous tissue, and possibly the calcification of the gelatinous nucleus, and frequently the separation and rupture of the fibrous lamellae of the anulus. The narrow dorsal part of the anulus is most vulnerable, and when degeneration is advanced, stretching or total rupture of this section allows disc material to protrude into the vertebral canal where it may press (through the meninges) upon the spinal cord and nerves producing various and often severe dysfunctions. Radiography may reveal narrowing of the affected intervertebral spaces; misinterpretation is easy if insufficient attention is paid to the geometry of image formation (see page 5).

There are both breed and regional differences in the incidence of disc pathology. Chondrodystrophic breeds, such as the Dachshund and Pekingese, in which the degenerative process is both precocious and accentuated, are particularly prone to protrusions. Cervical discs, and especially that at the cervicothoracic junction, are quite commonly affected, but the bulk of the protrusions involve the discs of the caudal thoracic and lumbar regions. The presence of intercapital ligaments at the joints T1–T2 to T9–T10 offers almost complete protection to the greater part of the thoracic cord. It should be emphasized that nuclear calcifications are often evident in radiographs obtained of dogs that present no signs of dysfunction or pain. The intervertebral discs of cats are not immune to degeneration but, for reasons that are obscure, affected animals very often fail to manifest any clinical signs.

The *nuchal ligament* (absent in cats) is an elastic ribbon that extends from the spinous process of the axis to the tip of the first thoracic spinous process; it is then continued by the supraspinous ligament that follows the tips of the remaining spinous processes. The nuchal ligament plays an important role in the support of the head and must be spared during surgery (see Fig. 2–8/3).

## THE MUSCLES ASSOCIATED WITH THE VERTEBRAL COLUMN

*(See also pp. 47–51.)*

The muscles directly associated with the vertebral column mainly extend betwen points on the vertebrae (and ribs), but some also attach to the skull, the ilium, and, where the psoas group is concerned, the femur. They are covered in the neck and thorax by muscles arising from the sternum and by others inserting in the forelimb, and in the pelvic area by the more superficial gluteal muscles. These have been described on pages 81 and 95, respectively.

The *epaxial muscles* (see Fig. 2–22/*B*,12) must be separated and detached when access to the vertebral column is necessary to relieve pressure on the spinal cord caused by disc protrusion. Since the details of these muscles are *not* of great general interest, some readers may choose to skip the following section. Others, concerned with their potential relevance to spinal surgery, may welcome a recapitulation and enlargement of the account given in an earlier chapter (p. 47). Both groups should be aware that the epaxial muscles lend themselves to intramuscular injection.

The epaxial muscles comprise three longitudinal systems—iliocostalis, longissimus, and transversospinalis. The *iliocostalis muscle* is relatively thin (see Fig. 2–23/*B*,17). Its bundles span several vertebral segments and, in general, run from caudomedial and dorsal to craniolateral and ventral. The muscle is easily identified over the ribs by its glistening tendons. It arises caudally from the wing of the ilium and by (lumbar) fascia also from the spinous processes of the lumbar vertebrae. It attaches to the lumbar transverse processes and angles of the ribs and, with its most cranial bundle, on the transverse process of the last cervical vertebra. The iliocostalis lies lateral to the longissimus, and in the thoracolumbar region it is covered by the dorsal serratus and the origins of the latissimus and the two abdominal oblique muscles.

The *longissimus muscle* is much thicker than the preceding muscle (see Fig. 2–23/*B*,16″). Its bundles are similarly oriented but are largely fused, giving it a uniform appearance in the lumbar and thoracic regions. The muscle arises caudally from the wing of the ilium and the spinous processes, against which it lies in the lumbar area, and extends with its most cranial component (longissimus capitis) all the way to the head. In the neck (longissimus cervicis) its bundles are long and separate (/16′); these connect transverse and articular processes of thoracic and cervical vertebrae, respectively, with transverse processes of the more cranial cervical vertebrae. The thoracolumbar portion (longissimus dorsi) is thickest and is credited with powerful extension (straightening) of the vertebral column during the propulsive phase of the gallop. It is related medially to the multifidus, and over the thoracic vertebrae it is covered dorsally by the spinalis et semispinalis, although separated from both by fibrous septa. The ventral edge of the vertical septum it shares with the multifidus ends near the transverse processes of the vertebrae and is a

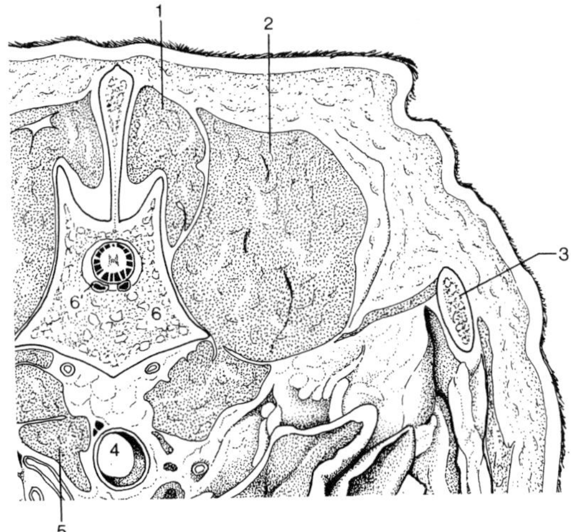


**Figure 12–6.** Transverse section of the back of a dog at the level of the first lumbar vertebra.

1, Multifidus and spinalis; 2, longissimus and iliocostalis; 3, last rib; 4, aorta; 5, right crus of diaphragm; 6, first lumbar vertebra; 6′, internal vertebral venous plexus.

landmark in the surgical approach to the intervertebral discs (Fig. 12–6/2,1).

The more complex *transversospinalis system* is most intimately related to the vertebrae (see Fig. 2–22/,21). Some fascicles connect one vertebra to the next, others span several vertebrae; most are oriented from caudoventral and lateral to craniodorsal and medial, in contrast to the direction taken by the preceding muscles. The transversospinalis system comprises spinalis et semispinalis thoracic et cervicis, semispinalis capitis, and several less important and more obviously segmental muscles (multifidi, intertransversarii, interspinales, and rotatores) that lie directly on the vertebrae.

The *spinalis et semispinalis thoracic et cervicis* extends from the midlumbar area to the spine of the axis and lies against the lateral surface of the spinous processes (see Fig. 2–24/*A*,2‴). Its fascicles connect spinous and mamillary processes with more cranial spinous processes. The *semispinalis capitis* is a more independent neck muscle lying between the splenius and the cervical components of the preceding muscle (see Fig. 2–23/*B*,15′). It is clearly divided into biventer and complexus, which contact their fellows, and the ligamentum nuchae in the median plane. The biventer is the more dorsal and more caudal of the two. It arises from and around the transverse processes of the first few thoracic vertebrae and ends on the occipital bone ventral to the external occipital protuberance. It can be identified by several tendinous inscriptions. The complexus arises from the articular processes of the more caudal cervical vertebrae and ends on the nuchal crest.

The *hypaxial muscles* comprise the longus colli and longus capitis in the neck and cranial thoracic areas, and the psoas muscles in the lumbar area. The former have already been described (p. 51). The latter consist of the psoas major and minor accompanied by a thin plate of muscle (quadratus lumborum) that lies directly below the lumbar transverse processes. The *psoas major* arises from the bodies of the lumbar vertebrae and passes caudally, medial to the wings of the ilium, where it fuses with the ilacus to form the iliopsoas (see Fig. 2–24/*B*,11). The iliopsoas attaches to the lesser trochanter of the femur; it flexes the lumbar vertebral column and advances the hindlimb. The *psoas minor* has a similar origin and lies medial to the psoas major. It inserts on the iliopubic eminence at the pelvic inlet. It flexes the lumbar vertebral column.

The four straight and two oblique muscles associated with the specialized atlanto-occipital and atlantoaxial joints form a group of their own, though they can be segregated into epaxial and hypaxial divisions. The *rectus capitis dorsalis major* (Fig. 12–7/2) comes from the spine of the

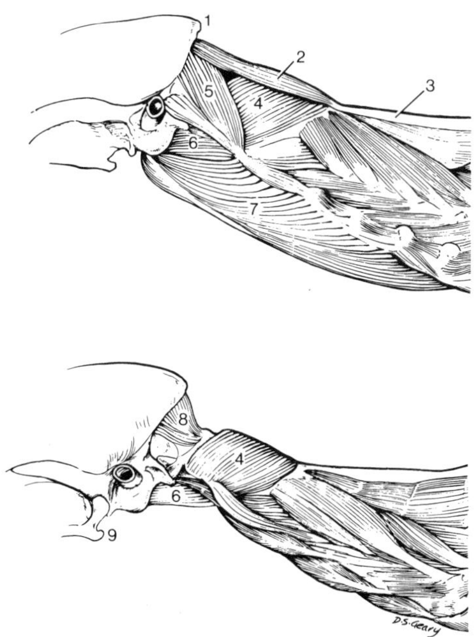


**Figure 12–7.** Muscles associated with the canine atlanto-occipital and atlantoaxial joints, lateral view.

1, External occipital protuberance; 2, rectus capitis dorsalis major; 3, nuchal ligament; 4, obliquus capitis caudalis; 5, obliquus capitis cranialis; 6, rectus capitis ventralis; 7, longus capitis; 8, rectus capitis dorsalis minor; 9, angular process of mandible.

axis and goes to the nuchal surface of the skull ventral to the insertion of the semispinalis capitis. The *rectus capitis dorsalis minor* (/8) lies deep to the preceding muscle; it comes from the dorsal arch of the atlas and goes to the skull. The *rectus capitis ventralis* (6) comes from the ventral arch of the atlas and goes to the ventral surface of the occipital bone. It lies dorsal to the much larger longus capitis, which goes to the same part of the skull but arises from more caudal cervical vertebrae (/7). The *rectus capitis lateralis* comes from the ventral arch of the atlas and goes to the paracondylar process of the occipital bone. The rectus muscles move the head up, down, and sideways. The *obliquus capitis cranialis* (/5) arises from the cranial surface of the wing of the atlas and inserts on the nuchal surface of the skull. The larger *obliquus capitis caudalis* (/4) arises from the lateral surface of the spine of the axis and inserts on the caudal surface of the wing of the atlas. The obliquus muscles are responsible for rotation of the head at the atlantoaxial joint.

## THE VERTEBRAL CANAL

*(See also pp. 298–302.)*

The dura mater adheres to the periosteum of the first two cervical vertebrae but separates thereafter, leaving a relatively narrower epidural space than is seen in the large animals (Fig. 12–4). The meninges, and indeed the cord, thus conform more closely to the dimensions of the vertebral canal. The cord is thickest in the atlas, where it measures about 1 cm. Elsewhere, except for the cervical and lumbar enlargements, it is approximately half that diameter. The cervical enlargement involves cord segments C6–T1, from which the nerves that give origin to the brachial plexus arise, while the lumbar enlargement, with a similar relationship to the lumbosacral plexus, involves cord segments L5–S1. The ascent of the cord (p. 298) within the vertebral column explains the topography of its segments (Plate 13/*G*). Most cervical segments lie about half a vertebra, and most thoracic segments a whole vertebra, cranial to the vertebra of the same designation, while the caudal thoracic and cranial lumbar segments occupy vertebrae with the same designations. Behind this the cord segments are markedly shorter, and this generally places the end of the cord over the last interlumbar joint (Figs. 12–8 and see 8–56/*B*). The cervical and lumbosacral enlargements lie in the sixth and seventh cervical and fourth and fifth lumbar vertebrae, respectively. The ascent is less marked in small dogs, in which the cord may reach the sacrum. The sacral canal contains only spinal nerves and the dural sheath, which extends about 2 cm beyond the cord. The termination of the cord is said to be very variable in *cats,* all levels from the caudal border of L7 to the caudal border of S3 being given by different authors. Some of this

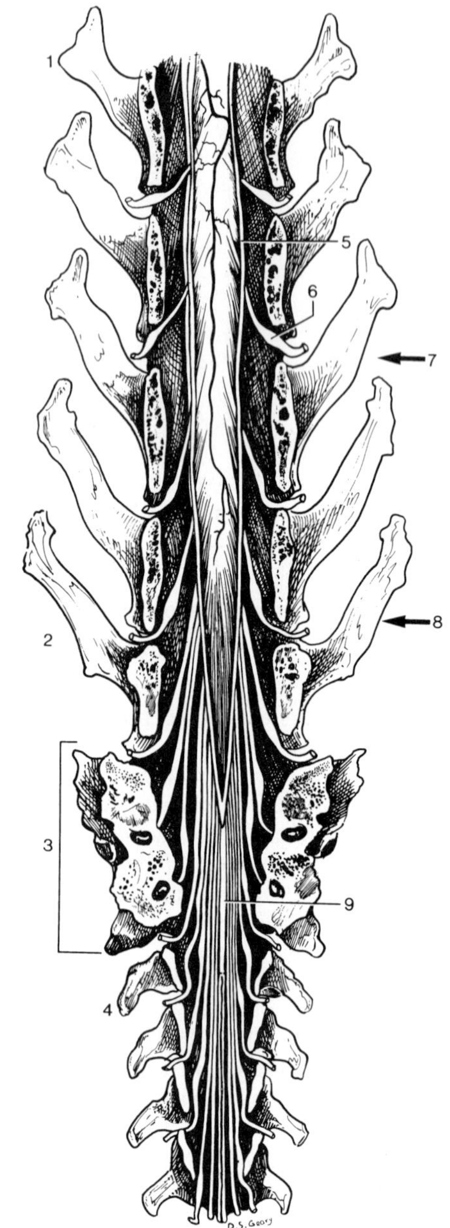


**Figure 12–8.** Caudal end of the canine spinal cord in situ, dorsal view.

1, Third lumbar vertebra; 2, last lumbar vertebra (L7); 3, sacrum; 4, first caudal vertebra; 5, dura mater; 6, dorsal root ganglion; 7, approximate level of L7 cord segment; 8, end of spinal cord; 9, cauda equina.

uncertainty may be due to individual and breed variation but there is a suspicion that the more cranial limit is likely to be nearer the mark in adults, the more caudal one in young kittens (*1A*). Possible puncture sites are located at the limits of this range and are relatively easily found. The lumbosacral space is located a little in front of the level of the cranial dorsal iliac spines (see Fig. 15–1). A misleading impression of its size may be obtained by failure to appreciate that the last lumbar spinous process is relatively short and fails to approach so closely to the skin as that of the preceding vertebra. The sacrocaudal space is smaller, and the defining features of the vertebrae are less salient, but compensation is found in the closeness of this space to the skin.

The cerebellomedullary cistern may be punctured through the atlanto-occipital space. For this procedure, the head is strongly flexed upon the neck and entry made midway between the cranial tip of the spinous process of the axis and the external occipital protuberance. These landmarks are more easily identified before flexion (Figs. 12–2/*A*, 12–3 and Plate 13/*F*). Epidural anesthetics are administered through the lumbosacral space or, for tail docking, at the sacrocaudal space.

As in other species, the internal vertebral venous plexus consists of two longitudinal valveless veins on the floor of the vertebral canal, where they are embedded in epidural fat (Fig. 12–6/6′; and p. 305). They anastomose frequently and receive blood from the spinal cord and vertebral bodies; they are linked to extensive but less regular external vertebral networks and to the adjacent great veins (caudal vena cava, azygous vein) by intervertebral veins. These veins, which may be double and triple, cushion the spinal nerve where they leave the vertebral canal.

At the foramen magnum the two veins of the internal plexus are continued by right and left basilar sinuses that lead to the system of venous sinuses on the floor of the cranial cavity.

Like many other mammals, the dog makes use of its tail to maintain balance when executing various energetic maneuvers, and for this, and other reasons, the routine cosmetic docking of the tails of puppies is hard to justify. However, it is sometimes necessary to amputate part of the tail of the adult following injury. The site of amputation will be determined by the lesion. Features relevant to the operation include the presence of the median caudal artery following a course below the vertebral bodies. The artery obtains no special protection where it follows the roof of the pelvis, but caudal to this it is partly shielded by processes of bone to each side. The protection takes the form of separate V-shaped hemal bones located below the fourth to sixth tail vertebrae, and by hemal processes projecting from the ventral aspect of the more distal vertebral bodies. Obviously amputation is simplest at the level of an intervertebral disc. It may be mentioned that these discs are not immune from the degenerative protrusion described earlier.

## Selected Bibliography


Adams, W.H., G.B. Daniel, A.D. Pardo, and R.R. Selcer: Magnetic resonance imaging of the caudal lumbar and lumbosacral spine in 13 dogs (1990–1993). Vet. Radiol. Ultrasound 36:3–13, 1995.

Autefage, A., P. Fayolle, and P.L. Toutain: Distribution of material injected intramuscularly in dogs. Am. J. Vet. Res. 51:901–904, 1990.

Boyd, J.S.: Color Atlas of Clinical Anatomy of the Dog and Cat. St. Louis, Mosby–Year Book, 1991.

Bradshaw, J., and C. Cameron-Beaumont: The signalling repertoire of the domestic cat and its undomesticated relatives. In Turner, D.C., and P. Bateson (eds): The Domestic Cat: The Biology of its Behaviour, 2nd ed. Cambridge, Cambridge University Press, 2000, pp. 67–93.

Burbidge, H.M., K.C. Tompson, and H. Hodge: Postnatal development of canine caudal cervical vertebrae. Res. Vet. Sci. 159:35–40, 1995.

Chambers, J.N., B.A. Selcer, T.W. Butler, et al: A comparison of computed tomography to epidurography for the diagnosis of suspected compressive lesions at the lumbosacral junction in dogs. Prog. Vet. Neurol. 5:30–34, 1994.

de Haan, J.J., S.B. Shelton, and N. Ackerman: Magnetic resonance imaging in the diagnosis of degenerative lumbosacral stenosis in four dogs. Vet. Surg. 22:1–3, 1993.

deLahunta, A., and R.E. Habel: Applied Veterinary Anatomy. Philadelphia, W.B. Saunders Company, 1986.

Feeney, D.A., P. Evers, T.F. Fletcher, et al: Computed tomography of the normal canine lumbosacral spine: A morphologic perspective. Vet. Radiol. Ultrasound 37:399–411, 1996.

Forsythe, W.B., and N.G. Ghoshal: Innervation of the canine thoracolumbar vertebral column. Anat. Rec. 208:57–63, 1984.

Gregory, C.R., J.M. Cullen, R. Pool, and P.B. Vasseur: The canine sacroiliac joint. Spine 11:1044–1048, 1986.

Horowitz A: The Fundamental Principles of Anatomy: Dissection of the Dog, Saskatoon, University of Saskatchewan, 1970. Published by the author.

Hudson, L.C., and W.P. Hamilton: Atlas of Feline Anatomy for Veterinarians. Philadelphia, W.B. Saunders Company, 1993.

Jones, J.C., R.E. Cartee, and J.E. Bartels: Computed tomographic anatomy of the canine lumbosacral spine. Vet. Radiol. Ultrasound 36:91–99, 1995.

Macpherson, J.M. and Y. Ye: The cat vertebral column: Stance configuration and range of motion. Exp. Brain Res. 119:324–332, 1998.

Ness, M.G.: Degenerative lumbosacral stenosis in the dog: A review of 30 cases. J. Small Anim. Pract. 40:185–190, 1994.

Palmer, R.H., and J.N. Chambers: Canine lumbosacral diseases. Part I. Anatomy, pathophysiology, and clinical presentation. Compend. Contin. Educ. Pract. Vet. 13:61–68, 1991.

Richards, M.W., and A.G. Watson: Development and variation of the lateral vertebral foramen of the atlas in the dog. Anat. Histol. Embryol. 20:363–368, 1991.

Selcer, R.R., W.J. Bubb, and T.L. Walker: Management of vertebral column fractures in dogs and cats: 211 cases (1977–1985). JAVMA 198:1965–1968, 1991.

Simoens, P., P. Poels, and H. Lauwers: Morphometric analysis of the foramen magnum in Pekingese dogs. Am. J. Vet. Res. 55:34–39, 1994.

Slijper, E.J.: Comparative biologic-anatomical investigations on the vertebral column and spinal musculature of mammals. Verh. Kl. Nederl. Akad. Wetensch. 42:1–128, 1946.

Smith, M.M., C.B. Carrig, D.R. Waldron, and P.B. Trevor: Direct cutaneous supply to the tail in dogs. Am. J. Vet. Res. 53:145–148, 1992.

Taga, A.T., Y. Tuara, T. Nishimoto, et al.: The advantage of magnetic resonance imaging in diagnosis of cauda equina syndrome in dogs. J. Vet. Med. Sci. 60:12 1345–1348, 1998.

Turner, W.D.: Fractures and fracture-luxations of the lumbar spine: A retrospective study in the dog. J. Am. Anim. Hosp. Assoc. 23:459–464, 1987.

Walter, M.C., G.K. Smith, and C.D. Newton: Canine lumbar spinal internal fixation techniques. A comparative biomechanical study. Vet. Surg. 15:191–198, 1986.

Watson, A.G., and A. de Lahunta: Atlantoaxial subluxation and absence of transverse ligament of the atlas in a dog. JAVMA 195:235–237, 1989.

Watson, A.G., and J.S. Stewart: Postnatal ossification centers of the atlas and axis in Miniature Schnauzers. Am. J. Vet. Res. 51:264–268, 1990.

Wisner, E.R., J.S. Mattoon, T. G. Nyland, and T.W. Baker: Normal ultrasonographic anatomy of the canine neck. Vet. Radiol. Ultrasound 32:185–190, 1991.

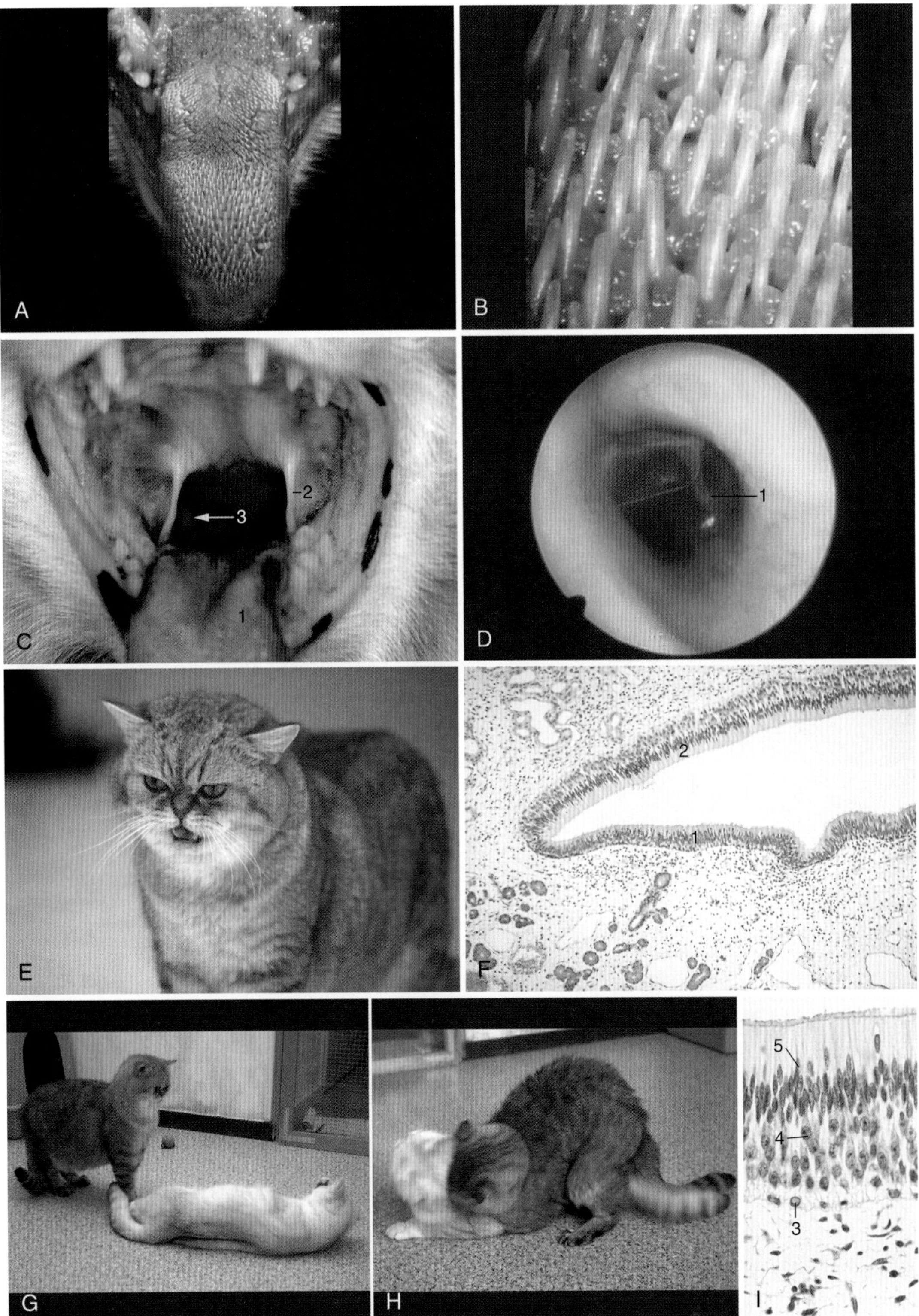


**Plate 17.** *A,* Tongue (cat). *B,* Enlargement showing caudally directed keratinized filiform papillae (cat). *C,* Oropharynx (cat): 1, tongue; 2, palatoglossal arch; 3, position of right palatine tonsil *(arrow). D,* Otoscopic view of the ear drum (cat): 1, malleus. *E,* Tomcat demonstrating Flehmen. *F,* Vomeronasal organ (pig) (HE) (70×): 1, ciliated pseudostratified columnar respiratory epithelium; (2), pseudostratified columnar epithelium of basal (3), ciliated sustentacular (4), and neurosensitive (5) cells. *G,* Flehmen by tomcat in presence of female in heat. *H,* Mating posture. *I,* Vomeronasal organ (pig) (HE) (279×); see *F* for label descriptions.

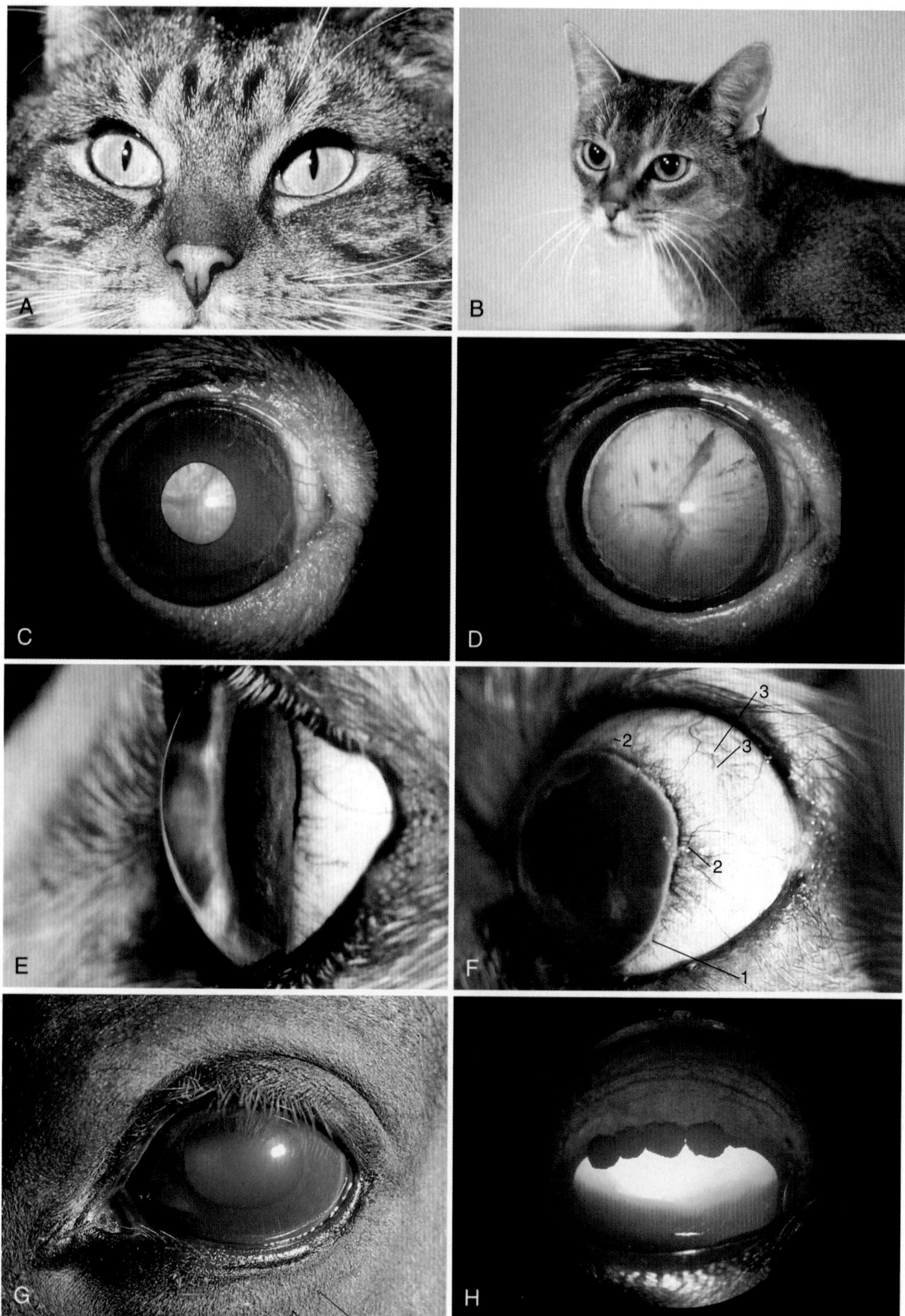


**Plate 18.** *A,* Slit form of constricted feline pupil. *B,* Round form of dilated feline pupil. *C,* Slightly constricted canine pupil with cataract. *D,* Canine pupil in mydriasis: lens, which is now totally visible, shows opacity due to cataract. *E,* Curvature of canine cornea. *F,* Exophthalmic canine eyeball and associated vascularization of bulbar conjunctiva and anterior sclera: 1, limbus corneae; 2, conjunctival vessels; 3, scleral vessels. *G,* Left equine eye; note implantation of eyelashes on lateral side of upper eyelid. *H,* Equine iris with characteristic iridic granules.

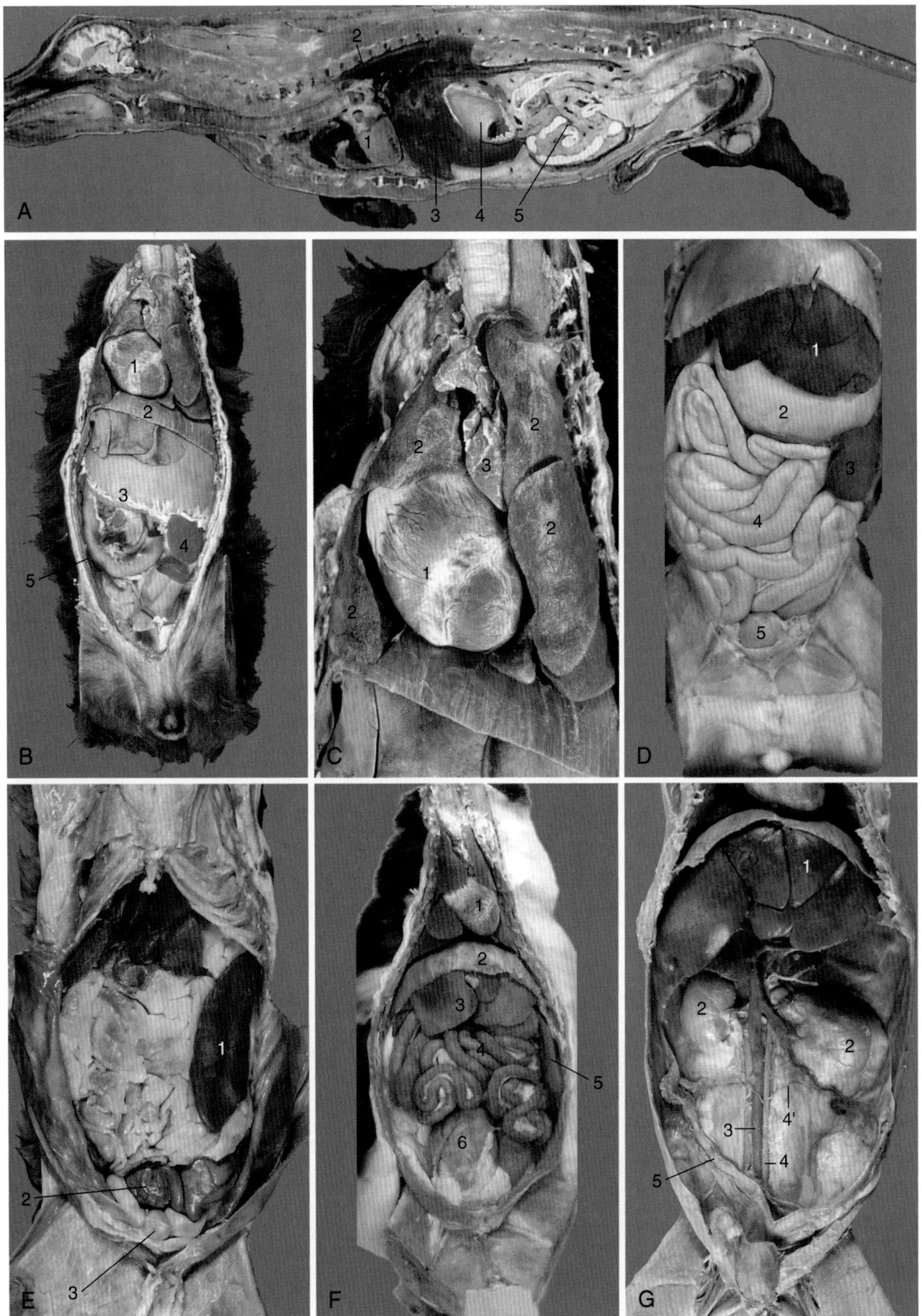


**Plate 19.** *A,* Median section of canine trunk, providing overview of viscera: 1, heart; 2, lung; 3, liver; 4, stomach; 5, intestine. *B,* Ventral view of canine trunk with overview of viscera: 1, heart; 2, diaphragm; 3, distended stomach (with attachment of greater omentum); 4, spleen; 5, duodenum. *C,* Enlargement of part of *B* showing thoracic viscera: 1, heart; 2, pulmonary lobes; 3, thymus. *D,* Abdominal viscera: 1, liver; 2, stomach; 3, spleen; 4, small intestine; 5, bladder. *E,* Ventral view of feline abdominal viscera; intestinal loops are concealed by fat-filled greater omentum: 1, spleen; 2, part of gravid uterus with two ampullae; 3, bladder. *F,* Ventral view of feline viscera after removal of omentum: 1, heart; 2, diaphragm; 3, liver; 4, intestine; 5, spleen; 6, bladder. *G,* Ventral view of feline abdominal roof: 1, liver; 2, kidneys (with stellate vv.); 3, caudal v. cava (injected); 4, aorta; 4′, ovarian a. (injected); 5, uterus.

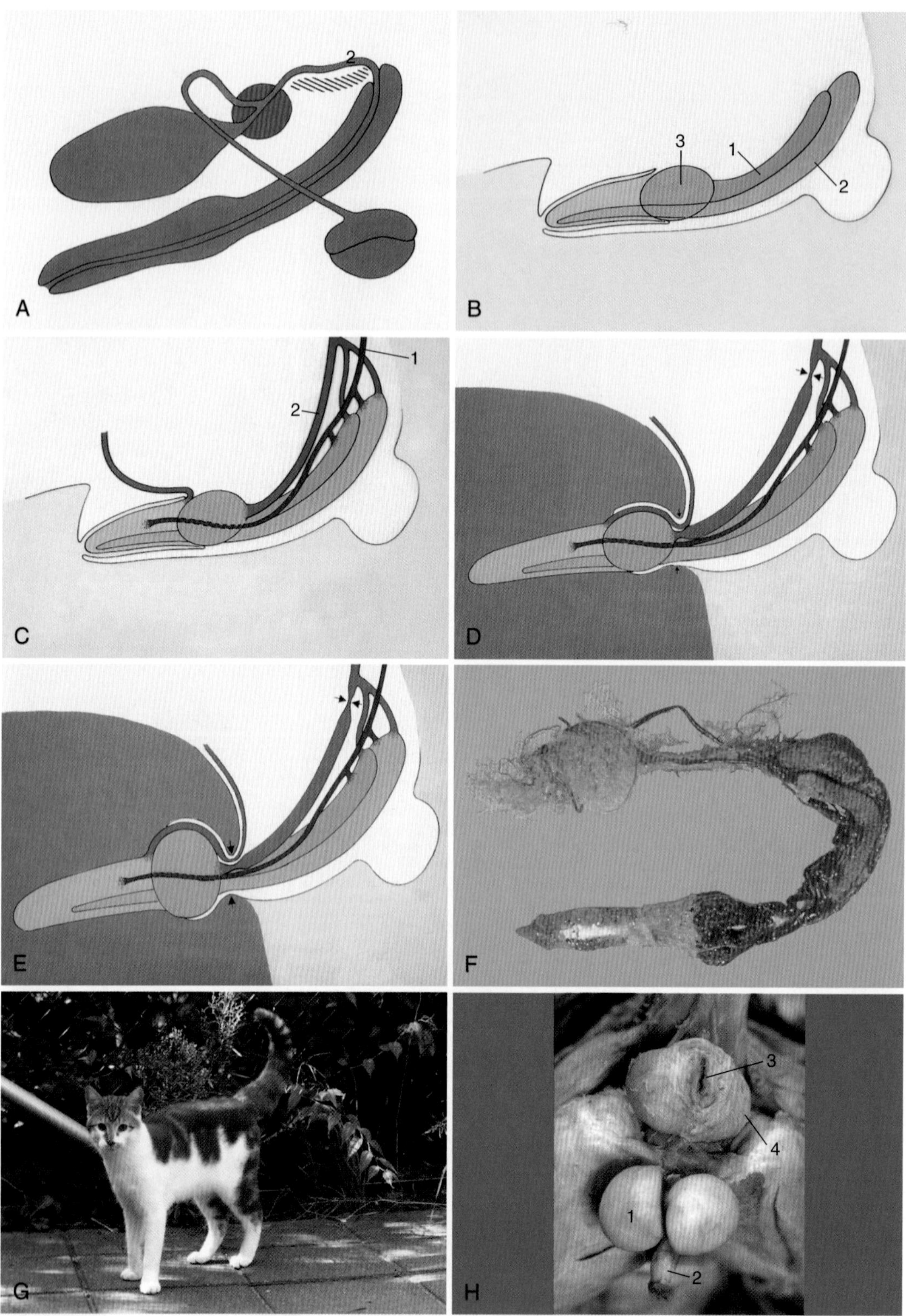


**Plate 20.** *A,* Schematic representation of canine male reproductive organs. *B,* Major vascular parts of canine penis: 1, corpus cavernosum; 2, corpus spongiosum; 3, bulbus glandis. *C, D,* and *E,* Stages in the erection process: 1, penile a.; 2, dorsal penile v. *F,* Corrosion cast of the arterial supply to prostate and penis. *G,* Tomcat spraying. *H,* Perineal area of tomcat: 1, testes; 2, penis; 3, anus; 4, anal sac.

CHAPTER 13

# The Thorax of the Carnivores*

## CONFORMATION AND SURFACE ANATOMY

The shape of the thorax varies greatly. It is laterally compressed and deep in certain breeds, of which the Borzoi is a good example, and broad and barrel-shaped in others, such as the Bulldog. These differencess are reflected in the form of the ribs, which are long and relatively straight in the Borzoi, and relatively short and strongly curved in the contrasting type. The small size of the cranial part of the bony thorax is masked by the long spinous processes of the first few thoracic vertebrae and the enclosure of the upper parts of the forelimbs within the skin of the cranial part of the trunk (Fig. 13–1). An obvious consequence of the barrel chest is lateral displacement of the lower end of the scapula; some allege an associated tendency to subluxation at the shoulder.

Despite the length of the thoracic spinous processes, the dorsal contours of the neck and thorax generally join without a noticeable elevation at the *withers.* The skin is loosely attached here, making this a suitable region for the subcutaneous infusion of large volumes of fluid when it is necessary to correct dehydration. The tips of the spinous processes are individually palpable, together with the spine and cranial and caudal angles of the scapula to each side. In the standing dog the dorsal scapular angles are placed opposite the spinous process of the first, and the bodies of the fourth and fifth thoracic vertebrae, respectively. The shoulder joint lies opposite the ventral end of the first rib with the point of the shoulder slightly behind the transverse level of the manubrium sterni. The olecranon is just below the ventral end of the fifth intercostal space. The gently curved *sternum* rises between the forelimbs to the thoracic inlet where the manubrium is easily palpated. The manubrium juts several centimeters cranial to the first pair of ribs. Breed and individual variation makes all these statements of projection approximate (Fig. 13–4).

The epaxial muscles provide a thick covering to the vertebrae and dorsal parts of the ribs. The angle between the scapula and humerus is filled by the fleshy triceps but the lateral parts of the ribs behind the limb are more thinly covered by the serratus ventralis, latissimus dorsi, scalenus and external abdominal oblique muscles. The outlines of some of these muscles may be palpable and, as they are mainly flat, it is usually possible to feel the ribs through them (see Fig. 2–53). Though the ventral surface of the thorax is covered by the pectoral muscles, the axilla is deep and permits palpation of the first five ribs, and of the axillary and accessory axillary (/10) lymph nodes when they are enlarged. The most extensive exposure of the lateral chest wall is obtained when the limb is drawn forward, which is possible in this relatively small and generally cooperative species.

The freedom with which the forelimbs of the cat may be shifted against the trunk deprives the projections of the various skeletal features of any great significance.

The thorax of young dogs and cats yields considerably to external pressure, which accounts for the often remarkable avoidance of major damage in traffic accidents. The costochondral joints of certain rib pairs can be brought together by manual compression in front of the heart.

## THE THORACIC WALL AND PLEURAL CAVITIES

*(See also pp. 51–53)*

The dog generally has 13 rib pairs of which 9 are sternal; 12 or 14 pairs are uncommon, and asymmetry of rib number is a recognized anomaly. The first three or four ribs are almost vertical; thereafter the ribs slope increasingly caudoventrally (Fig. 13–4). The ribs are relatively narrow, leaving wide intercostal spaces—an advantage in

*See introductory remarks on page 367.

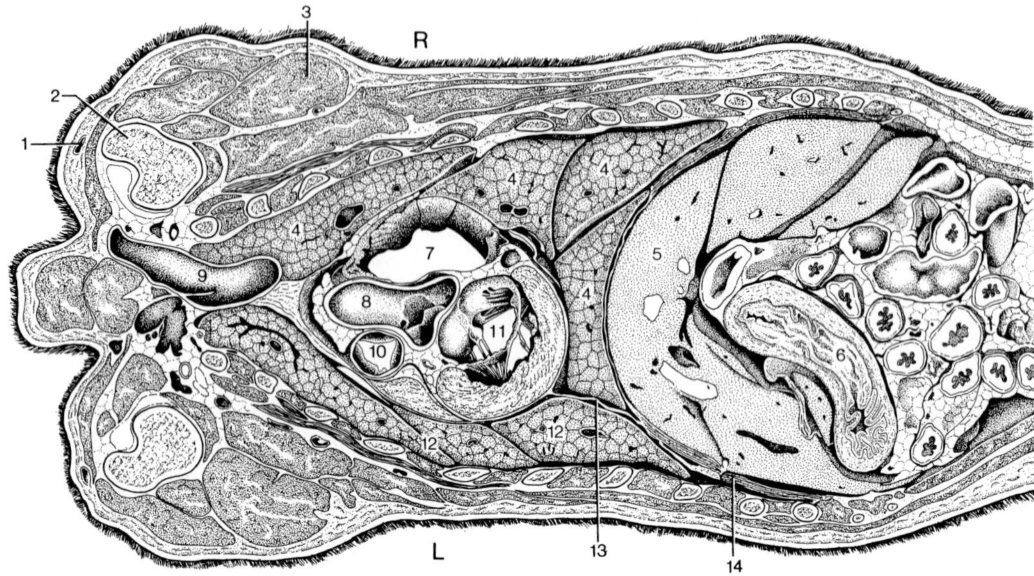


**Figure 13–1.** Dorsal section of the canine trunk level with the base of the heart, dorsal view.

1, Cephalic vein; 2, proximal end of humerus; 3, triceps; 4, cranial, middle, caudal, and accessory lobes of the right lung; 5, liver; 6, stomach; 7, right atrium; 8, aortic arch; 9, cranial vena cava; 10, pulmonary valve; 11, left atrioventricular valve; 12, divided cranial and caudal lobes of the left lung; 13, caudal mediastinum; 14, diaphragm.

thoracic surgery. The costal cartilages at first continue the direction of the ribs but then bend craniomedially, almost at right angles, forming the "knees" of the ribs. The cartilages of the four asternal ribs are joined by fascia and muscle to form the costal arch, which is easily palpated and may be followed to the vicinity of the xiphoid cartilage. The sternebrae are cylindrical and slender, though slightly thickened where the costal cartilages attach. Only a thin layer of compacta encloses the spongy bone and this, combined with their superficial position, makes them ideal for bone marrow biopsies (Fig. 13–11/11).

The intercostal spaces have the usual construction. The principal intercostal vessels and nerves lie caudomedial to the ribs, under the endothoracic fascia. Additional vessels arising from the internal thoracic trunks follow the cranial borders of the ribs in the ventral parts of the spaces. These locations must be borne in mind when contemplating incision or puncture (Fig. 13–2).

The *diaphragm* arises by right and left crura from the first few lumbar vertebrae and attaches to the medial surface of the ribs, close to the costal arch, and to the sternum. Its strong convexity brings its most cranial extent to the level of the sixth or seventh rib. It is largely fleshy; the tendinous center is small and trefoil-shaped and transmits the caudal vena cava a little to the right of the median plane. The openings for the esophagus and aorta lie in the fleshy lumbar part, the former opposite the upper palpable part of the 10th rib (Fig. 13–3). The major convexity of the ventral part of the diaphragm is continued dorsally by elongated paired elevations that present separate shadows in lateral radiographs (Fig. 13–6/*A*,4). In such radiographs, the more cranial outline of the double image is provided by the part of the diaphragm on the "lower" side, which is naturally subject to a greater forward pressure from the abdominal viscera against the less expanded, because lower, lung. The paired outlines are referred to by radiologists as right and left "crura"; because of lesser organ weights the "crura" are not as distinct in cats. Frequently a further guide is provided by a gas bubble in the stomach, which is related to the left part of the diaphragm. Sudden increase in abdominal pressure, commonly produced by compression in traffic accidents, may tear the diaphragm and allow abdominal viscera to enter the thoracic cavity (diaphragmatic hernia).

The cranial apex (cupula pleurae; Fig. 13–4/1) of each pleural sac projects a little beyond the first ribs, somewhat farther on the left than on the right. The cupulae may be injured in penetrating wounds sustained at the base of the neck, which may therefore cause lung collapse (pneumothorax).

The junction between costal and diaphragmatic pleurae, the line of pleural reflection (/4), is the most caudal extent of each pleural cavity. It runs from the sternum along the eighth costal cartilage, crosses the middle of the ninth cartilage, and then proceeds in a curve that extends from the costochondral junction of the 11th rib to the dorsal end of the 13th rib. The lowest point for puncture of a pleural cavity (thoracocentesis) is in the middle of the seventh or eighth intercostal space, just above the costochondral junction. The eighth space is optimal for this purpose in the cat (Fig. 13–5).

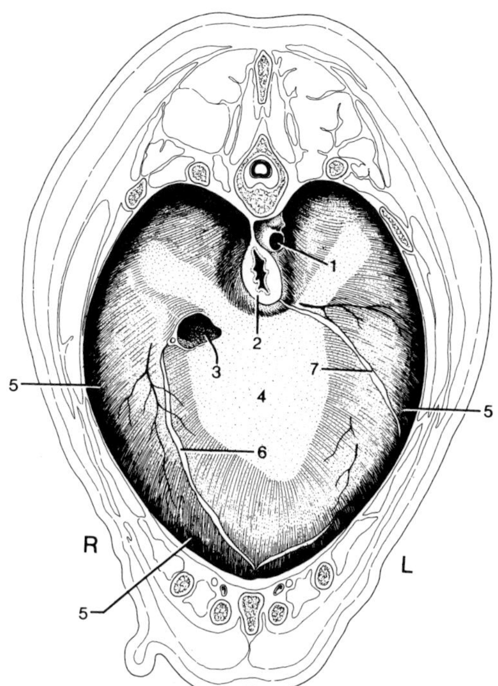


**Figure 13–3.** Cranial view of the canine diaphragm.

1, Aorta; 2, esophagus; 3, caudal vena cava; 4, tendinous center; 5, sternal and costal parts of diaphragm; 6, attachment of plica venae cavae; 7, attachment of caudal mediastinum.

# THE LUNGS

*(See also pp. 160–164.)*

The right lung is the larger of the two (Plate 19/*B,C*). It has cranial, middle, caudal, and accessory lobes; the left lung has a divided cranial and a single caudal lobe (Fig. 13–1/4,12). The lobes are so deeply divided by fissures that several are connected only by the bronchi and blood vessels. This permits occasional torsion of a lobe following diaphragmatic hernia or other trauma. In keeping with the difference in size, the cardiac impression on the medial surface of the left lung is shallow, while that of the right is deep. Though there is a small cardiac notch between the two parts of the cranial lobe opposite the ventral end of the third intercostal space, the left lung, for all practical purposes, covers the lateral surface of the heart. The right cardiac notch, between the cranial and middle lobes, is larger but still restricted to the ventral end of the fourth intercostal space; it is the recommended site for puncture of the heart (right ventricle; Fig. 13–4/at D).

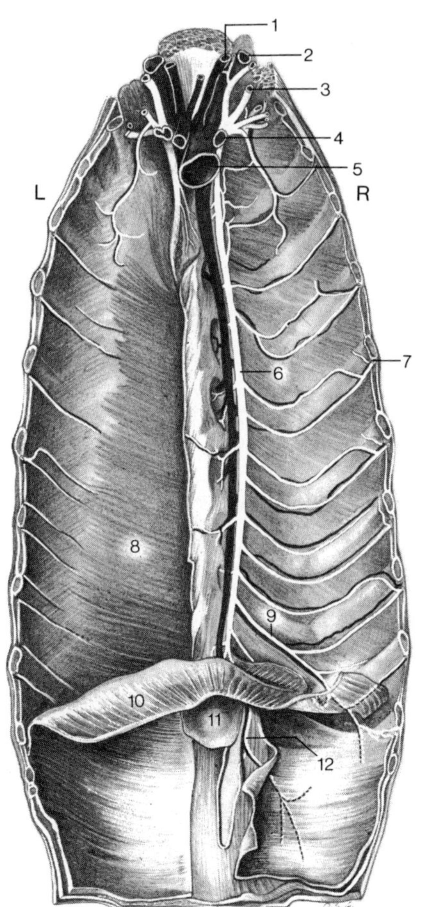


**Figure 13–2.** The vessels on the floor of the canine thorax; the transversus thoracis has been removed on the right.

1, Internal jugular vein; 2, external jugular vein; 3, vertebral artery; 4, right subclavian artery; 5, cranial vena cava; 6, internal thoracic artery; 7, intercostal artery; 8, transversus thoracis; 9, musculophrenic artery; 10, diaphragm; 11, xiphoid cartilage; 12, cranial epigastric artery.

The pulmonary lobules are not detectable by the naked eye through the covering pleura, which is continuous with the parietal pleura at the hilus and by the pulmonary ligament. The left ligament connects the medial surface of the lung caudal to the hilus to the aorta; the right one passes to the esophagus, extending to the level of the hiatus in the diaphragm.

The main contribution to the radiological features of the lungs is made by the blood within the pulmonary vessels. The arteries and veins, which cannot be immediately differentiated, form patterns of light streaks that radiate from the hilar region toward the periphery, branching and tapering as they go (Fig. 13–12/*A*). The bronchi, filled with air, provide dark streaks that contrast less definitely with the lung parenchyma. The bronchial walls may be invisible or appear as narrow whitish lines especially visible in older animals in which there is some calcification of bronchial cartilage. The relationships within the bronchial-vascular triads vary in different views and in different regions. The components are depicted best when viewed end-on; the dark circle of the bronchial lumen is then flanked to each side by the white circles representing the companion vessels. The subpleural connective tissue bordering the interlobar fissures may produce fine lines when penetrated tangentially. Both the bronchial tree and the vasculature can be more clearly depicted by appropriate techniques (contrast bronchography, Fig. 13–6; angiocardiography, Fig. 13–15).

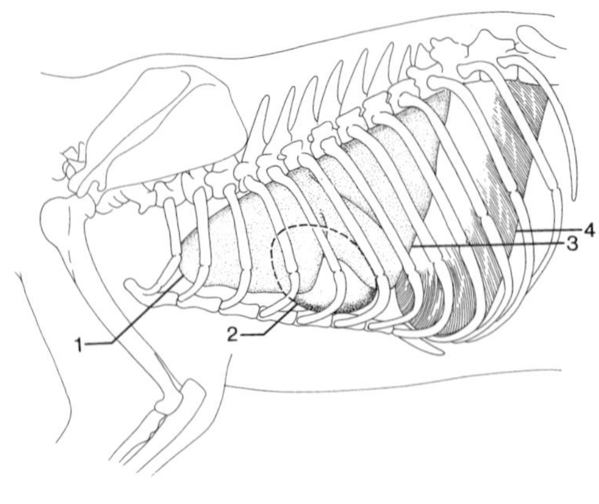


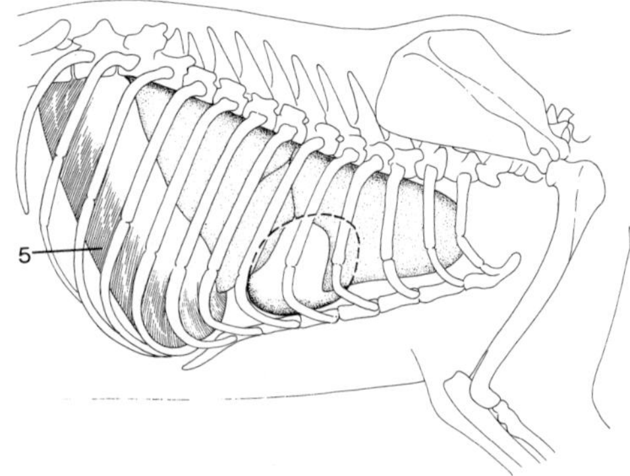


**Figure 13–5.** Left and right surface projections of the feline heart and lung.

1, Apex of left lung; 2, heart; 3, basal border of lung; 4, line of pleural reflection; 5, diaphragm.

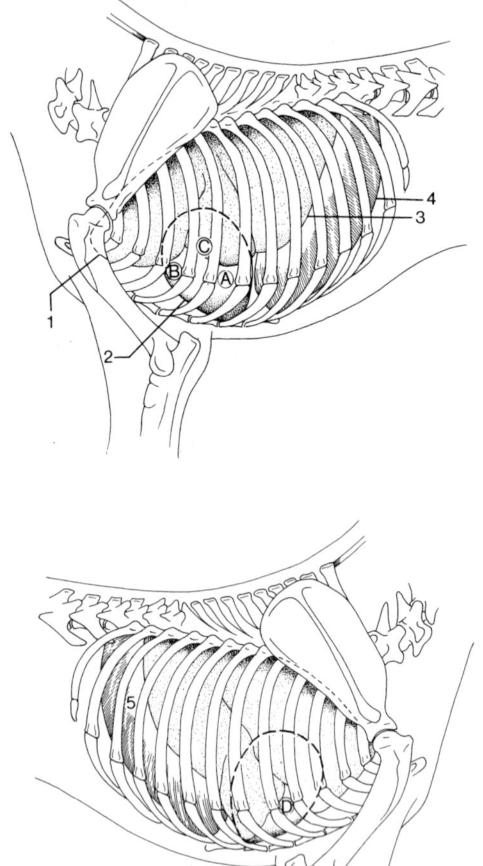


**Figure 13–4.** Left and right surface projections of the canine heart and lungs.

1, Apex of left lung *(broken line)* in cupula pleurae; 2, heart; 3, basal border of lung; 4, line of pleural reflection; 5, diaphragm.

*Circled letters on the heart:* Puncta maxima of left atrioventricular valve (A), pulmonary valve (B), aortic valve (C), and right atrioventricular valve (D).

Projection of the lungs on the lateral thoracic wall produces a triangular field for auscultation and percussion. The cranial border is the fifth rib (caudal border of triceps and teres major); the dorsal border is the palpable lateral margin of the back muscles (from the fifth rib to the 11th intercostal space); the caudoventral (basal) border (Fig. 13–4/3) extends from the costochondral junction of the sixth rib, through the middle of the eighth rib, to the dorsal end of the 11th intercostal space. The limb may be drawn forward to increase the accessible field by about the space of two ribs.

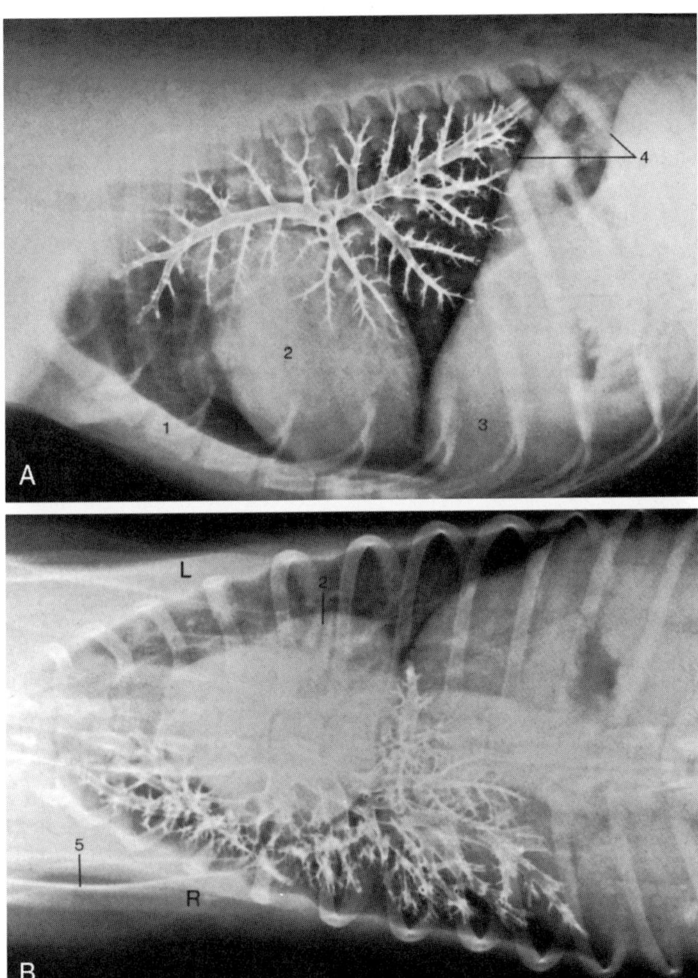


**Figure 13–6.** Lateral *(A)* and ventrodorsal *(B)* bronchograms of the right canine lung.

1, Sternum; 2, heart; 3, liver behind diaphragm; 4, paired shadows of the cranial extent of the diaphragm; 5, scapula.

## THE MEDIASTINUM

*(See also pp. 158–160.)*

The fibrous tissue associated with the thoracic organs and that between the pleural sacs is so scanty that the mediastinum is reduced in several places to a very delicate membrane consisting only of the apposed right and left pleural sheets.

The cranial mediastinum is wide dorsally, where it contains the trachea and esophagus lying side by side as they pass through the thoracic inlet; ventral to these the cranial vena cava and brachiocephalic trunk, with their respective branches, are embedded in generous quantities of fat. The ventral part of the cranial mediastinum contains lymph nodes, fat, the internal thoracic vessels, and, in the young animal, the thymus. This ventral part narrows after the regression of the thymus, allowing more room for the cranial lobes of the lungs (Fig. 13–7).

The dorsal part of the middle mediastinum is slightly narrower than the heart (Fig. 13–8). It contains the last part of the trachea, the esophagus, the aortic arch, the structures of the roots of the lungs, and lymph nodes. Its right surface is fairly flat, but the aorta (/4) bulges laterally on the left, indenting the left lung. The middle part of the mediastinum at this level contains the heart and pericardium. The ventral part, between the pericardium and sternum, is overample for the space it bridges and falls into folds somewhat resembling the greater omentum.

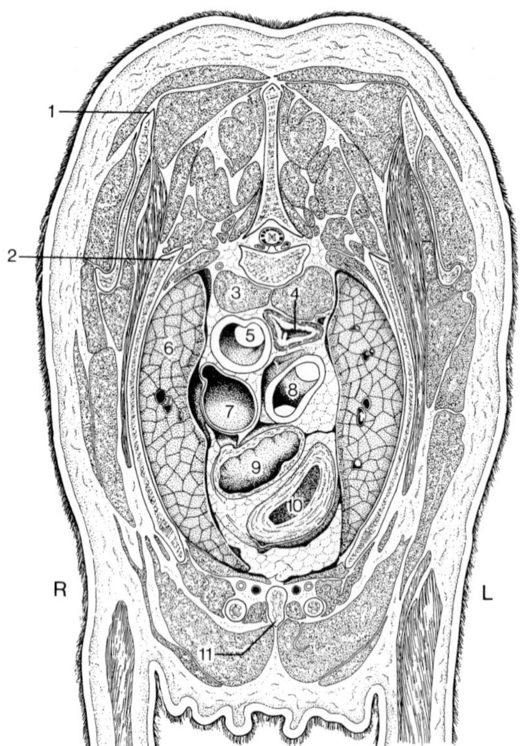


**Figure 13-7.** Transverse section of the canine trunk at the level of the fourth thoracic vertebra.

1, Dorsal border of scapula; 2, fourth rib; 3, longus colli; 4, esophagus; 5, trachea; 6, cranial lobe of right lung; 7, cranial vena cava; 8, aortic arch; 9, right auricle; 10, right ventricle; 11, sternum.

The triangular dorsal part of the caudal mediastinum contains the aorta and the right azygous vein and, more ventrally, the esophagus (Fig. 13–9). The delicate ventral part (/13) attaches to the caudal surface of the pericardium and to the diaphragm along a line that is displaced so far to the left that the mediastinum touches the lateral thoracic wall near the ninth costochondral junction (Fig. 13–3/7). The mediastinum is not visibly fenestrated, and, for practical purposes, the two pleural sacs may be regarded as enclosing independent cavities. However, most dogs with unilaterally induced pneumothorax showed bilateral pneumothorax on radiographs.

The rectangular infracardiac bursa (Fig. 13–10/2) lies against the right surface of the esophagus between the diaphragm and the root of the right lung. Portions of abdominal organs may enter it as a result of a congenital anomaly or trauma.

The plica venae cavae has the usual disposition and helps bound the large recess occupied by the accessory lobe of the right lung (Figs. 13–3/6 and 13–11; not caudal enough for accessory lobe, but caudal caval vein (/6) in dorsal border of plica venae cavae is shown. See also Fig. 13–10/5,6).

## THE HEART

*(See also pp. 219–224.)*

The canine heart is ovoid. Its long axis forms an angle of about 45 degrees with the sternum; the base thus faces craniodorsally and the blunt apex lies near the junction of the sternum and the diaphragm, a little to the left of the midline (Fig. 13–12). The angle varies with the shape of the thorax; it is larger in deep- than in barrel-chested dogs. The heart is also more conical in the deep-chested breeds. The heart is slightly biased toward the left and since a thinner layer of lung tissue intervenes, heart sounds are more pronounced on that side. The distance between the heart and the diaphragm is rather more variable than some accounts suggest—see Figures 13–6, 13–12, 13–15, and so forth.

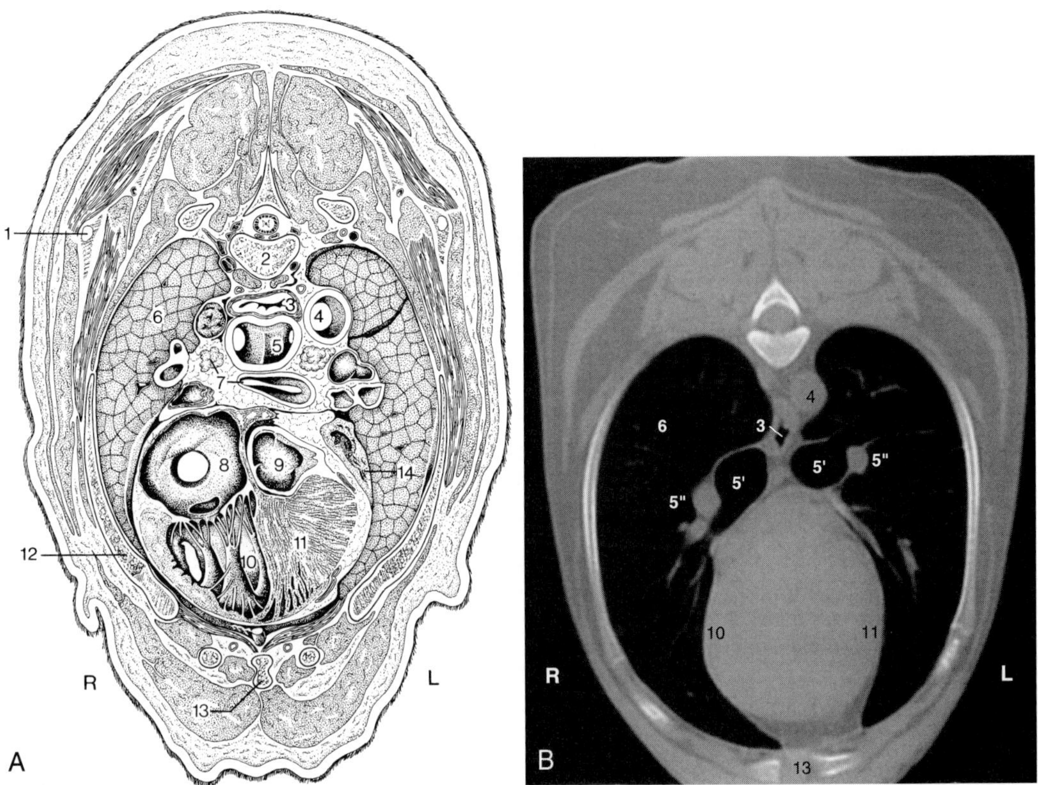


**Figure 13–8.** *A,* Transverse section of the canine trunk at the level of the sixth thoracic vertebra. *B,* Corresponding CT image at a slightly more caudal level.

1, Caudal angle of scapula; 2, sixth thoracic vertebra; 3, esophagus; 4, aorta; 5, tracheal bifurcation; 5′, principal bronchi; 5″, large blood vessels accompanying principal bronchi likely right and left pulmonary aa.; 6, right lung; 7, tracheobronchial lymph nodes and pulmonary a.; 8, right atrium; 9, origin of aorta; 10, right ventricle; 11, interventricular septum; 12, fifth rib; 13, sternum; 14, left auricle.

The relative weight is about 0.7% of body weight on average, but both absolute and relative heart weights vary considerably. Dogs trained for hunting or racing have hearts two or three times heavier than those of fat and less athletic individuals of comparable size.

The pericardium presents no special features beyond a long and relatively robust ligament (phrenicopericardiac in the carnivores) that connects with the sternal part of the diaphragm. This allows the apex more mobility than in the large species, in which the pericardium is firmly attached to the sternum.

The left surface presents the auricles embracing the pulmonary trunk and, below the level of the coronary groove, the paraconal interventricular groove (Fig. 13–9). The right surface presents the atria and the subsinuosal interventricular groove. Neither surface faces quite as its name indicates; the left surface is rotated a little more toward the sternum, while the right one faces a little more toward the vertebrae. Reading counterclockwise from the base, the periphery of the heart shadow on a left lateral radiograph therefore presents right auricle, right ventricle, left ventricle, and left atrium (Fig. 13–12/1–4); and on a ventrodorsal radiograph right atrium, right ventricle, left ventricle, and pulmonary trunk (/5,2,3,6). The apex is formed only by the wall of the left ventricle.

It is clearly important to know the relationships of the parts of the heart to external landmarks. The heart extends from the third rib to the sixth intercostal space, the latter limit roughly coinciding with the most cranial extent of the diaphragm *(/A).* The projection of the base intersects the middle of the fourth rib, and the most dorsal part of the heart reaches approximately to the line connecting the acromion with the ventral end of

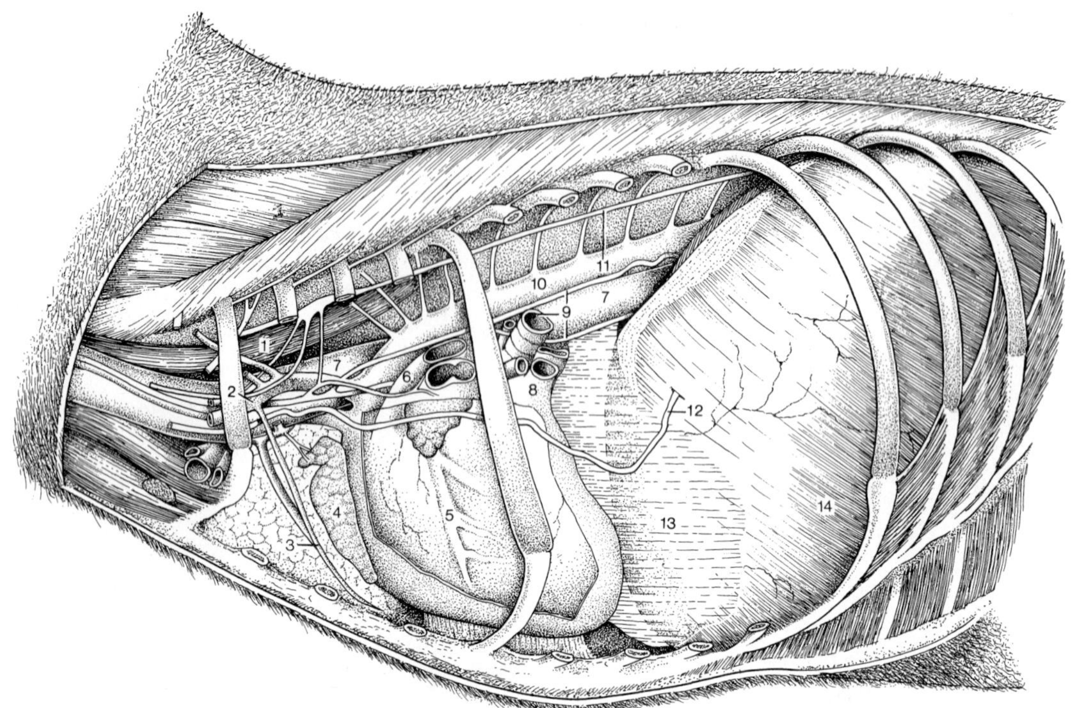


**Figure 13–9.** Left lateral view of the canine thoracic cavity; the lung and much of the pericardium have been removed.

1, Longus colli; 2, left subclavian artery; 3, internal thoracic vessels; 4, thymus; 5, vessels in paraconal interventricular groove; 6, pulmonary trunk; 7, esophagus; 8, pulmonary veins entering left atrium; 9, left principal bronchus and dorsal and ventral vagal trunks; 10, aorta; 11, sympathetic trunk; 12, phrenic nerve; 13, caudal mediastinum; 14, diaphragm.

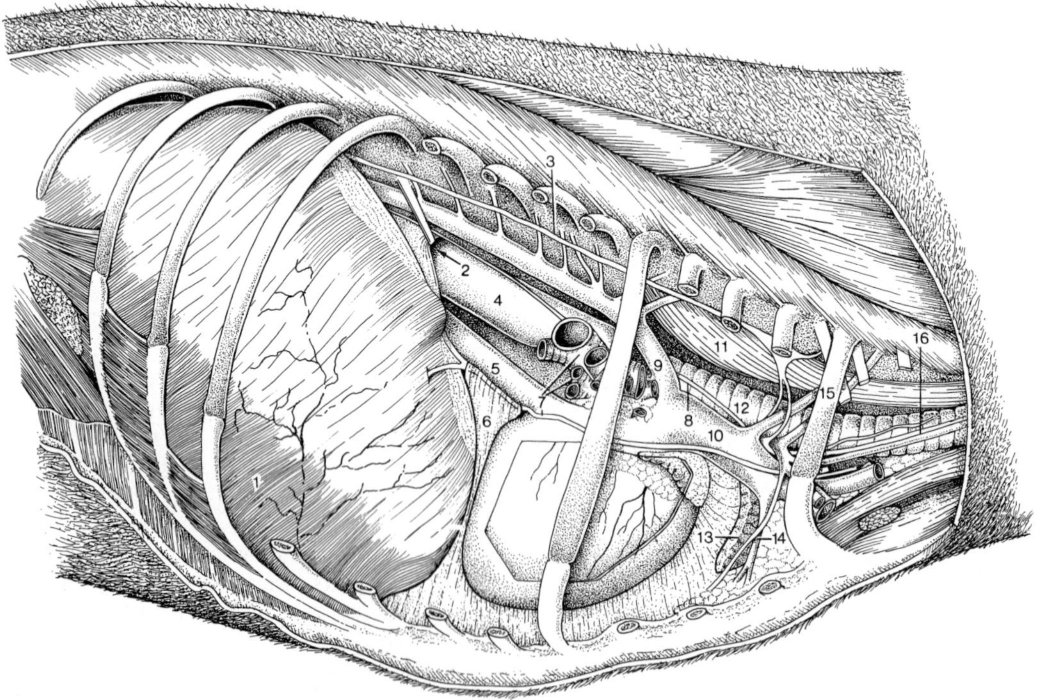


**Figure 13–10.** Right lateral view of the canine thoracic cavity; the lung and much of the pericardium have been removed.

1, Diaphragm; 2, infracardiac bursa; 3, sympathetic trunk; 4, esophagus; 5, caudal vena cava; 6, plica venae cavae; 7, root of lung and phrenic nerve; 8, right vagus; 9, right azygous vein; 10, cranial vena cava; 11, longus colli; 12, trachea; 13, thymus; 14, internal thoracic vessels; 15, first rib; 16, vagosympathetic trunk.

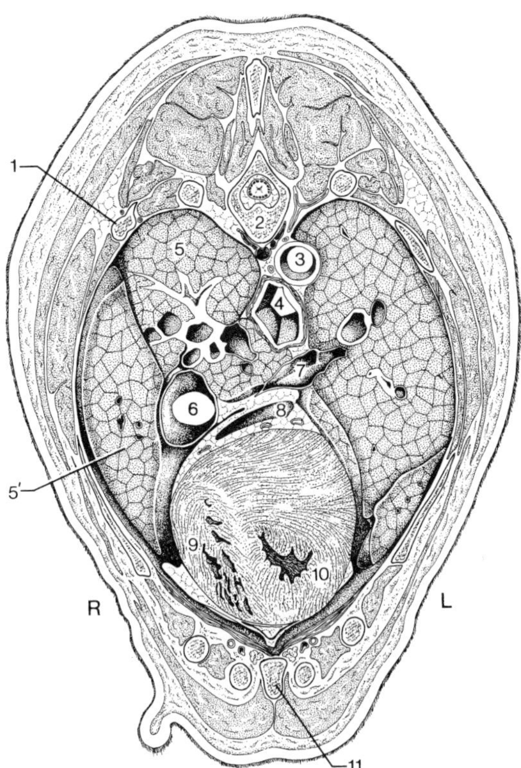


**Figure 13–11.** Transverse section of the canine trunk at the level of the seventh thoracic vertebra.

1, Sixth rib; 2, seventh thoracic vertebra; 3, aorta; 4, esophagus; 5, cranial lobe; 5′, middle lobe of right lung; 6, caudal vena cava; 7, pulmonary veins passing to left atrium; 8, great cardiac vein; 9, right ventricle; 10, left ventricle; 11, sternum.

the last rib. The apex lies just to the left of the second last sternebra (Fig. 13–4). The apex beat in the standing dog is palpable on each side low in the fifth or sixth intercostal space; the main contractions are said to be strongest in the lower third of the fourth or fifth spaces and to be a little more pronounced on the left. The position of the ligamentum arteriosum, which is located where the pulmonary trunk is intersected by the left vagus, is opposite the fourth rib (Fig. 13–9). This detail is relevant to the diagnosis and surgical treatment of the most common congenital anomaly of the canine cardiovascular system, persistent ductus arteriosus. Among other signs, this produces a characteristic machine murmur. The condition can be treated by ligation of the duct.

The heart makes contact with the ventral thoracic wall over a triangular area. The cranial base of the triangle crosses the sternum at the level of the fourth costal cartilages, while the apex lies near the left seventh costal cartilage. The thinner-walled right ventricle may be punctured in the right fourth or fifth intercostal spaces level with the costochondral junctions (Fig. 13–8/10). However, it should be noted that in obese dogs fat within the ventral mediastinum may force the heart away from the sternum.

The heart is easily auscultated because it is less covered by the forelimbs that in most other species, and the stethoscope can be introduced into the axilla. The puncta maxima for optimal perception of the sounds made at the valves may be summarized as follows: left atrioventricular

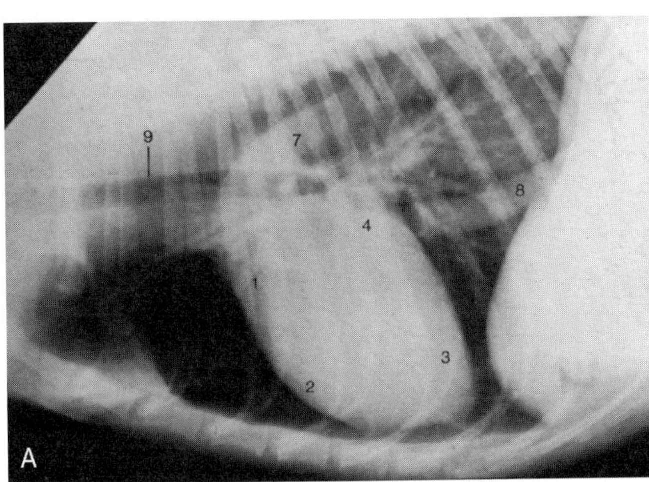


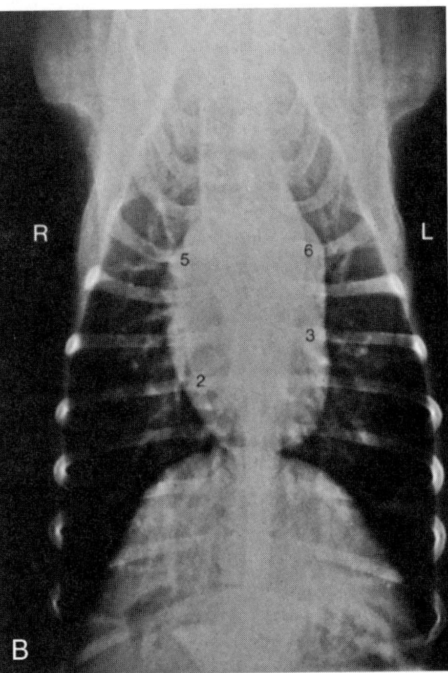


**Figure 13–12.** Lateral *(A)* and ventrodorsal *(B)* views of the position of the canine heart.

1, Right auricle; 2, right ventricle; 3, left ventricle; 4, left atrium; 5, right atrium; 6, pulmonary trunk; 7, aorta; 8, caudal vena cava; 9, trachea.

valve—low (at the costochondral junction) in the left fifth intercostal space; pulmonary valve—low in the left third space; aortic valve—high (just below the horizontal plane of the shoulder joint) in the left fourth space; and right atrioventricular valve—low in the right third or fourth space. These findings were confirmed from postmortem examination of dogs with valvular lesions; the auscultation points may not exactly coincide with the actual projections of the valves onto the chest wall (Fig. 13–4/*A–D*). Autopsy also reveals that the right atrioventricular valve possesses only two major cusps in many, perhaps most, dogs. No clinical significance attaches to the variation.

In North America many dogs are infested with large heartworms *(Dirofilaria immitis),* which occupy the pulmonary trunk and, in severe cases, the right ventricle, atrium, and caudal vena cava.

The heart of the *cat* extends from the third and fourth to the sixth and seventh ribs. Little is covered by the forelimb in the standing animal since the triceps reaches no farther than the fourth rib. The long axis of the heart forms a more acute angle with the sternum, resulting in a greater area of sternal contact. The contractions are strongest near the ventral ends of the fourth to sixth ribs on the left, and the fifth rib on the right (Fig. 13–13). The corresponding puncta maxima are as follows: for the left atrioventricular valve—over the left sixth costal cartilage; for the pulmonary and aortic valves—high in the left fourth intercostal space; and for the right atrioventricular valve—low in the right fifth space. Puncture is difficult because the organ is so small; a needle inserted from the right on either side of the fifth costochondral junction should enter a ventricle.

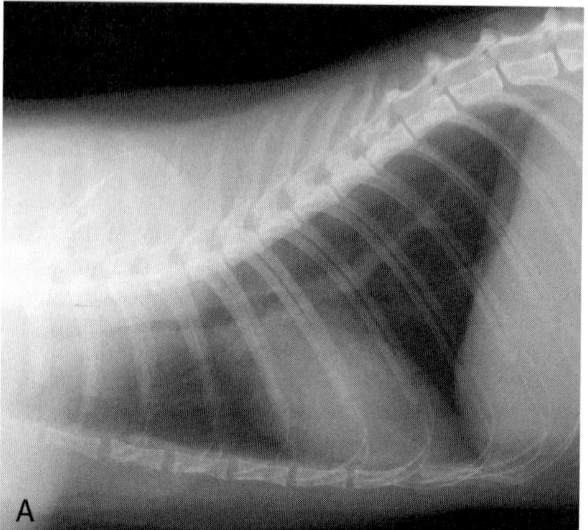


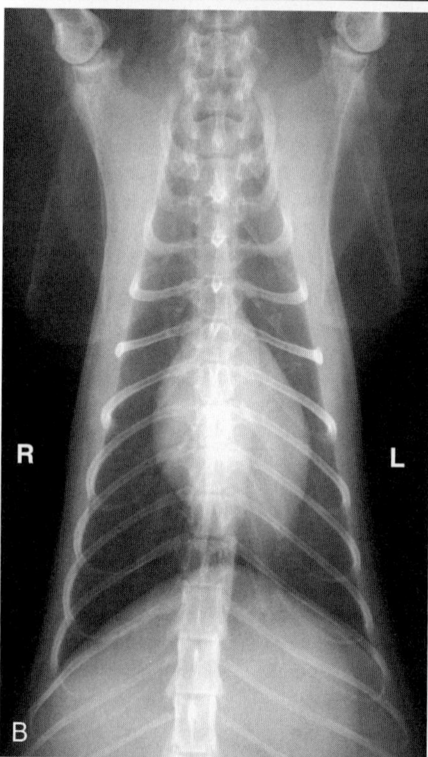


**Figure 13–13.** Lateral *(A)* and ventrodorsal *(B)* radiographic views of the position of the feline heart. The ventral ends of ribs 5, 6, and 7 lie on the heart shadow in *A*.

## THE ESOPHAGUS, TRACHEA, AND THYMUS

*(See also pp. 119, 156, and 258.)*

The *esophagus* enters the thoracic cavity to the left of the trachea and gradually assumes a more median position as it rises to the dorsal surface of the trachea within the cranial mediastinum. It is here related to the left subclavian artery, which intervenes between it and the left lung (Fig. 13–9/7,2). The esophagus crosses the heart on the dorsal surface of first the trachea and then the left bronchus, passing between the aortic arch (on the left) and the azygous vein (on the right). Its ability to expand is locally restricted by these vessels, and the slight rise it makes over the tracheal bifurcation also predisposes this part to obstruction by foreign bodies. A more serious disturbance to the esophagus (and trachea) results from the anomaly in which the right aortic arch persists as part of a constricting vascular ring composed of the aorta on the right and dorsally, the ligamentum arteriosum on the left, and the pulmonary trunk and right pulmonary artery ventrally (see Fig. 7–2/*D*). The condition is corrected by ligation and section of the ductus arteriosus (lig. arteriosum). Caudal to the tracheal bifurcation, the esophagus lies first on

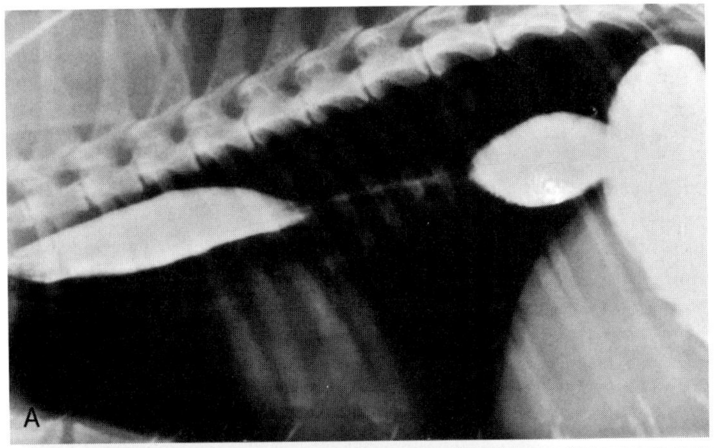


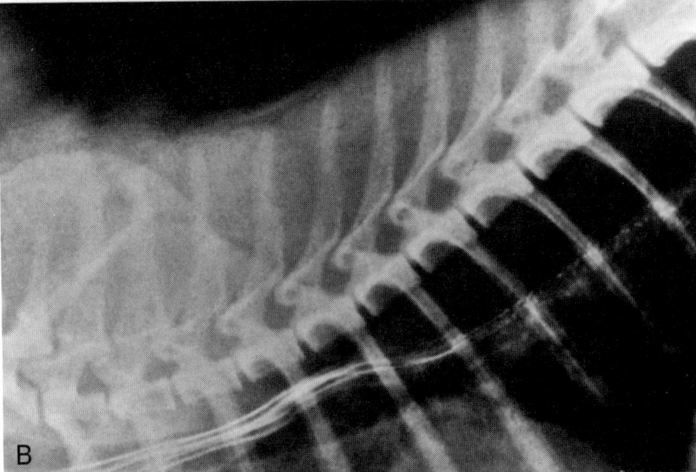


**Figure 13–14.** Contrast medium in the esophagus of the dog *(A)* and cat *(B)*. Note the herringbone pattern caused by the oblique folds in the caudal part of the feline esophagus.

the left atrium and then on the accessory lobe, enclosed between the caudal lobes of both lungs (Fig. 13–11/4). It penetrates the esophageal hiatus of the diaphragm ventral to the 10th thoracic vertebra; narrowing of the lumen makes this a further predilection site for obstruction.

The esophagus is extensively covered with serosa only caudal to the heart. Cranial to the heart the esophagus is more easily approached surgically from the left, but both sides are equally accessible caudal to the heart. Access from the right is preferred over the base of the heart because the azygous vein, unlike the aorta on the left, can be ligated without ill effects. The muscle is striated and mucous glands are present in the submucosa throughout the length of the esophagus of the dog (but not the cat). The mucosa is thrown into longitudinal folds; in the cat these are replaced by short oblique ones caudal to the heart. The longitudinal folds are responsible for the characteristic streaks seen on radiographs following a barium swallow; the oblique ones cause a herringbone pattern (Fig. 13–14). The blood supply to the thoracic part comes from the bronchoesophageal artery, complemented by direct branches of the aorta; the caudal segment also receives blood from the left gastric artery.

Little more need be said about the *trachea* (Plate 19/*A*). It lies against the longus colli at the thoracic inlet but shifts ventral to the esophagus by the level of the aortic arch (Fig. 13–8). This change in position produces an acute angle, open caudally, between the trachea and the vertebral column that is very obvious in lateral radiographs (Figs. 13–12/9 and 13–13). Changes in the angle betray abnormalities in adjacent mediastinal structures. In front of the heart the trachea is related ventrally to the great vessels, notably the brachiocephalic trunk, the common carotid arteries, and the cranial vena cava. The bifurcation over the base of the heart is ventral to the fifth or sixth vertebra. The left principal bronchus is slightly more dorsal than the right one, even though the esophagus rests on it.

In the dog, the *thymus* is confined to the thorax, where it occupies the ventral part of the cranial mediastinum, from the thoracic inlet to the pericardium upon which it is molded (Fig. 13–9/4 and Plate 19/*C*,3). A larger part extends onto the left surface of the pericardium than onto the right, producing a characteristic shadow (sail sign) in dorsoventral radiographs of dogs under 1 year of age. The thymus consists of right and left lobes, is pink when fresh, and is distinctly lobulated. The greatest development is at 6 to 8 weeks of age; regression begins about the fourth month (when the permanent teeth appear) but is never complete. Thymic neoplasms can compress the cranial vena cava and esophagus at the thoracic inlet.

## THE GREAT VESSELS AND NERVES WITHIN THE THORAX

*(See also pp. 237, 238, and 245–247.)*

The *aorta* arises from the center of the base of the heart between the pulmonary trunk to the left and the right atrium to the right. It is slightly expanded (bulbus aortae) at this level, providing room for the aortic valve in its interior (Fig. 13–15/4).

The aorta passes craniodorsally before turning back to follow the vertebrae toward the diaphragm (Fig. 13–9/10). The convexity of the arch gives rise to the *brachiocephalic trunk* and, a short distance farther on, to the left subclavian artery (/2). The trunk lies ventral to the esophagus and trachea, and detaches the two common carotid arteries that accompany these organs through the thoracic inlet. It is continued as the right subclavian artery, which shifts gradually to the right before winding around the cranial border of the first rib to enter the forelimb as the axillary artery. The aortic arch is a prominent feature on lateral radiographs (Fig. 13–12/7).

The *pulmonary trunk* arises from the craniosinistral aspect of the base of the heart, to the left of the aorta. It passes dorsocaudally before dividing into divergent left and right pulmonary arteries (Fig. 13–15/*A*,10,11). Shortly before its division, it is connected to the aorta by the ligamentum arteriosum.

The *cranial vena cava* passes ventral to the trachea to the right of the brachiocephalic trunk (Fig. 13–10/10). It is formed by the union of the two brachiocephalic veins, which receive tributaries corresponding to the branches of the subclavian arteries (see Fig. 7–42).

The *caudal vena cava* spans the short distance between the right atrium and the diaphragm within the plica venae cavae. It is a conspicuous feature on lateral radiographs of the chest (Fig. 13–12/8).

The dog has a *right azygous vein,* which joins the dorsal surface of the cranial vena cava near its junction with the right atrium (Fig. 13–10/9). It receives (most) dorsal intercostal and the first few lumbar veins and through these is connected with the internal vertebral plexus (p. 305).

There are no particular specific features of interest in the formation, course, or distribution of the phrenic, vagus, or sympathetic nerves.

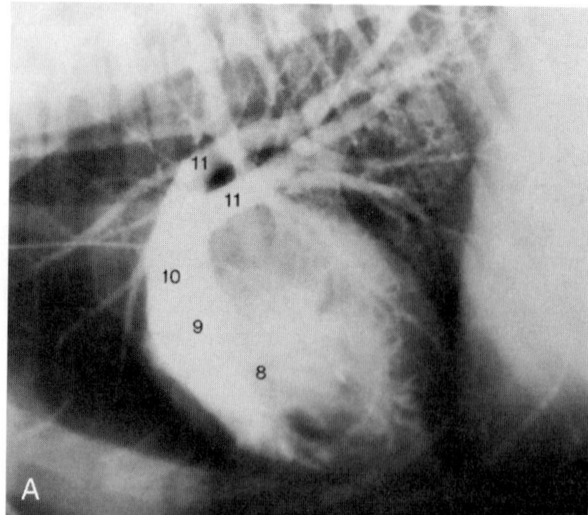


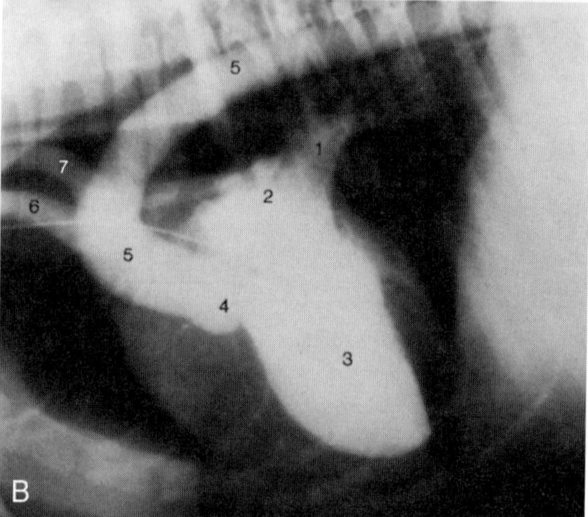


**Figure 13–15.** Contrast medium in the canine right *(A)* and left *(B)* ventricles and marking the great vessels. The catheter is in the cranial vena cava.

1, Pulmonary veins; 2, left atrium; 3, left ventricle; 4, position of aortic valve; 5, aorta; 6, brachiocephalic trunk; 7, left subclavian artery; 8, right ventricle; 9, position of pulmonary valve; 10, pulmonary trunk; 11, pulmonary arteries.

## LYMPHATIC STRUCTURES OF THE THORAX

*(See also pp. 253–254.)*

A single *intercostal lymph node* may be present under the pleura at the dorsal end of the fifth or sixth intercostal space. It drains the structures of the dorsal thoracic wall. The efferent vessels go to the cranial mediastinal nodes (see Fig. 7–52/6).

The *sternal lymph nodes* are large—up to 2 cm in length—and are embedded in fat beside the sternum at the level of the second rib. They receive lymph from the muscles of the ventral chest wall, the diaphragm, and the mediastinum and may collaborate with the axillary nodes in draining the first three pairs of mammary glands. Their efferent vessels go to the veins at the thoracic inlet (/10).

The *cranial mediastinal lymph nodes* are related variously to the large blood vessels in front of the heart. They drain structures in the mediastinum (including the tracheobronchial nodes) and the deep muscles at the base of the neck. Their outflow enters the veins at the thoracic inlet (/8).

The *tracheobronchial lymph nodes* (Figs. 13–8/7 and 7–53) are scattered about the termination of the trachea and the principal bronchi. They drain the lungs and also mediastinal structures and part of the diaphragm. Their efferent vessels pass to the cranial mediastinal nodes.

The thin-walled *thoracic duct* begins between the crura of the diaphragm as the continuation of the cisterna chyli. It accompanies the aorta and azygous vein forward and, level with the heart, passes obliquely to the left, crossing the esophagus to gain its left face within the cranial mediastinum. It follows the esophagus to the thoracic inlet, where it opens into one or other large vein. The duct, which has a diameter of 2 to 3 mm in a medium-sized dog, may be plexiform (see Fig. 7–54).

## Selected Bibliography


Amis, T.C., and B.C. McKiernan: Systematic identification of endobronchial anatomy during bronchoscopy in the dog. Am. J. Vet. Res. 47:2649–2657, 1986.

Bilbrey, S.A., and S.J. Birchard: Pulmonary lymphatics in dogs with experimentally induced chylothorax, J. Am. Anim. Hosp. Assoc. 30:86–92, 1994.

Birchard, S. J., and T. W. Fossum: Chylothorax in the dog and cat. Vet. Clin. North. Am. Small Anim. Pract. 17:271–283, 1987.

Boyd, J. S.: Color Atlas of Clinical Anatomy of the Dog and Cat. St. Louis, Mosby–Year Book, 1991.

Buchanan, J: Cardiac radiology. In Proceedings of 13th Forum of the American College of Veterinary Internal Medicine, 1995, pp. 191–195.

Buchanan J. W.: Changing breed predispositions in canine heart disease. Canine Pract. 18:12–24, 1993.

Buchanan, J.W. and J. Bücheler: Vertebral scale system to measure canine heart size in radiographs. JAVMA 206:194–199, 1995.

Coyne, B.E., and R.B. Fingland: Hypoplasia of the trachea in dogs: 103 cases (1974–1990). JAVMA 201:768–772, 1992.

Darke, P.G.G., J.D. Bonagura, and D.F. Kelly; Color Atlas of Veterinary Cardiology. Turin, Mosby-Wolfe, 1996.

deLahunta, A., and R.E. Habel: Applied Veterinary Anatomy. Philadelphia, W.B. Saunders Company, 1986.

Ellison, G.W.: Surgical correction of persistent right aortic arch. *In* Bojrab, M.J. (ed.): Current Techniques in Small Animal Surgery. Philadelphia, Lea & Febiger, 1990.

García, F., D. Prandi, T. Peña, et al.: Examination of the thoracic cavity and lung lobectomy by means of thoracoscopy in dogs. Can. Vet. J. 39:285–292, 1998.

Grandage, J.: The radiology of the dog's diaphragm. J. Small Anim. Pract. 15:1–17, 1974.

Hudson, L.C., and W.P. Hamilton: Atlas of Feline Anatomy for Veterinarians. Philadelphia, W.B. Saunders Company, 1993.

Kern, D.A., C.B. Carrig, and R.A. Martin: Radiographic evaluation of induced pneumothorax in the dog. Vet. Radiol. Ultrasound 35:411, 1995.

Kehmhuh, L.B., J.D. Bonagura, D.S. Biller, and W.M. Hartman: Radiographic evaluation of caudal vena cava size in dogs. Vet. Radiol. Ultrasound, 38:94–100, 1997.

Khurana, R.K., and J.M. Petras: Sensory innervation of the canine esophagus, stomach, and duodenum. Am. J. Anat. 192:293–306, 1991.

King, A.S.: The Cardiorespiratory System: Integration of Normal and Pathological Structure and Function. Oxford, Blackwell Science, 1999.

Litster, A.L., and J.W. Buchanan: Vertebral heart scale system to measure heart size in radiographs of cats. JAVMA, 216:210–214, 2000.

Losonsky, J.M., and S.K. Kneller: Misdiagnosis in normal radiographic anatomy: Eight structural configurations simulating disease entities in small animals. JAVMA 191:109–114, 1987.

Martin, R.A., D.L. Barber, D.L.S. Richards, et al.: A technique for direct lymphangiography of the thoracic duct system in the cat. Vet. Radiol. Ultrasound 29:116–121, 1988.

Moise, N.S.: Doppler echocardiographic evaluation of congenital cardiac disease. J. Vet. Intern. Med. 3:195–207, 1989.

Moon, M.L., Keene, B.W., Lessard, P., et al.: Age related changes in the female cardiac silhouette. Vet. Radiol. Ultrasound 34:315–320, 1993.

Nakakuki, S.: The bronchial tree and lobular division of the dog lung. J. Vet. Med. Sci. 56:455–458, 1994.

Piffer, C.R., M.I.S. Piffer, F.P. Santi, and M.C.O. Dayoub: Anatomic observations of the coronary sinus in the dog *(Canis familiaris).* Anat. Histol. Embryol. 23:301–308, 1994.

Puriton, P.T., J.N. Chambers, and J.L. Moore: Identification and categorization of the vascular patterns of the thoracic limb, thorax, and neck of dogs. Am. J. Vet. Res. 53:1435–1445, 1992.

Roudebush, P.: Tracheobronchoscopy. Vet. Clin. North Am. Small Anim. Pract. 20:1297–1314, 1990.

Samii, V.F., D.S. Biller, and P.D. Koblik: Normal cross-sectional anatomy of the feline thorax and abdomen: Comparison of computed tomography and cadaver anatomy. Vet. Radiol. Ultrasound 39:504–511, 1998.

Schebitz, H., and H. Wilkens: Atlas of Radiographic Anatomy of the Dog and Cat, 4th ed. Berlin, Paul Parey Verlag, 1986.

Smallwood, J.E., and T.F. George II: Anatomic atlas for computed tomography in the mesaticephalic dog: Thorax and cranial abdomen. Vet. Radiol. Ultrasound 34:65–84, 1993.

Stickle, R.L., and L.K. Anderson: Diagnosis of common congenital heart anomalies in the dog using survey and nonselective contrast radiography. Vet. Radiol. Ultrasound 28:6–12, 1987.

Suter, P.F.: Thoracic Radiography: A Text Atlas of Thoracic Diseases of the Dog and Cat. Davis, Calif., Stonegate Publishing, 1984.

Tangkawattana, P., M. Muto, T. Nakayama, et al.: Prevalence, vasculature, and innervation of myocardial bridges in dogs. Am. J. Vet. Res. 58:1209–1215, 1997.

Toombs, J.P., and P.N. Ogburn: Evaluating canine cardiovascular silhouettes: Radiographic methods and normal radiographic anatomy. Compend. Contin. Educ. Pract. Vet. 7:579–587, 1985.

van den Broek, A.H.M., and P.G.G. Darke: Cardiac measurements on thoracic radiographs of cats. J. Small Anim. Pract. 28:125–135, 1987.

van Grundy, T.: Vascular ring anomalies in the dog and cat. Compend. Contin. Vet. Pract. Educ. 11:36–46, 1989.

Venker-van-Haagen, A.J., M.W. Vroom, A. Heijn, and P.G. van Ooijen: Bronchoscopy in small animal clinics: An analysis of the results of 228 bronchoscopies. J. Am. Anim. Hosp. Assoc. 21:521–526, 1985.

Zook, B.C., R.A. Hitzelberg, and E.W. Bradley: Cross-sectional anatomy of the beagle thorax. Vet. Radiol. Ultrasound 30:277–281, 1989.

CHAPTER 14

# The Abdomen of the Carnivores*

## CONFORMATION AND SURFACE ANATOMY

The cranial boundary of the accessible abdominal wall is easily determined by palpation of the last rib and costal arch, but the caudal boundary is more difficult to discover, since only the ventral part (pecten pubis) of the bony ring about the pelvic inlet can be palpated between the thighs. The wings of the ilia, though prominent landmarks, rise above the level of the abdomen and pertain to the back. The thick muscles above the lumbar transverse processes are palpable but not the processes themselves; however, the tips of the spinous processes provide a guide to the identification of individual vertebrae.

The abdominal cavity is of course larger than these landmarks appear to indicate, since the diaphragm bulges far into the rib cage at its cranial end. The organs in this intrathoracic part of the abdomen are protected by the ribs and are in part overlain by the caudal lobes of the lungs. The abdominal cavity is relatively less voluminous than in the large domestic species and has, by and large, the shape of a cone with a bulbous cranial base (see Fig. 2–2). Its longitudinal axis inclines cranioventrally at an angle that varies considerably; it is steepest in deep-chested breeds. Except in fat subjects and heavily pregnant or lactating bitches, the ventral abdominal wall rises from the sternum to the pecten in a straight or even slightly concave line. Dog fanciers use the expression "tucked-up" to describe animals with an especially shallow body depth at the loin. The skin fold that connects the flank with the stifle tends to obscure the shallowness of this part. Superficial inguinal lymph nodes may be palpated in the groin, lateral to the bulbus glandis of the penis or in a comparable site in the bitch (Fig. 14–1/*B*, 6).

Advancing pregnancy enlarges the abdomen in both depth and breadth, and gives it a more cylindrical or even a barrel shape. The *mammary glands* contribute to the contours at this time. There are generally five pairs—though four or six are sometimes seen, and four is normal in the cat—spread along the ventral aspect of the trunk (see Fig. 10–30/*B,C*). The two cranial pairs are thoracic, the next two abdominal, and the caudalmost pair inguinal in position. Their pattern is often staggered, a favorable arrangement, since it makes all teats equally accessible to the pups when the bitch suckles lying on her side. The glands are very small in the virgin and regress greatly in the parous but nonpregnant and nonlactating bitch. They are covered by the hair, which may completely hide the teats, although these remain enlarged in parous bitches, in which they are superimposed on the abdominal organs in ventrodorsal radiographs. The teats, which occur in rudimentary form in males, are bare and perforated at their tips by 10 or 12 fine openings—half this number in the cat—through which milk is drawn.

The glands become very conspicuous toward parturition and during lactation; they are then swollen, pendulous, and confluent with their ipsilateral neighbors.

The blood supply to the mammary glands varies in detail but mainly originates from the lateral and internal thoracic, and the external pudendal, arteries; some assistance may be provided by lesser vessels from other sources. In most cases, the three cranial glands are supplied craniolaterally by the lateral thoracic artery (from the axillary) and deeply by the cranial superficial epigastric artery and perforating branches of the intercostal arteries (which all derive from the internal thoracic). The two caudal pairs are supplied from the caudal superficial epigastric artery (from the external pudendal) and deeply by branches from the cranial abdominal and deep circumflex iliac arteries. The veins are satellite. Both arteries and veins anastomose freely, forming arterial and venous plexuses (Fig. 14–1/*A*).

Lymph from the three cranial glands goes to the axillary, accessory axillary, and sternal nodes, and that from the two (occasionally three) caudal glands to the superficial inguinal nodes, which lie

*See introductory remarks on page 367.

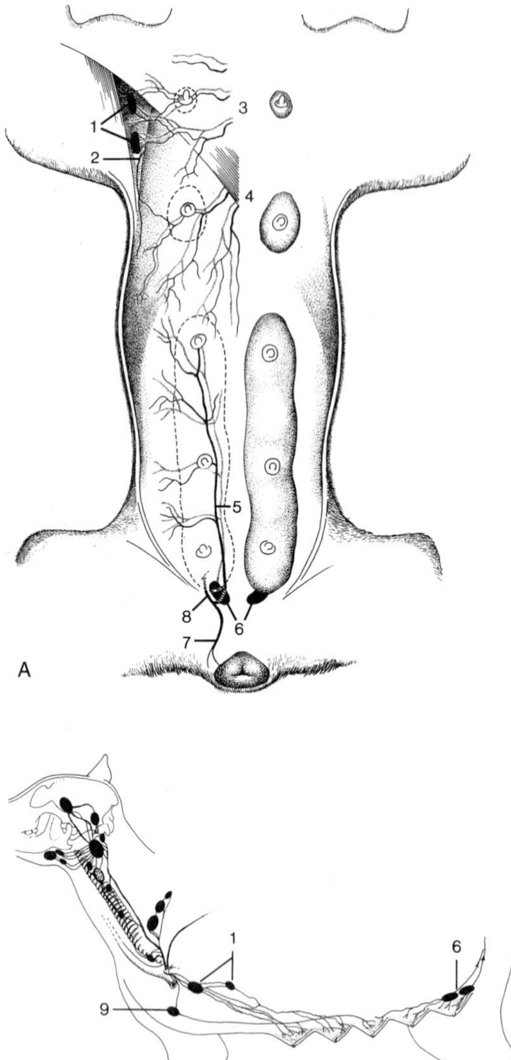


**Figure 14–1.** Blood vessels and lymphatics of the canine mammary glands. *A,* Ventral view of the mammary glands, blood vessels, and certain lymph nodes. *B,* Lateral view of regional lymph nodes.

1, Axillary and accessory axillary lymph nodes; 2, branch of lateral thoracic artery; 3, perforating branches of internal thoracic vessels; 4, branches of the cranial superficial epigastric vessels; 5, caudal superficial epigastric artery; 6, superficial inguinal lymph nodes; 7, ventral labial branch to vulva; 8, external pudendal artery; 9, sternal lymph node.

dorsal to the caudal border of the inguinal mammary gland. The pathways are erratic and some lymph may cross the midline. The superficial inguinal nodes and caudal glands are related to the vaginal process, which is vulnerable during surgical removal of a diseased gland; injury to the process may cause inadvertent opening of the peritoneal cavity. In the cat a few small nodes of this series may be found more widely spaced along the course of the caudal epigastric vessels (from which they occasionally receive a separate [caudal epigastric] designation). In both species the superficial inguinal nodes drain the adjacent part of the abdominal wall in addition to the caudal mammary glands. These details obtain importance from the prevalence of mammary tumors in both dogs and cats. In bitches they are the commonest of all tumors and show a disturbingly high (ca. 50%) incidence of malignancy. Though somewhat less common in cats, mammary tumors are even more likely to be malignant in this species.

## THE ABDOMINAL WALL

*(See also pp. 53–56.)*

The ventrolateral abdominal wall is constructed according to the common pattern, with only a few features of distinction; since abdominal surgery is so frequently performed in dogs and cats it is necessary to be familiar with the details, and it may be prudent to review the description previously given (p. 53). The principal distinctions concern the linea alba and rectus sheath, which are now described more fully because most abdominal incisions are median or paramedian. The description of the inguinal canal also bears recapitulation.

The *linea alba* is the fibrous seam in which the aponeuroses of the right and left oblique and transverse abdominal muscles come together. It extends from the xiphoid process to the pubis and includes the umbilicus at about the level of the third lumbar vertebra. The rectus muscle to each side is so loosely enclosed within its sheath that its medial border can easily be drawn laterally, away from the linea alba. The linea alba is about 1 cm* wide cranial to the umbilicus (Fig. 14–12/11) but gradually narrows behind this point and is reduced to a barely visible line in its caudal third (see Fig. 2–26). Incisions through the linea alba spare the muscles, vessels, and nerves; there is the additional advantage that the parietal peritoneum does not retract from the edges of a median incision as happens elsewhere. The falciform ligament (see further on) and the median ligament of the bladder attach to the dorsal surface of the linea alba, cranial and caudal to the umbilicus, respectively. Umbilical hernias, often associated with an overwide linea alba and hypoplastic rectus muscles, are common.

The *rectus sheath* is formed by the aponeuroses of the oblique and transverse abdominal muscles.

*Where we give an indication of weight or measure, we have in mind a subject of the size of a beagle, an animal weighing 15 to 20 kg or so. Cats, or course, vary less if we exclude such atypical breeds as the Maine Coon.

In the simplest arrangement (that seen in the large animals) the fused aponeuroses of the oblique muscles pass ventral to the rectus muscle, while that of the transverse muscle covers its dorsal surface. In the dog, the most cranial portion of the internal oblique aponeurosis detaches an additional lamina that passes dorsally, on the deep face of the rectus (see Fig. 2–23/*A*). At the other extremity of the abdomen, the most caudal portion of the transverse aponeurosis changes position to the ventral surface, leaving the dorsal surface of the rectus covered only by fascia and peritoneum (see Figs. 2–23/*B*, 14–2, and Plate 19/*A*). The rectus muscle is adherent to its sheath only at the tendinous inscriptions.

The ventral abdominal wall is supplied by four *arteries* on each side. Two enter from the sternal region, two from the vicinity of the pelvis. The cranial pair are branches of the internal thoracic artery; the cranial superficial epigastric artery runs between the abdominal muscles and the skin and supplies the region cranial to the level of the umbilicus (it is enlarged in the lactating bitch); the cranial epigastric artery runs deep to the rectus, between it and its sheath. The caudal superficial epigastric artery, a branch of the external pudendal, is distributed subcutaneously and also supplies the prepuce; the caudal epigastric artery arises from the pudendoepigastric trunk and passes forward, first along the lateral border and then on the deep surface of the rectus muscle (see Fig. 2–26). Cranial and caudal sets of vessels anastomose.

The abdominal wall is most safely punctured (paracentesis) a short distance caudolateral to the umbilicus; this site avoids both the fat-filled falciform ligament and risk of injury to a full bladder. The falciform ligament, carrying the round ligament of the liver in its free border, is the remnant of the ventral mesogastrium that conveyed the umbilical vein from the umbilicus to the liver in the fetus. The part adjacent to the liver survives, if at all, as a simple peritoneal fold. The part extending forward from the umbilicus over the abdominal floor commonly serves as a major fat storage depot and may become so thickened and enlarged that it complicates the opening and closure of a midline abdominal incision (Figs. 14–5 and 14–6). Part or all of this obstruction may be excised with no greater risk than minor bleeding.

The *inguinal canal* is a potential space between the external and internal abdominal oblique muscles that extends between deep and superficial openings (rings). The deep ring leads from the canal into the abdominal cavity, the superficial ring from the canal to the subcutaneous tissues of the groin. In both sexes the canal conveys the external pudendal vessels and the genitofemoral nerve; it also conveys the spermatic cord in the dog and tom, the vaginal process in the bitch and queen.

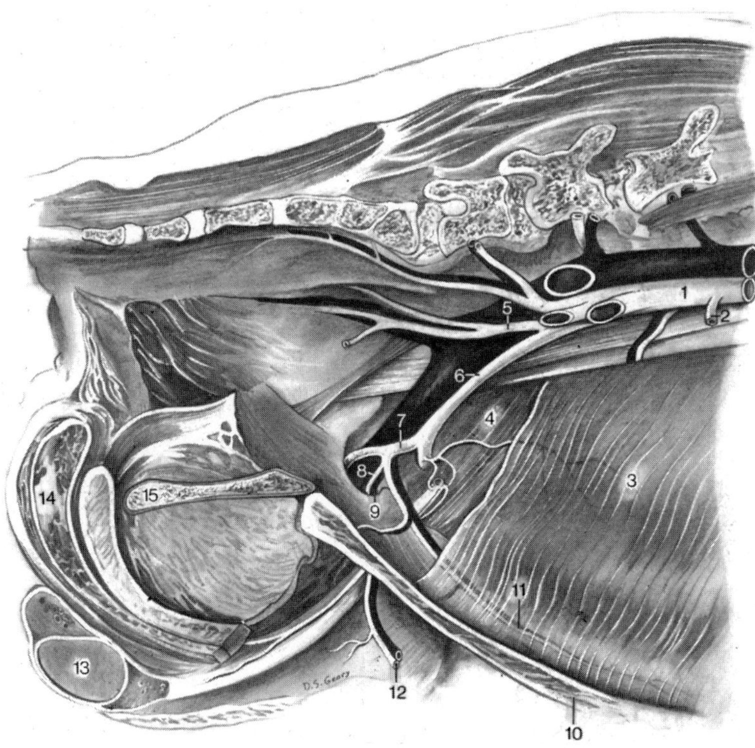


**Figure 14–2.** Abdominal wall and pelvic canal of the male dog, showing the breakup of the aorta; medial view.

1, Aorta; 2, caudal mesenteric a.; 3, transversus abdominis; 4, internal abdominal oblique m.; 5, internal iliac a.; 6, external iliac a.; 7, deep femoral a.; 8, pudendoepigastric trunk; 9, deep inguinal ring; 10, rectus abdominis m.; 11, caudal epigastric a.; 12, external pudendal a.; 13, left testis; 14, bulb of the penis; 15, pelvic symphysis.

These all emerge at the superficial inguinal ring, a nearly sagittal slit in the external abdominal oblique aponeurosis about 3 cm lateral to the linea alba, close to where this attaches on the pubis (see Fig. 2–27/*A*,4′). Only the caudal end of the ring is palpable. The narrow strip of aponeurosis (/*A* between 4′ and 6) lateral to the ring forms the only barrier between the structures issuing from the canal and the large femoral vessels as they enter the thigh through the vascular lacuna (/6).

The deep inguinal ring is visible only from within the abdomen (Fig. 14–2/9). It is bounded caudolaterally by the caudal border of the external abdominal oblique aponeurosis, cranially by the unattached border of the internal abdominal oblique muscle, and medially by the rectus muscle (see Fig. 2–27/*B*). None of these boundaries is palpable in the intact animal. The parietal peritoneum that covers the ring evaginates through the inguinal canal and, as the vaginal tunic, accompanies the spermatic cord into the scrotum. In the bitch and queen it envelops the round ligament of the uterus and is known as the vaginal process; the process is not present in females of other domestic species and is the occasional recipient of herniated abdominal organs (p. 440).

## GENERAL ASPECTS OF VISCERAL TOPOGRAPHY

Although the small intestine dominates the abdominal topography, it is not usually visible immediately when the cavity is opened, since it is separated from the abdominal floor by the especially well-developed greater omentum (Plate 19/*E*). The organs that are usually exposed on removal of the abdominal floor are the ventral part of the spleen projecting beyond the left costal arch, a fringe of liver behind the xiphoid process, and the bladder directly before the pubis (see Fig. 3–41 and Plate 19/*D,F*). In order to facilitate cross-reference to the accounts of other species, we adhere to a common sequence of description of the viscera despite the different order in which they claim attention in the ordinary course of dissection.

The diagnostic role of palpation through the abdominal wall of the intact subject is obviously very much greater in the small species than in the large, in which the comparable, but more limited, technique is supplied by rectal exploration. References to palpable features of the abdominal contents have been gathered together and, since they include attention to some reproductive organs, have been relegated to the following chapter (p. 451).

## THE SPLEEN

*(See also p. 257.)*

The spleen of the dog is an elongated, roughly dumbbell-shaped organ that lies more or less vertically against the left abdominal wall (Fig. 14–3/*A*,4). Its position is much influenced by the distention of the stomach (and by its own capacity to become engorged) but generally it is largely deep to the ribs. The dorsal end reaches the left crus of the diaphragm, passing between the gastric fundus and the cranial pole of the left kidney under cover of (usually) the last two ribs. The larger ventral end extends below the costal arch and may cross the ventral midline, to reach under the costal cartilages of the right side. It then provides a dense triangular shadow on the abdominal floor in lateral radiographs (Fig. 14–4/*A*,3). A similar shadow between the stomach and left kidney may reveal the position of the organ in ventrodorsal films. The parietal surface makes contact (in dorsoventral sequence) with the diaphragm, costal arch, and abdominal muscles. The visceral surface is divided by a hilar ridge into a cranial strip related to the stomach and a caudal strip related to the left kidney and intestine.

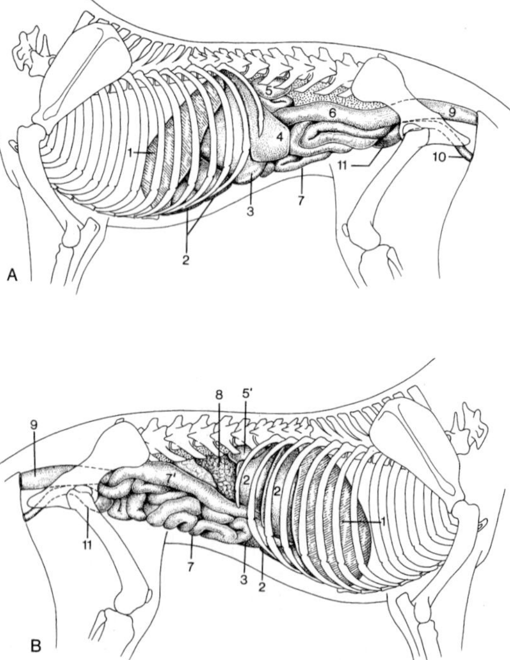


**Figure 14–3.** Visceral projections on the left *(A)* and right *(B)* canine abdominal walls.

1, Diaphragm; 2, liver; 3, stomach; 4, spleen; 5, 5′, left and right kidneys; 6, descending colon; 7, small intestine; 7′, descending duodenum; 8, pancreas; 9, rectum; 10, female urogenital tract; 11, bladder.

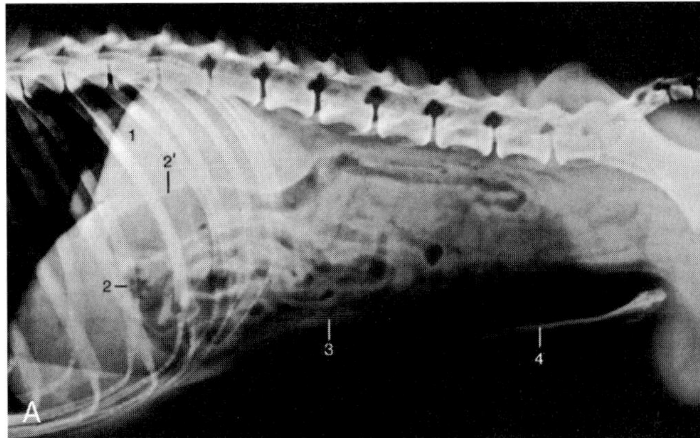


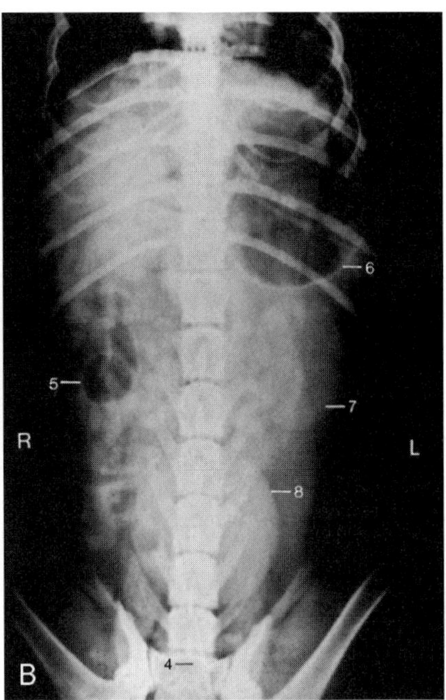


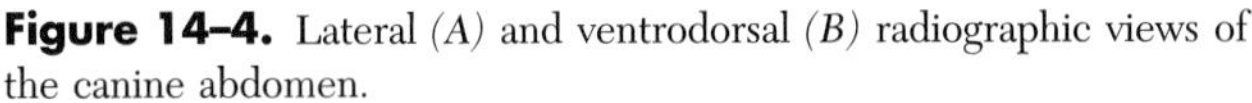
**Figure 14–4.** Lateral *(A)* and ventrodorsal *(B)* radiographic views of the canine abdomen.

1, Liver; 2, pyloric part of stomach; 2′, descending duodenum; 3, spleen; 4, os penis; 5, cecum; 6, fundus of stomach; 7, left kidney; 8, bladder.

The wide gastrosplenic ligament attaches the spleen to the greater curvature of the stomach. Though permitted considerable mobility, the spleen follows the movements of the stomach, and when this enlarges the spleen is displaced caudally and ventrally so that it may be palpated through the abdominal wall. Other restraining influences are provided by the tether of its blood vessels.

The splenic artery and vein pass (as several divergent branches) to the dorsal end of the spleen. The left gastroepiploic vessels are detached about the middle of the hilus and cross to the greater curvature of the stomach within the gastrosplenic ligament (Fig. 14–8/3,11). The splenic lymph nodes lie by the splenic vessels, a few centimeters distant from the organ.

The spleen serves as an important blood reservoir in the dog and cat, and its size and weight therefore vary widely (Plate 19/*F*). Rupture of the spleen is not uncommon following traffic accidents but fortunately the organ may be removed without risk to life. The relatively loose attachment of the spleen to the stomach facilitates access to the vascular supply at surgery (splenectomy*).

*In this operation it is necessary to divide the branches of the splenic artery that actually supply the spleen shortly before they enter the organ at the hilus. One or more of the branches will normally be found to contribute to the left gastroepiploic artery, a vessel essential to the integrity of the greater curvature of the stomach (see Figs. 3–39, and 14–8).

## THE STOMACH

*(See also pp. 125–129.)*

The dog has a simple stomach that exhibits the idealized form described on pages 125 and 126 only when moderately full. The fundus and body merge smoothly and are capable of great expansion, while the cylindrical and thicker-walled pyloric part is less able to enlarge. The fundus projects dorsally to the left of the cardia, against the liver. The cardia is generally wide, and this may be related to the ease with which dogs vomit. The pylorus, on the other hand, is narrow and pyloric stenosis is not uncommon in the young. When the organ is quite empty, the body also becomes more or less cylindrical with the fundus then forming a bulbous dorsal enlargement (Figs. 14–5/5 and 14–6/3). When the organ is greatly distended, all parts except the pyloric canal merge in a common sac. The capacity of the stomach ranges from 0.5 to 6.0 L, with an average stomach of about 2.5 L; it is thus relatively large in relation to body size.

The position and relations obviously depend on the degree of fullness, with the cardia providing a fixed point opposite the ninth intercostal space. The fundus and body lie mainly to the left of the median plane, in contact with the diaphragm and liver, respectively, but the ventral part of the body crosses to the right before being continued by the

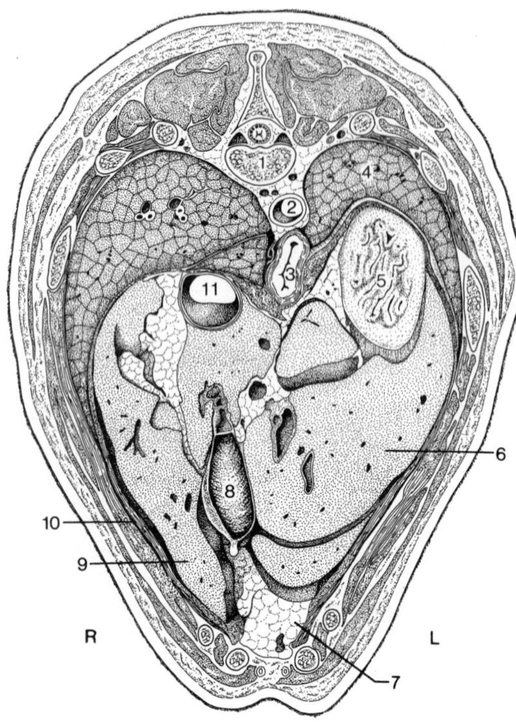


**Figure 14–5.** Transverse section of the canine trunk at the level of the 11th thoracic vertebra.

1, Eleventh thoracic vertebra; 2, aorta; 3, esophagus; 4, left lung; 5, fundus of stomach; 6, left lateral lobe of liver; 7, fat-filled falciform ligament; 8, gallbladder; 9, right medial lobe of liver; 10, diaphragm; 11, caudal vena cava.

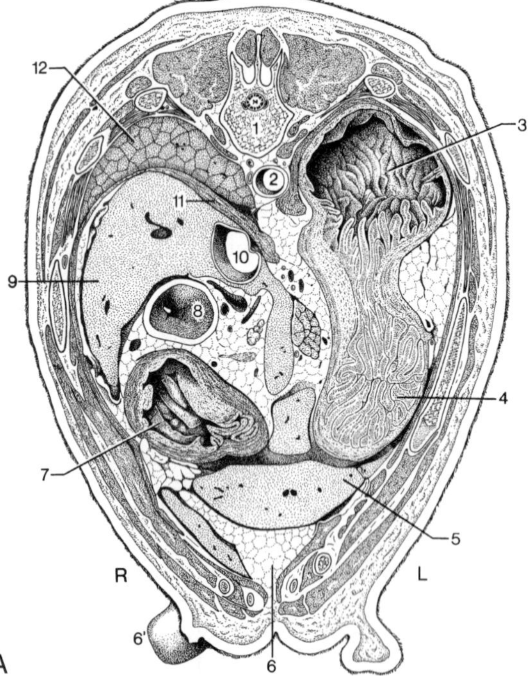


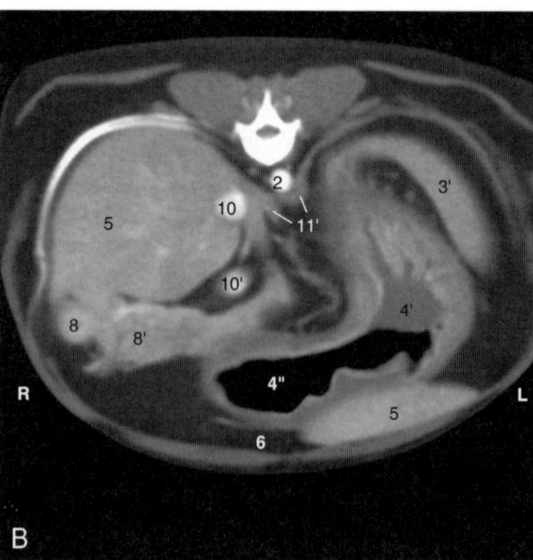


**Figure 14–6.** *A,* Transverse section of the canine trunk at the level of the 12th thoracic vertebra. *B,* Corresponding CT image slightly more caudal than *A;* the dog was lying on its back during the CT procedure.

1, Twelfth thoracic vertebra; 2, aorta; 3, fundus of stomach; 3′, spleen; 4, body of stomach; 4′ with fluid; 4″ with gas; 5, liver; 6, fat-filled falciform ligament; 6′, teat; 7, pyloric part of stomach; 8, descending duodenum; 8′, right lobe of pancreas; 9, caudate process of liver; 10, caudal vena cava; 10′, portal vein; 11, diaphragm; 11′, crura of diaphragm; 12, right lung.

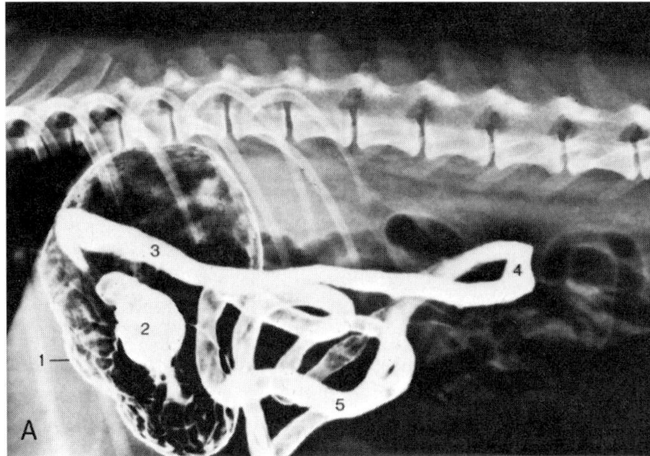


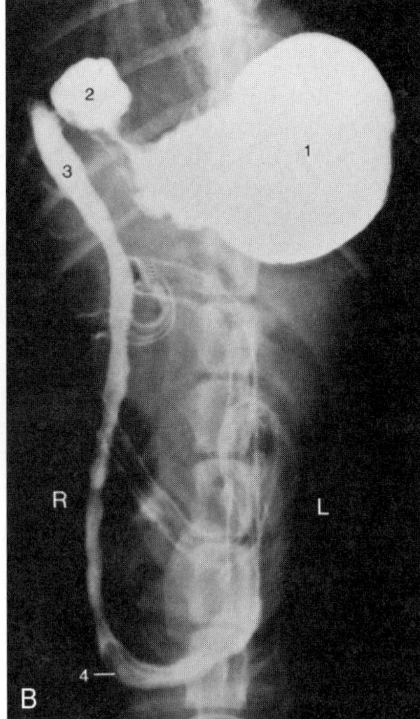


**Figure 14–7.** Lateral *(A)* and ventrodorsal *(B)* radiographic views of the canine abdomen after administration of a barium suspension.

1, Stomach; 2, pyloric part; 3, descending duodenum; 4, caudal flexure of duodenum; 5, jejunum.

pyloric part, which also lies against the liver; indeed, its lesser curvature is bound to the porta of the liver by the lesser omentum (Fig. 14–6/3,4,7). The greater curvature faces mainly to the left, toward the spleen, and ventrally, where it usually lies on the ventral fringe of the liver and on the falciform ligament (/6); it reaches the abdominal floor only when the stomach is greatly distended, and in these circumstances it may be palpated through the abdominal wall. Otherwise, the stomach is out of reach and aligned with the 9th to 12th ribs of the left side (or thereabouts; Fig. 14–7/A). As the stomach expands, its ventral parts (mainly the body) move caudoventrally into broad contact with the abdominal floor and left costal arch, displacing the jejunum from contact with the liver in the process. Excessive distention, not uncommon in this greedy species, may carry the stomach to a level behind the umbilicus. Such gross enlargement also alters its cranial relationships, pushing the liver to the right and the diaphragm forward, reducing the thoracic cavity.

The stomach of the *cat* is more sharply flexed upon itself, and the pyloric part reaches little, if at all, into the right half of the abdomen. Gross distention is also less common in cats which tend to moderate their appetites better than dogs.

Survey radiographs of the abdomen generally reveal few details of the stomach beyond the gas that naturally collects in the uppermost part of the organ—the fundus in the animal standing or in right lateral recumbency. This useful orientation feature is lost when the animal is placed in other positions. A more complete demonstration of the topography is obtained with the administration of a barium meal. The existence of the rugae may be revealed by defects in the outline of the contrast mass; the most satisfactory depiction is obtained after the evacuation of the bulk of the meal when the residual agent clings to the mucosa and fills the spaces between adjacent rugae. These folds are conspicuously fewer, and proportionately smaller, in cats than in dogs.

A number of structures join the stomach to neighboring parts. The fundus is directly bound to the left crus of the diaphragm (gastrophrenic ligament), while there are looser attachments between the cardia and the diaphragm, the lesser curvature and liver (lesser omentum), and the greater curvature and spleen (greater omentum). Except at these reflections, the stomach is completely covered with serosa.

The stomach receives blood from all three branches into which the celiac artery divides directly after leaving the aorta between the crura of the diaphragm. The branches to the stomach therefore approach from the right of the fundus and dorsal to the cardia (Fig. 14–8). The splenic artery supplies short branches as it crosses the caudal surface of the fundus before reaching the spleen. A more substantial branch (left gastroepiploic artery; /11) follows the greater curvature to an anastomosis with the right gastroepiploic artery (a branch of the hepatic artery). The left gastric artery (/5) supplies the fundus and cardiac region, and a branch to the esophagus before following the lesser curvature to an anastomosis with the right gastric artery (/8), a further branch of the hepatic artery. The arterial arcades that follow the curvatures supply fair-sized branches to adjacent parts of both surfaces. Large vessels are absent from the strips midway between the curvatures, which are therefore the preferred locations for incision. The parietal surface can be exposed and opened through a midline or paracostal incision (a common procedure for the recovery of foreign bodies), but the visceral surface is inaccessible unless the omental bursa is opened first (see p. 123).

Gastric volvulus is relatively common, especially in large deep-chested breeds. In this mishap the stomach rotates about the esophagus (usually in a clockwise direction as seen from behind), and this closes the esophagus at the cardia. The pyloric end of the stomach, less firmly held in place by the lesser omentum and bile duct, moves ventrally and to the left, stretching the cranial part of the duodenum across the ventral surface of the cardia. The twist compresses the veins, causing congestion of the stomach and engorgement of the spleen.

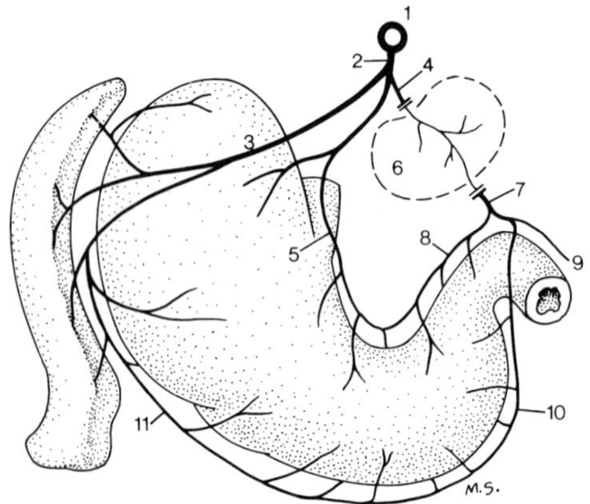


**Figure 14–8.** The blood supply of the stomach and spleen, caudal view; schematic.

1, Aorta; 2, celiac a.; 3, splenic a.; 4, hepatic a.; 5, left gastric a.; 6, indication of the liver; 7, gastroduodenal a.; 8, right gastric a.; 9, cranial pancreaticoduodenal a.; 10, right gastroepiploic a.; 11, left gastroepiploic a.

The *greater omentum* is extremely well developed and is folded on itself to form a flat sac with superficial and deep leaves that intervene between the intestinal mass and the abdominal floor (see Fig. 3–33). In consequence, only parts of the liver, spleen, and bladder come into view when the abdomen is opened in the usual dissection or autopsy procedure. The omental bursa exists as a potential space between the leaves.

The superficial leaf arises from the greater curvature of the stomach; the deep leaf arises from a line that begins at the esophageal hiatus, runs along the left crus of the diaphragm to the celiac artery, and then runs over the left lobe of the pancreas to reach the epiploic foramen on the right. The attachments of superficial and deep leaves come together on the left where the greater curvature of the stomach lies against the left crus of the diaphragm, and on the right in the vicinity of the duodenum, completing the circle of attachment.

The superficial leaf (/14) passes caudally from its origin, in direct contact with the ventral abdominal wall to reach the bladder, where it is reflected dorsally to become the deep leaf (/13). This runs forward between the superficial leaf and jejunal coils; at the cranial end of the jejunum it passes dorsally, against the caudal (visceral) surface of the stomach, to reach the left lobe of the pancreas, which it encloses and by means of which it gains the roof of the abdominal cavity. The right border of the omental sac is ventral to the descending duodenum; the left extends more dorsally to the level of the kidney and sublumbar muscles and is complicated by an attachment to the hilus of the spleen. The part of the omentum extending between the left crus of the diaphragm and the splenic hilus may be known as the phrenicosplenic ligament; the more generous part between the stomach and hilus forms the gastrosplenic ligament. As a further complication, a sagittal fold (omental veil) with a caudal free border connects the deep leaf with the left surface of the descending mesocolon.

The greater omentum always contains fat. This is first deposited along the small omental vessels, giving the structure a lacy appearance; however, in obese dogs (less so in cats) it forms a more or less continuous layer.

The *lesser omentum* is considerably wider than the short space it has to bridge between the lesser curvature of the stomach and the liver. It blends on the right with the mesoduodenum, the bile duct marking the boundary between the two.

The cat's stomach is similar to that of the dog; its topography and that of the intestines are shown in the radiographs of Figures 14–9 and 14–10, and on Plate 19/*F*).

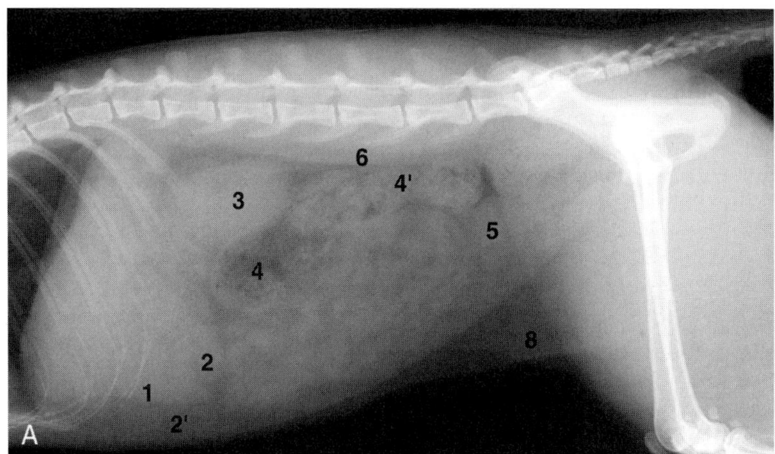


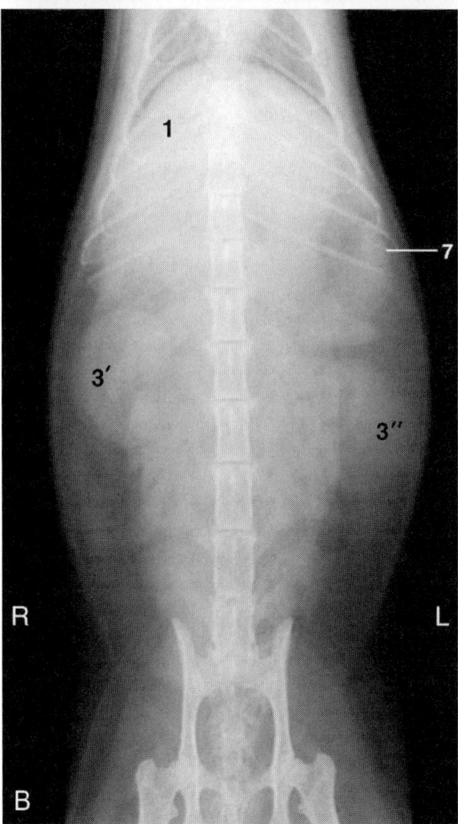


**Figure 14–9.** Lateral *(A)* and ventrodorsal *(B)* radiographic views of the feline abdomen.

1, Liver; 2, stomach; 2′, falciform fat; 3, superimposed right and left kidneys; 3′, right kidney; 3″, left kidney; 4, gas in transverse colon; 4′, gas and feces in descending colon; 5, bladder; 6, sublumbar muscles; 7, spleen; 8, flank fold.

## THE INTESTINES

*(See also pp. 129–135.)*

Since the general features of the intestinal tract have been described (p. 129) it is now permissible to concentrate on its relationships to other organs and to external landmarks, and on its attachments and blood supply.

The small intestine is relatively short, perhaps three or four times the body length. Of this, the *duodenum* contributes, on average, only 25 cm. The short cranial part of the duodenum passes dorsally and to the right, against the visceral surface of the liver, roughly opposite the ninth intercostal space. It is continued caudally beyond the porta as the descending duodenum, which follows the right abdominal wall to reach a point somewhere between the fourth and sixth lumbar vertebrae (Fig. 14–3/*B*,7′). In its passage it is related dorsally to the right lobe of the pancreas, ventrally to the jejunal mass, and medially to the ascending colon and cecum (Fig. 14–11/5). The mesentery of the descending duodenum begins by being relatively long but shortens toward the caudal flexure, where the gut is closely anchored to the abdominal roof. An additional (duodenocolic) fold with a free caudal border attaches the duodenum to the descending mesocolon at this level. The ascending duodenum (/6), which begins at the caudal flexure, is more tightly tethered than the preceding segment and runs forward, close to the midline, between the descending colon on the left and the root of the mesentery. It turns ventrally at the cranial limit of the root to be continued by the jejunum. Other relations of this part are the medial border of the left kidney dorsally and the jejunal mass ventrally (Figs. 14–4/*A* and 14–7/*B*).

The *jejunum* and short *ileum* form a mass occupying the ventral part of the abdomen between the stomach and the bladder (Fig. 14–12 and Plate 19/*A,D,F*). The coils of the jejunum are quite mobile and at first sight their disposition appears to be haphazard; closer inspection shows that there is some pattern to the arrangement. The mainly sagittal coils of the proximal part lie largely cranial to the more transverse coils of the distal part (Fig. 14–4/*A*). The suspending mesentery is relatively long and imposes little restraint, allowing the gut to slip freely over the floor in response to respiratory

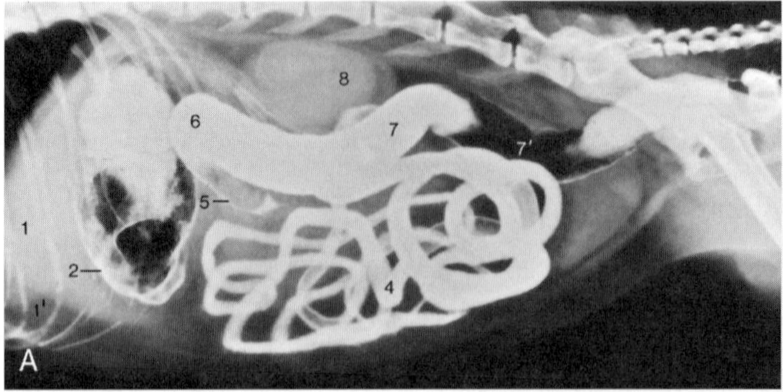


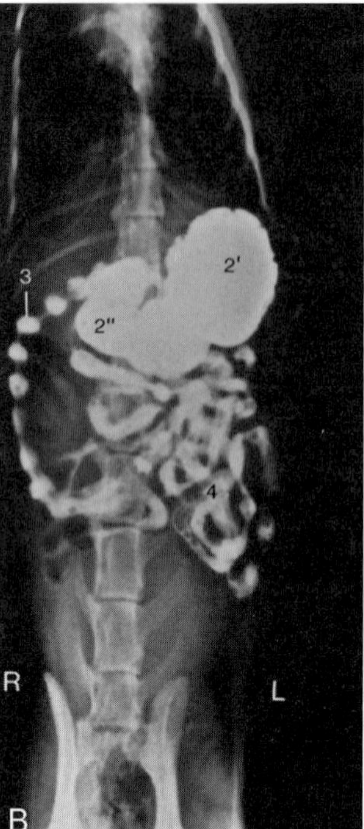


**Figure 14–10.** Lateral *(A)* and ventrodorsal *(B)* radiographic views of the feline abdomen after administration of a barium suspension.

1. Liver; 1′, fat-filled falciform ligament elevating the liver; 2, gas and barium in stomach; 2′, fundus; 2″, pyloric part of stomach; 3, descending duodenum—the striking "string-of-pearls" appearance (characteristic of cats) is due to segmental peristalsis; 4, jejunum; 5, ascending colon; 6, transverse colon; 7, descending colon; 7′, gas in descending colon; 8, kidneys (superimposed).

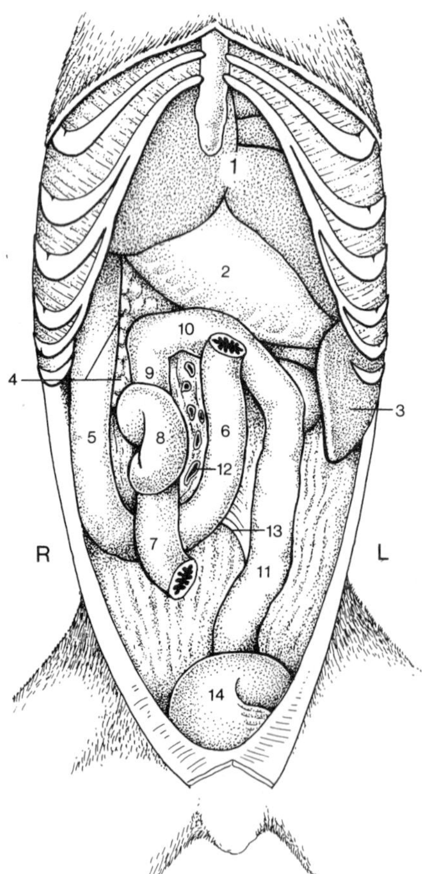


**Figure 14–11.** The canine duodenum, cecum, and colon in situ; ventral view.

1, Liver; 2, stomach; 3, spleen; 4, pancreas; 5, descending duodenum; 6, ascending duodenum; 7, ileum; 8, cecum; 9, 10, 11, ascending, transverse, and descending colon; 12, vessels in root of mesentery; 13, duodenocolic fold; 14, bladder.

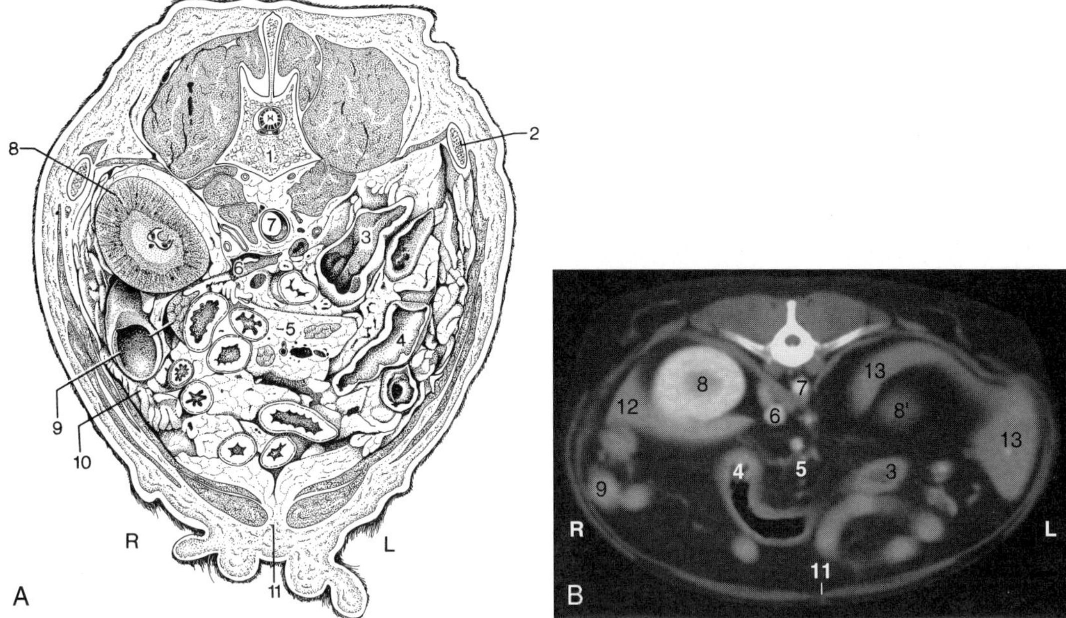


**Figure 14–12.** *A,* Transverse section of the canine abdomen at the level of the first lumbar vertebra. *B,* Corresponding CT image slightly more caudal than *A;* the dog was lying on its back during the CT procedure.

1, First lumbar vertebra; 2, last rib; 3, descending colon; 4, transverse colon; 5, lymph nodes and blood vessels in mesentery; ventral to them is the jejunum; 6, caudal vena cava; 7, aorta, between crura of diaphragm; 8, right kidney; 8′, cranial pole of left kidney; 9, descending duodenum and pancreas; 10, greater omentum; 11, linea alba; 12, liver; 13, spleen.

and other movements. This feature enables the surgeon to exteriorize much of the jejunum in order to improve the exposure of more dorsal organs. Dorsally, the jejunal mass extends to the descending duodenum on the right and the kidney and sublumbar muscles on the left. The jejunal coils are generally entirely related to the folded greater omentum ventrally; cranially only the deep leaf intervenes between them and the stomach. The *ileum* arises at the caudal end of the mass and passes forward and to the right to open into the ascending colon below the first or second lumbar vertebra.

Small patches of aggregate lymph nodules of varying sizes are present throughout the small intestine; the largest are said to be in the ileum.

In life the intestine is not uniformly full and at any moment most parts are flattened and molded by the pressures of adjacent viscera. The lumen may be locally obliterated and when a passage is retained it is, more often than not, reduced to a narrow channel along one margin—a "keyhole" section. This explains the narrow streaks that are the common representation of the small intestine in radiographs obtained after the administration of a barium meal. Segmental and peristaltic movements continually alter the configuration in life. Following the administration of a contrast medium, the duodenum of the cat often displays segmental contractions that are sufficiently pronounced to divide the gut content into a linear series of globular expansions separated by (more or less) empty regions; this creates the very striking "pearl necklace" effect (Fig. 14–10/*B*). A similar appearance in other regions of the cat's bowel, or in the duodenum of the dog, is probably evidence of abnormality.

The ileocecocolic junction is peculiar in that the ileum and colon are in line and form a continuous tube that is joined by the cecum to one side. (In the other species it is the cecum and colon that meet end to end.) The *cecum* is short—though of varying length—and twisted (Figs. 14–11/8 and 14–13/4). It is joined to the ileum by a short (ileocecal) fold and is oriented craniocaudally, although its rounded blind end may finally point in any direction. The cecum communicates with the ascending colon through the cecocolic orifice adjacent to the ileal orifice. The cecum lies to the right of the root of the mesentery and is related to the right kidney dorsally, the descending duodenum and pancreas laterally, and the jejunum ventrally. It lies below the second lumbar joint and thus is broadly level with the most caudal part of the costal arch.

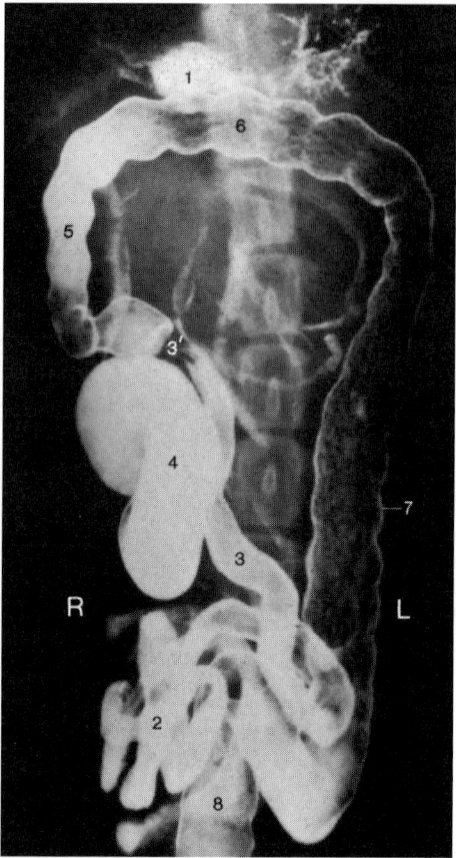


**Figure 14–13.** Ventrodorsal radiographic view of the canine abdomen after administration of a barium suspension.

1, Residue of barium in stomach; 2, jejunum; 3, ileum; 3′, ileocolic junction; 4, cecum; 5–7, ascending, transverse, and descending colon; 8, rectum.

The cecum of the cat is small and comma-shaped. Surprisingly, it can be located on palpation by reference to the firm ileocecocolic junction at the level of the fourth lumbar vertebra. The firmness can be mistaken for a tumor or intussusception (Fig. 14–15/4).

The *colon,* 65 cm long on average, is only slightly wider than the small intestine. It is easily recognized by its course cranial to the root of the mesentery and its nearly straight descent on the left toward the pelvis, which it enters dorsal to the bladder (and uterus) (see Figs. 3–44 and 14–13). The short ascending part lies to the right, between the descending duodenum and the root of the mesentery, and generally makes contact with the pyloric part of the stomach. Its narrow mesocolon permits it little mobility. The transverse colon runs from right to left, cranial to the root of the mesentery and ventral to the left lobe of the pancreas (Fig. 14–11). It is more loosely attached and sinks within the abdomen; usually it is the lowest part of the colon when depicted in lateral radiographs. The free attachment sometimes allows it to fold on itself to appear as no more than a flexure connecting the ascending with the descending colon. The descending colon is by far the longest segment. It passes caudally, to the left of the mesenteric root, to reach the pelvic cavity, where it continues as the rectum (Fig. 14–3/*A*,6). It is related dorsally to the left kidney and sublumbar muscles, and ventrally to the jejunal mass; it may lie against the left abdominal wall (Figs. 14–9/4′ and 14–14/4). The descending colon is the only segment of the large intestine of the dog that may easily be palpated.

The prominence of the cecum and colon in plain radiographs of the canine abdomen is determined by the amount of gas and the nature and volume of the digestive residues present (Fig. 14–13). The cecum almost always contains sufficient gas to provide a reminder of the twisted course of its lumen. This convenient identifying feature is not found in cats in which the simpler conformation rarely allows gas to be retained; see Figure 14–15 which also depicts the cat's colon.

The *blood supply* of the intestines comes mainly from the cranial and caudal mesenteric arteries, with a part of the duodenum supplied by

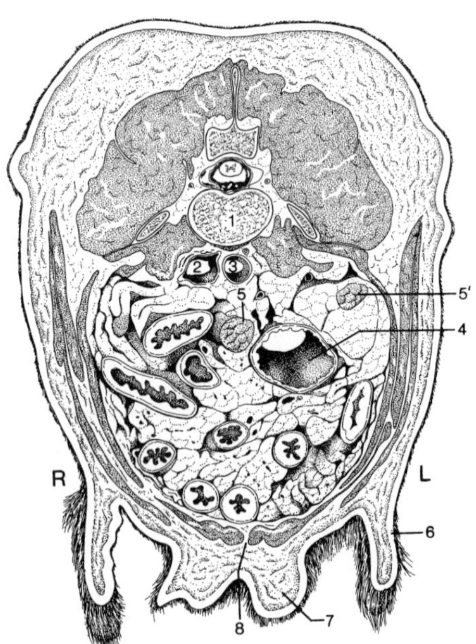


**Figure 14–14.** Transverse section of the canine abdomen at the level of the fourth or fifth lumbar vertebra.

1, Lumbar vertebra; 2, caudal vena cava; 3, aorta; 4, descending colon; 5, 5′, right and left uterine horns; 6, flank fold; 7, mammary gland; 8, linea alba.

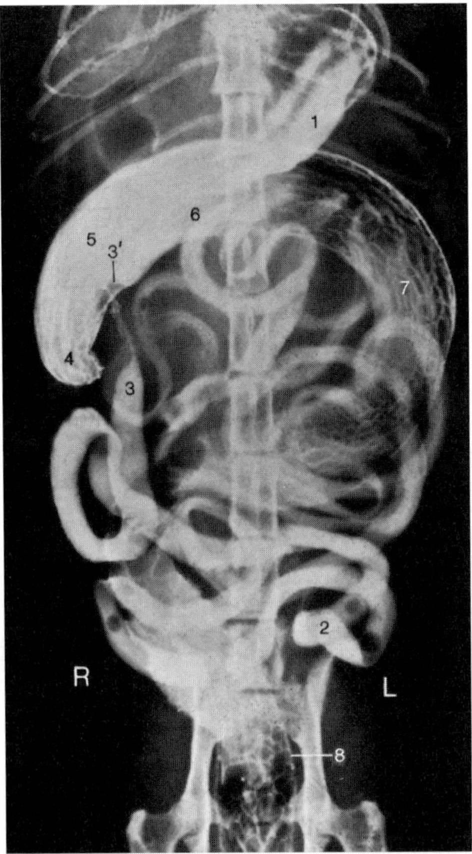


**Figure 14–15.** Ventrodorsal radiographic view of the feline abdomen after administration of a barium suspension.

1, Residue of barium in stomach; 2, jejunum; 3, ileum; 3′, ileal papilla; 4, cecum; 5–7, colon—the long descending part (7) has curved far to the right in this animal; 8, rectum.

the cranial pancreaticoduodenal branch of the gastroduodenal artery. The details are shown in Figure 14–16.

Several colic *lymph nodes* lie within the curvature of the ascending and transverse colon. The more prominent jejunal nodes lie high in the root of the mesentery; one, surprisingly large (perhaps 10 cm in the beagle), accompanies the jejunal arteries (Fig. 14–12/5). Several smaller caudal mesenteric nodes lie within the descending mesocolon, scattered about the branches of the caudal mesenteric artery.

## THE LIVER

*(See also pp. 135–138.)*

The liver is relatively large—weighing about 450 g on average—and accounts for 3% to 4% of the body weight. It is almost entirely intrathoracic, occupying a central position with only a slight bias to the right side (Figs. 14–3/2, 14–5, and Plate 2/*A,B*). The modest asymmetry is caused by the enlargement of the caudate process beneath the last ribs where it makes contact with the right kidney (Fig. 14–6/9). The ventral border extends across the costal arches and would be palpable were it not for the fat within the falciform ligament and the taut rectus muscles. Even so, it may be appreciated when significantly enlarged. The canine liver is deeply divided by fissures extending from the ventral margin; the pattern, the relative extents, and the names of the lobes may be obtained from Figure 3–51.

The cranial surface conforms to the curvature of the diaphragm with which it is in extensive contact and to which it is secured by the caudal vena cava embedded in the dorsal border. The attachment to the tendinous center of the diaphragm is completed by right and left coronary ligaments caudolateral to the vein. Most of the liver can therefore be

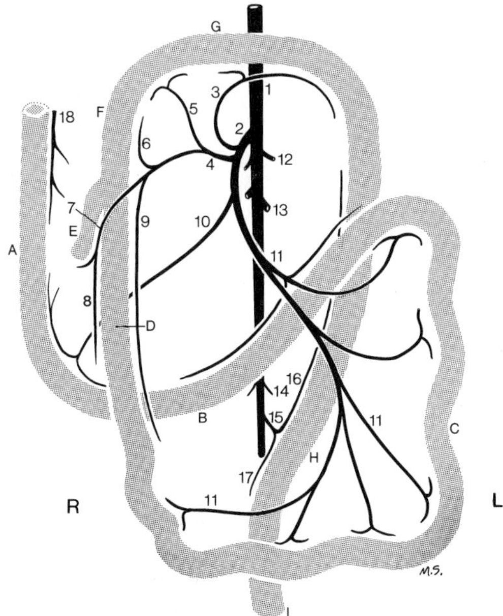


**Figure 14–16.** The blood supply of the intestinal tract, ventral view; schematic. A, Descending duodenum; B, ascending duodenum; C, jejunum; D, ileum; E, cecum; F, ascending colon; G, transverse colon; H, descending colon; I, rectum.

1, Abdominal aorta; 2, cranial mesenteric a.; 3, middle colic a.; 4, ileocolic a.; 5, right colic a.; 6, colic branch of ileocolic a.; 7, cecal a.; 8, antimesenteric ileal branch; 9, mesenteric ileal branch; 10, caudal pancreaticoduodenal a.; 11, jejunal aa.; 12, phrenicoabdominal aa.; 13, renal aa.; 14, testicular (ovarian) aa.; 15, caudal mesenteric a.; 16, left colic a.; 17, cranial rectal a.; 18, cranial pancreaticoduodenal a.

retracted at operation to expose the diaphragm. The gallbladder is sunk deeply between the lobes, just to the right of the median plane opposite the eighth intercostal space; it usually makes contact with the diaphragm and always appears at the visceral surface, although it is too short to reach the ventral border (Fig. 14–5/8).

The visceral surface, though concave, is made irregular by various visceral impressions. The largest of these is made by the body of the stomach to the left of the median plane; the pyloric part and duodenum produce a narrower impression leading away to the right (Fig. 14–6/7). The other prominent impression, involving the right lateral lobe and caudate process, is made by the right kidney. Other organs that may touch the liver, especially when the stomach is empty, leave no mark, except the pancreas, which attaches near the porta. Biopsy samples of liver tissue may be obtained by puncture caudal to the xiphoid process; the instrument is directed toward the large left lobe to avoid the gallbladder (see Fig. 3–41).

In survey radiographs of the abdomen the liver appears as a large, uniformly dense shadow from which its size, relative to the species norm, may be crudely assessed. In making such assessment, it is necessary to be mindful that the liver is more or less completely "intrathoracic" in large, deep-chested breeds, whereas a more appreciable portion projects beyond the costal arch in dogs of less extreme conformation. Dorsal displacement of the liver, away from the abdominal floor, may be encountered in cats that are overindulged; it is due to the deposition of excessive fat within the falciform ligament.

## THE PANCREAS

*(See also pp. 138–139.)*

The slender pancreas consists of two limbs or lobes that diverge from the vicinity of the pylorus. The left lobe is directed caudomedially and crosses the median plane behind the stomach to end against the left kidney (see Fig. 3–53/5). It divides the branches of the celiac artery from those of the cranial mesenteric and is enclosed within the deep leaf of the greater omentum where this passes dorsal to the transverse colon. Its dorsal surface is crossed by the portal vein, where it makes contact with the porta of the liver to the right of the median plane.

The longer right lobe is directed caudodorsally and follows the dorsal surface of the descending duodenum within the mesoduodenum. It is related dorsally to the visceral surface of the liver and, behind this, to the ventral surface of the kidney (Fig. 14–12/9). It lies lateral to the ascending colon and dorsal to the small intestine.

Two secretory ducts open into the duodenum where the two lobes diverge. The smaller and inconstant pancreatic duct joins the bile duct just before this opens on the major duodenal papilla, 3 to 6 cm distal to the pylorus. The accessory pancreatic duct, the main channel, opens on the minor duodenal papilla 3 to 5 cm farther down the gut. Both papillae can be detected with the unaided eye. The duct systems of the two lobes communicate internally.

## THE KIDNEYS AND ADRENAL GLANDS

*(See also pp. 175–179 and 215–216.)*

The kidneys are short, thick, and bean-shaped; they lie against the sublumbar muscles. The right kidney is usually said to lie below the first three lumbar vertebrae, the left one below the second to fourth (Fig. 14–17), but this may specify their positions too definitely and they may be found a full vertebral length more caudally. Though retroperitoneal, their positions (particularly that of the left kidney) vary with posture and respiration. The right kidney is more restricted by being deeply recessed within the liver. In obese subjects the kidneys are embedded within, though rarely concealed by, large amounts of fat.

The right kidney is related medially to the right adrenal gland and caudal vena cava, laterally to the last rib and abdominal wall, and ventrally to the liver and pancreas (Fig. 14–18). The left kidney is related cranially to the spleen (or stomach when enlarged), medially to the left adrenal gland and aorta, laterally to the abdominal wall, and ventrally to the descending colon. In the bitch the caudal poles of both kidneys are related to the fat-filled mesovaria and ovaries. The left kidney may be palpated in most dogs, the right one only exceptionally, in thin subjects.

The renal arteries and veins come directly from the aorta and caudal vena cava, respectively. The former usually branch before entering the kidney. Small arteries of aberrant origin may also be present (Fig. 14–19).

The cat's kidneys are relatively large and are given a distinctive appearance by capsular veins converging over the surface toward the hilus (Plate 19/*G*). They are more mobile than the kidneys of the dog, especially the left one, which can be displaced cranially or caudally from its usual position below the second to fifth lumbar

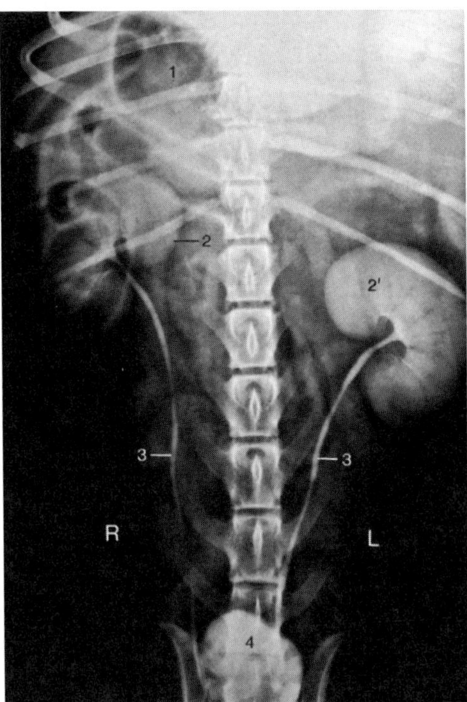


**Figure 14–17.** Urogram of a dog.

1, Gas in stomach; 2, 2′, right and left kidneys; 3, ureters; 4, bladder.

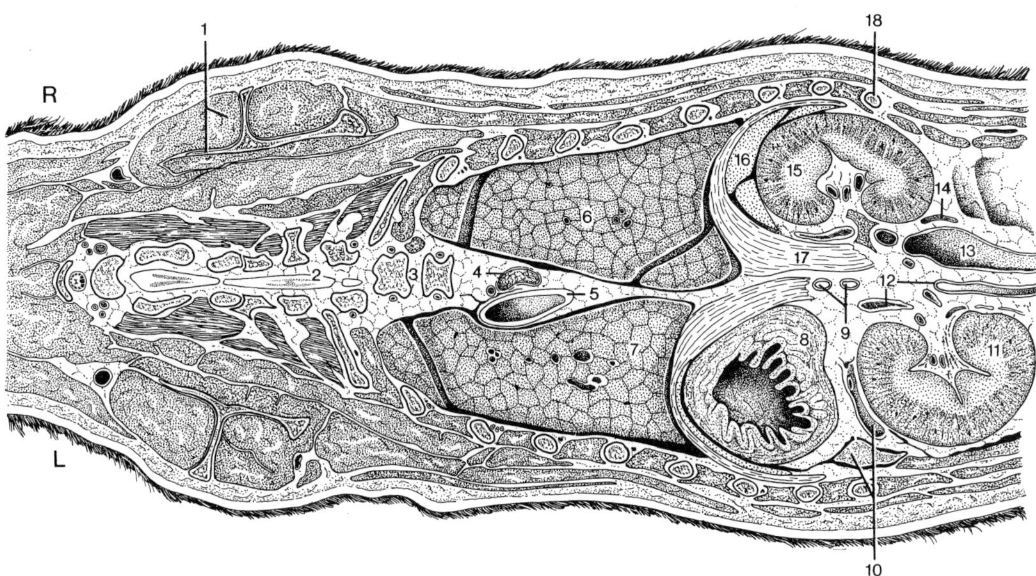


**Figure 14–18.** Dorsal section of the canine trunk at the level of the kidneys.

1, Supraspinatus and scapula; 2, spinal cord; 3, sixth and seventh thoracic vertebrae; 4, right azygous vein; 5, thoracic aorta; 6, 7, right and left lungs; 8, fundus of stomach; 9, celiac and cranial mesenteric arteries; 10, splenic vessels and spleen; 11, left kidney; 12, left adrenal gland and abdominal aorta; 13, caudal vena cava; 14, right ureter; 15, right kidney (the right adrenal gland is shown medial to the cranial pole); 16, liver; 17, right crus of diaphragm; 18, last rib.

vertebrae (Fig. 14–9); it has been taken for a pathological swelling. In cats, both kidneys are readily palpable.

In the dog (if not the cat) it is generally thought more prudent to expose a kidney by laparotomy when a biopsy specimen is required, rather than attempt a blind puncture.

The ureters are at risk in the common spay operation. They run caudally on the psoas muscles about 1 to 2 cm lateral to the median plane and thus closer to the aorta (or vena cava) than to the origin of the broad ligament in the female (Figs. 14–17/3, 14–19/11, and Plate 19/*G*). They cross the dorsal (lateral) surface of the gonadal vessels and the ventral surface of the deep circumflex iliac vessels and the large terminal branches of the aorta and vena cava. In the pelvis the ureters course in the base of the broad ligament or genital fold; those of the male dog cross over the dorsal surface of the deferent ducts before entering the bladder.

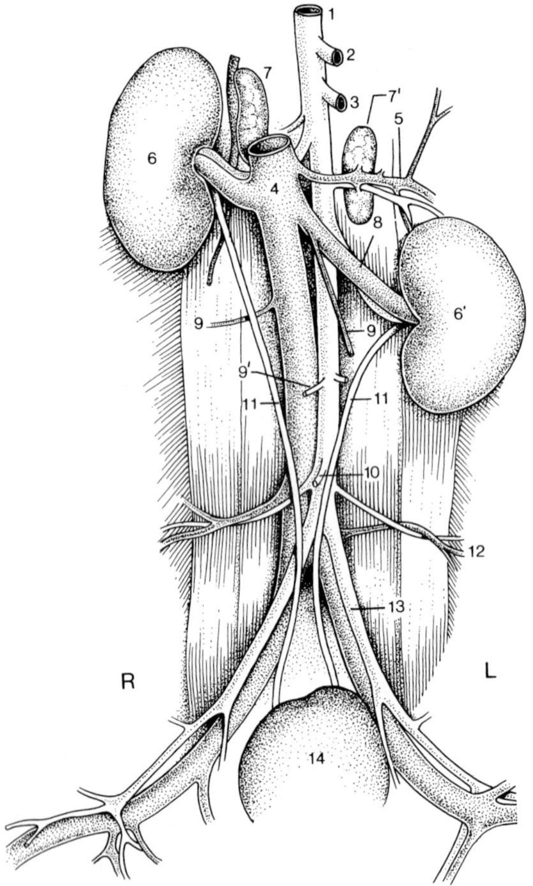


**Figure 14–19.** The canine urinary organs and adjacent blood vessels in situ.

1, Aorta; 2, celiac a.; 3, cranial mesenteric a.; 4, caudal vena cava; 5, phrenicoabdominal vessels; 6, 6′, right and left kidneys; 7, 7′, right and left adrenal glands; 8, left renal vessels; 9, ovarian vv.; 9′, ovarian aa.; 10, caudal mesenteric a.; 11, ureters; 12, deep circumflex iliac vessels; 13, external iliac vessels; 14, bladder.

Survey radiographs of the abdomen will adequately reveal the external anatomy of kidneys when, as is usually the case, they are enclosed in fat. (Deficiency of fat occurs in very young pups and in emaciated older subjects.) Visualization of internal features requires the intravenous injection of an appropriate contrast agent which is then excreted in the urine; suitably staged radiographs will show general opacification of the cortex and medulla of the kidney (Fig. 14–17), renal pelvic morphology (Fig. 5–25), and, later, the status of the ureters and of the bladder. Since the passage of urine is assisted by peristaltic contraction, a single radiograph does not usually depict a healthy ureter along its entire length.

The yellowish-white *adrenal glands* (Fig. 14–19/7,7′) are dorsoventrally flattened, about 2 to 3 cm long and 1 cm wide. Each occupies the space medial to the kidney, cranial to the renal vessels, and dorsolateral to the aorta (or vena cava). The ventral surface is crossed and indented by the phrenicoabdominal veins; on the left, this surface is also related to the pancreas. The left gland is more easily found, since the right one is wedged between the kidney, the caudate process of the liver, and the vena cava.

The glands are diffusely supplied by branches from adjacent vessels—the aorta and the renal, phrenicoabdominal, lumbar, and cranial mesenteric arteries. The nerve supply is derived from a dense network on the dorsal surface that appears continuous with the nearby celiac and mesenteric plexuses. The fibers that actually enter the glands are preganglionic and provided by the splanchnic nerves that enter the abdominal cavity close by. The adrenal glands of older cats are occasionally calcified and are then visible on radiographs.

As already described (p. 242) the aorta* continues a short distance beyond the origin of the

*In both companion species, but especially in the cat, the terminal segment of the aorta is commonly the location of a large thrombus, often known as a "saddle" thrombus from its disposition across the division, which may partially or wholly block the three terminal branches. The origin of the thrombus, the degree of obstruction it causes, and the rate at which it developed, determine the severity of the clinical signs, which may include complete paralysis of the hindlimbs.

Venography of the portal vein (Fig. 7–44) is occasionally employed to ascertain the existence (and condition) of portosystemic connections; a small intestinal tributary is chosen for the injection. The shunts most commonly revealed connect the portal system with the caudal caval tributaries at the abdominal roof, and with the azygous vein within the thorax.

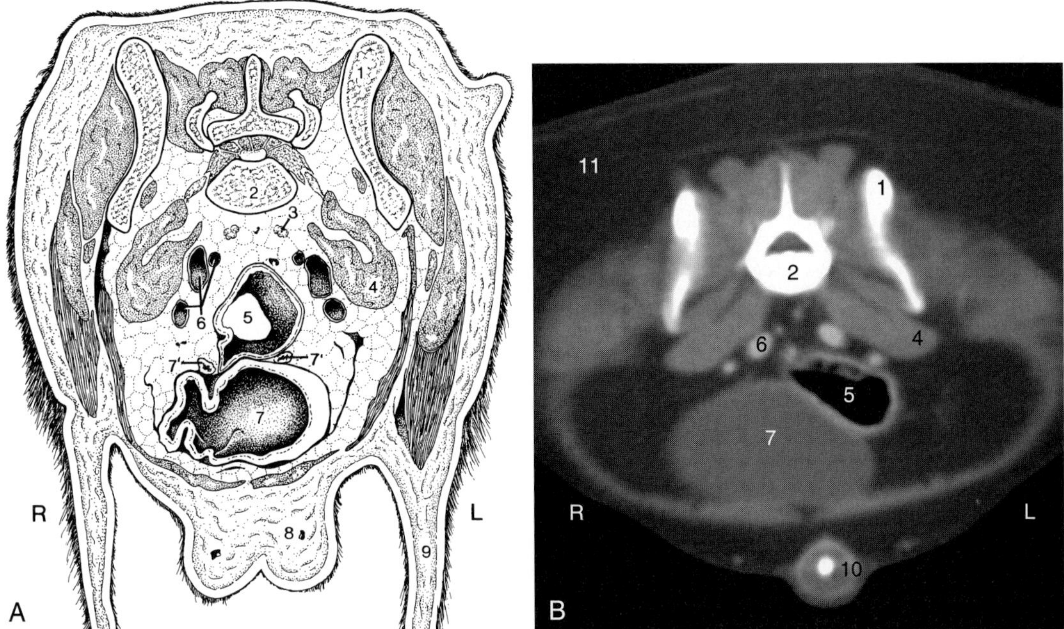


**Figure 14–20.** *A,* Transverse section of the canine abdomen at the level of the seventh lumbar vertebra. *B,* Corresponding CT image at about the same level.

1, Wing of ilium; 2, seventh lumbar vertebra; 3, sacral lymph nodes; 4, iliopsoas; 5, descending colon; 6, internal iliac artery (most dorsal), external iliac vein, and external iliac artery; 7, bladder; 7′, uterine horns; 8, mammary gland; 9, flank fold; 10, penis with os penis; 11, fat.

external iliac arteries before dividing into three: the paired internal iliac arteries and the small median sacral.

The lymph nodes at the breakup of the aorta can be palpated rectally in larger individuals (Fig. 14–20/3).

Though the ovaries and other reproductive organs are found within the abdomen, they are described in the following chapter.

References to the palpation of abdominal organs and to digital exploration per rectum will be found on p. 451.

## Selected Bibliography

Boothe, H.W.: Exploratory laparotomy in small animals. Compend. Contin. Educ. Pract. Vet. 12:1057–1066, 1990.

Bostwick, D.R., & D.C. Twedt: Intrahepatic and extrahepatic portal venous anomalies in dogs: 52 cases (1982–1992). JAVMA 206:1181–1186, 1995.

Boyd, J.S.: Color Atlas of Clinical Anatomy of the Dog and Cat. St. Louis, Mosby–Year Book, 1991.

Brockman, D.J., A.D. Pardo, M.G. Conzemius, et al.: Omentum-enhanced reconstruction of chronic nonhealing wounds in cats: Techniques and clinical use. Vet. Surg. 25: 99–104, 1996.

Bunch, S.E., Polak, D.M., and W.E. Hornbuckle: A modified laparoscopic approach for liver biopsy in dogs. JAVMA 187:1032–1035, 1985.

Cockett, P.A.: Radiographic anatomy of the canine liver: Simple measurements determined from the lateral radiograph. J. Small Anim. Pract. 27:577–589, 1986.

Dean, P.W., Bojrab, M.J., and G.M. Constantinescu: Canine ectopic ureter. Compend. Contin. Educ. Pract. Vet. 10:146–158, 1988.

deHaan, J.J., G.W. Ellison, and J.R. Bellah: Surgical correction of idiopathic megacolon in cats. Feline Pract. 20:6–11, 1992.

deLahunta, A., and R.E. Habel: Applied Veterinary Anatomy. Philadelphia, W.B. Saunders Company, 1986.

Ellison, G.W.: Gastric dilation-volvulus surgical prevention. Vet. Clin. North Am. Small Anim. Pract. 23:513–530, 1993.

Evans, H.E.: Miller's Anatomy of the Dog, 3rd ed. Philadelphia, W.B. Saunders Company, 1993.

Fletcher, T.F.: Applied anatomy and physiology of the feline lower urinary tract. Vet Clin. North Am. Small Anim. Pract. 26:181–196, 1996.

Glickman, L., T. Emerick, N. Glickman, et al.: Radiological assessment of the relationship between thoracic conformation and the risk of gastric dilation-volvulus in dogs. Vet. Radiol. Ultrasound 37:174–180, 1996.

Godshalk C.P., S.K. Kneller, R.R. Badertscher, and D. Essex-Sorlie: Quantitative noninvasive assessment of liver size in clinically normal dogs. Am. J. Vet. Res. 51:1421–1426, 1990.

Habel, R.E, and K.D. Budras: Anatomy of the prepubic tendon in the horse, cow, sheep, goat, and dog. Am. J. Vet. Res. 53:2183–2195, 1992.

Holt, P.E., and A. Hotston Moore: Canine ureteral ectopia: An analysis of 175 cases and comparison of surgical treatments. Vet. Rec. 136:345–349, 1995.

Hosgood, G: The omentum—the forgotten organ: Physiology and potential surgical applications in dogs and cats. Compend. Contin. Educ. Pract. Vet. 12:45–51, 1990.

Hosgood, G., Bone, D.L., Vorhees, W.D., III, and W.M. Reed: Splenectomy in the dog by ligation of the splenic and short gastric arteries. Vet. Surg. 18:110–113, 1989.

Hudson, L.C., and W.P. Hamilton: Atlas of Feline Anatomy for Veterinarians. Philadelphia, W.B. Saunders Company, 1993.

Johnston, D.E., and B.A. Christie: The retroperitoneum in dogs: Anatomy and clinical significance. Compend. Contin. Educ. Pract. Vet. 12:1027–1055, 1990.

Jones, B.D., Hitt, M., and T. Hurst: Hepatic biopsy. Vet. Clin. North Am. Small Anim. Pract. 15:39–65, 1985.

Kalt, D.J., and J.E. Stump: Gross anatomy of the canine portal vein. Anat. Histol. Embryol. 22:191–197, 1993.

Lamb, C.R., and R.N. White: Morphology of congenital intrahepatic portacaval shunts in dogs and cats. Vet. Rec. 142:55–60, 1998.

Lantz, G.C.: Treatment of gastric dilatation-volvulus syndrome. *In* Bojrab, M.J. (ed.): Current Techniques in Small Animal Surgery, 3rd ed. Philadelphia, Lea & Febiger, 1990.

Losonsky J.M., and S.K. Kneller: Misdiagnosis in normal radiographic anatomy: Eight structural configurations simulating disease entities in small animals. JAVMA 191:109–114, 1987.

Love, N.E.: The appearance of the canine pyloric region in right versus left lateral recumbent radiographs. Vet. Radiol. Ultrasound 34:169–170, 1993.

Martin, R.A.: Congenital portosystemic shunts in the dog and cat. Vet. Clin. North Am. Small Anim. Pract. 23:609–623, 1993.

McCrackin, M.A., R.C. DeNovo, R.M. Bright, and R.L. Toal: Endoscopic placement of percutaneous gastroduodenostomy feeding tube in dogs. JAVMA 203:792–797, 1993.

Patsikas, M.N., and A. Dessiris: The lymph drainage of the mammary glands in the bitch: A lymphographic study. Part I: The 1st, 2nd, 4th and 5th mammary glands. Anat. Histol. Embryol. 25:131–138, 1996.

Patsikas, M.N., and A. Dessiris: The lymph drainage of the mammary glands in the bitch: A lymphographic study. Part II: The 3rd mammary gland. Anat. Histol. Embryol. 25:139–143, 1996.

Poogird, W., and A.K.W. Wood: Radiologic study of the canine urethra. Am. J. Vet. Res. 47:2491–2497, 1986.

Richardson, E.F., and H. Mullen: Cryptorchidism in cats. Compend. Contin. Educ. Pract. Vet. 15:1342–1369, 1993.

Rosin, E.: Megacolon in cats: The role of colectomy. Vet. Clin. North Am. Small Anim. Pract. 23:587–594, 1993.

Scavelli, T.D., W.S. Hornbuckle, L. Roth, et al.: Portosystemic shunts in cats: Seven cases (1976–1984). JAVMA 189:317–325, 1986.

Schebitz, H., and H. Wilkens: Atlas of Radiographic Anatomy of the Dog and Cat, 4th ed. Berlin, Paul Parey Verlag, 1986.

Scrivani, P.V., D.J. Chew, T. Buffington, et al.: Results of retrograde urethrography in cats with idiopathic, nonobstructive lower urinary tract disease and their association with pathogenesis: 53 cases (1993–1995). JAVMA 211:741–748, 1997.

Slatter, D. (ed.): Textbook of Small Animal Surgery, 2nd ed. Philadelphia, W.B. Saunders Company, 1993.

Spaulding, D.K.: A review of sonographic identification of abdominal blood vessels and juxtavascular organs Vet. Radiol. Ultrasound 38:4–23, 1997.

Steyn, P.F., and D.C. Twedt: Gastric emptying in the normal cat: A radiographic study J. Am. Anim. Hosp. Assoc. 30:78–80, 1994.

Suter, P.F.: Portal vein anomalies in the dog, their angiographic diagnosis. J. Am. Vet. Radiol. Soc. 16:84, 1975.

Tisdall, P.L.C., G.B. Hunt, R.P. Borg, and R. Malik: Anatomy of the ductus venosus in neonatal dogs *(Canis familiaris).* Anat. Histol. Embryol. 26:35–38, 1997.

van Bree, H., V. Jacobs, and P. Vandekerckhove: Radiographic assessment of liver volume in dogs. Am. J. Vet. Res. 50:1613–1615, 1989.

White, R.N., and C.A. Burton: Anatomy of the patent ductus venosus in the dog. Vet. Rec. 146:425–429, 2000.

Wrigley, R.H., L.J. Konde, R.D. Park, and J.L. Lebel: Ultrasonographic diagnosis of portocaval shunts in young dogs. JAVMA 191:421–424, 1987.

# CHAPTER 15

# The Pelvis and Reproductive Organs of the Carnivores*

## GENERAL ANATOMY OF THE PELVIS AND PERINEUM

(*See also pp. 56–57.*)

The bony pelvis is formed by the pelvic girdle, sacrum, and first few caudal vertebrae—the caudal limit of the roof being, as always, difficult to define precisely. These bones were described in Chapter 2, and the surface landmarks they create are mentioned in Chapter 17. It will therefore be sufficient at this point to recapitulate a few general features.

The *pelvic cavity* is smaller than might be supposed from examination of the intact animal or the isolated girdle. The discrepancy between expectation and reality is due to the shallowness of the caudal part of the abdomen and to the acute angle (about 20 degrees) formed between the ilia and the vertebral column (Fig. 15–1). The pronounced obliquity of the inlet places the pubic brim level with, or even behind, the caudal limit of the sacrum. The iliac shafts are not quite parallel and the inlet is widest in its middle part, narrowest dorsally. Unusually among domestic species, the outlet is less confined than the inlet, and it possesses a considerable capacity for further enlargement through elevation of the tail behind the very short sacrum. Only a small part of the lateral wall is bony as neither the ischial spine nor the ischial tuber rises to any great height. In the dog the sacrotuberous ligament is reduced to a narrow cord extending (under cover of the superficial gluteal muscle) between the ischial tuber and the caudolateral corner of the sacrum (see Fig. 2–20/*A*).

The pelvic girdle of the cat shows some differences. Cranially, the ilia diverge slightly, producing a somewhat funnel-shaped entrance to the pelvis from the abdominal cavity. The wings of these bones are relatively smaller and shallower, which also eases the transition. The ischial tubers stand closer together than in the dog, giving the pelvis a more rectangular appearance in ventrodorsal view and a more confined exit (Fig. 15–2). In consequence of the last feature the perineum is narrow. There are no sacrotuberous ligaments in this species.

The axis of the short pelvic canal is almost straight and in general the conformation appears well adapted for easy parturition. Sexual dimorphism is not pronounced, and pelvic measurements have not been given much attention in small animal obstetrics. An ill match of the proportions of the fetus and the dam is most common when the litter is small (and the individual fetus relatively large), in toy dogs, and in those breeds in which a measure of achondroplasia is a feature of the conformation. On rectal examination the pelvic canal of young dogs is shaped like an hourglass, which may mistakenly suggest a pelvic fracture.

The perineum slopes somewhat ventrocaudally and is largely concealed when the tail is carried low. When the tail is raised, it exhibits a shield of naked integument about the anal orifice and, at some distance ventral to this, the vulva or root of the penis; these features are considered in more detail later. The *ischiorectal fossa* between the anus and the ischial tuber naturally varies in prominence with the character of the coat and the degree of obesity. The fossa is bounded by the sacrotuberous ligament and the deep face of the superficial gluteal muscle laterally and by the superficial face of the coccygeus medially. It is traversed by the large caudal gluteal vessels that run against the lateral wall and by the main trunks and certain branches of the internal pudendal vessels and pudendal nerve placed more medially, toward the floor (Fig. 15–13/2,3).

The *pelvic diaphragm* has the usual composition. The lateral muscle, the coccygeus, has a tendinous origin from the ischial spine and inserts

*See introductory remarks on page 367.

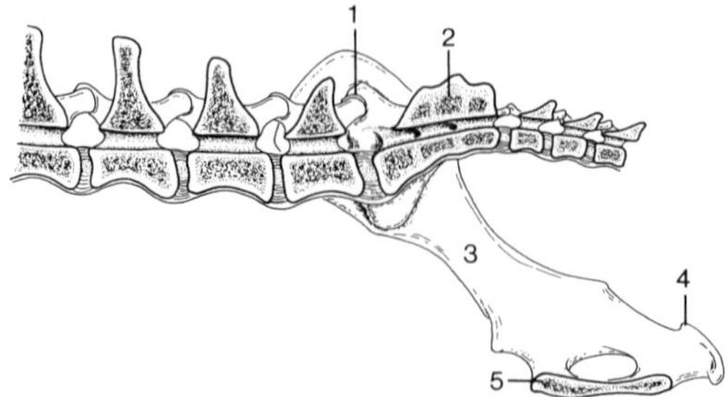


**Figure 15–1.** The right half of the canine bony pelvis, medial view.

1, Sacroiliac joint; 2, sacrum; 3, shaft of ilium; 4, ischial tuber; 5, symphysis.

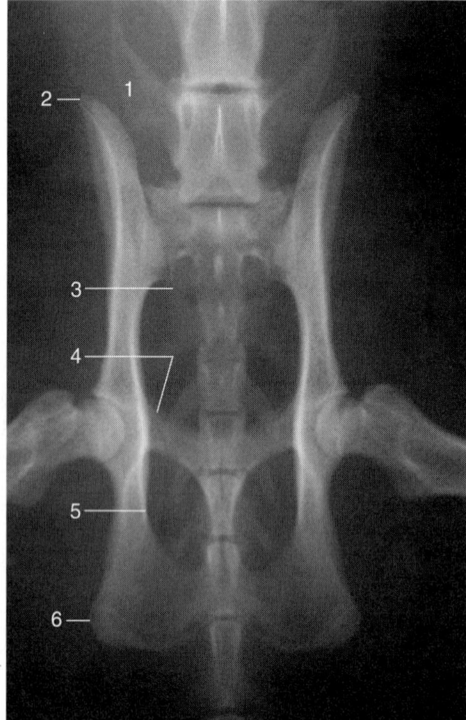


**Figure 15–2.** Radiograph of the feline pelvis.

1, Transverse process of last lumbar vertebra (L7); 2, iliac crest; 3, sacrum; 4, pecten of the pubis; 5, obturator foramen; 6, ischial tuber.

on the lateral aspect of the tail between the second and fifth vertebrae (see Fig. 3–47/1). The deeper and thinner levator ani (/2) has a wider origin, which extends from the iliac shaft onto the pelvic floor along which it runs, directly to the side of the symphysis (Fig. 15–3/7). The part arising from the pelvic floor closely embraces the pelvic viscera in its passage to its insertion on the tail, reaching as far caudally as the seventh vertebra. The levator fibers run more obliquely than those of the coccygeus, and part of the levator emerges superficially behind that muscle. The levator has only a passing fascial connection with the external sphincter of the anus and, like the coccygeus, it is primarily a depressor of the tail. However, its fascial attachment enables it to help fix the position of the anus during defecation. The tone of both muscles is important in retaining the pelvic viscera in place, and perineal hernia—in which pelvic organs are displaced to form a swelling to the side of the anus—may be a sequel to their paralysis or atrophy. Surgical repair of this condition involves suture of the external sphincter to the coccygeus, internal obturator, and sacrotuberous ligament about the margins of the space.

The pelvic blood vessels and nerves were sufficiently described in the general accounts (pp. 244 and 316). Since there are only three sacral spinal nerves, the origins of the pudendal, caudal rectal, and pelvic nerves are rather compressed; variations in the branching patterns of the first two are common. The pudendal and caudal rectal nerves supply afferent and efferent fibers to the perineum, and their integrity is necessary for the execution of the perineal reflex that provides a means of gauging the depth of narcosis. The modified skin about the anus is especially sensitive, and even a gentle touch evokes a brisk contraction of the anal sphincter of the conscious or lightly anesthetized animal.

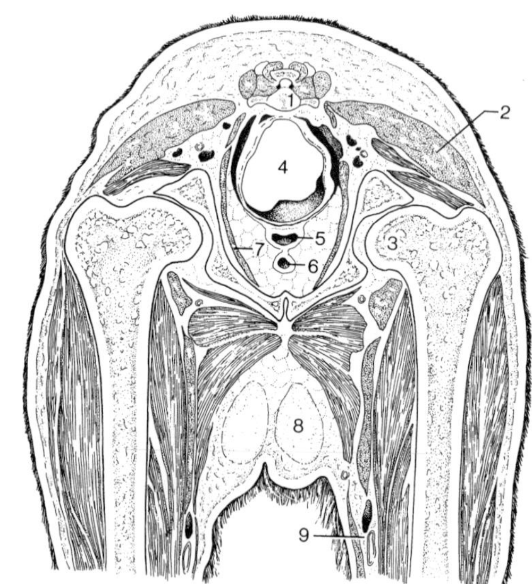


**Figure 15–3.** Transverse section of the canine pelvis at the level of the hip joint.

1, Caudal vertebra; 2, superficial gluteal muscle; 3, head of femur in acetabulum; 4, rectum suspended by a short mesorectum; 5, vagina; 6, urethra; 7, levator ani; 8, inguinal mammary gland; 9, femoral artery and vein.

## THE RECTUM AND ANUS

*(See also pp. 133 and 134.)*

The *rectum* joins the anal canal ventral to the second or third caudal vertebra. Its cranial part is intraperitoneal and joined to the pelvic roof by a short mesorectum (Fig. 15–3/4); the caudal part becomes entirely retroperitoneal once the serous covering has been reflected onto the pelvic walls and the dorsal surface of the reproductive tract (bitch) or prostate (dog). The dorsal relations of the rectum include the ventral muscles of the tail and certain smooth muscle bundles (rectococcygeus) that run caudally from the rectal wall to the undersurface of the tail; these bundles probably help draw the anus caudally when a column of feces descends from the colon. The ventral relations of the rectum of the bitch are the cervix, and possibly the body, of the uterus in addition to the vagina; in the dog they are the prostate and urethra. Laterally, the rectum is bounded by the levator muscle and crossed by the internal pudendal vessels (Fig. 15–13) and the sciatic, pelvic, pudendal, and caudal rectal nerves; cushioning by fat gives the rectum some freedom to deviate from its usual median course.

In most breeds the rectal lumen is sufficiently wide to permit digital exploration of the pelvic walls and contents. The structures that can be identified include much of the pelvic skeleton and the prostate or female tract. The rectal mucosa has a pitted appearance since the many lymph nodules with which it is strewn are each indented by a crypt.

The short (ca. 7 mm) initial columnar portion of the *anal canal* is fashioned by underlying vessels into a series of longitudinal ridges whose interdigitation helps maintain continence (see Figs. 3–46/2 and 15–4). These ridges end upon a scalloped line that represents the junction between the columnar intestinal epithelium and the stratified cutaneous epithelium. The outer cutaneous zone is of variable extent; the modified skin that lines this last part of the passage may be everted to appear as a purplish patch upon the perineal surface, especially when defecation impends. At this time the anal orifice takes on a triangular form in place of the transverse slit generally displayed (see Fig. 10–27/*A*).

All fissiped carnivores (other than bears) possess paired *anal sacs* enclosed between the external and internal anal sphincters. In the dog each is about 1 cm in diameter and discharges through a short duct that opens ventrolateral to the anal orifice, concealed or exposed on the perineal surface according to the physiological condition (see Fig. 3–46/1). The sacs, which are commonly

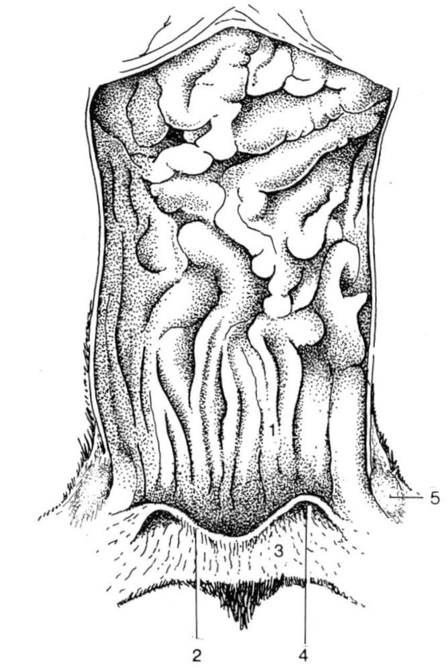


**Figure 15–4.** Feline anal canal opened dorsally.

1, Columnar zone; 2, anocutaneous line; 3, cutaneous zone; 4, opening of the right anal sac; 5, right anal sac.

blocked or infected in dogs, may be examined by palpation, either externally or after insertion of a finger into the rectum. The sacs store the sebaceous secretion of coiled glands massed in the fundic part of the lining; this evil-smelling material is normally extruded in the later stages of defecation and serves as a marker that identifies the animal to other members of its species. There are, in addition, small anal glands within the columnar zone and much larger and more numerous circumanal glands within the cutaneous zone; the latter increase greatly in amount with age.

Cats also possess these sacs but as they are infrequently diseased their presence tends to be forgotten, although the duct openings, one to each side of the anus, can be very conspicuous if occupied by inspissated secretion (Fig. 15–4/4,5).

A note on what may be examined on digital exploration per rectum is found on page 452.

## THE BLADDER AND FEMALE URETHRA

*(See also pp. 179–182.)*

Although the neck of the canine bladder extends a little way into the pelvic cavity, the bulk of the organ is visible as soon as the floor of the abdomen is removed since it is left uncovered by the greater omentum (Fig. 15–5/1). Its size varies greatly and when excessively distended, as in house-trained animals denied opportunity for relief, it may reach to or even beyond the umbilicus (Fig. 15–16). In dogs allowed freedom, the bladder is rarely very large since the frequent discharge of urine performs a social (scent-marking) as well as eliminative function.* The bladder may be identified on abdominal palpation when moderately (or more greatly) distended. Unless handled with care, a grossly distended bladder may be ruptured when compressed through the abdominal wall to induce micturition. Even cautious compression, if too long maintained, may overcome the protection afforded by the oblique passage of the ureters through the bladder wall, allowing the reflux of urine with the risk of contamination when there is infection of the bladder. Moderate increase in size is not accompanied by increased tension, and radiographs obtained with the (contrasted) bladder in this state show its contours molded to those of adjacent organs (see Fig. 5–26). The organ is globular when fully contracted.

The peritoneal covering, which extends onto the cranial part of the urethra, is reflected into the usual lateral and ventral median folds.

The *female urethra* is relatively long. It originates within the cranial part of the pelvis and follows the symphysis to open on the floor of the vestibule, immediately caudal to the vestibulovaginal junction. In the bitch, the orifice is raised on a tubercle that continues some way over the vestibular floor and is flanked by well-marked depressions. Though blind catheterization is difficult in small subjects, the procedure is possible in larger bitches, in which a finger may be introduced to locate the tubercle and guide the instrument.

*In addition to marking, ostentatious cocking of the leg by a male dog when passing urine may assert superiority. Cats also make a social use of micturition (see further on).

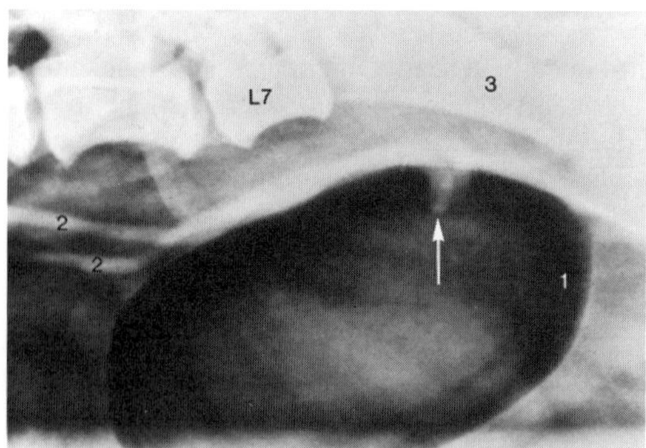


**Figure 15–5.** The canine bladder made visible by the introduction of air. The arrow indicates the terminations of the ureters in the dorsal wall of the bladder, superimposed here on the air-filled lumen.

1, Caudal end of bladder; 2, ureters; 3, shaft of ilium.

The bladder of the cat is more cranially placed than that of the dog and lies wholly within the abdomen at all times. In consequence of this, the urethra is unusually long and some authors have been tempted to interpret the intraabdominal part as a curiously drawn-out bladder neck (Fig. 15–6). The urethra of the queen is more or less uniformly wide (unlike its counterpart in the tom) and makes a more discrete entry into the vestibule than that of the bitch.

The male urethra of both species is considered with the reproductive organs (pp. 188–189).

## THE FEMALE REPRODUCTIVE ORGANS

### The Ovaries and Uterine Tubes

*(See also pp. 193–195.)*

The distal mesovarium and the mesosalpinx fuse extensively to create a bursa into which the ovary projects and within which it is entrapped. In bitches these folds contain much fat that largely conceals the ovary (see Fig. 5–49/*B*). When it is exposed, the ovary is found to be a firm, flattened, ellipsoidal body measuring about 15 × 10 × 6 mm in animals of Beagle size. Its contours are less regular in phases of the estrous cycle in which large follicles or corpora lutea are present (Plate 7/*C,D*). The walls of the ovarian bursae of cats commonly contain conspicuously less fat than those of the bitch and the ovaries are consequently more immediately visible.

The ovaries lie close to, or even in contact with, the caudal poles of the kidneys; in conformity with the asymmetrical position of the kidneys the left ovary is set a little caudal to its fellow. Though most spays (the removal of ovaries and uterine horns; ovariohysterectomy) are now performed by midline incision, an alternative lateral approach is available and is quite often used in cats. The flank incision is made midway between the iliac crest and the last rib in the confident expectation that the ovary will be within easy reach. The right ovary is usually found dorsal or dorsolateral to the ascending colon, the left one between the dorsal extremity of the spleen and the descending colon. Lengthening of the attachments in older animals, especially those that have borne young, allows the ovaries a greater mobility.

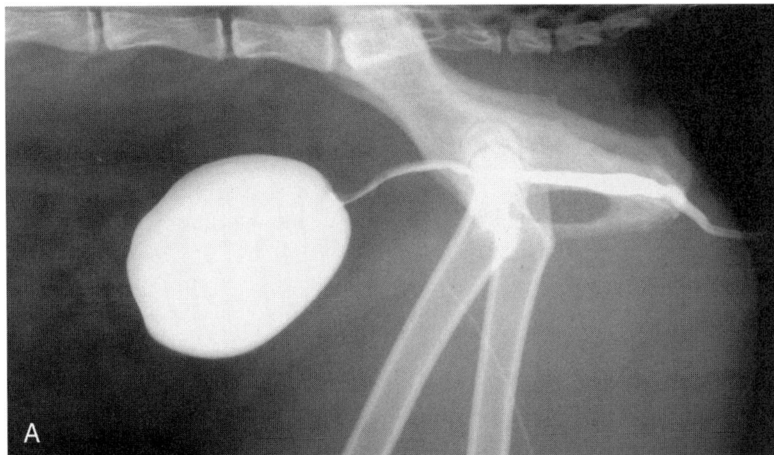


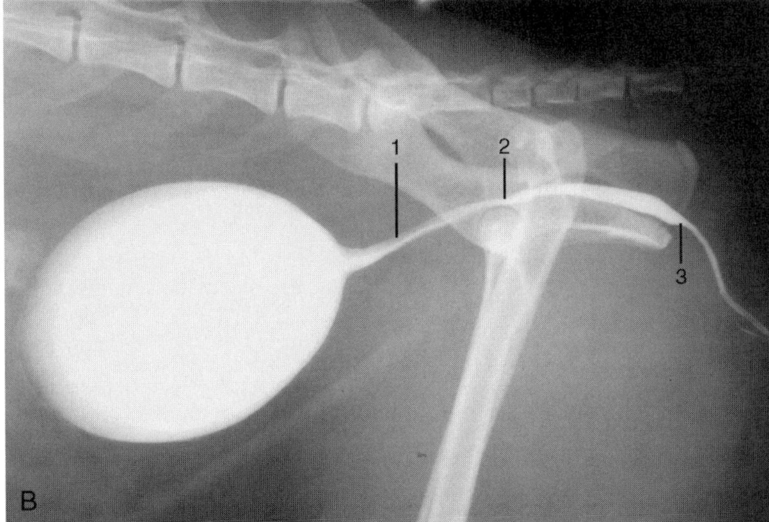


**Figure 15–6.** Radiographs of the feline bladder when moderately *(A)* and markedly *(B)* full.

1, Preprostatic urethra: the upper gray part is the urethral crest, the lower white part is the lumen filled with contrast medium; 2, slight dorsal dip marks the seminal colliculus; 3, isthmus, narrowing of lumen.

The ovary is fixed additionally by suspensory and proper ligaments. The former ligament is a peritoneal fold, thickened along its free margin, that attaches to the transverse fascia close to the last rib (Fig. 15–7/6); it is prolonged caudally as the proper ligament, which extends beyond the ovary to merge with the tip of the corresponding uterine horn. The anchorage provided by the suspensory ligament makes surgical exteriorization of the ovary difficult although its mobility is increased when the trunk is flexed ventrally.

The entrance to the ovarian bursa is reduced to a slit in the medial wall, which is usually made obvious by the protrusion of a few dark-hued infundibular fimbriae. The infundibulum is continued by the narrower part of the uterine tube, which is not obviously divided between ampulla and isthmus. These parts follow a tortuous course within the walls of the bursa; disregarding minor kinks and bends, the tube runs in a broad sweep that first passes forward in the distal mesovarium before crossing cranial to the ovary to continue caudally in the mesosalpinx (see Fig. 5–49). It ends in an abrupt junction with the horn of the uterus. Although in most subjects much of the tube is concealed by fat deposits, the terminal part is usually visible.

## The Uterus

*(See also pp. 195–196.)*

The uterus, which lies mainly dorsal to the small intestine, consists of a very short (ca. 2 to 3 cm) body from which two long and slender (ca. 12 × 1 cm) horns diverge (Fig. 15–7/8,7 and Plate 19/*G*). The body is near the pubic brim but may be

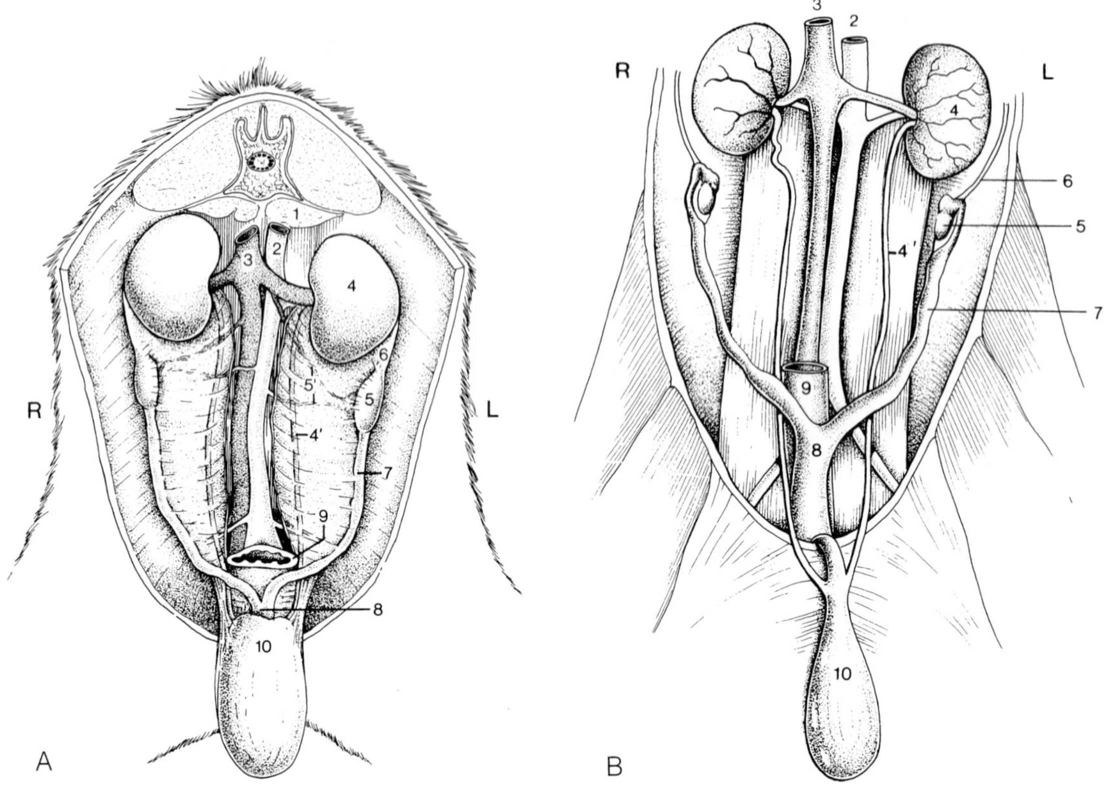


**Figure 15–7.** Canine *(A)* and feline *(B)* ovaries and uterus in situ, ventral view.

1, Psoas muscles; 2, aorta; 3, caudal vena cava; 4, 4′, left kidney and ureter; 5, ovary; 5′, ovarian vessels; 6, suspensory ligament of ovary; 7, uterine horn; 8, body of uterus; 9, rectum; 10, bladder, reflected caudally.

abdominal or pelvic in position. It is, in fact, even shorter than external inspection suggests since a short internal septum continues caudally from the junction of the horns. The cervix is also very short—the canal is barely 1 cm long—but the tissue thickening extends beyond the external ostium as a fold on the roof of the vagina (Fig. 15–8/3,3′). Transverse grooves frequently divide this fold into cranial, middle, and caudal tubercles; these become much swollen at certain stages of the cycle. The ostium of the cervix generally faces caudoventrally, and this orientation, combined with the asymmetry of the fornix and the fissuration of the cervical prolongation, may make its identification rather difficult, even with the aid of an endoscope.

The *broad ligaments* also commonly contain much fat. They are wider in their middle parts than toward their extremities and afford the horns of the uterus considerable mobility. An unusual feature is the detachment from the lateral surface of a peritoneal fold that extends toward, and in the bitch through, the inguinal canal to end variously between the groin and vulva. The fold is thickened at its free margin (the round ligament), and this slightly dilates the canal, predisposing to inguinal hernia, which is almost a male prerogative in other species. Since the uterine horn is the most likely organ to be herniated, the bizarre situation sometimes arises in which a portion of the pregnant uterus is trapped subcutaneously; a fetus developing in this situation must be delivered by separate section if the herniated part is not restored to the abdomen in good time.

The vascularization of the uterus depends on the branches of the ovarian artery and the uterine artery, a branch of the vaginal artery (Fig. 15–9/1,5). These vessels lie close to the extremities of the uterus but swing away in the intermediate part of the broad ligament. The proximity of the uterine artery to the cervix allows an arterial ligature to be securely anchored to the uterine stump to prevent slippage when the bulk of the uterus is removed surgically. Almost the entire uterus is drained by a large uterine branch of the ovarian vein.

## The Vagina, Vestibule, and Vulva

*(See also pp. 196–197.)*

The vagina is very long (ca. 12 cm) and extends horizontally through the pelvis before dipping beyond the ischial arch to join the vestibule (see Fig. 5–31/5,9). Apart from the prominent dorsomedian fold that continues the cervix for a short distance, the interior of the undistended organ is obstructed by the irregular folds into which the wall naturally falls. These end at the junction of the vagina with the vestibule (Fig. 15–8). The vestibule continues the downward slope of the vagina, which must be kept in mind when introducing a vaginal speculum or other instrument (see Fig. 5–2). This must be passed in a craniodorsal direction to clear the ischial arch before it can be advanced horizontally. During such examinations the dorsal fold combines with the lateral and ventral vaginal walls to simulate a cervix (pseudocervix).

The cranial part of the vestibular floor (of the bitch) displays the hummock and flanking depressions associated with the opening of the urethra, while the caudal part presents the fossa into which

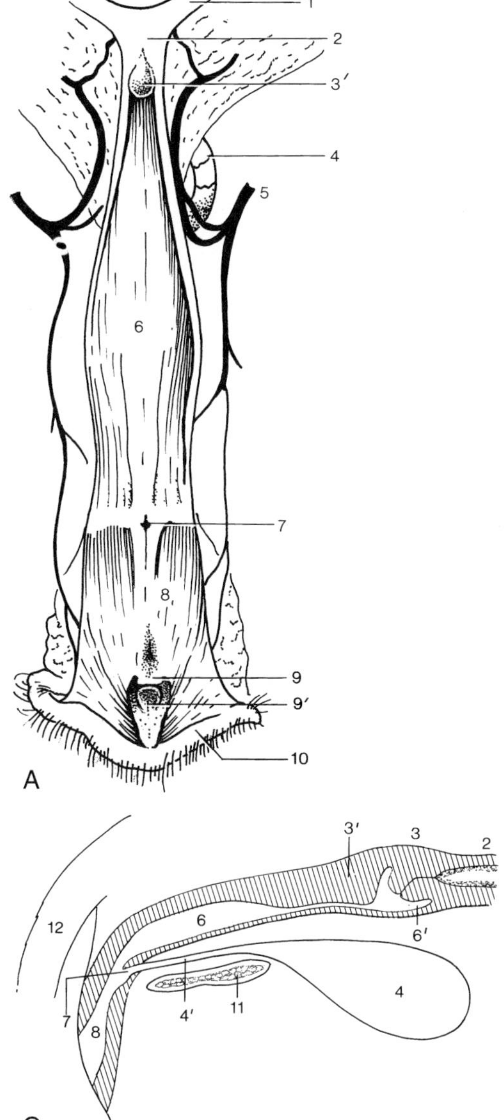


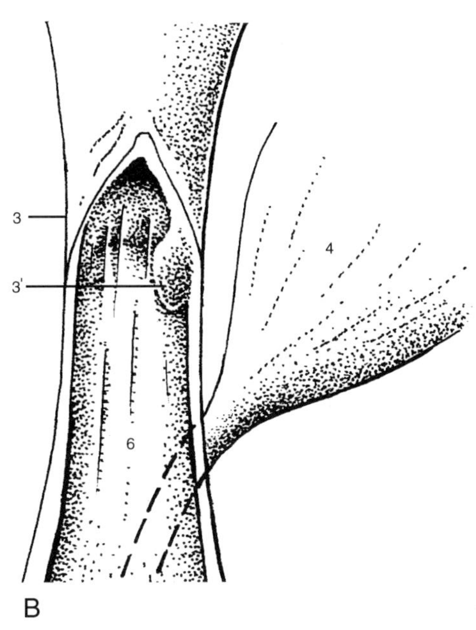


**Figure 15–8.** *A*, Canine vagina, vestibule, and vulva, opened dorsally. *B*, Enlarged view of the cervix. *C*, Schematic median section of the organs shown in *A*.

1, Right uterine horn; 2, body of uterus; 3, cervix; 3′, dorsal fold which may extend a considerable distance into the vagina; 4, bladder; 4′, urethra; 5, vaginal artery; 6, vagina; 6′, fornix; 7, external urethral orifice; 8, vestibule; 9, clitoris; 9′, clitoral fossa; 10, right labium of vulva; 11, pelvic symphysis; 12, tail.

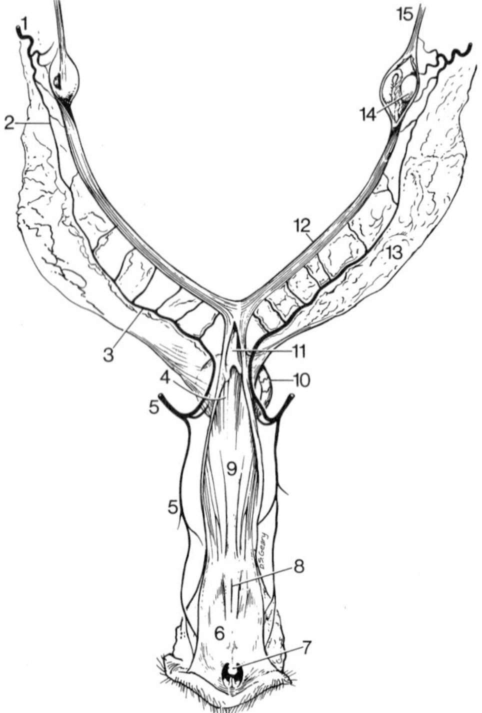


**Figure 15–9.** Blood supply of the reproductive organs of the bitch, dorsal view. The right ovarian bursa and the caudal parts of the tract have been opened.

1, Ovarian artery; 2, uterine branch of ovarian artery; 3, uterine artery; 4, dorsomedian fold continuing the cervix; 5, vaginal artery; 6, vestibule; 7, clitoris; 8, external urethral orifice; 9, vagina; 10, bladder; 11, cervix; 12, right uterine horn; 13, broad ligament; 14, right ovary; 15, suspensory ligament of ovary.

the glans of the clitoris projects (Fig. 15–8/9,9′). Darker patches of the lateral walls betray the positions of the vestibular bulbs, which are well developed in the bitch but slighter and more diffuse in the female cat. Vestibular glands are present only in the cat.

The thick labia of the vulva meet in a rounded dorsal and a pointed ventral commissure. More lateral folds that are sometimes apparent are believed to be homologous with the labia majora of human anatomy. The crura and body of the clitoris possess a little erectile tissue; the glans is largely of fatty fibrous tissue but sometimes contains a small bone, the os clitoridis.

## Functional Changes

It is often curtly stated that bitches come in heat twice a year—in spring and autumn. In fact, three heats are not uncommon, although even when this is so the greater part of the year is occupied by periods of anestrus. Cats are even less dependable in these matters, and even four cycles are possible in place of the usual two. The first heat occurs at the age of 6 to 9 months or thereabouts in bitches, and at 6 to 12 months in young queens depending on the season of their birth.

The reproductive organs, quiescent during anestrus, develop rapidly in proestrus when, over a period of a week, a batch of follicles enlarges. The uterus now increases in length and in thickness; its endometrium proliferates, and the entire reproductive tract becomes hyperemic. A thickened, edematous vulva discharges the serous uterine secretion, which is tinged with blood, the result of diapedesis from the widened endometrial vessels. Estrus also lasts about a week. The endometrial hypertrophy and hyperemia continue but the discharge gradually becomes less blood-stained. Ovulation, which occurs on about the second day, is succeeded by very rapid formation of corpora lutea, which may be mature by the end of estrus.* The separation of di- and metestrus is difficult to determine since there is often a period (2 to 8 weeks) of pseudopregnancy during which the bitch exhibits the usual physical and behavioral signs of pregnancy, even though fertilization has not occurred; pseudopregnancy can perhaps be likened to a greatly extended period of diestrus. The cervix is tightly closed during di- and metestrus, and secretions that would have been utilized for embryo nutrition then accumulate in amounts that may distend the uterus; infection often supervenes, producing a condition (pyometra) that may necessitate hysterectomy.

The responses of the vaginal epithelium to changes in hormonal levels are more pronounced than in other domestic species and smears taken from the vagina provide evidence of the stage within the cycle. Both cornified epithelial cells and erythrocytes are present in large numbers during proestrus, but while the former persist through estrus, the latter gradually become fewer as leukocytes begin to make a presence.

The stages of the cycle are also reflected in the gross appearance of the vaginal lining, including that covering the dorsomedian fold. In proestrus the lining becomes edematous and forms prominent soft folds. As estrogen levels drop rapidly during estrus, water is lost from the vaginal wall and the lining wrinkles until about 4 days after ovulation, when the surface resembles crepe paper. A few days later the mucosa becomes flat and

*Ovulation is not spontaneous in the cat but is induced by coitus.

patchy with the desquamation of the cornified superficial layer of epithelium; this allows the blood vessels to shine through once more.

Ova enter the uterus about the sixth day following their release. If fertilized, they implant after a further 10 days, and this delay allows them to find appropriately spaced stations. An omphalovitelline (yolk sac) attachment is first established but, though effective in early pregnancy, it is later supplanted by the definitive chorioallantoic placenta (Fig. 15–10/6). This develops through the invasion of the endometrium by villi growing from a broad band of the chorion encircling the trunk of the fetus, continuing a process of erosion begun earlier in the nonvascular (chorioamniotic) regions and about the yolk sac attachment. The erosion leads to the interdigitation of thin plates of fetal tissue, with endometrial lamellae reduced to little more than the maternal capillary endothelium (Plate 9/*F,G*). The tissue barrier of this basically chorioendothelial placenta is further reduced at the margins of the zonary band where blood extravasated from maternal vessels directly bathes the fetal tissue. Hemoglobin breakdown in these marginal hematomas is responsible for the brilliant green pigmentation that contrasts with the deep red

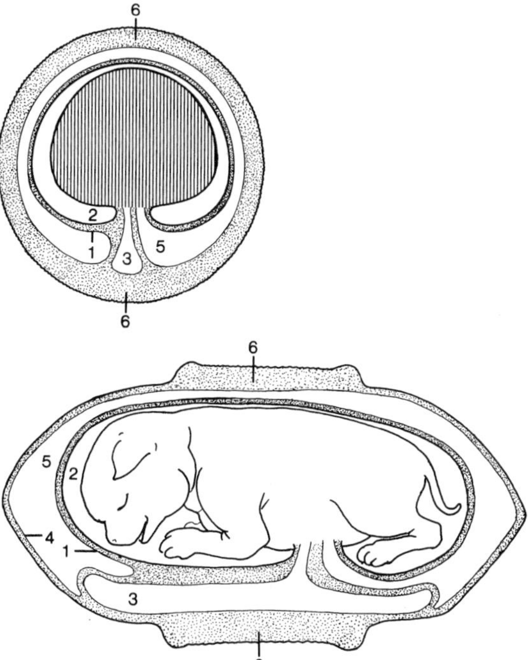


**Figure 15–10.** The feline fetal membranes in transverse and longitudinal section, schematic.

1, Amnion; 2, amniotic cavity; 3, yolk sac; 4, chorioallantois; 5, allantoic cavity; 6, zonary placenta.

of the major part of the placenta (Plate 8/*G*). Only a certain amount of the dam's antibodies penetrates the placenta; the greater share (about 75%) of the passive immunization of the newborn is dependent on the colostrum.

Initially the uterus enlarges locally, with each conceptus confined within a globular swelling that is bounded by regions of constriction. The separate ampullae persist until about the 40th day (in a gestation that averages 63 days, measured from the date of ovulation*) when there begins a gradual relaxation of the constrictions, eventually creating an almost uniformly expanded uterus. The positions of the individual fetuses are still obvious on inspection of the exposed organ since the whole thickness of the uterine wall is very vascular at the placental sites (Fig. 15–11/*A*). The uterine horns are relatively fixed at their extremities, and when they lengthen they are forced into loops that first bend cranially from the ovarian attachment before sweeping ventrally, then caudally, to join the body. The pattern of coiling is even more complicated when the litter is large, and radiographs obtained in later pregnancy (when there is mineralization of the fetal skeletons) sometimes show the puppies arranged in a confusing jumble (/*B*).

In the later stages of pregnancy such radiographs not only serve to determine the number of pups in the litter but also provide a means of assessing fetal age and thus predicting the date of parturition. Mineralization commences in the axial skeleton by about the 45th day, and is soon followed by the progressive mineralization of the appendicular skeleton in proximodistal sequence (Plate 10/*E–G*). Mineralization of the skeleton of kittens follows the same pattern but with each element making its appearance a few days earlier than in pups (Table 15–1).

Parturition is facilitated by pelvic rotation at the sacroiliac joints and by elevation of the tail, maneuvers that significantly increase the dimensions of the pelvis. In both dogs and cats some 60% to 80% of fetuses present the head toward the cervix, a bias that has yet to receive a satisfactory explanation of how it is achieved. Fetuses tend to be delivered from each horn in alternation and when each is delivered the emptied

*Successful service may precede or follow ovulation by an interval of several days, and gestation measured from the date of service consequently has the inconveniently wide range of 58 to 68 days. The practice—generally unavoidable—of measuring gestation in days after service explains the difficulty of precisely specifying the period of change in the form of the uterus or of specific development of the fetus. Prediction of the date of parturition in days subsequent to the appearance of certain features of skeletal mineralization is more exact.

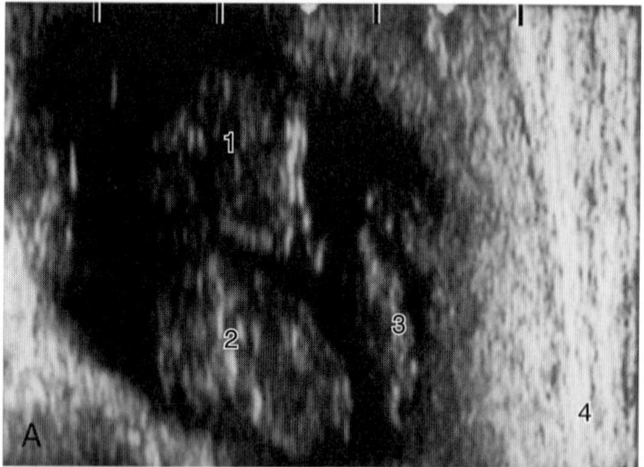


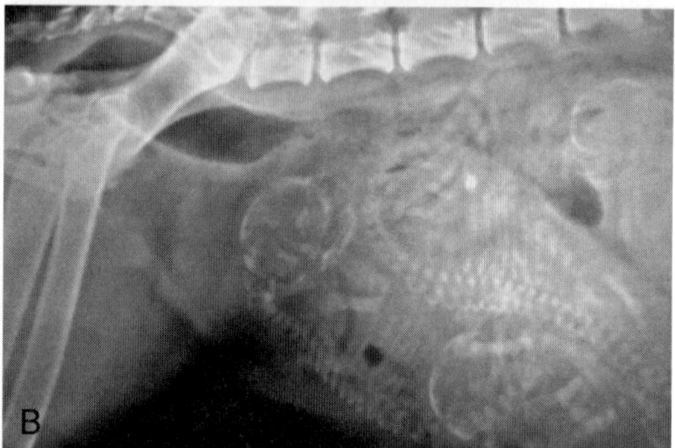


**Figure 15–11.** *A,* Ultrasonographic (transabdominal) view of a 33-day (after a single mating) Beagle fetus in its ampulla; the scale on top is in centimeters. *B,* Pregnant bitch with several almost full-term fetuses. Note the gas in the rectum.

1, Head of fetus; 2, thorax of fetus; 3, yolk sac; 4, uterine wall.

**Table 15–1.** Guide to the Mineralization of Dog Fetuses

| Days | Skeletal Elements |
|---|---|
| 45 | Skull, vertebrae, and ribs |
| 48 | Proximal long bones of limbs |
| 52 | Distal long bones of limbs |
| 54 | Pelvis |
| 60 | Minor bones of limbs |

Based on data from Concannon and Rendano, 1983; and Yaeger et al., 1992.

segment of the uterus contracts, bringing those littermates left behind closer to the exit. When expelled, each fetus is still attached to its placenta, from which it is freed by the dam's biting through the umbilical cord. The "afterbirth," with which considerable maternal tissue is shed, is normally consumed.

Although less often useful to the clinician, some information on the development of certain external features of fetuses will be found in Tables 15–2 and 15–3.

In recent years ultrasonography has provided an additional means of diagnosing pregnancy and predicting term. Its advantages and disadvantages for these purposes, when compared with radiography, are dependent to a large extent upon the stage

**Table 15–2.** Guide to the Aging of Dog Fetuses

| Weeks | Crown-Rump Length (cm) | External Features |
|---|---|---|
| 3 | ≈1 | Embryo C-shaped; limb buds forming |
| 4 | ≈2 | Hand plate present; shallow grooves between digits |
| 5 | ≈3 | Eyelids partly cover eye; pinna covers acoustic meatus; external genitalia differentiated; digits separated distally |
| 6 | ≈7 | Eyelids fused; hair follicles present on body; digits widely spread; claws formed |
| 7 | ≈11 | Hair almost completely covering body; color markings present |
| | | Full term: on average 63–64 days |

From Evans, H. E., and W. O. Sack: Prenatal development of domestic and laboratory animals. Growth curves, external features and selected references. Anat. Histol. Embryol. 2:11–45, 1973.

**Table 15–3.** Guide to the Aging of Cat Fetuses

| Weeks | Crown-Rump Length (cm) | External Features |
|---|---|---|
| 3 | ≈1 | Acoustic meatus forming; eye well formed and pigmented; forelimb hand plate notched |
| 4 | ≈3 | All digits widely spread; pinna almost covers acoustic meatus; claws forming; eyelids partly cover eyes |
| 5 | ≈5 | Eyelids fused; tactile hairs present on face |
| 6 | ≈7 | Fine hairs appearing on body; claws begin to harden |
| 7 | ≈10.5 | Fine hairs cover body; claws white and hard; color markings present |
| | | Full term: on average 65 days (counted from first mating) |

From Evans H. E., and W. O. Sack: Prenatal development of domestic and laboratory animals. Growth curves, external features and selected references. Anat. Histol. Embryol. 2:11–45, 1973.

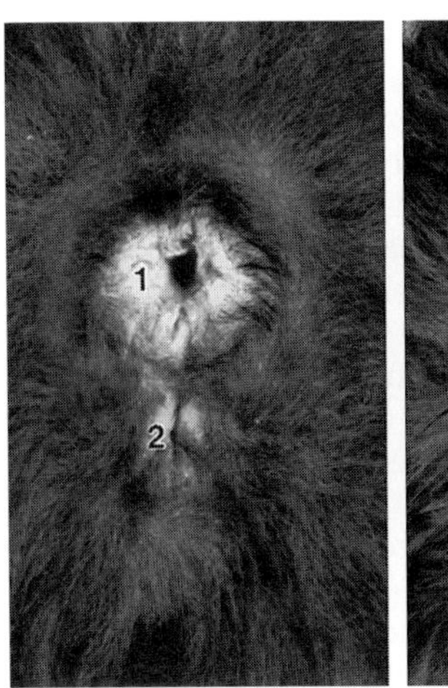


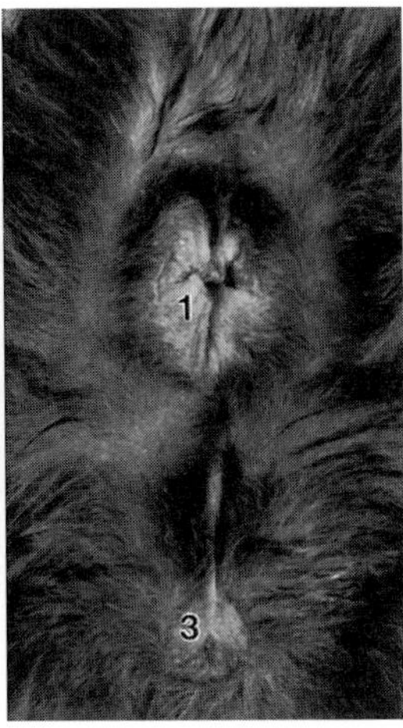


**Figure 15–12.** Perineum of 5-week-old littermate kittens.

1, Anus; 2, vulva; 3, prepuce.

of pregnancy when the examination is made. It has been claimed successful in recognizing uterine enlargement only a few days after fertilization; one report gives 4 days in a queen, 7 days in a bitch, but confident diagnosis requires a longer wait—perhaps till 25 days.

Potentially embarrassing mistakes in the determination of the sex of newborn kittens are relatively easily made. The difficulty arises from the orientation of the penis. This brings the anal and genital openings relatively close together in the tom, the spacing being inconveniently similar to that in the female (Fig. 15–12).

# THE MALE REPRODUCTIVE ORGANS

## The Scrotum and Testes

*(See also pp. 183–187.)*

The rather pendulous scrotum of the dog is globular and placed in a position intermediate between the perineum and the groin (Fig. 15–13/11). It is most easily inspected from behind and, since sparsely haired, its close molding upon the testes is obvious. A deep groove defines the boundary between the internal compartments occupied by the generally asymmetrical testes. The thin scrotal skin and underlying fasciae do not impede palpation, which normally allows recognition of the body and tail of the epididymis, the deferent duct, and the spermatic cord in addition to the testis itself. The scrotum of the cat is perineal, sessile, and commonly concealed by a dense covering of hair (Fig. 15–18/5).

The testes are relatively small in both species. They are carried horizontally in dogs but with their caudal extremities tipped toward the anus in cats. Each testis is roughly oval in outline, laterally compressed, and related to the epididymis along its dorsal (in cats, craniodorsal) margin. The head and tail of the epididymis adhere to the testis but the body is partly free, creating a testicular bursa. The constituents of the compact cord disperse at the internal inguinal ring. The canine deferent duct widens into a slight, glandular ampulla prior to penetrating the prostate before entering the urethra. There is no ampulla in the cat.

## The Urethra and Accessory Reproductive Glands

*(See also pp. 188–190.)*

The first part of the urethra of the dog is entirely surrounded by the prostate (see Fig. 5–1/9). Its lumen is indented by a dorsal ridge, locally raised to form a seminal colliculus that is perforated to each side by the narrow opening of the deferent duct and numerous pores that drain the prostate. The remaining part of the pelvic urethra is provided with a thin sleeve of cavernous tissue

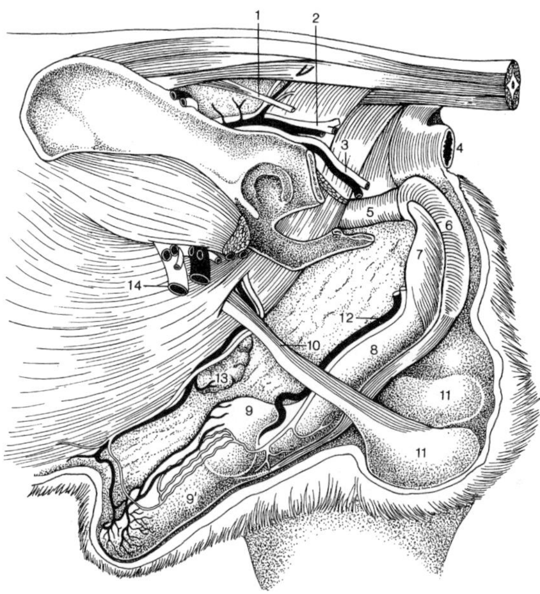


**Figure 15–13.** Deep dissection of the external reproductive organs of the dog.

1, Sacrotuberous ligament; 2, caudal gluteal vessels; 3, internal pudendal vessels; 4, anus; 5, pelvic urethra; 6, bulb of penis enclosed by bulbospongiosus; 7, ischiocavernosus over left crus; 8, body of penis; 9, 9′, bulbus and pars longa glandis; 10, spermatic cord; 11, testes in scrotum; 12, dorsal artery and vein of the penis; 13, superficial inguinal lymph nodes and caudal superficial epigastric vessels; 14, femoral vessels.

within the striated urethralis. The urethral lumen widens caudal to the prostate but narrows again at its exit from the pelvis over the ischial arch. The radiographic appearance of the above urethral features is shown in Figure 15–6/1,2,3 for the cat.

The ampullary glands and prostate provide the entire complement of accessory sex glands in the dog. The cat, which lacks ampullary glands, has small bulbourethral glands located on the urethra level with the ischial arch, but these are of very slight importance. In both species the prostate contributes the bulk of the seminal fluid; it comprises a large compact mass about the urethra and neck of the bladder, and a small disseminate part spread within the urethral mucosa. The compact part varies greatly in size, and this obviously affects its position and relations. It may be within the pelvic cavity when small, but more usually it is mainly if not entirely intra-abdominal in mature and older dogs (Fig. 15–14/2). A dorsal groove and internal septum divide it into right and left lobes, which are subdivided into lobules by finer septa that radiate outward to the capsule. The prostate is extremely sensitive to hormonal influences, and it is difficult to suggest normal dimensions since hyperplasia of the parenchymatous part commonly develops in early middle age, while fibrosis and shrinkage are common senile changes. The hyperplasia sometimes affects the different lobes unequally. An enlarged prostate may press on the large intestine, producing constipation and difficulties in defecation but, in contrast to the human experience, interference with micturition is unusual unless the condition is very gross. The state of the prostate—its size, firmness, and regularity of form—may be assessed by digital examination per rectum, a procedure facilitated by pushing the bladder toward the pelvis by pressure through the abdominal wall. The proportions of parenchyma and supporting tissue may be estimated from gross sections of autopsy specimens; connective tissue normally predominates in the prostate of the very young, glandular tissue in those from animals in their prime, while the relationship is inconstant in the glands of aged dogs. It has been reported that the prostate is proportionately much larger (by a factor of four) in the Scottish terrier than in other breeds.

Enlargement of the prostate is sometimes treated by castration. Alternatively, or if castration fails, surgical removal may be performed. It is then relevant to note that generally only the craniodorsal aspect of the gland has a peritoneal covering and that the lateral aspect is crossed by certain vessels and nerves that must be spared. The trunk of the prostatic artery continues over the gland as the supply to the bladder after detaching prostaticovesical and prostaticourethral branches. The other structure at risk is the plexus formed by the pelvic and hypogastric autonomic nerves.

In the cat the neck of the bladder is carried forward into the abdomen, and a relatively long preprostatic part of the urethra intervenes between this region and the prostate (Fig. 15–6). The prostatic part of the urethra is slightly constricted, and enclosed by the gland on all but its ventral side. Beyond the prostate, the urethra widens before narrowing on leaving the pelvis and becoming incorporated in the penis. It is narrowest just before opening to the exterior at the tip of the glans where urinary calculi, a frequent affliction of male cats, are often held up.

Little is known of age changes to the prostate of this species in which enlargement is a much less frequently encountered problem (Fig. 15–18/8).

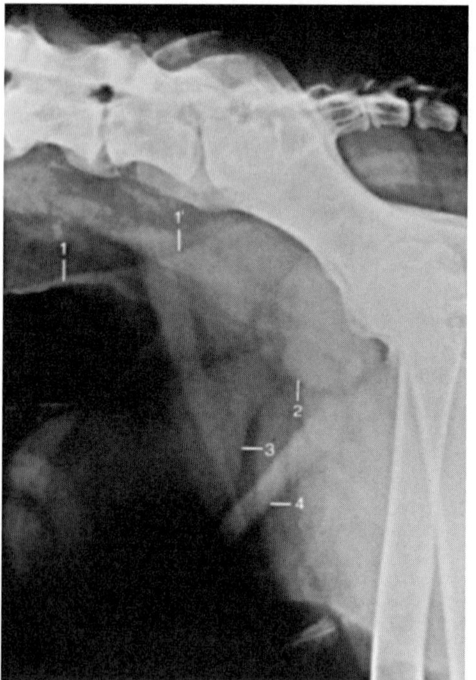


**Figure 15–14.** Lateral radiographic view of the canine caudal abdomen to show the position of the prostate.

1, 1′, Descending colon containing gas and feces; 2, prostate; 3, bladder; 4, abdominal floor.

## The Penis and Prepuce

*(See also pp. 190–191.)*

The penis of carnivores presents several unusual features, while additional differences between the organs of the dog and cat make separate description necessary.

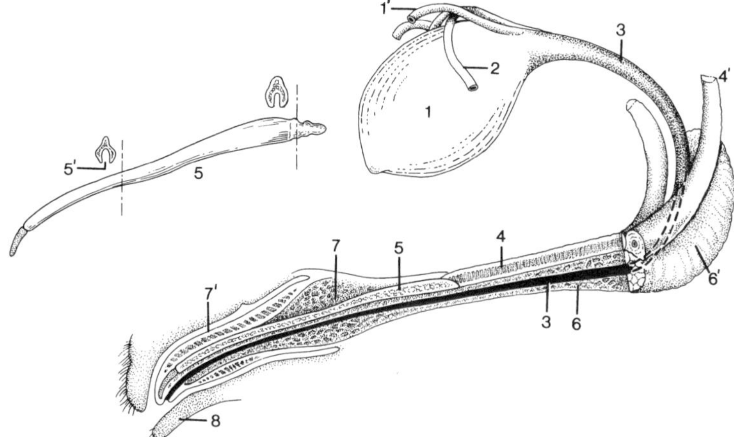


**Figure 15–15.** Canine bladder, urethra, and penis (in section).

1, Bladder; 1′, left ureter; 2, left deferent duct; 3, urethra; 4, corpus cavernosum; 4′, left crus; 5, os penis; 5′, urethral groove; 6, corpus spongiosum; 6′, bulb of penis; 7, bulbus glandis; 7′, pars longa glandis; 8, prepuce.

The penis of the dog is slung between the thighs, where it may be palpated along its whole length. The root is formed of two slender crura that arch forward from their ischial attachments to combine in a common body that is little stouter than either contributor (Fig. 15–15/4′). The urethra is incorporated at the same level and runs forward on the ventral surface of the body (/3); its erectile investment expands to form the glans, which is unusually extensive and clearly divided, both externally and internally, into a proximal expanded part (bulbus glandis; /7) and a distal cylindrical part (pars longa glandis; /7′), which provides the apex of the entire organ. About half the bulbus and the whole pars longa project into the preputial cavity, where they may be palpated. The proximal part of the body forms a corpus cavernosum (/4) with a tough outer fibrous covering and a substantial median septum; these give rise to radial trabeculae that divide and enclose relatively meager cavernous spaces. The corpus cavernosum comes to a premature end since its distal part is converted into a bone, the os penis, within the core of the organ (/5). This bone is grooved ventrally for the reception and protection of the urethra within its spongy covering; the bone tapers toward its distal extremity, which is prolonged by a short, ventrally deflected rod of fibrocartilage that reaches almost to the very apex of the penis. The fibrocartilage remains unossified even in aged animals. The partial enclosure of the urethra within the groove of the os penis impedes the passage of urethral calculi, which therefore tend to lodge at the caudal end of the bone.

The caudal (or proximal) part of the glans penis, the bulbus glandis, is considerably expanded, even in the quiescent state. It is firmly anchored to the bone and considerably overlapped by the elongated distal division, which presents the urethral orifice toward its tip. The pars longa is more loosely attached to the bone. Both contain

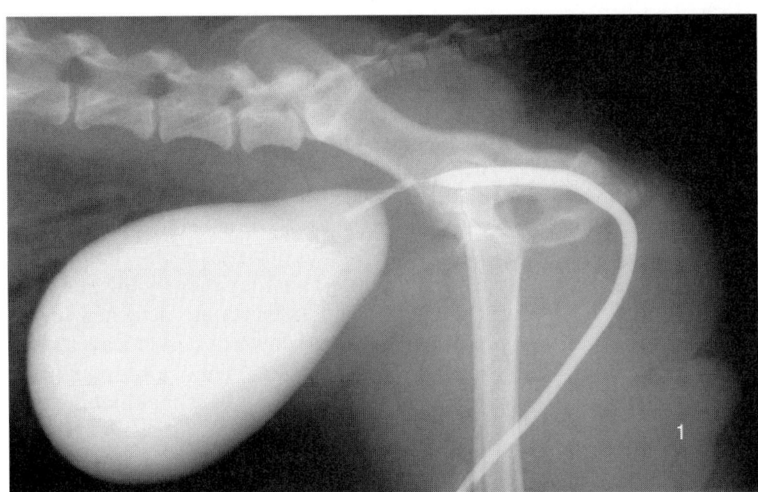


**Figure 15–16.** Contrast medium in the male canine bladder and urethra. The prostatic urethra appears to be less distensible.

1, Scrotum.

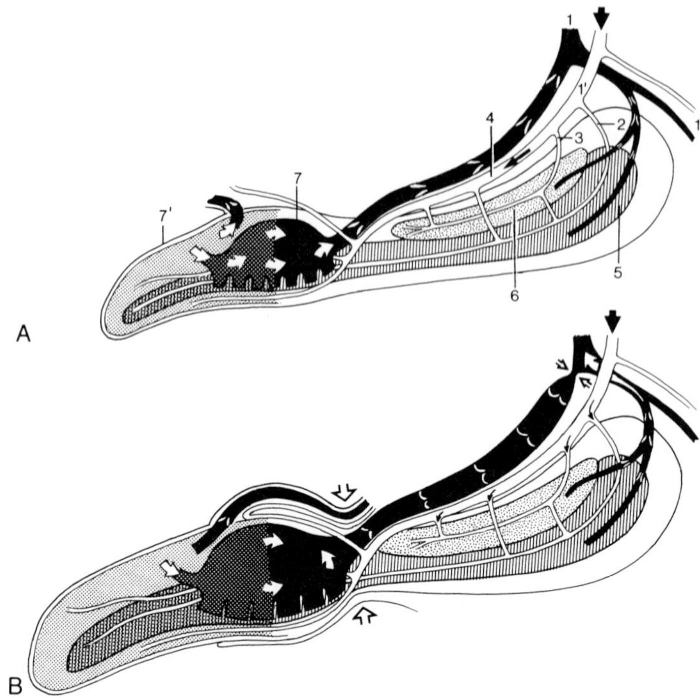


**Figure 15–17.** Schematic representation of the blood supply and the blood spaces of the quiescent *(A)* and erect *(B)* canine penis.

1, Internal pudendal vessels; 1′, artery of the penis; 1″, perineal branches; 2, artery of the bulb; 3, deep artery of the penis; 4, dorsal artery of the penis; 5, corpus spongiosum; 6, corpus cavernosum; 7, bulbus glandis; 7′, pars longa glandis.

large blood spaces enclosed by relatively weak trabeculae.

The structure and connections of the various erectile bodies and their relationships to the supplying and draining vessels require close attention if the mechanism of erection is to be understood (Fig. 15–17 and Plate 20/*A–F*). The penis is supplied by the continuation (beyond the origin of its perineal branch) of the internal pudendal artery, which now becomes the artery of the penis (/1′). The artery of the penis divides into three. One division, the artery of the bulb (/2), supplies the bulb (of the penis) and then runs distally within the organ to supply the corpus spongiosum about the urethra and later, on approaching the apex of the penis, the elongated portion of the glans. The second, the deep artery of the penis (/3), supplies several branches to both the tissues and the blood spaces of the corpus cavernosum. The third, the dorsal artery of the penis (/4), may be regarded as the direct continuation of the main trunk; it first runs on the dorsal aspect of the penis before sinking to the side prior to dividing close to the caudal limit of the bulbus; a superficial branch runs almost to the tip of the organ below the skin over the ventral aspect of the glans; a deep branch penetrates the bulbus to run apically on the os penis to enter the pars longa; a preputial branch forks into a division that runs over the dorsal aspect of the bulbus to supply the dorsal aspect of the pars longa and the prepuce.

The veins are broadly satellite to the arteries. The dorsal vein leaves the lateral aspect of the bulbus and runs caudally, gradually shifting toward the dorsal aspect of the penis, where it is joined by a common trunk formed of the veins corresponding to the deep artery and that of the bulb. The augmented dorsal vein then bends around the ischial arch to enter the pelvis, where it provides the main radicle of the internal pudendal vein. Other veins assist in the drainage of the glans. A superficial vein leaves the pars longa to wind around the fornix of the prepuce before joining the external pudendal vein. A deep vein within the glans drains blood from the pars longa to the bulbus; it is valved so that reflux of blood is impossible and is so arranged that it may either provide a through passage to the dorsal vein or open into the blood spaces of the bulbus, from which the blood then enters the dorsal vein.

The usual muscles are present. The retractor, largely composed of smooth muscle, loops to the side of the anal canal before converging on its fellow to form a band that runs along the urethral aspect of the penis to a termination by the preputial fornix. A few small fascicles are detached to the scrotum. Short but powerful ischiocavernosus muscles cover the crura. The bulbospongiosus forms a transverse covering over the urethra from the bulb to its incorporation in the penis. A small ischiourethralis passes from the ischial tuber to a fibrous ring that encloses the dorsal veins at their entry to the pelvis. The two large muscles at the root of the penis can be identified on palpation (Fig. 15–13/7,6).

The prepuce of the dog is rather pendulous toward its cranial extremity, where it is suspended below the abdomen by a fold of skin. It has a simple arrangement and the parietal part of its lining is studded with lymph nodules, which give it a rather irregular appearance. There are also small scattered preputial glands. Paired preputial muscles, detachments from the cutaneous trunci, run from the abdominal floor to meet and partially decussate in the skin of the prepuce caudal to the T-shaped orifice. Congenital or acquired narrowing of the preputial orifice may prevent protrusion of the penis (phimosis). Those acquired cases that are due to scar formation following an earlier inflammation may be treated surgically. The wisdom of surgical intervention may be questioned when the defect is congenital and possibly hereditary. Paraphimosis, in which the erect penis is unable to subside and be withdrawn into the prepuce, requires more urgent attention since the interruption of the circulation may cause tissue death within hours.

The *penis of the cat* is unique (among domestic species) in retaining the embryonic position in which the apex is directed caudoventrally and the urethral surface is uppermost (Fig. 15–18/6 and Plate 20/*H*). It is relatively much shorter than the penis of the dog but has a similar construction, including the transformation of the distal part of the corpus cavernosum into bone. The glans, however, is small, and its free surface is generously ornamented with small, keratinized spines in the tom; these develop during the first few months of postnatal life and regress to a very insignificant state in castrated animals (Figs. 15–19 and 15–20). The prepuce is thick but short and often much obscured by hair; its orifice faces caudally and urine is ejected in this direction. The spraying of urine by the tom is a social gesture marking territory (Plate 20/*G*). The sites are not always discreetly chosen and are often inconvenient to the owner, providing one reason for the common practice of castration.*

## Age and Functional Changes

Although there has been little detailed study of the postnatal development, it is known that the testes remain within the abdomen until about the third day after birth. Their descent through the inguinal canal then commences and, while it is completed within a couple of days, another 4 or 5 weeks are required before the testes occupy their definitive positions within the scrotum. The seminiferous tissue increases markedly in volume during this time, but spermatogenesis does not begin until about the sixth month. Since the testes attain their definitive locations so precociously, some have advocated castration of male kittens at much younger ages—6 to 14 weeks—than the 5 or 6 months conventionally adopted. It is claimed that

*Queens also sometimes spray, though generally they squat when passing urine, which they then seek to conceal by scratching dirt over it. It seems that spraying by females is most often performed far from home, at the bounds of a territory disputed with other cats; it is, in consequence, less commonly objectionable to the householder. In both sexes, the practice may have sexual connotations.

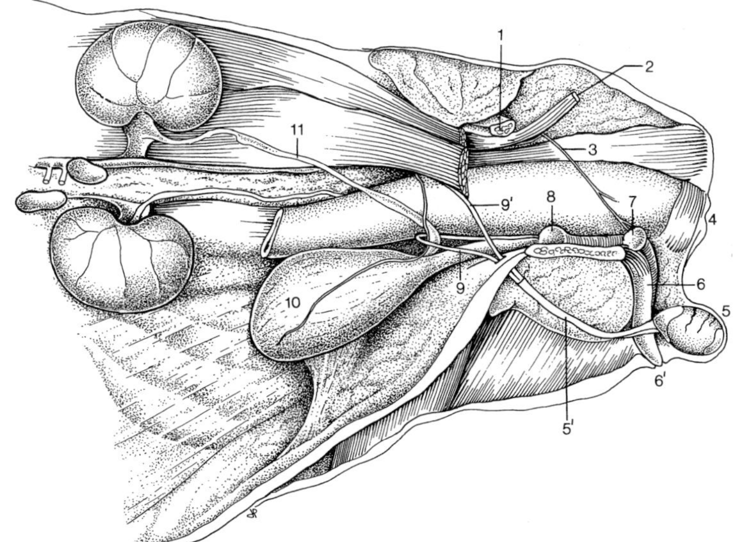


**Figure 15–18.** The reproductive organs of the tomcat in situ, left lateral view.

1, Shaft of ilium; 2, sciatic nerve; 3, pudendal nerve; 4, anus; 5, left testis in scrotum; 5′, spermatic cord; 6, penis; 6′, prepuce; 7, bulbourethral gland; 8, prostate; 9, deferent duct; 9′, testicular vessels; 10, bladder; 11, left ureter.

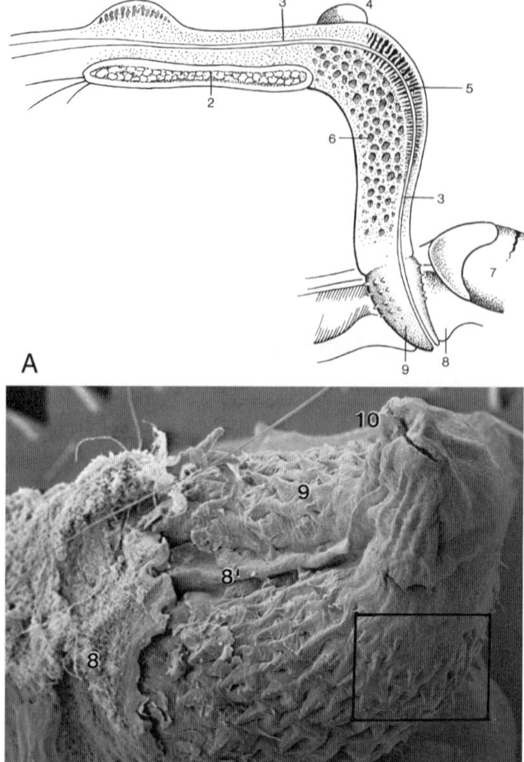


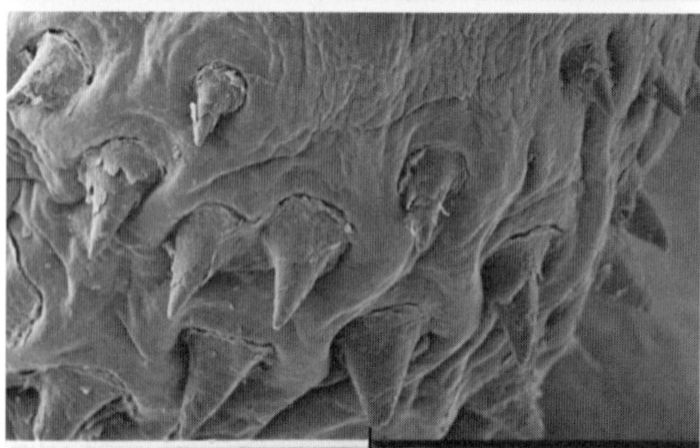

**Figure 15–19.** *A,* Median section of the feline penis, left lateral view. *B,* Scanning electron micrograph of a feline glans, and enlargement of the marked area (bar = 1 mm).

1, Prostate; 2, pelvic symphysis; 3, urethra; 4, right bulbourethral gland; 5, corpus spongiosum; 6, corpus cavernosum; 7, right testis; 8, prepuce; 8′, preputial frenulum; 9, glans (with spines); 10, external urethral orifice.

the operation is well tolerated by these very young animals.*

The mating behavior of dogs is most unusual. The dog mounts the bitch in the usual way but shortly after intromission he drops to her side and reverses so that the pair stand rear to rear during the remainder of the "tie" which may last for a further 45 minutes or even longer. There has been surprisingly little consideration of the anatomy of this process; the present account rests heavily upon the description by Grandage (1972!).

Although all erectile tissues of the penis become engorged when erection is complete, they attain very different degrees of expansion and turgidity (Plate 20/*A–C,F*). The corpus cavernosum swells least, and its construction allows it to remain flexible about a vertical, though not about a horizontal, axis even in this state. The bulbus glandis is most capable of expansion and swells to twice its resting thickness, becoming very tense in the process. The pars longa stiffens least but elongates considerably, which causes it to slide apically on the os penis to which it is only loosely attached; it then extends well beyond the fibrocartilaginous extension of the bone and presents an indentation about the urethral orifice in consequence of the tighter anchorage of this part.

Intromission necessarily occurs before the penis is markedly enlarged (Plate 20/*D,E*). The labia thrust the prepuce caudally when the dog mounts

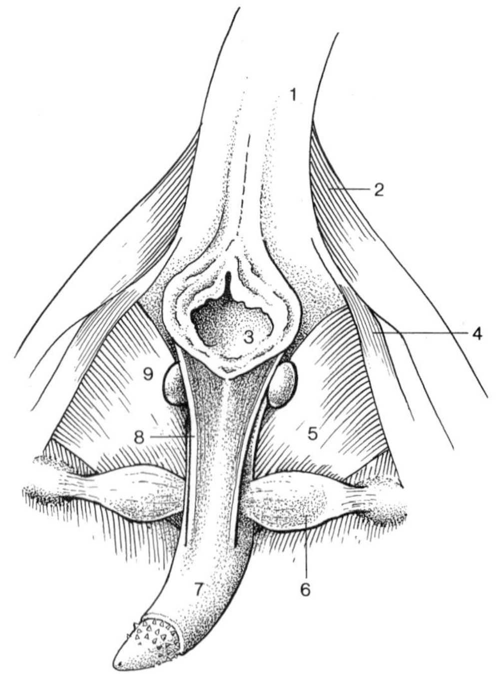


**Figure 15–20.** Feline penis in situ, caudal view.

1, Tail (raised); 2, gluteofemoralis; 3, anus; 4, coccygeus; 5, internal obturator; 6, ischiocavernosus; 7, penis; 8, left retractor penis; 9, left bulbourethral gland.

*It is also claimed that female kittens can be spayed at the same early age without unacceptably greater risk. Humane societies tend to be the strongest advocates of early neutering, before kittens are adopted by their permanent owners, since this avoids unwanted pregnancies with the inevitable consequence of abandoned animals contributing to feral populations.

and introduces the glans into the vagina. The slope of the female passage requires a dorsocranial penetration and the relatively soft tip of the glans is diverted ventrally by its impingement (through the soft tissues) on the pelvic roof. This deflection allows the penis to be advanced toward the fornix and perhaps explains the necessity for the softer nature of the pars longa and the early termination of its bony support. When the stud dog dismounts and turns through 180 degrees, the body of the penis is bent laterally and then caudally; withdrawal of the penis is prevented by the swollen bulbus glandis and the grip exerted on it by the engorged vestibular bulbs and muscles associated with the female tract. The reversal of position twists the prepuce, tightening the preputial muscles into a cord that presses on the veins draining the glans. The dorsal veins of the penis, buckled by the flexion of the penis, are further obstructed by being pressed against the ischial arch by the contraction of the ischiourethralis. Detumescence is probably eventually achieved by relaxation of the bulbospongiosus, which allows the spaces within the corpus spongiosum to provide alternative channels for the escape of blood from the engorged penis.

The initial, sperm-rich fraction of the ejaculate is discharged during the first stage of coitus when the dog is mounted in the fashion conventional for quadrupeds. The second stage is occupied in pumping out the much larger fraction—perhaps 30 mL—provided by the prostate; the tide sweeps the sperm-rich part through the cervix into the body of the uterus. It is known that short matings—in which only first-stage coitus occurs—may be fertile.

The *penis of the cat* increases considerably in length on erection and then curves downward and forward. This change in orientation, allied to a ventral flexion of the pelvic region, enables coitus to be performed in a fashion not greatly different from that usual in quadrupeds (Plate 17/*H*).

## THE ANATOMY OF ABDOMINAL AND RECTAL PALPATION

A number of abdominal organs may be identified and assessed by palpation through the abdominal wall. The procedure is most rewarding in cats and small dogs, and least rewarding in large well-muscled or obese dogs. An initial examination is usually performed with the subject standing and the converged, extended fingers of the examiner's hands placed over the flanks. For some purposes it is helpful to have the cranial part of the body raised, allowing the intrathoracic abdominal organs to slide caudally, and for others to have the subject laterally recumbent or supine. A one-handed approach, with the converged fingers opposed to the thumb, is useful with cats and small dogs. Whatever the technique, it is important to allay anxiety so that the animal relaxes its abdominal muscles; the recti then form a thick ventral median band, which may be initially disconcerting.

The normal *liver* projects only slightly, and variably, behind the costal arches and is difficult if not impossible to recognize using the bilateral approach. Greater success may be obtained if the fingertips are insinuated deep to the costal arch—a liberty permitted only when the flank muscles are fully relaxed. It may then be possible to identify the sharp free margin and narrow adjoining strip of the liver. The empty *stomach* is tucked under the ribs, out of reach on the left side, but when full of ingesta or distended with gas, it projects behind the costal cartilages. It is more easily found in narrow, deep-chested dogs than in those in which the trunk is barrel-shaped. The *spleen* occupies the same region against the left flank, but since its usual consistency is soft and deformable, it is not easily appreciated unless considerably enlarged and firmed.

Success in locating the *kidneys* is rather unpredictable in the dog. Most often only the caudal pole of the left kidney is within reach when it may be identified by its firm, rounded contours. The right kidney is commonly inaccessible. In some dogs, generally of the larger breeds, the left kidney is pendulous and "floats" at a more ventral level than usual; this is the normal condition in the cat, in which both kidneys can generally be found and may be steadied through the abdominal wall for biopsy puncture. The entire surface of a "floating" kidney, including the depression at the dorsally facing hilus, may be examined. As already remarked, the cat's bladder is located more cranially than that of the dog, well forward of the pubic brim.

The fluctuating *intestinal mass* occupies a large part of the abdomen, extending from the roof to the floor, and from one flank to the other. Identification of most individual parts is problematical. The descending duodenum may sometimes be identified on the right side if the fingers are first pressed against the abdominal roof and then drawn laterally. There is no difficulty in finding the jejunum, whose coils may be made to slip between the hands. In the dog the only part of the large intestine that may be sought with confidence is the descending colon on the left side. It is most readily identified when occupied by a column of hard or granular feces. The ascending colon and cecum may sometimes be identified, most readily when gas-distended, but the transverse colon is too deeply tucked under the ribs to be within reach. All parts of the large intestine are more readily found in cats, in which a useful guide to the positions of the cecum and ascending colon is provided by the firmness at the ileocecocolic junction. The lymph nodes associated with the intestine evade detection unless enlarged.

The *bladder* can be found extending forward from the pubic brim; when grossly distended it lies over a large part of the abdominal floor. Micturition may be induced by gentle compression through the abdominal wall—a procedure not free from risk if performed incautiously. The *prostate,* notoriously variable in size and position (p. 446), may sometimes be palpated between the pubic brim and the bladder.

The empty *uterus* cannot normally be palpated. The gravid uterus is readily identified at certain stages of pregnancy by its beaded form or general enlargement, or through the recognition of individual fetuses. The separate loculi (p. 443) within which the embryos initially develop reach a maximal size (ca. 15 mm) about the beginning of the sixth week (bitch), but this stage is soon followed by that in which the horns are uniformly swollen. A little later individual fetuses may be palpated, although it is not always possible to make an exact count when the litter is large.

*Digital examination* per rectum, a procedure possible only in subjects of a certain size, may provide some additional information. In addition to revealing the tone of the anal sphincter and the condition of the rectum and its mucosa, digital examination may be used to explore the pelvic skeleton for evidence of fracture or deformity. The anal sacs may be palpated and their content expressed with the aid of a finger within the rectum. The only other visceral organs that may usually be examined are the urethra and the prostate in the male, and the vagina in the female. Evaluation of the prostate requires consideration of its size, consistency, and symmetry. In large dogs the gland may be out of reach, but the prostate and the neck of the bladder may be made more accessible by coordinating the rectal examination with manipulation of the abdomen to press the caudal abdominal contents toward the pelvic entrance.

The *superficial inguinal ring* may be located in the laterally recumbent animal; the spermatic cord may then be traced toward the scrotum in the male. The location of the ring is determined by its relationship to the tense medial crus of the ring, which may be traced over the abdominal wall from the origin of the pectineus muscle (which forms the conspicuous swelling on the medial surface of the thigh). The superficial inguinal lymph nodes lie a little cranial to the ring. They are contained within the fold of skin that supports the prepuce in the male but are more difficult to find in the bitch, especially the parous bitch, since they lie deep to the inguinal mammary gland.

## Selected Bibliography


Ackerman, N.: Radiographic evaluation of the uterus: A review. Vet. Radiol Ultrasound 22:252–257, 1981.

Allen, W.E., and C. France: A contrast radiographic study of the vagina and uterus of the normal bitch. J. Small Anim. Pract. 26:153–166, 1985.

Aronsohn, M.G., and A.L. Fagella: Surgical techniques for neutering 6- to 14-week-old kittens. JAVMA 202:53–55, 1993.

Basinger, R.R., and C.A. Rawlings: Surgical management of prostatic diseases. Compend. Contin. Educ. Pract. Vet. 9:993–1000, 1987.

Baumans, V., G. Dijkstra, and C.J.G. Wensing: Testicular descent in the dog. Zentralbl. Vet. Med. C. 10:97–110, 1981.

Boyd, J.S.: Color Atlas of Clinical Anatomy of the Dog and Cat. St. Louis, Mosby–Year Book, 1991.

Cartee, R.A., P.F. Rumph, D.C. Kenter, et al.: Evaluation of drug-induced prostatic involution in dogs by transabdominal B-mode ultrasonography. Am J. Vet. Res. 51:1773–1778, 1990.

Christensen, G.C.: Angioarchitecture of the canine penis and the process of erection. Am. J. Anat. 95:227–262, 1954.

Concannon, P., and V. Rendano: Radiographic diagnosis of canine pregnancy: Onset of fetal skeletal radiopacity in relation to times of breeding, preovulatory leuteinizing hormone release, and parturition. Am. J. Vet. Res. 44:1506–1512, 1983.

Dean, P.W., C.S. Hedlund, D.D. Lewis, and M.J. Bojrab: Canine urethrotomy and urethrostomy. Compend. Contin. Educ. Pract. Vet. 12:1541–1554, 1990.

Del Campo, C.H., and O.J. Ginther: Arteries and veins of uterus and ovaries in dogs and cats. Am. J. Vet. Res. 35:409–415, 1974.

deLahunta, A., and R.E. Habel: Applied Veterinary Anatomy. Philadelphia, W.B. Saunders Company, 1986.

England, G.C.W., and W.E. Allen: Studies on canine pregnancy using B-mode ultrasound: Diagnosis of early pregnancy and the number of conceptuses. J. Small. Anim. Pract. 31:321–323, 1990.

England, G.C.W., W.E. Allen, and D.J. Porter: Studies on canine pregnancy using B-mode ultrasound: Development of the conceptus and determination of gestational age. J. Small Anim. Pract. 31:324–329, 1990.

Evans, H.E.: Miller's Anatomy of the Dog, 3rd ed. Philadelphia, W.B. Saunders Company, 1993.

Griffin, D.W., C.R. Gregory, and R.L. Kitchell: Preservation of striated-muscle urethral sphincter function with use of a surgical technique for perineal urethrostomy in cats. JAVMA 194:1057–1060, 1989.

Grandage, J.: The erect dog penis: A paradox of flexible rigidity. Vet. Rec. 91:141–147, 1972.

Gunn-Moore, D.A., P.J. Brown, P.E. Holt, and T.J. Gruffydd-Jones: Priapism in seven cats. J. Small Anim. Pract. 36:262–266, 1995.

Habel, R.E.: Uterine tube more appropriate term for mammals [letter]. Amer. J. Vet. Res. 58 no 1 (1997):4

Hosgood, G., and C.S. Hedlund: Perineal urethrostomy in cats. Compend. Contin. Educ. Pract. Vet. 14:1195–1207, 1992.

Hudson, L.C., and W.P. Hamilton: Atlas of Feline Anatomy for Veterinarians. Philadelphia, W.B. Saunders Company, 1993.

Janssens, L.A.A., and G.H.R.R. Janssens: Bilateral flank ovariectomy in the dog—surgical technique and in 72 animals. J. Small Anim. Pract. 32:249–252, 1991.

Johnston, G.R., Feeney, D.A., and C.A. Osborne: Urethrography and cystography in cats. I. Technique, radiographic anatomy, and artifacts. Compend. Contin. Educ. Pract. Vet. 4:823–835, 1982.

Johnston, G.R., Osborne, C.A., and C.R. Jessen: Effects of urinary bladder distention on the length of the dog and cat urethra. Am. J. Vet. Res. 46:509–512, 1985.

Johnston, G.R., C.A. Osborne, C.R. Jessen, and D.A. Feeney: Effects of urinary bladder distention on location of the urinary bladder and urethra of healthy dogs and cats. Am. J. Vet. Res. 47:404–415, 1986.

Komtebedde, J., and J. Hauptman: Bilateral ischiocavernosus myectomy for chronic urine spraying in castrated male cats. Vet. Surg. 19:293–296, 1990.

MacDonald, D.W.: Carnivores. *In* Brown, R.E., and D.W. MacDonald: Social Odours in Mammals. Oxford, Clarendon Press, 1985.

Mann, F.A., D.J. Nonneman, E.R. Pope, et al.: Androgen receptors in the pelvic diaphragm muscles of dogs with and without perineal hernia. Am. J. Vet. Res. 56:134–139, 1995.

Mattiesen, D.T.: Diagnosis and management of complications occurring after perineal herniorrhaphy in dogs. Compend. Contin. Educ. Pract. Vet. 11:797–822, 1989.

Ninomiya, H., T. Nakamura, I. Niizuma, and T. Tsuchiya: Penile vascular system of the dog, an injection-corrosion and histological study. Jpn. J. Vet. Sci. 51:765–773, 1989.

Orsher, R.J., and D.E. Johnston: The surgical treatment of perineal hernia in dogs by transposition of the obturator muscle. Compend. Contin. Educ. Pract. Vet. 7:233–239, 1985.

Raffan T.J.: A new surgical technique for repair of perineal hernias in the dog. J. Small Anim. Pract. 43:13–19, 1993.

Root, M.V., S.D. Johnston, and P.N. Olson: Estrous length, pregnancy rate, gestation and parturition lengths, litter size, and juvenile mortality in the domestic cat. J. Am. Anim. Hosp. Assoc. 31:429–433, 1995.

Roszel, J.F.: Anatomy of the canine uterine cervix. Compend. Contin. Educ. Pract. Vet. 14:751–760, 1992.

Salmeri, K.R., Olson, P.N., and M.S. Bloomberg: Elective gonadectomy in dogs: A review. JAVMA 198:1183–1192, 1991.

Salmeri, K.R., Bloomberg, M.S., Scruggs, S.L., et al.: Gonadectomy in immature dogs: Effects on skeletal, physical, and behavioral development. JAVMA 198:1193–1203, 1991.

Schebitz, H., and H. Wilkens: Atlas of Radiographic Anatomy of the Dog and Cat, 4th ed. Berlin, Paul Parey Verlag, 1986.

Scrivani, P.V., D.J. Chew, C.A.T. Buffington, et al.: Results of retrograde urethrography in cats with idiopathic, nonobstructive lower urinary tract disease and their association with pathogenesis: 53 cases (1993–1995). JAVMA 211:741–748, 1997.

van Ee, R.T., and A. Palminteri: Tail amputation for treatment of perianal fistulas in dogs. J. Am. Anim. Hosp. Assoc. 23:95–100, 1987.

van Sluijs, F.J., and B.E. Sjollema: Perineal hernia repair in the dog by transposition of the internal obturator muscle. Vet. Qt. 11:12–17, 1989.

Yeager, A.E., H.O. Mohammed, V. Meyers-Wallen, et al.: Ultrasonographic appearance of the uterus, placenta, fetus and fetal membranes throughout accurately timed pregnancy in beagles. Am. J. Vet. Res. 53:324–329, 1992.

# CHAPTER 16

# The Forelimb of the Carnivores*

Fractures and luxations resulting from traffic accidents contribute the bulk of the clinical work on the forelimb of dogs and cats. The bones and muscles have been sufficiently described (pp. 74 and 82), and it will suffice here, as in the following chapter, to concentrate attention on their surface and radiological anatomy and on those relations with vessels and nerves that have particular clinical significance. Details of the development of the forelimb skeleton are summarized in Table 16–1. There is considerable variation in the age at which different events occur, with a tendency for development to be more precocious in small breeds than in large. The figures presented in the text refer more particularly to dogs of medium size represented by the Beagle.

## THE SHOULDER REGION AND ARM

*(See also pp. 81 and 85.)*

The scapula and humerus form the skeletal basis of the shoulder and arm, including the shoulder joint. The most easily recognized skeletal features are the acromion on the distal end of the scapular spine and the greater tubercle of the humerus just distal to it. Deeper palpation also reveals the rest of the spine; the cranial border, angle, and dorsal border of the scapula; the tendon of origin of the biceps; the deltoid tuberosity; and the medial and lateral surfaces of the shaft of the humerus (the last by grasping the bone between the fingers of one hand). The attachment of the pectoral muscles to cranial parts of the bones near the shoulder joint prevents palpation of the medial surface of the joint and upper part of the humerus. The superficial cervical lymph nodes cranial to the scapula are most easily palpated with the limb retracted (see Fig. 2–53/4). The axillary lymph nodes, on the thoracic wall caudal to the shoulder joint, can be palpated with the limb protracted but only when they are enlarged. Both groups drain the forelimb. An accessory axillary node is occasionally present on the chest wall dorsal to the olecranon; it drains skin and muscles of the area and also the thoracic mammary glands (/10).

The scapula is covered laterally by the trapezius and the supra- and infraspinatus muscles (Fig. 16–1/*A*,4,7). The tendons of the spinatus muscles cross the joint for attachment to the humerus; the belly of the infraspinatus is suitable for intramuscular injections. The flexor aspect of the joint is covered by the deltoideus, which connects the scapular spine with the deltoid tuberosity. The shaft of the humerus is overlain laterally by the lateral head of the triceps and the brachialis, cranially by the biceps (itself partly covered by the brachiocephalicus), and caudally by the brachialis (winding around the shaft) and the remaining heads of the triceps. In contrast, the medial surface, once free of the pectoral muscles, is relatively uncovered; this allows the brachial vessels, and the nerve trunks for the distal portion of the limb, to lie close to the bone (Fig. 16–2).

In craniocaudal radiographs of the extended shoulder joint, the supraglenoid tubercle overlaps the head of the humerus; in lateral radiographs this tubercle is superimposed on the greater tubercle of the humerus (Fig. 16–3). In dogs younger than 3 to 5 months the supraglenoid tubercle is still separated by cartilage from the rest of the scapula. The proximal epiphysis for the tubercles and head of the humerus commonly fuses with the shaft at about 10 months (but several months later in larger breeds). A small ossicle representing the clavicle lies cranioventral to the shoulder joint. In cats, the vestigial clavicle is a slender rodlet, roughly 2 cm long, in the corresponding place; it is regularly depicted in radiographic films and may be palpated against the cranial aspect of the joint (/*C′*). The feline acromion is broadened by a flat, caudally directed (suprahamate) process (see Fig. 2–43/*D*); the coracoid process on the medial aspect of the supraglenoid tubercle is often also very prominent in this species (/11 in the dog).

The capsule of the shoulder joint envelops the biceps tendon where it crosses the cranial aspect of

*See introductory remarks on page 367.

**Table 16–1.** Development and Maturation of the Forelimb Skeleton

| Ossification Centers Present at Birth (After Birth) | Approximate Age at Growth Plate Closure Observed on Radiographs | |
|---|---|---|
| | Dog | Cat |
| Scapula | | |
| Body | | |
| Supraglenoid tubercle (7 wk) | 3–7 mo[2,5] | 3.5–4.0 mo |
| Humerus | | |
| Prox. epiphysis (head and tubercles) (1–2 wk) | 10–15 mo[2,5] | 18–24 mo |
| Diaphysis | | |
| Distal epiphysis | 5–8 mo[2,5] | 4 mo |
| Lat. part of condyle (2–3 wk) | 5 mo[4] | 3.5 mo |
| Med. part of condyle (2–3 wk) | 5 mo[4] | 3.5 mo |
| Med. epicondyle (6–8 wk) | 5–6 mo[4,6] | 4 mo |
| Lat. epicondyle | At birth | 3.5 mo |
| Radius | | |
| Prox. epiphysis (3–5 wk) | 5–11 mo[2,5] | 5–7 mo |
| Diaphysis | | |
| Distal epiphysis (2–4 wk) | 6–12 mo[2,5] | 14–22 mo |
| Ulna | | |
| Olecranon tubercle (6–8 wk) | 5–10 mo[2,4,5,6] | 9–13 mo |
| Diaphysis | | |
| Anconeal process (12 wk) | 3–5 mo[7] | |
| Distal epiphysis (6–8 wk) | 6–12 mo[2,5,6] | 14–25 mo |
| Carpus | | |
| Radial carpal (3–4 wk) | | |
| Three centers | 3–4 mo[1–3] | |
| Accessory carpal | | |
| Diaphysis (3 wk) | | |
| Epiphysis (7 wk) | 3–6 mo[1,2,4,5] | 4 mo |
| Other carpal bones | | |
| One center each | | |
| Metacarpus | | |
| Metacarpal I | | |
| Prox. epiphysis (5 wk) | 6–7 mo[3] | |
| Diaphysis | | |
| Metacarpals II–V | | |
| Diaphysis | | |
| Distal epiphysis (4 wk) | 5–7 mo[2,4,5] | 7–10 mo |
| Digit | | |
| Phalanges I and II | | |
| Prox. epiphysis (4–5 wk) | 5–7 mo[1,2,5,6] | 4.0–5.5 mo |
| Diaphysis | | |
| Phalanx III | | |
| One center | | |

[1]Based on Chapman, W. L.: Appearance of ossification centers and epiphyseal closures as determined by radiographic techniques. JAVMA 147:138–141, 1965.

[2]Based on Hare, W. C. D.: The age at which epiphyseal union takes place in the limb bones of the dog. Wien. Tierärztl. Monatsschr. 9:224–245, 1972.

[3]Based on Pomriaskynski-Kobozieff, N., and N. Kobozieff: Etude radiologique de l'aspect du squelette normal de la main du chien aux divers Stades de son évolution de la naissance à l'âge adult. Rec. Med. Vet. 130:617–646, 1954.

[4]Based on Smith, R. N., and J. Allcock: Epiphyseal fusion in the Greyhound. Vet. Rec. 72:75–79, 1960.

[5]Based on Sumner-Smith, G.: Observations on the epiphyseal fusion of the canine appendicular skeleton. J. Small Anim. Pract. 7:303–311, 1966.

[6]Based on Ticer, J. W.: Radiographic Technique in Small Animal Practice. Philadelphia, W. B Saunders Company, 1975, p. 101.

[7]Based on Van Sickle, D.: The relationship of ossification to elbow dysplasia. Anim. Hosp. 2:24–31, 1966.

Prox., proximal; Lat., lateral; Med., medial.

From deLahunta and Habel, 1986.

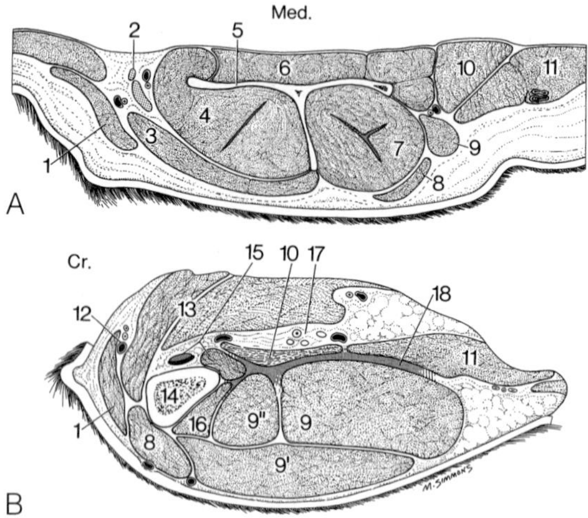


**Figure 16–1.** Transverse sections of the left canine forelimb at the level of the scapula *(A)*, and just distal to the shoulder joint *(B)*.

1, Brachiocephalicus; 2, superficial cervical lymph nodes; 3, omotransversarius; 4, supraspinatus; 5, scapula; 6, subscapularis; 7, infraspinatus; 8, deltoideus; 9, 9′, 9″, long, lateral, and accessory heads of triceps; 10, teres major; 11, latissimus dorsi; 12, cephalic vein; 13, pectoral muscles; 14, humerus; 15, biceps tendon and coracobrachialis; 16, brachialis; 17, brachial vessels and nerve trunks; 18, heavy intermuscular fascia.

the joint, bound down by a transverse ligament extending between the tubercles of the humerus. The joint may be punctured midway between the acromion and the greater tubercle by passing a needle medially through the deltoideus. It is useful to remember that the distal end of the acromion is opposite the joint space and that the glenoid concavity is considerably smaller than the head of the humerus. In sedated or anesthetized dogs it is possible to abduct the humerus at this relatively loose joint. Luxation of the joint and fractures of the scapula are both relatively rare; since the clavicle lacks a functional connection with the trunk, the entire joint apparently "rides with the blow" when subjected to sudden external force. Fractures of the humerus are much more common and occur mostly at midshaft level.

## THE ELBOW AND FOREARM

*(See also pp. 81 and 86.)*

Both medial and lateral aspects of the elbow joint are conveniently accessible because the arm is freer, and the axillary fossa correspondingly deeper, than in the larger species in which the medial approach is difficult. The summit of the olecranon, the most prominent palpable feature of the region, is located just below the ventral end of the fifth intercostal space in a dog standing squarely. The medial and lateral epicondyles and adjacent parts of the humerus are all easily palpated. The bundle of the brachial vessels and median nerve can be palpated against the medial surface of the bone, between the biceps and triceps. A smaller bundle formed by the collateral ulnar vessels and ulnar nerve may be located against the triceps tendon and olecranon (Fig. 16–12/5,6). The collateral ligaments arising from the epicondyles are also easily palpated. Though the condyle of the humerus projects forward from the long axis of the bone, a considerable covering of muscle makes it less accessible.

The entire medial border of the radius is subcutaneous; the cranial surface is palpable distally where it is only thinly covered by the extensor carpi obliquus and the tendons of the other extensors (Fig. 16–4/6). The ulna is more

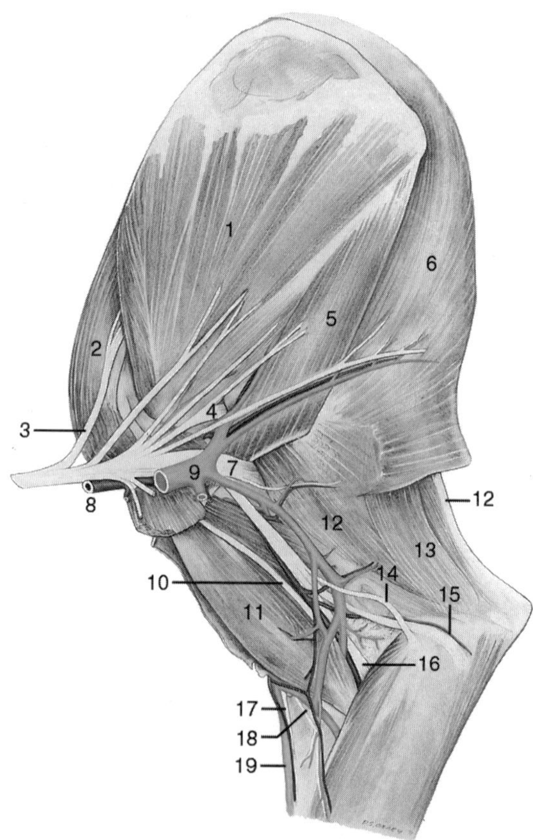


**Figure 16–2.** Medial surface of the right canine shoulder and arm.

1, Subscapularis; 2, supraspinatus; 3, suprascapular nerve; 4, axillary nerve; 5, teres major; 6, latissimus dorsi; 7, radial nerve; 8, axillary artery; 9, axillary vein; 10, musculocutaneous nerve; 11, biceps; 12, long head of triceps; 13, tensor fasciae antebrachii; 14, caudal cutaneous antebrachial nerve; 15, ulnar nerve and collateral ulnar artery; 16, median nerve and brachial artery; 17, medial branch of superficial radial nerve; 18, median cubital vein; 19, cephalic vein

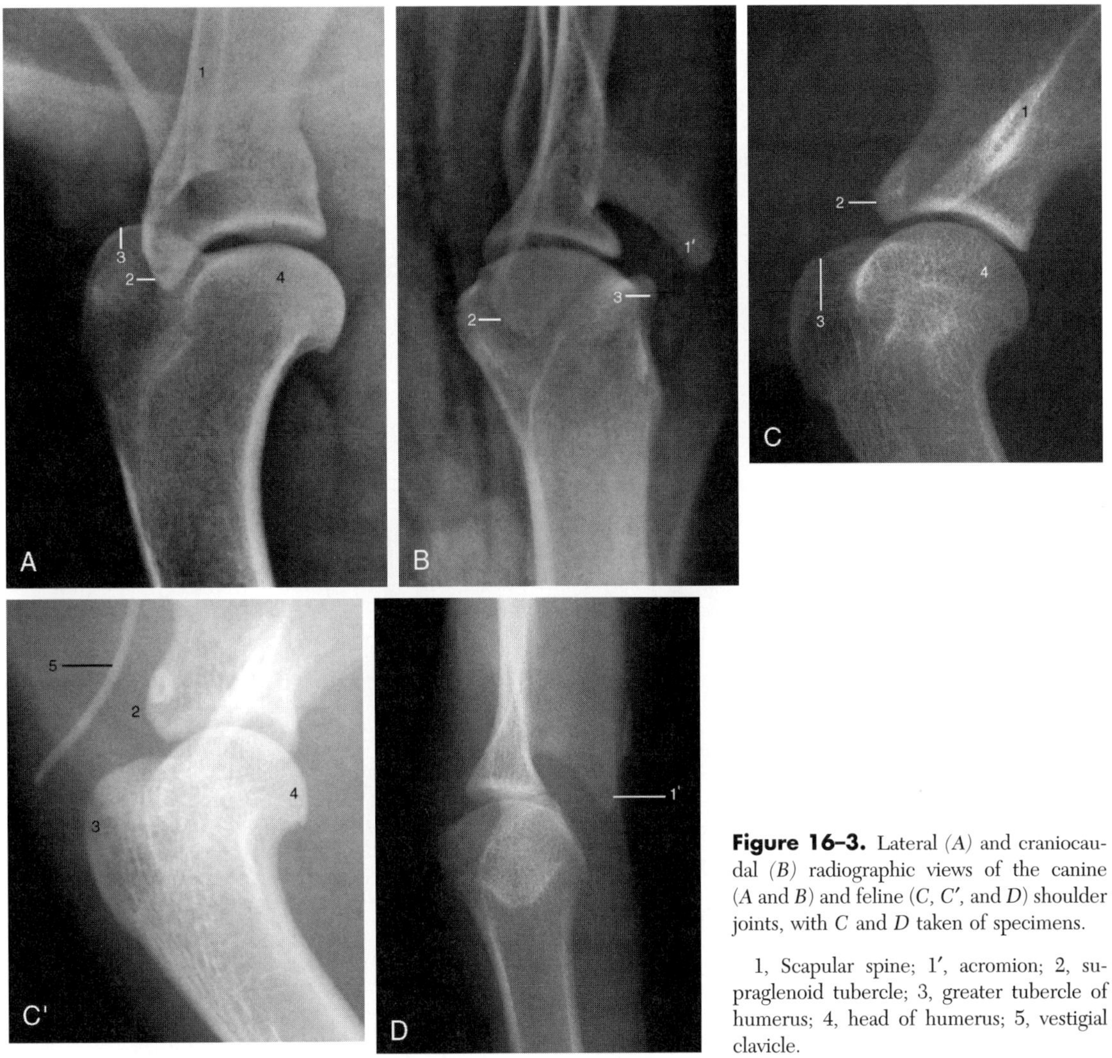

**Figure 16–3.** Lateral *(A)* and craniocaudal *(B)* radiographic views of the canine *(A* and *B)* and feline *(C, C′,* and *D)* shoulder joints, with *C* and *D* taken of specimens.

1, Scapular spine; 1′, acromion; 2, supraglenoid tubercle; 3, greater tubercle of humerus; 4, head of humerus; 5, vestigial clavicle.

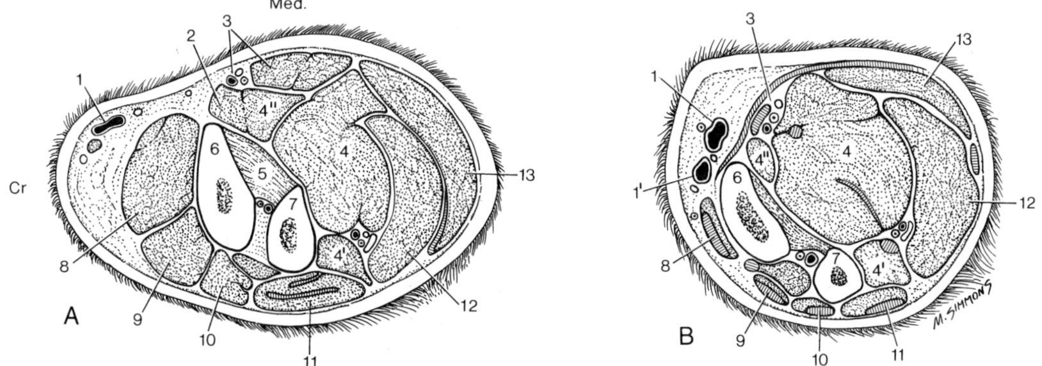


**Figure 16–4.** Transverse sections of the left canine forelimb just distal to the elbow joint *(A)*, and just proximal to the carpus *(B)*.

1, Cephalic vein and branches of superficial radial nerve; 1′, accessory cephalic vein; 2, pronator teres; 3, median vessels and nerve, and flexor carpi radialis; 4, 4′, 4″, humeral, ulnar, and radial heads of deep digital flexor; 5, pronator quadratus; 6, radius; 7, ulna; 8, extensor carpi radialis; 9, common digital extensor; 10, lateral digital extensor; 11, ulnaris lateralis; 12, flexor carpi ulnaris; its small ulnar head lies on its caudal, and the ulnar vessels and nerve on its cranial aspect; 13, superficial digital flexor.

deeply placed, except at its distal end, where its styloid process connects with the carpal bones. A deep depression behind this process is bounded by the prominent tendon of the flexor carpi ulnaris and the accessory carpal bone.

The *cephalic vein* (/1) is the most popular choice for intravenous injections. It follows the cranial border of the forearm, where it can be palpated when raised by pressure over the elbow; it sometimes produces a visible ridge even when not occluded. Since it sends an anastomosis (median cubital vein) to the deep system of veins at the elbow before continuing over the lateral surface of the arm, it is best compressed distal to the anastomosis (Fig. 16–5/2). The vein lies on the extensor carpi radialis, the largest of the extensor muscles that spring from the lateral epicondyle of the humerus and the more proximal crest. The carpal and digital flexors arise from the angular medial epicondyle, lie caudal to the radius, and cover the medial and caudal surfaces of the ulna (Fig. 16–4). The median vessels (/3) (continuations of the brachial) and nerve are embedded among these muscles, close to the medial border of the radius (Fig. 16–6).

In cats, a prominent medial (supracondylar) foramen at the distal end of the humerus (see Fig. 2–44/*C*,14) transmits the brachial artery and median nerve in the caudocranial direction. These structures are therefore vulnerable in fractures and surgery of this part.

Lateral radiographs show the humeral condyle deeply seated in the trochlear notch of the ulna (Fig. 16–7/*A*). The prominent medial epicondyle (/1′) is superimposed on the olecranon, while the anconeal process, at the proximal end of the notch (/4), is superimposed in turn on the medial epicondyle. The anconeal process has its own ossification center which fuses with the rest of the bone at 3 to 5 months of age. If it fails to do so, or if it becomes detached, the loose piece causes severe lameness; the condition ("un-united anconeal process") is mainly encountered in larger breeds. The medial coronoid process at the distal end of the trochlear notch (/5) is not formed from a separate ossification center, and the separation that sometimes occurs is therefore not due to a failure of fusion—as has been alleged—but to osteochondrosis. This process is superimposed on the proximal end of the radius in lateral radiographs of the normal joint.

The elbow joint is most easily punctured cranial to the lateral collateral ligament. A small sesamoid bone is occasionally associated with the ligament.

An understanding of luxation of the elbow joint may be assisted by fitting the three loose bones together. It will be found that the joint is most easily luxated (by lateral displacement of the radius and ulna) when it is flexed because the anconeal process is then withdrawn from the olecranon fossa of the humerus. Medial luxation is less frequent, probably because it is more difficult for the anconeal process to snap over the larger medial epicondyle. It follows that a dislocation will be most easily reduced if the joint is first strongly flexed to disengage the anconeal process from the humerus.

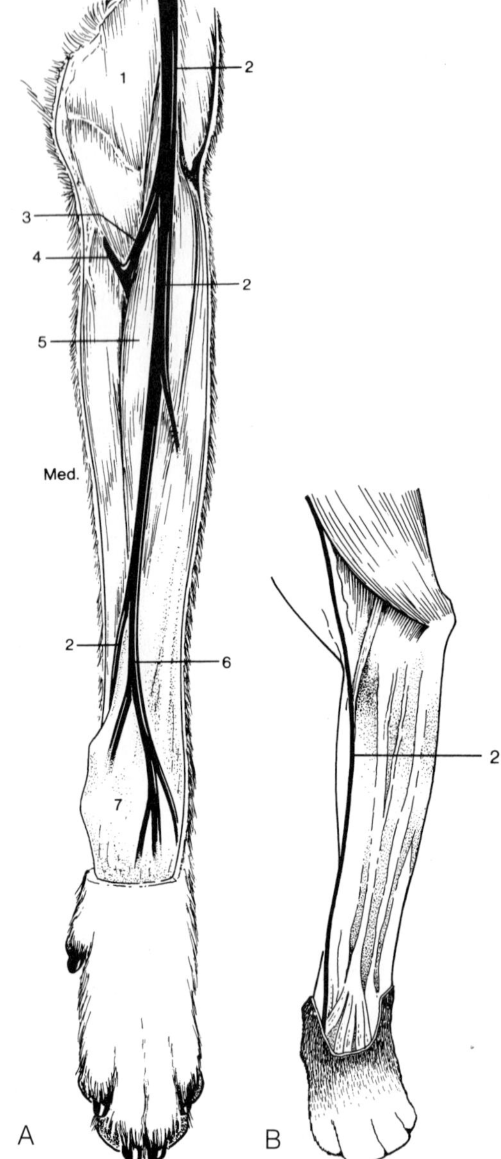


**Figure 16–5.** *A,* Superficial veins on the left canine forearm. *B,* The course of the cephalic vein on the left feline forearm.

1, Brachiocephalicus; 2, cephalic vein; 3, median cubital vein; 4, brachial vein; 5, extensor carpi radialis; 6, accessory cephalic vein; 7, carpus.

Repair of a torn collateral ligament may be required following reduction.

The distal epiphysis of the humerus fuses with the shaft at 5 to 8 months, considerably before closure at the proximal end. The proximal epiphysial cartilage of the radius and that of the tuber olecrani generally disappear at about the same time; the larger distal cartilages of the forearm bones disappear a little later, usually at about 6 to 9 months. Fully two thirds of the lengthening of the radius is due to growth at the distal cartilage; lengthening of the ulna (distal to the elbow joint) is almost entirely due to the growth at its V-shaped distal cartilage. The deformation sometimes found following unequal elongation of these bones results from "premature fusion" of one cartilage; the most prominent effect is deviation of the paw, which tenses the connective tissue connections of the bones, especially the radioulnar ligament at the distal end.

Forearm fractures are relatively common. They occur most often in the distal half and, as would be expected, generally involve both bones. Fracture of the olecranon is also fairly common.

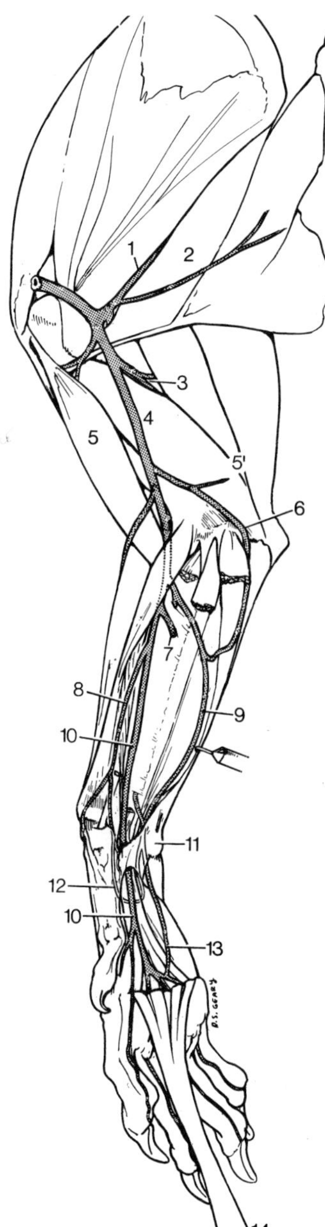


**Figure 16–6.** The topography of the major arteries of the right canine forelimb, medial view. The caudomedial muscles of the forearm have been removed.

1, Subscapular artery; 2, teres major; 3, deep brachial artery; 4, brachial artery; 5, biceps; 5′, triceps; 6, collateral ulnar artery; 7, deep antebrachial artery; 8, radial artery; 9, ulnar artery; 10, median artery; 11, accessory carpal bone; 12, deep palmar arch; 13, superficial palmar arch; 14, superficial digital flexor, reflected.

## CARPUS AND FOREPAW

*(See also pp. 82 and 354–358.)*

The carpal and metacarpal bones and the phalanges should be studied principally with a view to becoming familiar with their radiographic appearances.

The most obvious external features are the digital, metacarpal, and carpal pads, and the claws. At birth, a reduced first digit, or "dewclaw," is generally present below the carpus on the medial side of the paw. It is often removed routinely, even in city dogs, although the presumed purpose of this mutilation is to avoid the risk of injury should the dewclaws catch in scrub. It must be retained in puppies of certain breeds if there is a possibility that they will later be shown. The carpal pad, just distal to the palpable accessory carpal bone, is normally denied contact with the ground except in animals cornering at speed; it is occasionally injured in this way in racing Greyhounds (Fig. 10–13/4). The metacarpal and digital pads make ground contact and the small papillae that normally roughen their surfaces may be worn smooth in dogs regularly walked on paving. The metacarpal pad is molded over the flexor surface of the metacarpophalangeal joints (Fig. 16–9/8). The digital pads are centered over the flexor surfaces of the distal interphalangeal joints (/7). Webs of skin connecting the digits proximal to the pads are common sites of interdigital infections, and of cysts.

The wall of the claw is shaped to the dorsal and lateral surfaces of the curved unguicular process of

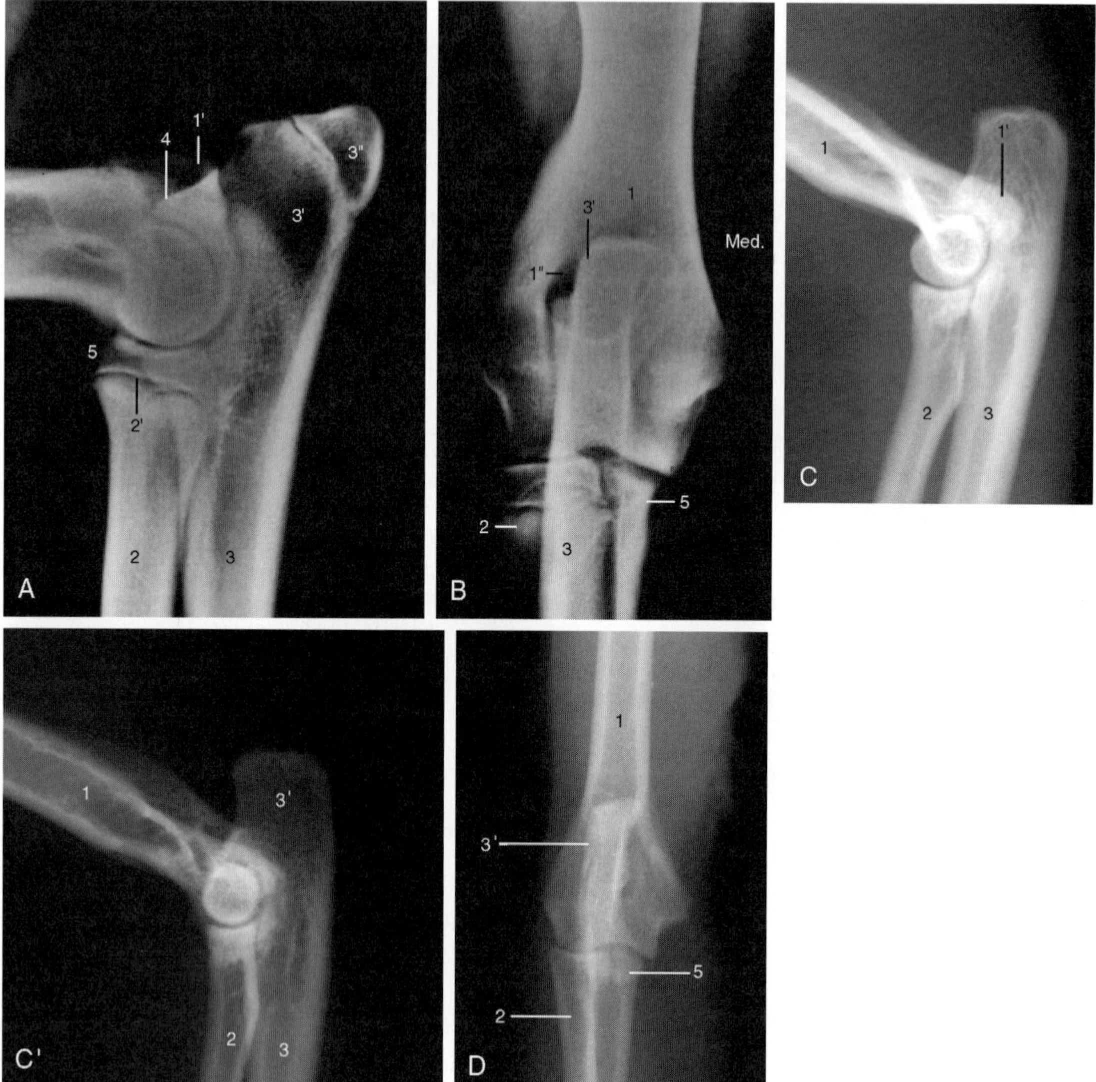


**Figure 16–7.** Lateral *(A)* and craniocaudal *(B)* radiographic views of the elbow joint of a young dog *(A* and *B)* and of a cat *(C, C'*, and *D)*. The (feline) supracondylar foramen is depicted on Figure 2–44/*C*.

1, Humerus; 1′, medial epicondyle; 1″, supratrochlear foramen; 2, radius; 2′, proximal epiphysial cartilage; 3, ulna; 3′, olecranon; 3″, apophysis of tuber olecrani; 4, anconeal process; 5, medial coronoid process.

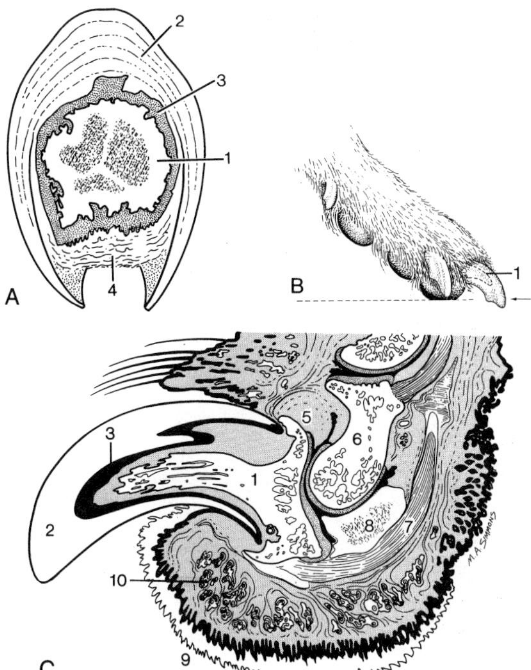


**Figure 16–8.** *A,* Transection of canine claw. *B,* Correct trimming of canine claws. *C,* Axial section of the canine digit.

1, Unguicular process of distal phalanx; 2, wall of claw; 3, laminar dermis; 4, crumbly sole of claw; 5, dorsal elastic ligament; 6, middle phalanx; 7, deep digital flexor tendon; 8, distal sesamoid (cartilaginous); 9, digital pad; 10, sweat glands.

the distal phalanx to which it is connected by a laminar dermis (Fig. 16–8/*B,C*). The sole of the claw (/4) covers the ventral surface of the process and appears as a crumbly whitish material between the edges of the wall. The claws, especially those of heavy city dogs, are generally worn level with the digital pads; they must be trimmed when there is insufficient wear, since if left unattended they would grow round to penetrate the pad. Special clippers should be used since the lateral pressure exerted by scissors or human nail clippers causes pain. The claw should be trimmed level with the ground surface of the pad but not so short that the vascular and sensitive dermis is damaged (/*A*). The pink dermis may be seen in nonpigmented claws, but when denied this guide a warning sign is provided by the appearance of a black dot on the cut surface just distal to the dermis. Elastic dorsal ligaments (/5) extend from the proximal end of the middle phalanx to the unguicular crest of the distal phalanx to keep the claws elevated. The deep digital flexor opposes the ligaments and protrudes the claws for scratching or digging.

The claws of the cat are laterally compressed, strongly curved, and drawn out to sharp points. They can be fully retracted into the fur of the paw, enabling cats to walk silently and without blunting the claws through ground contact. The elastic dorsal ligaments are of unequal length; long ones extend from the proximal interphalangeal joint to the sides of the distal phalanx, and a single short ligament extends between the distal end of the middle phalanx and the top of the unguicular crest (Fig. 16–9/3,12). This disposition, combined with the obliquity of the articular surfaces, allows the base of the claw to be drawn lateral to the corresponding middle phalanx (Fig. 16–10/*F*).

The ligaments keep the claws strongly retracted so that the digital flexors move only the metacarpophalangeal and proximal interphalangeal joints. The claws are protruded by simultaneous contraction of the deep digital flexor (which flexes the distal interphalangeal joints) and the digital extensors (which stabilize the more proximal joints of the paw). Cats use their protrusible claws for climbing trees and for initial prey contact—unlike dogs, which use their jaws for prey contact. The characteristic "clawing" on logs, rugs, or furniture, commonly thought to be performed in order to sharpen the claws, is actually related to territorial marking by sweat from the glands

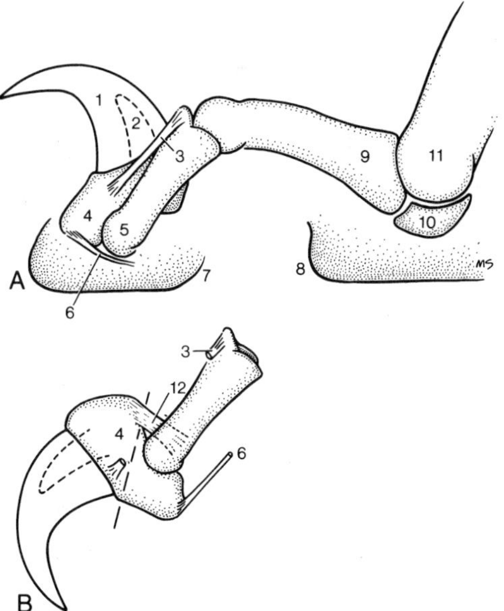


**Figure 16–9.** The feline claw, fully retracted *(A)* and protruded *(B)* shows the division *(broken line)* of the distal phalanx in declawing. The arrangement of the elastic ligaments has been greatly simplified.

1, Claw; 2, unguicular process of distal phalanx; 3, medial dorsal elastic ligament; 4, distal phalanx; 5, middle phalanx; 6, deep digital flexor tendon; 7, digital pad; 8, metacarpal pad; 9, proximal phalanx; 10, proximal sesamoid bone; 11, metacarpal bone; 12, lateral dorsal elastic ligament.

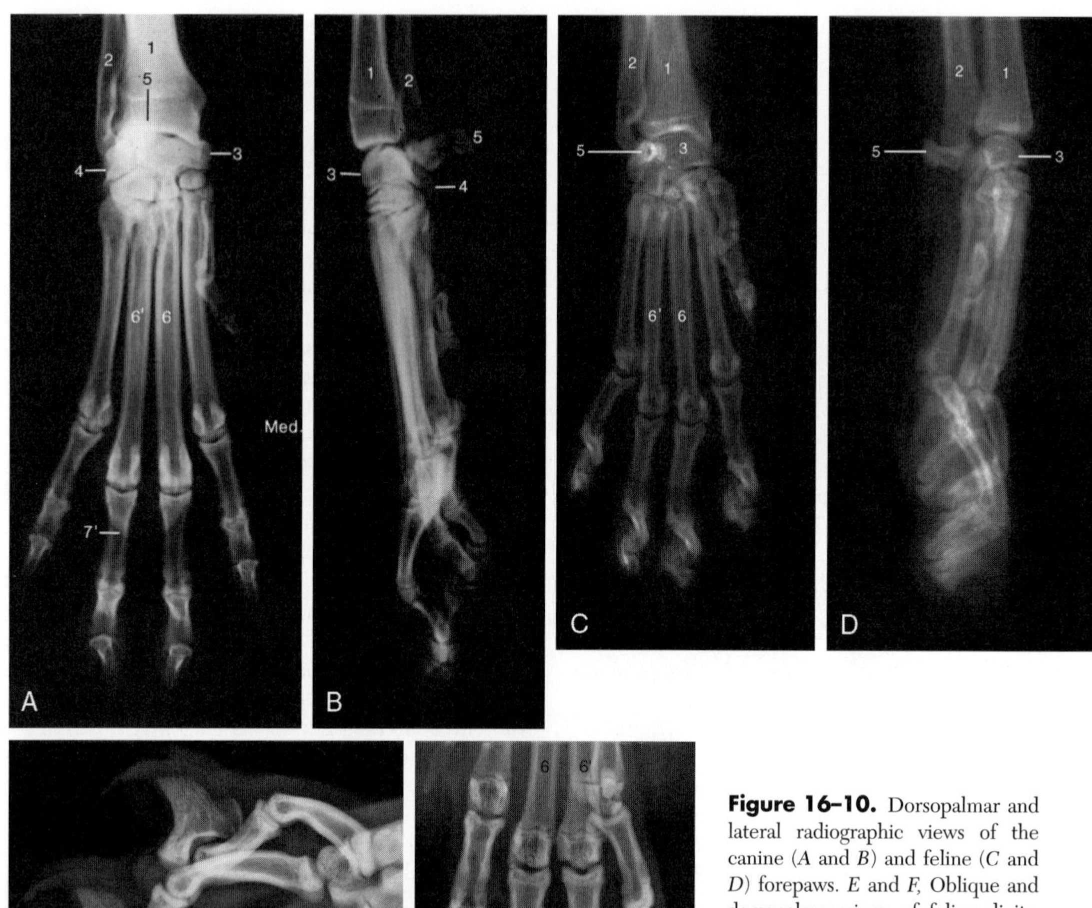


**Figure 16–10.** Dorsopalmar and lateral radiographic views of the canine (*A* and *B*) and feline (*C* and *D*) forepaws. *E* and *F*, Oblique and dorsopalmar views of feline digits; note how the distal phalanges slide next to the middle phalanges when the claws are retracted.

1, Radius; 2, ulna; 3, radial carpal; 4, ulnar carpal; 5, accessory carpal; 6, 6′, third and fourth metacarpals; 7, metacarpal pad; 7′, distal border of 7; 8, a digital pad.

concentrated in the digital pads. Clawing also promotes shedding of an outer, worn-out layer of a claw (Plate 15/*D*). Destructive cats can be declawed by transection of the distal phalanx; the base of the bone with the attachment of the deep digital flexor is left in place while the unguicular crest, enclosing the base of the claw, is removed (Fig. 16–9/*B*). An alternative procedure, simpler and causing less postoperative pain, consists in the resection of portions of the digital branches of the deep flexor tendon. Neither mutilation will be favored by those who value their cats above their furnishings. Forceful scraping of the ground by dogs after defecation or urination may have a similar marking purpose that utilizes the secretion of the sweat glands of their pads.

Except for the accessory, the individual carpal bones cannot be distinguished by palpation. Flexion of the joint widens the dorsal gap at the antebrachiocarpal level and facilitates appreciation of the tendons of the extensor carpi radialis and common digital extensor. The proximal compartment of the joint can be entered by passing a needle between these tendons; it does not communicate with the lower levels of articulation. The bones distal to the carpus are all readily identified by palpation since the metacarpals, though crowded together proximally, diverge distally. The extensor tendons can be rolled against the metacarpal bones, while the digital flexors and the interossei together form a soft package on the palmar aspect. The paired sesamoid bones on the palmar surface of the metacarpophalangeal joints are embedded in the metacarpal pad (/10,8).

Dorsopalmar radiographs show the carpal bones with a minimum of overlapping (Fig. 16–10). The large radial carpal (/3), which incorporates an intermediate element in both dogs and cats, lies distal to the radius; the oddly shaped ulnar carpal (/4) next to it extends distally (on the palmar surface) to be superimposed on the fourth carpal (and even on the corresponding metacarpal). The accessory carpal (/5) is superimposed on the junction of the radius, ulna, and ulnar carpal. On the medial side, carpals 1 and 2 are superimposed; the sesamoid in the extensor carpi obliquus also may be visible here opposite the midcarpal joint. The carpal pad produces a fainter shadow. The distal radial epiphysis has occasionally been mistaken for a carpal bone. It should be noted that in slightly oblique projections of the cat's carpus a wide space exists between the distal extremities of the radius and ulna; this could be misinterpreted as a subluxation.

The epiphysis of the accessory carpal fuses with the rest of the bone between 3 and 6 months. The three centers of the radial carpal fuse about 1 month before that. The distal epiphyses of the principal metacarpal bones fuse with the shafts at about 5 to 7 months. (The proximal metacarpal epiphyses fuse prenatally.)

The main arteries of the forelimb have been described (p. 238); their relations are shown in Figure 16–6. A branch of the radial artery may be used for taking the pulse of cats. It is to be found on the dorsomedial aspect of the distal carpus.

## THE MAJOR NERVES OF THE FORELIMB

This account is concerned only with the nerves in the free part of the limb. Since the main features conform closely to the common pattern (p. 312) it is now sufficient to concentrate attention on their relations and cutaneous distribution. The brachial plexus originates from C6–T1 in about 60%, from C5–T1 in 20%, from C6–T2 in about 20%, and from C5–T2 in a very small proportion (less than 3%) of dogs. The origins of the individual nerves are therefore subject to considerable variation; those described later refer to the most common arrangements. There is also considerable overlap between their cutaneous territories, which can be indicated only approximately. Figure 16–11 shows the much smaller autonomous zones used for testing the integrity of *individual* nerves. The courses and distributions of the nerves within the paw have little clinical application and can be dealt with summarily.

The *musculocutaneous nerve* (C6–C7) innervates the biceps, brachialis, and coracobrachialis. It descends on the medial surface of the arm between the biceps and the brachial artery, and at the elbow detaches a communicating branch to the more caudally placed median nerve. It is continued into the forearm by a cutaneous branch (medial cutaneous antebrachial nerve), which passes between the biceps and brachialis to become subcutaneous craniomedial to the elbow, before supplying skin over the medial surface of the forearm (Figs. 16–11/2 and 16–12/1,11). Although dysfunction of the nerve causes little change in gait, an affected animal is unable to respond to the invitation to "offer a paw" since flexion of the elbow requires activity of at least one of the biceps and brachialis muscles.

The *axillary nerve* (C7–C8) supplies the prime flexors of the shoulder joint. It leaves the axillary space by disappearing dorsal to the teres major (Fig. 16–2/4,5) and then winds around the caudal aspect of the joint to reach the deltoideus; the branches that continue beyond this point supply skin over the craniolateral region of the arm and a part of the forearm (Fig. 16–11/1). Paralysis of the nerve has little effect since the latissimus dorsi and the long head of the triceps are available to compensate for the loss of most shoulder flexors.

The *median nerve* (C8–T1) innervates the flexors of the carpus and digits. It descends on the medial surface of the arm just caudal to the brachial artery and passes the elbow cranial to the medial collateral ligament before dipping under the pronator teres and flexor carpi radialis muscles (Fig. 16–12/7). It detaches its muscular branches and then continues (under cover of the last-named muscle) near the medial border of the radius as a mainly sensory nerve. This accompanies the digital flexor tendons and the median artery through the carpal canal before dividing to supply the medial and caudal aspects of the paw in collaboration with the ulnar nerve. Dysfunction has little effect on the gait, but the carpus may become overextended when the dog is standing, resulting in the claws being slightly raised from their normal posture.

The *ulnar nerve* (C8–T1) innervates the remaining carpal and digital flexors. It first descends with the median nerve, but in the distal half of the arm it seeks a more caudal course, which takes it over the medial epicondyle of the humerus (where it is palpable) accompanied by the collateral ulnar vessels (/6). A cutaneous branch (caudal cutaneous antebrachial nerve; /5) that becomes subcutaneous on the medial aspect of the olecranon supplies the

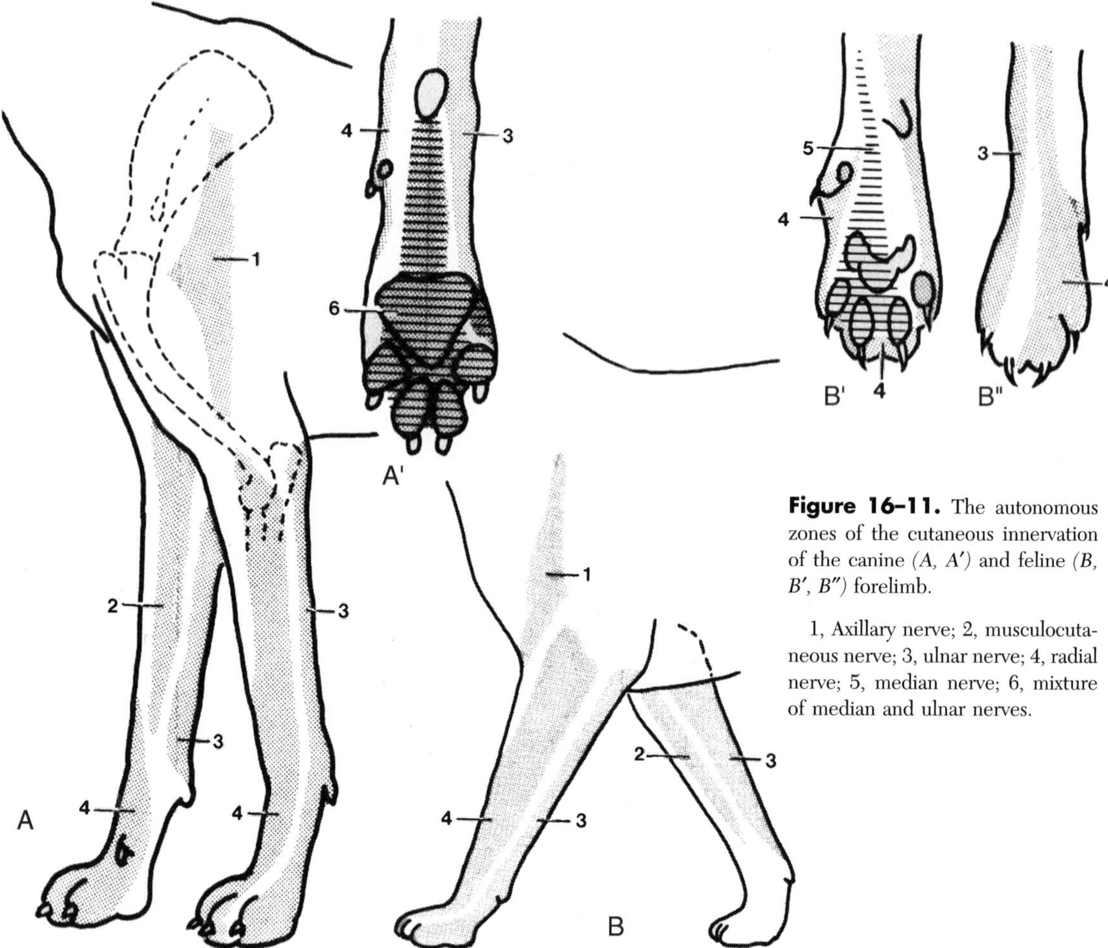


**Figure 16–11.** The autonomous zones of the cutaneous innervation of the canine *(A, A′)* and feline *(B, B′, B″)* forelimb.

1, Axillary nerve; 2, musculocutaneous nerve; 3, ulnar nerve; 4, radial nerve; 5, median nerve; 6, mixture of median and ulnar nerves.

caudal surface of the forearm. The main trunk dives into the caudomedial forearm muscles and, after supplying these, it re-emerges on the lateral side, where it joins the ulnar artery and vein before descending caudal to the ulna. It divides into dorsal and palmar branches in the distal half of the forearm. The dorsal branch comes to the surface in the large depression between the ulnaris lateralis and the flexor carpi ulnaris and innervates the skin on the caudolateral aspect of the paw. The palmar branch crosses the carpus with the flexor tendons and median nerve to supply the caudal aspect of the paw. Paralysis of the nerve has no obvious effect on gait or posture.

The important *radial nerve* (C7–T1) supplies the extensors of the elbow, carpal, and digital joints. It leaves the axilla by plunging into the triceps, at about the middle of the arm (Fig. 16–2/7). After detaching branches to the triceps, it accompanies the brachialis muscle around the lateral aspect of the humerus to gain the flexor surface of the elbow. In this part of its course it is eminently vulnerable in fractures and from the tumors that commonly affect the humerus. It divides into deep and superficial branches before leaving the arm. The former continues distally, first between the brachialis and extensor carpi radialis and then between the supinator and the joint capsule, to supply the carpal and digital extensors in the upper part of the forearm. The latter splits into medial and lateral branches that emerge from the cranial border of the lateral head of the triceps to run subcutaneously, one to each side of the cephalic vein; they enter the paw with the accessory cephalic vein (Fig. 16–4/1,1′). The superficial branch supplies skin on the dorsal surface of forearm and paw, sharing the most proximal part of this region with the axillary nerve (Fig. 16–11/4).

If the nerve is seriously injured proximal to the origin of the tricipital branches, the elbow cannot be fixed and the limb, unable to bear weight, is carried in the flexed position with the toes knuckled over and presenting their dorsal surfaces to the ground. More distal injury is less serious since dogs soon learn to compensate for loss of the

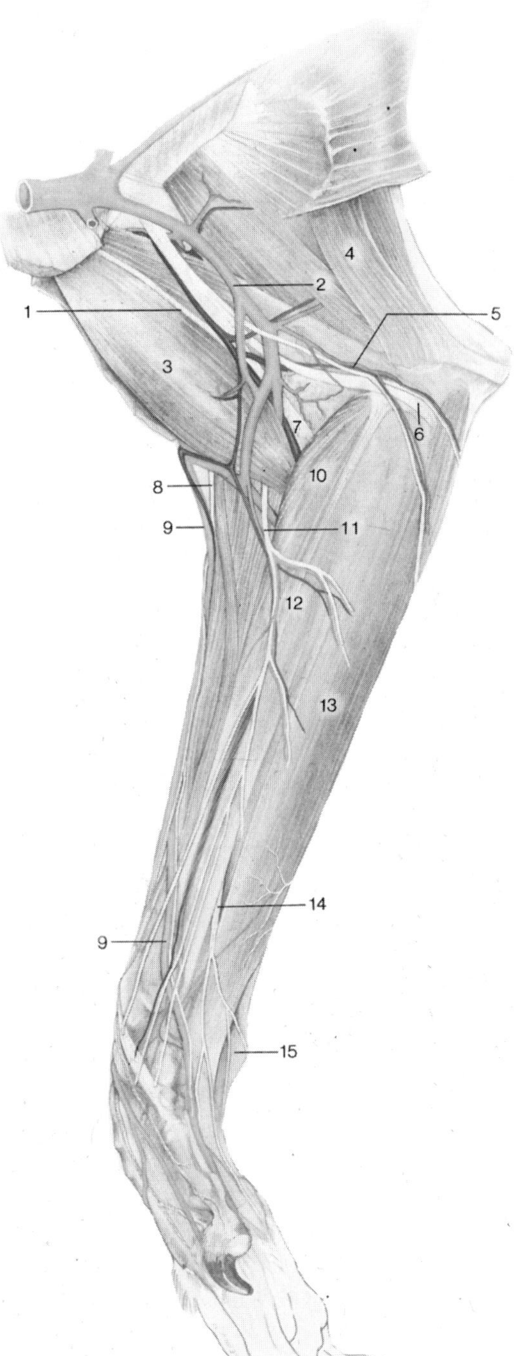


**Figure 16–12.** Superficial dissection of the right canine forelimb, medial view.

1, Musculocutaneous nerve; 2, brachial vein; 3, biceps; 4, tensor fasciae antebrachii; 5, caudal cutaneous antebrachial nerve and collateral ulnar vessels; 6, ulnar nerve; 7, median nerve and brachial artery; 8, medial branch of superficial radial nerve; 9, cephalic vein; 10, pronator teres; 11, medial cutaneous antebrachial nerve; 12, flexor carpi radialis; 13, superficial digital flexor; 14, inconstant cutaneous branch of ulnar nerve; 15, accessory carpal bone.

digital extensors by flicking the raised paw forward so that it lands on the pads.

## Selected Bibliography

Anderson, A., A.C. Stead, and A.R. Coughlan: Unusual muscle and tendon disorders of the forelimb in the dog. J. Small Anim. Pract. 34:313–318, 1993.

Bardet, J.F.: Arthroscopy of the elbow in dogs. Part I: The normal arthroscopic anatomy using the craniolateral portal. V.C.O.T. 10:1–5, 1997.

Bennett, R.A.: Contracture of the infraspinatus muscle in dogs: A review of 12 cases. J. Am. Anim. Hosp. Assoc. 22:481–487, 1986.

Boyd, J.S.: Color Atlas of Clinical Anatomy of the Dog and Cat. St. Louis, Mosby–Year Book, 1991.

Boulay, J.P.: Fragmented medial coronoid process of the ulna in the dog. Vet. Clin. North Am.: Small Anim. Pract. 28:1:51–74, 1998.

Bryant, H.N., A.P. Russell, R. Laroiya, and G.L. Powell: Claw retraction and protraction in the carnivora: Skeletal microvariation in the phalanges of the felidae. J. Morphol. 229:289–308, 1996.

Chalman, J.A., and B. Slocum: The caudolateral approach to the canine elbow joint. J. Am. Anim. Hosp. Assoc. 19:637–641, 1983.

Cross, A.R., and J.N. Chambers: Ununited anconeal process of the canine elbow. Compend. Contin. Educ. Pract. Vet. 19:349–361, 1997.

deLahunta, A., and R.E. Habel: Applied Veterinary Anatomy. Philadelphia, W.B. Saunders Company, 1986.

Denny, H.R.: The canine elbow. Br. Vet. J. 143:1–20, 1987.

Fox, S.M.: Premature closure of distal radial and ulnar physes in the dog, Part I. Pathogenesis and diagnosis. Compend. Contin. Educ. Pract. Vet. 6:128–140, 1984.

Fox, S.M., and A.M. Walker: OCD of the humeral head: Its diagnosis and treatment. A special symposium on osteochondrosis in dogs. Vet. Med. 88:123–131, 1993.

Fox, S.M., and A.M. Walker: Identifying and treating the primary manifestations of osteochondrosis of the elbow. A special symposium on osteochondrosis in dogs. Vet. Med. 88:132–146, 1993.

Guthrie, S., J.M. Plummer, and L.C. Vaughan: Post-natal development of the canine elbow joint: A light and electron microscopical study. Res. Vet. Sci. 52:67–71, 1992.

Hudson, L.C., and W.P. Hamilton: Atlas of Feline Anatomy for Veterinarians. Philadelphia, W. B. Saunders Company, 1993.

Jankowski, A.J., D.C. Brown, J. Duval, et al.: Comparison of effects of elective tenectomy or onychectomy in cats. JAVMA 213:370–373, 1998.

Johnston, S.A.: Articular fractures of the scapula in the dog: A clinical retrospective study of 26 cases. J. Am. Anim. Hosp. Assoc. 29:157–164, 1993.

Kriegleder, H.: Mineralization of the supraspinatus tendon: Clinical observations in seven dogs. Veterinary Comparative Orthopedic Traumatology 8:91–97, 1995.

Lewis, D.D., R.B. Parker, and D.A. Hager: Fragmented medial coronoid process of the canine elbow. Compend. Contin. Educ. Pract. Vet. 11:703–715, 1989.

Losonsky, J.M., and S.K. Kneller: Misdiagnosis in normal radiographic anatomy: Eight structural configurations simulating disease entities in small animals. JAVMA 191:109–114, 1987.

Lowry, J.E., L.G. Carpenter, R.D. Park, et al.: Radiographic anatomy and technique for arthrography of the cubital joint in clinically normal dogs. JAVMA 203:72–77, 1993.

Martinez, S.A., J. Hauptman, and R. Walshaw: Comparing two

techniques for onychectomy in cats and two adhesives for wound closure. Vet. Med. 88:516–525, 1993.

McCarthy, P.H., and A.K.W. Wood: Anatomic and radiologic observations of the clavicle in adult dogs. Am. J. Vet. Res. 956–959, 1988.

McLaughlin, R., Jr., and J.K. Roush: A comparison of two surgical approaches to the scapulohumeral joint in dogs. Vet. Surg. 24:207–214, 1995.

Mehumuza, L., J.P. Morgan, T. Miyabayashi, et al.: Positive contrast arthrography, a study of the humeral joints in normal beagle dogs. Vet. Radiol. Ultrasound 29:157–161, 1988.

Mikic, Z.D.: Blood supply of the articular disc of the antebrachiocarpal joint in dogs. J. Anat. 181:447–453, 1992.

Miyabayashi, T., M. Takiguchi, S.C. Schrader, and D.S. Biller: Radiographic anatomy of the medial coronoid process of dogs. J. Am. Anim. Hosp. Assoc. 31:125–132, 1995.

Muir, P.: Physical examination of lame dogs. Compend. Contin. Educ. Pract. Vet. 19:1149–1160, 1997.

Nordberg, C.C., and K.A. Johnson: Magnetic resonance imaging of normal canine carpal ligaments. Vet. Radiol. Ultrasound 40:128–136, 1999.

Ocal, M.K., R. Mutus, and H. Alpak: Classification of the vascular patterns of the thoracic limb muscles of cats. Ann. Anat. 178:83–89, 1996.

Puriton, P.T., J.N. Chambers, and J.L. Moore: Identification and categorization of the vascular patterns of the thoracic limb, thorax, and neck of dogs. Am. J. Vet. Res. 53:1435–1445, 1992.

Rife, J.N.: Deep digital flexor tendonectomy—an alternative to amputation onychectomy for declawing cats. J. Am. Anim. Hosp. Assoc. 24:73–76, 1988.

Schebitz, H., and H. Wilkens: Atlas of Radiographic Anatomy of the Dog and Cat, 4th ed. Berlin, Paul Parey Verlag, 1986.

Sharp, N.J.H.: Craniolateral approach to the canine brachial plexus. Vet. Surg. 17:18–21, 1988.

Snaps, F.R., M.H. Balligand, and J.H. Saunders: Comparison of radiography, magnetic resonance imaging, and surgical findings in dogs with elbow dysplasia. Am. J. Vet. Res. 58:1367–1370, 1997.

Suess, R.P., Jr., E.J. Trotter, D. Konieczynski, et al.: Exposure and postoperative stability of three medial surgical approaches to the canine elbow. Vet. Surg. 23:87–93, 1994.

Swalec, T.K.: Feline onychectomy at a teaching institution: A retrospective study of 163 cases. Vet. Surg. 23:274–280, 1994.

van Bree, H.: Comparison of the diagnostic accuracy of positive-contrast arthrography and arthrotomy in evaluation of osteochondrosis lesions in the scapulohumeral joint in dogs. JAVMA 203:84–88, 1993.

van Bree, H., H. Degryse, B. Van Ryssen, et al.: Pathologic correlations with magnetic resonance images of osteochondrosis lesions in canine shoulders. JAVMA 202:1099–1105, 1993.

Van Ryssen, B., H. van Bree, and P. Vyt: Arthroscopy of the shoulder joint in the dog. J. Am. Anim. Hosp. Assoc. 29:101–105, 1993.

Vannini, R., M.L. Olmstead, and D.D. Smeak: An epidemiological study of 151 distal humeral fractures in dogs and cats. J. Am. Anim. Hosp. Assoc. 24:531–536, 1988.

Vogelsang, R.L., P.B. Vasseur, J.R. Peauroi, et al.: Structural, material, and anatomic characteristics of the collateral ligaments of the canine cubital joint. Am. J. Vet. Res. 58:461–466, 1997.

Voorhout, G., and H.A.W. Hazewinkel: Radiographic evaluation of the canine elbow joint with special reference to the medial humeral condyle and the medial coronoid process. Vet. Radiol. 28:156–165, 1987.

Voorhout, G., R.C. Nap, and H.A.W. Hazewinkel: A radiographic study on the development of the antebrachium in Great Dane pups, raised under standardized conditions. Vet. Radiol. Ultrasound 35:271–276, 1994.

Welch, J.A., R.J. Boudrieau, L.M. DeJardin, and G.J. Spodnick: The intraosseous blood supply of the canine radius: Implications for healing of distal fractures in small dogs. Vet. Surg. 26:57–61, 1997.

Wood, A.K.W., P.H. McCarthy, and C.R. Howlett: Anatomic and radiographic appearance of a sesamoid bone in the tendon of origin of the supinator muscle of dogs. Am. J. Vet. Res. 46:2043–2047, 1985.

Wood, A.K.W., P.H. McCarthy, and I.C.A. Martin: Anatomic and radiographic appearance of a sesamoid bone in the tendon of origin of the supinator muscle of the cat. Am. J. Vet. Res. 56:736–738, 1995.

Worthman, R.P.: Demonstration of specific nerve paralyses in the dog. JAVMA 131:174–178, 1957.

# CHAPTER 17

# The Hindlimb of the Carnivores*

## THE CROUP, HIP, AND THIGH

*(See also pp. 91–92 and 94–97.)*

The habitual stance varies among breeds. The major differences are well illustrated by German Shepherds, which tend to crouch with the back and croup sloping down toward the tail (and the hip, stifle, and hock joints markedly flexed), and Boxers, which favor a stiffer, more upright posture (with the major joints, particularly the hock, significantly straighter). The more upright limb appears to predispose to several common stifle disorders. In Greyhounds and other lean, short-coated dogs, the contours of the croup may reproduce the form of the underlying muscles, the superficial gluteal especially; but such details are more often obscured by subcutaneous fat or a thick coat. The major skeletal landmarks are always palpable and reveal the small angle the ilium makes with the vertebral column.

The dorsal and ventral spines of the ilium are very prominent. The convex (iliac) crest joining these points can also be followed in its length and provides a convenient site for bone marrow biopsy in larger breeds; it is too thin to serve this purpose in smaller animals. A narrow strip of the pelvic floor bordering the ischial arch can usually be palpated between the salient tubers. In the dog the cordlike sacrotuberous ligaments, which are lacking in cats, can also be felt as they approach these projections from their origins on the sacrum. The greater trochanter of the femur is found cranial to the ischial tuber, and since its summit is very nearly level with the femoral head, it provides a good guide to the position of the joint, which is not itself palpable. Attention should be paid to the spacing of these features of the ilium, ischium, and femur since alteration may indicate luxation of the femur. This is a relatively frequent mishap; the femoral head is most often displaced dorsocranially (which widens the ischiofemoral gap) but may pass dorsocaudally or, though rarely, ventrocaudally when it may engage within the obturator foramen. Luxation may be confirmed by rotating the thigh outward while the thumb is pressed between the trochanter and the tuber; the movement normally forces the thumb from the recess, but a luxated femur is unable to exert the necessary leverage.

Though the hip joint is constructed according to the usual plan, it possesses greater range and versatility of movement in the dog and cat than in other domestic species. The enhanced potential for abduction is shown by the ease with which dogs cock their legs when urinating, while the general versatility, taken in combination with the suppleness of the trunk, enables both species to reach most parts of the head, neck, and thorax when scratching with the hindpaw. The articular surfaces reflect these abilities. The femoral head is an almost perfect hemisphere, marred only by the small central fovea where the intracapsular ligament (of the femoral head) inserts; it is deeply seated within the acetabular cup, which is only slightly extended by a labrum about its rim (see Fig. 2–60). There are no peripheral ligaments to limit movement. The intracapsular ligament, though variable in length and thickness, is generally lax enough to survive intact when the head is luxated. This is often the case when there is a preexisting dysplasia of the joint.

The most convenient access to the joint, for puncture and in surgery, is from the craniolateral direction. An approach between the tensor and biceps muscles exposes the proximal part of the vastus lateralis (whose origin runs from just below the greater trochanter) and the gluteal muscles that clothe the joint directly. The most important structures that are endangered are the sciatic nerve and caudal gluteal vessels but since these cross the dorsocaudal aspect of the joint as they proceed into the thigh, the risk is relatively remote.

The radiological anatomy is very relevant to the diagnosis of the two conditions that commonly affect the joint: luxation and dysplasia. For the standard ventrodorsal radiograph (Fig. 17–1/*A*), the supine animal must be placed with its limbs

*See introductory remarks on page 367.

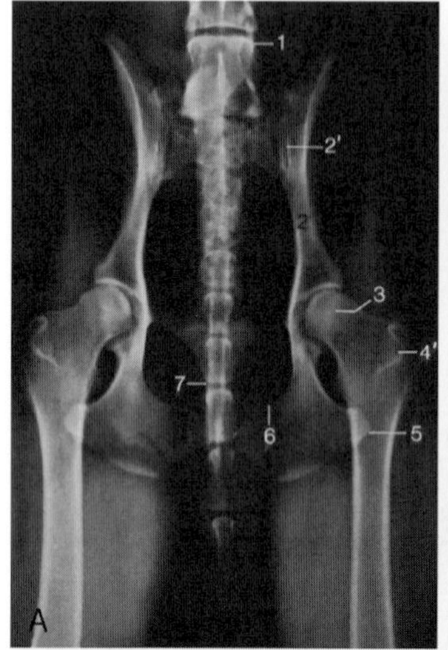


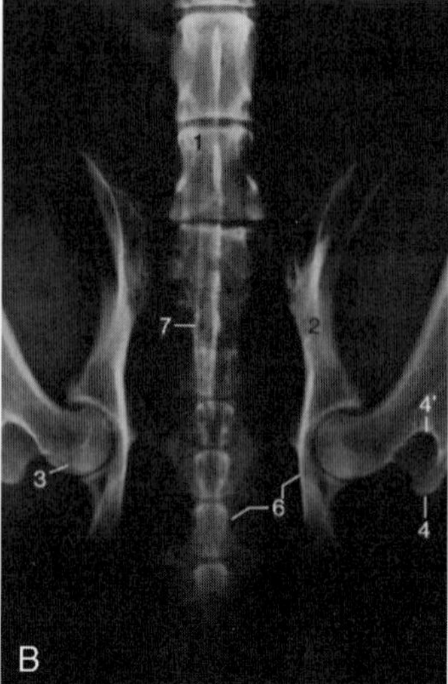


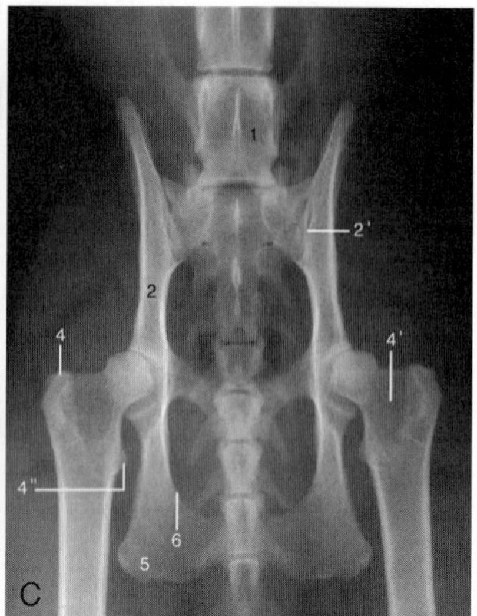


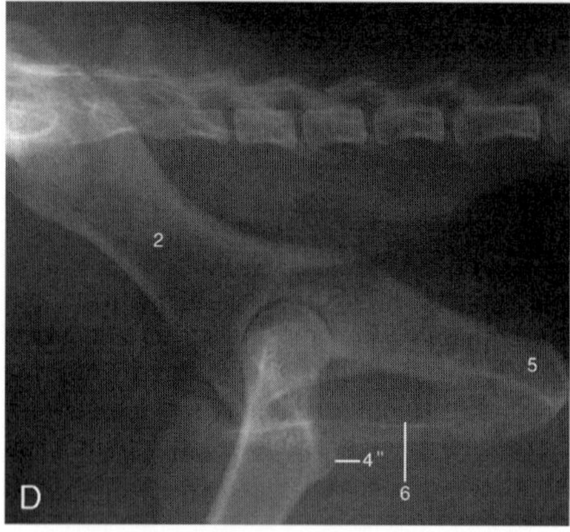


**Figure 17–1.** Ventrodorsal radiographic views of the canine pelvis with extended *(A)* and flexed *(B)* hip joints. *C* and *D*, Radiographs of the feline pelvis in ventrodorsal and lateral views, with *D* taken of a specimen.

1, Last lumbar vertebra (L7); 2, shaft of ilium; 2′, sacroiliac joint; 3, dorsal border of acetabulum superimposed on the femoral head; 4, greater trochanter; 4′, trochanteric fossa; 4″, lesser trochanter; 5, ischial tuber; 6, obturator foramen; 7, os penis superimposed on vertebrae.

drawn uniformly backward to ensure symmetrical depiction of bilateral structures. Though most features of the pelvis are too obvious to require comment, attention may be drawn to the slight lateral bowing of the canine ilia (in contrast to the parallel course of these bones in the cat). The relationship between the dorsal rim of the acetabulum and the femoral head upon which it is superimposed is of the greatest importance in determining the integrity of the joint (/3). Attention is also directed to the relative radiolucency of the region (corresponding to the trochanteric fossa) between the greater and lesser trochanters of the femur since it is sometimes misinterpreted. The less useful lateral view reveals the position of the hip joints below the first two caudal vertebrae (/*D*).

The maturation of the skeleton can be followed in radiographs obtained from young animals. In puppies there are primary ossification centers for the ilium, ischium, pubis, and acetabular bone, and secondary centers for the iliac crest, ischial tuber, and border of the ischial arch. The acetabular bone is the first to lose its independence, but this is followed by the merger of the other primary centers at a comparatively early age (4 to 6 months); the secondary centers remain distinct until much later (15 months to 5 years for the iliac crest, and 8 to 14 months for the ischial tuber). Fusion at the proximal extremity of the femur is completed between the 6th and 12th month (Table 17–1 and Plate 10/*E–G*).

A special position, in which the hindlimbs of the supine animal are rotated inward until the femoral trochleae and patellae face directly upward, is used for the better depiction of the contours of the femoral head when hip dysplasia is suspected. In this view it is easier to gauge the congruence of the femoral head with the acetabulum and to recognize any flattening or distortion of its contours. Progressive deformation of the head and worsening of fit characterize the progress of the condition.

The etiology of hip dysplasia, very common in certain larger breeds and with a familial tendency, is uncertain. Several once promising theories have been abandoned and much recent work has concentrated upon the belief that the dysplasia, which inevitably leads to osteoarthritic changes, is a consequence of the instability permitted by abnormally lax soft articular tissues. It has been shown that many affected dogs exhibit similar but milder features of the capsules of certain other joints. This prompts the suspicion that the dysplasia is not so much a unique affection of the hip as

**Table 17–1.** Development and Maturation of the Hindlimb Skeleton

| | Approximate Age at Growth Plate Closure Observed on Radiographs | |
|---|---|---|
| **Ossification Centers Present at Birth (After Birth)** | *Dog* | *Cat*[3] |
| Os coxae (hip bone) | | |
| Ilium | 4–6 mo[1, 2, 6] | |
| Ischium | 4–6 mo[1, 2, 6] | |
| Pubis | 4–6 mo[1, 2, 6] | |
| Acetabular bone (7 wk) | 4–6 mo[1, 2, 6] | |
| Iliac crest (4 mo) | 15 mo–5.5 yr[2] | |
| Ischial tuber, caudal border of ischium (3) | 8–14 mo[2, 6] | |
| Caudal pelvic symphysis, interischiadic bone (7 mo) | 15 mo–5 yr[2, 6] | |
| Pelvic symphysis closure (cranial to caudal) | 2.5–6.0 yr[2] | |
| Femur | | |
| Lesser trochanter (8 wk) | 8–13 mo[1, 2, 6] | 8–11 mo |
| Greater trochanter (8 wk) | 6–9 mo[2, 5] | 7–10 mo |
| Head (2 wk) | 6–9 mo[2, 5] | 7–10 mo |
| Diaphysis | | |
| Distal epiphysis (3 wk) | 6–12 mo[2, 5] | 13–19 mo |
| Trochlea (3 wk) | 3 mo[6] | |
| Patella (9 wk) | | |
| Tibia | | |
| Tibial tuberosity (8 wk) | 8–10 mo[2, 6] | |
| Proximal epiphysis (3 wk) | 6–15 mo[2, 5] | 12–18 mo |
| Diaphysis | | |
| Distal epiphysis (3 wk) | 5–11 mo[2, 5] | 10–13 mo |
| Medial malleolus (3 mo) | 4–5 mo[2, 6] | |
| Fibula | | |
| Proximal epiphysis (9 wk) | 6–12 mo[2, 6] | 13–18 mo |
| Diaphysis | | |
| Distal epiphysis (2–7 wk) | 5–13 mo[2, 5] | 10–14 mo |
| Sesamoids | | |
| Gastrocnemius (3 mo dog; 2.5–4.0 mo cat) | | |
| Popliteus (3 mo dog; 4–5 mo cat) | | |
| Tarsus | | |
| Calcaneus | | |
| Calcanean tuber (6 wk) | 3–8 mo[2, 4, 5, 6] | 7–13 mo |
| Diaphysis | | |
| Other tarsal bones (2–4 wk), 1 center each | | |
| Metatarsus | | |
| Diaphysis | | |
| Distal epiphysis (4 wk) | 5–7 mo[2, 5] | 8–11 mo |
| Digit similar to forelimb | | |

[1]Based on Chapman, W. L.: Appearance of ossification centers and epiphyseal closures as determined by radiographic techniques. JAVMA 147:138–141, 1965.

[2]Based on Hare, W. C. D.: The age at which epiphyseal union takes place in the limb bones of the dog. Wien. Tierärztl. Monatsschr. 9:224–245, 1972.

[3]Based on Smith, R. N.: Fusion of ossification centers in the cat. J. Small Anim. Pract. 10:523–530, 1969.

[4]Based on Smith, R. N. and J. Allcock: Epiphyseal fusion in the Greyhound. Vet. Rec. 72:75–79, 1960.

[5]Based on Sumner-Smith, G.: Observations on the epiphyseal fusion of the canine appendicular skeleton. J. Small Anim. Pract. 7:303–311, 1966.

[6]Based on Ticer, J. W.: Radiograpic Technique in Small Animal Practice. Philadelphia: W. B. Saunders Company, 1975, p. 101.

From deLahunta and Habel, 1986.

a particularly severe local manifestation of a more widespread developmental disorder.

The shaft of the femur is so deeply embedded among the muscles of the thigh that only a general impression of its presence may be obtained on palpation (Fig. 17–2/9). Despite this protection, the femur is the most commonly fractured bone, most breaks occurring about or below midshaft level. Such fractures are often complicated by considerable overriding, with the lower fragment commonly displaced caudally by the pull of the gastrocnemius. They are often repaired by intramedullary pinning, a procedure usually requiring direct exposure of the break. A lateral approach is most convenient: after incision of the fascia lata, the biceps, whose cranial margin is often palpable through the skin, is reflected, completing the exposure of the vastus lateralis; the path is now open to the bone along the attachment of the latter muscle (/8,10,9).

The cranial thigh muscles lend themselves to intramuscular injection.

The most important palpable structure of the thigh is the femoral artery (/2), which is subcutaneous on the medial aspect of the limb toward the groin. It lies within the femoral triangle, a pyramidal space whose base lies against the vascular lacuna (the passage to and from the abdomen for the femoral artery and vein) and which is closed distally by the convergence of the sartorius and pectineus muscles that form its cranial and caudal walls. The pectineus forms so obtrusive a fusiform swelling that it immediately guides the fingers to the adjacent artery, which is the first choice for the evaluation of the circulation. Pulsation may be perceived in a stretch of the artery after it has first dived more deeply among the muscles of the thigh. Its course leads it across the medial aspect of the femur to reach the popliteal fossa, where it is renamed the popliteal artery (Fig. 17–6/1,2). The accompanying vein is less conspicuous, but its constant relationship to the caudal border of the artery makes it easily found and convenient for intravenous injection in the supine, anesthetized subject. The saphenous artery (/4) branches from the concealed part of the femoral but soon becomes subcutaneous and runs over the medial aspect of the thigh toward the stifle. Both it and a large, more proximal branch (running caudally toward the gracilis) may be palpated.

Unlike the larger species, the dog and cat have no subiliac lymph nodes. However, the popliteal node is usually palpable within the popliteal fossa, between the distal parts of the biceps and semitendinosus as they diverge toward their insertions at the stifle (Figs. 17–3/10 and 17–5/6). This part of either muscle may be used for intramuscular injection and, since the sciatic nerve runs between them, it is a wise precaution to place a thumb into the fossa to ensure that the needle is directed away from the nerve.

## THE STIFLE JOINT AND LEG

*(See also pp. 92–93 and 97–99.)*

The stifle joint is flexed in the standing posture. Though it is more fully extended in certain phases of locomotion, the femur and tibia are never brought into line, and in dogs the caudal angle of the joint does not open beyond 150 degrees or so (considerably greater extension is permitted to cats). Some lateral or medial angulation of the joint may often be observed when the limb is viewed from in front or behind. In the "bow-legged" version common in certain toy breeds, the pull of the quadriceps does not coincide with the axis of the femoral trochlea, and there is a

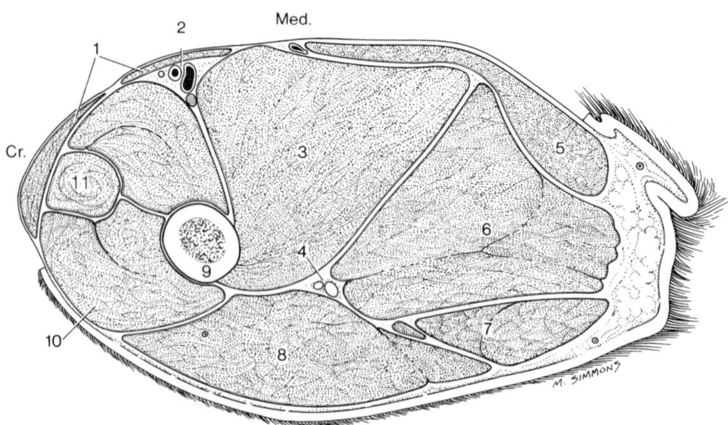


**Figure 17–2.** Transverse section of the canine left thigh.

1, Sartorius; 2, femoral vessels; 3, adductor; 4, sciatic nerve; 5, gracilis; 6, semimembranosus; 7, semitendinosus; 8, biceps; 9, femur; 10, vastus lateralis (of quadriceps); 11, rectus femoris.

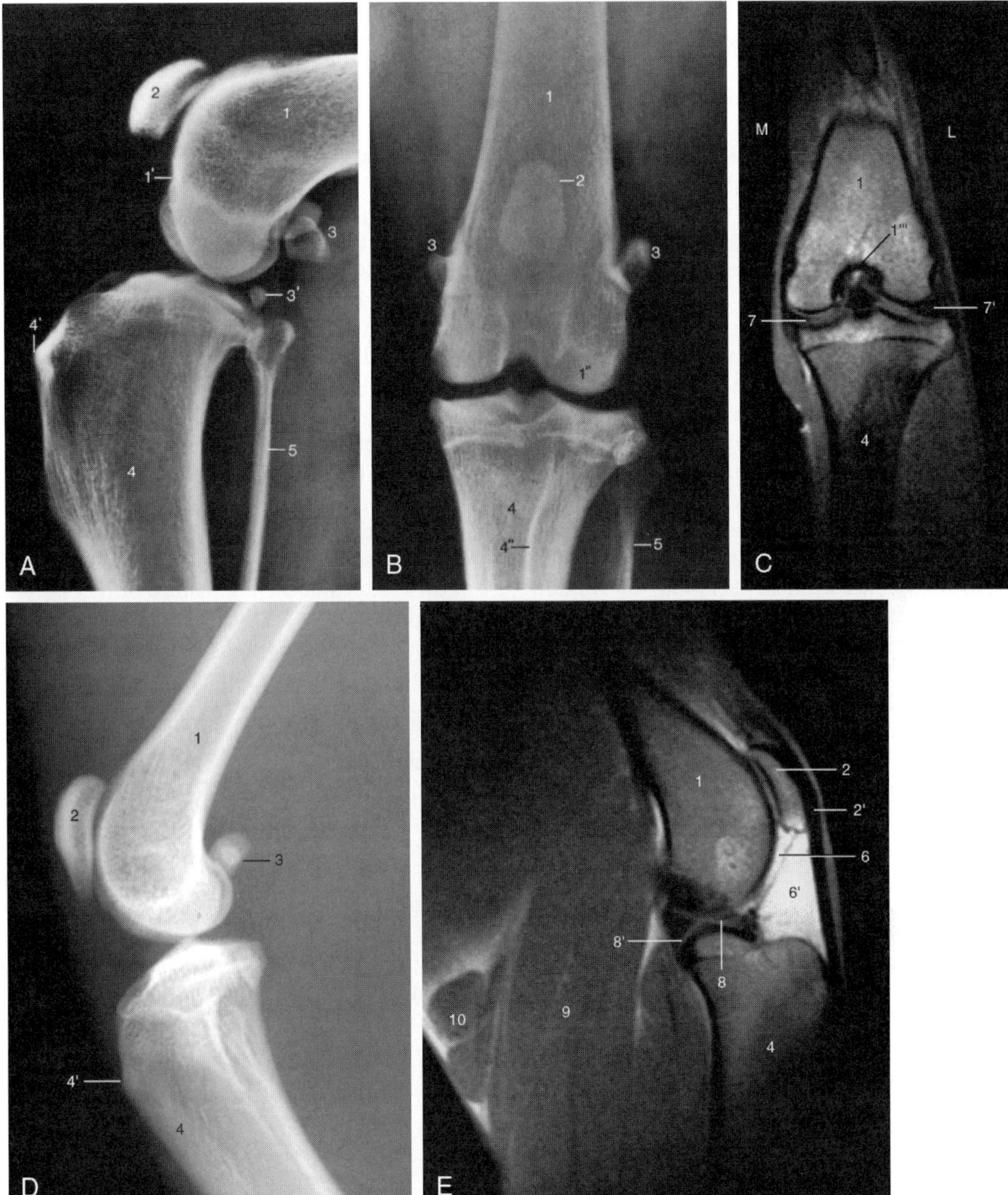


**Figure 17–3.** Lateral *(A)* and craniocaudal *(B)* radiographic views of the canine and feline (*D*, lateral only) stifles. *C* and *E*, Frontal and axial images of 4-mm-thick T1-weighted spin-echo magnetic resonance slices of the left canine stifle.

1, Femur; 1′, extensor fossa; 1″, lateral condyle; 1‴, intercondylar fossa; 2, patella; 2′, patellar ligament; 3, sesamoid bones in gastrocnemius; 3′, popliteal sesamoid bone; 4, tibia; 4′, tibial tuberosity; 4″, tibial crest; 5, fibula; 6, femoropatellar joint cavity; 6′, infrapatellar fat; 7, 7′, medial and lateral menisci; 8, 8′, cranial and caudal cruciate ligaments; 9, gastrocnemius; 10, popliteal lymph nodes.

tendency to medial luxation of the patella. The luxation, which may be intermittent or permanent, causes the limb to be carried and if left uncorrected leads to deformity of other parts.

Palpation of the stifle joint reveals the following features of the skeleton: the patella; the ridges of the trochlea, and the outer surfaces of the condyles of the femur; the sesamoid bones within the origin of the gastrocnemius; the head of the fibula; the edge of the lateral condyle adjacent to the fibula, the tuberosity, the extensor groove, and the medial surface of the tibia. The single patellar ligament and the medial and lateral collateral ligaments may also be distinguished but not the femoropatellar ligaments, which are overlain by the aponeuroses of the sartorius and semimembranosus on the medial side, and by that of the biceps (which extends over the tibialis cranialis in the upper part of the leg) laterally.

The most distinctive internal feature of the joint is the free communication of the various synovial compartments, which ensures that a single injection will reach all parts of the cavity. The most convenient entry is made from the lateral side, caudal to the thick pad of fat interposed between the patellar ligament (and adjoining retinaculum) and the synovial membrane. The cruciate ligaments are set well back (see Fig. 2–61/15,16). They assist the collateral ligaments in opposing rotation and medial or lateral deviation of the leg. They are most susceptible to injury when tautened. The cranial cruciate ligament, named (it will be recalled) for the relative position of its tibial attachment (/16), is therefore at highest risk when strained in overextension of the joint; its rupture allows abnormally free forward displacement of the tibia in relation to the femur (the "cranial drawer" sign). The caudal cruciate ligament is at greatest risk in the flexed position of the joint, and its rupture allows excessive caudal displacement of the tibia (the "caudal drawer" sign). Various surgical techniques for the restoration or replacement of these ligaments use fascial or artificial substitutes.

The menisci, joined cranially by an intermeniscal ligament in addition to the usual restraints, are also prone to traumatic injury. They are most vulnerable when torsion is imposed upon a limb in which the stifle is extended and the foot fixed—a combination of circumstances found when an abrupt change in direction is attempted by a dog traveling at speed.

Both lateral and craniocaudal radiographic projections are commonly used in the diagnosis of stifle injuries (Fig. 17–3). In the latter view, the patella is superimposed on the distal end of the femur, where it is flanked by the ridges of the trochlea, which appear as thin radiodense lines. The tibial condyles are relatively flat since they are not separated by conspicuous intercondyloid tubercles (present in the larger species). The head of the fibula falls short of the extremity of the tibia. In the lateral view, the femoral and tibial condyles are seen to have only limited, rather caudal contact and the joint appears unstable since the menisci that maintain its congruence are not revealed. The patellar ligament, the most prominent soft tissue shadow, runs at some distance from the femur, the space behind it being occupied by the infrapatellar fat cushion. This view best depicts the associated sesamoid bones. The pair within the heads of the gastrocnemius are large and well defined (/3); they articulate with small facets on the upper parts of the corresponding femoral condyles. That within the popliteus tendon is smaller, less sharply outlined, and occasionally duplicated; it is related to the margin of the tibia (/3′). A relatively radiolucent area between the trochlea and lateral femoral condyle marks the site of the extensor fossa (1′); it has occasionally been mistaken for an osteolytic lesion.

In dogs, both the distal epiphysis of the femur and the proximal epiphysis of the tibia generally fuse with their respective shafts between the 6th and 12th months. The center for the tibial tuberosity fuses between the 8th and 10th months; while it persists, the cartilage line between this center and the shaft is rather wide and irregular, presenting an appearance that simulates avulsion of the tuberosity. The onset and completion of these fusions are somewhat delayed in cats.

Few features of the leg require further comment. The subcutaneous surface of the tibia divides the cranial and caudal crural muscles medially, while the fibula makes the same division laterally (Fig. 17–4). In lean dogs the fibula may be palpated along its length, but in fatter and particularly well-muscled animals only the head and the distal half of the shaft may be felt with certainty. The superficial flexor and gastrocnemius components of the common calcaneal tendon may be identified separately, distal to the belly of the latter muscle. The lateral saphenous vein is a very conspicuous surface feature of the lateral aspect (Fig. 17–5/9). It runs proximocaudally over the lower part of the leg before following the gastrocnemius on the caudal border; it enters the popliteal fossa to join the femoral vein. The vein is much used for

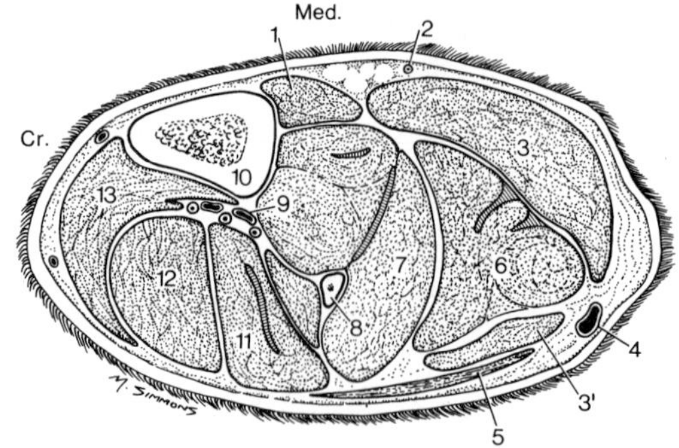


**Figure 17–4.** Transverse section of the canine left leg.

1, Popliteus; 2, saphenous artery; 3, 3′, medial and lateral heads of the gastrocnemius; 4, lateral saphenous vein; 5, biceps; 6, superficial digital flexor; 7, deep digital flexor; 8, fibula; 9, cranial tibial vessels; 10, tibia; 11, peroneus longus; 12, long digital extensor; 13, tibialis cranialis.

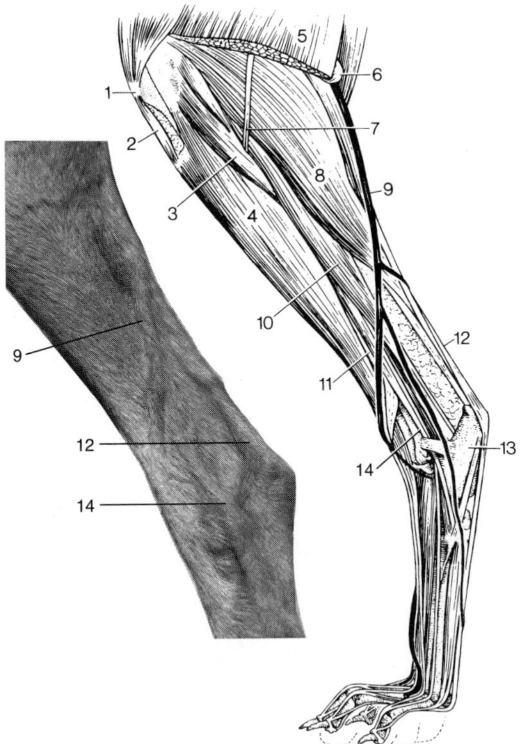


**Figure 17–5.** Left canine hindlimb; the inset shows the actual appearance of the lateral saphenous vein (9); lateral view.

1. Patella; 2, patellar ligament; 3, peroneus longus; 4, tibialis cranialis; 5, biceps; 6, popliteal lymph node; 7, common peroneal nerve; 8, lateral head of gastrocnemius; 9, lateral saphenous vein; 10, deep digital flexor; 11, superficial peroneal nerve; 12, calcanean tendon; 13, calcaneus; 14, peroneus longus tendon.

intravenous injections; its proximal part is better suited to this use since it is both relatively fixed and straight; the more mobile distal part undulates, dipping between the caudal crural muscles and the common calcanean tendon.

The vascularization of the leg and more distal parts depends on the cranial tibial and saphenous arteries since the caudal tibial is quite insignificant (Fig. 17–6/3,4). The cranial tibial continues the popliteal artery, which runs deep to the popliteal muscle on the caudal aspect of the stifle. The artery then passes between the tibia and fibula in the proximal part of the leg before penetrating the dorsal muscles. It reappears toward the hock and then follows the long extensor tendon across the joint into the paw. The saphenous artery, which broadly serves the territory assigned to the caudal tibial in many species, crosses the medial aspect of the stifle before dividing into cranial and caudal branches. The cranial branch (/6) remains superficial and continues into the paw, where it supplements the cranial tibial in supplying dorsal structures; the caudal branch (/5) accompanies the tibial nerve and, after supplying caudal crural muscles, follows the flexor tendons into the plantar aspect of the paw.

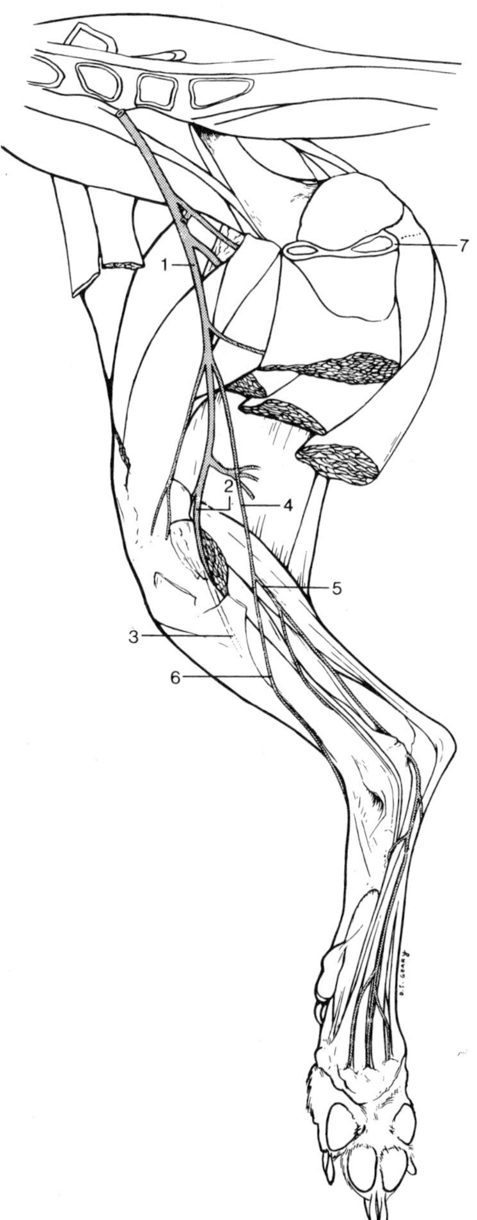


**Figure 17–6.** The principal arteries of the canine right hindlimb, medial view.

1, Femoral a.; 2, popliteal a.; 3, cranial tibial a. passing between tibia and fibula; 4, saphenous a.; 5, 6, caudal and cranial branches of saphenous a.; 7, pelvic floor.

## THE HOCK AND HINDPAW

*(See also pp. 91 and 93.)*

Inspection of the distal part of the limb reveals the distinctive conformation of the hock but little external difference between the fore- and hindpaws beyond the absence of any analogue of the carpal pad. A dewclaw is commonly present at birth but is routinely removed at an early age in puppies of many breeds. It is not found in the cat.

Although the hock skeleton is complete—there is no suppression or fusion of the standard elements—most bones cannot be individually identified on palpation. The most easily recognized feature is the long and rather slender calcaneus, which provides the leverage for the effective extension of the hock; the arrangement carries an intrinsic risk, and the bone is occasionally fractured by the force exerted by the powerful muscles attaching to its slightly swollen tip. The calcaneus also extends a medial process, the sustentaculum tali, over the plantar aspect of the talus, where it may be felt despite being covered by the deep flexor tendon (Fig. 17–7/3′). The more distal tarsal bones do not carry identifying surface features, but their locations and extents may be deduced after reference to a skeleton or to radiographs. The other prominent surface features of the region are the projections of the tibial and fibular malleoli at the lower limit of the leg and the equally prominent swellings at the proximal ends of the second and fifth metatarsal bones. A long collateral ligament may be traced from the malleolar to the metatarsal thickening on each side of the limb. The extensor tendons can be followed over the dorsal surface of the hock; the retinacula that hold them in place over the distal tibia and again at the proximal end of the metatarsus can also be appreciated in many dogs.

Only the tarsocrural joint is large enough to be punctured in the live animal. This is done on the lateral side just distal to the malleolus; the needle is directed distally toward the lateral surface of the palpable lateral trochlear ridge of the talus.

Similar impressions of the bones and soft structures of the paw are obtained as on palpation of the forelimb. Although a complete radiographic examination of the hock calls for exposures in dorsoplantar, mediolateral, and oblique projections, the most useful general picture is obtained from the dorsoplantar view since it permits identification of all the bones, some more easily than others, as there is considerable superimposition (Fig. 17–7/A). Both the talus and the calcaneus are well outlined despite the overlap of the

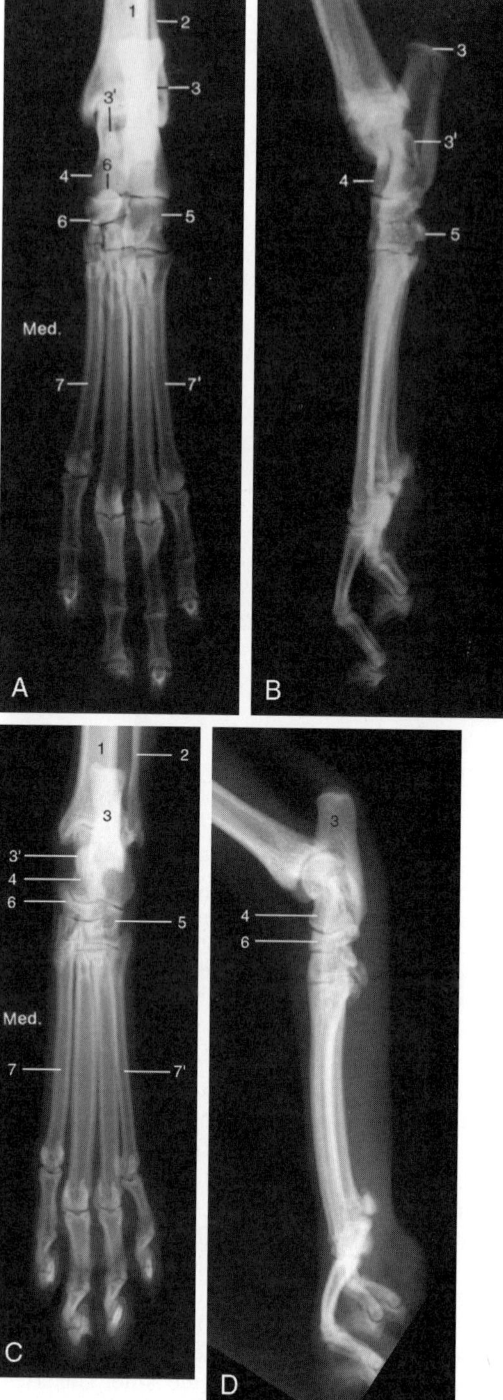


**Figure 17–7.** Dorsoplantar and lateral radiographic views of the canine (*A* and *B*) and feline (*C* and *D*) hocks and hindpaws.

1, Tibia; 2, fibula; 3, calcaneus; 3′, sustentaculum tali; 4, talus; 5, fourth tarsal bone; 6, central tarsal bone; 7, 7′, second and fifth metatarsal bones.

sustentaculum tali with the talus. The two bones in the subjacent tier—the fourth and central tarsals (/5,6)—are also generally well outlined, although the mediodistal part of the fourth is superimposed on the third. The second tarsal is clearly shown with the smaller first tarsal superimposed on it. The distal extremities of the tibia and fibula appear closely related in this projection; the gap between them appears unexpectedly wide in slightly oblique projections obtained of the cat's hock, a feature occasionally misinterpreted as evidence of luxation.

The lateral projection (*/B*) depicts the calcaneus and talus clearly, although they overlap toward the center of the field. The more distal bones are less easily identified in this view, apart from the fourth, which is betrayed by a protuberance on its plantar aspect (Fig. 17–8/4′). Since the central bone is occasionally dislocated, it is important to note the normal alignment of the dorsal borders of the bones of successive tiers. Two previously unrecorded sesamoid bones have recently been described in the Greyhound at the plantar aspect of the hock about the level of the tarsometatarsal joint. They would appear to have the usual significance of such sesamoids—potential misinterpretation as chips fractured from the major bones.

There are no distinctive features of the radiological anatomy of the metatarsal bones and phalanges.

## THE MAJOR NERVES OF THE HINDLIMB

It is only necessary to deal briefly with the course, relations, and distribution of those nerves that extend substantially into the free limb since a general account of the lumbosacral plexus (usually formed by the nerves L4–S2) and its divisions has been presented (p. 315).

The *femoral nerve* (L4–L6) has a very short course within the thigh before it ends by ramifying within the quadriceps femoris, the principal

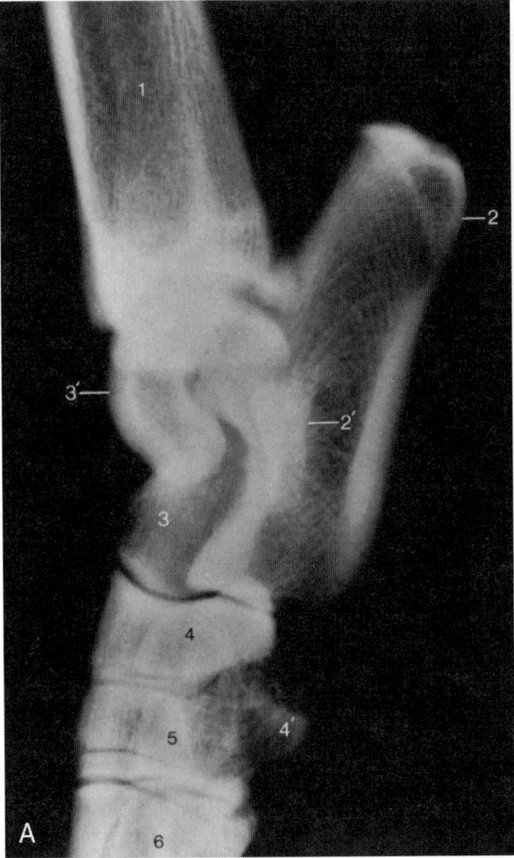


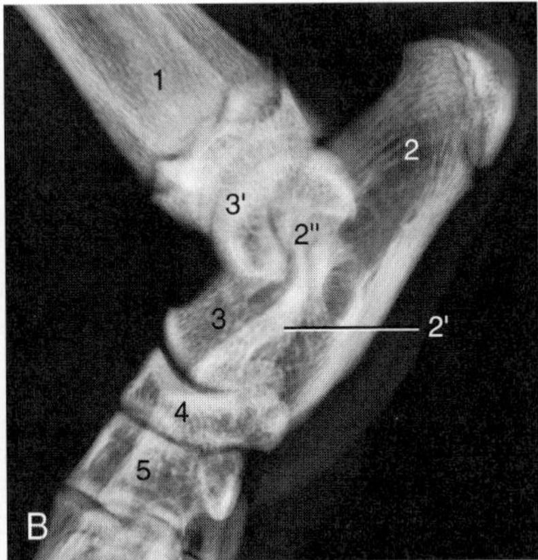


**Figure 17–8.** Lateral radiographic views of the canine *(A)* and young feline *(B)* hocks.

1, Tibia and fibula; 2, calcaneus; 2′, sustentaculum tali; 2″, coracoid process; 3, talus; 3′, trochlea of talus; 4, superimposed fourth and central tarsal bones; 4′, palmar tubercle on fourth tarsal bone; 5, distal row of tarsal bones; 6, metatarsal bones.

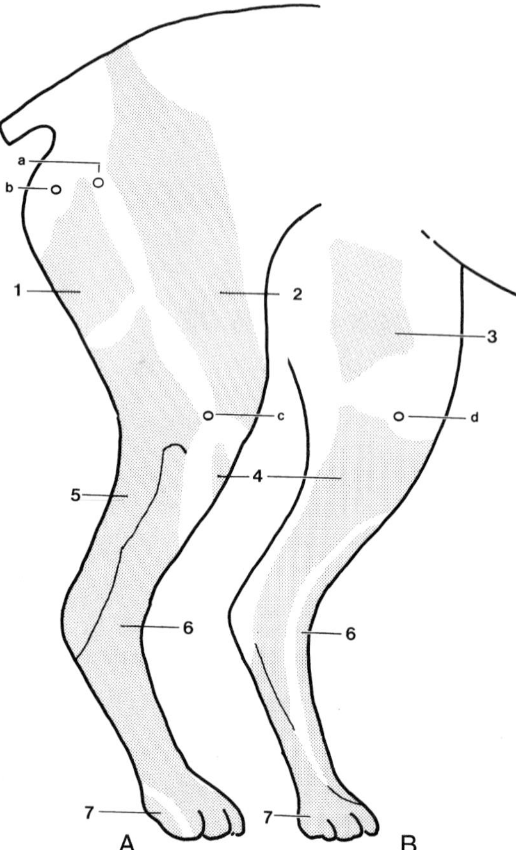


**Figure 17–9.** Autonomous zones of the cutaneous innervation on the lateral *(A)* and medial *(B)* surfaces of the canine hindlimb.

1, Caudal cutaneous femoral nerve; 2, lateral cutaneous femoral nerve; 3, genitofemoral nerve; 4, saphenous nerve; 5, sciatic nerve; 6, peroneal nerve; 7, tibial nerve.

a, Position of greater trochanter; b, ischial tuber; c, lateral tibial condyle; d, medial tibial condyle.

extensor of the stifle, and an ancillary flexor of the hip. Shortly before disappearing into this muscle it detaches the saphenous nerve, which descends superficially over the medial aspect of the limb accompanied by the (palpable) saphenous artery. Although the *saphenous nerve* supplies the sartorius, it is largely sensory, serving the skin of the medial surface of the thigh, stifle, leg, and hock (Fig. 17–9). Dysfunction of the femoral nerve paralyzes the quadriceps, resulting in the collapse of the stifle and disabling the entire limb. Compensation is not available. The skin of the medial surface of the limb is deprived of sensation.

The *sciatic nerve* (L6–S1) crosses the dorsal border of the hip bone to enter the limb together with the caudal gluteal vessels. After passing the dorsocaudal aspect of the hip joint, deep to the greater trochanter, where it is susceptible to injury in trauma or surgery of the joint, the nerve and vessel bundle supplies branches to the hamstring muscles. The nerve then continues distally in a central position within the thigh, caudal to the femur, and cushioned between the biceps laterally, the adductor, and later the semimembranosus, medially (Fig. 17–2/4). At a rather variable point it divides into common peroneal and tibial nerves that continue the course of the parent trunk until they diverge caudal to the stifle. The sciatic nerve and its peroneal and tibial branches collectively supply the skin of the entire limb distal to the stifle joint, with the minor exception of the medial strip claimed by the saphenous.

The *common peroneal nerve,* the more lateral of the terminal divisions of the sciatic, can be palpated in lean dogs, where it passes over the lateral head of the gastrocnemius (Fig. 17–5/7). It then dives deeply among the dorsal crural muscles (the extensors of the digits and flexors of the hock), which it supplies. It is continued by superficial and deep (peroneal) branches that enter the paw over the dorsal aspect of the hock; they supply the skin of the dorsal surface. Paralysis of the common peroneal nerve produces slight overextension of the hock and inability to extend the digits, which may be rested on their dorsal surfaces. In time, dogs learn to flick their paw forward, enabling the limb to support weight. The dorsal surface of the paw is without sensation.

The *tibial nerve* passes between the two heads of the gastrocnemius, where it detaches branches to the muscles behind the tibia (the flexors of the digit and extensors of the hock). The depleted nerve, now largely sensory but retaining a small motor component for the intrinsic muscles of the paw, continues distally within the web of skin between the caudal crural muscles and the common calcanean tendon. It crosses the hock beside the deep flexor tendon before branching to supply the plantar structures of the paw. Tibial nerve injuries cause the hock to be flexed and lowered closer to the ground when the limb bears weight. The paralysis of the digital flexors elevates the toes; their plantar aspect is without sensation.

## Selected Bibliography

Alexander J.W.: Coxofemoral luxations in the dog. Compend. Contin. Educ. Pract. Vet. 4:575–583, 1982.

Arnbjerg, J., and N.I. Heje: Fabellae and popliteal sesamoid bones in cats. J. Small Anim. Pract. 34:95–98, 1993.

Arnoczky, S.P.: Stifle surgery: An update. 1986. *In* Proceedings of the American Animal Hospital Association, 1986, pp 507–513.

Arnoczky, S.P.: The cruciate ligaments: The enigma of the canine stifle. J. Small Anim. Pract. 29:71–90, 1988.

Autefage, A., P. Fayolle, and P.L. Toutain: Distribution of material injected intramuscularly in dogs. Am. J. Vet. Res. 51:901–904, 1990.

Bailey, C.S., R.L. Kitchell, S.S. Haghighi, and R.D. Johnson: Spinal nerve root origins of the cutaneous nerves of the canine pelvic limb. Am. J. Vet. Res. 49:115–119, 1988.

Baird, D.K., J.T. Hathcock, P.F. Rumph, et al.: Low-field magnetic resonance imaging of the canine stifle joint: Normal anatomy. Vet. Radiol. Ultrasound 39:87–97, 1998.

Basinger, R.R., Aron, D.N., Crowe, D.T., and P.T. Purinton: Osteofascial compartment syndrome in the dog. Vet. Surg. 16:427–434, 1987.

Beale, B.S., and R.L. Goring: Exposure of the medial and lateral trochlear ridges of the talus in the dog. Part I: Dorsomedial and plantaromedial surgical approaches to the medial trochlear ridge. J. Am. Anim. Hosp. Assoc. 26:13–18, 1990.

Boyd, J.S.: Color Atlas of Clinical Anatomy of the Dog and Cat. St. Louis, Mosby–Year Book, 1991.

Cardinet, G.H., and G. Lust: The international symposium on hip dysplasia in dogs. JAVMA 210:1417–1418, 1997.

Cardinet, G.H., III, P.H. Kass, L.J. Wallace, and M.M. Guffy: Association between pelvic muscle mass and canine hip dysplasia. JAVMA 210:1466–1473, 1997.

Chambers, J.N., P.T. Puriton, S.W. Allen, and J.L. Moore: Identification and anatomic categorization of the vascular patterns of the pelvic limb muscles of dogs. Am. J. Vet. Res. 51:305–313, 1990.

deLahunta, A., and R.E. Habel: Applied Veterinary Anatomy. Philadelphia, W.B. Saunders Company, 1986.

Dew, T.L., and R.A. Martin: A caudal approach to the tibiotarsal joint. J. Am. Anim. Hosp. Assoc. 29:117–121, 1993.

Dupuis, J., J. Harari, M. Papageorges, et al.: Evaluation of fibular head transposition for repair of experimental cranial cruciate ligament injury in dogs. Vet. Surg. 23:1–12, 1994.

Farese, J.P., R.J. Todhunter, G. Lust, et al.: Dorsolateral subluxation of hip joints in dogs measured in a weight-bearing position with radiography and computed tomography. Vet. Surg. 27:393–405, 1998.

Gee, M., T.M. Lenehan, and G.B. Tarvin: Rotatory intra-articular dislocation of the patella in two dogs. JAVMA 209:2082–2084, 1996.

Goring, R.L., and B.S. Beale: Exposure of the medial and lateral trochlear ridges of the talus in the dog. Part II: Dorsolateral and plantarolateral surgical approaches to the lateral trochlear ridge. J. Am. Anim. Hosp. Assoc. 26:19–24, 1990.

Gregory, C.R., J.M. Cullen, R. Pool, and P.B. Vasseur: The canine sacroiliac joint. Preliminary study of its anatomy, histopathology, and biomechanics. Spine 11:1044–1048, 1986.

Harari, J.: Caudal cruciate ligament injury. Vet. Clin. North Am. Small Anim. Pract. 23:821–827, 1993.

Harasen, G.L.G.: A retrospective study of 165 cases of rupture of the canine cranial cruciate ligament. Can. Vet. J. 36:250–251, 1995.

Horowitz, A.: The Fundamental Principles of Anatomy; Dissection of the Dog. Saskatoon, University of Saskatchewan, 1970. Published by the author.

Hudson, L.C., and W.P. Hamilton: Atlas of Feline Anatomy for Veterinarians. Philadelphia, W.B. Saunders Company, 1993.

Ihemelandu, E.C., G.H. Cardinet, III, M.M. Guffy, and L. J. Wallace: Canine hip dysplasia: Differences in pectineal muscles of healthy and dysplastic German Shepherd dogs when two months old. Am. J. Vet. Res. 44:411–416, 1983.

Johnson, A.L., and M.L. Olmstead: Caudal cruciate ligament rupture—a retrospective analysis of 14 dogs. Vet. Surg. 16:202–206, 1987.

Lust, G., R.J. Todhunter, H.N. Erb, et al.: Comparison of three radiographic methods for diagnosis of hip dysplasia in eight-month-old dogs. JAVMA 219:1242–1246, 2001.

Lust, G., A.J. Williams, N. Burton-Wurster, et al.: Joint laxity and its association with hip dysplasia in Labrador Retrievers. Am. J. Vet. Res. 54:1990–1999, 1993.

Mahler, S., and T. Havet: Secondary ossification centre at the acetabular dorsal rim in a dog. Radiographic and MRI observations. Vet. Comp. Orthop. Traumatol. 12:70–73, 1999.

Mauterer, J.V., Jr., R.G. Prata, C.A. Carberry, and S.C. Schrader: Displacement of the tendon of the superficial digital flexor muscle in dogs: 10 cases (1983–1991). JAVMA 203:1162–1165, 1993.

McCarthy, P.H., and A.K.W. Wood: Anatomical and radiological observations of the sesamoid bone of the popliteus muscle in the adult dog and cat. Anat. Histol. Embryol. 18:58–65, 1989.

Moore, K.W., and R.A. Read: Rupture of the cranial cruciate ligament in dogs—Part I. Compend. Contin. Educ. Pract. Vet. 18:223–234, 1996.

Moore, K.W., and R.A. Read: Rupture of the cranial cruciate ligament in dogs—Part II. Diagnosis and management. Compend. Contin. Educ. Pract. Vet. 18:381–405, 1996.

Pavaux, C., Y. Lignereux, and J.Y. Sautet: Anatomie comparative et chirurgicale du tendon calcanéen commun des mammifères domestiques. Anat. Histol. Embryol. 12:60–69, 1983.

Payne, J.T., and G.M. Constantinescu: Stifle joint anatomy and surgical approaches in the dog. Vet. Clin. North Am. Small Anim. Pract. 23:691–701, 1993.

Pérez-Aparicio, F.J., and T.O. Fjeld: Coxofemoral luxations in cats. J. Small Anim. Pract. 34:345–349, 1993.

Piermattei, D.L., and R.G. Greeley: An Atlas of Surgical Approaches to the Bones of the Dog and Cat, 3rd ed. Philadelphia, W.B. Saunders Company, 1992.

Prose, L.P.: Anatomy of the knee joint of the cat. Acta. Anat. 119:40–48, 1984.

Reinke, J.D., A.J. Mughannam, and J.M. Owens: Avulsion of the gastrocnemius tendon in 11 dogs. J. Am. Anim. Hosp. Assoc. 29:410–418, 1993.

Saunders, J.H., T. Godefroid, F.R. Snaps, et al.: Comparison of ventrodorsal and dorsoventral radiographic projections for hip dysplasia diagnosis. Vet. Rec. 145:109–110, 1999.

Scavelli, T.D., and S.C. Schrader: Nonsurgical management of rupture of the cranial cruciate ligament in 18 cats. J. Am. Anim. Hosp. Assoc. 23:337–340, 1987.

Schebitz, H., and H. Wilkens: Atlas of Radiographic Anatomy of the Dog and Cat, 4th ed. Berlin, Paul Parey Verlag, 1986.

Sylvestre, A.M., M.J. Weinstein, C.A. Popovitch, and D.J. Brockman: The sartorius muscle flap in the cat: An anatomic study and two case reports. J. Am. Anim. Hosp. Assoc. 33:91–96, 1997.

Todhunter, R.J., T.A. Zachos, R.O. Gilbert, et al.: Onset of epiphyseal mineralization and growth plate closure in radiographically normal and dysplastic Labrador Retrievers. JAVMA, 210:1458–1462, 1997.

Updike, S.J.: A redescription of the gross anatomy of the canine extensor digitorum longus muscle. Anat. Histol. Embryol. 14:432–437, 1985.

Van Ryssen, B., H. van Bree, and P. Vyt: Arthroscopy of the canine hock joint. J. Am. Anim. Hosp. Assoc. 29:107–115, 1993.

Vasseur, P.B.: The stifle joint. *In* Slatter D.H.: Textbook of Small Animal Surgery, 2nd ed. Philadelphia, W.B. Saunders Company, 1993, pp. 1817–1866.

Wallace, J.: Canine hip dysplasia: Differences in pectineal muscles of healthy and dysplastic German Shepherd dogs when two months old. Am. J. Vet. Res. 44:411–416, 1983.

Whitehair, J.G., P.B. Vasseur, and N.H. Willits: Epidemiology of cranial cruciate ligament rupture in dogs. JAVMA 203:1016–1019, 1993.

Williams, J., Jr., J. Tomlinson, and G.M. Constantinescu: Diagnosing and treating meniscal injuries in the dog. Vet. Med. 89:42–47, 1994.

Worthman, R.P.: Demonstration of specific nerve paralysis in the dog. JAVMA 131:174–178, 1957.

Yahia, L.H., N.M. Newman, and M. St.-Georges: Innervation of the canine cruciate ligaments: A neurohistological study. Anat. Histol. Embryol. 21:1–8, 1992.

CHAPTER 18

# The Head and Ventral Neck of the Horse

HORSE

## CONFORMATION AND EXTERNAL FEATURES

The general character of the head is determined by the age, the sex, and the breed. In young foals the cranial vault is domed to match the contours of the brain and projects above a face that is both short and shallow (Fig. 18–1). The adult conformation develops as the face lengthens and deepens to accommodate the full complement of teeth and expanding paranasal sinuses; enlargement of the frontal sinus smoothes the dorsal profile at the junction of face with cranium. Sex and breed differences are not wholly separable from those due to age since the face is disproportionately increased in larger animals; a longer face is therefore characteristic of the adult compared with the juvenile, the stallion with the mare, and the heavy draft horse with the pony. The other very obvious breed difference concerns the dorsal profile; a relatively straight profile is generally preferred but some convexity ("ram's head") is characteristic of certain heavy breeds, while concavity ("dishing") is the rule in Arabs and common in horses with admixture of Arab blood (Fig. 18–1). The ventral margin of the lower jaw of young horses may be disfigured by one or more rounded swellings, each corresponding in position to the root of an unerupted permanent cheek tooth. The temporary irregularities, though unsightly, are part of a normal process (p. 492).

The skin is thinner and more firmly bound down than over most other parts of the body and is especially tight where it lies directly upon bone. The coat is generally short but a forelock continuing the mane may be prominent; a "mustache" is a feature of some animals, especially the larger breeds. Tactile hairs are numerous and widely scattered on the lips and chin and about the margins of the nostrils.

The *nostrils* are large and widely spaced, especially in Thoroughbreds (Fig. 18–2). Their peculiar form is imposed by the supporting alar cartilages (Fig. 18–3/*B*,1′,2′). The upper part of the opening leads to a blind nasal diverticulum (/1″) which occupies the nasoincisive notch (/6) and is without counterpart in other domestic species.* The lower part leads directly to the nasal cavity. It is therefore essential when passing a stomach tube to ensure that it is guided into this lower part. The margins of the nostril are very flexible and allow the opening to be dilated, both actively when breathing is strenuous and passively upon manipulation. The dilated nostril is rounded, the change in form being achieved by apposition of the walls of the diverticulum. The pliancy of the tissues facilitates examination of the nasal vestibule and exposure of the opening of the *nasolacrimal duct,* which is found on the floor, about 5 cm internal to the entrance and near the mucocutaneous junction. Occasionally the duct has more than one opening.

The entrance to the mouth is small with the commissure a little in front of the first cheek teeth (P2). The skin of the *lips* and adjacent part of the muzzle is sparsely covered by short, fine hairs that impart a velvety texture. The lips are both mobile and sensitive, and are used in the selection and prehension of food. The sensitivity of the upper lip is exploited when a twitch is applied to control a horse during procedures (e.g., injections) elsewhere on the body. The application of acupressure causes the animal to become somewhat sedated while its heart rate is lowered and endorphins are released. It is suggested that the endorphins activate a pain-decreasing mechanism. The lower lip surmounts the chin swelling, which is based on a pad of fatty fibrous tissue.

The *eyes* are prominent and placed to each side of the head, indicating that the horse, like other

*The barbaric custom of splitting the lateral wall of this diverticulum is known from Pharaonic times, and may still be encountered in the Middle East. It is of course completely without the intended effect on the efficiency of respiration.

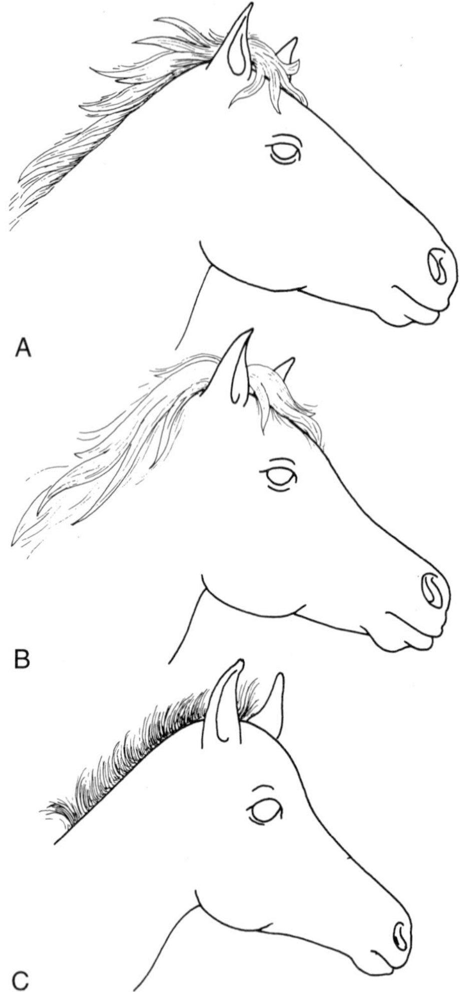


**Figure 18–1.** Variations in the profile of the equine head. *A,* The common straight profile. *B,* The dished Arabian profile. *C,* The domed contour of the foal.

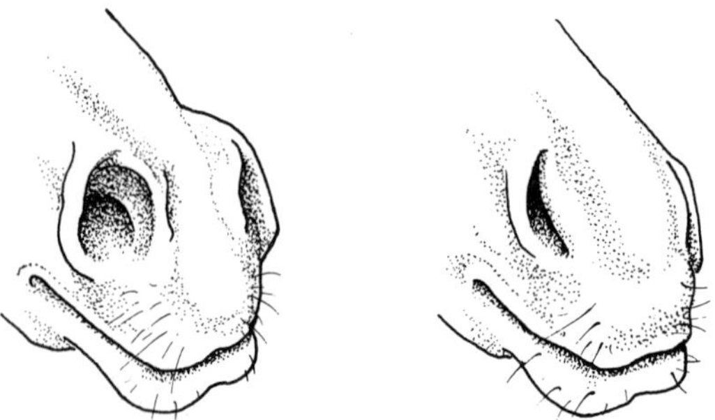

**Figure 18–2.** Functional variations in the form of the nostril.

herbivores, enjoys a panoramic field of vision. Indeed, horses may view almost all around by making only slight movements of the head. This ability to survey widely—perhaps through 330 degrees—is obtained at the expense of the binocular field, which is limited to some 65 degrees. The field of overlap is further reduced by the length and shape of the muzzle, which creates a blind area directly to the front (see Fig. 9–1).

The upper and lower *eyelids* and adjacent skin carry a few scattered tactile hairs. The palpebral skin is thin and, being loosely attached, is thrown into folds when the eye is open. The lid margins

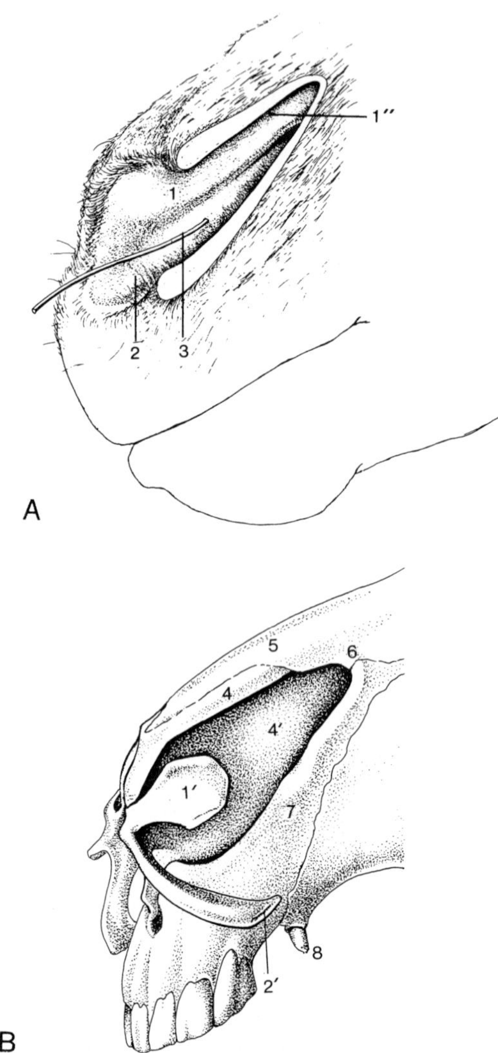


**Figure 18–3.** *A,* Left nostril opened laterally to expose nasal diverticulum. *B,* Nasal cartilages.

1, Alar fold, supported by the lamina (1′) of the alar cartilage; dorsal to the alar fold is the nasal diverticulum (1″); 2, floor of nostril supported by the cornu of the alar cartilage (2′)—the floor leads into the nasal cavity; 3, probe in nasolacrimal duct; 4, dorsal lateral nasal cartilage; 4′, nasal septum; 5, nasal bone; 6, nasoincisive notch; 7, incisive bone; 8, canine tooth.

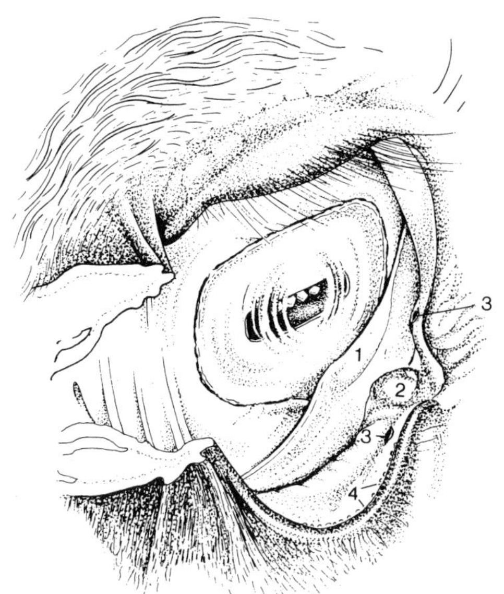


**Figure 18–4.** The right conjunctival sac.

1, Third eyelid; 2, lacrimal caruncle; 3, lacrimal puncta; 4, openings of the tarsal glands.

carry numerous lashes, longer and more prominent on the upper than on the lower lid (Plate 18/*G*). The *tarsal glands,* which open at the junction of the skin with the conjunctiva, number about 50 in the upper lid, rather fewer below, and are clearly visible in palisade formation when the lids are everted. The palpebral conjunctiva is well vascularized, the bulbar part less generously; the bulbar conjunctiva is strongly pigmented toward the corneoscleral region. The third eyelid (Fig. 18–4/1) in the medial angle can be exposed in the usual way by pressing upon the eyeball through the upper eyelid; a small accessory lacrimal gland is associated with it. The lacrimal caruncle is prominent. The features of the eyeball are considered later (p. 503).

A depression caudal to the eye (behind the palpable postorbital bar of bone) is prominent in the animal at rest. It disappears and reappears during feeding in rhythm with the movements of the jaws; the effects are due to the displacement of a pad of fat interposed between the temporalis and the periorbita. The fat is depleted in horses in poor condition when exaggeration of the hollow contributes significantly to the haggard appearance.

Little need be said concerning the external ears, which are prominent and capable of being swiveled when attempts are made to locate the origin of a sound. Their carriage is also very expressive of emotion.

# SUPERFICIAL STRUCTURES

## The Muscles of Facial Expression

Many clinically important features are revealed as soon as the skin is removed. Large areas of the skull are not covered by any considerable thickness of soft tissue and are therefore vulnerable to injury. These areas include the dorsal aspect of the nose, the forehead, and part of the temple, in addition to much of the mandible. Prominent landmarks include the facial crest, which runs parallel to the dorsum of the nose; it begins above the rostral margin of the fourth cheek tooth, continues into the zygomatic arch, which forms the lower margin of the orbit, and extends to the temporomandibular joint (Fig. 18–5/4). The joint itself is easily located by the salience of the lateral aspect of the condyle, directly before the palpable caudal margin of the mandible. The identification becomes more certain if the animal can be induced to perform chewing movements. The ventral margin of the mandible is also prominent, particularly the half that lies rostral to the masseter muscle. A shallow notch in the bone directly in front of the muscle conveys the facial vessels and parotid duct from the intermandibular space to the face.

The incomplete sheet of cutaneous muscle over the lateral aspect of the head is best developed where it merges with the orbicularis oris around the opening of the mouth.

A few individual mimetic muscles deserve notice. The *levator labii superioris* arises over the maxilla and runs dorsorostrally to form a common tendon with its fellow of the other side (Fig. 18–7/1′); the tendon, which is enclosed within a synovial sheath, descends between the nostrils to splay out within the upper lip. This muscle is responsible for the lip curl (Flehmen) seen in certain circumstances, including sexual excitement. The levator belly is easily palpated and since it covers the infraorbital foramen, it must be pushed dorsally in order to locate the emergent infraorbital nerve (/1). This foramen lies along the line joining the nasoincisive notch to the rostral end of the facial crest.

The *depressor labii inferioris* (/3′) arises with the buccinator from the alveolar margin and adjacent part of the mandible under cover of the masseter. It can be identified as a rounded cord running rostrally over the body of the bone. The tendon covers the mental foramen, located about 2 to 3 cm caudal to the angle of the mouth, and this is readily palpable when the muscle is slid aside (/3). The *buccinator* (/8) has a well-marked

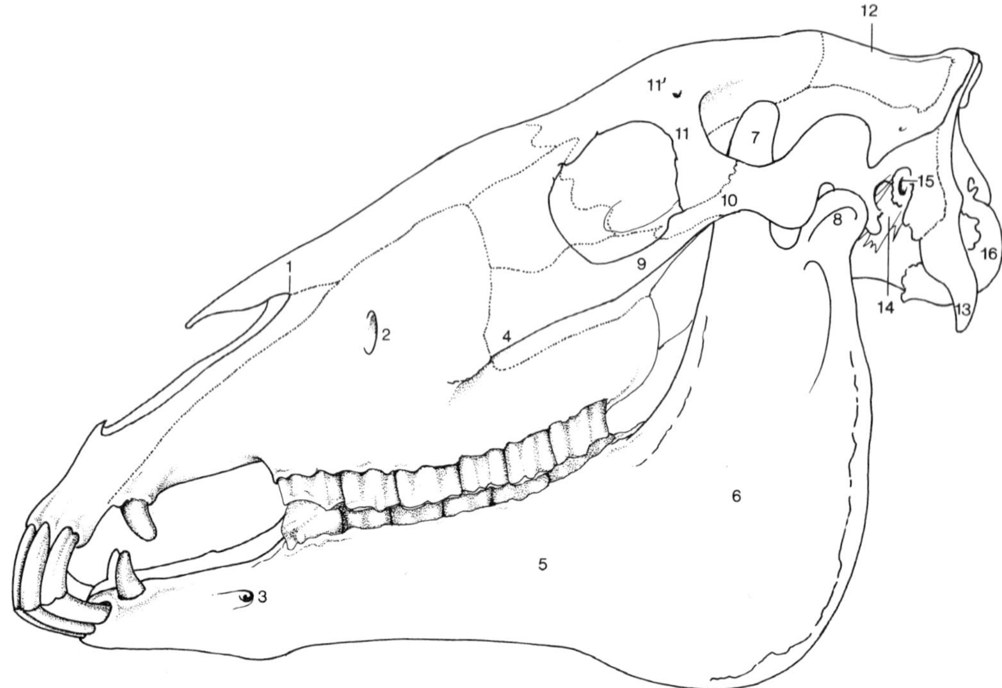


**Figure 18–5.** Lateral view of the skull.

1, Nasoincisive notch; 2, infraorbital foramen; 3, mental foramen; 4, facial crest; 5, body of mandible; 6, ramus of mandible; 7, coronoid process; 8, condylar process; 9, temporal process of zygomatic bone; 10, zygomatic process of temporal bone; 11, zygomatic process of frontal bone; 11′, supraorbital foramen; 12, external sagittal crest; 13, paracondylar process; 14, styloid process; 15, external acoustic meatus; 16, occipital condyle.

herringbone structure and is partly covered by the masseter. It is important in returning food to the central cavity of the mouth, preventing its accumulation in the oral vestibule.

## Superficial Vessels

The *facial artery* and *vein* enter the face in company with the parotid duct (Fig. 18–6/10,9). The artery is easily found where it is in contact with the bone and is convenient for taking the pulse (Fig. 18–37/7). The artery then ascends along the rostral margin of the masseter before terminating in divergent branches; although the pattern of collateral and terminal branches varies, it is usually possible to identify inferior and superior labial, lateral and dorsal nasal, and angularis oculi arteries.

The arrangement of the veins is similar, and their pattern may be visible in life in thin-skinned horses. Certain of the tributaries turn caudally, deep to the masseter, to anastomose with other veins of the head. The most dorsal connection, the *transverse facial vein* (Fig. 18–7/5), joins the superficial temporal vein. The rostral part lies deep to the masseter, but it then penetrates the muscle and in the caudal part of its course it lies superficially and follows the ventral edge of the zygomatic arch. This caudal stretch is accompanied by an artery (an alternative site for examination of the pulse) and nerve. Another site for pulse-taking is the subcutaneous segment of the masseteric artery (Fig. 18–6/15).

The second connection, the *deep facial vein* (Fig. 18–7/6), buries below the masseter and perforates the periorbita before passing through the orbital fissure to join the cavernous venous sinus within the cranial cavity. Two features of this vein are believed to possess functional significance. The discharge into the cavernous sinus contains relatively cool blood drained from the hard palate and nasal cavity; since the sinus envelops the internal carotid artery, this cools the arterial blood passing to the brain where the temperature is monitored as part of the heat control mechanism. Secondly, an expansion of the vein deep to the masseter may form the basis of a pumping mechanism. It is liable to compression by the masseter and it is asserted that this helps prevent stagnation of the venous return from the lowered head of the grazing animal.

There is a similar expansion on the third connection, the *buccal vein* (/7), which also runs deep to the masseter to join the superficial temporal tributary of the maxillary vein.

There are two superficial groups of lymph nodes. The parotid group under cover of the rostral part of the parotid gland is not usually palpable unless enlarged. The second group comprises numerous mandibular nodes arranged in a spindle within the intermandibular space. Together with their contralateral fellows, these nodes form a forward-pointing V that is always very distinctly palpable (Fig. 18–35/2). The course of the lymph flow is dealt with later (p. 507).

## Superficial Nerves

Only a few features of the superficial nerves require notice. The *facial nerve* detaches its *auriculopalpebral branch* before it enters the face (Fig. 18–25/19). This branch then takes an independent course across the zygomatic arch (where it is palpable), which leads it between the eye and the ear. The branch may be blocked by injection between the caudal end of the arch and the base of the ear. The procedure facilitates examination of the eye since it eliminates blinking and closure of the lids (p. 336).

The facial trunk divides into *dorsal* and *ventral buccal branches* before or, more commonly,

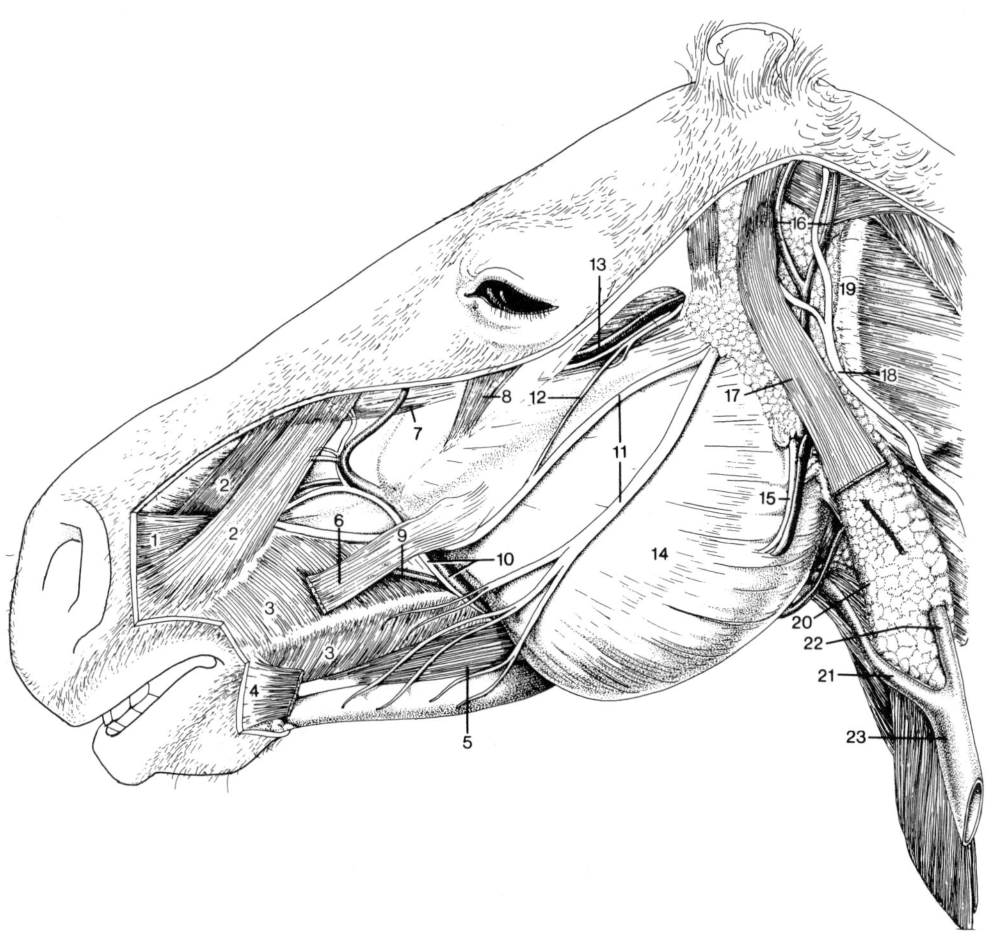


**Figure 18–6.** Superficial dissection of the head.

1, Caninus; 2, levator nasolabialis; 3, buccinator; 4, stump of cutaneous muscle joining orbicularis oris; 5, depressor labii inferioris; 6, zygomaticus; 7, levator labii superioris; 8, malaris; 9, parotid duct; 10, facial artery and vein; 11, buccal branches of facial nerve; 12, rostral communicating branch of auriculotemporal nerve; 13, transverse facial artery and vein and transverse facial branch of auriculotemporal nerve; 14, masseter; 15, masseteric artery and vein; 16, auricular veins; 17, parotidoauricularis; 18, great auricular nerve (C2); 19, wing of atlas; 20, parotid gland; 21, linguofacial vein; 22, maxillary vein; 23, external jugular vein.

shortly after emerging from under the protection of the parotid gland (Fig. 18–6/11). These branches, and the smaller divisions into which they soon assort, run forward over the masseter, where they are palpable and sometimes even visible through the skin. Blows over the masseter or pressure in prolonged recumbency may damage some or all of the divisions. The asymmetry of the face that results when the muscles of the lips, cheek, and nose are paralyzed is usually more striking than in other species. Since the auriculopalpebral branch is precociously detached, such trauma generally spares the muscles of the eyelids and external ear; their involvement points to injury at a more proximal level, which suggests a more sinister causation.

The sensory innervation of the face is the duty of the *trigeminal nerve.* It is an easy matter to locate some of the principal branches concerned—the *supraorbital, infraorbital,* and *mental nerves*—where they emerge from the corresponding foramina (Fig. 18–7/1,3). The supraorbital nerve leaves the supraorbital foramen within an easily located dimple in the root of the zygomatic process of the frontal bone. The nerve supplies the upper eyelid and adjacent part of the forehead skin. Directions for location of the infraorbital and mental nerves have already been given (pp. 65 and 481). Anesthetic deposited about the infraorbital nerve at its emergence will desensitize the skin of the upper lip, nostril, and much of the nose extending well caudal to the foramen. Blockage of the mental nerve desensitizes the skin of the lower lip and chin region. When blocking either of these nerves it is possible to insert the tip of the needle through the foramen into the bony canal within the jaw. If this is done, injection of anesthetic will also deaden the more rostral teeth (from P2 forward).

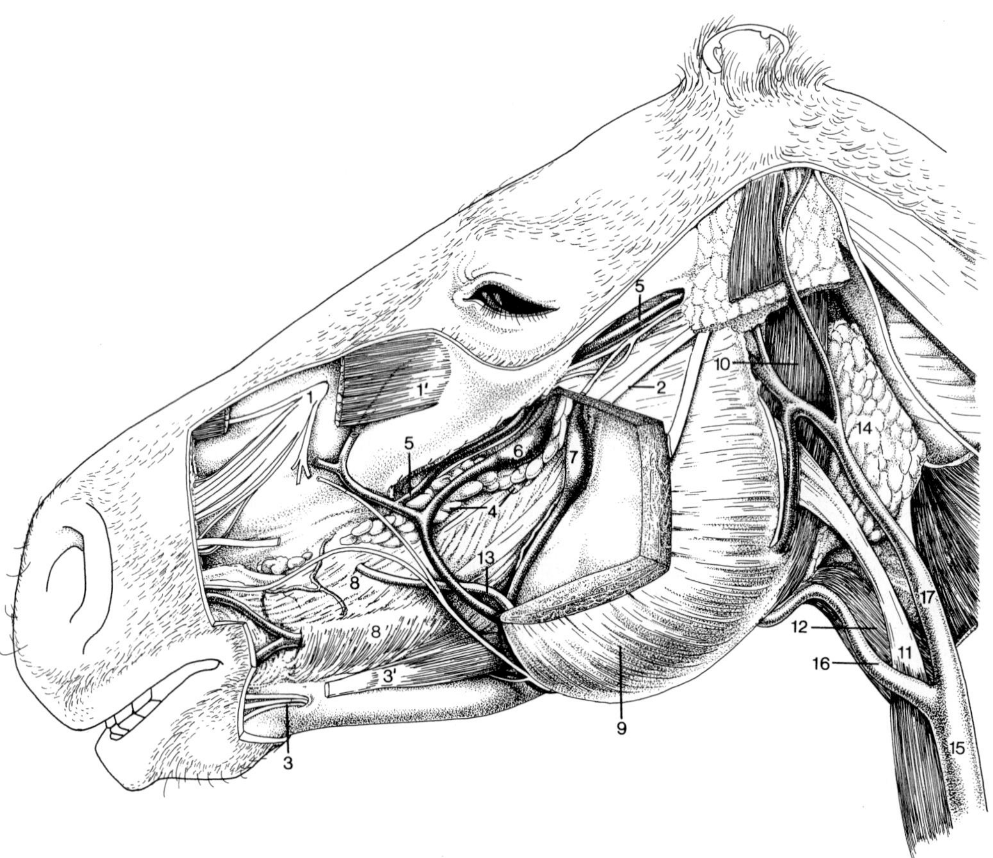


**Figure 18–7.** Deeper dissection of the head. Parts of the superficial muscles, masseter, and parotid gland have been removed.

1, Infraorbital nerve; 1′, levator labii superioris; 2, dorsal buccal branch of facial nerve; 3, mental nerve; 3′, depressor labii inferioris; 4, buccal glands; 5, transverse facial vein; 6, deep facial vein; 7, buccal vein; 8, buccinator; 9, masseter; 10, occipitomandibularis; 11, sternocephalicus; 12, fused omo- and sternohyoidei; 13, parotid duct; 14, mandibular gland; 15, external jugular vein; 16, linguofacial vein; 17, maxillary vein.

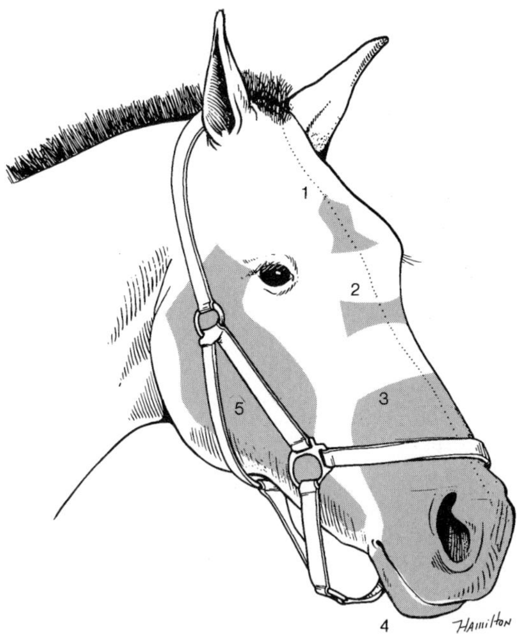


**Figure 18–8.** Five autonomous zones of the cutaneous innervation of the head.

1, Supraorbital nerve; 2, infratrochlear nerve; 3, infraorbital nerve; 4, mental nerve; 5, transverse facial branch of auriculotemporal nerve.

Figure 18–8 shows the autonomous zones of several of these nerves.

# THE NASAL CAVITY AND PARANASAL SINUSES

## The Nasal Cavity

Some features of the external nose have been described (p. 479). The ventral part of the nostril leads through a constricted vestibule into a nasal cavity considerably less roomy than might be supposed from the exterior. The factors that determine this are common to all species, but their importance is exaggerated in the horse by the reserve portions of the cheek teeth and the extensive development of the paranasal sinus system (see Fig. 3–16).

The dorsal and ventral conchae form delicate scrolls that coil in opposite directions from their lateral attachments (Fig. 18–9). The space enclosed within each is divided into two compartments by an internal septum. The caudal part of the dorsal concha is occupied by a rostral extension of the frontal sinus with which it enjoys free communication. The caudal space within the ventral concha communicates with the rostral maxillary sinus. The space within the rostral part of each major concha is in direct communication with the nasal cavity. Numerous small ethmoidal conchae projecting into the fundus serve to enlarge the olfactory area (Fig. 18–10/3).

The major *conchae* divide the cavity into the usual pattern of meatuses (Fig. 18–9). It may be presumed (for direct evidence is lacking) that the dorsal meatus leads air to the olfactory mucosa and the middle meatus to the sinuses, while the ventral and common meatuses supply the principal respiratory passage. The conjunction of the last two provides the widest and most convenient route for the introduction of a stomach tube, endoscope, or other instrument. The fragility of the ventral concha and the vascularity of the covering mucosa require that the procedure be performed with care.

Since breathing through the mouth is impossible, augmentation of the air intake in conditions of stress depends on reduction of the obstruction offered by the nose itself. The nostrils may be greatly widened by obliteration of the nasal diverticulum (Fig. 18–2), while contraction of the mucosal venous plexuses thins (and blanches) the membrane. Conversely, congestion of the mucosal vessels seriously impedes air flow. In infections, thickening of the mucosa around the slitlike entrance to the sinus system may obstruct its drainage, damming back a catarrhal exudate.

The *vomeronasal organ* does not communicate with the mouth in the horse but maintains the usual connection with the nasal cavity (Fig. 18–11/2).

## The Paranasal Sinuses

The extensive sinus system possesses considerable clinical interest since it is susceptible to infection that may spread from the nose or from an alveolar abscess. It also provides a means of access to the unerupted portions of the caudal cheek teeth (Fig. 18–12).

On each side there are frontal, caudal maxillary, and rostral maxillary sinuses of importance, and sphenopalatine and ethmoidal spaces of less account. The layout is complicated and in one important respect unique (among domestic species); the frontal sinus communicates with the nasal cavity indirectly via the caudal maxillary sinus.

The *frontal sinus* occupies the dorsal part of the skull medial to the orbit. It overlaps both cranial and nasal cavities, and since it also occupies the closed part of the dorsal concha, it is more

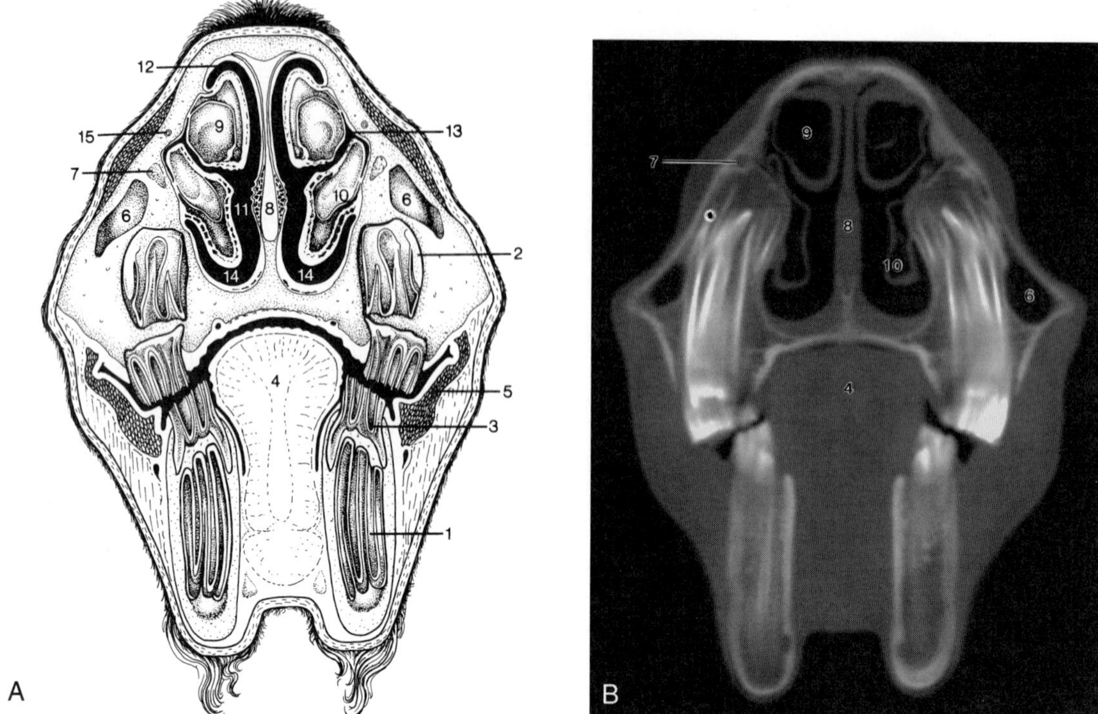


**Figure 18–9.** *A*, Transverse section of the head at the level of the rostral maxillary sinus. *B*, CT scan (bone window) at about the same level.

1, $P_4$; 2, $P^4$; 3, $p_4$; 4, tongue; 5, buccinator; 6, rostral maxillary sinus; 7, infraorbital nerve; 8, nasal septum; 9, dorsal nasal concha; 10, ventral nasal concha; 11, common nasal meatus; 12, dorsal nasal meatus; 13, middle nasal meatus; 14, ventral nasal meatus; 15, nasolacrimal duct.

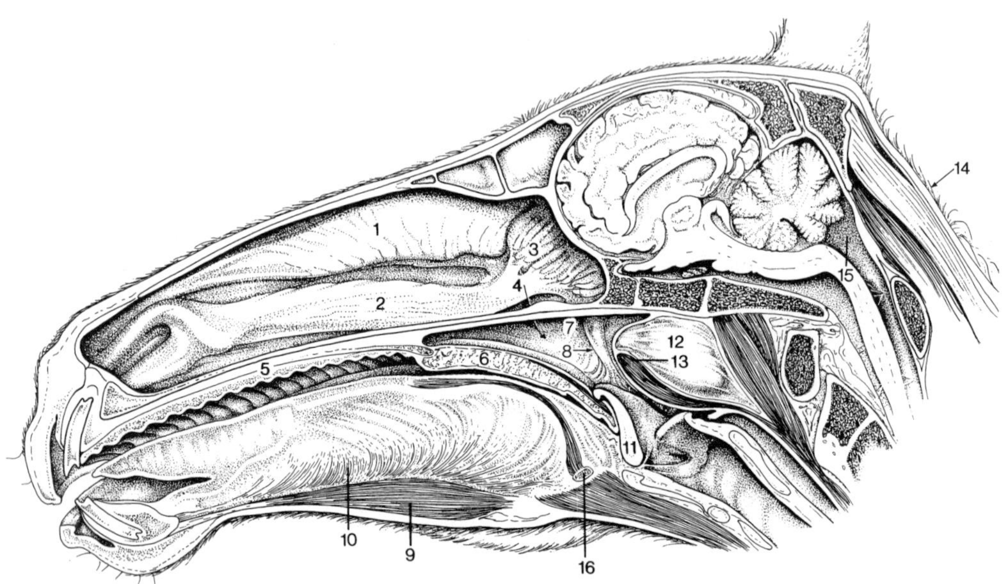


**Figure 18–10.** Median section of the head; most of the nasal septum has been removed.

1, Dorsal nasal concha; 2, ventral nasal concha; 3, ethmoidal conchae; 4, right choana *(arrow);* 5, hard palate with prominent ridges (rugae); 6, soft palate; 7, nasopharynx; 8, pharyngeal opening of auditory tube; 9, geniohyoideus; 10, genioglossus; 11, epiglottis; 12, medial wall of guttural pouch; 13, pharyngeal muscles; 14, site for tapping the cerebellomedullary cistern; 15, cerebellomedullary cistern; 16, basihyoid.

correctly known as the conchofrontal sinus. Its extent is shown in Figure 18–13/1,1′. From this it will be seen that the interior of the frontal part is incompletely divided by several bony lamellae. The floor of this part is molded over the ethmoid labyrinth and rostrolateral to these unevennesses it displays the large oval communication (frontomaxillary opening) with the caudal maxillary sinus. The opening normally allows easy natural drainage. A window may be opened, usually by trephination, in the roof of the sinus to allow for irrigation or for removal of a molar by repulsion,

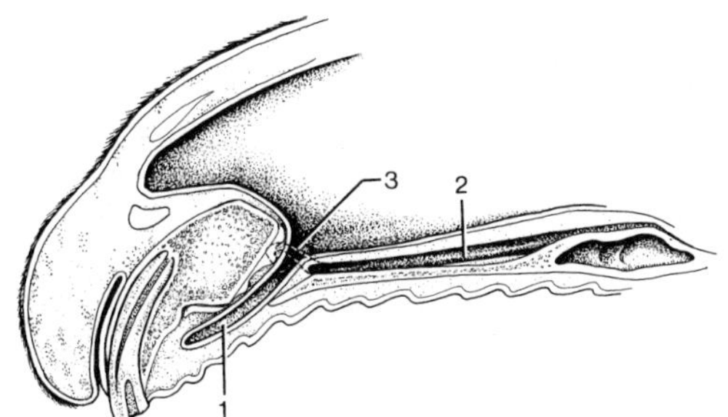


**Figure 18–11.** Paramedian section of the rostral end of the nose.

1, Incisive duct; 2, vomeronasal organ; 3, opening of the incisive duct into the nasal cavity and of the vomeronasal organ into the incisive duct.

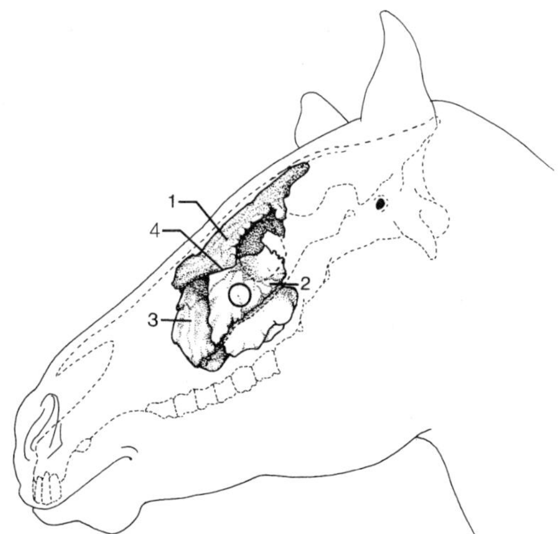


**Figure 18–12.** Topography of the conchofrontal and maxillary sinuses, which are filled with casting material. The circle indicates where the caudal maxillary sinus can be trephined.

1, Conchofrontal sinus; 2, caudal maxillary sinus; 3, rostral maxillary sinus; 4, position of frontomaxillary opening between 1 and 2.

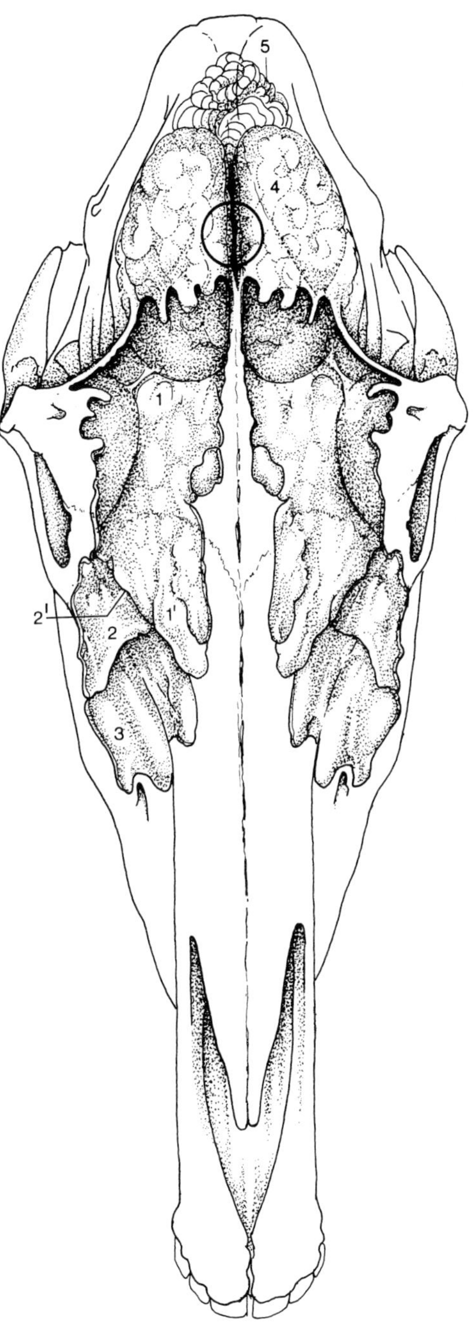


**Figure 18–13.** Projection of the brain and frontal and maxillary sinuses on the dorsal surface of the skull. The sinuses are filled with casting material. The frontal sinus extends caudally over the rostral part of the brain and rostrally beyond the level of the orbit. The circle indicates the center of the brain and the location where a horse may be shot.

1, 1′, Conchofrontal sinus; 1, frontal part; 1′, dorsal conchal part; 2, caudal maxillary sinus; 2′, position of frontomaxillary opening; 3, rostral maxillary sinus; 4, cerebrum; 5, cerebellum.

when a punch introduced through the frontomaxillary opening is brought to bear on the appropriate alveolus. Such a window allows also introduction of a fiber-optic endoscope to inspect the interior of this large sinus.

The two *maxillary sinuses* together occupy a large part of the upper jaw, where they have a critically important relationship to the embedded portions of the caudal cheek teeth. They share a slitlike communication (nasomaxillary opening) with the middle meatus of the nasal cavity but are otherwise completely divided by an oblique septum. This is variable in position but most commonly located about 5 cm caudal to the rostral end of the facial crest. The ventral part of each sinus is also divided into medial and lateral spaces by an upright longitudinal plate supporting the infraorbital canal and fused in young animals to the alveoli containing the roots and unerupted portions of the cheek teeth. The medial part of the caudal sinus continues into the irregular sphenopalatine sinus. The corresponding part of the rostral sinus extends into the ventral concha.

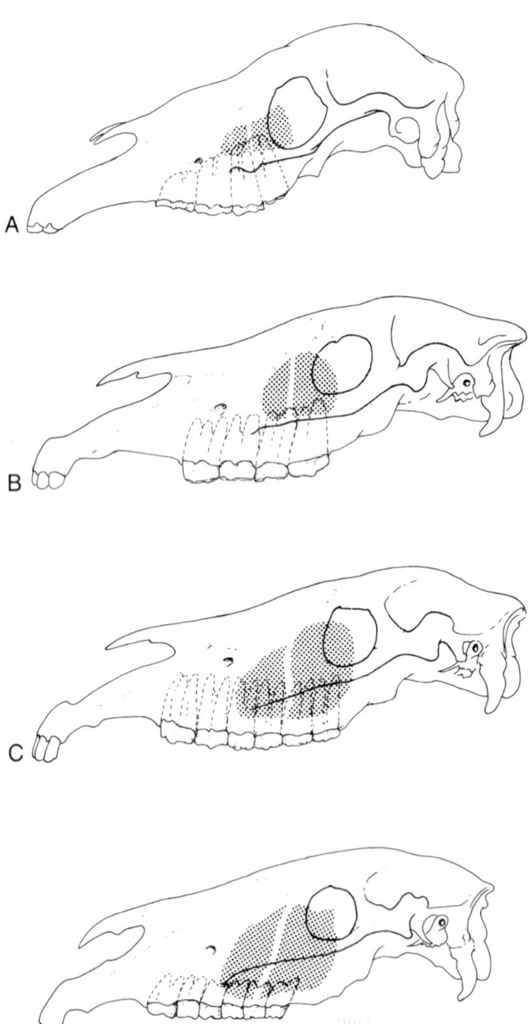


**Figure 18–14.** Projection of the maxillary sinuses at various ages. In older horses the cheek teeth are more rostrally placed. *A*, One month. *B*, One year. *C*, Four to six years. *D*, Over 12 years.

It is impossible to define the exact extent and projections of the maxillary sinuses, which enlarge considerably after birth as the teeth are extruded (Fig. 18–14). Their relationship to the teeth is also affected by the forward migration of the teeth as they develop and come into wear. As Figure 18–14 shows, the relationship is confined to the last premolar and first molar tooth in the newborn foal; it later extends to involve the last four teeth but finally retains contact only with the three molars. There is much variation and attention to the varying inclination of the embedded parts of different teeth is required.

The surface projection of the maxillary sinuses is considerably larger than the safe surgical field. The latter is determined by several factors, not least the routes followed by the very vulnerable nasolacrimal duct and infraorbital nerve. The potential operating area is defined by the following boundaries: (1) the vertical line tangential to the rostral limit of the orbit; (2) the facial crest; (3) the oblique line joining the rostral limit of the crest to the infraorbital foramen; and (4) the line parallel to the facial crest that intersects the infraorbital foramen. Entry to the sinus may be required to effect drainage, since the natural route—the nasomaxillary opening—is placed high in the wall, or to give access to certain teeth.

## THE MOUTH

The small size of the entrance makes it impossible to open the mouth wide; this limitation, coupled with the great depth of the cavity, severely hampers clinical inspection.

The *vestibule* communicates with the mouth cavity proper only between the incisor and cheek teeth (where the diastema may be interrupted by the canine) and by small gaps behind the last molars. The *hard palate* is therefore largely bounded by the alveolar processes and teeth. It is almost uniformly broad and is marked by two more or less symmetrical series of ridges (Fig. 18–10/5). The incisive papilla is found directly behind the central incisors; grooves that flank the

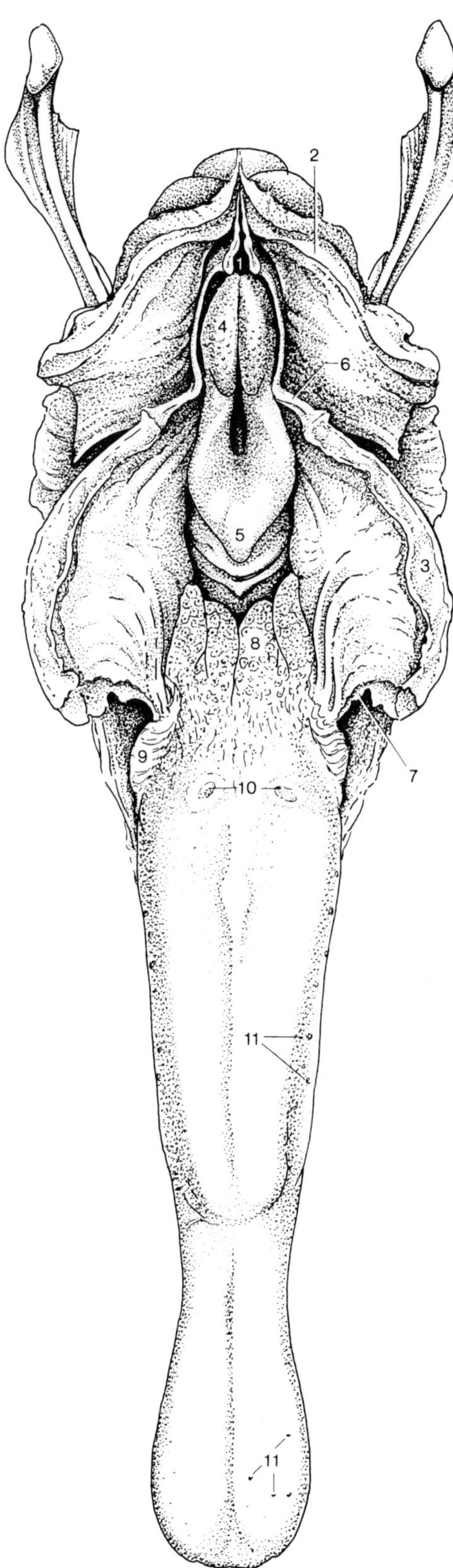


elevation end blindly and do not communicate with the nasal cavity and vomeronasal organs (Fig. 18–11). The mucosa of the hard palate is thick, particularly in its most rostral part, and incorporates a very generous venous plexus, which may become engorged (lampas) at the time of tooth replacement when it may project above the occlusal surfaces of the neighboring teeth. The appearance is striking and laypeople are sometimes alarmed by this purely physiological phenomenon.

The *soft palate* continues the hard palate opposite the second-to-last cheek teeth. It is remarkably long and in repose hangs down in front of the epiglottis with its free margin in contact with the base of the cartilage (Fig. 18–10/6). This relationship explains both the inability of horses to resort to oral breathing in respiratory distress and the course taken by ingesta on the rare occasions when they vomit; denied access to the mouth, the ingesta of necessity pass into the nasopharynx and thence the nasal cavity.*

The mucosa on the oral surface of the soft palate is marked by numerous pits where the palatine glands open. It also exhibits a rostral median tonsillar swelling (see Fig. 3–26).

The *tongue* is long, conforming to the shape of the cavity, and is spatulate at its apex, which is incompletely restrained by a narrow frenulum. Its upper surface is thickly strewn with delicate filiform papillae that confer a velvet-like texture; the larger papillae with gustatory function are less widely spread (Fig. 18–15/9,10,11). A scattering of

*However, displacement of the soft palate to the dorsal surface of the epiglottis is a recognized anomaly, most commonly encountered in horses worked at a fast pace. The displaced palate obstructs the nasopharynx to a degree that may make even moderate exertion impossible. The cause is not definitely known but it is suspected that excessive contraction of the ventral neck muscles draws the larynx so far caudally that the soft palate is released from its usual position rostral to the epiglottis. Softening or hypoplasia of the epiglottis may be a contributory factor.

**Figure 18–15.** The tongue and pharynx; the latter has been opened dorsally to expose the entrance to the larynx.

1, Entrance into esophagus; 2, dorsal wall of nasopharynx (split in median plane); 3, soft palate (split in median plane); 4, corniculate process of arytenoid cartilage; 5, epiglottis; 6, free border of soft palate, continued caudally by palatopharyngeal arch; 7, palatoglossal arch; 8, lingual tonsil; 9, foliate papillae; 10, vallate papillae; 11, examples of fungiform papillae.

lymphoid tissue over the root constitutes a diffuse lingual tonsil. Each of two low mucosal folds beneath the apex of the tongue carries a fleshy sublingual caruncle where the mandibular duct opens.

# THE DENTITION AND MASTICATORY APPARATUS

## The Dentition

The dentition of the horse is admirably suited to a diet of grass, a surprisingly abrasive material. The masticatory area is increased by the enlargement of the premolars and their assimilation to the molars with which they present a continuous grinding surface. Both cheek teeth and incisors have high crowns, which ensure a long working life, despite the considerable attrition that takes place at the occlusal surfaces. Delayed formation of the roots also allows the cheek teeth to grow for some years after they come into wear. Attrition wastes the cheek tooth by 2 to 3 mm each year; to allow for this the greater part of the crown is initially embedded within the jaw and only gradually extruded to compensate for this loss. The enamel casing of the incisor and cheek teeth is also folded, although in different ways in the incisor, upper cheek, and lower cheek teeth series. The folding increases the area of the durable enamel presented at the working surface where it stands proud of the neighboring dentine, the alternation of harder and softer tissues providing efficient grinding instruments (Fig. 18–18). The formula of the temporary dentition is

$$\frac{3\text{–}0\text{–}3}{3\text{–}0\text{–}3},$$

that of the permanent dentition,

$$\frac{3\text{–}1\text{–}3(4)\text{–}3}{3\text{–}1\text{–}3\text{–}3}.$$

The *incisor teeth* are ranked together to form a continuous arch in each jaw and are so implanted that their roots converge (Fig. 18–16). Each is curved lengthwise, presenting a labial convexity. When in occlusion the upper and lower incisors of the young animal form a continuous arch when viewed in profile. Later, as they wear, the upper and lower teeth meet at an increasingly pronounced angle. The occlusal surface recently brought into use is a broad transverse oval (Fig. 18–17/*B*) and presents an outer enamel casing and an inner enamel ring lining the infolding known as the infundibulum; this is partially filled with

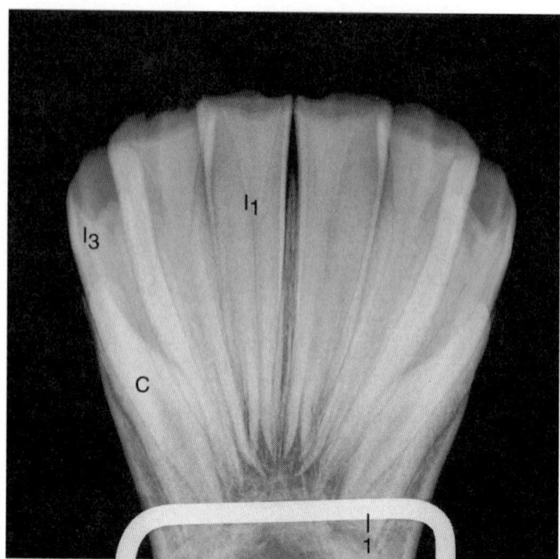


**Figure 18–16.** Root convergence of permanent lower incisors; radiograph of a bone specimen from a 5-year-old (estimated) horse. Note the funnel-shaped infundibulum visible in each of the first and second incisors.

$I_1$, $I_3$, Lower first and third incisors; C, lower canine tooth, present only in the male; 1, mounting wire of specimen.

cement, leaving a small cavity, the cup (/1). Since the enamel lining is more resistant, it projects above the surrounding dentine. Changes in the appearance of the occlusal surface provide the information principally used in aging older horses. The points to note are the depth of the infundibulum and its overlap with the dental cavity. Although it may appear that wear would eventually expose the pulp, this is prevented by the timely formation of secondary dentine, distinguishable from primary dentine by its darker color; this secondary dentine provides the feature known as the dental star (/3).

Although *canine teeth* generally form in both sexes, they are rudimentary and commonly fail to erupt in mares. In male animals they are low, laterally compressed cones placed within the diastemas rather closer to the corner incisors than to the cheek teeth. The embedded portions are disproportionately large in relation to the exposed crowns.

The *first premolar* ("wolf" tooth) often fails to develop and when present it is vestigial and almost invariably confined to the upper jaw. Though without functional significance, it does have a potential nuisance value since it may shift under the pressure of the bit and so irritate the gum. It is easily extracted.

The remaining *premolars* (P2–P4) form a continuous row with the *molars*. The first and last of the six cheek teeth are somewhat triangular in section, the others rectangular; but, that apart, each is so like its neighbors that only an expert may distinguish isolated teeth (Fig. 18–20). There are, however, important differences between the upper and lower sets; the upper teeth are much wider and exhibit a more complicated enamel folding, which creates two infundibula that fill with cement before eruption. The enamel of the lower teeth is also much folded but forms no infundibula (Fig. 18–18/*B*). Most teeth occlude with two members of the opposing set along a relatively narrow area of contact that follows the lingual edge of the upper, and buccal edge of the lower, teeth. The occlusal plane slopes ventrobuccally (Fig. 18–9). Irregular or incomplete chewing movements may cause the buccal edge of the upper, and the lingual edge of the lower, cheek teeth to escape wear (sharp teeth); the resulting protrusions must be filed down (floated) to prevent injury to cheeks and tongue.

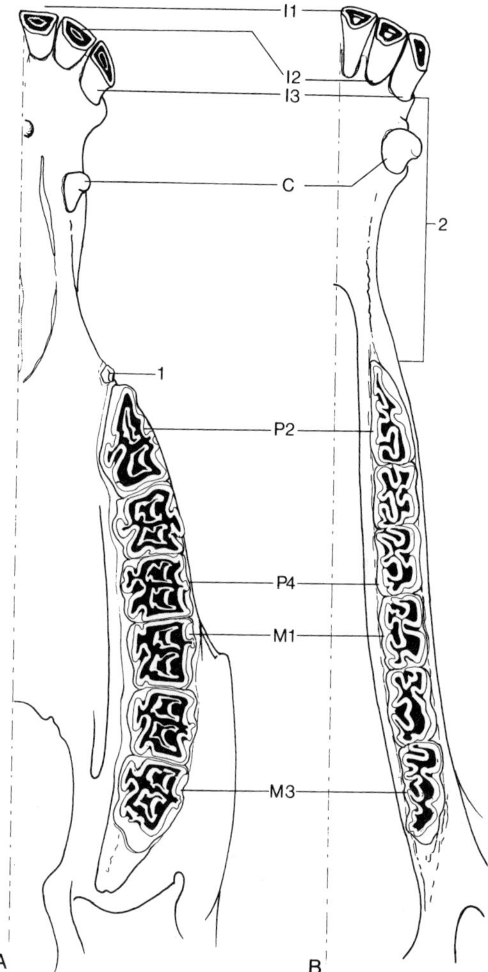


**Figure 18–18.** The permanent teeth of the upper *(A)* and lower *(B)* jaws.

1, "Wolf" tooth (P1); 2, diastema.

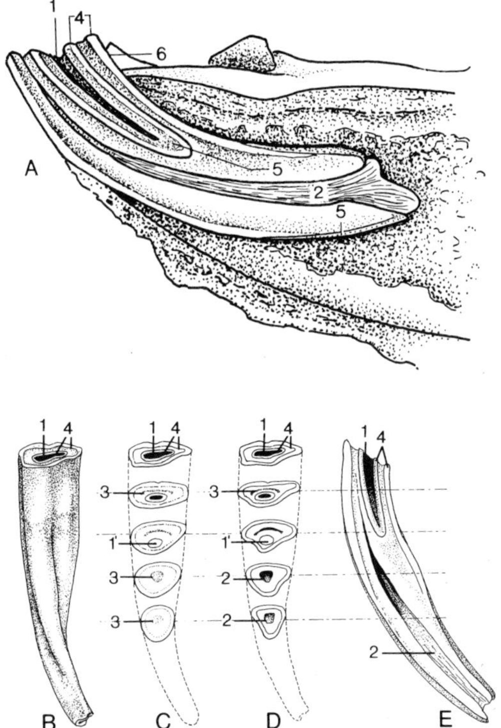


**Figure 18–17.** Structure of a lower incisor. *A,* In situ, sectioned longitudinally; the clinical crown is short in relation to the embedded part of the tooth. *B,* Caudal view; the junction between the clinical crown and the rest of the tooth is not marked. *C,* As a result of wear the occlusal surface changes; the cup gets smaller and disappears, leaving, for a time, the enamel spot; the dental star appears and changes from a line to a large round spot. *D,* These are sawn sections of a young tooth for comparison. *E,* Longitudinal section of incisor, showing the relationship between the infundibulum and dental cavity; the latter is rostral.

1, Cup, black cavity in center of infundibulum; 1′, enamel spot, proximal end of infundibulum; 2, dental cavity; 3, dental star, changing in shape from a linear to a rounded form; 4, outer and inner enamel rings; 5, cement; 6, lingual surface.

The structure of the cheek teeth is shown in Figure 18–19. The upper teeth are anchored by three or four roots and are so implanted that the reserve portions slope caudally at varying angles (Fig. 18–20). The relationship to the maxillary sinuses and other features of the skull is very helpfully revealed in radiographs. Only a thin plate of alveolar bone separates the molars from the sinus; in consequence, infection may easily spread to the sinus from tooth or alveolar abscesses. The

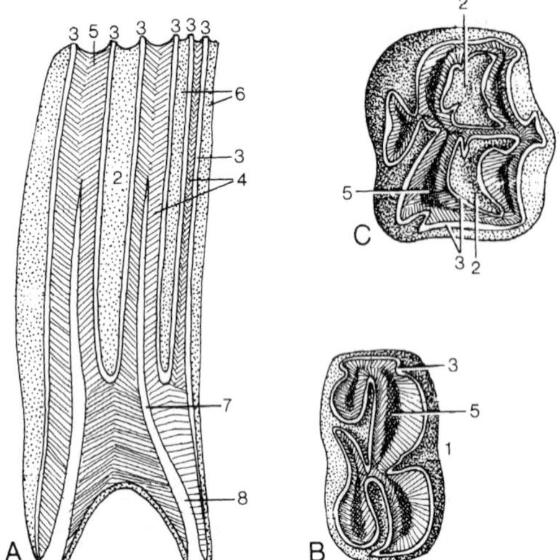


**Figure 18–19.** Structure of the cheek teeth shown in sagittal section *(A)* and by views of the occlusal surface of lower *(B)* and upper *(C)* molars.

1, Buccal (labial) surface; 2 infundibulum; 3, enamel; 4, dentine; 5, secondary dentine; 6, cement; 7, dental cavity; 8, root canal.

relationship changes with age, partly because gradual extrusion lowers the alveolar floor, enlarging the sinus, and partly because the teeth migrate rostrally (Fig. 18–14).

The transitory swellings occasionally seen on the ventral margin of the mandible of 2- to 4-year-old horses are produced by modeling of the mandible to accommodate the formation of the roots of permanent teeth which are prevented from rising within the jaw by remnants (caps) of deciduous predecessors blocking the way (Fig. 18–21). When the remnants are shed, their successors can move into place. Further modeling of the mandibular border erases the swellings.

Simple extraction of cheek teeth is more or less impossible. Their length, curvature, and close fit would hamper any effort to draw one out past its neighbor(s), even were the attempt permitted by the small size of the opening between the lips and the depth of the oral cavity. Instead, they must be removed by expulsion, by means of a punch brought to bear over the root in an operation of some severity and difficulty involving the opening of a window through bone. Accurate determination

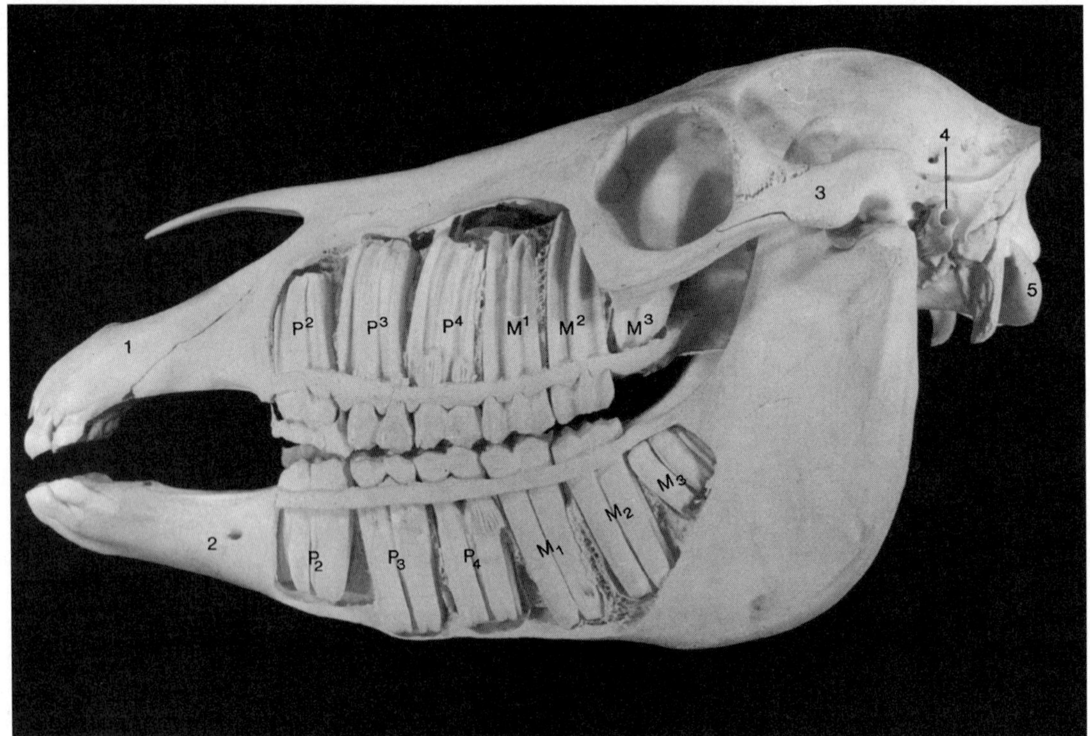


**Figure 18–20.** Exposed cheek teeth of a horse 2½ years old (estimated). *Upper jaw:* The deciduous premolars are still present, $Pd^2$ in the form of a cap; $M^3$ has not yet erupted. *Lower jaw:* The deciduous premolars 3 and 4 are still present in the form of caps; $M_3$ has not yet erupted.

1, Incisive bone; 2, mental foramen; 3, zygomatic arch; 4, external acoustic meatus; 5, occipital condyle.

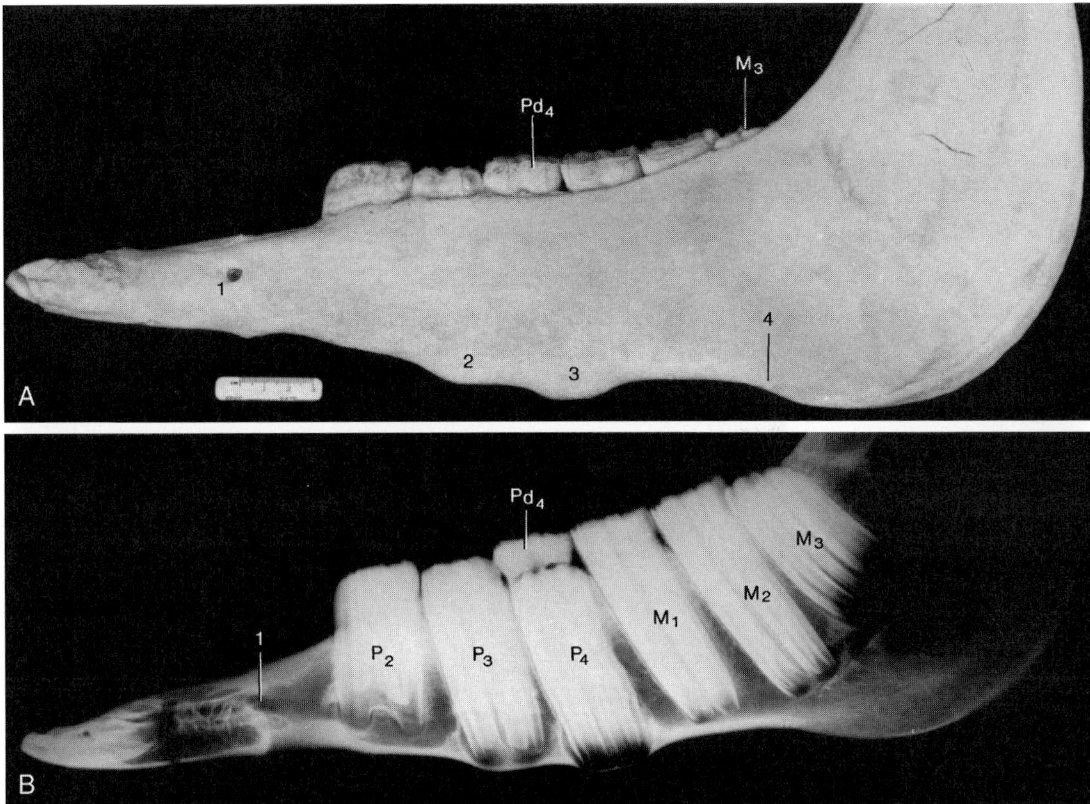


**Figure 18–21.** Photograph *(A)* and radiograph *(B)* of the left half-mandible of a horse 3 years old (estimated). Note the transitory tubercles on the ventral border, and the wedged-in cap ($Pd_4$) that retards the advance of $P_3$ and $P_4$.

1, Mental foramen; 2, 3, tubercles over the proximal ends of $P_3$ and $P_4$, respectively; 4, notch for facial artery and vein.

of the position of the root of the tooth involved is essential, and for this it is necessary to be mindful of how the dispositions of the teeth change with age. The approach to a caudal member of the upper cheek teeth series is made via the caudal maxillary sinus, or the frontal and caudal maxillary sinuses when $M^3$ is involved.

The deciduous teeth generally resemble the permanent teeth but are much smaller and significantly shorter in relation to their breadth. The deciduous incisors are constricted at the neck and much whiter than their replacements, the porcelain-like enamel being unobscured by the cement encrustation that gives permanent teeth a slightly yellow and porous appearance. Some longitudinal striation is apparent on the temporary incisor crown.

## The Estimation of Age from the Teeth

Examination of the teeth provides the traditional and sole convenient means of estimating age. Since there is a copious specialist literature the subject is treated very briefly (Table 18–1). The eruption dates and changes in appearance of the occlusal surfaces, specifically those of the lower incisors, are the main criteria. Neither is wholly dependable but the first is more reliable, although limited in application to younger animals; the second may be used throughout the life span but becomes increasingly inaccurate.

The initially oval occlusal surface of the incisors becomes rounded and finally forms a triangle elongated in the labiolingual direction. The enamel casing is intact when the tooth erupts, and the occlusal surface then presents a central depression (cup) that is soon stained by food debris. Wear first abrades the labial edge but quickly extends all around, isolating the infundibular from the external enamel; the tooth is then said to be level. Further wear reduces the depth of the cup, although its thick base (the enamel "spot") resists attrition for a considerable time. The dental star appears on the labial aspect of the cup meanwhile, and persists

**Table 18-1.** A Rough Guide for the Aging of the Horse by Its Teeth

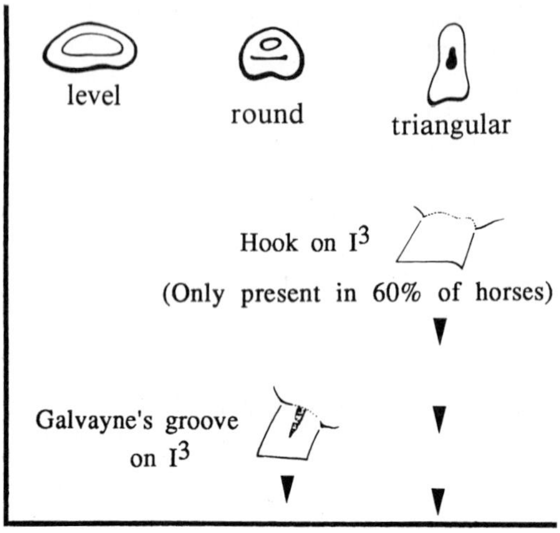

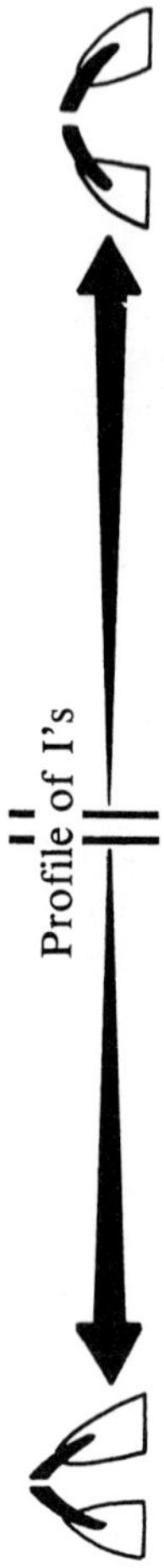

| | Age | Lower Incisors* | |
|---|---|---|---|
| FAIRLY ACCURATE (Based largely on eruption) | 6 d | $Di_1$ erupts | level / round / triangular |
| | 6 w | $Di_2$ erupts | |
| | 6 m | $Di_3$ erupts | |
| | 1 y | $Di_3$ in wear | Hook on $I^3$ |
| | 2 y | $Di_{1+2}$ level | (Only present in 60% of horses) |
| | 2½ | $I_1$ erupts | |
| | 3½ | $I_2$ erupts | Galvayne's groove on $I^3$ |
| | 4½ | $I_3$ erupts | |
| | 5 | all cups present; $I_1$, $I_2$ level | |
| | 6 | $I_1$ cup gone | |
| | 7 | $I_2$ cup gone; I's level; | |
| LARGELY SPECULATION (Based on wear) | 8 | $I_3$ cup gone; stars appear | |
| | 9 | $I_1$ becomes (round) | |
| | 10 | $I_2$ becomes (round); | |
| | 11 | maybe | |
| | 15 | enamel spots gone; | |
| | 16-18 | I's become (triangular); stars round | |
| | 20 | | |
| | 25 | | |
| | 30 | | |

Profile of I's

*It takes about 6 months for an erupted tooth to reach the height of its neighbors.
Di, I, I's: deciduous incisor, incisor, incisors.

after the cup and the enamel spot have been entirely lost.

Less reliable criteria are a "hook" on $I^3$ (Table 18–1) and Galvayne's groove on the labial surface of the same tooth. The hook is present when the horse is about 7 years old; unfortunately it may recur at 11 years. The appearance, progression, and disappearance of Galvayne's groove are also depicted in Table 18–1. Though unreliable by themselves, both features may enhance accuracy when combined with the appearance of the occlusal surfaces and the profile of the incisors. (See also Plates 21 and 22.)

It has to be emphasized that the variation in these (and in other undescribed) features is extremely large and in a horse more than 8 years old the assessment may be at fault by several years.

## The Muscles of Mastication and the Temporomandibular Joint

The muscles of mastication are well developed. The *masseter* takes origin along the whole length of the facial crest and zygomatic arch and inserts on the mandible between the vascular notch and condyle (Fig. 18–6/14). It is a multipennate muscle constructed so that the fibers of the superficial strata run caudoventrally, while those more deeply placed are nearly vertical. Its cranial margin produces a very prominent surface contour that serves as a guide to the location of the facial vessels and parotid duct; its caudodorsal part is overlain by the parotid gland but to a variable depth and extent, which affect the accessibility to palpation of the parotid lymph nodes; laterally, the masseter is traversed by buccal branches of the facial nerve.

The *temporalis* almost fills the temporal fossa, where it is easily palpated despite the partial covering of thin muscles concerned with the movement of the external ear (Fig. 18–22/1). It arises from the wall of the fossa, and from the sagittal crest that forms its median margin, and envelops the coronoid process of the mandible. On contraction it raises the mandible.

The *pterygoideus medialis* and *lateralis,* deep to the mandible, broadly correspond to the masseter in position, orientation, and attachments (/2,3). The medial muscle, as always the larger, extends from the pterygoid process to the mandibular margin. The lateral muscle runs more horizontally to insert close to the condyle. The masseter and contralateral pterygoid muscles act together to produce the horizontal shifts that supply the principal grinding movement.

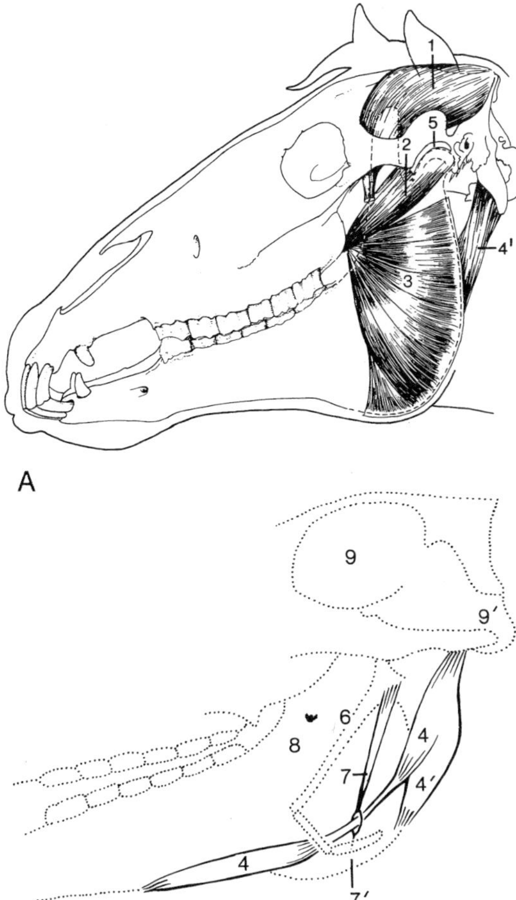


**Figure 18–22.** *A,* The deep masticatory muscles of the left side have been exposed by removal of the left mandibular ramus *(stippled). B,* Medial view of the right digastricus and some related structures.

1. Temporalis; 2, pterygoideus lateralis; 3, lateral surface of pterygoideus medialis; 4, digastricus; 4′, occipitomandibularis; 5, left temporomandibular joint; 6, stylohyoid; 7, stylohyoideus; 7′, insertion of 7 on thyrohyoid; 8, medial surface of right mandible and mandibular foramen; 9, cranial cavity; 9′, foramen magnum.

The *digastricus* and *occipitomandibularis* (strictly a part of the digastricus; /4,4′) are responsible for active opening of the mouth. Despite its much greater bulk, the latter may be regarded as a detachment from the caudal belly of the digastricus. It extends between the paracondylar process of the occipital bone and the caudal border of the mandible. The much more slender digastricus has a similar origin. It presents an intermediate tendon that passes through a split in the insertion of the stylohyoideus. The rostral belly attaches to the ventromedial part of the molar region of the mandible. When the mouth is closed, contraction of the digastricus raises the hyoid apparatus (by virtue of its association with the stylohyoideus) and thus the root of the tongue (Fig. 18–22/*B*).

A thick intra-articular disc is interposed between the expanded and rather flat facets of the mandibular condyle and articular tubercle of the temporal bone (Fig. 18–22/*A*,5). Hinge movements occur at the lower level, which is supported by a tight capsule; the lateral and slight protrusive movements occur at the upper level where the joint cavity is more capacious. The whole joint is supported by a fibrous lateral ligament and an elastic caudal one.

## THE SALIVARY GLANDS

The *parotid* is clearly lobulated with a firm texture and a yellow-gray or yellow-pink color. It is the largest salivary gland and extends ventrally from the base of the ear and wing of the atlas into the angle formed by the convergence of the maxillary and linguofacial veins, and possibly beyond since the maxillary vein frequently tunnels through the gland substance (Fig. 18–6/20). The cranial margin is largely contained by the caudal border of the mandible, but a thin flange extends some distance over the masseter directly ventral to the jaw joint, where it covers the parotid lymph nodes. The lateral surface is overlain by a well-developed fascia that gives attachment to the parotidoauricularis muscle (/17). The deep surface is related to the guttural pouch, the stylohyoid, the muscles that run to the corner of the jaw and open the mouth, and the combined insertion tendon of the brachiocephalicus and sternocephalicus, which separates it from the more deeply placed mandibular gland (Fig. 18–7).

The serous secretion of the parotid is drained by several sizable ducts that come together at the rostroventral angle of the gland to form a single channel. This crosses the tendon of the sternocephalicus before turning forward to run medial to the ventral border of the mandible. Accompanied by the facial vessels, it turns onto the face, where it ascends along the rostral margin of the masseter. It first lies caudal to the artery and vein but later shifts rostral to them (/13). It ends by opening into the vestibule opposite the third upper cheek tooth. The duct is relatively exposed in the last part of its course and may be damaged in superficial wounds. Leakage is most profuse when feeding stimulates the flow of saliva.

The much smaller and crescentic *mandibular gland* extends from the basihyoid to the atlantal fossa and is thus partly under cover of the mandible (Figs. 18–7/14 and 18–25/5). The superficial relations include the parotid gland and the medial pterygoid, sternocephalic, digastric, and occipitomandibular muscles. Its deep location puts it out of reach on palpation. The mandibular duct is formed along the concave rostral margin of the gland by the confluence of several ductules. It runs rostrally, covered by the mylohyoideus, and follows the medial aspect of the sublingual gland until it opens on the floor of the mouth at the small sublingual caruncle. The secretion is mixed.

The *sublingual gland* lies directly below the oral mucosa, between the body of the tongue and the medial surface of the mandible, extending as a thin strip from the symphysis to the level of the fifth cheek tooth (/1). It drains through numerous small ductules that open below the tongue.

Two rows of *buccal glands* are scattered along the dorsal and ventral margins of the buccinator (Fig. 18–7/4). The glands of the dorsal series are more considerable and clump together caudally. Small salivary glands are found in the lips, soft palate, and tongue.

## THE PHARYNX AND GUTTURAL POUCH

### The Pharynx

The pharynx lies wholly beneath the skull to which the rostral third of its roof is directly applied. The remaining part of the roof and the lateral walls are enveloped by the guttural pouches. The lumen is clearly divided into upper and lower compartments by the soft palate and the palatopharyngeal arches, which extend over the lateral walls to meet directly above the entrance to the esophagus (Fig. 18–10). The most prominent features of the *nasopharynx* are the flaps guarding the entrances to the auditory tubes. Each is about 3 cm long and is pressed against the pharyngeal wall, presenting an oblique and rather sinuous ventral free edge (/8 and Plate 3/*A*). It is stiffened by a flange of cartilage, the expansion of the medial cartilage that supports the auditory tube. The slitlike opening lateral to the flap is normally held closed but becomes patent when the animal swallows. This provides an opportunity for equalizing the pressure on the two sides of the tympanic membrane. The maneuver, which can be observed endoscopically, involves the flap swinging medially while the soft palate rises and momentarily narrows the lumen of the nasopharynx (Plate 3/*C*). The flap can also be elevated passively, and it is a relatively simple matter to introduce an endoscope in order to examine, or a catheter to drain or irrigate, the

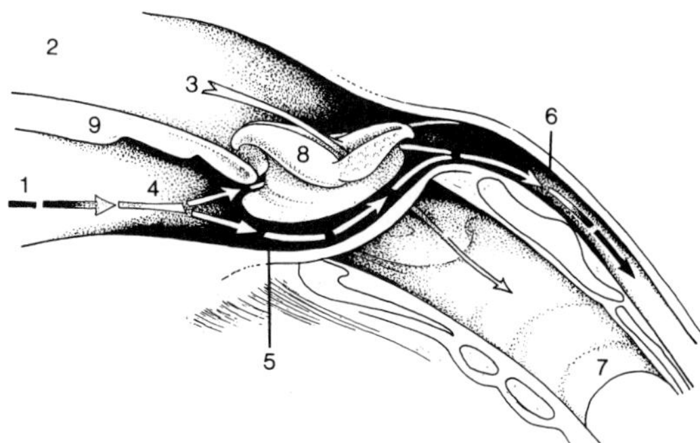


**Figure 18–23.** The communications of the pharynx, rostrally with the oral and nasal cavities, caudally with the esophagus; schematic. The broken arrows mark the digestive tract; the unbroken arrow marks the respiratory tract.

1, Oral cavity; 2, nasal cavity; 3, nasopharynx; 4, oropharynx; 5, laryngopharynx; 6, esophagus; 7, trachea; 8, epiglottis, laryngeal entrance; 9, soft palate.

guttural pouch. The entrance to the tube lies in the transverse plane of the lateral angle of the eye, a useful external guide to its position. An indication of the progress of the instrument through the ventral meatus and nasopharynx is provided by the resistance encountered; the firm support offered to its tip by the vertical lamina of the pterygoid bone is lost only a short distance rostral to the opening. Advancement of the instrument to this level generally provokes a swallowing movement when deflection of the cartilage flap facilitates entry to the pouch. When the procedure is performed blind, the absence of resistance to deeper penetration indicates that the pharyngotubal opening has been successfully passed.

The lower compartment of the pharynx is divided between the oropharynx and the laryngopharynx (Fig. 18–23/4,5). The narrow *oropharynx* extends between the attachment of the palatoglossal arches to the tongue and the epiglottis; its lateral walls and floor contain much diffuse tonsillar tissue, including the long palatine tonsil (see Fig. 3–26). The *laryngopharynx* is largely occupied by the projection of the larynx, and its floor is reduced to the narrow flanking piriform recesses. The laryngopharynx narrows abruptly to the origin of the esophagus.

The structure and musculature follow the common pattern (Fig. 18–24). Difficulties in swallowing sometimes arise from malfunction of palatine and pharyngeal muscles. The cause frequently lies in involvement of the relevant glossopharyngeal and vagus nerves in infections of the guttural pouch; since the nerves run together they are equally susceptible (Fig. 18–25/8,20).

## The Guttural Pouch

A diverticulum of the auditory tube, the guttural pouch, is found in the horse and other

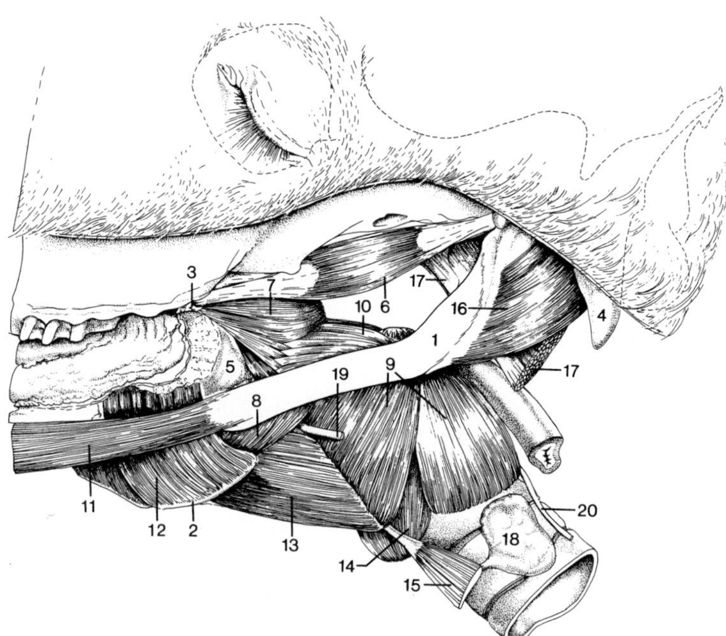


**Figure 18–24.** Muscles of the pharynx, soft palate, and hyoid apparatus.

1, Stylohyoid; 2, thyrohyoid; 3, hamulus of pterygoid bone; 4, paracondylar process; 5, buccopharyngeal fascia; 6, tensor veli palatini; 7, rostral pharyngeal constrictor; 8, middle pharyngeal constrictor; 9, caudal pharyngeal constrictor (thyro- and cricopharyngeus); 10, stylopharyngeus caudalis; 11, styloglossus; 12, hyoglossus; 13, thyrohyoideus; 14, cricothyroideus; 15, sternothyroideus; 16, occipitohyoideus; 17, longus capitis (stump); 18, thyroid gland; 19, cranial laryngeal nerve; 20, caudal (recurrent) laryngeal nerve.

Perissodactyla* (Fig. 18–26/9). It is formed by the escape of the mucosal lining of the tube through a ventral slit between medial and lateral supporting cartilages and attains a capacity of some 300 to 500 mL. It lies between the base of the skull and atlas dorsally, and the pharynx and commencement of the esophagus ventrally; it is covered laterally by the pterygoid muscles and parotid and mandibular glands; medially, the dorsal parts of the right and left sacs are separated by the ventral straight muscles of the head, but below this they meet, forming a thin median septum (Fig. 18–27). The floor lies mainly on the pharynx but also covers and is molded to the stylohyoid, which raises a ridge that incompletely divides medial and lateral compartments (Fig. 18–29).

More detailed relations include several cranial nerves and arteries that lie directly against the pouch as they pass to and from foramina in the caudal part of the skull. The glossopharyngeal, vagus, accessory, and hypoglossal nerves; the continuation of the sympathetic trunk beyond the cranial cervical ganglion; and the internal carotid artery are closely related for a stretch and together raise a mucosal fold that indents the medial compartment from behind; this is a conspicuous feature when the interior of the pouch is viewed endoscopically (Fig. 18–28/4 and Plate 23/*C*). The facial nerve has a more limited contact with the dorsal part of the pouch. The large external carotid artery passes ventral to the medial compartment

*And also in a small, strangely eclectic band of other species, including hyraxes, certain bats, and a South American mouse.

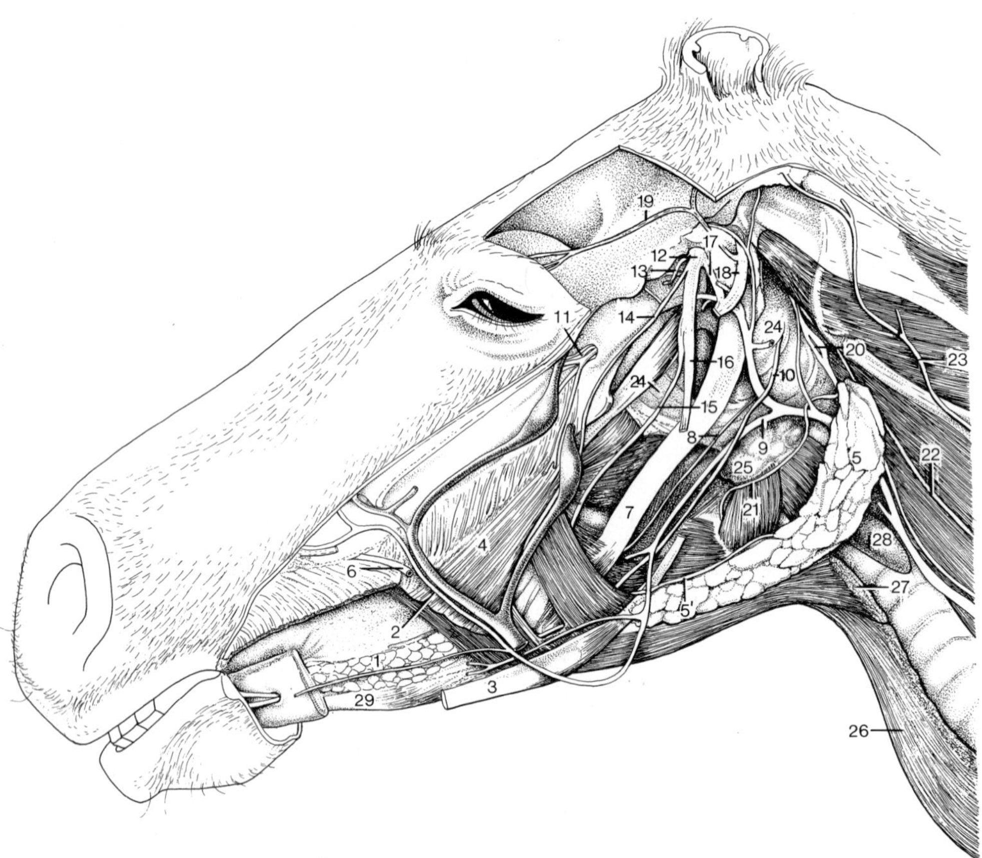


**Figure 18–25.** Deep dissection of the head. The mandible and masticatory muscles have been removed.

1, Sublingual gland; 2, facial artery and vein; 3, rostral belly of digastricus; 4, buccinator; 5, mandibular gland; 5′, mandibular duct; 6, parotid duct; 7, stylohyoid; 8, glossopharyngeal nerve; 9, linguofacial artery; 10, hypoglossal nerve; 11, maxillary artery and nerve in pterygopalatine fossa; 12, mandibular nerve; 13, masseteric nerve; 14, buccal nerve; 15, lingual nerve; 16, inferior alveolar nerve, cut where it enters the mandibular foramen; 17, auriculotemporal nerve; 18, facial nerve; 19, auriculopalpebral nerve; 20, vagus and sympathetic trunk; 21, cranial laryngeal nerve; 22, dorsal branch of spinal accessory nerve; 23, great auricular nerve; 24, guttural pouch; 25, medial retropharyngeal lymph nodes; 26, sternohyoideus; 27, stump of omohyoideus; 28, thyroid gland; 29, genioglossus.

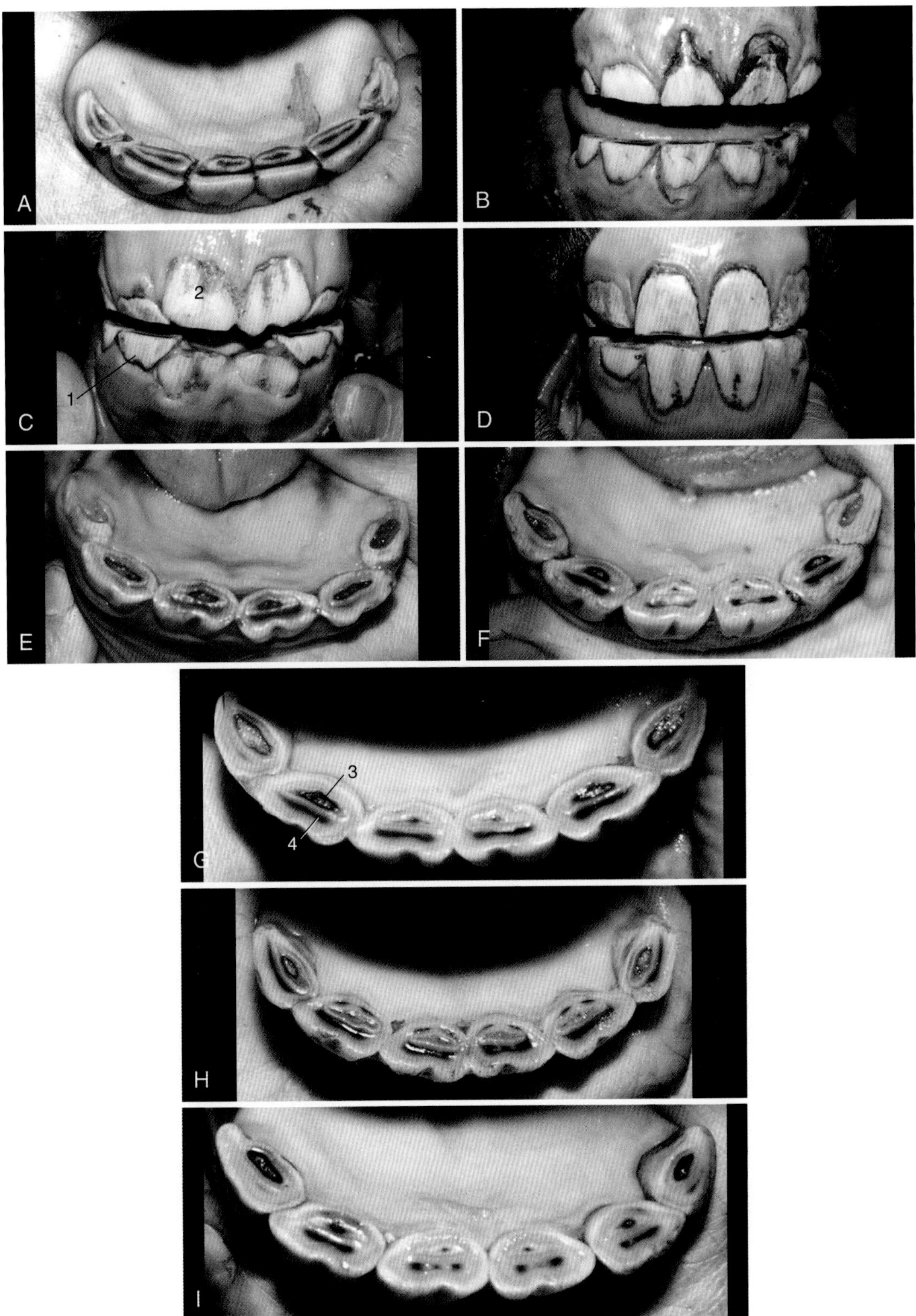


**Plate 21.** Characteristic appearance of lower incisors of Trotter horses of accurately known ages (see *I* for label descriptions). *A,* 1.5 years. *B,* 2.5 years. *C,* 3 years. *D,* 4 years. *E,* 5 years. *F,* 6 years. *G,* 7 years. *H,* 8 years. *I,* 9 years: 1, deciduous teeth; 2, newly erupted $I^1$; 3, dental cup; 4, dental star; 5, enamel spot. (prox. end of infundibulum).

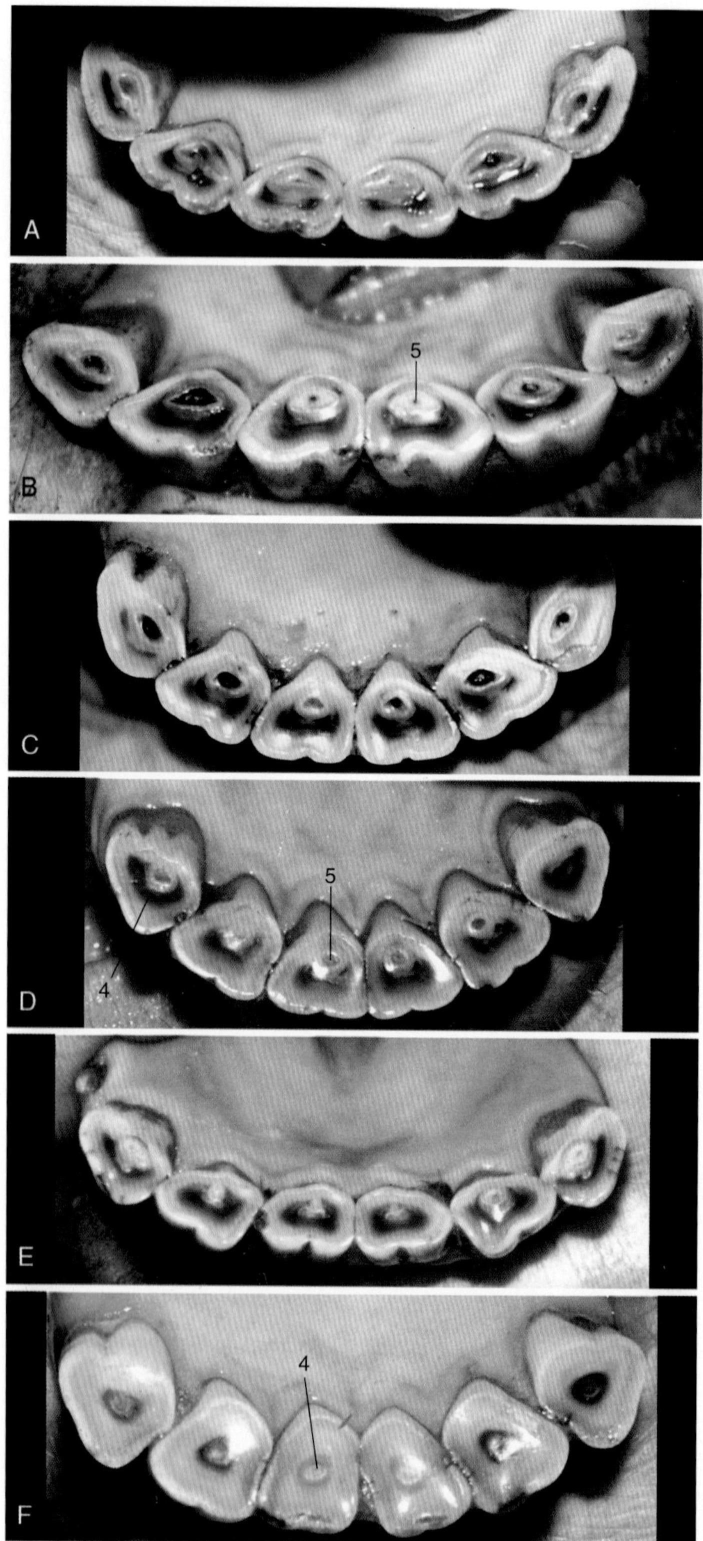


**Plate 22.** Characteristic appearance of lower incisors of Trotter horses of accurately known ages (see Plate 21/*I* for label descriptions). *A,* 11 years. *B,* 12 years. *C,* 14 years. *D,* 16 years. *E,* 17 years. *F,* 20 years. Note particularity of the changes in form of the occlusal surface—from oval, to round, to triangular.

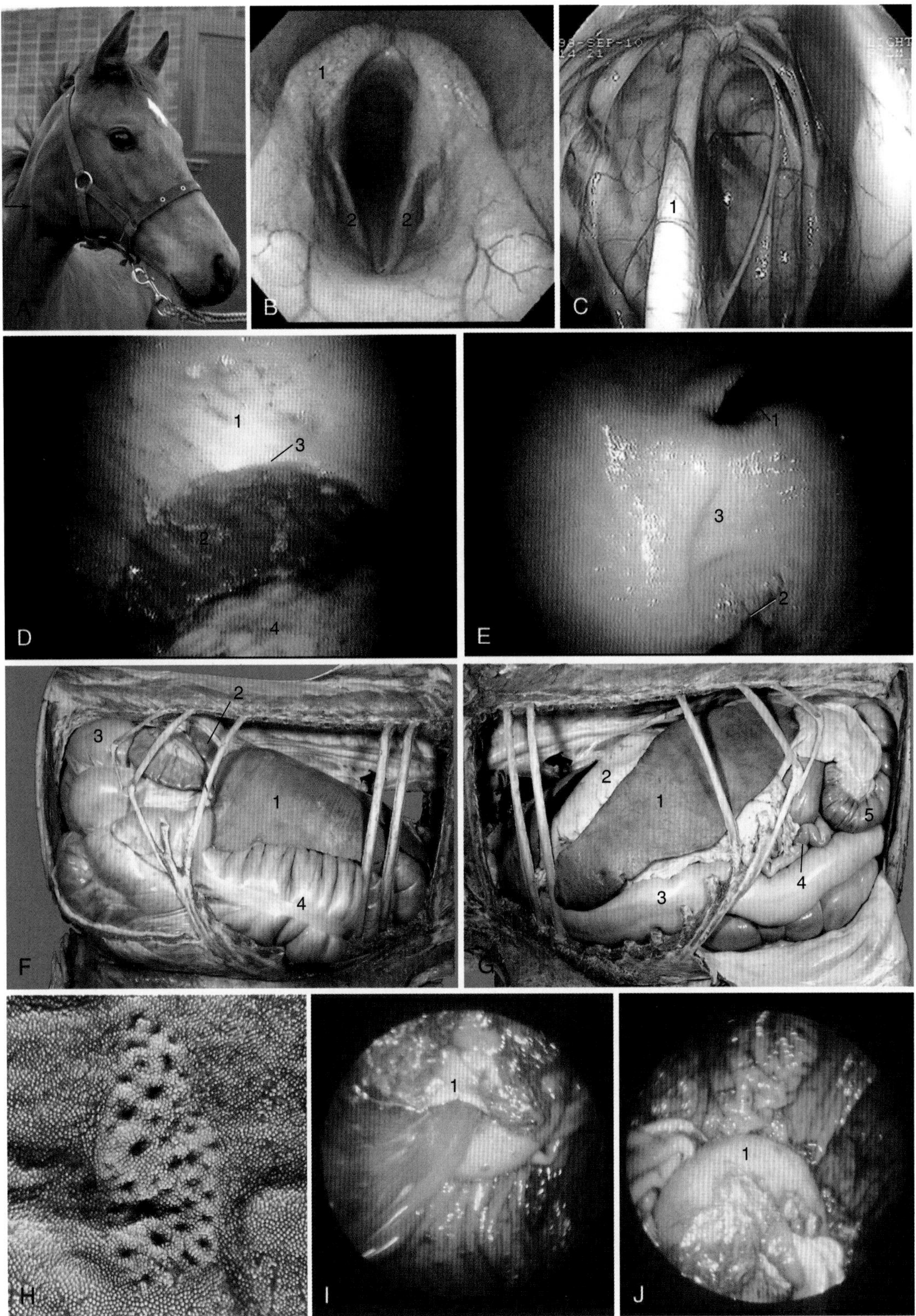


**Plate 23.** All photographs of horse. *A,* Tympany of the gutteral pouch *(arrow). B,* Endoscopic view of larynx: 1, arytenoid cartilage; 2, left and right vocal folds. *C,* Endoscopic view of interior of the guttural pouch: 1, stylohyoid dividing the pouch into two compartments. *D,* Endoscopic view of stomach: 1, nonglandular mucosa; 2, glandular mucosa; 3, margo plicatus; 4, ingesta. *E,* Endoscopic view of stomach: 1, fiber optic cable of endoscope entering through cardia; 2, pylorus; 3, lesser curvature. *F,* Right lateral view of abdominal viscera: 1, liver; 2, right kidney; 3, cecal base; 4, right ventral colon. *G,* Left lateral view of abdominal viscera: 1, spleen; 2, stomach; 3, left dorsal colon; 4, jejunal coils; 5, descending colon. *H,* Patch of aggregated lymph nodules in ileum. *I* and *J,* Endoscopic views of interior of the cecal base. In *I,* the ileal papilla (1) discharges fluid; in *J,* semisolid ingesta into the cecum.

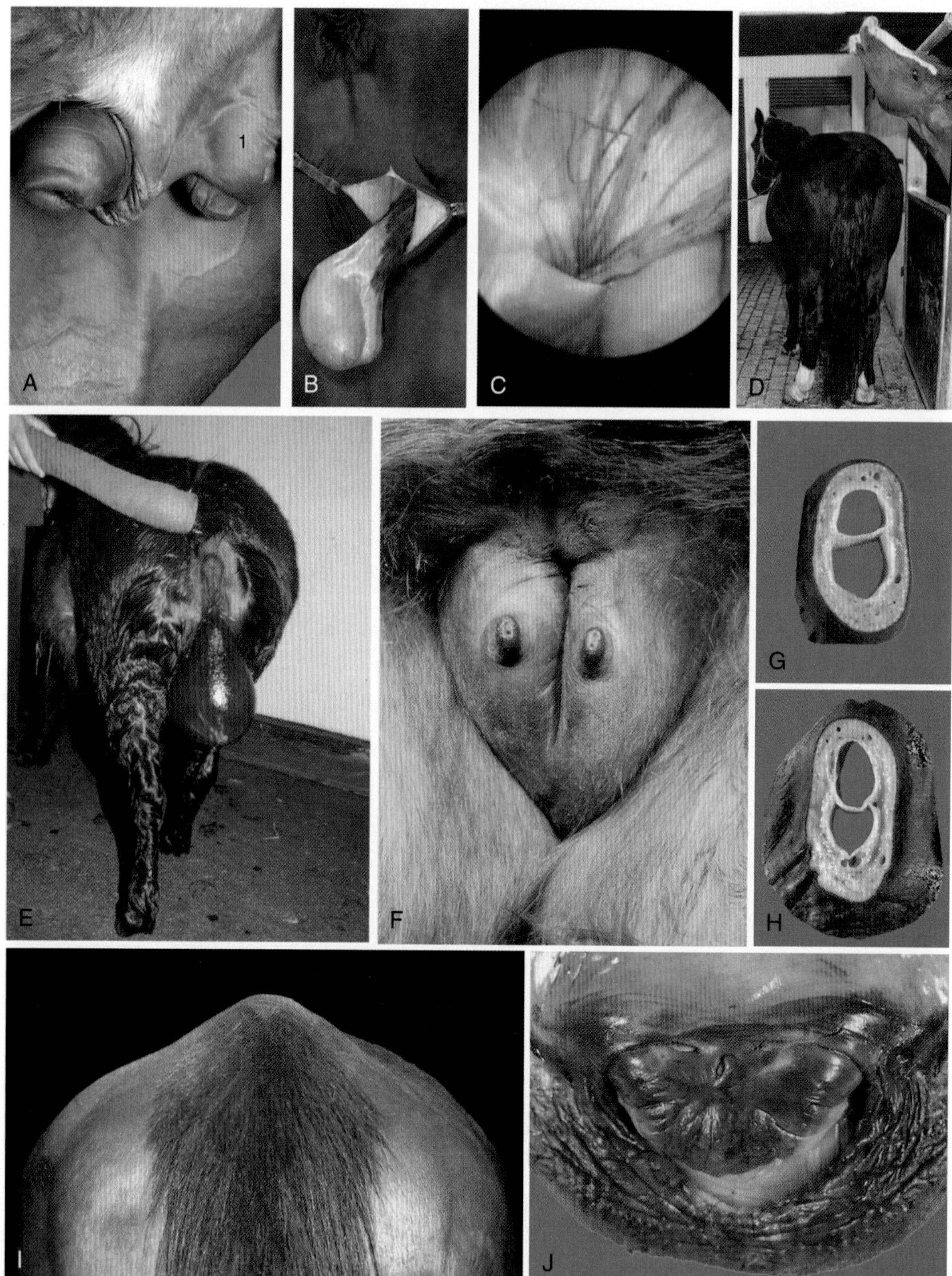


**Plate 24.** *A,* Inguinal area of stallion: 1, scrotum. *B,* Testis within exposed vaginal process. *C,* Endoscopic view of the vaginal ring. *D,* Stallion exhibiting Flehmen response to presence of mare in heat. *E,* Parturient mare: chorionic membrane with villiless "cervical star" clearly visible. *F,* Ventral view of udder of mare. *G* and *H,* Transected teats showing internal division. *I,* Sinking of hamstring muscles over relaxed sacrotuberal ligaments as parturition impends. *J,* Glans of clitoris in ventral commissure of vulva.

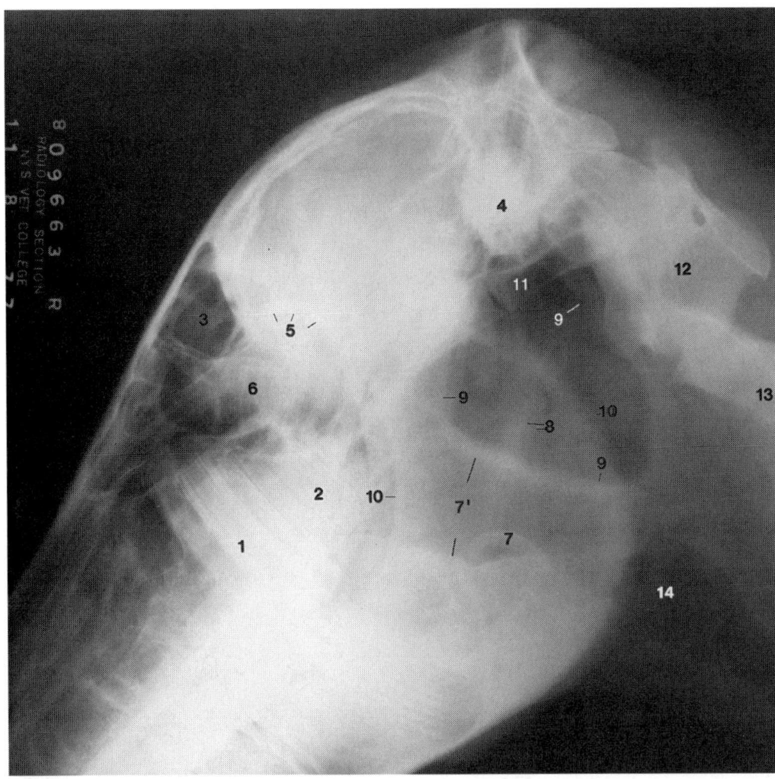


**Figure 18–26.** Lateral radiographic view of the head to show the position of the guttural pouches (9) in a horse $1\frac{1}{2}$ years old (estimated).

1, $M^1$; 2, unerupted $M^2$; 3, frontal sinus; 4, petrous temporal bone; 5, caudal border of orbit; 6, ethmoid labyrinth; 7, epiglottis; 7′, nasopharynx; 8, stylohyoid bones; 9, borders of guttural pouches; 10, rostral and caudal borders of mandible; 11, base of skull; 12, atlas; 13, axis; 14, larynx.

before crossing the lateral and then rostral walls of the lateral compartment (Fig. 18–28/6) in its approach (as the maxillary artery) to the alar canal. The pouch also directly covers the temporohyoid joint.

The mucous secretion of the lining normally drains into the pharynx through the pharyngotubal opening (Fig. 18–10/8) placed at the rostral end of the pouch, the most dependent part when the head is lowered. The connection opens when the horse swallows and grazing normally promotes drainage. When the exit is blocked or the secretion accumulates for any reason, the pouch distends, producing a palpable, often visible, swelling behind the jaw (Plate 23/ *A*). The exudate may be contaminated by microorganisms that invade along the tube or spread from infection of the neighboring retropharyngeal lymph nodes. Mycotic infections are common and often first establish where the mucosa overlies the temporohyoid joint; the trauma produced by minor movement is presumed to be a predisposing factor. Apart from such obvious signs as painful swelling of the parotid region, abnormal carriage of the head and neck, and nasal discharge, affected animals may exhibit a variety of specific abnormalities that result from involvement of structures directly related to the pouch. Fusion of the stylohoid with the adjacent portion of the petrous temporal bone, eliminating the intervening joint, may expose the complex to abnormal stress, for example, during movements of the tongue, and fractures of these bones have been reported. Other possible sequelae include inflammation of the middle ear (by extension of infection along the auditory tube); epistaxis (nasal bleeding) from erosion of the internal carotid artery; difficulty in swallowing following involvement of the glossopharyngeal and vagus nerves (or their pharyngeal branches); laryngeal hemiplegia (roaring) following vagus involvement; and various signs, collectively known as Horner's syndrome, that may result from involvement of the sympathetic nerve—nasal congestion, drooping of the upper eyelid, pupillary constriction, and sweating and increased skin temperature over the affected side of the head and neck. Signs of involvement of the facial nerve are relatively rare, while none suggestive of damage to the hypoglossal nerve have been recorded. The external carotid artery also seems to enjoy a relative immunity.

The pouch can be inspected or drained via the pharyngotubal opening or approached by open surgery. A favored route of access is provided by Viborg's triangle, bounded by the caudal border of the mandible (more deeply the occipitomandibularis), the tendon of the sternocephalicus, and the

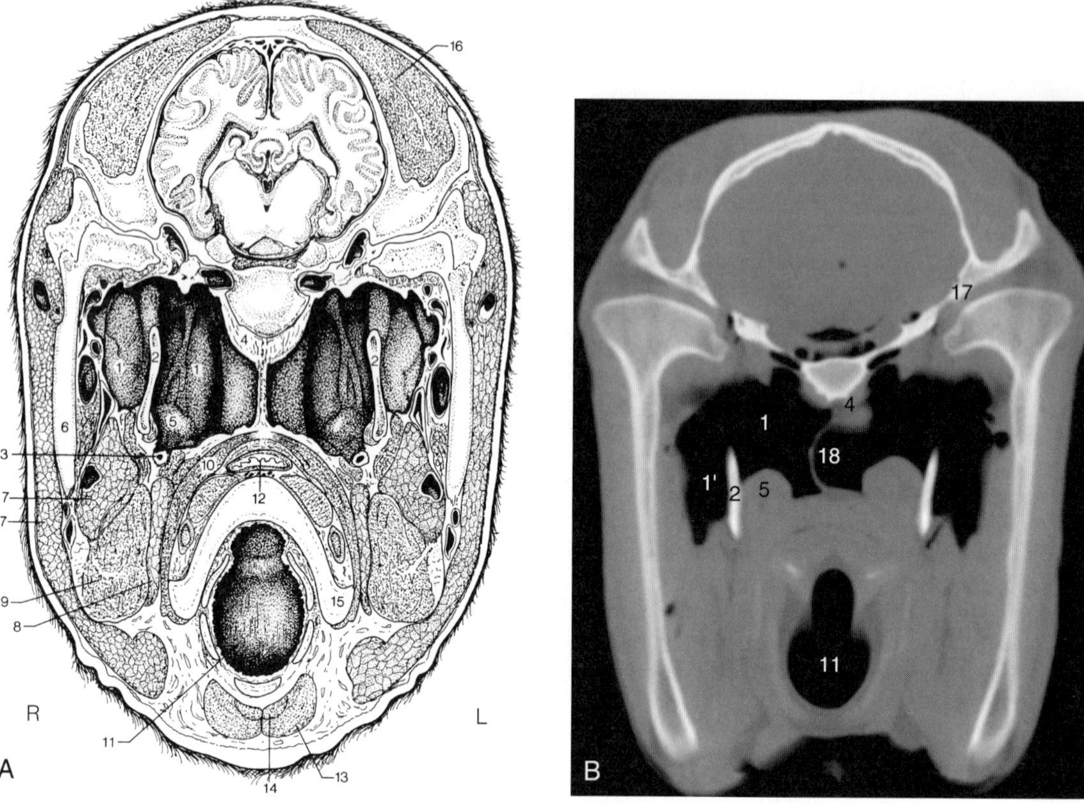


**Figure 18–27.** *A,* Transverse section of the head just caudal to the temporomandibular joint, looking caudally. *B,* CT scan (bone window) at about the same level.

1, 1′, Medial and lateral compartments of right guttural pouch; 2, stylohyoid; 3, external carotid artery; 4, rectus capitis ventralis; 5, medial retropharyngeal lymph nodes bulging into guttural pouch; 6, caudal border of mandible; 7, parotid gland; 8, mandibular gland; 9, occipitomandibularis; 10, cricopharyngeus; 11, larynx; 12, esophagus; 13, fused sterno- and omohyoideus; 14, sternothyroideus; 15, cricoid cartilage; 16, temporalis; 17, temporomandibular joints; 18, septum separating right and left guttural pouches.

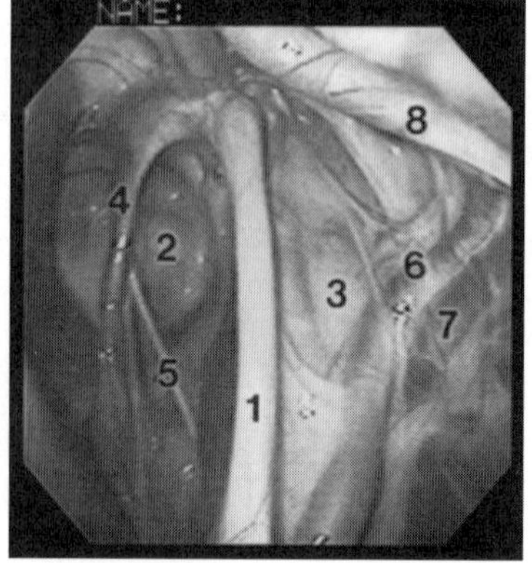


**Figure 18–28.** Endoscopic view of the dorsocaudal wall of the left guttural pouch.

1, Stylohyoid; 2, dorsocaudal recess of medial compartment; 3, lateral compartment; 4, fold containing internal carotid artery and cranial nerves IX, X, and XII; 5, glossopharyngeal (IX) and hypoglossal (XII) nerves passing rostrolaterally to accompany stylohyoid; 6, external carotid (and continuing maxillary) artery; 7, maxillary vein; 8, medial lamina of cartilage of auditory tube.

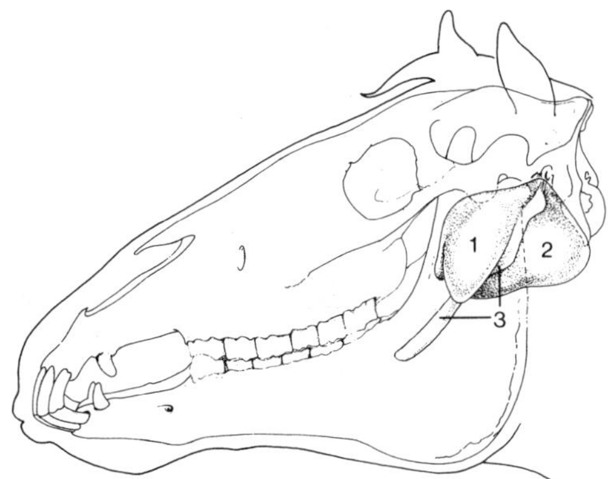


**Figure 18–29.** Position of the guttural pouch in relation to the skull and stylohyoid.

1, Lateral compartment of guttural pouch; 2, medial compartment of guttural pouch; 3, stylohyoid.

linguofacial vein (Fig. 18–30/1). The distance between the triangle and the pouch is greatly reduced when the pouch is enlarged. An alternative, more dorsal approach, involving reflection of the parotid gland, is also employed.

Hemorrhage from the internal carotid artery is frequently fatal unless treated in good time by closure of the vessel to each side of the leak. A proximal ligature is easily applied, but direct access to a site distal to the lesion may be impossible. Recourse may then be had to a balloon-tipped catheter, which is introduced beyond the proximal ligature and advanced into the siphon-like formation that the artery displays immediately before entering the cranial cavity. The catheter is left in place until it is judged that thrombosis will have sealed the damaged segment of the artery.

In foals, malfunction of the pharyngotubal opening may result in the pouch becoming distended with air to the extent that there is a swelling visible externally (Plate 23/*A*). It appears that there may be a redundancy of the mucosal fold (plica salpingopharyngea) that is normally present at the entry of the tube. In these individuals the excess mucosa creates a one-way valve that allows air to be drawn into, but not expelled from, the pouch. Unilateral tympany may be relieved by forcing an opening in the median septum so that both pouches communicate with the pharynx through a single opening. When swelling is bilateral, parts of the flaps guarding the openings may have to be removed.

Although the clinical importance of the guttural pouch has long been appreciated, its functional significance has resisted convincing explanation until very recently. Inevitably, the absence of hard fact has prompted speculative interpretations of different degrees of plausibility. These speculations can be disregarded following recent experimental investigations which identify the pouch as a mechanism for cooling the cerebral blood supply, a mechanism that is peculiar to the horse (at least among domestic species) and additional to other devices found in mammals generally (pp. 303, 482). These studies emphasize the relevance of the extensive contact between the extracranial part of the internal carotid artery and the exceedingly thin pouch wall. That this intimacy provides the potential for cooling the major, that is internal carotid, contribution to the cerebral blood supply was revealed in these experiments in which thermocouples were implanted at various points along the course of the vessel. No local differences in blood temperature were registered in the resting animal but a significant drop in temperature (of about 2°C) at the distal end of the artery was demonstrated in horses engaged in 15 minutes of strenuous exercise. Physical activity of course raises body temperature, ultimately to a level that could endanger brain function unless effective countermeasures exist. The transfer of heat from internal carotid blood to adjacent air is facilitated by the more vigorous ventilation of the pouch that accompanies exertion.

## THE LARYNX

The larynx is suspended by the hyoid apparatus and is partly contained within the intermandibular space (see Fig. 4–8). Though few distinguishing features of the cartilages are important, attention

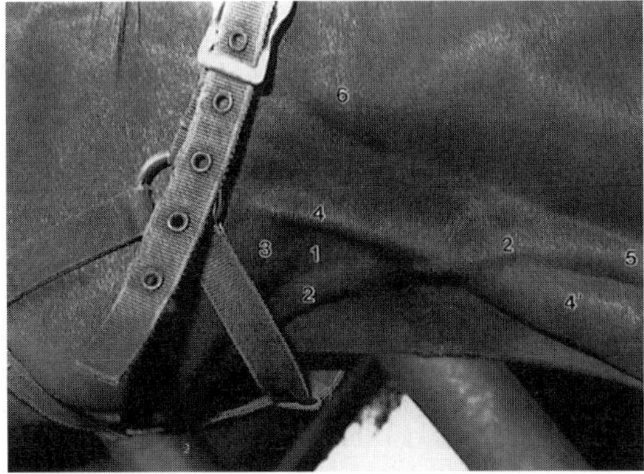


**Figure 18–30.** Retromandibular region showing Viborg's triangle.

1, Viborg's triangle; 2, linguofacial vein; 3, caudal border of mandible; 4, tendon of sternocephalicus, the muscle belly at 4′; 5, external jugular vein in jugular groove; 6, wing of atlas.

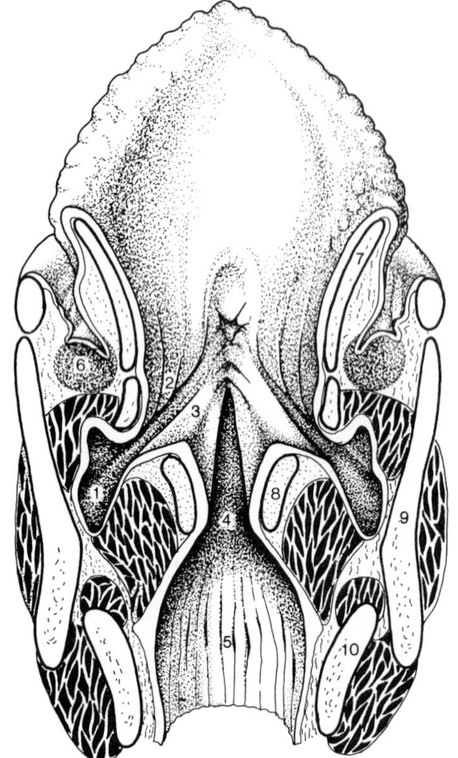


**Figure 18–31.** Dorsal section of the larynx.

1, Laryngeal ventricle; 2, vestibular fold with ventricularis; 3, vocal fold with vocalis; 4, glottic cleft; 5, infraglottic cavity; 6, caudal end of palatine tonsil; 7, epiglottic cartilage; 8, arytenoid cartilage; 9, thyroid cartilage; 10, cricoid cartilage.

must be drawn to the deep notch in the ventral part of the thyroid cartilage since this provides very convenient access to the interior after incision of the cricothyroid ligament. A prominence rostral to the notch and the ventral part of the cricoid arch provide the necessary landmarks (see Fig. 4–13/7). A prudent operator will also identify the basihyoid to confirm the site before making the initial skin incision. The normally retrovelar position of the leaf-shaped epiglottis has been pointed out (Fig. 18–10/11 and Plate 3/*B*).

The mucosa forms outpouchings (ventricles) that pass laterally between the vocal and vestibular folds but remain within the protection of the thyroid lamina. The ventricular entrance is sufficiently large to admit the burr that is used to evert the sac in one of the "roaring" operations (Fig. 18–31/1).

The term *roaring* is applied to a strident sound produced at inspiration in affected animals. The sound is caused by the flow of air passively vibrating a lax, adducted vocal fold (Fig. 18–32/4; see also Plates 3/*A* and 23/*B*). The laxity results from paralysis of certain muscles. For reasons that are not yet clear, the paralysis is almost always limited to the left side, and though it initially affects the cricoarytenoideus dorsalis—abductor of the arytenoid cartilage and vocal fold (see Fig. 4–14/5)—other muscles may later become involved. Several unsubstantiated theories have been advanced in explanation of the condition.

The asymmetry in incidence directs attention to differences in the courses and relations of the right and left recurrent laryngeal nerves. The left nerve loops around the aortic arch and has a closer relationship to tracheobronchial and other lymph nodes within the chest. Since the condition often follows a respiratory infection, the relationship to the nodes is perhaps the more relevant; it is not a complete explanation since laryngeal muscular atrophy has been recognized in unborn foals. Wastage of the cricoarytenoideus dorsalis alters the contours of the larynx in a manner that can be appreciated on external palpation; it hollows the space above the arytenoid cartilage, which makes the muscular process of that cartilage more prominent. One of the operations for the relief of roaring is the reinforcement of the wasted dorsal cricoarytenoideus muscle by a suture tightened to fix the arytenoid cartilage in permanent abduction. An older alternative was the eversion and exci-

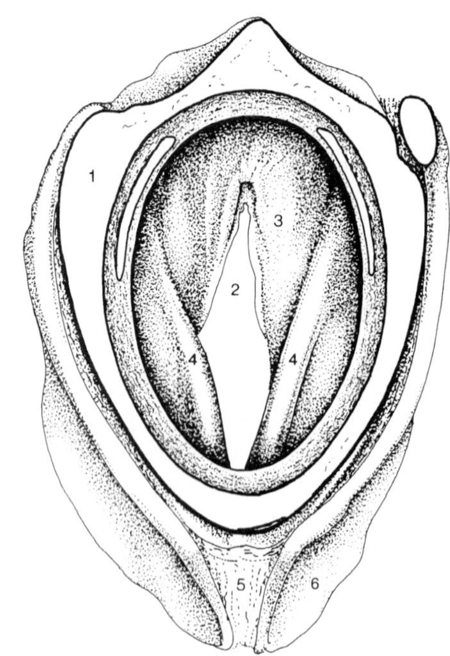


**Figure 18–32.** Interior of the larynx, caudal view.

1, Cricoid cartilage; 2, glottic cleft; 3, arytenoid cartilage, covered with mucosa; 4, vocal fold; 5, cricothyroid ligament; 6, thyroid cartilage.

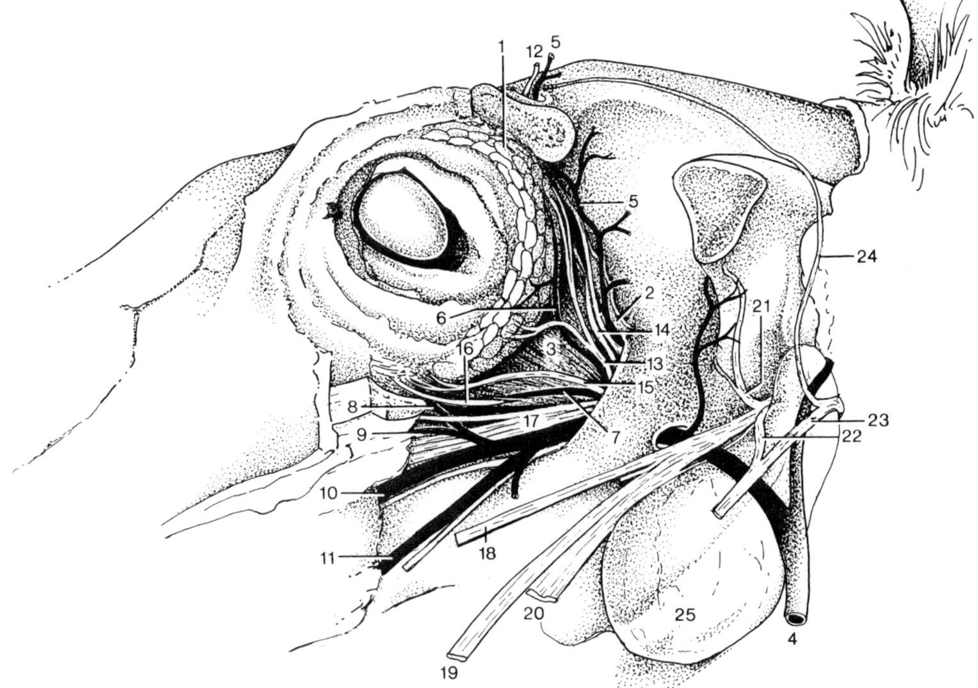


**Figure 18–33.** Dissection of the orbit; the zygomatic arch and periorbita have been removed.

1, Lacrimal gland; 2, periorbita; 3, lateral rectus; 4, maxillary a.; 5, supraorbital a.; 6, lacrimal a.; 7, muscular branch of external ophthalmic a.; 8, malar a.; 9, infraorbital a.; 10, major palatine a.; 11, buccal a.; 12, supraorbital n.; 13, lacrimal n.; 14, trochlear n.; 15, zygomatic n.; 16, oculomotor n.; 17, rostral branches of maxillary n.; 18, buccal n.; 19, lingual n.; 20, inferior alveolar n.; 21, masticatory n.; 22, auriculotemporal n.; 23, facial n.; 24, auriculopalpebral n.; 25, guttural pouch.

sion of the lateral laryngeal ventricle in the expectation that the resulting scar tissue would bind this cartilage to the thyroid cartilage. Both operations result in tightening the vocal fold and widening the glottic cleft. Neither operation effects a cure of the condition, which has human and canine parallels.

## THE EYE

Some account has been given of the external features (p. 479). The adnexa call for little comment. The *lacrimal gland* is relatively large and placed over the dorsolateral aspect of the bulbus, where it is protected by the adjacent part of the orbital rim (Fig. 18–33/1). A small accessory lacrimal gland is associated with the deep part of the cartilage of the third eyelid.

The *nasolacrimal duct,* already mentioned in relation to surgical access to the maxillary sinus, provides a conspicuous feature where it opens on the floor of the nostril (Fig. 18–3). The extraocular muscles show little that is distinctive; as is common in ungulates, the retractor bulbi is relatively large (see Fig. 9–13/7).

The eyeball shows significant departure from the spheroidal form—it is compressed from front to back and is higher than it is wide—which is relevant to the concept of the ramp retina (see further on). It is constructed of the usual layers. The *sclera* is relatively thin toward the equator, where it obtains a bluish tint from the pigmentation of the underlying choroid. The *cornea* is relatively small and ovoid, the pointed end being lateral.

The *choroid* exhibits a triangular green or bluish-green tapetum dorsal to the optic disc (Plate 14/*F*). The ciliary muscle is poorly developed, a second point adduced in support of the theory of the ramp retina as the means of accommodation. The iris is generally dark brown; in the absence of pigmentation (a not uncommon occurrence) it is a rather unattractive bluish color ("walleye"). Both the iris and the pupillary opening within it are oval (with the long axes horizontal) but the pupil becomes rounder when contracted. The pupil of the newborn is almost round. Both margins of the pupil, but particularly the upper one, carry irregular granular excrescences interpreted as "shades" that limit the entry of light (see Fig. 9–6/3).

The *optic disc,* very prominent on ophthalmoscopic examination of the fundus, is placed ventral to the tapetum and ventrolateral to the posterior pole of the bulb (Plate 14/*F*). The macula is said to comprise both round and elongated parts; it is asserted that the former is concerned with binocular, the latter with monocular vision. The central artery of the retina is poorly developed, and the few straight branches that radiate from the margins of the disc soon fade. Much the larger part of the retina is nourished by the vessels of the middle tunic. There is nothing noteworthy in the refractive media.

It is believed that the poor development of the ciliary muscle compels the horse to rely on the distorted form of the bulb for accommodation. The upper part of the retina, which is at a greater distance from the lens, serves for near vision; the lower part, closer to the lens, serves for distance vision. The animal therefore adjusts the carriage of the head—and thereby the location of the image on the retina—as a means of focusing. The technique is sometimes well illustrated by a horse approaching and jumping an obstacle.

## THE VENTRAL PART OF THE NECK

The ventral part of the neck contains the visceral space occupied by the esophagus, trachea, and

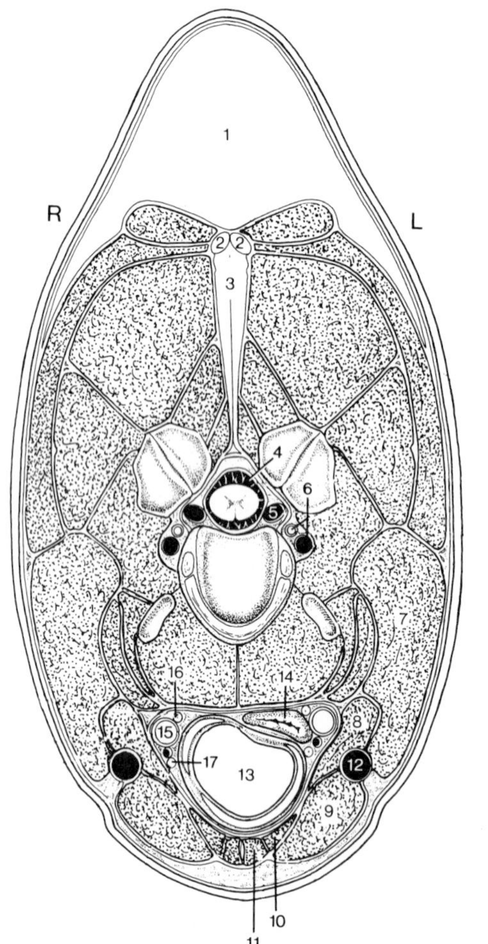


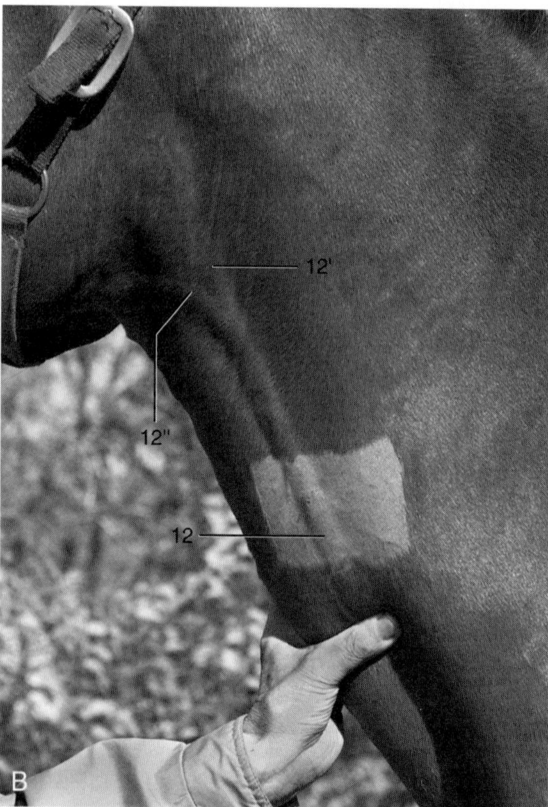


**Figure 18–34.** *A,* Transection of the neck at the level of the fourth cervical vertebra. *B,* The external jugular vein is raised by occluding it in the jugular groove. (The shaved patch is from a previous placement of an indwelling catheter.)

1, Crest; 2, 3, funicular and laminar parts of nuchal ligament; 4, subarachnoid space; 5, internal vertebral venous plexus; 6, vertebral artery and vein; 7, brachiocephalicus; 8, omohyoideus; 9, sternocephalicus; 10, sternothyroideus; 11, sternohyoideus; 12, external jugular vein; 12′, maxillary vein; 12″, linguofacial vein; 13, trachea; 14, esophagus; 15, common carotid artery; 16, vagosympathetic trunk; 17, recurrent laryngeal nerve.

other structures passing between the head and the thorax. This space is bounded dorsally by the muscles below the vertebrae and laterally and ventrally by flatter muscles united by stout fasciae. The foremost lateroventral muscles are the brachiocephalicus and sternocephalicus, which bound the groove occupied by the (external) jugular vein (Fig. 18–34/12). The caudal part of this groove is covered by the cutaneous muscle of the neck, which radiates from a manubrial origin; the muscle thins as it passes from its origin, which increases the prominence of the cranial part of the vein, the obvious target when the vein is raised for puncture (Fig. 18–35/9,11). The brachiocephalicus is described on page 569.

The right and left *sternocephalicus muscles* arise from the manubrium side by side but diverge toward their mandibular insertions (/8). This leaves a median space through which the trachea may be palpated, although it is still covered by the thin *sternothyroideus* and *sternohyoideus* (/6). These are combined at their origin from the sternum but branch into slips that diverge to attach to the thyroid cartilage and the basihyoid. The omohyoideus (/7), which extends between the medial aspect of the shoulder and the basihyoid, forms the floor of the jugular groove. It is said, unconvincingly, to protect the more deeply placed common carotid artery in unskillful venipuncture (Fig. 18–34/8). The muscles ventral to the trachea constitute the "strap muscles" that are resected in Forsell's operation for cribbing, a stable vice in which a horse hangs onto the crib with its teeth and dilates the pharynx to swallow air. The best results appear to be obtained by combining resection of the sternothyroideus, sternohyoideus, and omohyoideus muscles with section of the ventral branch of the accessory nerve, easily found where it enters the sternocephalicus close to the musculotendinous junction; the section of the muscles and nerve is of course bilateral.

The *trachea* occupies a median position in the visceral space. Its size bears no constant relation to that of the body—an important point when selecting an endotracheal tube since the generous size of the glottis is not a limiting factor. The tracheal lumen is slightly flattened dorsoventrally and is, of course, maintained patent by the tracheal rings (Fig. 18–36). It is therefore customary to completely transect as few cartilages as possible in order to avoid collapse of the wall in tracheotomy operations, such as those performed to allow the air intake to bypass an obstructed larynx.

The *esophagus* begins dorsal to the trachea but slips to the left side by the middle of the neck (Fig. 18–34/14). It then slowly creeps back toward a

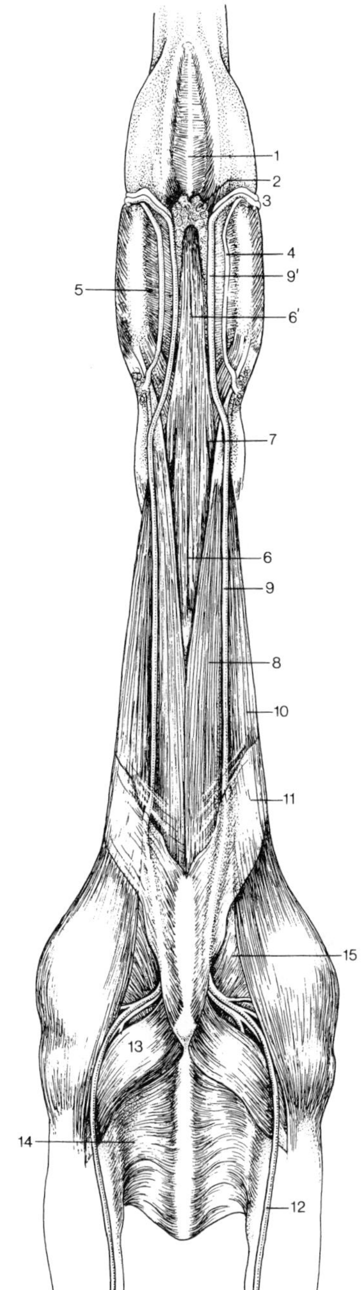


**Figure 18–35.** Ventral view of the neck and intermandibular space.

1, Mylohyoideus; 2, mandibular lymph nodes; 3, facial artery and vein; 4, parotid duct; 5, medial pterygoid; 6, sternohyoideus and -thyroideus; 6′, combined sterno- and omohyoideus; 7, omohyoideus; 8, sternocephalicus; 9, external jugular vein; 9′, linguofacial vein; 10, brachiocephalicus; 11, cutaneus colli; 12, cephalic vein; 13, pectoralis descendens; 14, pectoralis transversus; 15, subclavius.

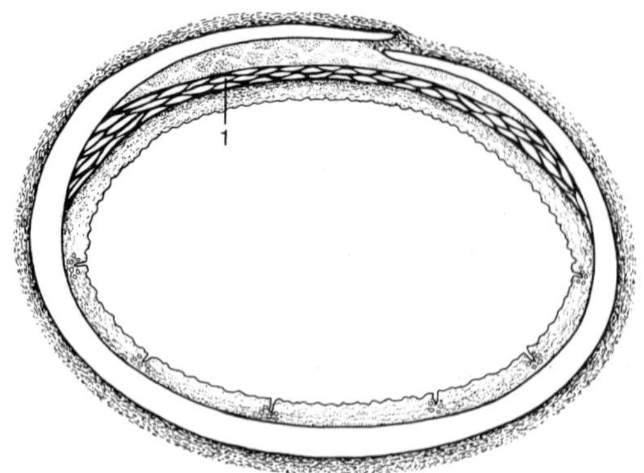


**Figure 18–36.** Transverse section of the trachea.

1, Trachealis.

median position, though it is often ventral to the trachea just before it enters the chest. It takes a more direct course when the neck is extended. The esophagus is too soft to identify easily on palpation but its position is revealed when the animal swallows.

The *common carotid artery* lies ventral to the trachea at the base of the neck but gradually ascends to a more dorsal position (/15); it divides above the pharynx into occipital, internal carotid, and external carotid arteries. The internal carotid supplies the brain, and the occipital supplies the region of the poll. The clinically relevant branches of the external carotid have been noted in previous contexts; the overall pattern of distribution is shown in Figure 18–37. Pulsations of the common carotid may sometimes be felt in the middle of the neck when the artery is pressed against the subvertebral muscles. The artery is enclosed in a thick fascial sheath shared with the vagosympathetic trunk, which follows its dorsal border. The recurrent laryngeal nerve lies ventral to it in the tracheal fascia (Fig. 18–34/16,17).

The *deep cervical lymph nodes* are scattered in packets—cranial, middle, and caudal—along the course of the tracheal lymph duct. The caudal group receives the outflow from the superficial cervical nodes (Fig. 18–38).

The *external jugular vein* is supplemented by the vertebral vein, and the plexus within the vertebral canal, in the drainage of the head. It is formed at the caudoventral angle of the parotid gland by the confluence of maxillary and linguofacial veins. It stands out very prominently, and very

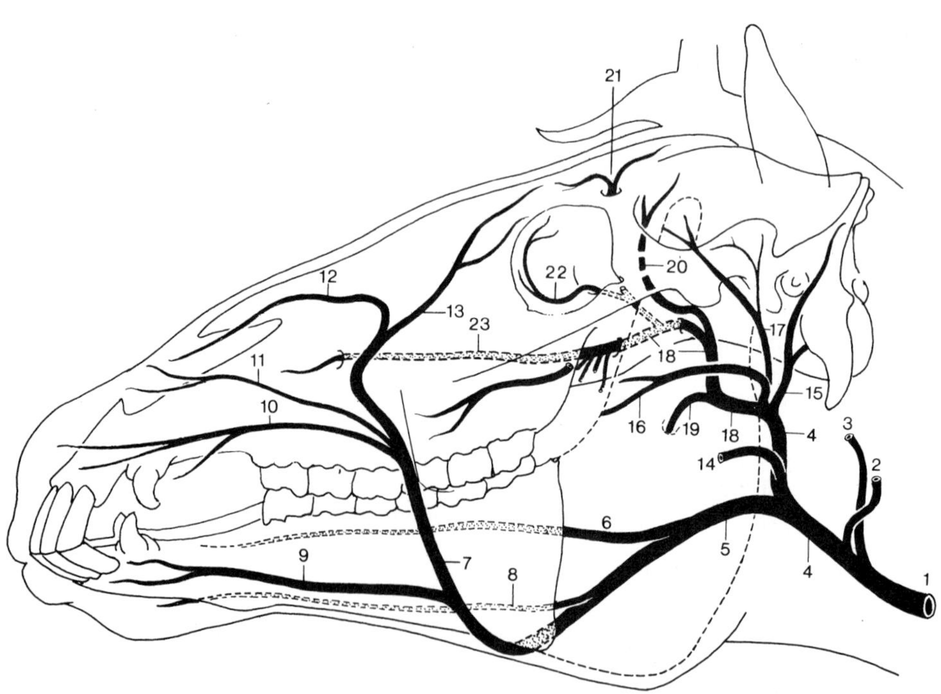


**Figure 18–37.** Principal arteries of the head, schematic.

1, Common carotid a.; 2, occipital a.; 3, internal carotid a.; 4, external carotid a.; 5, linguofacial a.; 6, lingual a.; 7, facial a.; 8, sublingual a.; 9, inferior labial a.; 10, superior labial a.; 11, lateral nasal a.; 12, dorsal nasal a.; 13, angularis oculi a.; 14, masseteric a.; 15, caudal auricular a.; 16, transverse facial a., displaced ventrally for clarity; 17, superficial temporal a.; 18, maxillary a.; 19, inferior alveolar a.; 20, caudal deep temporal a.; 21, supraorbital a.; 22, malar a.; 23, infraorbital a.

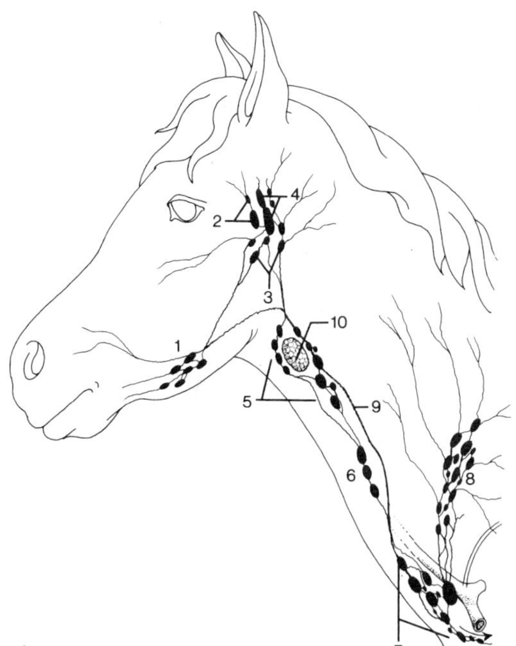


**Figure 18–38.** Lymphatic structures of the head and neck, schematic.

1, Mandibular lymph nodes; 2, parotid lymph nodes; 3, medial retropharyngeal lymph nodes; 4, lateral retropharyngeal lymph nodes; 5, 6, 7, cranial, middle, and caudal deep cervical lymph nodes; 8, superficial cervical lymph nodes; 9, tracheal duct; 10, thyroid gland.

conveniently for injection and sampling, when raised by pressure over the jugular groove.

The lobes of the *thyroid gland* can be recognized on palpation as soft ovoid structures placed dorsolateral to the first part of the trachea (Fig. 18–25/28). They are joined ventrally by a narrow isthmus.

Though rarely as well developed as in the calf, a cervical part of the *thymus* may extend beside the trachea in the caudal part of the neck. It is often separated from the thoracic part and may be broken into several masses.

## THE LYMPHATIC STRUCTURES OF THE HEAD AND NECK

The parotid, mandibular, and deep cervical lymph nodes have been encountered (p. 483 and 506). The superficial cervical nodes are described on page 599.

The *retropharyngeal nodes* are arranged in clumps upon the pharyngeal wall (Figs. 18–25/25 and 18–27/5). The lateral group is also related to the guttural pouch, lying caudal to it within the atlantal fossa. Infection of these nodes, frequently leading to abscess formation (strangles), may be followed by contamination of the guttural pouch with the potential sequelae already mentioned (p. 499). The pattern of drainage is such that the medial retropharyngeal nodes serve as the collecting center for all lymph emanating from the upper part of the head (Fig. 18–38).

## Selected Bibliography

Ahern, T.J.: A review of the anatomical components, and the process of entrapment of the epiglottis in the horse, with a comparative synopsis of surgical treatments. J. Equine Vet. Sci. 16:408–414, 1996.

Anderson, B.G., and M. Wyman: Anatomy of the equine eye and orbit: Histological structure and blood supply of the eyelids. J. Equine Med. Surg. 3:4–9, 1979.

Arencibia, A., J.M. Vázquez, R. Jaber, et al.: Magnetic resonance imaging and cross sectional anatomy of the normal equine sinuses and nasal passages. Vet. Radiol. Ultrasound 41:313–319, 2000.

Ashdown, R.R., and S. Done: Color Atlas of Veterinary Anatomy: The Horse. Philadelphia, J.B. Lippincott, 1987.

Baptiste, K.E.: Functional anatomy observations of the pharyngeal orifice of the equine guttural pouch (auditory tube diverticulum). Vet. J. 153:311–319, 1997.

Baptiste, K.E.: A preliminary study on the role of the equine guttural pouches in selective brain cooling. Vet. J. 155:139–148, 1998.

Baptiste, K.E., S.D. Holladay, and L.E. Freeman: Alterations in equine guttural pouch morphology with head position: Observations. Anat. Rec. 246:579–584, 1996.

Baptiste, K.E., J.M. Naylor, J. Bailey, et al.: A function for guttural pouches in the horse. Nature 403:382–383, 2000.

Behrens, E., J. Schumacher, and E. Morris: Contrast paranasal sinusography for evaluation of disease of the paranasal sinuses of five horses. Vet. Radiol. Ultrasound 32:105–109, 1991.

Bell, B.T.L., G.J. Baker, L.C. Abbott, et al.: The macroscopic vascular anatomy of the equine ethmoidal area. Anat. Histol. Embryol. 24:39–45, 1995.

Blythe, L.L., B.J. Watrous, G.M.H. Shires, et al.: Prophylactic partial stylohyoidostectomy for horses with osteoarthropathy of the temporohyoid joint. J. Equine Vet. Sci. 14:32–37, 1994.

Boyd, J.S.: Selection of sites for intramuscular injections in the neck of the horse. Vet. Rec. 121:197–200, 1987.

deLahunta, A., and R.E. Habel: Applied Veterinary Anatomy. Philadelphia, W.B. Saunders Company, 1986.

De Schaepdrijver, L., P. Simoens, H. Lauwers, and J.P. De Geest: Retinal vascular patterns in domestic animals. Vet. Sci. 47:34–42, 1989.

Dik, K.J., and I. Gunsser: Atlas of Diagnostic Radiology of the Horse. Parts 1–3. Philadelphia, W.B. Saunders Company, 1988–1990.

Ducharme, N.G., and R.P. Hackett: The value of surgical treatment of laryngeal hemiplegia in horses. Compend. Contin. Educ. Pract. Vet. 13:472–475, 1991.

Freeman, D.E., M.W. Ross, W.J. Donawick, and A.N. Hamir: Occlusion of the external carotid and maxillary arteries in the horse to prevent hemorrhage from guttural pouch mycosis. Vet. Surg. 18:39–47, 1989.

Freeman, D.E., P.G. Orsini, M.W. Ross, and J.B. Madison: A large frontonasal bone flap for sinus surgery in the horse. Vet. Surg. 19:122–130, 1990.

Gibbs, C., and J.G. Lane: Radiographic examination of the facial, nasal and paranasal sinus regions of the horse. II. Radiological findings. Equine Vet. J. 19:474–482, 1987.
Greet, T.R.C.: Windsucking treated by myectomy and neurectomy. Equine Vet. J. 14:299–301, 1982.
Greet, T.R.C.: Outcome of treatment in 35 cases of guttural pouch mycosis. Equine Vet. J. 19:483–487, 1987.
Hakansson, A., P. Franzen, and H. Pettersson: Comparison of two surgical methods for treatment of cribbing in horses. Equine Vet. J. 24:494–496, 1992.
Hammer, E.J., E.P. Tulleners, E.J. Parente, and B.B. Martin, Jr.: Videoendoscopic assessment of dynamic laryngeal function during exercise in horses with grade-III left laryngeal hemiparesis at rest: 26 cases (1992–1995). JAVMA 212: 399–403, 1998.
Hardy, J., M.T. Robertson, and D.A. Wilkie: Ischemic optic neuropathy and blindness after arterial occlusion for treatment of guttural pouch mycosis in two horses. JAVMA 196:1631–1634, 1990.
Harrison, I.W., and C.W. Raker: Sternothyrohyoideus myectomy in horses: 17 cases (1984–1985). JAVMA 193:1299–1302, 1988.
Hawkins, J.F., E.P. Tulleners, L.H. Evans, and J.A. Orsini: Alar fold resection in horses: 24 cases (1979–1992). JAVMA 206:1913–1916, 1995.
Heffron, C.J., G.J. Baker, and R. Lee: Fluoroscopic investigations of pharyngeal function in the horse. Equine Vet. J. 11:148–152, 1979.
Holcombe, S.J., F.J. Derksen, J.A. Stick, and N.E. Robinson: Effects of bilateral hypoglossal and glossopharyngeal nerve blocks on epiglottic and soft palate position in exercising horses. Am. J. Vet. Res. 58:1022–1026, 1997.
Holcombe, S.J., F.J. Derksen, J.A. Stick, and N.E. Robinson: Effect of bilateral blockade of the pharyngeal branch of the vagus nerve on soft palate function in horses. Am. J. Vet. Res. 59:504–508, 1998.
Honnas, C.M., and J.D. Wheat: Epiglottic entrapment—a transnasal surgical approach to divide the aryepiglottic fold axially in the standing horse. Vet. Surg. 17:246–251, 1988.
Hoyt, S.C., R.S. Pleasant, R.M. Dabareiner, and R.O. Carolan: Detachable latex balloon occlusion of an internal carotid artery with an aberrant branch in a horse with guttural pouch (auditory tube diverticulum) mycosis. JAVMA 216:888–891, 2000.
Judy C.E., Chaffin, M.K., and Cohen, N.D.: Empyema of the guttural pouch (auditory tube diverticulum) in horses: 91 cases (1977–1997). JAVMA 215:1666–1670, 1999.
Kainer, R.A.: Clinical anatomy of the equine head. Vet. Clin. North Am. Equine Pract. 9:1–23, 1993.
Kirkland, K.D., G.J. Baker, S.M. Marretta, et al.: Effects of aging on the endodontic system, reserve crown and roots of equine mandibular cheek teeth. Am. J. Vet. Res. 57:31–38, 1996.
Lane, J.G.: The management of guttural pouch mycosis. Equine Vet. J. 21:321–324, 1989.
Lane, J.G., C. Gibbs, S.E. Meynink, and F.C. Steele: Radiographic examination of the facial, nasal and paranasal sinus regions of the horse: I. Indications and procedures in 235 cases. Equine Vet. J. 19:466–473, 474–482, 1987.
Latimer, C.A., and M. Wyman: Atresia of the nasolacrimal duct in three horses. JAVMA 184:989–992, 1984.
Lindsay, F.E., and H.M. Clayton: An anatomical and endoscopic study of the nasopharynx and larynx of the donkey *(Equus asinus)*. J. Anat. 144:123–132, 1986.
Lindsay, W.A., and E.B. Hedberg: Performing facial nerve blocks, nasolacrimal catheterization, and paranasal sinus centesis in horses, Vet. Med. 86:72–83. 1991.
Littauer, M.A.: Slit nostrils of equids. Z. Saugetierkd. 34:183–186, 1969.
Lowder, M.Q., and P.O.E. Mueller: Dental embryology, anatomy, development, and aging. Vet. Clin. North Am. Equine Pract. Dent. 14:227–245, 1998.
Martin, G.S., R.E. Beadle, P.F. Haynes, and J.W. Watters: Cross-sectional area of the aditus laryngis and rima glottidis before and after transection of the left recurrent laryngeal nerve in the horse. Am. J. Vet. Res. 47:422–425, 1986.
McCarthy, P.H.: Galvayne: The mystery surrounding the man and the eponym. Anat. Histol. Embryol. 16:330–336, 1987.
McCarthy, P.H.: Anatomy of the laryngeal and adjacent regions as perceived by palpation of clinically normal standing horses. Am. J. Vet. Res. 51:611–618, 1990.
McCarthy, P.H.: Subcutaneous part of the masseteric ramus of the external carotid artery as a proposed site of pulse-taking in Thoroughbreds. JAVMA 197:751, 1990.
McCarthy, P.H.: The triangle of Viborg *(Trigonum viborgi)* and its anatomical relationship in the normal standing horse. Anat. Histol. Embryol. 19:303–313, 1990.
McCarthy, P.H.: The zygomatic branch of the auriculopalpebral nerve: Can it be normally palpated in the live horse? Anat. Histol. Embryol. 25:7–10, 1996.
McCue, P.M., D.E. Freeman, and W.J. Donawick: Guttural pouch tympany: 15 cases (1977–1986). JAVMA 194:1761–1763, 1989.
Muylle, S., P. Simoens, and H. Lauwers: Ageing horses by an examination of their incisor teeth: An (im)possible task? Vet. Rec. 138:295–301, 1996.
Muylle, S., P. Simoens, H. Lauwers, and G. Van Loon: Ageing Arab horses by their dentition. Vet. Rec. 142:659–662, 1998.
Orsini, P., C.W. Raker, C.F. Reid, and P. Mann: Xeroradiographic evaluation of the equine larynx. Am. J. Vet Res. 50:845–849, 1989.
Rakestraw, P.C., R.P. Hackett, N.G. Ducharme, and G.J. Nielan: Arytenoid cartilage movements in resting and exercising horses. Vet. Surg. 20:122–127, 1991.
Richardson, J.D., J.G. Lane, and K.R. Waldron: Is dentition an accurate indication of the age of a horse? Vet. Rec. 135:31–34, 1994.
Richardson, J.D., P.J. Cripps, M.H. Hillyer, et al.: An evaluation of the accuracy of ageing horses by their dentition: A matter of experience? Vet. Rec. 137:88–90, 1995.
Ruggles, A.J., M.W. Ross, and D.E. Freeman: Endoscopic examination of normal paranasal sinuses in horses. Vet. Surg. 20:418–423, 1991.
Russell, A.P., and D.E. Slone: Performance analysis after prosthetic laryngoplasty and bilateral ventriculectomy for laryngeal hemiplegia in horses: 70 cases (1986–1991). JAVMA 204:1235–1241, 1994.
Samuelson, D., P. Smith, and D. Brooks: Morphologic features of the aqueous humor drainage pathways in horses. Am. J. Vet. Res. 50:720–727, 1989.
Simoens, P., S. Muylle, and H. Lauwers: Anatomy of the ocular arteries in the horse. Equine Vet. J. 28:360–367, 1996.
Smyth, D.A., K.E. Baptiste, A.M. Cruz, et al.: Primary distension of the guttural pouch lateral compartment secondary to empyema. Can. Vet. J. 40:802–804, 1999.
Sweeney, C.R., and E.J. Parente: The transverse facial vein: An alternate site for venipuncture in the horse. Equine Pract. 18:7–9, 1996.
Sweeney, C.R., A.D. Maxson, and L.R. Soma: Endoscopic findings in the upper respiratory tract of 678 Thoroughbred racehorses. JAVMA 198:1037–1038, 1991.
Tietje, S., M. Becker, and G. Böckenhoff: Computed tomographic evaluation of head diseases in the horse: 15 cases. Equine Vet. J. 28:98–105, 1996.
Trotter, G.W.: Paranasal sinuses. Vet. Clin. North Am. Equine Pract. 9:153–169, 1993.

Turner, A.S., N. White, and J. Ismay: Modified Forsell's operation for crib biting in the horse. JAVMA 184:309–312, 1984.

Wheat, J.D.: Sinus drainage and tooth repulsion in the horse. Proc. Am. Assoc. Equine Pract. 19:171–176, 1973.

Williams, J.W., J.R. Pascoe, D.M. Meagher, and W.J. Hornof: Effects of left recurrent laryngeal neurectomy, prosthetic laryngoplasty, and subtotal arytenoidectomy on upper airway pressure during maximal exertion. Vet. Surg. 19:136–141, 1990.

CHAPTER 19

# The Neck, Back, and Vertebral Column of the Horse

This chapter is concerned with the dorsal part of the neck, the back, the loins, and the tail. The ventral part of the neck was considered with the head; the croup is considered with the hindlimb.

## CONFORMATION AND SURFACE FEATURES

The neck and back vary considerably in conformation according to breed, sex, age, and condition. The dorsal contour of the back and loins closely reflects the course of the vertebral column, but that of the neck, where the vertebrae are more deeply buried, depends largely upon the nuchal ligament and crest (see further on).

The neck may be arched, straight, or hollowed in the natural standing posture. The arched form, known to horsemen as a swan- or peacock-neck, is characteristic of certain breeds, including the Lipizzaner. The concave form or ewe-neck is not prized and for most breeds it is the straight neck that is held in greatest esteem. The transition between the neck and withers may be smooth or marked by a dip. In saddle horses the neck deepens considerably toward the chest but the change is usually less marked in the heavier draft breeds. Viewed from above, the neck is relatively narrow and of even width, except immediately before the shoulder where the mergence with the trunk is eased by the presence of the subclavius, which fills out the hollow along the cranial margin of the scapula. The heavy neck of the stallion is mainly due to the strong development of the fatty fibrous tissue (crest) dorsal to the nuchal ligament (Fig. 18–34/1).

The course of the cervical vertebrae may not be evident on simple scrutiny, although the wing of the atlas is almost always a prominent visible and palpable landmark. The positions of the transverse and articular processes of the third to sixth neck vertebrae may be visible in animals that are lean or in poor condition. These features are usually detectable on palpation, although in fat or particularly well-muscled horses it may be impossible to gain more than a general impression of the course of the vertebrae (Fig. 19–1). In thin-skinned horses certain of the superficial muscles (especially the trapezius and rhomboideus) stand out as individual surface features when tensed (Fig. 19–2/1,8).

The characteristic prominence of the withers is due to the great length of the spinous processes of the second to ninth thoracic vertebrae, but the region also embraces the scapular cartilages and associated muscles. The withers vary considerably, and in saddle animals it is preferred that they be both high and long, and of moderate width; excessive narrowness may make a proper fit of the saddle difficult.

Behind the withers the line of the back is more or less straight, and though it slopes up somewhat toward the croup, this is only occasionally so exaggerated that the horse can be said to be "croup-high." There is, however, a tendency for the back to sag in older animals, those in poor condition, and mares advanced in pregnancy. The cranial part of the back merges smoothly with the lateral chest and abdominal wall.

The caudal part (the loins) tends to be broader and flatter, and merges with the flanks without the sharp change in contour that is so striking in ruminants. The transverse processes of the lumbar vertebrae are not palpable. The spinous processes of the lumbar and caudal thoracic vertebrae may be palpated, though rarely so easily that they can be separately identified and counted. A median groove between the muscles of the loins and croup is most marked in draft animals.

The dorsal contour of the croup is convex and slopes toward the root of the tail, sometimes—commonly in the Lipizzaner and Belgian breeds—so steeply as to merit the description "goose rump."

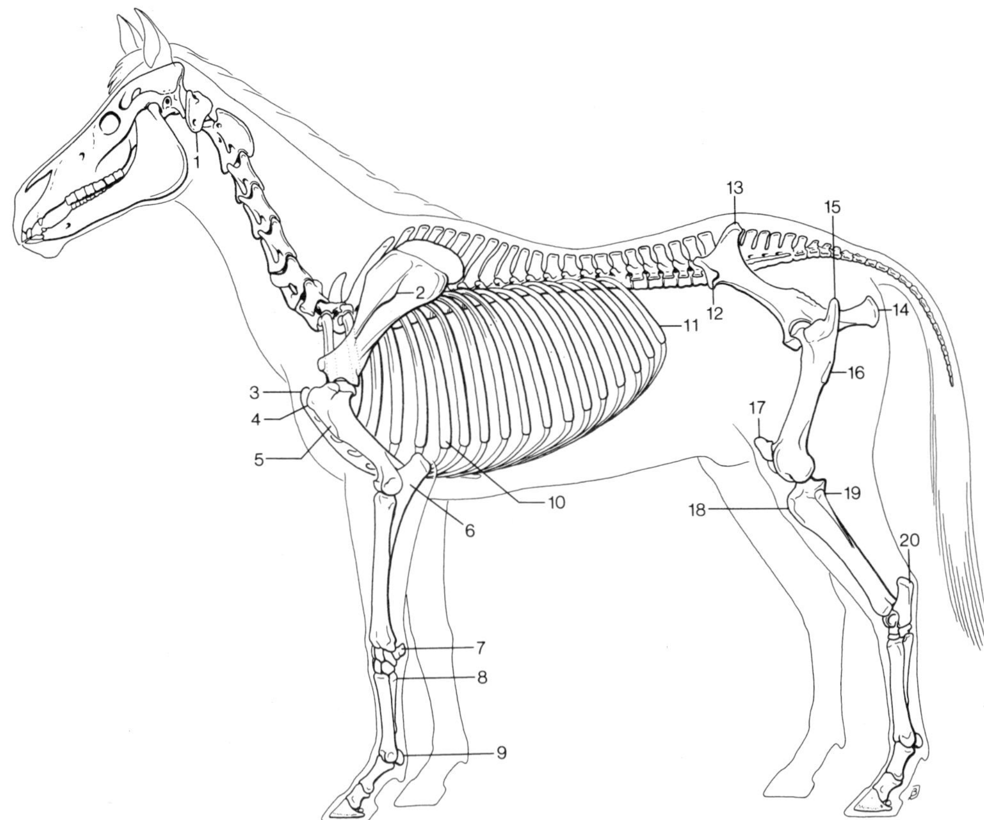


**Figure 19–1.** The equine skeleton. The features labeled are among those normally palpable.

1, Wing of atlas; 2, tuber of scapula; 3, manubrium; 4, greater tubercle; 5, deltoid tuberosity; 6, olecranon; 7, accessory carpal bone; 8, proximal end (base) of lateral splint bone; 9, proximal sesamoid bone; 10, rib 6; 11, last (18th) rib; 12, coxal tuber; 13, sacral tuber; 14, ischial tuber; 15, greater trochanter; 16, third trochanter; 17, patella; 18, tibial tuberosity; 19, head of fibula; 20, calcanean tuber.

## THE VERTEBRAL COLUMN

The vertebral column comprises 7 cervical, 18 thoracic, 6 lumbar, 5 sacral, and about 20 caudal vertebrae. Variations in number are not uncommon; the most frequent is the reduction of the lumbar vertebrae to five, especially in the Arab. The impression of shortness in the loins in other breeds is more often due to a marked caudal inclination of the last ribs.

The vertebral column inclines ventrally below the withers to reach its lowest point at the cervicothoracic junction, although the external elevation creates a contrary impression. It then changes direction abruptly and as it ascends toward the poll it shifts closer to the dorsal contour (Fig. 19–1).

The cervical vertebrae are individually long. Those behind the axis have rudimentary spinous processes, large divided transverse processes, and broad articular surfaces. The thoracic vertebrae are unremarkable apart from the great length of the spinous processes that form the basis of the withers. Independent centers of ossification develop for the summits of the first 12 or so spinous processes, and these may not fuse until comparatively late (10 or more years)—if at all. The lumbar vertebrae have long horizontal transverse processes; synovial joints sometimes develop between those of the fourth and fifth bones, and are constant between the fifth and sixth bones, and between the sixth and the wings of the sacrum. In saddle horses exostoses sometimes develop on the summits of the lumbar spinous processes, bringing these into painful contact with their neighbors ("kissing spines") and resulting in minor local deflections of the vertebral axis.

The *intervertebral discs* are relatively thin, collectively accounting for only 10% to 11% of the length of the vertebral column. Each consists of a peripheral anulus fibrosus and central nucleus pulposus, but the boundary between these parts is less distinct than in many species. Age changes

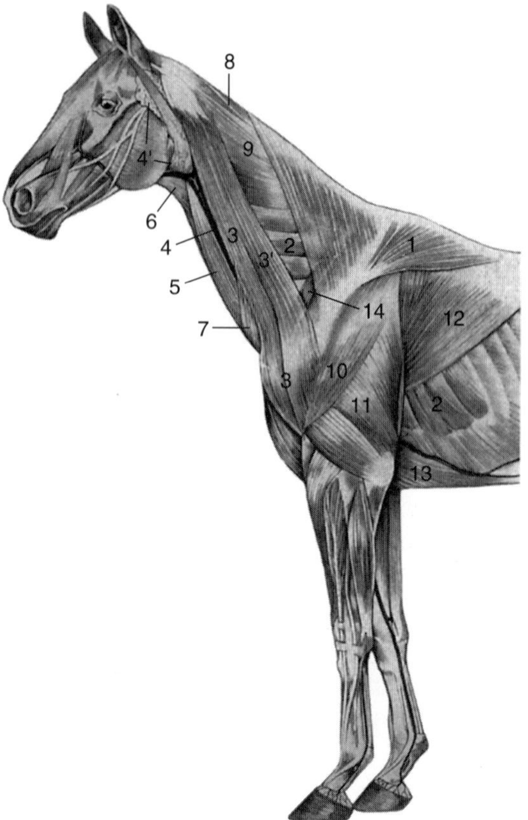


**Figure 19–2.** Superficial dissection of the neck and shoulder region.

1, Trapezius; 2, serratus ventralis; 3, brachiocephalicus; 3′, omotransversarius; 4, external jugular vein; 4′, parotid gland; 5, sternocephalicus; 6, omohyoideus; 7, cutaneus colli; 8, rhomboideus cervicis; 9, splenius; 10, deltoideus; 11, triceps; 12, latissimus dorsi; 13, pectoralis ascendens; 14, subclavius.

include dehydration and fragmentation of the outer fibrous part, but rarely calcification of the center. The discs most severely affected tend to be those of the neck and that between the last lumbar vertebra and the sacrum—regions where movement is greatest. Such changes do not appear to have much clinical importance.

The *nuchal ligament,* which divides the dorsal cervical muscles into right and left groups, is massively developed and supports much of the burden of the head without interfering with the ability to lower the neck when grazing (Fig. 19–3). It consists of two clearly defined parts, each paired. The dorsal (funicular) part is a thick cord extending between the highest spines of the withers and the external occipital protuberance of the skull. It is flattened at its cranial attachment, becomes rounded shortly behind this, and flattens again as it nears the withers, where it forms a broad flange extending almost to the scapular cartilage. It is continued behind the withers as the narrower supraspinous ligament. The second (laminar) part forms a fenestrated sheet closely applied to its fellow. It fills the space between the funicular part and the cervical vertebrae and consists of bundles of elastic fibers that run cranioventrally from the funicular part and the spines of T2 and T3 to attach to C2–C7. Synovial bursae are interposed between the funicular part and certain bony saliences to minimize pressure. One, the nuchal bursa, is constantly present above the dorsal arch of the atlas; a second is sometimes found above the spine of the axis; a third, the supraspinous bursa, is constantly present over the most prominent processes of the withers (Fig. 19–3/2,2′,2″). Infections of the first and third—leading to conditions known as "poll evil" and "fistulous withers," respectively—were formerly frequent and required extensive surgery for their eradication.

The complicated arrangement of the powerful epaxial muscles of the back and neck conforms, but only in a general way, to the account given in Chapter 2 (pp. 47–51). The many features of difference are fortunately not of clinical importance and illustration of their arrangement in transverse sections of the neck and back will suffice for a description (see Figs. 18–34 and 19–4). One specific feature of the associated deep fascia does, however, require notice. In the horse this thoracolumbar fascia possesses, opposite the scapula, an additional superficial lamina of importance. This, the *dorsoscapular ligament* (Fig. 19–3/5,5′), has an origin, in common with the deeper layers, from the supraspinous ligament over the highest spines of the withers. In its ventral passage it is applied to the deep surface of the rhomboideus and gradually transforms from a purely fibrous to a largely elastic nature. It detaches a number of side branches that insert upon the deep face of the scapula, alternating with divisions of the serratus ventralis muscle. The arrangement provides an elastic mechanism that helps absorb shock when the foot strikes the ground, limiting the dorsal shift of the scapula that would otherwise occur.

As always, the cervical part of the vertebral column is most mobile; the mouth may be brought around to reach the flank on full lateral flexion of the neck and ventrally to reach the pasture on ventral flexion. The latter movement is not always so easy for draft animals, which have relatively short necks; these animals may adopt a spreading posture of the forelimbs and lean forward when grazing. Only small movements are permitted to the back and loins except at the very mobile lumbosacral joint.

## THE VERTEBRAL CANAL

The relationships of the segments and cervical and lumbar swellings of the spinal cord to the vertebrae are shown in Figure 8–15. The first three sacral segments occur within the last lumbar vertebra, and the cord terminates within the cranial quarter of the sacrum of the adult (Fig. 19–5).

The meninges remain separate to a more caudal level than in other species, and there is still a substantial subarachnoid space at the lumbosacral level. A communication exists in this species between the lumbar part of the space and a local widening (ventriculus terminalis) of the central canal of the spinal cord.

Both lumbosacral and caudal sites of injection are commonly employed to obtain epidural anesthesia. The procedure at the former level utilizes the divergence of the spinous process of the last lumbar and sacral vertebrae for identification of the injection site (Fig. 19–5). Although the interarcuate space is quite large, its distance (8 to 10 cm) from the skin makes it relatively easy to miss. "Low" epidural anesthesia is performed between the first and second caudal vertebrae; the joint between these bones is very mobile, and the site for injection is readily discovered by "pumping" the tail up and down. The needle is inserted with a cranial inclination so that its point enters the canal within the first tail vertebra.

The vascularization of the spinal cord appears to be relevant to the etiology of a relatively frequent form of ataxia ("wobbles") that occurs in foals and young horses. This has its origin in congenital maldevelopment and subsequent exostoses of the

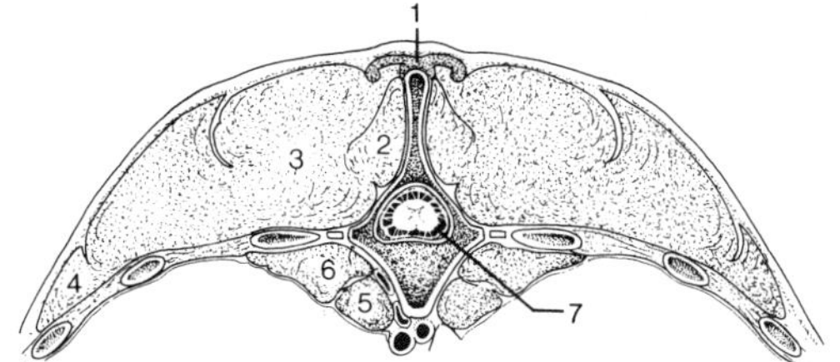


**Figure 19–4.** Transverse section of the back showing the principal muscle groups.

1, Supraspinous ligament; 2, transversospinalis group; 3, longissimus dorsi; 4, iliocostalis; 5, psoas minor; 6, psoas major; 7, vertebral canal and contents.

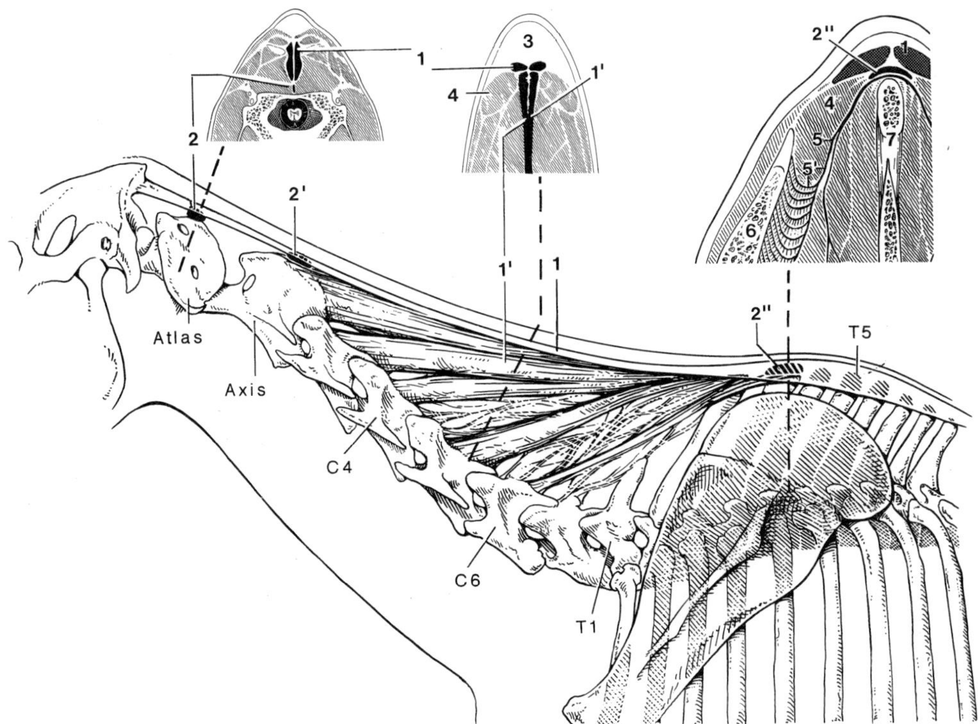


**Figure 19–3.** The nuchal ligament and associated bursae in lateral view and in three transverse sections.

1, 1′, Funicular and laminar parts of nuchal ligament; 2, 2′, 2″, cranial nuchal, caudal nuchal (inconstant), and supraspinous bursae; 3, fatty "crest" dorsal to nuchal ligament; 4, rhomboideus; 5, dorsoscapular ligament connecting spinous processes of the withers with the scapula; 5′, elastic part of 5; 6, scapula; 7, spinous processes.

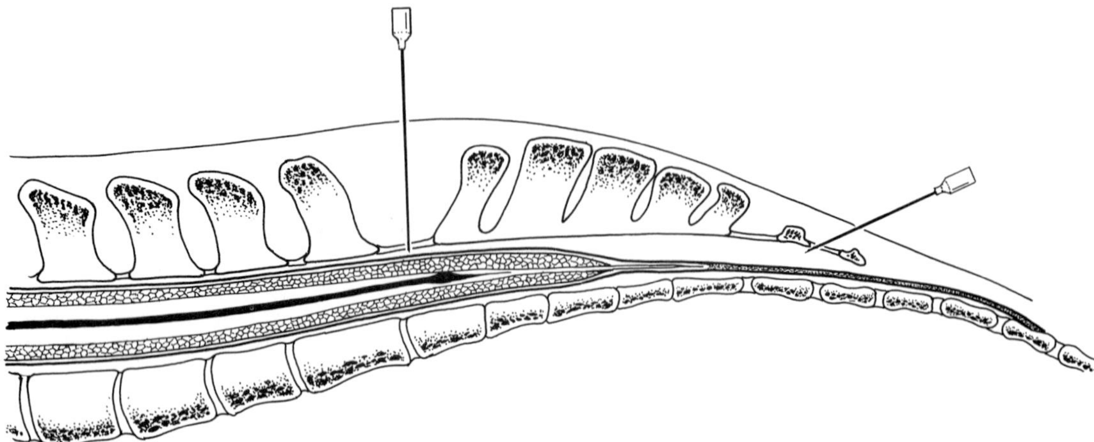

**Figure 19–5.** Median section of the equine vertebral canal and spinal cord. The lumbosacral interarcuate space and the space between the first and second caudal vertebrae are indicated by hypodermic needles placed at the common "high" and "low" sites for epidural anesthesia.

cervical articular processes that narrow the vertebral canal at the intervertebral levels. These exert pressure on the cord, although it is said that the cord lesions are secondary to interference with the venous drainage. In this context it should be known that the spinal arteries and veins are arranged in two sets, connected by relatively ineffectual anastomoses. One set enters the cord by way of the ventral fissure and supplies (and drains) the central gray substance and a thin surrounding shell of white. The second clambers over the lateral aspect to detach branches at intervals; these enter to supply (and drain) the bulk of the white matter (Fig. 19–6). It is the veins of the second set that are supposedly compressed, leading to venous congestion and subsequent degeneration of the nervous tissue. It is claimed that the condition may develop in the fetus.

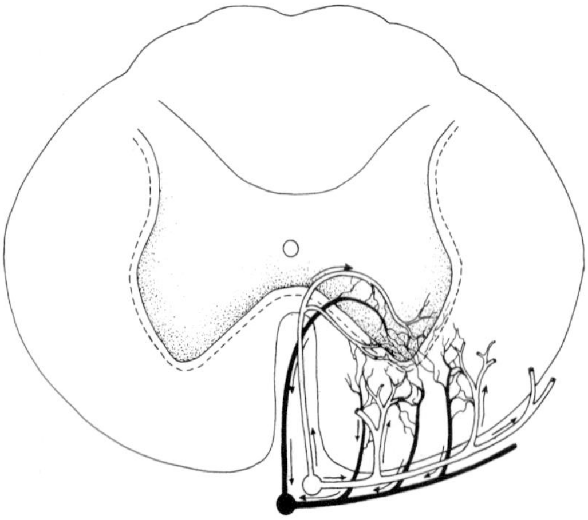

**Figure 19–6.** Blood circulation in the ventral part of the spinal cord, schematic. The blood supply to the gray substance, and to the adjacent layer of the white, is more or less independent of that to most of the white substance.

## Selected Bibliography


Boyd, J.S.: Selection of sites for intramuscular injection in the neck of the horse. Vet. Rec. 121:197–200, 1987.

Cohen, N.D., W.C. McMullan, and G.K. Carter: Fistulous withers: The diagnosis and treatment of open and closed lesions. Vet. Med. 86:416–426, 1991.

Cohen, N.D., G.K. Carter, and W.C. McMullan: Fistulous withers in horses: 24 cases (1984–1990). JAVMA 201:121–124, 1992.

Dalin, G., and L.B. Jeffcott: Sacroiliac joint of the horse 1. Gross morphology. Anat. Histol. Embryol. 15:80–94, 1986.

Denoix, J.M.: Ultrasonography evaluation of back lesions. Vet. Clin. North Am. Equine Pract. 15:131–159, 1999.

Dik, K.J., and I. Gunsser: Atlas of Diagnostic Radiology of the Horse. Parts 1–3. Philadelphia, W.B. Saunders Company, 1988–1990.

Garrett, P.D.: Anatomy of the dorsoscapular ligament. JAVMA 196:446–448, 1990.

Gaughan, E.M., L. Fubini, and A. Dietze: Fistulous withers in horses: 14 cases (1978–1987). JAVMA 193:964–966, 1988.

Haussler, K.K.: Anatomy of the thoracolumbar vertebral region. Vet. Clin. North Am. Equine Pract. 15:13–26, 1999.

Haussler, K.K., and S.M. Stover: Stress fractures of the vertebral lamina and pelvis in Thoroughbred racehorses. Equine Vet. J. 30:374–381, 1998.

Haussler, K.K., S.M. Stover, and N.H. Willits: Developmental variation in lumbosacropelvic anatomy of Thoroughbred racehorses. Am. J. Vet. Res. 58:1083–1091, 1997.

Haussler, K.K., S.M. Stover, and N.H. Willits: Pathologic changes in the lumbosacral vertebrae and pelvis in Thoroughbred racehorses. Am. J. Vet. Res. 60:143–153, 1999.

Heath, E.H., and V.S. Myers: Topographic anatomy for caudal anesthesia in the horse. Vet. Med. 67:1237–1239, 1972.

Jeffcott, L.B., and G. Dalin: Natural rigidity of the horse's backbone. Equine Vet. J. 12:101–108, 1980.

Jeffcott, L.B., and G. Dalin: Bibliography of thoracolumbar conditions in the horse. Equine Vet. J. 15:155–157, 1983.

LeBlanc, P.H., J.P. Caron, J.S. Patterson, et al.: Epidural injection of xylazine for perineal analgesia in horses. JAVMA 193:1405–1408, 1988.

Martin, B.B., and A.M. Klide: Physical examination of horses with back pain. Vet. Clin. North Am. Equine Pract. 15:61–70, 1999.

Moon, P.F., and C.M. Suter. Paravertebral thora columbar anaesthesia in 10 horses. Equine Vet. J. 25:304–308, 1993.

Rendano, V.T., and C.B. Quick: Equine radiology—the cervical spine. Med. Vet. Pract. 59:921–927, 1978.

Schebitz, H., and H. Wilkens: Atlas of Radiographic Anatomy of the Horse, 4th ed. Berlin, Paul Parey Verlag, 1986.

Skarda, R.T., and W.W. Muir III: Caudal analgesia induced by epidural or subarachnoid administration of detomidine hydrochloride solution in mares. Am. J. Vet. Res. 55:670–680, 1994.

Stecher, R.M.: Anatomical variations of the spine in the horse. J. Mammal. 43:205–208, 1962.

Townsend, H.G.G., and D.H. Leach: Relationship between intervertebral joint morphology and mobility of the equine thoracolumbar spine. Equine Vet. J. 16:461–465, 1984.

# CHAPTER 20

# The Thorax of the Horse

## CONFORMATION AND SURFACE ANATOMY

In the horse the difficulties in obtaining a reliable impression of the thoracic cavity from simple inspection of the exterior are increased by the height of the withers and the caudal prolongation of the rib cage. The narrow cranial part of the thorax is completely covered by the shoulder and arm. Some variation in the projection of the limb bones on the thoracic skeleton is due to the inconstant slope of the scapula. As a general guide, the caudal angle of this bone lies over the upper end of the seventh rib, while the supraglenoid tubercle projects in front of the first rib, a little above the manubrium of the sternum (Figs. 20–1 and 20–2). The humerus forms a lesser angle with the horizontal than in the smaller species and this brings the elbow within the skin of the trunk. The precise position of the elbow joint is not immediately apparent but may be inferred from its relation to the olecranon whose summit (point of elbow) lies over the lowest part of the fifth rib or succeeding intercostal space. The triangle between the scapula and humerus is completely occupied by the massive triceps muscle, which severely restricts clinical access to the cranial part of the thorax.

There are 18 pairs of ribs. Those behind the triceps, that is, those from the seventh rib caudally, are individually identifiable on palpation even though covered in varying degree by certain muscles: cutaneous trunci, latissimus dorsi, serratus ventralis, and obliquus externus abdominis. The most caudal ribs may even provide visible landmarks; this is most often true of the upper part of the last rib, which prominently marks the cranial limit of the flank. Palpation of the ribs reveals their changing orientation. The last two or three, which are relatively short, have a pronounced caudal inclination; the half-dozen or so (R9–15) in front of these are longer and of equal length and curvature; the more cranial ribs are both shorter and less strongly curved. The first rib, the shortest of all, is almost vertical. The increasing slope of the ribs as the series is followed caudally brings the last rib remarkably close to the coxal tuber (see Fig. 19–1).

Between the forelimbs the thorax is covered by the powerful pectoral muscles that form paired swellings separated by a prominent groove along the line of the sternum (see Fig. 23–4). The cranial part of this bone—the manubrium—projects as a readily found landmark. The caudal xiphoid process is also palpable, though not quite so easily; it is broad and flexible and is enclosed between the converging costal arches. External inspection fails to suggest the tilt of the sternum, which slopes upward toward the manubrium; this, in combination with the ventral slope of the cranial thoracic vertebrae, reduces the depth of the cranial part of the thoracic cavity.

An exact appreciation of the position of the diaphragm is essential for the clinician. The vertex is level with the sixth intercostal space (or even the sixth rib) and thus comes to within a short distance of the point of the elbow in an animal standing square (Fig. 20–3). The inexperienced find it particularly hard to accept this crucial fact.

There are naturally considerable breed and individual variations in conformation. Without considering these in detail it may be said that a deep chest is generally favored. In saddle horses it is desirable that the ribs slope caudally without excessive lateral bowing since too pronounced a "barrel" makes for an uncomfortable seat.

## THE THORACIC WALL

Removal of the forelimbs exposes the contrasting form of the cranial and caudal parts of the thorax. The cranial part (formed by the sternal ribs) is narrow and bilaterally compressed and shows little movement; the caudal part (formed by the asternal ribs) is conspicuously wider and more rounded, and makes a substantial contribution to the respiratory excursions (Fig. 20–9). In comparison with the bovine chest, the ribs are narrow and the intercostal spaces conspicuously wide, especially in their ventral parts. The arrangement of the structures within the spaces follows the usual pattern.

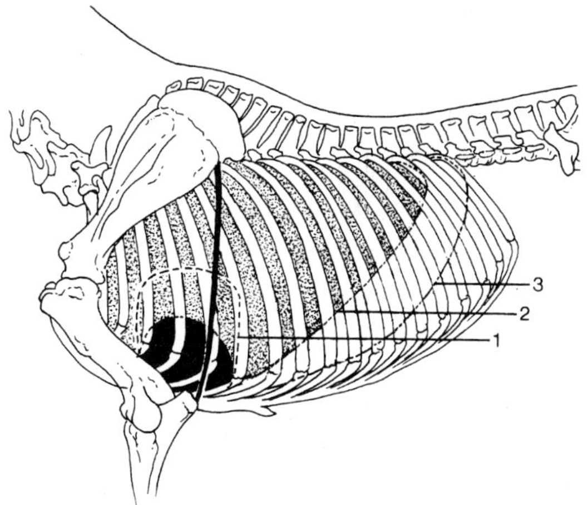


**Figure 20–1.** Projections of the heart and lung on the left thoracic wall. The heavy line indicates the caudal border of the triceps.

1, Outline of heart; 2, basal border of lung; 3, line of pleural reflection.

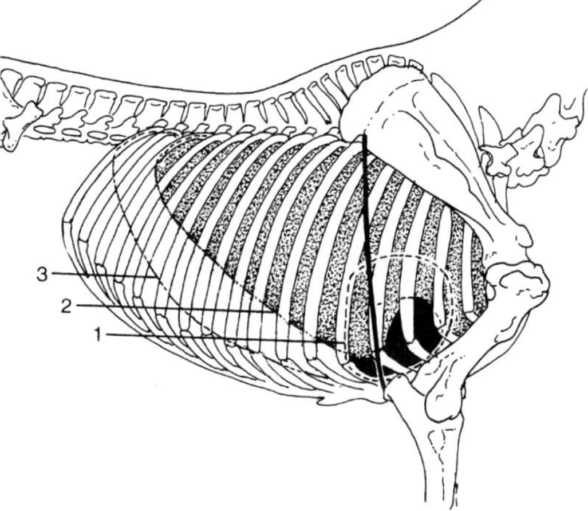


**Figure 20–2.** Projections of the heart and lung on the right thoracic wall. The heavy line indicates the caudal border of the triceps.

1, Outline of heart; 2, basal border of lung; 3, line of pleural reflection.

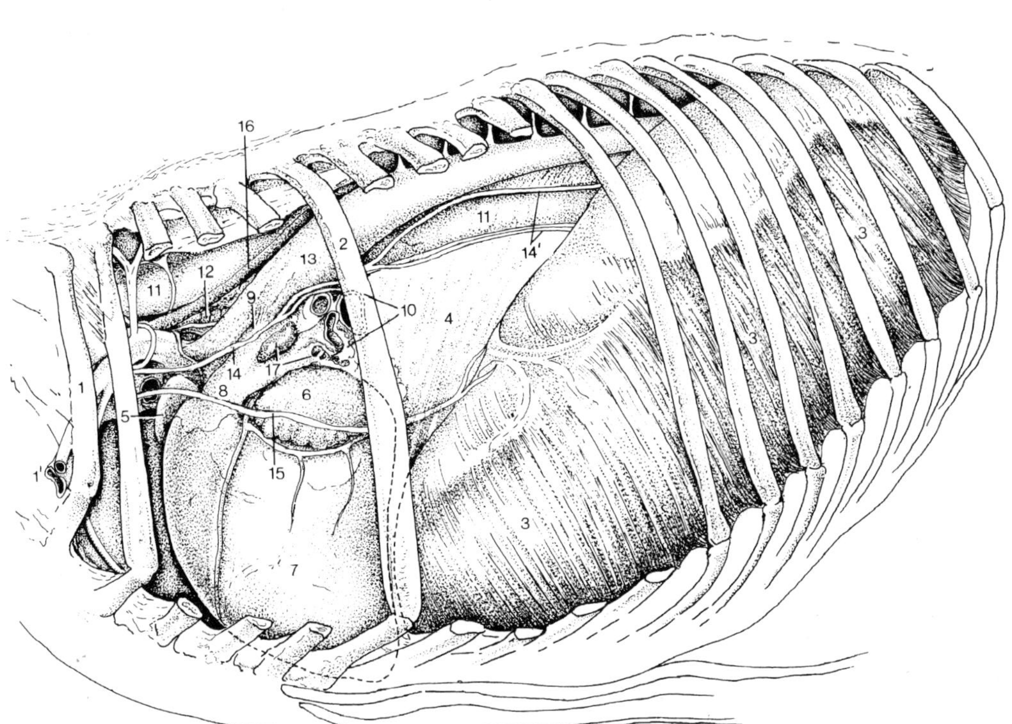


**Figure 20–3.** Structures within the mediastinum. The mediastinal pleura cranial to the heart has been removed, exposing the cranial lobe of the right lung.

1, First rib; 1′, axillary vessels; 2, sixth rib; 3, diaphragm; 4, caudal mediastinum covering right lung; 5, right auricle; 6, left auricle; 7, left ventricle; 8, pulmonary trunk; 9, ligamentum arteriosum; 10, root of lung; 11, esophagus; 12, trachea; 13, aorta; 14, vagus; 14′, dorsal and ventral vagal trunks; 15, phrenic nerve; 16, thoracic duct; 17, tracheobronchial lymph nodes.

The short, stout first rib is almost immobile, as it is stabilized by tight joints with the vertebral column and sternum, and by anchorage to the cervical vertebrae through the scalenus. The brachial plexus divides this muscle into ventral and (small) middle parts, while the axillary vessels emerge ventral to it. These vessels wind around the cranial margin of the first rib where the artery may be palpated against the bone. It is punctured at this site when a sample of arterial blood is required (Fig. 20–3/1′).

In conformity with the length of the thorax the diaphragm is more oblique than in other domestic species. It has the same general form and bulges forward from its peripheral attachments to the lumbar vertebrae, ribs, and sternum. Its most cranial part, the vertex, is situated directly above the sternum and, as already emphasized, projects upon the lower part of the sixth space or preceding rib. The dorsal part of the diaphragm is molded to present right and left elevations between which the median portion is retracted by the crura to form a recess. The middle and ventral parts are uniformly curved from side to side. The openings within the diaphragm show no important specific features (Fig. 20–4).

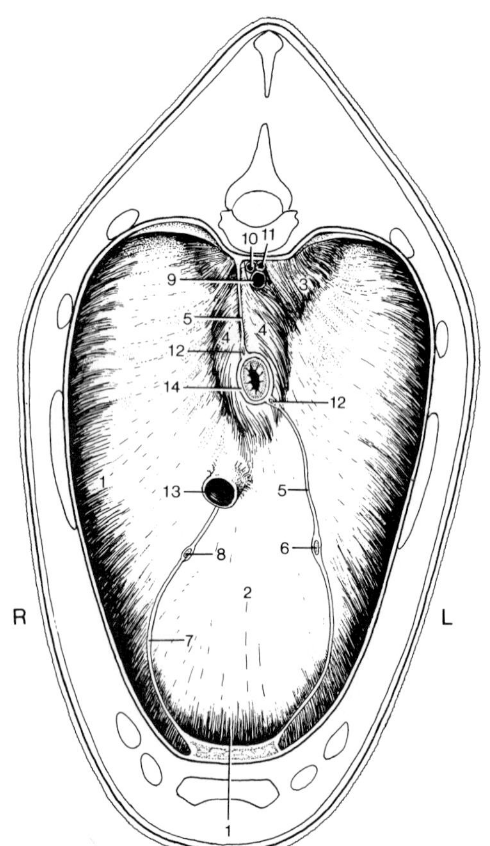


**Figure 20–4.** Cranial surface of the diaphragm.

1, Sternal and costal parts of diaphragm; 2, tendinous center; 3, left crus; 4, right crus; 5, caudal mediastinum; 6, left phrenic nerve; 7, plica venae cavae; 8, right phrenic nerve; 9, aorta; 10, right azygous vein; 11, thoracic duct; 12, dorsal and ventral vagal trunks; 13, caudal vena cava; 14, esophagus.

## THE PLEURAL CAVITIES

The arrangement of the pleura follows the usual pattern with the thoracic interior divided into two pleural cavities by an intermediate septum, the mediastinum. The subpleural connective tissue is poorly developed and in consequence of this the mediastinum is weak.

The projection of the pleural cavities upon the chest wall is always a matter of clinical significance. The mediastinal pleura is reflected onto the thoracic wall within the costovertebral gutter, and the costal pleura thus extends above the ventral border of the vertebral bodies; the ventral limit of the costal pleura follows an irregular line that passes over the costal cartilages. Cranially, the pleural sac extends medial to the first rib, and beyond this on the right side where an outpouching (cupula pleurae) passes several centimeters into the neck; this prolongation of the right sac is of potential importance since it may be punctured by penetrating wounds that appear to spare the thorax. The caudal reflection of the costal pleura onto the diaphragm has an unusual line. It begins at the vertebral end of the 17th rib and is then deflected caudally to reach the middle of the last rib before turning forward. It then follows a more conventional course that intersects successive ribs at progressively lower levels until it continues along the eighth rib cartilage to the sternum. This line traces a slight dorsocranial concavity (Figs. 20–1 and 20–2/3).

As always, the pleural cavities are considerably larger than the lungs even when there is maximal inflation. There thus exist potential spaces along the ventral and caudal margins of the lung that are never utilized. The breadth of these spaces (the costomediastinal and costodiaphragmatic recesses) varies with the phase of respiration. The costodiaphragmatic recess lies over the intrathoracic part of the abdomen and provides a potential route for the puncture of certain abdominal organs. Obviously the risk of injury to the lung is minimized if the needle is introduced during full expiration (Fig. 20–9/13′).

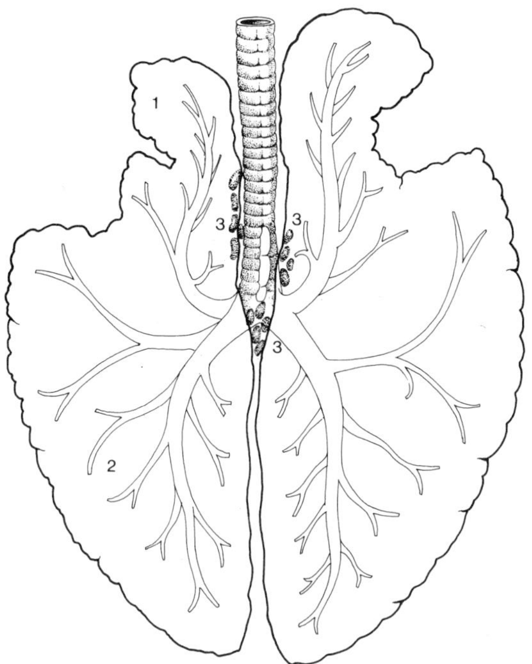


**Figure 20–5.** Dorsal view of the lungs and bronchial tree, schematic.

1, Apex (cranial lobe) of left lung; 2, base (caudal lobe) of left lung; 3, tracheobronchial lymph nodes.

# THE LUNGS

The lungs are elongated and shallow, corresponding to the general form of the pleural cavities. The right and left lungs are more nearly equal in size than in other species (Fig. 20–5) and, since the difference lies mainly in the greater thickness of the right lung, the asymmetry that does exist may easily escape notice (Figs. 20–6, 20–7, and 20–8). There is no external evidence of lobation other than the presence of the accessory lobe appended to the base of the right lung. However, the cranial part of each lung is somewhat separated from the caudal mass by a relatively attenuated region (see Figs. 4–23 and 20–1). The two lungs are extensively joined by connective tissue caudal to the bifurcation of the trachea.

The left lung exhibits a deep cardiac notch that allows the pericardium extensive contact with the chest wall between the third and sixth ribs (Fig. 20–1). The notch is margined by a thinned region so that the lung provides little cover to the pericardium over a much larger area (Fig. 20–7). The arrangement on the right side is similar, although the asymmetry of the heart reduces the size of the cardiac notch, which extends from the third rib to the fourth intercostal space (Fig. 20–2). When moderately expanded, the base of each lung reaches to a line passing through the upper part of the 16th, the middle of the 11th, and the costochondral junction of the sixth rib; the upper part of this line is almost vertical, the lower part sweeps cranioventrally. This margin of the lung is separated from the line of pleural reflection by about 5 cm dorsally and ventrally but by as much as 15 cm in its middle part (Figs. 20–1 and 20–2). In young foals the extent of the lung is more restricted and the caudal limit is at about the 13th rib.

The projection of the lung on the chest wall is considerably larger than the clinically useful area for percussion and auscultation since examination of the thin margins of the lung will not provide useful information. The area for such examination is triangular and is defined by the caudal angle of the scapula, the point of the elbow, and the upper end of the 16th rib. Two sides of this triangle are

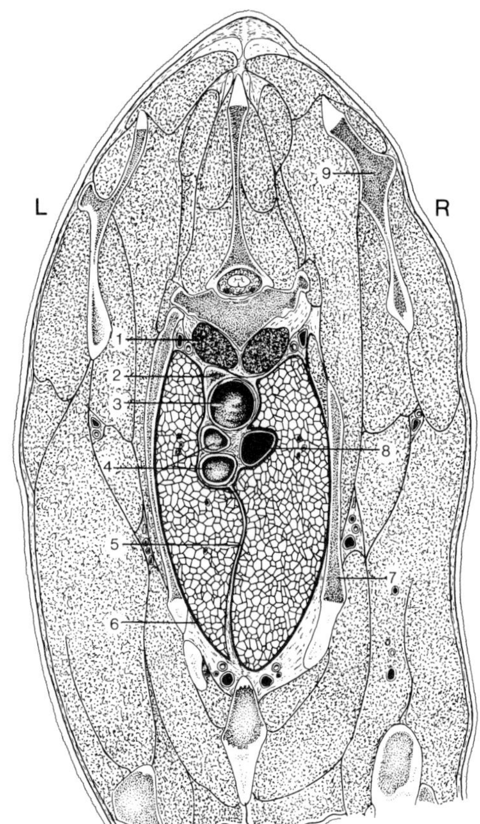


**Figure 20–6.** Transverse section of the thorax at the level of T2.

1, Longus colli; 2, esophagus; 3, trachea; 4, brachiocephalic trunk and left subclavian artery; 5, cranial mediastinum; 6, left pleural cavity; 7, second rib; 8, cranial vena cava; 9, scapula.

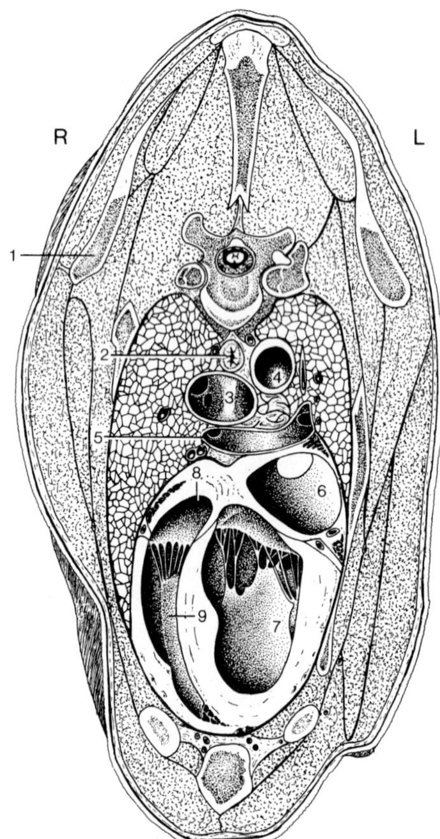


**Figure 20–7.** Transverse section of the thorax at the level of T5.

1, Caudal angle of scapula; 2, esophagus; 3, bifurcation of the trachea; 4, aorta; 5, bifurcation of the pulmonary trunk; 6, left atrium; 7, left ventricle; 8, right atrium; 9, right ventricle.

more or less straight but the caudoventral side—the hypotenuse—is slightly bowed.

Tapping of pleural fluid is most safely performed in the lower part of the seventh intercostal space, ventral to the margin of the lung. Care is required to avoid puncturing the superficial thoracic ("spur") vein that crosses the site (see Fig. 23–3/11″).

The lobulation of the lungs is not obtrusive but can be detected on careful examination of the expanded lung. It is less obvious in the collapsed state when the covering pleura is wrinkled. It is also evident on section. However, it is accepted that the septa are incomplete and that the possibility of collateral ventilation between neighboring lobules exists.

The chief bronchus, the pulmonary artery, and the pulmonary vein combine to form the root of the lung before entering at the hilus in a region deprived of pleura and directly adherent to the same part of the other lung. The chief bronchus divides within the lung into a small cranial division that passes toward the cranial lobe, and a larger caudal division that attends to the ventilation of the remainder of the organ. There are difficulties in homologizing the bronchi of lower orders with those in other domestic species but at the present time these details are not of great importance; lung surgery is rarely performed in horses.

In standing animals the ventilation and perfusion of different regions and lobes of the lungs are reasonably well matched, although in larger species, such as the horse, there must be some tendency for gravity to favor the perfusion of more ventral parts. The spatial relationship of ventilation and perfusion is disturbed in animals placed in dorsal or lateral recumbency, and the disturbance becomes significant when the recumbent posture is long maintained—as during major surgery. In these circumstances there is compression of whichever part of the lung is at the bottom. This reduces the tensile forces that ordinarily hold airways open in that part of the lung. The ensuing airway closure

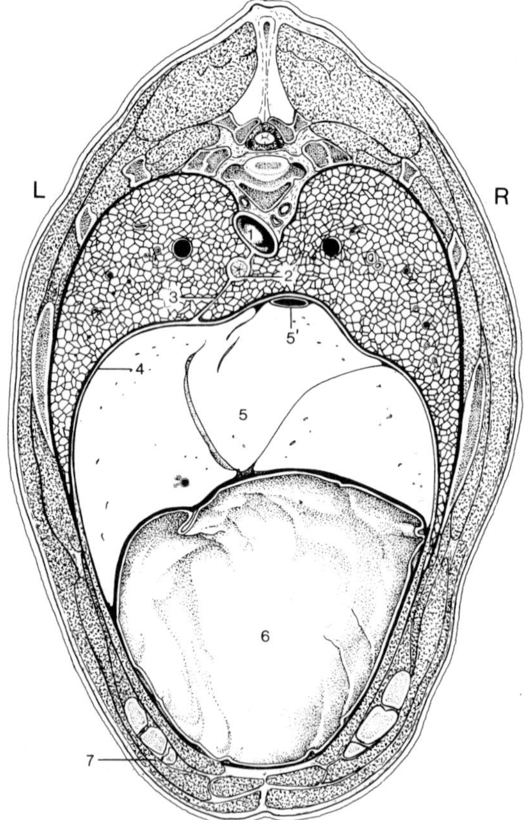


**Figure 20–8.** Transverse section of the trunk at the level of T12 and the middle of the ninth rib.

1, Aorta; 2, esophagus; 3, caudal mediastinum; 4, diaphragm; 5, liver; 5′, caudal vena cava; 6, diaphragmatic flexure of the ascending colon; 7, costal arch.

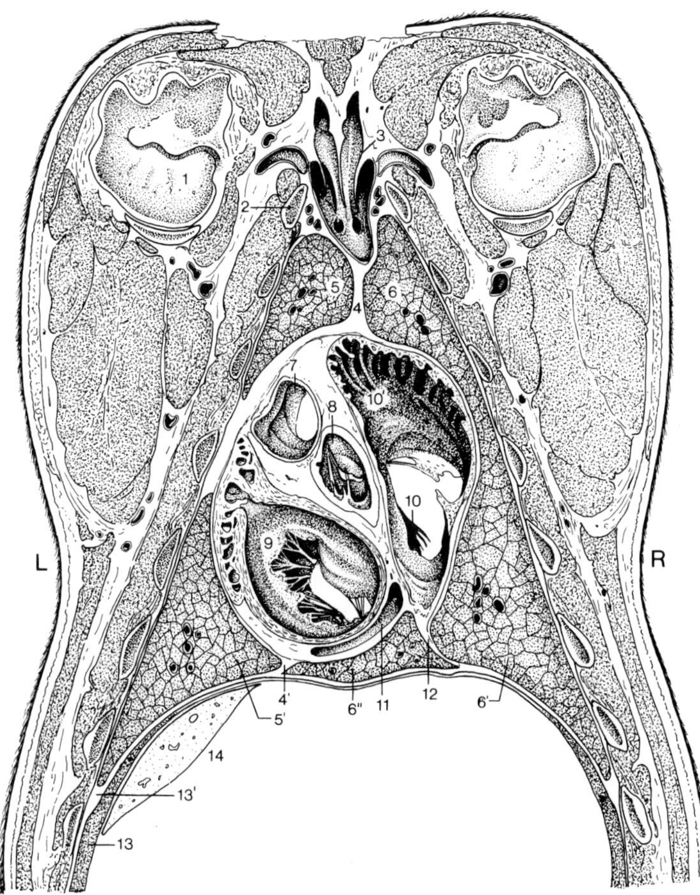


**Figure 20–9.** Dorsal section of the thorax at the level of the atrioventricular valves.

1, Head of humerus; 2, first rib; 3, formation of cranial vena cava; 4, 4′, cranial and caudal mediastinum; 5, 5′, cranial and caudal lobes of the left lung; 6, 6′, 6″, cranial, caudal, and accessory lobes of the right lung; 7, pulmonary valve; 8, aortic valve; 9, left atrioventricular valve; 10, right atrioventricular valve; 10′, right auricle; 11, coronary sinus; 12, plica venae cavae; 13, diaphragm; 13′, costodiaphragmatic recess; 14, part of the liver.

permits complete collapse of the alveoli served by such airways; blood perfusing these alveoli cannot take part in respiratory gas exchange.

The pattern of division of the pulmonary artery corresponds to that of the bronchi. A separate bronchial artery attends to the supply of the bronchial and peribronchial tissue, but the blood is returned by the single set of pulmonary veins.*

*The hemorrhage from the pulmonary vasculature that is induced by severe exercise is a major concern of the horseracing industry. Though the existence of the condition is rarely made evident by loss of blood externally, or by abnormal distress during or immediately after a race, tracheobronchial endoscopy at the latter time reveals some loss of blood from the lungs of most (some would say all) Thoroughbreds subjected to the extreme demands of racing. There is some dispute concerning the origin of the blood leakage—whether it is from branches of the bronchial or the pulmonary arteries, and whether it results from preexisting structural abnormality of the vessel wall. The condition impairs performance, worsens progressively, and is responsible for the premature retirement from racing of many horses. It is not known to occur in horses exposed to more moderate stress, although similar exercise-induced hemorrhage is recognized in racing Greyhounds, camels, and some elite human athletes.

The lymphatic drainage leads first through very small pulmonary nodes embedded in the substance of the organ and then to larger tracheobronchial nodes about the bifurcation of the trachea (Fig. 20–3/17). From here most lymph is drained via the cranial mediastinal nodes.

The nerves that enter at the hilus derive from the pulmonary plexus to which both sympathetic and parasympathetic fibers contribute (pp. 319 and 321).

## THE MEDIASTINUM

The heart divides the mediastinum into the familiar parts (Fig. 20–9/4,4′).

The cranial part is markedly asymmetrical; it attaches to the left first rib and gradually shifts to reach a more or less median situation directly in front of the heart. The dorsal part is thick, the ventral part much thinner, especially after the thymus has regressed. The dorsal part occupies about half the transverse diameter of the thorax and includes the esophagus and trachea, the brachiocephalic trunk and cranial vena cava with their respective branches and tributaries, the cranial mediastinal lymph nodes, the thoracic duct, and the phrenic, vagus, and sympathetic nerves (Fig. 20–6). The interstices between these structures are occupied by fat, sometimes present in large amounts. The thymus is the sole content of the ventral portion.

The ventral part of the middle mediastinum is very broad since it contains the heart and pericardium (Fig. 20–7). The dorsal part is paper-thin except where it contains the esophagus, the continuation of the trachea to its bifurcation, the aorta, and certain nerves that include branches of the vagi.

In lateral view the caudal mediastinum is triangular (Fig. 20–3/4). It is divided into two parts by adhesion between the lungs about and caudal to their roots. The ventral part, whose sole occupant is the left phrenic nerve, is diverted far to the left before it merges with the pleura covering the diaphragm (Fig. 20–4/5). The dorsal part is thin except where it encloses the esophagus and aorta.

Except in foals, small openings in the mediastinum place the two pleural cavities in communication. Apart from these fenestrations, the mediastinum is very fragile, and exposure during dissection inevitably increases the number of the openings; this happens so readily that most believe that the fenestrations exist when the thorax is intact. From this, the mediastinum would appear to be an ineffectual partition. However, small openings in the thoracic wall such as are made for the purpose of endoscopy (when the influx of air can be controlled) result in incomplete unilateral pneumothorax and are survived without obvious adverse effect.

## THE HEART

The heart lies in the ventral part of the middle mediastinum, directly cranial to the diaphragm and largely covered by the forelimbs (Fig. 20–1). It forms an irregular and laterally compressed cone, with the larger part lying left of the median plane, and is so disposed that the axis slopes caudoventrally and to the left (Fig. 20–3). There is significant variation in heart size, with that of a Thoroughbred conspicuously larger than that of a draft animal. The difference is partly inherited, partly conditioned by training. Such variation inevitably affects the topography. Most commonly the heart extends between the planes of the second to sixth intercostal spaces, which places the apex directly caudal to the level of the point of the elbow. The cranial margin is strongly curved and is arranged with its upper part vertical, while its lower part follows the dorsal surface of the sternum. The caudal border, though sinuous in profile, is more or less upright (Fig. 20–3). The flattened lateral surfaces are related through the pericardium to the mediastinal surfaces of the lungs except where the cardiac notches allow direct contact with the thoracic wall; as already stated, this contact is greater on the left side. A strong sternopericardiac ligament attaches the pericardium to the sternum and this, with the anchorage of the great vessels, limits the displacement allowed to the heart. A slight shift, however, does occur with the movement of the diaphragm.

Apart from the general form there is little of significance to distinguish the heart of the horse. Mention should be made, however, of two features of the aortic and pulmonary valves, the former especially. The cusps commonly develop nodules at the free margins, and these can be quite striking in older animals; in addition, fenestrations often appear in the middle region of the cusps. Neither development appears to have much, if any, functional significance. The puncta maxima, the sites at which the valve sounds are most clearly heard, do not correspond exactly to the projections of the openings on the chest wall. The left atrioventricular valve is auscultated to most advantage in the fifth intercostal space, a little caudodorsal to the point of the elbow; the aortic valve at a somewhat higher level in the fourth space; and the pulmonary valve lower within the third space—all, of course, on the left side. The right atrioventricular valve is best heard in the lower parts of the third and fourth right intercostal spaces. These directions are perhaps overprecise since the skeletal topography is not always easy to appreciate in practice. It is perhaps more useful to be aware that the puncta lie within a band of a few centimeters' depth about midway between the horizontal planes that intersect the points of the shoulder and of the elbow. Within this band the punctum maximum of the left atrioventricular valve is at the intersection of the vertical line that falls a couple of fingerbreadths behind the point of the elbow. The approach to the other valves follows from the relative positions indicated and requires the introduction of the stethoscope between the limb and the chest wall.

The coronary arteries share the supply of the heart wall in more equal fashion than in many other species since the right one ends by descending within the right (subsinuosal) interventricular groove (see Fig. 7–17/*B*).

## THE ESOPHAGUS, TRACHEA, AND THYMUS

Although the *esophagus* still lies partly to the left on entering the chest, it quickly regains a position dorsal to the trachea and thereafter it pursues a median course apart from slight deflections as it passes the aortic arch and again just before the esophageal hiatus. The striated muscle of the cranial part of the esophagus is gradually replaced by smooth muscle as the heart is approached; the color change makes the transformation obvious. The muscle is somewhat thicker immediately before the diaphragm, and this part of the tube is commonly contracted in the dead specimen. There is no evidence that the diaphragm embraces the esophagus tightly at the hiatus as sometimes alleged. Indeed, the free movement of the diaphragm over the esophagus is facilitated by the peritoneum pouching through the hiatus on the right and ventral side of the esophagus.

The *trachea* is median soon after entering the thorax. It then lies against the longus colli muscles but soon diverges to run lower within the mediastinum. After passing over the left atrium, it bifurcates at about the level of the fifth rib (or space) (Figs. 20–6/3 and 20–7/3). The bifurcation is not symmetrical; the right bronchus is larger.

The *thymus* is prominent in early life but soon regresses. Its formation from right and left parts is not obvious since they are closely applied together. In the young foal it completely fills the ventral part of the mediastinum cranial to the heart and may even extend over the left side of the pericardium; part may also pass into the neck beside the trachea, very occasionally reaching the thyroid gland. At this stage the thymus is clearly lobulated and bright pink. It is largest about 2 months after birth and thereafter regresses, though the rate is variable. Usually little remains after 3 years when the vestige consists largely of fatty fibrous tissue. At its apogee the thymus makes contact with most structures within the cranial mediastinum.

## THE GREAT VESSELS AND NERVES WITHIN THE THORAX

The pattern of arterial branching is shown in Figure 7–35 and need not be further described since the details are altogether without clinical significance. Rupture of the aortic wall in the sinus region, or at the origin of the brachiocephalic trunk, is not too uncommon in conditions of stress; the resulting hemorrhage is rapidly fatal. It appears to indicate inherent weakness at these sites since pathological change is rarely evident.

The presence of a single right azygous vein may be used to distinguish the equine from the bovine heart.

The formations, the courses, and the ramifications of the phrenic, sympathetic, and vagus nerves conform to the usual patterns; certain details, none of great practical importance, are illustrated in

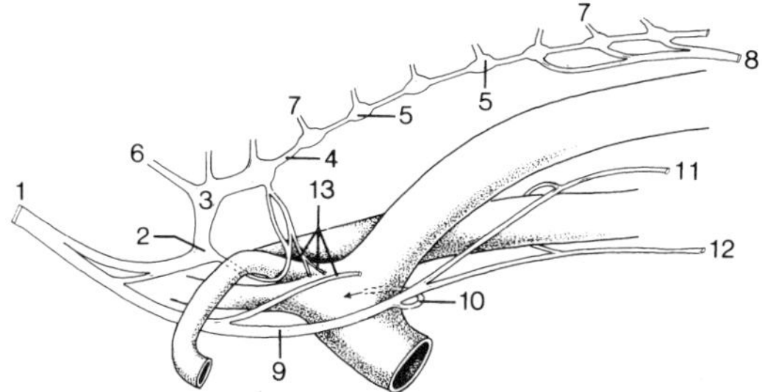


**Figure 20–10.** Distribution of the sympathetic and vagus nerves on the left side of the thorax, schematic.

1, Vagosympathetic trunk; 2, middle cervical ganglion; 3, cervicothoracic ganglion; 4, sympathetic trunk; 5, sympathetic ganglia; 6, vertebral nerve; 7, communicating branches; 8, major splanchnic nerve; 9, left vagus; 10, recurrent laryngeal nerve; 11, dorsal vagal trunk; 12, ventral vagal trunk; 13, cardiac nerves.

Figure 20–10. The relationship of the *left recurrent laryngeal nerve* to the aortic arch, though not specific to the horse, deserves emphasis since intermittent stretching of the nerve with the pulsation of the vessel has been postulated as a factor in the etiology of laryngeal hemiplegia (roaring). The closer association of the left nerve to the tracheobronchial lymph nodes is a second factor of alleged but unproven significance (p. 502).

## THE LYMPHATIC STRUCTURES OF THE THORAX

There are very numerous lymph nodes within the thorax. Though most are collected in groups, these are sometimes less discrete than is suggested, and the provenance of the more scattered nodes may be difficult to determine. The following are the principal groups.

Small *intercostal nodes* lie in the dorsal part of some intercostal spaces. They receive lymph from the vertebrae and the adjacent muscles, the dorsal part of the diaphragm, and the local costal and mediastinal pleura. The efferent flow is to the thoracic duct.

The *cranial mediastinal nodes* are numerous and scattered about the esophagus, trachea, and vessels at the entrance to the thorax; usually some form a discontinuous chain that joins the caudal deep cervical nodes within the neck. The most caudal members reach the pericardium, where they overlap the nodes about the tracheal bifurcation that are assigned to the tracheobronchial and caudal mediastinal groups. Most efferent vessels pass to the thoracic duct; those from the most cranial nodes in the series may first perfuse deep cervical nodes.

The *tracheobronchial group* is scattered about the caudal part of the trachea and the chief bronchi (Fig. 20–3/17); left, middle, and right subdivisions are commonly distinguished. Small nodes within the peribronchial tissue of the lung may be regarded as members of this series. Most lymph passing through this group has origin within the lungs but some comes from the pericardium, the heart, and the caudal mediastinal nodes. The efferent vessels are divided between those that go directly to the thoracic duct and those that first perfuse the cranial mediastinal nodes.

A number of small *caudal mediastinal nodes* lie directly in front of the diaphragm and between the esophagus and aorta. Lymph is received from the esophagus, the diaphragm, the liver, the mediastinal and diaphragmatic pleura, and, apparently, the lungs. The efferent lymph flow is divided between the thoracic duct and the tracheobronchial and cranial mediastinal lymph nodes.

The few ventral mediastinal lymph nodes are without significance.

The thoracic duct exhibits no important distinctive features. It drains into one or another of the large veins at the entrance to the thorax, most commonly the cranial vena cava.

## Selected Bibliography


Beech, J: Evaluation of the horse with pulmonary disease. Vet. Clin. North Am. Large Anim. Pract. 1:43–58, 1979.

Cobb, M.A., W.A. Schutt, Jr., and J.W. Hermanson: Morphological, histochemical, and myosin isoform analysis of the diaphragm of adult horses, *Equus caballus*. Anat. Rec. 238:317–325, 1994.

Cobb, M.A., W.A. Schutt, Jr., J.L. Petrie, and J.W. Hermanson: Neonatal development of the diaphragm of the horse, *Equus caballus*. Anat. Rec. 238:311–316, 1994.

Dik, K.J., and I. Gunsser: Atlas of Diagnostic Radiology of the Horse. Parts 1–3. Philadelphia, W.B. Saunders Company, 1988–1990.

Farrow, C.S.: Equine thoracic radiology. JAVMA 179:776–781, 1981.

Littlewort, M.C.G.: The clinical auscultation of the equine heart. Vet. Rec. 74:1247–1259, 1962.

Mackey, V.S., and J.D. Wheat: Endoscopic examination of the equine thorax. Equine Vet. J. 17:140–142, 1985.

Miller, P.J., and J.R. Holmes: Observations on structure and function of the equine mitral valve. Equine Vet. J. 16:457–460, 1984.

Nakakuki, S.: The bronchial tree and lobulur division of the horse lung. J. Vet. Med. Sci. 55:435–438, 1993.

Roudebush, P., and C.R. Sweeney: Thoracic percussion. JAVMA 197:714–718, 1990.

Sanderson, G.N., and M.W. O'Callaghan: Radiographic anatomy of the equine thorax as a basis for radiological interpretation. N.Z. Vet. J. 31:127–130, 1983.

Savage, C.J.: Evaluation of the equine respiratory system using physical examination and endoscopy. Vet. Clin. North Am. Equine Pract. 13:443–462, 1997.

Schebitz, H., and H. Wilkens: Atlas of Radiographic Anatomy of the Horse, 4th ed. Berlin, Paul Parey Verlag, 1986.

Smetzer, D.L., and C.R. Smith: Diastolic heart sounds of horses. JAVMA 146:937–944, 1965.

Smith, B.L., E. Aguilera-Tejero, W.S. Tyler, et al.: Endoscopic anatomy and map of the equine bronchial tree. Equine Vet. J. 26:283–290, 1994.

Sweeney, C.R.: Equine bronchoscopy: Help, where am I? *In* Proceedings of the 14th ACVIM Forum, 1996, pp. 320–321.

Sweeney, C.R., J.L. Baez, and S.R. Lindborg: Bronchoscopy of the horse. Am. J. Vet. Res. 53:1953–1956, 1992.

Vachon, A.M., and A.T. Fischer: Thoracoscopy in the horse: Diagnostic and therapeutic indications in 28 cases. Equine Vet. J. 30:467–475, 1998.

Voros, K., J.R. Homres, and C. Gibbs: Anatomical validation of two-dimensional echocardiography in the horse. Equine Vet. J. 22:392–397, 1992.

Wilson, J.H.: Tips for assessment of the respiratory tract: Percussion of the upper and lower respiratory tracts and guttural pouch catheterization. Am. Assoc. Equine Pract. 38:489–494, 1992.

CHAPTER 21

# The Abdomen of the Horse

## CONFORMATION AND SURFACE ANATOMY

Like other herbivores that subsist on a diet rich in roughage, the horse has a capacious gastrointestinal tract and a correspondingly bulky abdomen. However, the extent of the abdomen is not immediately apparent since a large part is concealed within the rib cage. The olecranon and the lower end of the sixth rib are handy guides to the cranialmost extent of the diaphragm (see Fig. 20–3). The flank is reduced in size by the caudal inclination of the ribs, the last of which may be within a few fingerbreadths of the coxal tuber (see Fig. 22–24/*A*, 1″,3).

Abdominal conformation varies much with age, condition, and the amount and nature of the rations. The ventral contour is especially variable; it slopes gradually between the sternum and the pubic brim in animals in hard condition but dips to reach its lowest point behind the xiphoid process in those in softer condition, in pregnant mares, and in ponies generally. In the latter groups the most caudal part of the floor ascends very steeply. These differences are not always obtrusive since the most caudal part of the abdomen is covered laterally by the skin fold that passes between the flank and the thigh (/6), and ventrally by the prepuce or udder.

The trunk is broadest at the last ribs. The upper part of the flank sinks in to form a paralumbar fossa, but the relative shortness of the region behind the ribs makes this feature much less obvious than in cattle. The lower part of the belly is rounded from side to side, except in foals, in which the whole abdomen is slab-sided and shallow (see Fig. 23–2). The usual symmetry may be disturbed in late pregnancy or by accumulation of gas in parts of the gastrointestinal tract.

The position of the last rib is often visible, but most other skeletal boundaries of the flank and floor are less easily found. The transverse processes of the lumbar vertebrae are usually too deeply buried under muscle to be palpable. The dorsal part of the coxal tuber is very conspicuous, but the ventral part, which gives origin to the internal oblique and tensor fasciae latae, is not visible, although it is easily palpable.

Soft features that may be recognized include the internal oblique muscle, which raises a ridge along the caudoventral boundary of the paralumbar fossa (Fig. 21–4/*B*) and the superficial thoracic ("spur") vein, which runs over the ventral part of the abdominal wall toward the axilla, following the dorsal border of the deep pectoral muscle. The subiliac lymph nodes can usually be identified and rolled below the fingers; they are arranged in a spindle against the cranial margin of the thigh, midway between the coxal tuber and patella. They are more easily found if drawn forward. The superficial ring of the inguinal canal can be found on deep palpation of the groin, a procedure sometimes resented and therefore to be performed with care (/*A*,3).

The usual system of reference to abdominal regions is applicable to the horse, although little favored by clinicians (see Fig. 3–35).

## THE VENTROLATERAL ABDOMINAL WALL

### Structure

The skin is thick over the flank but thins ventrally, particularly in heavy draft animals. It is especially thin in the cleft between the abdomen and thigh where it is sparsely haired and glistens with the secretion of the sebaceous glands concentrated here. In contrast, sweat glands are most abundant over the flank.

A large subcutaneous bursa, a postnatal development, is present over the coxal tuber. Elsewhere the skin is closely adherent to the cutaneous trunci, which cover most of the flank, though not the abdominal floor. The upper border of the cutaneous muscle follows a line drawn from the withers to the stifle. The muscle is thickest cranially where it extends into the fascia over both the lateral and the medial aspects of the shoulder and arm. Caudally, it continues within the flank fold to end on the lateral femoral fascia. The cutaneous muscle is employed to twitch the skin to dislodge flies and other irritants. No detached bundles are associated with the prepuce as in many species.

The loose fascia deep to the muscle conveys the cutaneous nerves and superficial vessels and encloses the subiliac lymph nodes.

The deeper fascia consists largely of elastic tissue and, being yellowish, is also known as the tunica flava. It is well adapted to the passive support of the viscera and is thickest ventrally where the burden is greatest. The dorsal part is easily dissected from the underlying muscle, but its ventral part exchanges fibers with the aponeurosis of the external oblique and is more tightly adherent. Bands detached from the tunic help support the prepuce or the udder. Careful suturing of this layer is necessary after abdominal surgery since its elastic nature tends to evert and draw apart the edges of a wound in the underlying muscle.

Before considering the muscles of the abdominal wall it is necessary to pay attention to the linea alba and prepubic tendon since these and the associated structures have a particular importance in the horse. The *linea alba,* mainly formed from the aponeuroses of the flank muscles, is considerably strengthened by longitudinal fibers. It is unequally developed along its length, being widest where it carries the umbilical scar (Fig. 21–1/d). It

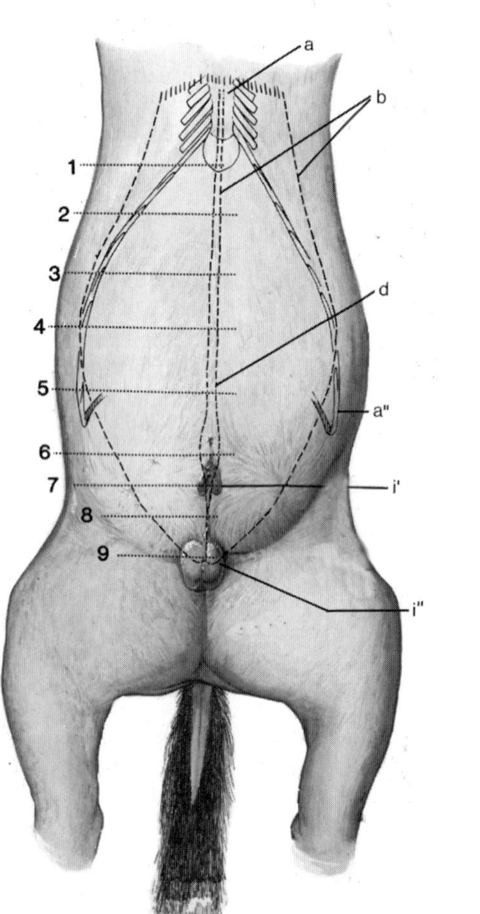


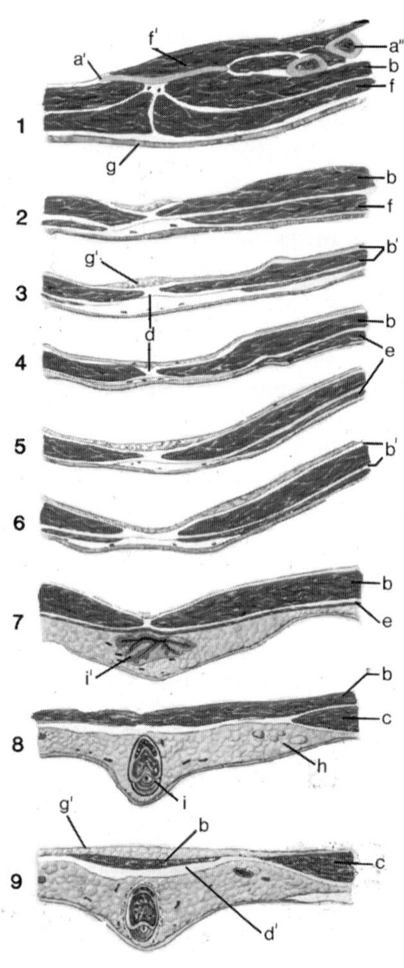


**Figure 21–1.** Changes in the structure of the abdominal floor shown by means of a series of transverse sections (1–9) of a gelding.

a, Sternum; a′, xiphoid cartilage; a″, costal arch; b, rectus abdominis; b′, rectus sheath; c, internal oblique; d, linea alba; d′, prepubic tendon; e, cutaneus trunci; f, pectoralis ascendens; f′, diaphragm; g, skin; g′, fat; h, superficial inguinal lymph nodes; i, penis; i′, prepuce; i″, scrotum.

finally combines with the insertion tendons of the right and left rectus abdominis muscles to form a broad plate. This may be regarded as the initial formation of the *prepubic tendon** through which the abdominal muscles find attachment to the pelvic skeleton (Fig. 21–2/5). The tendon once formed ascends almost vertically toward the pelvic brim, but before reaching this it is augmented by a strong transverse thickening. This thickening is mainly formed by the tendons of origin of the pectineus muscles (of the thighs), which arise from both the ipsi- and contralateral pubic bones (from and medial to the iliopubic eminences) and which thus partly decussate across the midline. Additional but lesser contributions to the prepubic tendon are made by the caudal margins of the oblique abdominal muscles and the cranial part of the gracilis. A feature of great interest, peculiar to the horse, is the detachment from the caudolateral aspects of the prepubic tendon of the stout rounded cords that furnish accessory ligaments to the hip joints (/5′ and Fig. 21–3). Each accessory ligament crosses the ventral surface of the pubis, heading toward the acetabulum, which it enters through the notch in the rim; it ends by inserting on the head of the femur beside the intracapsular ligament (of the head of the femur) that is found in all species. Each accessory ligament is predominantly composed of fibers from the two rectus muscles, many fibers having decussated from the contralateral side. The ligaments appear to be the principal insertions of these muscles. Their existence partly explains the restrictions on the movements permitted at the equine hips. It is postulated that the accessory ligaments are tensed by the weight of the abdominal contents and that this tension helps secure the femoral heads in place.

Since the main weight of the abdominal organs is carried by the prepubic tendon it follows that its rupture has the most dire consequences. This mishap, fortunately rare, is for obvious reasons most common in heavily pregnant mares.

The *external abdominal oblique* (Fig. 21–4/1) is the most extensive muscle of the flank. It arises from the lateral aspect of the thoracic wall (from the fifth rib caudally) by a series of digitations that engage with those of the serratus ventralis, and also from the thoracolumbar fascia. The majority of its fascicles run caudoventrally to a broad aponeurosis that succeeds the fleshy part of the muscle along a line that sweeps from the coxal tuber toward the ventral end of the fifth rib.

Before insertion, the aponeurosis splits into a large abdominal tendon that continues over the rectus to reach and insert on the linea alba, and a small pelvic tendon that inserts on the coxal tuber, the fascia over the iliopsoas and sartorius muscles, and the prepubic tendon (Fig. 21–2). The split between the two tendons constitutes the superficial ring of the inguinal canal (Fig. 21–4/3). (The margins of the tendons are known as crura where they bound the opening, but the term is often misapplied to the tendons themselves.)

The unnecessary term *inguinal ligament* confuses many descriptions of these structures. It is sometimes specifically applied to the thickened caudodorsal edge of the pelvic tendon. In fact, the prominence of this edge (/4) owes less to thickening than to tension through its connection with the fascia covering the iliopsoas and sartorius.

The *internal oblique muscle* (/5) radiates from an origin concentrated on the coxal tuber but extending onto the dorsocaudal edge of the pelvic tendon of the external oblique. Most bundles run cranioventrally to insert on the last costal cartilages or, via an aponeurosis that fuses with that of the external oblique, into the linea alba. Some pass ventrally and caudoventrally, and these cover the superficial inguinal ring on its internal aspect (Fig. 21–5/4). A caudal slip provides the cremaster, which passes onto the spermatic cord. The junction of the fleshy and aponeurotic parts of this muscle occurs more than halfway down the abdominal wall.

The *transversus abdominis* (Fig. 21–4/7) takes origin from the lumbar vertebrae and the medial aspect of the last ribs, ventral to the origin of the diaphragm. The fleshy part is continued by an aponeurosis that passes deep to the rectus abdominis to reach the linea alba. The transversus, the least extensive of the three muscles of the flank, does not extend caudal to the level of the coxal tuber; the internal lamina of the rectus sheath is thus deficient caudally.

The *rectus abdominis* (/8) arises from the fourth to ninth costal cartilages and the adjacent part of the sternum. It inserts by way of the prepubic tendon and accessory ligaments. The muscle,

*Although all agree that the prepubic tendon is the means by which the abdominal muscles obtain a principal attachment to the pelvic skeleton, opinions are divided on what constitutes the essential elements of this structure (and what are to be regarded as secondary augmentations). We adhere to the view that it is primarily formed of the linea alba and rectus tendons and secondarily complicated by the incorporation of other elements, especially the decussation of the pectineus tendons. Others have regarded it as primarily a transverse structure attaching to and lying in front of the right and left pubic bones and strengthened by giving attachment to the linea alba and recti (and other components). Interpretation is complicated by interspecific differences. The interweaving of the fibers of the various contributors makes analysis of the construction difficult, but fortunately most readers may safely disregard the details.

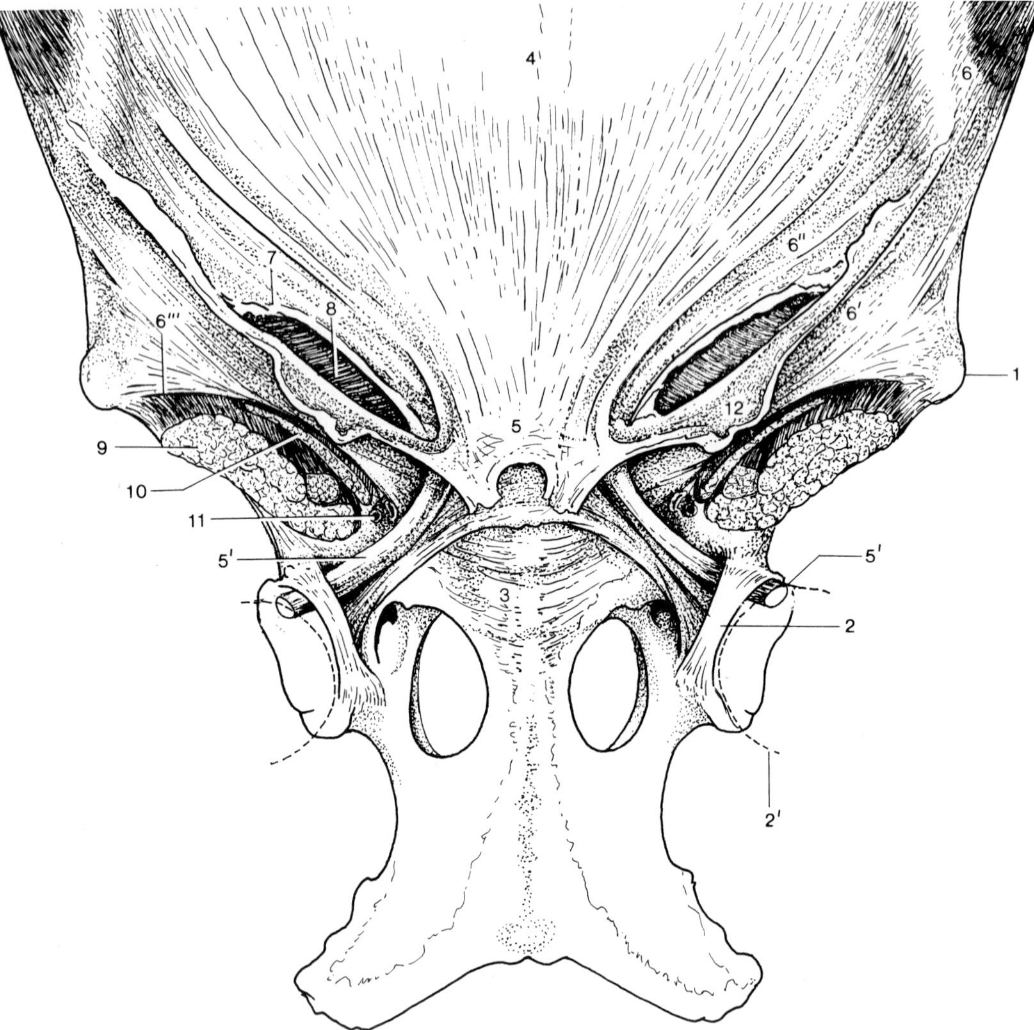


**Figure 21–2.** The attachment of the abdominal muscles on the pelvis and the prepubic tendon.

1, Coxal tuber; 2, transverse acetabular ligament; 2′, femoral head; 3, pubis; 4, tunica flava over linea alba; 5, prepubic tendon; 5′, accessory ligament; 6, external abdominal oblique; 6′, 6″, pelvic and abdominal tendons of external oblique aponeurosis; 6‴, attachment of pelvic tendon of external oblique aponeurosis on sartorius and iliopsoas ("inguinal ligament"); 7, superficial inguinal ring; 8, internal abdominal oblique; 9, iliopsoas; 10, sartorius; 11, vascular lacuna containing femoral vessels; 12, femoral fascia (lamina).

relatively narrow over the thorax, widens considerably over the abdomen before again narrowing toward its insertion (Fig. 21–1/b).

Although the functions of the abdominal muscles are the same in all species, the expiratory role is relatively more important in the horse because the elasticity of the lungs is frequently reduced in older horses (resulting in heaves). Contraction of the abdominal musculature is then more necessary to return the viscera, and thus the diaphragm, from the inspiratory position. In this action the junction between the fleshy and aponeurotic parts of the external oblique muscle becomes visible as the so-called heave line.

The fascia that supports the peritoneum is often heavily but unequally infiltrated with fat. This layer, which may be 6 cm or more thick in horses in good condition, must be taken into account when making and closing a surgical incision.

## The Inguinal Canal

The inguinal canal follows the general pattern but merits a full description because of its relevance to castration, which is performed on the vast majority of male horses. It is the opening in the caudal part of the abdominal wall through which the testis travels in its descent into the scrotum, a process usually completed shortly before or shortly after birth in this species. The canal contains the spermatic cord of the colt and stallion; a stump frequently remains in the gelding. In addition, the external pudendal artery and the genitofemoral nerve travel through the canal.

The term *inguinal canal* suggests a roomier passage, but the canal is no more than a potential space between the flesh of the internal and the aponeurosis of the external abdominal oblique. The entrance (deep inguinal ring) lies along the free caudal edge of the internal abdominal oblique muscle, which determines its oblique orientation (Fig. 21–5/5); the origin of the internal abdominal oblique from the external abdominal oblique and the convergence of the two muscles on the lateral edge of the prepubic tendon determine its length (generally ca. 15 cm).

The exit (superficial inguinal ring), between the two tendons into which the external oblique aponeurosis splits, is more or less horizontal (/4). It

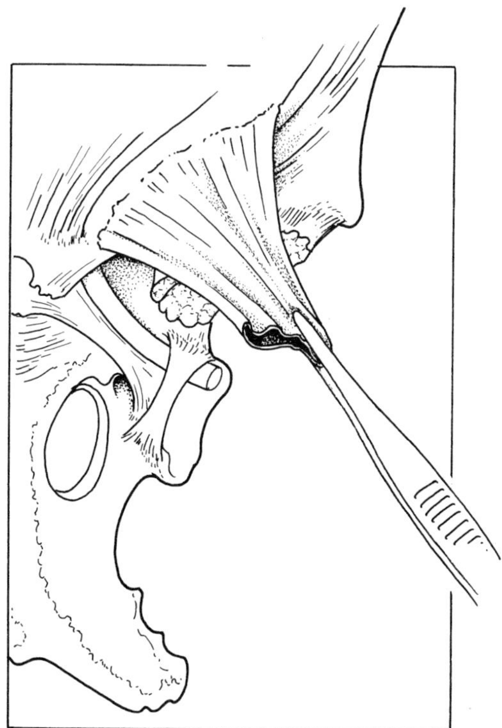

**Figure 21–3.** The origin of the external spermatic fascia and femoral lamina from the margin of the superficial inguinal ring. (See Fig. 21–2 for orientation.)

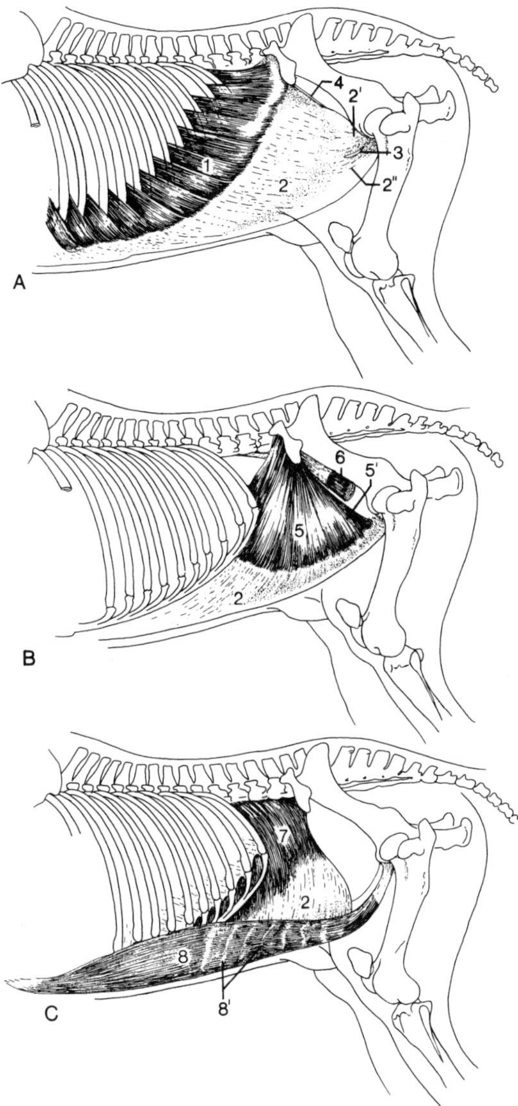


**Figure 21–4.** The abdominal muscles and their skeletal attachments.

1, External abdominal oblique, muscular part; 2, aponeurotic parts of 1, 5, and 7; 2′, 2″, pelvic and abdominal tendons of aponeurotic part; 3, superficial inguinal ring; 4, attachment of pelvic tendon of external oblique aponeurosis on iliopsoas and sartorius ("inguinal ligament"); 5, internal abdominal oblique, muscular part; 5′, free caudal border forming the cranial margin of the deep inguinal ring; 6, iliopsoas, partly enclosed by iliac fascia; 7, transversus abdominis, muscular part; 8, rectus abdominis; 8′, tendinous inscriptions.

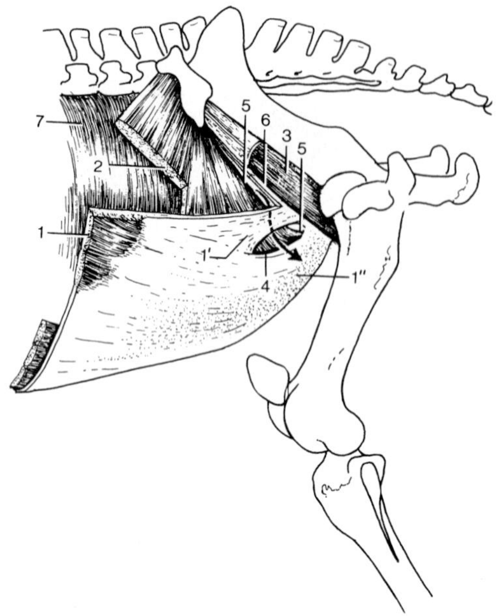


**Figure 21–5.** The muscles of the inguinal region. The arrow passes through the inguinal canal.

1, External abdominal oblique; 1′, 1″, pelvic and abdominal tendons of external oblique aponeurosis; 2, internal abdominal oblique; 3, iliopsoas partly enclosed by iliac fascia; 4, superficial inguinal ring; 5, cranial border of deep inguinal ring; 6, attachment of pelvic tendon of external oblique aponeurosis on iliopsoas and sartorius ("inguinal ligament"); 7, transversus abdominis.

is limited laterally by the exchange of fibers between the two tendons where they part company and medially by the tendons meeting and fusing with the edge of the prepubic tendon. The margins of the opening are less clearly defined than many accounts suggest. The lateral (dorsal) crus gives origin to the external spermatic fascia and femoral lamina, which appear to continue the lateral crus directly (Fig. 21–3). The medial (ventral) crus is somewhat frayed but can be identified on palpation through the skin. This is best performed by placing the palm against the belly and advancing the fingers into the cleft between the thigh and abdominal wall. The lateral crus is passed unnoticed, but the medial crus is recognized as a firm edge. The fingers pass into the outer part of the canal most readily with the thigh abducted (when the femoral fascia [lamina] draws the lateral crus outward). It follows from the orientation of the deep and superficial rings that the canal has a triangular outline; it is relatively long cranially, very short caudally where the two openings butt against the prepubic tendon (Fig. 21–5).

The peritoneal sheath (vaginal tunic) of the spermatic cord contains a cavity that places the space about the testis in free communication with the peritoneal cavity of the abdomen. The communication occurs through the vaginal ring (ca. 3 cm long) situated midway in the deep inguinal ring (see Fig. 22–20/12 and Plate 24/*C*); the vaginal ring, with the constituents of the spermatic cord converging on it, can be identified per rectum in the stallion. The vaginal cavity provides a possible route for the herniation of intestines that may even reach the scrotum. This occurrence (indirect inguinal hernia) is a comparatively common sequel to castration. Direct inguinal hernia, in which a loop of intestine forces an entry into the canal beside the vaginal tunic, is rare in horses.

Incomplete descent of one or both testes (cryptorchidism) is common in the horse (p. 560). The testis may be retained within the abdomen or may enter but fail to leave the canal. Surgical correction may be indicated. It is therefore necessary to be aware that while the spermatic cord occupies a central position within the canal, the external pudendal artery, which must be treated with respect, occupies the caudomedial corner. The artery is accompanied by the genitofemoral nerve and a small vein; the larger (accessory) external pudendal vein makes a separate passage between the pectineus and gracilis muscles.

## Innervation and Vascularization

The segmental innervation of the abdominal wall corresponds to the common pattern, and the minor variations are of little importance since paravertebral anesthesia is rarely practiced in the horse. The vascularization also follows the common pattern in the main. Mention may be made of a cranial branch of the deep circumflex iliac artery, which extends forward from the region of the coxal tuber between the muscles of the flank; it is susceptible to injury during surgery in this region. The artery of the right side is also at risk in trocarization, which is occasionally performed to relieve tympany of the cecal base. The abdominal floor and lower flank are served in the usual way by the cranial and caudal epigastric arteries and their superficial branches. Paradoxically, these vessels are at less risk when the classic procedures are employed than in laparoscopic surgery in which stab wounds are blindly made to create the necessary instrument portals. No warning of the exact position of the vessels is available and, should vascular damage occur, control of the resulting hemorrhage may be troublesome and time-consuming. It is said that the caudal epigastric artery is the vessel most often traumatized. The superficial thoracic or spur vein runs toward the axilla in the superficial fascia at the ventral edge of the cutaneous muscle. Connections with tributaries of the external pudendal vein make it available as an alternative drainage route from the prepuce or udder.

## GENERAL ASPECTS OF ABDOMINAL TOPOGRAPHY

The influences on abdominal topography common to all species have been discussed (p. 125). Pathological adhesions of the peritoneum are common in the horse; most result from the migration and encapsulation of the larvae of the nematode worms that infest all horses. Arterial aneurysms and thickenings are also almost universal and have the same causation. Their significance varies greatly but those involving the cranial mesenteric artery are usually both the most obvious and potentially the most important.

Except in advanced pregnancy, when the uterus has an even greater influence, the topography of the equine abdomen is dominated by the large intestine. The cecum and ascending colon are the seat of the microbial fermentation that makes the cellulose constituents of the diet available, and their significance is therefore comparable to that of the forechambers of the ruminant stomach. The large intestine is so voluminous that it is almost always encountered immediately when the abdomen is opened, whether the incision is made in the flank or in the floor. Its disposition is complicated, and although it is necessary to give a systematic account of each individual part, a first impression may be obtained from such illustrations as Figures 21–6, 21–7, 21–11, and Plate 23/*F,G*.

## THE SPLEEN

The spleen lies within the left dorsal part of the abdomen where it is largely, if not wholly, protected by the caudalmost ribs from which it is separated only by the diaphragm. The broad dorsal base lies under the last three ribs, although a small corner may project against the flank. The pointed ventral apex reaches forward to about the 9th or 10th rib, a handbreadth above the costal arch (Fig. 21–6/4). The cranial margin is concave, the caudal margin convex, and the organ thus approximately sickle-shaped. The parietal surface is generally smooth, though sometimes marked by depressions that may even perforate to the visceral surface. It lies against the diaphragm but is not joined to this. The visceral surface presents three parts. A small dorsal region fits against the left crus of the diaphragm and left kidney and is bound to these by phrenicosplenic and renosplenic ligaments (Fig. 21–8/7,6). The remainder of the visceral surface is

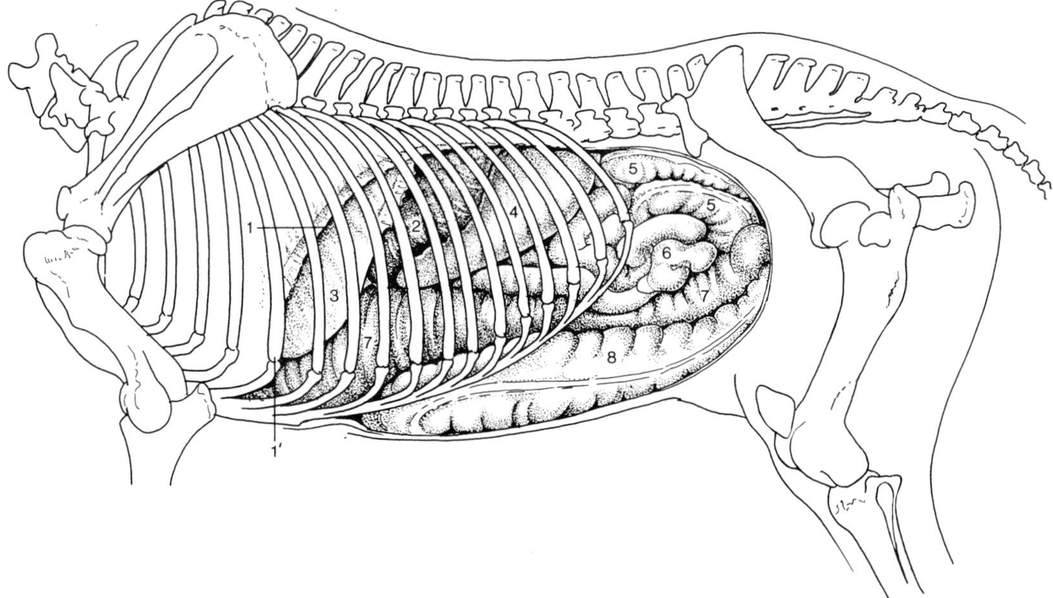


**Figure 21–6.** Visceral projections on the left abdominal wall (including the diaphragm).

1, Cut edge of diaphragm; 1′, rib 6; 2, stomach; 3, liver; 4, spleen; 5, descending colon (banded); 6, jejunum (smooth); 7, left dorsal colon; 8, left ventral colon.

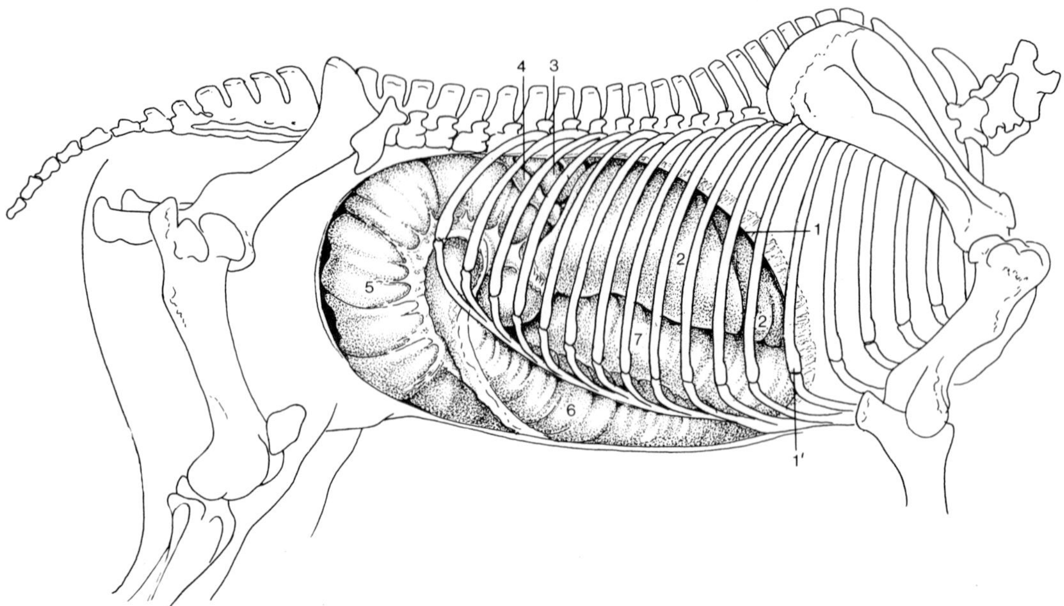


**Figure 21–7.** Visceral projections on the right abdominal wall (including the diaphragm).

1, Cut edge of diaphragm; 1′, rib 6; 2, liver; 3, right kidney; 4, descending duodenum; 5, body of cecum; 6, right ventral colon; 7, right dorsal colon.

divided by a ridge along which the splenic artery runs and to which the greater omentum attaches. The narrow strip cranial to the ridge, the gastric surface, is applied to the greater curvature of the stomach (Fig. 21–21); the larger area caudal to the ridge, the intestinal surface (/1), is related to various parts of the intestinal mass.

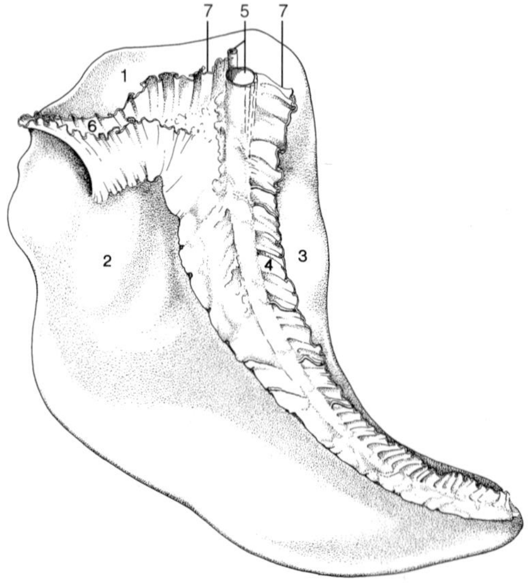


**Figure 21–8.** Visceral surface of the spleen.

1, Renal surface; 2, intestinal surface; 3, gastric surface; 4, greater omentum (gastrosplenic ligament); 5, splenic artery and vein; 6, renosplenic ligament; 7, phrenicosplenic ligament.

The thick capsule contains a considerable amount of smooth muscle, allowing much variation in volume since the spleen becomes engorged when the capsule is relaxed. This occurs in certain diseases and is very obvious in animals that have succumbed to anthrax. The organ is steel blue on first removal from the fresh carcass but turns reddish brown on exposure to the air. This color is derived from the red pulp that forms the bulk of the parenchyma. The white pulp that flecks the red is not normally visible to the naked eye.

The position of the spleen naturally varies with respiration. Usually only the caudal margin is within reach on rectal exploration (see Fig. 22–25/3); a greater part becomes accessible when the stomach is distended.

## THE STOMACH

The most remarkable feature of the stomach is its small size in relation to the animal and to the volume of fodder consumed. It is probably flattered by the figure of 5 to 15 L commonly quoted as the physiological capacity. It is relatively larger in the unweaned foal.

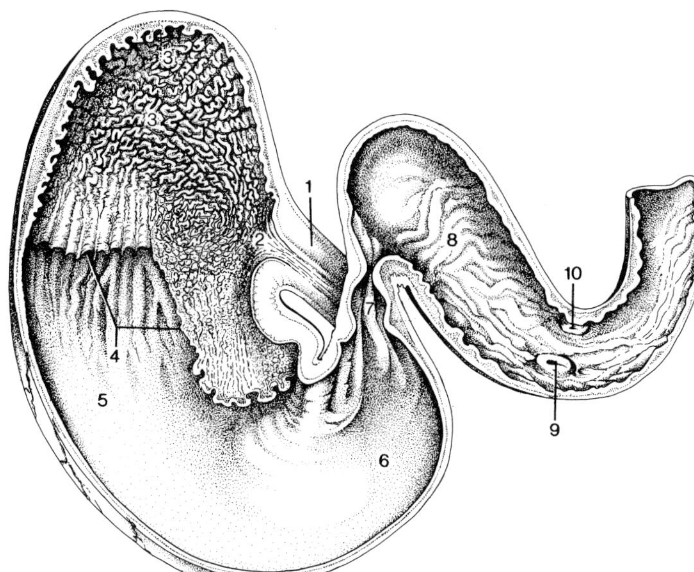


**Figure 21–9.** Interior of the stomach and cranial part of the duodenum.

1, Esophagus; 2, cardiac opening; 3, fundus (blind sac); 4, margo plicatus; 5, body; 6, pyloric part; 7, pylorus; 8, cranial part of duodenum; 9, major duodenal papilla within hepatopancreatic ampulla; 10, minor duodenal papilla.

The equine stomach lies mainly within the left half of the abdomen (Fig. 21–10/2). Like other simple stomachs, it consists of two limbs that meet at a ventral angle. The left limb comprises the fundus (unusually large and often termed *saccus cecus* [blind sac] in this species) and the body; the right limb or pyloric part is much narrower and extends across the midline to join the duodenum (Fig. 21–9/6). Although the situation naturally varies with the degree of distention, the stomach remains within the protection of the rib cage even when grossly distended; it is, therefore, inaccessible by the ordinary methods of clinical examination, either through the flank or per rectum. Gross overdistention may be revealed by a raising of the overlying ribs on the left side, which destroys the normal symmetry of the trunk. When moderately distended the fundus extends under the upper part of the 15th rib (or thereabouts), and the lowest part of the body reaches the ventral parts of the 9th and 10th ribs. The cardia provides a relatively fixed point—opposite the upper part of the 11th rib—and enlargement after feeding is therefore mainly downward and forward (Fig. 21–6/2).

The cranial surface is directed against the diaphragm above, the left lobe of the liver more ventrally; it faces cranially, dorsally, and laterally. The caudal surface faces in the opposite direction and makes contact with various viscera, including coils of small intestine and descending colon dorsally, the dorsal diaphragmatic flexure of the ascending colon ventrally. The left part of the greater curvature is followed by the hilus and adjoining gastric surface of the spleen (Fig. 21–21).

A stepped edge (margo plicatus; /2″) divides the interior between a large nonglandular region, occupying the fundus and part of the body, and a glandular region. The nonglandular part resembles the mucosa of the esophagus and is dirty white and harsh to the touch. The softer glandular region consists of cardiac, proper gastric, and pyloric glandular zones; although the borders between these zones are ill-defined, the zone occupied by the proper gastric glands is somewhat darker and redder than the yellowish cardiac and pyloric zones in the fresh specimen (Plate 23/*D,E*). Both the cardiac and pyloric regions are commonly parasitized by botfly *(Gastrophilus)* larvae; when these relinquish their hold to pupate in the soil they may leave the mucosa densely pocked by small focal ulcerations. These, when semihealed, can be misinterpreted as normal features.

The cardiac sphincter is exceptionally well developed and this, coupled with the oblique entrance of the esophagus, is held responsible for the horse's reputed inability to eructate or vomit; vomiting, though rare, is, however, possible. The canal or distal portion of the pyloric part is more muscular than the remainder of the organ and is bounded by proximal and distal thickenings that converge at the lesser curvature. Even when the second of these, the pyloric sphincter, is fully relaxed, the actual exit is remarkably narrow (Fig. 21–21/5).

# THE INTESTINES

The intestines occupy the greater part of the abdominal cavity. The small intestine is unremarkable, but the large intestine is greatly modified and enlarged. It provides the reservoir for microbial fermentation and assumes a form and disposition that make it difficult to recognize the homologies of its parts with those of the gut of other species. However, these may be deduced from the attachments and arterial supply and confirmed by reference to the development.

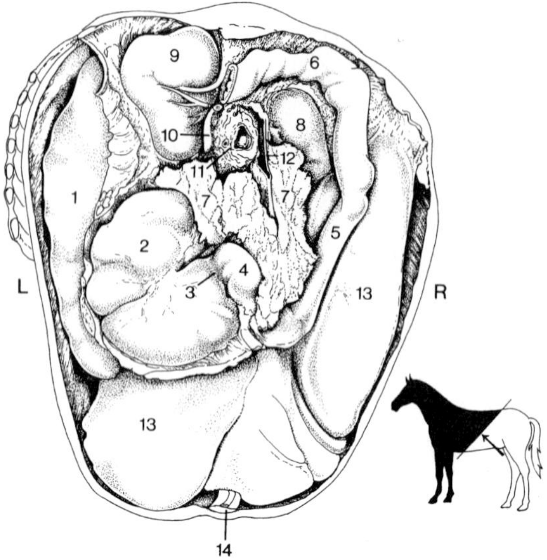


**Figure 21–10.** The organs in the craniodorsal part of the abdominal cavity of a young horse, caudoventral view (see *inset*).

1, Spleen; 2, stomach; 3, pylorus; 4, 5, cranial and descending parts of duodenum; 6, caudal flexure of duodenum; 7, pancreas; 8, right kidney; 9, left kidney; 10, left adrenal gland; 11, cranial mesenteric artery and vein; 12, portal vein; 13, liver; 14, falciform ligament.

## The Small Intestine

The small intestine measures about 25 m in the carcass, though probably much less in life. The duodenum is relatively short, and since closely tethered it is more or less constant in position. It commences ventral to the liver where the initial (cranial) part forms a sigmoid flexure of which the first curve is convex dorsally, the second convex ventrally. The second (descending) part then runs caudally, still below the liver, until it reaches the lateral margin of the right kidney, which it follows to the caudal pole; it then bends medially behind the root of the mesentery (Figs. 21–10/6 and 21–11/2,3). The descending duodenum is also related to the right lobe of the pancreas and crosses above the last part of the right dorsal colon and the base of the cecum to which it is attached (Fig. 21–15). This relationship permits the formation of a temporary duodenocecal anastomosis in the treatment of gastroduodenojejunitis, obviating the reflux of fluid and consequent overloading of the stomach that characterizes this condition. The third (ascending) part runs forward against, and adherent to, the left face of the mesentery; it bends ventrally below the left kidney to continue as the jejunum. The caliber of the duodenum is uniform except at its commencement where the first bend of the sigmoid flexure is somewhat widened. The bile and pancreatic ducts open here. The bile and major pancreatic ducts discharge through a single papilla within an enclosure (ampulla hepatopancreatica) bounded by a circular mucosal rampart. This is situated on the convex margin of the flexure, while the accessory pancreatic duct opens on a small papilla on the facing margin (Fig. 21–21/7,8).

The position and restricted mobility of the duodenum make its access difficult through the usual surgical exposures; fortunately, indications for duodenal surgery are largely restricted to the condition recently mentioned.

The remainder of the small intestine lies within the free margin of the great mesentery, which is sufficiently long to allow the coils considerable latitude in position. Most are piled into the left dorsal part of the abdomen where they mingle with those of the descending colon; however, some insinuate themselves between the large intestine and the flanks, while others may reach the abdominal floor between the body of the cecum and the ventral parts of the ascending colon. The ileum (according to the convention we employ [p. 130]) is very short, and in most circumstances it is distinguished from the remainder of the small intestine by its much thicker wall and firmer consistency. It approaches the left side of the cecal base from below and ends by protruding into the cecal interior, raising a papilla on which it opens (Fig. 21–16/1 and Plate 23/*I,J*).

The mobility of the small intestine may be blamed for the incarceration of a part within one of several openings such as the epiploic foramen,* vaginal ring, or even a rent in the mesentery. Intussusception is also relatively common, especially in the young horse. A form peculiar to the horse involves the passage of the terminal part of

*Perhaps surprisingly, this is not a particularly rare accident.

the small intestine into the interior of the cecal base. Necrosis of the intruded part follows quickly unless surgical correction is undertaken.

## The Large Intestine

In addition to its enormous capacity, the large intestine is also characterized by having a sacculated form. The sacculations or haustra result from the shortening of the teniae, bands formed by the concentration of the external longitudinal muscle and elastic fibers at certain (from one to four) positions on the circumference. Semilunar folds project internally where grooves divide adjacent haustra externally (Fig. 21–11). The haustral segmentation is not constant but is constantly modified in life—by gradual "haustral flow" and by intermittent disappearance of the contractions with re-formation in a different pattern.

The arrangement of the large intestine of the horse predisposes to various forms of obstruction and displacement, conditions collectively known as colic (although this term is widely used to include any painful abdominal disorder).

### *The Cecum*

The cecum incorporates an initial portion of the ascending colon as is revealed by its extending distally beyond the entrance of the ileum. It follows that the so-called cecocolic orifice is actually a constriction of the ascending colon set some distance distal to its true origin. However, the conventional terminology pays no regard to such considerations and is based entirely on the form of the adult organ (Fig. 21–12).

The cecum consists of an expanded dorsal base, a curved tapering body, and a blind ventral apex; these parts merge smoothly, and the organ is often likened to a comma (Fig. 21–13). In large horses it may have a capacity in excess of 30 L and may measure a meter or more between extremities. The base lies in the right dorsal part of the abdomen, partly against the flank, partly under cover of the ribs. It has an extensive contact with the abdominal roof and sublumbar organs from the 15th rib (or thereabouts) to the coxal tuber, but the direct dorsal adhesion is confined to the region of the pancreas and right kidney. This retroperitoneal attachment extends caudally to the level of the second lumbar vertebra. The base also fuses with the root of the mesentery medially and with the right dorsal colon cranially. The cranial part of the base forms an overhanging enlargement that at first sight appears to be blind (Fig. 21–16); closer inspection reveals the origin of the colon from the middle of the caudal wall of this overhang. The caudal part of the base merges imperceptibly with the body of the cecum. Microbial fermentation

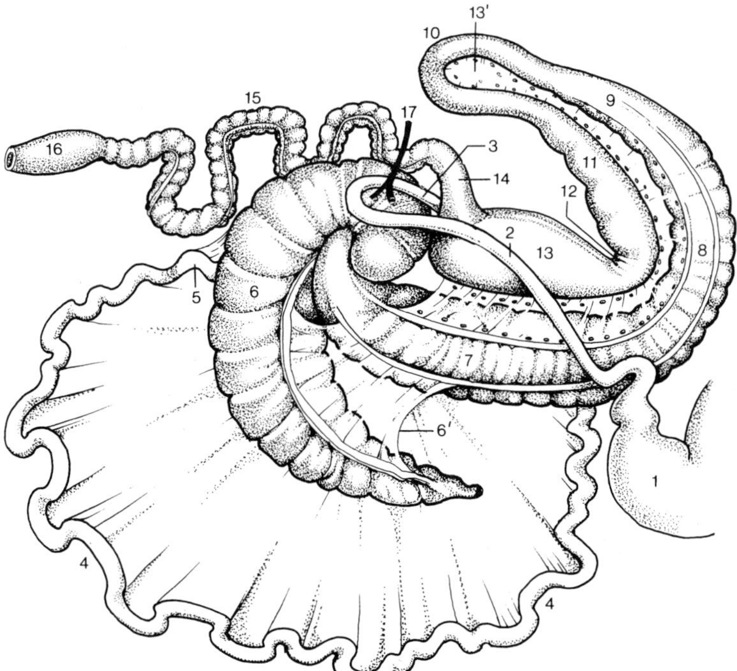


**Figure 21–11.** The intestinal tract seen from the right, schematic. The caudal flexure of the duodenum and the cranial mesenteric artery (17) have been displaced to the right of the animal to lie over the base of the cecum.

1, Stomach; 2, 3, descending and ascending duodenum; 4, jejunum; 5, ileum; 6, cecum; 6′, cecocolic fold; 7, right ventral colon; 8, ventral diaphragmatic flexure; 9, left ventral colon; 10, pelvic flexure; 11, left dorsal colon; 12, dorsal diaphragmatic flexure; 13, right dorsal colon; 13′, ascending mesocolon; 14, transverse colon; 15, descending (small) colon; 16, rectum; 17, cranial mesenteric artery.

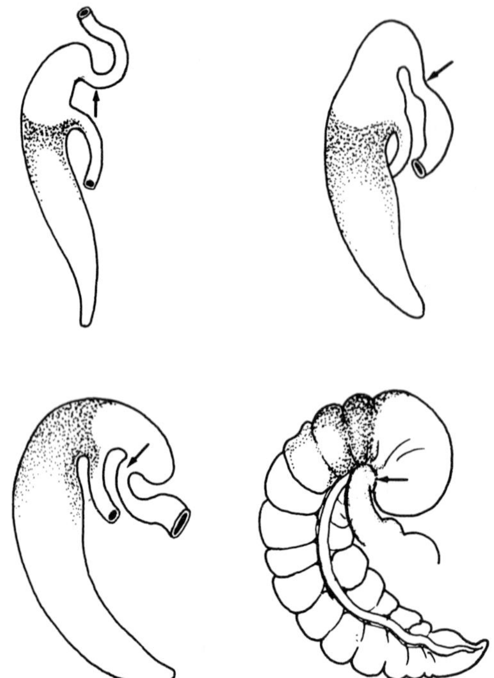

**Figure 21–12.** Development of the equine cecum, schematic. The stippled part of the cecum is homologous with the cecum of other species. The nonstippled part is the annexed first part of the colon. The cecocolic orifice is a constriction of the ascending colon *(arrows).*

within the cecum produces gas that is normally discharged at intervals into the right ventral colon. Occasionally, gas is produced excessively, causing the overhanging part of the base to press on the origin of the right ventral colon, interfering with the normal mechanism. The resulting tympany of the base can only be relieved by needle decompression through the paralumbar fossa.

The body runs ventrally before turning cranially (Fig. 21–13/2). At first it lies against the right flank, following the caudal border of the right ventral colon, but as it sinks within the abdomen it is displaced medially, and when it reaches the abdominal floor it lies between the ventral parts of the ascending colon. It terminates in the apex, close to the xiphoid cartilage. There are four teniae over most of the organ but the number diminishes toward the apex. Retroflexion of the apical part of the cecum is occasionally encountered in apparently healthy subjects.

The interior is marked by numerous folds corresponding to the external divisions of the haustra. These folds are impermanent, but a larger and more persistent fold at the level of the ileal papilla partially separates the cranial expansion from the remainder of the base (Fig. 21–16). The ileal papilla is variable in form. In most postmortem specimens it is a low conical projection whose summit carries a slitlike opening bounded by lax folds of mucosa (/1). In life, it is usually much more salient and more cylindrical and has a rounded orifice circumscribed by a firm and thickened rim. The erection of the papilla is caused by the tonus of the muscle and engorgement of a mucosal venous plexus (Plate 23/*I,J*).

Although the exit from the cecum by the cecocolic orifice (/2) lies at some distance from the ileal papilla, the curvature of the cecal base brings it more or less into the same transverse plane. In the dead specimen it is a transverse slit that scarcely admits a couple of fingers, but in life it generally allows the passage of a hand.

## The Colon

The colon consists of the usual ascending, transverse, and descending parts (see Fig. 3–44). The first two together constitute the "large colon" of common usage, the third the "small colon" (Fig. 21–11/15). The ascending colon is arranged in four parallel limbs separated by three flexures, each separately named. The sequence runs right ventral colon (/7), ventral diaphragmatic flexure, left ventral colon, pelvic flexure, left dorsal colon, dorsal diaphragmatic flexure, right dorsal colon (/13). The right dorsal colon leads to the short transverse colon (/14); this is followed in its turn by the descending colon, which is long and thrown into coils (/15).

The *cecocolic transitional region* forms a sigmoid flexure; the convexity of the first bend (provided by the overhanging part of the cecal base) is directed ventrally; that of the second bend

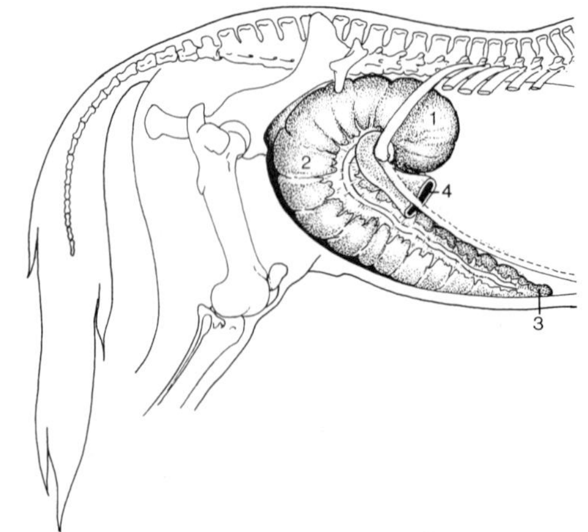


**Figure 21–13.** The cecum in situ.

1, Base of cecum; 2, body of cecum; 3, apex of cecum; 4, right ventral colon.

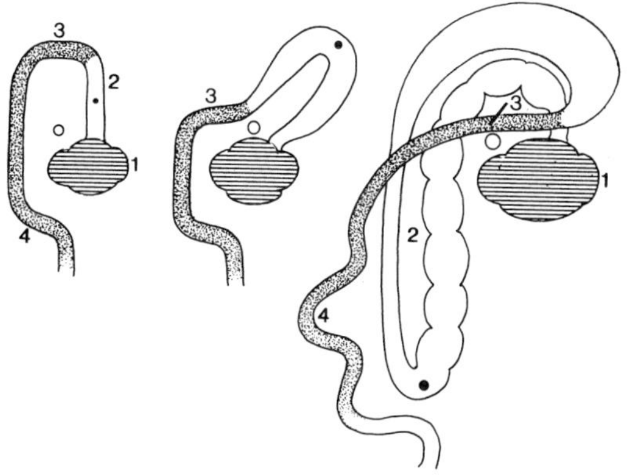


**Figure 21–14.** The development of the ascending colon, dorsal view. The dot indicates the position of the pelvic flexure, the circle that of the cranial mesenteric artery.

1, Cecum; 2, ascending colon; 3, transverse colon; 4, descending colon.

(provided by the first part of the colon) is directed dorsally (Figs. 21–15 and 21–16). This conformation appears to be caused by the looser attachment of the medial and lateral teniae at this level; they run as chords across the arcs into which the bowel is drawn. The *right ventral colon* (/4) is narrow when it emerges from this siphon-like arrangement but soon expands to continue, first ventrally, then cranially on the abdominal floor, as a wide (ca. 20 cm) tube of uniform caliber (Plate 23/*F*). It is deflected across the midline on reaching the diaphragm (ventral diaphragmatic flexure) and then becomes known as the left ventral colon. The *left ventral colon* runs toward the pelvis, still on the abdominal floor (Fig. 21–17/6 and Plate 23/*G*) until a sharp flexure through 180 degrees marks its junction with the following, left dorsal, part. The *pelvic flexure* is also distinguished by a reduction in caliber (Fig. 21–11) and by the disappearance of three of the four bands found on the ventral parts with a consequent loss of the haustrations. Although there is no evidence of a conventional sphincter, the pelvic flexure marks the boundary between two distinct functional units of the colon. The decrease in the fluidity of the ingesta, the sudden alteration in course, and the reduction in caliber explain why impaction is common at this level. The location of the flexure varies with the fullness of the rectum, bladder, and uterus but, since it is usually just within or in front of the pelvic cavity, it is easily found on rectal examination.

The *left dorsal colon* is narrow and smooth-walled where it emerges from the pelvic flexure, but it gradually widens; the teniae increase from one to three and the sacculations return. It runs cranially above the left ventral colon, below the coils of small intestine and descending colon, to reach the liver where it joins the right dorsal colon at the dorsal diaphragmatic flexure. Toward its termination it is related to the spleen and the stomach (Fig. 21–6/7). The *right dorsal colon* is both the shortest and, at its termination, by far the widest part (ca. 30 cm) of the ascending colon (Fig. 21–18/7). It ascends below the liver to meet the cranial part of the cecal base by which it is deflected medially to become the transverse colon (/8). The right dorsal colon is also the best-fixed part and is adherent to the abdominal roof, the

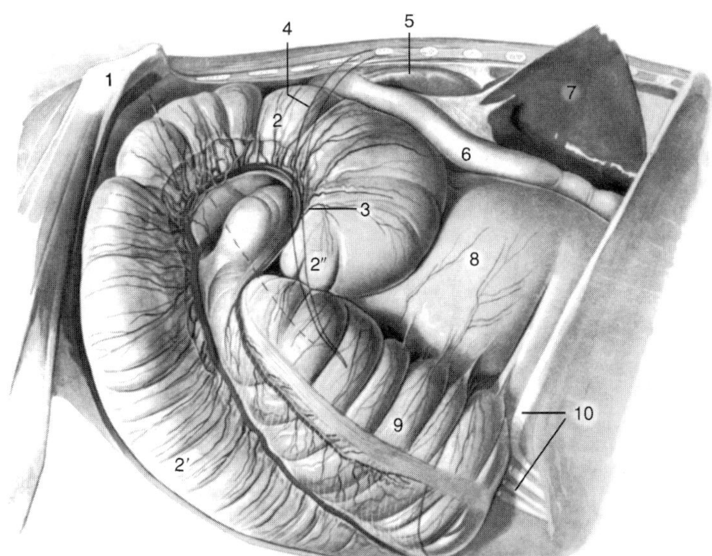


**Figure 21–15.** Cecum and related organs lying against the right abdominal wall and flank. The broken line indicates the position of the cranial branch of the deep circumflex iliac artery crossing the flank.

1, Coxal tuber; 2, 2′, base and body of cecum; 2″, overhanging part of cecal base; 3, position of cecocolic orifice; 4, position of last rib; 5, right kidney; 6, descending duodenum; 7, right lobe of liver, elevated; 8, right dorsal colon; 9, right ventral colon; 10, 10th rib and costal arch.

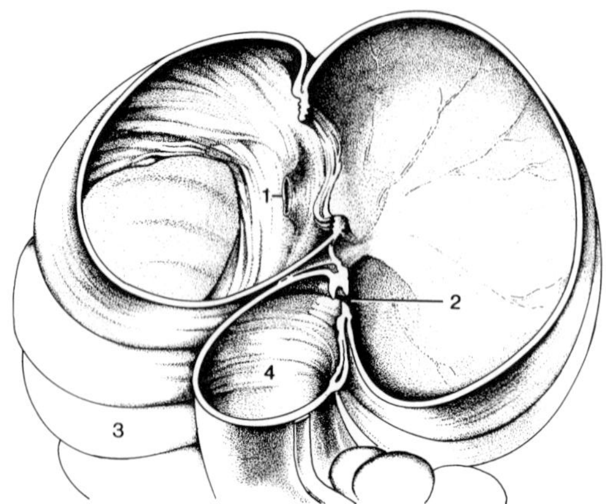


**Figure 21–16.** The interior of the base of the cecum, right lateral view.

1, Termination of ileum at ileal papilla; 2, cecocolic orifice; 3, body of cecum; 4, right ventral colon.

cecal base, and the root of the mesentery. It carries three bands.

The *transverse colon* is very short and is situated according to the common mammalian pattern, passing from right to left in front of the root of the mesentery. It carries two bands and rapidly funnels to the much smaller caliber of the descending colon (/9) by which it is succeeded in the region of the left kidney. The transverse colon also has a direct retroperitoneal attachment to the abdominal roof.

Except at its origin and termination the ascending colon is free within the abdomen, although its great bulk ensures that it does not change much in position. The folding it undergoes in development transforms the original mesentery into a short peritoneal sheet (ascending mesocolon) passing between adjacent portions of the dorsal and ventral limbs (Fig. 21–11/13′). Through continuity with the cecum and transverse colon it is anchored by the retroperitoneal attachments of these parts. The loose attachment between the left limbs allows the dorsal part to slip some way to the side (generally the right side) of the ventral part as a common and probably temporary variant of the usual topography. When the rotation of these parts about their common axis is pronounced there arises the condition known as twist (volvulus), which is one of the most severe abdominal catastrophes to which the horse is subject. Volvulus initially narrows the lumen but may proceed to close it and then to interrupt the blood flow in the vessels that follow the bowel. Another malposition of the ascending colon that has been increasingly recognized in recent years involves the lodgment of the left limbs above the spleen. Although the cause of this painful condition is not known with certainty, it is postulated that the accumulation of gas raises the left limbs against the abdominal wall until they pass over the base of the spleen, to be trapped on the shelf formed by the phrenicosplenic and renosplenic ligaments. The spontaneous restoration of normal topography is unlikely. Restoration may be achieved by rolling and maneuvering the recumbent (anesthetized) animal but, this failing, surgical intervention (decompression) is required.

Occasionally a portion of the large colon may become incarcerated within the epiploic foramen.

The *descending colon* (/15), much narrower than the other parts, is several meters long, and alone hangs within a conventional mesentery. These features account for its alternative names, small colon and floating colon. It lies mainly within the dorsal, caudal, and left part of the abdomen, largely dorsal to the small intestine, and ends in the rectum (Fig. 21–6/5). The distinction between the descending colon and rectum is based entirely on the pelvic location of the latter, and no immediate change in structure or appearance occurs. The descending colon is drawn by two prominent bands into a linear series of sacculations occupied by the familiar dry fecal balls. The rectum is considered with the pelvic organs.

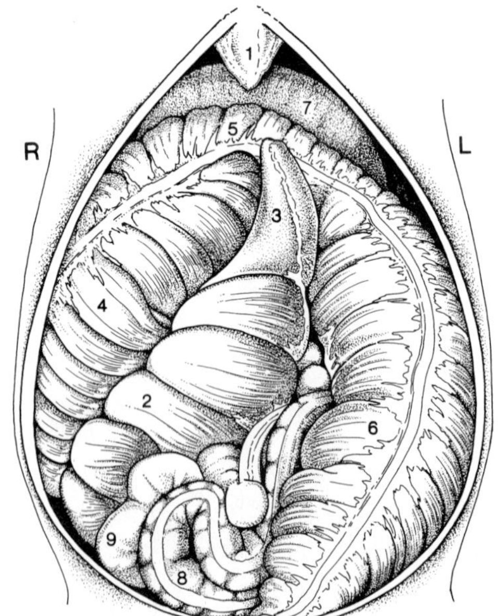


**Figure 21–17.** Visceral projection on the ventral abdominal wall. The position of the apex of the cecum is variable.

1, Xiphoid cartilage; 2, body of cecum; 3, apex of cecum; 4, right ventral colon; 5, ventral diaphragmatic flexure; 6, left ventral colon; 7, dorsal diaphragmatic flexure; 8, descending colon (banded); 9, jejunum (smooth).

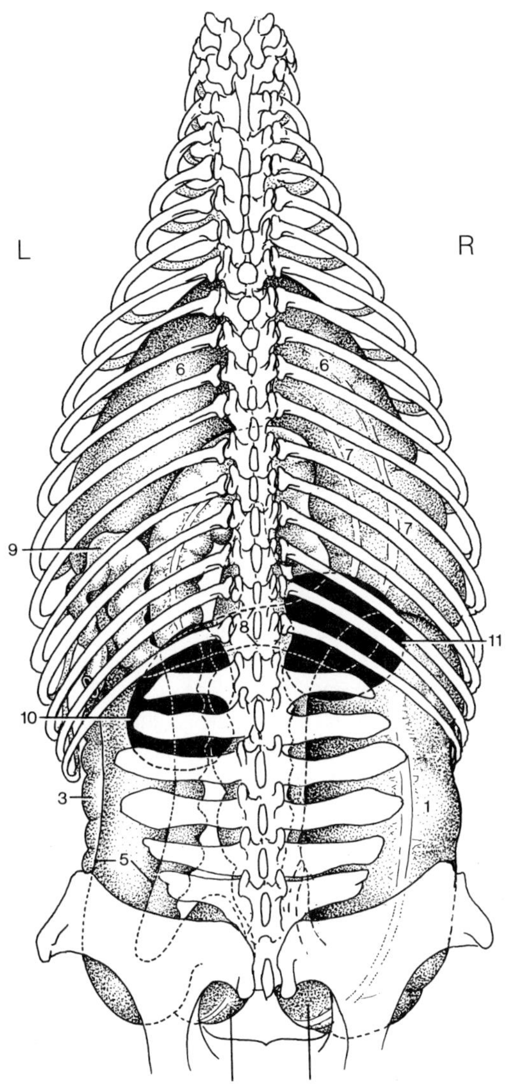


**Figure 21–18.** Position of the large intestine and the kidneys, dorsal view.

1, Base of cecum; 2, body of cecum; 3, left ventral colon; 4, pelvic flexure; 5, left dorsal colon; 6, dorsal diaphragmatic flexure; 7, right dorsal colon; 8, transverse colon; 9, proximal part of descending colon, cut; 10, left kidney; 11, right kidney.

## VASCULARIZATION, LYMPH DRAINAGE, AND INNERVATION OF THE GASTROINTESTINAL TRACT

The vascularization of the equine abdominal viscera is of great clinical importance because of the almost universal occurrence of vascular pathology caused by migrant nematode larvae. The fact that these lesions are not often fatal is due to the extensive system of anastomoses between the arteries supplying successive parts of the gastrointestinal tract. The pathology is often most serious in the cranial mesenteric artery and its major branches; these may be so greatly enlarged by aneurysm formation and by connective tissue reaction that the normal structure and topography are grossly disturbed. Paradoxically, obstruction of one of the large branches may have much less serious consequences than closure of a smaller one; the anastomoses of the major arteries are large and constant, those of the minor arteries small and often dangerously deficient. The caudal mesenteric artery, specifically concerned with the descending colon, is also commonly affected.

The branching and distribution of the two mesenteric arteries are shown in Figure 21–19. The celiac artery has essentially the same distribution to stomach, liver, and spleen as in other species. The venous drainage parallels the arterial supply, the portal vein being ultimately formed by the union of the caudal mesenteric, cranial mesenteric, and splenic tributaries.

Lymph from the regional nodes of the stomach, spleen, liver, pancreas, and diaphragm drains to a lymph center about the celiac artery and thence to the cisterna chyli via a celiac trunk.

The very numerous nodes that receive lymph from the intestines (with the exception of the caudal part of the descending colon) are scattered at the root of the mesentery and along the arteries of the cecum and colon. Lymph is collected and conveyed to the cisterna chyli by an intestinal trunk. The nodes scattered along the remainder of the descending colon send lymph to a center at the root of the colic mesentery and then to the lumbar trunk; this route is also followed by most of the lymph draining the rectum and anus.

The abdominal viscera are supplied by nerves that pass through plexuses associated with the mesenteric ganglia (Fig. 21–24/18,20). The nervous structures about the celiac and cranial mesenteric arteries may be involved in the reaction provoked by the nematode larvae and are difficult to display satisfactorily except in juvenile animals. It is often asserted, although it remains unproven, that the "colic" pain and functional disturbance associated with helminth infestations are caused by secondary involvement of the nerves rather than by the primary vascular lesions.

## THE LIVER

The liver is quite variable in form and size but on average weighs about 5 kg in a saddle horse and thus accounts for about 1.5% of the body weight, a much smaller proportion than in carnivores.

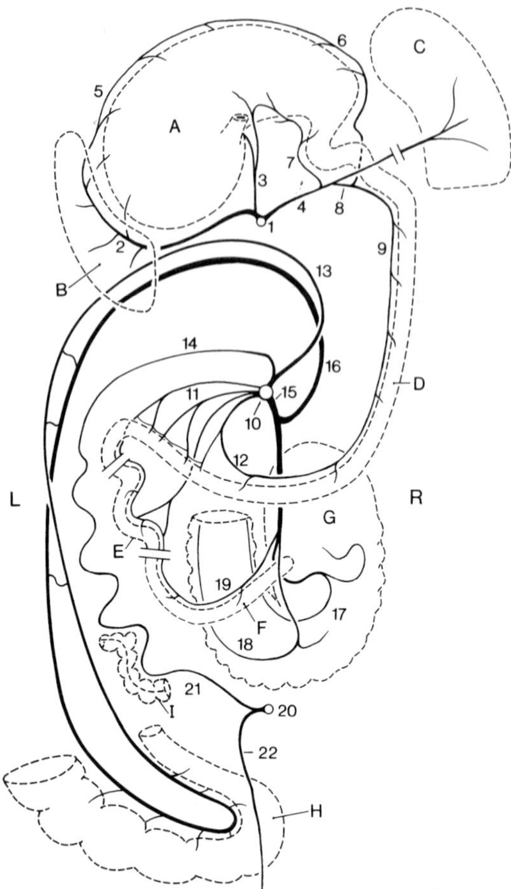


**Figure 21–19.** The major arteries of the gastrointestinal tract, schematic dorsal view. The structures have been stretched craniocaudally for clarity.

A, Stomach; B, spleen; C, liver; D, duodenum; E, jejunum; F, ileum; G, cecum; H, pelvic flexure; I, descending colon. 1, Celiac a.; 2, splenic a.; 3, left gastric a.; 4, hepatic a.; 5, left gastroepiploic a.; 6, right gastroepiploic a.; 7, right gastric a.; 8, gastroduodenal a.; 9, cranial pancreaticoduodenal a.; 10, cranial mesenteric a.; 11, jejunal aa.; 12, caudal pancreaticoduodenal a.; 13, right colic a.; 14, middle colic a; 15, ileocolic a.; 16, colic branch of ileocolic a.; 17, lateral cecal a.; 18, medial cecal a.; 19, mesenteric ileal a.; 20, caudal mesenteric a.; 21, left colic a.; 22, cranial rectal a.

It is situated in the most cranial part of the abdomen directly against the diaphragm. It is markedly asymmetrical in the healthy young subject, in which about two thirds lie to the right of the median plane (Fig. 21–7/2). The most caudal part, which is also the most dorsal, lies ventral to the vertebral extremities of the 16th and 17th ribs of the right side; the most cranial and most ventral part lies against the left part of the vertex of the diaphragm (Fig. 21–6/3 and Plate 23/*F,G*); the long axis thus runs obliquely. In the newborn foal the liver is relatively much larger and extends onto the abdominal floor behind the costal arch; it is also more symmetrical. In older subjects atrophy is common; this is most obvious in the right lobe and results from chronic pressure from the right dorsal colon and cecal base; less often, the left lobe atrophies under pressure from the stomach.

The parietal surface is joined to the diaphragm by a complicated system of ligaments. The visceral surface lies against and is impressed by the stomach, duodenum, dorsal diaphragmatic flexure of the colon, and cecal base (Fig. 21–10). The porta is central, within an area made rough by the direct attachment of the pancreas. The dorsal fixed margin of the liver extends between the right and left triangular ligaments and is very irregular (Fig. 21–20 and Plate 2/*F*). Its right part is thick and excavated to receive the cranial pole of the right kidney; a sulcus medial to this transmits the caudal vena cava (/7). Its left part is much thinner and does not extend nearly so far dorsally; it carries the impression of the esophagus close to the midline (/6). The long free margin is much sharper and is interrupted by a series of fissures of which the largest divide named lobes. The current nomenclature recognizes left, quadrate, right, and caudate lobes. The first two are separated by the fissure carrying the round ligament of the liver (vestige of the umbilical vein; /4), but the boundaries of the

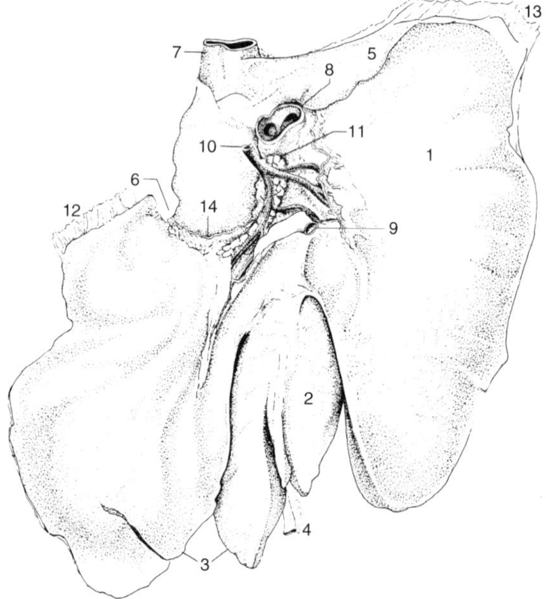


**Figure 21–20.** Visceral surface of the liver.

1, Right lobe; 2, quadrate lobe; 3, left lobe; 4, round ligament; 5, caudate process; 6, esophageal notch; 7, caudal vena cava; 8, portal vein; 9, bile duct; 10, hepatic artery; 11, hepatic lymph nodes; 12, left triangular ligament; 13, right triangular ligament; 14, lesser omentum.

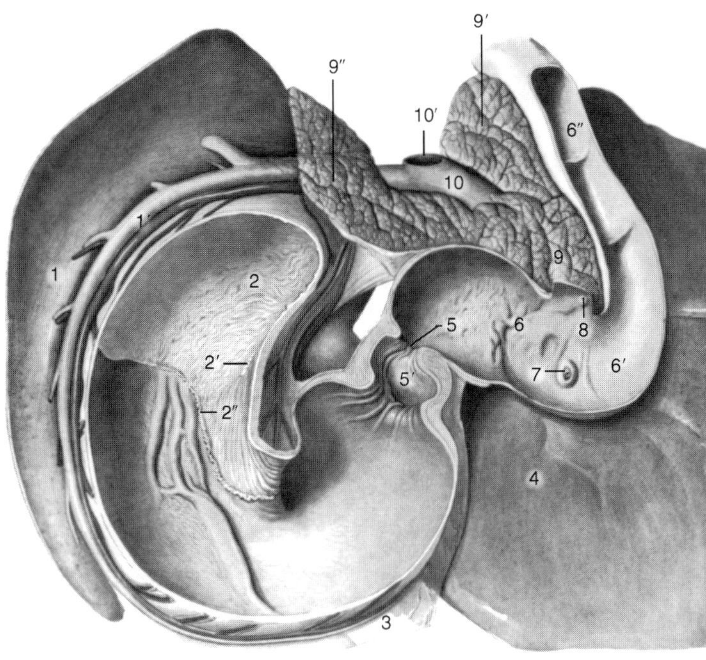


**Figure 21–21.** Topography of spleen, stomach, pancreas, and liver, caudoventral view.

1, Intestinal surface of spleen; 1′, splenic a. and v.; 2, fundus (blind sac) of stomach; 2′, cardia; 2″, margo plicatus; 3, greater omentum; 4, liver; 5, pyloric orifice; 5′, pyloric antrum; 6, S-shaped cranial part of duodenum; 6′, cranial flexure of duodenum; 6″, descending duodenum; 7, major duodenal papilla; 8, minor duodenal papilla; 9, body of pancreas; 9′, 9″, left and right lobes of pancreas; 10, portal v; 10′, stump of cranial mesenteric v.

others are more arbitrary and are of doubtful morphological significance.

The duct system is remarkable for the absence of a gallbladder, but its wide caliber compensates for this. The bile duct (/9) opens into the cranial duodenum on the papilla shared with the major pancreatic duct (Fig. 21–21/7). The oblique passage of the duct through the duodenal wall serves as a sphincter and prevents the influx of ingesta.

## THE PANCREAS

The pancreas lies largely to the right and is pressed against the abdominal roof and sublumbar organs (Fig. 21–10/7). It is triangular in outline with its apex fitted into the second concavity of the duodenal sigmoid flexure. The right border follows the descending duodenum; the left border passes obliquely toward the left kidney. The portal vein (Fig. 21–21/10) perforates the pancreas close to the caudal border. The ventral surface is directly bound to the right dorsal colon and cecal base, the dorsal surface to the right kidney and liver. The openings of its two ducts (/7,8) are described with the duodenum.

## THE KIDNEYS AND ADRENALS

The kidneys lie against the diaphragm and psoas muscles dorsally, each enclosed within a capsule of fat. The right kidney lies ventral to the last two or three ribs and first lumbar transverse process; the left one lies ventral to the last rib and first two or three processes and is thus about half a kidney length caudal to the level of its fellow (Fig. 21–18/10,11). Each kidney weighs about 700 g. The right one is shaped like the heart on a playing card, but the left one has a more conventional form. Both are dorsoventrally flattened (Fig. 21–22).

The cranial pole of the right kidney fits into the renal impression of the liver; caudal to this it is ventrally attached to the pancreas and the base of the cecum (Fig. 21–15/5,2). The duodenum winds around the lateral margin and adjoining part of the ventral surface, the only region sometimes covered with peritoneum. The short medial border is indented by the hilus and is related to the caudal vena cava and the right adrenal gland (Fig. 21–22).

The ventral surface of the left kidney has a more complete covering of peritoneum and is related to coils of small colon and small intestine, generally including the duodenojejunal junction. Cranioventrally it lies against the spleen; it may make contact with a distended stomach (Fig. 21–10). The medial border is related to the aorta and the left adrenal gland (Fig. 21–22).

The kidneys are of a modified unipyramidal type; the numerous constituent pyramids are completely fused, their former boundaries being revealed only by the arrangement of the interlobar arteries. A clearer indication of the lobation, with some external fissuration, is common in the foal. The structure is best revealed in section

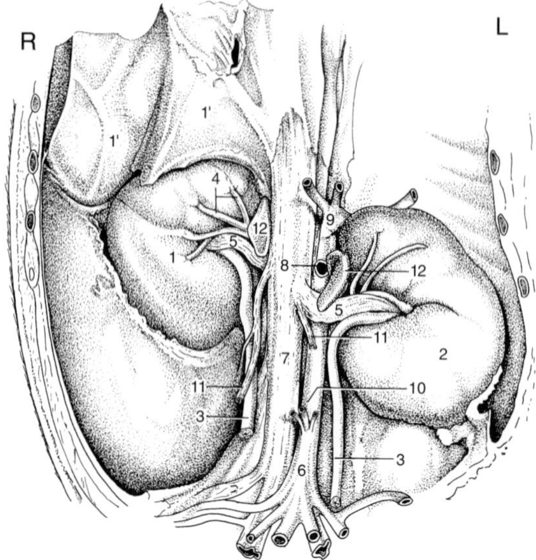


**Figure 21–22.** Kidneys and adrenal glands in situ, ventral view.

1, Right kidney; 1′, liver; 2, left kidney; 3, ureter; 4, renal artery; 5, renal vein; 6, aorta; 7, caudal vena cava; 8, cranial mesenteric artery; 9, celiac artery; 10, caudal mesenteric and testicular arteries; 11, testicular veins; 12, adrenal glands.

(Fig. 21–23). The strong external fibrous capsule can normally be easily stripped away, except within the renal sinus where it merges with the adventitia of the structures entering and leaving. The division of the parenchyma between cortex and medulla is indicated by a color change and by the sectioned arcuate arteries. The cortex is brownish red and granular. The peripheral part of the medulla is dark red, the inner part pale; both show radial striations. The apices of the fused medullary pyramids form a common renal crest that projects into the pelvis. This has a curious form consisting of a central expansion (/4) at the origin of the ureter and two terminal recesses toward the poles (/5); most papillary ducts open into the recesses. The pelvic mucosa produces a mucous secretion, and as a result the unfiltered urine normally contains some protein (physiological albuminuria).

The renal vessels are short and wide. The artery often splits before reaching the hilus, and a number of branches may enter the ventral surface independently (/8).

The ureters are wide at their origin but soon reduce to a narrow, more uniform caliber. They bend caudally on emerging from the renal sinus and thereafter pursue a tortuous course over the roof of the abdomen to reach the pelvis. Here they follow the lateral parts of the broad ligaments (genital fold in the male) before inclining medially to pierce the bladder wall close to its neck.

The elongated and irregular *adrenal glands* lie against the cranial parts of the medial borders of the corresponding kidneys (Fig. 21–22/12). Each consists of an outer bright-yellow cortex and an inner brownish-red medulla. The glands are relatively large in juvenile animals.

## THE ROOF OF THE ABDOMEN

The bodies of the lumbar vertebrae, the sublumbar muscles, and the diaphragm furnish the roof of the abdomen. The aorta and caudal vena cava lie within the cleft between the two psoas minor muscles, the artery to the left, the vein to the right (/6,7). The branches of the aorta and the tributaries of the vein are, in principle, the same as in other species.

The autonomic nerves and ganglia show some specifically equine features, although these are matters of detail rather than of substance. The general pattern is shown in Figure 21–24. The fused celiac and cranial mesenteric ganglia lie ventral to the aorta, to each side of the celiac and cranial mesenteric arteries. The right and left ganglia are joined by bridges cranial and caudal to

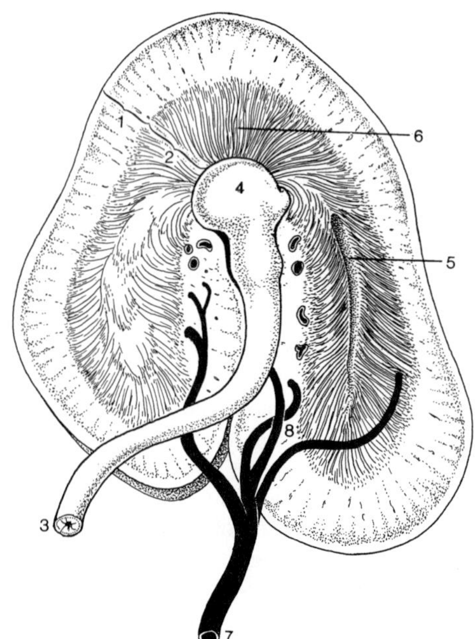


**Figure 21–23.** Dorsal section through the kidney, semischematic.

1, Renal cortex; 2, renal medulla; 3, ureter; 4, pelvis; 5, terminal recess; 6, papillary ducts; 7, renal artery; 8, interlobar arteries.

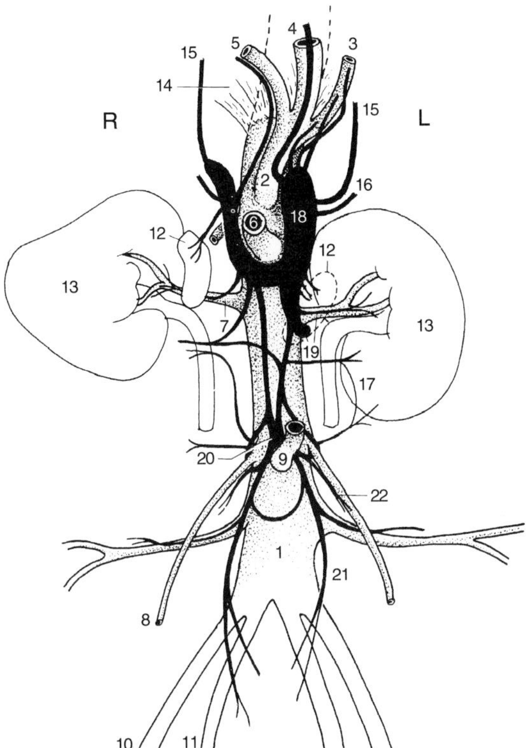


**Figure 21-24.** Schema of the abdominal autonomic nerves and branches of the abdominal aorta, ventral view.

1, Aorta; 2, celiac a.; 3, splenic a.; 4, left gastric a.; 5, hepatic a.; 6, cranial mesenteric a.; 7, renal a.; 8, testicular (ovarian) a.; 9, caudal mesenteric a.; 10, external iliac a.; 11, internal iliac a.; 12, adrenal glands; 13, kidneys; 14, crus of diaphragm; 15, major splanchnic nn.; 16, minor splanchnic nn.; 17, lumbar splanchnic nn.; 18, combined celiac and cranial mesenteric ganglia; 19, renal plexus; 20, caudal mesenteric ganglion; 21, hypogastric n.; 22, testicular (ovarian) plexus.

the latter artery. They are sizable structures, 5 cm or so long, and are generally unequal, the left complex being larger and more regular than the right one (/18). Each is joined by a major splanchnic nerve and, in varying fashion, by parasympathetic fibers from the dorsal vagal trunk. The nerves that leave the ganglia follow the arteries, branching where these branch and forming a dense plexus in which the sympathetic and parasympathetic contributions mingle. The whole plexiform arrangement that radiates from the major ganglia is known as the celiacomesenteric (solar) plexus. Additional small renal ganglia occur on the nerves about the renal arteries.

The celiacomesenteric complex is joined to the caudal mesenteric plexus by a plexus on the aorta and an additional trunk that runs at a more ventral level within the colic mesentery.

The caudal mesenteric ganglion lies cranial to the origin of the like-named artery (/20,9). It gives rise to nerve plexuses that follow this vessel and the gonadal vessels to the small colon and reproductive organs, respectively, and to the hypogastric nerves (/21) that pursue a retroperitoneal course on the roof of the pelvis. Lumbar splanchnic nerves join the major ganglia and the aortic plexus in an erratic fashion.

The usual direct detachment of preganglionic fibers from the splanchnic nerves to the medullary parts of the adrenal glands exists.

## Selected Bibliography

Alexander, R.M.: The relative merits of foregut and hindgut fermentation. J. Zool. 231:391–402, 1993.

Archer, R.M., W.A. Lindsay, D.F. Smith, et al.: Vascular anatomy of the equine small colon. Am. J. Vet. Res. 50:893–897, 1989.

Bernard, W.V., V.B. Reef, J.M. Reimer, et al.: Ultrasonographic diagnosis of small intestinal intussusception in three foals. JAVMA 194:395–397, 1989.

Bertone, A.L., T.S. Stashak, and K.E. Sullins: Large colon resection and anastomosis in horses. JAVMA 188:612–617, 1986.

Bertone, A.L., T.S. Stashak, K.E. Sullins, and S.L. Ralston: Experimental large colon resection at the cecocolic ligament in the horse. Vet. Surg. 16:5–12, 1987.

Blikslager, A.T., K.F. Bowman, M.L. Haven, et al.: Pedunculated lipomas as a cause of intestinal obstruction in horses: 17 cases (1983–1990). JAVMA 201:1249–1252, 1992.

Boure, L., M. Marcoux, and S. Laverty: Laparoscopic abdominal anatomy of foals positioned in dorsal recumbency. Vet. Surg. 26:1–6, 1997.

Burns, G.A.: The teniae of the equine intestinal tract. Cornell Vet. 82:187–212, 1992.

Burns, G.A., and J.F. Cummings: Equine myenteric plexus with special reference to the pelvic flexure pacemaker. Anat. Rec. 230:417–424, 1991.

Byars, T.D., L.W. George, and D.S. Beisel: A laboratory technique for teaching rectal palpation in the horse. J. Vet. Med. Educ. 7:80–82, 1980.

Campbell, M.L., N. Ackerman, and L.C. Peyton: Radiographic gastrointestinal anatomy of the foal. Vet. Radiol. Ultrasound 25:194–204, 1984.

Collatos, C., and S. Romano: Cecal impaction in horses: Causes, diagnosis, and medical treatment. Compend. Contin. Educ. Pract. Vet. 15:976–981, 1993.

Dart, A.J., J.R. Snyder, and F.A. Harmon: Microvascular circulation of the descending colon in horses. Am. J. Vet. Res. 53:1001–1006, 1992.

Dart, A.J., J.R. Snyder, D. Julian, and D.M. Hinds: Microvascular circulation of the cecum in horses. Am. J. Vet. Res. 52:1545–1550, 1991.

Dart, A.J., J.R. Snyder, D. Julian, and D.M. Hinds: Microvascular circulation of the small intestine in horses. Am. J. Vet. Res. 53:995–1000, 1992.

Dik, K.J., and I. Gunsser: Atlas of Diagnostic Radiology of the Horse, Parts 1–3. Philadelphia, W.B. Saunders Company, 1988–1990.

Dyce, K.M., and W. Hartman: An endoscopic study of the cecal base of the horse. Tijdschr. Diergeneeskd. 98:957–962, 1973.

Dyce, K.M., W. Hartman, and R.H.G. Aalfs: A cinefluoroscopic study of the cecal base of the horse. Res. Vet. Sci. 20:40–46, 1976.

Fischer, A.T., and D.M. Meagher: Strangulating torsions of the equine large colon. Compend. Contin. Educ. Pract. Vet. 8:S25–S30, 1986.

Fischer, A.T., and A.M. Vachon: Laparoscopic intra-abdominal ligation and removal of cryptorchid testes in horses. Equine Vet. J. 30:105–108, 1998.

Foerner, J.J., M.J. Ringle, D.S. Junkins, et al.: Transection of the pelvic flexure to reduce incarceration of the large colon through the epiploic foramen in a horse. JAVMA 203:1312–1313, 1993.

Fontaine, G.L., D.H. Rodgerson, R.R. Hanson, et al.: Ultrasound evaluation of equine gastrointestinal disorders. Compend. Contin. Educ. Pract. Vet. 21:253–262, 1999.

Ford, T.S., D.E. Freeman, M.W. Ross, et al.: Ileocecal intussusception in horses: 26 cases (1981–1988). JAVMA 196:121–126, 1990.

Galuppo, L.D., J.R. Snyder, and J.R. Pascoe: Laparoscopic anatomy of the equine abdomen. Am. J. Vet. Res. 56:518–531, 1995.

Galuppo, L.D., J.R. Snyder, J.R. Pascoe, et al.: Laparoscopic anatomy of the abdomen in dorsally recumbent horses. Am. J. Vet. Res. 57:923–931, 1996.

Gift, L.J., E.M. Gaughan, R.M. DeBowes, et al.: Jejunal insussusception in adult horses: 11 cases (1981–1991). JAVMA 202:110–112, 1993.

Habel, R.E., and K.D. Budras: Anatomy of the prepubic tendon in the horse, cow, sheep, goat, and dog. Am. J. Vet. Res. 53:2183–2195, 1992.

Hackett, M.S., and R.P. Hackett: Chronic ileocecal intussusception in horses. Cornell Vet. 79:353–361, 1989.

Hackett, R.P.: Nonstrangulated colonic displacement in horses. JAVMA 182:235–240, 1983.

Hance, S.R., and R.M. Embertson: Colopexy in broodmares: 44 cases (1986–1990). JAVMA 201:782–787, 1992.

Hance, S.R., R.M. DeBowes, M.F. Clem, and R.D. Welch: Umbilical, inguinal, and ventral hernias in horses. Compend. Contin. Educ. Pract. Vet. 12:862–871, 1990.

Harrison, I.W.: Equine large intestinal volvulus. Vet. Surg. 17:77–81, 1988.

Huskamp, B.: Diagnosis of gastroduodeno-jejunitis and its surgical treatment by a temporary duodenocaecostomy. Equine Vet. 17:314–316, 1985.

Jakowski, R.M.: Right hepatic lobe atrophy in horses: 17 cases (1983–1993). JAVMA 204:1057–1061, 1994.

Janis, C.: The evolutionary strategy of the Equidae and the origins of rumen and caecal digestion. Evolution 30:757–774, 1976.

Kiper, M.L., J. Traub-Dargatz, and C.R. Curtis: Gastric rupture in horses: 50 cases (1979–1987). JAVMA 196:333–336, 1990.

Kotze, S.H.: Arterial blood supply to the ileocaecal junction in the horse J. S. Afr. Vet. Assoc. 61:2–4, 1990.

McCarthy, P.H.: Eyes at the tips of your fingers: The anatomy of the abdominal and pelvic viscera of the narcotized horse as perceived by palpation during exploratory laparotomy. The Australian Equine Research Foundation, 1986. [c/o Peat, Marwick, Mitchell & Co., 500 Bourke St., Melbourne, Victoria 3000, Australia.]

Murray, J.M.: Gastric ulceration in horses: 91 cases (1987–1990). JAVMA 201:117–120, 1992.

Popesko, P.: Atlas of Topographic Anatomy of the Domestic Animals, vol. 2: Thoracic and Abdominal Cavities. Philadelphia, W.B. Saunders Company, 1971.

Ragle, C.A., and R.K. Schneider: A ventral abdominal technique for laparoscopic ovariectomy in equids. Vet. Surg. 24:492–497, 1995.

Ragle, C.A., L.L. Southwood, and R.K. Schneider: Injury to abdominal wall vessels during laparoscopy in three horses. JAVMA 212:87–89, 1998.

Ross, M.W., W.J. Donawick, A.F. Sellers, and J.E. Lowe: Normal motility of the cecum and right ventral colon in ponies. Am. J. Vet. Res. 47:1756–1762, 1986.

Santschi, E.M., D.E. Slone, Jr., and W.M. Frank, II: Use of ultrasound in horses for diagnosis of left dorsal displacement of the large colon and monitoring its nonsurgical correction. Vet. Surg. 22:281–284, 1993.

Schebitz, H., and H. Wilkens: Atlas of Radiographic Anatomy of the Horse, 4th ed. Berlin, Paul Parey Verlag, 1986.

Schusser, G.F., and N.A. White: Morphologic and quantitative evaluation of the myenteric plexus and neurons in the large colon of horses. JAVMA 210:928–934, 1997.

Sellers, A.F., and J.E. Lowe: Review of large intestinal motility and mechanisms of impaction in the horse. Equine Vet. J. 18:261–263, 1986.

Sellers, A.L., J.E. Lowe, C.J. Drost, et al.: Retropulsion-propulsion in equine large colon. Am. J. Vet. Res. 43:390–396, 1982.

Sivula, N.J.: Renosplenic entrapment of the large colon in horses: 33 cases (1984–1989). JAVMA 199:244–246, 1991.

Snyder, J.R., W.S Tyler, J.R. Pascoe, et al.: Microvascular circulation of the ascending colon in horses. Am. J. Vet. Res. 50:2075–2083, 1989.

Steenhaut, M., I. Vandenreyt, and M. van Roy: Incarceration of the large colon through the epiploic foramen in a horse. Equine Vet. J. 25:550–551, 1993.

Stickle, P.L., and J.F. Fessler: Retrospective study of 350 cases of equine cryptorchidism. JAVMA 172:343–346, 1978.

Vachon, A.M., and A.T. Fischer: Small intestinal herniation through the epiploic foramen: 53 cases (1987–1993). Equine Vet. J. 27:373–380, 1995.

Wallace, K.D., B.A. Selcer, and J.L. Becht: Transrectal ultrasonography of the cranial mesenteric artery of the horse. Am. J. Vet. Res. 50:1699–1703, 1989.

White, N.A., II: Surgical exploration of the equine intestinal tract for acute abdominal disease. Compend. Contin. Educ. Pract. Vet. 10:955–966, 1988.

White, N.A.: The Equine Acute Abdomen. Philadelphia, Lea & Febiger, 1990.

CHAPTER 22

# The Pelvis and Reproductive Organs of the Horse

This chapter is concerned with the pelvic cavity and its contents, and with the extrapelvic parts of the reproductive organs of both sexes. It also includes a brief account of the udder. The general conformation of the region and the surface landmarks created by the pelvic skeleton are dealt with in Chapter 24.

## GENERAL ANATOMY OF THE PELVIS AND PERINEUM

The pelvic cavity is roofed by the sacrum and first two or three caudal vertebrae—it is impossible to be more specific since an arbitrary element exists in the definition of the outlet. The roof narrows from front to back and is slightly concave in its length. The ischial tuber and spine are both less prominent than in cattle, and the contribution of the substantial sacrosciatic ligament to the lateral wall is therefore relatively greater (Fig. 22–1/7). The floor is solid since the symphysis is firmly fused in mature animals. It is more or less horizontal and flat in its length, though somewhat hollowed from side to side. The pubic region presents a median swelling or ridge in young animals, but while it retains this conformation in the stallion, the bone thins and the upper surface becomes markedly excavated in mares, especially those that have carried several foals.

The entrance to the pelvic cavity faces cranioventrally; its slope places the pubic brim below the third, or even fourth, sacral vertebra in the mare but only the second in the stallion. Viewed from the front, the inlet to the female pelvis is wide and rounded while that of the male is more angular and cramped, particularly ventrally (Fig. 22–2). In both sexes, the outlet from the cavity is much smaller than the inlet; it is bounded by a caudal vertebra, the free edges of the sacrosciatic ligaments, and the ischial tubers and arch.

The cavity has the approximate form of a truncated cone with the longitudinal axis almost straight between the entrance and the exit (Fig. 22–3). The pelvis of the mare is thus more favorably formed for ease of parturition than that of the cow; the entrance is wide, the exit less confined, the cavity generally more capacious, the axis without marked deflection, and a greater part of the lateral walls composed of soft tissue.

The reader is referred to page 43 for a general account of the structure of the pelvis and to Figures 22–9 and 22–20 for an indication of the topography and peritoneal relationships of the viscera.

The most distinctive feature of the perineum is its confinement between the semimembranosus muscles, which extend ventrally from their vertebral heads of origin. These muscles cover the ischial tubers and also the ischiorectal fossae, which therefore do not contribute to the surface contour. Since the muscles bury the caudal borders of the sacrosciatic ligaments they hamper recognition of the softening that is so useful an indication of the approach of parturition in cattle.

The thin, sparsely haired, and deeply pigmented perineal skin obtains a surface sheen from the secretion of sebaceous glands. It is raised over the caudal part of the anal canal, forming a projection whose shape and salience vary with the functional state. The unusual outline of the vulva and its variable position are the subject of a later comment (p. 553). In the male the urethra may be palpated where it bends around the ischial arch.

The deeper structures of the perineum closely resemble their bovine counterparts, to which reference may be made (p. 695); differences in detail, though numerous, are not of practical significance.

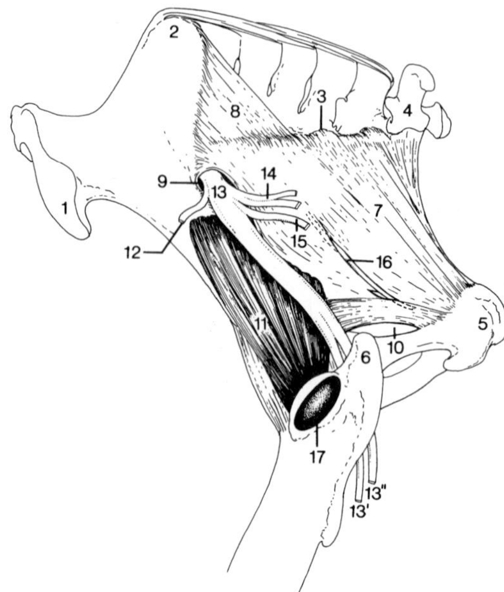


**Figure 22–1.** Lateral view of the bony pelvis and sacrosciatic ligament.

1, Coxal tuber; 2, sacral tuber; 3, lateral border of sacrum; 4, Cd1; 5, ischial tuber; 6, caudal part of greater trochanter; 7, sacrosciatic ligament; 8, dorsal sacroiliac ligament; 9, greater sciatic foramen; 10, lesser sciatic foramen; 11, gluteus profundus; 12, cranial gluteal nerve; 13, sciatic nerve; 13′, common peroneal nerve; 13″, tibial nerve; 14, caudal gluteal nerve; 15, caudal cutaneous femoral nerve; 16, pudendal nerve; 17, trochanteric bursa.

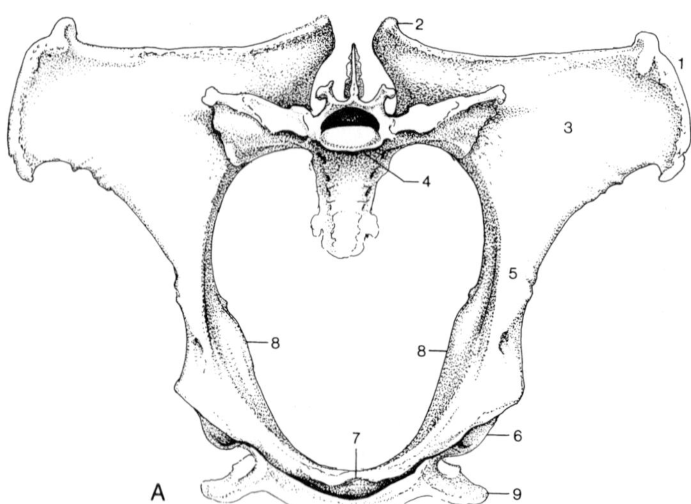


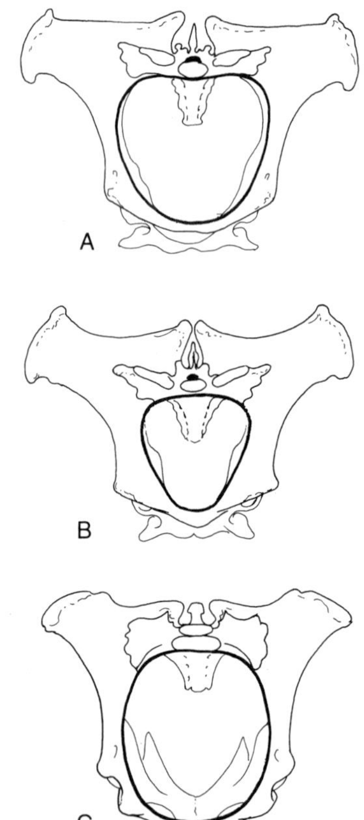


**Figure 22–2.** Cranial view of the pelves of the mare *(A)*, stallion *(B)*, and cow *(C)*. The terminal line is emphasized in the smaller pictures; observe the differences in the shape of the pelvic inlet and position of the ischial spines.

1, Coxal tuber; 2, sacral tuber; 3, wing of ilium; 4, promontory; 5, shaft of ilium; 6, acetabulum; 7, brim of pubis; 8, ischial spines; 9, ischial tuber.

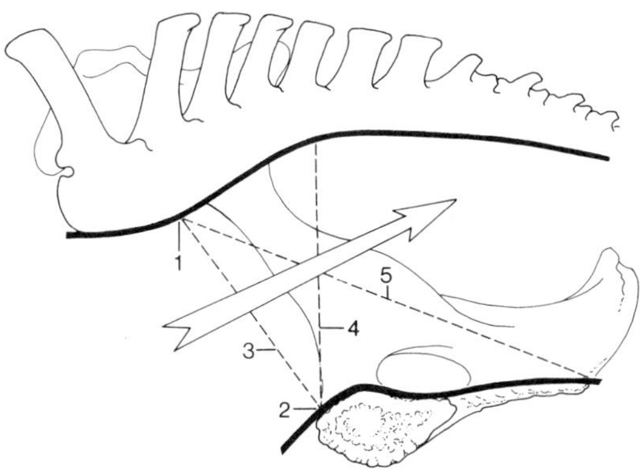


**Figure 22–3.** Schematic median section of the mare's pelvis illustrating certain obstetrical terms.

1, Promontory; 2, cranial end of the pelvic symphysis; 3, conjugata; 4, vertical diameter; 5, diagonal conjugata. The arrow indicates the axis of the pelvic canal.

## Innervation, Vascularization, and Lymph Drainage of the Pelvic Walls

The branches of the *lumbosacral plexus* that traverse the pelvis are considered at length on page 315 and only a few features are mentioned here. The obturator nerve follows the usual course over the medial aspect of the shaft of the ilium to reach the obturator foramen, and this exposes it to risk of injury in fractures of the bone or by compression when the mare is giving birth (Fig. 22–4/15). The nervous web from which the cranial gluteal, sciatic, and caudal gluteal nerves arise is exposed to similar risk where it lies against the ventral aspect of the sacrum, en route to the greater sciatic foramen (/13).

The pudendal nerve (/12) arises from the middle sacral nerves (S[2]3–4) and heads in the direction

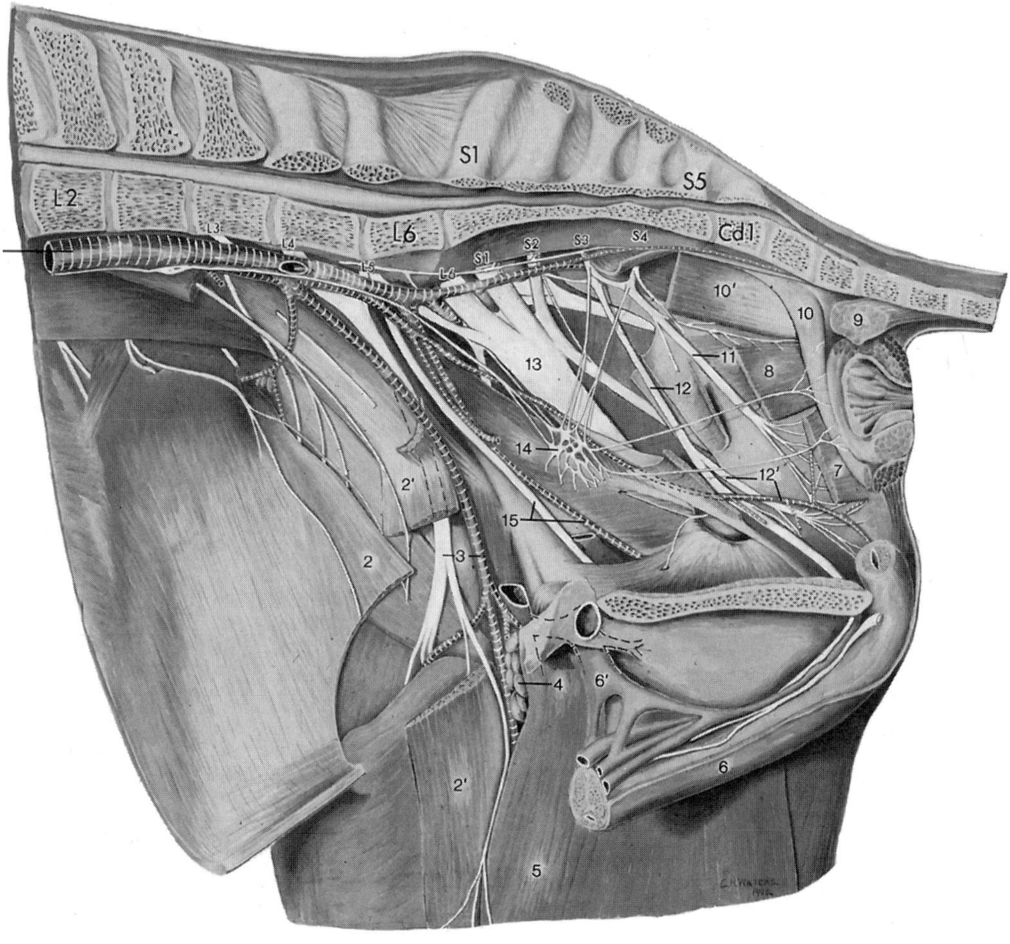

**Figure 22–4.** Dissection of the pelvic wall; medial view.

1, Aorta; 2, internal abdominal oblique; 2′, sartorius, resected; 3, femoral a. and n.; 4, deep inguinal lymph nodes; 5, gracilis; 6, penis; 6′, (accessory) external pudendal v.; 7, levator ani, resected; 8, coccygeus; 9, rectococcygeus; 10, retractor penis; 10′, ventral tail muscle; 11, caudal rectal n.; 12, pudendal n.; 12′, deep perineal n. and internal pudendal a.; 13, sciatic n.; 14, pelvic plexus; 15, obturator n., and vessels.

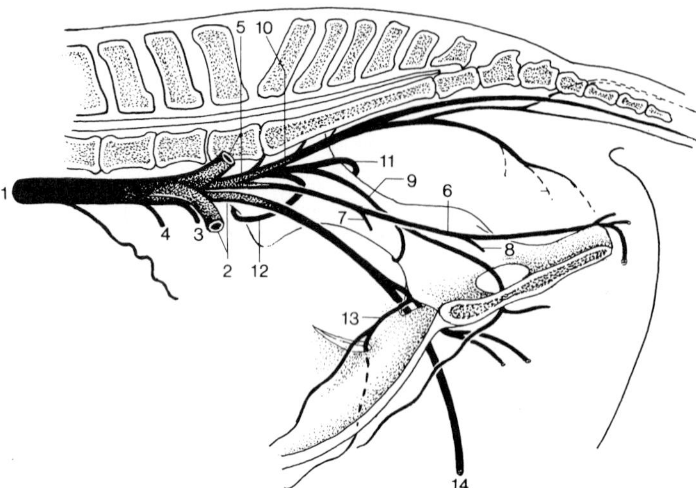


**Figure 22–5.** The principal arteries on the right wall of the pelvic cavity, medial view.

1, Aorta; 2, external iliac a. (and left stump); 3, uterine a.; 4, deep circumflex iliac a.; 5, internal iliac a. (and left stump); 6, internal pudendal a.; 7, umbilical a.; 8, prostatic (vaginal) a.; 9, obturator a.; 10, caudal gluteal a.; 11, cranial gluteal a.; 12, iliolumbar a.; 13, pudendoepigastric trunk; 14, femoral a.

of the ischial tuber. The nerve first runs internal to the sacrosciatic ligament but later becomes embedded within its substance. As the nerve passes the lesser sciatic foramen it exchanges fibers with the caudal cutaneous nerve of the thigh through the opening. It later splits into several branches of which the most important is the deep perineal nerve (/12′). The main trunk continues to the clitoris or penis. The deep perineal is concerned with the innervation of the striated musculature of the perineum. The superficial branch is sensory to the anus, vulva, and perineal skin as far ventrally as the udder (or scrotum and prepuce).

The caudal rectal nerve (/11), which arises from the same sacral nerves (S[2]3–4), is motor to the striated muscles of the dorsal part of the perineum and sensory to the rectum, wall of the anal canal, and adjacent skin.

The pelvic nerves (/14) are deployed in the usual fashion and are composed of parasympathetic fibers from the second, third, and fourth sacral nerves.

The *blood supply* to the pelvic contents and walls is attended to by the internal iliac arteries, terminal branches of the abdominal aorta (Fig. 22–5/5). The very short internal iliac artery passes below the wing of the ilium and soon divides into internal pudendal and caudal gluteal arteries. The internal pudendal artery (/6) has a mainly visceral distribution. It runs caudoventrally on the deep face of the sacrosciatic ligament, close to the pudendal nerve, before swinging medially to divide about the level of the ischial spine. Its branches include the umbilical artery, which conveys a little blood to the vertex of the bladder (and the adjacent part of the deferent duct in the male) and a much more important branch that supplies the bulk of the intrapelvic reproductive organs. This is known as the vaginal artery (/8) in the female, in which it supplies the greater part of the bladder, the urethra, the caudal part of the uterus, the vagina, and, by way of the middle rectal artery, a substantial part of the rectum. The homologous prostatic artery supplies the bladder, the urethra, the accessory genital glands, and the corresponding part of the rectum. End branches of the internal pudendal include the caudal rectal artery to rectum and anus, a (ventral) perineal artery for the tissues between anus and vulva, and branches to the vestibule and the vestibular bulb; the male counterpart of the last-named is the artery of the penis, which anastomoses with divisions of the obturator (/9).

The caudal gluteal artery (/10) passes caudally in the dorsolateral wall of the pelvis; it branches off the obturator and cranial gluteal arteries. The trunk pierces the sacrosciatic ligament before supplying the hamstring muscles and the tail. The obturator artery leaves the pelvis through the obturator foramen, the cranial gluteal artery through the greater sciatic foramen.

The veins largely mirror the patterns of the arteries.

The *lymph nodes* associated with the pelvic walls display the usual species characteristics, comprising numerous, closely packed, and individually small nodes that aggregate to form sizable masses. The major groupings are related to the termination and parietal branches of the aorta. Sacral nodes lie between the divergent internal iliac arteries, medial iliac nodes at the origin (from the external iliac) of the deep circumflex iliac arteries, and lateral iliac nodes at the terminal division of the latter.

Other, anorectal, nodes lie over the caudal part of the rectum. In the horse the deep inguinal nodes

(Fig. 22–4/4) lie outside the pelvic cavity, within the femoral triangle and at no great distance from the superficial inguinal nodes. The latter are interposed between the prepuce and scrotum (or udder) and the trunk. They drain lymph from the external reproductive organs (and udder), and from the skin and deeper structures over a considerable part of the ventral trunk. This lymph is then channeled to the deep inguinal nodes, which also receive most lymph from the hindlimb, a part after prior filtration through the nodes in the popliteal fossa. The outflow goes to the medial iliac nodes, which constitute the collecting center for lymph emanating from the caudal abdominal and pelvic walls, and from the pelvic viscera. Much of this lymph has already passed through anorectal, sacral, or lateral iliac nodes. The outflow is either to the aortic lumbar nodes of the abdominal roof or directly to an erratically formed lumbar trunk.

## THE RECTUM AND ANAL CANAL

The principal features of visceral topography and peritoneal disposition are shown in Figures 22–6, 22–7, and 22–8.

The rectum continues the descending colon beyond the pelvic inlet. Initially it resembles the colon in structure and in relationship to the peritoneum, but as it proceeds caudally the mesentery shortens and the peritoneal covering is gradually lost (commencing with the dorsal aspect); finally the rectum is wholly retroperitoneal and embedded in a fat-rich connective tissue. The proportion of the rectum that is retroperitoneal appears to vary between individuals. Perforations of the wall of the rectum are the unfortunate and highly embarrassing mishaps that occasionally complicate rectal exploration. The terminal part of the rectum loses the sacculated character and forms a wide flasklike expansion (ampulla) just before it joins the anal canal. The ampulla stores feces prior to evacuation. A change of lesser importance is the regrouping of the dorsal and lateral longitudinal muscle into bundles that break free, pass above the anus, and anchor the rectum to the fourth or fifth caudal vertebra; these bundles constitute the smooth rectococcygeus (Fig. 22–4/9).

The relations of the rectum depend on its fullness and on the sex. In the mare, the rectum lies on the uterus and vagina unless, as often happens, these are displaced to one side and the rectum is enabled to make contact with the bladder. In male animals the ventral surface lies on the bladder, the urethra, and the accessory reproductive glands; the extents of the individual contacts depend on the state of the bladder and the development of the glands, which are naturally smaller in the gelding.

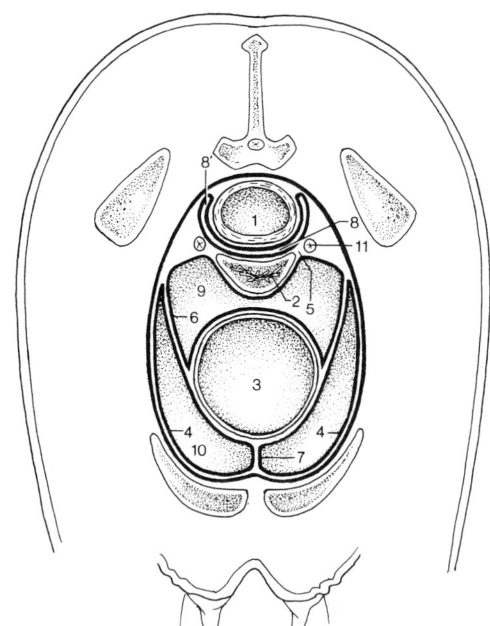


**Figure 22–7.** The disposition of the peritoneum in the pelvis of the mare (transverse section).

1, Rectum; 2, vagina; 3, bladder; 4, parietal peritoneum; 5, broad ligament; 6, lateral ligament of bladder; 7, median ligament of bladder; 8, rectogenital pouch; 8′, pararectal fossa; 9, vesicogenital pouch; 10, pubovesical pouch; 11, ureter.

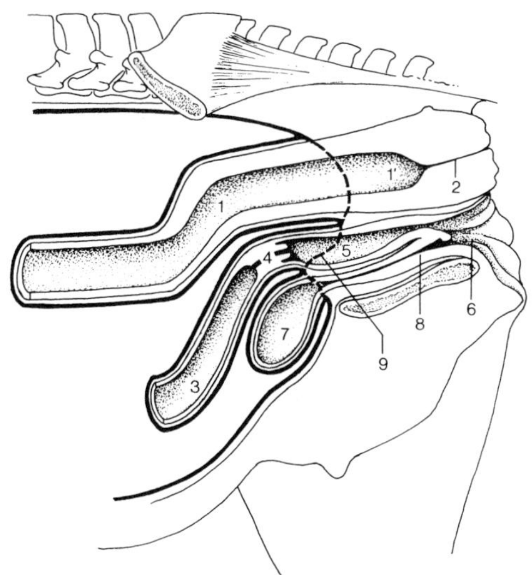


**Figure 22–6.** Schematic median section of the pelvis of the mare.

1, 1′, Peritoneal and retroperitoneal parts of the rectum; 2, anal canal; 3, uterus; 4, cervix; 5, vagina; 6, vestibule; 7, bladder; 8, urethra; 9, caudal extent of peritoneum.

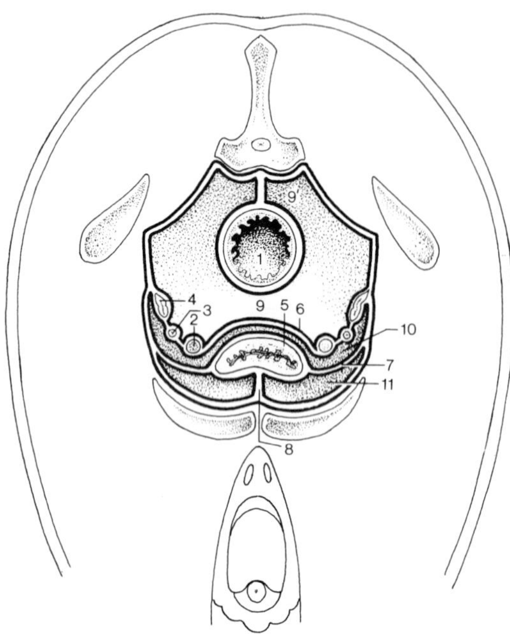


**Figure 22–8.** The disposition of the peritoneum in the pelvis of the stallion (transverse section).

1, Rectum; 2, deferent duct; 3, ureter; 4, vesicular gland; 5, bladder; 6, genital fold; 7, lateral ligament of bladder; 8, median ligament of bladder; 9, rectogenital pouch; 9′, pararectal fossa; 10, vesicogenital pouch; 11, pubovesical pouch.

The anal canal continues the rectum but, unlike this, is generally empty of feces. It is closed by the apposition and interdigitation of longitudinal mucosal folds and by the contraction of the internal and external anal sphincters. The extent of the canal is sharply defined by anorectal and anocutaneous lines marking the limits of epithelial specialization. The canal is embraced by the pelvic diaphragm (/7,8); the part caudal to the pelvic diaphragm projects as a cylindrical eminence within the perineal region.

## THE BLADDER AND FEMALE URETHRA

The neck region of the bladder lies directly on the pelvic floor, and when the organ is fully contracted it forms a firm, globular swelling about the size of a clenched fist; it is so far withdrawn into the pelvic cavity that it is almost wholly retroperitoneal. As the bladder fills it gradually assumes a more ovoid form and extends cranially over the abdominal wall.

The relations of the bladder depend on the degree of filling and on the sex. When empty, its vertex is generally in contact with the pelvic flexure of the colon, but as the bladder enlarges, the vertex and adjacent parts obtain a more extensive and more varied relationship to the intestine. In the mare the dorsal surface is in contact with the cranial part of the vagina, the cervix, a variable part of the body of the uterus, and sometimes the rectum (Fig. 22–9). The corresponding relations in the male are the genital fold, the deferent ducts, the vesicular glands, the prostate, and the rectum.

The relatively large neonatal bladder is entirely intra-abdominal. It slowly adjusts to the adult proportions and position with the postnatal enlargement of the pelvis and the development of the intestines. Leakage at the navel from a still-patent urachus is not uncommon in the first period after birth and provides a potential portal for infection.

The female urethra is very short, only 6 cm or thereabouts, and opens into the vestibule, immediately caudal to the transverse fold of the hymen. It is rather wide; it admits one finger without difficulty and by gentle manipulation may be persuaded, with low epidural anesthesia, to accept a small hand—convenient when returning a bladder prolapse or removing a kidney or bladder stone from the bladder. The shortness, wide caliber, and dilatable nature of the urethra permit occasional prolapse of the bladder into the vestibule.

The male urethra is described with the reproductive organs.

## THE FEMALE REPRODUCTIVE ORGANS

The anatomy of the female reproductive organs is strongly influenced by age, present status, and previous reproductive history. The initial description refers to the mature, parous but nongravid mare (Fig. 22–10).

### The Ovaries

The ovaries scarcely descend from the sites where they develop initially, and they commonly lie in the dorsal part of the abdomen, cranioventral to the iliac wings, approximately in the plane of the fifth lumbar vertebra. Each is suspended by a thick mesovarium that allows the ovary considerable latitude in position (Fig. 22–9/16). The length of the mesovarium is such that the ovary may generally be brought into, but not through, a flank incision.

In comparison with those of other species, the ovaries of the mare are conspicuously large;

indeed, in a large draft mare they may measure as much as 8 to 10 cm along the major axis. They are also remarkable for their shape since the free border is deeply indented to form an "ovulation fossa," the site of rupture of the mature follicles (Fig. 22–11/4 and Plate 7/*G*). The internal structure also shows a departure from the usual arrangement. The follicles and corpora lutea are scattered within the central part of the organ and toward the ovulation fossa. They are enclosed within a dense, richly vascularized connective tissue casing that corresponds to the medulla of the ovary of other species. Because of this, even large follicles and corpora lutea do not form prominent surface elevations, and their identification on rectal exploration is more difficult than in the cow. A change in hue marks the boundary between the covering of the fossa and the common peritoneum that clothes the remainder of the organ. The position, the form, the consistency, and the general absence of marked surface projections characterize the ovaries sufficiently to allow them to be easily recognized on rectal examination; even so, notorious incidents are recorded in which feces-filled pouches of small colon were mistakenly removed in the blind ovariectomy procedure that is performed per vaginam.

## The Uterine Tubes

The uterine tube measures about 20 cm when extended but in nature follows a tortuous course that brings its beginning and end close together.

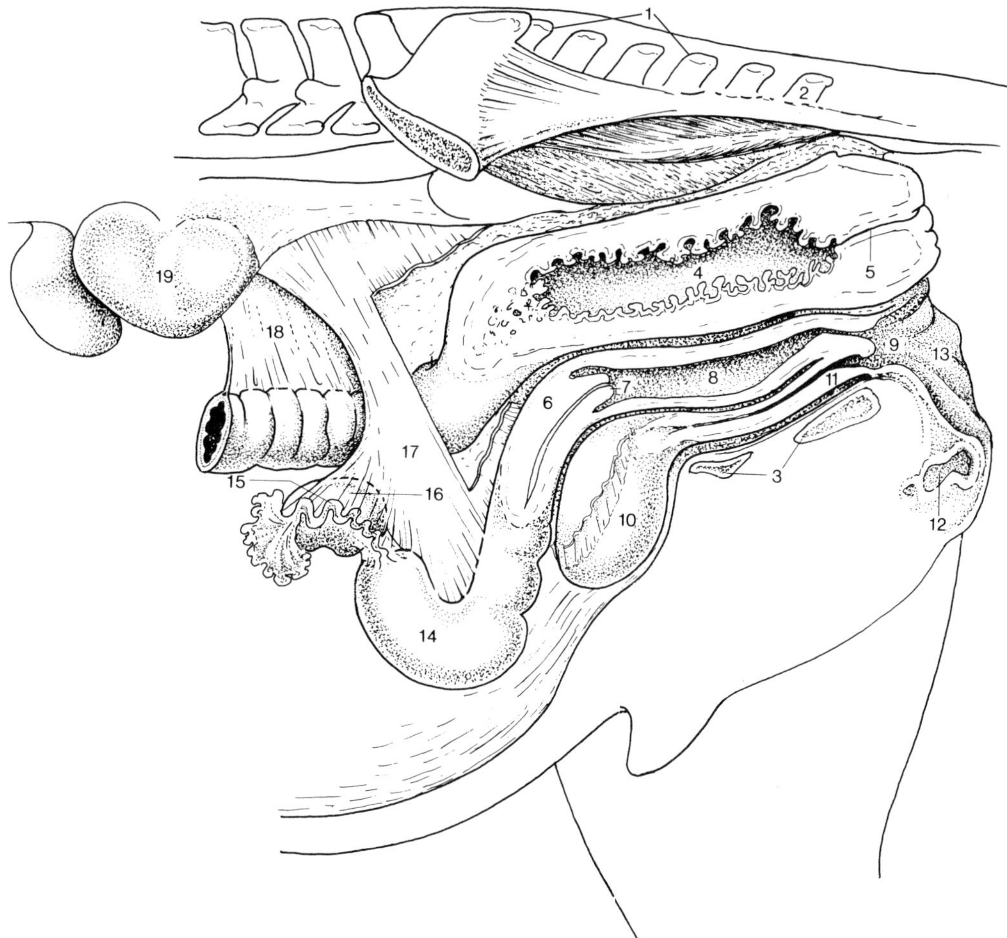


**Figure 22–9.** Caudal abdominal and pelvic organs of the mare in situ; the organs have been sectioned in a paramedian plane with the pelvis. Because of the absence of the intestines the ovaries hang much lower than they would in the intact animal.

1, Sacrum; 2, Cd2; 3, floor of pelvis; 4, rectum; 5, anal canal; 6, cervix; 7, vaginal part of cervix; 8, vagina; 9, vestibule; 10, bladder; 11, urethra; 12, clitoris; 13, vulva; 14, left uterine horn; 15, uterine tube; 16, ovary; 17, broad ligament (largely cut away); 18, descending mesocolon; 19, left kidney.

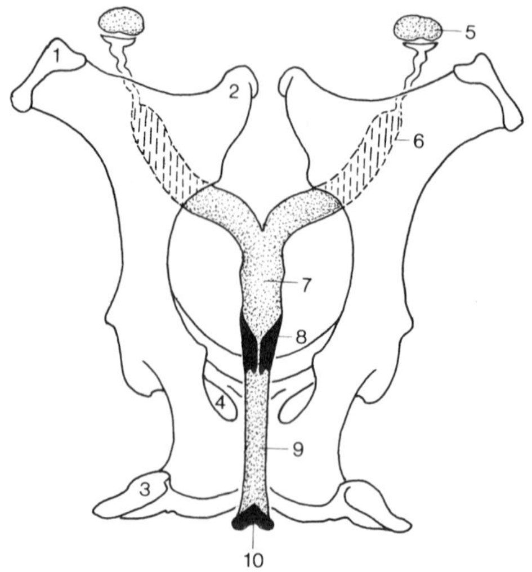


**Figure 22–10.** The female reproductive organs in relation to the pelvis, dorsal view.

1, Coxal tuber; 2, sacral tuber; 3, ischial tuber; 4, obturator foramen; 5, ovary; 6, uterine horn; 7, body of uterus; 8, cervix; 9, vagina; 10, vulva.

The infundibulum is margined by ragged fimbriae that spread over the surface of the ovary where some make permanent attachment (Fig. 22–12/2). A small opening in the depth of the infundibulum leads to the ampulla (/3), which is approximately 10 cm long and about 6 mm wide; its caliber at all stages of the cycle is greater than that of the isthmus, which is only half as wide. The isthmus (/4), also about 10 cm long, opens into the apex of the uterine horn through a small orifice on the summit of an eccentrically placed papilla. Strangely, this uterotubal junction is able in some way to distinguish between fertilized and infertile ova; the former are admitted to the uterus after the appropriate delay, the latter are denied entry. The tubal mucosa is plicated, especially within the ampulla where the elaborate major folds carry secondary and even tertiary ridges. The mesosalpinx, which supports the tube, branches from the lateral surface of the mesovarium and with this encloses a large but shallow ovarian bursa (/9 and see Fig. 5–49/*A*,5).

## The Uterus

The uterus has a large body and two divergent horns. The horns, which are about 25 cm long, lie wholly within the abdomen and diverge sharply from each other. They are suspended from the abdominal roof by the broad ligaments whose width varies so that the extremities of each horn are more tightly tethered than the intermediate part (Fig. 22–9/14). However, in life, the horns are usually raised toward the abdominal roof on the mass of intestines. The body of the uterus is a little shorter (≈20 cm) than the horns and lies in part within the abdomen, in part within the pelvis. Although its relations vary, they always include the terminal part of the descending colon and rectum dorsally, the bladder and various parts of the gut ventrally. The body is often displaced to one side by a distended bladder or by pressure from the gut. When the uterus is empty both horns and body are flattened and the lumen almost obliterated.

The cervix (/6) is rather short (≈6 cm). Although its position and extent are not readily distinguishable on visual inspection, they are at once revealed on palpation since the cervix has a somewhat firmer consistency. The caudal part of the cervix projects into the lumen of the vagina where it is surrounded by an annular space (fornix) of more or less uniform depth. This intravaginal part (/7) has a lobed appearance created by the extension through the external ostium of the mucosal folds lining the cervical canal. These folds continue onto the vaginal wall where they gradually subside. Except at estrus and parturition the cervical canal is closed, but not so tightly that it does not admit a finger on gentle probing (Fig. 22–13).

## The Vagina

The vagina is about as long as the body of the uterus. It lies ventral to the rectum, dorsal to the bladder and urethra, and in lateral contact with the pelvic wall (Figs. 22–9 and 22–14/8). Although it is largely retroperitoneal, the extent of the covering depends on the degrees of filling of the bladder and rectum (Fig. 22–6). A small cranial part of the ventral and a somewhat larger part of the dorsal aspect are always clad in peritoneum. This arrangement is useful since incision of the dorsal part of the vaginal fornix provides a convenient means of access to the peritoneal cavity; the approach is used mainly for operations on the ovaries.

The vagina is thin walled, and although its lumen is normally closed by the dorsal and ventral walls falling together, the organ is remarkably distensible in length and circumference. The vaginal mucosa is ridged lengthwise, although the ridges are readily effaced on distention. The mucosa is normally pale pink but darkens when suffused with blood, as tends to happen on prolonged exposure to air during vaginoscopy. A transverse fold cranial to the opening of the urethra represents the remains of the hymen; although very variable, it is generally more prominent than in other domestic species.

## The Vestibule and Vulva

The dorsal wall of the vestibule only gradually departs from the line of the rectum and anal canal; the longer ventral wall slopes more steeply downward beyond the ischial arch (Fig. 22–9/9). Noteworthy features are the urethral opening at the cranial limit and the clitoris within the ventral commissure of the vulva. The clitoris varies much in development and is largely covered by a transverse preputial fold that attaches to the dorsal surface of its glans (Fig. 22–14/12,12′). The fold and ventral commissure together constitute the prepuce. The clitoris is very prominent in mares in heat when exposed by "winking" movements of the labia. Laterally and ventrally it is separated from the labia by a clitoral fossa (/12″). Several sinuses (/13) of varying depth invade the glans (Plate 24/*J*). These may harbor the organism responsible for contagious equine metritis and, on this account, the clitoris must be partially excised in brood mares intended for importation into the United States. Further mucosal recesses (/13′) are present in the ventral parts of the clitoral fossa and labia. Although no major vestibular glands exist, numerous minor glands discharge within small depressions, ranked in ventral and dorsolateral rows. The mucosa overlying the vestibular bulb, situated in the lateral wall toward the vulva, is more darkly colored.

The vulva is unusual in having rounded ventral and pointed dorsal commissures, a reversal of the

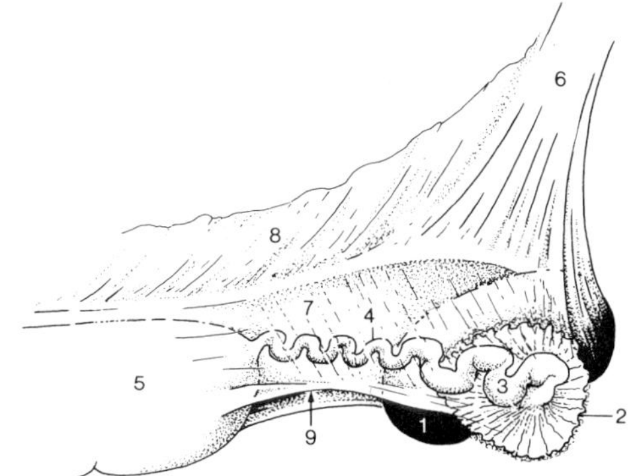


**Figure 22–12.** The right ovary, uterine tube, and uterine horn; lateral view.

1, Ovary; 2, infundibulum with fimbriae; 3, ampulla of uterine tube; 4, isthmus of uterine tube; 5, uterine horn; 6, mesovarium; 7, mesosalpinx; 8, mesometrium; 9, entrance to the ovarian bursa.

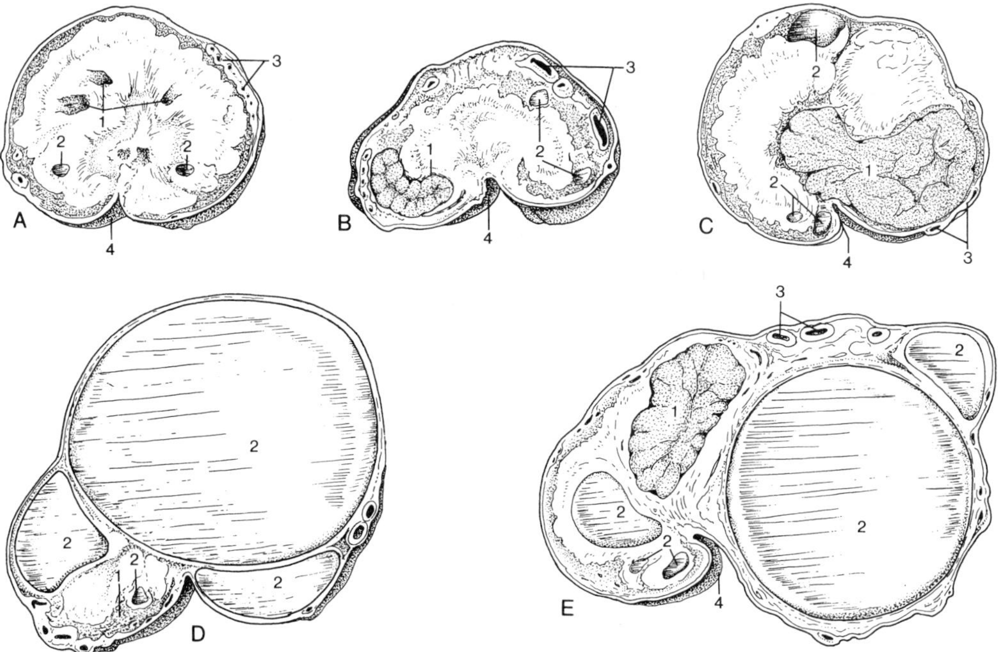


**Figure 22–11.** Sections of ovaries in various functional states. *A*, Ovary with corpora lutea and small follicles. *B*, Ovary with developing corpus luteum. *C*, Ovary with fully developed corpus luteum. *D*, Ovary with mature follicle. *E*, Ovary with follicles of various sizes and a rather large corpus luteum. The corpus luteum of the mare does not protrude from the ovary as in other species.

1, Corpora lutea; 2, follicles; 3, blood vessels; 4, ovulation fossa.

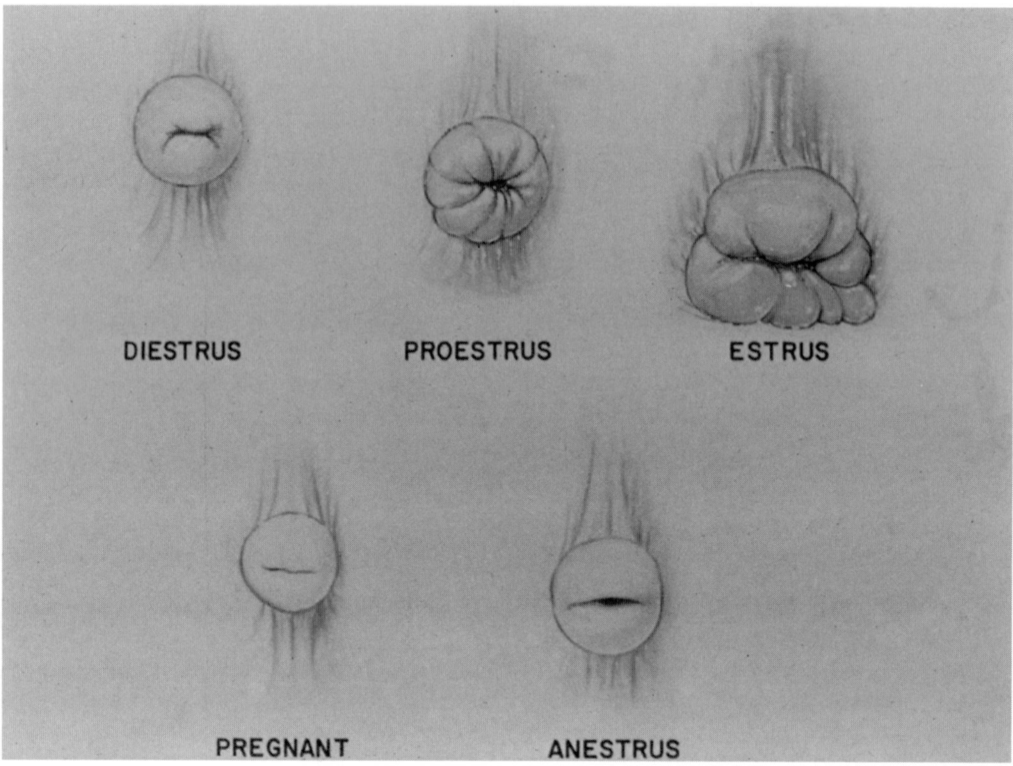


**Figure 22–13.** The changing appearance of the cervix.

usual arrangement (Fig. 22–15/3). The relationship of the vulva to the pelvic skeleton varies considerably and significantly. Usually it is largely ventral to the pelvic floor and the opening is closed. Sometimes, and quite commonly in Thoroughbreds, the opening is more dorsal and closure is less effective; in this circumstance, air may be drawn into or expelled from the tract with each change in intra-abdominal pressure. Bacteria may be introduced and the contamination may spread to the endometrium, with sterility resulting. The same fault (wind-sucking) may be due to laceration of the vulva at a previous parturition.

## Vascularization and Innervation

The reproductive organs are principally supplied by the ovarian, uterine, and vaginal arteries. The ovarian artery, a direct branch from the aorta, divides into uterine and ovarian branches. The ovarian branch pursues a tortuous course within the mesovarium before dividing into several branches that spread over the surface of the ovary; this contrasts with the arrangement in other species, in which the vessels penetrate the ovary immediately on arrival. The other branch passes to the cranial part of the horn. The corresponding vein is disproportionately large and drains much of the uterus in addition to the ovary. Little transfer of prostaglandins from venous to arterial blood occurs in the mare, a fact that may be correlated with the less intimate relationship of the ovarian artery and vein than exists in many other species.

The uterine artery, a branch of the external iliac, is the foremost supply to the uterus. It divides into several branches within the broad ligament, and these approach the mesometrial border of the horn and body separately. The antimesometrial aspect is reached only by small vessels and thus lends itself to relatively bloodless incision. Anastomoses with branches of the ovarian and vaginal arteries are present.

The vaginal artery takes origin from the internal pudendal in common with the middle rectal artery. It passes through the retroperitoneal tissue lateral to the vagina before bending forward to divide and supply the larger part of the vagina, the cervix, the caudal part of the body of the uterus, the bladder, and the urethra. The remaining part of the vagina and the vestibule are supplied from the vestibular branch of the internal pudendal artery.

The veins draining the genital organs are satellite to the arteries. The innervation displays no noteworthy special features.

## Growth and Cyclical Changes in the Reproductive Organs

At midgestation the fetal ovaries are much larger than those of the dam but they later regress, and by birth they are reduced to one tenth of their greatest fetal size. They then grow slowly until puberty when a sudden spurt occurs. The first estrus is generally at the beginning of a breeding season, and the age at which it occurs therefore varies with the date of the individual's birth as well as with breed and nutrition. It usually occurs sometime between the 18th and 27th months. The neonatal ovary is ellipsoidal; the peculiar indented adult form develops during the first two or three years (Fig. 22–16). In the mature ovary the larger follicles are concentrated near the ovulation fossa to which they migrate as they enlarge (Fig. 22–11/2). Two or three (perhaps spread between the two ovaries) reach full size in each cycle, but usually only one ruptures; its diameter is then about 5 cm. After rupture, the cavity contains some blood, and for a time the soft clot may be appreciated on rectal examination. It then gradually fills with luteal cells, but even when mature the corpus luteum hardly projects above the surrounding surface. The corpus luteum is initially brick-red but becomes ocherous as it matures. Its regression begins about the tenth day and is more or less complete when its successor forms. The cycle averages 22 days. The left ovary is generally the more active; despite this the right uterine horn is slightly more favored by conceptuses. Transuterine migration by a conceptus must be common.

Ultrasonic examination may be used to follow the stages of follicular development, to determine the occurrence of ovulation, and to trace the fate of the resulting follicular cavity. It is generally successful in determining the course of events a little before this is possible by palpation per rectum. It may allow the prediction of ovulation by

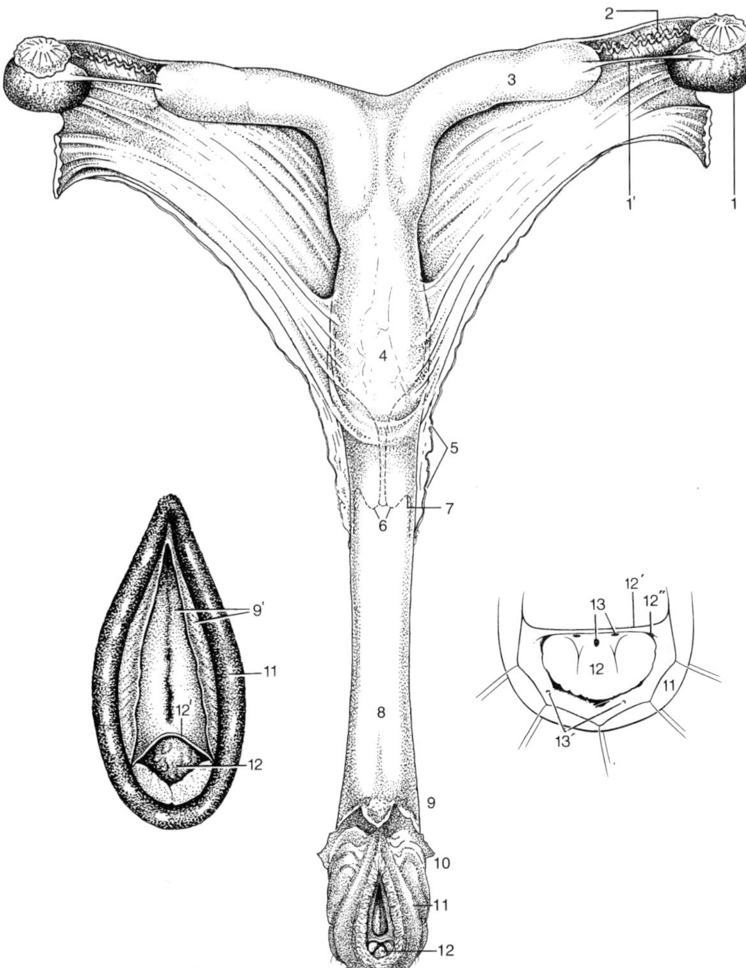


**Figure 22–14.** Dorsal view of the female reproductive organs. The *left inset,* an enlargement of the vulva, shows the glans of the clitoris within the ventral commissure. The *right inset* is a further enlargement of the clitoral glans (12).

1, Right ovary; 1′, proper ligament of ovary; 2, uterine tube; 3, horn of uterus; 4, body of uterus; 5, cervix; 6, vaginal part of cervix; 7, fornix; 8, vagina; 9, vestibule; 9′, wall of vestibule; 10, vulva; 11, right labium; 12, glans of clitoris; 12′, transverse preputial (frenular) fold; 12″, clitoral fossa, exposed by stay sutures; 13, median and right lateral sinuses, often filled with smegma; 13′, labial and ventral mucosal recesses (not in fixed positions).

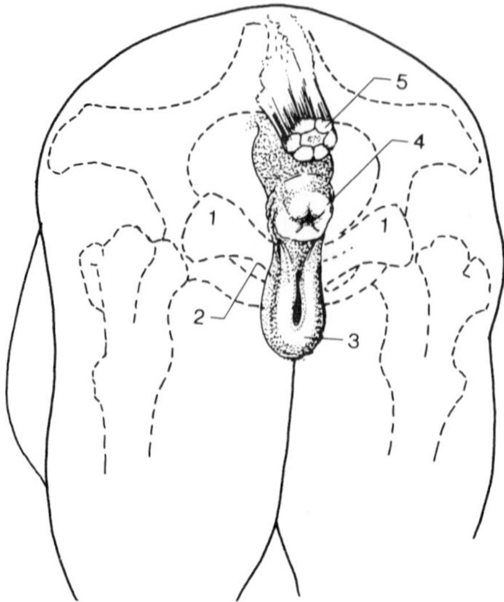


**Figure 22–15.** The anus and vulva superimposed on the outline of the bony pelvis. Note the relationship of the ischial arch and tubers to the vulva.

1, Ischial tuber; 2, ischial arch; 3, vulva; 4, anus; 5, tail (section).

about a day through revealing the change in the form—from spherical to pyriform—of the ripening follicle. A further advantage lies in its success in recognizing the parallel maturation of the multiple follicles that may result in twin pregnancy.

The juvenile reproductive tract is small, symmetrical, and thin walled. The endometrium is pale, and the layers of the uterine wall are difficult to differentiate with the naked eye. The broad ligaments are thin and transparent and the blood vessels narrow and relatively inconspicuous. Growth is initially isometric—it keeps pace with growth of the body as a whole—until a prepuberal acceleration occurs. Cyclical changes in the uterus broadly resemble those in other species with increased retention of water, a greater blood flow, and activation of the glands thickening the wall in preparation for the reception of the blastocyst. If pregnancy does not result, these changes recede with the regression of the corpus luteum. Cyclical changes in muscular tonus are the subject of some controversy, but most authorities hold that tonus is greatest about a week after ovulation.

The cervix softens during estrus when the intravaginal part droops so that its orifice is lost to view on vaginoscopic examination. When stimulated by handling, it becomes firmer, returns to the horizontal, and may exhibit rhythmic contractions. It is also moist, swollen, and pink at this time. It is paler in appearance and firmer during metestrus and diestrus when the lumen is closed by a plug of thick mucus (Fig. 22–13). Although the vaginal wall is pink and moist during estrus, its liability to change color on prolonged exposure to air denies diagnostic significance to its appearance. Cytological changes in the vaginal epithelium are slight and also of little diagnostic value.

## The Reproductive Tract During Pregnancy

The ovaries continue to show cyclical activity during the first months of pregnancy. Although the first corpus luteum does not persist beyond the usual term, it is replaced by a succession of other corpora over the next 5 months; some are formed after rupture of follicles, others apparently by direct luteinization. The accessory corpora lutea survive longer than the original one and are a rich source of progesterone. The growth, ripening, and luteinization of the new follicles are controlled by gonadotrophic hormones derived from the endometrial cups that are so distinctive a feature of the species. After 5 months the accessory corpora lutea also regress and pregnancy is then maintained by progesterone of placental origin. The enormous enlargement of the fetal gonads, peculiar to the

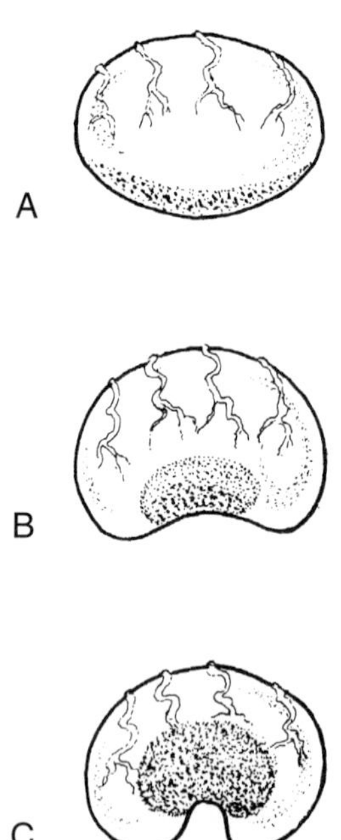


**Figure 22–16.** The postnatal development of the ovary. The more rapid growth at the poles confines the germinal epithelium (stippled) to a small central area.

*A*, At birth; the germinal epithelium is widespread over the surface. *B*, At 6 months of age. *C*, Adult; the germinal epithelium surrounds an indentation known as the ovulation fossa.

horse among domestic species, reaches a peak between 6 and 8 months. Despite recent assertions that fetal hypophysial luteinizing hormone (LH) is responsible for the enlargement, unpublished information indicates that the enlargement continues in the decapitated fetus; this points to the endometrial gonadotrophins as a contributing if not sole source (Plate 8/*F,* and see p. 558). The temporary enlargement of the fetal testes influences the timing and the success of their descent, which is normally completed about full term.

The proliferative changes of the endometrium that occur with each cycle continue and intensify if pregnancy has occurred. The early diagnosis of pregnancy and, because of the prevalence of early embryonic death, the confirmation of its continuation through the critical early stages have a particular importance in equine practice. An additional significance is provided by the desirability of recognizing twin pregnancies at an early stage. Twin pregnancies are rarely completed successfully, and the clinician and client may choose the prompt abortion of twins to lessen the risk of losing a breeding season. Though various laboratory methods of pregnancy diagnosis exist, the principal reliance remains on careful internal examination per rectum, supplemented by ultrasonography (Fig. 22–17). The experienced clinician may recognize a loss of uterine tone at the location of a conceptus, compared with the tone of neighboring parts, as early as the 20th day—possibly even a day or two before this. The location of the conceptus at this time is within the part of a uterine horn adjacent to the junction with the body of the organ; at this stage the conceptus has a diameter of approximately 30 to 40 mm, and a slight bulge of the ventral aspect of the pregnant horn should be detectable. Ultrasonic examination may bring forward the time of recognition of the presence of a conceptus to as early as the 11th or 12th day, occasionally even the 9th day. Since at this stage the conceptus has a diameter of only a few millimeters, it is clear that very systematic examination is required in order to detect, or confidently to exclude, its presence. The identification of the body of the embryo becomes possible a week or so later (about day 19), and this removes any lingering suspicion that a cavity identified at an earlier examination might be attributable to an endometrial cyst. The differentiation of pregnancy from pathology will probably receive additional confirmation from a shift in location of a conceptus, which is still mobile, unlike a lesion.

The early conceptus enjoys considerable mobility before adopting a fixed location within the uterus. There is evidence to suggest that, though most equine conceptuses are located within the

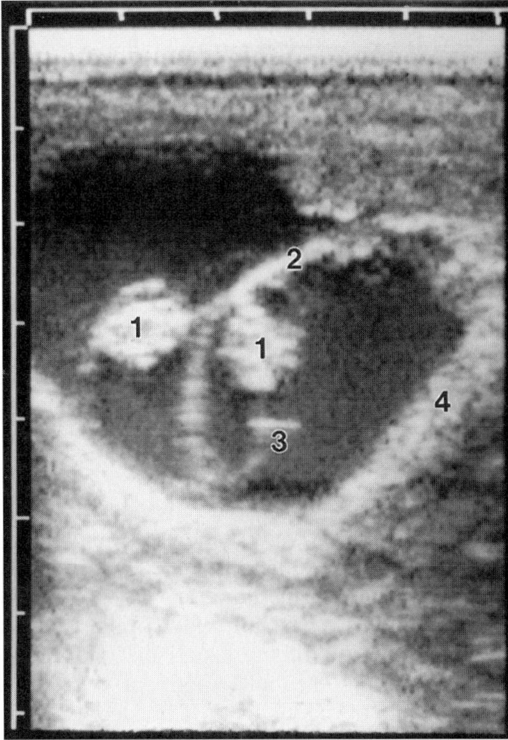


**Figure 22–17.** Ultrasonographic view of 31-day equine twin embryos. The scale is in centimeters.

1, Twin embryos; 2, junction of the two conceptuses; 3, developing allantoic membrane; 4, uterine wall.

body of the uterus about the 10th day, they will have settled within a horn a week or so later.

Ultrasonography may be employed at a somewhat later stage of pregnancy in order to determine the sex of the fetus, which is revealed by the location of the genital tubercle; it is found close to the umbilical cord in the male, nearer the tail in the female. Such examinations are best deferred to 7 or 8 months.

The whole pregnant horn (which is more commonly the right one) then gradually enlarges, followed by the body and, though in lesser degree, the nonpregnant horn. As the uterus enlarges it sinks into the abdomen, dragging the body and the cervix out of the pelvis (Fig. 22–18). The broad ligaments exert constraint on the mesometrial margins, and the horns therefore enlarge asymmetrically and become more flexed on themselves; the ovaries are drawn ventrocranially. The uterine arteries, which are pulled in the same direction, develop a characteristic vibration (fremitus or thrill) in the pregnant mare. This feature may be appreciated on rectal examination and its diagnostic value is greatest at that stage of pregnancy (between the third and fifth month) when the

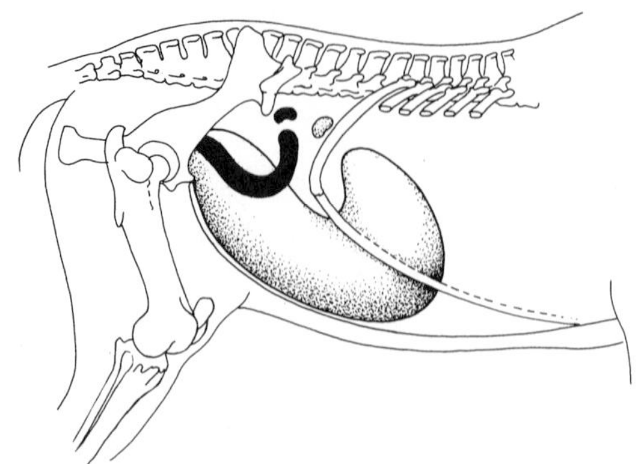

**Figure 22–18.** Changes in the topography of the uterus and ovary between the beginning *(black)* and the end *(stippled)* of pregnancy.

uterus has sunk out of reach. The position of the foal adapts to the form of the uterus; by midpregnancy it has come to lie with its back against the greater curvature of the horn (and thus ventrally), and with its head generally (99%) raised toward the cervix. In the circumstances that most favor easy parturition, the bulky body of the foal is preceded into the cervix by the extended forelimbs upon which rest the relatively small head and slender neck. The foal is delivered with its back uppermost. Because of the general enlargement and considerable size of the body of the uterus, it is possible for the occasional fetus to lie transversely, extending from one horn into the other; clearly this bodes ill for parturition. Enlargement of the uterus displaces the other abdominal contents forward and upward; in later pregnancy the uterus dominates the entire abdominal topography, extending forward on the abdominal floor and under the rib cage, but it generally remains to the left of the cecum.

A prominent feature of the uterus in early months of pregnancy is the presence of a ring or horseshoe formation of scablike structures, disfiguring the endometrium of the caudal part of the horn, the location where the young conceptus comes to rest. These, the so-called endometrial cups (Plate 8/*F*) are unique to Equidae and are the source of equine chorionic gonadotropin (formerly known as pregnant mare's serum gonadotropin [PMSG]), the hormone responsible for the unusual activity of the ovary of the pregnant mare (p. 556) and the even more remarkable, though temporary, enlargement of the gonads of equine fetuses of both sexes. The cups have their origin in cells that invade the endometrium from a limited region of the chorion—the (allanto-) chorionic girdle that marks the boundary between the allanto- and omphalochorionic (yolk-sac) portions of the embryonic vesicle and provides the area of initial adhesion of the conceptus to the uterus (Plate 8/*E*). The migration of chorionic cells begins about the 35th day and the cups soon become visible as low endometrial elevations. They continue to grow, forming irregular centrally depressed saliences that reach their zenith about the 60th day, only to enter upon a process of degeneration and necrosis shortly thereafter. The process culminates in their separation and sloughing from the endometrium, events largely concluded by the 120th day (or thereabout), though a few may persist much longer. The fetal (chorionic) cells penetrate some way into the endometrial stroma, and though they provide the essential endocrine components of the cups, they become admixed with connective tissue cells, blood vessels, and glandular debris and secretion contributed by the endometrium. Some detached cups come to lie between the endometrium and chorion; other detachments of this material push into the allantoic cavity, enclosed within pedunculated sacs of allantochorion, and these protrusions may be the origin of some of the hippomanes mentioned shortly.

The cervix of the pregnant mare is firm and closed by a plug of mucus (Fig. 22–13). The pale vaginal wall is also coated with mucus that becomes stickier and more inspissated as pregnancy progresses. The connective tissues of the cervix, vagina, and vulva, and the sacrotuberal ligaments (Plate 24/*J*), soften shortly before birth, which is generally speedily executed, assisted by the generous dimensions of the pelvic cavity. It is necessary that it should be so, since rupture of the membranes with loss of fetal fluids (Plate 24/*E*) allows separation of the loose attachment between the chorion and the endometrium, jeopardizing fetal respiration.

Puerperal changes follow the same pattern as in other species but run a rapid course. Involution of the uterus is completed sooner than in the cow and, since there is no endometrial damage to repair, mares covered at the "foal heat"—about two weeks after giving birth—often conceive.

## Placentation and Prenatal Development

In the horse, unlike other domestic species, a choriovitelline (or omphalo-) placenta provides the principal organ of exchange for the first third or so of intrauterine life. Thereafter, with the establishment of the chorioallantoic placenta, the yolk-sac wanes (Fig. 22–19/4). The definitive chorioallantoic placenta is of the epitheliochorial type and is commonly described as diffuse. The outer surface of the chorion carries innumerable branched villi that penetrate into crypts of the endometrial surface to form a loose attachment that is reinforced by the radial pressure exerted by the fetal fluids. Although the villi are widely spread, their distribution is not uniform, and they are clumped together in groups sometimes known as microcotyledons (because they resemble on a smaller scale the cotyledonary arrangement in ruminants). Small spaces between the microcotyledons face the openings of the uterine glands and fill with their secretions (Plate 9/*B*).

The capillaries of both fetal and maternal parts of the placenta reach directly below the corresponding epithelia, and only a thin tissue layer separates the two blood streams. Even so, the passage of large molecules, including antibodies, is impossible, and the passive transfer of immunity from mother to offspring is dependent on the foal ingesting colostrum.

A peculiar feature is the presence of so-called hippomanes in the allantoic (and, to a lesser extent, amniotic) fluid. These are soft brownish bodies; most are formed by the deposition of organic material upon nuclei provided by solid particles within the fluids, but some have their origin in material flaked from endometrial cups when these have completed their role. The latter are sometimes found anchored to the chorioallantoic membrane by attenuated stalks. Hippomanes have no clinical (or residual physiological) importance, but lay people sometimes credit them with the most fantastic origins and various—often rather lurid but wholly mythical—properties.

Although detailed information must be sought elsewhere, it may be useful to have this bare guide to the estimation of fetal age (Table 22–1). Crown-rump measurements are of limited value in this species with its wide range of body size.

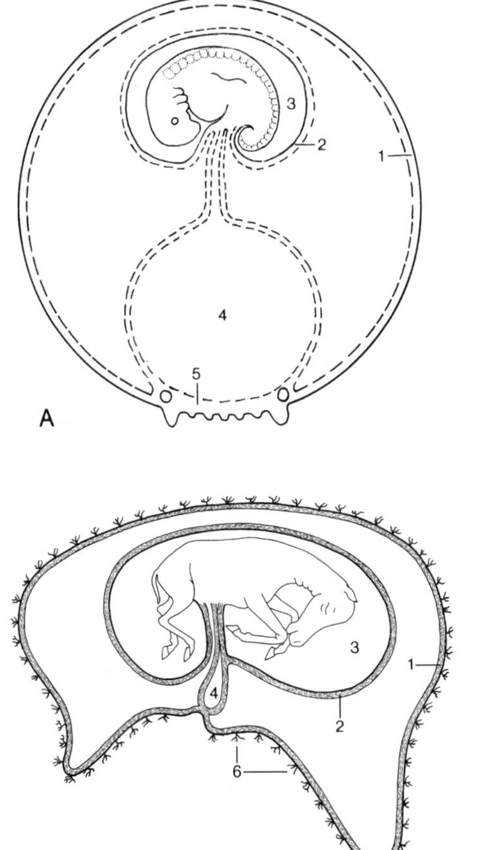


**Figure 22–19.** Schema of the choriovitelline (yolk-sac) placenta (*A*) and the definitive chorioallantoic placenta (*B*).

1, Chorioallantois; 2, amnion; 3, amniotic cavity; 4, yolk sac; 5, yolk-sac placenta; 6, microcotelydons.

**Table 22–1.** Guide to the Aging of Horse Fetuses

| Month | Crown-Rump Length | External Features |
|---|---|---|
| 1 | — | The embryo is about 1–1.5 cm long |
| 2 | ≈7 cm | The species is recognizable and the sex determinable from the external genitalia |
| 3 | ≈14 cm | The parts of the hoof are distinct |
| 4 | ≈25 cm | Some hair is present around the mouth |
| 5 | ≈36 cm | Hairs are present above the eyes |
| 6 | ≈50 cm | Eyelashes are present |
| 7 | ≈65 cm | Hair is present at the tail tip |
| 8 | ≈80 cm | Hair has appeared along the back and on the limbs |
| 9 | ≈95 cm | Fine hair covers most of the body (the belly excepted) |
| 10 | ≈110 cm | The body is completely haired |
| 11 | | Full term (generally in the range of 330–345 days) |

From Evans, H.E., and W.O. Sack: Prenatal development of domestic and laboratory animals. Growth curves, external features and selected references. Anat. Histol. Embryol. 2:11–45, 1973.

# THE MALE REPRODUCTIVE ORGANS

## The Scrotum and Testes

The scrotum lies below the pubic brim where it is concealed from lateral inspection by the thigh (Plate 24/*A*). It is broadly globular, commonly asymmetrical, and divided by an external raphe that extends cranially onto the prepuce and caudally onto the perineum. The scrotal skin is thin, supple, and sparsely haired and is usually deeply pigmented; it glistens from sebaceous secretion. The deeper layers of the scrotal wall are constructed in the usual fashion.

The testes are imperfectly ellipsoidal, being slightly compressed from side to side (Plate 24/*B* and Fig. 5–34). They generally lie with their long axes horizontal but become almost vertical on strong contraction of the cremaster muscles that attach to the vaginal tunic near the cranial poles. The tunica albuginea is less thick than in ruminants, and the testes yield on gentle compression; even so, the grayish pink parenchyma is contained under some pressure and bulges through any incision of the tunic. The septa that extend inward from the capsule do not join to form a visibly distinct mediastinum. The epididymis lies along the dorsal border and projects a little beyond the poles of the testis where it is most firmly attached. It leaves a distinct testicular bursa that opens laterally. The ligament of the tail of the epididymis (/8) is quite thick and must be severed in castration by the "open" method. Wartlike growths (appendices testis) on the testis near the head of the epididymis are very common; they are remnants of the paramesonephric duct.

The spermatic cord is broad and thin where it attaches to the testis but rounds when followed toward the superficial inguinal ring. The cranial vascular part (/5) is clearly distinguished from the caudal part that carries the deferent duct. The constituents diverge in the usual manner on entering the abdomen (Fig. 22–20/12 and Plate 24/*C*). The course of the deferent duct then takes it across the dorsal face of the bladder, beside the medial border of the vesicular gland, before it penetrates the prostate to reach the urethra. The subterminal part (≈20 cm) of the duct is widened to form an ampulla (/14), an inappropriate term since it is the wall and not the lumen that is enlarged. The ampulla is less distinct in geldings, particularly those castrated early.

The wide inguinal canal makes inguinal hernia a relatively common occurrence.

Although the process of testicular descent may be presumed to be governed by the same factors (pp. 173–175) as in other species, it is marked by one circumstance unique among domestic mammals. The testes of the fetal colt exhibit an inordinate though temporary increase in size between the 100th and 250th days of gestation, attaining a peak on about the 215th day. (A comparable enlargement affects the ovaries of the fetal filly.) In consequence, although each testis arrives in the vicinity of the vaginal ring on about the 120th day it is delayed here and does not resume its migration until it has shrunk to a fraction of its maximal size. It does not arrive in the scrotum until close to the time of birth, or even after this event—say within 2 weeks either way.

Not infrequently a testis fails to reach the scrotum even then but remains hidden within the abdomen or delayed within the inguinal canal. Retention may be temporary or permanent, confined to one side or bilateral, and if bilateral the sites of lodgement may be asymmetrical. The condition, known as cryptorchidism, may resolve spontaneously with the testis making a delayed appearance in the scrotum at some time within the first year of postnatal life, or possibly even later. In such cases it may be assumed that the testis was held up within the inguinal canal since the vaginal ring normally contracts shortly after birth, preventing a late entry to the canal from the abdomen. Testes that fail to make an appearance within a reasonable time require surgical removal, for which a variety of techniques is available depending on the location of the arrest. The diagnosis of cryptorchidism is sometimes less obvious than might be supposed. Cryptorchid animals that have changed hands may be presented in good faith as geldings, suspicion only arising when stallion characters of conformation and behavior develop. Moreover, in young horses of nervous disposition, successfully descended testes may initially escape detection by being withdrawn into the groins, against the superficial inguinal rings, when the scrotum and inguinal regions are palpated.

## The Pelvic Reproductive Organs

The short (≈12 cm) pelvic urethra lies directly over the pelvic symphysis. Though generally remarkably wide (≈6 cm), its lumen is narrowed in two places, one level with the body of the prostate, the other where the urethra crosses the ischial arch (Fig. 22–21). The *deferent ducts* (/2) penetrate the urethral wall close to the origin of the urethra from the bladder. Each combines with the duct of the neighboring vesicular gland to form a common passage, the ejaculatory duct. This is only a few millimeters long and opens into the urethra to the side of the dorsal thickening, the seminal colliculus.

The *vesicular glands* (/3) of the horse merit the alternative name "seminal vesicles" since they take the form of smooth-surfaced, pear-shaped bladders, approximately 12 cm long, with large central lumina. Each is contained within the genital fold.

The *prostate* (/4) is largely retroperitoneal and entirely compact. It consists of two lateral lobes joined by a narrow isthmus that crosses the dorsal

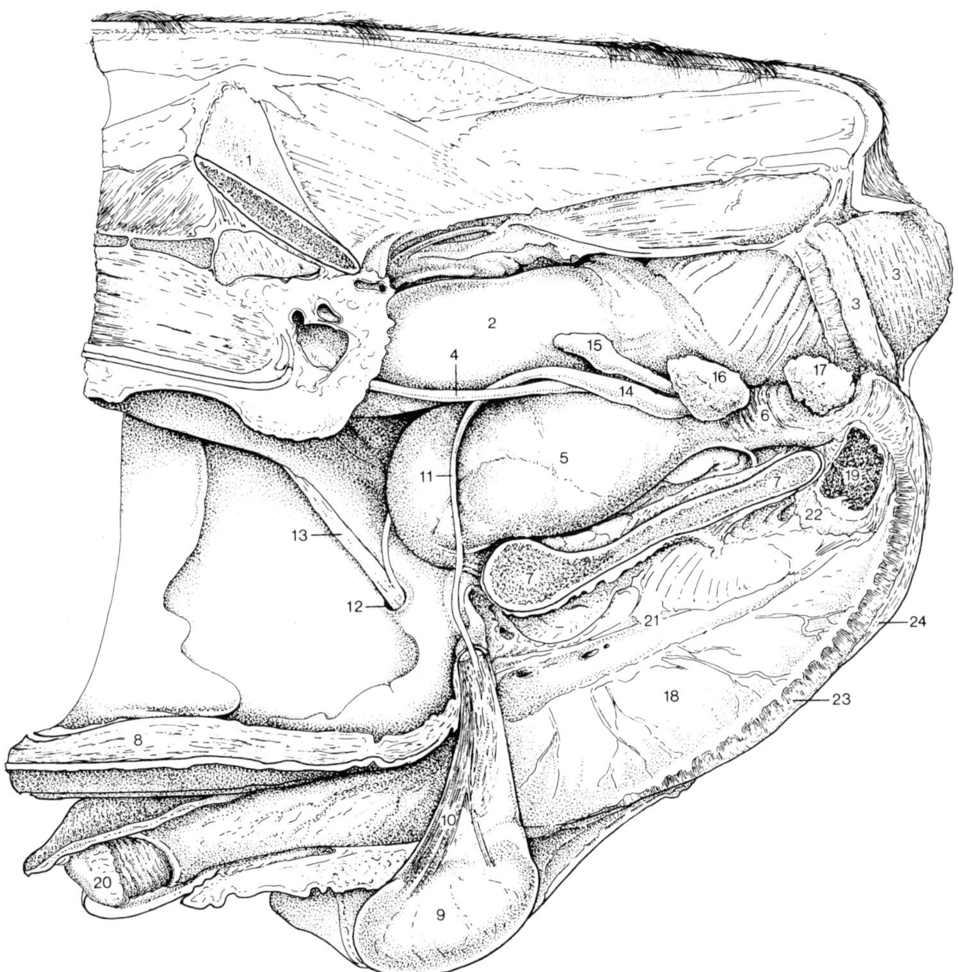


**Figure 22–20.** The reproductive organs of the stallion in situ.

1, Wing of ilium; 2, rectum; 3, external anal sphincter; 4, ureter; 5, bladder; 6, urethra; 7, floor of pelvis; 8, floor of abdomen; 9, testis within tunica vaginalis (shown rotated through 180 degrees into an unusual but not aberrant posture); 10, cremaster; 11, left deferent duct; 12, vaginal ring; 13, right testicular artery and vein; 14, ampulla of deferent duct; 15, vesicular gland; 16, prostate; 17, bulbourethral gland; 18, penis; 19, left crus (in section); 20, glans penis; 21, suspensory ligament of penis; 22, ischiocavernosus; 23, bulbospongiosus; 24, retractor penis.

aspect of the urethra close to the bladder neck. Each lateral lobe is pressed against the border of the urethra and extends cranially along the caudolateral edge of the adjacent vesicular gland. Since the prostate is firm and lobulated the two glands are easily distinguished on rectal examination. Numerous ductules drain from the prostate to discharge into the urethra through tiny slits beside the colliculus (see Fig. 5–39/7).

The paired *bulbourethral glands* lie dorsolateral to the urethra at the pelvic outlet. They are thinly covered by striated muscle (bulboglandularis), about 4 cm long, and so oriented that their pointed caudal ends converge (Fig. 22–21/6). These glands discharge through numerous small pores that open into the urethra where it leaves the pelvis.

All accessory reproductive glands are, of course, much reduced in geldings.

## The Penis and Prepuce

The penis of the horse is composed of the usual triad of structures and is of the musculocavernous variety. The two dorsal elements—the crura penis—arise from the ischial arch, bend forward between the thighs, and soon unite in a single corpus cavernosum, which is divided in its proximal part by a median septum that reflects the compound origin (Fig. 22–22). The septum fades and finally disappears when followed toward the apex. The corpus cavernosum is somewhat compressed laterally and carries ventrally a groove into which the third erectile body, the corpus spongiosum, fits.

The corpus spongiosum expands over the apex of the organ to form the distinctively shaped *glans* (Fig. 22–23/*A*,1). This has a resemblance to a mushroom; the widest part, the corona, is some distance proximal to the apex where the terminal part of the urethra protrudes into a central fossa (/3). The glans is constricted to form a neck behind the corona and is then prolonged in a tapering process over the dorsal aspect of the body; this feature is not visible externally (Fig. 22–22/7).

A considerable portion of the quiescent penis projects into the preputial cavity. The equine prepuce (sheath) is peculiar in being thrown into an additional fold that allows for the considerable lengthening of the penis on erection (Fig. 22–23/*B*). The entrance (preputial ring; /15′) to this inner sleeve lies just within the preputial orifice. Sometimes as a congenital defect the ring is unduly tight and prevents protrusion of the penis (phimosis). The condition may be corrected by section of the responsible encircling band of muscle that is included within the ring. The preputial lining contains many glands and is commonly fouled by their secretion, the smegma. An inspissated mass of this dark material—the "bean" of the penis is the stable term—commonly fills a small (urethral) sinus above the urethral process (/3′).

The penis of the horse obtains blood from the obturator and external pudendal arteries in addition to the usual internal pudendal source.

Unusually, the bulbospongiosus continues along the ventral aspect of the penis well beyond the point of incorporation of the urethra (Fig. 22–22/5). The muscle, which is the direct continuation of the urethralis, bridges the ventral groove of the corpus cavernosum and on contraction compresses the corpus spongiosum (and urethra), assisting in the expulsion of urine and semen. The ischiocavernosus muscles are powerful but in no way remarkable. The smooth retractor penis muscles loop round the rectum before passing onto the ventral surface of the penis (/6). They continue forward, gradually weaving through the transverse fibers of the bulbospongiosus to find attachment on the glans.

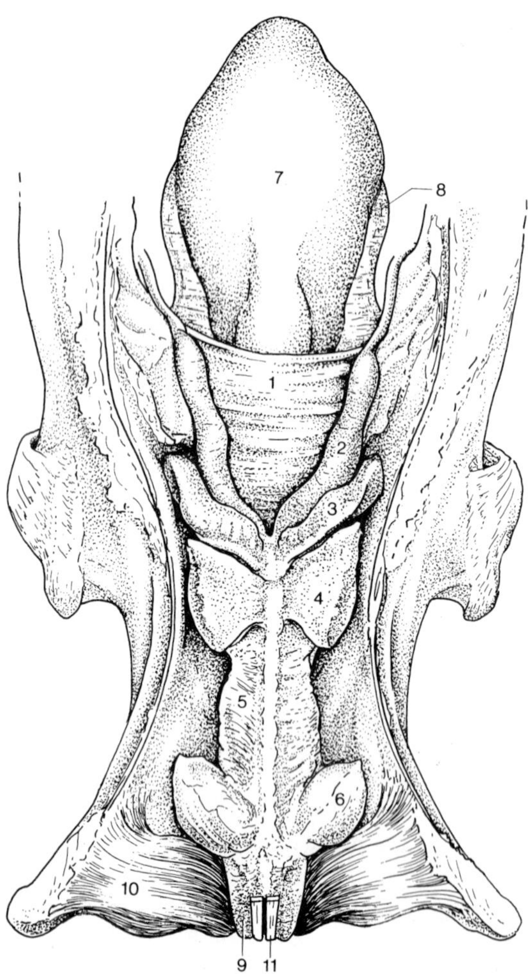


**Figure 22–21.** Dorsal view of the pelvic urethra and accessory reproductive glands (in situ).

1, Genital fold; 2, ampulla of deferent duct; 3, vesicular gland; 4, prostate; 5, urethralis; 6, bulbourethral gland; 7, bladder; 8, lateral ligament of bladder; 9, bulbospongiosus; 10, ischiocavernosus; 11, retractor penis.

## Erection

Since the penis is of the musculocavernous type it becomes considerably engorged with blood when erect. When erection is complete, a process requiring some little time and achieved by the relaxation of the helicine arteries* and the pumping action of the ischiocavernosi, the organ is much enlarged in both length and girth (Fig. 22–23/*C*). A very considerable pressure, perhaps as much as 3700 mm Hg, is attained within the blood spaces of the corpus cavernosum and, as in other species, this occasionally results in rupture of the fibrous capsule. The ejaculate is relatively large (≈65 mL on average) and is mainly the product of the vesicular glands.

Dismounting after service is often followed by a

*Terminal arteries that open directly into the cavernous spaces of the erectile tissue of the penis. Their myoepithelial walls cause them to be coiled (helicine) and closed in the flaccid penis. Sexual stimulation relaxes them, allowing blood to engorge the erectile tissue.

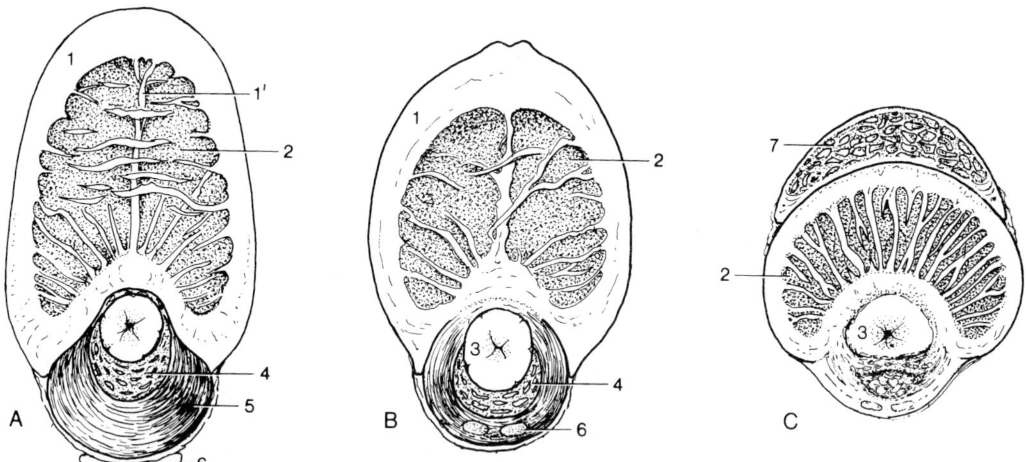


**Figure 22–22.** Transections of the penis, directly distal to the root *(A),* midshaft *(B),* and in its free part *(C).*

1, Tunica albuginea; 1′, incomplete septum penis; 2, corpus cavernosum; 3, urethra; 4, corpus spongiosum; 5, bulbospongiosus; 6, retractor penis; 7, dorsal process of glans.

remarkable "flaring" or enlargement of the glans in which the corona may briefly attain a diameter of 12 cm or so before it subsides. The return of the flaccid penis to the sheath is effected by the retractor muscles assisted by the smooth muscle component of the walls of the cavernosus spaces. Indeed, the resting posture of the penis is dependent on the tonus of this muscle. If this is reduced or lost—a relatively common occurrence in horses that are fatigued or in poor condition—the penis limply droops from the prepuce. It is vulnerable to injury when exposed in this way. The resistance of the muscle may also be overcome by sustained traction when it is necessary to expose the organ for clinical examination or for washing as part of routine stable hygiene.

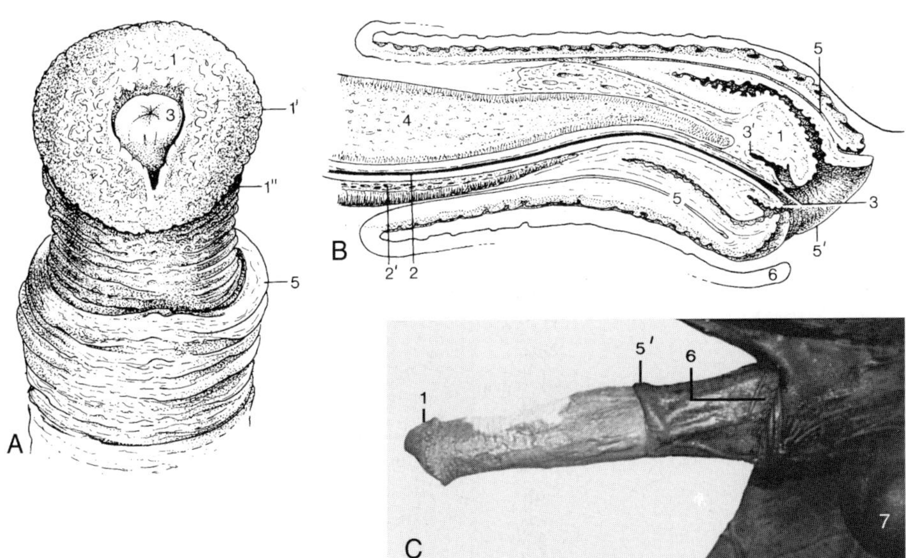


**Figure 22–23.** Extremity of penis exposed *(A)* and within prepuce in median section *(B);* and the entire organ in state of erection *(C).*

1, Glans; 1′, corona glandis; 1″, collum glandis; 2, urethra; 2′, corpus spongiosum; 3, urethral process within fossa glandis; 3′, urethral sinus; 4, corpus cavernosum; 5, preputial fold; 5′, preputial ring; 6, prepuce, forming preputial orifice with the body wall; 7, scrotum.

## THE ANATOMY OF RECTAL EXPLORATION

Exploration per rectum is an important diagnostic technique in the horse. A hand can very easily be introduced into the rectum and descending colon and then passed in various directions to examine the pelvic and caudal abdominal wall, the pelvic contents, and a variable amount of the abdominal contents (Fig. 22–24/7). Rectal examinations are not free from risk of injury to the mucosa or even, in extreme cases, of perforation of the intestinal wall—a mishap most likely to occur when invasion of the rectum induces straining. The novice should not attempt the procedure without appropriate supervision. Some organs can always be identified with certainty, others less consistently, for the results of the investigation depend not only on the relative sizes of the investigator and patient but also on the condition of the organs. It is one thing to palpate an organ through the gut wall, quite another to recognize enough of its nature to be confident of identification. The greater part of the pelvic skeleton can be identified with absolute certainty, although the part of the floor about the symphysis may be made inaccessible by overlying organs. The caudal part of the abdominal wall is also within reach, although it rarely reveals much of interest other than the caudal margin of the internal oblique muscle bordering the deep inguinal ring (/8), and the vaginal ring within that opening. The vaginal ring can be recognized most easily in the stallion, in which the deferent duct may be picked up where it lies on the bladder and traced to its disappearance.

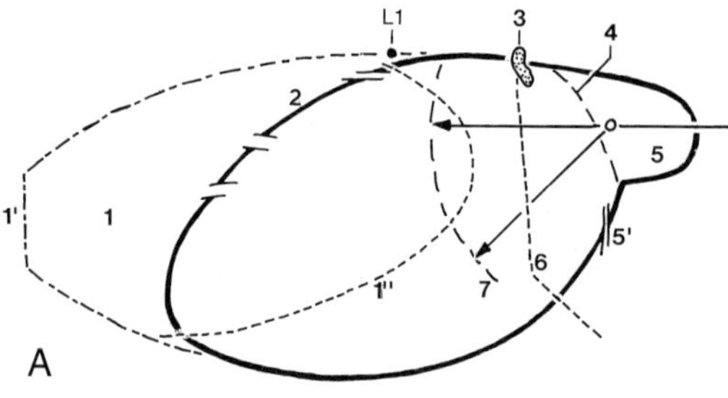


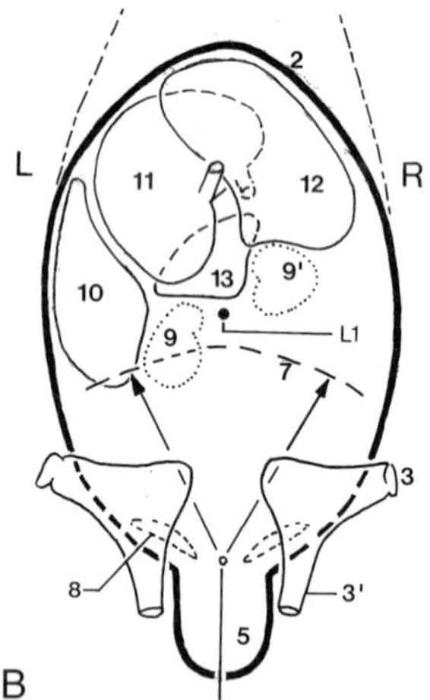


**Figure 22–24.** Drawings of the abdominal and pelvic cavities in left lateral *(A)* and dorsal *(B)* outline indicating the scope of rectal exploration. The dorsal outline encloses a ring of the relatively fixed organs (9, 9′, 10, 11, 12) with the pancreas (13) in the center.

1, Thoracic cavity; 1′, thoracic inlet; 1″, costal arch; 2, diaphragm; 3, coxal tuber; 3′, shaft of ilium; 4, terminal line; 5, pelvic cavity; 5′, inguinal canal; 6, thigh and stifle; 7, approximate range in rectal palpation in the median plane *(A)* and directly ventral to the kidneys *(B)*; 8, deep inguinal ring; 9, 9′, left and right kidneys; 10, spleen; 11, stomach; 12, liver; 13, pancreas.

Of the viscera, the small colon is the most easily recognized since its identity is betrayed by the chain of sacculations that are usually filled with firmish feces; even when empty this part of the gut can be distinguished by the teniae, one following the mesenteric attachment, the other the facing margin. Although the small colon has a mobile disposition, a mass of coils is generally found just in front of the pelvic inlet and mainly to the left. A considerable part of the ascending colon is also within reach. The pelvic flexure, the part most easily identified, is usually found immediately before or even within the pelvic cavity. Most often it lies just to the left of the median plane but it may cross to the right. The adjoining parts of the left ventral and dorsal parts of the ascending colon can be followed for some distance. They are most easily recognized when gas-filled, as this emphasizes the contrast between the sacculations of the wide ventral part and the smooth surface of the narrower dorsal part. Although the names of these parts are indicative, it must not be assumed that they necessarily lie directly one above the other. The dorsal diaphragmatic flexure and right parts of the colon are out of the reach of even the longest arm, although sometimes it is just possible for the finger tips to touch and trace the junction of the ascending and transverse parts of the colon. The base and the dorsal part of the body of the cecum (Fig. 22–25/9) are consistently within reach, although unless they are inflated little beyond position exists to identify them. The cranial mesenteric artery, adherent to the left face of the cecal base, may sometimes be identified when thickened by reaction to nematode larval

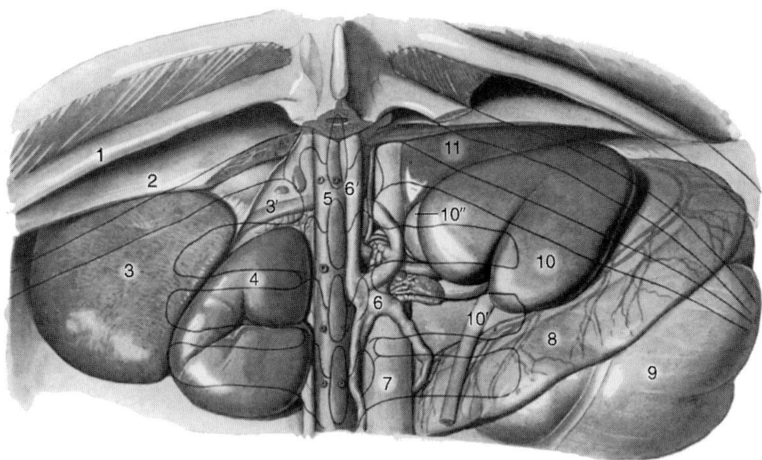


**Figure 22–25.** Kidneys and related organs exposed after removal of certain ribs, lumbar vertebrae, and associated muscles, dorsocaudal view.

1, Seventeenth rib; 2, diaphragm; 3, base of spleen; 3′, splenic v.; 4, left kidney, under first three lumbar transverse processes; 5, aorta; 6, cisterna chyli; 6′, thoracic duct; 7, caudal vena cava; 8, duodenum, caudal flexure; 9, base of cecum; 10, right kidney, under last two ribs and first lumbar transverse process; 10′, ureter; 10″, adrenal gland; 11, right lobe of liver.

invasion. Even in the most favorable circumstances it is barely within reach.

Although much of the small intestine is accessible, it is usually impossible to identify it with certainty, the exception being the firmer terminal part of the ileum, which may be picked up as it approaches the medial aspect of the cecal base; identification is easiest when it is impacted. When distended with gas the caudal flexure of the duodenum may be identified as it crosses the root of the mesentery.

A small horse and a long arm are the prerequisites if any of the contents of the cranial part of the abdomen are to be reached. The caudal pole of the left kidney (/4) may usually be felt, and it is theoretically possible to trace both ureters over the abdominal roof; in practice, healthy ureters cannot be identified. The caudal margin of the spleen (/3) is also accessible, although it may not always be appreciated; a greater part of this organ may be brought within reach when the stomach is distended. The fundus of the stomach may then also be identifiable.

An emergency means of euthanasia, probably of little relevance today, is available in transection of the abdominal aorta per rectum.

The bladder is invariably identifiable, regardless of its degree of filling and despite the fact that it is partly overlain by reproductive organs. In the mare, the vagina is distinguishable as a rather lax organ interposed between rectum and bladder; if followed forward it leads to the somewhat firmer cervix. Beyond the cervix, the body of the uterus may be traced to its bifurcation and the horns then followed laterally toward the ovaries. The dimensions and the texture of the uterus vary greatly with its state, and the experienced equine clinician can date an early pregnancy with quite remarkable precision by palpating the uterus. The ovaries are among the easiest organs to identify since they have a very characteristic shape and consistency. They are rather movable and are not always found exactly where expected. Only the largest follicles may be appreciated individually.

The pelvic urethra of the stallion is easily identified as a wide slack tube, although its outline is partly concealed by the associated glands (Fig. 22–21). The bulbourethral glands at the pelvic exit, the smooth pear-shaped vesicular glands, the more knobby prostate, and the fusiform enlargements of the ampullae of the deferent ducts are almost always individually distinctive. Manipulation may stimulate the urethral muscle, firming the urethra and causing it to exhibit rhythmic contractions.

## THE UDDER

The mammary glands are consolidated in a rather small udder situated below the caudal part of the abdominal floor and cranial part of the pelvis, and they are concealed from casual inspection by the thigh (Plate 24/*F* and Fig. 22–26). The form and size of the udder vary with the present state and previous history of the mare; it is very small in young virgin animals. A prominent external groove indicates its formation from right and left halves; each half has the form of a laterally compressed cone and, though carrying a single teat, is composed of two (occasionally three) separate duct systems.

The skin over the udder is thin, strongly pigmented, and sparsely haired; it is supplied with many sweat and sebaceous glands and usually glistens. The teat is small and cylindrical, except in the lactating mare, in which it is both larger and

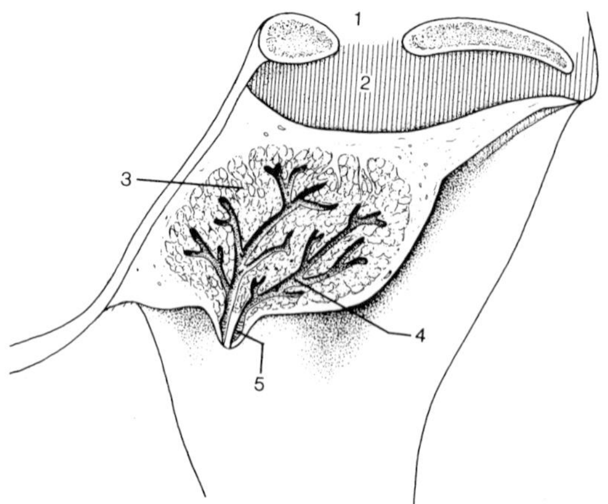


**Figure 22–26.** Sagittal section of the udder.

1, Obturator foramen; 2, adductor muscles; 3, glandular tissue; 4, lactiferous ducts; 5, teat sinus.

more conical. Two (or three) openings perforate the apex; each leads through a short papillary duct to a small lactiferous sinus (/5) spread between the teat and gland mass and associated with an independent set of lactiferous ducts (/4; and Plate 24/*G,H*). The tissues of the individual glands of each side interdigitate, and it is impossible to demonstrate their independence on dissection. Though much less developed, the suspensory apparatus resembles that of the cow's udder and combines medial elastic and lateral fibrous ligaments, which together encapsulate the udder and supply the lamellae that support the parenchyma. The medial ligaments provide a cleavage plane between the apposed surfaces of the udder halves.

The blood supply comes from the external pudendal artery, and the principal venous return is by the corresponding vein, which does not follow the usual course through the inguinal canal (p. 530). As in the cow, a subcutaneous venous connection with a superficial vein of the thoracic wall develops as an alternative drainage route during the first pregnancy. Lymph drains to the mammary (superficial inguinal) nodes. The cutaneous innervation is divided between the nerves of the flank and a descending (mammary) branch of the pudendal nerve; the contributing spinal nerves are thus those of cord segments L2–4 and S2–4. The substance of the gland is supplied by the genitofemoral nerve (L3–4). The glands develop rapidly during the second half of the first pregnancy and commence secretion before birth. Sebaceous secretion, epithelial debris, and possibly colostrum that escape through the teat openings during the last days of pregnancy dry to give the apex a waxy covering, which is a useful indication that parturition impends.

## Selected Bibliography

Amann, R.P.: A review of anatomy and physiology of the stallion. J. Equine Vet. Sci. 1:83–106, 1981.

Amoroso, E.C., J.L. Hancock, and J.E. Rowlands: Ovarian activity in the pregnant mare. Nature 161:355–356, 1948.

Barber, S.M.: Castration of horses with primary closure and scrotal ablation. Vet. Surg. 14:2–6, 1985.

Bartels, J.E., S.D. Beckett, and B.G. Brown: Angiography of the corpus cavernosum penis in the pony stallion during erection and quiescence. Am. J. Vet. Res. 45:1464–1468, 1984.

Beckett, S.D., R.S. Hudson, D.F. Walker, T.M. Reynolds, and R.I. Vachon: Blood pressure and penile muscle activity in the stallion during coitus. Am. J. Physiol. 225:1072–1075, 1973.

Boure, L., M. Marcoux, and S. Laverty: Laparoscopic abdominal anatomy of foals positioned in dorsal recumbency. Vet. Surg. 26:1–6, 1997.

Caslick, E.A.: The vulva and vulvo-vaginal orifice and its relation to genital health of the Thoroughbred mare. Cornell Vet. 27:178–187, 1937.

Colbern, G.T., W.A. Aanes, and T.S. Stashak: Surgical management of perineal lacerations and rectovestibular fistulae in the mare: A retrospective study of 47 cases. JAVMA 186:265–269, 1985.

Colbern, G.T., and W.J. Reagan: Ovariectomy by colpotomy in mares. Compend. Contin. Educ. Pract. Vet. 9:1035–1041, 1987.

Curran, S., and O.J. Ginther: Ultrasonic determination of fetal gender in horses and cattle under farm conditions. Theriogenology 36:809–814, 1991.

deLahunta, A., and R.E. Habel: Applied Veterinary Anatomy. Philadelphia, W.B. Saunders Company, 1986.

Desjardins, M.R., D.R. Trout, and C.B. Little: Surgical repair of rectovaginal fistulae in mares: Twelve cases (1983–1991). Can. Vet. J. 34:226–231, 1993.

Dik, K.J., and I. Gunsser: Atlas of Diagnostic Radiology of the Horse. Parts 1–3. Philadelphia, W.B. Saunders Company, 1988–1990.

Fischer, A.T., and A.M. Vachon: Laparoscopic intra-abdominal ligation and removal of cryptorchid testes in horses. Equine Vet. J. 30:105–108, 1998.

Ginther, O.J.: Equine pregnancy: Physical interactions between the uterus and conceptus. AAEP Proceedings 44:73–104, 1998.

Ginther, O.J.: The nature of embryo reduction in mares with twin conceptuses. Deprivation hypothesis. Am. J. Vet. Res. 50:45–53, 1989.

Ginther, O.J.: Reproductive Biology of the Mare, 2nd ed. Cross Plains, Wisconsin, Equiservices, 1992.

Ginther, O.J., M.C. Garcia, E.L. Squireys, and W.P. Steffenhagen: Anatomy of vasculature of uterus and ovaries in the mare. Am. J. Vet. Res. 33:1561–1568, 1972.

Ginther, O.J., and R.A. Pierson: Ultrasonic anatomy and pathology of the equine uterus. Theriogenology 21:505–516, 1984.

Ginther, O.J., and R.A. Pierson: Ultrasonic anatomy of the equine ovaries. Theriogenology 21:471–483, 1984.

Goetz, T.E., C.H. Boulton, and J.R. Coffman: Inguinal and scrotal hernias in colts and stallions. Contin. Educ. 3:S272–S277, 1981.

Guglick, M.A., C.G. MacAllister, P.J. Ewing, and A.W. Confer: Thrombosis resulting in rectal perforation in a horse. JAVMA 209:1125–1127, 1996.

Habel, R.E.: The perineum of the mare. Cornell Vet. 43:247–278, 1953.

Hallowell, A.L., and G.L. Woods: Management of twin

pregnancy. *In* Robinson, N.E. (ed.): Current Therapy in Equine Medicine, vol 3. Philadelphia, W.B. Saunders, 1992.

Leith, G.S., and A.K. Allen: Ultrasonography for reproductive management in the mare. *In* Nyland, T.G., and J.S. Mattoon (eds.): Veterinary Diagnostic Ultrasound. Philadelphia, W.B. Saunders, 1995, pp. 305–320.

Leith, G.S., and O.J. Ginther: Characterization of intrauterine mobility of the early equine conceptus. Theriogenology 22:401–408, 1984.

Lieux, P.: Relationship between the appearance of the cervix and the heat cycle in the mare. Vet. Med. [SAC] 65:879–886, 1970.

Little, T.V., G.R. Holyoak: Reproductive anatomy and physiology of the stallion. Vet. Clin. North Am. Equine Pract. 8:1–29, 1992.

Love, C.C.: Ultrasonographic evaluation of the testis, epididymis, and spermatic cord of the stallion. Vet. Clin. North Am. Equine Pract. 8:167–182, 1992.

McAllister, R.A., and W.O. Sack: Identification of anatomic features of the equine clitoris as potential growth sites for Taylorella equigenitalis. JAVMA 196:1965–1966, 1990.

McCarthy, P.H.: Eyes at the tips of your fingers: The anatomy of the abdominal and pelvic viscera of the narcotized horse as perceived by palpation during exploratory laporatomy. Melbourne, Peat, Marwick, Mitchell, 1986.

McKinnon, A.O., and J.L. Voss: Equine reproduction. Philadelphia, Lea & Febiger, 1993.

Moll, H.D. et al.: A survey of equine castration complications. J. Equine Vet. Sci. 15:522–526, 1995.

Morrow, D.A.: Current Therapy in Theriogenology 2. Diagnosis, Treatment and Prevention of Reproductive Diseases in Animals. Philadelphia, W.B. Saunders Company, 1986.

Palmer, S.E.: Standing laparoscopic laser technique for ovariectomy in five mares. JAVMA 203:279–283, 1993.

Pascoe, J.R., and D.R. Pascoe: Displacements, malpositions and miscellaneous injuries of the mare's urogenital tract. Vet. Clin. North Am. Equine Pract. 4:439–450, 1988.

Perkins, N.R., J.T. Robertson, and L.A. Colon: Uterine torsion and uterine tear in a mare. JAVMA 201:92–94, 1992.

Schebitz, H., and H. Wilkens: Atlas of Radiographic Anatomy of the Horse, 4th ed. Berlin, Paul Parey Verlag, 1986.

Sullins, K.E., J.L. Traub-Dargatz: Endoscopic anatomy of the equine urinary tract. Compen. Cont. Ed. 6:S663–S668, 1984.

Taylor, T.S., T.E. Blanchard, D.D. Varner, W.L. Scrutchfield, M.T. Martin, R.G. Elmore: Management of dystocia in mares: Uterine torsion and cesarian section. Compend. Contin. Educ. Pract. Vet. 11:1265–1273, 1989.

Threlfall, W.R., C.L. Carleton, J. Robertson, T. Rosol, A. Gabel: Recurrent torsion of the spermatic cord and scrotal testis in a stallion. JAVMA 196:1641–1643, 1990.

Van der Velden, M.A., and L.J.E. Rutgers: Visceral prolapse after castration in the horse: A review of 18 cases. Equine Vet. J. 22:9–12, 1990.

Waldow, D.: Management of twin pregnancy in mares. The Compendium on Continuing Education for the Practicing Veterinarian. 18:808–811, 1996.

Weber, J.A., R.T. Geary, and G.L. Woods: Changes in accessory sex glands of stallions after sexual preparation and ejaculation. JAVMA 196:1084–1089, 1990.

CHAPTER 23

# The Forelimb of the Horse

In the Western world horses are now mainly bred for use in sport and recreation, pursuits that often make heavy demands on their speed and endurance and expose their limbs to continual strain and repeated risk of injury. Even relatively minor incapacity may unfit a horse for this work, and the importance of soundness of limb is crisply stated by the old adage "no foot, no horse." Since lameness accounts for much of the work of equine practitioners, it follows that they have need of a more detailed knowledge of the anatomy of the limbs than is necessary for those who deal with other species.

The limbs of the horse display extreme adaptations for fast running with a concomitant loss of versatility. Although both fore- and hindlimbs find their main, indeed almost exclusive, employment in supporting the body when at rest and in driving it forward when in motion, they do manifest significant division of labor. It is the forelimbs that carry the greater part (some 55% to 60%) of the body weight at rest; they also supply the principal shock absorbers that are necessary in the faster gaits and especially when landing from a jump. The hindlimbs are less committed to these tasks and furnish the main propulsive thrust. However, this distribution of duties is not invariable; in particular, the share of the load that is supported by each limb may be altered by varying the posture to shift the center of gravity. The most obvious maneuver is to raise the head, so shortening the lever arm of the neck and displacing the center caudally; the reciprocal movement brings the center of gravity cranially. These alterations in the carriage of the head may be pronounced in a lame animal, which lifts the head when a painful forelimb is placed on the ground and lowers it when the sound limb bears weight. Since it is the latter movement that usually strikes an observer with more force, a horse with forelimb lameness is said to "nod on the sound foot." When there is a painful condition of a hindlimb the head is lowered as the affected limb assumes support.

A forelimb with good conformation is straight when viewed from the front. A line dropped from the point of the shoulder bisects the limb and passes through the center of the hoof; the digit continues the cannon (metacarpus) in a straight line, neither "toeing-in" nor "toeing-out" (Fig. 23–1). Much of the limb should also be straight when viewed from the side; a line dropped from the tuberosity of the scapular spine should bisect it to the fetlock and then pass just behind the hoof whose slope should parallel that of the digit. Deviations from the normal conformation can result in abnormal movements, with interference between the feet, unequal and abnormal hoof wear, and development of lameness.

The more common deviations seen when viewing from the front are categorized as "base-wide," in which the limbs slope laterally, and "base-narrow," in which they slope medially. Deviations seen from the side include "standing under," in which the limbs slope caudally, and "camped," in which they slope cranially. Cranial, caudal, medial, and lateral deviations of the carpus are also recognized; the last two faults are "knock-knees" and "bowlegs."

Retention of the full length of the shaft of the ulna is a congenital anomaly that is fairly common in Shetland ponies. It is associated with a valgus deformity*—sometimes very severe—of the limb.

The distinctive "leggy" appearance of the young foal must be familiar to every reader (Fig. 23–2). The acquisition of the adult shape involves changes in the ratios of the lengths of the limbs (taken as a whole) to that of the trunk, and in the ratios between the lengths of successive segments of the limbs—arm (thigh), forearm (leg), and metacarpus (metatarsus). According to one source, in the newborn Thoroughbred the ratio of the humerus (femur) to the metacarpus (metatarsus) is approximately 4:5 (4:5); in the adult the ratio is approximately 6:5 (6.5:5). These changes are achieved through a postnatal growth in length of the metacarpal (metatarsal) bones

*A lateral deviation of a part of a limb distal to a joint. The opposite varus deformity is a similar deviation but angulated medially.

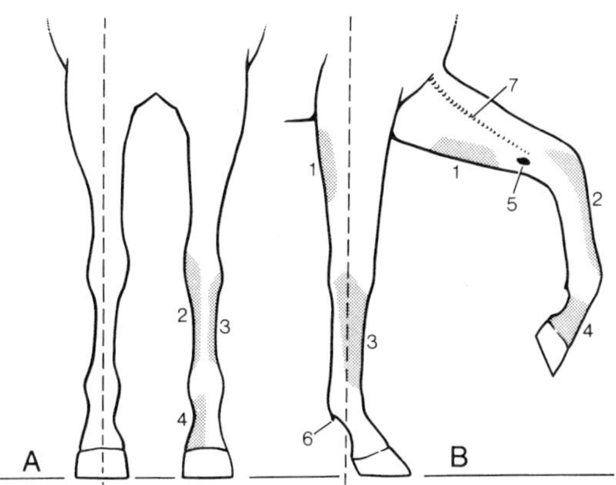


**Figure 23–1.** Desirable conformation and autonomous zones of cutaneous innervation of the forelimb. *A*, Cranial view; a vertical broken line dropped from the point of the shoulder bisects the limb. *B*, Right lateral view; a vertical line dropped from the tuberosity of the scapular spine bisects the limb down to the fetlock. The autonomous zones represent skin areas innervated solely by the nerves below.

1, Caudal cutaneous antebrachial nerve (ulnar); 2, medial cutaneous antebrachial nerve (musculocutaneous); 3, ulnar nerve; 4, median nerve; 5, chestnut; 6, ergot; 7, cephalic vein.

of about 20% and of the humerus and femur of about 100%.

The cutaneous features known as chestnuts and ergots are described on page 357.

## THE GIRDLE MUSCLES

The same muscles join the limb to the trunk as in other species but there are certain differences in detail. The *trapezius* arises from the dorsal midline, extending almost from the poll to beyond the withers. Both cervical and thoracic parts insert upon the spine of the scapula, and when they act in unison they raise this bone against the trunk. The cervical part acting alone swings the scapula forward, advancing the limb, while the thoracic part acting alone swings it in the opposite direction. Both parts may be visibly outlined through the skin when contracted. The nerve supply is the accessory nerve.

The *brachiocephalicus* (Fig. 23–3/4) arises from the mastoid region of the skull and inserts upon a ridge of the humerus that extends distally from the deltoid tuberosity. It is intimately joined in the neck to the *omotransversarius* (/6), which takes origin from the transverse processes of the more cranial cervical vertebrae and ends at the clavicular intersection that divides the brachiocephalicus into cervical (cleidomastoideus) and brachial (cleidobrachialis) parts. The dorsal edge of the omotransversarius is connected to the trapezius by the superficial fascia. The ventral edge of the brachiocephalicus is clearly delineated, at least in its

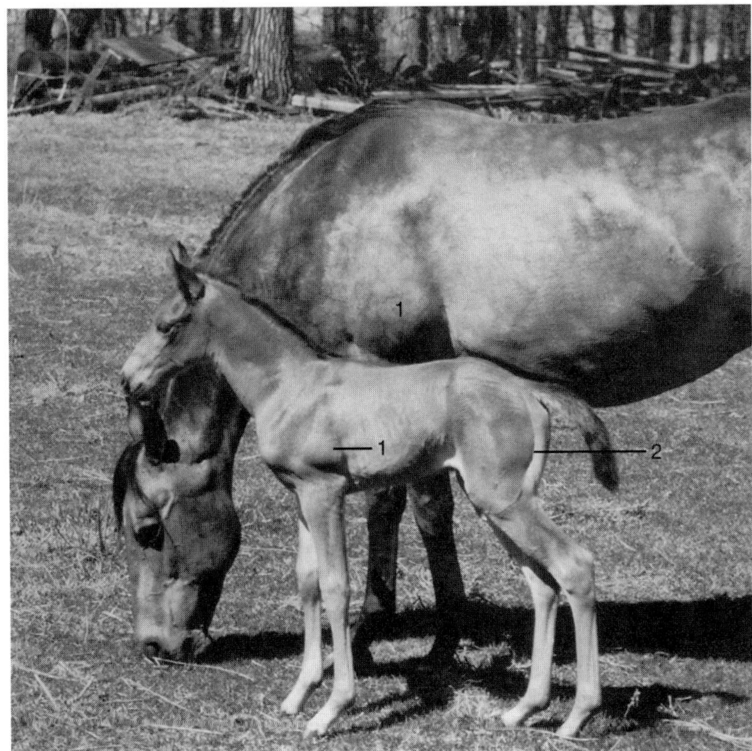


**Figure 23–2.** This photograph of a 10-day-old foal with its dam illustrates the proportions of the limbs and trunk that account for the "leggy" appearance of the young foal.

1, Flaccid long and medial heads of triceps; 2, "poverty" line between biceps femoris and semitendinosus.

cranial half, since it forms the upper margin of the jugular groove (see Fig. 18–34/*B*).

The muscle is broadest over the shoulder joint where it covers the origin of the biceps and the insertions of the supra- and infraspinatus. Bilateral action flexes the neck ventrally when that part is free to move. Unilateral action in the same circumstances bends the neck toward the active side; when the neck is fixed and it is the limb that is free, unilateral action advances the limb. The innervation is shared by the accessory, cervical, and axillary nerves.

The *latissimus dorsi* (/13) arises from the supraspinous ligament and thoracolumbar fascia and converges to an insertion upon the teres tuberosity of the humerus. The cranial strip covers the caudal angle of the scapula and holds it against the trunk. This muscle is commonly described as a retractor of the limb and thus as an antagonist of the brachiocephalicus; in fact, its most important role, especially in draft animals, may be to pull the trunk forward onto an advanced limb. It is supplied by the thoracodorsal nerve.

The superficial layer of girdle muscles is completed by the two superficial pectoral muscles. The cranial *pectoralis descendens* arises from the manubrium and divides its insertion between the humerus and fascia of the arm (Fig. 23–4/4). It is well developed and clearly outlined in life; a median groove separates it from its contralateral

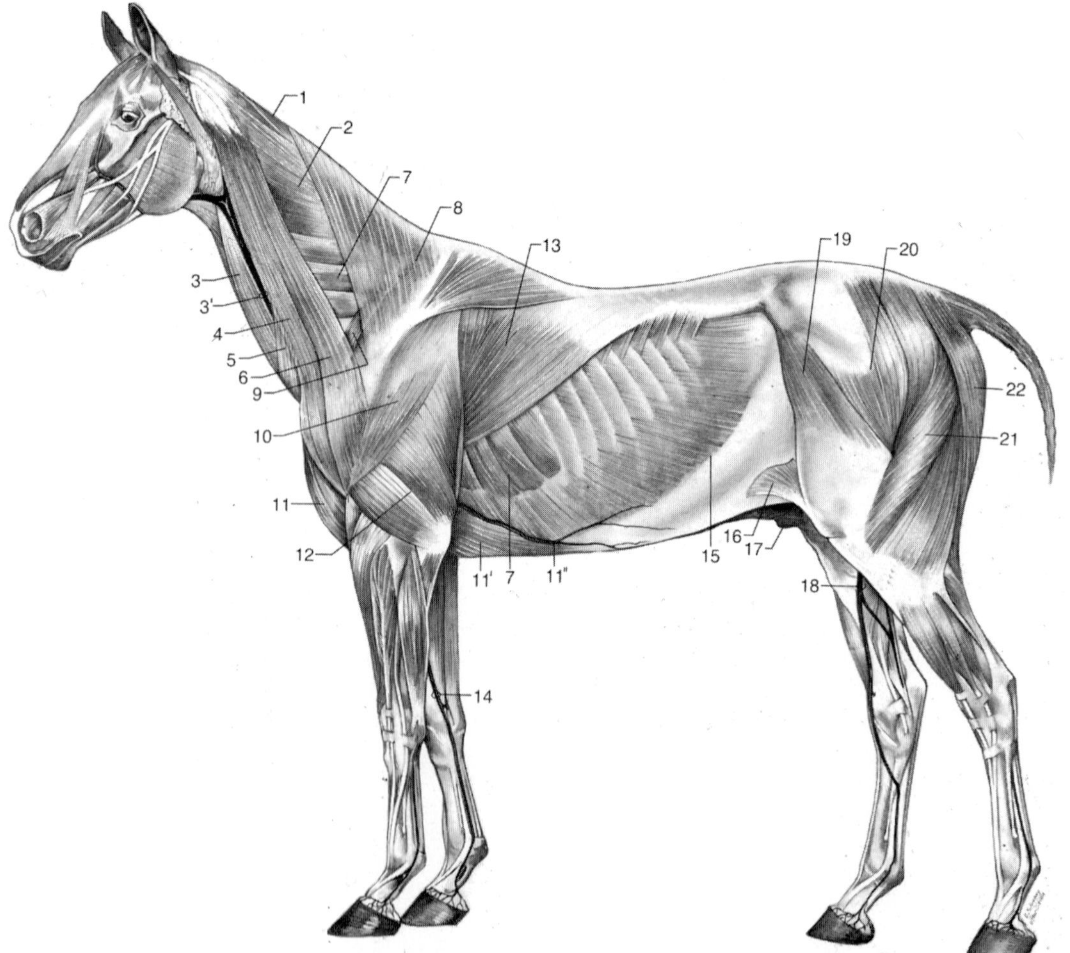


**Figure 23–3.** The superficial muscles and veins. The cutaneous muscles except for the cutaneous colli have been removed.

1, Rhomboideus; 2, splenius; 3, sternocephalicus; 3′, jugular vein; 4, brachiocephalicus; 5, cutaneous colli; 6, omotransversarius; 7, serratus ventralis; 8, trapezius; 9, subclavius; 10, deltoideus; 11, pectoralis descendens; 11′, pectoralis ascendens; 11″, superficial thoracic vein; 12, triceps; 13, latissimus dorsi; 14, cephalic vein; 15, external abdominal oblique; 16, stump of cutaneus trunci forming flank fold; 17, sheath; 18, medial saphenous vein; 19, tensor fasciae latae; 20, gluteus superficialis; 21, biceps femoris; 22, semitendinosus.

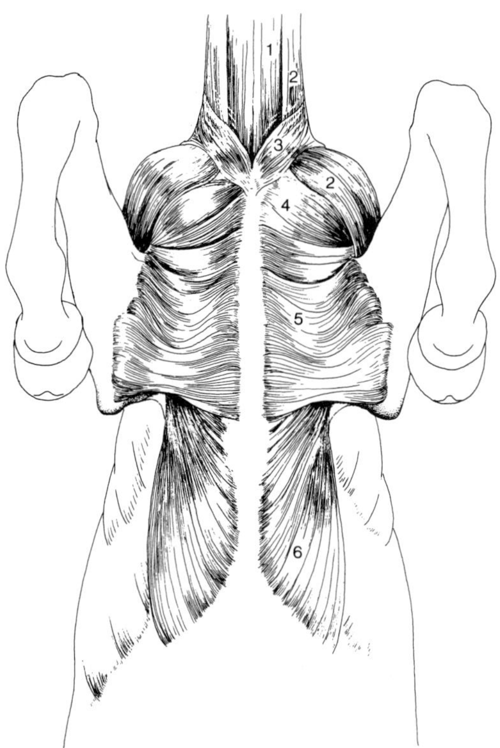


**Figure 23–4.** Muscles on the ventral surface of the thorax.

1, Sternocephalicus; 2, brachiocephalicus; 3, cutaneus colli; 4, pectoralis descendens; 5, pectoralis transversus; 6, pectoralis profundus.

fellow. The lateral groove that marks its boundary with the brachiocephalicus is occupied by the cephalic vein. It is primarily an adductor.

The caudal *pectoralis transversus* (/5) arises from the cranial sternebrae and inserts into the fascia over the medial aspect of the upper part of the forearm. The transverse course of its fibers makes it clear that it is essentially an adductor, a term that embraces the lateral shifting of the trunk toward a previously abducted limb. Both superficial pectoral muscles are supplied by pectoral branches of the brachial plexus.

Although the *rhomboideus* lies deep to the trapezius, it may, when contracted, form a visible surface feature. Its origin from the nuchal and supraspinous ligaments extends between the second cervical and seventh thoracic vertebrae. The entire muscle inserts upon the deep face and dorsal edge of the scapular cartilage (Fig. 23–5/4). Although it serves to raise the scapula, the course of the thoracic fascicles enables them to rotate the bone so that the ventral angle is carried caudally. The innervation is by dorsal branches of caudal cervical nerves.

The *serratus ventralis* (/1) is very strong, both actively because of its extent and bulk and passively because it is covered and inter-shot by stout connective tissue sheets. The origin spreads from the fourth cervical vertebra to the tenth rib. The insertion is confined to the scapular cartilage and to two triangular areas on the adjacent part of the medial surface of the scapula. The dominant function of the serratus is support of the trunk. However, the cervical and thoracic parts each have an additional (and antagonistic) function in rotating the scapula. The cervical part rotates the bone so that the ventral angle is carried caudally and so retracts the limb; contraction of the thoracic part advances this angle and thus the limb. The serratus ventralis is supplied by the long thoracic nerve.

The *pectoralis profundus* has a widespread origin from the caudal part of the sternum and adjacent area of the abdominal floor (/3). The fascicles converge, and the muscle thickens as it passes craniolaterally to a restricted insertion on the greater and lesser tubercles of the humerus. The relative heights of the origin and insertion suggest that the deep pectoral muscle may assist the serratus in supporting the weight of the trunk; the catastrophic results of rupture of the serratus suggest the limited effectiveness in this capacity (Plate 27/*A*). Its foremost uses are probably adduction, retraction of the limb when this is free to move, and advancement of the trunk onto an advanced and fixed limb. It is supplied by pectoral nerves.

The *subclavius* (/2), to the front of the deep pectoral, takes origin from the cranial part of the sternum. It then bends dorsally to follow the cranial surface of the supraspinatus, over which it tapers to an extended insertion on the epimysium. Its presence along the leading edge of the scapula helps smooth the transition from the narrow neck to the greater breadth between the shoulders. The actions of the subclavius complement those of the deep pectoral (of which it was formerly regarded as a part). It too is supplied by pectoral nerves.

## THE SHOULDER REGION AND UPPER ARM

The bases of the shoulder region and upper arm are the scapula and humerus, both wholly included within the skin of the trunk. The slope of the *scapula,* of interest to horsemen and -women, varies considerably and is revealed by the orientation of its spine. A more sloping shoulder is preferred in saddle horses. The thickened middle portion (tuber spinae) of the spine is readily

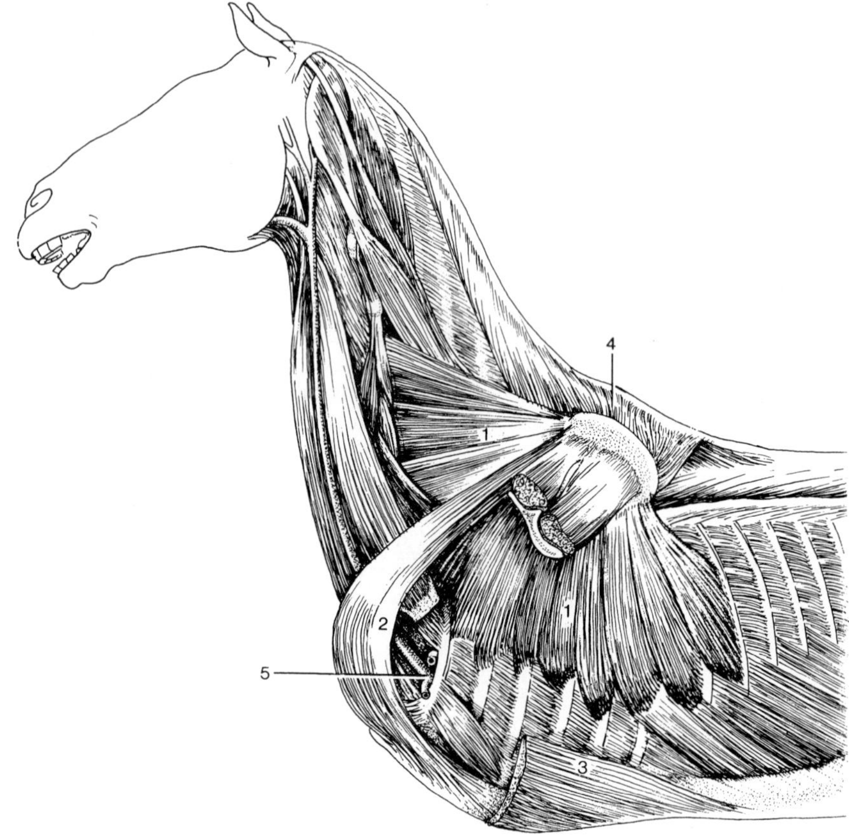


**Figure 23–5.** Deep muscles attaching the forelimb to the trunk.

1, Serratus ventralis; 2, subclavius; 3, pectoralis profundus; 4, rhomboideus; 5, axillary vessels turning around first rib into limb.

recognized on palpation and may even provide a visible landmark (Fig. 23–6/*A*,3). The distal part of the spine subsides gradually and does not form an acromion. The bone is extended beyond its dorsal border by a large scapular cartilage that is incorporated within the withers. The margin of the cartilage and the cranial and caudal angles of the bone may be palpated in most subjects. The caudal angle is often quite prominent even though it is covered by the latissimus (Fig. 23–3/13).

The *humerus* forms a right angle with the scapula and slopes less steeply than in the smaller species. Its surface relief is marked, and many features may be felt through the skin and musculature. The greater and lesser tubercles of the proximal extremity are both well developed and are more nearly equal than in most species. Each is divided into cranial and caudal parts. The cranial parts are separated by an intertubercular groove that is interrupted by an intermediate tubercle; there are thus five processes that together enclose the head on all but its caudal aspect. Although both parts of the greater tubercle are easily palpated, it is the cranial division that provides the surface feature known as the "point of the shoulder" (Fig. 23–6/*A*,8). Distal to this, the deltoid tuberosity furnishes another easily found landmark (/10).

The *shoulder joint* has the attributes of a spheroidal joint and is theoretically capable of considerable versatility of movement (Fig. 23–7). In practice, it generally functions as a hinge joint whose excursions take place in a sagittal plane. The restriction upon transverse movements, imposed by collateral ligaments at most hinge joints, is here provided by the tendons of the muscles that closely surround the shoulder, notably the infraspinatus (and, to a lesser degree, the supraspinatus) laterally, and the subscapularis medially. The cavity is relatively capacious. It may be tapped by inserting a needle at the cranial margin of the palpable infraspinatus tendon 2 cm or so proximal to the caudal part of the greater tubercle. The needle is directed ventromedially and must be introduced about 4 or 5 cm before its tip penetrates the capsule. The procedure requires some care since a cranial deflection may cause the needle to enter a quite separate synovial sac, the bursa that protects the biceps tendon within the intertubercular groove. This intertubercular bursa corresponds to the diverticulum of the joint capsule found in the dog and sheep.

The muscles that act primarily on the shoulder may be considered as being arranged in lateral and medial groups, although they enclose the joint on all sides. The lateral group comprises the supraspinatus, infraspinatus, deltoideus, and teres minor (Fig. 23–6/*B*).

The *supraspinatus* (/8) arises from and occupies the supraspinous fossa of the scapula; it bulges beyond the bone cranially where its covering epimysium provides insertion to the subclavius. It splits before its insertion, forming two short tendons that straddle the origin of the biceps before attaching to the cranial parts of the tubercles of the humerus. The muscle is placed to extend the shoulder joint, but its most important function may be stabilization of the joint.

The *infraspinatus* (/9) has a similar relationship to the infraspinous fossa. Its insertion crosses the lateral aspect of the shoulder joint before separating into deep and superficial tendons. The short deep tendon attaches to the edge of the caudal part of the greater tubercle. The superficial tendon crosses this projection to attach at a more distal level and is protected by a synovial bursa where it lies against the bone. Inflammation of the bursa may be painful and may cause the animal to stand with the affected limb abducted at the shoulder, a posture that relieves the pressure at the site. The infraspinatus is primarily a shoulder fixator whose

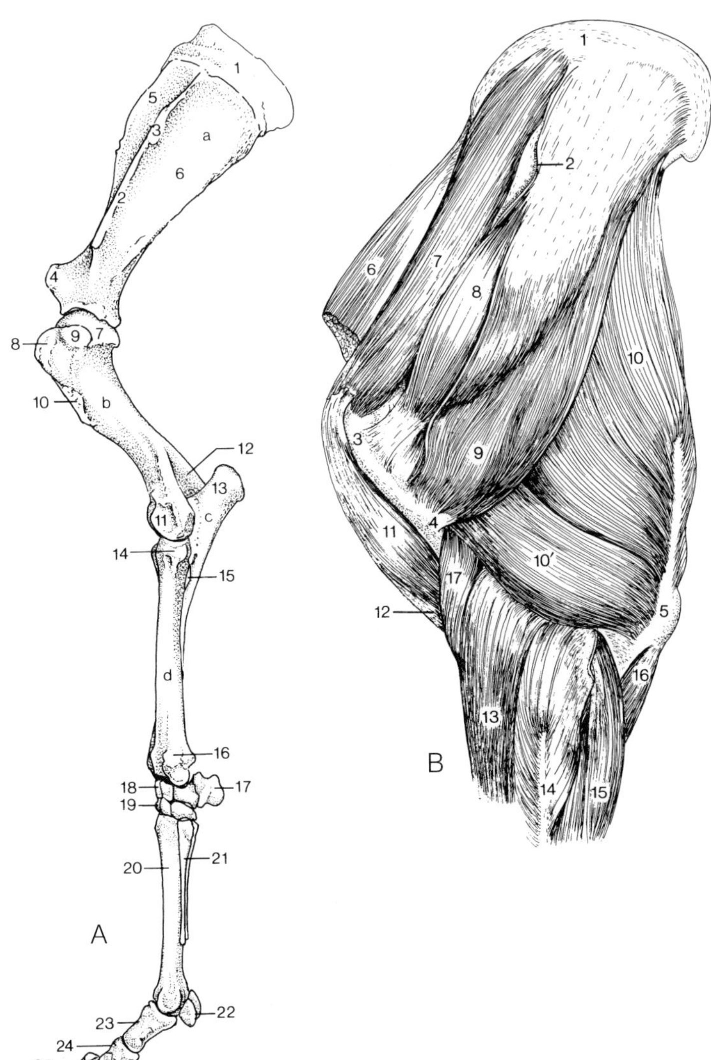


**Figure 23–6.** *A*, Skeleton of the left forelimb; lateral view.

a, Scapula; b, humerus; c, ulna; d, radius; 1, scapular cartilage; 2, scapular spine; 3, tuberosity of scapular spine; 4, supraglenoid tubercle; 5, 6, supra- and infraspinous fossae; 7, head of humerus; 8, 9, cranial and caudal parts of greater tubercle; 10, deltoid tuberosity; 11, condyle; 12, olecranon fossa; 13, olecranon; 14, tubercle for lateral collateral ligament; 15, interosseous space; 16, lateral styloid process; 17, accessory carpal; 18, 19, proximal and distal row of carpal bones; 20, large metacarpal (cannon) bone; 21, small metacarpal (splint) bone; 22, proximal sesamoid bones; 23, proximal phalanx; 24, middle phalanx; 25, distal phalanx.

*B*, Muscles associated with shoulder and elbow joints; lateral view.

1, Scapular cartilage; 2, scapular spine; 3, greater tubercle of humerus; 4, deltoid tuberosity of humerus; 5, olecranon; 6, subclavius; 7, supraspinatus; 8, infraspinatus; 9, deltoideus; 10, long head of triceps; 10′, lateral head of triceps; 11, biceps; 12, lacertus fibrosus; 13, extensor carpi radialis; 14, common digital extensor; 15, ulnaris lateralis; 16, ulnar head of deep digital flexor; 17, brachialis.

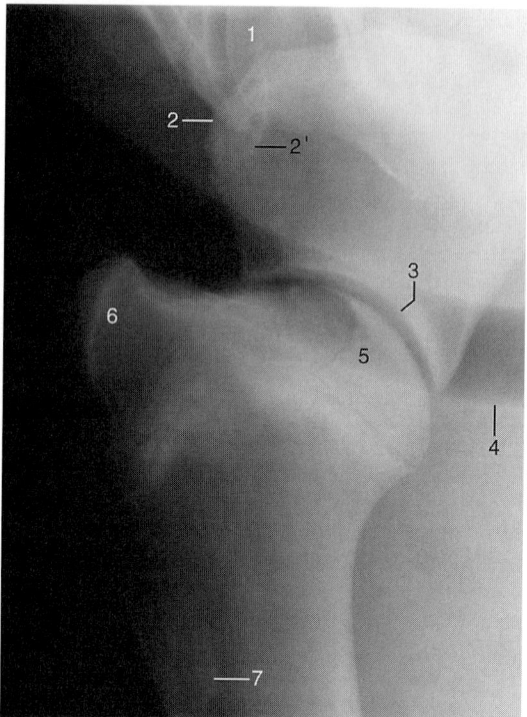


**Figure 23–7.** Lateral radiograph of a shoulder joint.

1, Sixth cervical vertebra; 2, supraglenoid tubercle of scapula; 2′, coracoid process; 3, glenoid cavity; 4, trachea; 5, head of humerus; 6, superimposed greater, lesser, and intertubercular tubercles; 7, deltoid tuberosity.

tendon substitutes for a lateral collateral ligament. It has a secondary abductor action. Both supraspinatus and infraspinatus are supplied by the suprascapular nerve.

The *deltoideus* (/10) arises from the caudal border and spine of the scapula, the latter origin being indirect and effected by way of an aponeurosis that covers the infraspinatus. The insertion is to the deltoid tuberosity. This muscle may be identified by first referring to that landmark and then following the belly proximally. It is partly recessed within a depression of the triceps, and the line between the muscles is sometimes visible in thin-skinned animals. The deltoideus is a shoulder flexor with a secondary role as abductor of the arm. Innervation is by the axillary nerve.

The unimportant teres minor is buried by the deltoideus over the caudolateral aspect of the shoulder joint.

The medial muscle group comprises the subscapularis, teres major, coracobrachialis, and capsularis—the last of trivial significance. The *subscapularis* arises from and occupies the subscapular fossa (Fig. 23–9/3). It inserts upon the lesser tubercle and, though primarily employed to stabilize the joint, may also function as an adductor of the arm. It is supplied by the subscapular nerve.

The *teres major* (/6) arises from the caudal angle of the scapula. It is contained between the subscapularis and the latissimus dorsi and inserts in common with the latter. It is chiefly a flexor of the shoulder but may also adduct the arm. It is supplied by the axillary nerve as are all the true flexors of the shoulder.

The *coracobrachialis* (/11) arises from the coracoid process on the medial aspect of the supraglenoid tubercle and inserts upon the proximal part of the shaft of the humerus. It is an adductor of the arm but is of little consequence. It is supplied by the musculocutaneous nerve.

## THE ELBOW JOINT AND THE MUSCLES OF THE ARM

The skeletal basis of the *elbow joint* is provided by the distal end of the humerus and proximal parts of

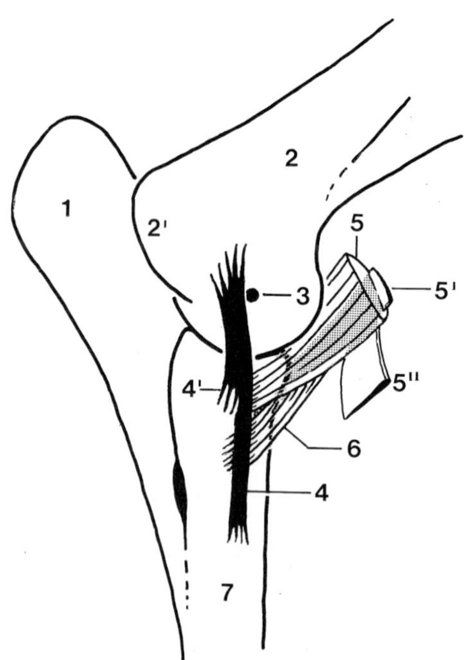


**Figure 23–8.** Medial view of left elbow joint to show the eccentrically placed collateral ligament and the insertions of biceps and brachialis. The internal tendon (5′) of the biceps splits off the lacertus fibrosus (5″) from the surface of the muscle.

1, Olecranon; 2, humerus; 2′, medial epicondyle; 3, axis of rotation; 4, 4′, long superficial and short deep parts of medial collateral ligament; 5, biceps; 5′, internal tendon of biceps; 5″, lacertus fibrosus; 6, brachialis; 7, radius.

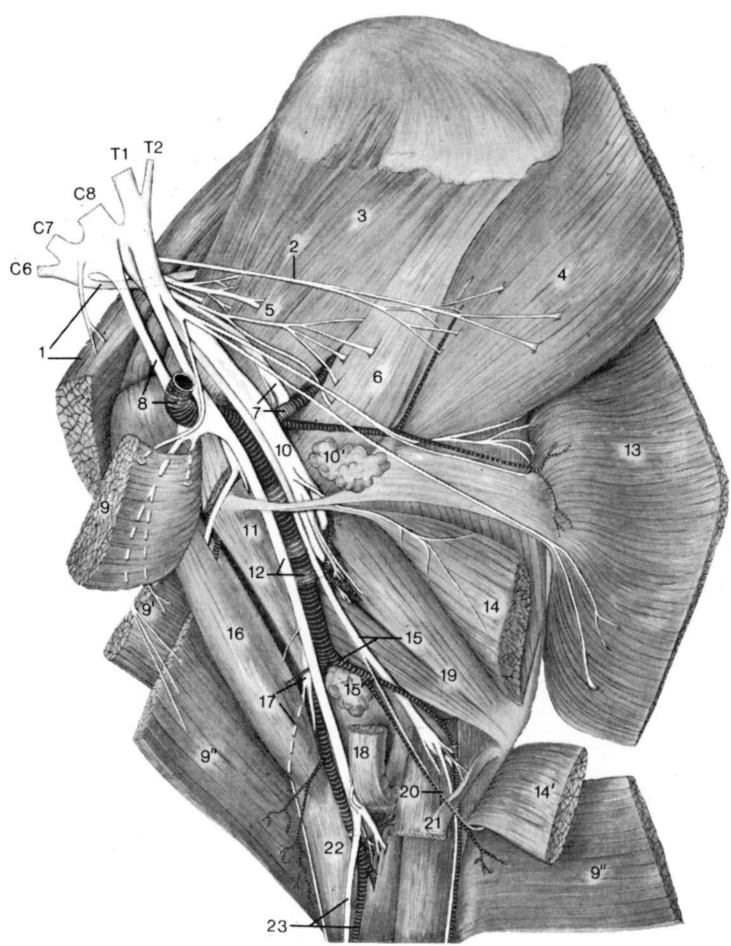


**Figure 23–9.** Nerves and arteries on the medial surface of the right shoulder and arm.

1, Suprascapular n. and subclavius; 2, thoracodorsal n.; 3, subscapularis; 4, latissimus dorsi; 5, subscapular n.; 6, teres major; 7, axillary n. and subscapular a.; 8, musculocutaneous n. and axillary a.; 9, 9′, 9″, pectoralis profundus, descendens, and transversus; 10, radial n.; 10′, axillary lymph nodes; 11, coracobrachialis; 12, median n. and brachial a.; 13, cutaneus trunci; 14, 14′, stumps of tensor fasciae antebrachii; 15, ulnar n. and collateral ulnar a.; 15′, cubital lymph nodes; 16, biceps; 17, musculocutaneous and medial cutaneous antebrachial nn.; 18, flexor carpi radialis; 19, triceps; 20, caudal cutaneous antebrachial n.; 21, flexor carpi ulnaris; 22, lacertus fibrosus; 23, median n. and a.

the radius and ulna (Fig. 23–6/*A*). Both epicondyles of the humerus may be palpated without much difficulty, but the medial one is especially prominent and projects to the inner aspect of the olecranon. The condyle may be identified more distally; it presents a deep fossa into which fits the anconeal process of the olecranon (Fig. 23–10/4,6). A shallow radial fossa occupies the corresponding site on the cranial aspect.

The powerful olecranon rises high above the joint to project upon the lower part of the fifth rib (or following space) and is therefore a less direct guide to the position of the articulation. The shaft of the ulna is much reduced. It tapers distally to fusion and ultimate submergence within the shaft of the radius, but it leaves open an interosseous space in the proximal forearm. The proximal extremity of the radius is expanded. It carries an articular surface that engages with the cylindrical humeral condyle and, just distal to this, medial and lateral eminences that furnish attachment to the collateral ligaments. The radial tuberosity is present to the front (/8). Both collateral ligaments may be palpated, although the medial one is covered by the relatively thick pectoralis transversus. A cranial division of this ligament represents a vestige of the pronator teres.

The shape of the articular surfaces and the presence of stout collateral ligaments restrict movement of the elbow joint to flexion and extension in a sagittal plane. The equine elbow is a good example of the "snap" joint, which abruptly moves from a stable to a more mobile position. This character depends on two features of its construction. The first is the unequal curvature of the humeral surface; the radius of curvature of the central part is longer than those of the parts in front and behind, which are in contact with the radius in the more flexed and more extended positions of the joint. The second is that the collateral ligaments insert eccentrically on the humerus and are taut only in the intermediate position (Fig. 23–8).

The joint is most conveniently punctured by passing a needle between the lateral epicondyle

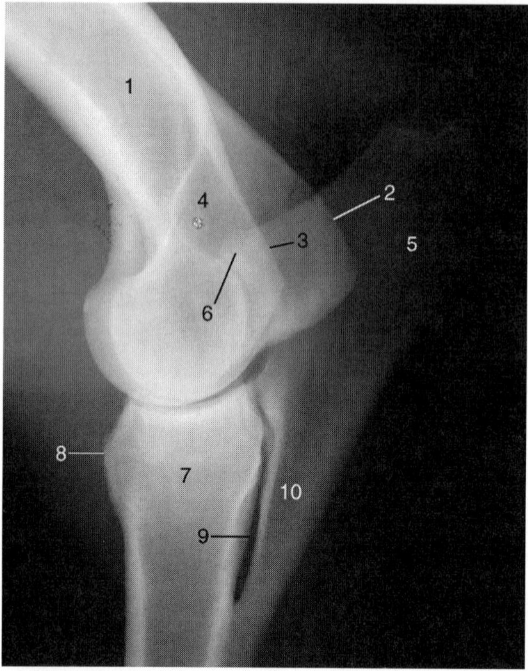


**Figure 23–10.** Lateral radiograph of an elbow joint.

1, Humerus; 2, medial epicondyle; 3, lateral epicondyle; 4, olecranon fossa; 5, olecranon; 6, anconeal process of olecranon; 7, radius; 8, radial tuberosity; 9, interosseous space; 10, ulna.

and the olecranon into a caudal pouching of the joint capsule within the olecranon fossa.

The muscles of the arm that operate the elbow joint are arranged in flexor and extensor groups.

## The Flexor Muscles

The flexor muscles comprise the biceps brachii and brachialis. Though largely under cover of the brachiocephalicus, the belly of the *biceps* is palpable as it lies against the cranial face of the humerus. The biceps takes origin from the supraglenoid tubercle of the scapula by means of a short, broad, and largely fibrocartilaginous tendon that is molded upon the intertubercular groove. The (intertubercular) bursa that protects the tendon spreads from the groove onto the cranial aspect of the humerus; it may be a cause of shoulder lameness when inflamed. The bursa may be reached, certainly if overdistended, by inserting a needle between the muscle and the bone, slightly above the level of the deltoid tuberosity, and then directing it proximally (Fig. 23–11/3).

The biceps inserts mainly on the radial tuberosity, but a branch of the attachment passes beneath the medial collateral ligament to the adjoining parts of the radius and ulna. A more important peculiarity is the existence within its belly of a fibrous strand (internal tendon; Fig. 23–8/5′) that joins the tendons of origin and insertion; a part splits away to emerge on the surface and blend more distally with the epimysium of the extensor carpi radialis. The bridging band, known as lacertus fibrosus, is easily found as a firm structure crossing the flexor aspect of the elbow (/5″; Fig. 23–9/22). It is taut in the standing animal but slackens as the joint is flexed. The internal tendon and the lacertus help maintain the carpal joint in extension when the biceps resists collapse of the shoulder under the weight of the trunk (Fig. 23–38/*A*,2,6).

The biceps is a fixator, and potentially an extensor, of the shoulder; the construction and form of the tendon of origin suggest its particular fitness for the first task. Though it is regarded as the most important flexor of the elbow, the fibrous

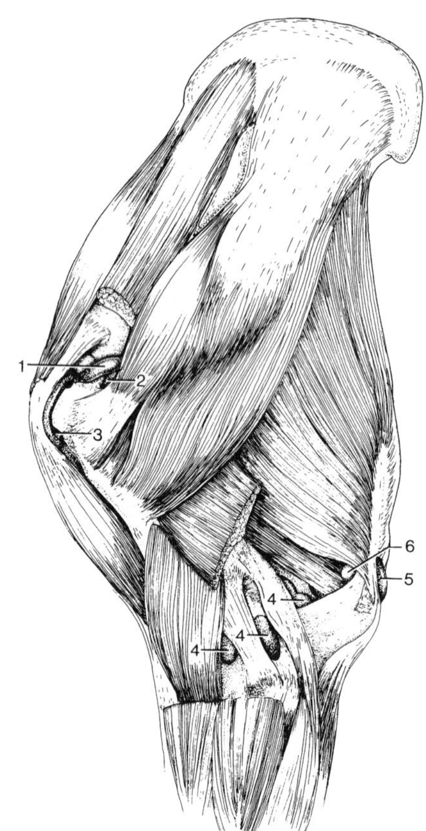


**Figure 23–11.** Synovial structures of the left shoulder and elbow regions; lateral view.

1, Shoulder joint capsule; 2, infraspinatus bursa; 3, intertubercular bursa (between biceps tendon and humerus); 4, elbow joint capsule; 5, subcutaneous olecranon bursa; 6, subtendinous olecranon bursa. (For identification of the muscles see Figure 23–6/*B*.)

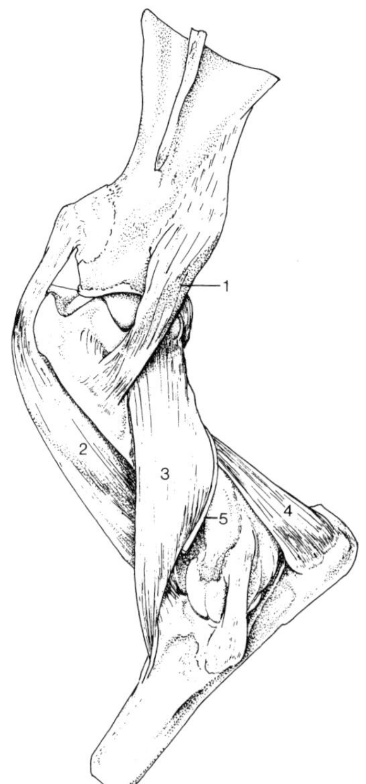


**Figure 23–12.** Deep muscles of the left shoulder and elbow joints; lateral view.

1, Teres minor; 2, biceps; 3, brachialis; 4, anconeus; 5, radial nerve.

arrangements imply that its passive role may be more significant at this joint also. Its nerve supply comes from the musculocutaneous nerve.

The *brachialis* is purely fleshy and crosses only one joint, the elbow. It arises from the caudoproximal part of the humerus, winds laterally within a spiral groove, and then crosses the flexor aspect of the elbow to insert upon the craniomedial part of the proximal radius (Fig. 23–12/3). Proximally, the muscle is covered by the triceps, but its distal part is superficial and may be palpated. The brachialis is purely an elbow flexor. It is supplied by the musculocutaneous nerve with, rather surprisingly, a contribution from the radial nerve.

## The Extensor Muscles

The extensor muscles constitute a large mass that fills the triangle between the scapula and humerus. The group comprises the triceps, tensor fasciae antebrachii, and anconeus.

The *triceps* is by far the most important extensor of the elbow. It presents three heads (Fig. 23–6/*B*,11,11′). The long head arises from the caudal border of the scapula by a short aponeurosis, the lateral and medial heads from the shaft of the humerus. Together they insert on the olecranon where a small bursa is inserted between the tendon and the bone. The division between the long and lateral heads is sometimes visible in thin-skinned animals. A second, acquired (adventitious) bursa is commonly found subcutaneously, over the triceps insertion and expanded part of the olecranon tuber ("capped elbow"; Fig. 23–11/5).

The triceps is extensor to the elbow. Since the long head spans the shoulder joint it is theoretically available to flex this joint; it is probably little used for that purpose.

The *tensor fasciae antebrachii* (Fig. 23–9/14,14′) is a broad, thin sheet covering the medial aspect of the triceps. Its origin is from the caudal border of the scapula and the tendon of the latissimus, while its insertion is spread between the olecranon and forearm fascia. Since it crosses both shoulder and elbow joints it must be considered as having a potential action at each; neither is likely to be of great importance.

The much smaller *anconeus* lies within the olecranon fossa, embedded within the deep face of the lateral head of the triceps and directly related to the capsule of the elbow joint. It may be supposed that its principal action is to tense the capsule, so preventing it from being pinched between the humerus and ulna (Fig. 23–12/4).

The radial nerve supplies all muscles of the extensor group.

# THE FOREARM AND CARPUS

## The Skeleton and Carpal Joint

The shaft of the radius is flattened from front to back and is covered by muscle on all but its subcutaneous medial border. The distal extremity broadens to meet the expanded carpus (commonly known as the "knee"). On each side it carries a styloid process and, proximal to this, an eminence for the attachment of a collateral ligament. The cranial aspect is grooved for the passage of the extensor tendons. These tendons, the adjacent molding of the bone, the styloid processes, and the eminences for ligamentous attachment are all very distinctly palpable.

The carpal skeleton is arranged in the usual two rows (Fig. 23–20/*A*). The proximal row comprises radial, intermediate, and ulnar carpal bones, concerned in weight-bearing, together with a laterally flattened, discoidal accessory bone that projects backward in a very conspicuous fashion. The accessory bone articulates with the lateral styloid process and the ulnar carpal but bears no weight. The distal row is also deep; in addition to three constant elements—second, third, and fourth carpal bones—there is often a pea-shaped first carpal. This bone is frequently isolated from the remainder of the skeleton, embedded in the palmar carpal ligament behind the second carpal; it may be mistaken for a bone fragment when shown in radiographs (Fig. 23–13/6 and Plate 25/*A*).

The *carpal joint* is maintained in full extension in the standing posture but is capable of very considerable flexion. It presents three levels of articulation. Movement is most free at the radiocarpal (antebrachiocarpal) level where as much as 90 or 100 degrees of flexion is allowed. The midcarpal articulation is also mobile, allowing perhaps 45 degrees of flexion, but no significant movement is possible at the carpometacarpal level (Fig. 23–13/*B*).

The articular surfaces of the bones reflect these differences (Fig. 23–14/*A*). The radial articular surface shows some demarcations corresponding to the three proximal carpal bones but overall presents a caudal hemicylindrical ridge and narrow cranial gutter. The upper surfaces of the proximal carpal bone row have the reciprocal conformation. Their lower surfaces are convex in front and concave behind. The surfaces at the distal joint are broadly flat. Figure 23–15/*A* illustrates these features and the two axes of rotation. The fronts of the bones are driven together in full extension of the joint and may splinter ("chip fractures"*) during the fast gaits.

The carpus is mainly supported by the cannon bone but also makes contact with the bases of the splint bones. Indeed, so large a part of the second carpal bone rests on the second metacarpal that it may tend to drive that bone away from its larger neighbor, inducing the painful acute inflammation mentioned later. Certainly the condition known as "splints" is more common at the medial intermetacarpal joint.

The three levels of articulation share a common fibrous capsule, but the synovial compartments are separate except for a narrow communication between the middle and distal levels (Fig. 23–14). The fibrous capsule (Fig. 23–15/*A*,3), which has extensive connections with all the bones involved in the joint, is of very unequal thickness. It is weakest dorsally where it is rather loose in the extended position of the joint. It is much thicker

*Similar fractures rarely occur also on the palmar surface of these bones; they are given a poor prognosis.

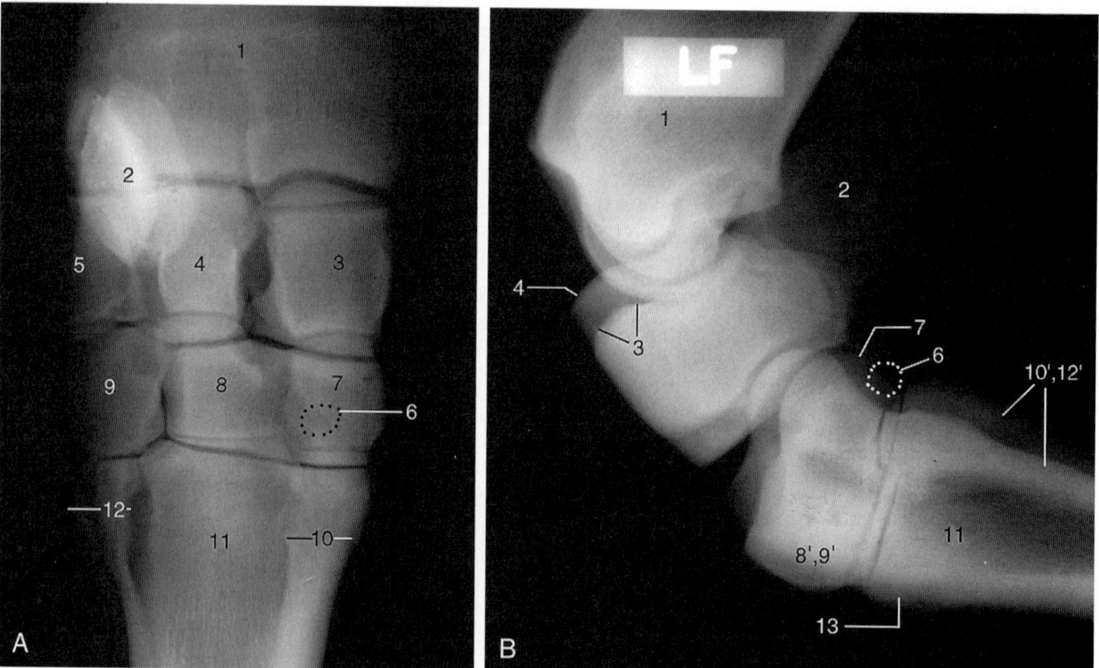


**Figure 23–13.** Dorsopalmar *(A)* and lateral *(B)* radiographs of the carpus.

1, Radius; 2, accessory carpal (faint); 3, radial carpal; 4, intermediate carpal; 5, ulnar carpal; 6, position of first carpal, when present; 7, 8, 9, second, third, and fourth carpals; 8′, 9′, superimposed third and fourth carpals; 10, 11, 12, second, third, and fourth metacarpals; 10′, 12′, superimposed second and fourth metacarpals; 13, metacarpal tuberosity.

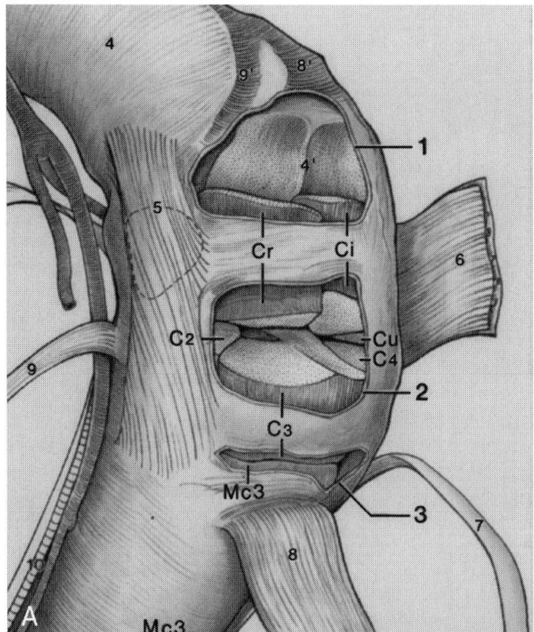


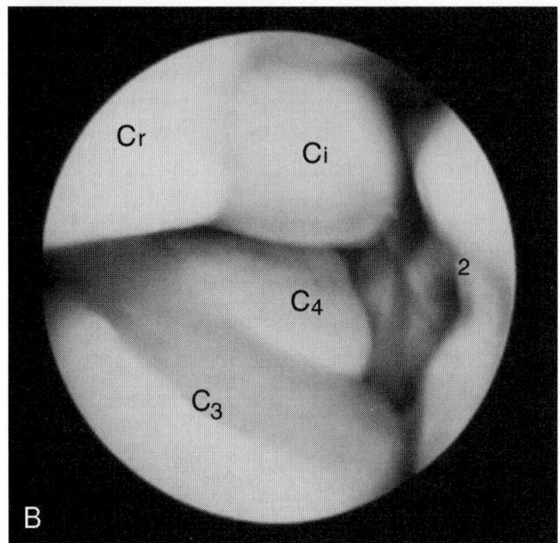


**Figure 23–14.** *A,* Flexed left carpus, dorsomedial view. The articular surfaces are stippled. *B,* Arthroscopic medial-to-lateral view of the left midcarpal joint. Cr, Ci, Cu, radial, intermediate, and ulnar carpal bones; C2, C3, C4, second, third, and fourth carpal bones; Mc3, third metacarpal (cannon) bone.

1, Radiocarpal joint capsule, fenestrated; 2, midcarpal joint capsule, fenestrated in *A*; 3, carpometacarpal joint capsule, fenestrated; 4, 4′, radius and its distal articular surface; 5, position of bursa between medial collateral ligament and extensor carpi obliquus (9); 6, extensor retinaculum, reflected; 7, common digital extensor; 8, 8′, extensor carpi radialis and its groove on radius; 9, 9′, extensor carpi obliquus and its groove on radius; 10, medial palmar nerve, artery, and vein.

over the palmar aspect (/7) where it opposes overextension. This part, the palmar carpal ligament, fills the irregularities of the bones and smoothes the backward facing aspect of the carpal skeleton. Medial and lateral collateral ligaments extend between the lower end of the radius and the upper part of the metacarpus. They have intermediate attachments to the carpal bones and ensure that movement is confined to the sagittal plane. There are numerous additional ligaments. Some merely join adjacent bones in the same row, or distal bones to the metacarpus, and though they help stabilize the joint, they are not individually of interest. Others secure the accessory bone; one that runs obliquely from its distal edge to the metacarpus forms a conspicuous ridge. A larger transverse ligament (flexor retinaculum; /22) extends from the palmar edge of the accessory bone to attach at the mediopalmar aspect of the joint. It completes the enclosure of a space, the carpal canal, through which pass the flexor tendons and other structures en route from the forearm to the distal part of the limb.

Distention of the radiocarpal joint capsule is not uncommon. The capsule pouches where support is weak, dorsally between the extensor tendons and proximally, above the accessory bone, just caudal to the lateral digital extensor tendon (Fig. 23–16/1). It may be punctured here, but a more convenient approach is from the dorsal aspect. Flexion of the carpus opens up the joint space, facilitating the entry of a needle between the extensor tendons. A similar approach may be made to the middle compartment (Plate 25/*B,C*).

## The Muscles of the Forearm

### *The Extensor Group*

With one exception, the extensor carpi obliquus, all carpal and digital extensors arise from the craniolateral aspect of the distal end of the humerus and occupy the craniolateral part of the forearm. Their insertion tendons begin a little above the carpus and are secured in their passage over the joint by condensed deep fascia known as the extensor retinaculum (Fig. 23–15/*B*,11). Each is also individually protected by a synovial sheath, from just above to well below the carpus (Fig. 23–16).

Except for the ulnaris lateralis, all are extensor to the carpus; the longer muscles also extend the joints of the digit. In addition, their origin provides them with some capacity to flex the elbow, although they are probably little used in this role. All are supplied by the radial nerve. They may each be identified on palpation, and several provide quite conspicuous visible features of the forearm of thin-skinned animals.

The *extensor carpi radialis* (Fig. 23–17/5), the most medial member of the group, runs directly to the front of the subcutaneous border of the radius.

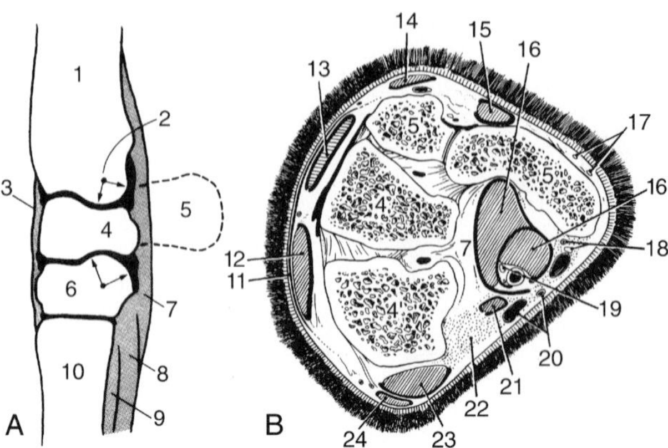


**Figure 23–15.** *A,* Axial section of the carpus. *B,* Transverse section of the right carpus, proximal surface. Both joints face to the left.

1, Radius; 2, axis of rotation; 3, fibrous joint capsule; 4, 4′, intermediate and radial carpal; 5, 5′, accessory and ulnar carpal; 6, third carpal; 7, palmar carpal ligament; 8, accessory (check) ligament of deep digital flexor; 9, interosseus; 10, large metacarpal; 11, extensor retinaculum; 12, extensor carpi radialis; 13, common digital extensor; 14, lateral digital extensor; 15, long tendon of ulnaris lateralis; 16, 16′, deep and superficial flexor tendons in carpal canal; 17, dorsal branch of ulnar nerve; 18, palmar branch of median artery and lateral palmar nerve; 19, median artery and medial palmar nerve; 20, radial artery and vein; 21, flexor carpi radialis; 22, flexor retinaculum; 23, medial collateral ligament; 24, extensor carpi obliquus.

Its epimysial covering is joined by the lacertus fibrosus that enables it passively to prevent flexion of the carpal joint when weight is on the limb.

The *common digital extensor* (/6) possesses a rather slight radial head in addition to the more substantial origin from the humerus. The radial head is never fully incorporated in the main mass and separates in the lower part of the forearm; its tendon joins that of the lateral digital extensor within the cannon. The main tendon continues down the dorsal aspect to the metacarpus and digit to insert upon the extensor process of the distal phalanx. Just before this, it is joined by branches of the interosseus that wind around the sides of the digit from the palmar aspect (/13).

The slighter *lateral digital extensor* (/7) creates a prominent ridge on the lateral aspect of the forearm. It is joined by the contribution from the common extensor in the upper part of the cannon and then gently inclines toward the dorsal aspect of the limb to insert on the proximal end of the proximal phalanx.

The *ulnaris lateralis* (/9) runs down the caudal aspect of the forearm. Its short tendon of insertion splits above the accessory carpal bone; a part at once inserts on this bone, while a longer branch descends over the lateral aspect of the bone, tunnels under the collateral ligament, and ends upon the head of the lateral splint bone. The longer division requires the protection of a synovial sheath (Fig. 23–16/8).

The *extensor carpi obliquus* is distinguished by arising from the shaft of the radius. It runs in a mediodistal direction to insert upon the medial splint bone. Though largely covered by the other muscles, its tendon becomes superficial to that of the extensor carpi radialis (Fig. 23–17/8).

## The Flexor Group

The muscles of the flexor group also share several attributes. They arise from the caudomedial aspect of the humerus, occupy the caudal part of the forearm, obtain their innervation from the median and ulnar nerves, and are flexor to the carpal joint; those that proceed beyond this level are also flexor to the digital joints.

The *flexor carpi radialis* (Fig. 23–18/8) follows the subcutaneous border of the radius and covers the important median vessels and nerve. The tendon of insertion tunnels through the flexor retinaculum where it obtains the necessary protection of a synovial sheath before attaching to the medial splint bone.

The *flexor carpi ulnaris* (/9) lies on the medial aspect of the forearm, partly under cover of the flexor carpi radialis. It arises by two heads—from the humerus and the ulna—and inserts upon the proximal margin of the accessory carpal bone by means of a short tendon that has no need of synovial protection.

The *superficial digital flexor* occupies a central position within the flexor group, between the larger mass of the deep flexor and the flexor carpi ulnaris (Fig. 23–19/9). A purely tendinous head, usually known as an accessory or check ligament (/4), arises from the caudal surface of the radius to join the main tendon in the lower part of the forearm; it is a component of the passive stay-apparatus (see further on). The superficial and deep flexor tendons share a common synovial sheath, the carpal sheath, in their passage through the carpal canal.

The tendon is superficial to that of the deep tendon in the metacarpus, but at the fetlock it obtains the deeper position necessary for its insertion on neighboring parts of the proximal and middle phalanges (Fig. 23–18/13).

The *deep digital flexor* is by far the largest of the flexors, although this is not apparent without dissection (Fig. 23–19/9′). In addition to the humeral head there are lesser heads of origin from the upper parts of the radius and ulna. The common tendon passes through the carpal canal and continues down the palmar aspect of the limb to find insertion upon the palmar surface of the distal phalanx. In the metacarpus the tendon is joined by a stout tendinous band that arises from the thick fibrous joint capsule on the palmar aspect

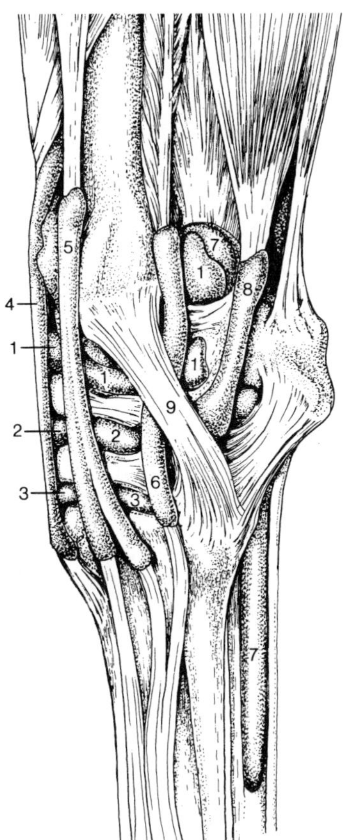


**Figure 23–16.** Synovial structures of the left carpus; lateral view.

1, Radiocarpal joint capsule; 2, midcarpal joint capsule; 3, carpometacarpal joint capsule; 4, tendon sheath of extensor carpi radialis; 5, tendon sheath of common digital extensor; 6, tendon sheath of lateral digital extensor; 7, tendon sheath of superficial and deep digital flexors (carpal sheath); 8, tendon sheath of ulnaris lateralis; 9, lateral collateral ligament.

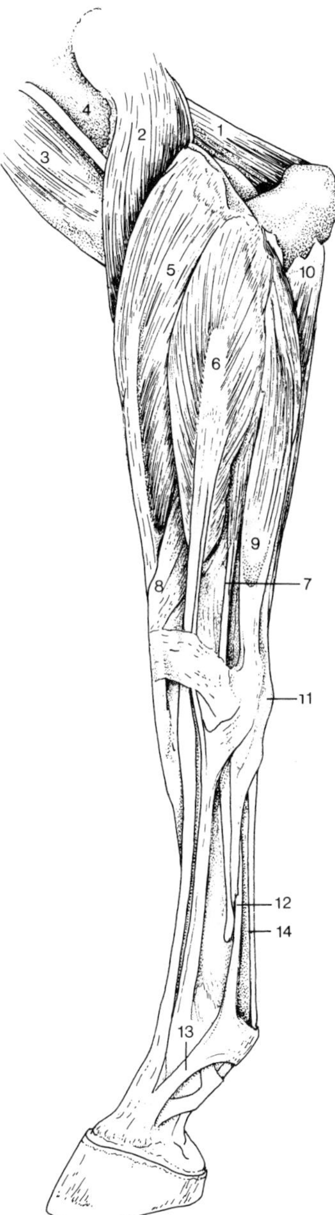


**Figure 23–17.** Distal muscles of the left forelimb; lateral view.

1, Anconeus; 2, brachialis; 3, biceps; 4, deltoid tuberosity of humerus; 5, extensor carpi radialis; 6, common digital extensor; 7, lateral digital extensor; 8, extensor carpi obliquus; 9, ulnaris lateralis; 10, ulnar head of deep digital flexor; 11, accessory carpal bone; 12, interosseus; 13, extensor branch of interosseus; 14, flexor tendons.

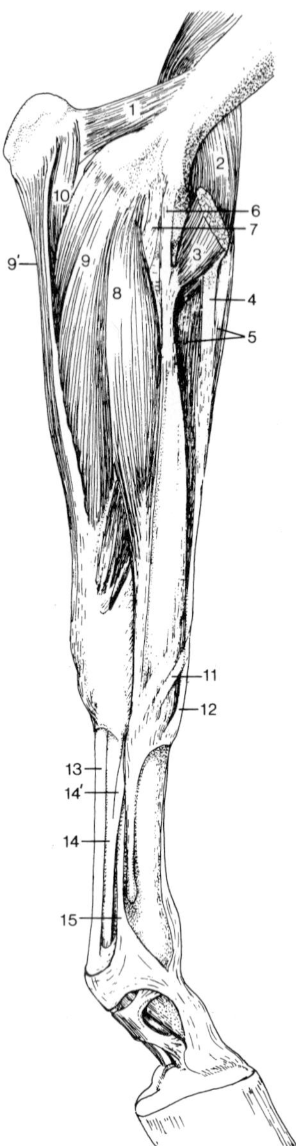


**Figure 23–18.** Distal muscles of the left forelimb; medial view.

1, Anconeus; 2, brachialis; 3, biceps; 4, lacertus fibrosus; 5, extensor carpi radialis; 6, long part of medial collateral ligament (pronator teres); 7, short part of medial collateral ligament; 8, flexor carpi radialis; 9, 9′, humeral and ulnar heads of flexor carpi ulnaris; 10, ulnar head of deep digital flexor; 11, tendon of extensor carpi obliquus; 12, tendon of extensor carpi radialis; 13, tendon of superficial digital flexor; 14, tendon of deep digital flexor; 14′, accessory (check) ligament; 15, interosseus.

of the carpal joint (Fig. 23–18/14,14′). This is almost invariably known as an accessory or check ligament; it provides an important element of the passive stay-apparatus, one that is of far greater significance than the analogous contribution to the superficial tendon.

## THE DISTAL PART OF THE LIMB

The more distal structures of the limb not only have the greatest propensity to injury but also show many and important specific differences.

### The Skeleton and Joints

The skeleton comprises the metacarpal bones and the proximal, middle, and distal phalanges. The metacarpophalangeal and the proximal and distal interphalangeal joints linking these bones are commonly referred to as the fetlock, pastern, and coffin joints. A pair of proximal sesamoid bones

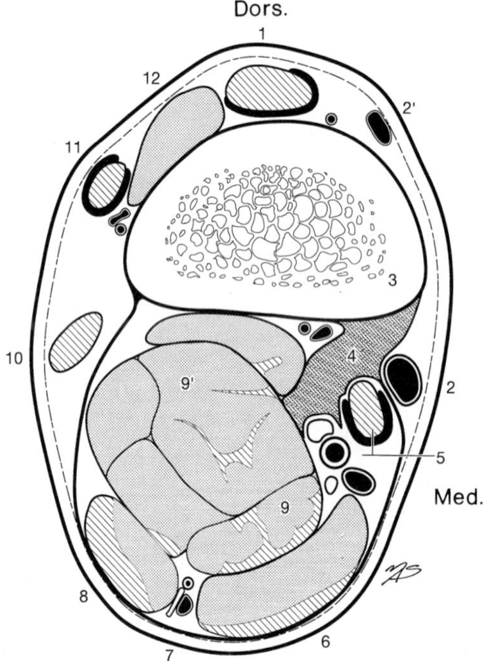


**Figure 23–19.** Transverse section of the left forearm 6 cm proximal to the proximal border of the accessory carpal, to demonstrate the topography of the accessory (check) ligament (4) of the superficial digital flexor; looking distally. The *hatched areas* are tendons or tendinous tissue, and the *gray areas* are muscle tissue.

1, Extensor carpi radialis; 2, 2′, cephalic and accessory cephalic veins; 3, radius; 4, accessory (check) ligament of superficial digital flexor; 5, flexor carpi radialis, median artery, and medial and lateral palmar nerves; 6, flexor carpi ulnaris; 7, ulnar nerve and collateral ulnar vessels; 8, ulnaris lateralis; 9, 9′, superficial and deep digital flexors; 10, 11, 12, lateral, common, and oblique extensors.

enlarges the concavity of the fetlock joint, a single distal sesamoid bone that of the coffin joint.

The metacarpal skeleton comprises second, third, and fourth *metacarpal bones*. The third bone, the cannon bone, is much stronger than the other two and is the functional element. It carries a prominent tuberosity on its dorsal surface just distal to the joint. The bones to each side, generally known as the splint bones, are much reduced in size. Each has a small proximal base that continues into a tapering shaft. In young animals the splint and cannon bones are joined by fibrous tissue; this generally later ossifies and the upper parts of the shafts are then fused together. The process is often accompanied by an acute inflammation (a condition known as "splints"), which leaves a palpable—and often visible—blemish on the dorsal surface.

The tapering second and fourth metacarpals end in slight but easily palpable buttons three quarters of the way down the cannon (see Fig. 2–49/*D*). The lower parts of their shafts are free, and when a break occurs it is a simple matter to remove the fragment below the fracture line.

The third metacarpal bone is exceptionally robust. It is oval in cross section (which distinguishes it from the longer but more rounded cannon bone of the hindlimb), and its thick compacta attests to its tremendous strength; it is in fact one of the strongest elements of the skeleton (Fig. 23–45/1).

The distal extremity presents an axially keeled condyle that articulates with the proximal phalanx and the paired sesamoid bones. When viewed from the side, the condyle encompasses some 220 degrees of a circle, evidence of the great range of flexion and extension, the only movements allowed. The articular surface to each side of the keel is interrupted by a slight ridge that separates the more strongly curved palmar area from the larger dorsal one. Despite the obvious strength of the cannon bone, longitudinal fractures of the distal extremity are common racing injuries, more often involving the lateral than the medial side and the fore- rather than the hindlimb. The degree of involvement of the joint surface is an important factor in prognosis.

The *proximal sesamoid bones* are three-sided pyramids whose bases face distally (Fig. 23–20/10). The dorsal (articular) surface of each lies against the condyle, the palmar (flexor) surface tilts axially and faces the flexor tendons that ride over it, and the abaxial surface is hollowed for the reception of the thick branch of the interosseous (see further on). The palmar aspects of the bones are converted by thick fibrous tissue (palmar ligament) into a single bearing surface over which

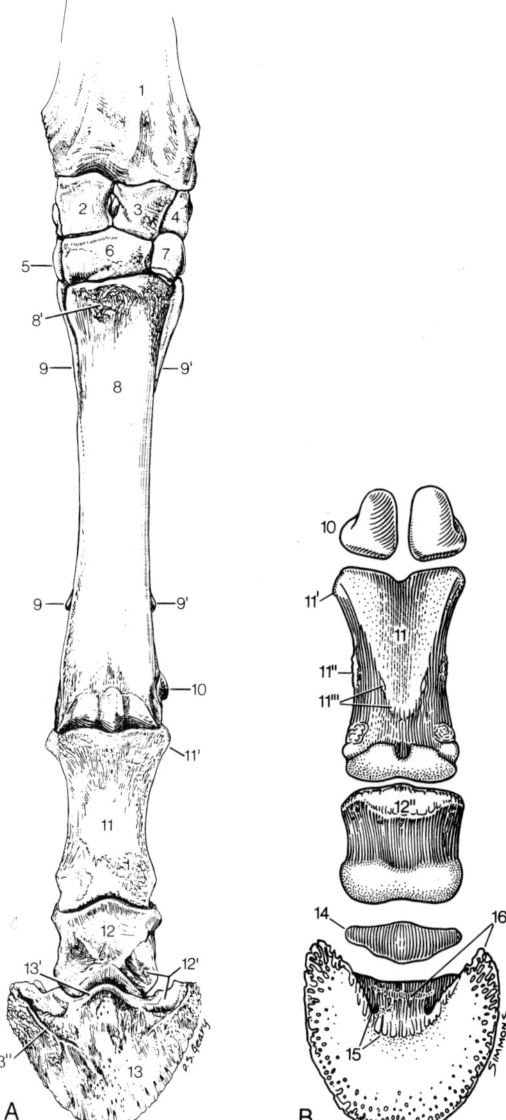


**Figure 23–20.** Skeleton of the distal part of the forelimb. *A*, Left limb, dorsal view. *B*, Palmar view.

1, Radius; 2, radial carpal; 3, intermediate carpal; 4, ulnar carpal; 5, 6, 7, second, third, and fourth carpals; 8, large metacarpal bone; 8′, metacarpal tuberosity; 9, 9′, medial and lateral splint bones; 10, proximal sesamoid bones; 11, proximal phalanx; 11′, proximal tubercle; 11″, attachment of distal digital annular and abaxial palmar ligaments; 11‴, attachment of axial palmar and oblique sesamoidean ligaments; 12, middle phalanx; 12′, attachments of collateral ligament of coffin joint; 12″, bearing surface for deep flexor tendon; 13, distal phalanx; 13′, extensor process; 13″, parietal groove; 14, navicular bone; 15, sole foramen and semilunar crest for attachment of deep flexor tendon; 16, palmar process and attachment of distal navicular ligament.

the flexor tendons change direction. Though close to the proximal phalanx, the sesamoid bones do not articulate with it.

The proximal sesamoids fracture most often of all the bones in the forelimb, followed in frequency by the metacarpal and carpal bones. These fractures are known in racetrack practice as "the big three" for which, when serious, horses pay with their lives.

The strong *proximal phalanx* (PI for short) is compressed from front to back and wider proximally than distally. Its proximal extremity is hollowed and deepened axially by a groove to conform to the condyle of the large metacarpal bone. Palpable tubercles to each side receive the collateral ligaments of the fetlock joint. The distal end is shaped as two condyles separated by a shallow axial groove and presents similar but smaller tubercles for the collateral ligaments of the pastern joint. The palmar surface of the bone is roughened for the attachment of several ligaments; a large triangular area, and various smaller ones to each side, stand out (/11,11′,11″,11‴).

The *middle phalanx* (PII) is on the whole similar to PI but, being only half as long, is proportionately very robust. Both extremities are of equal width. The proximal articular surface—hollowed with a slight axial ridge—is the reciprocal of the lower end of PI, while the distal one—two condyles separated by a groove—mimics that of PI. The distal articular surface extends onto the palmar aspect where it articulates with the distal sesamoid bone. There are proximal collateral tubercles on middle phalanx for the collateral ligaments of the pastern joint; the corresponding distal sites from which the collateral ligaments of the coffin joint arise, are excavated. The proximopalmar border presents a smooth area (/12″) that is enlarged in the natural state by a complementary fibrocartilage, forming a bearing surface for the deep flexor tendon (see further on). The fibrocartilage enlarges the articular surface of the pastern joint and gives attachment to several ligaments.

The *distal phalanx* (PIII, coffin bone) generally conforms to the interior of the hoof in which it resides "as in a coffin." It is wedge-shaped—sharp distally and to the sides, blunt proximally and toward the back. The dorsal (parietal) surface is convex from side to side and lies against the dermis that unites it to the inner surface of the hoof wall. It tapers caudally into medial and lateral palmar processes that are notched (or perforated) and grooved for the dorsal terminal branches of the digital arteries and accompanying nerves (Fig. 23–20/13″). Depressions for the collateral ligaments of the coffin joint are present proximodorsal to the processes. The palmar (sole) surface is slightly concave to fit the domed sole of the hoof. Both parietal and sole surfaces are very porous to allow the passage of numerous small arteries from the interior of the bone into the overlying dermis. The articular surface faces proximally; it is very similar to the proximal articular surface of PII, consisting of two fossae separated by an axial ridge. Its dorsal border tapers to an extensor process, the highest point of the bone, where the common digital extensor tendon is attached. The palmar border is extended by a narrow articular zone for the distal sesamoid bone which, in contrast to the proximal sesamoids, articulates with both major bones of the joint. Just distal to this, two prominent foramina lead to a U-shaped canal within the bone; this contains the anastomosis of the terminal palmar branches of the digital arteries. The deep flexor tendon ends on the semilunar crest just distal to the foramina (/15).

The flat cartilages (of the hoof), which surmount and continue the palmar processes, lie mainly against the inner wall of the hoof, but their proximal borders are free, subcutaneous, and palpable to each side of the pastern joint (Fig. 23–21/4 and Plate 25/*I*).

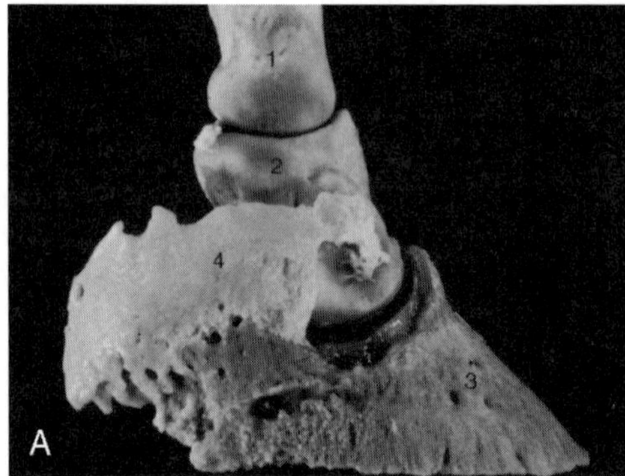


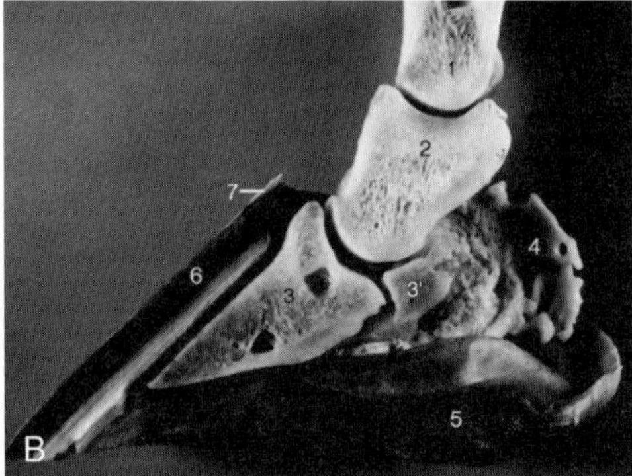


**Figure 23–21.** *A*, Hoof cartilage attaching to palmar process of distal phalanx. *B*, Position of distal phalanx and navicular bone within hoof, axial section.

1, 2, 3, Proximal, middle, and distal phalanges; 3′, navicular bone; 4, hoof cartilage; 5, frog; 6, wall; 7, periople.

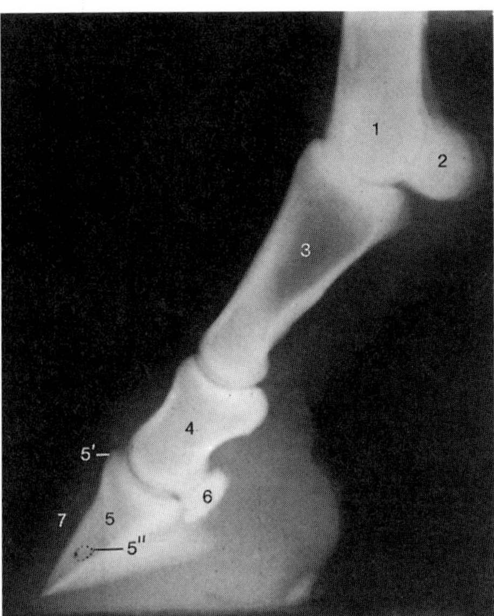


**Figure 23–22.** Lateral radiograph of fetlock joint and digit.

1, Large metacarpal bone; 2, proximal sesamoid bones; 3, proximal phalanx; 4, middle phalanx; 5, distal phalanx; 5′, extensor process; 5″, canal containing terminal arterial arch; 6, navicular bone; 7, wall of hoof.

The *distal sesamoid (navicular) bone* (/3′) is boat shaped with straight proximal and convex distal borders. Its dorsal (articular) surface contacts the distal end of PII; a narrow distal facet touches PIII. The palmar (flexor) surface faces the wide tendon of the deep flexor, providing it with yet another bearing surface as it bends toward the semilunar crest on the undersurface of PIII. The navicular bone enlarges the distal articular surface of the coffin joint (Fig. 23–24/7′,7″).

The *fetlock joint* is formed between the large metacarpal bone, PI, and the proximal sesamoid bones (Fig. 23–22). The large bones are connected by medial and lateral collateral ligaments, while additional smaller and triangular (collateral) ligaments anchor the sesamoid bones to the sides of the metacarpal condyle and the proximal tubercles of PI. A series of sesamoidean ligaments connects the bases of the sesamoid bones to the first phalanx and ensures that the sesamoids move against the metacarpal condyle in unison with PI. The deepest ligaments are short and pass to the proximopalmar border of PI; they are overlain by rather longer cruciate ligaments that end a little more distally, and these in turn are overlain by oblique ligaments that attach broadly to the central triangular area of the palmar surface of the same bone. Finally, an additional straight sesamoidean ligament, arising from the bases of the sesamoids, connects with the complementary fibrocartilage of PII (Fig. 23–23/4). The cruciate, oblique, and straight ligaments are mentioned again in connection with the action of the interosseus.

The sesamoid bones are connected to each other by a thick palmar ligament that extends the bearing surface for the flexor tendons proximally by about 2 cm (/2). This extension supports the tendons when the sesamoids themselves slip below the condyle in maximal overextension of the fetlock joint (when the dorsal angle can be as small as 90 degrees). When the joint is fully flexed, the sesamoid bones lose contact with the condyle and ride up on the back of the metacarpal bone where bone-to-bone contact is prevented by the proximal extension of the palmar ligament.

The joint capsule is capacious, and to allow for the region's mobility it extends large dorsal and

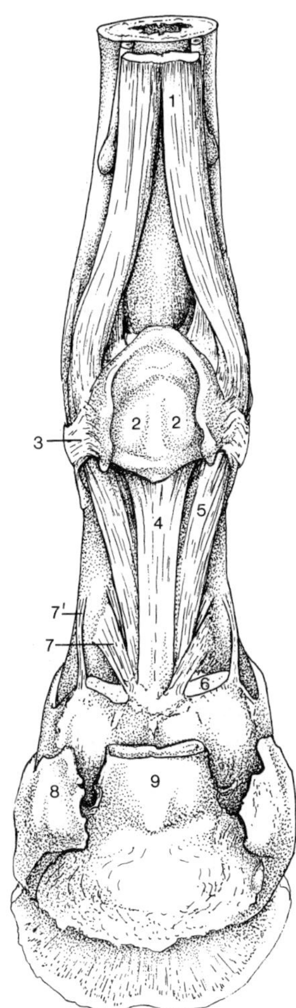


**Figure 23–23.** Structures supporting the fetlock joint.

1, Interosseus; 2, proximal sesamoid bones connected by thick palmar ligament; 3, collateral sesamoidean ligament; 4, straight sesamoidean ligament; 5, oblique sesamoidean ligament; 6, stump of superficial flexor; 7, 7′, axial and abaxial palmar ligaments of pastern joint; 8, hoof cartilage; 9, stump of deep flexor.

palmar pouches proximally (Fig. 23–27/7). These lie against the shaft of the metacarpal bone and are easily punctured from the side; the end of the splint bone, the interosseus, and the sesamoid bone are convenient (almost visible) landmarks for entry into the palmar pouch (Fig. 23–26/11 and Plate 25/*D*[*arrow*],*F*). Distentions of the joint known as "wind puffs" or "galls" manifest themselves at this site. The interior of the dorsal pouch contains a so-called capsular fold (Fig. 23–27/7′). This arises from the shaft of the metacarpal bone and projects distally into the center of the pouch; its inflammation and enlargement can cause lameness. Short distal palmar pouches are palpable as small depressions in the angles between PI and the bases of the sesamoid bones.

The movement of the *pastern joint* is much more restricted. Paired (axial and abaxial) palmar ligaments connect the palmar aspect of PI with the complementary fibrocartilage of PII (Fig. 23–23/7,7′); together with the straight sesamoidean ligament (/4) they limit overextension. The capsule is similar to that of the fetlock joint, but the pouches are smaller and only the dorsal one is accessible for puncture, again from the side. The radiographic appearance of the pastern and coffin joints is shown in Figure 23–24/*A*).

The *coffin joint* allows flexion and extension to about the same degree as the pastern joint. The collateral ligaments are short and thick and are solidly anchored at both ends to depressions in the bones. The navicular bone, an integral part of the joint, is suspended from the distal extremity of PI by the collateral navicular ligaments (Fig. 23–25/2). These cross the medial and lateral borders of PII and attach to the ends and proximal border of the navicular bone in a U-shaped fashion. A very short but wide distal navicular

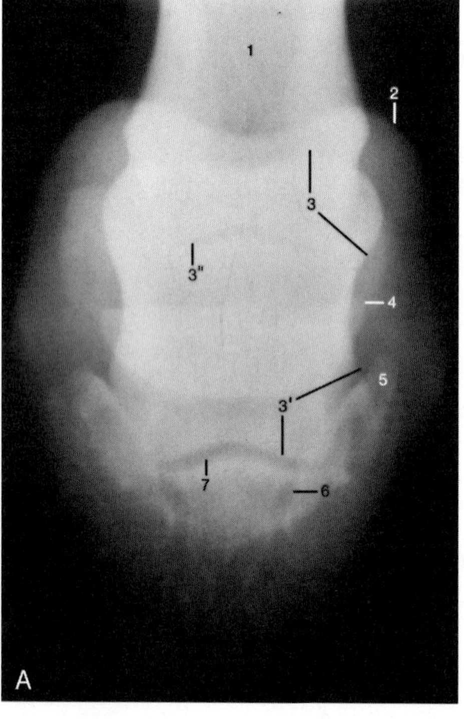


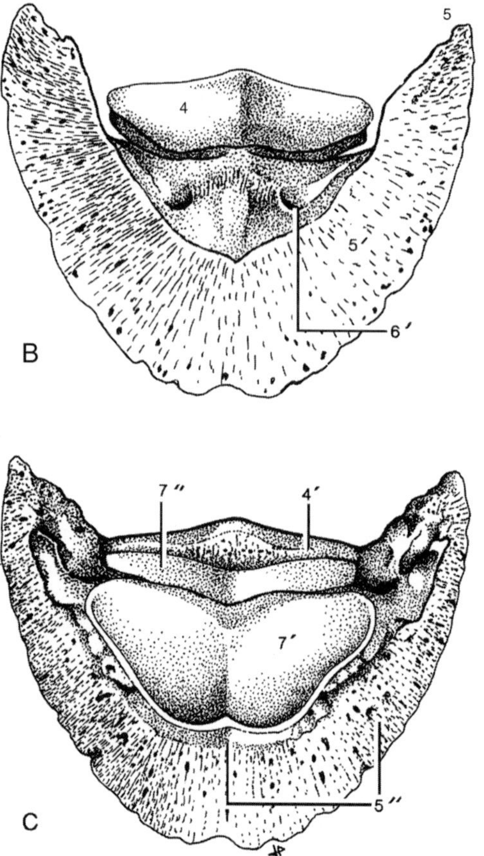


**Figure 23–24.** *A*, Dorsopalmar radiograph of hoof. *B* and *C*, Palmar and dorsal surfaces of distal phalanx (PIII) and navicular bone.

1, Proximal phalanx; 2, bulb of heel; 3, 3′, proximal and distal contours of middle phalanx; 3″, pastern joint; 4, navicular bone (its flexor surface in *B*); 4′, proximal border of navicular bone; 5, palmar process of PIII; 5′, palmar (sole) surface of PIII; 5″, extensor process and dorsal (parietal) surface of PIII; 6, canal containing terminal arterial arch, 6′, sole foramen (entrance to 6); 7, coffin joint; 7′, articular surface of PIII; 7", articular surface of navicular bone.

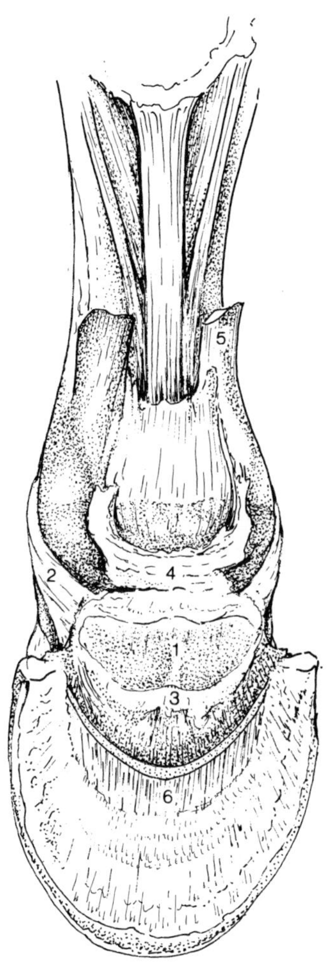


**Figure 23–25.** Ligaments of the navicular bone; palmar view.

1, Navicular bone; 2, collateral ligament of navicular bone; 3, distal navicular ligament; 4, connective tissue between coffin joint, digital sheath, and navicular bursa (see Fig. 23–27/15); 5, stump of superficial digital flexor; 6, stump of deep digital flexor.

ligament (/3) connects the distal border of the bone with PIII, attaching proximal to the prominent sole foramina. The capsule attaches to the articular margins of the three bones and resembles those of the other digital joints in having dorsal and palmar pouches. The pouches are small, and only the dorsal one is accessible for puncture (at the proximal border of the hoof); the procedure is not easy (Plate 25/*H,G*).

The incorporation of sesamoid bones in the fetlock and coffin joints divides the weight pressing onto the lower part of each joint over two bones, phalanx and sesamoid. The elasticity of the sesamoid ligaments and of the flexor tendons behind them allows the joint to yield slightly during foot impact. This is but one of several mechanisms designed to dissipate the concussion generated by so heavy and swift an animal. The concussive effects may be accentuated by poor conformation, upright pasterns and small feet (in relation to body size) being a combination encountered frequently in animals afflicted with navicular disease, a relatively common cause of lameness. This condition is characterized by erosion at the margins of the navicular bone where its ligaments attach, and by inflammation and degeneration of the navicular bursa (Fig. 23–27/10) and related part of the deep flexor tendon (/13). But the exact pathogenesis is still debated and different authorities give quite contradictory explanations.

## The Tendons, Annular Ligaments, and Interosseus Muscle

The tendons of the common and lateral digital extensors enter the foot to the front of the metacarpal bone, those of the superficial and deep flexors behind it. A third very important element in the support of the fetlock, the tendinous interosseus muscle, is situated on the palmar aspect, between the bone and the flexor tendons. The structures on the palmar surface of the cannon are enclosed within a deep fascia that extends from one splint bone to the other (Fig. 23–46/8′). The fascia is thickest immediately below the carpus but gradually thins when followed distally, and toward the fetlock it offers little hindrance to the palpation of deeper structures.

The *common extensor tendon* is protected by a synovial bursa as it passes over the dorsal pouch of the fetlock joint. Broadening, it makes limited attachments at the proximal borders of PI and PII before receiving the extensor branches of the interosseus that wind around the digit. It ends on the extensor process of PIII (Figs. 23–26/1 and 23–27/17).

The *lateral extensor tendon* descends on the metacarpal bone lateral to the common tendon, crosses the fetlock joint, and ends on a roughening on the dorsal aspect of PI. Both extensor tendons, though easily palpated in the metacarpus, evade recognition beyond the fetlock joint where they become broader and thinner. The extensor branches of the interosseus are more prominent below the skin.

The *superficial digital flexor tendon* becomes subcutaneous (but for the fascial investment of distally decreasing thickness) after emerging from the carpal canal and provides the caudal border of the cannon. It forms a sleeve around the deep flexor tendon at the level of the proximal sesamoid

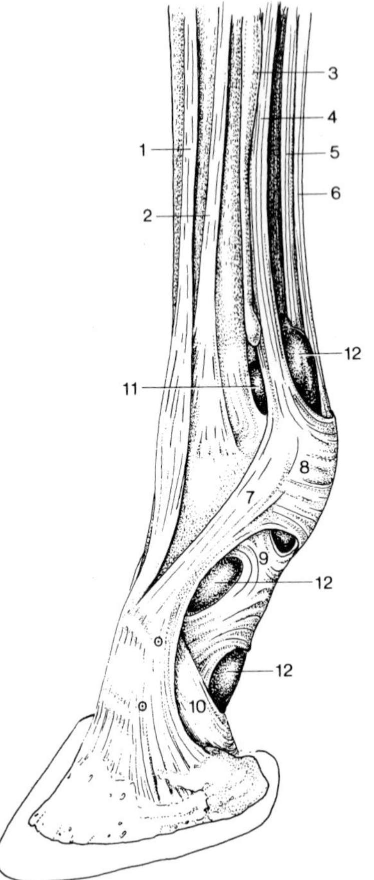


**Figure 23–26.** Tendons and annular ligaments of the left digit; dorsolateral view. The two *dotted circles* indicate the sites for injecting the pastern and coffin joints.

1, Common digital extensor; 2, lateral digital extensor; 3, lateral splint bone; 4, interosseus; 5, deep digital flexor; 6, superficial digital flexor; 7, extensor branch of interosseus; 8, palmar annular ligament; 9, proximal digital annular ligament; 10, distal digital annular ligament; 11, palmar pouch of fetlock joint; 12, digital sheath.

bones (Fig. 23–28/*B*). The deep part of the sleeve splits opposite the middle of PI to allow the superficial flexor to attach to the distal tubercles of PI and the adjacent complementary fibrocartilage of PII. The palmar part of the sleeve ends at about the same level to allow the deep flexor tendon to gain the superficial position where it is palpable for a few centimeters before it enters the hoof.

Only the medial and lateral borders of the *deep flexor tendon* can be palpated above the fetlock. The tendon is most easily separated and distinguished from that of the superficial flexor muscle when the fetlock joint is flexed to relieve tension, but even in these circumstances it is usually impossible to identify the very strong accessory (check) ligament that arises from the palmar carpal ligament to join the deep face of the tendon toward the middle of the cannon (Fig. 23–18/14′). The tendon then passes the fetlock in the sleeve formed by the superficial tendon, and beyond the middle of PI it rides over the bearing surface provided by the complementary fibrocartilage of PII. It then widens before passing over the navicular bone to terminate on PIII.

The flexor tendons are held in place by three *annular ligaments,* which are local thickenings of the deep fascia. The first, the palmar annular ligament, arises from the abaxial borders of the proximal sesamoid bones; since it adheres to the superficial flexor tendon the potential for movement between the tendon and the sesamoids is clearly restricted. The second, the proximal digital annular ligament, resembles an X when viewed from behind (Fig. 23–29/6). The proximal margin of the X and the four corners, which attach near the proximal and distal tubercles of PI, are most easily distinguished since the body and the distal margin fuse with the superficial tendon. The third, the distal digital annular ligament, arises from the medial and lateral borders of PI together with the abaxial palmar ligaments of the pastern joint. It provides a sling that fuses with the palmar surface of the deep tendon, continuing to the insertion on PIII within the hoof; it separates the tendon from the digital cushion. Usually, only its free upper border can be demonstrated (/7).

The navicular (podotrochlear) bursa protects the deep flexor tendon from excessive friction and pressure against the navicular bone (Fig. 23–27/10). More proximally the tendon shares a complex synovial (digital) sheath (/14) with the superficial flexor tendon. The sheath begins a few centimeters proximal to the fetlock joint and ends level with the middle of PII (Plate 25/*E*). It lubricates the passage of the tendons over the bearing surfaces and under the free parts of the annular ligaments and facilitates their movements against each other where they exchange position. It is a common site of inflammation and when distended bulges most noticeably above the proximal sesamoid bones. Though the sheath is in close proximity to the fetlock, pastern, and coffin joints and to the navicular bursa, these cavities do not communicate, except for a connection between the sheath and the coffin joint in the foal. Despite this, anesthetics injected into the coffin joint of adult horses reach the navicular bursa by diffusion.

The *interosseus muscle* is a strong, flat, predominantly tendinous band, long better known as the suspensory ligament. Though it includes a small contingent of muscle fibers, there is little evidence that these fibers are gradually replaced by tendinous tissue as the animal becomes older and heavier. The interosseus arises from the palmar carpal ligament and adjacent part of the large metacarpal bone, descends between the splint bones, and divides a short distance above the fetlock. The two divisions are substantial—and easily palpable—and insert on the abaxial surface of the proximal sesamoid bones. Each detaches a weak (extensor) branch that winds around PI to join the common extensor tendon at the level of the pastern joint (Figs. 23–23/1 and 23–26/7).

A functional continuation of the interosseus beyond the sesamoid bones is provided by the cruciate, oblique, and straight sesamoidean ligaments (Fig. 23–23/4,5). These support the normally overextended fetlock joint; the inclusion of the sesamoids permits frictionless movement over the flexor aspect of the joint (Fig. 23–27/11,5,12). Energy, stored within the apparatus (and in the flexor tendons) by stretching on hoof impact, is released at the end of the stride, allowing the joint to flex and impart forward impetus.

## The Hoof

The distal extremity of the limb is protected by the hoof, which is formed by epithelial keratinization over a greatly modified dermis*; this is continuous with the common dermis of the skin at the coronet (the term applied to the junction between skin and hoof). The hoof is conveniently divided into wall, periople, sole, and frog; the last is an integral part of the hoof capsule, although homologous with the digital pad of other species (see Fig. 10–16).

The *wall* is the part of the hoof visible in the standing animal (see Fig. 10–18). It is highest at its dorsal segment (toe) and decreases in height over the sides (quarters) until it is reflected upon itself, forming the rounded heels at the back of the hoof. The inflected parts continue forward for a short distance as the bars that are visible beside the frog when the hoof is raised (Fig. 23–30/1‴ and Plate

*Formerly, and still commonly, termed the *corium.*

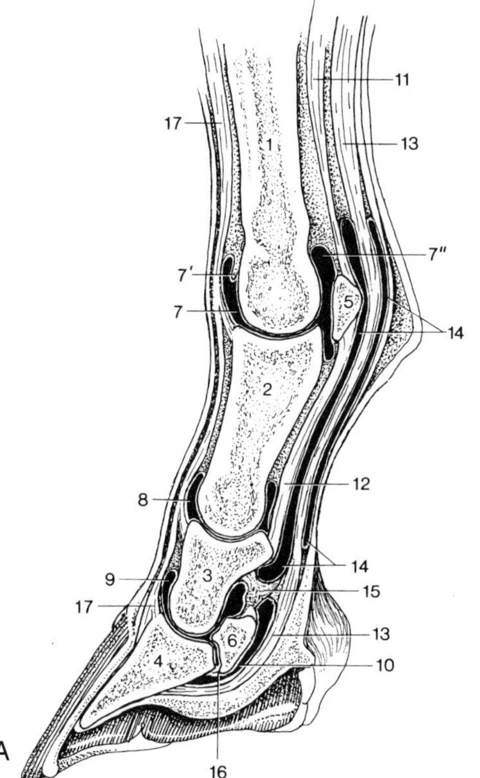


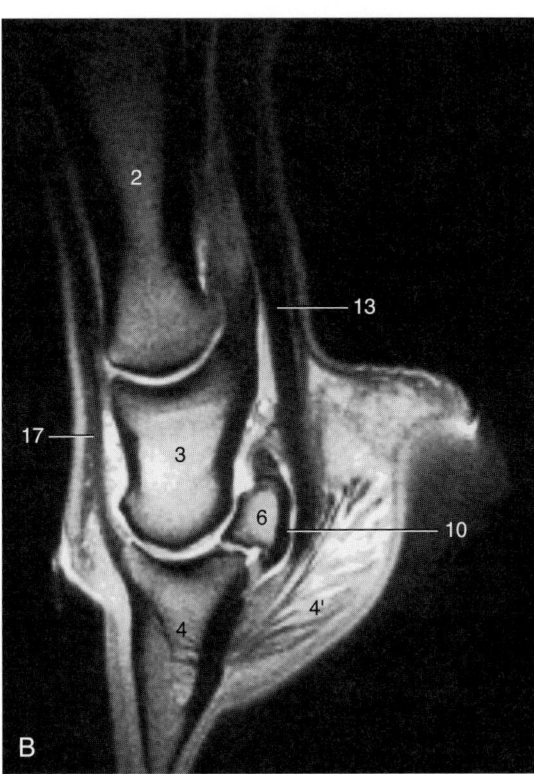


**Figure 23–27.** *A*, Axial section of digit, semischematic. *B*, Corresponding magnetic resonance image.

1, Large metacarpal bone; 2, proximal phalanx; 3, middle phalanx; 4, distal phalanx; 4′, digital cushion; 5, proximal sesamoid bone; 6, distal sesamoid (navicular) bone; 7, dorsal pouch of fetlock joint; 7′, capsular fold; 7″, palmar pouch of fetlock joint; 8, 9, dorsal pouch of pastern and coffin joints; 10, navicular bursa; 11, interosseus; 12, straight sesamoidean ligament; 13, deep flexor tendon; 14, digital sheath; 15, connective tissue bridge; 16, distal navicular ligament; 17, common digital extensor tendon.

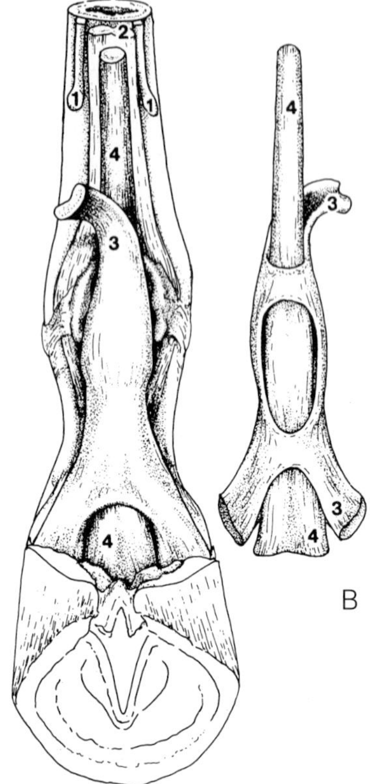


**Figure 23–28.** Relations and topography of the superficial and deep flexor tendons. *A*, Palmar view, in situ. *B*, Dorsal view, isolated.

1, Splint bones; 2, interosseus; 3, superficial digital flexor; 4, deep digital flexor.

26/*G*). The angle that the toe makes with the ground is about 50 degrees in the forelimb, slightly more in the hindlimb; the quarters descend toward the ground more steeply, especially on the medial side. The wall is thickest at the toe and gradually thins toward the bars—an important point for farriers to bear in mind when rasping or driving nails.

The wall grows from the epithelium covering the coronary dermis (Fig. 23–31/2) (which almost surrounds the digit at the coronet). It consists of horn tubules embedded in less structured intertubular horn and slides over the dermis covering the coffin bone and hoof cartilages to be worn away by contact with the ground. The greater part forms the generally pigmented stratum medium. The deeper, nonpigmented stratum internum comprises about 600 (horny) laminae that interdigitate with the sensitive laminae of the underlying laminar dermis (/5 and Plate 15/*F,G*). Trauma affecting the coronary dermis causes horn defects that descend with the wall, reaching the ground in about 8 months (a rate of growth of less than 1 cm per month).

The *periople* contributes the stratum externum of the wall (/6,6′). It consists of a band of soft, rubbery horn a few millimeters thick near the coronet but dries to a thin glossy layer distally. The band widens toward the palmar aspect where it covers the bulbs of the heels and blends with the

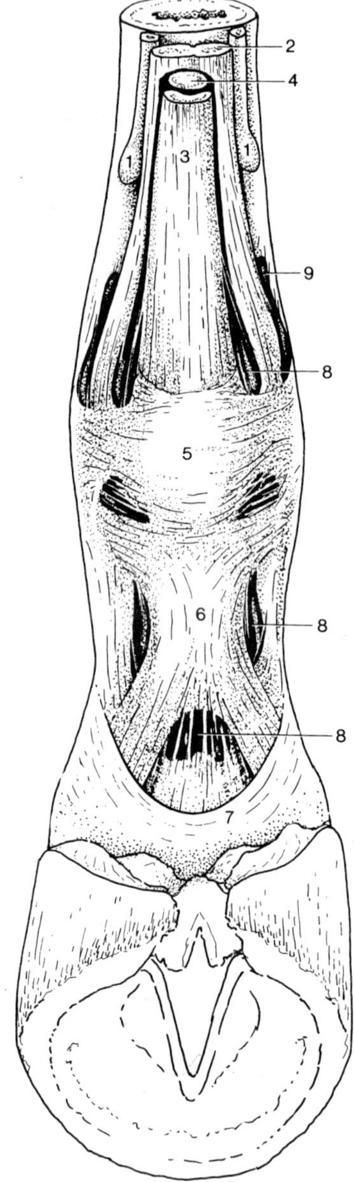

**Figure 23–29.** Annular ligaments of the digit.

1, Splint bones; 2, interosseus; 3, superficial digital flexor; 4, deep digital flexor; 5, palmar annular ligament; 6, proximal digital annular ligament; 7, distal digital annular ligament; 8, digital sheath; 9, palmar pouch of fetlock joint.

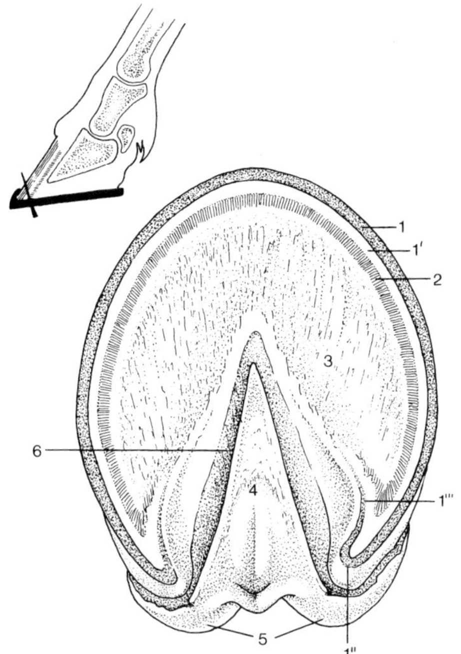


**Figure 23–30.** Ground surface of the hoof. The inset shows the direction of hoof nails started at the white line.

1, Wall; 1′, unpigmented part of wall; 1″, heel; 1‴, bar; 2, white line (union of wall and sole); 3, sole; 4, frog; 5, bulbs of the heels; 6, paracuneal groove.

base of the frog. The periople, which also consists of an admixture of tubular and intertubular horn, is produced over the narrow perioplic dermis (/1) directly proximal to the coronary dermis.

The *sole* fills the space between the wall and frog and forms most of the undersurface of the hoof (Fig. 23–32/*B*,11). It is slightly concave so that only the distal edge of the wall and the frog make contact on firm ground. The parts between the bars and quarters, known as the angles of the sole (/11′), are the seat of "corns," blood-soaked flecks resulting from trauma to the underlying dermis. Sole horn, though softer than that of the wall, again consists of an admixture of tubules and intertubular horn; it tends to become spongy and to flake in animals required to stand on soiled bedding.

The junction between the sole and the wall is known as the white line (zona alba; /3′). It includes some of the nonpigmented stratum medium of the wall, the distal ends of the horny laminae (stratum internum), and, between these, pigmented horn produced over the terminal papillae of the laminar dermis (these project distally, level with the dermal papillae above the sole) (Fig. 23–33/3). The startlingly white streak within the broad, so-called white line is provided by "cap horn" produced over the distal third of the dermal laminae. The

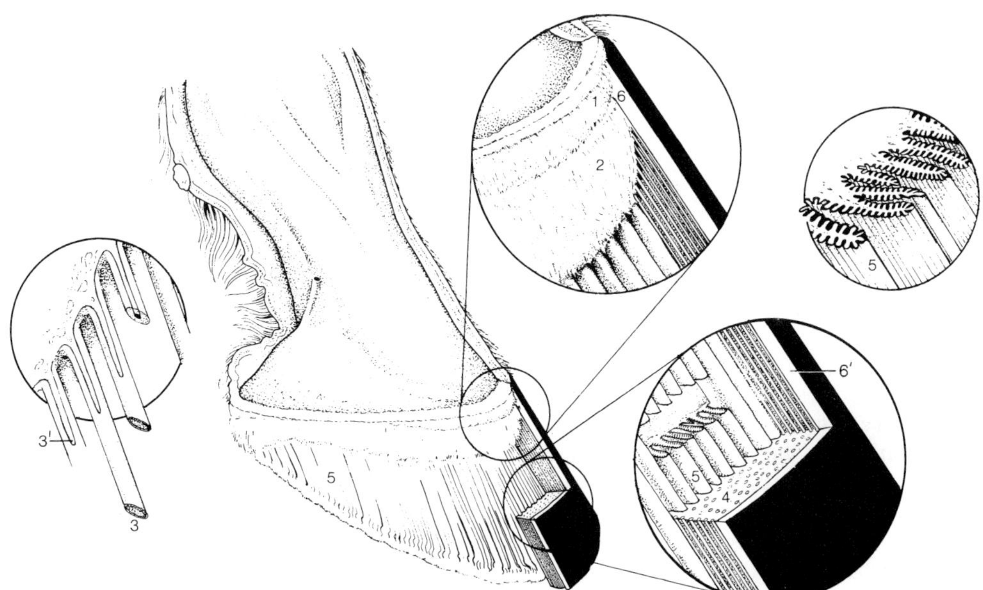


**Figure 23–31.** The structure of the hoof wall and of the underlying laminar dermis.

1, Perioplic dermis; 2, coronary dermis; 3, horn tubules growing from epithelium over papillae (3′) of the coronary dermis (enlarged in left inset); 4, stratum medium of wall consisting of horn tubules embedded in less structured intertubular horn; 5, dermal laminae that interdigitate with the horny laminae of the hoof wall (see also insets to the right); 6, periople; 6′, stratum externum of wall (dried periople).

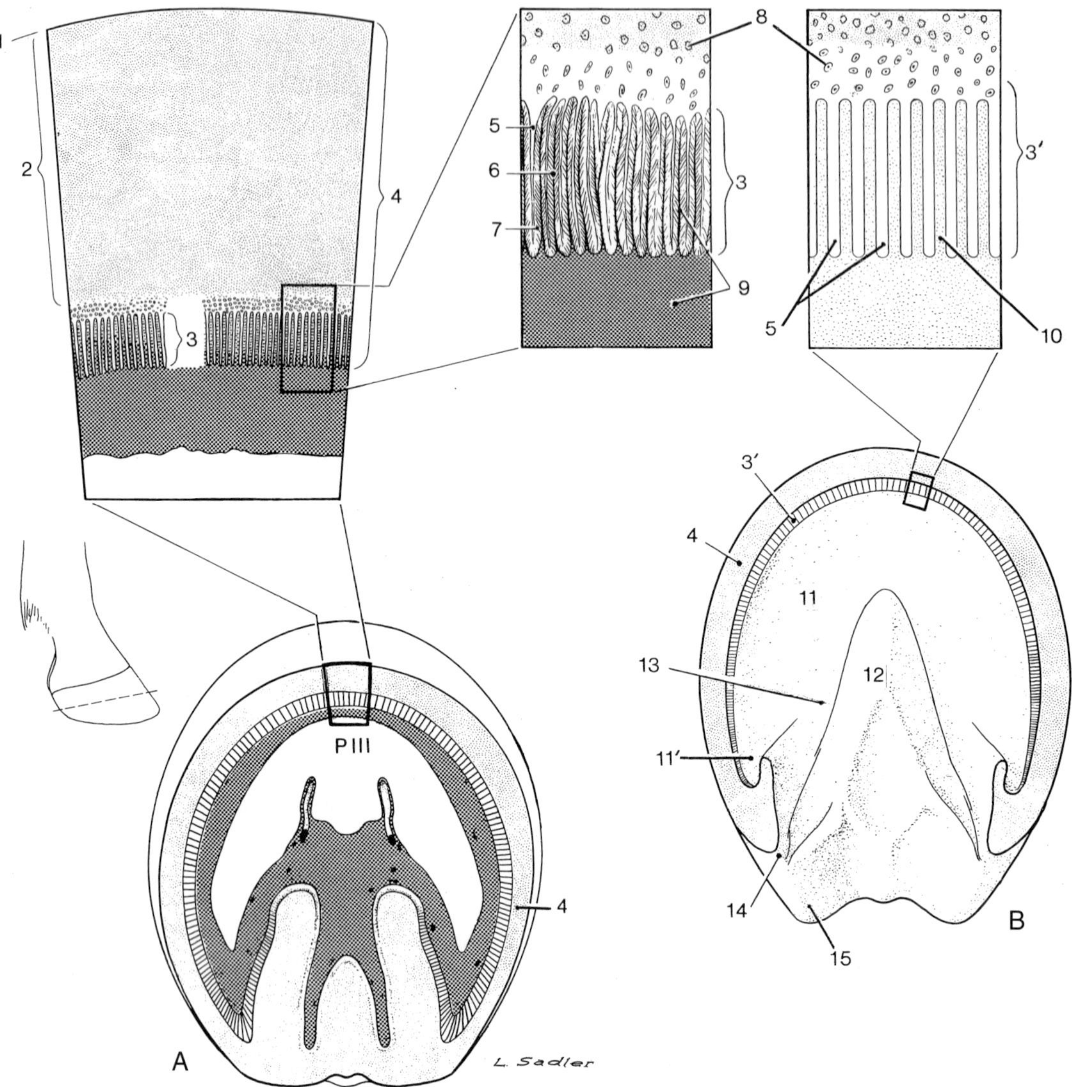


**Figure 23–32.** *A*, Transverse section of the digit at the level of PIII, proximal surface. *B*, Ground surface of the hoof. Schematic.

1, 2, 3, Stratum externum, medium, and internum; 3′, white line; 4, wall; 5, primary horny laminae; 6, primary dermal laminae; 7, interdigitating secondary laminae; 8, horn tubules; 9, laminar dermis; 10, pigmented horn produced by terminal papillae; 11, sole; 11′, angles of sole; 12, frog; 13, paracuneal groove; 14, heel; 15, bulb of heel.

internal rim of the white line is where farriers place nails when shoeing; the nails pass obliquely through the wall to emerge a few centimeters above the shoe where they are cut and clinched (Fig. 23–30).

The wedge-shaped *frog* (cuneus ungulae) projects into the sole from behind. Its wide base closes the gap between the heels where it furnishes the palmar part of the hoof (/4) and spreads upward to end in thickenings, the bulbs of the heels, that overhang the heels of the wall. Its external surface is marked by a central groove to which corresponds an internal spine (frog-stay) that juts proximally into the digital cushion (see further on). The frog is separated from the bars and the sole by deep (paracuneal) grooves (/6) that accentuate its medial and lateral borders; the grooves are convenient for the application of hoof testers (large "pincers" used to detect soreness in deeper structures). The projection of these structures is shown in Figure 23–33. In horses stood on damp bedding, the grooves are often the site of "thrush," a foul-smelling infection that may spread to deeper, sensitive tissues.

The frog horn is tubular and fairly soft and elastic, being kept pliable by the fatty secretion of glands in the underlying digital cushion. Though horses can be shod with the "frog off the ground" (as were city draft horses formerly), a sound hoof requires the frog pressure that is obtained through ground contact.

The *dermis* deep to the hoof capsule can be divided into five parts: perioplic, coronary, and laminar dermis and those of the sole and frog that are associated with the like-named segments of the hoof. Both the coronary and laminar dermis are associated with the wall.

The entire dermis (other than the laminar part) carries papillae that run parallel to each other and to the dorsal surface of the hoof, directed toward the ground. It is richly supplied with vessels and nerves, and an ill-directed farrier's nail that penetrates the dermis ("quick") therefore draws blood and causes pain. Since nerves are absent from the hoof capsule, the apposing dermal and epidermal tissues are often designated sensitive and insensitive, respectively.

The *subcutis,* generally thin, attaches the dermis to such deeper structures as the coffin bone, the hoof cartilages, and the tendons. It is greatly thickened in two places: beneath the coronary dermis (the coronary cushion), and beneath the frog dermis (the digital cushion). These cushions consist of a feltwork of collagenous and elastic fibers interspersed with small islands of fat and cartilage.

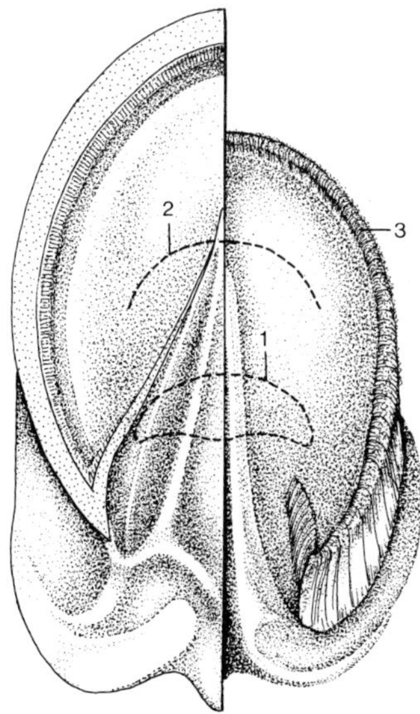


**Figure 23–33.** Ground surface of the hoof. Half of the hoof has been removed to expose the dermis.

1, Position of navicular bone; 2, position of the insertion of the deep flexor tendon; 3, terminal papillae.

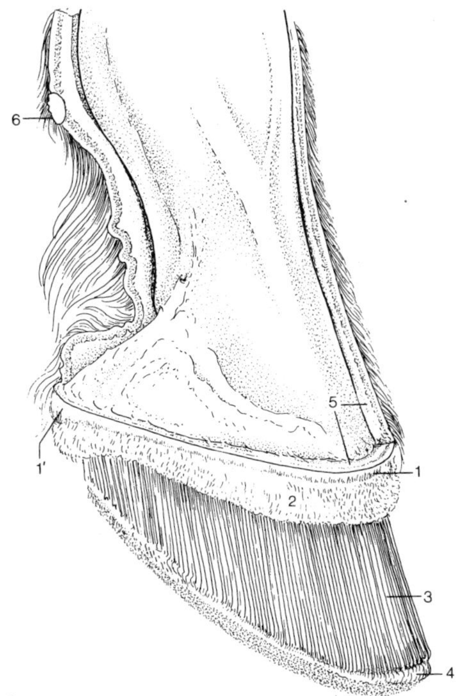


**Figure 23–34.** Dermis exposed by removal of the hoof.

1, Perioplic dermis; 1′, widened perioplic dermis at the bulb of the heels; 2, coronary dermis; 3, laminar dermis; 4, terminal papillae on the ends of the dermal laminae; 5, cut edge of skin; 6, ergot.

The narrow, raised *perioplic dermis* embraces the digit at the coronet. Studded with short papillae, it widens caudally where it covers the bulbs of the heels (Fig. 23–34/1,1′).

The wider elevation of the *coronary dermis* (/2) is separated from the perioplic dermis by a shallow groove. Its prominence is due to the rounded underlying coronary cushion. The coronary dermis also follows the coronet but, like the hoof wall, it folds upon itself above the heels. It is widely known as the coronary band, although many clinicians interpret this term more widely to include the (external) coronet. The epithelium over most of its surface produces the bulk of the wall; that over the tucked-in distal margin produces most of the unstructured horn of the horny laminae.

The *laminar dermis* is composed of about 600 sensitive (dermal) laminae that interdigitate with the insensitive (horny) laminae on the deep surface of the wall (Fig. 23–32/5–7 and Plate 15/*E–H*). Both sets bear numerous secondary laminae that further secure the wall to the dermis, and ultimately to the coffin bone, while leaving it possible for the horn to slide over the bone.

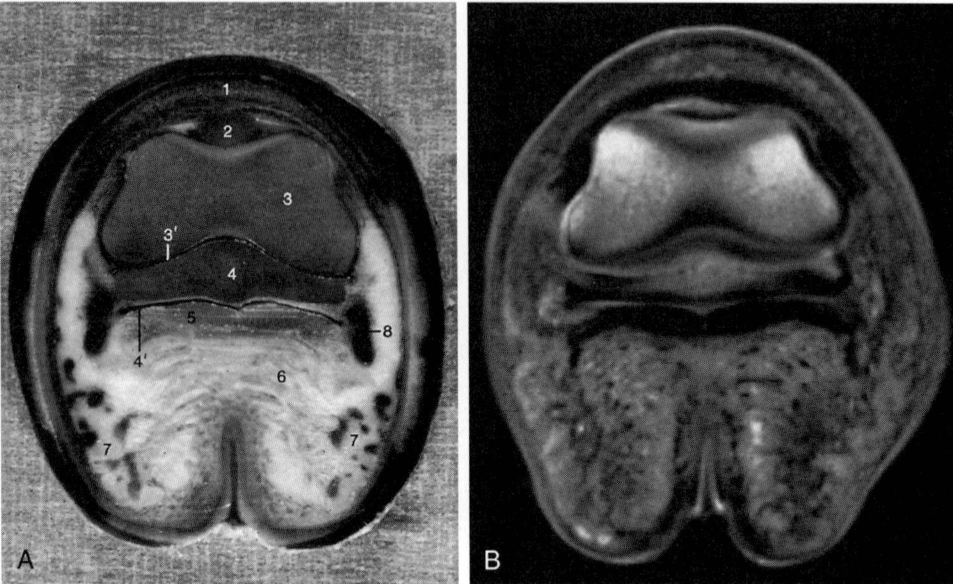


**Figure 23–35.** *A*, Transverse section of the digit at the level of the navicular bone, proximal surface. *B*, Magnetic resonance image taken at the same level.

1, Coronary dermis; 2, extensor process of PIII; 3, distal end of PII; 3′, coffin joint; 4, navicular bone; 4′, navicular bursa; 5, deep flexor tendon; 6, digital cushion; 7, cartilage of hoof and venous plexus; 8, position of digital vessels and nerve.

Normally the epithelium covering the sensitive laminae proliferates just sufficiently to allow the wall to slide past. But it has the capacity to produce additional amounts of (scar-) horn when a defect in the wall must be closed. This potential is utilized even more dramatically in chronic laminitis (founder), a disease in which the normal attachment is loosened and the coffin bone rotates away from the wall; the space in front of the bone becomes filled with irregular horn produced over a new set of sensitive laminae that form near the dorsal surface of the bone.

The *dermis of the sole* is firmly attached to the undersurface of the coffin bone.

The *dermis of the frog* lies between the frog and the digital cushion, which occupies the space below the deep flexor tendon and between the cartilages of the hoof (Fig. 23–35/6).

The blood supply of the dermis comes from three sets of vessels, all branches of the digital arteries that descend into the hoof to each side of the flexor tendons. Those that arise at the level of the coronet supply the perioplic and coronary dermis, those that arise opposite the pastern joint supply branches to the digital cushion and the dermis of the caudal aspect of the hoof, including the frog; the vessels of the third set arise from the dorsal and palmar terminal branches (mentioned in connection with the sole foramina of PIII) and go to the laminar and sole dermis. Veins do not accompany the arteries but instead form extensive interconnected networks in the dermis* and underlying subcutis, particularly in the coronary band, in the laminar dermis, and under the palmar aspect of the hoof (the coronary, dorsal, and palmar plexuses, respectively). They combine to form medial and lateral digital veins that become satellite to the arteries at the level of the pastern joint.

The hoof is a flexible structure, yielding under pressure on impact with the ground and so dissipating much of the attending concussion. The load that presses on the coffin joint is split between PIII and the navicular bone. The force on PIII is transmitted by the interdigitating laminae to the wall of the hoof, whose distal border is thus a principal weight bearer, especially in horses shod with the frog off the ground. The force retracts the slanted toe while the heels are spread by the distortion of the wall. The force exerted on the navicular bone presses into the yielding "sling" provided by the deep flexor tendon, which in turn compresses the digital cushion and frog (Fig. 23–27). These redirect the force sideways,

*It is known that certain regions of the hoof dermis are generously provided with epithelioid arteriovenous anastomoses (of a rather unusual character). It has been postulated that these anastomoses may be affected by vasoactive peptides released in certain pathologies of various organs remote from the limbs. According to the theory, the resulting dilation of these channels, when prolonged, may prejudice the normal capillary circulation, and this may sometimes be a predisposing factor in the development of acute laminitis.

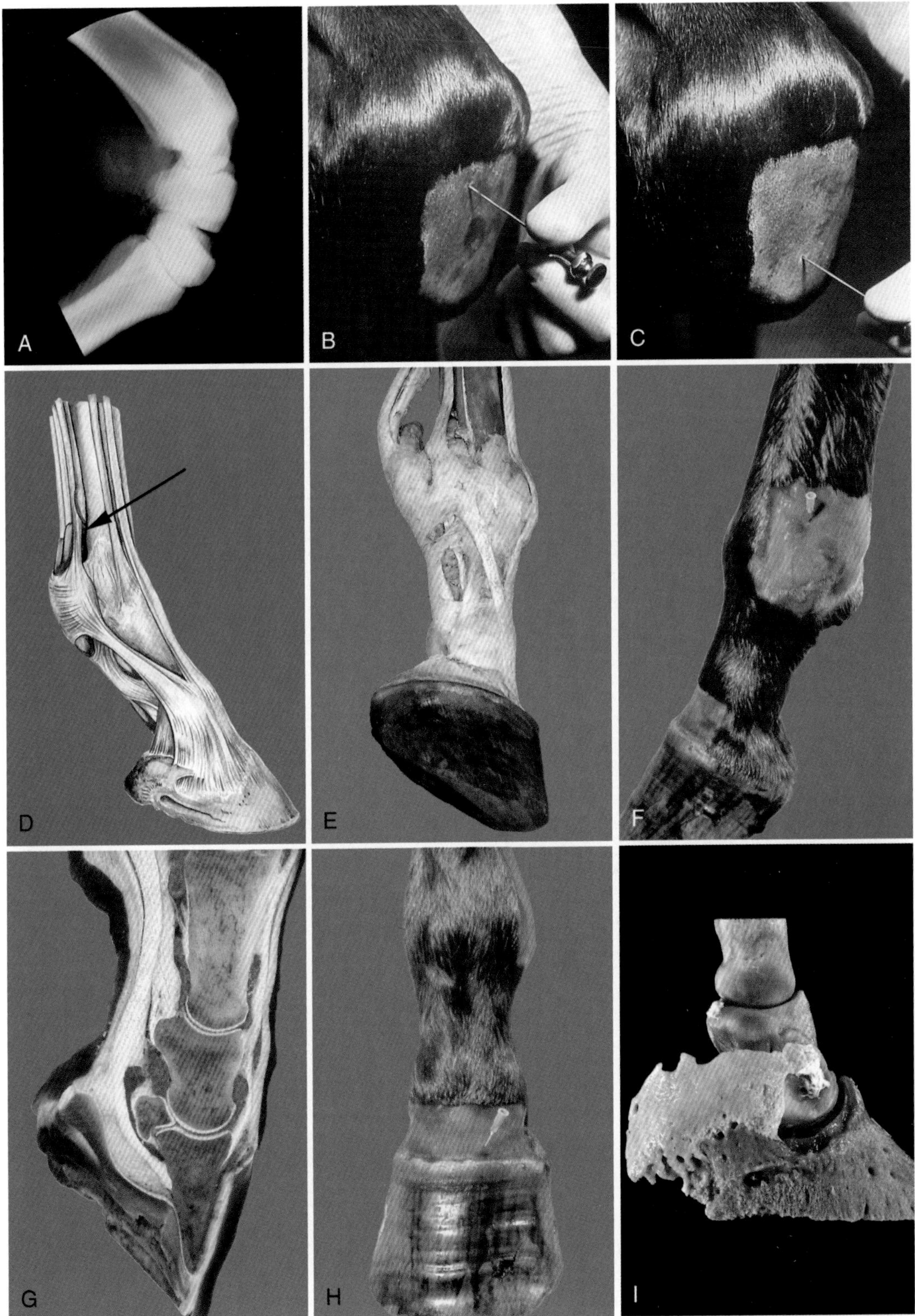


**Plate 25.** All illustrations of horse. *A*, Radiograph of flexed carpus. *B*, Puncture of radiocarpal joint. *C*, Puncture of midcarpal joint. *D*, Schematic drawing of right digit showing digital sheath (green) and palmar pouch of fetlock joint *(arrow)*. *E*, Digital sheath injected with pink, fetlock joint with blue latex. *F*, Puncture of fetlock joint. *G*, Axial section of digit with latex injected fetlock, pastern, and coffin joints. *H*, Puncture of coffin joint. *I*, Hoof cartilage attached to palmar process of distal phalanx.

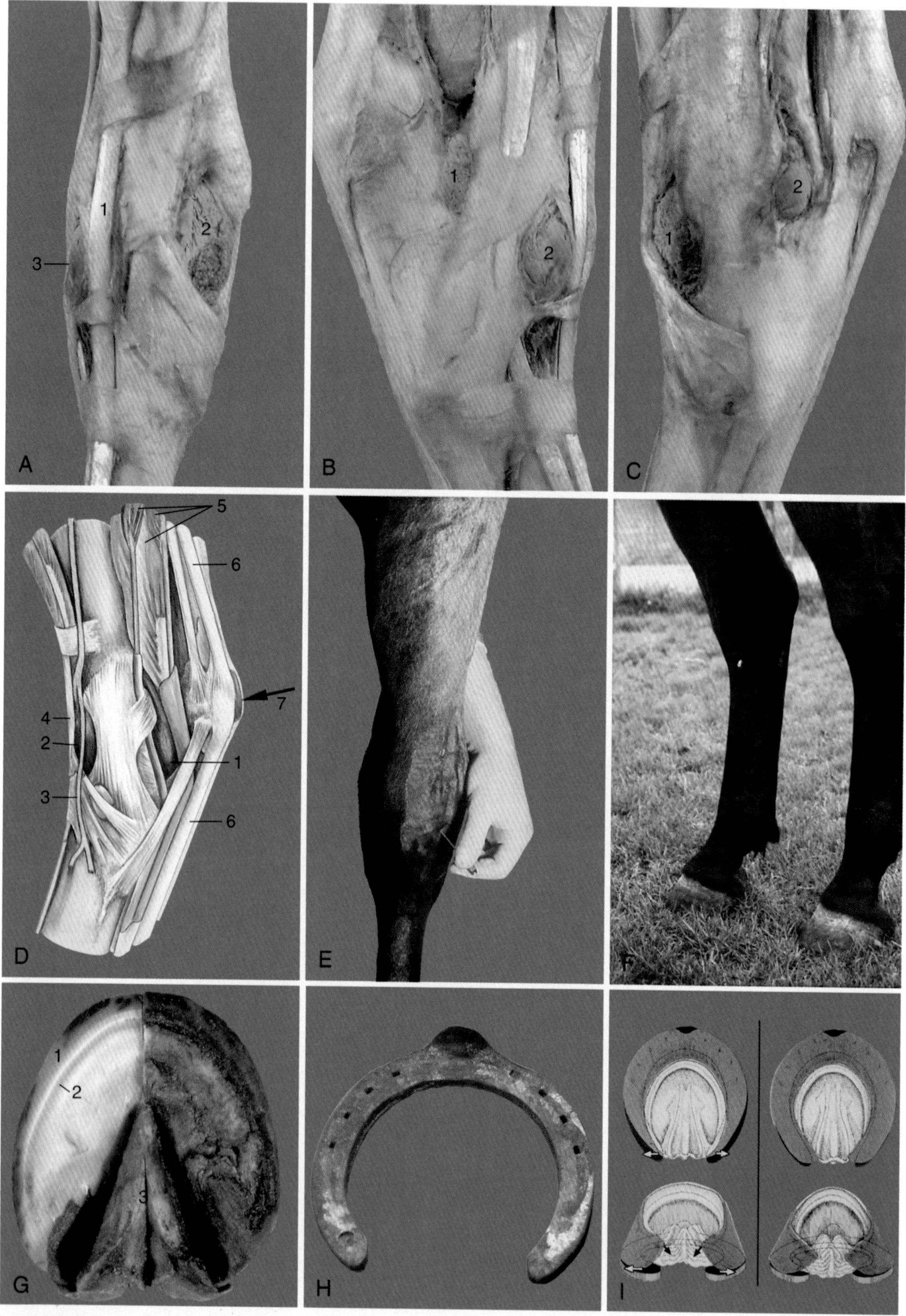


**Plate 26.** All illustrations of horse. *A,* Dorsal view of right hock: 1, long digital extensor; 2, 3, mediodorsal and laterodorsal pouches of tarsocrural joint, respectively, are filled with latex. *B,* Lateral view of right hock: 1, 2, lateral plantar and laterodorsal pouches of tarsocrural joint, respectively, filled with latex. *C,* Medial view of right hock: 1, 2, mediodorsal and medioplantar pouches of tarsocrural joint, respectively. *D,* Right hock, medial side: 1, medioplantar extension of talocrural joint; 2, mediodorsal pouch; 3, cran. br. of saphenous v.; 4, peroneus tertius; 5, deep digital flexors; 6, superficial flexor tendon; 7, subcutaneous calcanean bursa *(arrow)*. *E,* Puncture of the laterodorsal pouch of the tarsocrural joint. *F,* Puncture of the mediodorsal pouch. *G,* Ground surface of hoof: 1, wall; 2, white line; 3, frog. *H,* Shoe showing the heel part polished by movement of the hoof heel. *I,* Changes in the form of the hoof during locomotion.

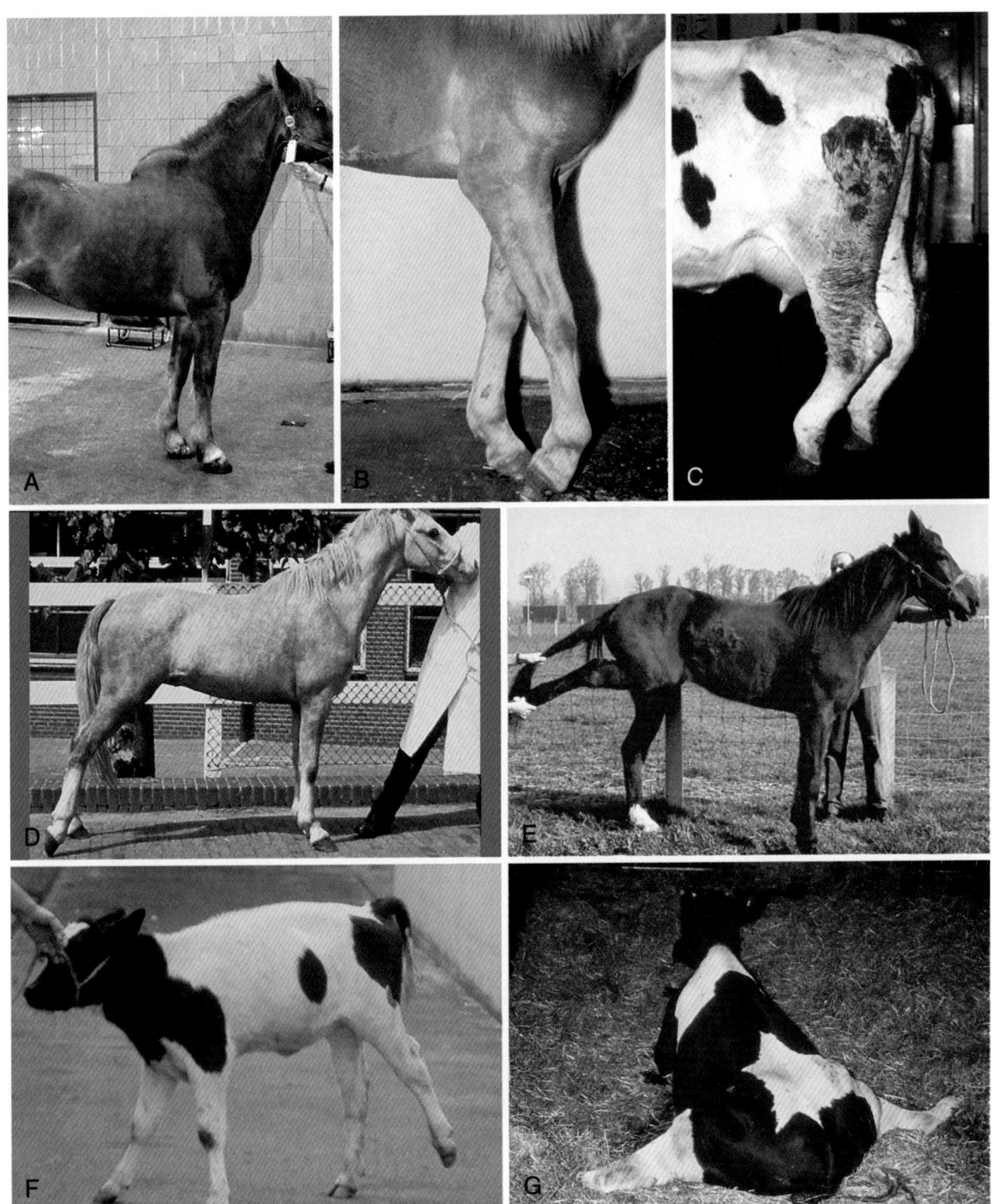


**Plate 27.** *A*, Rupture of serratus ventralis muscle. *B*, Lower radial paralysis. *C*, Peroneal paralysis. *D*, Locked patella. *E*, Rupture of peroneus tertius. *F*, Spastic paresis. *G*, Bilateral obturator paralysis.

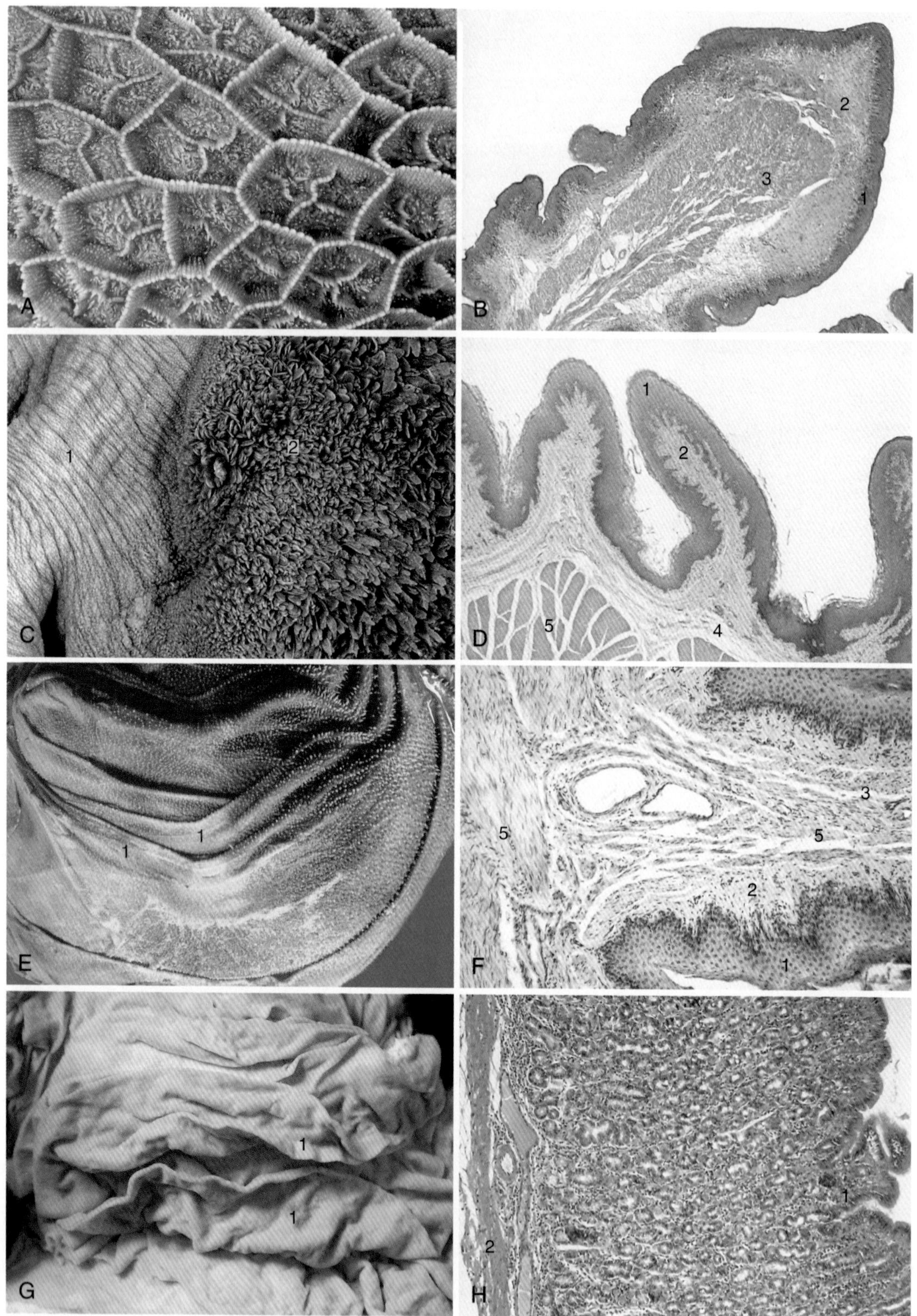


**Plate 28.** *A*, Internal surface of reticulum (cow). *B*, Reticulum (goat) (28×): 1, stratif. squam. epithelium; 2, lam. propria; 3, lam. muscularis mucosae; 4, submucosa; 5, muscularis interna. *C*, Internal surface of rumen (cow): 1, pillar; 2, papillae. *D*, Rumen (goat) (28×) (see *B* for label descriptions). *E*, Internal surface of omasum (cow): 1, omasal laminae. *F*, Omasum (goat) (70×) (see *B* for label descriptions). *G*, Internal surface of abomasum (cow): 1, spiral folds. *H*, Abomasum (goat) (70×): 1, gastric pit; 2, lam. muscularis mucosae.

the cushion pressing against the cartilages, the frog against the bars and sole thus assisting the outward movement of the heels (Plate 26/*I*).

The to-and-fro movement of the heels is not obvious to the eye but, as any farrier can verify, polishes the upper surface of the related parts of the shoe. It is to avoid interfering with this mechanism that farriers do not nail these parts of the shoe to the wall; if this precaution is neglected, the horse develops "contracted heels" and eventually goes lame (Plate 26/*H*).

The mechanism explains why the coffin bone is continued caudally by cartilage, rather than by bone (Fig. 23–21/4). Progressive calcification of the cartilage with subsequent replacement by bone is a common aging process known as "sidebone," yet another cause of lameness.

The movements of the heels have a further benefit, aiding venous return. The dense plexuses on both sides of the cartilages (Fig. 23–35/7) are compressed at each step and deliver blood into the valved digital veins. This has been shown experimentally by cannulating a digital vein under local anesthesia; blood is squirted at every step the horse takes. (In other species, contractions of striated muscles within the foot compress the veins and assist the venous return.)

Apart from minor differences in conformation, the fore and hind hoofs are identical (Fig. 23–36). In conformity with its larger weight-bearing role the fore hoof is somewhat wider and therefore more rounded in outline than the narrower, more pointed hind hoof (/*C,D*). But the distinction is less than the adjectives suggest, and the provenance—fore or hind—of a single specimen is not always obvious.

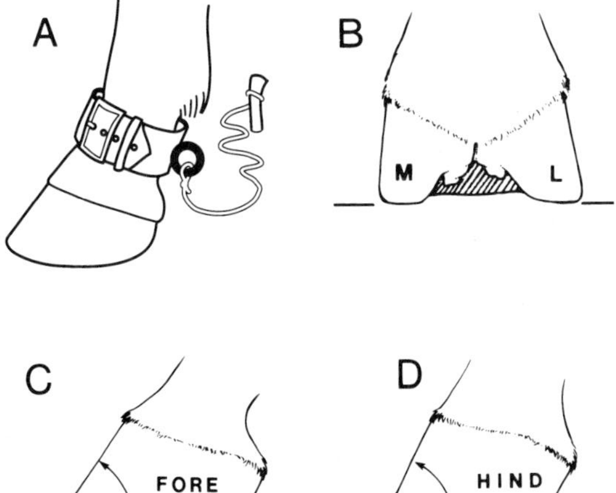


**Figure 23–36.** *A,* In former days horses at pasture were hobbled with a "pastern"; this is why the narrow part of the limb above the hoof is known today as the pastern. *B,* Palmar (plantar) view of the foot; the lateral (L) angle of the wall (with the ground) is more acute than the medial (M). *C* and *D,* The angle at the toe is more acute in the forelimb than in the hindlimb.

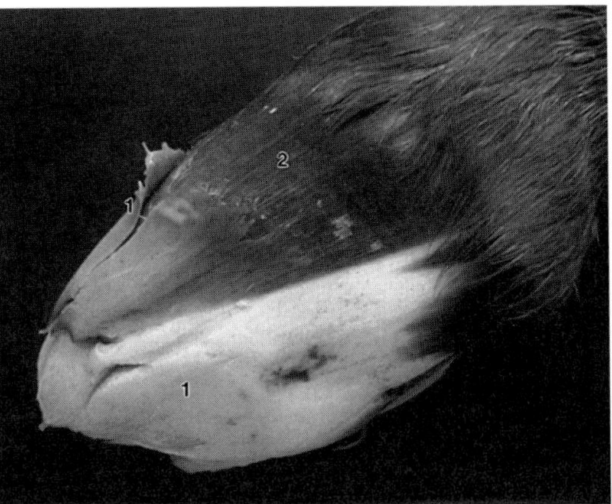


**Figure 23–37.** Hoof of a newborn foal.

1, Mass of soft, primary horn covering the ground surface and distal half of the hard, permanent hoof wall; 2, pigmented permanent hoof wall.

When the hoof capsule first forms early in fetal life, it consists of horn that is soft, unpigmented, and of uniform composition. Later, new hard and more structured horn is produced that pushes the soft horn distally where it becomes a rather misshaped mass covering the entire ground surface of the hoof and (thinly) an adjoining strip of the hoof wall. When exposed to air at term, the soft mass soon dries and sloughs away. The soft mass over the hard horn of the fetal hoof is said to prevent injury to the fetal membranes and birth canal (Fig. 23–37).

## THE PASSIVE STAY-APPARATUS

It is well known that horses can remain on their feet for much longer than other domestic animals. In fact, they are thought by many to sleep while standing. This is not quite true: they may rest or doze standing, but for a refreshing sleep they lie down, often only at night when unobserved. When horses stand quietly, most weight is carried by the tendons, ligaments, and deep fascia of the stay-apparatus, which do not tire; only a minimum of muscular energy is expended.

The bony column of the forelimb supports the cranial end of the trunk at the attachment of the serratus ventralis muscle to the medial surface of the scapula (Fig. 23–38/*A*,1). A vertical line dropped from the center of this attachment passes caudal to the shoulder, through the elbow, through or slightly cranial to the carpal joint, and cranial to the fetlock and pastern joints. If unsupported, the

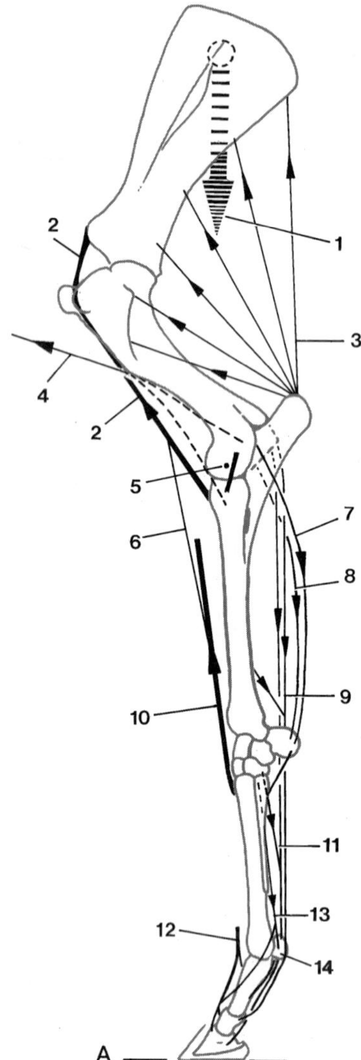


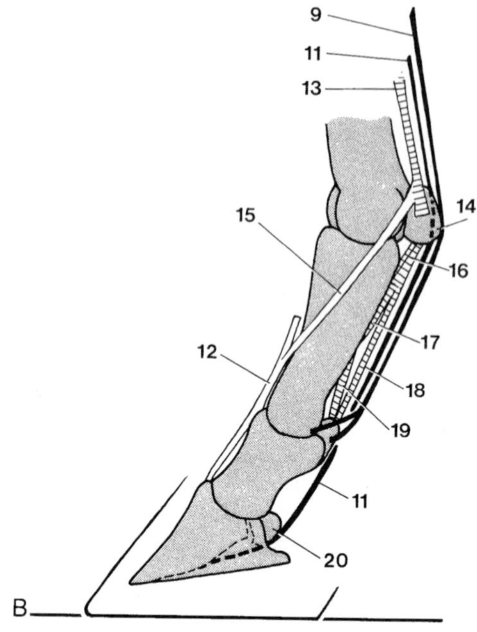


**Figure 23–38.** *A,* The stay-apparatus of the left forelimb; lateral view. *B,* Detail of digit; lateral view.

1, Weight of trunk; 2, internal biceps tendon; 3, triceps; 4, brachiocephalicus and brachial fascia to elbow joint; 5, axis of elbow rotation, next to eccentric collateral ligament; 6, lacertus fibrosus; 7, ulnaris lateralis; 8, flexor carpi ulnaris; 9, superficial digital flexor and accessory (check) ligament; 10, extensor carpi radialis; 11, deep digital flexor and accessory (check) ligament; 12, common digital extensor; 13, interosseus; 14, proximal sesamoid bones; 15, extensor branch of interosseus; 16, 17, 18, cruciate, oblique, and straight sesamoidean ligaments; 19, axial palmar ligament; 20, navicular bone.

column would collapse by flexion of the shoulder and elbow joints, by overextension (or possibly flexion [buckling forward]) of the carpal joint, and by overextension of the fetlock and pastern joints. (The coffin joint actually flexes when the fetlock sinks under weight and can be disregarded in this discussion.)

The *shoulder joint* is prevented from flexion by the strong internal biceps tendon (/2) that connects the supraglenoid tubercle of the scapula with the radius. The latter attachment can be regarded as fixed because it is very close to the axis of rotation of the elbow joint (/5), which is stabilized by the weight on the limb. Tension in the wide biceps tendon puts great pressure on the intertubercular groove of the humerus. Indeed, some believe that the molding of the tendon to the intermediate tubercle actually causes the joint to lock. At its other end, the pull of the biceps is transmitted via the lacertus and extensor carpi radialis (/6,10) to a second fixed point at the upper end of the large metacarpal bone. This pull augments the action of the extensors of the *carpal joint* and prevents that joint from buckling forward and collapsing the limb; any tendency toward overextension is prevented by close packing of the carpal bones in front and by the strong palmar carpal ligament behind (Fig. 23–15/*A,B,*7).

The *fetlock joint* is prevented from overextension principally by the suspensory apparatus (comprising the interosseus, proximal sesamoid bones, and distal sesamoidean ligaments), which is tensed under load (Fig. 23–38/13,14,16–18). The effect is reinforced by tension in the accessory (check) ligaments and distal parts of the superficial and deep flexor tendons (/9,11).

Tension in the deep flexor tendon tends to flex the coffin joint, causing the toe of the hoof to dig into the ground. The extensor branches of the interosseus (/15), pulling on the extensor process of the bone at impact, counteract this and keep the hoof level.

Overextension of the *pastern joint* is opposed by the axial and abaxial palmar and straight sesamoidean ligaments (/19,18), which span its palmar aspect. The taut deep flexor tendon gives additional support. (Buckling forward is prevented by the superficial flexor that attaches on the palmar aspect of the joint.)

With the shoulder joint fixed (by the biceps tendon), the weight of the trunk rests on the upper end of the nearly vertical radius. Therefore, unless the horse sways markedly forward, only small forces are requird to prevent the elbow joint from flexing. These are mainly supplied by passive tension of the tendinous components of the carpal and digital flexors (the superficial digital flexor especially) and the eccentrically placed collateral ligaments (/5,7–9). Recent information indicates that because of their muscle fiber composition—characteristic of postural muscles—the anconeus and the medial head of the triceps may also oppose flexion of the elbow joint. The large mass of the long and lateral heads of the triceps—the principal extensor of the elbow joint—remains flaccid even when the other forelimb is picked up to make the horse stand three-legged (see Fig. 23–2/1 and the effects of radial paralysis on page 600.

## THE BLOOD VESSELS AND LYMPHATIC STRUCTURES OF THE FORELIMB

The *axillary artery,* the main supply of the limb, enters the axillary space after crossing the cranial border of the first rib where it may be punctured (p. 518). It descends on the medial aspect of the arm in company with the median and ulnar nerves and shortly becomes known as the *brachial artery.* The trunk releases several branches to the muscles of the shoulder and arm, the most prominent being the subscapular artery, which follows the caudal border of the scapula, and the deep brachial, which disappears between the heads of the triceps (Fig. 23–9). Just proximal to the elbow joint, lesser cranial and caudal branches (transverse cubital and collateral ulnar arteries, respectively) are detached for the muscles in the forearm; their further courses and connections are shown in Figure 23–39/12,11. The brachial artery crosses the elbow cranial to the medial collateral ligament where it

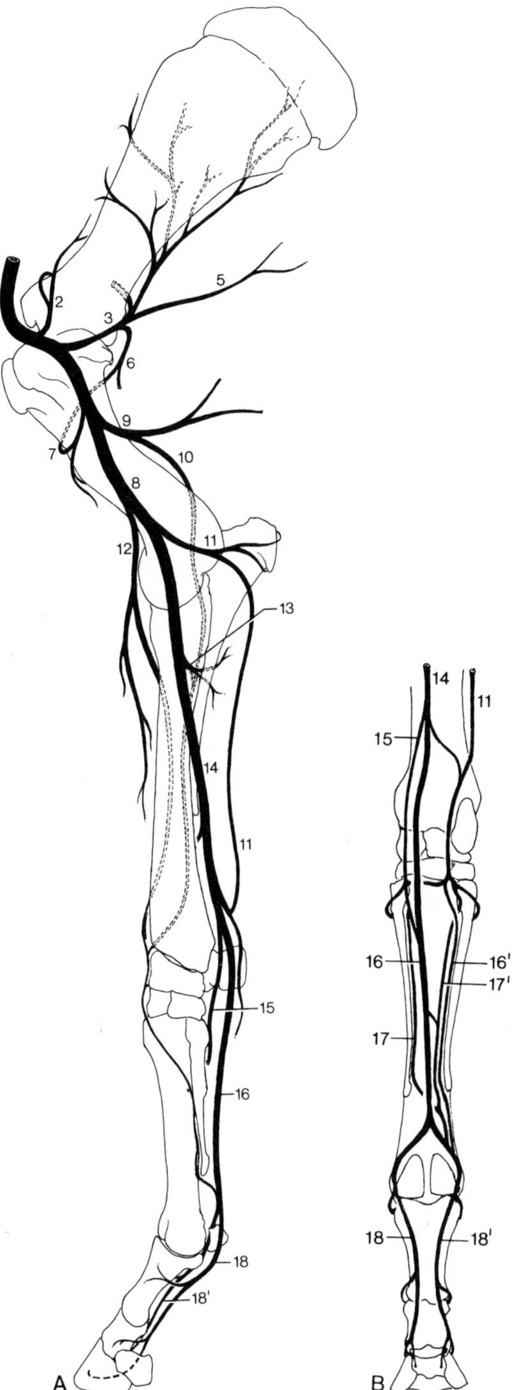


**Figure 23–39.** The major arteries of the right forelimb. *A,* Medial view. *B,* Palmar view.

1, Axillary a.; 2, suprascapular a.; 3, subscapular a.; 5, thoracodorsal a.; 6, 7, caudal and cranial circumflex humeral aa.; 8, brachial a.; 9, deep brachial a.; 10, collateral radial a.; 11, collateral ulnar a.; 12, transverse cubital a.; 13, common interosseous a.; 14, median a.; 15, radial a.; 16, 16′, medial and lateral palmar aa.; 17, 17′, medial and lateral palmar metacarpal aa.; 18, 18′, medial and lateral digital aa.

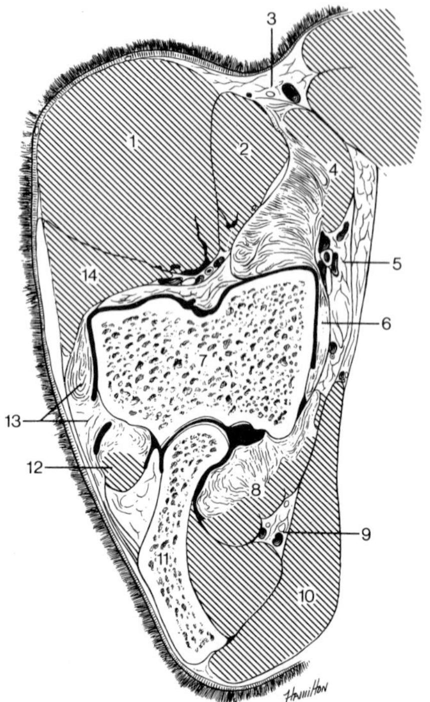


**Figure 23–40.** Transverse section of the left elbow.

1, Extensor carpi radialis; 2, brachialis; 3, medial cutaneous antebrachial nerve and cephalic vein lying on lacertus fibrosus; 4, biceps; 5, brachial vessels and median nerve; 6, medial collateral ligament; 7, humerus; 8, flexors arising from medial epicondyle of humerus; 9, ulnar nerve and collateral ulnar vessels; 10, tensor fasciae antebrachii; 11, olecranon; 12, ulnaris lateralis; 13, lateral collateral ligament; 14, common digital extensor.

can be palpated, and the pulse evaluated, through the pectoralis transversus (Fig. 23–40/5). Together with the median nerve it dips under the flexor carpi radialis caudal to the radius and soon gives off the common interosseous artery, which passes through the interosseous space to reach the craniolateral muscles of the forearm.

The main trunk, now redesignated the *median artery* (Fig. 23–41/12), gradually works its way to the caudal surface of the forearm before dividing into three above the carpus. The lesser branches (palmar branch of median, radial artery) contribute the small palmar metacarpal arteries that accompany the interosseus muscle, while the main trunk passes through the carpal canal with the digital flexor tendons (Fig. 23–15/*B*,19). It continues with these in the cannon where it becomes the medial palmar artery, the main artery to the digit and hoof. This inclines axially before splitting into the medial and lateral digital arteries above the fetlock. The digital arteries pass over the abaxial surfaces of the sesamoid bones (where they are palpable) and continue into the digit on each side of the flexor tendons; the lateral artery is reinforced by the small metacarpal arteries that join above the sesamoid bone (Fig. 23–39/18′). The branches of the digital arteries distal to the fetlock are symmetrical. Dorsal and palmar branches are given off opposite PI, and these supply adjacent structures while forming a circle about the bone. A branch to the digital cushion is detached level with the pastern joint before the digital artery disappears by passing deep to the hoof cartilage. Dorsal and palmar branches detached opposite the middle of PII comport themselves similarly to the branches about PI but also take part in the supply of the dermis of the hoof. The dorsal and palmar terminal branches (to PIII) have been described (pp. 584 and 594); the palmar branches anastomose to form a terminal arch within the bone.

Most *veins* of the forelimb are satellite, though often duplicated or further replicated where they

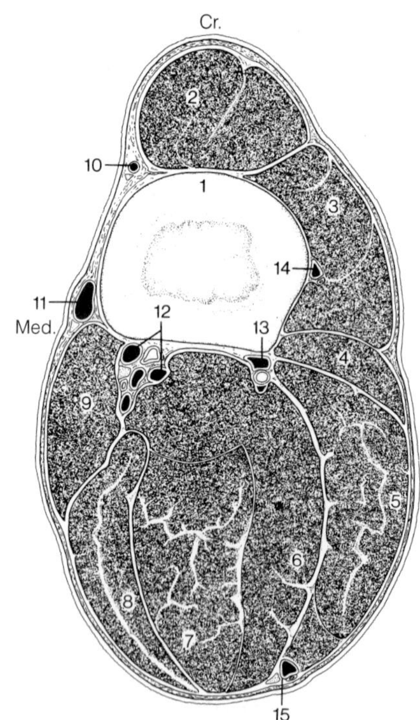


**Figure 23–41.** Transverse section of the right forearm at the level shown in Figure 23–42.

1, Radius; 2, extensor carpi radialis; 3, common digital extensor; 4, lateral digital extensor; 5, ulnaris lateralis; 6, deep digital flexor; 7, superficial digital flexor; 8, flexor carpi ulnaris; 9, flexor carpi radialis; 10, accessory cephalic vein and medial cutaneous antebrachial nerve (from musculocutaneous); 11, cephalic vein; 12, median artery, veins, and nerve; 13, muscular branches of median vessels; 14, cranial interosseous vessels; 15, ulnar nerve and collateral ulnar vessels.

accompany the larger arteries (Fig. 23–42/1). Some superficial veins seek independent courses, and those coming from the hoof have already been mentioned. The superficial veins include the cephalic and accessory cephalic veins, which are prominent and palpable in the forearm (/10,10′). The cephalic vein is joined to the brachial vein via the median cubital at the elbow and continues to ascend in the groove between brachiocephalicus and pectoralis descendens, where it is at risk in "staking" injuries. It joins the external jugular vein at the base of the neck.

Two clusters of *lymph nodes* drain the free part of the limb. The cubital nodes lie on the medial aspect of the humerus just proximal to the elbow joint (Fig. 23–9/15′). They drain more distal parts of the limb and channel their outflow to the axillary nodes. These lie medial to the shoulder joint in the angle between the axillary and subscapular arteries (/10′) and drain the arm and shoulder, together with a part of the thoracic wall caudal to the limb. Their efferent vessels go to the caudal deep cervical nodes, and thence the lymph flows directly or indirectly to the veins at the thoracic inlet. The superficial cervical nodes are arranged in a long chain that crosses the deep surface of the omotransversarius and brachiocephalicus (see Fig. 18–38/8). The group consists of many small nodes, and since these are embedded in fat and do not form a firm compact mass, the group is not always easily located. Palpation should be directed to drawing the nodes forward, away from the subclavius against which they lie. The superficial cervical nodes mainly drain skin over the upper part of the limb but also receive some lymph from deeper structures.

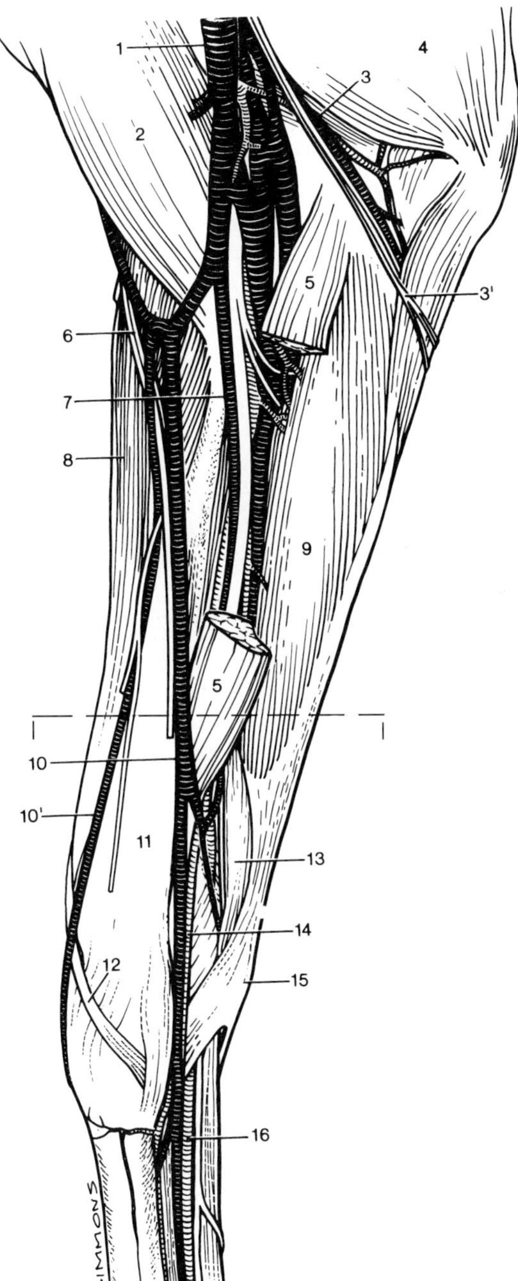


**Figure 23–42.** Dissection of the medial surface of the right forearm. (The *broken transverse line* indicates level of section in Figure 23–41.)

1, Multiple brachial veins; 2, biceps; 3, ulnar nerve and collateral ulnar vessels; 3′, caudal cutaneous antebrachial nerve; 4, triceps; 5, flexor carpi radialis, resected; 6, medial cutaneous antebrachial nerve; 7, median nerve and vessels; 8, extensor carpi radialis; 9, flexor carpi ulnaris; 10, 10′, cephalic and accessory cephalic veins; 11, radius; 12, extensor carpi obliquus; 13, superficial digital flexor; 14, radial artery and vein; 15, accessory carpal bone; 16, medial palmar nerve and vessels.

# THE NERVES OF THE FORELIMB

## The Branches of the Brachial Plexus

With few exceptions, the structures of the forelimb are innervated from the brachial plexus formed by contributions from the last three cervical and first two thoracic nerves (C6–T2). The plexus reaches the axilla as a broad band that emerges between the parts of the scalenus, but this soon divides into the usual dozen or so trunks. The major trunks, of clinical interest because of their vulnerability to injury or availability for nerve-blocking techniques, are described even though there are few specific features of significance above the carpus.

The *suprascapular nerve* (C6–7) leaves the axilla by sinking between the subscapular and supraspinatus muscles. It then winds around the neck of the scapula before expending itself in the

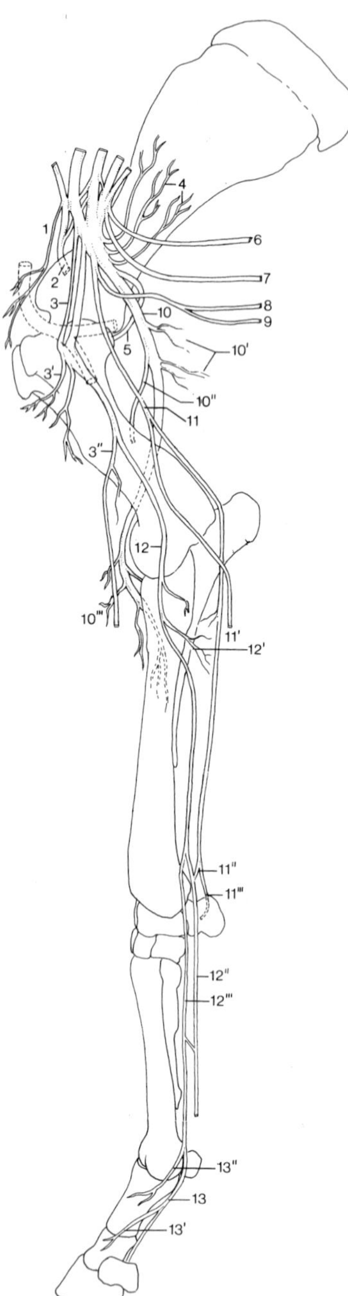


**Figure 23–43.** Distribution of the nerves in the right forelimb; medial view. The axillary artery at the shoulder joint is *stippled*.

1, Cranial pectoral nn.; 2, suprascapular n.; 3, musculocutaneous n.; 3′, proximal branches; 3″, distal branches with medial cutaneous antebrachial n.; 4, subscapular n.; 5, axillary n.; 6, long thoracic n.; 7, thoracodorsal n.; 8, lateral thoracic n.; 9, caudal pectoral nn.; 10, radial n.; 10′, proximal muscular branches (triceps); 10″, lateral cutaneous antebrachial n.; 10‴, distal muscular branches; 11, ulnar n.; 11′, caudal cutaneous antebrachial n.; 11″, palmar branch; 11‴, dorsal branch; 12, median n.; 12′, muscular branches; 12″, lateral palmar n.; 12‴, medial palmar n.; 13, medial palmar digital n.; 13′, 13″, dorsal branches.

supra- and infraspinatus (Fig. 23–43/2). A direct relationship to bone always carries a risk of injury, and the suprascapular nerve may be damaged where it lies against the scapula; apparently this is usually the result of pulling on the nerve as the animal stumbles with the limb stretched back. Injury is therefore most frequent in horses worked over uneven ground. Even serious damage to the nerve may have little immediate effect, although an observer stationed in front of an affected horse may notice a lateral deviation of the shoulder joint at each stride. After a time, muscular atrophy markedly alters the conformation of the shoulder region, causing the scapular spine to project above the wasted muscles. Suprascapular paralysis is commonly known as sweeny or shoulder slip.

The *musculocutaneous nerve* (C7–8) (/3,3′,3″) first runs craniolateral to the axillary artery before turning below the vessel to unite with the median nerve. A branch to the coracobrachialis and biceps is detached before the union. The part incorporated in the median trunk separates in the distal arm and supplies the brachialis and a medial cutaneous antebrachial nerve that crosses the lacertus fibrosus, where it is easily palpated, before being distributed to the skin over the cranial and medial aspects of the forearm and carpus. Damage to the musculocutaneous nerve cannot be common, but, should such occur, it is unlikely that loss of activity by the principal elbow flexors would greatly affect the gait.

The *axillary nerve* (C7–8) (/5) has the usual course and distribution—to the principal flexors of the shoulder and the skin over the lateral aspect of the arm and forearm. There appear to be no records of traumatic damage to this nerve in the horse; it is known that in other species section does not impair the gait since other muscles are potentially able to flex the shoulder.

The *radial nerve* (C8–T1) is one of the larger branches of the plexus (/10). It follows the caudal border of the brachial artery in the upper arm and later sinks between the medial and long heads of the triceps, rounding the caudal surface of the humerus to gain the lateral aspect of the limb. The nerve detaches branches to the triceps group in the proximal part of the arm; more distally, where it is covered by the lateral head of the triceps, it detaches other branches to the extensor muscles of the carpus and digit. A purely sensory continuation (lateral cutaneous antebrachial nerve) supplies skin over the lateral aspect of the forearm; contrary to the pattern in other species, this branch fades at carpal level.

The radial nerve is the sole supply to the extensor muscles of all joints distal to the shoulder; the effects of damage are therefore proportionately severe. When injury is proximal to the origin of the tricipital branches, the animal is unable to support weight upon the affected limb. It stands with the joints uncharacteristically flexed; the angle between scapula and humerus is enlarged, and the elbow is dropped in relation to the trunk; the hoof is rested on its dorsal aspect. High radial paralysis may arise from injury to or disease of the humerus, or from damage to the brachial plexus itself. If other components of the plexus are affected the signs may be complicated by simultaneous paralysis of the flexor muscles of the distal joints.

The results of injury distal to the origin of the tricipital branches are naturally less severe. Normal stances of the shoulder and elbow are maintained (Plate 27/*B*). The animal may rest the dorsal surface of the hoof on the ground but supports weight on the limb if the hoof is first restored to the normal position. Many horses learn to compensate for this disability by setting the hoof down before the impetus, gained when the limb is swung forward during the stride, is lost; the gait may appear almost normal when the terrain is flat, but unevenness quickly brings an affected animal into difficulties. Low radial paralysis may be simulated by the ischemia that sometimes results from prolonged lateral recumbency.

The *median nerve* (C8–T2) is the largest branch of the brachial plexus (/12). It follows the cranial border of the brachial artery for most of its course through the arm but shifts to the caudal margin on approaching the elbow. It is covered by the pectoralis transversus as it crosses this joint but, even so, the nerve and artery together form a palpable cord (Fig. 23–42/7). The two structures continue together as they descend the forearm, buried within the flexor mass of muscle; they divide at the same level, a little above the radiocarpal joint. The end branches, known as the medial and lateral palmar nerves, are described in the next section. The muscular branches to the flexor muscles of the carpus and digit are detached in the very proximal part of the forearm; beyond these detachments the nerve is purely sensory.

The *ulnar nerve* (T1–2) follows the caudal border of the brachial artery in the proximal part of the arm (Fig. 23–43/11). It then diverges caudally, detaches the caudal cutaneous antebrachial nerve (for the caudal aspect of the forearm) and passes over the medial epicondyle of the humerus before entering the forearm. As it does so it releases branches to the flexor muscles. The much depleted and now purely sensory nerve follows the ulnar head of the deep flexor at the caudal margin of the limb, under cover of deep fascia (Fig. 23–41/15). A few centimeters above the carpus it divides into dorsal and palmar branches. The dorsal branch comes to the surface a short distance proximal to the accessory carpal bone and can be palpated against the ulnaris lateralis tendon attaching here; it passes over the lateral aspect of the carpus to expend itself in the skin over the lateral surface of the metacarpus. The palmar branch passes the carpus within the flexor retinaculum where it exchanges fibers with the lateral palmar nerve, one of the terminal branches of the median (Fig. 23–44/3,5′).

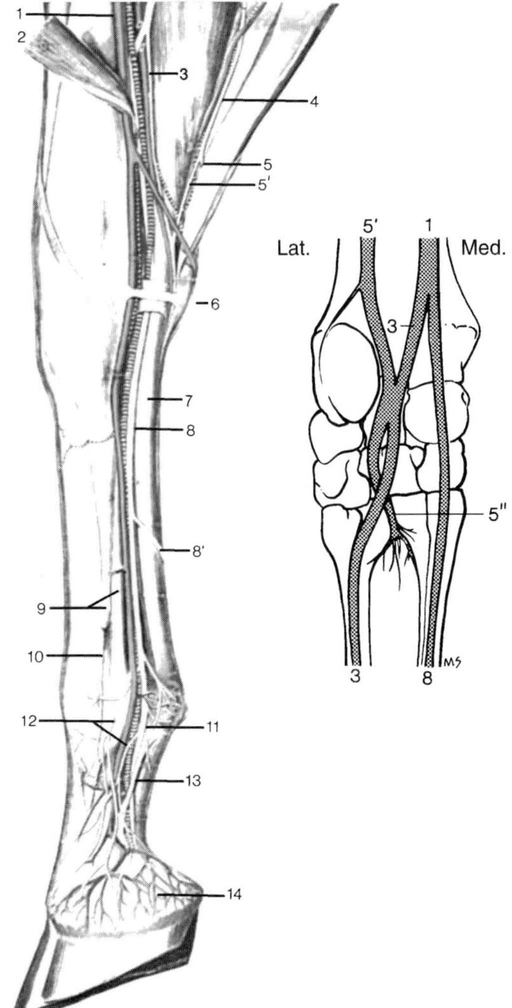


**Figure 23–44.** Vessels and nerves of the right forefoot; medial view. The inset gives a caudal view of the exchange of fibers between median and ulnar nerves at the (left) carpus.

1, Median vessels and nerve; 2, flexor carpi radialis; 3, lateral palmar nerve; 4, ulnar nerve; 5, 5′, dorsal and palmar branches of ulnar nerve; 5″, deep branch to interosseus and giving rise to the palmar metacarpal nerves; 6, flexor retinaculum; 7, flexor tendons; 8, medial palmar nerve and vessels; 8′, communicating branch; 9, interosseus and distal end of splint bone; 10, medial palmar metacarpal nerve; 11, digital nerve and vessels; 12, dorsal branches of digital nerve; 13, ligament of the ergot; 14, coronary venous plexus.

The overlap of the median and ulnar nerves in their motor distribution makes it unlikely that damage restricted to either one would much affect the gait.

## Innervation of the Forefoot

Four nerves attend to the innervation of most of the structures distal to the carpus: the medial and lateral palmar nerves from the median nerve, and the palmar and dorsal branches of the ulnar nerve. All but the dorsal branch of the ulnar lie palmar to the large metacarpal bone. The medial palmar nerve (/8) lies in the groove between the interosseus and the flexor tendons. In midcannon it detaches a communicating branch that crosses obliquely over the superficial flexor tendon (where it is palpable) to join the lateral palmar nerve. A little above the fetlock the medial palmar becomes the medial digital nerve, which immediately gives rise to one or two dorsal branches that ramify over the dorsomedial aspect of the digit and coronet. The main trunk of the digital nerve continues with the like-named artery over the outer aspect of the proximal sesamoid bone, passes under the ligament of the ergot (/13), and then disappears into the hoof. The neurovascular bundle may be palpated against the sesamoid bone. Small branches supply the structures caudal to the phalanges. The nerve ends by supplying the laminar and sole dermis.

The lateral palmar nerve (/3), it will be recalled, exchanged fibers with the palmar branch of the ulnar nerve at the carpus. It emerges from the short (1 to 2 cm) union and takes a course and has a distribution similar to those of the medial palmar nerve, including the ramifications in the digit. The first branch of this composite nerve arises at the carpus and soon splits into thin medial and lateral palmar metacarpal nerves that descend, deeply embedded, along the axial surface of the splint bones. These nerves supply the interosseus and the palmar pouch of the fetlock joint before becoming subcutaneous at the distal ends of the splint bones (/10). They now supply the dorsal pouch of the joint before mingling with the dorsal branches of the digital nerves; they do not reach the coronet.

All of these nerves can be blocked at various levels—mainly for the diagnosis of lameness. The rationale of the procedure is that a lame horse temporarily becomes sound when the area that contains the undetected lesion is desensitized. A sequence of injections, in which increasingly larger territories are desensitized, is therefore required. Four sites are commonly used.

1. The palmar digital blocks have as their targets the digital nerves, level with the pastern joint and just proximal to the hoof cartilage (the digital artery lies next to the nerve). The block desensitizes all structures in the hoof except the dorsal part of the coronary band.

2. Blocks at the level of the proximal sesamoid bones have as their targets the digital nerves and their dorsal branches (the digital artery and vein lie dorsal to the nerve adjacent to the dorsal branches). The block desensitizes the digit except the dorsal aspect of the pastern.

3. In the distal metacarpal blocks the injections are made level with the distal extremities of the splint bones. The target combines the palmar nerves (the palmar vein lies dorsal to the nerve, the artery lies deep to it) and branches of the palmar metacarpal nerves (subcutaneous, distal to splint bone; deep, between splint bone and interosseus; Fig. 23–45). The block desensitizes the digit, including the fetlock joint, with the possible exception of its dorsal pouch.

4. In the proximal metacarpal block the injections are made on the axial surface of the proximal end of the splint bones. The targets are the medial and lateral palmar nerves and the origin of the metacarpal nerves from the latter (large vessels accompany especially the medial palmar nerve;

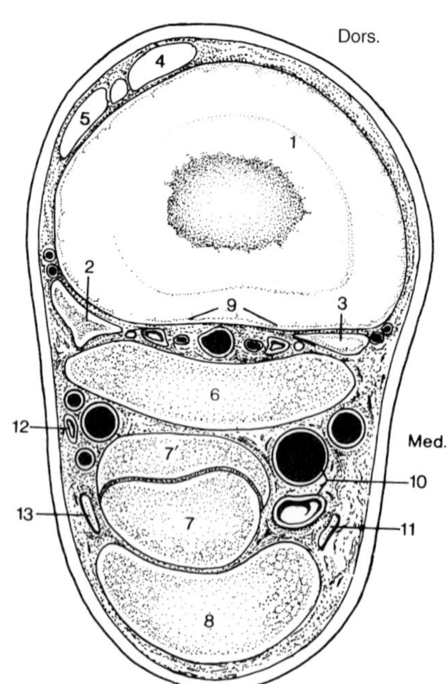


**Figure 23–45.** Transverse section of the middle of the left metacarpus.

1, 2, 3, Large and small metacarpal bones; 4, common digital extensor; 5, lateral digital extensor; 6, interosseus; 7, deep digital flexor; 7′, accessory (check) ligament; 8, superficial digital flexor; 9, palmar metacarpal vessels and nerves; 10, medial palmar artery and vein; 11, medial palmar nerve; 12, lateral palmar artery; 13, lateral palmar nerve.

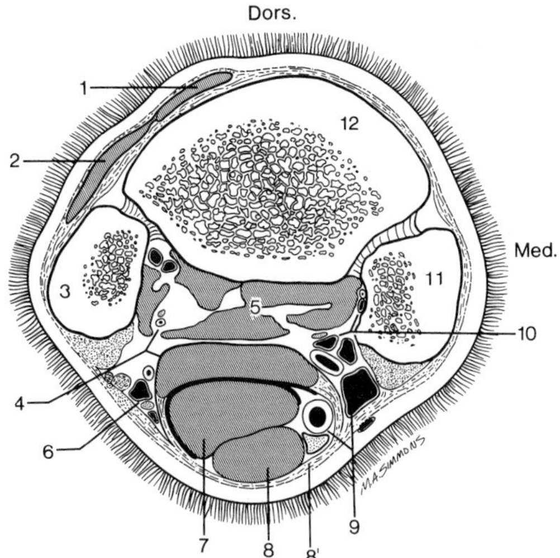


**Figure 23–46.** Transverse section of the left metacarpus about 3 cm distal to the carpometacarpal joint.

1, Common digital extensor; 2, lateral digital extensor; 3, lateral splint bone; 4, lateral palmar metacarpal artery and nerve, and accessory ligament of the deep flexor tendon; 5, interosseus; 6, lateral palmar nerve and vessels; 7, deep digital flexor; 8, superficial digital flexor; 8′, deep fascia; 9, medial palmar nerve and vessels; 10, medial palmar metacarpal nerve and superficial palmar branch of radial artery, and medial palmar metacarpal vessels; 11, medial splint bone; 12, large metacarpal (cannon) bone.

Fig. 23–46). The block desensitizes the digit, including the fetlock joint (with the possible exception of its dorsal pouch), and most structures in the caudal metacarpus; because of distopalmar outpouchings of the nearby carpometacarpal joint, this and the midcarpal joint may also be desensitized.

The *autonomous zones of skin innervation* are shown in Figure 23–1. A skin prick in the center of a zone tests for the integrity of the particular nerve.

## Selected Bibliography


Adams, M.N. and Tracy Turner: Endoscopy of the intertubercular bursa in horses. JAVMA 214:221–225, 1999.

Bassage, L.H., and D.W. Richardson: Longitudinal fractures of the condyles of the third metacarpal and metatarsal bones in racehorses: 224 cases (1986–1995). JAVMA 212:1757–1764, 1998.

Bowker, R.M., S.J. Rockershouser, K.B. Vex, I.M. Sonéa, J.P. Caron, and R. Kotyk: Immunocytochemical and dye distribution studies of nerves potentially desensitized by injections into the distal interphalangeal joint or the navicular bursa of horses. JAVMA 203:1708–1714, 1993.

Bowker, R.M., K. Linder, I.M. Sonéa, and R.E. Holland: Sensory innervation of the navicular bone and bursa in the foal. Equine Vet. J. 27:60–65, 1995.

Bowker, R.M., K. Linder, K.K. Van Wulfen, and I.M. Sonéa: Anatomy of the distal interphalangeal joint of the mature horse: Relationships with navicular suspensory ligaments, sensory nerves and neurovascular bundle. Equine Vet. J. 29:129–135, 1997.

Bowker, R.M., K.K. Van Wulfen, S.E. Springer, and K.E. Linder: Functional anatomy of the cartilage of the distal phalanx and digital cushion in the equine foot and a hemodynamic flow hypothesis of energy dissipation. Am. J. Vet. Res. 59:961–968, 1998.

Buchner, H.H.F., H.H.C.M. Savelberg, H.C. Schamhardt, and A. Barneveld: Head and trunk movement adaptations in horses with experimentally induced fore- and hindlimb lameness. Equine Vet. J. 28:63–70, 1996.

Budras, K.D., R.L. Hullinger, and W.O. Sack: Light and electron microscopy of keratinization in the laminar epidermis of the equine hoof with reference to laminitis. Am. J. Vet. Res. 50:1150–1160, 1989.

Budras, K.D., C. Schiel, and C. Mülling: Horn tubules of the white line: An insufficient barrier against ascending bacterial invasion. Equine Vet. Educ. 10:81–85, 1998.

Caron, J.P., R.M. Bowker, R.H. Abhold, and P.G. Orsini: Synovial innervation of equine middle carpal joint. Equine Vet. J. 23:364–366, 1992.

Cornelissen, B.P.M., A.B.M. Rijkenhuizen, W. Kersten, and F. Nemeth: Nerve supply of the proximal sesamoid bone in the horse. Vet. Quart. (Suppl. 2) 2:566–569, 1994.

Crabill, M.R., M.K. Chaffin, and D.G. Schmitz: Ultrasonographic morphology of the bicipital tendon and bursa in clinically normal Quarter Horses. Am. J. Vet. Res. 56:5–10, 1995.

Crevier-Denoix, N., C. Collobert, M. Sanaa, et al.: Mechanical correlations derived from segmental histologic study of the equine superficial digital flexor tendon, from foal to adult. Am. J. Vet. Res. 59:969–977, 1998.

Denoix, J.M.: Functional anatomy of tendons and ligaments in the distal limbs (manus and pes). Vet. Clin. North Am. Equine Pract. 10:273–322, 1994.

Denoix, J.M.: The equine distal limb: Atlas of clinical anatomy and comparative imaging. London, Mason Publishing/ Veterinary Press, 2000.

Denoix, J.M., and V. Busoni: Ultrasonographic examination of the accessory ligament of the superficial digital flexor tendon. Equine Vet. J. 31:186–191, 1999.

Denoix, J.M., N. Crevier, B. Roger, and J.F. Lebas: Magnetic resonance imaging of the equine foot. Vet. Radiol. Ultras. 34:405–411, 1993.

Derksen, F.J.: Diagnostic local anesthesia of the equine front limb. Equine Pract. 2:41–47, 1980.

Dik, K.J., S. Boroffka, and P. Stolk: Ultrasonographic assessment of the proximal digital annular ligament in the equine forelimb. Equine Vet. J. 26:59–64, 1994.

Dik, K.J., and I. Gunsser: Atlas of Diagnostic Radiology of the Horse. Parts 1–3. Philadelphia, W.B. Saunders Company, 1988–1990.

Dyson, S.J., and L. Kidd: A comparison of response to analgesia of the navicular bursa and intra-articular analgesia of the distal interphalangeal joint in 59 horses. Equine Vet. J. 25:93–98, 1993.

Ellenberger, W., and H. Baum: Handbuch der vergleichenden Anatomie der Haustiere, 18th ed. Berlin, Springer, 1943.

Ford, T.S., M.W. Ross, and P.G. Orsini: Communications and boundaries of the middle carpal and carpometacarpal joints in the horse. Am. J. Vet. Res. 49:2161–2164, 1988.

Ford, T.S., M.W. Ross, and P.G. Orsini: A comparison of methods for proximal palmar metacarpal analgesia in horses. Vet. Surg. 18:146–150, 1989.

Gabriel, A., S. Yousfi, J. Detilleux, et al.: Morphometric study of the equine navicular bone: Comparisons between fore and rear limbs. J. Vet. Med. A44:579–594, 1997.

Garrett, P.D.: Anatomy of the dorsocapular ligament. JAVMA 196:446–448, 1990.

Genovese, R.L., N.W. Rantanen, M.L. Hauser, and B.S. Simpson: Diagnostic ultrasonography of equine limbs. Vet. Clin. North Am. Equine Pract. 2:145–226, 1986.

Gibson, K.T., L.W. McIlwraith, and R.D. Park: A radiographic study of the distal interphalangeal joint and navicular bursa of the horse. Vet. Radiol. 31:22–25, 1990.

Gray, B.G., H.N. Engel, Jr., P.F. Rumph, J. LaFaver, B.G. Brown, and J.S. McKibben: Clinical approach to determine the contribution of the palmar and palmar metacarpal nerves to the innervation of the equine fetlock joint. Am. J. Vet. Res. 41:940–943, 1980.

Hassel, D.M., S.M. Stover, T.B. Yarbrough, et al.: Palmar-plantar axial sesamoidean approach to the digital flexor tendon sheath in horses. JAVMA 217:1343–1347, 2000.

Hermanson, J.W., and M.A. Cobb: Four forearm flexor muscles of the horse, *Equus caballus:* Anatomy and histochemistry. J. Morphol. 212:269–280, 1992.

Hermanson, J.W., and K.J. Hurley: Architectural and histochemical analysis of the biceps brachii muscle of the horse. Acta Anat. 137:146–156, 1990.

Hickman, J.: Navicular disease. What are we talking about? Equine Vet. J. 21:395–398, 1989.

Hurtig, M.B., and P.B. Fretz: Arthroscopic landmarks of the equine carpus. JAVMA 189:1314–1321, 1986.

Jansson, N., H.V. Sonnichsen: Acquired flexural deformity of the distal interphalangeal joint in horses: Treatment by desmotomy of the accessory ligament of the deep digital flexor tendon. J. Equine. Vet. Sci. 15:353–356, 1995.

Kainer, R.A.,: Functional anatomy of equine locomotor organs. *In* Stashak, T.L.: Adam's Lameness in Horses, 4th ed. Philadelphia, Lea & Febiger, 1987.

Kaser-Hotz, B., and G. Ueltschi: Radiographic appearance of the navicular bone in sound horses. Vet. Radiol. Ultras. 33:9–17, 1992.

Kaneps, A.J., P.D. Koblik, D.M. Freeman, et al.: A comparison of radiology, computed tomography, and magnetic resonance imaging for the diagnosis of palmar process fractures in foals. Vet. Radiol. Ultras. 36:467–477, 1995.

Keegan, K.G., D.A. Wilson, J.M. Kreeger, et al.: Local distribution of mepivacaine after distal interphalangeal joint injection in horses. Am. J. Vet. Res. 57:422–426, 1996.

Keg, P.R., H.C. Schamhardt, P.R. van Weeren, and A. Barneveld: The effect of diagnostic regional nerve blocks in the forelimb on the locomotion of clinically sound horses. Vet. Quart. 18:S106–S109, 1996.

Keg, P.R., P.R. van Weeren, H.C. Schamhardt, and A. Barneveld: Variations in the force applied to flexion tests of the distal limb of horses. Vet. Rec. 141:435–438, 1997.

Kneller, S.K., and J.M. Losonsky: Misdiagnosis in normal radiographic anatomy: Nine structural configurations simulating disease entities in horses. JAVMA 195:1272–1282, 1989.

Kneller, S.K., and J.M. Losonsky: Variable locations of nutrient foramina of the proximal phalanx in forelimbs of Thoroughbreds. JAVMA 197:736–738, 1990.

Leach, D.H.: Structural changes in intercellular junctions during keratinization of the stratum medium of the equine hoof wall. Acta Anat. 147:45–55, 1993.

Leach, D., R. Harland, and B. Burko: The anatomy of the carpal tendon sheath of the horse. J. Anat. 133:301–307, 1981.

Losonsky, J.M., and S.K. Kneller: Variable locations of nutrient foramina of the proximal phalanx in forelimbs of Standardbreds. JAVMA 193:671–673, 1988.

Martinelli, M.J., G.J. Baker, R.B. Clarkson, et al.: Equine metacarpophalangeal joint: Correlation between anatomy and magnetic resonance imaging. Vet. Surg. 23:425, 1994.

Mitten, L.A., and A.L. Bertone: Angular limb deformities in foals. JAVMA 204:717–720, 1994.

Molyneux, G.S., C.J. Haller, K. Mogg, and C.C. Pollitt: The structure, innervation and location of arteriovenous anastomoses in the equine foot. Equine Vet. J. 26:303–312, 1994.

Nicoll, R.G., A.K.W. Wood, and I.C.A. Martin: Ultrasonographic observations of the flexor tendons and ligaments of the metacarpal region of horses. Am. J. Vet. Res. 54:502–506, 1993.

Nixon, A.J.: Endoscopy of the digital flexor tendon sheath in horses. Vet. Surg. 19:266–271, 1990.

Nyrop, K.A., J.R. Coffman, R.M. DeBowes, and L.C. Booth: The role of diagnostic nerve blocks in the equine lameness examination. Compend. Contin. Educ. 5:S669–S676, 1983.

Parente, E.J., D.W. Richardson, and P. Spencer: Basal sesamoidean fractures in horses: 57 cases (1980–1991). JAVMA 202:1293–1297, 1993.

Poulos, P.W., and M.F. Smith: The nature of enlarged vascular channels in the navicular bone of the horse. Vet. Radiol. 29:60–64, 1988.

Rijkenhuizen, A.B.M., F. Nemeth, K.J. Dik, and S.A. Goedegebuure: The arterial supply of the navicular bone in adult horses with navicular disease. Equine Vet. J. 21:418–424, 1989.

Rose, P.L.: Villonodular synovitis in horses. Compend. Contin. Educ. Pract. Vet. 10:649–654, 1988.

Rose, R.J.: Navicular disease in the horse. J. Equine Vet. Sci. 16:18–24, 1996.

Ryan, J.M., M.A. Cobb, and J.W. Hermanson: Elbow extensor muscles of the horse: Postural and dynamic implications. Acta Anat. 144:71–79, 1992.

Sams, A.E., C.M. Honnas, W.O. Sack, and T.S. Ford: Communication of the ulnaris lateralis bursa with the equine elbow joint and evaluation of caudal arthrocentesis. Equine Vet. 25:130–133, 1993.

Schebitz, H., and H. Wilkens: Atlas of Radiographic Anatomy of the Horse, 4th ed. Berlin, Paul Parey Verlag, 1986.

Smallwood, J.E., S.M. Albright, M.R. Metcalf, and I.D. Robertson: A xeroradiographic study of the developing equine foredigit and metacarpophalangeal region from birth to six months of age. Vet. Radiol. 30:98–110, 1988.

Smallwood, J.E., S.M. Albright, M.R. Metcalf, P.W. Poulos, and I.D. Robertson: A xeroradiographic study of the developing Quarterhorse foredigit and metacarpophalangeal region from six to twelve months of age. Vet. Radiol. 31:254–259, 1990.

Soana, S., G. Gnudi, G. Bertoni, and P. Botti: Anatomic-radiographic study on the osteogenesis of carpal and tarsal bones in horse fetus. Anat. Histol. Embryol. 27:301–305, 1998.

Southwood, L.L., T.S. Stashak, and R.A. Kainer: Tenoscopic anatomy of the equine carpal flexor synovial sheath. Vet. Surg. 27:150–157, 1998.

Specht, T.E., P.W. Poulos, M.R. Metcalf, and I.D. Robertson: Vacuum phenomenon in the metacarpophalangeal joint of a horse. JAVMA 197:749–750, 1990.

Squire, K.R.E., S.B. Adams, W.R. Wimer, et al.: Arthroscopic removal of a radial osteochondroma causing carpal canal syndrome in a horse. JAVMA 201:1216–1218, 1992.

Stashak, T.S.: Adam's Lameness in Horses, 4th ed. Philadelphia, Lea & Febiger, 1987.

Stephens, P.R., D.W. Richardson, and P.A. Spencer: Slab fractures of the third carpal bone in Standardbreds and Thoroughbreds: 155 cases (1977–1984). JAVMA 193:353–358, 1988.

Trumble, T.N., S.P. Arnoczky, J.A. Stick, and R.L. Stickle: Clinical relevance of the microvasculature of the equine proximal sesamoid bone. Am. J. Vet. Res. 56:720–724, 1995.

Vázquez de Mercado, R., S.M. Stover, K.T. Taylor, et al.: Lateral approach for arthrocentesis of the distal interphalangeal joint in horses. JAVMA 212:1413–1418, 1998.

Verschooten, F., B.V. Waerebeek, and J. Verbeeck: The ossification of cartilages of the distal phalanx in the horse: An anatomical, experimental, radiographic and clinical study. J. Equine Vet. Sci. 16:291–305, 1996.

Vollmerhaus, B.: *In* Nickel, R.A., A. Schummer, and E. Seiferle: The Anatomy of the Domestic Animals, Vol. 3, Berlin, Paul Parey Verlag, 1981.

Weaver, J.C.B., S.M. Stover, and T.R. O'Brien: Radiographic anatomy of soft tissue attachments in the equine metacarpophalangeal and proximal phalangeal region. Equine Vet. J. 24:310–315, 1992.

Wilke, M., A.J. Nixon, J. Malark, and G. Myhre: Fractures of the palmar aspect of the carpal bones in horses: 10 cases (1984–2000). JAVMA 219:801–804, 2001.

Wilson, D.A., G.J. Baker, G.J. Pijanowski, M.J. Boero, and R.R. Badertscher: Composition and morphologic features of the interosseous muscle in Standardbreds and Thoroughbreds. Am. J. Vet. Res. 52:133–139, 1991.

Wright, I.M., L. Kidd, and B.H. Thorp: Gross, histological and histomorphometric features of the navicular bone and related structures in the horse. Equine Vet. J. 30:220–234, 1998.

Wright, I.M., and P.J. McMahon: Tenosynovitis associated with longitudinal tears of the digital flexor tendons in horses. Equine Vet. J. 31:12–18, 1999.

# CHAPTER 24

# The Hindlimb of the Horse

## CONFORMATION OF THE CROUP

Although the hindlimbs support little more than 40% of the body weight, they supply by far the greater part of the forward impetus in locomotion. This thrust is delivered through the hip and sacroiliac joints, which are intrinsically more stable than the shoulder and scapulothoracic synsarcosis, the corresponding "joints" of the forelimb. The sacroiliac joint is strengthened by tight ligaments, and both it and the hip joint are well supported by the muscles of the croup and thigh. These muscles are particularly massive in the horse, in which they round the contours in a distinctive fashion. In consequence, it is more difficult to appreciate the features and orientation of the pelvis of the horse than those of the pelves of other domestic species.

Despite the muscular development, the coxal tuber remains a conspicuous landmark that is palpable in its whole extent and visible in its upper part (Fig. 24–1/2). The sacral tuber (/2′), difficult to palpate in most animals, rises a little above the level of the adjacent spinous processes. The ischial tuber (/3) is also not always easy to appreciate, although its location and a general impression of its form may be obtained on deep palpation over the muscles that form the caudal contour of the croup and thigh. If this is done, the slope of the pelvis may be estimated by visualizing the line joining the coxal and ischial projections. In the standard, generally approved conformation, this line forms an angle of about 30 degrees with the horizon; from this it may be inferred that the sacrum is more or less horizontal. When the angle is significantly smaller—and the two tubers come close to sharing the same horizontal plane—the tail appears to be set high. When the angle is significantly greater, the animal is said to be goose-rumped. The croup is short in such animals, and the hamstring muscles are reduced in length and in the leverage they may exert. Although this is clearly disadvantageous, some compensation is obtained from the more stable support the limbs afford the trunk, and many horsemen and -women find a gently sloping croup acceptable in a saddle horse. Undue prominence of the sacral tubers ("hunter's bumps") sometimes develops, especially in show jumpers and other horses subjected to similar repeated stress. The deformity is commonly ascribed to subluxation of the sacroiliac joints.

The position of the hip joint cannot be determined directly but may be deduced from its relationship to the greater trochanter of the femur. This protuberance is divided into low cranial and high caudal parts, separately identifiable on palpation (/5,5′). At more distal levels, the third trochanter (prominent only in this species) and the lateral epicondyle are easily distinguished and may be used to reveal the orientation of the femur. This bone is more nearly vertical than is often supposed (see Fig. 19–1).

## THE HIP JOINT

The stability of the hip joint owes much to the depth and extent of the acetabulum, which is considerably increased by a fibrocartilaginous rim; it embraces a large part of the femoral head (Fig. 24–1/4). The head is additionally secured against luxation by two ligaments. One, the *ligament of the femoral head,* is short and stout but is in no important way peculiar. The other, the *accessory ligament,* is unique to the horse (and donkey) among domestic species. It begins as a detachment from the prepubic tendon and reaches the joint by following a shallow groove on the ventral aspect of the pubis; this leads it to the acetabular notch through which it passes to insert on the head (see Fig. 21–2/5′). The two ligaments together restrict both the range and the versatility of movement permitted to the joint. The restrictions on rotation and abduction are most severe; in practice, movement is almost confined to flexion and extension in a sagittal plane, a much more limited repertory than the geometry of the articular surfaces suggests. The stability of the joint is partly dependent on the tension exerted by the weight of the abdominal viscera pulling on the prepubic tendon and thus on the accessory ligament (p. 527).

Although the joint capsule is quite capacious, its deep location makes it relatively difficult of

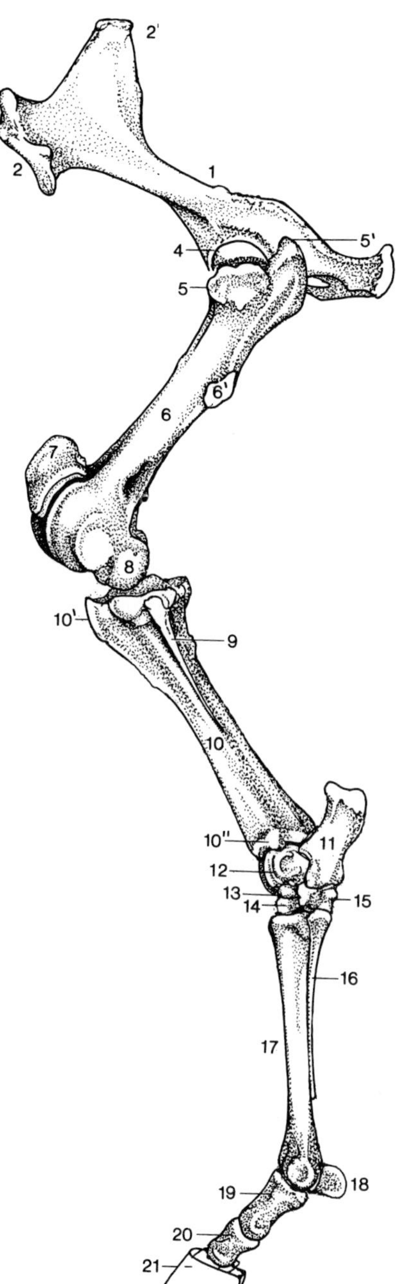


**Figure 24–1.** The skeleton of the left hindlimb, lateral view.

1, Hip bone (os coxae); 2, coxal tuber; 2′, sacral tuber; 3, ischial tuber; 4, head of femur; 5, 5′, cranial and caudal parts of greater trochanter; 6, femur; 6′, third trochanter; 7, patella; 8, femoral condyle; 9, fibula; 10, tibia; 10′, tibial tuberosity; 10″, lateral malleolus; 11, calcaneus; 12, talus; 13, central tarsal; 14, third tarsal; 15, fourth tarsal; 16, metatarsal IV (lateral splint bone); 17, metatarsal III (cannon bone); 18, proximal sesamoid bones; 19, 20, 21, proximal, middle, and distal phalanges, the last within the hoof.

access. When it must be punctured, the needle is introduced between the two parts of the greater trochanter and is directed horizontally and craniomedially, at an angle of about 40 degrees to the transverse plane.

## THE MUSCLES OF THE HIP AND THIGH

These are conveniently regarded as comprising gluteal, hamstring, medial, and cranial groups.

### The Gluteal Muscles

The superficial and deep fasciae of the croup and thigh continue the corresponding coverings of the loins. The deep fascia detaches various septa that find anchorage on the pelvic girdle and the caudal edge of the sacrosciatic ligament after passing between certain muscles. The most substantial of these separate the gluteus superficialis and biceps femoris, the biceps and semitendinosus, and the semitendinosus and semimembranosus, and so mold the muscles that their individual contours are often clearly visible through the skin; this is especially so in animals in "hard" training and when the muscles are contracted. The inner surface of this fascia, including the sides of the septa, itself gives origin to many fascicles of the muscles it covers.

The *tensor fasciae latae* (Fig. 24–2/3) radiates from its origin on the coxal tuber to end by a broad aponeurosis (fascia lata) that inserts on the patella, the lateral patellar ligament, and the cranial border of the tibia. The cranial border of the fleshy part is related to the subiliac lymph nodes. The tensor is a flexor of the hip that helps to advance the limb during the swing phase of the stride. It is supplied by the cranial gluteal nerve.

The *gluteus superficialis* lies between the tensor and biceps (/4). It has separate origins from the coxal tuber and the gluteal fascia, but the two parts combine to a common insertion on the third trochanter. Occasionally, this projection is broken off and it is then displaced dorsally by the attaching muscle. The gluteus superficialis is potentially a flexor of the hip and abductor of the thigh. Its two parts are separately supplied by the cranial and caudal gluteal nerves.

The *gluteus medius* is a muscle of exceptional size and power (/*B*,2′). Its wide origin spreads from a depression scooped in the surface of the longissimus dorsi, over the coxal tuber and iliac wing, to the sacrum and adjacent part of the

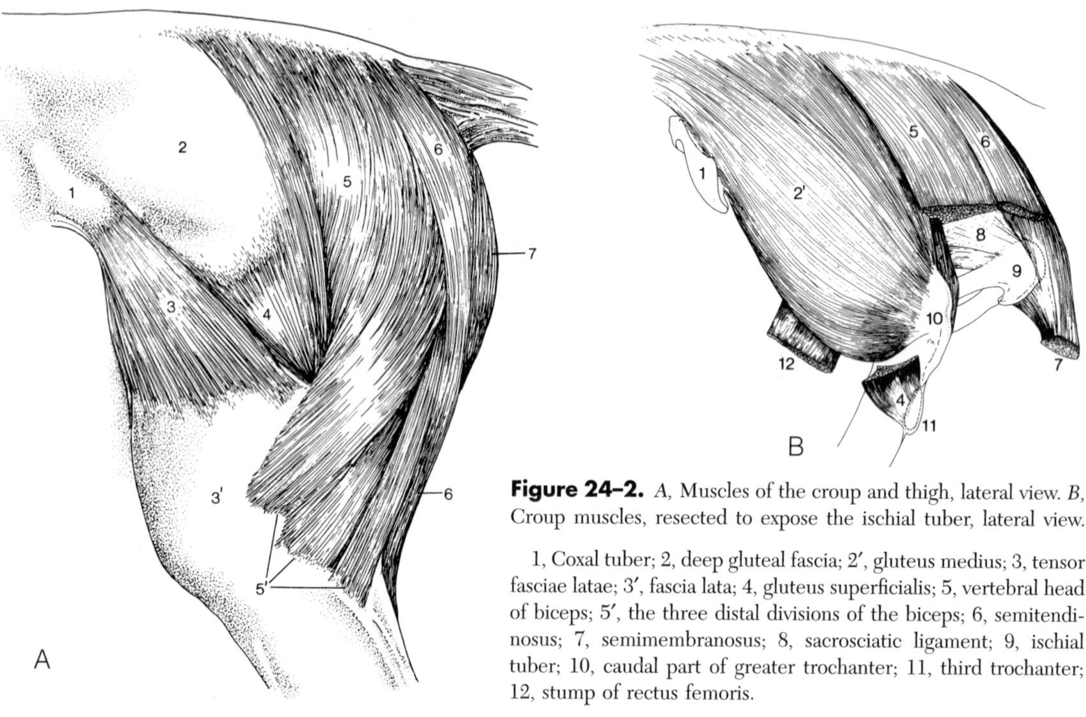


**Figure 24–2.** *A*, Muscles of the croup and thigh, lateral view. *B*, Croup muscles, resected to expose the ischial tuber, lateral view.

1, Coxal tuber; 2, deep gluteal fascia; 2′, gluteus medius; 3, tensor fasciae latae; 3′, fascia lata; 4, gluteus superficialis; 5, vertebral head of biceps; 5′, the three distal divisions of the biceps; 6, semitendinosus; 7, semimembranosus; 8, sacrosciatic ligament; 9, ischial tuber; 10, caudal part of greater trochanter; 11, third trochanter; 12, stump of rectus femoris.

sacrosciatic ligament. The principal insertion is to the caudal part of the greater trochanter, but a deep division—gluteus accessorius—has a separate aponeurotic attachment to the intertrochanteric line of the femur. This aponeurosis passes over the cranial part of the trochanter where its passage is eased by the interposition of a synovial (trochanteric) bursa. This bursa may become inflamed, a condition detectable by the animal's flinching when pressure is exerted over it. Horses so afflicted obtain relief by standing with the affected limb somewhat abducted; when they move, they tend to adopt an oblique doglike gait, swinging the limb in an arc.

This muscle is primarily an extensor of the hip, but it has a secondary use as an abductor of the thigh. Its association with the longissimus dorsi makes it an effective participant in rearing. It is supplied by the cranial gluteal nerve.

The *gluteus profundus* lies deep to the caudal part of the gluteus medius. It arises from and around the ischial spine and passes more or less transversely to insert on the cranial part of the greater trochanter. An abductor of the thigh, it is supplied by the cranial gluteal nerve.

## The Caudal (Hamstring) Muscles

In the horse, the three muscles of this group possess well-developed vertebral heads of origin (in addition to the usual pelvic heads); it is these vertebral heads that account for the characteristic filling and rounding of the croup (Fig. 24–2/5,6; but compare with Plate 24/*I* showing these muscles from the rear in a pregnant mare close to parturition). The vertebral head of the *biceps* arises from the sacrum and adjacent part of the sacrosciatic ligament. It descends behind and partly covers the gluteal muscles before it crosses the ischial tuber to be joined by the smaller pelvic head that arises from that process. The muscle inserts by three divisions (/5′), the first in the fascia lata and on the patella, the second on the lateral patellar ligament and tibial crest, while the third, the tarsal tendon, joins the common calcanean tendon. The vertebral head is supplied by the caudal gluteal nerve, the pelvic head by the sciatic nerve.

The vertebral head of the *semitendinosus* (/6) has an origin adjoining that of the biceps. After this merges with the pelvic head, the combination edges medially to insert on the medial aspect of the tibia and the crural fascia. It also detaches a tarsal tendon that joins the common calcanean tendon. The vertebral and pelvic heads are supplied by the caudal gluteal and sciatic nerves, respectively.

The *semimembranosus* (/7) is included in the hamstring group, although topographically it is a muscle of the medial aspect of the thigh. The vertebral head is relatively weak, the pelvic head more substantial. The combined muscle is largely covered by the gracilis and follows the caudal margin of the adductor to which it is closely bound. It inserts by two divisions. The cranial division inserts on the medial epicondyle of the femur and the medial collateral ligament of the stifle joint; the caudal division proceeds distally to the medial condyle of the tibia. The principal nerve supply is from the sciatic nerve.

The actions and uses of the hamstring muscles are complicated and in certain respects enigmatic. It is clear that all three units are well placed to extend the hip. In considering the actions on the stifle it is more useful to divide the hamstring group into two functional units, one that inserts proximal to the axis of rotation of the joint, the other distal to it, rather than to consider the three muscles individually. The "proximal unit" comprises parts of the muscles that are potentially extensor since they may straighten the stifle by drawing the femur caudally when the limb bears weight. The "distal unit" will flex the stifle when the hoof is raised from the ground but extend it when the hoof is firmly planted. The contributions of the biceps and semitendinosus to the common calcanean tendon must not be forgotten; these parts are extensor to the hock.

Some of these actions are clearly incompatible since the movements of the stifle and hock joints are linked in their actions by the reciprocal mechanism (see p. 619). It follows that the entire hamstring group, which includes parts that may flex the stifle, cannot always contract en masse.

## The Medial Muscles

The medial muscles are disposed in the same three layers as in other species. The superficial layer comprises the *gracilis* and *sartorius* (Fig. 24–3/14,8). The gracilis exhibits no specific features that require notice. The sartorius arises from the psoas fascia and the insertion tendon of the psoas minor and gains the thigh by passing through the gap between the caudal margin of the flank and the ilium. It is related to the deep inguinal lymph nodes where it forms the cranial margin of the femoral triangle. The sartorius inserts on medial structures of the stifle joint, including the condyle of the tibia. Both muscles may adduct the thigh, but the sartorius is probably more important as a hip flexor. The gracilis is supplied by the obturator nerve, the sartorius by the saphenous nerve.

The pectineus and adductor constitute the middle layer. The *pectineus* (/13) is a small fusiform muscle that arises from the margin of the pubis and inserts on the medial surface of the femur. A part of the tendon of origin is from the contralateral side, and the resulting decussation contributes a transverse strengthening to the prepubic tendon (p. 527). The pectineus is placed to flex the hip and adduct the thigh. It is supplied by the obturator nerve.

The much larger *adductor* (/15) fills the space between pectineus and semimembranosus. It arises from the floor of the pelvis and symphysial tendon, and inserts on the caudal surface and medial epicondyle of the femur and the medial collateral ligament of the stifle. Although adduction of the thigh is the primary function, a subsidiary extensor action is possible. Innervation is from the obturator nerve.

The small muscles of the hip—quadratus femoris, gemelli, obturator internus, and obturator externus—are of little importance. The tendon of the obturator internus crosses the margin of the ischium as in the dog. The first three are supplied by the sciatic nerve, the obturator externus by the obturator.

## The Cranial Muscles

This group comprises the *quadriceps femoris,* which possesses the usual four individually named heads of origin, and the insignificant capsularis.

The four heads of the quadriceps combine in a common insertion on the patella, with the interme-

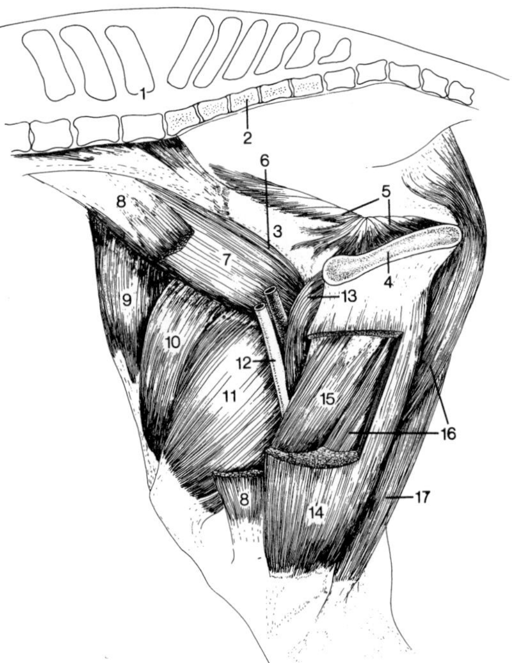


**Figure 24–3.** Muscles of the thigh, medial view.

1, Last lumbar vertebra; 2, sacrum; 3, shaft of ilium; 4, pelvic symphysis; 5, internal obturator; 6, psoas minor; 7, iliopsoas; 8, sartorius, resected; 9, tensor fasciae latae; 10, rectus femoris; 11, vastus medialis; 12, femoral vessels in femoral triangle; 13, pectineus; 14, gracilis, fenestrated; 15, adductor; 16, semimembranosus; 17, semitendinosus.

diate patellar ligament (Fig. 24–4/8) supplying the functional continuation to the tibial tuberosity. The rectus femoris is a potential flexor of the hip, but the principal action of the group is extension of the stifle. Extension, of course, embraces stabilization of the joint to prevent its collapse when the limb bears weight during the support phase of the stride. It can be observed, and confirmed by palpation, that the muscle appears relaxed when the animal stands quietly. This suggests that, once the patella has been brought into its resting position, no considerable further effort is required of the quadriceps. Quadriceps paralysis is a very severe handicap. The animal is unable to stabilize the stifle; it is also unable to stabilize the hock joint whose movements are linked to those of the stifle

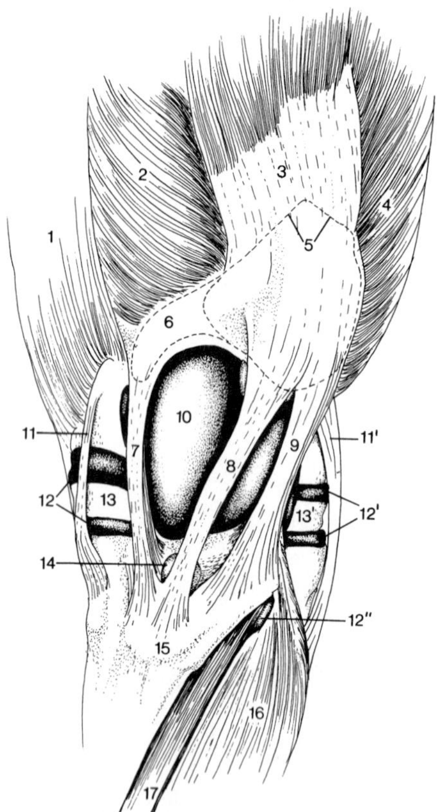


**Figure 24–4.** The left stifle joint, cranial view.

1, Adductor; 2, vastus medialis; 3, rectus femoris; 4, vastus lateralis; 5, outline of patella; 6, outline of patellar fibrocartilage; 7, 8, 9, medial, intermediate, and lateral patellar ligaments; 10, joint capsule over medial ridge of femoral trochlea; 11, 11′, medial and lateral collateral ligaments; 12, 12′, medial and lateral femorotibial joint capsules; 12″, recess of 12′ under combined tendon of peroneus tertius and long digital extensor; 13, 13′, medial and lateral menisci; 14, distal infrapatellar bursa; 15, tibial tuberosity; 16, long digital extensor; 17, tibialis cranialis.

by the reciprocal mechanism (p. 619). The group is supplied by the femoral nerve.

## THE STIFLE JOINT

Although generally conforming to the common pattern, the equine stifle also exhibits several important features of distinction. The most remarkable provide the means of "locking" the joint so that one hindlimb may support a disproportionate part of the body weight and allow the other to be rested while the animal remains standing. The arrangement is a major component of the passive stay-apparatus (p. 618).

The locking mechanism relies upon certain peculiarities of the articular surfaces. The femoral trochlea is markedly asymmetrical. The medial ridge is larger than the lateral one and is prolonged proximally to a terminal protuberance that is easily identifiable on palpation (Figs. 24–4/10, 24–5/4, and 24–6/2). The trochlear surface comprises two distinct areas. The larger one, known as the gliding surface, corresponds to the whole trochlea of most species and faces in a predominantly cranial direction; the smaller one, known as the resting surface, forms a narrow shelf above the gliding surface, from which it is sharply angled to face proximally (Fig. 24–15/18). The patella is broadly diamond-shaped when viewed from in front (*/B,2*); in the fresh state it is extended medially by a *patellar fibrocartilage* (/3). The articular surface of the patella is also divided. The more extensive backward-facing area engages with the trochlea during the greater part of the normal range of movement; a narrow strip at the apex is directed distally and makes contact with the femur only at the limit of extension.

In this species there are three *patellar ligaments* joined by a retinaculum in which the insertion tendons of several thigh muscles merge. The intermediate ligament (Fig. 24–4/8), the homologue of the single structure of the smaller species, runs from the apex of the patella to the tibial tuberosity. The lateral and medial ligaments run from the angles of the patella or, more accurately where the medial one is concerned, from the parapatellar cartilage. The three ligaments are thus quite widely separated at their origins but converge distally and insert close together. The gap between the proximal parts of the medial and intermediate ligaments is especially wide and is occupied by the medial ridge of the trochlea (/10).

The patella slides up and down over the femoral trochlea during the greater part of the normal excursions of the joint. Only in extreme extension, as momentarily during the support phase of a

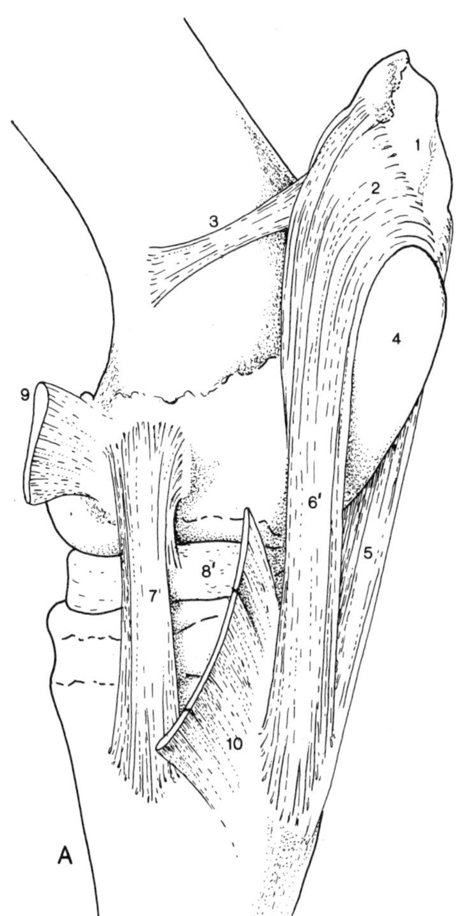


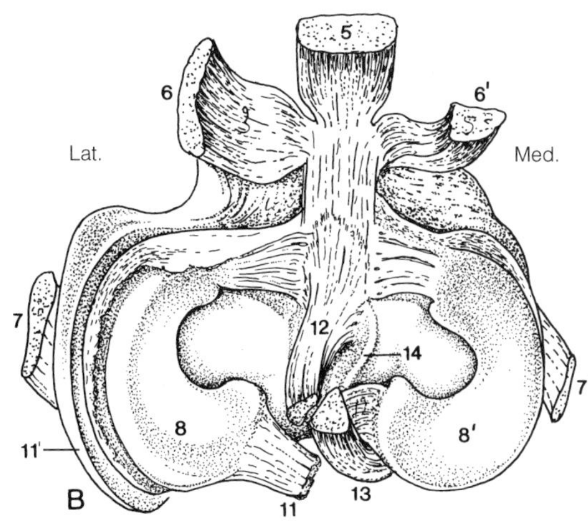


**Figure 24–5.** The ligaments of the left stifle joint. *A,* Medial view. *B,* Proximal view of the left tibia and the menisci.

1, Patella; 2, patellar fibrocartilage; 3, medial femoropatellar ligament; 4, medial ridge of trochlea; 5, intermediate patellar ligament; 6, 6′, lateral and medial patellar ligaments; 7, 7′, lateral and medial collateral ligaments; 8, 8′, lateral and medial menisci; 9, insertion of semimembranosus; 10, insertion of gracilis and sartorius; 11, meniscofemoral ligament; 11′, tendon of popliteus; 12, 13, cranial and caudal cruciate ligaments; 14, intercondylar eminence.

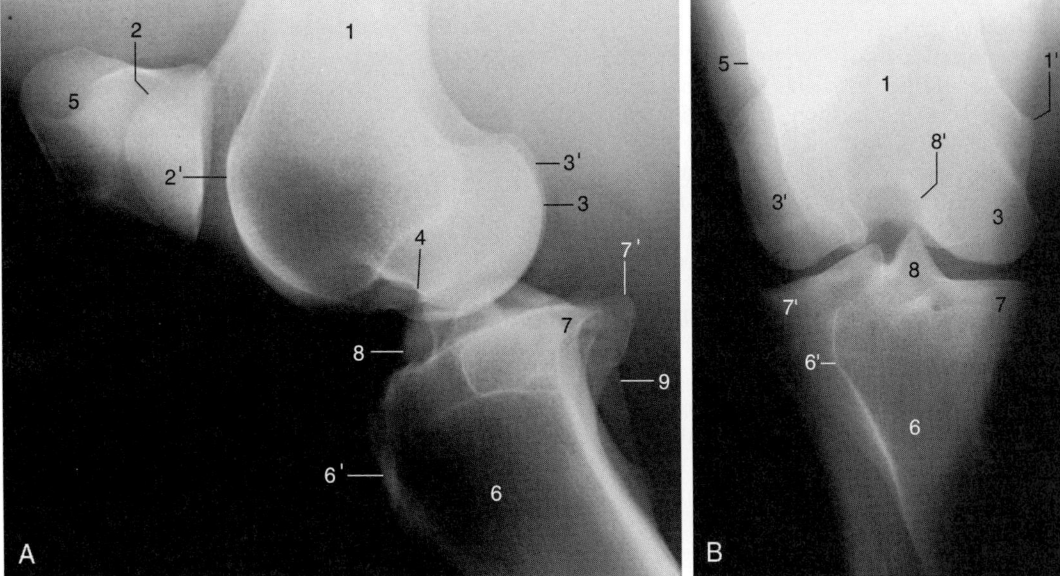


**Figure 24–6.** Lateral *(A)* and caudocranial *(B)* radiographs of the stifle joint.

1, Femur; 1′, medial epicondyle; 2, 2′, medial and lateral ridges of the trochlea; 3, 3′, medial and lateral condyles; 4, extensor fossa; 5, patella; 6, tibia; 6′, tibial tuberosity; 7, 7′, medial and lateral condyles; 8, intercondylar eminence; 8′, intercondylar fossa; 9, fibula.

walking stride, do the resting surfaces engage. The resting position is also adopted when the animal is standing squarely with its weight evenly distributed over the two hindlimbs. That this is so is easily verified on palpation; it can be found that the medial ligament then runs even with the edge of the corresponding ridge of the trochlea. This position is maintained without the assistance of the main extensor (quadriceps femoris) of the stifle, but does require some effort on the part of the muscles that converge on the medial and lateral patellar ligaments—the biceps and tensor fasciae latae laterally, the gracilis and sartorius medially. The position is unstable and the patella is easily dislodged—it then slips back onto the gliding surface of the trochlea.

The joint cavity is capacious and its division into compartments is relatively complete. The extensive femoropatellar compartment is mainly contained between the femur, the patella, and the quadriceps. The part distal to the patella is more accessible, though separated from the patellar ligaments (and retinaculum) by a thick cushion of fat. It communicates with the medial femorotibial compartment in the large majority of horses but with the corresponding lateral compartment in far fewer, perhaps 25%. The partition between the medial and lateral compartments is almost always imperforate. The inconstancy of these arrangements has considerable practical importance; it must be assumed that any infection spreads readily among the three compartments, while prudence dictates that therapeutic substances be separately injected into each.

Such injections require familiarity with the disposition of the ligaments and the ability to recognize them on palpation. The medial collateral ligament can be picked out close to its origin from the femoral epicondyle and provides a convenient landmark in puncture of the medial femorotibial compartment. The needle is introduced close to its cranial border, between it and the medial patellar ligament (Figs. 24–4/11,7 and 24–5/7′,6′). The lateral collateral ligament is palpable along its whole length but is most easily found close to its insertion upon the head of the fibula. The lateral femorotibial compartment is punctured between this ligament and the more cranial, and also palpable, tendon of origin of the long digital extensor (Fig. 24–4/11′,16). The femoropatellar compartment is also easily entered from the side, behind the proximal part of the lateral patellar ligament (/9). Alternatively, this compartment can be approached from in front, between the patellar ligaments, but this requires that the needle be passed through a considerable thickness of fat.

## THE SKELETON OF THE LEG AND HOCK; THE HOCK JOINT

The tibia is the only functional component of the skeleton of the leg. Its shaft is thickly covered by muscle on its craniolateral and caudal aspects but is subcutaneous medially (Fig. 24–7/1). The distal articular surface, known as the cochlea, comprises two grooves separated by a ridge, all with a craniolateral inclination. The cochlea is flanked by medial and lateral malleoli (Fig. 24–8/2,2′).

The fibula is much reduced. The proximal extremity or head forms a tight articulation with the lateral condyle of the tibia (Fig. 24–1/9). The head usually continues into a short and rodlike shaft, but sometimes a band of soft tissue intervenes; this may simulate a fracture when depicted in a radiograph. In later embryonic life the isolated distal extremity of the fibula becomes assimilated within the tibia to which it furnishes the lateral malleolus (see Fig. 2–57/*D,E*,6″). The independence of the malleolar center of ossification is clearly evident in radiographs of young animals, and the line of union may be evident in the adult bone.

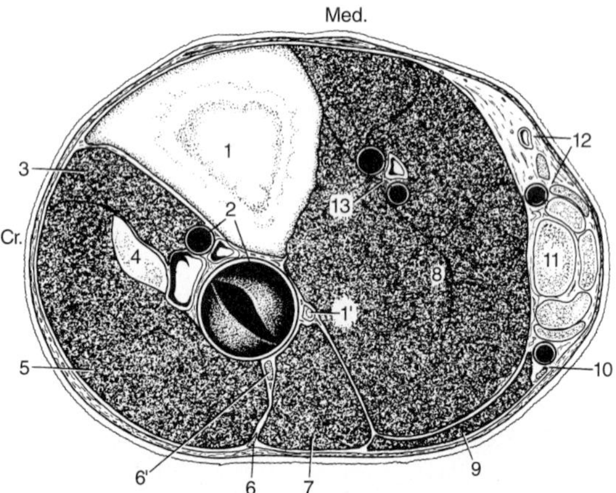


**Figure 24–7.** Transverse section of the left leg slightly above its middle.

1, Tibia; 1′, fibula; 2, cranial tibial vessels; 3, tibialis cranialis; 4, peroneus tertius; 5, long digital extensor; 6, 6′, superficial and deep peroneal nerves; 7, lateral digital extensor; 8, deep digital flexors; 9, soleus; 10, lateral saphenous vein and caudal cutaneous sural nerve; 11, superficial digital flexor surrounded by the other components of the common calcanean tendon (gastrocnemius and tarsal tendons of semitendinosus and biceps); 12, caudal branch of medial saphenous vein, tibial nerve, and saphenous artery; 13, caudal tibial vessels.

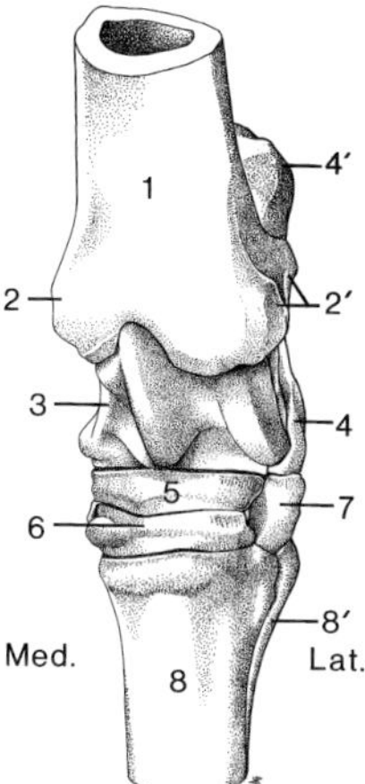


**Figure 24–8.** Dorsal view of the left hock.

1, Tibia; 2, 2′, medial and lateral malleoli; 3, talus with trochlea; 4, calcaneus; 4′, calcanean tuber (point of hock); 5, central tarsal bone; 6, third tarsal bone; 7, fourth tarsal bone; 8, third metatarsal (cannon) bone; 8′, fourth metatarsal (lateral splint) bone.

The hock (Fig. 24–8) comprises the following elements: talus and calcaneus in the proximal row, a central tarsal bone in the intermediate row, and fused first and second bones and separate third and fourth bones in the distal row. The proximodorsal surface of the talus (/3) carries an oblique trochlea corresponding to the cochlea of the tibia. The distal surface is more or less flat and rests on the central bone. The calcaneus (/4,4′) lies largely to the plantar aspect of the talus; the tuber surmounting the calcanean process rises about 5 cm above the tarsocrural joint space and serves as a rough guide to that feature. The composite bone formed by the first and second tarsal bones is relatively small and lies mainly behind the much larger, wedge-shaped third tarsal (/6). The fourth bone (/7; on the lateral side) is cuboidal, unlike the other bones in the distal row, which are flattened; its greater depth causes it to occupy both the intermediate and the distal tiers. The bones of the distal row articulate with the metatarsal bones—the third (cannon) bone centrally and the much smaller second and fourth (splint) bones to the sides.

Even cursory examination of the tarsal skeleton is sufficient to make it plain that while free movement is allowed at the tarsocrural joint, there can be almost no play at any other level. The obliquity of the articular surfaces of the tibia and talus ensures that the distal part of the limb is carried outward as well as forward when the hock joint is flexed.

The fibrous layer of the joint capsule extends from the tibia to the metatarsus. It is firmly attached over various parts of the skeleton but is free elsewhere and then varies considerably in strength; the weaker parts (pouches) bulge when the synovial sac is distended. Numerous ligaments are associated with the hock, but the majority are short and are conveniently regarded as mere local thickenings of the capsule. Three that are larger and more discrete are of greater importance. Paired collateral ligaments extend from the malleoli to the corresponding splint bones and may be palpated along their whole lengths (Fig. 24–10/11,11′ and Plate 26/*C,D*). They have intermediate attachments to the bones they cross, and these help ensure that movements of the hock are restricted to flexion and extension at the tarsocrural level. A long plantar ligament (/14) follows the plantar aspect of the calcaneus, passes over the fourth tarsal, and then continues distally onto the proximal part of the metatarsus. It is largely covered by the tendon of the superficial digital flexor but may be palpated to each side of this. It is not uncommonly strained about the middle of its length, and in lateral view the resulting thickening gives a convex profile to the plantar aspect of the hock. The condition is known as a curb (from the French *courbe,* curve, contour).

The hock is a compound joint with three joint sacs, one common to the tarsocrural and proximal intertarsal levels, one for the distal intertarsal level, and one for the tarsometatarsal level (Fig. 24–9/10–13). The two more distal sacs are small and occasionally communicate; the distal intertarsal sac may be punctured from the medial side, while access to the tarsometatarsal sac may be gained between the fourth tarsal and the head of the splint bone; the novice will find neither technique very reliable. The proximal part of the talocrural sac is capacious and is prone to overdistention, which causes the capsule to pouch at its weakest points. There are three such pouches. One, at the dorsomedial aspect of the hock, is bounded by the tendon of the peroneus tertius, the medial collateral ligament, the medial malleolus, and the medial branch of the tendon of the tibialis cranialis (Fig. 24–10/10 and Plate 26/*E,F*). The sac is easily punctured here, even when it is not distended; care must be taken to avoid the cranial branch of the medial saphenous vein, which crosses the site. The second and third pouches are on the plantar aspect. One is found between the medial collateral ligament and the deep flexor tendon at the level of the medial malleolus (/10′); the other is behind the lateral collateral ligament, between the calcaneus and the lateral malleolus. Unless the joint sac is

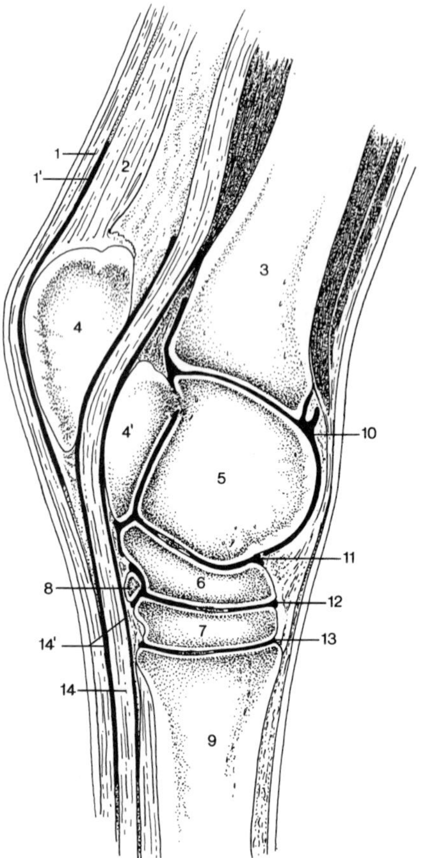


**Figure 24–9.** Sagittal section of the hock joint.

1, Superficial digital flexor; 1′, subtendinous calcanean bursa; 2, gastrocnemius; 3, tibia; 4, calcaneus; 4′, sustentaculum tali; 5, talus; 6, central tarsal; 7, third tarsal; 8, fourth tarsal (mainly on lateral side); 9, large metatarsal (cannon) bone; 10, tarsocrural joint; 11, proximal intertarsal joint (communicates with 10); 12, distal intertarsal joint; 13, tarsometatarsal joint; 14, deep digital flexor; 14′, tarsal sheath.

considerably distended, puncture at either of these sites may prove difficult.

Swelling of the joint sac may be confused with swelling of the synovial (tarsal) sheath around the deep flexor tendon (/3″). The differential diagnosis is simple. When the joint sac is distended, pressure applied to either plantar pouch is transmitted to the dorsal pouch (and vice versa). Swelling of the tarsal sheath is transmitted from plantaromedial to plantarolateral (or vice versa) if local pressure is applied; it is not transmitted to the dorsal aspect of the joint. Moreover, the swelling of the tendon sheath is evident about 5 cm proximal to the plantar swelling of the joint.

Arthritic changes (spavin) commonly affect the bones of the hock. The changes most commonly begin on the medial aspect, near the meeting of the third and central tarsal and third metatarsal bones. This region, the "seat of spavin," is crossed by the medial branch of the tibialis cranialis tendon (the cunean tendon of clinical authors) (/8′) en route to its insertion on the combined first and second tarsal bones. The tendon is a useful reference point since it is palpable. A portion is sometimes resected with the object of reducing pressure over the lesion and by eliminating movement between the distal tarsal elements. The treatment is often effective in reducing pain, although obviously it does not cure the condition.

## THE MUSCLES OF THE LEG

The leg is enveloped by three layers of fascia. The superficial layer continues the corresponding fascia of the thigh. The middle layer is formed by the aponeuroses of the tensor fasciae latae, biceps, semitendinosus, gracilis, and sartorius. Its lateral and medial parts combine on the caudal aspect to form a stout plate that bridges the space between the deep flexor and the common calcanean tendon. The plate receives the tarsal tendons of the biceps and semitendinosus and attaches to the calcaneus as part of the common calcanean tendon formation. The saphenous artery, medial and lateral saphenous veins, and lateral and caudal sural nerves are enclosed between the superficial and middle fasciae. The deep fascial layer extends septa that pass between the muscles to attach to the tibia. It thus divides the leg into a number of osteofascial compartments.

### The Craniolateral Muscles

This group comprises the tibialis cranialis, peroneus tertius, and the long and lateral digital extensors. All are flexors of the hock, and those that proceed farther are extensors of the digit. The *tibialis cranialis* arises from the lateral condyle and tuberosity of the tibia and continues distally, closely applied to the bone (Fig. 24–7/3). The insertion tendon begins just above the level of the hock and passes through a split in the tendon of the peroneus tertius before itself dividing. The larger dorsal branch continues to the metatarsal tuberosity. The smaller medial branch diverges to cross the medial collateral ligament before inserting upon the combined first and second tarsal bones (Fig. 24–10/8,8′ and Plate 26/*C*). When the muscle contracts it presses on the "seat of spavin" (see this page, top). Though the tibialis cranialis appears to be a flexor of the hock, it is difficult to be certain of its function. According to one view, its prime role is to counteract the bending moment applied to the tibia by the action of other muscles and by gravity.

The *peroneus tertius* is almost exclusively tendinous (Fig. 24–7/4). It arises from the lower end of the femur together with the long extensor; for much of its course it is recessed in the deep surface of that muscle. It bifurcates at the hock; the lateral branch inserts on the calcaneus and fourth tarsal bone, the dorsal one on the proximal part of the third tarsal and third metatarsal bones (Fig. 24–12/1 and Plate 26/*A*). The tendon links the actions of the stifle and hock joints, a function convincingly demonstrated should it be ruptured; there then appears an ability to extend the hock while retaining a flexed stifle, a combination of movements normally impossible.

The *long digital extensor,* the largest muscle of the group, arises in common with the peroneus tertius by a short tendon. This is soon succeeded by a broad belly that covers the tibialis cranialis (Fig. 24–13/5). The insertion tendon begins in the lower leg and continues to the extensor process of the distal phalanx, with passing attachments to the proximal and middle phalanges. It is joined by the smaller tendon of the lateral extensor (/6) near the middle of the cannon. As it descends on the dorsal surface of the limb it is surrounded by a synovial sheath from midtarsal level to the tendon union, and is held in place by three retinacula where it crosses the hock. This muscle is capable of flexion of the hock and extension of the digit.

The *lateral digital extensor* runs between the long extensor and the deep flexor on the lateral aspect of the limb. It arises from the lateral

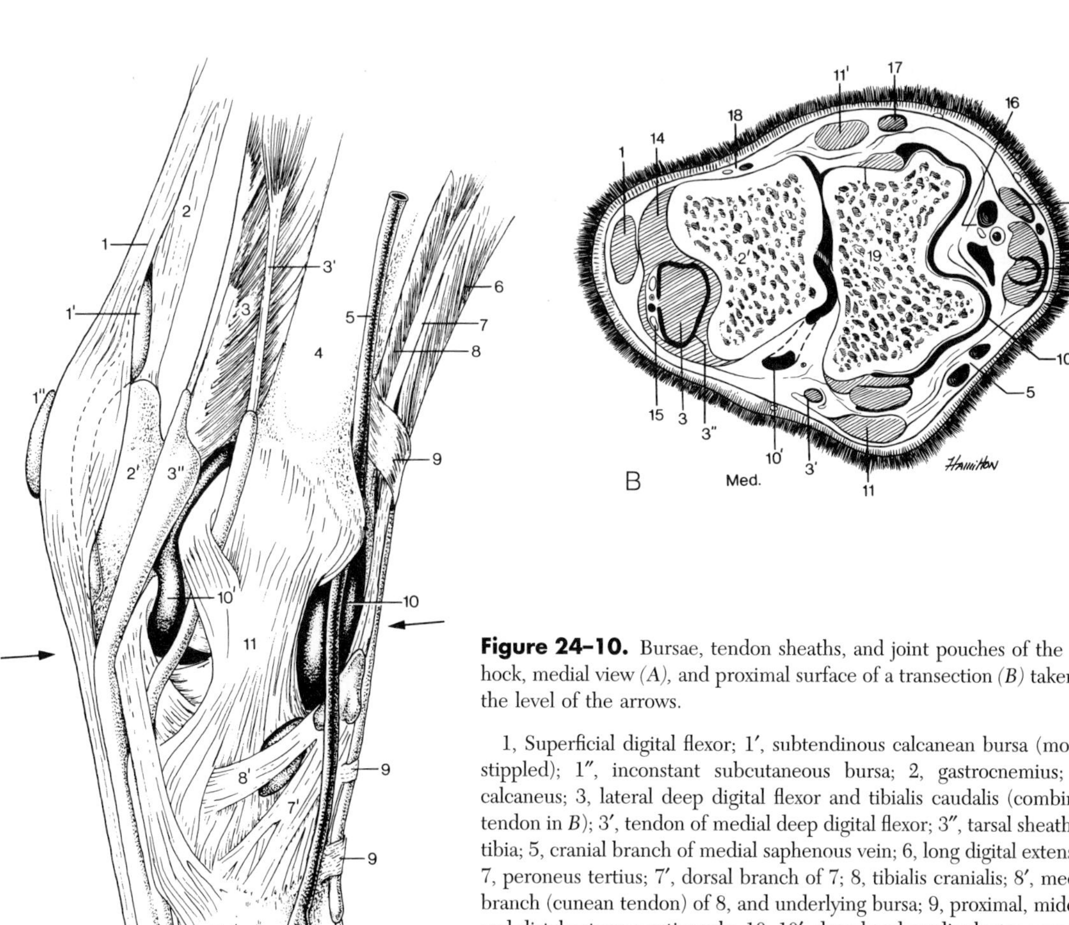


**Figure 24–10.** Bursae, tendon sheaths, and joint pouches of the left hock, medial view *(A),* and proximal surface of a transection *(B)* taken at the level of the arrows.

1, Superficial digital flexor; 1′, subtendinous calcanean bursa (mostly stippled); 1″, inconstant subcutaneous bursa; 2, gastrocnemius; 2′, calcaneus; 3, lateral deep digital flexor and tibialis caudalis (combined tendon in *B*); 3′, tendon of medial deep digital flexor; 3″, tarsal sheath; 4, tibia; 5, cranial branch of medial saphenous vein; 6, long digital extensor; 7, peroneus tertius; 7′, dorsal branch of 7; 8, tibialis cranialis; 8′, medial branch (cunean tendon) of 8, and underlying bursa; 9, proximal, middle, and distal extensor retinacula; 10, 10′, dorsal and medioplantar pouches of tarsocrural joint; 11, 11′, medial and lateral collateral ligaments (superficial parts); 12, medial splint bone; 13, cannon bone; 14, long plantar ligament; 15, plantar nerves and saphenous vessels; 16, cranial tibial vessels and deep peroneal nerve; 17, lateral digital extensor; 18, caudal cutaneous sural nerve and lateral saphenous vein; 19, talus.

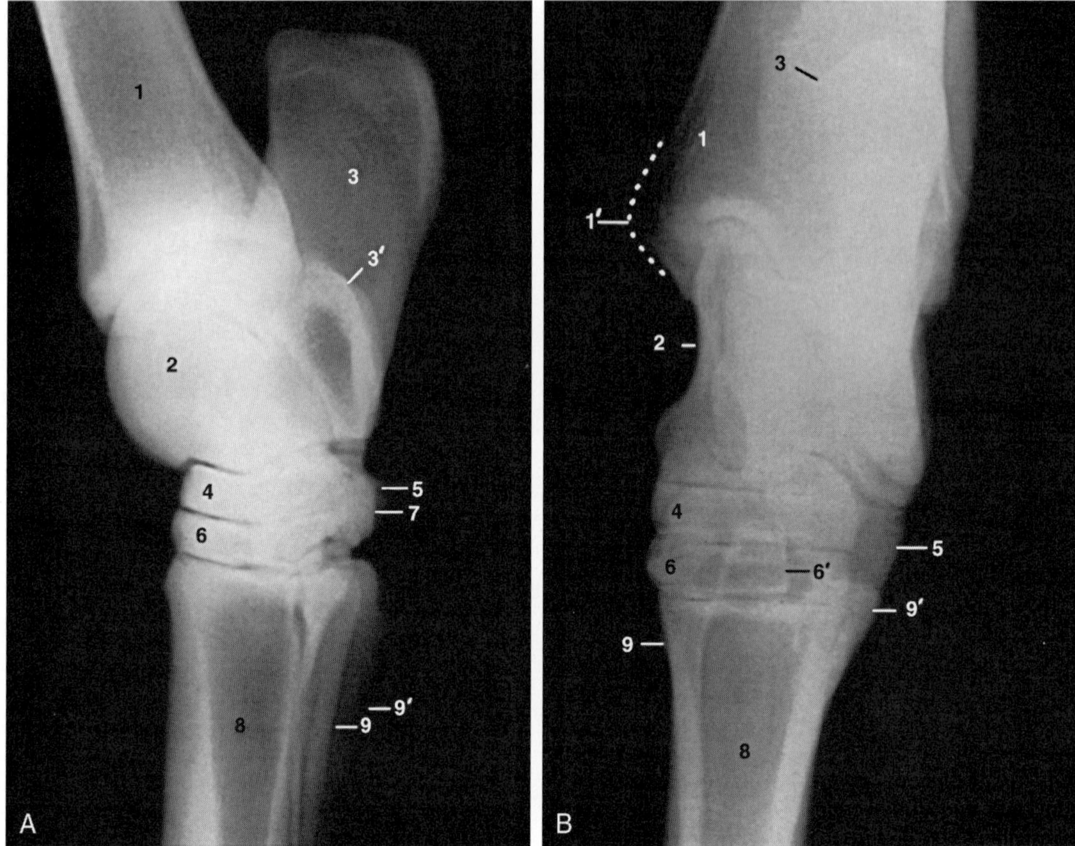


**Figure 24–11.** Lateral *(A)* and dorsoplantar *(B)* radiographs of the hock joint.

1, Tibia; 1′, medial malleolus *(outlined)*; 2, talus; 3, calcaneus; 3′, sustentaculum tali; 4, central tarsal; 5, fourth tarsal; 6, third tarsal (in *B* superimposed on tarsal 1 and 2); 6′, plantar projection of third tarsal; 7, tarsal 1 and 2; 8, large metatarsal bone; 9, 9′, medial and lateral splint bones.

collateral ligament of the stifle, and adjacent parts of both tibia and fibula, and ends by joining the long extensor tendon. Its tendon is also held down by retinacula and protected by a synovial sheath where it crosses the hock. A very small, short digital extensor muscle (extensor digitalis brevis) occupies the angle between the converging tendons of the larger muscles (/10). It is of no importance.

All muscles of the craniolateral group are supplied by the peroneal nerve.

## The Caudal Muscles

This group comprises the popliteus, whose action is confined to the stifle, and the gastrocnemius, soleus, and superficial and deep digital flexors, which all extend the hock; the last two also flex the digit.

The *popliteus* is a relatively small triangular muscle placed directly over the caudal aspect of the stifle joint (Fig. 24–14/*B*,7). It arises from the lateral condyle of the femur and inserts on the caudomedial border of the tibia. The popliteus flexes the stifle and rotates the leg inward.

The *gastrocnemius,* the most superficial and largest muscle of the group, arises by two heads from the supracondylar tuberosities of the femur (/1). The heads, which are first covered by the hamstring muscles, soon unite in a single strong tendon that is a major component of the calcanean tendon. The gastrocnemius tendon inserts upon the point of the hock where it is covered by the tendon of the superficial flexor. In order to attain this deep position it must first wind round the lateral border of the flexor tendon where it is cushioned by the interposition of a synovial bursa (see below). Theoretically, the gastrocnemius is a flexor of the stifle and extensor of the hock, but since the tendons of the peroneus tertius and superficial flexor ensure that these joints extend or flex together, it is difficult to envisage its action. It has been asserted that its prime function is comparable to that of the tibialis cranialis—adjustment of the load upon the tibia. A ribbon-like soleus runs from the head of the fibula to the gastrocnemius tendon but is of no importance.

The *superficial digital flexor* (/B,3) is largely tendinous, although it has a slightly greater content of flesh than the peroneus tertius. It arises from the supracondylar fossa of the femur under cover of the gastrocnemius, and, twisting around the medial surface of the tendon of that muscle, passes toward the calcanean tuber where it expands to form a cap; the medial and lateral edges attach here, but the main part continues over the plantar aspect of the hock to enter the cannon. It inserts on the first and second phalanges in similar fashion to the superficial flexor of the forelimb. A considerable synovial bursa protects the expanded tendon where it caps the tuber; the bursa also extends proximally between the flexor and gastrocnemius tendons where they wind around each other (Fig. 24–10/1′). A second, smaller, subcutaneous bursa (/1″) may form over the expanded tendon where it caps the calcaneus ("capped hock"). Both bursae are liable to inflammation and distention. The proximal part of the muscle is a main constituent of the so-called reciprocal mechanism (p. 619). The distal part supports the fetlock and pastern joints in similar fashion to the superficial flexor of the forelimb.

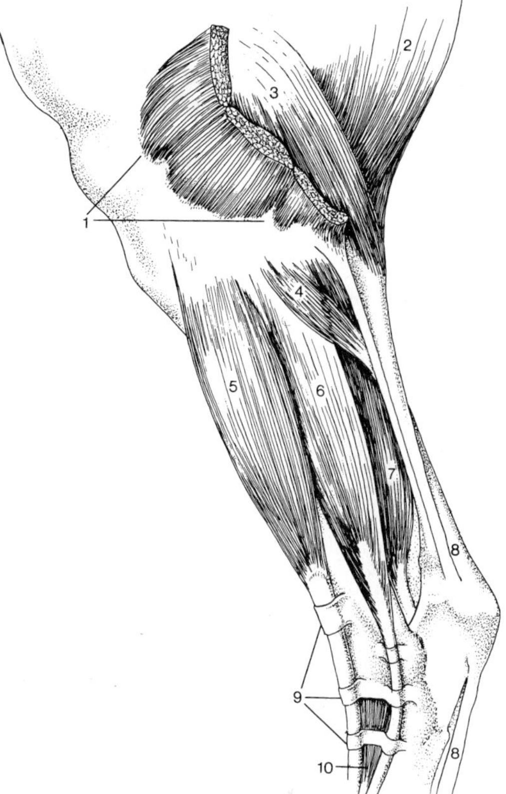


**Figure 24–13.** The stifle and leg, lateral view.

1, Distal divisions of biceps; 2, semitendinosus; 3, gastrocnemius; 4, soleus; 5, long digital extensor; 6, lateral digital extensor; 7, deep digital flexors; 8, superficial digital flexor; 9, proximal, middle, and distal extensor retinacula; 10, extensor digitalis brevis.

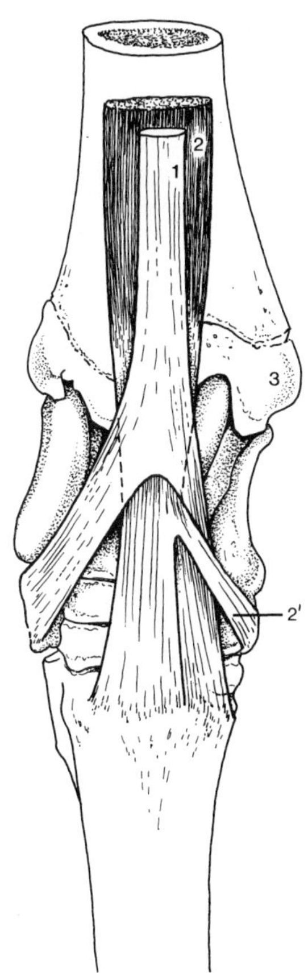


**Figure 24–12.** The insertion of the flexors of the right hock, dorsal view.

1, Peroneus tertius, splitting into dorsal and lateral branches; 2, tibialis cranialis, splitting into dorsal and medial (cunean 2′) branches; 3, medial malleolus.

The deep digital flexor arises by three separate and individually named heads—lateral digital flexor, medial digital flexor, and tibialis caudalis—which later unite to form a single stout tendon of insertion. The medial flexor arises from the lateral condyle of the tibia but soon swings to the medial

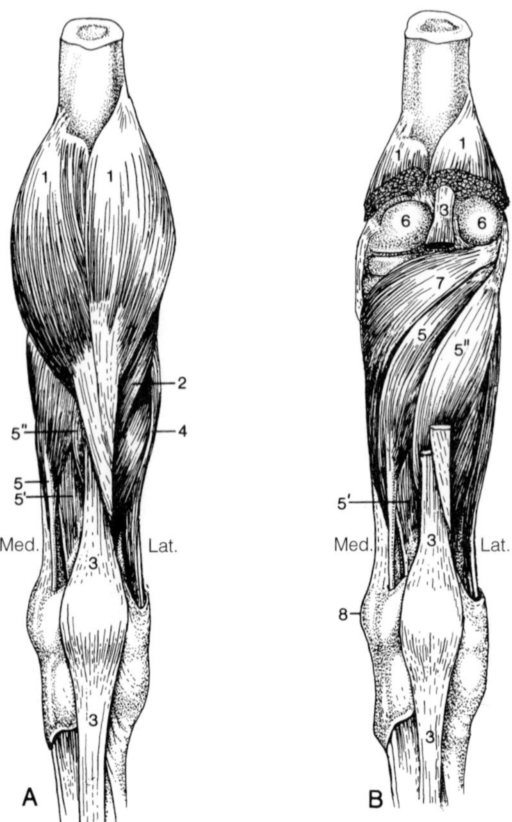


**Figure 24–14.** Superficial *(A)* and deep *(B)* muscles of the right leg, caudal view.

1, Gastrocnemius; 2, soleus; 3, superficial digital flexor; 4, lateral digital extensor; 5, 5′, 5″, medial and lateral deep digital flexors and tibialis caudalis; 6, femoral condyles; 7, popliteus; 8, medial malleolus.

side of the leg (Fig. 24–14/5). The narrow tendon passes the hock resting within a groove on the medial malleolus and medial collateral ligament where it is protected by a synovial sheath. Once past the hock, the tendon unites with the tendon common to the other two muscles.

The lateral flexor and the tibialis caudalis have extensive origins from the caudal surface of the tibia, distal to the attachment of the popliteus (/5′,5″). They are difficult to separate, and there is little merit in attempting the distinction since the tendons combine in the lower part of the leg. The common tendon crosses the plantar aspect of the hock over the sustentaculum tali of the calcaneus. A synovial (tarsal) sheath invests the tendon from the distal part of the leg to its junction with the tendon of the medial flexor in the upper part of the cannon (Fig. 24–10/3″). A further tendinous slip (the accessory ligament) that passes from the joint capsule to join the common tendon is analogous to the forelimb formation but is usually less developed. The distal part of the tendon comports itself similarly to the corresponding part of the deep digital flexor of the forelimb.

The deep plantar metatarsal fascia resembles the corresponding forelimb fascia and offers the same obstruction to palpation of the flexor tendons in the proximal half, and more, of the cannon.

The tibial nerve supplies all muscles of the caudal group.

The remaining structures of the metatarsus and digit closely resemble the corresponding parts of the forelimb. Certain quantitative differences have been mentioned (p. 568 and Fig. 23–36).

## THE PASSIVE STAY-APPARATUS

The caudal end of the trunk rests on the head of the femur. A vertical line dropped from the center of the support passes caudal to the stifle joint and cranial to the hock, fetlock, and pastern joints before intersecting the hoof (Fig. 24–15/*A*). If unsupported, the bony column of the hindlimb would collapse by flexion of the stifle and hock and overextension of the fetlock and pastern joints. The tendons and ligaments of the passive stay-apparatus enable the horse to prevent this collapse using only a minimum of muscular effort.

The supportive mechanisms below the hock are very similar to those of the forelimb (p. 596). However, the accessory ligament of the deep digital flexor tendon, which arises from the caudal aspect of the hock, is weak and occasionally absent. This is compensated by the firm, intermediate attachment of the superficial digital flexor tendon to the point of the hock, which is broadly comparable in function to the accessory ligament of the corresponding tendon of the forelimb. The part of the superficial flexor tendon between its attachments proximal and distal to the fetlock joint is tensed when weight is on the limb and assists the interosseus in supporting the fetlock.

Fixation of the stifle and hock joints depends on the locking mechanism of the former joint and the existence of the so-called reciprocal mechanism, which associates the movements of the two joints. In order to "lock" the stifle, the patella is first brought into the resting position (by extending the joint) and then fixed by being rotated medially through about 15 degrees (/*E,* arrow). This hooks the parapatellar cartilage and medial patellar ligament securely over the protuberance of the medial trochlear ridge (/17); palpation confirms that the medial ligament now runs more caudally than before, being displaced as much as 2 cm behind the crest of the medial ridge. Secured in this position, the patella firmly resists displacement, and a larger part of the body weight can be lowered onto the locked joint, enabling the other hindlimb to be rested with only the toe of the hoof on the ground. The "unlocking" is effected quite briskly: the patella is rotated laterally and snaps back into its usual place; the joint may now be flexed.

The reciprocal mechanism is provided by two tendinous cords—the peroneus tertius and the superficial flexor—that pass between the distal end of the femur and the hock, one on the cranial, the other on the caudal aspect of the tibia (/7,9; Plate 27/*E* demonstrates the result of the rupture of the peroneus tertius.) These ensure that the two joints move in unison; flexion or extension of one necessitates a similar movement of the other joint. However, some looseness in the system renders it unnecessary for the angular changes at the two joints to be exactly the same, especially during fast gaits when large forces must be absorbed by the tendons.

When the stifle is locked, the weight of the hindquarters tends to flex the hock joint; this is opposed by tension in the superficial flexor caudal to the tibia. The peroneus tertius is not involved at this time, and it seems that it is superfluous in the animal standing quietly.

The stifle joint is fully locked only when the horse takes most of the weight on that limb and rests the other on the toe of the hoof. It should be emphasized that while the arrangement conserves energy, it does not eliminate muscular effort; every few minutes the animal shifts its support from one side to the other as muscles tire, or perhaps as tension in the passive supporting structures becomes uncomfortable.

Sometimes a neuromuscular disorder makes

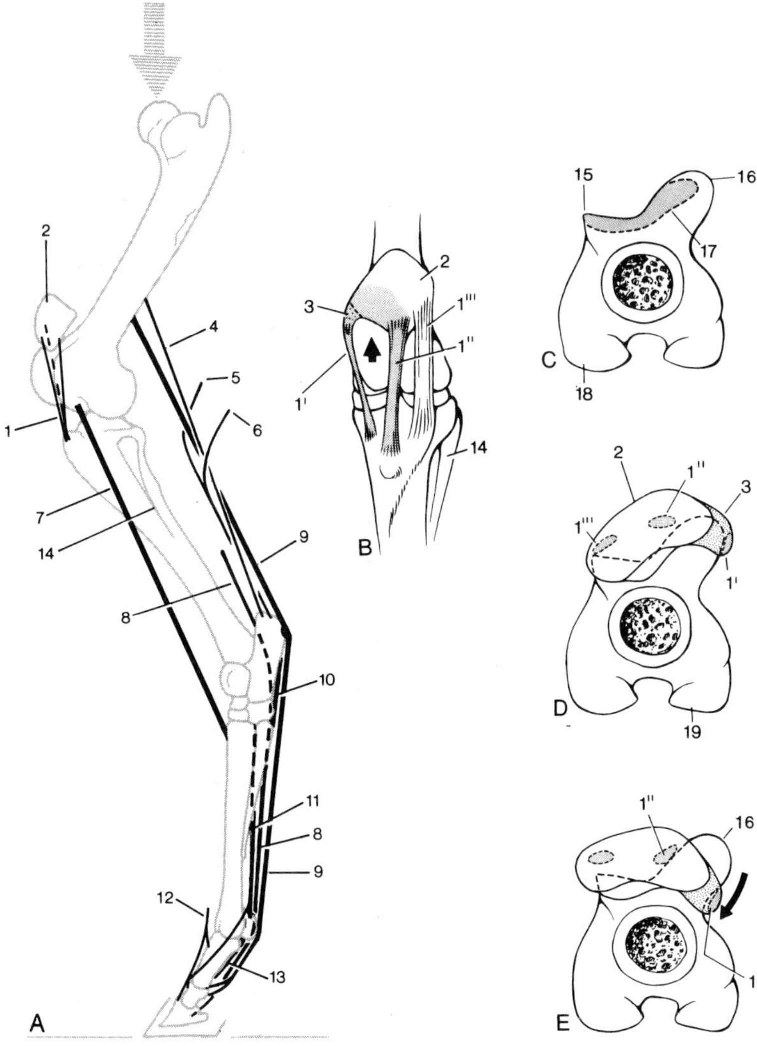


**Figure 24–15.** *A,* Stay-apparatus of the left hindlimb, lateral view. *B,* Left stifle joint, cranial view. *C–E,* Distal end of left femur, looking distally; in *D,* position of patella in horse standing square; in *E* the stifle is locked.

1′, Medial; 1″, intermediate; 1‴, lateral patellar ligaments; 2, patella; 3, parapatellar fibrocartilage; 4, fibrous band associated with gastrocnemius; 5, tarsal tendon of semitendinosus; 6, tarsal tendon of biceps; 7, peroneus tertius; 8, deep digital flexor; 9, superficial digital flexor; 10, long plantar ligament; 11, interosseus; 12, long digital extensor; 13, sesamoidean ligaments; 14, fibula; 15, lateral trochlear ridge; 16, tubercle on proximal end of medial trochlear ridge; 17, resting surface on proximal end of trochlea; 18, lateral condyle; 19, medial condyle.

unlocking of the stifle difficult or even impossible (Plate 27/*D*). A temporary "lock" may be broken by startling a horse into sudden movement; a persistent "lock" may be alleviated by section of the medial ligament to break the retention loop (/*B*,1′). The operation is easily and safely performed since a considerable thickness of fat lies deep to the ligament, protecting the synovial membrane.

## VASCULARIZATION OF THE HINDLIMB

The chief artery of the limb, the *femoral artery,* directly continues the external iliac artery (Fig. 24–16/1,3). It reaches the femoral triangle, traveling in company with the femoral vein and nerve. Almost at once, it detaches the saphenous artery and several larger muscular branches. The saphenous artery (/8) pursues a superficial course down the medial aspect of the limb where it may be traced almost to the hock.

The muscular branches include deep and caudal femoral arteries (/4,9) that anastomose with each other and with other more proximal and more distal arteries, forming an alternative pathway available when the chief trunk is obstructed. The femoral artery then passes obliquely over the femur to gain the caudal aspect of the stifle where it passes between the heads of the gastrocnemius. The segment at the stifle, known as the popliteal artery, divides into cranial and caudal tibial arteries in the upper part of the leg.

The larger *cranial tibial artery* (/11) passes through the interosseous space between the fibula and tibia to gain the dorsolateral aspect where it turns distally between the muscles and the bone. It comes to the surface at the hock and continues as the dorsal pedal artery and then, on entering the groove between the cannon and lateral splint bones, as the dorsal metatarsal artery. A perforating branch (/13) of the dorsal pedal passes between the tarsal bones to reach the plantar aspect of the limb where it anastomoses with branches of the saphenous artery. The dorsal metatarsal artery, the major supply to the foot, is well placed at the proximal end of the cannon for evaluation of the pulse. Toward the fetlock, it passes under the free end of the splint bone to gain the plantar aspect of the cannon where it is reinforced by small branches from the saphenous. It ends by dividing into medial and lateral digital arteries (/17,17′) that replicate the pattern of the forelimb vessels.

The *caudal tibial artery* first runs distally in the deep flexor (/12). Toward the hock it enters the space before the calcanean tendon and sends a short S-shaped anastomosis to the nearby saphenous artery and a longer branch that reascends the leg to join the caudal femoral. The saphenous artery, thus reinforced, divides into medial and

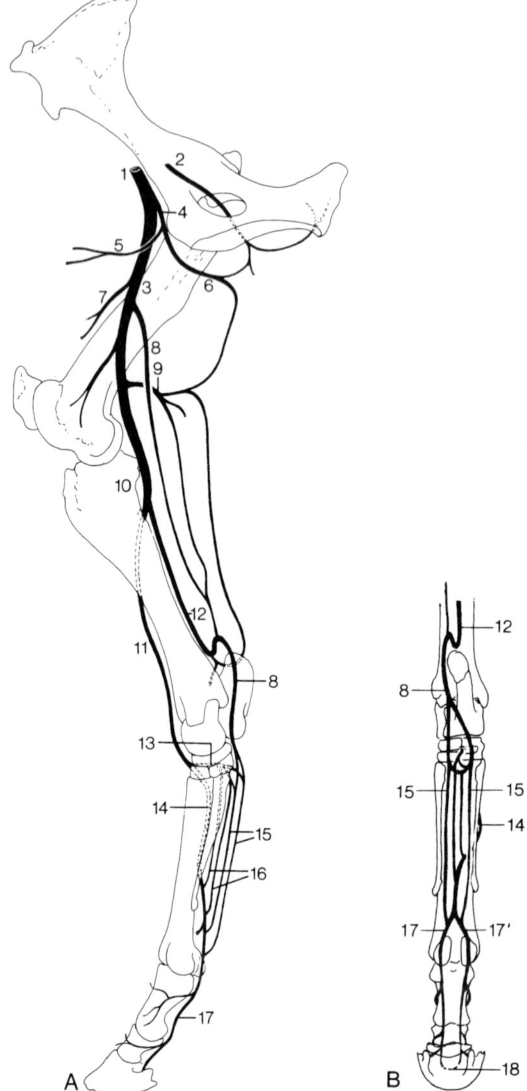


**Figure 24–16.** The principal arteries of the right hindlimb, medial view *(A),* caudal view *(B).*

1, External iliac a.; 2, obturator a.; 3, femoral a.; 4, deep femoral a.; 5, pudendoepigastric trunk; 6, medial circumflex femoral a.; 7, lateral circumflex femoral a.; 8, saphenous a.; 9, caudal femoral a.; 10, popliteal a.; 11, cranial tibial a.; 12, caudal tibial a.; 13, perforating tarsal a.; 14, dorsal metatarsal a.; 15, medial and lateral plantar aa.; 16, medial and lateral plantar metatarsal aa.; 17, 17′, medial and lateral digital aa.; 18, terminal arch, anastomosis of digital aa. within the distal phalanx.

lateral plantar arteries that descend toward the fetlock (/15). These and the deeper plantar metatarsal arteries are individually of no great importance and may eventually fade away or join the dorsal metatarsal artery or its digital divisions.

The deep *veins* are largely satellite to the arteries. As in the forelimb, certain superficial trunks run alone; they include the medial and lateral saphenous veins. A branch of the former is often prominent where it crosses the dorsal aspect of the hock; the swelling ("blood spavin") may occasionally be mistaken for a distention of the dorsal joint pouch (Fig. 24–10/5,10). Within the leg, the saphenous veins run between the calcanean tendon and the caudal muscle mass, one to each side (Fig. 24–7/10,12). The medial vein later crosses the medial aspect of the thigh to open into the femoral vein. The lateral vein joins the caudal femoral vein at the stifle.

Lymph draining from the distal part of the limb passes mainly to the group of *popliteal nodes* tucked within the popliteal fossa between the biceps and semitendinosus. Efferent vessels from this group, and additional vessels that arise within the thigh, proceed mainly to the *deep inguinal nodes* within the femoral triangle. Some lymph from superficial structures passes to the *subiliac nodes,* which drain into the lateral and middle iliac nodes. The courses of certain lymphatic vessels may be manifested as cords visible through the skin in some lymph-borne infections.

## THE NERVES OF THE HINDLIMB

The formation and ramification of the lumbosacral plexus and the distribution of its peripheral branches follow the common pattern in broad outline; important species differences are confined to the innervation of the foot.

The *cranial* and *caudal gluteal nerves* attend to the innervation of the lateral muscles of the croup, including vertebral heads of the hamstring muscles; the details have been given.

The distributions of the femoral, obturator, and sciatic nerves have greater clinical relevance. The *femoral nerve* (L4–L6) (Fig. 24–17/1) passes through and also supplies the sublumbar muscles before entering the thigh by way of the vascular lacuna. It then splits into several branches, most of which at once enter the quadriceps. The one branch of more extended course, the saphenous nerve (/1′), continues within the femoral triangle before penetrating the medial femoral fascia to obtain a more superficial position. It continues through the thigh, leg, and upper cannon, supplying skin over the medial aspect of the limb from thigh to fetlock. It also supplies the sartorius. Extensive damage to the femoral nerve is uncommon, but when it does occur the consequences are severe; paralysis of the quadriceps removes the ability to fix the stifle and therefore the ability to support weight upon the affected limb. In addition, skin sensibility is lost over a considerable area.

The *obturator nerve* (L4–L6) (/2) leaves the pelvis by way of the obturator foramen and innervates the adductor muscles (pectineus, gracilis, adductor, and obturator externus). Injury, which generally follows foaling or pelvic fracture, results in partial or complete inability to adduct the limb. The severity of the dysfunction is rather unpredictable; it appears to depend on the weight of the animal and the nature of the terrain as well as on the extent of the lesion.

The *sciatic nerve* (L6–S2) (/4) leaves the pelvis by the greater sciatic foramen and after a short course over the sacrosciatic ligament turns distally caudal to the hip joint to enter the thigh under cover of the biceps. It divides about the level of the joint into tibial and peroneal nerves that initially run together. They part company a little above the stifle when the peroneal nerve moves laterally to pass between the biceps and the lateral head of the gastrocnemius; the tibial nerve holds its course and runs between the two heads of the gastrocnemius. Both divisions detach cutaneous branches while still within the thigh. That from the peroneal (lateral cutaneous sural nerve; /5′) becomes subcutaneous by piercing the biceps and then spreads to supply skin over the lateral aspect of the leg. The corresponding tibial branch (caudal cutaneous sural nerve; /6′) descends in the fascial plate between the calcanean tendon and deep flexor, following for part of its course the lateral saphenous vein. It supplies branches to the skin over the plantarolateral aspect of the hock and cannon, reaching to the fetlock.

The *peroneal nerve* divides caudal to the lateral collateral ligament of the stifle into deep and superficial branches. The superficial branch (/5″) continues down the leg, slightly sunken within the groove between the long and lateral extensors, where it can be palpated below the middle of the leg. It supplies the lateral extensor and the skin over the lateral aspect of the leg and more distal segments of the limb. The deep branch takes a parallel course after sinking deeply between the same two muscles to follow the cranial face of the intervening septum (/5‴ and Fig. 24–7/6′). It supplies branches to the remaining muscles of the dorsolateral group and then continues under cover of the long extensor tendon as a purely sensory nerve that splits into medial and lateral branches over the hock. These, the medial and lateral dorsal

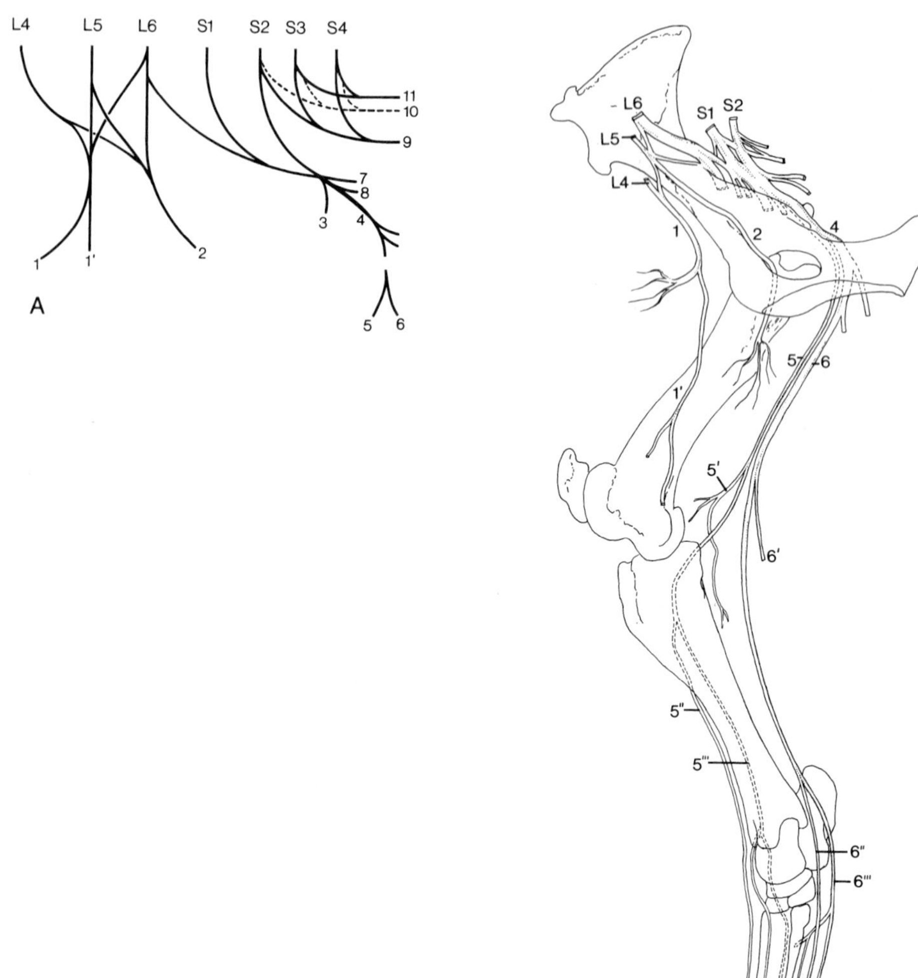


**Figure 24–17.** The nerves of the hindlimb. *A,* The lumbosacral plexus, schematic. *B,* The principal nerves, medial view.

1, Femoral n.; 1′, saphenous n.; 2, obturator n.; 3, cranial gluteal n.; 4, sciatic n.; 5, common peroneal n.; 5′, lateral cutaneous sural n.; 5″, 5‴, superficial and deep peroneal nn.; 6, tibial n.; 6′, caudal cutaneous sural n.; 6″, 6‴, medial and lateral plantar nn. (the lateral nerve gives rise to the plantar metatarsal nn.); 7, caudal gluteal n.; 8, caudal cutaneous femoral n.; 9, pudendal n.; 10, pelvic n.; 11, caudal rectal n.

metatarsal nerves, edge toward the grooves between the cannon and splint bones (Fig. 24–18/3,3′). The lateral nerve follows the palpable dorsal metatarsal artery (Fig. 24–19/8). After detaching twigs to the skin and the fetlock and pastern joints, both finally fade within the hoof.

Complete section of the peroneal nerve results in inability to extend the digit actively; the hoof rests upon its dorsal surface unless the ground surface is passively set down. The posture invites comparison with that which occurs in radial paralysis. Afflicted animals may learn to compensate in a similar manner—they flick the foot forward and plant the hoof before the impetus is lost. In addition to the motor disability, skin sensation is lost over the dorsolateral aspect of the lower part of the limb. Peroneal lesions are most frequent in two circumstances: intrapelvic damage to the sciatic nerve (which is likely also to involve the tibial division), and as the result of trauma in the region of the fibula where the nerve is superficial (Plate 27/*C*, shown on a cow).

The *tibial nerve* dives between the two heads of the gastrocnemius and crosses the stifle on the surface of the popliteus. It detaches branches to these muscles and to other muscles of the caudal group before continuing as a sensory trunk in the space between the calcanean tendon and the deep flexor where it is easily palpated (Fig. 24–7/12). When level with the calcaneus, it divides into medial and lateral plantar nerves that pass over the sustentaculum tali beside the deep flexor tendon. The lateral nerve diverges laterally and, just distal to the hock, it detaches the common trunk of the medial and lateral plantar metatarsal nerves (Fig. 24–18/2′). These supply the interosseous muscle and associated structures and the plantar pouch of the fetlock joint (/4,4′). The medial plantar nerve follows the line of the parent trunk. Although the plantar nerves generally resemble the palmar nerves of the forelimb, the communicating branch is relatively slight or even absent; when present, it can usually be palpated as it slopes in a laterodistal direction over the superficial aspect of the flexor tendons (/1′).

There is one other difference. The dorsal and plantar metatarsal nerves play a rather larger role in the sensory innervation of the hoof contents than do the corresponding forelimb trunks—the dorsal branch of the ulnar nerve and the palmar metacarpal nerves—which commonly fail to reach the coronet.

Tibial paralysis is manifested by a slight sagging of the hock when weight is borne on the affected limb. Despite the inability to flex the distal joints, the gait is not seriously disturbed. The sensory deficit is very considerable.

Lesions that affect the sciatic trunk involve the hamstring as well as the leg muscles. Despite this, the consequences are less disastrous than might well be supposed. Retention of activity by the quadriceps enables the animal to fix the stifle and, through the reciprocal apparatus, the hock. It is thus able to support weight upon the limb. Cutaneous and deep sensations are lost below the stifle, except in the province of the saphenous nerve.

Both superficial and deep branches of the peroneal nerve can be blocked by injecting, subcutaneously and then deeply from the same point of entry, between the long and lateral extensors a handbreadth or so proximal to the tarsocrural joint (Fig. 24–7/6,6′). Apart from this, the local anesthetic techniques for surgical and diagnostic purposes generally resemble those prescribed for the forelimb; the one distinction of relevance is the distal extension of the dorsal metatarsal nerves. It is possible to block the

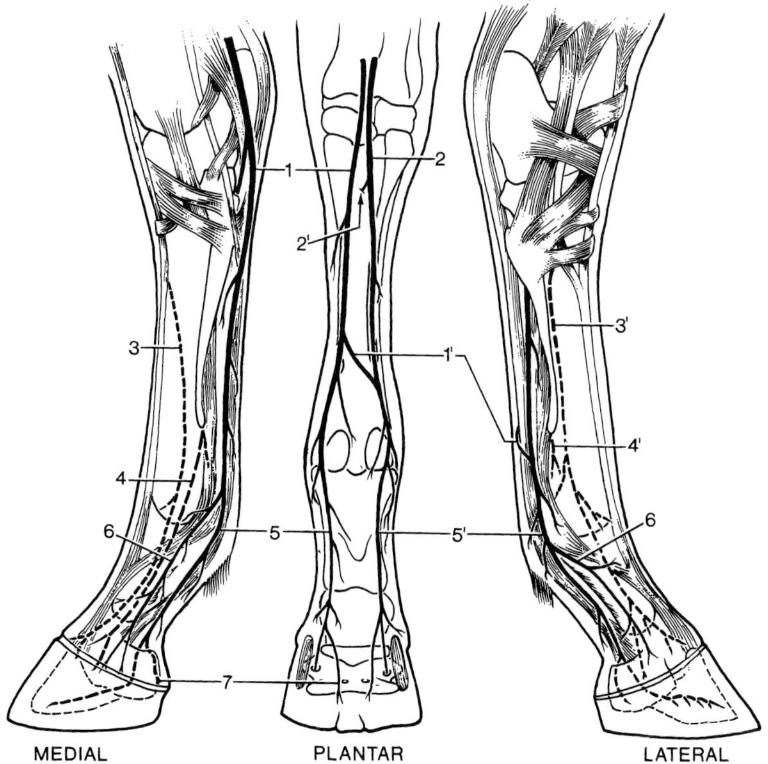


**Figure 24–18.** The nerves of the right hindfoot.

1, 2, Medial and lateral plantar nn. (from tibial); 1′, communicating branch; 2′, deep branch (for plantar metatarsal nn.), cut; 3, 3′, medial and lateral dorsal metatarsal nn. (from deep peroneal); 4, 4′, medial and lateral plantar metatarsal nn. (from lateral plantar, 2′); 5, 5′, medial and lateral digital nn.; 6, dorsal branch of digital n.; 7, branch to digital cushion.

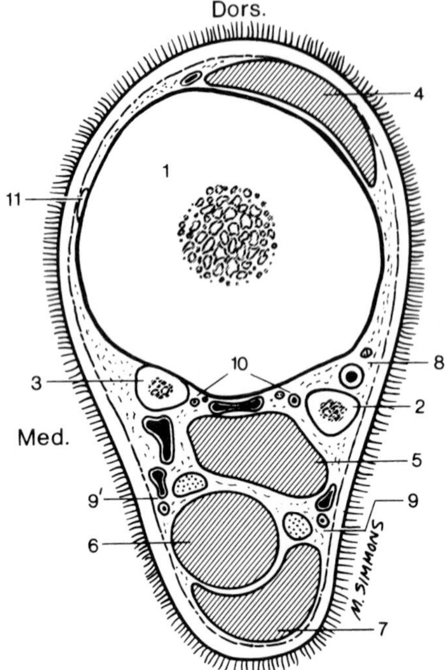


**Figure 24–19.** Transverse section of the middle of the right metatarsus.

1–3, Large and small metatarsal bones; 4, long digital extensor; 5, interosseus; 6, deep digital flexor; 7, superficial digital flexor; 8, dorsal metatarsal a. and lateral dorsal metatarsal n.; 9, 9′, lateral and medial plantar vessels and n.; 10, plantar metatarsal vessels and nn.; 11, medial dorsal metatarsal n.

undivided tibial nerve (level with the point of the hock) as an alternative to the plantar nerves (/12).

## Selected Bibliography

Adams, W.M., and J.P. Thilsted: Radiographic appearance of the equine stifle from birth to 6 months. Vet. Radiol. Ultrasound 26:126–132, 1985.

Bell, B.T.L., G.J. Baker, J.H. Foreman, and L.C. Abbott. *In vivo* investigation of communication between the distal intertarsal and tarsometatarsal joints in horses and ponies. Vet. Surg. 22:289–292, 1993.

Bohanon, T.C.: Contrast arthrography of the distal intertarsal and tarsometatarsal joints in horses clinically affected with osteoarthrosis. *In* Proceedings of the 40th Annual Convention of the American Association of Equine Practitioners, 1994, pp. 193–194.

Crabill, M.R., C.M. Honnas, D.S. Taylor, et al.: Stringhalt secondary to trauma to the dorsoproximal region of the metatarsus in horses: 10 cases (1986–1991). JAVMA 205:867–869, 1994.

Denoix, J.M.: Functional anatomy of tendons and ligaments in the distal limbs (manus and pes). Vet. Clin. North Am. Equine Pract. 10:273–322, 1994.

Dik, K.J., and I. Gunsser: Atlas of Diagnostic Radiology of the Horse. Parts 1–3, Philadelphia, W.B. Saunders Company, 1988–1990.

Dyson, S., I. Wright, S. Kold, and N. Vatistas: Clinical and radiographic features, treatment and outcome in 15 horses with fracture of the medial aspect of the patella. Equine Vet. J. 24:264–268, 1992.

Dyson, S.J., and J.M. Romero: An investigation of injection techniques for local analgesia of the equine distal tarsus and proximal metatarsus. Equine Vet. J. 25:30–35, 1993.

Genovese, R.L., N.W. Rantanen, M.L. Hauser, and B.S. Simpson: Diagnostic ultrasonography of equine limbs. Vet. Clin. North Am. Equine Pract. 2:145–226, 1986.

Henrickson, D.A., and A.J. Nixon: A lateral approach for synovial fluid aspiration and joint injection of the femoropatellar joint of the horse. Equine Vet. J. 24:399–401, 1992.

Hendrickson, D.A., and A.J. Nixon: Comparison of the cranial and a new lateral approach to the femoropatellar joint for aspiration and injection in horses. JAVMA 205:1177–1179, 1994.

Holcombe, S.J., A.L. Bertone, D.S. Biller, and V. Haider: Magnetic resonance imaging of the equine stifle. Vet. Radiol. Ultrasound 36:119–125, 1995.

Honnas, C.M., D.T. Zamos, and T.S. Ford: Arthroscopy of the coxofemoral joint of foals. Vet. Surg. 22:115–121, 1993.

Imschoot, J., M. Seenhaut, A. De Moor, and F. Verschooten: Partial tibial neurectomy and neurectomy of the deep peroneal nerve as a treatment of bone spavin in 24 horses. Equine Pract. 17:8–13, 1994.

Jansson, N.: Treatment for upward fixation of the patella in the horse by medial patellar desmotomy: Indications and complications. Equine Pract. 18:24–29, 1996.

Jeffcott, L.B.: Pelvic lameness in the horse. Equine Pract. 4:21–47, 1982.

Jeffcott, L.B.: Interpreting radiographs. 3: Radiology of the stifle joint of the horse. Equine Vet. J. 16:81–88, 1984.

Kainer, R.A.: Functional anatomy of equine locomotor organs. *In* Stashak, T.L.: Adam's Lameness in Horses, 4th ed., Philadelphia, Lea & Febiger, 1987.

Kneller, S.K., and J.M. Losonski: Misdiagnosis in normal radiographic anatomy: Nine structural configurations simulating disease entities in horses. JAVMA 195:1272–1282, 1989.

Kraus-Hansen, A.E., H.W. Jann, D.V. Kerr, and G.E. Fackelman: Arthrographic analysis of communication between the tarsometatarsal and distal intertarsal joints of the horse. Vet. Surg. 21:139–144, 1992.

Lindsay, W.A., D.M. Fantov, and T. Miyabayshi: A practitioner's guide to dissecting the equine stifle. Vet. Med. Equine Pract. 84:406–413, 1989.

Martin, G.S., and C.W. McIlwraith: Arthroscopic anatomy of the equine femoropatellar joint and approaches for treatment of osteochondritis dissecans. Vet. Surg. 14:99–104, 1985.

Mathew, J.R., and G.W. Trotter: Reciprocal apparatus dysfunction as a cause of severe hindlimb lameness in a horse. JAVMA 199:1047–1048, 1991.

McCarthy, P.H.: The anatomic features of the normal tarsus of the live horse as perceived by the sense of sight. Anat. Histol. Embryol. 23:239–256, 1994.

Nickels, F.A., and R. Sande: Radiographic and arthroscopic findings in the equine stifle. JAVMA 181:918–924, 1982.

Pankowski, R.L., and K.K. White: Fractures of the patella in horses. Compend. and Contin. Educ. Pract. Vet. 7:S566–S573, 1985.

Pilsworth, R.C., M.C. Shepherd, B.M.B. Herinckx, and M.A. Holmes: Fracture of the wing of the ilium, adjacent to the sacroiliac joint. *In* Thoroughbred racehorses. Equine Vet. J. 26:94–99, 1994.

Poland, J.W., C.W. McIlwraith and G.W. Trotter: Arthroscopic surgery for osteochondritis dissecans of the femoropatellar joint of the horse. Equine Vet. J. 24:419–423, 1992.

Prades, M., B.D. Grant, T.A. Turner, et al.: Injuries to the cranial cruciate ligament and associated structures: Summary of clinical, radiographic, arthroscopic and pathological findings from 10 horses. Equine Vet. J. 21:354–357, 1989.

Reeves, M.J., and G.W. Trotter: Reciprocal apparatus dysfunction as a cause of severe hind limb lameness in a horse. JAVMA 199:1047–1048, 1991.

Reeves, M.J., G.W. Trotter, and R.A. Kainer: Anatomical and functional communications between the synovial sacs of the equine stifle joint. Equine Vet. J. 23:215–218, 1991.

Schebitz, H., and Wilkens, H.: Atlas of Radiographic Anatomy of the Horse, 4th ed. Berlin, Paul Parey Verlag, 1986.

Schneider, R.K., P. Jenson, and R.M. Moore: Evaluation of cartilage lesions on the medial femoral condyle as a cause of lameness in horses: 11 cases (1988–1994). JAVMA 210: 1649–1652, 1997.

Shoemaker, R.S., G.S. Martin, D.J. Hillmann, et al.: Disruption of the caudal component of the reciprocal apparatus in two horses. JAVMA 198:120–122, 1991.

Smallwood, J.E., J.A. Auer, R.J. Martens, et al.: The developing equine tarsus from birth to six months of age. Equine Pract. 6:7–47, 1984.

Stashak, T.S.: Adam's Lameness in Horses, 4th ed. Philadelphia, Lea & Febiger, 1987.

Stick, J.A., L.A. Borg, F.A. Nickels, et al.: Arthroscopic removal of an osteochondral fragment from the caudal pouch of the lateral femorotibial joint in a colt. JAVMA 200:1695–1697, 1992.

Tietje, S.: Computed tomography of the stifle region in the horse: A comparison with radiographic, ultrasonographic and arthroscopic evaluation. Pferdeheilkunde 13:647–658, 1997.

Trumble, T.N., J.A. Stick, S.P. Arnockzy, and D. Rosenstein: Consideration of anatomic and radiographic features of the caudal pouches of the femorotibial joints of horses for the purpose of arthroscopy. Am. J. Vet. Res. 55:1682–1690, 1994.

Updike, S.J.: Functional anatomy of the equine tarsocrural collateral ligaments. Am. J. Vet. Res. 45:867–874, 1984.

Updike, S.J.: Anatomy of the tarsal tendons of the equine tibialis cranialis and peroneus tertius muscles. Am. J. Vet. Res. 45:1379–1382, 1984.

Updike, S.J.: Fascial compartments of the equine crus. Am. J. Vet. Res. 46:692–696, 1985.

Vacek, J.R., S.F. Troy, and C.M. Honnas: Communication between the equine femoropatellar and medial and lateral femorotibial joints. Am. J. Vet. Res. 53:1431–1434, 1992.

van Weeren, P.R., A.J. van den Bogert, A. Barneveld, et al.: The role of the reciprocal apparatus in the hindlimb of the horse investigated by a modified CODA-3 opto-electronic kinematic analysis system. Equine Vet. J., Suppl. Equine Exerc. Phys. 95–100, 1990.

van Weeren, P.R., M.O. Jansen, A.J. van den Bogert, and A. Barneveld: A kinematic and strain gauge study of the reciprocal apparatus in the equine hindlimb. J. Biomech. 25:1–11, 1992.

# CHAPTER 25

# The Head and Ventral Neck of the Ruminants

The account contained in this and the following chapters (Chapters 26–33) is predominantly of bovine anatomy. Sheep and goats differ from one another and, more obviously, from cattle in many features of their anatomy, but it seems unnecessary to include any but the most significant and clinically relevant distinctions.

## CONFORMATION AND EXTERNAL FEATURES

### Conformation and External Features in Cattle

The features of the bovine head that first attract notice are the angular, pyramidal form, the bare muzzle, and the horns (when these are present). The form owes much to the late development of the frontal sinuses that invade the bones of the cranial vault, transforming the domed contours of the calf's head into the broad, flattened forehead and upright nuchal surface of the adult (Figs. 25–1, 25–2, and 25–3). The proportions are also much altered after birth by the greater growth of the facial part than of the neurocranium.

The modified skin around the nostrils extends to the margin of the upper lip, forming the slightly cobbled naked *nasolabial plate*. This is kept moist by the watery secretion of a thick layer of eccrine glands massed below the skin. The surface is marked by numerous fine grooves that outline a pattern said to be individual and sometimes used as a means of identification ("noseprinting") (Fig. 25–4).

The naked integument continues through the large oval nostril into the nasal vestibule where it blends with the mucosa. The opening of the nasolacrimal duct is placed just caudal to the mucocutaneous junction. It is concealed on the ventromedial side of the fold that prolongs the ventral concha rostrally but may be uncovered for cannulation by bending the wing of the nostril outward; this procedure is made possible by the pliancy of the fibrous and cartilaginous skeleton of the muzzle.

The lips are thick, relatively immobile, and insensitive; they take little part in prehension of food. The upper one is the larger and overlaps the lower lip to the front and sides when at rest.

The size and conformation of the *horns* depend upon breed, age, and sex. The horns are based upon much smaller cornual processes that grow from the frontal bones at the caudolateral angles of the forehead. The cornual process has a ridged and porous surface and is covered by a papillated dermis that also serves as periosteum. The specialized dermis blends with that of the surrounding skin at the base of the projection. The major part of the horn wall or sheath grows from the epithelium that covers the dermis over the horn process; the softer outermost layer (epiceras) is produced by an irregular epithelial strip at the base that is transitional to the ordinary epidermis. The horn sheath represents a modification of the cornified stratum of the epithelium and consists chiefly of tubules formed over the dermal papillae; the tubules run lengthwise and are welded together by irregular, intertubular horn produced by the interpapillary regions of the epithelium. Since the whole epithelial surface is productive, and the older horn is thrust apically by that of more recent origin, it follows that the horn sheath increases in thickness toward the tip (Fig. 25–5). Although horn growth is continuous, the rate of production varies according to the stresses to which the animal is subjected, and it is usual to find the horns marked by alternating rings of greater and lesser thickness. The latter represent periods when production was less active and the horn that was produced was softer and more prone to wear. In cows these periods commonly correspond to calvings. Since the first calf is generally born when the cow is aged about 2 years, and subsequent calves are born at yearly intervals thereafter, the number of rings is commonly onc fewer than the animal's age in years (Fig. 25–6).

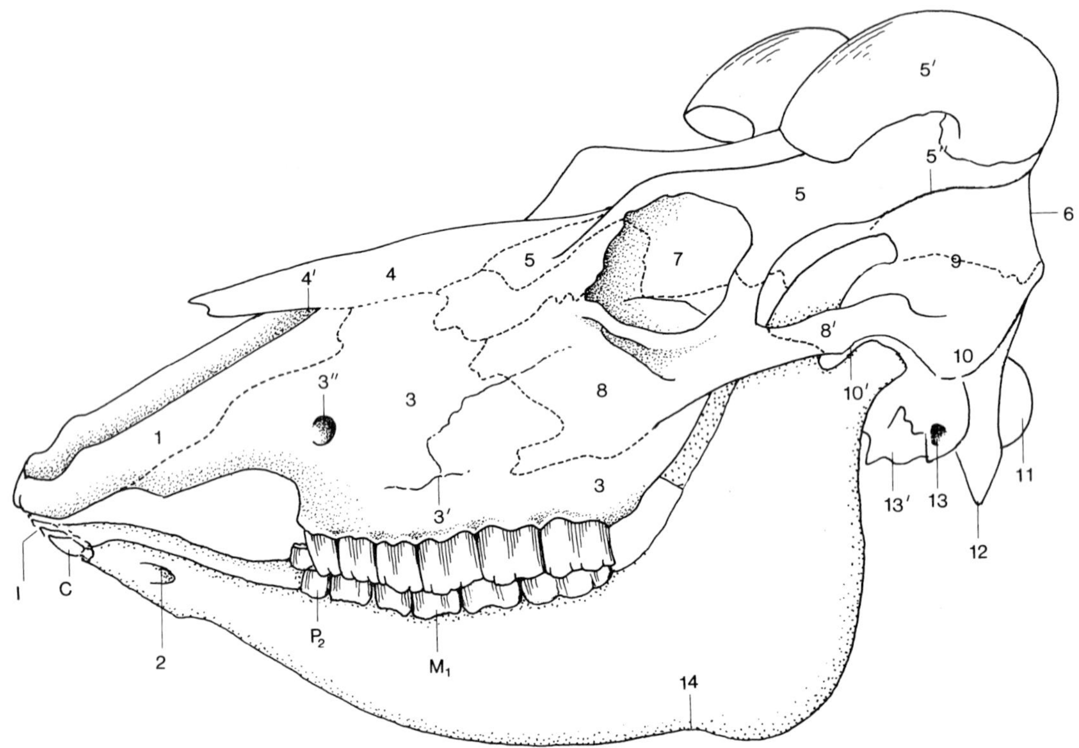


**Figure 25–1.** Lateral view of bovine skull.

1, Incisive bone; 2, mental foramen; 3, maxilla; 3′, facial tuberosity; 3″, infraorbital foramen; 4, nasal bone; 4′, nasoincisive notch; 5, frontal bone; 5′, horn surrounding cornual process of frontal bone; 5″, temporal line; 6, nuchal surface; 7, orbit; 8, zygomatic bone; 8′, zygomatic arch; 9, temporal fossa; 10, temporal bone; 10′, temporomandibular joint; 11, occipital condyle; 12, paracondylar process; 13, external acoustic meatus; 13′, tympanic bulla; 14, vascular notch.

The sensitive dermis of the horn is supplied mainly by the cornual nerve (Fig. 25–2/8), a branch of the zygomaticotemporal division of the maxillary nerve. The cornual nerve arises within the orbit and then passes backward through the temporal fossa where it is sheltered by the prominent ridge of the temporal line. The nerve later divides into two or more branches that wind around this ridge and approach the horn separately under cover of the thin frontalis muscle. The cornual nerve is often blocked for dehorning operations and is then sought where it crosses the ridge, roughly midway between the postorbital bar and the horn (Fig. 25–7/1). The anesthetic technique is not always successful; among the explanations advanced to account for its failure are variation in the relationship of the nerve to the bony ridge, precocious division into divergent branches, and the existence of unusually substantial contributions from the supraorbital or infratrochlear nerves. Since the nerve to the frontal sinus may extend to the diverticulum within the horn, even infiltration around the horn base does not ensure complete loss of sensibility.

The cornual nerve is accompanied by a considerable artery and vein that branch from the superficial temporal vessels within the temporal fossa. The artery ramifies before it reaches the horn. Its smaller branches run in the grooves and canals of the cornual process and retract when severed so that they cannot be easily grasped with hemostats; because of this, dehorning is accompanied by spurting arterial hemorrhage unless the cut is made close to the skull where the arteries are still embedded in soft tissue.

The horns are barely indicated in the newborn calf, and their development can be prevented by cauterization of the germinal epithelium at an early age (2 to 4 weeks). The surrounding epidermis, which spreads to heal the wound, lacks the specialized inductive capacity of the original covering. An extension from the frontal sinus invades the cornual process when the calf is about 6 months old.

## Conformation and External Features in Sheep and Goats

The shape and appearance of the head show many specific, breed, sex, and age differences, but while they determine the "character" of the animal, they are for the most part of no great clinical interest. It is, however, important to note that the dorsal profile of the skull, unlike that of adult cattle, is domed over the cranial cavity and slopes caudally toward the nuchal plane; this feature is commonly masked by the location and size of the horns. A Roman nose is a feature and requirement in certain sheep breeds (Fig. 25–8).

The goat's head has a fairly long coat of hair, but that of sheep is shorter, and in some breeds wool extends considerably onto the face. The nasal plate resembles that of the dog but has a more limited extent, particularly in goats. It is confined to a narrow strip to each side of the deep median philtrum, with lateral prolongations along the upper edges of the long, slitlike nostrils.

The horns arise close behind the orbits in a parietal position quite unlike the temporal one of cattle (see Fig. 26–2). Each is based upon a separate ossification center that makes a secondary fusion to a projection of the skull quite close to its contralateral fellow. In both sheep and goats the frontal sinus later excavates the horn core at the

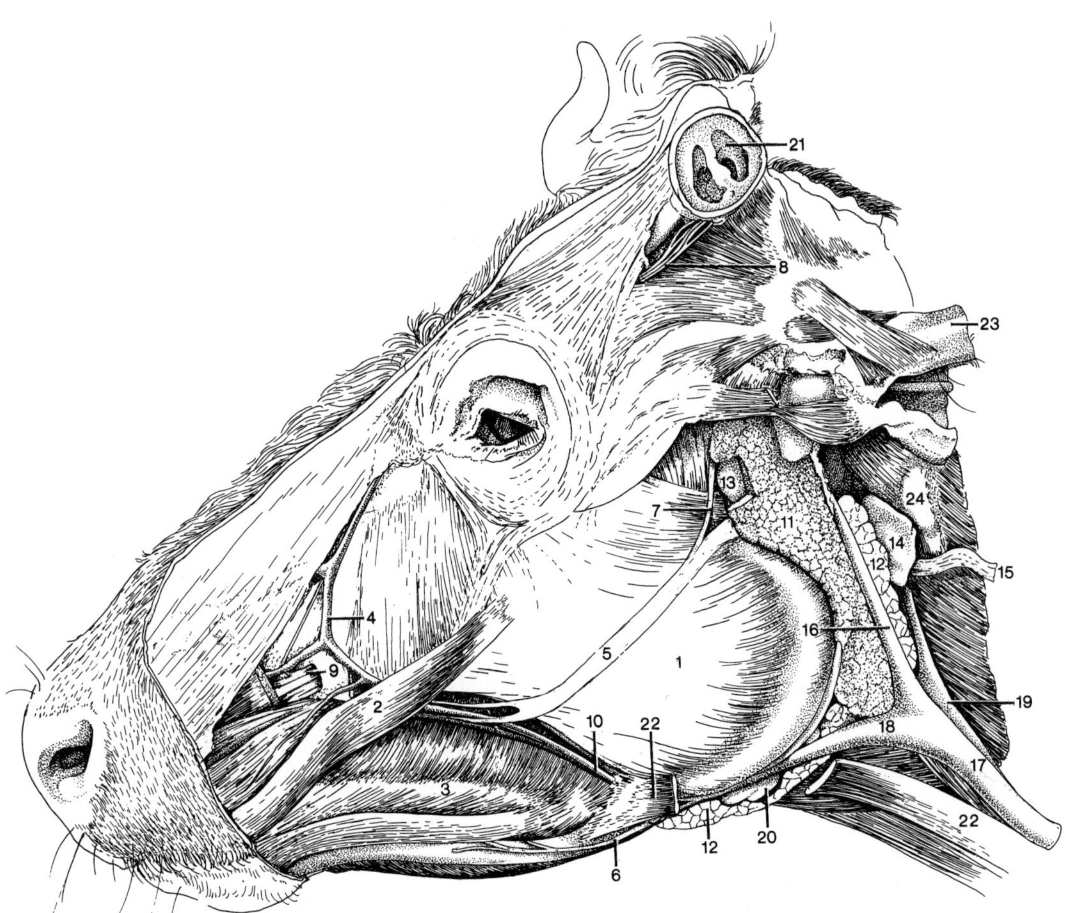


**Figure 25–2.** Superficial dissection of the head.

1, Masseter; 2, zygomaticus; 3, buccinator; 4, facial vein, 5, 6, dorsal and ventral buccal branches of facial nerve; 7, auriculotemporal nerve; 8, cornual nerve; 9, infraorbital nerve; 10, parotid duct and facial artery and vein; 11, parotid gland; 12, mandibular gland; 13, parotid lymph node; 14, lateral retropharyngeal lymph node; 15, spinal accessory nerve; 16, maxillary vein; 17, external jugular vein; 18, linguofacial vein; 19, common carotid artery; 20, mandibular lymph node; 21, cornual diverticulum of frontal sinus; 22, sternomandibularis, resected; 23, stump of ear; 24, wing of atlas.

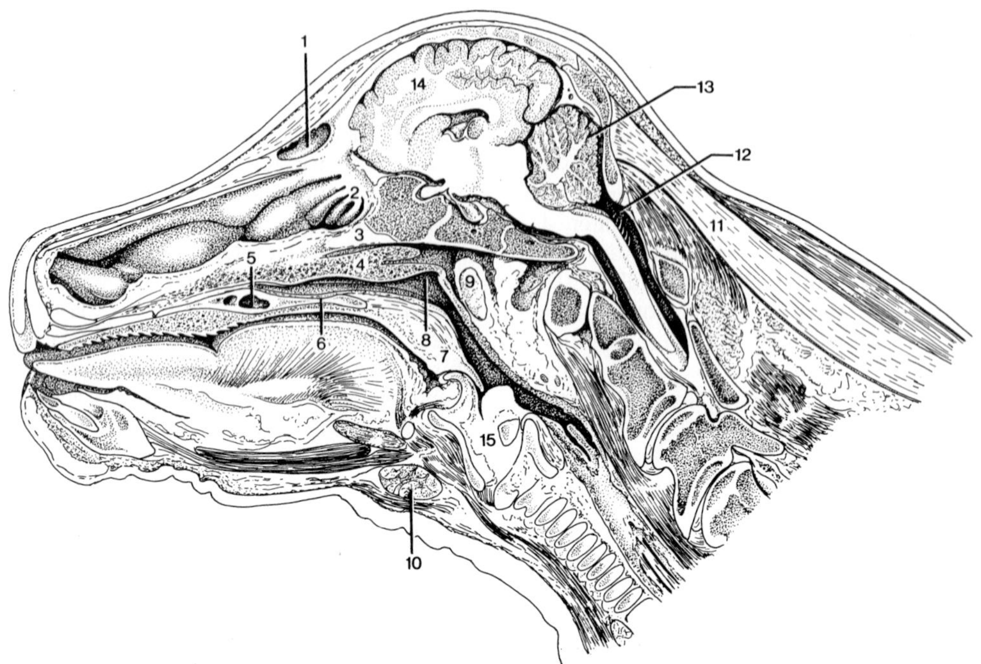


**Figure 25–3.** Paramedian section of the head of a 2-week-old calf. Note the rounded vault.

1, Frontal sinus; 2, ethmoidal conchae; 3, vomer; 4, pharyngeal septum; 5, palatine sinus; 6, hard palate; 7, soft palate; 8, nasopharynx; 9, medial retropharyngeal lymph node; 10, mandibular gland; 11, nuchal ligament; 12, cerebellomedullary cistern; 13, cerebellum; 14, cerebrum; 15, larynx.

base but does not reach so far toward the tip as in cattle. Polled breeds are common, but when horns occur they are generally present in both sexes, though those of males are more strongly formed. In a few rare breeds two, in rams occasionally three, pairs may exist. The multiple-horn (polycerate) condition is frequently associated with defects of cranial sutural closure and of the eyelids.

The horns of goats generally have an oval section and grow caudally over the skull. Those of sheep are triangular in section and pursue a helical course that carries them first caudally, then ventrally and dorsally in a form of increasing complexity. This growth sometimes carries the inner surface of the horn close to the skin of the face, which may suffer from pressure necrosis if contact is made. Shepherds of flocks of the vulnerable breeds are on watch for this occurrence and often remove a surface slice from the horn in treatment or in prevention. The operation can be performed without anesthetic if only "horn" is sawn away; on occasion sensitive dermis and bone must also be removed.

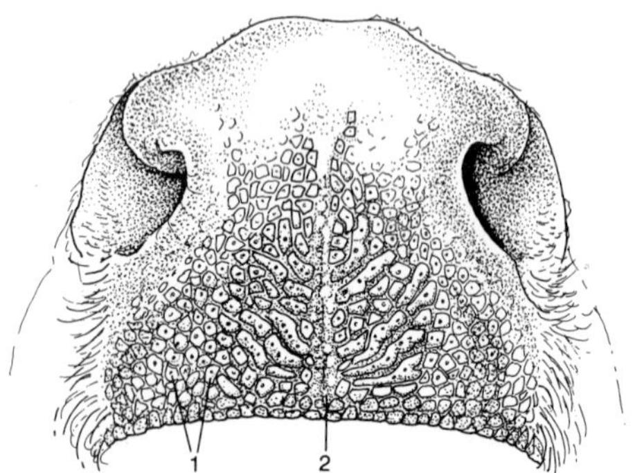


**Figure 25–4.** The upper lip and the borders of the nostrils combine to form the nasolabial plate in cattle. Note the orifices of the nasolabial glands (1) and the philtrum (2).

The horns of the sheep and goat are placed so close to the orbit that the supplying structures ascend directly behind the zygomatic process where the nerve may be blocked. The horn of the goat receives a subsidiary supply through branches of the infratrochlear nerve; these can be reached by a second injection at the dorsomedial margin of the orbit.

Intermittent growth of the horn substance produces a very corrugated external surface; there are usually several or even many minor variations in production rate in any year, but these are much less marked than the major ridges that reflect the seasons.

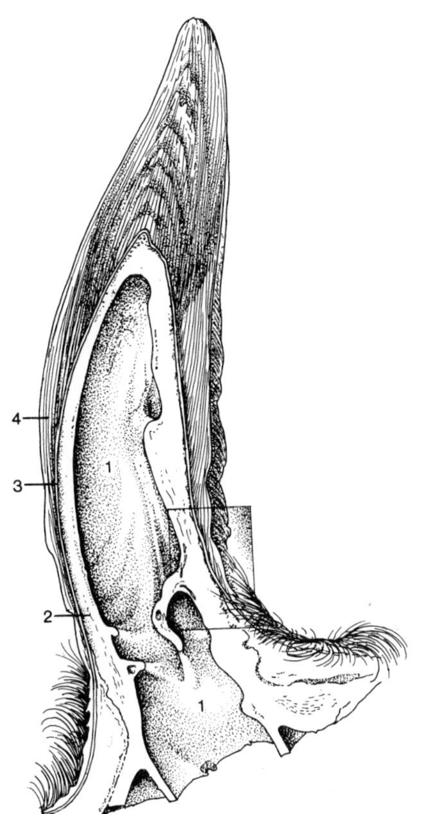


**Figure 25–5.** Longitudinal section of a bovine horn. The rectangle refers to the inset in Figure 10–20, which shows the production of the horn tubules over dermal papillae.

1, Cornual diverticulum of frontal sinus; 2, cornual process; 3, periosteum, dermis, and epidermis; 4, horn tubules.

Certain other special features of the skin are mentioned in Chapter 10; the most important are the presence in sheep of an infraorbital (preorbital) cutaneous pouch from which secretion escapes to stain the face in front of the eye (p. 360) and the groups of glands at the base of the horns of goats (p. 360). The wattles (tassels) that are often suspended from the throat region in goats are cylindrical skin appendages containing a cartilaginous rod and some vessels and nerves; their significance is unknown.

## SUPERFICIAL STRUCTURES

Other organs that are visible or palpable in life may be identified with the assistance of Figure 25–2. Relatively little of the skull lies directly below the skin, but large areas have thin coverings of fascia and cutaneous muscle that offer little obstacle to palpation. In addition to the broad forehead and dorsum of the nose, the temporal line, zygomatic arch, facial tuberosity, nasoincisive notch, and ventral border of the mandible are all easily identified. The supraorbital, infraorbital, and mental foramina can also be palpated (Figs. 25–1, 25–13, and 25–8).

Few specific features of the mimetic musculature are important. It is supplied by the *facial nerve* (VII), which divides into its principal terminal branches under cover of the parotid gland. The auriculopalpebral nerve supplies muscles of the external ear and eyelids. It reaches these by crossing the zygomatic arch directly in front of the temporomandibular joint where its superficial position makes it vulnerable (Fig. 25–7/3). Damage to the nerve may be evidenced by drooping of the ear and sagging of the eyelids, particularly the lower one. Paralysis of the orbicularis makes it impossible to close the eye. It is therefore clear that it may be advantageous to block the nerve to eliminate the blink reflex when examining the eye. It is most easily palpated where it passes over the zygomatic arch.

The dorsal buccal branch continues the parent trunk, crossing the masseter muscle in an exposed

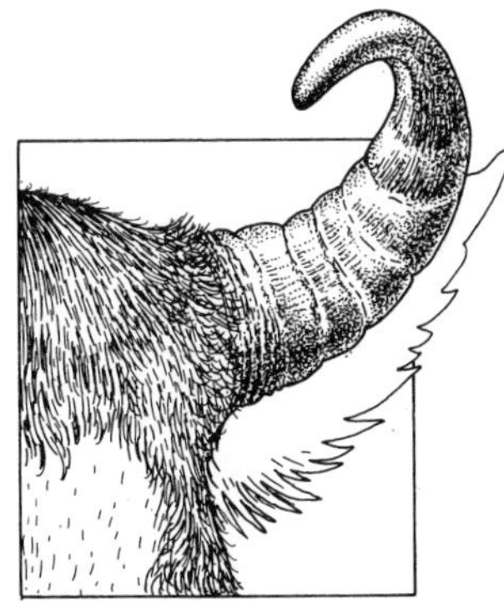

**Figure 25–6.** Horn rings resulting from variation in horn production and wear in cattle.

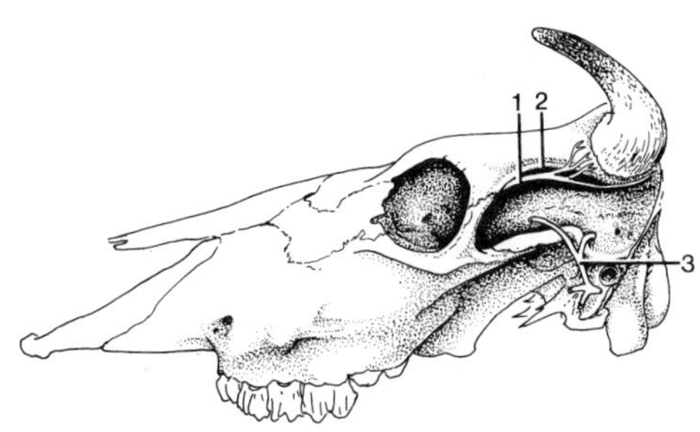


**Figure 25–7.** Bovine skull with cornual nerve (1) and auriculopalpebral nerve (3). The cornual nerve follows the temporal line (2) to the base of the horn. The auriculopalpebral nerve is palpable where it crosses the zygomatic arch.

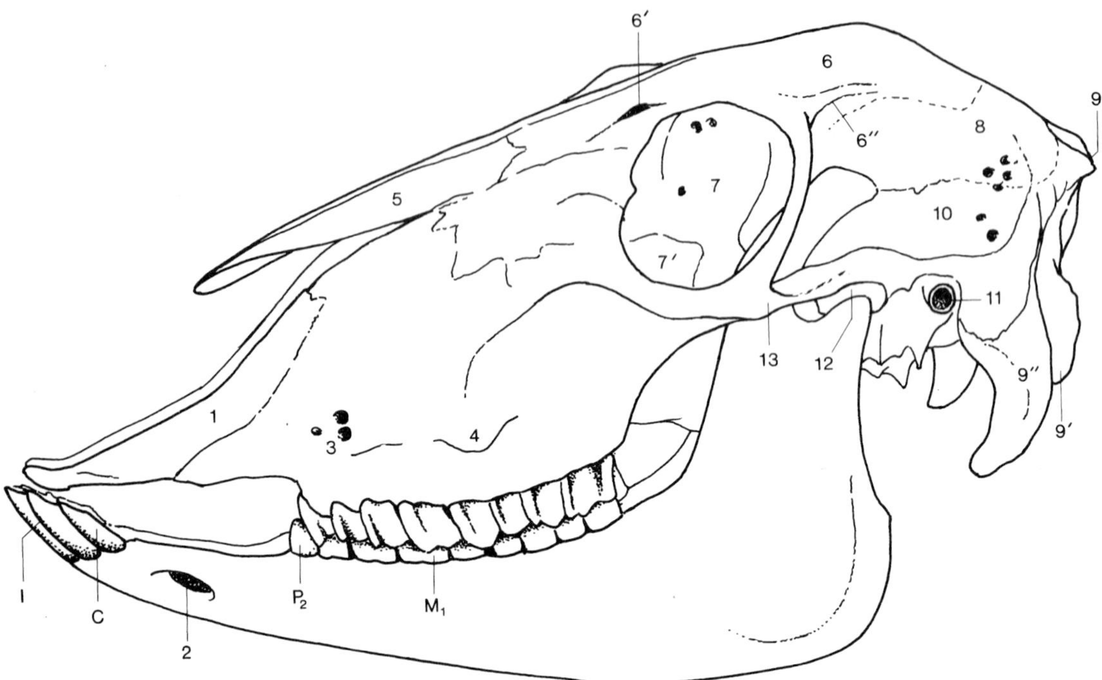


**Figure 25–8.** Lateral view of the skull of a sheep.

1, Incisive bone; 2, mental foramen; 3, infraorbital foramina; 4, facial tuberosity; 5, nasal bone; 6, frontal bone; 6′, supraorbital foramen and groove; 6″, temporal line; 7, orbit; 7′, lacrimal bulla; 8, parietal bone; 9, external occipital protuberance; 9′, occipital condyle; 9″, paracondylar process; 10, temporal fossa; 11, external acoustic meatus; 12, temporomandibular joint; 13, zygomatic arch.

position that carries considerable risk of injury. The effects of such injury include loss of innervation to the muscles of the nose and upper lip and to the buccinator. The first loss leads to slight distortion of the face, which is drawn toward the unaffected side; the second allows food to collect in a wad within the oral vestibule. The ventral buccal branch takes a more protected course caudomedial to the ramus of the mandible and reaches the face in company with the facial artery and vein. It has a limited distribution, and the visible effects of injury are minimal (Fig. 25–2/5,6).

The distribution of the *cutaneous nerves* is shown in Figure 25–9. The greater part of the skin of the head is supplied by trigeminal branches, although the first two cervical nerves supply a caudal strip over the angle of the jaw while the vagus innervates some skin of the external ear. Specific "blocks" of certain of these nerves are occasionally attempted. The large infraorbital nerve can be palpated where it leaves the infraorbital foramen, about 3 cm dorsal to the first cheek tooth. The mental nerve is found where it leaves the mental foramen of the mandible, about 3 to 4 cm caudal to the lateral incisor tooth.

The *facial artery* and *vein* are the most important superficial vessels. They cross the ventral margin of the mandible in front of the masseter muscle and are distributed to the lips, cheeks, muzzle, and periocular structures. The pulse may be examined where the artery lies on the side of the bone; it is less easily located in the notch of the ventral border.

The position of the *frontal vein* should also be noted since this fair-sized vessel is at some risk in trepanation of the caudal frontal sinus. The vein takes a caudorostral course in a palpable groove over the frontal bone to enter the supraorbital foramen; it then traverses a canal in the lateral part of the sinus. The foramen is located about 2 cm medial to the temporal line and about 2 cm caudal to the lateral angle of the eye (Fig. 25–13/4). A system of veins on the external surface of the pinna becomes engorged and prominent when a tourniquet is applied around the base of the ear. The central member of the set is sometimes used as an alternative to the jugular vein for the placement of an indwelling catheter. Neither site is free from problems.

The ventral end of the *mandibular gland* forms a conspicuous swelling in the intermandibular space. When palpated, this gland is often mistaken for the adjacent *mandibular lymph node;* its larger size, softer consistency, and more medial and more rostral extent make confusion unnecessary. The lymph node can be separately identified on the medial aspect of the sternomandibularis tendon (Fig. 25–2/20,22). Normally the parotid lymph node is also palpable rostroventral to the temporomandibular joint.

In the last part of its course along the rostral margin of the masseter, the *parotid duct* accompanies the facial vessels and ventral buccal nerve. The duct penetrates the cheek opposite the fifth upper cheek tooth.

## THE NASAL CAVITY AND PARANASAL SINUSES

The nasal cavity is much smaller than would be supposed from the exterior since its walls are widened and hollowed by air sinuses, while much of the internal space is occupied by the conchae. The nasal septum caudally fails to reach the floor, resulting in the formation of a single median channel that continues the paired nasal passages into the nasopharynx (Figs. 25–10 and 25–11).

Each nasal passage is divided by the major conchae into dorsal, middle, and ventral meatuses that branch from the common meatus located against the nasal septum. The lumen of the deeper part of the cavity is further subdivided by the numerous ethmoidal conchae; the largest of these projects rostrally and is known as the middle concha. The dorsal meatus leads to the ethmoidal meatuses and is especially concerned with olfaction; the middle meatus communicates with certain sinuses; the ventral meatus is the principal respiratory pathway. The nasal route is occasionally chosen for the passage of a sound when the instrument is directed to follow the largest space, formed at the junction of the ventral and common meatuses (Fig. 25–11/9).

The walls of the nasal passages are clothed by a thick, generously vascularized mucous membrane. The mucosa covers the *vomeronasal organ* within the floor of the cavity; the organ communicates with the ventral meatus and with the mouth via the incisive duct.

The paranasal sinus system is very poorly developed in the young calf, and several years must elapse before it attains full size. Even in the mature animal, the maxillary compartment continues to adjust to extrusion of the cheek teeth (Figs. 25–3/1,5 and 25–10/9,9′,10).

The complete set of sinuses is very complicated. It comprises frontal compartments within the bones of the cranial roof and side walls; a palatomaxillary complex within the caudal part of the hard palate and the face, both before and below the orbit; a lacrimal sinus within the medial orbital wall; sphenoidal sinuses that extend past the orbit into the rostral part of the cranial floor; and conchal sinuses within the nasal conchae. Any of these may be infected or otherwise become an object of clinical interest, but in practice attention

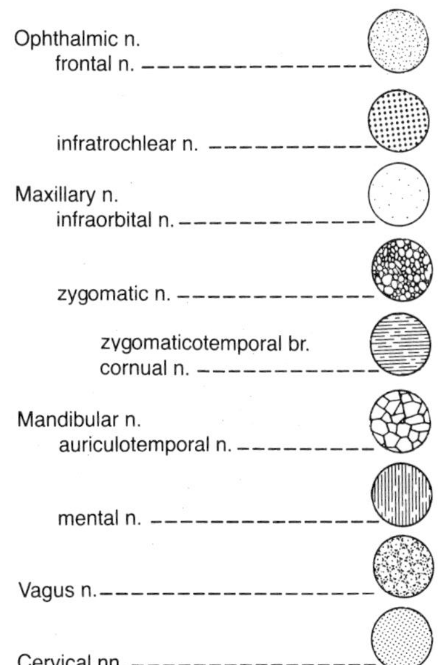


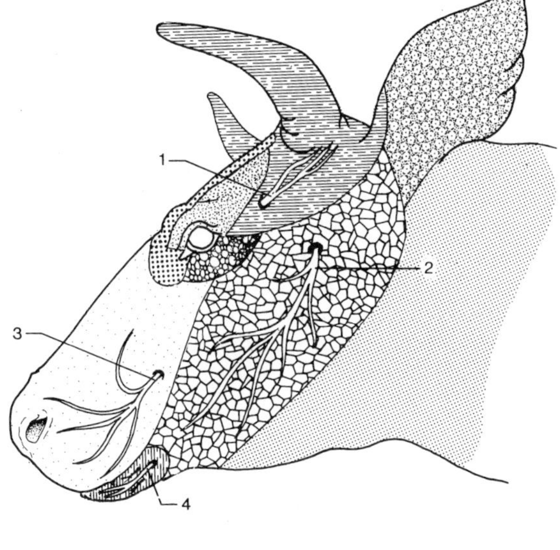


**Figure 25–9.** Skin innervation of the head.

1, Cornual n.; 2, auriculotemporal n.; 3, infraorbital n.; 4, mental n.

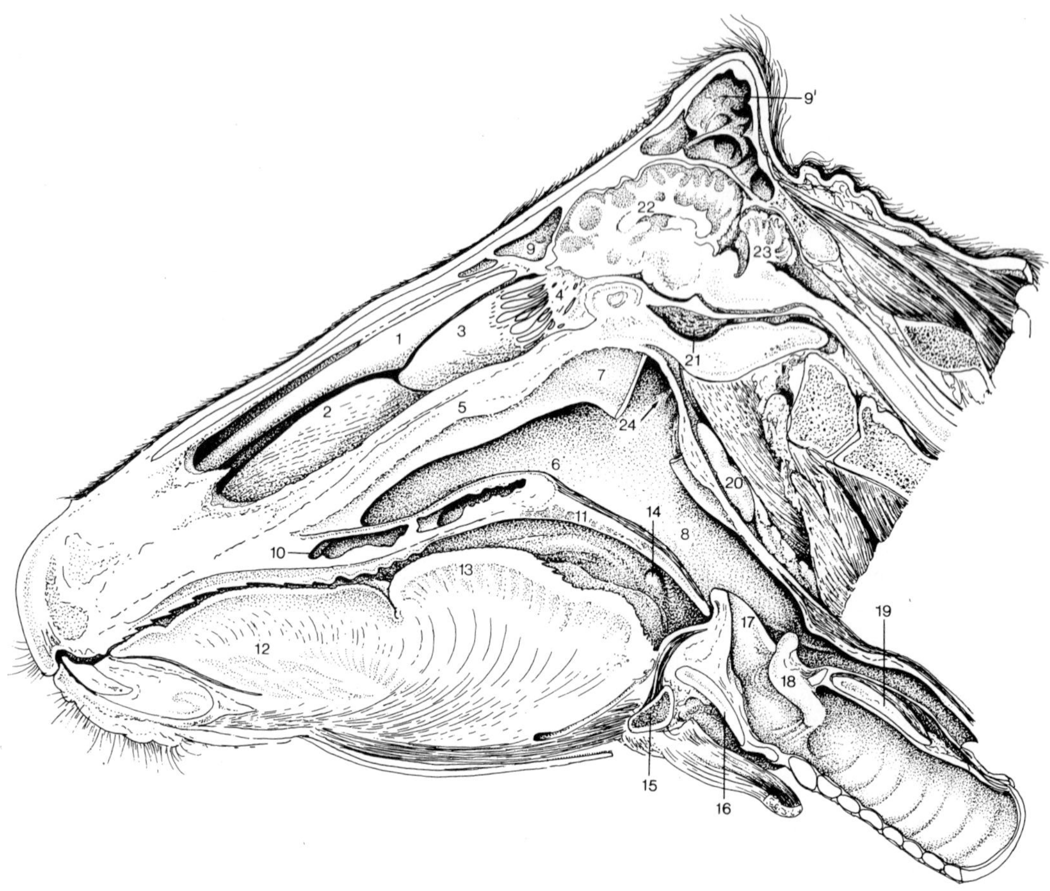


**Figure 25–10.** Paramedian section of the head.

1, Dorsal nasal concha; 2, ventral nasal concha; 3, middle nasal concha; 4, ethmoidal conchae; 5, vomer; 6, choana; 7, pharyngeal septum, resected; 8, nasopharynx; 9, rostral frontal sinus; 9′, caudal frontal sinus; 10, palatine sinus; 11, soft palate; 12, apex of tongue; 13, torus linguae; 14, entrance to tonsillar sinus; 15, basihyoid; 16, thyroid cartilage; 17, epiglottis; 18, arytenoid cartilage; 19, cricoid cartilage; 20, medial retropharyngeal lymph node; 21, venous plexus surrounding hypophysis; 22, cerebrum; 23, cerebellum; 24, to pharyngeal opening of auditory tube.

is concentrated upon the maxillary and caudal frontal sinuses. The surface projections over which these spaces may be percussed are illustrated in Figures 25–12 and 25–13.

The *maxillary sinus* occupies much of the upper jaw above the alveoli of the cheek teeth. It communicates with the nasal cavity via a large nasomaxillary opening but natural drainage of pus or other fluid is hindered by the location of this opening high in the medial wall. The maxillary sinus is continuous with the palatine sinus over the plate of bone that carries the infraorbital nerve in its free margin (Fig. 25–11/6). It also extends caudally (as the lacrimal sinus in front of the orbit) and within the fragile lacrimal bulla that intrudes into the ventral part of the orbit.

The *frontal sinus* comprises several compartments that communicate separately with ethmoidal meatuses. The two, occasionally three, small rostral compartments are of little clinical interest. The caudal compartment, by far the largest and most important, spreads mainly within the frontal bone. It covers the dorsal part of the brain case and also extends into the lateral and nuchal walls and into the horn core. It is separated from its fellow and from the smaller homolateral compartments by partitions of rather variable position (Fig. 25–13). The openings in these partitions, visible in dry skulls, are closed by mucosa in the fresh state. The major cavity, which continues to increase throughout life, is further subdivided by irregular and perforate septa. Inflammation of its mucosa is a common sequel to surgical dehorning.

The protection that the frontal sinus affords the *cranial cavity* makes it impossible to predict the extent of the latter by simple inspection of the head. The cranial cavity is in fact surprisingly small, rather globular, and so tilted that its rostral extremity is placed above as well as behind the nasal cavity (Fig. 25–10). It is protected above, behind, and to the sides by the pneumatized bones of the cranial vault. The topography is relevant to the usual humane slaughter technique. The target spot is defined by the intersection of the diagonals joining the lateral angles of the eyes to the nearest parts of the opposite horn bases (or equivalent points in polled breeds). The bolt or bullet then has to pass through the shallowest part of the frontal sinus en route to the brain.

The maxillary sinus is shallower and simpler in the *sheep* and *goat*. It does not communicate with the lacrimal sinus, which may open into the nasal cavity separately or via the lateral frontal sinus. The frontal sinus comprises separate medial and lateral compartments in both these species. They lie medial to the orbit (and extend slightly beyond this, both rostrally and caudally) and are of irregular form. The lateral compartment corresponds to the caudal sinus of cattle and provides the extension into the horn core.

The most common clinical involvement of the sinuses of sheep is that caused by invasion of the

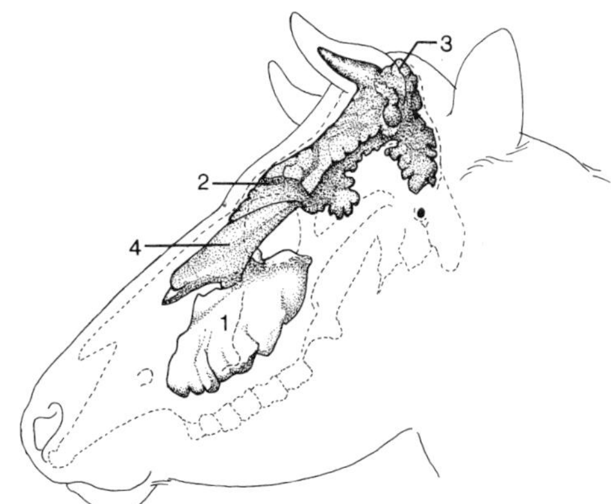


**Figure 25–12.** Topography of the paranasal sinuses, which are filled with casting material.

1, Maxillary sinus; 2, rostral frontal sinuses; 3, caudal frontal sinus; 4, dorsal conchal sinus.

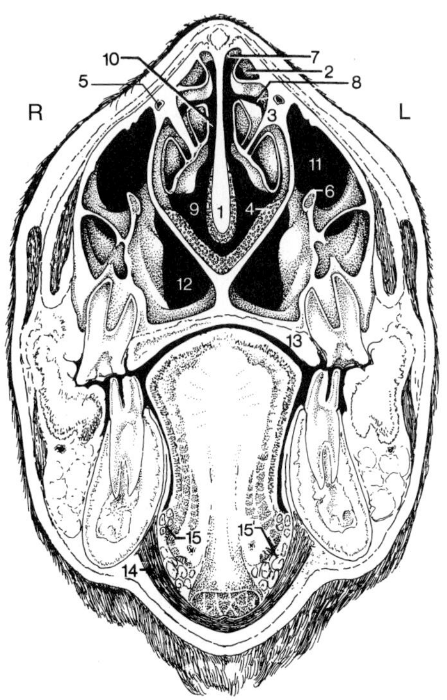


**Figure 25–11.** Transverse section of a bovine head at the level of the last premolars.

1, Nasal septum; 2, dorsal nasal concha; 3, ventral nasal concha; 4, thick nasal mucosa containing venous plexus; 5, nasolacrimal duct; 6, infraorbital canal with infraorbital nerve; 7, dorsal nasal meatus; 8, middle nasal meatus; 9, ventral nasal meatus; 10, common nasal meatus; 11, maxillary sinus; 12, palatine sinus; 13, hard palate; 14, mylohyoideus; 15, polystomatic sublingual gland; 15′, monostomatic sublingual gland.

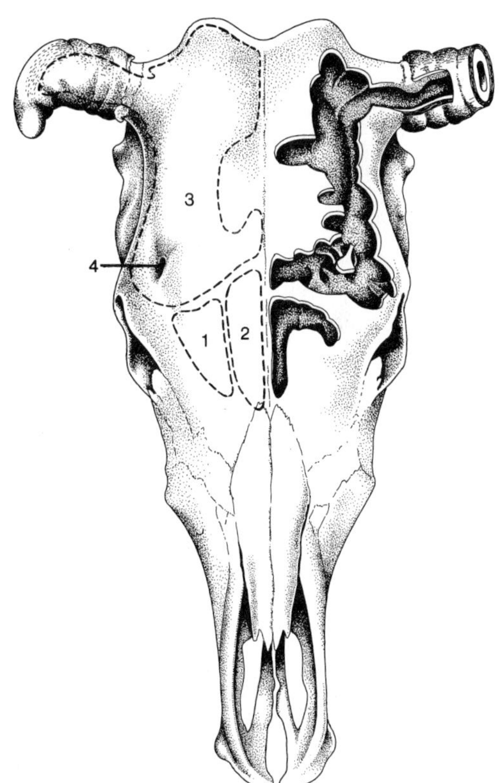


**Figure 25–13.** Dorsal projection of the frontal sinuses.

1, Lateral rostral frontal sinus; 2, medial rostral frontal sinus; 3, caudal frontal sinus with cornual diverticulum; 4, supraorbital foramen.

frontal sinus by larvae of oestrid flies. Treatment involves surgical puncture, the preferred sites being rostral to the horn or medial to the middle of the orbital rim where there is no risk of injury to the frontal vein.

## THE MOUTH

Since cattle do not ingest large mouthfuls, the small size of the oral opening is no disadvantage to the animal; it is a considerable hindrance to clinical inspection of the mouth parts and pharynx. The vestibule between the cheeks and the margin of the jaws is surprisingly roomy; the inner surface of the lips and cheeks bears large, backward-pointing papillae that are most prominent toward the corners of the mouth (Fig. 25–14/6).

The mouth cavity proper is long and narrow and is largely occupied by the tongue. The hard palate is most constricted directly in front of the cheek teeth. It is sculpted to display a dozen or more transverse ridges that progressively decrease in prominence and at last fade out toward the back of the mouth; their crests carry numerous papillae (Fig. 25–15). The region occupied in other species by the upper incisor teeth here carries the paired dental pads; these are crescentic elevations that are pliant when compressed, though cornified on the surface (/2). Cattle do not graze by edge-to-edge biting but, after drawing a tuft into the mouth with the assistance of the tongue, sever it by pressing the incisor blades against these pads; the risk of injury to the pads is reduced by their tough covering and pliant consistency and by the procumbent arrangement and rather loose implantation of the incisors (Figs. 25–17 and 25–19). The incisive papilla behind the pads is flanked by the small openings of the incisive ducts.

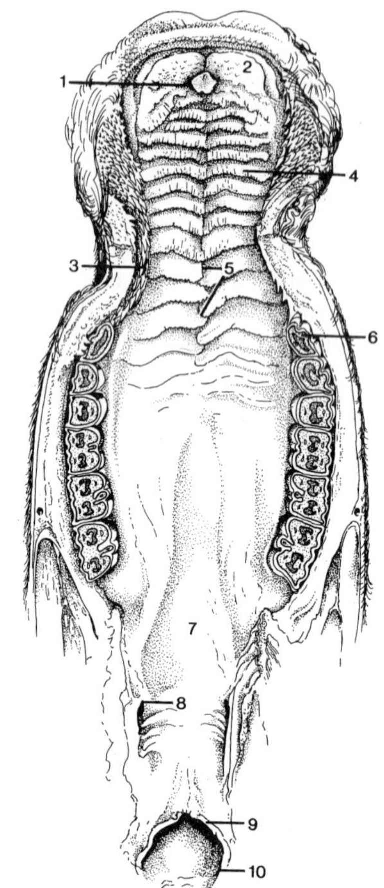


**Figure 25–15.** The roof of the bovine oral cavity.

1, Incisive papilla; 2, dental pad; 3, buccal papillae; 4, palatine ridges; 5, palatine raphe; 6, first upper cheek tooth ($P^2$); 7, soft palate; 8, opening of tonsillar sinus; 9, free border of soft palate; 10, palatopharyngeal arch.

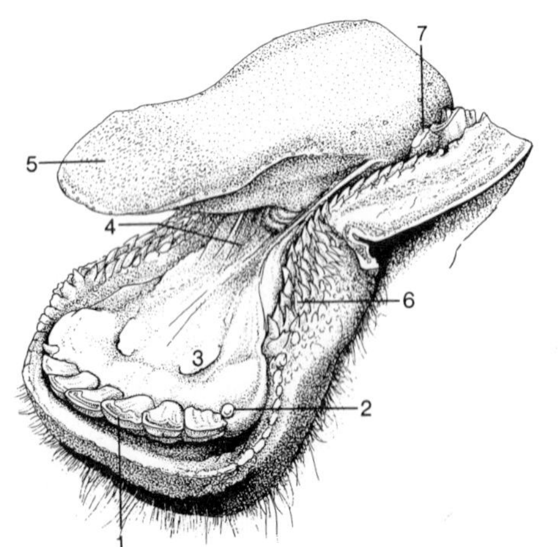


**Figure 25–14.** Floor of the bovine mouth and tongue.

1, Central incisor; 2, remnant of worn fourth deciduous incisor ($i_4$); 3, sublingual caruncle; 4, frenulum; 5, apex of tongue; 6, buccal papillae; 7, first cheek tooth ($P_2$).

The lips of small ruminants are much more mobile than those of cattle. They are the principal organs of prehension and enable these species to crop a pasture closely.

In cattle it is the pointed *tongue* that is the principal organ of prehension. Its caudal part is raised to form a large torus that is marked off in front by a transverse lingual fossa in which food tends to collect; it is a potential portal for infection since the epithelium, quite delicate within the fossa, is easily pricked by sharp particles (Fig. 25–16/5). The papillae that give the surface of the tongue a characteristic roughness are concentrated over the dorsum and toward the apex. Harsh, caudally directed, filiform papillae are freely spread over the apex, while conical and flat lenticular papillae are present upon the torus (/4′,4″); all of these have a purely mechanical function. As usual, it is the fungiform papillae scattered upon the apex and the numerous vallate papillae (/3) present toward the root that carry the sensory receptors concerned with taste. An accumulation of lymphoid tissue toward the root constitutes the diffuse lingual tonsil.

The oral floor below the apex of the tongue presents a fleshy sublingual caruncle to each side; the ducts of the mandibular and monostomatic sublingual glands open beside this (Fig. 25–14).

The orientation of the projections upon the cheeks, palate, and tongue encourages the backward movement of material within the mouth; this, combined with the general insensitivity of the mouth parts and the copious salivary secretion, may explain the frequency with which cattle swallow foreign bodies concealed within their forage.

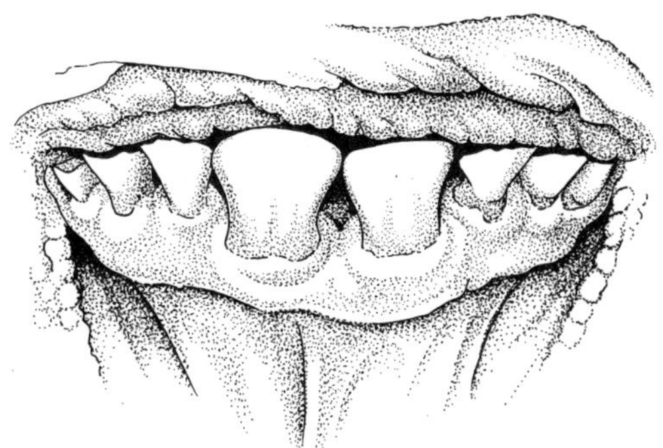

**Figure 25–17.** Front view of the incisors of a 2-year-old cow. The central incisors are permanent, the others deciduous.

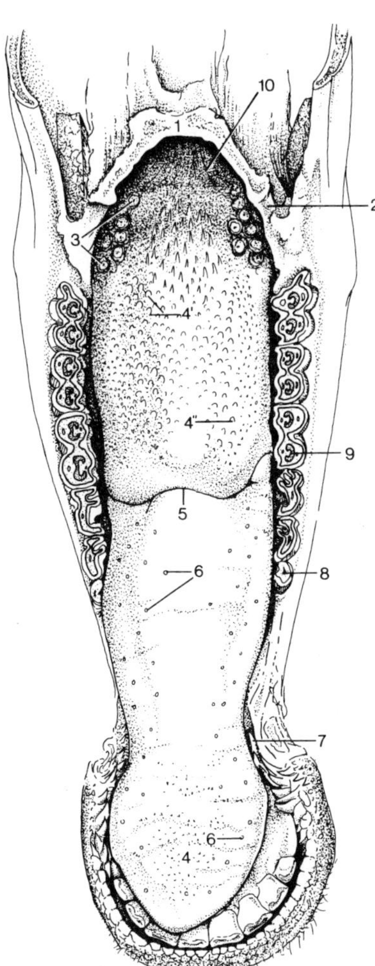


**Figure 25–16.** Bovine tongue and lower jaw.

1, Soft palate, cut; 2, palatoglossal arch; 3, vallate papillae; 4, filiform papillae; 4′, lenticular papillae; 4″, conical papillae; 5, lingual fossa; 6, fungiform papillae; 7, buccal papillae; 8, first lower cheek tooth ($P_2$); 9, $M_1$; 10, diffuse lingual tonsil.

## THE DENTITION AND MASTICATORY APPARATUS

The most unusual features of the dentition are the absence of incisor and canine teeth in the upper jaw and the assimilation of the canines to the incisors in the lower one. Since both upper and lower first premolar teeth fail to develop, the dental formulae read $\frac{0\text{-}0\text{-}3}{3\text{-}1\text{-}3}$ for the temporary, $\frac{0\text{-}0\text{-}3\text{-}3}{3\text{-}1\text{-}3\text{-}3}$ for the permanent set. It is customary to refer to the canine tooth as the fourth or corner incisor.

The eight *incisor teeth* toward the front of the lower jaw are arranged in a continuous crescent that is opposed to the dental pads when the mouth is closed. Each tooth presents a wide spatulate crown abruptly joined to a narrow, peglike root; the crown is asymmetrical, and in young animals it overlaps the lingual aspect of its medial neighbor (Fig. 25–17). The convex labial and concave lingual surfaces initially meet at a ridge, but this becomes increasingly broadened and the dentine increasingly exposed with continuing use (Figs. 25–18/*D,E* and 25–19). The crowns are sometimes wholly eroded in old animals, and then only narrow but widely spaced roots remain in the margin of the jaw. Often the incisors are shed before this state is reached.

The wide gap or diastema that separates the front from the cheek teeth makes it easy to grasp the tongue to force the animal to permit examina-

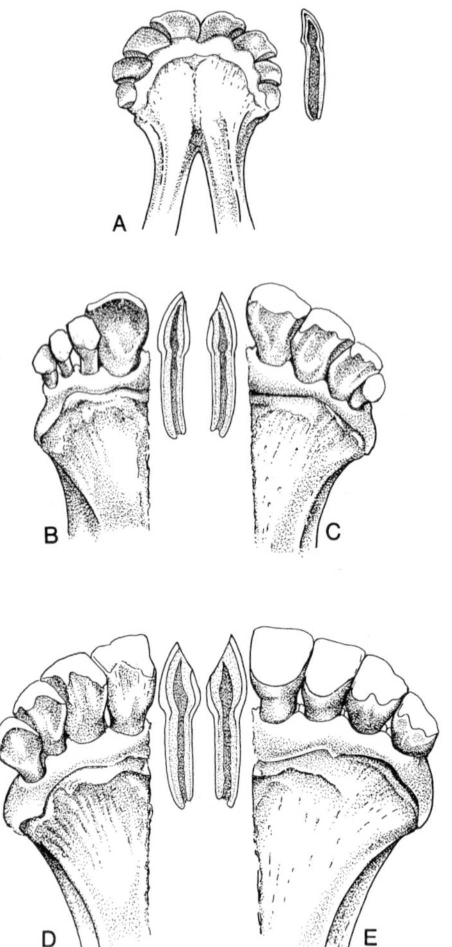


**Figure 25–18.** Changes in the bovine incisors with increasing age.

*A,* Deciduous incisors in the newborn calf. In the longitudinal section of $i_1$ the enamel still surrounds the crown. *B,* Two years: $i_1$ has been replaced. The other incisors are deciduous. The distal border of $I_1$ is slightly worn, and the dentine is exposed. *C,* Three and a half years: $I_1$, $I_2$, and $I_3$ are permanent; $i_4$ is deciduous. The occlusal surface of $I_2$, wider than that of $I_3$, is shown in the longitudinal section. *D,* Five years. *E,* Eight years. Note the size of the occlusal surface in the longitudinal section. The lingual edge of the occlusal surface of $I_1$ and $I_2$ is smooth; these two teeth are said to be "level."

tion of its mouth. The six *cheek teeth* in each jaw increase in size from front to back and are so arranged that most occlude with two opponents. The upper tooth rows are more widely separated than those of the lower jaw; consequently, only narrow strips of opposing teeth are in contact when the mouth is closed in central occlusion (Fig. 25–11). The tables slope transversely; the buccal edge is raised on the maxillary teeth, the lingual edge on those in the mandible. The masticatory surfaces of unworn teeth bear a series of crescentic enamel cusps arranged in two rows parallel to the axis of the jaw; the premolars have one, the molars two pairs of these cusps. Once wear has exposed the dentine, the alternation of softer and more resistant tissues creates an uneven surface that is a very efficient shredding mechanism when the lower teeth are swung inward across their upper counterparts (Fig. 25–20). Attrition of the crowns is for a time compensated by their continuing

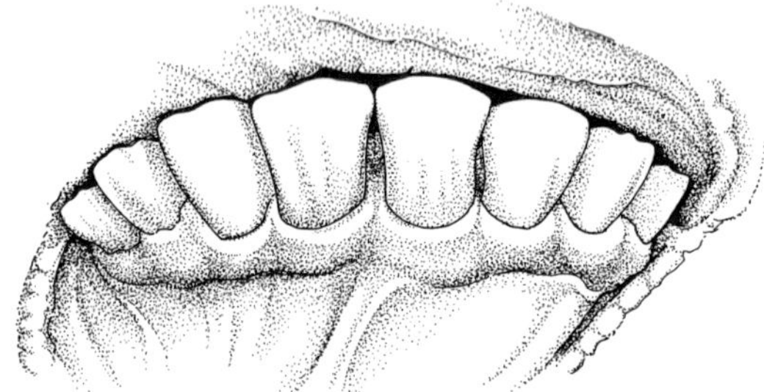

**Figure 25–19.** Front view of the incisors of a 4½- to 5-year-old cow. The fourth incisors have reached the height of their neighbors and are coming into wear.

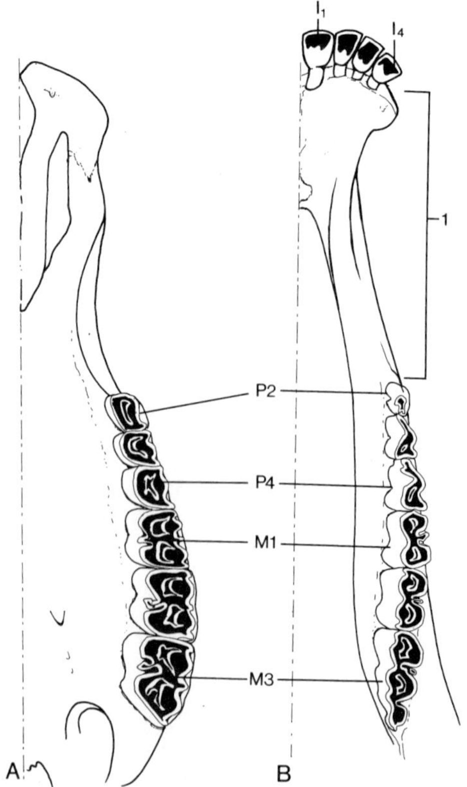


**Figure 25–20.** Left half of upper and right half of lower jaw of cattle. Note the different shapes of the upper and lower cheek teeth and the large diastema (1).

**Table 25-1.** Eruption Dates of the Teeth of Cattle

| | Temporary Tooth (wk) | Permanent Tooth (mo) |
|---|---|---|
| Incisor 1 | Birth–2 | 18–24 |
| Incisor 2 | Birth–2 | 24–30 |
| Incisor 3 | Birth–2 | 36–42 |
| Incisor 4 | Birth–2 | 42–48 |
| Premolar 2 | Birth–1 | 24–30 |
| Premolar 3 | Birth–1 | 18–30 |
| Premolar 4 | Birth–1 | 20–36 |
| Molar 1 | | 6 |
| Molar 2 | | 12–18 |
| Molar 3 | | 24–30 |

growth; when growth eventually ceases, the roots are formed, and the height of the exposed part is then maintained only by gradual extrusion of the embedded portion. The crowns are eventually consumed in animals that survive to very advanced age.

Most *temporary teeth* closely resemble their replacements but the temporary premolars, which initially bear the full burden of mastication, are larger and more complicated than those that succeed them.

The eruption dates of the teeth are given in Table 25–1.

Estimation of age is based on these dates and on the state of wear of the incisors. Neither factor is very reliable. The dates of eruption are influenced by breed and reflect differences in the general rate of maturation. The rate of wear provides a somewhat more useful criterion, though it obviously depends upon the nature of the fodder. Wear converts the cutting edge into a gradually broadening surface. The lingual edge of this surface is originally jagged (due to the ridging of the distal part of the lingual surface of the crown) but becomes smooth when the tooth is worn down; the change in character occurs at 6 years on the first incisor and at 7, 8, and 9 years on the second, third, and fourth incisors, respectively. The teeth are then said to be "level." Exposure of the root coincides with this alteration in the crown (Fig. 25–18/*E*). The changes at later ages are too unreliable to be of value.

The dentition of the *small ruminants* broadly resembles that of cattle. The teeth of sheep are often exposed to very rough wear, and tooth loss ("broken mouth") is a frequent reason for culling older animals. Some experiments with prosthetic replacements have been performed, but with only limited success. The dates of tooth eruption and replacement in sheep and goats are given in Table 25–2.

Because of the unequal width of the upper and lower dental arcades, mastication is unilateral, and though both sides are used in alternation, most animals tend to favor one. The usual action comprises three phases. In the first, the jaw is dropped and carried laterally; in the second, it is raised while displaced farther to the side; and in the third, which is performed much more swiftly and vigorously, it is carried upward and medially so that the tooth crescents of the lower row engage between those of the upper row as the jaw is returned to its resting position.

The pterygoids of the active side, the masseter of the passive side, are the most important muscles in the work stroke. The powerful *masseter* is divided into two layers; the fibers of the superficial layer run predominantly horizontally, those of the deep part almost vertically; both divisions are intersected by tendon sheets. The small lateral and powerful medial *pterygoid muscles* broadly correspond to the two divisions of the masseter in the orientation of their fibers. The *temporalis,* which raises the jaw without displacement to either side, is relatively weak; in adult cattle it is confined to the temporal fossa on the lateral aspect of the skull.

## THE SALIVARY GLANDS

Cattle produce an enormous volume of saliva—perhaps as much as 100 L a day—which contributes to the fermentation medium within the forechambers of the stomach where it helps to buffer the fatty acids that are produced. Interference with the normal flow to the stomach results in

**Table 25-2.** Eruption Dates of the Teeth of Sheep and Goats

| | Temporary Tooth (wk) | Permanent Tooth (mo) |
|---|---|---|
| Incisor 1 | Before birth–1 (at birth) | 12–18 |
| Incisor 2 | Before birth–1 (at birth) | 18–24 |
| Incisor 3 | Before birth–1 (at birth) | 30–36 |
| Incisor 4 | Birth–1 wk (1–3) | 36–48 |
| Premolar 2 | Birth–4 wk (3) | 18–24 |
| Premolar 3 | Birth–4 wk (3) | 18–24 |
| Premolar 4 | Birth–4 wk (3) | 18–24 |
| Molar 1 | | 3 (3–4) |
| Molar 2 | | 9 (8–10) |
| Molar 3 | | 18 (18–24) |

From Habermehl, K.H.: Altersbestimmung bei Haus- und Labortieren, 2nd ed. Berlin, Blackwell Wissenschafts-Verlag, 1975.

serious depletion of the electrolytes that are normally reabsorbed and recycled.

Though the *parotid gland* is almost continuously active, it is smaller than might be expected. It lies ventral to the ear along the caudal border of the masseter where it partly covers the parotid lymph node. A spurt in its growth is coordinated with the initiation of ruminant digestion by the calf. The duct was encountered in the description of the face (Fig. 25–2/10).

The *mandibular gland* is considerably larger. It produces a mixed secretion but only when the animal is actually feeding or remasticating; the flow is most copious when the fodder is dry. The gland extends in an arc on the inner aspect of the lower jaw. Its palpable ventral end projects below the mandible and often almost meets its fellow in the midline; its dorsal end is within the atlantal fossa. The duct runs below the oral mucosa to open by the sublingual caruncle (Fig. 25–14/3).

The *sublingual gland* has the usual two divisions. The polystomatic part lies in the mouth floor, lateral to the tongue, and drains through many small openings beside the frenulum. It is overlapped by the more compact rostral part whose single duct opens close by, or together with, that of the mandibular gland (Fig. 25–11/15,15′).

Many minor salivary glands are scattered below the labial, buccal, palatine, and lingual mucosae; those in the cheeks are particularly well developed. In the aggregate, these lesser glands must contribute a considerable volume of secretion.

There are no important differences in the salivary glands of the small ruminants.

## THE PHARYNX

The pharynx is divided in the customary fashion.

The *nasopharynx* extends the nasal cavity caudally. In the ruminants it is incompletely divided by a median membranous fold (pharyngeal septum) that prolongs the nasal septum to the dorsal pharyngeal wall (Fig. 25–10/7). The caudal end of this septum is thickened by a mass of lymphoid tissue, the pharyngeal tonsil. Other lymphoid aggregations are found around the slitlike entrances to the auditory tubes on the lateral pharyngeal walls (see Fig. 3–26).

The *oropharynx* is narrow, and this significantly restricts the size of the morsels that can be swallowed. It contains within its lateral wall the palatine tonsil, which projects away from the lumen around a deep, branching tonsillar sinus. The entrance to this sinus (Fig. 25–10/14), but not the tonsil itself, is visible on the surface.

The *laryngopharynx* tapers caudally before joining the esophagus, and its lumen is normally held closed by the investing muscles; the muscle principally involved, the cricopharyngeus, is sometimes described as the cranial sphincter of the esophagus. The piriform recesses to each side of the entrance to the larynx allow a continuous dribble of saliva to reach the esophagus without need for active swallowing (Fig. 25–22/7).

The pharynx may be examined by palpation, externally or through the mouth, and its interior may also be inspected using an oral speculum. Swelling of lymphoid tissue in the pharyngeal wall may intrude upon the food and air pathways. The pharynx may also be compressed when the adjacent medial retropharyngeal lymph nodes are inflamed (Fig. 25–21/12).

The pharynx receives and transmits to the mouth the regurgitated cud. It also receives the gas that is eructated from the stomach in large amounts; some of this gas is lost to the exterior but a significant portion is directed to the lungs when the communication with the nasopharynx is shut off. The significance of this phenomenon is not fully understood; in animals on certain rations, absorption of eructated gas may lead to tainting of the milk and to pathology of the lung.

## THE LARYNX

The larynx is largely situated between the mandibular rami but extends into the upper part of the neck where it may be felt. The appreciation of its palpable features requires the correct identification of three midline skeletal structures: the basihyoid and the thyroid and cricoid cartilages. Those familiar with the surface anatomy of the horse may experience an initial uncertainty when first examining cattle. The different spacing of the ventral prominences is due to the shape of the bovine thyroid cartilage, which is complete ventrally and most salient toward its caudoventral point.

The bovine larynx shows few other peculiarities of note. The *entrance,* which may be inspected with the assistance of a laryngoscope, is bounded by the low, curled margin of the epiglottis and the prominent corniculate extensions of the arytenoid cartilages (Fig. 25–22/4,5). Intubation is made difficult by a slight caudal deflection of the entrance (Fig. 25–10).

The *vestibule* possesses neither median nor lateral ventricles, and its side walls shelve smoothly to the glottis. (A small median ventricle is present in sheep and goats.) The size of the *glottic cleft* varies with the phase of respiration,

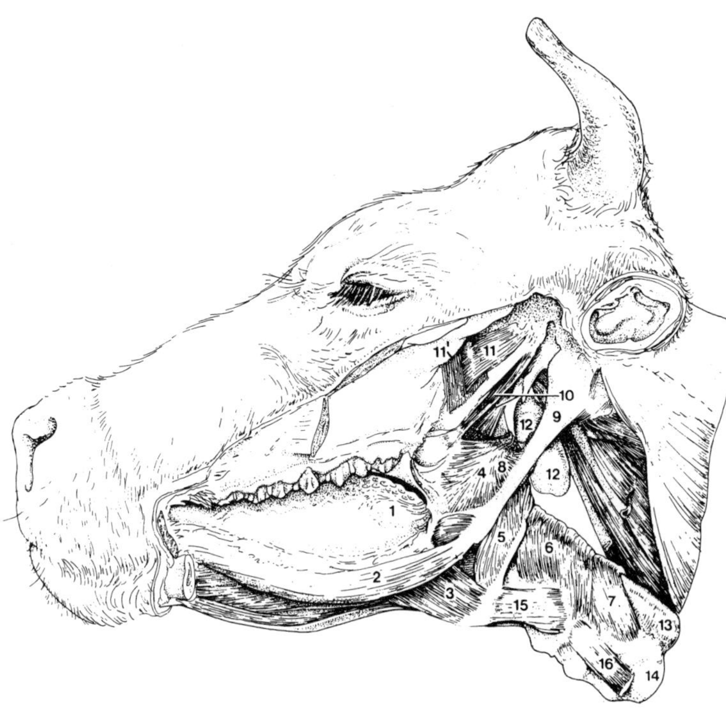


**Figure 25–21.** Connections of the pharynx and larynx with the base of the skull and the tongue.

1, Root of tongue; 2, styloglossus; 3, hyoglossus; 4, rostral pharyngeal constrictor; 5, middle pharyngeal constrictor; 6, 7, caudal pharyngeal constrictors (thyropharyngeus and cricopharyngeus); 8, stylopharyngeus caudalis; 9, stylohyoid; 10, tensor and levator veli palatini; 11, pterygoideus lateralis; 11′, remnants of pterygoideus medialis; 12, medial retropharyngeal lymph node; 13, esophagus; 14, trachea; 15, thyrohyoideus; 16, sternothyroideus.

but the changes are not pronounced during quiet breathing. It is narrower than might be supposed, and this limits the caliber of the endotracheal tube that may be passed. The relationship to the medial retropharyngeal lymph nodes is important; when much enlarged, these may seriously compress the larynx as well as the pharynx (/20).

## THE EYE

The orbital rim projects above the surrounding surfaces. The *orbital cavity* is capacious, although reduced ventrorostrally by the fragile, thin-walled swelling of the lacrimal bulla into which the maxillary sinus extends. The orbital axes diverge upward, outward, and forward and together subtend an angle of approximately 120 degrees. It is therefore clear that, as is usual in ungulates, the field of monocular vision is large, the binocular one small.

The *eyelids* are supported by dense fibrous plates or "tarsi." The skin adheres tightly over the orbicularis muscle, but elsewhere its attachment is looser and the lid becomes furrowed when the eye is open. The lashes are long and are more densely spread on the upper lid (Fig. 25–23). The muscles of the lids include the frontalis, which extends from the forehead into the upper lid, and the malaris, which radiates from the lower lid onto the face. These are supplied by the facial nerve, mainly through the auriculopalpebral nerve. The levator, supplied as always by the oculomotor nerve, remains active in facial paralysis, mitigating the effects of this injury.

The conjunctiva contains considerable scattered lymphoid accumulations in its palpebral part. The usual glands are present within the eyelids. The largest, the tarsal (Meibomian) glands, occupy the deeper layers of the tarsi; they may be visible through the conjunctiva of the everted lid.

The medial corner of the palpebral opening forms a bay containing the fleshy lacrimal caruncle. The *third eyelid* covers a variable part of the bulb. The supporting cartilage sinks medial to the eyeball where it is associated with superficial and deep accessory lacrimal glands. Only a small part of the third eyelid is normally visible (/10). A larger part is brought into view when the eyeball is withdrawn or pressed into its socket; this maneuver displaces the retrobulbar fat, which in turn pushes the cartilage, and therefore the fold, outward.

The lobulated, bipartite *lacrimal gland* lies dorsolaterally upon the eyeball. It drains by numerous ducts of varying caliber into the upper conjunctival fornix. The tears collect by the lacrimal caruncle before entering the slitlike puncta lacrimalia that lead to the lacrimal sac. The sac lies within a depression of the cranial part of

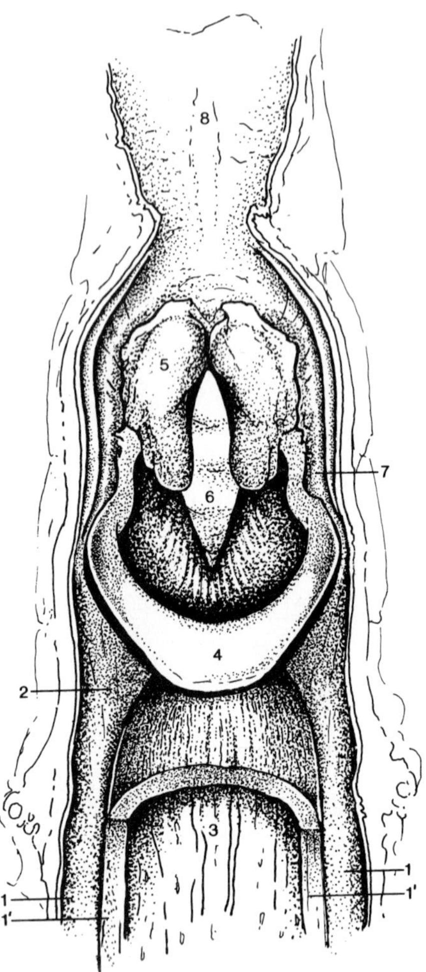


**Figure 25–22.** Rostrodorsal view of the bovine larynx.

1, Soft palate (the greater part has been resected to expose the tongue); 1′, cut edge of soft palate; 2, palatopharyngeal arch; 3, root of tongue; 4, epiglottis; 5, corniculate process of arytenoid cartilage; 6, glottic cleft allowing view of infraglottic cavity; 7, piriform recess; 8, esophagus, opened.

the orbital wall. It tapers to the nasolacrimal duct, which first traverses the maxillary sinus and then runs on the lateral nasal wall to discharge within the nasal vestibule.

The *extrinsic muscles,* which exhibit no especially notable features, are shown schematically in Figure 9–13.

The eyeball is small in relation to the orbit. The *sclera* is thin and locally obtains a bluish tinge from the dark underlying choroid. Some pigmentation is common, especially toward the junction with the cornea, and tends to increase with age. The cornea is ovoid with the pointed end lateral. It is rather thick, especially toward its margin.

The bovine pupil is widened from side to side when constricted but becomes circular on dilation. Its upper and lower margins are broken by irregular projections, the iridic granules, which are smaller than in the horse; they are more prominent along the upper margin. The ciliary muscles are poorly developed, and the capacity for accommodation is limited accordingly. The vascular and choroidocapillary layers of the choroid are separated in the caudal part of the bulb by the brilliantly colored reflective *tapetum* (Plate 14/*D,E*). The tapetum is triangular with its base directly above the optic disc. Its peripheral parts are most colorful and display an array of metallic blues and greens, while the area close to the optic disc is reddish, especially in the calf. Ophthalmoscopic examination of the tapetum reveals scattered dark flecks where capillaries enter, while larger vessels appear as red lines. Four pairs of arteries and veins radiate in cruciate fashion from the optic disc which is lateroventral to the posterior pole of the eye. The dorsal vein is especially large and is entwined by a spiraling artery. A clear spot in the center of the disc indicates the vestige of the hyaloid artery; as would be expected, the remnant is more obvious in the newborn calf. The macula of the retina consists of two rather ill-defined parts: a rounded area placed dorsolateral to the optic disc is concerned with

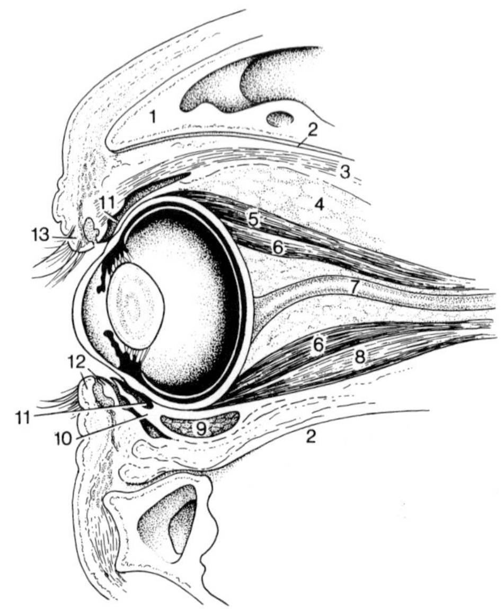


**Figure 25–23.** Section of the bovine orbit.

1, Frontal bone with rostral frontal sinus; 2, boundaries of the orbit; 3, levator of upper lid; 4, fat; 5, dorsal rectus; 6, retractor bulbi; 7, optic nerve; 8, ventral rectus; 9, ventral oblique; 10, third eyelid; 11, conjunctival sac; 12, lower lid; 13, upper lid.

binocular vision; a horizontal strip below the tapetum is concerned with monocular vision. Their extents are suggested by their relatively poor vascularization.

Evisceration of the orbit is sometimes performed, usually under the local anesthetic technique devised by Peterson. In cattle the ophthalmic and maxillary nerves enter the orbit with those to the extraocular muscles, sharing a single opening that corresponds to the combined orbital and round foramina of other species. To block the nerves a needle is entered in the angle between the temporal and frontal processes of the zygomatic bone and pushed horizontally to graze past the rostral border of the coronoid process of the mandible. Penetration to a depth of about 7 cm brings the needle tip to the foramen orbitorotundum where the agent is deposited. A second deposit, sometimes made by redirecting the needle from the point of first insertion, is placed about the auriculopalpebral nerve where it crosses the zygomatic arch (Fig. 25–7/3).

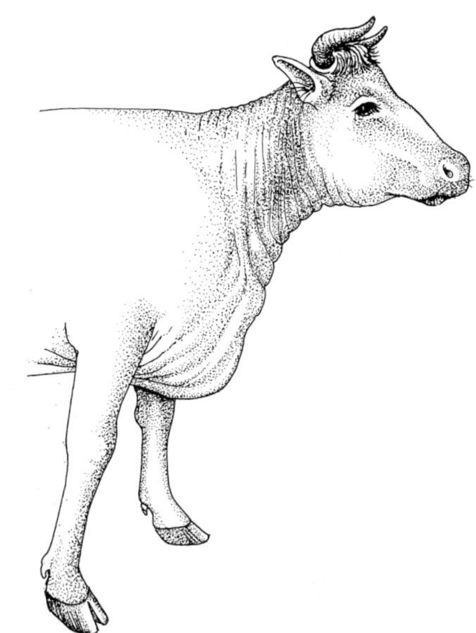

**Figure 25–24.** Large median skin fold (dewlap) at the caudal end of the neck.

## THE VENTRAL PART OF THE NECK

Dorsal cervical structures are described with the vertebral column (Chapter 26). The skin of the ventral aspect is freely movable and redundant in amount; it becomes folded and creased when the head is lowered to the ground. In addition, the caudal part of the neck carries the large dewlap that continues onto the brisket (breast) between the forelimbs (Fig. 25–24). There is scant evidence for the belief that this increase in surface area is important in heat dissipation as is sometimes claimed, for the zebu in particular. Zebu cattle do possess, here and elsewhere, more numerous, larger, and more saclike sweat glands than are found in cattle of European origin.

The *groove* over the course of the external jugular vein is generally obvious, at least in cows. It is bounded dorsally by the brachiocephalicus (cleidomastoideus) extending from the arm to the skull, and ventrally by the part (sternomandibularis) of the sternocephalicus that runs between the manubrium of the sternum and the angle of the jaw. Except in the most caudal part of the neck, a second part of the sternocephalicus (sternomastoideus) forms the floor of the groove and provides a substantial separation between the vein and the common carotid artery (Fig. 25–25/7). The *external jugular vein* is easily raised for injection and blood sampling since only the caudal part is covered by the cutaneous muscle and even this is rather weak. The vein is formed caudal to the parotid gland by the confluence of maxillary and linguofacial radicles (Fig. 25–2). It is the principal drainage of the head and neck but is assisted by the internal jugular vein, the vertebral vein, and the internal vertebral plexus.

The superficial muscles enclose the space that contains the cervical viscera and the vessels and nerves that make their way between the thorax and the head (Fig. 25–25). All of these organs are enclosed within tough fascial investments joined by looser tissue.

The *trachea* may be identified on deep palpation and is most easily appreciated toward the upper end of the neck, between the diverging sternocephalic muscles; even here it is not directly subcutaneous since the thin straplike sternothyrohyoid muscles follow its whole length. The trachea (/14) is small in section and slightly deeper than it is wide; its form makes it susceptible to narrowing by local pressure. The symmetry of its relations is disturbed by the devious course of the esophagus. Its structure is mainly remarkable for the concentration of lymphoid tissue in the dorsal retromucosal space (external to the tracheal muscle but within the cartilage rings).

Although the *esophagus* cannot be identified by palpation, its position is made evident by the swift movement along its track when the animal swallows. In its cervical course the esophagus gradually slips to the left of the trachea only to creep back to a more dorsal position as the thorax is approached. However, its position varies with posture; its course is considerably straightened when the neck is extended. The relations in the middle of the neck are shown in Figure 25–25.

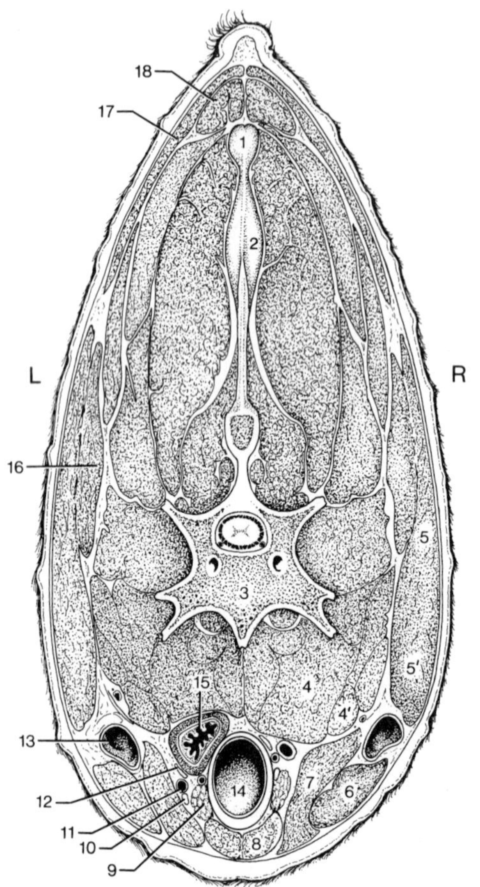


**Figure 25–25.** Transverse section through the middle of the bovine neck.

1, 2, Nuchal ligament (funiculus and lamina nuchae); 3, vertebra; 4, longus colli; 4′, longus capitis; 5, 5′, brachiocephalicus; 5, cleido-occipitalis; 5′, cleidomastoideus; 6, 7, sternocephalicus; 6, sternomandibularis; 7, sternomastoideus; 8, combined sternohyoideus and sternothyroideus; 9, thymus and internal jugular vein; 10, recurrent laryngeal nerve; 11, common carotid artery; 12, vagosympathetic trunk; 13, external jugular vein; 14, trachea; 15, esophagus; 16, omotransversarius; 17, trapezius; 18, rhomboideus.

The ruminant esophagus is very distensible, and the appearance that is common in the cadaver, when the lumen is very wide and the wall thin and slack, gives a misleading impression of the usual condition in life. The mucosa is remarkably insensitive, one reason why cattle rarely appear to be distressed by the passage of a stomach tube or probang. Although transport is normally rapid in both directions, chunks of food quite commonly become lodged in the esophagus. The predilection sites are at the origin from the pharynx, at the thoracic inlet, and level with the tracheal bifurcation.

The *thyroid gland* is almost completely divided into two lobes, each shaped like an inverted pyramid and placed laterally over the cricoid cartilage. They are tenuously joined by an isthmus that crosses the second tracheal ring ventrally. They are finely granular and brick-red in the adult but paler in the calf (see Fig. 6–4/*C*).

The *parathyroid glands* are small (ca. 8 to 10 mm) and, because irregular in shape and inconstant in position, are frequently difficult to find. They may be embedded in other structures—usually the thyroid, thymus, or mandibular gland. The external parathyroid most often lies cranial to the thyroid but caudal to the carotid bifurcation; the internal one is perhaps most often embedded in the thyroid or located between this and the trachea. They have been confused with lymph nodes, which they resemble superficially.

The *thymus* is large and lobulated and extends from the larynx to the pericardium in young animals (Fig. 25–26/1,2). Its cervical part is connected to the thoracic thymus by a narrow isthmus ventral to the trachea. The cervical part divides into two horns that taper over the lateral aspects of the trachea, possibly reaching the larynx; the cranial tip may be, or appear to be, detached and fragmented and more closely associated with the medial retropharyngeal lymph node and the mandibular and parathyroid glands. The thymus grows rapidly during the first 6 or 9 months of postnatal life, although it attains its greatest relative size much earlier. Indeed, involution may begin as early as the eighth week after birth. The tempo of regression varies, and the thymus, particularly its thoracic part, may still be quite large in animals several years old. Ultimately the isthmus and neck part disappear almost completely. The thymus of young calves is bright pink or even red but the organ lightens with age; its consistency also firms as the active tissue is progressively replaced by fatty fibrous tissue.

The *common carotid artery* runs dorsolateral to the trachea within a fascial sheath shared with the vagosympathetic trunk. The internal jugular vein and the recurrent laryngeal nerve are closely related to the sheath on the right side; the esophagus intervenes on the left. The artery ends over the lateral pharyngeal wall where it detaches a small occipital artery; the parent trunk is continued (without alteration of course) as the external carotid artery. In the fetus an internal carotid artery arises with the occipital artery, but the part proximal to the rete mirabile (see Fig. 7–33) begins to close even before birth; complete obliteration is usually achieved a few months after birth, although a residual lumen sometimes persists for a year or two (Fig. 25–27/4). The common carotid artery detaches no branches of individual consequence before its termination. Pulsation in the common carotid may sometimes be detected when the artery is pressed against the transverse processes of the vertebrae.

At this point brief mention may be made of the blood supply to the brain, less because of any clinical significance than on account of its relevance to the controversial Jewish and Muslim slaughter techniques, in which the animals are killed by a deep ritual slash of the neck without preliminary stunning.

The brain is supplied by a combination of vessels that feed very intricate arterial plexuses within the cranial cavity, external to the dura mater and submerged within the cavernous and associated venous sinuses. These plexuses, the retia mirabilia, are formed by many closely wound, anastomosing arteries. The retia are entered on their peripheral aspect from several sources (see Fig. 7–33); on the distal or cerebral side the network narrows to one emissary trunk that pierces the dural membrane to form the cerebral arterial circle with its fellow. The circle lies on the ventral aspect of the brain and gives off branches according to the conventional pattern. The basilar artery, which runs caudally over the medulla and continues down the spinal cord, is a contributor to the circle in cattle but leads blood from it in sheep. Though difficult to explain on hemodynamic grounds, all parts of the bovine brain are supplied by a mixture of carotid and vertebral blood, whereas in sheep the vertebral blood is restricted to the caudal part of the brainstem. These differences are germane to the ritual slaughter technique since the vertebral arteries are spared when the common carotid trunks are severed. The suggestion that abrupt reduction of the pressure within the cerebral arteries produces almost immediate loss of consciousness has been questioned.

The *vagosympathetic trunk* exhibits no particular features of note. The vagus and sympathetic components loosen their association and part company before entering the thorax. Their further courses and connections are described elsewhere. The recurrent laryngeal nerves resemble those of other species.

## THE LYMPHATIC STRUCTURES OF THE HEAD AND NECK

The most important lymph nodes of the head were mentioned in their topographical contexts; other smaller nodes that are usually found medial to the

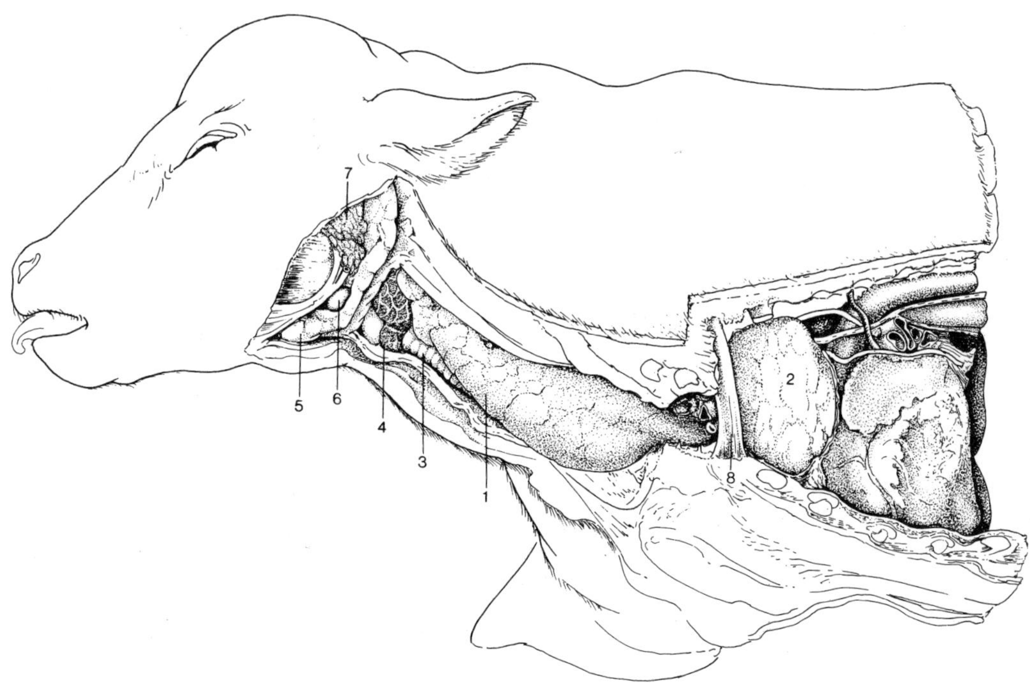


**Figure 25–26.** The thymus in the newborn calf.

1, Cervical part of thymus; 2, thoracic part of thymus; 3, trachea; 4, thyroid gland; 5, mandibular gland; 6, mandibular lymph node; 7, parotid gland; 8, first rib.

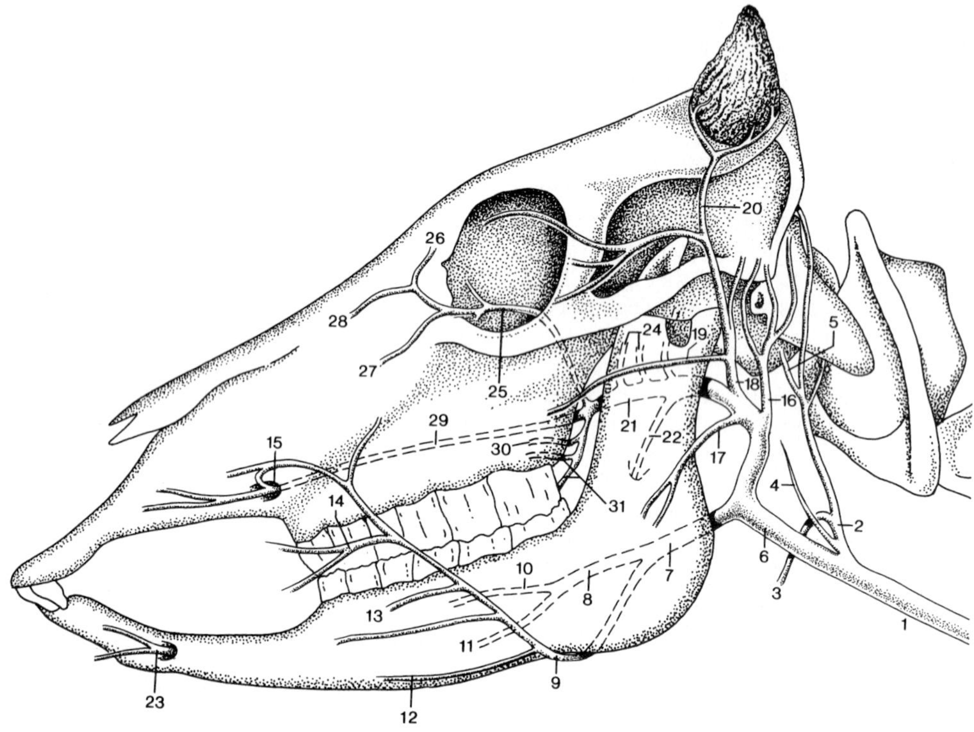


**Figure 25–27.** Branching of the left common carotid artery.

1, Common carotid a.; 2, occipital a.; 3, ascending palatine a.; 4, remnant of internal carotid a.; 5, medial meningeal a.; 6, external carotid a.; 7, linguofacial trunk; 8, lingual a.; 9, facial a.; 10, deep lingual a.; 11, sublingual a.; 12, submental a.; 13, inferior labial aa.; 14, superior labial a.; 15, infraorbital foramen; 16, caudal auricular a.; 17, masseteric branch; 18, superficial temporal a.; 19, transverse facial a.; 20, cornual a.; 21, maxillary a.; 22, inferior alveolar a.; 23, mental a; 24, rostral and caudal branches to rete mirabile; 25, malar a.; 26, angular a. of the eye; 27, caudal lateral nasal a.; 28, dorsal nasal a.; 29, infraorbital a.; 30, sphenopalatine a.; 31, major and minor palatine aa.

ramus of the mandible are of slight practical concern.

The *parotid node* (Fig. 25–2/13) receives lymph from the skin covering most of the head, especially the more dorsal areas. It also collects from the upper jaw, temporomandibular joint, masticatory muscles, nasal cavity, hard palate, orbit, and the region about the external ear. The efferent vessels pass to the lateral retropharyngeal node.

The territory of the *mandibular node* (/20) overlaps those of the parotid and medial retropharyngeal nodes. The chief afferent vessels come from the skin and underlying structures of the ventral part of the head and from the rostral part of the mouth, including the apex of the tongue. The efferent vessels pass to the lateral retropharyngeal node.

The large *medial retropharyngeal node* lies embedded in fat between the pharynx and the muscles below the cranial base (Figs. 25–10/20

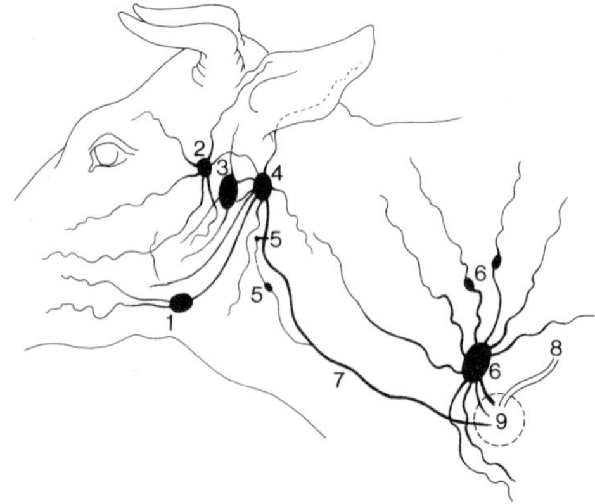


**Figure 25–28.** The lymph drainage of the head and neck.

1, Mandibular lymph node; 2, parotid lymph node; 3, medial retropharyngeal lymph node; 4, lateral retropharyngeal lymph node; 5, deep cervical lymph nodes; 6, superficial cervical lymph nodes; 7, tracheal duct; 8, thoracic duct; 9, area within which lymphatic vessels enter veins.

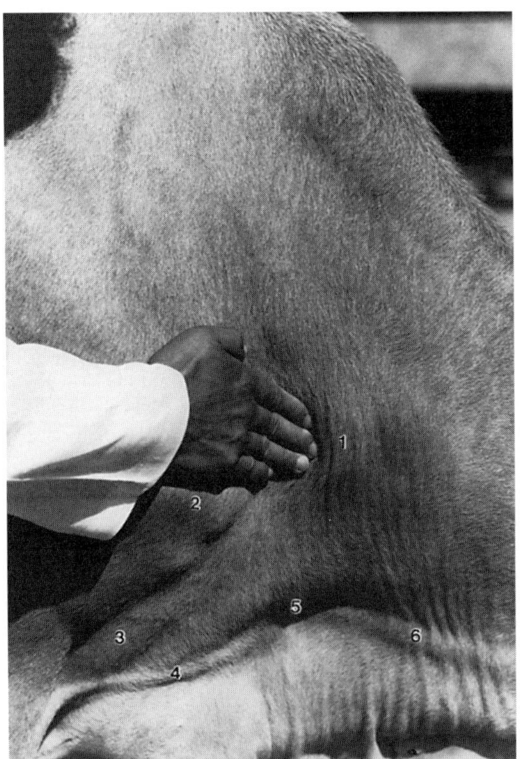


**Figure 25–29.** Palpation of the right superficial cervical lymph node in a cow with its head lowered; cranial is to the right.

1, Superficial cervical lymph node; 2, greater tubercle of humerus; 3, biceps; 4, cephalic vein; 5, caudal end of jugular groove; in its depth the carotid and axillary arteries may be palpated, the latter as it winds around the first rib; 6, external jugular vein.

and 25–21/12). It collects lymph from most of the deeper structures of the head, including the nasal and oral cavities, pharynx, larynx, cranium, and jaw muscles, and from the ventral part of the upper end of the neck. The efferent vessels once again drain into the *lateral retropharyngeal node,* which is the collecting center for the entire head (Fig. 25–28/4). This lateral node, which is placed below the atlantal wing (Fig. 25–2/14), also acts as a primary center for additional lymph vessels draining deeper structures of the head. It channels its outflow into a single large vessel, the tracheal duct, that runs down the neck within the fascia covering the lateral aspect of the trachea. The duct ends by joining the thoracic duct or by opening into one or another vein at the thoracic inlet; most usually the left tracheal duct opens into the thoracic duct while the right one drains directly into a major tributary of the cranial vena cava (Fig. 25–28/9).

A series of small *deep cervical lymph nodes* is spread along the course of each tracheal duct. These are supposedly divided into cranial, middle, and caudal clusters and receive lymph from the structures within the cervical visceral space. They transmit this lymph to the tracheal duct, sometimes directly, sometimes after serial passage through several nodes within the group. Usually one or more of the most caudal of these nodes receive the efferent vessels of the axillary lymph center of the forelimb, as well as smaller trunks coming directly from the brisket.

A single, much larger node lies in the lower part of the neck in front of the scapula. This is the *superficial cervical* (prescapular) *node,* which rests on the deep muscles over the cervical vertebrae; it is easily palpated, though covered by the omotransversarius (Fig. 25–29/1). It collects from the skin and underlying muscles over a very wide area extending from the middle of the neck to the caudal part of the thorax, including the proximal part of the forelimb. The flow through the node is compartmentalized, particular portions of the node being related to different parts of the drainage field. The large efferent vessels open variously into the major lymph and venous trunks in the vicinity.

Any of the major nodes may be duplicated.

## Selected Bibliography

Anderson, D.E., R.M. DeBowes, E.M. Gaughan, et al.: Endoscopic evaluation of the nasopharynx, pharynx, and larynx of Jersey cows. Am. J. Vet. Res. 55:901–904, 1994.

Ashdown, R.R., and S. Done: Color Atlas of Veterinary Anatomy: The Ruminants. Baltimore: University Park Press, 1984.

Bowen, J.S.: Dehorning the mature goat. JAVMA 171:1249–1250, 1977.

Brown, P.J., J.G. Lane, and V.M. Lucke: Developmental cysts in the upper neck of Anglo-Nubian goats. Vet. Rec. 125:256–258, 1989.

Butler, W.F.: Innervation of the horn region in domestic ruminants. Vet. Rec. 80:490–492, 1967.

Dehghani, S.N., C.J. Lischer, U. Iselin, et al.: Sialography in cattle: Technique and normal appearance. Vet. Radiol. Ultrasound 35:433–439, 1994.

De Schaepdrijver, L., P. Simoens, H. Lauwers, J.P. De Geest: Retinal vascular patterns in domestic animals. Vet. Sci. 47:34–42, 1989.

Diesem, C.: Gross anatomic structure of the equine and bovine orbit and its contents. Am. J. Vet. Res. 29:1769–1781, 1968.

Freeman, L.E., and H.F. Troutt: Lymph drainage of the conjunctiva: Topographic anatomic study in calves. Am. J. Vet. Res. 46:1967–1970, 1985.

Hague, B.A., and R.N. Hooper: Cosmetic dehorning in goats. Vet. Surg. 26:332–334, 1997.

Hoffsis, G.: Surgical (cosmetic) dehorning in cattle. Vet. Clin. North Am. Food Anim. Pract. 11:159–169, 1995.

Hull, B.L.: Dehorning the adult goat. Vet. Clin. North Am. Food Anim. Pract. 11:183–185, 1995.

Lambooy, E., and W. Spanjaard: Effect of the shooting position on the stunning of calves by captive bolt. Vet. Rec. 109:359–361, 1981.

Levinger, I.M.: Jewish method of slaughtering animals for food and its influence on blood supply to the brain and on the normal functioning of the nervous system. Anim. Reg. Stud. 2:111–118, 1979.

McCormack, J.E.: Variations of the ocular fundus of the bovine species. Scope 18:21–28, 1974.

Mitchell, B.: Local analgesia of the bovine horn and horn base. Vet. Rec. 79:133–136, 1966.

Pavaux, C.: A Color Atlas of Bovine Visceral Anatomy. London, Wolfe Publishing, 1983.

Rebhun, W.C.: Diseases of the bovine orbit and globe. JAVMA 175:171–175, 1979.

Ross, M.W., D.W. Richardson, R.P. Hackett, et al.: Nasal obstruction caused by cystic nasal conchae in cattle. JAVMA 188:857–860, 1986.

Roussel, A.J., L. Talioferra, C.B. Navarre, and R.N. Hooper: Catheterization of the auricular vein in cattle: 68 cases (1991–1994). JAVMA 208:905–907, 1996.

Soana, S., G. Bertoni, G. Gnudi, and P. Botti: Anatomo-radiographic study of prenatal development of bovine fetal teeth. Anat. Histol. Embryol. 26:107–113, 1997.

Verschooten, F., and W. Oyaert: Radiological diagnosis of esophageal disorders in the bovine. J. Am. Vet. Radiol. Soc. 18:85–89, 1977.

Ward, J.L., and W.C. Rebhun: Chronic frontal sinusitis in dairy cattle: 12 cases (1978–1989). JAVMA 201:326–328, 1992.

Williams, C.S.F.: Routine sheep and goat procedures. Vet. Clin. North Am. Food Anim. Pract. 6:737–758, 1990.

Wright, H.J., D.S. Adams, and F.J. Trigo: Meningoencephalitis after hot-iron disbudding of goat kids. Vet. Med. 78:599–601, 1983.

# CHAPTER 26

# The Neck, Back, and Tail of the Ruminants

## CONFORMATION AND SURFACE FEATURES

The back and loins are shaped over the framework of the thoracic and lumbar vertebrae. The loins are sharply divided from the flanks by the prominent tips of the lumbar transverse processes, but the boundaries of the back cannot be defined so precisely since the back blends smoothly with the lateral thoracic wall and incorporates the upper parts of the shoulder blades with their cartilages and covering muscles. It is convenient to include in this chapter the few observations that are necessary on the dorsal sacral region, which merges with the quarters and root of the tail.

In the animal standing quietly the dorsal contour is slightly raised over the withers, but otherwise it follows a fairly straight line from immediately behind the skull to the tail root (Fig. 26–1).* The line of the neck, which is based on the funicular part of the nuchal ligament, varies, of course, with the carriage of the head.

The dorsal contour of the trunk is prescribed by the summits of the spinous processes of the vertebrae, many of which can be palpated separately. Identification of individual bones is most reliable if begun at the wide space between the upright process of the last lumbar vertebra and the sloping cranial margin of the median sacral crest. The sacral crest can be followed caudally until it is succeeded by the separate projections of the spinous processes of the caudal vertebrae; any doubt about the identity of these processes may be resolved by pumping the tail up and down to discover the very mobile joint between the first and second tail bones (Fig. 26–3/6). Certainty in identifying the first intercaudal space has a special importance since this is the site for injection of local anesthetic when producing "low" epidural anesthesia (p. 652). The tail root is sometimes elevated, especially in cows during estrus.

Working cranially from the lumbosacral space, the lumbar spinous processes are easily distinguished in lean animals. Enumeration becomes more difficult over the caudal part of the chest where several processes converge, and the count is completely lost where the vertebrae become enclosed between the scapular cartilages. The first thoracic spine lies cranial to the scapulae where it can be felt on deep palpation even though it fails to approach close to the skin. The cervical vertebrae cannot be reached from above but their general position is detectable on palpation from the side. The transverse processes are well developed and divided into two parts, of which the ventral one is quite large; this is very obvious at the sixth cervical vertebra. Despite this, the individual identification of these bones is difficult until the wing of the atlas provides an unmistakable landmark.

Additional features that may be picked out in the region of the hindquarters include the salient sacral tubers of the pelvis, which lie to each side of the lumbosacral space, and the strong iliac crests, which join these projections to the coxal tubers. The crests are raised above their surroundings and are crossed by cranial prolongations of the gluteal musculature.

The head is carried higher in sheep and goats; these species also slope at the croup.

## THE VERTEBRAL COLUMN

The vertebral axis runs parallel to the skin line in the loins and caudal part of the back but more cranially it is deflected ventrally. It reaches its lowest level at the entrance to the thorax; an abrupt flexure there places it on a path that gradually returns closer to the dorsal border as it ascends the neck (Fig. 26–1).

The vertebral skeleton and articulations follow the usual pattern, and few features need be

*The description refers to cattle of European origin. The pronounced hump in cattle of the zebu *(Bos indicus)* line (and their crosses) is mainly due to enlargement of the rhomboideus muscles.

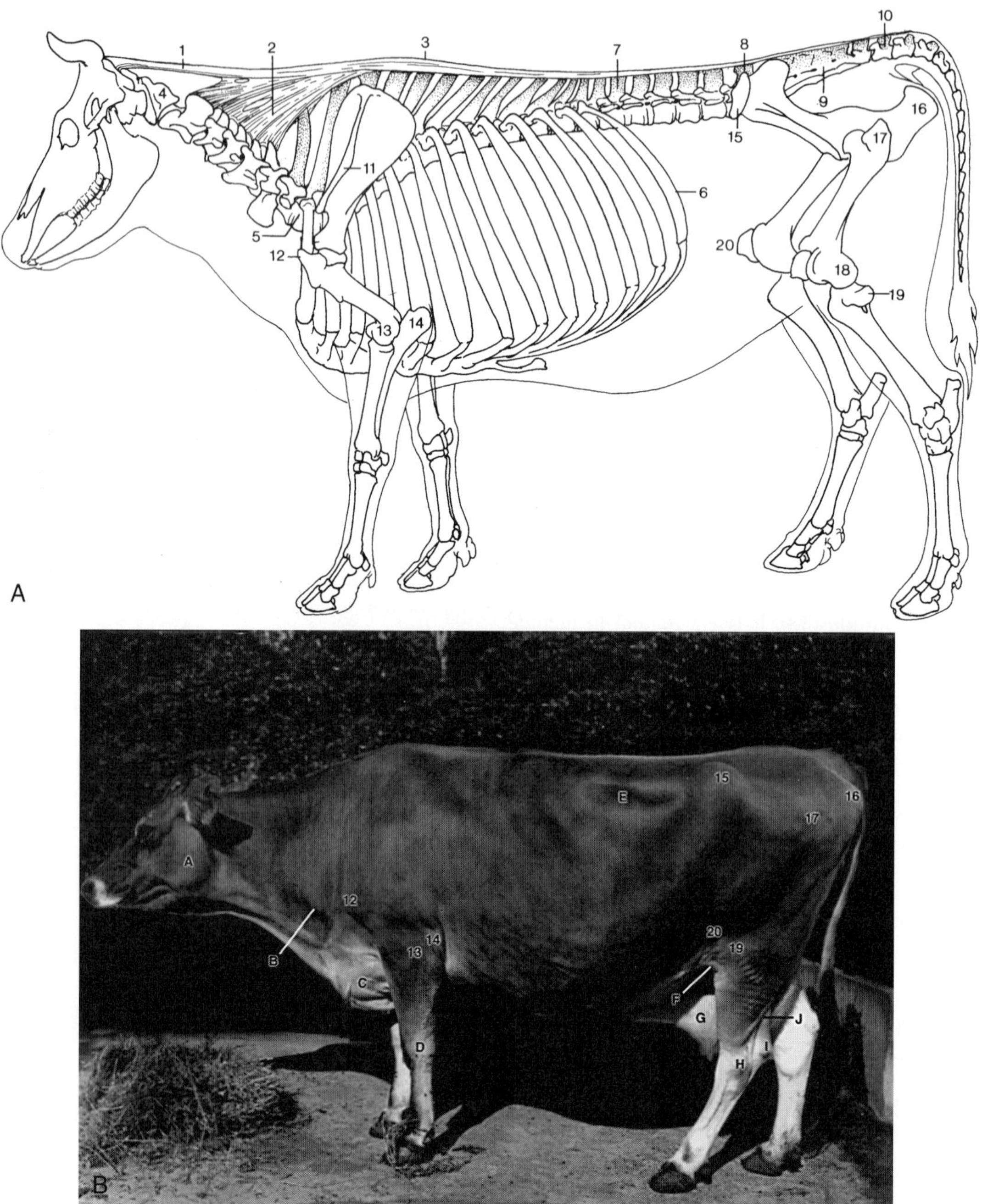


**Figure 26–1.** *A*, Skeleton with nuchal and supraspinous ligaments; most labeled parts are palpable. *B*, Cow in good condition.

1, 2, Nuchal ligament; 1, funiculus nuchae; 2, lamina nuchae; 3, supraspinous ligament; 4, atlas; 5, last cervical vertebra (C7); 6, 13th rib; 7, first lumbar vertebra (L1); 8, last lumbar vertebra (L6); 9, sacrum; 10, first caudal vertebra; 11, spine of scapula; 12, greater tubercle; 13, 14, palpable features at elbow joint; 13, lateral epicondyle; 14, olecranon; 15, coxal tuber; 16, ischial tuber; 17, greater trochanter; 18, 19, 20, palpable features of stifle joint; 18, lateral condyle; 19, lateral condyle of tibia and remnant of fibula; 20, patella.

A, Masseter; B, prominent lamina of C6; C, brisket; D, carpus; E, paralumbar fossa; F, flank fold; G, udder; H, hock joint; I, calcaneus (point of the hock); J, lateral saphenous vein.

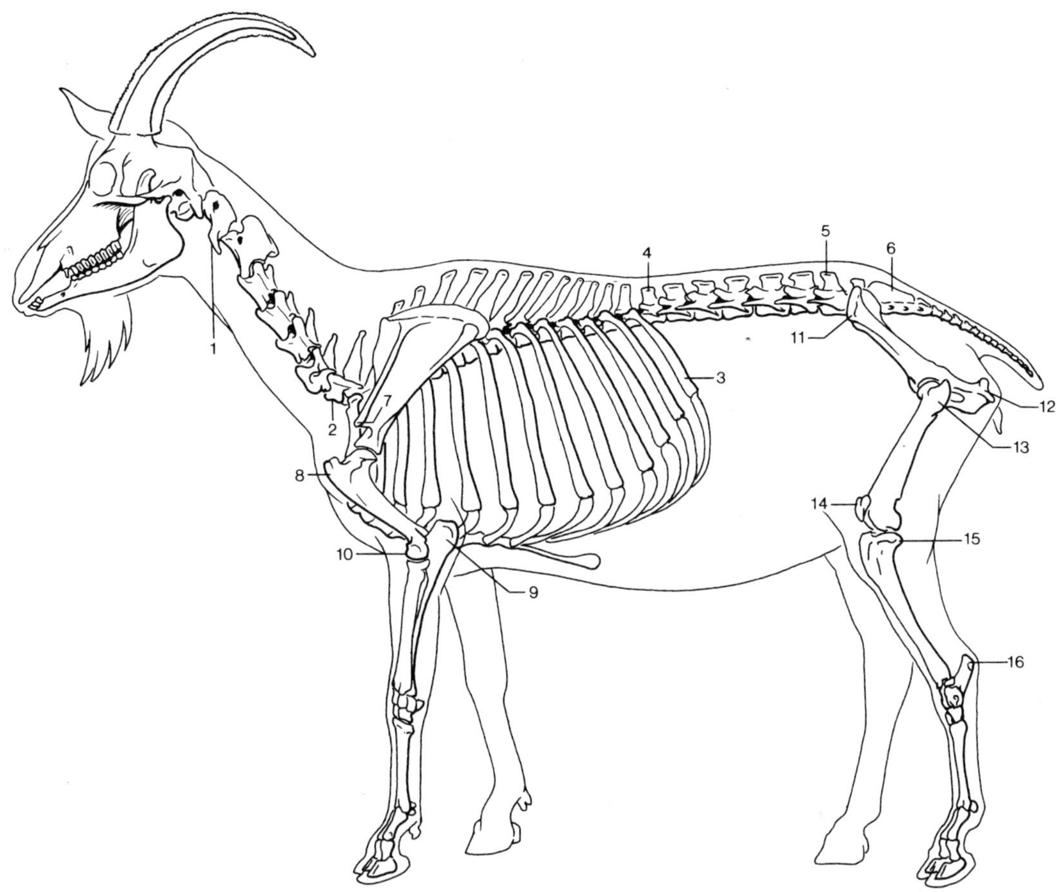


**Figure 26–2.** The skeleton of the goat. Most labeled parts of the skeleton are palpable.

1, Atlas; 2, last cervical vertebra (C7); 3, last rib; 4, first lumbar vertebra (L1); 5, last lumbar vertebra (L7); 6, sacrum; 7, acromion; 8, greater tubercle; 9, olecranon; 10, lateral epicondyle; 11, coxal tuber; 12, ischial tuber; 13, greater trochanter; 14, patella; 15, lateral condyle of tibia; 16, calcaneus.

mentioned. The vertebral formula is C7, T13, L6, S5, Cd18–20 in cattle; and C7, T13, L6(7), S4 (sheep) or S5 (goat), Cd16–18 in small ruminants. The great mobility of the neck allows the animal to raise and lower its head and to reach its side with its tongue. Most cervical movements represent the summation of small changes at several joints, but the adoption of the grazing position requires a more considerable straightening at the cervicothoracic joint where the neck vertebrae are brought into line with those of the chest. Although movements of the thoracic region are limited by the presence of the rib cage, the greatest flexibility of the trunk is found cranial to the level of the diaphragm. Behind this, movement is greatly restricted, especially in the lateral direction, by the close fit of the articular processes and the tightness of the capsules that embrace them. Greater mobility is again found at the lumbosacral joint.

The generally rather limited flexibility of the spine is suggested by the relative shortness of the intervertebral discs, which in cattle contribute only 10% of the length of the column. The discs have the usual construction and are subject to the same degenerative changes as occur in other species—progressive dehydration and collagenization of the nuclei with fragmentation of the enclosing fibrous bundles. These phenomena, which are part of the normal aging process, shade by imperceptible degrees into more severe and frankly pathological changes. While it appears that all discs are equally susceptible to degeneration, it is the lumbosacral disc that is most commonly grossly damaged because of the greater stress to which it is subjected by the special mobility of the lumbosacral articulation. Disc lesions are sometimes accompanied by changes in the lumbosacral synovial articulations and by the formation of abnormal bony outgrowths (osteophytes) from the ventral margins of the vertebral bodies. Certain of these common changes have a particular importance in bulls since they may lead to inability to serve.

The elastic *nuchal ligament* is the only ligamentous structure that needs to be described (Fig. 26–1/1,2). It consists of two parts, as in the horse. The funicular part, which runs between the occiput and the highest spines of the withers, is a paired cord that is rounded in cross section at its occipital attachment but widens as it passes caudally. It attaches to the sides of the first few thoracic spines, close to their summits; caudal to this it approaches and fuses with its fellow to form the supraspinous ligament that caps the bone processes. The rhomboideus and trapezius muscles cover the funicular part of the ligament, in contrast to the arrangement in the horse (see Fig. 25–25/1,2). The laminar part of the nuchal ligament lies in the median plane between the symmetrical dorsal muscles of the neck; it is divided into a cranial paired web that extends between the funicular part and the second to the fourth cervical bones, and an unpaired sheet that fills the triangle between the first thoracic and last one or two cervical spinous processes. In addition to relieving the cervical muscles, the nuchal ligament has an occasional significance in determining the track followed by infection. No cranial nuchal bursa exists, but a supraspinous bursa frequently is present between the ligament and the first few thoracic spinous processes.

## THE VERTEBRAL CANAL

The vertebral canal is widest within the atlas and tapers rapidly within the sacrum; in between, it is most expanded where it contains the swellings of the spinal cord that give rise to the nerves that form the limb plexuses. Access to the vertebral canal is frequently necessary to withdraw cerebrospinal fluid from the subarachnoid space or to introduce local anesthetic into the epidural space. Therapeutic agents are also occasionally injected into these spaces. Examination of the skeleton shows that while entry is theoretically possible through any of the interarcuate spaces, it is easiest at the wider gaps between the atlas and the skull, at the lumbosacral joint, and between the first two vertebrae of the tail (Fig. 26–3). The first intercaudal space is conveniently large, measuring about 2 × 2 cm. Most other interarcuate spaces measure only a few millimeters in each direction, and since they lie at a considerable depth below the skin they are not easily located when probing with a needle. Epidural injections through the cranial (especially the first) interlumbar interarcuate spaces are occasionally made to obtain local anesthesia of the flank. A slightly oblique approach from a point of entry a little lateral and caudal to the target space is usually adopted, as it gives the least risk of impingement of the needle on bone.

The cord reaches more or less through the first sacral vertebra in adult cattle and considerably farther in young calves, perhaps into the caudal half of the sacrum. It may occupy almost the whole sacrum in the small ruminant species.

It is divided into 8 cervical, 13 thoracic, 6 lumbar, 5 sacral, and (usually) 5 caudal segments. The eight cervical segments are accommodated within the seven neck vertebrae, while each of the thoracic and cranial lumbar segments shows an almost exact correspondence with the bone of the same designation. The cranial shift of the more caudal part of the cord leaves the canal within the last lumbar vertebra available for occupation by

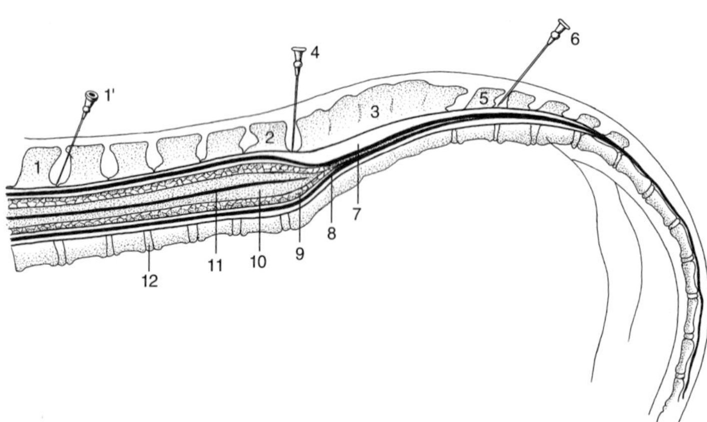


**Figure 26–3.** Caudal part of the bovine vertebral canal and its contents, schematic. Epidural injection sites are indicated by the needles.

1, First lumbar vertebra; 1′, needle in position for flank anesthesia; 2, last lumbar vertebra (L6); 3, sacrum; 4, needle in lumbosacral space; 5, first caudal vertebra; 6, needle between first and second caudal vertebrae (tail block); 7, epidural space; 8, dura mater; 9, subarachnoid space; 10, spinal cord; 11, central canal; 12, intervertebral disc.

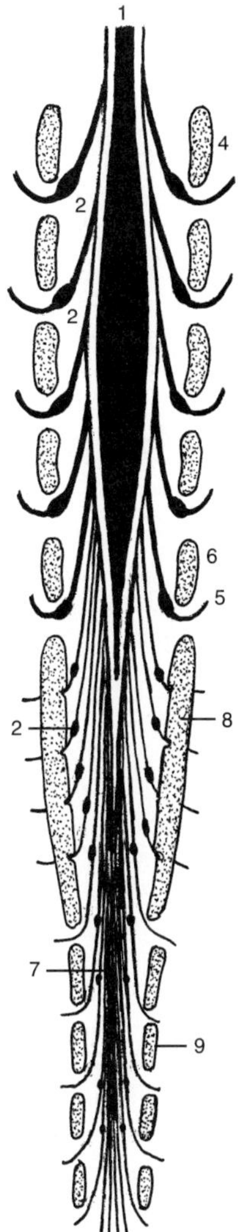


**Figure 26–4.** The relationship to the vertebrae of the caudal end of the spinal cord and its branches, schematic dorsal view. Note the position of the spinal ganglia (2). The schema indicates the situation in adult cattle. The cord extends to the second or even third sacral vertebra in the newborn calf and in adult sheep and goats.

1, Spinal cord; 2, spinal ganglia; 3, second lumbar spinal nerve; 4, section of arch of second lumbar vertebra; 5, sixth lumbar nerve; 6, section of arch of sixth lumbar vertebra; 7, cauda equina; 8, section of sacrum; 9, section of arch of second caudal vertebra.

the five short and telescoped sacral segments (Fig. 26–4). The subarachnoid space extends well into the sacrum and its dimensions are sufficiently generous to make subarachnoid puncture a relatively simple procedure at the lumbosacral level (Fig. 26–3/4).

The *internal vertebral plexus* (Fig. 26–5/1) has the same general organization and functions as in other species but presents two features of particular clinical interest. The first consists in the possibility of the plexus conveying blood that has been diverted from the caudal vena cava when this is narrowed or obstructed by ruminal tympany; compression of the vena cava may be direct or exerted indirectly by a shearing displacement of the liver against the diaphragm (Fig. 26–6). The second significant feature lies in the risk of hemorrhage in the performance of subarachnoid or epidural puncture.

## THE VESSELS OF THE TAIL

The median artery and vein of the tail require brief notice. The artery, which continues the median sacral, is ventral to the vein for most of the length of the tail and is commonly used for pulse-taking; the usual site is about 18 cm from the root of the tail. The vessels lie side by side in the most proximal part of the tail (Cd2 or Cd3) where both artery and vein are available for obtaining blood, although this site is an unwise choice because of

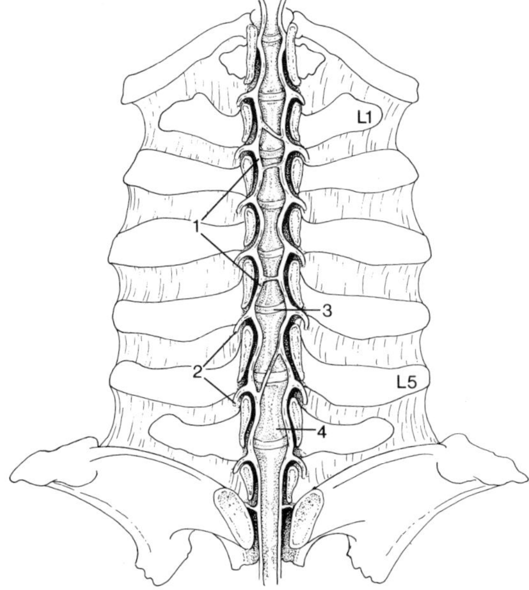


**Figure 26–5.** Dorsal view of the venous drainage in the bovine vertebral canal. The internal vertebral plexus, with its internal connections and its lateral segmental branches, has been exposed.

1, Internal vertebral plexus; 2, intervertebral veins; 3, an intervertebral disc; 4, a vertebral body.

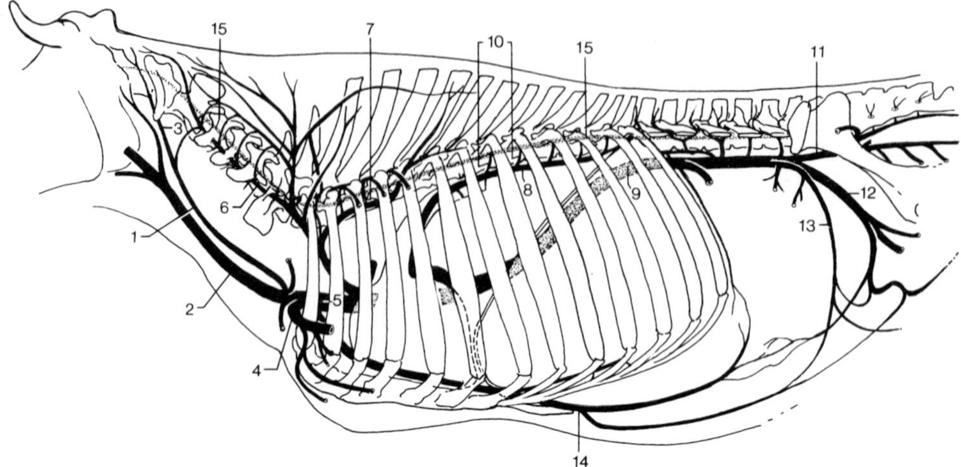


**Figure 26–6.** The connections of the major veins with the vertebral plexus–azygous system. Note specifically the connections between the internal vertebral plexus (15) and the intercostal veins (10) and between the plexus and the branches of the vertebral vein (6).

1, Internal jugular v.; 2, external jugular v.; 3, occipital v.; 4, axillary v.; 5, cranial vena cava; 6, vertebral v.; 7, supreme intercostal v.; 8, left azygous v.; 9, caudal vena cava; 10, intercostal vv.; 11, internal iliac v.; 12, external iliac v.; 13, deep circumflex iliac v.; 14, cranial epigastric v.; 15, internal vertebral plexus, stippled in the vertebral canal.

the inevitable fecal contamination of this portion of the tail (Plate 29/*A*). At this level both vessels lie against the ventral aspect of the caudal vertebrae where they are protected by the hemal processes (Fig. 26–7). Since these processes unite to form hemal arches on the first few tail vertebrae (see Fig. 2–12/*E*,9), the vessels are accessible only at the intervertebral level in the proximal part of the tail.

It is usual to dock the tail of lambs.

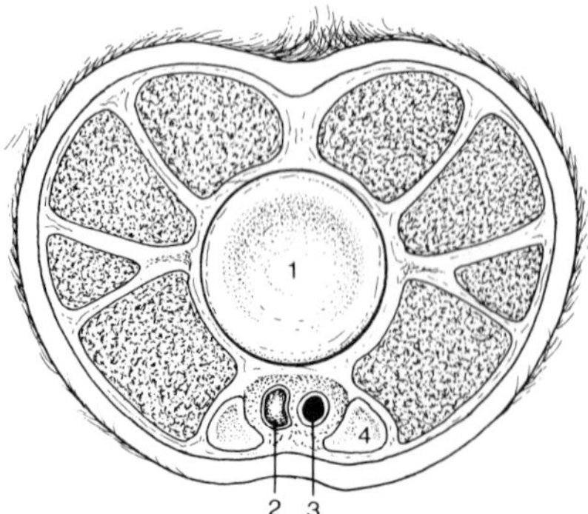


**Figure 26–7.** Transverse section of the bovine tail between Cd3 and 4.

1, Intervertebral disc; 2, median caudal vein; 3, median caudal artery; 4, hemal process.

## Selected Bibliography


Agerholm, J.S., A. Basse, and J. Arnbjerg: Vertebral fractures in newborn calves. Acta Vet. Scand. 34:379–384, 1993.

Almquist, J.O., and R.G. Thomson: Relation of sexual behavior and ejaculation frequency to severity of vertebral body osteophytes in dairy and beef bulls. JAVMA 163:163–168, 1973.

Ashdown, R.R., and S. Done: Color Atlas of Veterinary Anatomy: The Ruminants. Baltimore, University Park Press, 1984.

Bane, A., and H.J. Hansen: Spinal changes in the bull and their significance in serving inability. Cornell Vet. 52:362–384, 1962.

Caulkett, N.A., D.G. MacDonald, E.D. Janzen, et al.: Xylazine hydrochloride epidural analgesia: A method of providing sedation and analgesia to facilitate castration of mature bulls. Compend. Contin. Educ. Pract. Vet. 15:1155–1159, 1993.

Caulkett, N., P.H. Cribb, and T. Duke: Xylazine epidural analgesia for cesarean section in cattle. Can. Vet. J. 34:674–676, 1993.

Davis, L.E., H.E. Dale, and B.A. Westfall: Effects of ruminal insufflation on the venous return in the goat. Am. J. Vet. Res. 25:1166–1174, 1964.

Farquharson, J.: Paravertebral lumbar anesthesia in bovine species. JAVMA 97:54–57, 1940.

Hansen, H.J.: Studies on the pathology of the lumbosacral disc in female cattle. Acta Orthop. Scand. 25:161–165, 1956.

Kirk, E.J., R.L. Kitchell, and R.D. Johnson: Lumbosacral plexus in the sheep. Anat. Histol. Embryol. 15:174–175, 1986.

Skarda, R.T.: Local and regional anesthesia in ruminants and swine. Vet. Clin. North Am. Food Anim. Pract. 12:579–625, 1996.

Skarda, R.T., and W.W. Muir: Segmental lumbar epidural analgesia in cattle. Am. J. Vet. Res. 40:52–57, 1979.

Skarda, R.T., W.W. Muir, and J.A.E. Hubbell: Comparative study of continuous lumbar segmental epidural and subarachnoid analgesia in Holstein cows. Am. J. Vet. Res. 50:39–44, 1989.

Slijper, E.J.: Comparative biologic-anatomical investigations on the vertebral column and spinal musculature of mammals. K. Ned. Akad. Wet. 2:1–128, 1946.

Smuts, M.M.S.: The foramina of the cervical vertebrae of the ox. Part I: Atlas and axis; part II: Cervical vertebrae 3–7. Zentralbl. Vet. Med. C 3:289–295, 1974; C 4:24–37, 1975.

Smuts, M.M.S.: Venous drainage of the cervical vertebrae of the ox. Onderstep. J. Vet. Res. 44:233–248, 1977.

St. Jean, G., R.T. Skarda, W.W. Muir, and G.F. Hoffsis: Caudal epidural analgesia induced by xylazine administration in cows. Am. J. Vet. Res. 51:1232–1236, 1990.

Welker, B., and P. Modransky: Performing anesthesia of the paralumbar fossa in ruminants. Vet. Med. 89:163–169, 1994.

Zaugg, J.L., and M. Nussbaum: Epidural injection of xylazine: A new option for surgical analgesia of the bovine abdomen and udder. Vet. Med. 85:1043–1046, 1990.

# CHAPTER 27

# The Thorax of the Ruminants

## CONFORMATION AND SURFACE ANATOMY

The shape and extent of the thoracic cavity do not correspond to the expectations raised by the conformation of the living animal. This is for the usual reasons—the inclusion of the upper parts of the forelimbs in the skin of the trunk (Plate 29/*B*), the divergence of the lines of the back and brisket (the lower part of the thorax cranial to the forelimbs) from the internal boundaries of the thorax, and the forward projection of the diaphragm (Fig. 27–1).

The shoulder and arm fit snugly against the thoracic wall. Only a few features of the limb skeleton are directly palpable. The orientation of the scapula is revealed by the location of its spine—marked by a ridge—and by palpation of its cranial and caudal angles of which the latter lies over the vertebrae dorsal to the sixth rib. The dorsal margin of the scapular cartilage is also palpable; it is almost level with the ridge of the withers. The point of the shoulder lies above and in front of the first sternochondral joint (Fig. 27–2). The humerus slopes caudoventrally between the shoulder and the elbow. The position of the lower joint may be deduced from its relation to the olecranon process whose summit lies over the fifth intercostal space, just dorsal to the costochondral joints (Fig. 27–1). The forelimb can be rotated against the thoracic wall and may also be shifted bodily for some distance, but the range of movement is not sufficient to uncover the whole thorax, and parts of the heart and lungs cannot be made accessible for auscultation and percussion.

Cranial and caudal to the limb, much of the thorax is covered by the girdle muscles converging on their scapular and humeral insertions and by the external oblique and rectus muscles of the abdomen. It is not possible to palpate all the ribs, or the whole lengths of those that can be reached, but normally it is not difficult to identify the ribs from the 13th forward to the 6th. This enumeration discloses the increasing obliquity of the caudal bones and their great breadth, especially toward their lower ends. The costal cartilages slope increasingly forward from their unions with the ribs as the series is followed caudally. The first eight meet the sternum directly; the five following join to complete the costal arch, which furnishes the boundary of the flank (Fig. 27–1).

## THE THORACIC WALL

The structure of the lateral walls of the bovine thorax is mainly remarkable for the great breadth of the ribs. The reduction of the spaces between them hampers surgery, and access to the thorax, although only occasionally indicated, generally requires resection of one or more ribs. The ribs of the smaller ruminants are relatively narrower. The various respiratory muscles need not be listed, but note should be taken of the way in which the thick longissimus dorsi and the iliocostalis cover the vertebral extremities of the ribs and so limit the area of the lung available for percussion and auscultation.

In the ventral parts of the spaces intercostal vessels follow both margins of the ribs, a point to bear in mind when contemplating puncture of the pleural or pericardial cavity.

The sternal ribs have a tight connection with the sternum and form a part of the thorax that is narrow and rather rigid (Fig. 27–3). The asternal ribs are more strongly bowed and enclose a much wider space; their movements account for almost all the pulmonary ventilation not attributable to the diaphragm.

As in other species, the diaphragm is attached to the lumbar vertebrae by the tendons of the thick dorsal crural portions, and laterally and ventrally to the ribs and sternum by the fleshy sternocostal part. The salient centrum tendineum reaches as far forward as the sixth rib, only a little caudal to the point of the elbow in the animal standing square. Because of the shorter thorax, the slope of the diaphragm is steeper in ruminants than in the horse (Fig. 27–4/22).

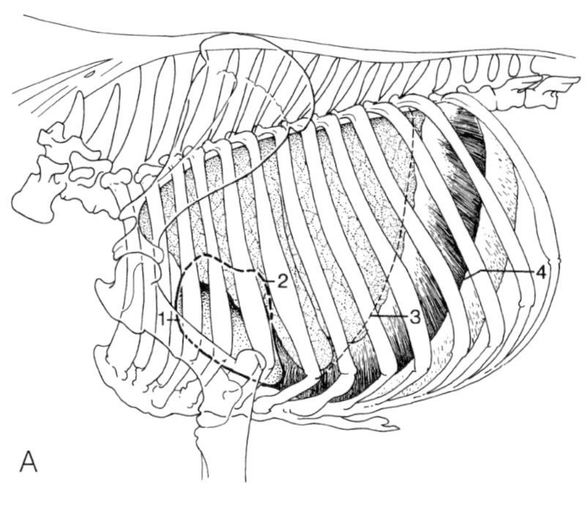


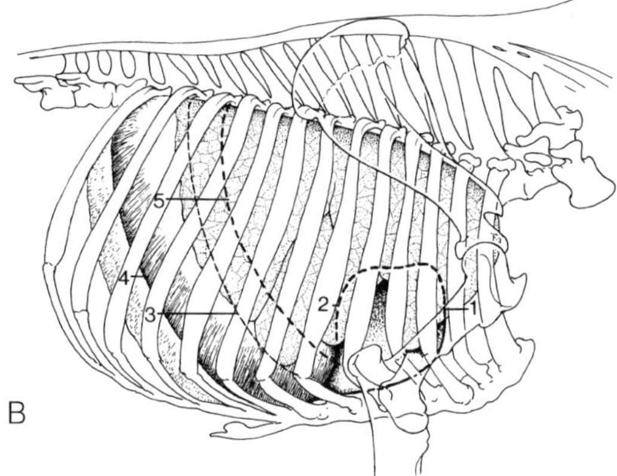


**Figure 27–1.** Left *(A)* and right *(B)* projections of the bovine heart and lungs on the thoracic wall. The basal border of the lung and the line of pleural reflection are also shown.

1, Cranial extent of heart; 2, caudal extent of heart; 3, basal border of lung; 4, line of pleural reflection; 5, caudal border of lung percussion area, shown on right side.

Although the activity of the diaphragm predominates in normal breathing, cattle can survive diaphragmatic paralysis but suffer greater disturbance than is usual in smaller animals.

## THE PLEURAL CAVITIES

Although each *pleural sac* resembles one half of a truncated cone, the asymmetry is more pronounced than in most species.

The external relationships of the pleural sacs are of great significance since they influence the approach to different thoracic and abdominal organs. Three features of pleural topography are of particular clinical interest. The first is situated cranially where the right costal pleura extends into the neck for a space of 3 to 5 cm in front of the middle part of the first rib before turning medially to join the mediastinum. The *cupula pleurae* formed in this way contains the tip of the cranial lobe of the right lung. The cupula always extends across the midline in conformity with the greater development of the right lung (Fig. 27–1/*B*). The main significance of the arrangement lies in the possibility of entry to the right pleural sac following penetrating wounds to the base of the neck.

The *caudal reflection of the pleura* from the thoracic wall to the diaphragm is more important. This follows a cranially concave line that ascends steeply in its caudal part; the path runs through the eighth costochondral junction, the middle of the 11th rib, and reaches the 12th rib a little below the lateral margin of the iliocostalis (Fig. 27–1/4). Behind this line the diaphragm is attached to the intercostal tissues and ribs, and the abdomen may be approached without risk of injury to the pleura.

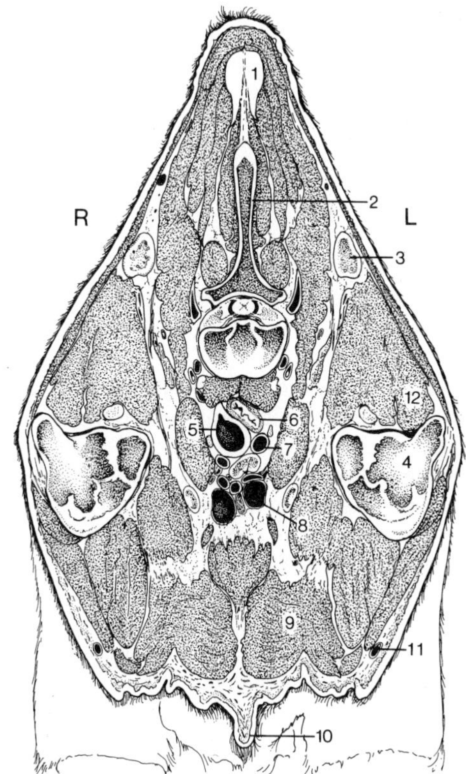


**Figure 27–2.** Transverse section of the bovine neck just cranial to the thoracic inlet.

1, Funicular part of nuchal ligament; 2, spinous process of seventh cervical vertebra; 3, superficial cervical lymph node; 4, proximal end of humerus; 5, trachea; 6, esophagus; 7, common carotid artery; 8, external jugular vein; 9, pectoralis descendens; 10, dewlap; 11, cephalic vein; 12, supraspinatus.

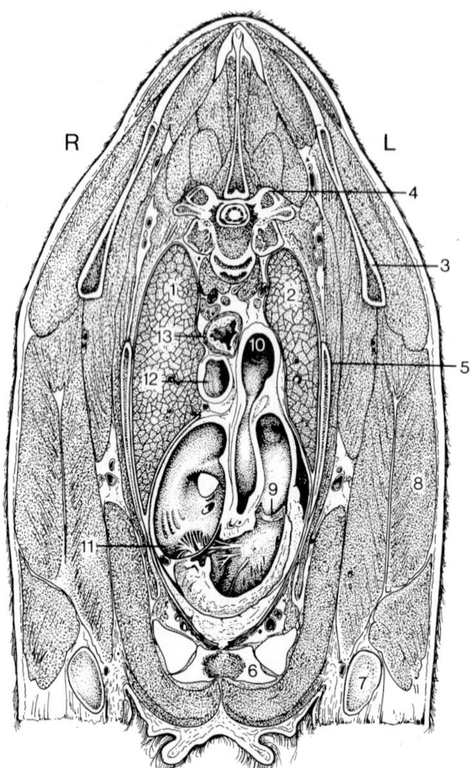


**Figure 27–3.** Transverse section of the bovine thorax at the level of the fourth thoracic vertebra. Note the asymmetry of the lungs.

1, 2, Cranial lobes of right and left lungs; 3, scapula; 4, fourth thoracic vertebra; 5, third rib; 6, sternum; 7, olecranon; 8, long head of triceps; 9, pulmonary valve; 10, aortic arch; 11, right atrioventricular valve; 12, trachea; 13, esophagus.

A rather exaggerated idea of the extent of the costodiaphragmatic recess may be obtained from the dead animal, in which collapse of the lungs and the accumulation of ruminal gas post mortem may thrust the diaphragm abnormally far into the thorax. It should be noted that in the small ruminant species the pleural sacs extend significantly farther caudally—even beyond the upper end of the last rib into the corner of the flank.

The third significant detail concerns the attachment of the *mediastinum* to the diaphragm. Although the mediastinum lies more or less in the median plane for much of its extent, the ventral half of the caudal part is deflected by the larger size of the base of the right lung and comes to lie far to the left. Although asymmetrical in relation to the thorax, its projection roughly bisects the reticulum within the abdomen, a point of great relevance when considering the probable course taken by a foreign body penetrating the diaphragm from the reticulum (Figs. 27–5 and 27–7; see also Fig. 28–17).

Thoracocentesis is best performed in the standing animal by puncture of the sixth or seventh intercostal space directly dorsal to the costochondral junctions. Pericardiocentesis is most safely performed at the same level of the fifth space, on the left side.

The pleura—or, more accurately, the subpleural fascia—of cattle has greater thickness and strength than that of most other species, and the mediastinum is able to withstand considerable lateral pressure, even where it is reduced to little more than two apposed pleural membranes. As a result, collapse of one lung is not inevitably followed by collapse of the other.

## THE LUNGS

The lungs of cattle possess the usual roughly pyramidal shape but are distinguished by their pronounced lobation, very evident lobulation, and marked asymmetry.

The *left lung* is divided into cranial and caudal lobes, but the former is itself divisible into two parts: one extends forward toward the apex of the pleural sac, the other ventrally over the pericardium (Fig. 27–6/7). It is unnecessary to describe each surface and margin of the lung. Most interest attends the form of the ventral and basal borders since the former determines the accessibility of the heart, the latter the caudal limit for examination. The ventral border is sinuous, but its main feature is the notch (between the two parts of the cranial lobe) that extends from the third intercostal space to the fifth rib and allows the heart to come into contact with the chest wall (Fig. 27–1/*A*). The basal border changes its position according to the phase of respiration; as a compromise between the inspiratory and expiratory positions, it may be regarded as following an almost straight line from the junction of the 6th rib with its cartilage to the upper part of the 11th rib (/3). It will not escape notice that the marginal part of the lung is very thin and that little information can normally be obtained from auscultation of this strip. The heart also reduces the lung field. In practice, therefore, the useful caudal area for auscultation of the lung is reduced to a surprisingly small triangle bounded by the triceps, the edge of the muscles of the back, and, as hypotenuse, the line joining the olecranon summit to the upper part of the 11th rib. It extends a little farther caudally on the right side because of the pressure exerted on the diaphragm by the stomach on the left. A small prescapular area (where the right lung is related through the mediastinum to the left chest wall!) is of very minor clinical importance.

The *right lung* is larger than the left in the proportion 3:2. In addition to cranial and caudal lobes it possesses a middle lobe and a small accessory lobe that springs from the medial aspect of the base (Fig. 27–6). The topographical consequences of the larger size of the right lung were considered with the mediastinum. It should also be observed that the cardiac notch, smaller than that on the left, is restricted to the lower parts of the third and fourth spaces and is thus wholly under cover of the arm (Fig. 27–1/*B*). The right cranial lobe is ventilated by a (tracheal) bronchus that arises independently from the trachea a few centimeters cranial to its bifurcation (Plate 3/*F*). Percussion of the basal border of the lung is more accurately performed on the right side where an abrupt transition occurs from the hollow lung sound to the dull sound of the liver; on the left side the gas-filled upper part of the rumen makes percussion unreliable.

The bovine lungs are distinguished by the very thick connective tissue septa that demarcate areas on the surface and extend inward to divide the lung substance into segments. The septa, which may help to localize infection, become even more obvious in certain diseases in which they are thickened and edematous (see Fig. 4–24).

The capacity for respiratory exchange is limited, when compared with that in other species, by the relatively small total alveolar surface area and lesser density of capillaries. A large part is required for basal needs and little reserve is available for more stressful circumstances.

The lungs of sheep and goats are similar in gross form but show a lesser degree of lobulation. The

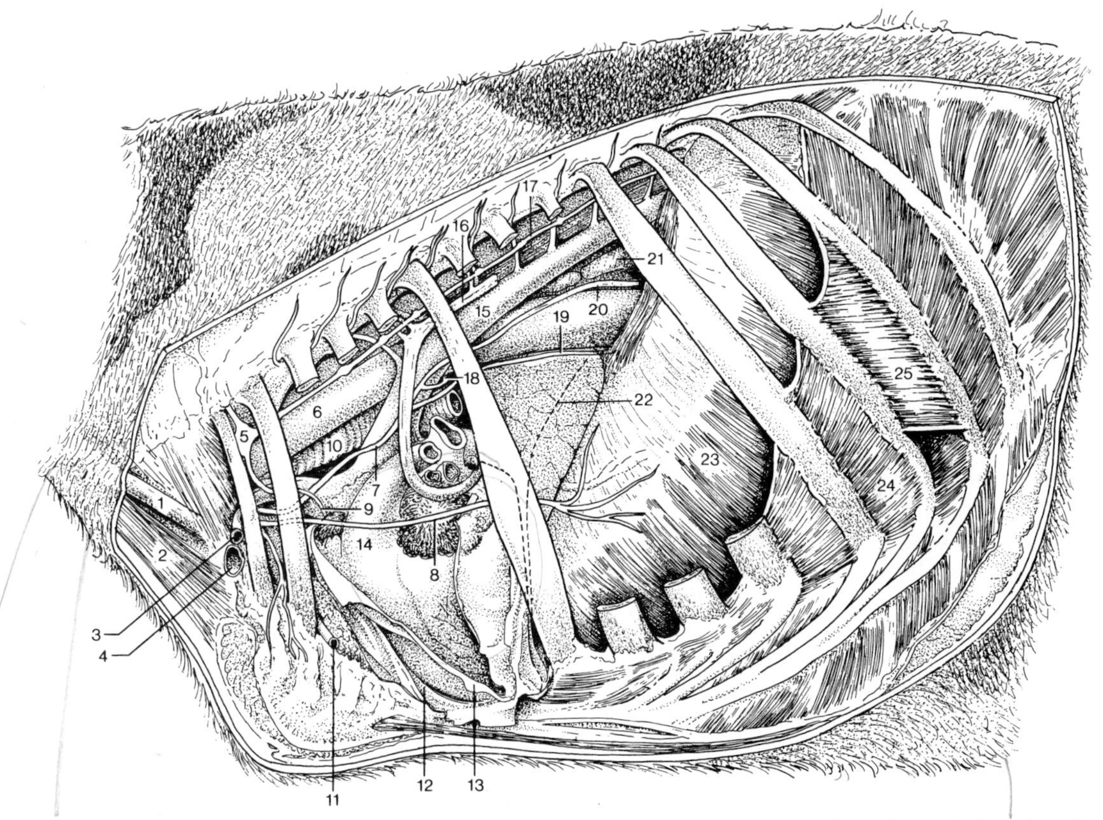


**Figure 27–4.** Left lateral view of the bovine thoracic cavity. The left lung and part of the mediastinal pleura have been removed.

1, External jugular vein; 2, sternocephalicus; 3, axillary artery; 4, axillary vein; 5, cervicothoracic ganglion; 6, esophagus; 7, vagus; 8, phrenic nerve; 9, one of the cardiac nerves; 10, trachea; 11, internal thoracic artery; 12, mediastinal pleura; 13, pericardium, reflected; 14, pulmonary trunk; 15, aorta; 16, left azygous vein; 17, greater splanchnic nerve; 18, recurrent laryngeal nerve; 19, ventral vagal trunk; 20, dorsal vagal trunk; 21, caudal mediastinal lymph nodes; 22, cranial extent of diaphragm; 23, diaphragm; 24, internal intercostal muscle; 25, external intercostal muscle.

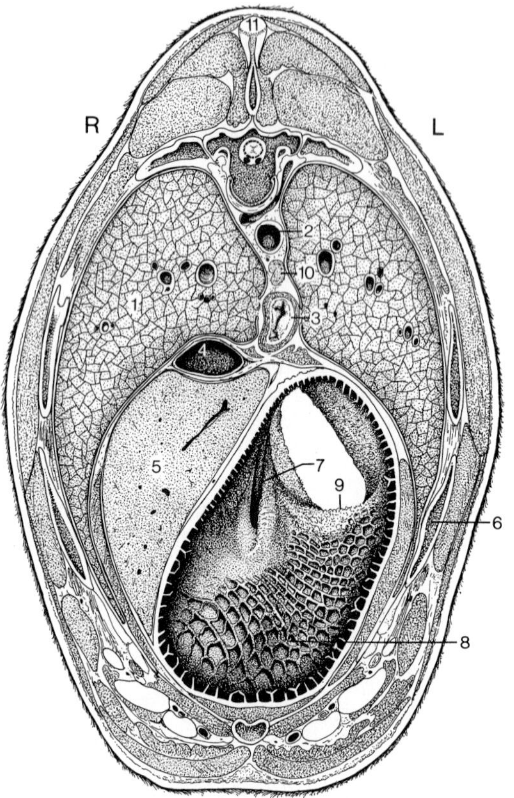


**Figure 27–5.** Transverse section of the bovine trunk at the level of the eighth thoracic vertebra. Note the cover to abdominal viscera provided by the ribs.

1, Caudal lobe of right lung; 2, aorta; 3, esophagus; 4, caudal vena cava; 5, liver; 6, seventh rib; 7, reticular groove; 8, reticulum; 9, ruminoreticular fold; 10, caudal mediastinal lymph node; 11, supraspinous ligament.

pattern in sheep often varies between parts of the lung, some of which may clearly show the connective tissue septa through the visceral pleura, while others may be almost unmarked.

The circulation through the lungs is maintained by the pulmonary and bronchial arteries and by the pulmonary veins. Numerous peripheral anastomoses are present between the bronchial and pulmonary systems, and all the blood returning to the heart is carried by a single set of veins. The pulmonary veins, although variable, are generally grouped in three clusters where they enter the left atrium.

Two lymphatic plexuses drain the lungs and converge on the nodes placed about the bronchial bifurcation. One plexus lies directly below the pleura and drains this and the adjoining connective tissue; the second runs more deeply in the peribronchial tracts. The courses of the deeper vessels are interrupted by small pulmonary lymph nodes situated on the bronchial tree within the substance of the lungs (Fig. 27–6/11); these nodes are never conspicuous and cannot always be found. Both deep and superficial vessels normally enter the tracheobronchial nodes, but a few circumvent these and pass to the next node in the chain.

The *tracheobronchial lymph nodes* (/9,10) are sometimes regarded as forming a separate lymph center and sometimes assigned to the mediastinal center. Each node is concerned with a limited territory, but the boundaries between adjacent drainage areas are not clear-cut. In general the cranial node receives lymph from the right cranial lobe and transmits it to the cranial mediastinal group; the right tracheobronchial node receives lymph from the middle and caudal parts of the right lung and transmits it to the middle mediastinal nodes; the middle node drains the accessory and both caudal lobes; and the left node receives lymph from all lobes of the left lung, and from the medial parts of the right lung, and sends its efferent vessels either directly to the thoracic duct or to the caudal mediastinal nodes. It is probable that connections between the various

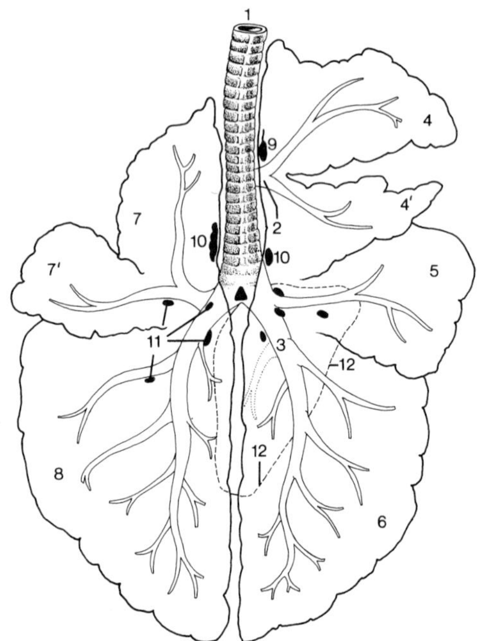


**Figure 27–6.** Lobation and bronchial tree of the bovine lungs, schematic dorsal view.

1, Trachea; 2, tracheal bronchus; 3, right principal bronchus; 4, 4′, divided right cranial lobe; 5, middle lobe; 6, right caudal lobe; 7, 7′, divided left cranial lobe; 8, left caudal lobe; 9, cranial tracheobronchial lymph node; 10, tracheobronchial lymph nodes; 11, pulmonary lymph nodes; 12, outline of accessory lobe of right lung.

nodes about the tracheal bifurcation establish alternative pathways.

## THE MEDIASTINUM

The thick dorsal part of the *cranial mediastinum* contains the esophagus and trachea, the great vessels passing to and from the neck and forelimbs, a considerable collection of lymph nodes, the thoracic duct, and various nerves (Fig. 27–4). In older animals the ventral part is thin and contains only the vestige of the thymus and the internal thoracic vessels; the difference in thickness is less striking in the younger animal, in which the thymus has not wholly regressed (Fig. 27–7/*A*,10″; see also Fig. 25–26/2). The cranial mediastinum is pushed across to lie against the left ribs by the greater size of the cranial lobe of the right lung, and its cranial border attaches to the left chest wall.

The *middle mediastinum* is occupied by the heart and pericardium ventrally; dorsally it numbers among its contents the termination of the trachea, esophagus, pulmonary vessels, aortic arch, thoracic duct, left azygous vein, middle mediastinal and tracheobronchial lymph nodes, and vagus trunks (Figs. 27–3 and 27–4). It thus forms a septum of very irregular thickness, being reduced in some places to a double pleural sheet. It is very wide ventral to the heart where it contains the sternopericardiac ligament. This breadth makes possible a transsternal approach to the pericardium, which avoids opening a pleural sac.

The *caudal mediastinum* is generally thin. The dorsal part extends far caudally below the vertebrae and contains the further courses of the esophagus, aorta, vagus trunks, and caudal mediastinal lymph nodes (Fig. 27–4). The septum is very short where it is level with the base of the heart but lengthens again ventrally where it is diverted to the left by the larger size of the right lung base (Fig. 27–7/10).

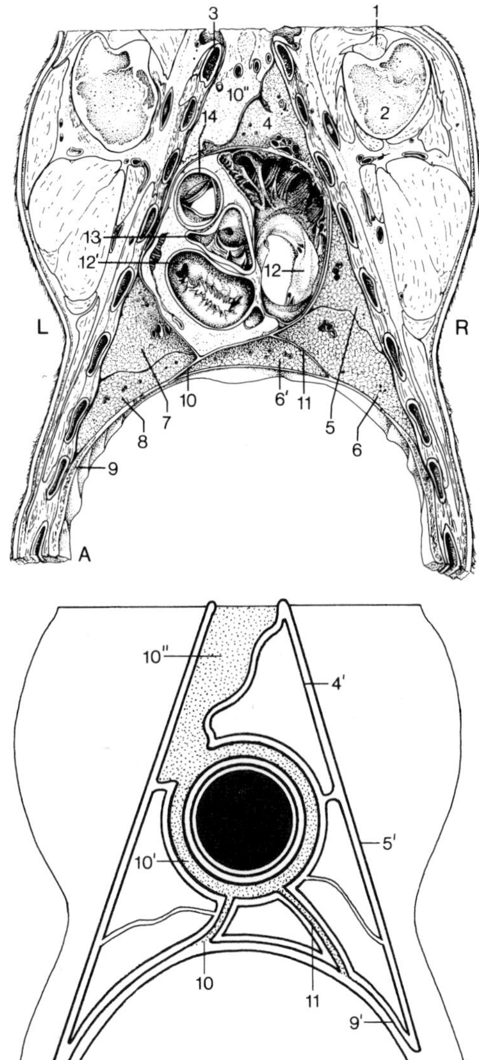


**Figure 27–7.** Dorsal section of the bovine thorax directly ventral to the shoulder joint. *A*, Actual. *B*, Schematized to show the asymmetry of the cranial and caudal parts of the mediastinum *(stippled)*.

1, Biceps tendon; 2, humerus; 3, first rib; 4, cranial lobe of right lung; 4′, pulmonary pleura; 5, middle lobe of right lung; 5′, costal pleura; 6, 6′, caudal and accessory lobes of right lung; 7, caudal part of cranial lobe of left lung; 8, caudal lobe of left lung; 9, diaphragm; 9′, diaphragmatic pleura; 10, 10′, 10″, caudal, middle, and cranial mediastinum, the last occupied by the thymus; 11, plica venae cavae; 12, 12′, right and left atrioventricular valves; 13, left coronary artery arising from aortic valve; 14, pulmonary valve.

## THE HEART

There are no detailed studies of the position of the heart in living cattle, but it is probable that individual differences as well as alterations due to respiratory and other activities exist. The conventional projections of the outline and orifices of the heart on the skeleton should therefore be applied with caution in clinical practice. The heart (within the pericardium) is placed asymmetrically within the thorax, 60% or more lying to the left of the midline, and it extends from the second intercostal space (or following rib) into the fifth space. It thus lies mainly under cover of the limbs in the animal standing square (Fig. 27–1). The base lies approximately in the horizontal plane of the last costochondral joint, while the apex lies opposite the sixth costal cartilage, a couple of centimeters dorsal to the sternum. The axis that joins the center of the base to the apex inclines somewhat caudally and to the left. The caudal border is more or less vertical.

Although the *general form* is conical, a certain amount of lateral compression defines right and left surfaces that are related to the medial aspects of the lungs and to the thoracic wall. It is relatively deeper than in the horse. While direct contact with the thoracic wall is restricted (Fig. 27–1), the lungs are so deeply excavated around the cardiac notches that auscultation over a wider area is possible.

In the young animal the cranial border of the pericardium is in contact with the thymus (Fig. 27–7/*A*, 10″); the caudal border is related to the diaphragm and through this to the liver and reticulum, a relationship of importance in connection with the penetration of foreign bodies from the reticulum (see Plate 29/*B* and Fig. 28–17). The base is crossed by the trachea, principal bronchi, and pulmonary vessels and is related to the tracheobronchial nodes (Fig. 27–4).

The hearts of sheep and goats vary much in size and form according to breed. In some breeds the heart is relatively long and narrow, in others much wider and shorter. In the absence of more absolute criteria, the isolated sheep heart is most easily identified by the quality of the fat. The bovine heart is constructed according to the general mammalian plan and exhibits few specific characters of importance. The *right atrium* is entered by the cranial and caudal venae cavae and by the coronary sinus, which also receives the left azygous in this species. A fossa, corresponding to the foramen ovale of fetal life, is found between the intervenous crest and the caudal caval orifice; an opening into the left atrium may still be present and patent to a probe in many younger animals but rarely has significance.

The *right ventricle,* crescentic in section, is wrapped around the right and cranial aspects of the left chamber (Figs. 27–3, 27–7/*A*, and Plate 11/*E*). The right atrioventricular valve is composed of three cusps whose free margins are thick and irregular, especially in later life. The cusps of the pulmonary valve are also thickened toward their margins, sometimes forming pronounced nodules in older animals.

The only feature of the *left atrium* worthy of note is the fibrous scar generally present at the former site of the valve of the foramen ovale.

The extent of the *left ventricle* is indicated by the interventricular grooves. The caudal aspect is marked by an almost equally prominent intermediate groove occupied by a branch of the left coronary artery. The left artrioventricular valve is comparable to that of the right side but possesses only two major cusps (Fig. 27–7/*A*, 12′). Nodular thickenings of the aortic valve are more common than those of the pulmonary valve.

As a rough guide to their positions, the pulmonary and aortic valves may be regarded as being placed under the third rib (and following space) and the fourth rib, respectively, each about 10 cm above the costochondral junctions, although the slope of the heart raises the aortic valve above, and lowers the pulmonary valve a little below, the suggested level. The left atrioventricular valve lies under the fourth space and fifth rib (see Fig. 28–5/3), the right one under the fourth rib and space, each at a slightly more ventral level than the associated arterial valve (see Fig. 28–27/1).

The *skeleton* of connective tissue that surrounds the atrioventricular and arterial openings contains a pair of ossicles (ossa cordis) (see Fig. 7–13/5). The larger of these bones, and normally the first to appear, is related to the origin of the septal aortic cusp; the second forms in relation to the attachment of the left cusp of this valve.

The left coronary artery is considerably larger than the right one, which is limited to a circumflex course.

It is worth mentioning that pathologists find the isthmus of the aorta (the stretch between the origin of the brachiocephalic trunk and the junction with the ductus arteriosus) greatly constricted in the newborn calf; the appearance may erroneously suggest to the casual observer an origin of the aorta from the right ventricle. The usual proportions are exhibited in calves that survive birth by a few days.

## THE ESOPHAGUS, TRACHEA, AND THYMUS

The esophagus and trachea enter the thorax surrounded by a loose fascia that continues the connective tissue of the neck between the two pleural sacs, providing a pathway for the spread of fluids and infection that is particularly important in connection with leaking wounds of the esophagus. The changing relations of the two organs in the neck are described elsewhere (p. 643); the esophagus lies dorsolateral to the trachea on the left side where it passes between the first ribs, but it soon obtains a more symmetrical position (Fig. 27–4/6). Other important relations of the esophagus are the cranial mediastinal and costocervical lymph nodes and the vagus and sympathetic nerves at the entrance to the chest; the thoracic duct (which crosses its left face very obliquely), left azygous vein, and aorta more caudally; the tracheobronchial and middle mediastinal lymph nodes where it crosses above the bifurcation of the trachea; and the dorsal and ventral vagal trunks and the caudal mediastinal lymph nodes in the last part of its course. The last relationship is especially important since an enlarged node may press on the esophagus and impede the eructation of gas from the rumen (Fig. 27–5/3,10).

Post mortem, the esophagus is normally seen in a relaxed condition when its diameter may reach 6 cm. The muscle is striated along its whole length. No anatomical evidence has been found for the existence of the functional sphincter that is described as existing directly before the diaphragm. The part embraced by the diaphragm is constricted in specimens embalmed in situ, but the examination of the hiatus in the living animal does not suggest that the diaphragm exerts a firm grip; a considerable amount of adventitial tissue is always present in this region.

The *trachea* is deep and laterally compressed; in life it is without the prominent dorsal ridge characteristic of the fresh specimen. It lies above the tributaries of the cranial vena cava where it enters the thorax and continues in this relative position to its termination, passing over the cranial vena cava and the right atrium. A separate bronchus for the right cranial lobe is detached a few centimeters before the bifurcation, level with the fourth rib or following space (Fig. 27–6/2). Other important relations are to the sympathetic, vagus, recurrent laryngeal, and phrenic nerves; to various lymph nodes at the thoracic entrance; and to the aorta, azygous vein, and tracheobronchial lymph nodes more caudally.

The *thymus* has already been encountered in the neck. The thoracic part of the thymus fills the ventral part of the cranial mediastinum when at its apogee, extending over the cranial surface of the pericardium and reaching some distance over the origin of the pulmonary trunk and the aortic arch (see Figs. 25–26/2 and 27–7/*A*, 10″). Involution of the thoracic part is rarely complete, and some vestige, consisting mainly of fatty fibrous tissue, normally persists even in aged animals. In the calf the phrenic nerves and other structures in this region may be buried between the lobules through which they thread their way.

## THE GREAT VESSELS AND NERVES WITHIN THE THORAX

Few details of the great vessels within the chest are clinically important. The branches of the thoracic aorta resemble those of the horse.

The *cranial vena cava* is formed just within the thorax by the union of a bijugular trunk with the two subclavian veins (see Fig. 7–42). Its tributaries include the internal thoracic veins, which receive the "milk veins" that run forward from the udder (see Fig. 31–7). The *caudal vena cava* passes within the plica venae cavae accompanied by the right phrenic nerve.

The *left azygous vein* drains the greater part of the dorsal part of the chest wall and the structures about the vertebrae. It curves ventrally within the mediastinum, crossing in front of the root of the left lung; after piercing the pericardium it winds caudally over the surface of the left atrium to enter the right atrium at the coronary sinus (Fig. 27–4/16). It has important connections with the venous channels within the vertebral canal by way of the intercostal and first lumbar veins (see Fig. 26–6). A right azygous vein is also present but overshadowed in significance.

The pressure within the caval veins reflects various events in the cardiac cycle. It rises on atrial systole, again when the cusps of the atrioventricular valve float into place at the beginning of ventricular systole, and yet again as the atrial chamber becomes increasingly filled preparatory to a new contraction. In cattle these pressure changes are frequently betrayed by pulsations in the external jugular vein in the lower part of the neck.

The cervical parts of the *vagus nerves* were noted earlier. The thoracic continuations take the usual course and have the usual collateral branches. They end by dividing into dorsal and ventral branches that join their partners of the other side to constitute dorsal and ventral vagal trunks that follow the corresponding borders of the esophagus into the abdomen. The dorsal trunk is the larger. Branches from both supply the esophageal wall, while a connection over the left surface of the esophagus seems to indicate further rearrangement of the fibers preparatory to entering the abdomen; the gross appearance sometimes suggests an increase of the dorsal trunk at the expense of the ventral, sometimes the reverse. The relationship of the dorsal trunk to the caudal mediastinal lymph nodes is of considerable importance (see further on).

Nothing need be added to the general accounts of the sympathetic nervous system and the phrenic nerves.

## THE LYMPHATIC SRUCTURES OF THE THORAX

The lymphatic drainage of the thorax is both complicated and variable. Since not all the many nodes described are found in every specimen, and since the boundaries between neighboring centers

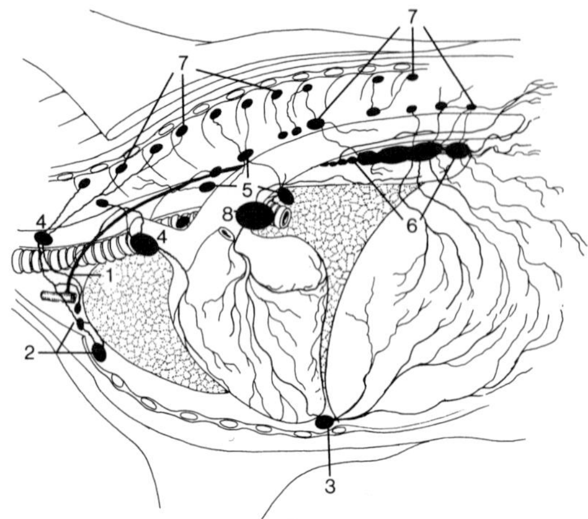


**Figure 27–8.** Lymph drainage of the bovine thoracic wall and mediastinum.

1, Thoracic duct; 2, cranial sternal lymph nodes; 3, caudal sternal lymph node; 4, cranial mediastinal lymph nodes; 5, middle mediastinal lymph nodes; 6, caudal mediastinal lymph nodes; 7, intercostal and thoracic aortic lymph nodes; 8, tracheobronchial node.

are sometimes indistinct, it is not always possible confidently to assign individual nodes to a particular group.

The dorsal part of the thorax is provided with small *intercostal nodes* that are found immediately below the pleura at the dorsal ends of certain spaces (Fig. 27–8/7). These receive their afferent vessels from structures about the vertebrae and from the dorsal part of the chest wall; their efferent vessels lead mainly to the cranial mediastinal nodes at the thoracic entrance. Some of this lymph may pass through a second row of small nodes situated about the aorta and companion vessels.

The caudal *sternal nodes* are concealed by the transversus thoracis, while the larger cranial node lies in front of this (/3,2). These nodes drain the ventral part of the thoracic and cranial abdominal walls and also receive some lymph from the overlying muscles of the limbs. The efferent vessels converge on the cranial mediastinal node, and from here the lymph passes to the thoracic or left tracheal duct; direct passage to these ducts is also possible.

Other more important nodes occupy more central positions in the mediastinum. The *cranial mediastinal* group consists of a large number of nodes scattered about between the trachea, esophagus, and major vessels just inside the thoracic inlet (/4). They receive lymph from the cranial mediastinum, the dorsal thoracic centers, and the lungs. The efferent vessels pass to the thoracic or one or other tracheal duct. One node, transitional to the caudal deep cervical nodes, may be individually named the costocervical node.

The *middle mediastinal nodes* lie mainly to the right of the aortic arch (/5). They receive lymph from adjacent structures and some of the tracheobronchial nodes. The outflow is divided between direct tributaries to the thoracic duct and the cranial and caudal mediastinal groups.

The *tracheobronchial nodes* are described with the lung (/8). Their outflow is spread among various mediastinal nodes. In some cattle additional (pulmonary) nodes are found on the bronchial tree within the lung. They are of no importance. The nodes associated with the lungs are fewer and less constant in the small ruminants.

The *caudal mediastinal* group consists of only one or two nodes (/6). The largest, and possibly solitary, node may attain a length of 20 cm or more and is flexed to fit over the terminal part of the esophagus and against the diaphragm dorsal to the hiatus. The group collects lymph from tracheobronchial nodes, the caudal mediastinal contents, the diaphragm, and adjacent sections of the liver, spleen, and stomach. The efferent vessels pass to the thoracic duct. Both the esophagus and the dorsal vagal trunk may be involved in conditions affecting these nodes.

The lymph from the skin and most superficial structures of the thoracic wall divides itself between the large superficial cervical node cranial to the scapula and the subiliac node far to the rear.

The *thoracic duct* into which most of this lymph eventually flows takes origin from the cisterna chyli and enters the thorax to the right of the aorta. It then inclines ventrally over the right face of the aortic arch and crosses the left aspect of the trachea to end by opening into the cranial vena cava or one of its tributaries of the left side. The duct is often duplicated for all or part of its course.

## Selected Bibliography

Alexander, A.F., and R. Jensen: Normal structure of bovine pulmonary vasculature. Am. J. Vet. Res. 24:1083–1093, 1963.

Ashdown, R.R., and S. Done: Color Atlas of Veterinary Anatomy: The Ruminants. Baltimore, University Park Press, 1984.

Cegarra, I.J., and R.E. Lewis: Bronchography in the goat *Capra hircus*. Am. J. Vet. Res. 38:1133–1136, 1977.

Curtis, R.A., L. Viel, S.M. McGuirk, et al.: Lung sounds in cattle, horses, sheep and goats. Can. Vet. J. 27:170–172, 1986.

deLahunta, A., and R.E. Habel: Applied Veterinary Anatomy. Philadelphia, W.B. Saunders Company, 1986.

Ducharme, N.G., S.L. Fubini, W.C. Rebhun, and K.A. Beck: Thoracotomy in adult dairy cattle: 14 cases (1979–1991). JAVMA 200:86–90, 1992.

Fowler, M.E.: Intrathoracic surgery in large animals. JAVMA 162:967–973, 1973.

Habel, R.E.: Guide to the Dissection of the Domestic Ruminants, 4th ed. Ithaca, 1989, Published by the author.

Lodge, D.: A survey of the tracheal dimensions in horses and cattle in relation to endotracheal tube size. Vet. Rec. 85:300–302, 1969.

McKibben, J.S., and R. Getty: A comparative morphologic study of the cardiac innervation in domestic animals: Cattle. Anat. Rec. 165:141–151, 1969.

Nakakuki, Shoichi: The bronchial tree and blood vessels of the cow (Holstein) lung. J. Vet. Med. Sci. 56:676–679, 1994.

Pavaux, C.: A Color Atlas of Bovine Visceral Anatomy. London, Wolfe Publishing, 1983.

Popesko, P.: Atlas of Topographic Anatomy of the Domestic Animals; vol. 2: Thoracic and abdominal cavities. Philadelphia, W.B. Saunders Company, 1971.

Tyler, J.W., K.L. Angel, H.D. Moll, and D.F. Wolfe: Something old, something new: Thoracic acoustic percussion in cattle. JAVMA 197:52–57, 1990.

Veit, H.P., and R.L. Farrell: The anatomy and physiology of the bovine respiratory system relating to pulmonary disease. Cornell Vet. 68:555–581, 1978.

# CHAPTER 28

# The Abdomen of the Ruminants

## CONFORMATION AND SURFACE ANATOMY

The form of the abdomen varies with age, obesity, and physiological condition. In adult animals it is both deep and wide, and the floor, which dips behind the sternum, ascends very steeply in its caudal part to join the pubic brim. This marked contraction is not obvious on first inspection because the caudal part of the abdomen is covered by the thighs and by the skin folds that pass between the flanks and stifle joints and is overlain ventrally by the udder or the prepuce. The cranial extent of the abdomen under cover of the more caudal ribs and cartilages is concealed but can be deduced from the description of the diaphragm (p. 656). The abdomen is usually bilaterally symmetrical, although advanced pregnancy or excessive distention of the rumen may cause one side to bulge more markedly. The upper part of the flank is dished, forming the paralumbar fossa beside the loins (see Fig. 26–1/*E*), while the lower convex part merges with the floor.

In the younger calf the abdomen is shallower and laterally compressed, and the floor slopes more gradually to the pelvis; the spreading of the caudal ribs, the deepening of the trunk, and the depressions beside the vertebral column develop concurrently with growth of the rumen.

The lateral and ventral abdominal walls are bounded by the last rib and costal arch, the extremities of the lumbar transverse processes, the coxal tuber, and the terminal line of the pelvic inlet (see Fig. 26–1). Not all of these are palpable, although identification of the margin of the thoracic cage, the coxal tuber, and most transverse processes normally presents no problem. Palpation should be performed with care since correct identification of the bones is important in certain anesthetic techniques. There are six lumbar vertebrae in cattle. Recognition of the second to fifth vertebrae is easy and may even be possible without palpation in lean cattle; the first process cannot always be located since it is short, tucked into the angle between the last rib and the spine, and generally overlain by a pad of fat; the last one always eludes the fingers since it lies medial to the coxal tuber below a thick covering of muscle (see Fig. 26–5). There are occasionally seven lumbar vertebrae in sheep and goats.

## THE VENTROLATERAL WALL OF THE ABDOMEN

### Structure

The ventrolateral wall of the abdomen is composed of as many as 9 or 10 layers, although not all cover the entire extent. The skin is freely movable except over the coxal tuber. The *cutaneous muscle* is thick over the lower parts of the flank but thins dorsally and does not extend over the paralumbar fossa; it also leaves the abdominal floor bare except for detached fascicles that supply the male animal with cranial and caudal muscles of the prepuce. The cutaneous muscle extends through the flank fold to end in an aponeurosis over the lateral surface of the thigh (Fig. 28–1/*A*).

The loose *superficial fascia* provides pathways for the cutaneous nerves and encloses certain lymph nodes. The elongated subiliac node lies vertically within the skin fold, pressed against the cranial margin of the thigh some distance above the patella; it can always be found on palpation. It drains the more superficial layers of the body wall as far forward as the caudal part of the thorax and also receives lymph coming from the skin and superficial muscles of the thigh and croup (see Fig. 31–9/2). A number of smaller nodes within the paralumbar fossa drain the surrounding parts; they normally escape notice but appear as circumscribed swellings when enlarged. The subcutaneous "milk" (abdominal) vein runs forward over the abdominal floor from the udder (Figs. 28–10/11 and 31–7/1).

The *deep fascia* is transformed into an elastic tunica flava, attached to the underlying muscle and

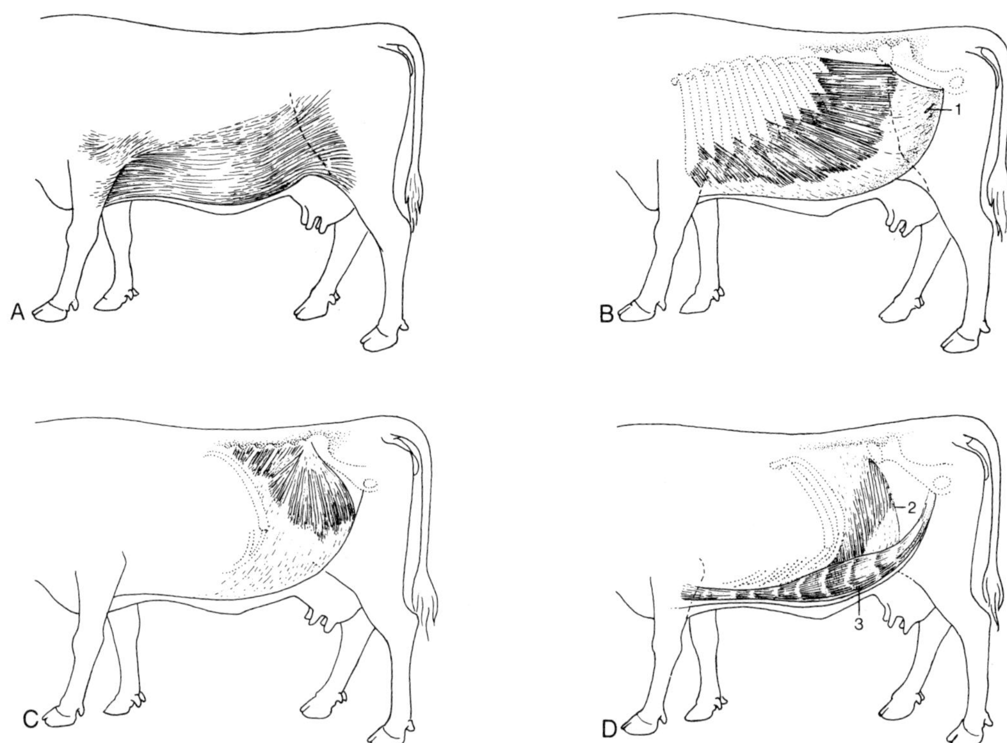


**Figure 28–1.** Cutaneus trunci and abdominal muscles. *A*, Cutaneus trunci, especially well developed ventrally. *B*, External abdominal oblique with superficial inguinal ring (1) in its aponeurosis. *C*, Internal abdominal oblique. *D*, Transversus abdominis (2) and rectus abdominis (3). Note the reduction in the thickness of the wall along the caudal part of the rectus margin.

sharing in supporting the viscera. Ventrally it gives origin to the external spermatic fascia or the medial lamina of the suspensory apparatus of the udder.

The *muscle layer* is broadly arranged as in other species. In the flank it consists of a triple layer of flat muscles that take origin from the ribs, lumbar transverse processes, and ilium (Fig. 28–1). These are continued over the abdominal floor by aponeurotic tendons that enclose the rectus muscles to each side of the linea alba where the aponeuroses attach (see Fig. 1–37). The linea alba runs from the xiphoid process of the sternum to the center of the prepubic tendon where it blends with the end tendons of the recti.

Ideally, though less frequently in practice, surgical incisions of the flank follow a gridiron pattern in which the fibers of each layer are parted rather than transected. A knowledge of the fiber course as well as of the relative extent of the fleshy and aponeurotic parts of these muscles is therefore of value to the surgeon.

The most superficial muscle of the flank, the *external oblique,* arises by fleshy serrations from the outer surfaces of the last eight ribs. Its most dorsal fibers run more or less horizontally toward the coxal tuber, but the greater number slope caudoventrally to find attachment to the linea alba (Fig. 28–1/*B*). The gap that intervenes between the dorsal border and transverse processes is closed by a sheet of fascia. The fleshy part is succeeded by an aponeurotic tendon, the transformation occurring along a line that first drops vertically, from a point roughly level with the coxal tuber, before sweeping cranially. A split within the aponeurosis provides the superficial opening (ring) of the inguinal canal.

The second muscle, the *internal oblique,* has a tendinous origin from the coxal tuber and the pelvic tendon of the external oblique, and several independent fleshy origins from the tips of the lumbar transverse processes. It radiates to insert on the last rib and into the linea alba. Most fibers run cranioventrally, but the thicker, most caudal fascicles pass slightly behind the plane of the tuber. The muscle-tendon junction slopes caudoventrally, and only the most caudal strip is fleshy where the muscle crosses the margin of the rectus (Fig. 28–1/*C*). The aponeuroses of the two oblique muscles become increasingly interwoven where they pass ventral to the rectus and together furnish the external layer of the rectus sheath. The flesh of the internal oblique forms the inner wall of the inguinal canal.

The third, the *transversus abdominis,* arises from the last ribs and the extremities of the lumbar transverse processes. Its craniodorsal triangle is tendinous, but most of the part covering the flank is fleshy; before reaching the edge of the rectus the flesh gives way to an aponeurosis that crosses the dorsal face of the rectus to gain the linea alba and thus form the inner layer of the rectus sheath. Most fibers run transversely, and none pass behind the plane of the coxal tuber; the dorsal surface of the rectus is thus left uncovered in its most caudal part (Fig. 28–1/*D*).

The *rectus abdominis* muscle is interrupted in the usual way by several tendinous intersections indicative of its multisegmental origin (/3). It arises from the outer surfaces of the lower ends of the last 10 ribs and continues as a wide band separated from its neighbor by the flattened linea alba; it narrows suddenly as it approaches the pubic brim and the tendon that succeeds the flesh twists to form with its fellow and the linea alba a V-shaped trough that continues as the central part of the prepubic tendon. Before reaching the pubic brim, which it approaches almost vertically from below, the prepubic tendon is strengthened by joining the decussation formed by the contralateral parts of the pectineus muscles (each of which arises from both pubic bones) and by additional contributions from the aponeuroses of the abdominal oblique muscles. Ultimately, and after partial decussation, the rectus tendons end in common on the symphysial crest of the pelvis and on the medial symphysial tendon that arises here. A rounded median depression of the internal surface of the prepubic tendon is ascribed to the drag of the udder upon the symphysial tendon (see Fig. 31–4).

A thin fascia covers the abdominal muscles internally and supports the parietal peritoneum. Deposits of fat in the subperitoneal tissues are most frequently encountered toward the pelvic inlet. The wholly tendinous nature of a region of the abdominal wall, along the border of the rectus in front of the stifle, merits emphasis.

The inguinal canal resembles that of the horse (p. 529) so closely that a separate description is unnecessary. Inguinal hernia is infrequent in cattle but common in male sheep, though there are no obvious differences in the adult anatomy. It is probable that the frequent incidence in rams is connected with inherited anomalies in gubernacular development.

## Innervation and Vascularization

The most important nerves of the abdominal wall are the last thoracic (T13) and the first and second lumbar nerves, although the floor ventral to the costal arch is served by continuations of the caudal intercostal nerves. A knowledge of the topography and distribution of the nerves to the flank is of practical importance in obtaining local anesthesia.

The skin of the abdomen is supplied by branches from both dorsal and ventral primary rami, but the muscles and other deep structures are supplied by ventral rami alone (see Fig. 1–37). The skin is divided into bands (dermatomes) that encircle the trunk, each the territory of a particular spinal nerve. These territories overlap, and every area of skin is normally reached by twigs from at least two successive nerves. The peritoneal regions supplied by the same spinal nerves correspond very closely to the dermatomes in position and extent.

The *dorsal rami* (/4) of the thoracic and lumbar nerves supply the epaxial muscles and the strip of skin extending from the dorsal midline roughly to the level of the patella. Below this line the skin is supplied by two tiers of branches from the ventral rami (/5).

The *ventral rami* are much widened where they enter the flank between the internal oblique and transverse muscles. Each possesses a rather constant relationship to the skeleton that is a useful guide when blocking the nerves with anesthetics. These nerves do not run transversely but obliquely, deviating in an increasingly caudal direction (Fig. 28–2). The last thoracic ventral branch usually passes below the tip of the first lumbar transverse process, the first lumbar branch (iliohypogastric n.) below the tip of the second lumbar vertebra, and the second lumbar branch (ilioinguinal n.) below the tip of the fourth bone (Fig. 28–3). Most variations affect the last of these three nerves, which sometimes passes less obliquely than usual and crosses below the transverse process of the third lumbar vertebra.

An exception to the general pattern of innervation of the abdominal wall is provided by the nerve to the cutaneous muscle; this is supplied by a branch from the brachial plexus.

It can now be appreciated that incisions of the upper flank require blockage of both dorsal and ventral branches. Anesthesia is most conveniently obtained by paravertebral injection of the relevant nerves close to their foramina of emergence from the vertebral canal. Anesthesia of the lower flank and abdominal floor requires blockage of the ventral branches only, and these are most conveniently reached where they pass close to the tips

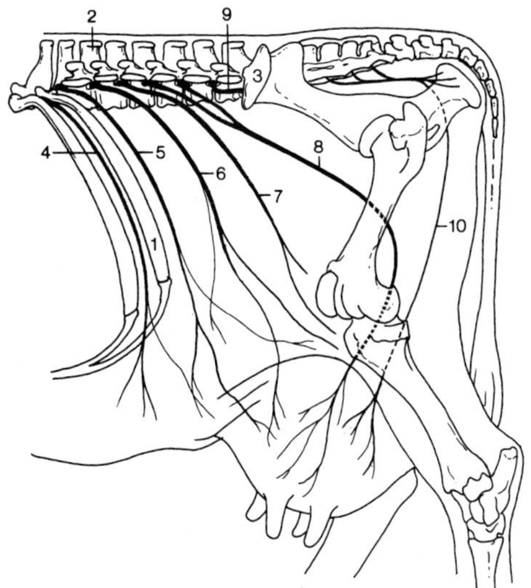


**Figure 28–2.** Topography of the nerves to the flank and udder, simplified. The dorsal branches of the spinal nerves to the upper part of the flank are not shown.

1, Last rib; 2, spinous process of L2; 3, coxal tuber; 4, 12th intercostal n. (T12); 5, T13 (costoabdominal n.); 6, L1 (iliohypogastric n.); 7, L2 (ilioinguinal n.); 8, L3, L4 (genitofemoral n.); 9, L5; 10, ventral perineal n.

of the lumbar transverse processes (paralumbar block). Variation in topography makes the procedure less reliable than might be wished unless the anesthetic agent is diffused rather widely. Lumbar epidural injection provides an alternative procedure. The specific innervation of the cutaneous muscle must be kept in mind whatever method is chosen.

The abdominal wall receives *blood vessels* from several sources. The ventral part obtains its supply through the cranial and caudal epigastric arteries, branches of the internal thoracic and external pudendal arteries, respectively. The flanks are supplied from parietal branches of the aorta, the most important surgically being the deep circumflex iliac artery, which comes from the external iliac to pierce the flank a little cranial to the coxal tuber. The veins are initially satellite, but in the parous cow the arrangement is modified with the formation of the "milk vein" whose special importance is considered later (p. 726).

# THE SPLEEN

A general impression of the visceral topography should be obtained from Figures 28–4 and 28–14 before the individual organs are considered.

The flat oblong spleen is situated over the craniodorsal part of the rumen, against the left half of the diaphragm, and attached to both of these organs. Its upper end lies under the dorsal ends of the last few ribs, and its axis extends ventrally, with a slight cranial inclination, across the line of the ribs to end in the region of the seventh costochondral joint (Figs. 28–4/*A*,2 and 28–5/6). In most animals the lower end passes onto the reticulum, which brings risk of involvement in the common abscesses and perforations of that organ. The upper part of the spleen is retroperitoneal, the line of serosal reflection running cranioventrally over both parietal and visceral surfaces. The hilus is confined to the dorsocranial angle of the medial side and to reach this site the splenic vessels must first pass over the roof of the rumen (Fig. 28–23/11).

The capsule contains little muscle, and physiological variation in spleen size is therefore more restricted than in certain other species. Occasionally an enlarged spleen may extend behind the last rib in the angle between this and the lumbar spine, but for practical purposes the spleen may be regarded as out of reach for palpation or percussion. Access for the purpose of biopsy is normally made through the upper end of the 11th intercostal space and involves little risk of injury to the lung, particularly if the needle is introduced during expiration.

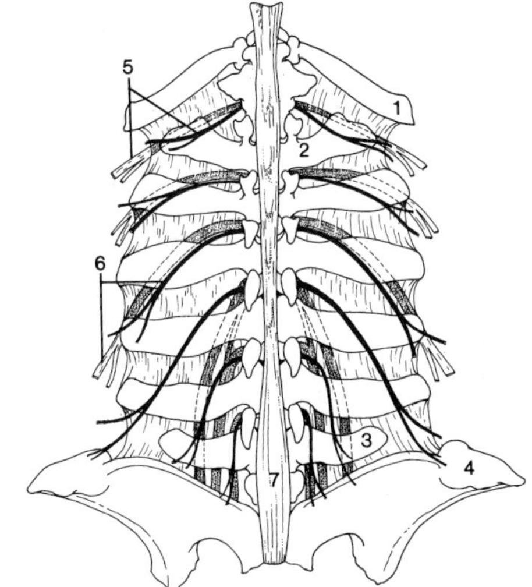


**Figure 28–3.** Relationship of the lumbar spinal nerves to the transverse processes of the bovine lumbar vertebrae.

1, Last rib; 2, first lumbar vertebra; 3, sixth lumbar vertebra; 4, coxal tuber; 5, dorsal and ventral branches of 13th thoracic nerve (the ventral branch is partly stippled); 6, dorsal and ventral branches of second lumbar nerve; 7, supraspinous ligament.

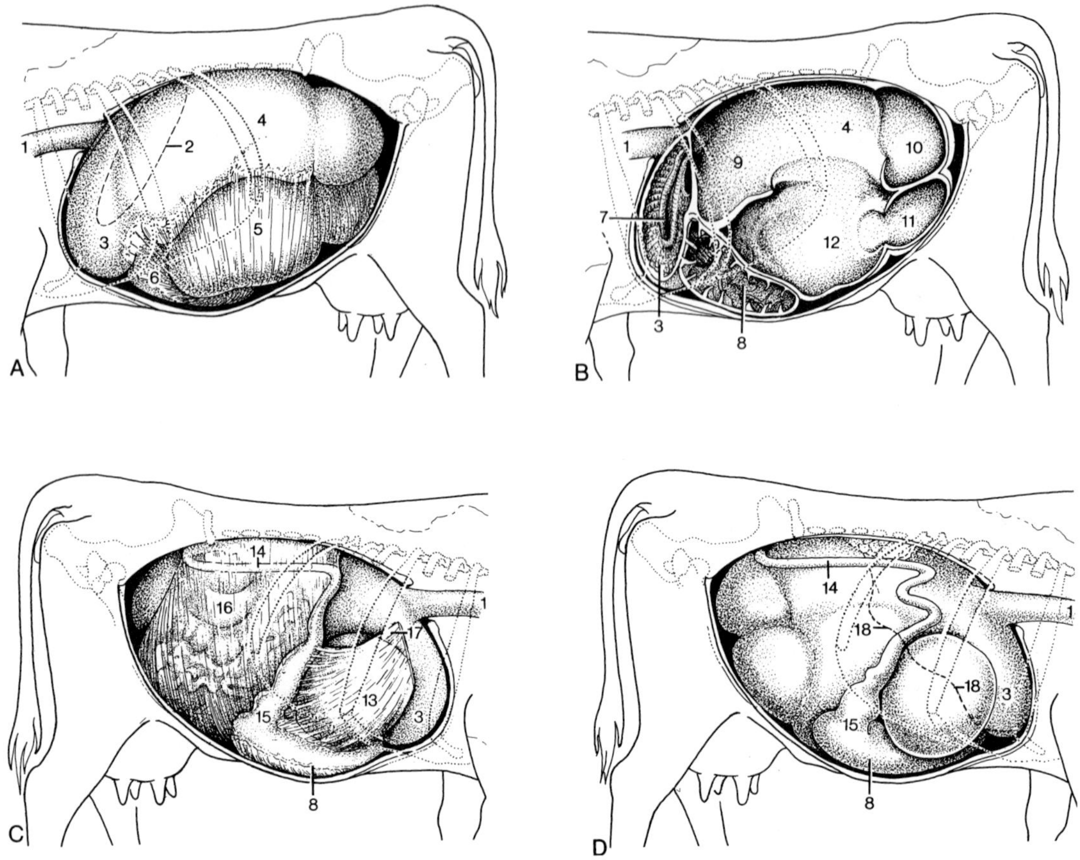

**Figure 28–4.** Topography of the abdominal viscera. *A,* Relationship of abdominal viscera to the left abdominal wall. *B,* The interior of the stomach seen from the left. *C,* Relationship of abdominal viscera to the right abdominal wall; the liver has been removed. *D,* Position of the parts of the stomach seen from the right.

1, Esophagus; 2, outline of spleen; 3, reticulum; 4, dorsal sac of rumen; 5, ventral sac of rumen, covered by superficial wall of greater omentum; 6, fundus of abomasum, covered by superficial wall of greater omentum; 7, reticular groove; 8, body of abomasum; 9, atrium ruminis; 10, caudodorsal blind sac; 11, caudoventral blind sac; 12, ventral sac of rumen (opened); 13, omasum, covered by lesser omentum; 14, descending duodenum; 15, pyloric part of abomasum; 16, greater omentum covering the intestinal mass; 17, lesser omentum cut away from the liver; 18, position of caudoventral border of liver.

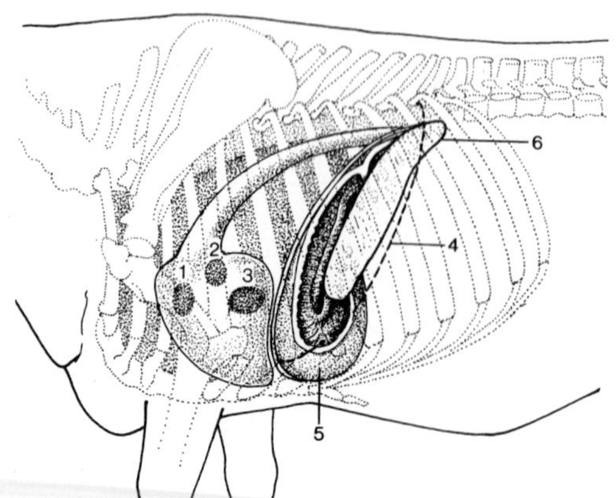


**Figure 28–5.** Left lateral projection of certain organs upon the bovine thoracic wall.

1, Pulmonary valve; 2, aortic valve; 3, left atrioventricular valve; 4, position of basal border of the lung; 5, reticulum, opened (note position of reticular groove); 6, spleen.

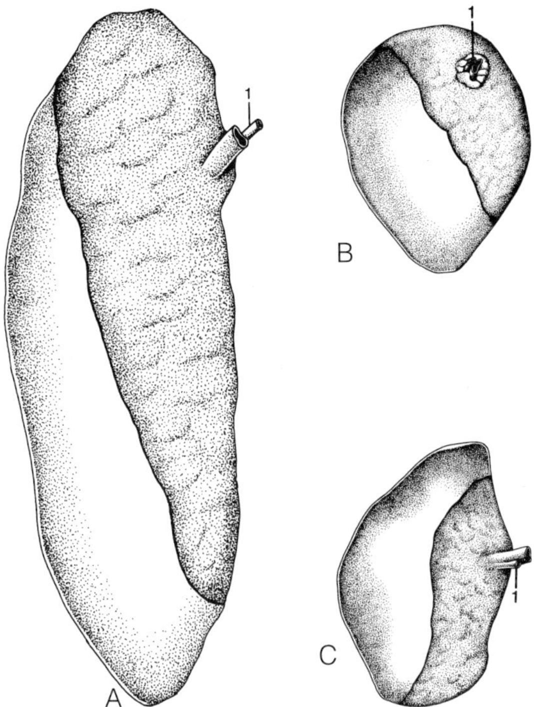


**Figure 28–6.** The spleens of cattle *(A)*, sheep *(B)*, and goat *(C)*, visceral surface. The craniodorsal area is bare. The splenic artery (1) is indicated.

The spleen has a relatively soft consistency. Its color varies considerably, tending to be steel blue in cows, more reddish in males and younger animals. The division of the pulp into red and white areas is very obvious, the white corpuscles being somewhat larger than pinheads.

The spleen is relatively small in *sheep* and *goats,* in which its form, position, and attachments resemble those of the dorsal extremity of the bovine organ. It is roughly triangular in sheep, quadrilateral in goats (Fig. 28–6/*B,C*).

# THE STOMACH

## General Considerations

The stomach is composed of four chambers—rumen, reticulum, omasum, and abomasum—through which the food passes successively (Plate 29/*C,D*). The first three, collectively known as the forestomach (proventriculus), are developed to cope with the complex carbohydrates that form so large a part of the normal diet of ruminants, and only the last chamber is comparable in structure and function to the simple stomach of most other species. All are derived, however, from the gastric spindle of the embryo without the assistance of a contribution from the esophagus (Fig. 28–7).

The topography of the ruminant abdomen is dominated by the enormous development of the stomach, which in adult cattle almost fills the left half of the cavity and occupies a substantial portion of the right (Plate 29/*B* and Figs. 28–8, 28–9, 28–10, and 28–11). Its capacity measures about 60 L. This figure, which is much more modest than many estimates, may be apportioned between the various chambers as follows: rumen, 80%; reticulum, 5%; omasum, 8%; and abomasum, 7%. The proportions in *small ruminants* are somewhat different, being perhaps rumen, 75%; reticulum, 8%; omasum, 4%; and abomasum, 13%. The relative volumes are fairly constant in the short term since the enormous storage capacity of the first chambers and the more or less continuous passage of ingesta into the distal parts minimize the effects of intermittent feeding.

The different chambers are identifiable as expansions of the foregut spindle in the early embryo. They increase at unequal rates throughout the embryonic and fetal periods, first one taking the lead and then another. At one stage the fetal stomach has an almost adult configuration, but during the last months of intrauterine life the abomasum outstrips the others, and at birth it accounts for more than half the weight and capacity of the entire organ—which is appropriate since it is

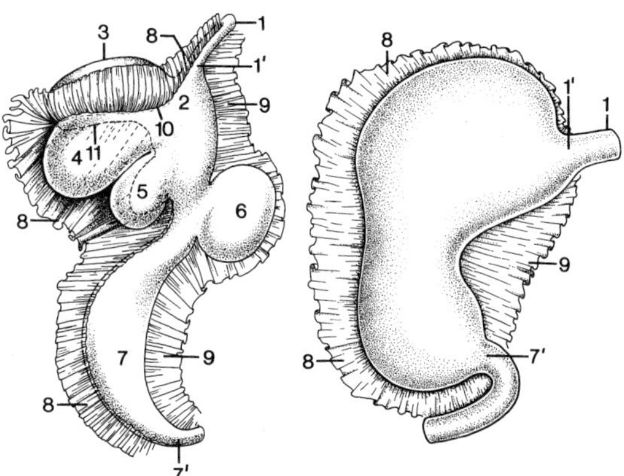


**Figure 28–7.** The attachments of the greater and lesser omenta on the developing ruminant stomach. The simple stomach to the right shows the correspondence of its parts to the compartments of the ruminant stomach.

1, Esophagus; 1′, cardia; 2, atrium ruminis; 3, dorsal sac of rumen; 4, ventral sac of rumen; 5, reticulum; 6, omasum; 7, abomasum; 7′, pylorus; 8, greater omentum; 9, lesser omentum; 10, part of greater curvature corresponding to the right longitudinal groove of the rumen; 11, part of greater curvature corresponding to the left longitudinal groove of the rumen.

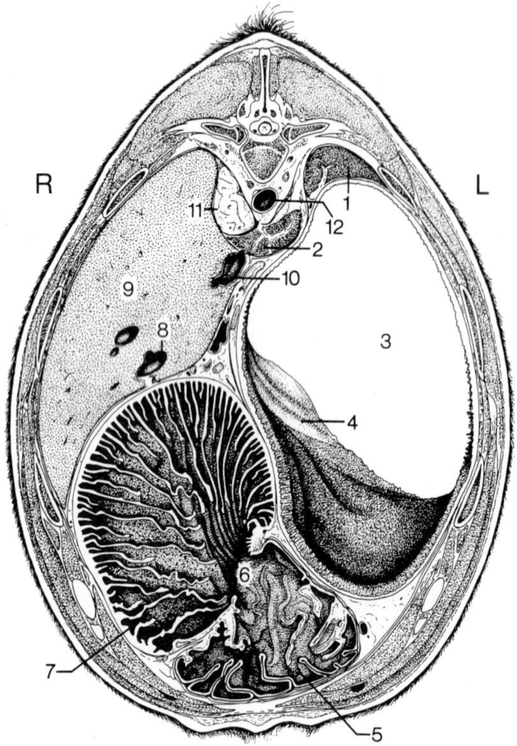


**Figure 28–8.** Transverse section of the bovine trunk at the level of the 10th thoracic vertebra.

1, Spleen; 2, crura of diaphragm; 3, atrium ruminis; 4, cranial pillar; 5, abomasum; 6, omasoabomasal opening; 7, omasum; 8, portal vein; 9, liver; 10, caudal vena cava; 11, right lung; 12, aorta.

the only part that has an immediate function to perform. The postnatal changes through which the adult proportions and topography are acquired are described later (p. 682).

## The Rumen and Reticulum

The rumen and reticulum together form the vessel in which the unpromising food material, invulnerable to attack by mammalian digestive enzymes, is reduced by processes of microbial fermentation. Some of the simpler products are assimilated directly, while others are susceptible to conventional digestion lower in the digestive tract.

The rumen is laterally compressed and extends from the cardia—which lies a little way above the middle of the seventh intercostal space or eighth rib—to the pelvic inlet, from the abdominal roof to the floor, and from the left body wall across the midline, especially caudally and ventrally where it may reach the lower right flank (Figs. 28–11 and 28–14/11). The much smaller reticulum lies cranial to the rumen under cover of ribs 6 to 8 and mainly to the left of the median plane. It reaches from the cardia to the most forward part of the diaphragm and occupies the full height of this shallower part of the abdomen; it also passes across the midline, especially ventrally where it lies above the xiphoid process of the sternum (see Figs. 27–5/8 and 28–4/3). This position allows the application of external pressure in the expectation of eliciting pain when the reticulum is diseased.

The rumen and reticulum are so intimately related in structure and function that many now prefer to describe a combined ruminoreticular compartment. There is much in favor of this convention. The division of the rumen from the reticulum, though more complete, is achieved in exactly the same way as the *subdivision* of the rumen, namely by the inflection of the walls to form a series of pillars (pilae) that project internally. The whole thickness of the stomach wall, except the peritoneum, participates in these formations. The divisions and the pillars that bound them are illustrated in Figure 28–4/*B*. The rumen and reticulum communicate over the U-shaped *ruminoreticular fold.* The principal *ru-*

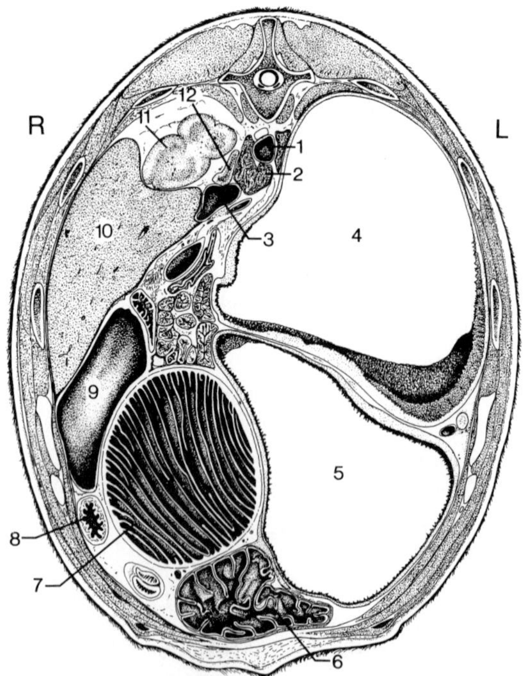


**Figure 28–9.** Transverse section of the bovine trunk at the level of the 13th thoracic vertebra.

1, Aorta; 2, right crus of diaphragm; 3, caudal vena cava; 4, dorsal sac of rumen; 5, ventral sac of rumen; 6, abomasum; 7, omasum; 8, duodenum; 9, gallbladder; 10, liver; 11, cranial pole of right kidney; 12, right adrenal gland.

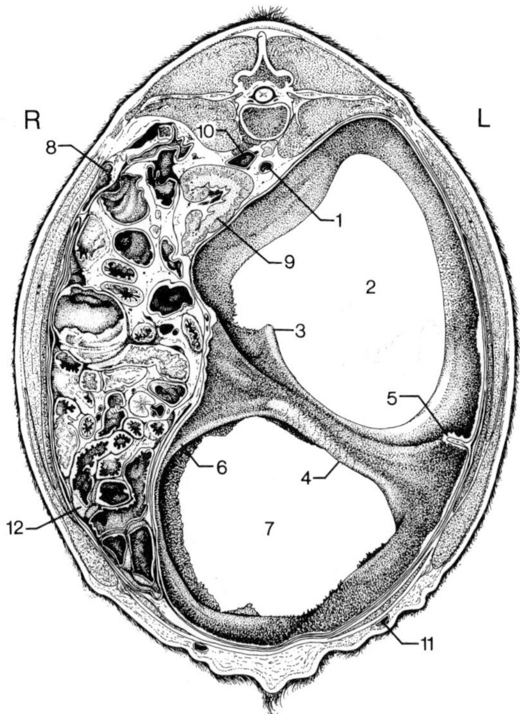


**Figure 28–10.** Transverse section of the bovine trunk at the level of the third lumbar vertebra.

1, Aorta; 2, caudodorsal blind sac; 3, dorsal coronary pillar; 4, caudal pillar; 5, left longitudinal pillar; 6, ventral coronary pillar; 7, caudoventral blind sac; 8, descending duodenum; 9, left kidney; 10, caudal vena cava; 11, milk vein; 12, intestinal mass.

*minal pillars* encircle the organ, dividing dorsal and ventral major sacs, while lesser *coronary pillars* mark off the caudal blind sacs. The cranial pillar has an oblique direction that partially divides the cranial extremity from the remainder of the dorsal sac, emphasizing the association of the former part *(atrium ruminis)* with the reticulum. External grooves correspond to the positions of all these folds. The relative proportions of the compartments vary among the domestic ruminants. The smaller size of the dorsal sac and the extensive caudal projection of the ventral blind sac give the rumen of sheep and goats an unbalanced appearance when compared with the more symmetrical bovine rumen. There are also differences in the development of the grooves visible externally, but these are altogether without practical significance.

The serosa covers the entire surface of the rumen and reticulum, except dorsally where the ruminal wall is directly adherent to the abdominal roof from the esophageal hiatus of the diaphragm to the level of the fourth lumbar vertebra (Fig. 28–21/12), and over certain grooves where it is reflected to continue into the greater omentum. This limitation of the direct attachment allows the ruminoreticulum the freedom necessary for the incessant and reciprocal contractions and enlargements of its various parts that characterize its normal state.

The *relationships* are most easily studied by reference to the illustrations (Figs. 28–4/*A,B;* 28–9; and 28–14). The most important points are contact between the reticulum and the diaphragm and liver cranially; insinuation of the abomasum between the two chambers (ventral sac of rumen and reticulum) ventrally; relation of the right surface of the rumen to the intestinal mass, omasum, abomasum, pancreas, and kidneys; and the intrusion of the superficial wall of the greater omentum between the ventral sac of the rumen and the abdominal wall. The rumen also has a variable relationship to the uterus and other organs at the entrance to the pelvis where the dorsal sac may be palpated per rectum. The direct contact of the dorsal sac with the upper part of the left flank makes auscultation and palpation simple. It also facilitates trocarization for the relief of tympany.

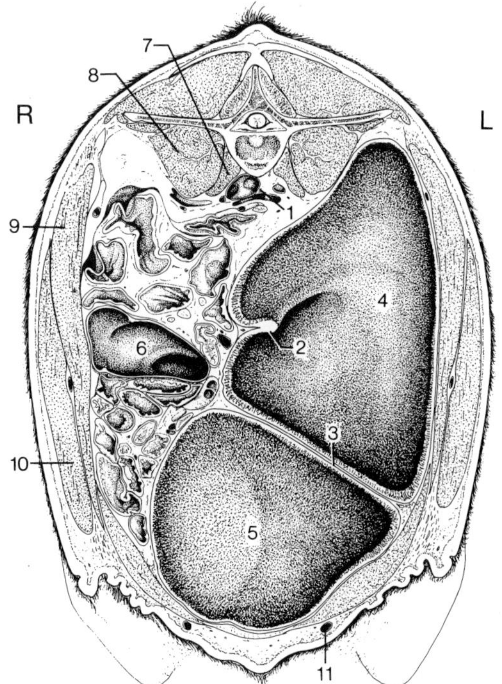


**Figure 28–11.** Transverse section of the bovine trunk at the level of the fifth lumbar vertebra.

1, Bifurcation of aorta and formation of caudal vena cava; 2, right dorsal coronary pillar; 3, caudal pillar; 4, caudodorsal blind sac; 5, caudoventral blind sac; 6, colon; 7, psoas minor; 8, psoas major; 9, internal abdominal oblique; 10, external abdominal oblique; 11, milk vein.

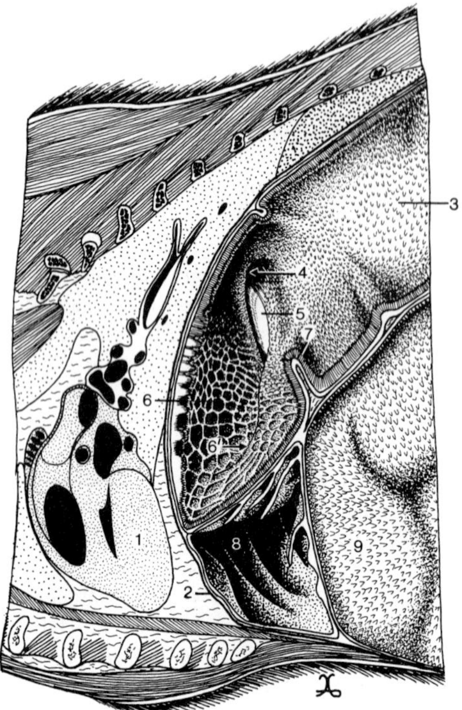


**Figure 28–12.** Paramedian section of part of the trunk of a goat.

1, Heart; 2, diaphragm; 3, atrium ruminis; 4, 5, 6′, reticular groove; 4, cardia; 5, floor of groove; 6′, reticulo-omasal orifice; 6, reticulum; 7, ruminoreticular fold; 8, abomasum; 9, ventral sac of rumen.

The *interior* of the ruminoreticulum communicates with the esophagus and omasum through openings placed at the extremities of the *reticular* (formerly esophageal) *groove,* a prominent gutter that descends from the cardia over the right face of the reticulum toward the fundus (Fig. 28–12/4,5,6′). The groove is bounded by spiral fleshy lips; the upper end of the left (cranial) lip is expanded to overhang the slitlike cardiac opening, while a similar thickening of the lower end of the right (caudal) lip partly conceals the round exit into the omasum (Fig. 28–15/1,2). The cardia is placed at the junction of the rumen and reticulum and discharges into both chambers. In the unweaned animal the reticular groove may be converted into a closed tube, forming a channel that conveys milk directly from the esophagus to the omasal canal, whence it drops into the abomasum. The muscular contractions that draw the lips together are reflexly stimulated by sucking from the dam or by the presentation of suitable bucket feeds. As the animal matures, alterations in diet and feeding regimen result in decreasing use of this route although even in the adult a portion of the soluble nutrients released into the saliva during mastication succeeds in bypassing the ruminoreticulum. The groove reflex is stimulated by antidiuretic hormone (ADH), indicating that the reflex may have some function in adult life. ADH is produced in response to dehydration or increase in plasma osmolality. ADH is associated with thirst, and its effect on the reticular groove may cause a portion of the water drunk by dehydrated animals to bypass the ruminoreticulum. Closure of the groove can be stimulated by certain chemicals (e.g., copper sulfate). This provides a useful stratagem when it is desirable to introduce drugs to the abomasum without prior dilution in the forechambers.

The *ruminoreticular mucosa* is lined by a harsh stratified cutaneous epithelium (Plate 28/*B,D*) that is stained a greenish brown; the floor of the reticular groove, however, is smooth and pale. The reticular mucosa has a distinctive pattern formed by ridges about 1 cm high that outline four-, five-, and six-sided "cells" (see Fig. 27–5/8, 28–13/*B*, and Plate 28/*A*). These ridges, and the cell floors between them, carry low papillae. The reticulate pattern becomes less regular toward the junction with the rumen and gradually modifies to merge with the papillated surface of this chamber. The epithelium of the reticular mucosa is stratified

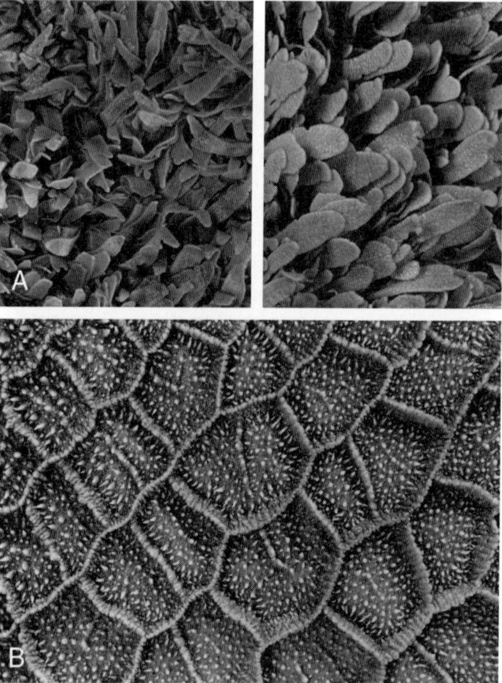


**Figure 28–13.** *A,* Rumen papillated mucosa taken from a Waterbuck *(left)* and a lesser Kudu. *B,* Reticulum: mucosal ridges outlining "cells" characteristic of the reticular mucosa.

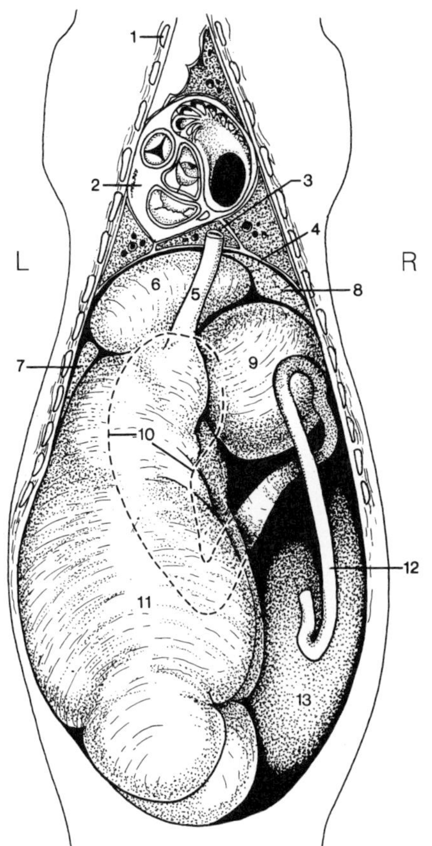


**Figure 28–14.** Dorsal section of the thorax, and dorsal view of the stomach and intestinal mass to illustrate the topography of the bovine thoracic and abdominal organs.

1, First rib; 2, heart sectioned at the level of the valves; 3, accessory lobe of right lung; 4, diaphragm; 5, esophagus; 6, reticulum; 7, spleen; 8, liver; 9, omasum; 10, outline of abomasum; 11, dorsal sac of rumen; 12, descending duodenum; 13, intestinal mass.

squamous. The upper keratinized layer protects against abrasion by the rough, fibrous diet, whereas the deeper layers metabolize volatile short-chain fatty acids. Histologically, the epithelium shows many similarities with the epidermis. The lamina propria-submucosa, formed by a network of collagen and elastic fibers, includes bands of smooth muscle within the distal parts of the reticular folds (Plate 28/*B*). The ruminal papillae vary in prominence according to age, diet, and location (Fig. 28–13/*A* and Plate 28/*C*). Normally they are largest and most densely strewn within the blind sacs, fewer and less prominent in the ventral sac, and least developed over the center of the roof and toward the free margins of the pillars. Individual papillae vary from low rounded elevations through conical and tonguelike forms to flattened leaves about 1 cm long. The ruminal epithelium resembles that of the reticulum. A thick lamina propria beneath the epithelium forms the core of the papilla; apart from collagen, elastic, and reticular fibers, it includes a dense capillary network. There is no muscularis mucosae. The looser submucosa is located directly against the lamina propria and also contains a vascular network (Plate 28/*D*).

The rugose nature of the ruminoreticular lining was formerly interpreted as an adaptation for the mechanical disruption of the macerating ingesta. Since it became known that the volatile fatty acids produced by microbial fermentation are absorbed in the rumen and reticulum it has been regarded as primarily a device to increase the epithelial surface. Papillary development is stimulated by these acids (especially butyric) and their absorption is facilitated by the very rich subepithelial capillary plexus. In wild ruminants striking changes in papillary prominence and size, and thus in the ruminal surface area (Fig. 28–13/*A*), accompany seasonal changes in forage quality. Changes in papillary development tend to be more restrained in domestic species whose diet is subject to human influence to a greater or lesser degree.*

The reticulum of the *small ruminants* is relatively larger than that of cattle. Though it extends farther caudally, its contact with the abdominal floor is subject to much functional variation (Fig. 28–12/6). There are conspicuous species differences in its lining. The ridges that bound the reticular "cells" are relatively much lower and have more prominently serrated margins in sheep and goats. The papillated "ruminal" mucosa also extends over a larger part of the reticular wall in these species.

The smooth muscle of the ruminoreticular wall is arranged in two coats that continue the striated muscle of the esophagus. The thin outer coat runs craniocaudally over the rumen but has an oblique course on the reticulum. Most bundles of the much thicker inner layer run more or less at right angles to the superficial coat and thus encircle the long axis of the rumen. They extend into the pillars and form the bases of these structures. The thicker parts of the ruminoreticular muscle are sold for consumption as tripe.

The regular sequence of *ruminoreticular contractions* mixes and redistributes the stomach contents. The cycle consists of a biphasic reticular contraction (relaxation between contraction phases is more consistent in cattle than in sheep), which

*In wild ruminants striking changes in the total mass of the salivary glands are correlated with the ruminal response to the fibrous content of the forage.

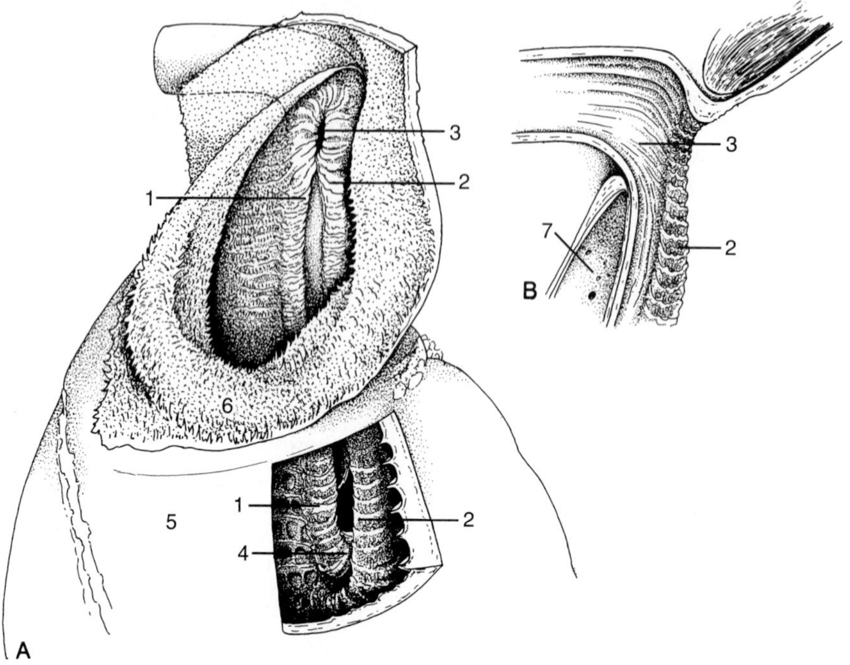


**Figure 28–15.** Opening of esophagus into stomach with the course of the (slightly untwisted) reticular groove *(A)*, and detail of the cardiac orifice *(B)*.

1, Left (cranial) lip of reticular groove; 2, right lip of reticular groove; 3, cardiac orifice; 4, reticulo-omasal orifice; 5, wall of reticulum; 6, ruminoreticular fold; 7, liver.

throws the reticular contents into the atrium ruminis, followed by contraction of first the dorsal and later the ventral rumen sacs. The wave of contraction passes over each in a craniocaudal direction. The process is centrally regulated, and the tempo and vigor are adjusted according to information supplied by intramural receptors that are stimulated by stretching of the wall and by contact with floating fragments. Both the sensory and the motor pathways travel within the vagus nerves.

Regurgitation of food for remastication requires the coordination of the stomach movements with those of the thoracic wall and throat. It is preceded by an additional reticular contraction that floods the cardiac region; the ingesta are drawn into the esophagus upon expansion of the thorax with a closed upper airway and are then carried orally by an antiperistaltic wave. The heavy remasticated cud, now further sodden and divided, tends to drop from the cardia into the reticulum.

In eructation (the discharge of gas through the esophagus), ruminal contractions in which the reticulum does not participate are substituted for the normal pattern of activity. These contractions originate in the ventral sac and generally spread to the dorsal sac where they begin caudally and extend cranially; they force the ruminal gas forward to the cardiac area whence it is aspirated into the esophagus, through which it is hurried orally by an antiperistaltic wave. It then passes through the relaxed pharyngoesophageal sphincter into the pharynx. Some escapes from the mouth but, as already discussed, part is directed to the lungs.

The content of the rumen shows some stratification with food of recent ingestion piled above the heavier, more sodden remasticated material. It is therefore the lighter material that is most liable to be regurgitated for further mastication and insalivation (Fig. 28–16).

Cattle are notoriously careless feeders and often ingest foreign bodies, especially pieces of wire, with their forage. These bodies tend to collect within the reticulum and, when sharp, may be driven through the reticular wall by the contractions of this organ (traumatic reticulitis—"hardware disease"). Common sequelae include abscessation of the liver and possibly other abdominal organs and, more critically, a purulent pericarditis when the object penetrates the diaphragm. Some of these bodies corrode, while others may be immobilized by introducing a magnet through the mouth (Fig. 28–17/2 and inset).

## The Omasum

The omasum lies within the intrathoracic part of the abdomen to the right of the midline, between the rumen and reticulum to the left and the liver and body wall to the right (Figs. 28–8/7 and 28–14/9). It is bilaterally flattened and displays a long convex border that faces dextrocaudally and a much shorter lesser curvature that looks in the opposite direction. The long axis is more or less vertical in the cadaver, but the position and orientation of the living organ alter constantly. Most of the omasum lies under cover of ribs 8 to 11, but in cattle the lower pole generally projects onto the abdominal floor below the costal arch (Fig. 28–27/5). Although its position places most of the omasum beyond direct manual reach, the organ may be examined by auscultation and percussion. The lower pole of the omasum has an extensive attachment to the fundic region of the abomasum around the omasoabomasal orifice. Much of its right surface is covered by and partly connected to the lesser omentum (Fig. 28–4/*C*,13).

The omasum is relatively smaller in sheep and goats, in which it is bean-shaped. It maintains an almost vertical position when the stomach is at rest. It projects upon the eighth and ninth ribs but, because of the intervention of the liver, makes no direct contact with the body wall.

The *interior* is occupied by about a hundred crescentic laminae that arise from the sides and greater curvature and project toward the lesser curvature where there is a more open passage, the *omasal canal* (Fig. 28–8). The laminae are of several lengths, and those of different sizes alternate so as to divide the lumen into a series of narrow and fairly uniform recesses (Plate 28/*E*). The *reticulo-omasal orifice* is situated at the upper end of the short canal; the large, oval *omasoabomasal opening* (/6) at the other extremity is partly occluded by the prolapse of abomasal folds. The floor of the canal (known as the omasal groove) is smooth except for a few low ridges that run along its length and a scattering of clawlike projections that guard the upper opening.

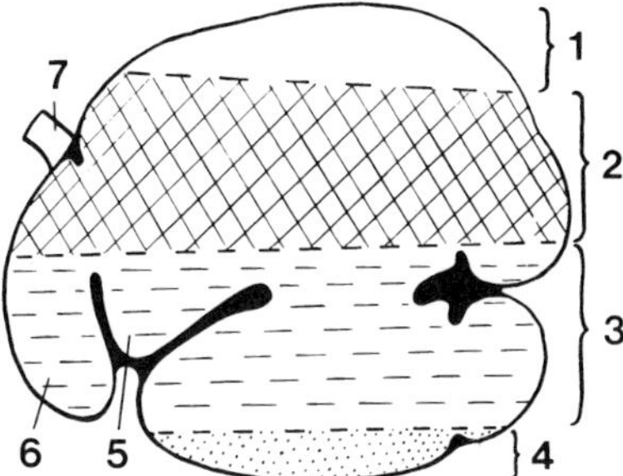


**Figure 28–16.** Stratification of ingesta in the ruminoreticulum, left lateral view.

1, Gas bubble; 2, coarse forage ("floating mat"); 3, more finely ground material with higher specific gravity than 2; 4, liquid zone; 5, atrium ruminis; 6, reticulum; 7, esophagus.

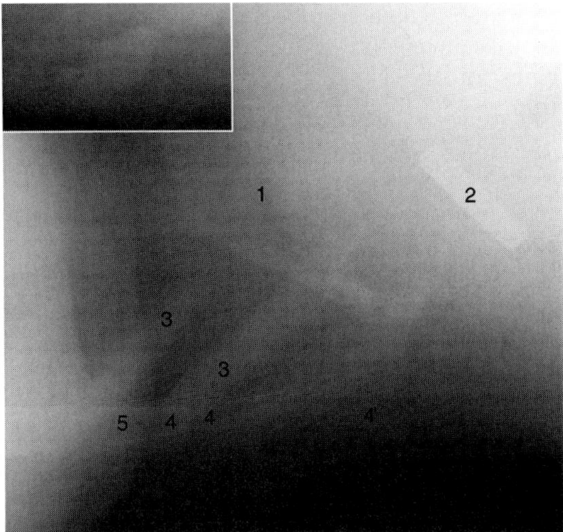


**Figure 28–17.** Lateral radiograph of the vicinity of the reticulum of a young cow (cranial is to the left). The inset shows a close-up of a magnet with adhering metal objects.

1, Cranial wall of reticulum with sediment in its "cells"; 2, magnet; 3, costal cartilages; 4, sternebrae; 4′, xiphoid cartilage; 5, proximal epiphysis of ulna (olecranon).

The keratinized stratified squamous epithelium over the laminae is raised to cover numerous papillae. Most of these are small and lenticular, but there are a few larger, conical projections that point distally and perhaps promote the onward movement of the ingesta. The mucosa is further characterized by a lamina propria including a dense subepithelial capillary network and enclosing a thick muscularis mucosae consisting of a thin outer longitudinal layer and a thicker inner circular layer. The inner layer is continuous with the muscle of the omasal wall (Plate 28/*F*). The contents of the omasal recesses are finely divided and rather dry; they impart a firmness to the organ that allows it to be readily recognized on palpation at laparotomy, directly, or after incision of the rumen wall.

Omasal contractions are biphasic. The first phase squeezes ingesta from the omasal canal into the recesses between the laminae; the second phase is a mass contraction of the omasum. The principal effect is to squeeze fluid from the material within the recesses, a process essential to the continuing movement of ingesta to the abomasum. These contractions occur at a much slower and more deliberate tempo than those of the ruminoreticulum. Although the rough surfaces and muscular cores of the laminae suggest that these folds triturate the food by rubbing against each other, there is no evidence of such activity. Absorption is continued in the omasum.

## The Abomasum

The abomasum lies flexed upon the abdominal floor, embracing the lower pole of the omasum from behind (Fig. 28–14/10). The larger of the two limbs forms a piriform sac that reaches forward to the left to make contact with the body wall between the reticulum and the atrium and ventral sac of the rumen (Fig. 28–4/*A*,6). This limb is divided by analogy with the simple stomach into *fundus* and *body,* but the boundary between these parts is imprecise. In fact, the location of the omasoabomasal opening in the living animal is not known with certainty; it is possible that it is terminal, and in that case no blind diverticulum, and therefore no true fundus, exists. The cranial part of the fundus is extensively connected to the reticulum, atrium, and ventral sac by muscle bundles.

The narrower and more uniform distal limb constitutes the *pyloric part* of the organ. It passes transversely, or with a slightly cranial inclination, toward the right body wall and ascends to terminate at the pylorus, caudal to the lower part of the omasum (/*D*,15 and Plate 29/*D*). The abomasum does not usually come into contact with the liver in adult cattle.

The abomasum of the sheep and the goat is relatively large but, this apart, shows no important features of distinction. In contrast to the situation in adult cattle, it is usually allowed direct contact with the liver by the smaller size of the omasum.

The position and relations of the abomasum depend upon the fullness of the different parts of the stomach, intrinsic abomasal activity, and, most important, the contractions of the rumen and reticulum to which the abomasum is attached. Age and pregnancy are other important factors influencing its extent and topography (Fig. 28–19). Though it is difficult to specify abomasal relations exactly, it is vital to appreciate that there are limits to the normal variations beyond which deviations produce digestive disturbance and may endanger life. Abomasal displacement, which may be to the right or left, is a well-recognized disorder, particularly in dairy cows (see further on).

The abomasum is lined by a pink, slime-covered, *glandular mucosa* that is in striking contrast to the harsh lining of the forestomach. At the omasoabomasal junction the epithelium changes abruptly to a simple columnar epithelium with occasional goblet cells. The lamina propria is less dense than that of the omasum and, frequently, solitary lymph nodules are observed at the junction with the epithelium. The mucosa of the abomasum has all the characteristics of that of the simple stomach (Plate 28/*H*). The mucosal area is increased about sixfold by the presence of large folds, upward of a dozen in number, that arise around the entrance and course spirally over the walls of the fundus and body before subsiding as the flexure is approached (Fig. 28–18/2 and Plate 28/*G*). Approximation of the proximal ends of these folds forms a mucosal valve or "plug" that discourages the reflux of ingesta into the omasum. The mucosa of the pyloric part bears a few low rugae and is most remarkable for the large swelling or *torus* that projects from the lesser curvature to narrow the pyloric passage (/6). The vascular arrangements within the torus suggest that it is capable of a form of erection, but the possible functional significance of this (and of the entire structure, for that matter) is unknown. The dark mucosa of the body and fundus contains true peptic glands; the glands of the lighter pyloric part secrete mucus alone.

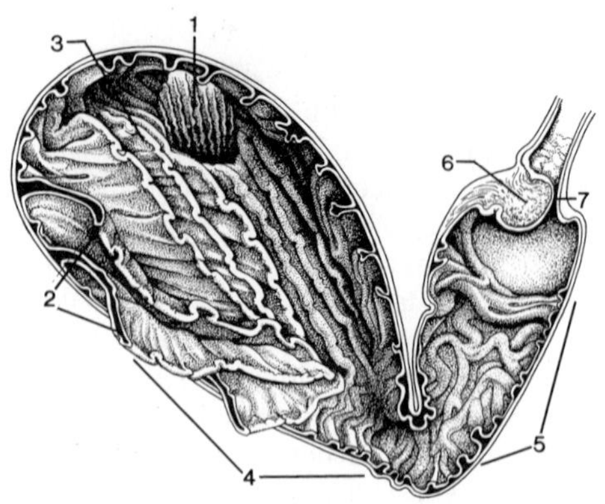


**Figure 28–18.** Opened abomasum as seen from behind, above, and slightly from the left.

1, Omasoabomasal opening through which the omasal laminae can be seen; 2, spiral folds; 3, fundus; 4, body; 5, pyloric part; 6, torus pyloricus; 7, pylorus.

The abomasal wall is relatively thin. The serous covering is deficient only at the attachment to the other stomach chambers and along the origins of the omenta. The muscle coat consists of longitudinal and circular strata. The longitudinal muscle is confined to the curvatures of the fundus and body but forms a thicker and wider covering to the pyloric part. The circular fibers provide a more powerful and more complete layer but are also better developed over the pyloric part, especially distally.

The *movements* of the adult abomasum are rather sluggish. They consist of general contractions of the proximal limb and more forceful peristalsis confined to the pyloric part. The latter activity often appears to be prompted by the tipping of the ingesta toward the pylorus when the fundic region is elevated by reticular contraction. It is possible that these normal alterations in position facilitate morbid displacements of the abomasum. Atony, with the accumulation of gas in the fundus, is a constant finding in these cases, and it may be that a slight initial displacement is worsened because this gas is denied its usual escape through the omasoabomasal opening when this comes to lie below the gas bubble.

*Displacements* are commonly related to the high proportion of concentrates to roughage in the ration of stabled cows, which leads to atony of the abomasum and accumulation of liquid ingesta and gas. Pregnancy may be a predisposing factor (Fig. 28–19/*C*). Since the abomasum is well fixed proximally to the heavy omasum and distally by the cranial part of the duodenum and lesser omentum to the liver, it is its middle part that travels farthest from its usual position on the abdominal floor. Contractions of the ruminoreticulum may allow the abomasum, buoyed by the gas within, to work its way under the atrium of the rumen and up on the left side. The loop formed by the middle part of the abomasum eventually comes to lie between the rumen and the left abdominal wall, deep to last three or four ribs where it can be identified by simultaneous percussion and auscultation (left displacement of the abomasum; LDA). In right displacement (RDA) the loop formed by the middle part of the abomasum slides to the right and lies between the right abdominal wall and the intestines and the liver. Displacements to the right are often complicated by twisting of the loop. Treatment of uncomplicated displacements consists of returning the abomasum to its normal position by placing the cow on its back, by deflating the organ through a paramedian incision of the abdominal wall, and by including its muscular coat in the closing of the incision (abomasopexy). Omentopexy is done in the standing cow through an incision in the right paralumbar fossa. The abomasum is deflated via a large hypodermic needle attached to a tube, then swept into its ventral position and held in place by including nearby omentum in the closing of the incision.

## The Omenta

The attachment of the *greater omentum* begins dorsal to the esophagus. The two serosal sheets of

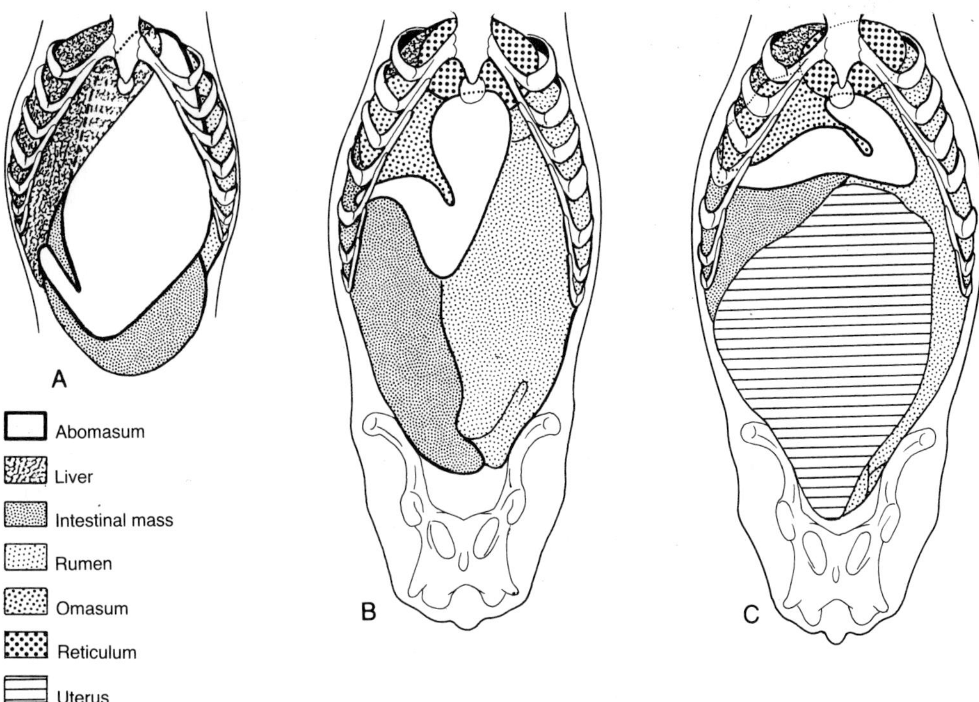


**Figure 28–19.** Ventral views of the abdominal viscera of a newborn calf (*A*), a 5-year-old cow (*B*), and a 6-year-old heavily pregnant cow (*C*) based on reconstructions of transverse sections of animals frozen in the standing position.

which it is composed pass directly onto the rumen but are so widely separated that the immediately postcardiac part of the rumen roof is enabled to attach directly to the abdominal roof (Fig. 28–21/12). This retroperitoneal space is closed caudally where the two serosal sheets come together halfway along the right longitudinal groove to form a conventional duplicature attaching to the stomach. The attachment of this fold may be traced along the right longitudinal groove, through the caudal groove between the caudal blind sacs, and then forward along the left longitudinal groove. It now crosses the atrium ruminis and widens to make a broad attachment to the reticulum before bending sharply to the right, ventral to the ruminoreticulum, to reach the greater curvature of the abomasum (Figs. 28–4/*A,C* and 28–7/8). It follows this to the pylorus and continues onto the caudal aspect of the first (vertical) part of the duodenum from which it extends onto the descending duodenum and later the mesoduodenum. The omental attachment is reflected where the duodenum turns cranially, and it retraces its attachment along the descending duodenum until carried back to the cranial duodenal flexure at the porta of the liver. It then returns to the right face of the rumen via the pancreas.

The *lesser omentum* arises from the visceral surface of the liver, between the porta and the esophageal impression (Fig. 28–26), and passes to the region of the reticular groove, the right face of the omasum, and thence along the lesser curvature of the abomasum to the first part of the duodenum, which returns it to the liver (Fig. 28–4/*C*).

The omental sheets enclose a space, the *omental bursa,* which is completely divided from the greater peritoneal cavity except at the epiploic foramen near the porta of the liver. The bursa is a mere capillary cleft in life, but it is simpler for descriptive purposes to envisage it as distended. A first impression of its topography may be obtained from the schema in which it can be seen that the ventral sac of the rumen projects into it (Fig. 28–20/*B*/6,2′). The omental sheets that run transversely across the abdomen lie one against the abdominal wall, the other against the viscera (chiefly intestines) (Fig. 28–21/3,4). The superficial and deep sheets pass into each other caudally and in this way close the bursa behind (Fig. 28–20/*A*). The omasum, abomasum, and lesser omentum provide most of the cranial bursal wall. The entrance to the bursal cavity, the epiploic foramen, is situated dorsocranially between the liver and the duodenum or, more precisely, between the caudal vena cava dorsally and the portal vein ventrally.

The greater omentum is an important store of fat that is first deposited along the small vessels that ramify and anastomose between the peritoneal layers; usually the fat is present in such large amounts that the whole omentum becomes thickened and opaque. (In many cows one such thickening forms a short offshoot near the pylorus known as "pig's ear"; it can be palpated during surgery and serves as a landmark for the position of the pylorus.) The superficial sheet screens the ventral sac of the rumen from view when the lower left flank is opened, and both superficial and deep sheets intervene between the organs that lie ventral to the duodenum and the right flank (Fig. 28–4/*A,C*). The intestines are closeted in the space above the bursa, and to the right of the rumen, which is known as the supraomental recess; it is freely open behind and is often entered by the pregnant uterus (Figs. 28–20/7 and 28–21/11).

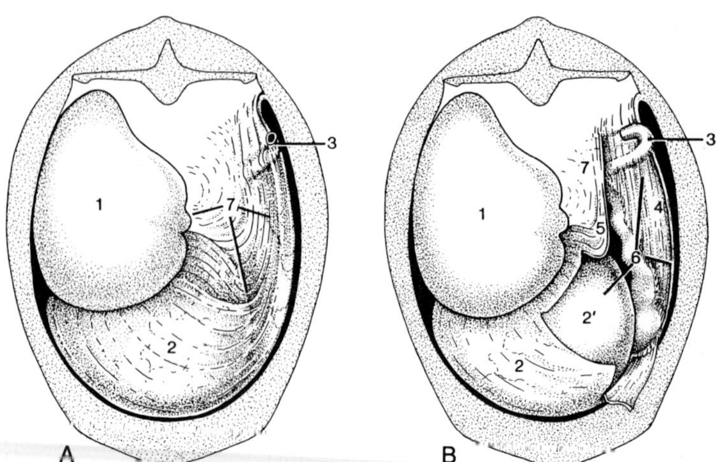


**Figure 28–20.** Attachment of the greater omentum to the stomach and the dorsal body wall. *A,* Caudal view of intact greater omentum. *B,* Caudal view of greater omentum fenestrated to permit a view into omental bursa.

1, Dorsal sac of rumen; 2, ventral sac of rumen, covered by superficial wall of greater omentum; 2′, ventral sac of rumen projecting into omental bursa; 3, caudal flexure of duodenum; 4, superficial wall of greater omentum; 5, deep wall of greater omentum; 6, omental bursa; 7, supraomental recess.

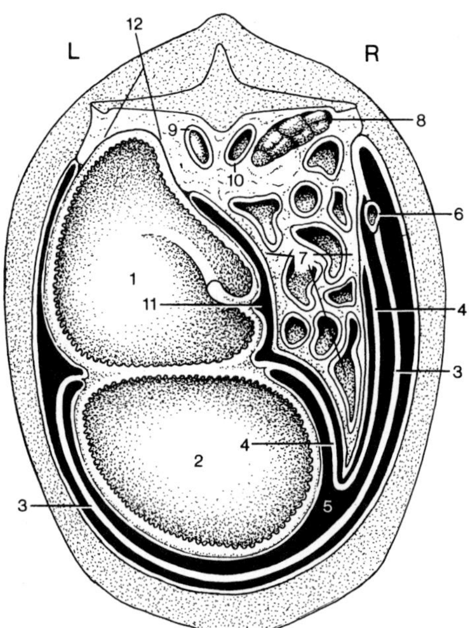


**Figure 28-21.** Schematic transverse section of the abdominal cavity to show the disposition of the greater omentum.

1, Dorsal sac of rumen; 2, ventral sac of rumen; 3, superficial wall of greater omentum; 4, deep wall of greater omentum; 5, omental bursa; 6, descending duodenum; 7, intestinal mass; 8, right kidney; 9, aorta; 10, caudal vena cava; 11, supraomental recess; 12, retroperitoneal attachment of rumen.

## Innervation and Vascularization

The principal gastric nerves, parasympathetic efferent and afferent, run in the trunks formed along the esophagus by the regrouping of vagal fibers (see Fig. 27–4/19,20). The sympathetic nerves that reach the stomach through periarterial plexuses have a subordinate role.

The *dorsal vagal trunk* is extensively connected with the celiac plexus but also supplies direct branches to the rumen wall, the region of the reticular groove, the reticulo-omasal orifice, the omasum, and the abomasum. The *ventral trunk* has a less substantial and indirect celiac connection; it detaches branches to the atrium ruminis and reticulum, again including the region of the groove and the reticulo-omasal orifice, and to the omasum and right face of the abomasum. An additional long branch reaches the pylorus independently after traveling through the lesser omentum (Fig. 28–22).

Section of both trunks abolishes all motor activity of the forechambers. Section of the dorsal trunk alone results in almost complete, but not necessarily permanent, paralysis of the rumen, while the effect on the reticulum is generally less marked. The effects of division of the ventral trunk are unpredictable and range from little or no discernible change to almost complete paralysis of the forechambers. It is presumed that these inconstant results can be explained by differences in the regrouping of fibers where the vagus nerves combine to form the dorsal and ventral trunks, and by the later assumption of part of these functions by association neurons in the stomach wall.

Abomasal contractions are greatly reduced following bilateral vagal section but are not wholly interrupted, possibly because some intrinsic control is vested in a submucosal nerve plexus present in the wall of this chamber alone. Division of the splanchnic nerves brings only slight alteration to the gastric movements. Clinically, disturbances of stomach function may follow involvement of the vagus nerves at any point along their courses from the brainstem; the most common causes are mediastinal infections and traumatic reticulitis.

The stomach is supplied with blood through several branches of the *celiac artery* (Fig. 28–23/3). The large right ruminal artery (/14) runs caudally in the right longitudinal groove and continues into the left groove by passing between the dorsal and ventral blind sacs. It supplies most of the rumen wall and ends in anastomosis with the left ruminal artery (/12), which follows the cranial groove (between atrium and ventral sac) to supply adjoining parts of the rumen and reticulum. The latter organ also receives a direct branch (/13) from the parent trunk. The omasum and abomasum are supplied by the left gastric and left gastroepiploic arteries (/4,5) that follow their curvatures; these

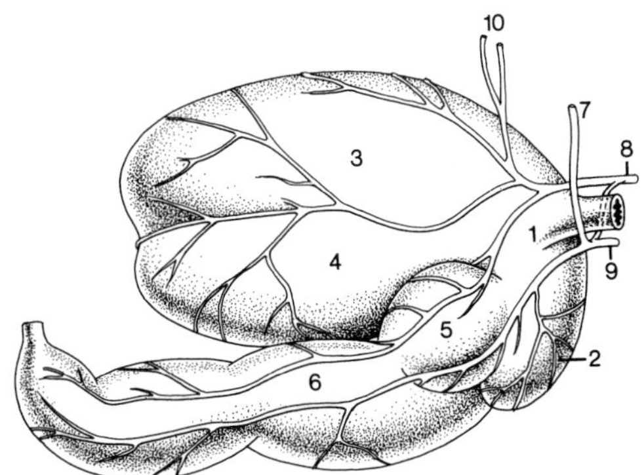


**Figure 28-22.** The pattern of parasympathetic innervation of the ruminant stomach. The dorsal vagal trunk (8) is of special importance for the innervation of the rumen, the ventral trunk (9) for the innervation of the reticulum, omasum, and abomasum.

1, Cardia; 2, reticulum; 3, 4, dorsal and ventral sacs of the rumen; 5, omasum; 6, abomasum; 7, branch of ventral vagal trunk to liver and pylorus; 8, dorsal vagal trunk; 9, ventral vagal trunk; 10, branches to celiacomesenteric ganglion.

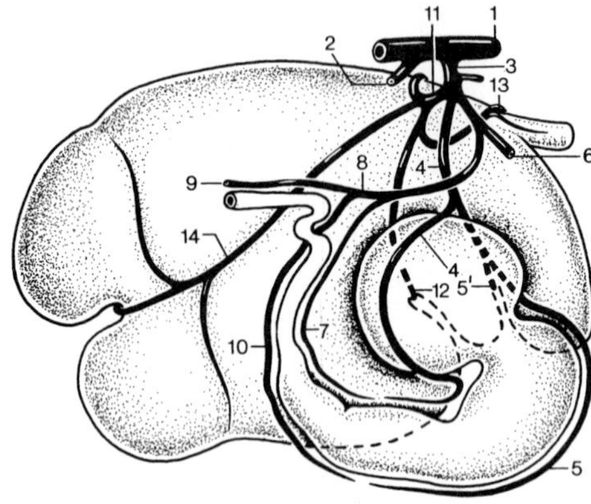


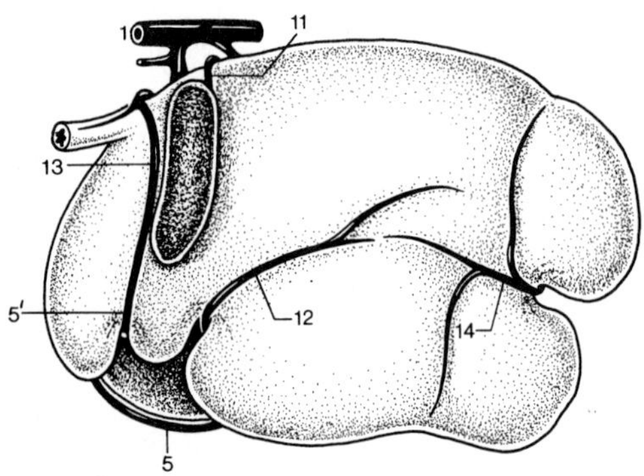


**Figure 28–23.** Arteries of the ruminant stomach.

1, Aorta; 2, cranial mesenteric a.; 3, celiac a.; 4, left gastric a.; 5, left gastroepiploic a.; 5′, accessory reticular a.; 6, hepatic a.; 7, right gastric a.; 8, gastroduodenal a.; 9, cranial pancreaticoduodenal a.; 10, right gastroepiploic a.; 11, splenic a.; 12, left ruminal a. (often from the left gastric); 13, reticular a.; 14, right ruminal a.

eventually unite with like-named branches of the hepatic artery that descend on the cranial part of the duodenum (/7,10).

The *veins* are mainly satellite to the arteries. The left ruminal vein joins the emissary vessels of the reticulum, omasum, and abomasum; the right one, the veins leading from the spleen; their union produces a major radicle (splenic vein) of the portal vein.

Many small *lymph nodes* are scattered over the stomach, particularly in the ruminal grooves and over the omasal and abomasal curvatures. Lymph from the forechambers leads, after serial passage through these peripheral nodes, to a number of large atrial nodes situated between the cardia and omasum and thence to the visceral root of the cisterna chyli. The nodes placed along the abomasal curvatures direct their efferent vessels to the hepatic lymph nodes.

## Postnatal Development

At the time of birth the ruminant stomach is prepared for the digestion of milk. The abomasum predominates and is remarkable not only for its size, which surpasses the combined capacity of the other chambers, but also for the degree of structural maturity that it has attained. Its full extent is apparent directly after the consumption of a generous feed. At such times the abomasum extends from the liver and diaphragm to the pelvic entrance, from one flank to the other, and from the floor well into the upper half of the abdomen (Figs. 28–19/*A* and 28–24/4). Its capacity may already exceed 60% of the adult measure. So large an organ inevitably impinges upon almost all other abdominal contents, but only the extensive contact with the liver, which in the neonatus reaches far across the median plane, need be mentioned. The abomasal mucosa is at first not quite mature, and a few days elapse before the fundic glands become fully active; presumably this is a provision to allow the absorption of unaltered antibodies from the colostrum during the first 24 hours of extrauterine life.

In contrast to the abomasum, the rumen and reticulum of the newborn calf are very small. They are confined to the left dorsal and cranial corner of the abdomen and are generally found crumpled and collapsed (/2,3); they are bypassed by milk feeds and normally contain only a small amount of fluid—secretions of the respiratory tract (swallowed in utero) in the youngest animals, saliva in those a little older. The omasum is also retarded in development, though less so than in the smaller ruminant species, and forms a relatively inconspicuous bridge between the reticulum and the abomasal fundus. The walls of the forechambers are thin and deficient in muscle and, while their mucosae possess the characteristic adult features, these are present in subdued form, especially in the rumen where the papillae project barely 1 mm above the surrounding surface and are fused together at their bases.

No striking changes in proportions and structure are to be observed before the young calf shows serious interest in solid food, generally from the time it is 2 or 3 weeks old. Thereafter the abomasum continues to increase at a slow but steady rate while the rumen and reticulum enter upon a period of spectacular growth. They have generally overtaken the abomasum by 8 weeks, and at 12 weeks they are more than twice as large. This unequal growth continues, but more slowly, until the time when the definitive topography and proportions are established. It is difficult to specify this age, for many variable factors are involved, and while some authors assert that the conformation is virtually adult after 3 months, others believe that it does not become so until near the end of the first year.

Normal development depends upon the availability of a normal diet of solid forage, but there remain some uncertainties concerning the precise stimuli that are involved. At one time it was thought that the physical characteristics of the diet were all-important and that roughage not only stretched the stomach wall and stimulated its muscular growth but also promoted the differentiation of the mucosa. Later it was shown that many gross and microscopic features of the mucosa develop only with exposure to certain end products of microbial fermentation, notably butyric acid. Exposure to these stimuli must be continued for some time if development is to follow its normal course, and the return of a young, partly weaned calf to a wholly milk diet may result in the arrest and sometimes even reversal of the maturation processes.

The abomasum is initially the most vigorous chamber, but its activity diminishes as the ruminoreticulum, first inert and then only spasmodically active, establishes a regular cycle of contraction by the second month. The feeding habits, the structural changes, and the motor and chemical activities of the stomach, when taken in conjunction, define three phases of development. A neonatal period, in which milk forms the sole diet, may last for 2 or at most 3 weeks and be followed by a transitional period when the stomach is adapting to solid food. From the eighth week onward the anatomy and the processes of digestion may be essentially those of the adult. The chronology will clearly be different in dairy and suckler calves.

Changes in abdominal topography are not confined to the stomach. In the newborn the liver is relatively large and lies across the midline, extensively related to the abomasum. As the rumen and reticulum increase in size the liver is pressed toward the right and dorsally, and it rotates so that its left lobe comes to lie cranioventral to the right one and out of the reach of the abomasum. The intestines are simultaneously pushed away from the left flank and become confined to the right side; the expansion of the dorsal ruminal sac also displaces the left kidney, thrusting it across the midline until it comes to rest below and caudal to its fellow (Figs. 28–10/9 and 29–10/10).

## THE INTESTINES

The intestines lie almost entirely to the right of the midline, packed mainly into the dorsal part of the abdomen and in part lying under cover of the ribs.

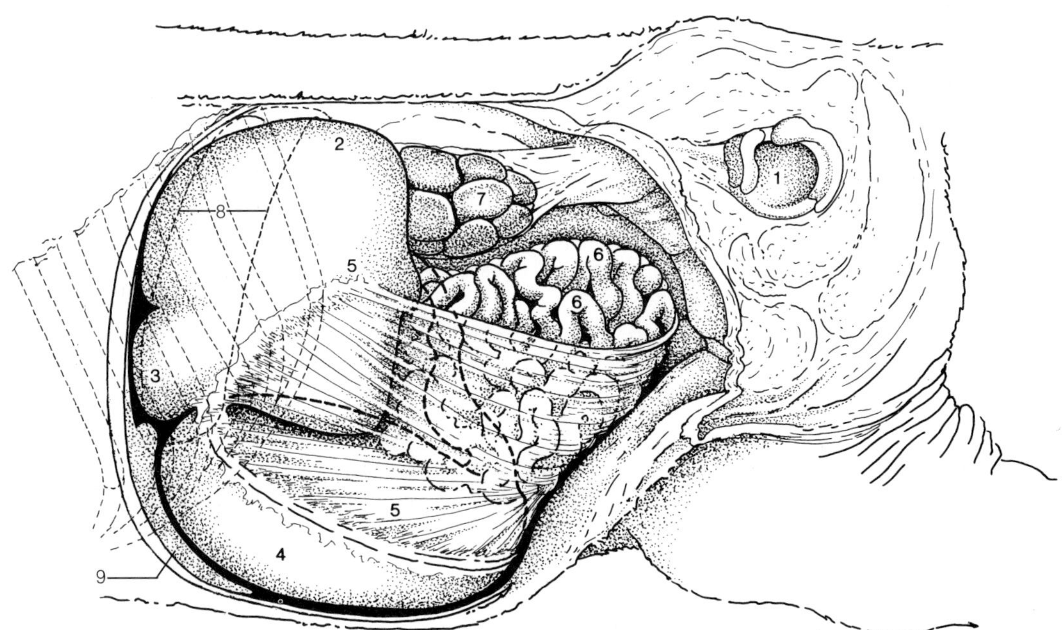


**Figure 28–24.** Topography of the abdominal organs in a newborn calf, left lateral view. The left abdominal wall and the left hindlimb have been removed.

1, Left acetabulum; 2, rumen; 3, reticulum; 4, abomasum; 5, greater omentum; 6, small intestine; 7, left kidney; 8, position of spleen; 9, liver.

Though measuring as much as 50 m in adult cattle, their capacity is relatively slight, a feature correlated with the efficiency of gastric digestion. Adhesion of the mesenteries of the small intestine and ascending colon during the fetal period results in these parts of the intestine sharing a common support in which they are flexed and coiled in a complex arrangement, easily traced in a schema (Fig. 28–25) or in an isolated specimen, but difficult to unravel in situ where the gut is bunched and partially concealed by fat.

The *duodenum* takes origin below the ribs. Its first part rises almost vertically toward the visceral surface of the liver against which it forms several bends in close succession. It then runs toward the pelvis as the descending duodenum but turns when almost level with the coxal tuber. The ascending part then returns toward the liver, passing to the left of the cranial mesenteric artery, to enter the fringe of the mesentery. It is continued by the jejunum. The first part of the duodenum is joined to the liver by the lesser omentum. The other border of the first and descending parts gives attachment, directly or at slight remove, to both walls of the greater omentum (Figs. 28–4/*C* and 28–20). Only the descending duodenum is immediately visible on opening the right flank.

The *jejunum* forms many short coils within the free margin of the mesentery. Their general course takes them ventrally, then caudally, and finally dorsally toward the large bowel. The position of these coils depends upon the fullness of the rumen and the size of the uterus; usually most lie within the supraomental recess, but some may spill from this to insinuate themselves behind the rumen and so appear against the left flank. The extent of the short *ileum* is defined by the ileocecal fold (Fig. 28–25/4,6).

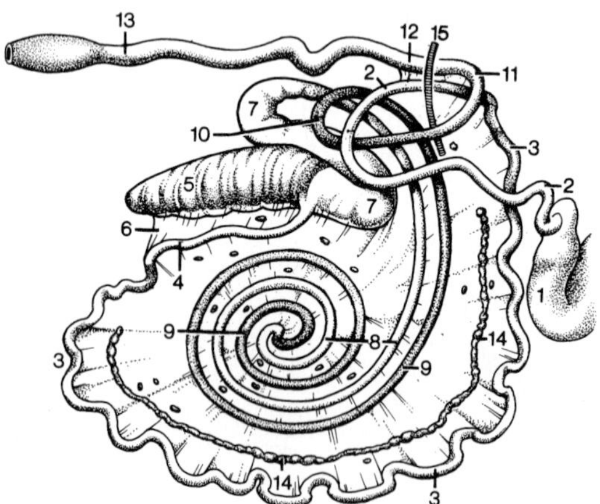


**Figure 28–25.** Right lateral view of the bovine intestinal tract, schematic.

1, Pyloric part of abomasum; 2, duodenum; 3, jejunum; 4, ileum; 5, cecum; 6, ileocecal fold; 7–10, ascending colon; 7, proximal loop of ascending colon; 8, centripetal turns of spiral colon; 9, centrifugal turns of spiral colon; 10, distal loop of ascending colon; 11, transverse colon; 12, descending colon; 13, rectum; 14, jejunal lymph nodes; 15, cranial mesenteric artery.

The *cecum* continues into the colon without obvious change in diameter, the junction being marked only by the entrance of the ileum. Though the widest part of the gut, it is rather featureless. Its rounded blind tip projects caudally from the supraomental recess and floats high when gas-filled but sinks when its contents are heavier. When greatly distended with gas for protracted periods it must be deflated surgically. Rotation of the cecum together with the proximal loop of the colon (/7) is common, compromises its function and blood supply, and requires surgical correction.

The *colon* is divided into the usual ascending, transverse, and descending parts (see Fig. 3–44/Ru). The first of these is wound in a very elaborate manner. On leaving the cecum it forms a flattened sigmoid flexure (/11) before narrowing and turning ventrally to trace a double spiral attached to the left side of the mesentery. Two centripetal turns are succeeded by two centrifugal turns that restore the colon toward the periphery of the mesentery where it continues into a distal loop that carries it first toward and then away from the pelvis (/11′). Beyond this it joins the short transverse colon (/4) that crosses the midline in front of the mesenteric artery and leads directly into the descending colon. This part runs toward the pelvic entrance within a mesentery that is thickened by fat and fused with neighboring parts of the gut. The mesentery of the descending colon is at first short but lengthens in front of the sacrum where the colon forms a sigmoid flexure before continuing as the rectum. This looseness gives the hand of the veterinarian considerable range in rectal exploration (p. 710). The rectum is described with the pelvic viscera.

The ascending colon of cattle presents one and one-half to two centripetal turns and the same number of centrifugal turns; in *small ruminants* there are three or four turns in each direction. A more significant difference lies in the pearl necklace appearance of the centrifugal turns of the small ruminants, in which the contents are already segmented into the pellets so characteristic of the feces. The linear string of these pellets in the ascending colon is replaced by their massing in a thicker column in the wider descending colon and rectum.

Few features of the *interior* of the intestines call for comment. In cattle the accessory pancreatic duct opens far down the descending duodenal limb, the bile duct more proximally where the duodenum lies against the liver. In the small ruminants the greater pancreatic duct is usually present. The ileum projects into the cecum, and a low rampart is thus present around the ileal orifice. Lymphoid tissue is generously spread through the mucosa, especially in the small intestine where both solitary and aggregated nodules occur. The aggregated nodules may reach lengths of 25 cm and are distinguished by their irregular cribriform surfaces. Usually one of these patches extends through the ileal orifice into the large gut.

The bulk of the intestines is supplied by the *cranial mesenteric artery,* but the first part of the duodenum is supplied from the celiac artery and the descending colon from the caudal mesenteric artery. The intestinal veins combine to form the cranial mesenteric radicle of the portal vein. Very many jejunal lymph nodes are found within the mesentery where they form a more or less continuous chain of giant nodes placed between the peripheral festoons of small intestine and the more central coils of the spiral colon (Fig. 28–25/14). The largest may be as much as a meter in length. In the small ruminants this chain of nodes lies central to the last centrifugal turn of the spiral colon. Other small nodes are scattered beside the cecum, colon, and rectum. The efferent stream from the mesenteric nodes joins the cisterna chyli. The nerves that reach the gut along the cranial mesenteric artery consist of both sympathetic and vagal fibers.* The parasympathetic nerves to the last part of the colon are derived from the sacral outflow.

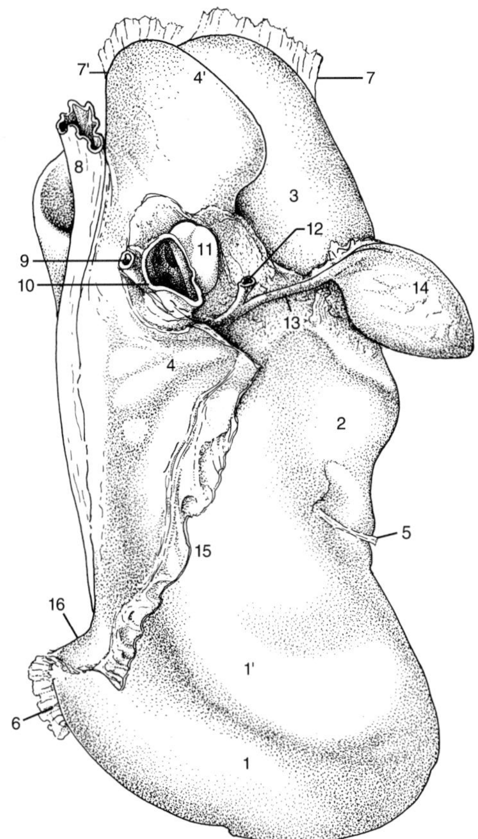


**Figure 28–26.** Visceral surface of the bovine liver.

1, Left lobe; 1′, omasal impression; 2, quadrate lobe; 3, right lobe; 4, 4′, papillary and caudate processes of caudate lobe; 5, round ligament; 6, left triangular ligament; 7, right triangular ligament; 7′, hepatorenal ligament; 8, caudal vena cava; 9, hepatic artery; 10, portal vein; 11, hepatic lymph node; 12, bile duct; 13, cystic duct; 14, gallbladder; 15, lesser omentum; 16, esophageal impression.

## THE LIVER

The liver of the adult animal lies almost entirely within the right half of the abdomen, related to the caudal face of the diaphragm and under cover of the ribs (Fig. 28–8/9). Its projection extends between the ventral third of the sixth intercostal space to the upper part of the last (Fig. 28–27/4). The visceral surface is related to the reticulum, atrium ruminis, omasum, duodenum, gallbladder, and pancreas, most of which impress their form upon the living organ; the indentations are retained by the specimen hardened in situ (Fig. 28–26). The thick dorsal border extends farthest caudally and is partly fashioned by the blunt caudate process; this is separated from the main mass by a recess into which fits the cranial pole of the right kidney. The medial (originally dorsal) border follows the midline rather closely; toward its lower end it is marked by an impression (/16) that gives passage to the esophagus, and below this a small part spreads across into the left half of the abdomen. The caudal vena cava (/8) tunnels through this edge of the liver and in its course receives its hepatic tributaries (Fig. 28–8/10).

The thin lateral border is marked by the fissure that divided the right and left "halves" of the fetal organ, and in most adult cattle this provides entrance for the round ligament, the remains of the umbilical vein (Fig. 28–26/5). The blind vertex of the piriform gallbladder (/14) projects beyond the lateral margin of the right lobe; it lies against the

*There is evidence that the infective (prion protein) agents responsible for the transmissible spongiform encephalopathies (e.g. bovine spongiform encephalopathy) reach the central nervous system by transport from the gut along the splanchnic and vagal nerves.

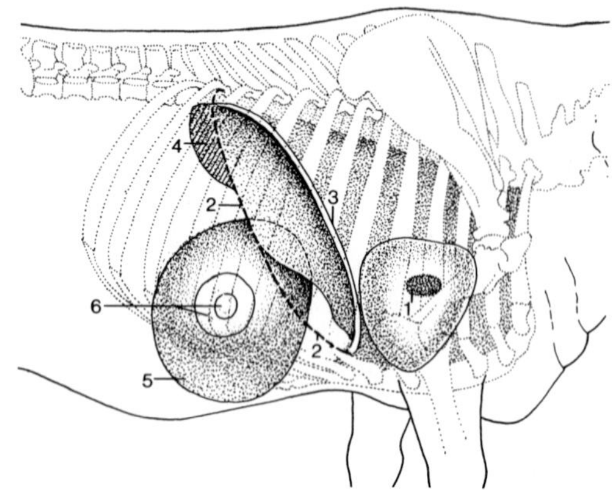


**Figure 28–27.** Right lateral projection of certain organs on the bovine thoracic wall.

1, Right atrioventricular valve; 2, position of basal border of lung; 3, cranial extent of diaphragm and liver; 4, field of liver percussion; 5, omasum; 6, field for percussion and auscultation of omasum.

diaphragm opposite the ventral part of the 10th or 11th rib.

The liver is retained in position by certain ligaments attaching it to the diaphragm and, more important, by visceral pressure. Its position may be verified by dullness on percussion over an area centered on the dorsal part of the 11th rib and 11th intercostal space. The percussion area is small in relation to the size of the organ and corresponds to the area of direct contact with the body wall (Fig. 28–9/10). A detectable increase in its extent generally signifies a disproportionate enlargement of the organ.

The relationship of the liver to the right pleural sac should be noted so that biopsy specimens may be obtained with the least risk (Fig. 28–27/2,4). The preferred site for puncture is through the 11th intercostal space in the plane of the lower part of the coxal tuber. The trocar is directed to meet the diaphragm, and thus the liver, at right angles to ensure a clean puncture; this route avoids the larger vessels. The relatively larger size of the liver of the young calf may allow the organ to be palpated behind the last rib.

The structure of the liver shows no species-specific features of importance. The organ is enclosed within a tough fibrous capsule, but the extensions into the parenchyma do not outline obvious lobules as in the liver of the pig. The hepatic ducts join together in the portal region to form a single channel from which the cystic duct branches to the gallbladder. The continuation beyond this junction constitutes the bile duct, which enters the duodenum. The most superficial hepatic ducts may be visible through the covering liver tissue, especially when thickened by disease; in many countries most ostensibly normal animals show this evidence of fluke infestation (distomiasis).

The liver receives its blood through the *hepatic artery* and *portal vein,* which enter at the porta. Blood from both these sources mixes within the hepatic sinusoids and returns to the general circulation through the hepatic veins, which enter the embedded portion of the caudal vena cava. The openings of the major hepatic veins are arranged in two widely separated clusters; intrahepatic anastomoses between the two sets provide a potential collateral pathway that becomes important when the intervening stretch of the caudal vena cava is obstructed.

The efferent lymphatic vessels pass mainly to the hepatic group of *nodes* scattered about the porta; the lymph thence drains into the visceral radicle of the cisterna chyli. Some lymph is routed via accessory hepatic (on the caudal vena cava) and caudal mediastinal nodes.

Though the livers of the *sheep* and the *goat* generally resemble that of cattle, size alone prohibits confusion of the adult organs. They are distinguished from the liver of the calf by the much deeper umbilical fissure, narrower and less bluntly shaped caudate process, more elongated gallbladder, and absence of the sizable vestige of the umbilical vein that is evident on the liver of the young calf. An extensive contact with the abomasum is retained throughout life.

## THE PANCREAS

The pancreas is a soft, lobulated gland of irregular form and pinkish-yellow color. The pancreas of the calf is consumed as a delicacy, together with thymus, under the title of sweetbread. For descriptive purpose it may be regarded as consisting of two lobes that join in a body located cranial to the portal vein where the gland is adherent to the liver. The left lobe extends across the abdomen, insinuated between the liver, diaphragm, and great vessels dorsally and the intestinal mass and dorsal ruminal sac ventrally; it thus enters the retroperitoneal area above the rumen. The right lobe has a more complete peritoneal covering and follows the mesentery of the descending part of the duodenum, ventral to the right kidney and against the flank.

Although developed from dorsal and ventral primordia, the excretory system is usually reduced in cattle to a single (accessory) duct when the ventral outgrowth loses its direct connection to the gut. The surviving duct enters the descending duodenum about 20 to 25 cm past the entry of the bile duct. Its orifice is raised on a slight papilla.

The pancreas of *small ruminants* is very similar in form and topography to that of cattle. A single duct that in these species represents the ventral duct is present; it opens into the duodenum with the bile duct, usually by means of a common trunk—a feature that suits these species to experimental studies of the effects of diverting bile into the pancreatic duct system.

## THE KIDNEYS AND ADRENAL GLANDS

The kidneys of adult cattle retain much of their fetal lobation and are each divided by surface fissures into about a dozen lobes (Plate 4/*E*). The right kidney has a flattened ellipsoidal form and lies in a conventional position with a dorsal retroperitoneal attachment to the sublumbar musculature. It is received cranially into the renal impression of the liver. The left kidney is less regular, being flattened at its cranial pole and thickened caudally (Fig. 28–28). Its position below and behind its fellow is unusual and is the consequence of the postnatal growth of the rumen (see Fig. 29–10/10). Although surrounded by considerable accumulations of fat (capsula adiposa), both kidneys vary in position with the phase of respiration and according to the pressure exerted by other viscera. In the cadaver the right kidney is commonly found below the last rib and first two or three lumbar transverse processes, while the left one lies at a more ventral level under the second to fourth lumbar vertebrae. The left kidney is thus within easy reach on rectal exploration, but contact with the right one is not usually attainable. The left kidney may return to the left side when the pressure on it is relieved—by fasting in life or following evisceration in the course of an autopsy.

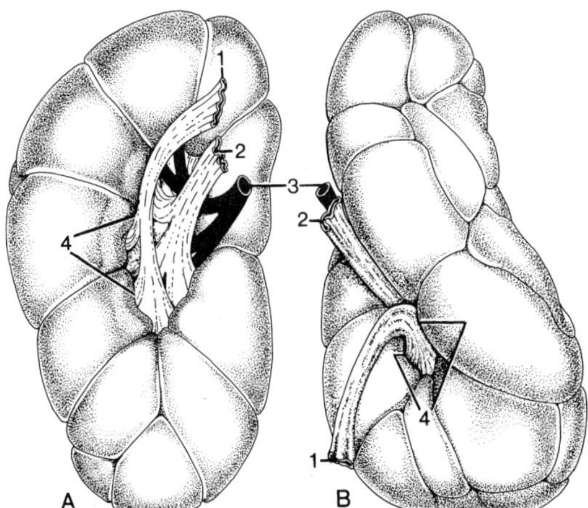

**Figure 28–28.** Ventral views of the right *(A)* and left *(B)* bovine kidneys.

1, Ureter; 2, renal vein; 3, renal artery; 4, renal sinus.

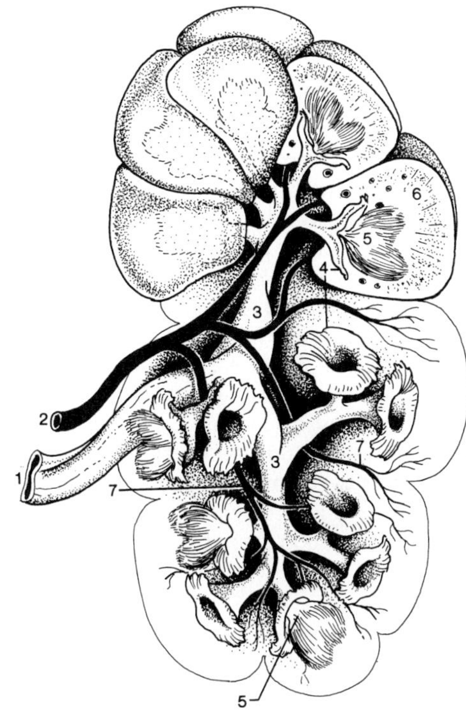

**Figure 28–29.** Bovine kidney dissected to show its interior, semischematic.

1, Ureter; 2, renal artery; 3, principal branches of ureter; 4, calices; 5, renal papilla; 6, renal cortex; 7, interlobar arteries.

The numerous relations of the right kidney need not be described at length. They include the liver, pancreas, duodenum, colon, and, in most animals, the adrenal gland. The hilus is widely open and lies ventromedially; the ureter runs from it, crossing the medial margin to follow a winding retroperitoneal course below the abdominal roof that carries it into the pelvis. The ureter may be palpated per rectum but is generally not appreciated unless distended.

The left kidney is swung through about 90 degrees around the axis of the aorta in moving from its fetal (Fig. 28–24) to its adult location against the right face of the dorsal sac; it hangs in a relatively long fold, rests upon the intestinal mass, and is flattened by contact with the rumen. The left ureter crosses the dorsal aspect of the kidney to regain the left half of the abdomen. Its later course is similar to that of the right duct.

In *structure* the bovine kidneys are of the multipyramidal type (Fig. 28–29). The separate medullary pyramids are capped by a continuous cortex, although on casual inspection this also appears fragmented by fissures extending inward from its surface. The cortex (/6) is clothed in a tough capsule that is easily stripped from the healthy organ, except toward the hilus where it blends with the wall of the ureter. The cortical and medullary regions are distinguishable in gross sections by the much lighter color of the former and by the cut vessels that mark their mutual boundary. The glomerular vascular tufts scattered through the cortex may be visible to the naked eye. The apex (papilla; /5) of each medullary pyramid fits into a calyx or cup formed by one of the terminal branches of the ureter; these branches eventually unite to form two major channels that converge from the cranial and caudal poles to yield a single ureter (Plate 4/*F*). There is thus no large central expansion corresponding to a renal pelvis.

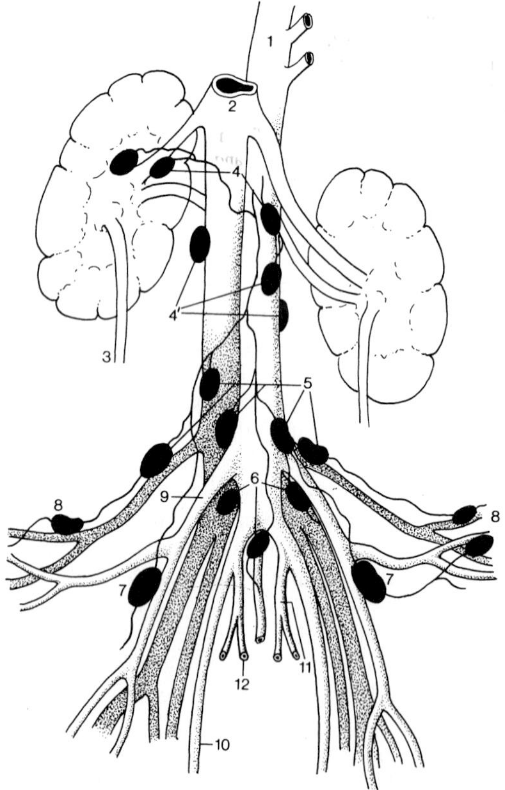


**Figure 28–30.** The lymph nodes associated with the caudal part of the abdominal aorta and caudal vena cava in cattle, ventral view.

1, Aorta; 2, caudal vena cava; 3, ureter; 4, renal lymph nodes; 4′, lumbar aortic lymph nodes; 5, medial iliac lymph nodes; 6, sacral lymph nodes; 7, deep inguinal lymph nodes; 8, lateral iliac lymph nodes; 9, external iliac artery; 10, internal iliac artery; 11, umbilical artery; 12, uterine artery.

The *renal arteries* (/2) are derived from the aorta and are unusually large in relation to the organs they supply. The *renal veins* join the caudal vena cava. Lymphatic vessels, present in generous profusion, lead to the renal nodes, enlarged members of the lumbar aortic series, and these in turn drain into the lumbar lymph trunk (Fig. 28–30/4,4′).

The *kidneys of the sheep and goat* are quite unlike those of cattle but conform closely in external appearance and internal structure to those of the dog (see Fig. 5–22). They are more regular in shape than the dog's, being protected from distorting pressures by enclosure in thick masses of fat. The fat cushion makes the left kidney less subject to displacement by the rumen.

The *adrenal glands* are located close to the kidneys. The right gland is heart-shaped and usually lies against the medial margin of the cranial extremity of the corresponding kidney (Fig. 28–9/12). The left one is less regular in form and less constant in position; generally it is found within the perirenal fat some centimeters cranial to the left kidney. The division into cortex and medulla is very evident in gross sections. The adrenal glands, and especially the cortices, are relatively larger in fetal and juvenile animals.

## THE LYMPH NODES OF THE ABDOMINAL ROOF

A number of important lymph nodes are scattered about the bifurcation of the aorta and between its terminal branches. Most belong to the medial iliac group, which collects lymph from the hindlimbs, pelvic walls, and pelvic viscera (Fig. 28–30/5). The large deep inguinal (iliofemoral) node, in the angle between the external and deep circumflex iliac arteries, receives the flow from the udder; when enlarged it can be palpated per rectum near the cranial border of the ilium (/7). The efferent stream forms the lumbar trunk, which runs forward over the aorta to enter the cisterna chyli, a large, thin-walled lymph sac occupying the space between the aorta and vena cava, close to the aortic hiatus in the diaphragm.

A few much smaller (lumbar aortic) nodes spread along the psoas musculature are concerned with the lymphatic drainage of the vertebrae and neighboring muscles. The renal nodes belong to this series (/4,4′).

## Selected Bibliography

Alexander, R.M.: The relative merits of foregut and hindgut fermentation. J. Zool. 231:391–402, 1993.

Anderson, D.E., E.M. Gaughan, and G. St.-Jean: Normal laparoscopic anatomy of the bovine abdomen. Am. J. Vet. Res. 54:1170–1176, 1993.

Ashdown, R.R., and S. Done: Color Atlas of Veterinary Anatomy: The Ruminants. Baltimore, University Park Press, 1984.

Baker, J.S.: Abomasal impaction and related obstructions of the forestomachs in cattle. JAVMA 175:1250–1253, 1979.

Baxter, G.M.: Umbilical masses in calves: Diagnosis, treatment, and complications. Compend. Contin. Educ. Pract. Vet. 11:505–513, 1989.

Braun, U., R. Eicher, and K. Hausammann: Clinical findings in cattle with dilatation and torsion of the caecum. Vet. Rec. 125:265–267, 1989.

Braun, U., M. Flückiger, and M. Götz: Comparison of ultrasonographic and radiographic findings in cows with traumatic reticuloperitonitis. Vet. Rec. 135:470–478, 1994.

Braun, U., M. Flückiger, and F. Nägeli: Radiography as an aid in the diagnosis of traumatic reticuloperitonitis in cattle. Vet. Rec. 132:103–109, 1993.

Campbell, M.E., and S.L. Fubini: Indications and surgical approaches for cesarean section in cattle. Compend. Contin. Educ. Pract. Vet. 12:285–292, 1990.

Cegarra, I.J., and R.E. Lewis: Contrast study of the gastrointestinal tract in the goat *(Capra hircus)*. Am. J. Vet. Res. 38:1121–1132, 1977.

Comline, R.S., L.A. Silver, and D.H. Stevens: Physiological anatomy of the ruminant stomach. *In* Handbook of Physiology, Section 6. Alimentary Canal, Vol. 5. Washington, D.C., American Physiological Society, 1968.

Constable, P.D., G.F. Hoffsis, and D.M. Rings: The reticulorumen: Normal and abnormal motor function. Part 1. Primary contraction cycle. Compend. Contin. Educ. Pract. Vet. 12:1008–1014, 1990.

Constable, P.D., G.F. Hoffsis, and D.M. Rings: The reticulorumen: Normal and abnormal motor function. Part II. Secondary contraction cycles, rumination, and esophageal groove closure. Compend. Contin. Educ. Pract. Vet. 12: 1169–1174, 1990.

Constable, P.D., D.M. Rings, B.L. Hull, et al.: Atresia coli in calves: 26 cases (1977–1987). JAVMA 195:118–123, 1989.

deLahunta, A., and R.E. Habel: Applied Veterinary Anatomy. Philadelphia, W.B. Saunders Company, 1986.

Dirksen, G.U., and F.B. Garry: Diseases of the forestomachs in calves—Part I. Compend. Contin. Educ. Pract. Vet. 9:F140–F146, 1987.

Dirksen, G.U., and F.B. Garry: Diseases of the forestomachs in calves—Part II. Compend. Contin. Educ. Pract. Vet. 9:F173–F179, 1987.

Dreyfuss, D.J., and E.P. Tulleners: Intestinal atresia in calves: 22 cases (1978–1988). JAVMA 195:508–513, 1989.

Ducharme, N.G., M. Arighi, D. Horney, et al.: Colonic atresia in cattle: A prospective study of 43 cases. Can. Vet. J. 29:818–824, 1988.

Ducharme, N.G., M. Arighi, D. Horney, et al.: Surgery of the bovine forestomach compartments. Vet. Clin. North Am. Food Anim. Pract. 6:371–397, 1990.

Ducharme, N.G., S.G. Dill, and V.T. Rendano: Reticulography of the cow in dorsal recumbency: An aid in the diagnosis and treatment of traumatic reticuloperitonitis. JAVMA 182:585–588, 1983.

Franco, A., A. Robina, S. Regodon, et al.: Histomorphometric analysis of the omasum of sheep during development. Am. J. Vet. Res. 54:1221–1229, 1993.

Fubini, S.L.: Surgery of the bovine large intestine. Vet. Clin. North Am. Food Anim. Pract. 6:461–471, 1990.

Fubini, S.L.: Surgical management of gastrointestinal obstruction in calves. Compend. Contin. Educ. Pract. Vet. 4:591–598, 1990.

Fubini, S.L., N.G. Ducharme, J.P. Murphy, and D.F. Smith: Vagus indigestion syndrome resulting from a liver abscess in dairy cows. JAVMA 186:1297–1300, 1985.

Fubini, S.L., H.N. Erb, W.C. Rebhun, and D. Horn: Cecal dilatation and volvulus in dairy cows: 84 cases (1977–1983). JAVMA 189:96–99, 1986.

Fubini, S.L., Y.T. Gröhn, and D.F. Smith: Right displacement of the abomasum and abomasal volvulus in dairy cows: 458 cases (1980–1987). JAVMA 198:460–464, 1991.

Fubini, S.L., D.F. Smith, P.K. Tithof, et al.: Volvulus of the distal part of the jejunoileum in four cows. Vet. Surg. 15:150–152, 1986.

Fubini, S.L., A.E. Yeager, H.O. Mohammed, and D.F. Smith: Accuracy of radiography of the reticulum for predicting surgical findings in adult dairy cattle with traumatic reticuloperitonitis: 123 cases (1981–1987). JAVMA 197: 1060–1064, 1990.

Habel, R.E.: A study of the innervation of the ruminant stomach. Cornell Vet. 46:555–633, 1956.

Habel, R.E.: Guide to the Dissection of the Domestic Ruminants, 4th ed. Ithaca, 1989. Published by the author.

Habel, R.E., and K.D. Budras: Anatomy of the prepubic tendon in the horse, cow, sheep, goat, and dog. Am. J. Vet. Res. 53:2183–2195, 1992.

Habel, R.E., and D.F. Smith: Volvulus of the bovine abomasum and omasum. JAVMA 179:447–455, 1981.

Hendrickson, D.A., P.C. Rakestraw, and N.G. Ducharme: Surgical repair of atresia jejuni in two calves. JAVMA 201:594–596, 1992.

Henninger, R.W.: Anterior abdominal pain in cattle. Compend. Contin. Educ. Pract. Vet. 6:S453–S464, 1984.

Hofmann, R.R.: How ruminants adapt and optimize their digestive system "blueprint" in response to resource shifts. *In* Weibel, E.R., C.R. Taylor, and L. Bolis (eds): Principles of Animal Design. Cambridge, Cambridge University Press, 1998.

Kelton, D.F., J. Garcia, C.L. Guard, et al.: Bar suture (toggle pin) vs open surgical abomasopexy for treatment of left displaced abomasum in dairy cattle. JAVMA 193:557–559, 1988.

Lauwers, H., L. Ooms, P. Simoens, and N.R. De Vos: The functional structure of the pylorus in the ox. Zentralbl. Vet. Med. C. Anat. Histol. Embryol. 8:56–78, 1979.

Levine, S.A., D.F. Smith, N.J. Wilsman, and D.S. Kolb: Arterial and venous supply to the bovine jejunum and proximal part of the ileum. Am. J. Vet. Res. 48:1295–1299, 1987.

Lowden, S., and T. Heath: Lymph pathways associated with Peyer's patches in sheep. J. Anat. 181:209–217, 1992.

Lowden, S., and T. Heath: Lymphatic drainage from the distal small intestine in sheep. J. Anat. 183:13–20, 1993.

Maala, C.P., and W.O. Sack: The venous supply of the cecum, ileum, and the proximal loop of the ascending colon in the ox. Zentralbl. Vet. Med. C. Anat. Histol. Embryol. 12:154–166, 1983.

Martens, A., F. Gasthuys, M. Steenhaut, and A. De Moor: Surgical aspects of intestinal atresia in 58 calves. Vet. Rec. 136:141–144, 1995.

McCarthy, P.H.: Surface rippling of the lower left flank of the cow: Mirror of ruminal motility. Am. J. Vet. Res. 42:225–228, 1981.

McCarthy, P.H.: Transruminal palpation and surface projection of the abomasum in the permanently fistulated cow. Am. J. Vet. Res. 42:1927–1932, 1981.

McCarthy, P.H.: Transruminal and transreticular palpation of abdominal viscera of the permanently fistulated dairy cow. Am. J. Vet. Res. 45:1413–1420, 1984.

Partington, B.P., and D.S. Biller: Radiography of the bovine cranioventral abdomen. Vet. Radiol. Ultrasound 32:155–168, 1991.

Pavaux, C.: A Color Atlas of Bovine Visceral Anatomy. London, Wolfe Publishing, 1983.

Popesko, P.: Atlas of Topographic Anatomy of the Domestic Animals, vol. 2: Thoracic and Abdominal Cavities. Philadelphia, W.B. Saunders Company, 1971.

Rebhun, W.C.: Differentiating the causes of left abdominal tympanitic resonance in dairy cattle. Vet. Med. 86:1126–1134, 1991.

Rebhun, W.C.: Right abdominal tympanitic resonance in dairy cattle: Identifying the causes. Vet. Med. 86:1135–1142, 1991.

Rebhun, W.C.: Vagus indigestion. JAVMA 176:506–510, 1980.

Rebhun, W.C., S.L. Fubini, T.K. Miller, et al.: Vagus indigestion in cattle: Clinical features, causes, treatments, and long-term follow-up of 112 cases. Compend. Contin. Educ. Pract. Vet. 10:387–391, 1988.

Rehage, J., M. Kaske, N. Stockhofe-Zurwieden, and E. Yalcin: Evaluation of the pathogenesis of vagus indigestion in cows with traumatic reticuloperitonitis. JAVMA 207:1607–1611, 1995.

Ruckebusch, Y., and P. Thivend: Digestive Physiology in Ruminants. Westport, Conn., AVI Publishing, 1980.

Sack, W.O.: Abdominal topography of a cow with left abomasal displacement. Am. J. Vet. Res. 29:1567–1576, 1968.

Sargison, N.D., K.J. Stafford, and D.M. West: Fluoroscopic studies of the stimulatory effects of copper sulphate and cobalt sulphate on the oesophageal groove of sheep. Small Ruminant Res. 32:61–67, 1999.

Smart, M.E., and M.J. Northcote: Liver biopsies in cattle. Compend. Contin. Educ. Pract. Vet. 7:S327–332, 1985.

Smith, D.F.: Bovine gastrointestinal surgery: Abomasal volvulus. Bovine Pract. 19:230–235, 1984.

Smith, D.F.: Bovine intestinal surgery [7 parts]. Mod. Vet. Pract. 65:705–710, 853–857, 909–914, 1984; 66:277–281, 405–409, 443–446, 995–999, 1985.

Smith, D.F.: Surgery of the bovine small intestine. Vet. Clin. North Am. Food Anim. Pract. 6:449–460, 1990.

Staller, G.S., E.P. Tulleners, V.B. Reef, and P.A. Spencer: Concordance of ultrasonographic and physical findings in cattle with an umbilical mass or suspected to have infection of the umbilical cord remnants: 32 cases (1987–1989). JAVMA 206:77–82, 1995.

Steiner, A., C.J. Lischer, and C. Oertle: Marsupialization of umbilical vein abscesses with involvement of the liver in 13 calves. Vet. Surg. 23:184–189, 1993.

Trent, A.M.: Surgery of the bovine abomasum. Vet. Clin. North Am. Food Anim. Pract. 6: 399–448, 1990.

Yamamoto, Y., N. Kitamura, J. Yamada, et al.: Morphological study of the surface structure of the omasal laminae in cattle, sheep and goats. Anat. Histol. Embryol. 23:166–176, 1994.

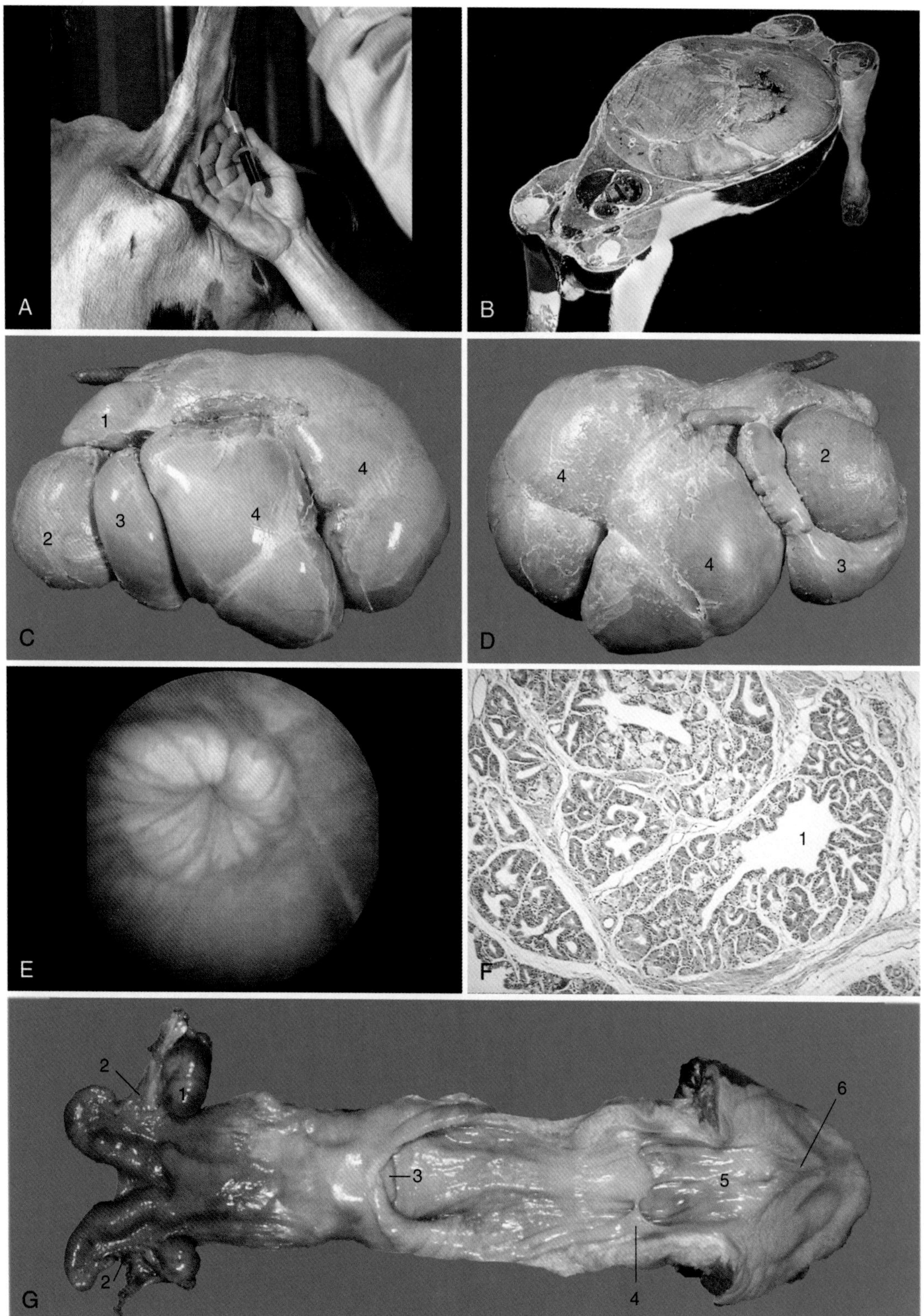


**Plate 29.** *A,* Collection of blood from tail vein (cow). *B,* Horizontal section at the level of the shoulder and stifle joints (cow). Note the relative volumes of the thoracic and abdominal cavities. *C,* Bovine stomach, left side: 1, reticulum; 2, omasum; 3, abomasum; 4, rumen. *D,* Bovine stomach, right side: (see *C* for label descriptions). *E,* Endoscopic view of bovine cervix. *F,* Bulbourethral gland (goat) (HE), a compound tubular gland lined with a columnar secretory epithelium (70×): 1, collecting duct. *G,* Uterus and opened vagina of the cow: 1, ovary; 2, uterine tube; 3, cervix; 4, hymen; 5, vestibulum; 6, glans of clitoris.

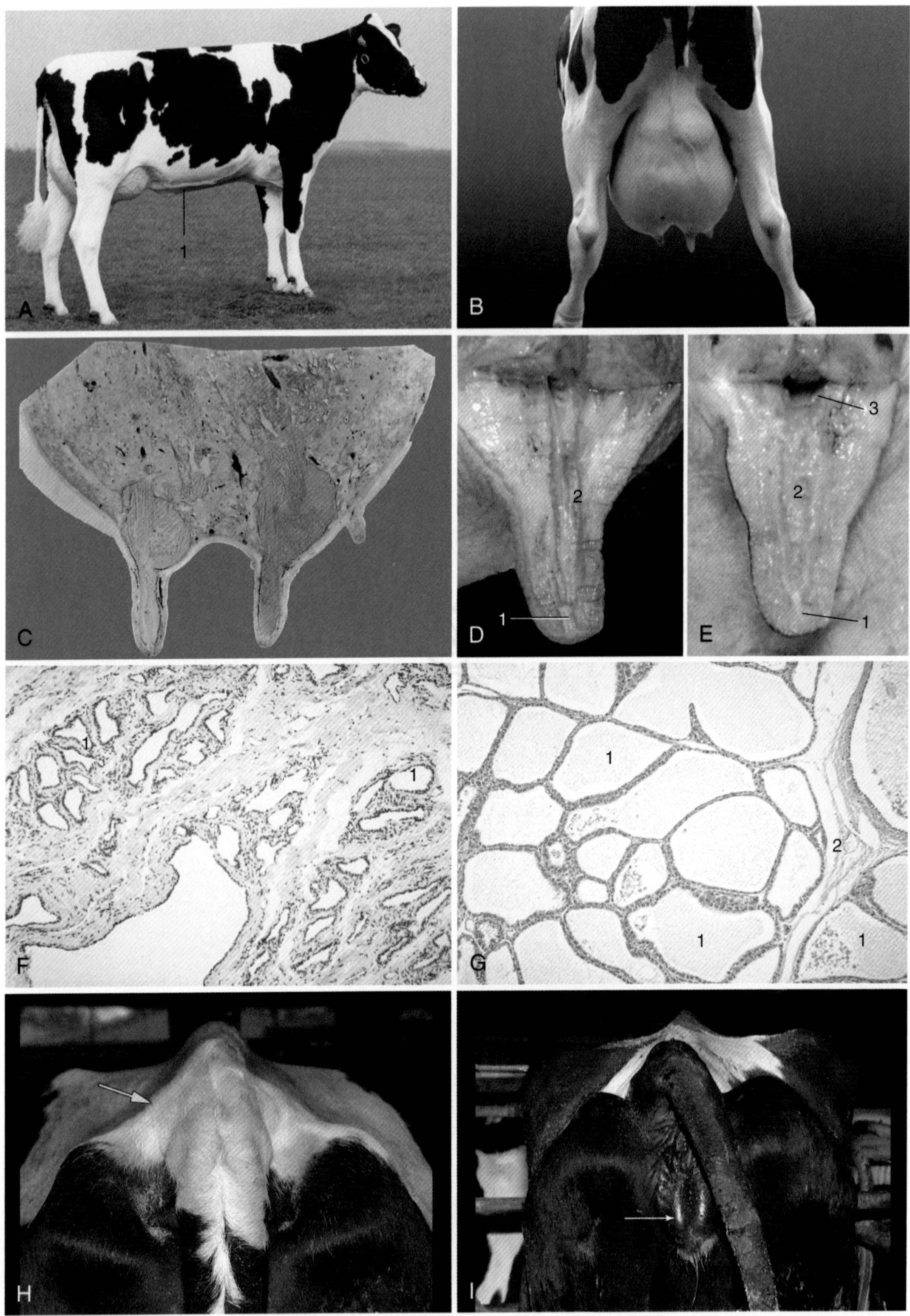


**Plate 30.** *A,* Holstein cow with well-developed udder: 1, mammary v. *B,* Enlarged mammary lymph nodes. *C,* Sagittal section of udder, showing teat and gland sinuses and lactiferous ducts filled with latex (cranial quarter, green; caudal quarter, blue). *D* and *E,* Sections of teat: 1, papillary duct; 2, teat sinus; 3, mucosal fold between teat and gland sinuses. *F* and *G,* Sections of nonlactating and lactating mammary glands; a compound tubuloalveolar gland (70×): 1, alveolus; 2, interlobular septum. *H,* Edge of the sacrotuberal ligament *(arrow)*. *I,* Relaxation of sacrotuberous ligament, and swelling of the vulva, as parturition impends *(arrow)*.

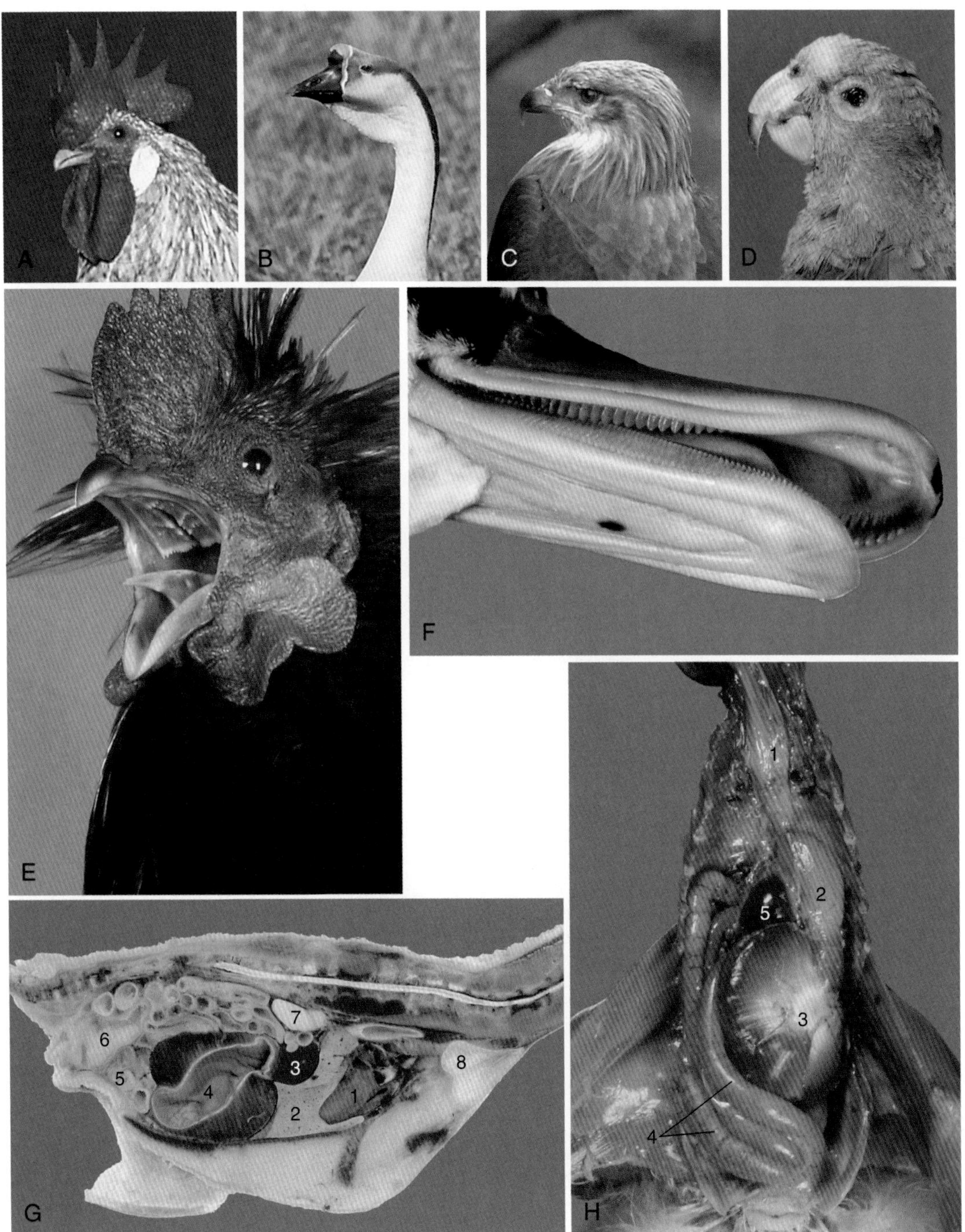


**Plate 31.** *A, B, C* and *D,* Differences in the form of the avian head. *E,* Male chicken; note median cleft (choana) in palate and tongue. *F,* Beak of duck with filter mechanism. *G,* Median section of male chicken: 1, heart; 2, liver; 3, proventriculus; 4, opened gizzard; 5, intestines; 6, coprodeum; 7, testis; 8, crop. *H,* Ventral view of the viscera after removal of the liver: 1, esophagus; 2, proventriculus; 3, gizzard; 4, descending and ascending duodenum; 5, spleen.

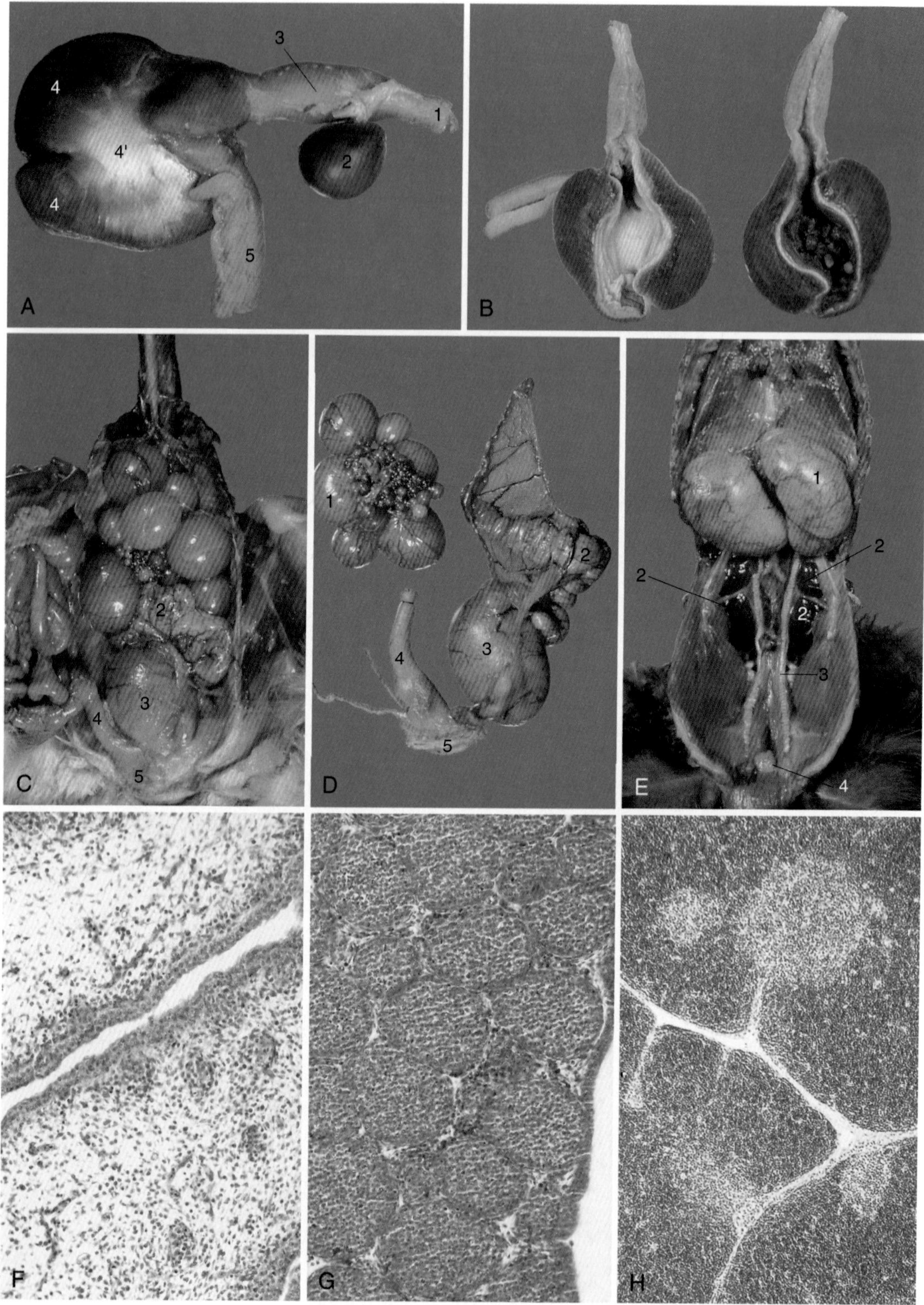


**Plate 32.** *A,* Stomach of chicken: 1, esophagus; 2, spleen; 3, proventriculus; 4, gizzard with aponeurosis (4′); 5, duodenum. *B,* Opened stomach: note grit inside gizzard *(right)*. *C,* Ventral view of reproductive organs of female chicken: 1, ovary with follicles in different stages of development; 2, oviduct; 3, uterus; 4, colon; 5, cloaca. *D,* Isolated female reproductive organs (see *C* for label descriptions). *E,* Ventral view of the male reproductive organs: 1, testis; 2, kidney; 3, deferent duct; 4, cloaca. *F* and *H,* Bursa cloacae (bursa Fabricius) located in the dorsal cloaca. *F,* Bursa of 15-day-old embryo (HE); some infiltrating lymphocytes are present (70×). *G,* Bursa of 18-day-old embryo (Azan) showing developing epithelial buds (70×). *H,* Bursa of 6-week-old chick (HE) showing developed bursa follicles (70×).

CHAPTER 29

# The Pelvis and Reproductive Organs of Female Ruminants

## THE PELVIC CAVITY

The surface landmarks of the *pelvic skeleton* are considered with the surface anatomy of the back and gluteal regions (p. 749). The pelvic roof, formed by the sacrum and first few caudal vertebrae, narrows from front to back. The sacrum, which supplies the greater part, is slightly concave in its length, and this line is first followed by the caudal vertebrae, which later turn sharply ventrally into the free tail. The sacrum articulates with the wing of the ilium cranially, and the stout, obliquely placed shaft of this bone forms the adjoining part of the lateral pelvic wall. Behind this, most of the side wall is membranous, although the ischial spine projects dorsally above the acetabulum, and the ischial tuber thrusts up from the floor to narrow the exit (Fig. 29–1). The two halves of the girdle meet at a symphysis, which is cartilaginous in the heifer but later ossifies. The floor is hollowed from side to side and also in its length, the ischial portion sloping steeply upward toward the exit (Fig. 29–2/8). In heifers a crest is formed over the most cranial part of the symphysis, but in aged cows this region is level or even sunken. The lateral parts of the floor are perforated by the large obturator foramina, while the caudal margin is deeply cut away by the ischial arch.

The membranous part of the lateral wall consists of the *sacrosciatic ligament* (/11), a broad sheet extending between the lateral margin of the sacrum and the dorsal borders of the ilium and ischium. It leaves open the greater and lesser sciatic foramina. In cattle the so-called lesser foramen is in fact by far the larger of the two (/10).

The *entrance* to the pelvic cavity is bounded by the terminal line formed in succession by the sacral promontory, the iliopectineal line of the ilium, and the cranial margin of the pubis (Fig. 29–3). The obliquity of the plane bounded by the terminal line places the pecten of the pubis below the second intersacral joint (Fig. 29–2). The entrance is comparatively narrow. The iliac shafts run parallel to the median plane except in heifers and young cows, in which the inlet narrows ventrally.

The *exit* is considerably narrower than the entrance. It is roughly triangular with a blunt dorsal apex formed by the third caudal vertebra, diverging lateral walls provided by the thickened edges of the sacrosciatic ligaments, and a base formed by the salient tubers and incised arch of the ischia (Fig. 29–12).

The *articulations* between the sacrum and the girdle are of a mixed character—the synovial joints are complemented by wide areas directly joined by ligaments—and are well adapted to the transmission to the vertebral column of the thrust from the hindlimbs. Longer ligaments bridge the gap between the sacral tubers of the ilia and the lateral margins and spinous processes of the sacrum. Normally little or no movement occurs at the sacroiliac joints; the pelvic movements seen during ordinary progression occur at the relatively mobile lumbosacral joint.

The relevance of the pelvic anatomy to parturition is considered later (p. 707).

Certain spaces within the bony pelvic ring are isolated from the pelvic cavity by the pelvic and urogenital diaphragms. These are the *ischiorectal fossae,* which lie one to each side of the anus and vestibule. They are normally filled with fat, but in older animals, and in others in poor condition, the fat is reduced in amount and the positions of the fossae are made more obvious by deep insinkings of the skin (/12).

The pelvic girdle of the small ruminants has a less robust construction than that of the cow. The iliac shafts are relatively long and incline at a smaller angle to their articulations with the vertebral column. These features, combined with the shorter sacrum (only four sacral vertebrae are present in sheep, although five are present in goats), cause the vertical diameter to intersect the tail (see Fig. 26–2).

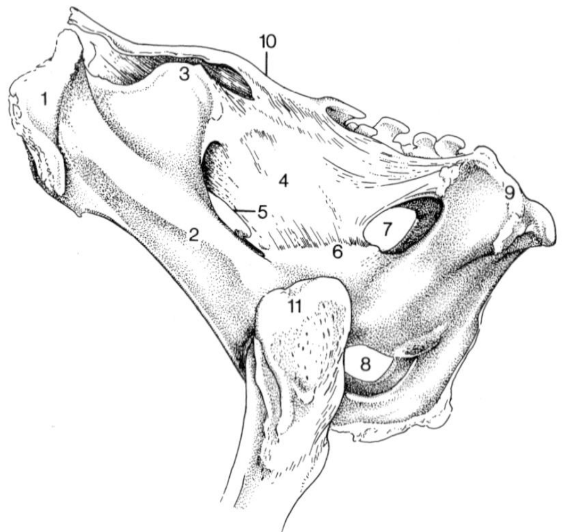


**Figure 29–1.** Lateral view of the bony pelvis of a cow.

1, Coxal tuber; 2, shaft of ilium; 3, sacral tuber; 4, sacrosciatic ligament; 5, greater sciatic foramen; 6, ischial spine; 7, lesser sciatic foramen; 8, right and left obturator foramina; 9, ischial tuber; 10, sacrum; 11, greater trochanter.

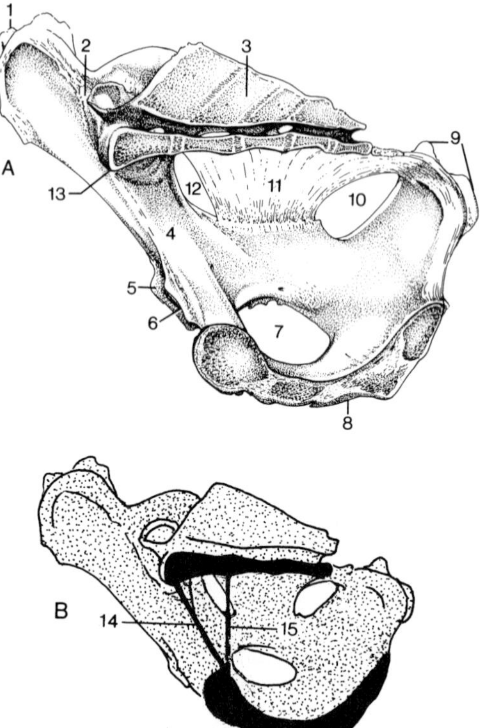


**Figure 29–2.** Median section of the bony pelvis of a cow. In *B* the roof and floor of the pelvic cavity are indicated in black. The line connecting the promontory with the pecten is the conjugata (14); the vertical line between the pecten and the roof is the vertical diameter (15).

1, Coxal tuber; 2, sacroiliac joint; 3, sacrum; 4, shaft of ilium; 5, cranial border of acetabulum; 6, pecten pubis; 7, obturator foramen; 8, symphysis; 9, ischial tuber; 10, lesser sciatic foramen; 11, sacrosciatic ligament; 12, greater sciatic foramen; 13, promontory; 14, conjugate; 15, vertical diameter.

## THE TOPOGRAPHY OF THE PELVIC WALLS

The pelvic blood supply is assured by the *median sacral* and internal iliac arteries (Fig. 29–4). The first of these runs below the sacrum, where it detaches the segmental vessels that enter the ventral sacral foramina, and then continues into the tail as the median caudal artery (p. 653) (see Fig. 26–7/3).

The *internal iliac artery* does not divide into visceral and parietal trunks as in some species but continues as a single vessel that detaches collateral branches to the viscera and to the gluteal muscles overlying the pelvic walls.

The artery crosses the terminal line close to the sacroiliac joint and proceeds over the ilium to reach the lower part of the sacrosciatic ligament where it divides into internal pudendal and caudal gluteal branches in the vicinity of the ischial spine (Fig. 29–5/10,10′,12). The only important collateral parietal branch of the internal iliac is the *cranial gluteal artery,* which turns out through the greater sciatic foramen. The *caudal gluteal artery* leaves the pelvis through the lesser sciatic foramen. The first visceral branch of the internal iliac is the *umbilical artery,* which is the origin of the large uterine artery that enters the broad ligament (p. 703); beyond this, the umbilical artery, so important in the fetus, is transformed into a largely fibrous cord with a vestigial lumen; it runs to the

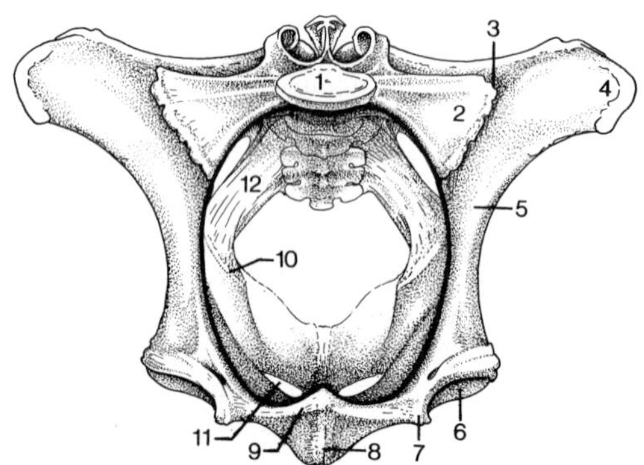


**Figure 29–3.** Cranial view of the bony pelvis of a cow. The terminal line *(black)* is indicated.

1, Body of first sacral vertebra; 2, wing of sacrum; 3, sacroiliac joint; 4, coxal tuber; 5, shaft of ilium; 6, acetabulum; 7, iliopubic eminence; 8, symphysis; 9, pecten pubis; 10, ischial spine; 11, obturator foramen; 12, sacrosciatic ligament.

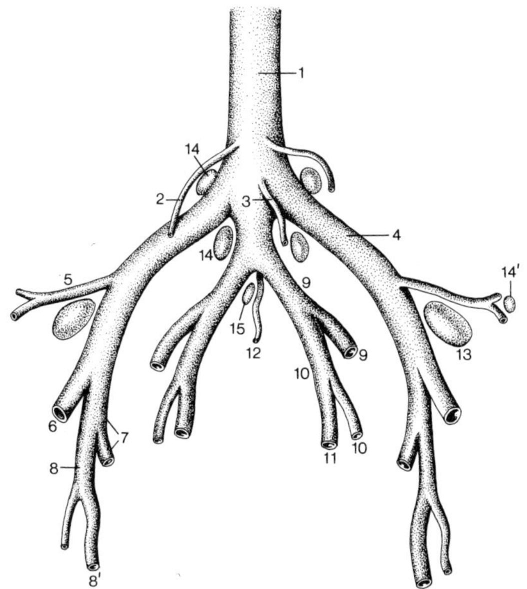


**Figure 29-4.** Branching pattern of the caudal part of the bovine abdominal aorta.

1, Aorta; 2, ovarian artery; 3, caudal mesenteric artery; 4, external iliac artery; 5, deep circumflex iliac artery; 6, femoral artery; 7, deep femoral artery; 8, pudendoepigastric trunk; 8′, external pudendal artery; 9, internal iliac artery; 10, umbilical artery; 11, uterine artery; 12, median sacral artery; 13, deep inguinal (iliofemoral) lymph node; 14, 14′, medial and lateral iliac lymph nodes; 15, sacral lymph nodes.

bladder within the free edge of the lateral vesical ligament. The other visceral branch is the *vaginal artery* (/11) for the reproductive tract within the pelvis.

The *internal pudendal artery* continues the course of the parent trunk, first passing by the lesser sciatic foramen, and later running over the lateral and ventral walls of the vestibule. It furnishes branches to the caudal part of the vagina, the vestibule, and the perineum. The perineal branches include one that reaches the caudodorsal part of the udder.

The arteries are accompanied by satellite veins. The visceral vessels are described with the organs they supply.

The *nerves* that follow the pelvic wall can be arranged in two overlapping groups. The first comprises the lumbosacral and obturator trunks, branches of the lumbosacral plexus that pass through the pelvis in their journeys to the limb. The second comprises the nerves derived from the sacral plexus that supplies pelvic and perineal parts (Fig. 29–6).

The large *lumbosacral trunk* (L6–S2) is the common origin of the sciatic, cranial and caudal gluteal, and caudal cutaneous femoral nerves that issue from the pelvis through the greater sciatic foramen (/4). The lumbar contribution to the sciatic nerve passes directly ventral to the wing of the sacrum, a relationship that brings risk of damage by compression at parturition.

The *obturator nerve* (L4–L6) enters the pelvis after making its way through the psoas muscles and courses over the shaft of the ilium to pass through the obturator foramen (Fig. 29–5/6). It ramifies in the adductor muscles of the thigh. The pelvic part of the obturator nerve is vulnerable in fractures and through compression during parturition where it lies against the bone.

The *pudendal nerve* (S2–S4) runs over the inner aspect of the sacrosciatic ligament dorsal to the internal pudendal artery (/7). It is primarily a somatic nerve to the voluntary muscles of the anus and vestibule and to perineal skin, but it also supplies twigs to the walls of the urethra, vagina, vestibule, and anus. The nerve-blocking technique that formerly made a detailed knowledge of the course and branching of the pudendal nerve necessary has now been largely superseded by low epidural anesthesia.

One or more *caudal rectal nerves* (S4–S5) run between the rectum and the internal face of the pelvic diaphragm (/8). They are compounded of somatic motor fibers destined for the pelvic diaphragm and voluntary anal musculature, parasympathetic motor fibers for the smooth muscle of the rectum, and sensory fibers for the anal and vestibular mucosae. The terminal divisions share their territory with the deep perineal branch of the pudendal nerve.

The so-called *pelvic nerve* (/9) has the same roots as the pudendal but consists of parasympathetic fibers that attend to the innervation of the pelvic viscera (p. 319). The sympathetic supply to the pelvic viscera constitutes the *hypogastric nerve*.

## GENERAL VISCERAL TOPOGRAPHY

The general topography of the pelvic viscera may be studied with the aid of the median and transverse sections (Figs. 29–7, 29–8, and 29–9). Of course, frequent movements of organs occur across the boundary between the abdomen and pelvis, and no single disposition of the viscera can be described as the normal pattern. The amount of the reproductive tract that lies within the pelvis is especially variable, depending on the age, the present status, and the past history of the cow; in the short term, however, it is the bladder that is least constant since it extends cranially along the

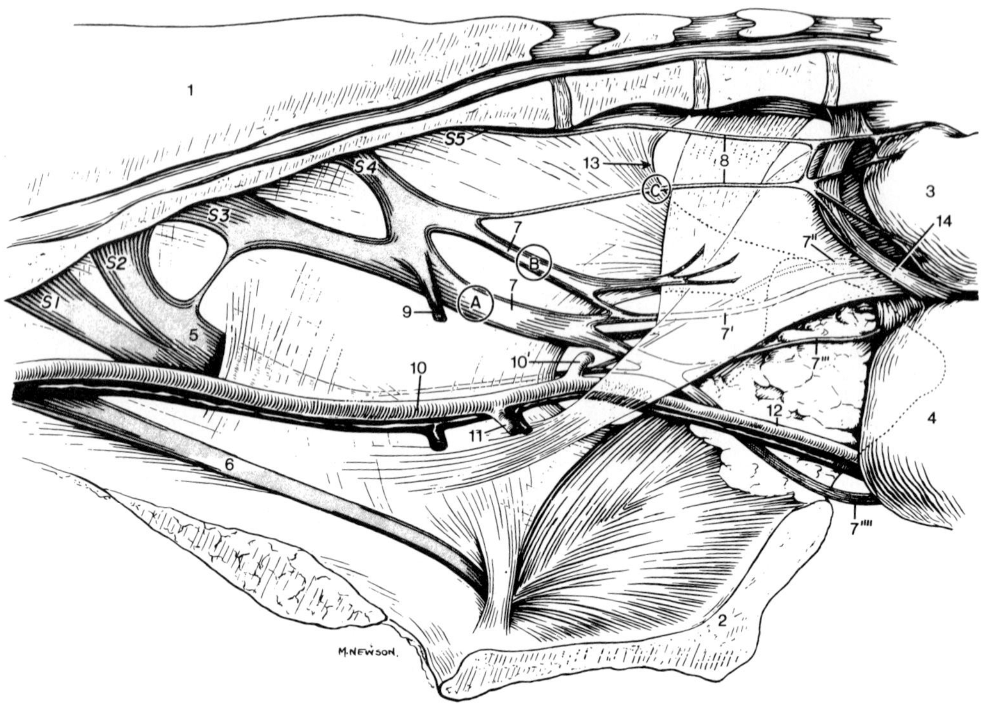


**Figure 29–5.** Nerves and vessels on the medial surface of the bovine pelvic wall. Local anesthesia of the pudendal nerve can be obtained by injections at A and B; anesthesia of the caudal rectal nerves is possible by an injection at C.

1, Sacrum; 2, pelvic symphysis; 3, rectum (reflected); 4, vagina (reflected); 5, sciatic n.; 6, obturator n.; 7, pudendal n.; 7′, distal cutaneous branch of pudendal n.; 7″, proximal cutaneous branch of pudendal n.; 7‴, deep perineal n.; 7⁗, continuation of pudendal n. to clitoris; 8, caudal rectal nn.; 9, pelvic n.; 10, internal iliac a.; 10′, caudal gluteal a.; 11, vaginal a.; 12, internal pudendal a.; 13, caudal border of sacrosciatic ligament; 14, retractor clitoridis.

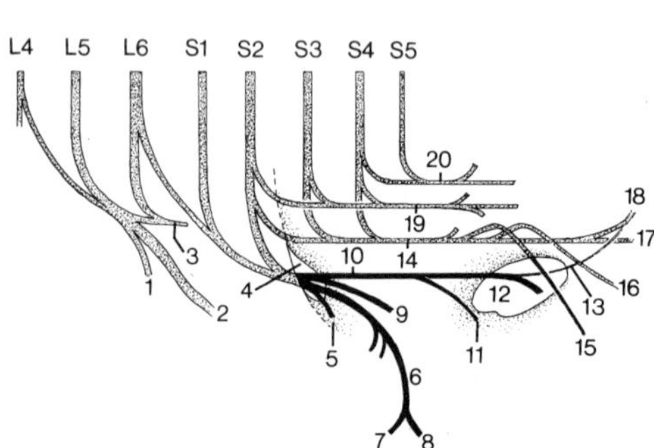


**Figure 29–6.** Schema of the lumbosacral plexus formed by the ventral branches of the caudal lumbar and sacral nerves. The deeper-lying nerves are stippled; those outside the bony pelvis are black.

1, Saphenous n.; 2, femoral n.; 3, obturator n.; 4, greater sciatic foramen; 5, cranial gluteal n.; 6, sciatic n.; 7, peroneal n.; 8, tibial n.; 9, caudal gluteal n.; 10, caudal cutaneous femoral n.; 11, cutaneous branch of 10; 12, lesser sciatic foramen; 13, communication between 10 and 18; 14, pudendal n.; 15, 16, proximal and distal cutaneous branches of 14; 17, superficial perineal n., 18, deep perineal n.; 19, pelvic nn.; 20, caudal rectal n.

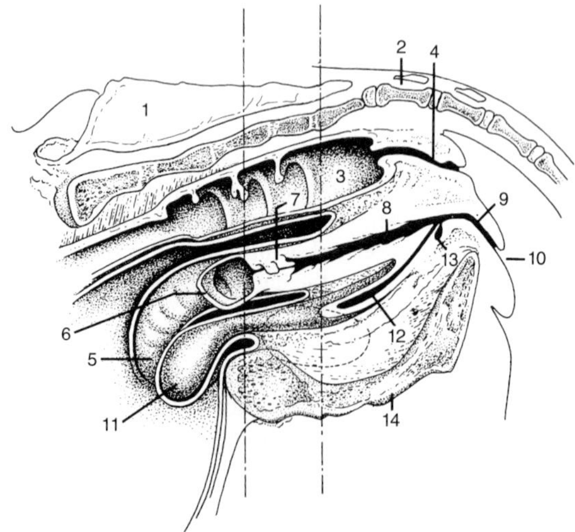


**Figure 29–7.** Median section of the bovine pelvis. The two vertical broken lines indicate the levels of the transverse sections in Figures 29–8 and 29–9. The position of the obturator foramen is indicated by a broken outline.

1, Sacrum; 2, first caudal vertebra; 3, rectum; 4, anal canal; 5, right uterine horn; 6, left uterine horn, mostly removed; 7, cervix; 8, vagina; 9, vestibule; 10, vulva; 11, bladder; 12, urethra; 13, suburethral diverticulum; 14, symphysis.

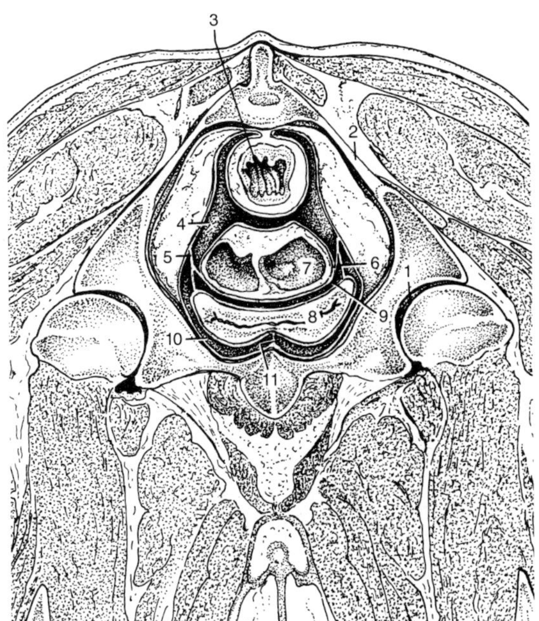


**Figure 29–8.** Transverse section of the bovine pelvis at the level of the hip joint (cranial surface). Note the large amount of retroperitoneal fat in the pelvis. (See Fig. 29–7 for the level of this section.)

1, Hip joint; 2, sacrosciatic ligament; 3, rectum; 4, rectogenital pouch; 5, broad ligament of uterus; 6, lateral ligament of bladder; 7, uterus sectioned where the two horns are conjoined; 8, bladder; 9, vesicogenital pouch; 10, pubovesical pouch; 11, median ligament of bladder.

abdominal floor when much distended and retires within the pelvis when voided of urine. Certain abdominal organs may also trespass across the terminal line. The most common offender is the apex of the cecum, which often may be found nestling against the uterus within the entrance to the pelvic cavity.

The *peritoneal cavity* extends almost to the sacrocaudal plane. The line of reflection is curved, and the cavity extends most deeply between the rectum and the vagina. The parietal and visceral parts of the peritoneum are also joined by various folds that pass between certain organs and the walls; these partially divide the cavity into the usual series of pouches (Figs. 29–7 and 29–8).

## THE RECTUM, ANUS, AND PELVIC DIAPHRAGM

Although the origin of the rectum is arbitrarily defined, its most caudal part is distinguished from the colon by a wider caliber and thicker, more muscular wall. The interior of the rectum is marked by impermanent transverse folds; it is generally distended with feces (Fig. 29–11/8).

The mesentery of the descending colon continues as the mesorectum, which at once shortens to a mere 3 cm. It continues to decrease when followed caudally and eventually disappears, bringing the rectum into broad contact with the pelvic roof and walls (Fig. 29–9/4). More and more of the rectal circumference then becomes denuded of serosa until finally the ventral surface alone faces into the *rectogenital pouch* (/5). The last part of the rectum is embedded in fat, which, with the other masses within the ischiorectal fossae, provides the cushion that allows the gut to adjust to varying degrees of fullness. The close connection with the pelvic walls and roof is a handicap to rectal explorations, and for many examinations the hand must be carried forward into the much more mobile colon (p. 710) (Fig. 29–10).

Some bundles (rectococcygeus) of the longitudinal muscle of the rectal wall pass dorsal to the anus to insert on the caudal vertebrae, while smaller fascicles invade the perineal body between the ventral margin of the anus and the vestibule.

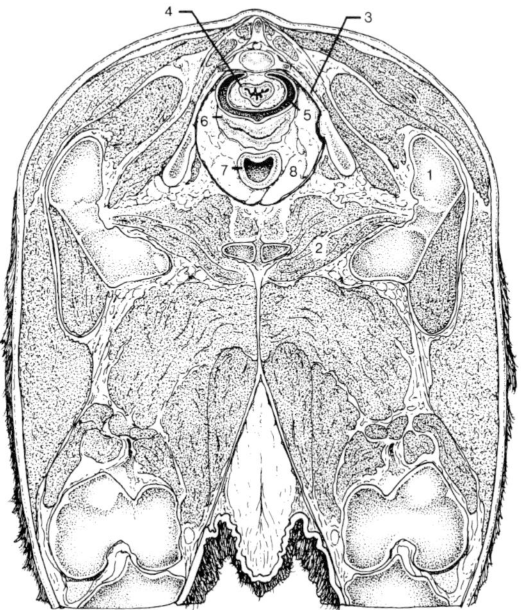


**Figure 29–9.** Transverse section of the bovine pelvis at the level of the first caudal vertebra (cranial surface). The section passes through the obturator foramen. Note that the peritoneum covers only the dorsal surface of the vagina; the lateral and ventral surfaces are retroperitoneal at this level. (See Fig. 29–7 for the level of this section.)

1, Greater trochanter; 2, obturator foramen; 3, sacrosciatic ligament; 4, rectum; 5, rectogenital pouch; 6, vagina; 7, neck of bladder; 8, retroperitoneal fat.

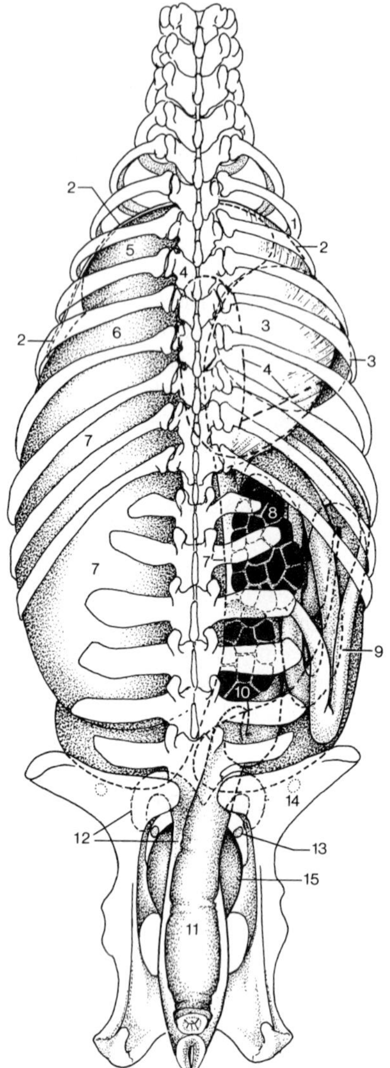


**Figure 29–10.** Relationship of the principal abdominal and pelvic organs to the bovine skeleton, dorsal view.

1, Sixth rib; 2, cranial extent of diaphragm; 3, omasum, most of it covered by the liver; 4, outline of abomasum; 5, reticulum; 6, atrium ruminis; 7, dorsal sac; 7′, right face of rumen; 8, right kidney; 9, descending duodenum; ventral to it is the intestinal mass; 10, left kidney; 11, rectum; 12, uterus; 13, ovary; 14, lateral iliac lymph node; 15, bladder.

The *anal canal* is embraced by the pelvic diaphragm; the postdiaphragmatic part forms a low cylindrical eminence below the skin. The anal opening is a short transverse slit through which the skin continues to provide the last stretch of the canal with a cutaneous epithelial covering. Most of the lining of the passage is molded to form a series of interdigitating columns and depressions that seal the lumen (Fig. 29–11/4).

The *anus* is guarded by two sphincters. The internal sphincter is merely a thickening of the circular muscle of the bowel. The external sphincter, striated and under voluntary control, forms a band about 3 cm wide, directly below the skin. Many fascicles encircle the lumen; a few attach to the caudal vertebrae, and a large proportion continue into the constrictor vulvae, generally after decussation in the perineal body (Fig. 29–12/5).

The major *blood supply* to the rectum is furnished by the cranial rectal artery, a branch of the caudal mesenteric artery, which runs within the mesorectum and then over the dorsal rectal wall. The caudal section, the anal canal, and the anal region generally are supplied by twigs from the caudal rectal artery, an indirect branch of the vaginal artery. The cranial rectal veins lead to the portal circulation through the mesenteric trunk, while those from the anal region drain into the systemic system through the internal pudendal veins.

The *pelvic diaphragm* consists of two parts that edge medially so gradually that they are almost parallel. Each half consists of two striated muscles, the coccygeus and the levator ani, sandwiched between inner and outer fascial sheets (Figs. 29–11/7,6 and 29–12/3,4).

These striated muscles share a common origin from the medial aspect of the ischial spine and adjacent part of the sacrosciatic ligament. The coccygeus passes obliquely beside the rectum to attach to the transverse processes of the first three vertebrae of the tail and has no direct connection with the anus. The greater part of the thinner and wider levator lies caudal and ventral to the

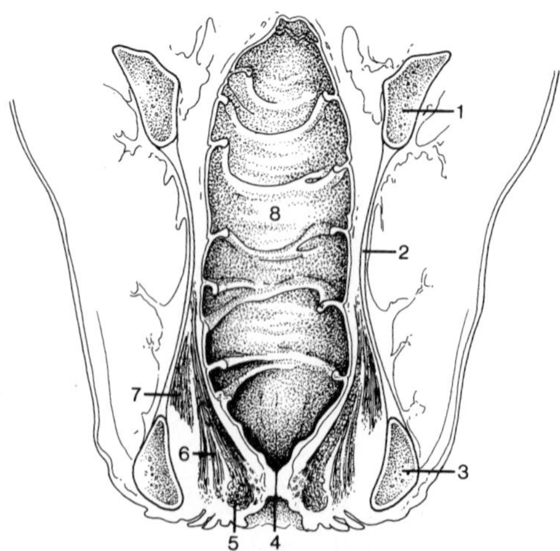


**Figure 29–11.** Dorsal section of the bovine rectum and adjacent structures. Note especially the topography of the pelvic diaphragm (6, 7).

1, Shaft of ilium; 2, sacrosciatic ligament; 3, ischial tuber; 4, anus; 5, external anal sphincter; 6, levator ani; 7, coccygeus; 8, rectum.

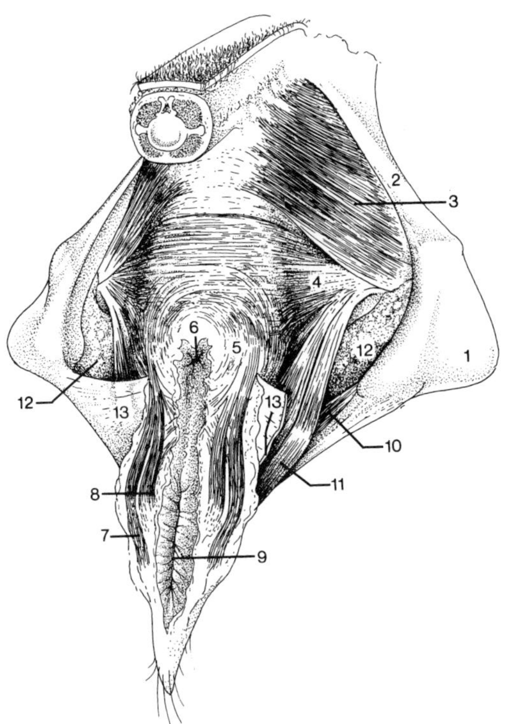


**Figure 29–12.** The perineal muscles of a cow.

1, Ischial tuber; 2, sacrosciatic ligament; 3, coccygeus; 4, levator ani; 5, external anal sphincter; 6, anus; 7, retractor clitoridis; 8, constrictor vulvae; 9, vulva; 10, urogenital diaphragm; 11, constrictor vestibuli; 12, fat in ischiorectal fossa; 13, perineal fascia (partly removed on the right side).

coccygeus and spreads toward its insertion; most bundles blend with the external anal sphincter, but some from the ventral border continue into the constrictor vestibuli without a break. The muscles of the pelvic diaphragm are supplied by twigs from the caudal rectal nerves and the main pudendal trunk (Fig. 29–5).

The fascia forms an essential part of the arrangement. The inner layer is a direct continuation of the parietal pelvic fascia and spreads over the two muscles to merge with the visceral fascia of the rectum, the rectovaginal septum (the deep continuation of the perineal body), and the fascia overlying the ventral muscles of the tail. The outer sheet diverges from the inner surface of the sacrosciatic ligament caudal to the origin of the muscles; it covers the lesser sciatic foramen and forms the medial wall of the ischiorectal fossa. The outer and inner sheets fuse together above and below the muscles of the diaphragm. The lower edge of the pelvic diaphragm is continuous with the urogenital diaphragm that completes the closure of the caudal pelvic aperture.

Although the muscles of the pelvic diaphragm undoubtedly help to retain the viscera within the pelvis, continuous activity is not required. When the animal is standing placidly the intrapelvic pressure is slightly subatmospheric, and any tendency toward visceral displacement must be inward, away from the perineum.

## THE BLADDER AND URETHRA

The piriform *bladder* is generally confined to the pelvic cavity and only when considerably distended does it extend forward over the abdominal floor. The neck lies far within the pelvis and is the only part of the organ without a peritoneal covering; in place of this, it is attached to the pelvic floor and to the ventral surface of the vagina by fat and loose connective tissue (Fig. 29–7). Urine that escapes from a ruptured bladder—a not infrequent mishap, although more common in steers—passes into the peritoneal cavity or infiltrates the pelvic fascia, according to the site of the tear. The body and the vertex rest on a bed of fat. They are smooth except where a scar marks the site of the connection with the fetal urachus. The peritoneal covering is continuous with the usual lateral and median bladder ligaments (Fig. 29–8/8,6,11).

The relations of the bladder naturally vary with its distention and with the condition of neighboring organs. It is always in contact with the cranial part of the vagina and cervix and often lies below the body and horns of the uterus. When it reaches into the abdomen, it makes contact with the caudodorsal blind sac of the rumen and with the intestines. The fetal bladder merges with the urachus (which extends through the umbilicus); the organ is still largely intra-abdominal in the young calf.

In the goat, the ruminant species in which these matters have been most studied, the bladder possesses no internal sphincter, and the first part of the urethra, that cranial to the striated urethral muscle, forms part of the reservoir.

The *urethra* is narrow (especially in comparison with that of the mare) and runs below the vagina, to which it becomes increasingly attached as it proceeds caudally. It opens into the vestibule through a median slit that is shared with the *suburethral diverticulum* (Fig. 29–7/13). This is a blind pouch that extends cranially below the last part of the urethra; it is big enough to admit the end joint of a finger and can be a nuisance when attempting catheterization. The opening is also guarded cranially by the mucosal fold (hymen) that marks the boundary between the vagina and the vestibule. The striated *urethralis,* or external bladder sphincter, covers only the caudal part of the tube, which more cranially is anchored to the pelvic floor by a short but strong symphysial

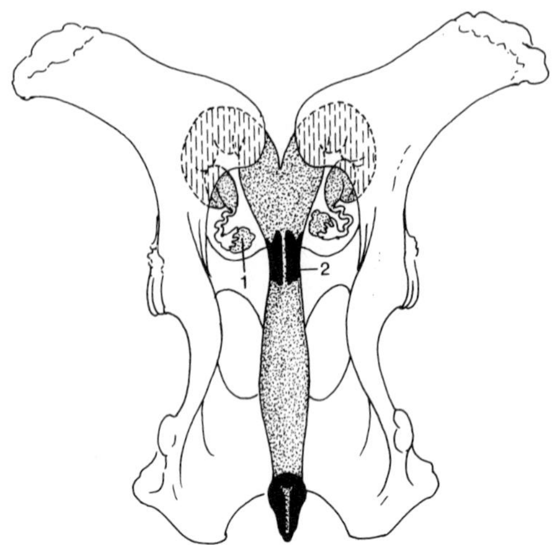


**Figure 29–13.** Dorsal view of the bony pelvis and related (nongravid) bovine reproductive organs. Note position of ovaries in relation to the pecten pubis.

1, Ovary; 2, cervix.

ligament. The cranial fascicles of the muscle insert into a median raphe dorsal to the urethra, but more caudally they form a U that attaches on each side of the vaginal and vestibular walls. The suburethral diverticulum is included within this sphincter.

The blood supply to these organs is derived from vesical and urethral twigs of the umbilical and vaginal arteries.

# THE REPRODUCTIVE ORGANS

Since the anatomy of the reproductive organs changes considerably with age and physiological activity, the initial description deals with the tract of the mature, parous but nongravid cow. The more important developmental and functional alterations are considered later.

The principal topographical peculiarities of the reproductive organs of the female ruminant are the consequence of the descent of the fetal ovaries, which is more considerable than in other domestic animals. The adult ovaries lie in the most caudal part of the abdomen; as a result the uterine horns are drawn back toward their ovarian attachments and, except in advanced pregnancy, do not range far into the abdominal cavity (Fig. 29–13/1).

## The Ovary and Uterine Tube

The bovine *ovary,* a firm irregular body with a basically ovoid form, is surprisingly small (4 × 2.5 × 1.5 cm) for the size of the animal. It is joined to the body wall immediately before the pelvic inlet, and to the reproductive tract by its inclusion in the broad ligament. The ovary is generally to be found related to the ventral part of the iliac shaft, about level with the bifurcation of the uterus, but its position is influenced by past history.

Follicles and corpora lutea may project from any part of the surface (Fig. 29–14 and Plate 7/*B*).

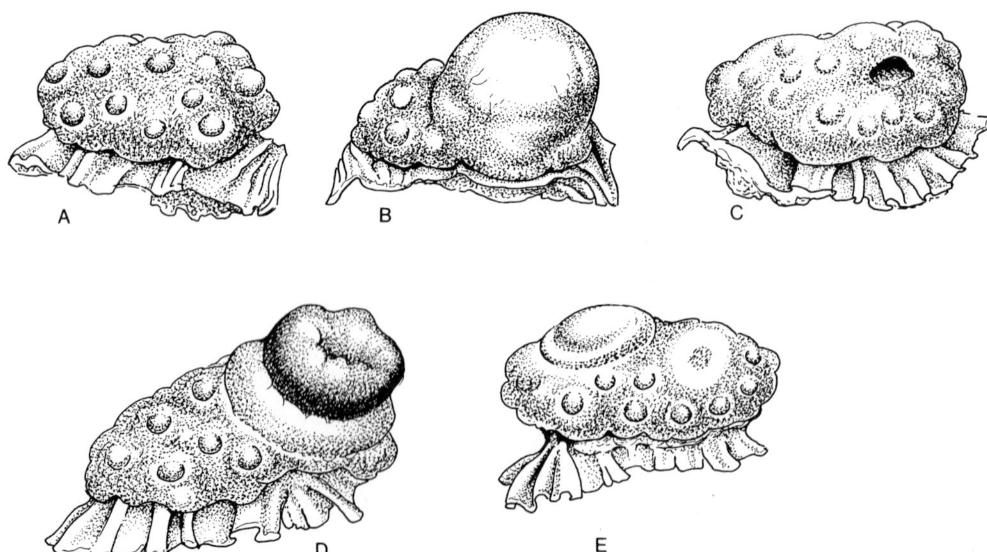


**Figure 29–14.** Various functional stages of the bovine ovary. *A,* Ovary with small secondary follicles. *B,* Ovary with mature follicle ready to rupture. *C,* Ovary with recently ruptured follicle; the scar is small and round. *D,* Ovary with mature corpus luteum. *E,* Ovary with regressing corpus luteum.

Their presence may be confirmed on palpation per rectum when those as small as 5 mm in diameter may be distinguished. The largest follicles attain a diameter of 2 cm and therefore distort the ovary in their neighborhood; any that are even larger are probably abnormal. The estrous cycle is quite short (generally 21 days), and mature follicles and large corpora lutea may be present at the same time (Plate 7/*F*).

The *uterine tube* is rather long but, as it pursues a very flexuous course, its beginning and end lie close together (Fig. 29–15/2). The thin-walled *infundibulum* lies over the lateral part of the ovary in the free margin of the mesosalpinx. The narrower succeeding part of the tube winds within the lateral wall of the ovarian bursa to reach the tip of the uterine horn; it is divided into ampulla and isthmus, approximately in the ratio 2:1. The ampulla is somewhat wider than the isthmus, but the difference is obvious only at certain phases of the cycle. The transition from tube to uterine horn is gradual and marked by muscular thickening.

The ovaries of the sheep and goat are similar to those of the cow apart from those functional changes associated with the wide occurrence of twin and multiple pregnancies. The uterine tube is relatively very long.

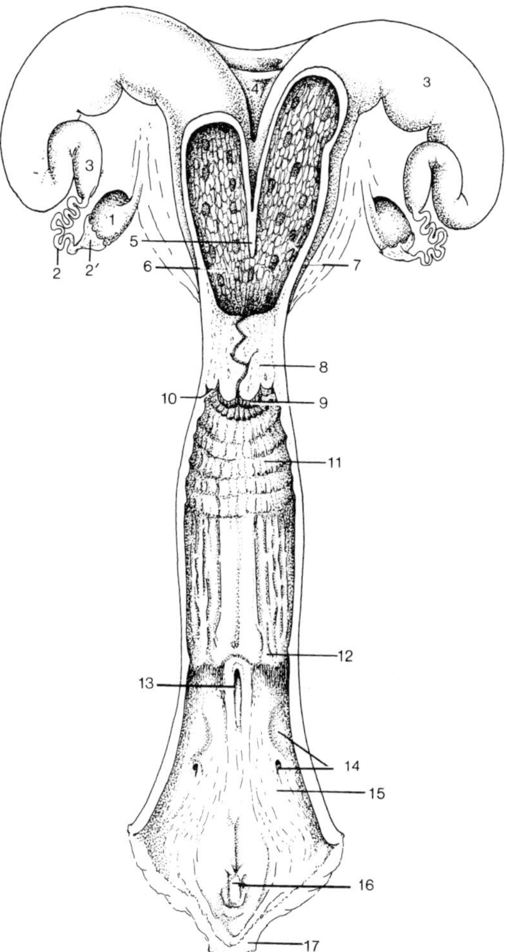


**Figure 29–15.** The bovine reproductive organs, dorsal view. The uterus, cervix, vagina, and vestibule have been opened.

1, Ovary; 2, uterine tube; 2′, infundibulum; 3, uterine horn; 4, intercornual ligament; 5, wall of uterus dividing the two horns; 6, body of uterus with caruncles; 7, broad ligament; 8, cervix; 9, vaginal part of cervix; 10, fornix; 11, vagina; 12, position of former hymen; 13, external urethral orifice and suburethral diverticulum; 14, major vestibular gland and its excretory orifice; 15, vestibule; 16, glans of the clitoris; 17, right labium.

## The Uterus

At first sight the bovine uterus appears to consist of a relatively long body succeeded by two tapering and divergent horns, each coiled ventrally on itself (Fig. 29–16). This impression is misleading. In the first place, most of the so-called body is formed by the incomplete fusion of the caudal parts of the horns that lie side by side, sharing common serosal and muscular coats. The true arrangement is suggested by a dorsal groove that becomes more pronounced toward the bifurcation and is of course very obvious in section. Where the horns at last diverge, the superficial tissues bridge the space between them, forming dorsal and ventral (intercornual) ligaments (/5) that bound a small pocket, open cranially and very conveniently arranged to allow the organ to be fixed by the insertion of a finger during rectal examination.

Secondly, the tight winding of the *horns* is not constant but results from stimulation of the muscle of the uterine wall and broad ligament. The stimulus is provided by handling in the living animal, and for this reason the form of the uterus sometimes appears to become more obvious, and its consistency firmer, in the course of a rectal examination. The effect is most noticeable during estrus, and some believe it to be restricted to this period.

The true *body* is very short (Fig. 29–15/6). The external appearance is not informative, and the cranial limit is difficult to determine on inspection or palpation. The caudal limit is more easily decided by the firmness of the cervix, which projects caudally into the vagina where it is surrounded by an annular fornix (/10). The arrangement of these parts becomes obvious when

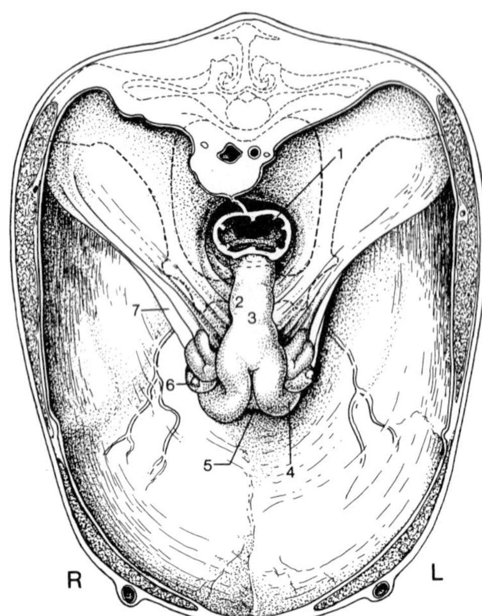


**Figure 29–16.** The reproductive organs of a cow in situ, cranial view. The bony pelvis is indicated by broken lines. The uterus sags within this largely eviscerated abdomen.

1, Rectum; 2, cervix; 3, body of uterus; 4, left uterine horn; 5, intercornual ligament; 6, right ovary; 7, broad ligament.

the organ is laid open; each horn is then found to measure about 35 cm, with the caudal third incorporated in the pseudobody; the true body is a bare 3 cm and the cervix about 8 or 10 cm long.

The thickness and color of the endometrium vary with the phase of the cycle. The surface carries low folds, both longitudinal and circular, but its most characteristic features are the uterine *caruncles,* the attachment sites of the fetal membranes in the pregnant state (Fig. 29–17 and Plate 8/*C,D*). The caruncles of the mature but nongravid cow are each about 15 mm long and project well above the surrounding surface. About forty are arranged in four more or less regular rows in the wider parts of each horn, reducing to a double line toward the tip. The mucosa of the body is smoother and leads into the cervix through the constriction of the internal uterine orifice (Fig. 29–15).

The lumen of the *cervix* is closed by the interlocking of irregular surface projections, the remains of the three or four circular folds that bar the passage in the heifer. The last of these rings projects into the vagina (Figs. 29–23/5 and 29–18). The cervical mucosa also carries longitudinal ridges that intersect the rings; when these reach the external opening of the cervical canal their divergence produces an appearance reminiscent of a peeled orange with its radial arrangement of segments (Plate 29/*E*). The cervical canal is most easily passed by an instrument during estrus and at parturition, but the difficulties experienced at other times can be overcome, indeed must be overcome, to perform embryo transfer. The cervical mucosa produces a mucous secretion at estrus; it is also the origin of the mucous plug that seals the canal of the pregnant animal.

Embryo transfer is important in bovine reproduction. The eggs are flushed from the uterus via the cervical canal 7 to 10 days after fertilization. They are then transferred to recipient cows that are

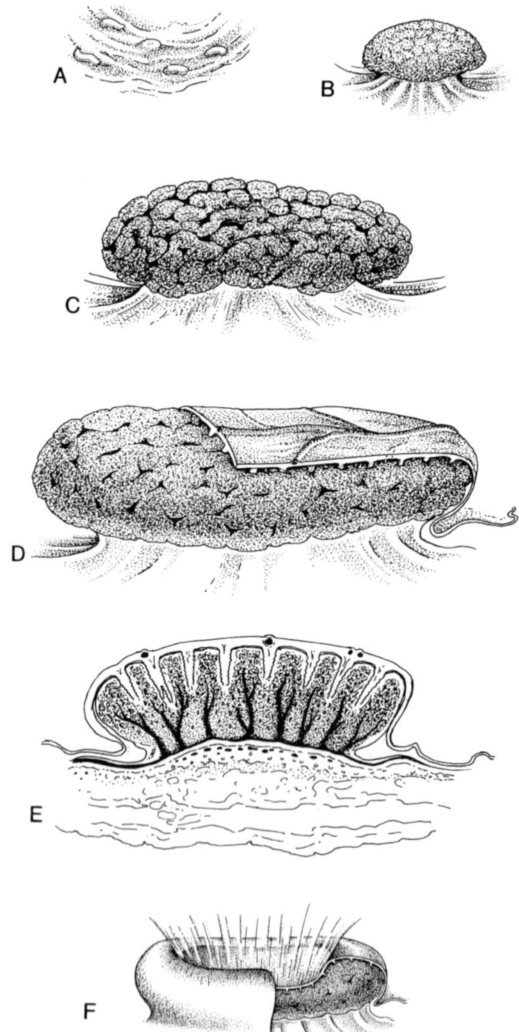


**Figure 29–17.** *A–E,* Development of caruncles in the wall of the bovine uterus. *A,* Caruncle in a nongravid uterus. *B,* Caruncle in a 2-week gravid uterus. *C,* Caruncle in a 6-month gravid uterus. *D,* Caruncle near term, covered in part by a cotyledon (fetal tissue). *E,* Section of a placentome. *F,* Placentome of a sheep.

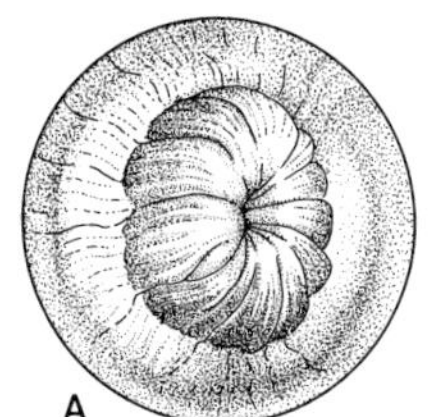


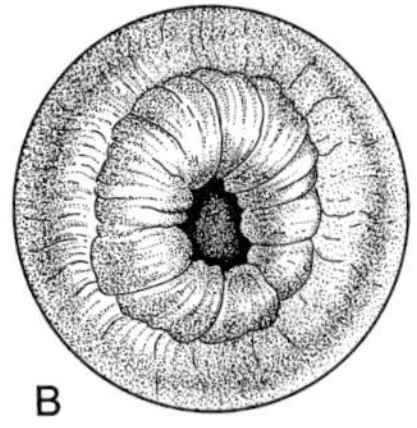


**Figure 29–18.** The appearance of the vaginal part of the bovine cervix during pregnancy *(A)* and during estrus *(B)*.

in the same stage of the estrous cycle as the donor. Overcoming the cervical barrier at this stage does not pose any problems.

Several features distinguish the uterus of the *small ruminants* but have little practical importance. The free surfaces of the uterine caruncles are concave, most obviously in the ewe (Fig. 29–17/*F*) in which the endometrium is generally, but very variously and irregularly, pigmented. Certain distinctions of the cervix are more significant. A larger number of irregular circular folds project into the canal and closely fit together; the final fold, which forms the vaginal portion of the cervix, is normally sunken within a recess of the vaginal wall. In combination, these features make catheterization of the uterus very difficult, if not impossible, in most stages of the cycle.

## The Vagina

The remaining part of the genital tract is divided between the vagina and the vestibule, approximately in the ratio 3:1. The boundary lies at the entrance of the urethra, which pierces the floor of the tract a couple of centimeters cranial to the ischial arch (Fig. 29–7).

The vagina is a rather featureless organ whose lumen is normally closed by the falling together of the dorsal and ventral walls (Fig. 29–9/6). The dimensions in the passive state have relatively little significance since the organ is capable of great expansion, both transversely and in length. It is usual to find the most caudal part narrowed, especially in younger, though not necessarily maiden, animals. The constriction usually involves only the ventral part, and since its extent corresponds with the caudal U-shaped portion of the urethral muscle it seems likely that it is due to this. It is not to be confused with the membranous hymen, which, rarely prominent, lies at the junction of the vagina and the vestibule (Fig. 29–15/12).

Externally the vagina has a very partial covering of peritoneum. The cranial two thirds of the dorsal surface face into the rectogenital pouch (Fig. 29–7). Caudal to this, the rectum and vagina are united by a wedge of tissue. The ventral surface has a less complete peritoneal covering and is related to the bladder and urethra and to the packing tissues that surround the urethra. The lateral vaginal walls are largely without peritoneum, being first included in the thickness of the broad ligament and more caudally sharing in the general retroperitoneal arrangement (Fig. 29–9/6). They are, in part, in direct contact with the pelvic walls. The relationship to the peritoneum is relevant to the prognosis of wounds of the vaginal wall. The serosal covering of the fornix region provides the surgeon with an alternative entry into the peritoneal cavity. The route is most often used for operations on the ovary; the dorsal wall is opened since this provides convenient access to the ovary while avoiding the major vessels that lie below and to the sides of the vagina (Fig. 29–19).

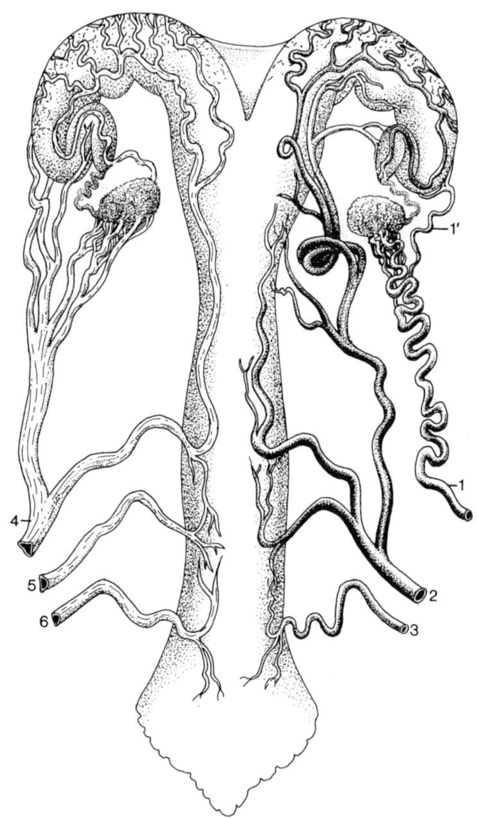


**Figure 29–19.** Semischematic ventral view of the blood supply to the bovine reproductive tract (cow). The arteries are depicted on the right side, the veins on the left.

1, Ovarian artery; 1′, uterine branch; 2, uterine artery; 3, vaginal artery; 4, ovarian vein; 5, accessory vaginal vein; 6, vaginal vein.

Apart from the features already mentioned, the interior is distinguished only by low folds that appear when the organ is collapsed. Most of these run lengthwise, but the cranial part may also carry a number of circular ridges. Vestiges of the mesonephric ducts run below the mucosa of the floor near the junction with the vestibule; they may be the origin of cysts.

The vagina is almost absent in the freemartin (p. 709), whose abnormally short reproductive tract is evident on examination of the vestibule. Aplasia or constriction of the vagina also occurs in white heifer disease, another congenital anomaly. Other constrictions may result from trauma at previous calvings.

## The Vestibule, Vulva, and Urogenital Diaphragm

The *vestibule* slopes ventrally to the opening between the labia of the vulva (Fig. 29–7/9). It is less distensible than the vagina, and its side walls are normally in contact. When they are drawn apart the median opening of the urethra is exposed at its cranial limit. At the other extremity, between the labia, a fossa containing the glans of the clitoris is present (Fig. 29–15/16). Closer inspection may disclose the sunken openings of the vestigial mesonephric ducts, one to each side of the urethral orifice; caudolateral to the orifice is a larger depression into which the duct of the *major vestibular gland* opens (/14). The gland, which is about 3 cm long, lies lateral to the vestibule, enclosed within the fascia of the urogenital diaphragm. The vestibular mucosa normally has a yellowish tinge, darkened laterally over the erectile tissue of the *vestibular bulb.*

The rounded labia are not very salient and vary in their outline according to the age and obstetrical experiences of the cow. The *clitoris* is long, slender, and arranged in a sigmoid flexure. It is rarely possible to make out much of its anatomy from external inspection since much of the glans remains fused with its prepuce (/16). The vulva of the freemartin is markedly small and surrounded by abnormally long hair.

The vestibule penetrates the *urogenital diaphragm (perineal membrane),* which closes the hiatus between the rectovaginal septum and the caudal margin of the pelvic floor. The strong fascia of the diaphragm arises from the ischial arch and bends dorsally around the vestibule to which it fuses; it completes its attachments by merging with the rectovaginal septum, the ventral edge of the pelvic diaphragm, and the parietal pelvic fascia. It firmly anchors the genital tract and opposes the forward drag of the pregnant uterus when this sinks into the abdomen and the backward pull on the tract during calving (Fig. 29–23).

The *constrictor vestibuli* (Fig. 29–12/11) arises from the lower margin of the levator ani and from the muscular decussation between the anus and the vulva. It runs over the lateral wall of the vestibule, immediately caudal to the diaphragm. Its tendon passes under the vestibule to join its fellow of the other side. Contraction narrows the genital passage and raises a ridge in its floor.

The *constrictor vulvae* (/8) is less important. It consists of several weak fascicles that continue from the anal sphincter to end by inserting on the vulvar and circumvulvar skin. Their contraction makes the vulvar opening gape.

## Vascularization and Innervation

The relatively small *ovarian artery* supplies the ovary, the uterine tube, and the adjoining part of the uterine horn; its uterine division anastomoses with cranial branches of the uterine artery. The ovarian artery is distinguished by the extraordinary convolutions it performs in its passage through the more cranial part of the broad ligament (Fig. 29–19/1). This coiling resembles that of the homologous testicular artery, and its extensive contact with the plexiform ovarian vein (Fig. 29–20) facilitates the

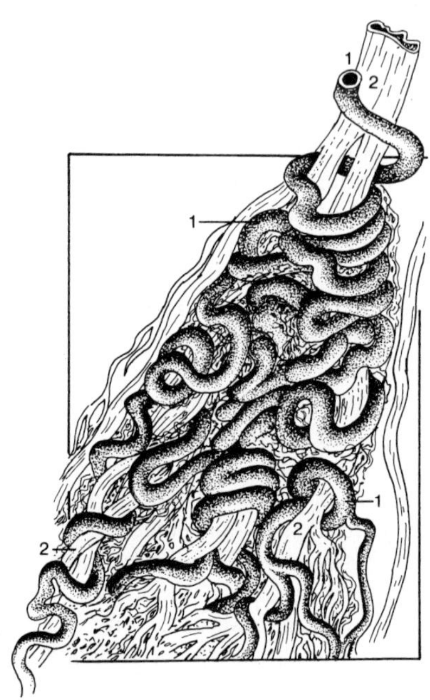


**Figure 29–20.** Relationship of the bovine ovarian artery and its branches (1) to the tributaries of the ovarian vein (2). The intertwining ensures a large area of contact.

transfer of prostaglandins from the venous to the arterial blood (p. 207).

The *uterine artery* arises from the internal iliac together with the umbilical artery (Fig. 29–4/11,10). This, by far the largest of the three genital arteries, enters the pelvic cavity within the broad ligament. Its mobility, which distinguishes it from neighboring parietal arteries, allows it to develop the striking vibration (fremitus or thrill) diagnostic of pregnancy. The vibration is evident from the third month and is a particularly useful diagnostic aid in that period when the uterus is out of reach (see further on). Before reaching the uterus the uterine artery divides into cranial and caudal branches from which about half a dozen stem vessels arise. These supply the uterine wall through a series of branches that run transversely over the dorsal and ventral aspects of the body and horns; the largest branches coincide in position with the ranks of the caruncles. The arrangement leaves the antimesometrial border of the uterine horns less well supplied than other parts of the circumference, a point of considerable surgical importance since an incision over this curvature is comparatively bloodless. The caudalmost branches anastomose within the broad ligament with divisions of the vaginal artery (Fig. 29–19/2,3).

The *vaginal artery* leaves the internal iliac in the caudal part of the pelvis and first runs onto the dorsolateral surface of the vagina before swinging forward over the lateral vaginal wall. It may be palpated through the rectum of the pregnant animal at this level. In its passage it detaches many branches to the vaginal and vestibular tissues as well as others that supply the urethra and the bladder. Rupture of the vaginal wall—a relatively common catastrophe in heifers calving for the first time—may involve destruction of this artery, with fatal intraperitoneal hemorrhage resulting.

A very large and conspicuous *venous plexus* lies in the parametrial tissues of the broad ligament and over the ventral aspect of the uterus and vagina where it is partly covered by the outer layer of uterine muscle. The plexus constitutes a blood pool that can drain in several directions (Fig. 29–19). The largest emissary vessel is the ovarian vein (/4), which runs in the cranial margin of the broad ligament; the vaginal veins, usually two on each side, are second in importance and run to the internal iliac trunk; the middle vein is actually known as the accessory vaginal vein since the vein that closely accompanies the uterine artery is very insignificant.

Both sympathetic and parasympathetic *nerves* supply the genital tract.

## THE LYMPHATIC STRUCTURES OF THE PELVIS

The lymph nodes within the pelvis are rather small and inconstant in occurrence and distribution; most of the lymph formed within the pelvic organs passes directly to the medial iliac and sacral nodes situated about the bifurcation of the aorta (see Fig. 28–30/5,6).

Anorectal and caudal mesenteric nodes lie scattered on the wall of the rectum and anal canal.

Hypogastric and other small inconstant nodes are sometimes found on the inner aspect of the sacrosciatic ligament. The hypogastric nodes may merge with those of the medial iliac group; when distinct, they appear to have the special responsibility of collecting lymph from the dorsal part of the pelvic walls, the tail, the lumbar and gluteal muscles, and the genital and urinary organs.

The entire pelvic lymphatic outflow is funneled through the medial iliac center to enter the lumbar lymphatic trunk at its origin.

The deep inguinal (iliofemoral) node (p. 688) receives lymph from the gluteal and thigh muscles, from the mammary and popliteal nodes, and possibly from the reproductive organs (Fig. 29–4/13).

## GROWTH AND CYCLICAL CHANGES IN THE REPRODUCTIVE ORGANS

The *juvenile reproductive organs,* disproportionately small, are soft to the touch. The ovaries contain follicles of different sizes but, as none have ripened, no corpora lutea are present. The uterus is symmetrical, thin-walled, and slack; its outer surface is rosy and smooth and its mucosa bright pink with the caruncles scarcely raised above their surroundings and more evident on account of their pallor. The cervix is soft, its folds regular, and its canal distensible. The broad ligaments are short, thin, and translucent. The vagina is narrow, and in the majority of young animals the mesonephric ducts run through the full length of the mucosa. In about 1 in 20 heifer calves the hymen persists in the form of a prominent fold. The vestibular mucosa often appears congested.

Before puberty the growth of the reproductive organs is isometric, but with the initiation of the *estrous cycle,* as a rule when the heifer is between 8 and 10 months of age, a response occurs to the ovarian hormones that are now produced. The cumulative effects of a few cycles result in a striking increase in dimensions with clearer differentiation of the component parts of the tubular organs. The uterine horns become more curved, the ovaries become firmer, and corpora lutea may be found.

The ripe follicle projects from the ovarian surface, and from the 16th day of the *cycle* it may be identified on rectal examination. Its full size (2 cm) is attained by the 18th day (Figs. 29–14/*B*, 29–21 and Plate 7/*B*). Rupture is preceded by a reduction in the internal pressure, recognized by fluctuation of its wall on palpation; it is sometimes followed by a moderate hemorrhage, but any clot is soon replaced by a corpus luteum that continues to grow for about 1 week. When at its maximum the corpus luteum is little smaller than the follicle that it replaced (Plate 7/*F* and Fig. 29–22). The corpus luteum then begins to regress, and by the 21st day, when the following estrus occurs, it has contracted to about one third of its greatest diameter. It continues to shrink and eventually disappears or becomes replaced by scar tissue. The bovine corpora lutea exhibit striking color changes, passing from brown to ocher as they mature and shading through orange and brick-red to grayish white in regression. The new crop of follicles begins to enlarge between the 12th and 14th days of the cycle.

Macroscopic cyclical changes in the tubes are not pronounced, although they are important functionally. The ampulla is noticeably wider than the isthmus following ovulation when the distal part of the tube acts as a sphincter that delays for some days the passage of the egg into the uterus.

The cyclical changes in the uterus (p. 200) commence in proestrus and continue into metestrus; hyperemia and edema thicken the endometrium, and their subsidence is often accompanied by local hemorrhages below the mucosal surface. This appears to be the origin, in part at least, of the increasing pigmentation of the uterine wall, for the intact older organ acquires a grayish or yellowish external tinge while the mucosa commonly turns reddish brown. The mobility of the uterine muscle—both spontaneous and in response to external stimuli—is greatest immediately before and during estrus.

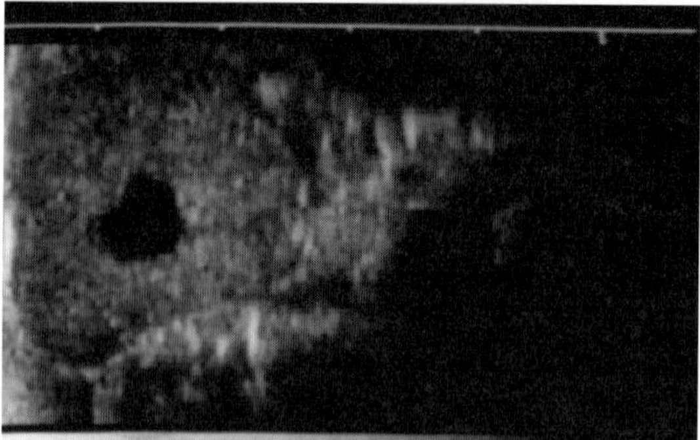

**Figure 29–22.** Ultrasonographic transrectal scan of a corpus luteum of a cycling cow; the corpus is marked by a cavity (black spot).

The cervical mucosa shows increased activity during estrus (Fig. 29–18/*B*) and this activity, which later spreads to the epithelium lining the cranial part of the vagina, produces a transparent mucus of low viscosity. The cervical (and vaginal) secretion is eventually discharged from the vulva, and when metestrus bleeding is considerable the mucus becomes stained with blood. Other endometrial changes, involving increase in the size, complexity, and activity of the glands, culminate a week or so after ovulation.

No pronounced cycle of cornification occurs in the vaginal epithelium.

The estrous cycle is repeated at intervals of 21 days. The small ruminants are seasonally polyestrous (largely in the fall and early winter); the cycle lasts 16 to 17 days in sheep, 20 days in goats.

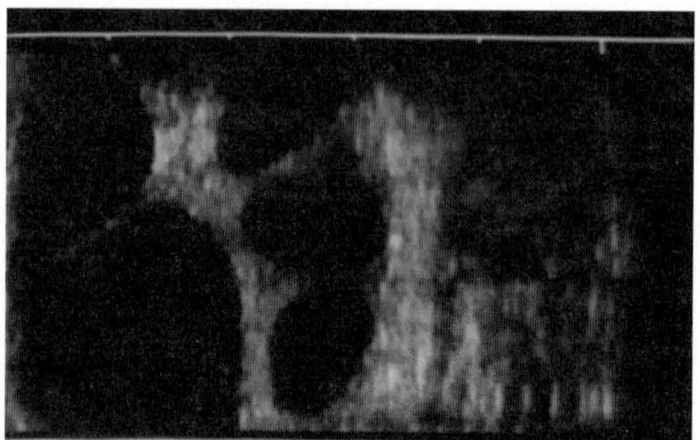

**Figure 29–21.** Ultrasonographic transrectal scan of the ovary of a cow that was stimulated with gonadotropin to induce superovulation. The black spots represent sections of large tertiary follicles.

## THE REPRODUCTIVE TRACT DURING PREGNANCY

Gestation lasts for 40 weeks (280 days) in cattle (but only about 147 days in sheep and 154 days in goats). During this time every part of the reproductive system shows some changes, but those that are most striking occur naturally in the uterus, which increases its weight 15-fold, indeed 100-fold if its content is included (Fig. 29–23).

The *ovary* of the pregnant animal is distinguished by the presence of the corpus luteum of pregnancy, which can be recognized by its persistence after the time when the periodic body of the infertile cycle would have begun to regress. Its survival is not always accompanied by a total suppression of all follicular activity; a few cows may come into heat and ovulate during the early stage of pregnancy. The corpus luteum is not necessary to maintain pregnancy during the last 3 months and normally begins to regress about 1 month before term.

The progestational changes in the *endometrium* that are part of the normal reproductive cycle persist and intensify in the presence of an embryo. This response is evident from about 30 days after fertilization (p. 207). The blastocyst is first confined to one horn, and since ovulation is commoner from the right ovary (60%) the same preference for this side is present. The membranes soon spread into the other horn, but the embryo, and later the fetus, is almost always confined unilaterally; a pronounced asymmetry of the gravid uterus is therefore the rule. Indeed, a developing inequality in the size of the horns is one of the first clinically detectable signs of pregnancy in the cow. The distended amnion is palpable from 30 days, and the fetus itself may be palpated around day 70.

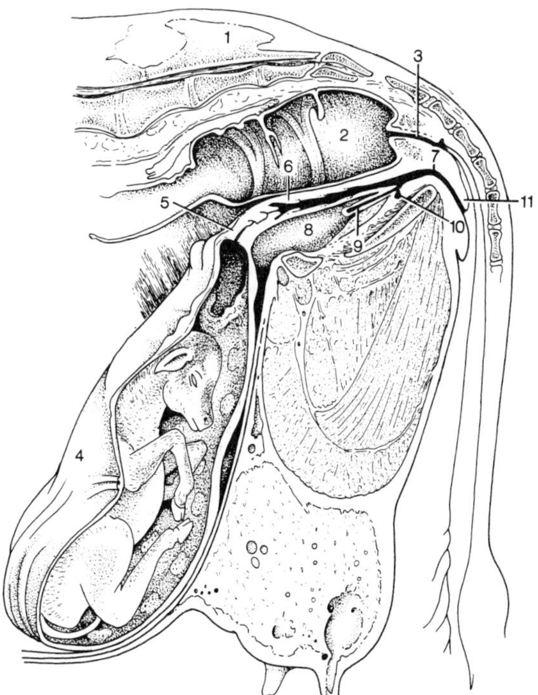


**Figure 29–23.** Paramedian section of the caudal abdomen and pelvis of a pregnant cow. The section is not quite vertical since it cuts through the vertebral canal and obturator foramen. Note the large placentomes.

1, Sacrum; 2, rectum; 3, anal canal; 4, uterus; 5, cervix; 6, vagina; 7, vestibule; 8, bladder; 9, urethra; 10, suburethral diverticulum; 11, vulva.

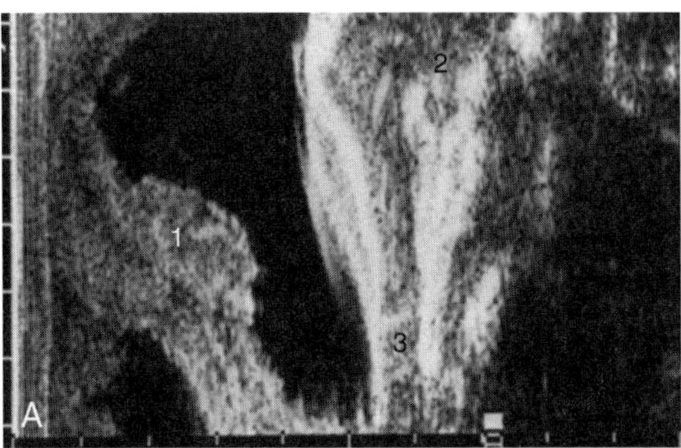


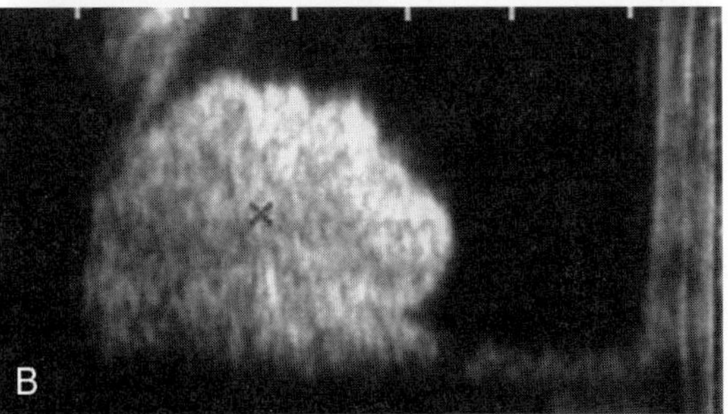


**Figure 29–24.** *A*, Transrectal ultrasonic view of a placentome (1) and fetal head (2) at 3 months' gestation. The two lower jaws of the fetus are at 3. *B*, Transrectal ultrasonic view of a placentome (+) at 5 months' gestation. Ultrasonic views of placentomes are diagnostic of pregnancy if the fetus itself cannot be visualized.

The *caruncles* in the gravid horn increase in size and become converted from low, smooth-surfaced "bumps" on the mucosa to large sessile swellings with a surface pitted for the reception of the chorionic villi (Figs. 29–17, 29–24 and Plate 8/*C,D*). Later, those in the nongravid horn enlarge but to a lesser degree. At term the largest caruncles are the size of a clenched fist. The stretching and enlargement do not affect all parts of the horn equally, and the lesser curvature, being tethered by the broad ligament, is most resistant to expansion; as a result, the pregnant horn alters its shape with the greater curvature and flanking parts growing away from the attachments.

The tissues within the broad ligament also hypertrophy and for a time restrain the uterus from sinking into the abdomen; by the third month, however, the ligament is fully streteched and the uterus then begins to slip downward over the abdominal floor (Fig. 29–23).

A great increase occurs in the *blood flow* through the pregnant uterus to which all the arteries contribute. The greatest change is seen in the uterine artery of the pregnant side, which increases its diameter from a few millimeters to the thickness of an index finger. The artery loses its flexuous character and runs directly through the tensed broad ligament, now passing forward across the shaft of the ilium against which it can be palpated through the rectal wall; the characteristic vibration (fremitus) is appreciated at this time. Similar but lesser and more delayed changes occur in the uterine artery of the nongravid side and in the vaginal and ovarian arteries.

The *topography* of the uterus is not the same in every pregnancy. Usually the enlarging uterus enters the supraomental recess between the right face of the rumen and the double layer of the greater omentum. As it grows, it sinks toward the abdominal floor, and by the end of the fourth month it lies almost entirely within the abdomen with the cervix carried across or even beyond the pubic brim. It enlarges rapidly during the next 2 months and passes cranially below the right costal arch, pressing the rumen to the left and the intestines dorsally (Fig. 29–25). The vagina becomes stretched in the process, and as the cervix slides down the caudal part of the abdominal floor the uterus passes out of reach of the hand within the colon. Inability to palpate the uterus for a space of time around the fifth month is as diagnostic of pregnancy as its palpable enlargement at earlier or later stages. Further increase in size soon restores the uterus to reach, and eventually it extends forward to come into contact with the diaphragm and liver, pushing the diaphragm toward the thorax and demonstrably reducing the space available to the lungs. Toward term the pregnant uterus occupies most of the ventral and right sections of the abdomen and has raised the rumen from the abdominal floor and crushed the intestines upward.

In other pregnancies the uterus fails to become confined within the supraomental recess and instead slips forward against the right or, less frequently, the left flank. If it passes to the left, it forces the rumen cranially and away from the left body wall; if to the right, it displaces the omentum and intestines from the flank.

During the first months of gestation the calf may move freely within the surrounding fluid but later it generally assumes a position in which its back is directed dorsally and often somewhat to one—most often the right—side, toward the greater curvature of the uterus, and through this toward its mother's flank. Some time passes before its attitude stabilizes, and the proportion presenting the head toward the cervix fluctuates, sinking to a minimum (ca. 45%) about the seventh month and thereafter gradually rising to a 95% predominance at term.

The *cervical canal* is closed by a mucous plug, developing from the first month and later projecting through the external cervical opening; this is less tightly contracted than in those species that have an upright posture. The first changes in the *vagina* are caused by the traction exerted on it, but later the wall becomes increasingly elastic and the potential lumen roomier in preparation for the passage of the calf. Enlargement of the *vulva*

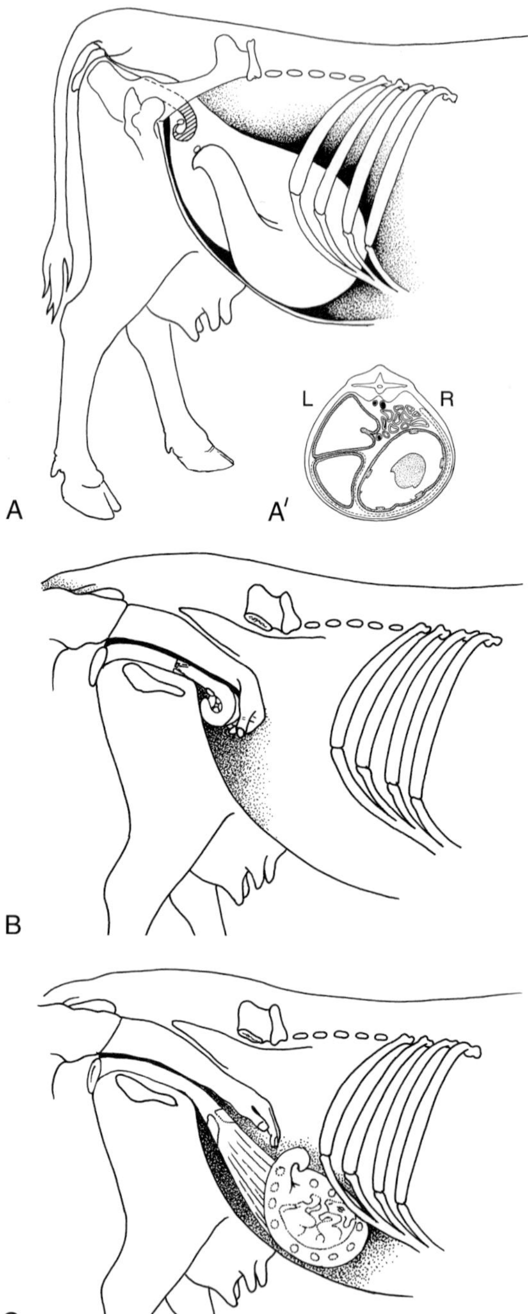


**Figure 29–25.** The position of the nongravid, and various stages of the gravid uterus in lateral view. *A,* Nongravid and 6-months gravid uterus; *A′,* The topography of the 6-months gravid uterus in transverse section. *B,* At 2 to 3 months the uterus has begun to slide down the caudal abdominal wall, but it can be scooped up by the hand in the colon. *C,* At 5 months the uterus is temporarily out of reach.

is apparent in primipara from the end of the first trimester, but in multipara, in which the vulva is often permanently thickened, no obvious changes may occur until shortly before birth.

Gestational effects on *other systems* have already been mentioned or implied. The stomach and intestines are displaced and compressed, pulmonary ventilation decreased following pressure on the thorax, the tissues of the abdominal wall stretched and hypertrophied, and the circulation in the abdominal veins embarrassed with increasing call on the alternative internal vertebral channels and adjustment of the mammary venous flow. Asymmetry of the abdomen, with bulging of the right ventral part, usually develops in the last months. The concurrent changes in the mammary glands are described later (p. 729).

## PARTURIENT AND PUERPERAL CHANGES

Certain other changes that signal the approach of parturition are probably mainly due to relaxin. Softening of the sacrosciatic ligament causes an insinking beside the tailhead (Plate 30/*H,I*). Similar changes also occur in the other pelvic ligaments, in the connective tissue of the cervix and caudal reproductive tract, and in the vulvar and perineal skin. The sacroiliac joints are loosened, but the effects on the pelvic symphysis are slight. These changes are spread over several weeks but are generally much accelerated in the last few days before birth. When parturition is actually impending, edema of the soft parts may cause the labia to gape.

Most features of pelvic anatomy that are of practical concern to the obstetrician have already been mentioned, but it may be useful to recapitulate certain points. The bovine bony pelvis is particularly unfavorable to easy parturition. It has a narrow inlet that is ventrally constricted in heifers; it is even more constricted farther caudally by the high, inflected ischial spines and the very salient ischial tubers; the axis of the "birth canal" is broken where it passes over the pelvic brim and again where the ischia turn dorsally toward the exit. The location of the pecten pubis below the middle of the sacrum makes it impossible to enlarge the height by raising the tailhead. While a modest increase may be obtained by rotating the pelvis ventrally about the slackened sacroiliac joints, this relief is denied to the standing cow, in which the body weight forces the girdle in the opposite direction. To these skeletal hazards are added certain potential obstructions represented by the less distensible soft parts; the principal impediments are the cervix, a tight region at the caudal end of the vagina, and the vulvar rim. Normally these are loosened by the hormonal influences just described.

The umbilical cord is ruptured when the cow gives birth and, being relatively short, often before delivery is complete; if not, it breaks when the calf drops from the vulva or the cow rises to her feet. Its constituents part at different levels, the urachus close to the bladder, the vessels at the umbilical opening in the abdominal musculature. The only constituent that remains visible externally, hanging from the navel, is the remnant of the amnion sheath. Critically, the arteries divide at predetermined levels where the longitudinal muscle of their walls is weak and the circular muscle exceptionally strong, facilitating sealing of the stumps. Despite frequent statements to the contrary, the arteries do not retract significantly, if at all, into the abdomen. The fetal membranes ("afterbirth" or "cleansings") may part from the uterus and be expelled shortly after delivery of the calf. The process may be hastened by secretion of oxytocin stimulated by suckling. Membranes that fail to separate and which corrupt in utero may require human intervention for their eventual removal.

Following parturition, the organs tend to return to their former state. Restoration may be more or less complete in the older multipara, but the first pregnancy leaves a permanent legacy in the form of increased size and thickening of the entire tract, loss of the virgin symmetry and neatness, and replacement of the trim cervical folds by irregular interlocking wedges. The uterus contracts as soon as it is emptied and undergoes a very rapid atrophy in which a third of its weight is lost within a couple of days, and a second third before the week is out. The decline thereafter is slower, and when the cow remains "empty" this phase may be succeeded by a period of superinvolution ("lactation atrophy") in which the size of the uterus drops below the resting norm.

Involution of the vagina, vestibule, and vulva is slower in execution and is never complete. The ligamentous structures are generally quickly, though sometimes incompletely, restored.

It is difficult to separate true *aging* changes from the effects of repeated pregnancy since most cows have a fairly active reproductive life. The tract of older animals is distinguished by its larger size; greater toughness; asymmetry; thickened and lengthened broad ligaments; thickened, more coiled, and more prominent arteries; and often by evidence of cervical and vulvar trauma. The ovaries do not sustain injury in pregnancy, but in older animals they are frequently distorted, showing adventitious adhesions.

# SOME ASPECTS OF PRENATAL DEVELOPMENT

## Early Development and Placentation

Ovulation in the cow occurs about 10 to 20 hours after the cessation of estrus.

*Cleavage* of the fertilized ovum begins as it passes down the tube and leads to the solid morula stage. The accumulation of fluid between the morular cells produces a blastocyst about the eighth or ninth day, 4 or 5 days after the conceptus arrives within the uterus. The delay is due to the temporary sphincter action of the isthmic region of the tube. The bovine blastocyst is first spherical but grows rapidly to form a very elongated vesicle.

A single conceptus normally remains within the horn it first enters, but when twins are produced from ova released by the same ovary, one may, with the help of uterine contractions, shift through the body to reach the other horn. No pronounced decidual reaction occurs in this species, and it is difficult to decide when *implantation* takes place; some writers believe the blastocyst is already implanted by the end of the second week, others that this event is delayed until late in the fifth week.

The amnion and chorion are defined by folding of the extraembryonic part of the trophoblast when the amnion comes to enclose the embryo directly. Their formation is followed (about the third week) by the outgrowth of the vascularized allantois from the hindgut. This soon extends two tubular processes that reach almost, but not quite, to the ends of the chorionic sac. The allantois vascularizes the chorion and amnion, except the chorionic tips which, left unlined, degenerate (Fig. 29–26 and Plate 8/*C,D*). The *placenta* develops by the interaction of the chorion with the endometrium of the caruncles and thus consists of scattered parts or *placentomes* formed largely over the chorioallantoic part of the fetal membranes. Each placentome consists of a maternal caruncular and a fetal cotyledonary part (Fig. 29–17/*D,E*). The membranes grow very rapidly in the early weeks of pregnancy and soon come to fill both horns.

Villous projections that grow from the chorion overlying the caruncles invade the pits in the endometrial surface after the fourth week. Later,

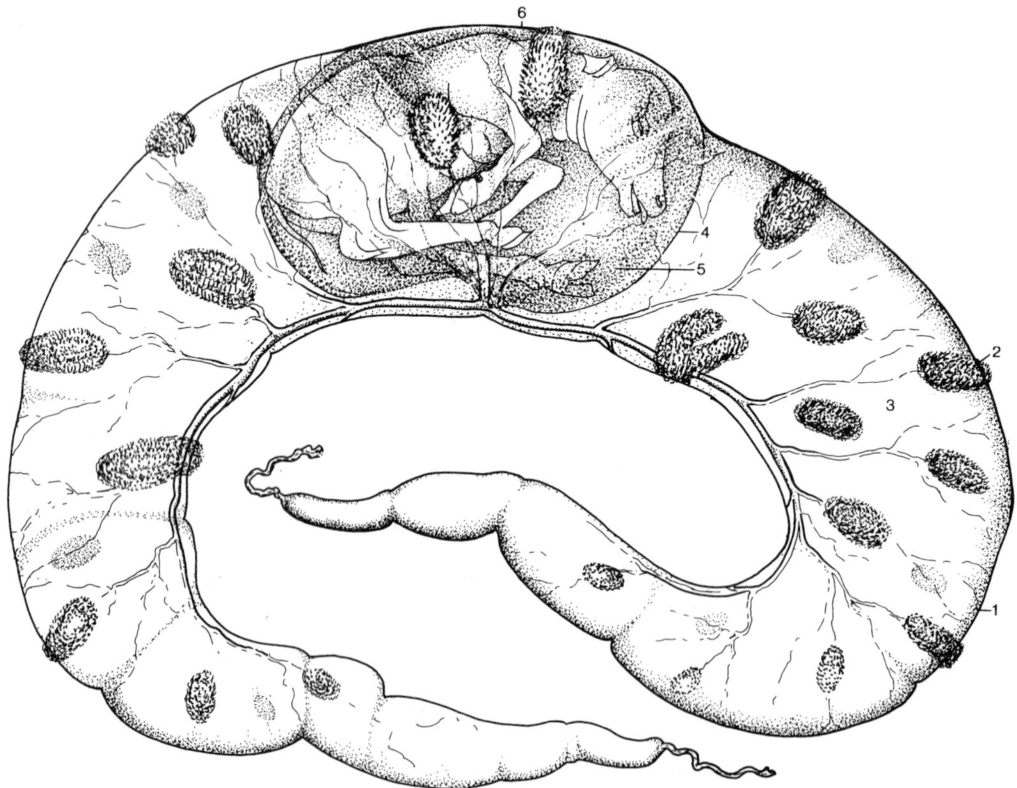


**Figure 29–26.** A bovine fetus within its membranes. The villi are mainly restricted to the cotyledons.

1, Chorioallantois; 2, cotyledon; 3, allantoic cavity; 4, amnion; 5, amniotic cavity; 6, chorioamnion.

**Table 29–1.** Guide to the Aging of Cattle Fetuses

| Age (mo) | Crown–Rump Length (cm) | External Features |
|---|---|---|
| 1 | 1 | Head and limb buds are distinguishable |
| 2 | 6 | Digits are distinguishable |
| 3 | 10 | Scrotal (male) or mammary (female) swelling is distinct |
| 4 | 20 | First hairs appear about the eyes; horn buds are present |
| 5 | 30–40 | Hairs appear about the mouth; testes are within the scrotum |
| 6 | 40–60 | Hair is present on the tail extremity |
| 7 | 50–70 | Hair is present on the proximal parts of the limbs |
| 8 | 60–80 | The haircoat is general but still short and sparse over the belly |
| 9 | 70–90 | The appearance is mature and the body is well haired; the incisors have erupted |
| Full term (278–290 days) | | |

From Evans and Sack, 1973.

similar formations create accessory intercaruncular placental areas related to the openings of the uterine glands. The villi that penetrate the crypts of the caruncular endometrium first establish only a loose relationship to the uterine surface. They increase in number over the next 3 months or so and become longer, branched, and firmly anchored. The chorionic and uterine epithelia are now believed to remain intact, and the placenta is classified as epitheliochorial. The placenta is a barrier to the exchange of immune bodies in utero, and the calf relies for its early immunological protection on absorption of antibodies from the colostrum during the first 24 hours of extrauterine existence.

Although the incidence of *twin pregnancy* in cattle is not high (1% to 4%, according to breed), the phenomenon has attracted rather more than its share of attention because of the frequency with which—indeed virtual certainty that—the female partner of a male calf exhibits intersex characteristics. This anomaly results from the fusion of the two sets of membranes with anastomoses of their vessels. The masculinization of the female partner (the so-called freemartin) was once thought to be due to exposure to androgens passing over from its male twin. This is now thought to be of little importance. More significant are the passing of antimüllerian hormone (causing regression of the müllerian ducts) and descendine (causing gubernacular regression) from male to female and the exchange of cells between the two embryos, which are in fact chimeras (Plate 5/*F*). Support for this interpretation can be obtained from the discovery that most cattle twins—presumably all that shared a common placental circulation—accept grafts of their partners' tissues in adult life, indicating the occurrence of cellular interchange at a time when they were immunologically tolerant. There is reason to believe that germ as well as somatic cells are exchanged.

Twins and triplets are of course common in sheep and goats. The incidence varies with the breed and reflects the clemency or severity of the environment for which that breed has evolved. Freemartins—although not unknown—are very uncommon.

## The Estimation of Fetal Age

It is often necessary (or at least convenient) to be able to make an approximate estimation of the age of an aborted embryo or fetus in the field. Many published tables record crown–rump lengths, fetal body weight, and so forth at different stages of gestation; all of these suffer from the disadvantage of recording average values for parameters that vary widely according to breed, nutritional status, "litter size," and other factors. One of the most popular guides, since most easily memorized, appears to be as reliable as any; it allows 1.0 cm of crown–rump length for each of the first 12 weeks of development and 2.5 cm for each week thereafter. Except with the very youngest embryos the resulting estimate is rarely much more than 2 weeks off when normal specimens from the larger breeds are concerned. A greater degree of accuracy is hardly to be expected from any rule-of-thumb method.

Qualitative methods which regard the external and internal anatomy of the fetus are more dependable but more difficult to commit to memory. Complete information on these matters can be found in any of the larger texts of veterinary embryology or obstetrics, and the very abbreviated guides (Tables 29–1 and 29–2) given here are for quick reference only.

Maturity, in the sense of the capacity to make the integrated physiological response necessary for survival outside the uterus, is not achieved until relatively late in gestation. In lambs the mortality

**Table 29–2.** Guide to the Aging of Sheep Fetuses

| Age (mo) | Crown–Rump Length (cm) | External Features |
|---|---|---|
| 1 | 2 | Pinna triangular; eyelids forming; tactile hair follicles beginning to appear around eyes; principal forelimb digits prominent |
| 1.5 | 6 | Eyelids fused; external genitalia differentiated; teats present |
| 2 | 11 | Hair begins to cover the body |
| 3 | 24 | Tactile hairs appear on face; testes in upper part of scrotum |
| 4 | 38 | Woolly hair begins to grow; eyes open again |
| Full term (147–155 days) | | |

From Evans and Sack, 1973.

is very high in those delivered prematurely at 140 days and is 100% at 135 days. Although no very reliable figures are available for cattle, premature calves appear to be relatively more viable (but still contrast unfavorably in survival potential with the human premature infant). Information on these matters, which are of such obvious economic importance and scientific interest, is sadly lacking and defective.

## THE ANATOMY OF RECTAL PALPATION IN CATTLE*

As in the horse, rectal exploration in cattle is not free from risk of injury to the mucosa or even, in extreme cases, perforation of the intestinal wall—a mishap most likely to occur when invasion of the rectum induces straining. The novice should not attempt the procedure without appropriate supervision. Although rectal examinations of cows are most frequently performed to obtain information on the functional or pathological status of the reproductive organs, it is necessary to be familiar with the larger anatomy that can be appreciated using this procedure. The territory that can be explored when the hand is carried forward into the descending colon is more extensive than might be supposed.

The parts of the pelvic and abdominal walls that are accessible include the bones bounding the pelvic cavity, and a part of the abdominal wall including the regions of the deep inguinal rings. Dorsally, the caudal segment of the aorta and its bifurcation are within reach, and, scattered about the vessels, the larger lymph nodes of the medial iliac and deep inguinal groups (Fig. 29–4/14,13) can be palpated. The deep inguinal nodes are particularly important in connection with mastitis. The caudal part of the rumen is very obvious directly before the pelvic inlet, and it can be confirmed that ventrally the rumen extends into the right half of the abdomen. The caudodorsal blind sac may even intrude into the pelvic cavity when distended with gas. However, much of the rumen and the remaining compartments of the stomach are inaccessible, as are the liver and the spleen. The one necessary qualification of this statement refers to the abomasum, part of which is brought into reach in certain displacements. The right dorsal quadrant of the abdomen is occupied by small intestine, cecum, and colon, which together form a soft, fluctuating mass in which individual parts are mostly not identifiable when normal; the most common exception is the rounded tip of the gas-filled cecum.

Most of the left kidney, pushed to the right by the rumen and suspended from the abdominal roof, may be palpated; only the caudal pole of the right kidney is within reach, and then only in smaller subjects. Healthy ureters are not detectable unless the initial portion of the left one can be appreciated where it passes over the surface of the kidney. The impression made by the bladder varies greatly since it forms a firm mass over the most cranial part of the pelvic floor when contracted but extends well forward into the abdomen as a fluctuating structure when distended. The intervention of the female reproductive tract makes this organ far less accessible in cows than in male animals.

Passing attention has already been given to the inspection per rectum of the reproductive organs, and we gather together here only the principal features. A systematic examination is best begun by locating the cervix, easily recognized by its firmness and dimensions, although its location varies greatly according to the present status and past history of the animal. The short body of the uterus lies forward of the cervix, and the uterus

*Except for digital explorations, rectal palpation is not routinely performed in small ruminants.

may be fixed by the insertion of a finger between the intercornual ligaments to allow examination and comparison of the horns that diverge to each side. Frequently these manipulations stimulate contraction, sometimes quite powerful, of the uterine muscle. The reader is reminded that in certain circumstances the uterus passes far into the abdomen. If not too much enlarged, it may be retrieved by passing the hand forward and downward into the ventral part of the abdomen on the right side and then withdrawing the hand with the fingers flexed toward the palm to enclose the uterus. The broad ligaments proceeding to the horns of the uterus are distinct, but the uterine tubes, which run near the free cranial margins of the ligaments, are less certainly discoverable since, although fairly firm, they are only about 2 mm wide. The free margins of the broad ligaments also provide a guide to the location of the ovaries, which lie on the floor of the pelvic cavity in the young virgin animal but are displaced cranially and ventrally into the abdomen in older, more sexually experienced cows. An indication has already been given of the features of the follicles and corpora lutea that may be appreciated by examination of the ovarian surface (p. 698). The reader is also reminded that the forward and downward movement of the reproductive organs in pregnancy may carry them out of reach for a time (Fig. 29–25). The direction taken by the uterine artery is then revealing; it is easily found as it passes forward across the shaft of the ilium and the identification confirmed by the characteristic fremitus.

## Selected Bibliography


Abusineina, M.E.: Effect of parity and pregnancy on the dimensions and weight of the cervix uteri of cattle. Br. Vet. J. 125:12–24, 1969.

Ashdown, R.R., and S. Done: Color Atlas of Veterinary Anatomy: The Ruminants. Baltimore, University Park Press, 1984.

Basset, E.G.: The anatomy of the pelvic and perineal region in the ewe. Aust. J. Zool. 13:201–241, 1961.

Belling, T.H.: The look and feel of normal bovine ovaries. Vet. Med. 81:455–463, 1986.

Betteridge, K.J.: Embryo Transfer in Farm Animals. A Review of Techniques and Applications. Monograph 16. Ottawa, Dept. of Agriculture, 1977.

Betteridge, K.J.: The normal genital organs. *In* Laing, J.A. (ed.): Fertility and Infertility in the Domestic Animals, 3rd ed. London, Baillière-Tindall, 1979.

Bowen, R.A., R.P. Elsden, and G.E. Seidel: Embryo transfer for cows with reproductive problems. JAVMA 172:1303–1307, 1978.

Cattell, J.H., and H. Dobson: A survey of caesarean operations on cattle in general veterinary practice. Vet. Rec. 127:395–399, 1990.

Dawson, F.L.M.: The normal bovine uterus: Physiology, histology and bacteriology. Vet. Rev. Annotations 5:73–81, 1959.

deLahunta, A., and R.E. Habel: Applied Veterinary Anatomy. Philadelphia, W.B. Saunders Company, 1986.

Deutscher, G.H.: Pelvic measurements. Key to reducing incidents of bovine dystocia. Norden News 63:18–25, 1988.

Drost, M., J.D. Savio, C.M. Barros, et al.: Ovariectomy by colpotomy in cows. JAVMA 200:337–339, 1992.

El-Banna, A.A., and E.S. Hafez: Profile analysis of the oviductal wall in rabbits and cattle. Anat. Rec. 166:469–478, 1970.

Evans, H.E., and W.O. Sack: Prenatal development of domestic and laboratory animals. Growth curves, external features and selected references. Anat. Histol. Embryol. 2:11–45, 1973.

Franco, O.J., M. Drost, M.-J. Thatcher, V.M. Shille, and W.W. Thatcher: Fetal survival in the cow after pregnancy diagnosis by rectal palpation. Theriogenology 27:631–644, 1987.

Ginther, O.J.: Utero-ovarian relationships in cattle: Physiologic aspects. JAVMA 153:1656–1664, 1968.

Ginther, O.J., and C.H. Del Campo: Vascular anatomy of the uterus and ovaries and the unilateral luteolytic effect of the uterus: Cattle. Am. J. Vet. Res. 35:193–203, 1974.

Habel, R.E.: The topographic anatomy of the muscles, nerves and arteries of the bovine female perineum. Am. J. Anat. 119:79–95, 1966.

Habel, R.E.: Guide to the Dissection of Domestic Ruminants, 5th ed. Ithaca, 1992. Published by the author.

Hartman, W., and C.C. Van de Watering: The function of the bladder neck in female goats. Zentralbl. Veterinarmed. [A] 21:430–435, 1974.

Hunter, R.H. F.: Physiology and Technology of Reproduction in Female Domestic Animals. London, Academic Press, 1980.

Jost, A., B. Vigier, and J. Prepin: Freemartins in cattle: The first steps of sexual organogenesis. J. Reprod. Fertil. 29:349–379, 1972.

Kirk, E.J., and R.L. Kitchell: Neurophysiological maps of the cutaneous innervation of the external genitalia of the ewe. Am. J. Vet. Res. 49:522–526, 1988.

Lamond, D.R., and M. Drost: Blood supply to the bovine ovary. J. Anim. Sci. 38:106–112, 1974.

Loen, A. v.: A Contribution to the Knowledge of the Double Cervix Condition in Cattle. Utrecht. Acad. Proefschrift, 1961.

Lyngset, O.: Studies on reproduction in the goat. I. The normal genital organs of the nonpregnant goat. II. The genital organs of the pregnant goat. Acta. Vet. Scand. 9:208–222; 242–256, 1968.

Mapletoft, R.J., M.R. Del Campo, and O.J. Ginther: Local venoarterial pathway for uterine-induced luteolysis in cattle. Proc. Soc. Exp. Biol. Med. 153:289–294, 1976.

Miller, R.I., and R.S.F. Campbell: Anatomy and pathology of the bovine ovary and oviduct. Vet. Bull. 48:737–753, 1978.

Morrow, D.A.: Current Therapy in Theriogenology 2. Philadelphia, W.B. Saunders Company, 1986.

Noakes, D.E.: The normal breeding animal. *In* Laing, J.A. (ed.): Fertility and Infertility in Domestic Animals, 3rd ed. London, Baillière-Tindall, 1979.

Pavaux, C.: A Color Atlas of Bovine Visceral Anatomy. London, Wolfe Publishing, 1983.

Popesko, P.: Atlas of Topographic Anatomy of the Domestic Animals, vol. 3: Pelvis and Limbs. Philadelphia, W.B. Saunders Company, 1971.

Roberts, S.J.: Veterinary Obstetrics and Genital Disease (Theriogenology), 3rd ed. Ann Arbor, Mich., Edwards Brothers, Inc. (Distr.). 1986. Published by the author.

Robinson, T.J.: Reproduction in cattle. *In* Cupps, P.T. (ed.): Reproduction in Domestic Animals, 4th ed. New York Academic Press, 1991.

Seidel, G.E., Jr.: Superovulation and embryo transfer in cattle. Science 211:351–357, 1981.

Sloss, V., and J.H. Duffy: Handbook of Bovine Obstetrics. Baltimore, Williams & Wilkins, 1980.

Stevens, D.H.: Comparative Placentation. London, Academic Press, 1975.

Thurmond, M.C., and J.P. Picanso: Fetal loss associated with palpation per rectum to diagnose pregnancy in cows. JAVMA 203:432–435, 1993.

Troyer, D., and H.W. Leipold: Rectovaginal constriction in Jersey cattle. Zentralbl. Veterinarmed. [A] 32: 752–759, 1985.

Walker, D.F., and J.T. Vaughan: Bovine and Equine Urogenital Surgery. Philadelphia, Lea & Febiger, 1980.

White, M.E., N. LaFaunce, and H.O. Mohammed: Optimal time postbreeding for pregnancy examination in dairy cattle. Can. Vet. J. 30:147–149, 1989.

# CHAPTER 30

# The Pelvis and Reproductive Organs of Male Ruminants

## GENERAL FEATURES OF THE PELVIS

Sex differences in the skeleton are quite marked in adult cattle, although difficulties may sometimes arise with the identification of the girdle of the castrate. The male bones are larger and more rugged than those of the female, and they enclose a canal that is conspicuously more cramped. The cranial part of the male pelvis floor is domed, not level as in the mature cow, while the caudal part slopes steeply dorsally. The appearance of the section through the symphysis is therefore sometimes recommended as a guide to the sex of the split carcass, but it is unreliable, especially in younger animals. The exit from the male pelvis is also narrowed by a greater inflection of the dorsal processes of the ischial tubers.

Ankylosis of the sacroiliac joints and spondylosis occur regularly in aging bulls—but not cows—and although usually without clinical significance may, when severe, lead to inability to mount for service.

The perineal region extends to the scrotum. The urogenital part is bisected by a raphe that follows the course of the urethra. The powerful bulbospongiosus and ischiocavernosus muscles that cover the urethra and the crura of the penis are palpable through the skin. They do not extend beyond the point where the components of the penis merge, and the body of the organ is therefore directly palpable both behind and in front of the scrotum. The skin of the urogenital region is supplied by cutaneous branches of the pudendal nerve; twigs corresponding to mammary branches reach the caudal scrotal wall.

The visceral topography in the dorsal part of the pelvic cavity is the same in both sexes. In the narrower ventral part, the male urethra is surrounded by considerable amounts of fat and connective tissue where it lies on the pelvic floor; only a narrow median strip faces directly into the rectogenital pouch, which extends to the level of the first caudal vertebra (Fig. 30–1/11).

## THE REPRODUCTIVE ORGANS

### The Scrotum

The pendulous scrotum is situated between the cranial parts of the thighs and may reach the level of the hock joints. It is molded on the testes and is marked by a median groove corresponding to the internal division. A constricted neck is formed at the junction of the scrotum with the body wall, between and slightly caudal to the superficial inguinal rings. The thin and supple scrotal skin is sparingly covered with fine hair and firmly attached to the underlying dartos. A mass of fat (“cod fat”) around the inguinal part of the cord is especially well developed in castrated animals. When present in excessive quantity it dilates the inguinal canal, producing a *pseudohernia inguinalis.*

Small rudimentary teats are located on the cranial face of the scrotum (Fig. 30–2). Attention is given to their number and spacing in the selection of bulls of dairy breeds since these characters are likely to be conveyed to their female offspring.

The scrotum receives its sensory nerve supply from three sources: the ventral branches of the first two lumbar nerves, the genitofemoral nerve, which passes through the inguinal canal, and long descending branches from the pudendal nerve. The genitofemoral nerve also supplies the cremaster.

The scrotum of the ram is sometimes concealed by wool, a possible cause of infertility since it impairs the dissipation of heat. Rudimentary teats

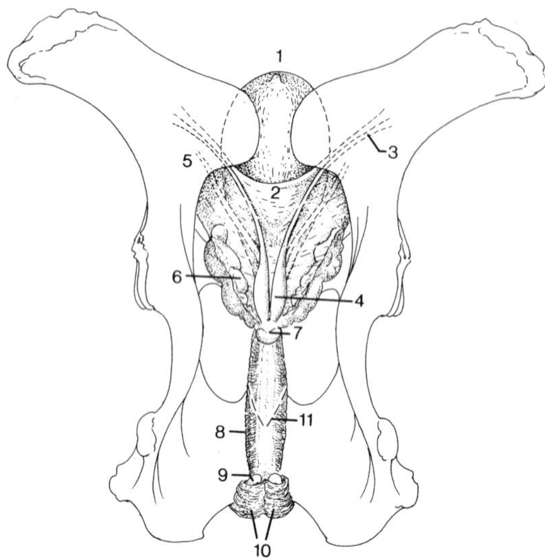


**Figure 30–1.** Dorsal view of the bull's pelvis and related urogenital organs.

1, Bladder; 2, genital fold; 3, right deferent duct; 4, ampulla of deferent duct; 5, left ureter; 6, vesicular gland; 7, body of prostate; 8, urethralis (surrounding urethra); 9, bulbourethral gland; 10, bulbospongiosus; 11, caudal extent of the rectogenital pouch *(broken line)*.

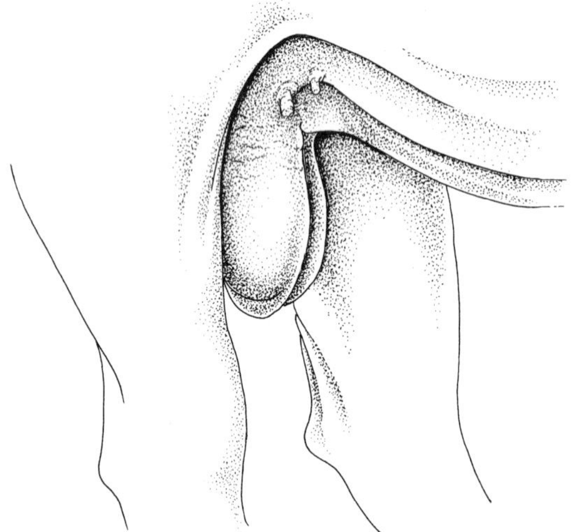

**Figure 30–2.** Craniolateral view of the bull's scrotum and nearby rudimentary teats.

are common on the scrotum of both rams and bucks.

## The Testis and Epididymis

The testes of the ruminants are large, elongated ellipsoids that hang almost vertically within the scrotum where they may be palpated. They should be freely movable—adhesions may be evidence of inflammatory disease—and plump; relatively small testes, which tend to be more cylindrical, are often associated with reduced fertility. The epididymis follows the caudomedial border of the testis that is turned toward its fellow and is tightly joined to the testis at the poles. Its head continues some distance over the free border of the testis before doubling back on itself. The tail projects ventrally, forming a conspicuous conical swelling; generally firm, the tail is softer for a time following ejaculation. The smooth external surface of the testis is remarkable only for the winding pattern of the intracapsular vessels (Fig. 30–3). The testes in relation to the body and the epididymides in relation to the testes are relatively larger in small ruminants.

Incision of the capsule exposes the yellow parenchyma that is contained under slight pressure

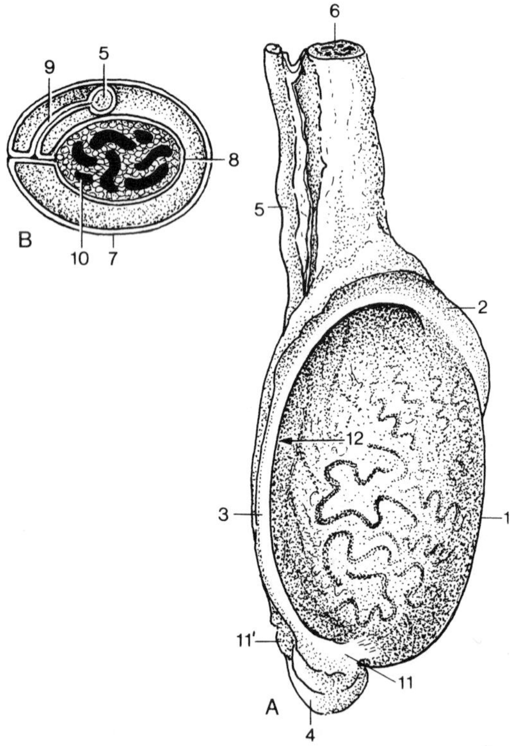


**Figure 30–3.** Caudal view of the bull's right testis *(A)* and schematic transection of the spermatic cord *(B)*.

1, Free border of testis; 2, head of epididymis; 3, body of epididymis; 4, tail of epididymis; 5, deferent duct; 6, vascular part of spermatic cord consisting of testicular artery and pampiniform plexus; 7, parietal vaginal tunic; 8, visceral vaginal tunic; 9, mesoductus deferens; 10, pampiniform plexus and testicular artery; 11, proper ligament of testis; 11′, ligament of the tail of the epididymis, cut; 12, testicular bursa.

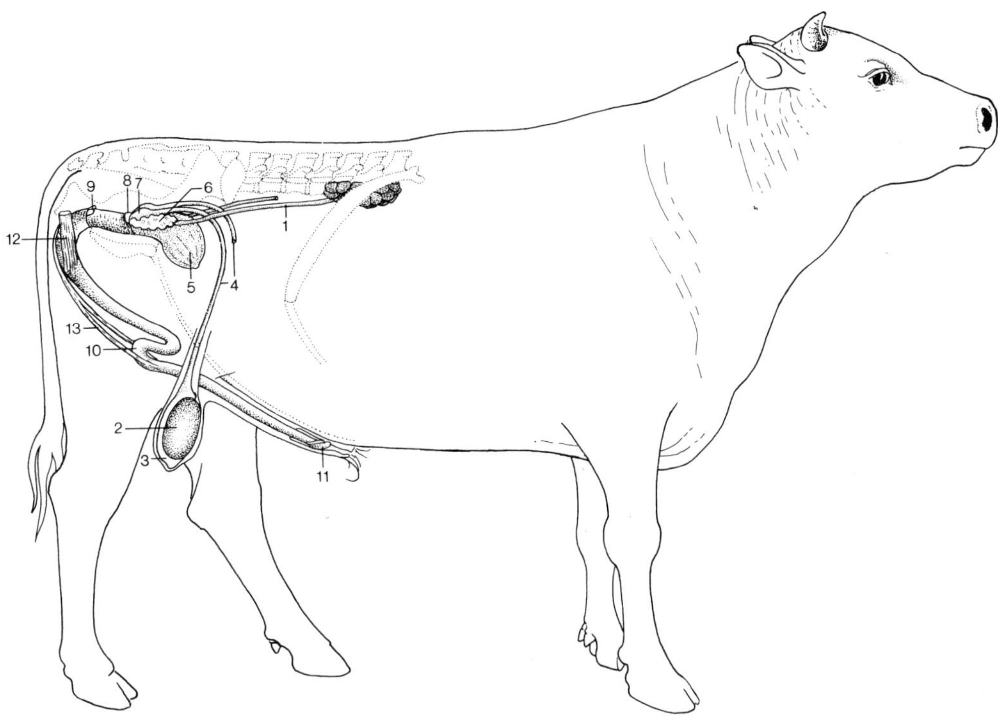


**Figure 30–4.** Disposition of the urogenital organs of a bull.

1, Ureter; 2, right testis; 3, epididymis; 4, deferent duct; 5, bladder; 6, vesicular gland; 7, ampulla of deferent duct; 8, body of prostate; 9, bulbourethral gland; 10, sigmoid flexure of penis; 11, glans penis; 12, ischiocavernosus; 13, retractor penis.

within delicate partitions that converge on a prominent central mediastinum (Plate 6/*B*).

The deferent duct ascends on the medial side of the testis where it follows the cranial margin of the epididymis after emerging from the tail; it is easily recognized on palpation as a firm but narrow strand (/5).

The spermatic cord may be identified within the scrotal neck. It is sought here to be crushed in the Burdizzo method of castration; the approach is most conveniently made from behind. The bulk of the cord is composed of the testicular vessels, which give it a conical, dorsally tapering form. The artery is even more convoluted than in other species, and its coils are embedded among the many veins that constitute the pampiniform plexus (see Figs. 5–36 and 5–37). Arteriovenous anastomoses exist; while their functional significance is uncertain, they may be the origin of the varicoceles that are occasionally found in the stump of the cord of the castrate (Plate 6/*C,D*).

The lymphatics of the cord carry a substantial fraction of the testosterone produced within the testes. These vessels pass directly to the medial iliac lymph nodes, while lymph coming from the scrotum goes to the superficial inguinal (scrotal) nodes, placed caudal to the scrotal neck.

## The Pelvic Reproductive Organs

The constituents of the spermatic cord disperse at the vaginal ring, which is easily identified on rectal exploration. The *deferent duct* is directed caudally and loops medial to the ureter to gain the dorsal aspect of the bladder (Fig. 30–4/4). It passes through the substance of the prostate before entering the urethra (Fig. 30–5); in the last part of its course it is joined by the duct of the vesicular gland to form a very short common passage.

The subterminal stretch (≈10 to 12 cm) of the duct lies beside its fellow within the genital fold. It is swollen to form the cylindrical ampulla or ampullary gland (Fig. 30–1/4), an enlargement entirely due to glandular proliferation within the mucosa. A median vestige (uterus masculinus) of the fused paramesonephric ducts is sometimes present between the ampullae.

The pelvic part of the *urethra* lies over the symphysis. Its relatively small lumen is further narrowed by a dorsal ridge continuing from the bladder and by longitudinal mucosal folds. Caudal to the ischial arch the lumen presents a dorsal diverticulum related to the excretory ducts of the bulbourethral glands; this feature makes catheterization of the bladder almost impossible since the

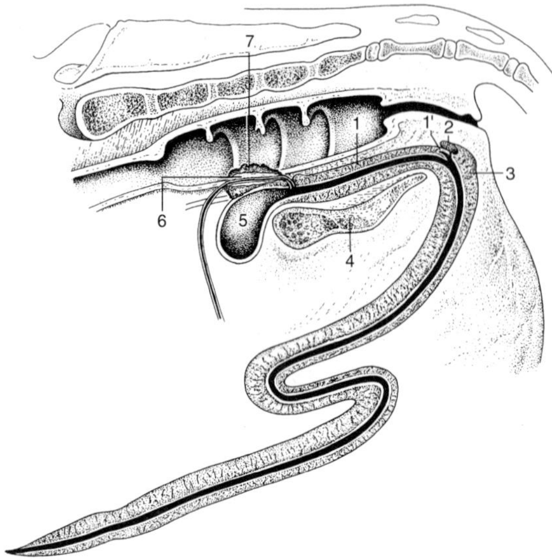


**Figure 30–5.** Median section through the bovine pelvis.

1, Pelvic part of urethra; 1′, dorsal diverticulum of urethra; 2, bulbourethral gland; 3, bulbospongiosus; 4, symphysis; 5, bladder; 6, ampulla of deferent duct (schematic); 7, vesicular gland.

tip of the instrument consistently engages the diverticulum* (Fig. 30–5/1′). The powerful striated urethralis appears crescentic in section since its dorsal part is replaced by a dense aponeurotic plate (Fig. 30–6/4,4′). The disseminate part of the prostate extends along the whole length of the pelvic urethra but diminishes in thickness when followed caudally; most lies dorsal to the lumen (/3). A thin sleeve of spongy tissue around the urethral lumen is expanded caudally to form the bilobed bulb of the penis. The penile urethra is reduced in caliber and is further constricted at the sigmoid flexure, close to the attachment of the retractor penis. Urinary calculi tend to lodge here, especially in castrated animals, in which the passage is narrower than in bulls. The urethra reaches to the very end of the penis where it finally appears as a surface ridge (urethral process) to one side of the glans (Fig. 30–10/*A*,2).

The *prostate* of bulls (unlike those of small ruminants) has a second, compact part (body) consisting of paired lobes that have broken through the aponeurosis of the urethralis. These form a narrow bar (4 cm wide and 1 cm long) across the first part of the urethra (Fig. 30–1/7).

The paired *vesicular glands* are very large (≈10 to 15 × 3 to 5 cm) and contribute the bulk of the seminal fluid (/6). They lie largely lateral to the ampullae of the deferent ducts and are covered by peritoneum of the genital fold except over their lateral edges. These glands are flexed on themselves, grossly lobulated, irregular, and more or less solid with narrow branching lumina (see Fig. 5–40/*B*).

The *bulbourethral glands* are small, dorsoventrally flattened, and situated almost level with the ischial arch (Fig. 30–1/9). They are largely covered by the thick and powerful bulbospongiosus and drain into the dorsal diverticulum (Figs. 30–5/2 and 30–7/5). Their watery secretion is discharged before the main ejaculate and flushes the penile urethra in advance of the passage of the sperm-rich fraction.

## Rectal Exploration

In bulls most pelvic reproductive organs may be palpated on *rectal exploration.* The ampullae are about 1 cm in diameter and are conspicuously softer than the adjoining parts of the deferent ducts. The vesicular glands are identified by their lobulated surface; a certain asymmetry is usual but is sometimes difficult to evaluate since inflammation and cyst formation are both common. Their consistency varies and tends to harden with age. The pelvic urethra may be felt along its length;

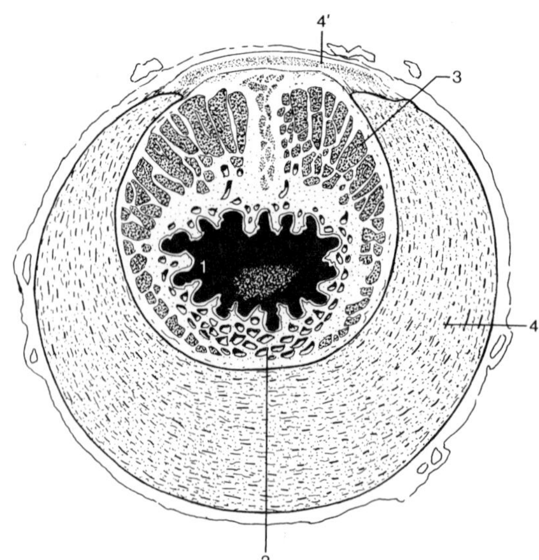


**Figure 30–6.** Transverse section of the bovine pelvic urethra immediately caudal to the body of the prostate.

1, Urethra; 2, spongy tissue (stratum spongiosum); 3, disseminate part of prostate; 4, urethralis; 4′, dorsal aponeurosis of urethralis.

*Catheterization would in any case be difficult without previous relaxation of the penis to eliminate the sigmoid flexure.

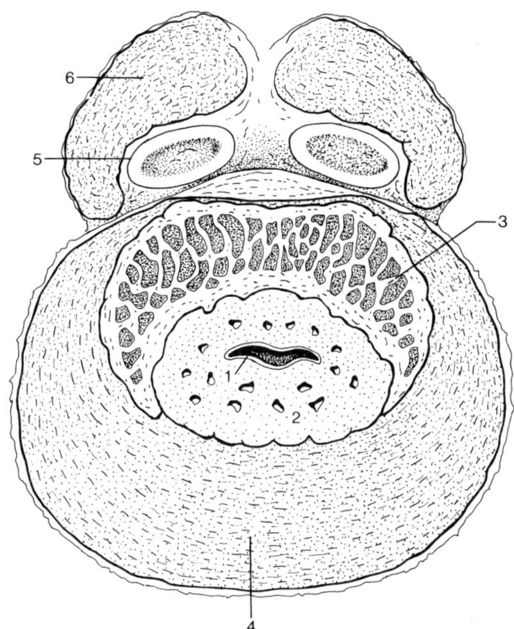


**Figure 30–7.** Transverse section of the bovine pelvic urethra immediately cranial to the ischial arch.

1, Urethra; 2, stratum spongiosum; 3, disseminate part of prostate; 4, urethralis; 5, bulbourethral gland; 6, bulbospongiosus, which also covers the bulbourethral gland (5).

manipulation often stimulates rhythmic contractions of its muscular covering. The body of the prostate is palpable, but the bulbourethral glands cannot usually be identified. Apart from the references to reproductive organs, the description of rectal exploration given for the cow (p. 710) is applicable to the male.

## The Penis and Prepuce

The penis of an adult bull is almost 1 m long, but about a quarter of its length is occupied by the sigmoid flexure located above and behind the scrotum (Fig. 30–4). The penis is of the fibroelastic type and is therefore relatively rigid even when nonerect. The crura are rodlike, laterally compressed, and almost surrounded by the powerful ischiocavernosus muscles (Fig. 30–8). They contain cavernous spaces that are more generously developed than those of other parts of the penis. The crus and associated muscle together deeply indent the muscles of the thigh, a useful pointer to the sex of the dressed carcass.

The body of the penis is more or less circular in section and is formed by the fusion of the crura and the incorporation of the spongy part of the urethra. This construction is not obvious externally since the three parts are enclosed by a common fibrous tunic (Fig. 30–9/4). The caudal part of the body is suspended from the symphysial tendon by the bilateral but closely spaced suspensory ligaments; these (often though inaccurately described as a single structure) occasionally rupture, allowing the penis to sag.

The free extremity of the quiescent penis lies within the caudal part of the preputial cavity (Fig. 30–4). It is capped by a small cushion of softer tissue forming the asymmetrical, ventrally bent, and slightly spiraled glans. The urethra follows a seam or raphe along the right aspect of the free part and ends in a low projection with a slitlike orifice at its tip (Fig. 30–10/*A*,2).

The free extremity of the penis is very distinctive in small ruminants in which the urethral process is continued for some centimeters (≈2 to 3 cm in bucks, 3 to 4 cm in rams) beyond the glans (/*D*,*C*). The process is slender and somewhat

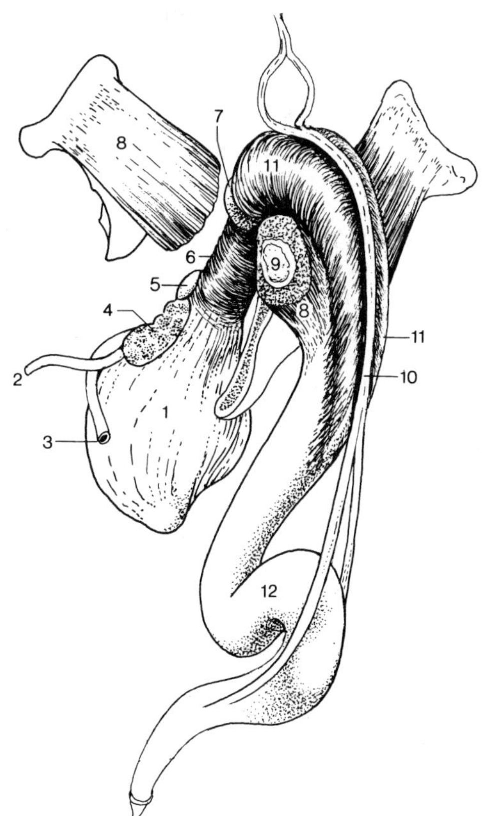


**Figure 30–8.** The bovine penis and its muscles; caudolateral view.

1, Bladder; 2, ureter; 3, deferent duct; 4, vesicular gland; 5, body of prostate; 6, urethralis; 7, bulbourethral gland; 8, ischiocavernosus; 9, crus of penis (in transverse section); 10, retractor penis; 11, bulbospongiosus; 12, sigmoid flexure.

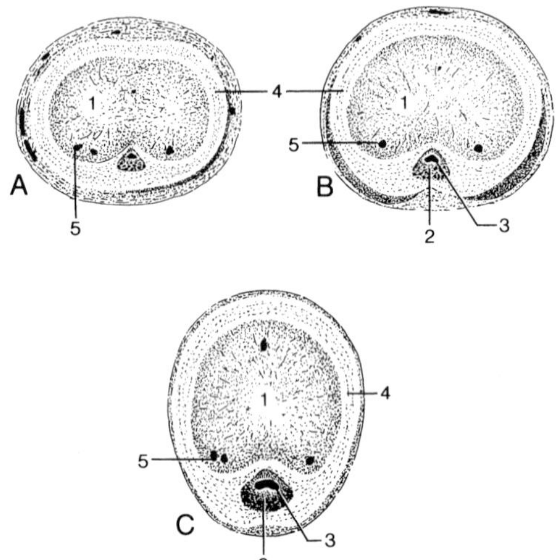


**Figure 30–9.** Transverse sections of the bovine penis, 18 cm caudal to the glans *(A)*, and 5 cm cranial *(B)* and 8 cm caudal *(C)* to the sigmoid flexure.

1, Corpus cavernosum; 2, corpus spongiosum; 3, urethra; 4, tunica albuginea; 5, thick-walled veins.

artery.) These arteries are accompanied by satellite veins that drain both the blood spaces and the tissues of the penis. The crura and corpus cavernosum penis form a continuous vascular unit into which extra blood is transferred during erection, first by elevation of the blood pressure after dilation of the vessels, and secondly by the contractions of the ischiocavernosus muscles. Venous blood draining from the crura and corpus cavernosum passes to the systemic circulation via pelvic channels. The bulb of the penis, the corpus spongiosum, and the glans also drain to veins within the pelvic area but an alternative route to more cranially located veins exists. Consequently, drainage of the spongiosum system is not completely arrested by the contraction of the bulbospongiosus muscle. The dorsal nerves of the penis, which run with the dorsal arteries, are paired but exhibit considerable overlap in their distribution. Since stimulation of the apex of the penis is necessary for the achievement of full erection, the integrity of these nerves is essential for reproductive competence.

sinuous and tapers to its tip where the urethra opens. This process is erectile and in former times, as in primitive societies today, was amputated with the design of depriving rams of their fertilizing capacity.

The preputial cavity is long (≈40 cm) and narrow; only the deepest part is normally occupied by a retracted penis. The skin of the free part of the penis is smooth and tightly adherent over the apex of the penis; it becomes less regular caudally where a looser attachment allows it to change its disposition when the penis is protruded or withdrawn. The internal lamina of the prepuce carries low longitudinal folds toward the orifice and scattered lymphoid elevations more deeply within the cavity. Externally, the cranial part of the prepuce droops caudal to the umbilicus, most conspicuously in bulls of beef breeds in which it may be vulnerable to injury by sharp grasses. The orifice is marked by a tuft of coarse long hair. The prepuce is relatively short in the smaller species.

The penis is supplied with blood through branches that arise from the internal pudendal arteries within the pelvis. One branch, the artery of the bulb, supplies the bulb and the corpus spongiosum. A second branch, the deep artery of the penis, enters the crus. A third, the dorsal artery, runs along the upper border toward the glans, which it supplies; it also detaches many twigs that feed the prepuce. (In small ruminants the external pudendal artery may supplement or replace the internal pudendal as the source of the dorsal

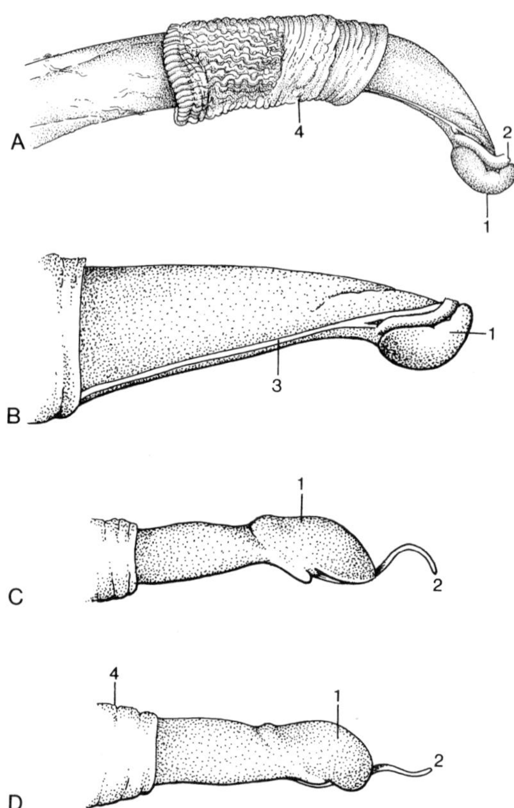


**Figure 30–10.** Right lateral view of the distal end of the bull's penis, flaccid *(A)* and erect *(B)*; and the distal end of the ram's *(C)* and buck's *(D)* penis.

1, Glans; 2, urethral process; 3, raphe; 4, preputial skin.

The preputial skin, including that covering the free part of the penis, is supplied by twigs from ventral abdominal (T13, L1–4) and pudendal (S2–4) nerve trunks.

The cranial preputial muscles arise from the xiphoid region and insert beside and behind the preputial opening; they draw the pendent part of the prepuce forward and upward and help to constrict the orifice. Caudal preputial muscles are generally also present but are slighter and of uncertain importance. Both groups are detachments of the cutaneous muscle of the trunk and receive their innervation from the brachial plexus.

The urethralis and bulbospongiosus muscles have already been mentioned. The bulbospongiosus follows the urethra over the ischial arch and onto the penis, diminishing in size as it extends distally (Fig. 30–8/11).

The retractor penis (/10) is much better developed than the homologous retractor clitoridis. It arises from the caudal vertebrae, passes to the side of the rectum, and then continues under the perineal skin to reach the penis at the second bend of the sigmoid flexure. Some fibers attach here, but most proceed to a more distal and diffuse insertion. Local contractions of this muscle that are normally evident help maintain the flexure. Contraction is controlled by the sympathetic innervation which, though of lumbar origin, is conveyed by the pudendal and caudal rectal nerve trunks. Because of this, anesthesia of the penis and relaxation of the retractor muscles cannot conveniently be achieved by epidural anesthesia, which would remove the ability to stand. The pudendal and caudal rectal trunks may, however, be blocked where they run medial to the sacrosciatic ligament; this procedure allows the penis to be withdrawn for inspection or treatment. The pudendal nerve is palpated per rectum against the medial surface of the sacrosciatic ligament, where it passes caudoventrally to the lesser sciatic foramen whose cranial border may be palpated, as shown in Figure 29–5/7. The figure also shows the relationship of the nerve to the internal iliac artery (/10), which may be identified by its pulse. A 12.5-cm needle is inserted medial to the palpable caudal border of the sacrosciatic ligament and guided to the nerve by the hand in the rectum. After blocking the pudendal nerve at *A* and *B* the infiltration is continued during withdrawal of the needle to block also the caudal rectal nerves (/13) at *C*. Relaxation of the penis may also be achieved by administration of an antiadrenergic tranquilizer. If anesthesia is also required, the sacral nerves must be blocked by "low epidural" infiltration. Elastic fibers in the corpus cavernosum passively assist the retractor muscles to re-create the flexure when the penis is later returned to the sheath. Anomalies of the retractor muscles are recorded; some appear to prevent protrusion of the erect organ, while others impair the ability to return the penis.

The lymphatics from the preputial region pass to superficial inguinal nodes about the scrotal neck; drainage is then to nodes placed at the bifurcation of the aorta.

## POSTNATAL DEVELOPMENT OF THE REPRODUCTIVE ORGANS

The bovine testes descend through the inguinal canal early in the fetal period, and at birth they lie in the upper part of the scrotum. Although large in the midterm fetus, the scrotum is a rather insignificant pouch in the newborn when the components of its wall are still poorly differentiated. The dartos muscle later increases in amount and becomes arranged in coarser bundles; it becomes sensitive to temperature changes about the seventh or eighth postnatal month.

The neonatal testes are very small—they increase their weight 50-fold before maturity—and lack the full, ellipsoid form of the adult organs. From the first week, they increase more rapidly than the body as a whole, and their development is further accelerated between the fourth and eighth months when the young bull approaches puberty. Although growth then for a time keeps pace with general somatic development, the testes later show a relative decrease in size; in older bulls an actual shrinkage occurs. The enlargement of the testes is accompanied by the differentiation and maturation of their histological structure; normal spermatogenesis is usually achieved by the 10th or 11th month, although a fully developed spermatogenic epithelium is sometimes already found at 8 months. Libido may develop before spermatogenesis is complete, and in these circumstances the ejaculate contains no sperm. Sperm production is said to be at its maximum by about the sixth or seventh year.

Growth of the epididymides is less striking, and these parts appear to lag a little behind the testes. The main functional divisions are established by the time spermatogenesis is achieved.

Progress in the development and differentiation of the accessory sex glands is testosterone-dependent and therefore follows on the maturation of the testes. The bulbourethral and ampullary glands appear to mature at a more even pace than the others. The bulbourethral glands are small and pear-shaped in the newborn; as their subsequent increase affects their length and breadth more than their depth, they appear to flatten against the urethra as they enlarge. The ampullary glands increase steadily but retain their initial shape.

More striking changes occur in the vesicular glands. In the newborn they are simple sprouts from the caudal ends of the deferent ducts, and it is only after they have grown considerably that the characteristic flexures appear. The first flexure becomes evident within a few weeks, but the second is not formed until the sixth month. Lobulation commences at the blind extremity and gradually spreads toward the duct; it is accompanied by a darkening of hue, softening of consistency, and enlargement of the lumen. Secretion commences as the second flexure is established.

The external part (body) of the prostate is initially confined within the aponeurotic shield but later bursts through this, just caudal to the bladder neck. Both external and disseminate parts of the prostate continue to grow during the first year and even, although more slowly, for some time thereafter.

The neonatal penis is very slender and less—often considerably less—than half the length of the adult penis. It is without a sigmoid flexure and contains only a small amount of erectile tissue. Its apex has not yet separated from its sheath, and the preputial cavity, which is shallow since it does not extend beside the penis, is occupied by irregular mucosal folds. Increase in length throws the penis into the characteristic curves that begin to form about the third month. Growth of the penis is relatively slow and, while it quickens at puberty, the final size is not attained until well into the second year, some time after the other reproductive organs have completed their development. Separation of the penis from the sheath begins about the fourth week according to some authors—others describe a much longer delay. It is first confined to the left aspect of the glans but later spreads around the whole circumference and extends proximally along the sides of the organ. A narrow frenulum persists for some time and, although separation is usually complete at about eight months, in many young bulls tags of this connection remain to join the penis to the internal lamina of the prepuce. These may be retained until first service when their rupture is accompanied by bleeding. The raphe along the apex of the adult organ provides evidence of the former connection. A complete frenulum occasionally persists to cause a ventral deflection of the apex of the erect penis.

Castration frustrates normal development or, if performed later, may lead to regression to a more infantile state. The accessory reproductive glands are especially sensitive to the endocrine status. The penis fails to develop normally in the castrate; it remains short and since its apex fails to become free, the animal must urinate deep within the sheath.

The reactions of the male organs to the artificial administration of estrogens have attracted attention since it became the custom in certain countries to administer preparations of these hormones to calves in order to promote growth. The practice, although rewarding to the farmer, is unsound since hormone residues in the carcass may constitute a danger to human health. The abnormalities of the testes and accessory reproductive organs produced by these hormones may be detected on histological examination. The prostate is most commonly employed to provide evidence of the practice, which has been made unlawful in many countries.

## ERECTION AND EJACULATION

It was said that the penis of the bull is of the fibroelastic type. This implies that erection involves only slight increase in diameter and length and that protrusion results from a stiffening of the organ with effacement of preexisting flexures as the internal pressure rises (Fig. 30–10/*B*). Since the cavernous spaces are relatively small, little additional engorgement is required and erection may be rapidly achieved.

In the first phase of erection relaxation of the supplying arteries occurs. This raises the pressure within the corpus spongiosum and corpus cavernosum from the resting level (5 to 16 mm Hg) to the arterial pressure (75 to 80 mm Hg); the pressures within these bodies then fluctuate with the heartbeat. The apex of the penis protrudes at this stage, although the muscles of the penis—the ischiocavernosi and bulbospongiosus—are not yet active. Contractions of the ischiocavernosi now raise the pressure further and at the same time occlude both the arteries and the veins by compressing them against the ischial arch. These contractions impel blood forward through thick-walled dorsal and ventrolateral veins of the corpus cavernosum to discharge within the sigmoid flexure (Fig. 30–9/*C*). The increase in pressure effaces the bends and straightens the penis, causing it to protrude about 25 to 40 cm from the prepuce. After intromission, contact with the vaginal wall stimulates receptors in the integument of the free part, reflexly stimulating completion of erection. During a short period pressure in the corpus cavernosum can rise remarkably, even to 60 to 100 times the arterial pressure.

Ejaculation now follows. The semen is transported through the urethra by contractions of the urethralis and bulbospongiosus muscles. These

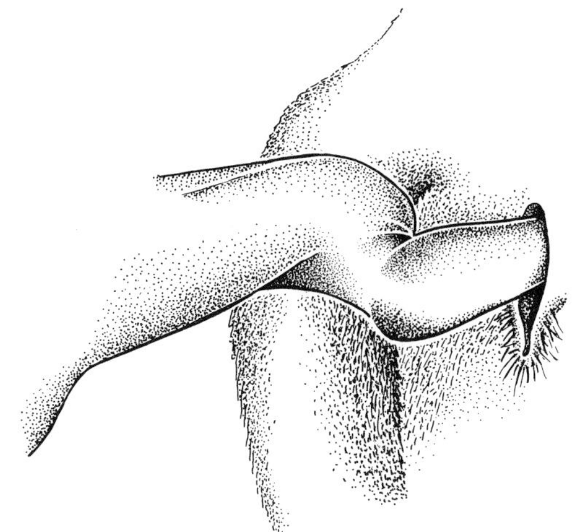

**Figure 30–11.** Spiraling of the free part of the bovine penis in full erection.

compress the spaces of the corpus spongiosum and, since these spaces and the spongy tissue in the glans constitute an open system, pressure waves run forward to assist the movement of the semen.

In the later stages of erection the free part of the penis spirals, following a left-hand thread around the raphe (Fig. 30–11). Spiraling is induced by the particular distribution of inextensible collagen fibers in the tunica albuginea where a local condensation constitutes the so-called apical ligament. Since precocious or exaggerated spiraling may make intromission impossible, occasional indications for the surgical division of the ligament occur. The extreme pressures developed in the later stages of erection sometimes result in bursting of the penis capsule; the most common site of rupture is on the dorsal surface, at the distal bend of the sigmoid flexure.

## Selected Bibliography


Ashdown, R.R., and S. Done: Color Atlas of Veterinary Anatomy: The Ruminants. Baltimore, University Park Press: and London, Gower Medical Publishing Ltd., 1984.

Ashdown, R.R., and Z. Majeed: The shape of the free end of the bovine penis during erection and protrusion. Vet. Rec. 99:354–356, 1976.

Ashdown, R.R., and H. Pearson: Anatomical and experimental studies on the eversion of the sheath and protrusion of the penis in the bull. Res. Vet. Sci. 15:13–24, 1973.

Ashdown, R.R., and J.A. Smith: The anatomy of the corpus cavernosum penis of the bull and its relationship to spiral deviation of the penis. J. Anat. 104:153–159, 1969.

Ashdown, R.R., J.S.E. David, and C. Gibbs: Impotence in the bull. 1. Abnormal venous drainage of the corpus cavernosum penis. Vet. Rec. 104:423–428, 1979.

Ashdown, R.R., H. Gilanpour, J.S.E. David, and C. Gibbs: Impotence in the bull. 2. Occlusion of the longitudinal canals of the corpus cavernosum penis. Vet. Rec. 104:598–603, 1979.

Aubry, J.N., and R.M. Butterfield: The structure and function of the prepuce in the bull. J. Anat. 106:192, 1970.

Beckett, S.D., R.S. Hudson, D.F. Walker, and R.C. Purohit: Effect of local anesthesia of the penis and dorsal penile neurectomy on the mating ability of bulls. JAVMA 173:838–839, 1978.

Beckett, S.D., T.M. Reynolds, and J.E. Bartels: Angiography of the crus penis in the ram and buck during erection. Am. J. Vet. Res. 39:1950–1954, 1978.

Beckett, S.D., T.M. Reynolds, D.F. Walker, R.S. Hudson, and R.C. Purohit: Experimentally induced rupture of corpus cavernosum penis of the bull. Am. J. Vet. Res. 35:765–767, 1974.

Beckett, S.D., D.F. Walker, R.S. Hudson, T.M. Reynolds, and R.I. Vachon: Corpus cavernosum penis pressure and penile muscle activity in the bull during coitus. Am. J. Vet. Res. 35:761–764, 1974.

Betteridge, K.J.: The normal genital organs. *In* Laing, J.A. (ed.): Fertility and Infertility in the Domestic Mammals, 3rd ed. London, Baillière, Tindall and Cassel, 1979.

Blockey, M.A. de B., and E.G. Taylor: Observations on spiral deviation of the penis in beef bulls. Aust. Vet. J. 61:141–145, 1984.

Blom, E., and N.O. Christensen: Studies on pathological conditions in the testis, epididymis and accessory sex glands in the bull. I. Normal anatomy technique of the clinical examination and a survey of the findings in 2000 Danish slaughter bulls. Skand. Vet. Tidekr. 37:1–47, 1947.

Bovee, K.C.: Physical examination of the urinary system. Vet. Clin. North Am. 1:119–128, 1971.

Caulkett, N.G., D.G. MacDonald, E.D. Janzen, et al.: Xylazine hydrochloride epidural analgesia: A method of providing sedation and analgesia to facilitate castration of mature bulls. The Compendium 8:1155–1159, 1993.

Claxton, M.S.: Methods of surgical preparation of teaser bulls. Compend. Cont. Edu. 11:974–990, 1989.

deLahunta, A., and R.E. Habel: Applied Veterinary Anatomy. Philadelphia, W.B. Saunders Company, 1986.

Garrett, P.D.: Urethral recess in male goats, sheep, cattle, and swine. JAVMA 191:689–691, 1987.

Gilbert, R.O., and S.S. van den Berg: Communication between the corpus cavernosum penis and the corpus spongiosum penis in a bull diagnosed by modified contrast cavernosography: A case report. Theriogenology 33:557–581, 1990.

Glossop, C.E., and R.R. Ashdown: Cavernosography and differential diagnosis of impotence in the bull. Vet. Rec. 118:357–360, 1986.

Hullinger, R.L., and C.J.G. Wensing: Descent of the testis in the fetal calf: A summary of the anatomy and the process. Acta. Anat. 121:63–68, 1985.

Kirk, E.J., R.L. Kitchell, and D.H. Carr: Neurophysiological maps of cutaneous innervation of the external genitalia of the ram. Am. J. Vet. Res. 48:1162–1166, 1987.

Larson, L.L.: Examination of the reproductive system of the bull. *In* Morrow, D.A. (ed.): Current Therapy in Theriogenology. Philadelphia, W.B. Saunders Company, 1986, pp. 101–116.

Larson, L.L.: The pudendal nerve block for anesthesia of the penis and relaxation of the retractor penis muscle. JAVMA 123:18–27, 1953.

Lewis, J.E., D.F. Walker, S.D. Beckett, and R.I. Vachon: Blood pressure within the corpus cavernosum penis of the bull. J. Reprod. Fertil. 17:155–156, 1968.

Mather, E.C.: Puberty in the bull. *In* Morrow, D.A. (ed.): Current Therapy in Theriogenology, 2nd ed. Philadelphia, W.B. Saunders Company, 1986.

Memom, M.A., L.J. Dawson, E.A. Usenik, et al.: Preputial

injuries in beef bulls: 172 cases (1980–1985). JAVMA 193:481–485, 1988.

Musser, J.M.B., G. St. Jean, J.G. Vestweber, and T.G. Pejsa: Penile hematoma in bulls: 60 cases (1979–1990). JAVMA 201:1416–1418, 1992.

Pavaux, C.: A Color Atlas of Bovine Visceral Anatomy. London, Wolfe Publishing, 1983.

Popesko, P.: Atlas of Topographic Anatomy of the Domestic Animals; Vol. III: Pelvis and Limbs. Philadelphia, W.B. Saunders Company, 1971.

Rumph, P.F., and P.D. Garret: The apical ligament of the penis of the goat and sheep. Anat. Histol. Embryol. 21:40–47, 1992.

Seidel, G.E., and R.H. Foote: Motion picture analysis of ejaculation in the bull. J. Reprod. Fertil. 20:313–317, 1969.

Setchell, B.P.: The Mammalian Testis. London, Elek. Books, 1978.

Singh, K.B.: Pelvic urethrotomies in bulls. Vet. Rec. 105:137–141, 1979.

Van Metre, D.C., J.K. House, B.P. Smith, et al.: Obstructive urolithiasis in ruminants: Medical treatment and urethral surgery. Comp. Contin. Educ. Pract. Vet. 18:317–328, 1996.

Watson, J.W.: Mechanism of erection and ejaculation in the bull and ram. Nature 204:95–96, 1964.

Wensing, C.J.G.: Testicular descent in some domestic mammals. I. Anatomical aspects of testicular descent. Proc. K. Ned. Akad. C. 71:423–434, 1968.

Wrobel, K.H., and N. Abu-Ghali: Autonomic innervation of the bovine testis. Acta. Anat. 160:1–14, 1997.

CHAPTER 31

# The Udder of the Ruminants

## EXTERNAL FEATURES

The four mammary glands of the cow are consolidated in a single mass, the udder. The bulk of this is placed below the caudal part of the abdomen, but part extends below the pelvic floor and thus lies between the thighs (Plate 30/*A*). The appearance of the udder varies greatly, depending on maturity and functional status as well as on individual and breed characteristics. In many dairy cows it is extremely large, sometimes weighing as much as 60 kg. However, size is not a reliable pointer to productivity as, apart from other considerations, wide differences exist in the proportions of gland parenchyma and of fat and other connective tissues. Also, little dependable evidence exists to support popular beliefs relating milk production to peculiarities of conformation. Certain features of conformation—in particular the size, shape, and position of the teats—do have a practical importance in determining the suitability of the udder to hand or machine milking (Fig. 31–1).

The udder is divided into quarters that correspond to the four glands. Each bears one of the principal teats. Accessory teats, sometimes associated with functional glandular tissue, are very common, particularly on the hindquarters (Fig. 31–2). They are undesirable and if, as sometimes happens, they are very close to or even fused with the principal teats, they can complicate milking. A prominent median intermammary groove generally marks the division of the udder into right and left halves; the boundary between the fore- and hindquarters of the one side is rarely distinct, as the parenchyma of one gland butts against the parenchyma of the other gland without evidence of internal septation (Plate 30/*C*). The dorsal surface of most of the udder is shaped to fit against the belly wall, but the part below the pelvis is less regular and narrower since it is laterally compressed between the thighs (Fig. 31–4). A certain amount of fat is interposed between the base and the structures lying above.

The skin covering the udder is thin, supple, and freely movable over the underlying fascia, except on the teats where it is bound to the deeper layers of the wall. It tends to fall into folds over the caudal part of the udder that ascends toward the perineum. It is sparsely covered by hair that is silkier than that found on neighboring parts; the teats, however, are naked.

## THE SUSPENSORY APPARATUS

The udder is suspended by strong fascial sheets that surround and enclose the gland substance and extend inward to fuse with the connective tissue framework that permeates the entire organ. Although careful examination shows that the fasciae that cover the inner and outer aspects of each udder half form a continuous investment, it is usual to describe medial and lateral laminae as though these were independent. The medial lamina is the more important (Figs. 31–3/9 and 31–4/5). It is largely composed of elastic tissue and, although its chief origin is from the tunica flava bordering the linea alba, it also reaches onto the beginning of the symphysial tendon that divides, and gives origin to, the medial muscles of the thighs. Since the udder continues below the pelvis it follows that many fibers of this lamina must radiate from the caudal end of the attachment. The right and left medial laminae are separated by a small amount of loose connective tissue, an arrangement that made possible the clean amputation of one half of the udder, an operation that is now more or less obsolete.

The lateral lamina is of dense connective tissue. Its cranial part arises from the lateral crus of the external inguinal ring; behind this, the origin inclines medially and a large part springs from the symphysial tendon (Figs. 31–3 and 31–4). The lateral lamina is found to split if followed ventrally; the outer sheet is prolonged as the medial femoral fascia, while the inner one continues over the surface of the mammary glands. The lamina protects the mammary vessels that pass through the inguinal canal and also covers the mammary (superficial inguinal) lymph nodes situated above the caudal part of the udder.

Both medial and lateral laminae are thick dorsally and become progressively thinner when traced ventrally; they are quite insubstantial when

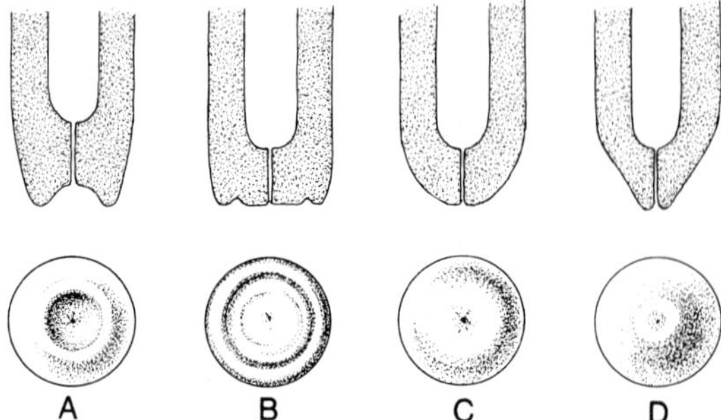


**Figure 31–1.** Variations in the form of the bovine teat extremity. *A*, Funnel-shaped. *B*, Dish-shaped. *C*, Rounded. *D*, Pointed.

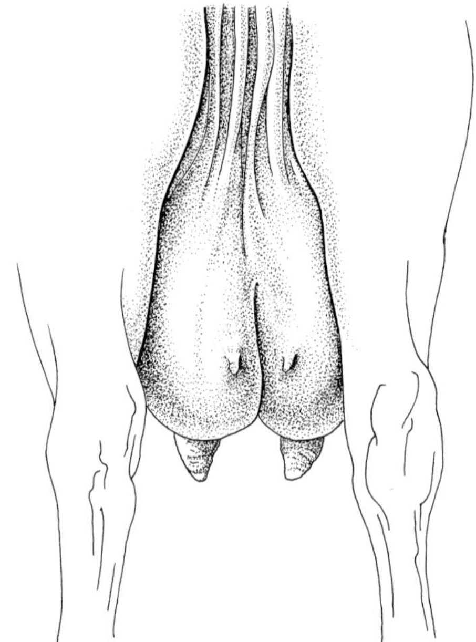

**Figure 31–2.** Supernumerary teats on the caudal surface of the bovine udder.

they reach the ventral aspect of the udder where they merge. Their attenuation is explained by the detachment of numerous lamellae that penetrate obliquely into the quarters to interleave with correspondingly oriented layers of gland tissue. The medial and lateral laminae also merge over the cranial and caudal borders of the udder halves. The difference in the structure of the laminae accounts for the sagging of the medial part of the heavily laden udder, an effect that is made more obvious by the teats diverging to the sides (Fig. 31–3).

A minor contribution to the support is made by a few ribbons of elastic tissue that arise from the tunica flava and dive into the adjacent part of the udder base.

Demands, some would say unreasonable demands, for ever-greater milk production place an increasing and sometimes unsustainable burden on the suspensory apparatus of the udder. Occurrences of rupture—a disastrous happening—are now commonly reported in some countries.

## THE STRUCTURE OF THE GLANDS AND TEATS

The substance of the udder consists of gland parenchyma and connective tissue intermingled in proportions that can sometimes be estimated by palpation through the skin. The udder in which the parenchyma predominates has a softer consistency when empty and a more turgid "feel" when distended with milk than the "fleshy" udder that is rich in connective tissue and is firm at all times. Each gland is constructed about a branching duct

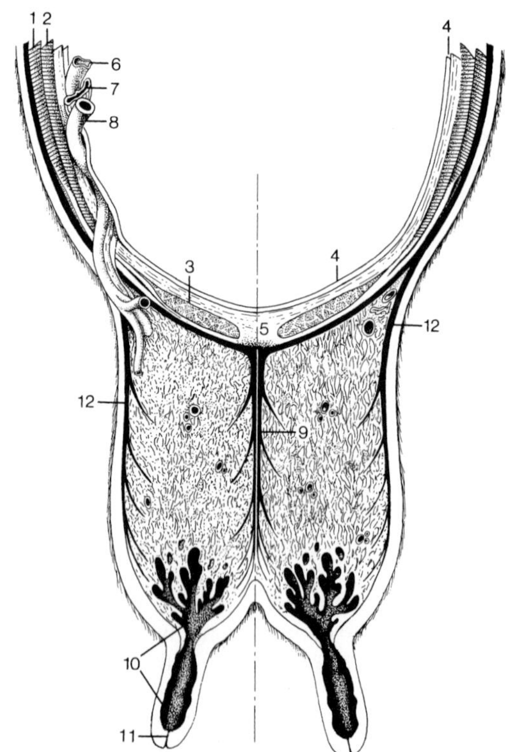


**Figure 31–3.** Transverse section of the abdominal floor and cranial quarters of the bovine udder.

1, External abdominal oblique; 2, internal abdominal oblique; 3, rectus abdominis; 4, peritoneum; 5, linea alba; 6, lymph vessel; 7, external pudendal vein; 8, external pudendal (mammary) artery; 9, medial lamina of suspensory apparatus; 10, lactiferous sinus; 11, papillary duct; 12, lateral laminae of suspensory apparatus.

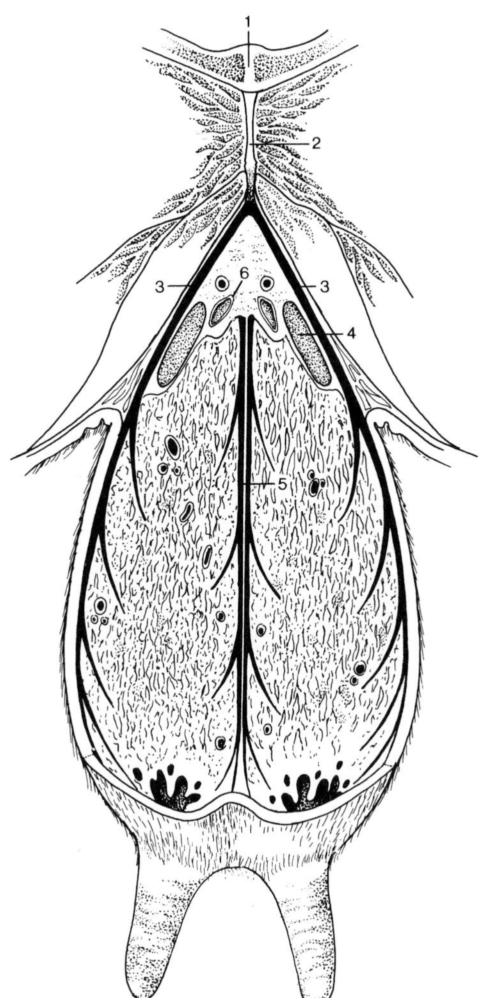


**Figure 31–4.** Transverse section of the pelvic floor and caudal quarters of the bovine udder.

1, Pelvic symphysis; 2, symphysial tendon; 3, lateral suspensory laminae; 4, mammary (superficial inguinal) lymph node; 5, medial suspensory laminae; 6, tributary of external pudendal vein.

system, and its peripheral sections are divided from each other by connective tissue lamellae that continue from the coverings. The secretory units within these sections take the form of microscopic alveoli that lead to small excretory ducts (Fig. 31–10 and Plate 30/*F,G*). Neighboring ducts combine, and after several successive unions about a dozen wide lactiferous ducts are produced that converge on a large lactiferous sinus situated in the lower part of the quarter and extending into the teat (see Fig. 10–31/4). Most ducts of the forequarter approach the corresponding sinus from the lateral side, while those of the hindquarter lie mainly toward the caudal aspect. The lactiferous ducts (/3) are unusual in being very irregular since dilatations and narrower sections alternate. Some of the more superficial wider parts, which may be 3 cm or more in caliber, are palpable when occupied by milk and are then known as "milk knots." The convergence of the ducts on the sinus gives the lower part of the sectioned quarter a spongy appearance (Fig. 31–5). The duct systems of the four quarters are independent, having no connection with each other (Plate 30/*C*). Despite this, infection may spread directly between the tissues of the quarters of the same side.

The lactiferous sinus has a capacity of several hundred milliliters (Fig. 31–5/1,2). It is very imperfectly divided by a mucosal fold into a part within the gland substance (gland sinus) and a part within the teat (teat sinus). The fold varies greatly in prominence, partly because of the varying engorgement of a submucosal ring of veins (/4). It may be sufficiently pronounced to impede the flow of milk from the gland sinus to the teat sinus, and its position is sometimes recognizable on palpation of the milk-laden udder (Plate 30/*D,E*).

The position, orientation, size, and form of the teats are all very variable, but usually these

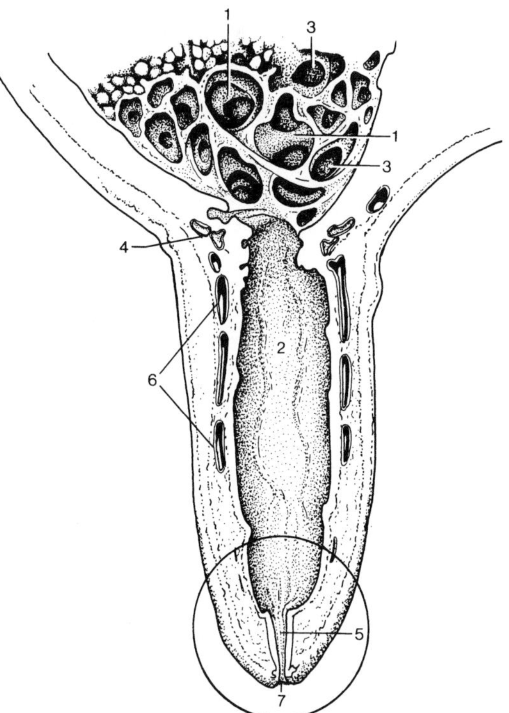


**Figure 31–5.** Section of a cow's teat and lactiferous sinus. The circled area is shown in Figure 31–6.

1, 2, Lactiferous sinus; 1, gland sinus; 2, teat sinus; 3, openings of lactiferous ducts; 4, submucosal venous ring; 5, papillary duct; 6, venous plexus in teat wall; 7, teat orifice.

structures are more or less cylindrical and about 8 cm long. The teat wall is generally about 6 mm thick but increases toward 1 cm at the lower end where it is traversed by the papillary duct (teat canal), misnamed the streak canal in much clinical literature; this narrow passage leads to the exterior (Fig. 31–6). Variations in the form of the teat apex are common (Fig. 31–1).

The teat wall consists of three strata, although a subdivision of the middle layer is sometimes made. The outer layer is provided by the dry, naked skin that lacks the usual glands; it is extremely sensitive. The middle layer consists of connective tissue mingled with a certain amount of smooth muscle. It contains many veins that constitute a form of erectile tissue, which becomes congested when the teat is manipulated. The plexus is spread through much of the wall, but many of the larger vessels lie directly below the mucosa and are evident when the teat is opened (Fig. 31–5/6). The mucosa constitutes the third layer. In the upper part of the teat it often forms permanent folds that run in all directions, producing a pitted surface. Folds are rarely prominent in the lower part; when present they run more or less vertically and tend to be effaced when the teat sinus is distended. The mucosa is yellowish except in the papillary duct. The white lining of this passage is marked by many fine longitudinal ridges, which, when followed proximately radiate from the internal opening. They form the so-called rosette of Fürstenberg, a structure that is rarely so conspicuous as most accounts suggest. If excessively developed, the rosette may form a plug that blocks the opening, interfering with ease of milking. Desquamation of the epithelium of the duct produces a fatty material that helps occlude the passage; it has a bactericidal effect and assists in preventing infection from spreading into the interior. The duct is normally held closed by a sphincter formed by a localized thickening of the smooth muscle of the teat wall; the action of the muscle is reinforced by a condensation of elastic tissue around the teat orifice (Fig. 31–6).

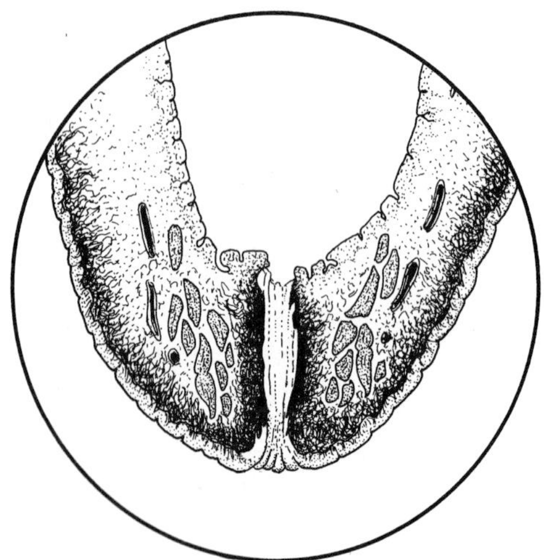

**Figure 31–6.** Section of the teat extremity showing the smooth muscle encircling the papillary duct.

## VASCULARIZATION AND INNERVATION

Since it is estimated that some 500 L of blood must flow through the udder for every liter of milk secreted, it is clear that the vascular arrangements must be generously conceived. The main artery to the udder continues the external pudendal artery beyond the detachment of branches to the abdominal wall and thigh. It is complemented by a small mammary branch of the ventral perineal artery. The main artery, which may exceed 1.5 cm in diameter, enters the udder after passing through the inguinal canal where it is accompanied by a satellite vein, lymphatics, and nerves (Fig. 31–3/6,7,8). The artery first forms a sigmoid flexure—a safeguard against stretching when the udder is laden—before dividing into a large cranial mammary artery that is directed ventrocranially and a much smaller caudal mammary artery that runs toward the caudal part of the udder. Both are partially or wholly embedded in the udder substance to which they supply many branches. Certain of the largest of these approach the lactiferous sinuses from all sides; they give rise to twigs that unite around the bases of the teats to form plexuses from which the teat walls are supplied.

The distribution of the mammary branch of the ventral perineal artery is normally restricted to a small part of the hindquarter and the mammary lymph nodes, but anastomoses with the larger caudal mammary artery provide potential collateral pathways.

The mammary arteries from the left and right halves of the udder are interconnected caudal to the medial laminae.

The pattern of the veins is more complicated. A venous ring is formed above the base of the udder by transverse connections between paired veins (Fig. 31–8/*B*). Drainage is effected by the external pudendal veins, which lead through the inguinal canals, and the subcutaneous abdominal ("milk") veins, which pursue flexuous subcutaneous courses over the ventral abdominal wall (Fig. 31–7/5,1 and Plate 30/*A*). Blood enters the caudal part of the

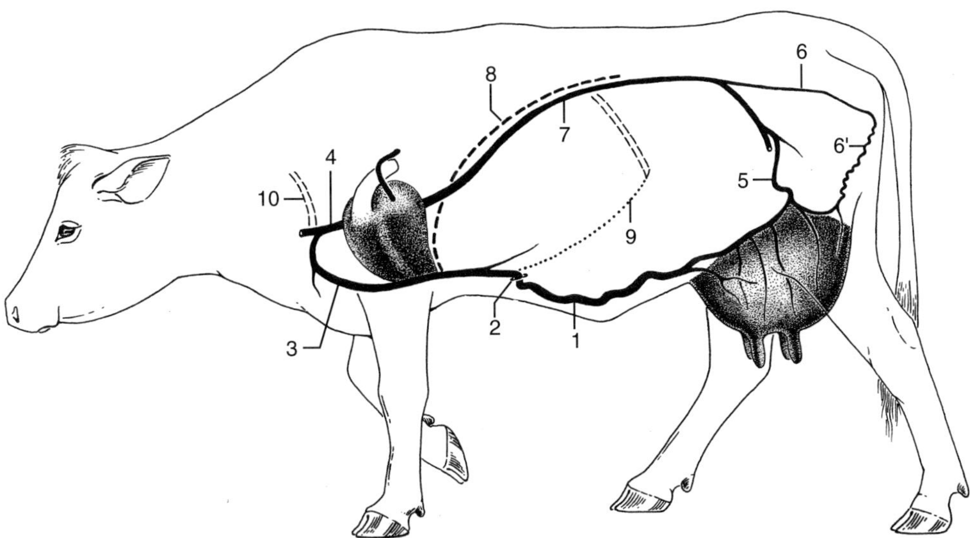


**Figure 31–7.** The venous drainage of the udder.

1, Subcutaneous abdominal (milk) v.; 2, milk "well"; 3, internal thoracic v.; 4, cranial vena cava; 5, external pudendal v.; 6, internal pudendal v.; 6′, ventral labial v. (connecting ventral perineal v. with caudal mammary veins); 7, caudal vena cava; 8, diaphragm; 9, costal arch; 10, first rib.

ring through one or two ventral labial veins (the arrangement is irregular), which descend over the perineum (/6′), and elsewhere through many tributaries from the udder itself. The latter may be divided into a deep set that penetrates the udder base, and superficial veins that pierce the covering fascia to run over the outer surface of the gland. Some are evident through the skin and can be distinguished from the subcutaneous lymphatic trunks by their dorsocranial direction. They are connected with the venous plexuses draining the teats and with the rings encircling the junctions of the teat and gland sinuses.

The main importance of this arrangement lies in the choice of routes available to blood leaving the udder, a necessary provision if the flow is not to be impeded in the recumbent animal. Examination of the valves shows that the caudal part of the ring, and the ventral labial veins that feed it, can pass blood only toward the external pudendal vein of the same or of the opposite side. The valves are less regular in the veins over the remainder of the udder base and are often few and clearly incompetent. In general, those situated close to the external pudendal vein direct blood toward this vessel; free movement in either direction is possible in the more cranial part of the ring, although this normally drains to the subcutaneous abdominal vein (Fig. 31–7). The angles formed by the tributary vessels at their entrances support this interpretation.

The subcutaneous abdominal vein has a strikingly tortuous course, a varicosed structure, and incompetent valves. It is formed during the later stages of the first pregnancy by the opening of a passage between the caudal and cranial superficial epigastric veins (Fig. 31–8). In the calf these form two very tenuously connected systems concerned with the drainage of the abdominal wall. The caudal superficial epigastric vein drains into the external pudendal vein as the orientation of the valves suggests and the directions taken by the entering radicles confirm. The cranial superficial epigastric vein is a minor vessel that penetrates the abdominal wall to join the cranial epigastric or, if the passage is made more cranially, the internal thoracic vein. Later, with the growth of the mammary glands in pregnancy and the vastly increased flow of blood through them, the mammary veins become congested, their tributaries engorged, and their valves progressively broken down until a connection is established with the cranial vessels over the former "watershed."

The adult subcutaneous abdominal vein sometimes possesses additional or alternative connections with the deeper veins at several levels. Occasionally it runs forward to join the superficial thoracic vein and can then be traced into the axilla. The opening through the body wall (the "milk well"), which it normally follows, is readily identified on palpation. Although the vein is sometimes employed for intravenous injection or

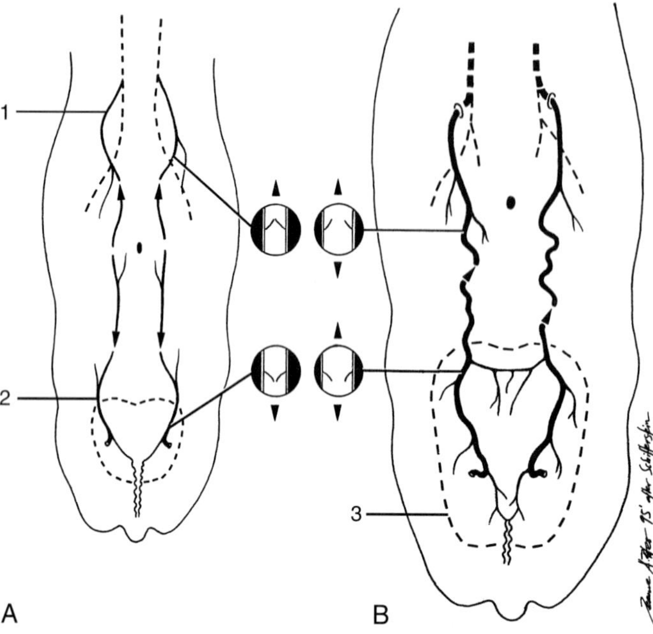


**Figure 31–8.** Development of the subcutaneous abdominal veins (schematic dorsal view). *A,* The region drained by the cranial superficial epigastric vein (1) is separated from that of the caudal superficial epigastric vein (2) in the calf and heifer. The valves in the cranial superficial epigastric vein direct blood cranially, while those in the caudal superficial epigastric vein direct blood caudally. *B,* The subcutaneous abdominal vein is formed during pregnancy. The increased blood flow through the enlarging udder (3) causes the veins to distend, the valves to become inefficient, and the two drainage regions to unite, allowing blood to flow in both directions.

blood sampling, it is not a wise choice since its structure predisposes to potentially troublesome leakage.

It is difficult to assess the significance of the perineomammary connection. In the young animal the orientation of the valves in the ventral section is such that the flow must be toward the udder, but sometimes it seems that the dorsal part drains toward the perineum and thus to the internal pudendal veins. In animals that have lactated the ventral labial vein is varicosed and open to the flow of blood in either direction.

A very rich, valveless lymphatic plexus extends through the teat wall and the connective tissue supporting the parenchyma. Most of the trunks that emanate from this plexus are superficial and, being unusually large, they may be apparent through the skin. They are distinguished from the subcutaneous veins by their dorsocaudal courses, which lead them to the mammary lymph nodes placed above and to the side of the caudal part of the udder but deep to the lateral suspensory sheet. The largest of the nodes may be detected in the living animal by deep palpation from behind, between the udder and the thigh (Figs. 31–4/4 and 31–9/1 and Plate 30/*B*).

The development and number of the nodes show considerable variation. In the most common arrangement only two nodes are present on each side: one is large (≈8 cm), kidney shaped, and superficial; the other is smaller, ovoid, and too deeply placed to be palpable. The superficial vessels are mainly directed to the lateral node, while most of the deeper lymphatics pass to the smaller medial one. But it is unlikely that the distribution is always so precise, and some lymph appears to pass through two or more nodes in

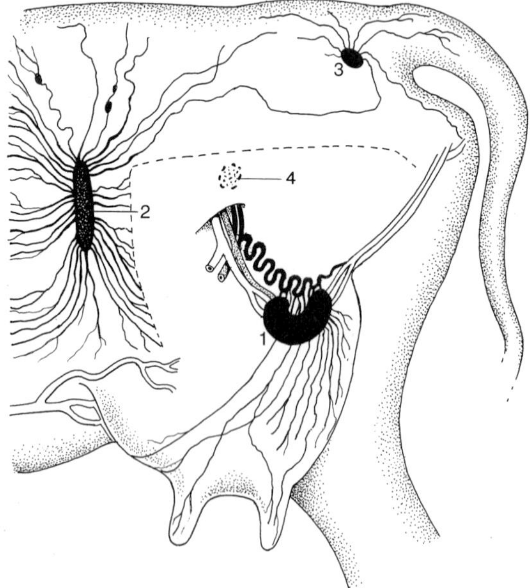


**Figure 31–9.** Lymph drainage of the udder. The *broken line* indicates where the left limb was removed to expose the udder.

1, Mammary (superficial inguinal) lymph node; 2, subiliac lymph node; 3, ischial lymph node; 4, position of deep inguinal (iliofemoral) node.

succession. The medial nodes usually collect from both halves of the udder. The efferent vessels—which may exceed 1 cm in diameter—pass cranially to enter the abdomen through the inguinal canal. They pass to the deep inguinal (iliofemoral) node, placed in the angle between the deep circumflex and external iliac arteries (see Figs. 28–30/7 and 31–9/4). When enlarged, this node is palpable per rectum. The lymph then passes through one or more of the medial iliac nodes lying about the aortic bifurcation before entering the lumbar trunk that runs forward to the cisterna chyli. The mammary contribution accounts for a substantial part of the total flow in this vessel.

The mammary nodes also collect from the perineal region and superficial structures of the adjacent part of the thigh. It is probable that a fraction of the lymph emanating from the udder by-passes these nodes and goes directly to the deep inguinal node. It has been claimed that some mammary lymph occasionally passes to the subiliac node within the flank fold. Small intramammary nodes are described but are not easily found.

The udder receives a multiple innervation from lumbar and sacral spinal nerves. The gland substance and the deeper parts of the teat wall are served by the genitofemoral nerve alone, but the skin covering the udder is supplied from three directions. The ventral branches of the first and second lumbar nerves pass caudoventrally over the abdominal wall to supply the skin over the cranial parts of the forequarters; the genitofemoral nerve passes through the inguinal canal and sends superficial branches to the skin over the middle section of the udder. The mammary branches of the pudendal nerve descend through the perineum to supply the skin over the caudal aspect of the hindquarters. This diffuse arrangement complicates local anesthesia techniques for major surgery of the udder; anesthesia for teat surgery is fortunately much simpler since the nerves run more or less vertically within the teat wall.

The genitofemoral nerve contains sympathetic efferent and afferent fibers. The former supply the smooth muscle of the teats and blood vessels and the myoepithelial cells of the gland substance. Stimulation of afferent fibers in the teat wall plays a role in the neurohumoral reflex of milk "let-down," initiating the release of oxytocin. Despite earlier assertions, it is not now believed that the udder receives a parasympathetic nerve supply.

## AGE AND FUNCTIONAL CHANGES

Development of the mammary glands commences in the young embryo and by birth has proceeded to the stage in which short but well-formed teats, small sinuses, and the first branchings of the duct systems are present (p. 363). The bulk of the udder—if this word may be used for so unimpressive a structure—consists of adipose tissue. During the first three postnatal months, increase of the udder barely keeps pace with general somatic growth and is entirely due to the accumulation of fat.

Thereafter, and thus commencing well before puberty, the rate of growth quickens. The duct system and glandular tissue develop more rapidly than the body as a whole during the remainder of the first year, although growth gradually slackens off and becomes isometric by the 12th month or thereabouts.

It is probable that the very rapid growth of the prepuberal period is due to the cyclical production of estrogens by the ovaries since spurts of activity occur directly before ovulation when estrogen levels are at their maxima. These waves of activity create a well-developed and much branched system of ducts by the time the heifer first becomes pregnant. Duct growth continues through the first half of pregnancy, while growth of the secretory units predominates in the second half. As the parenchyma increases, the fat diminishes and this process continues into the ensuing lactation.

Growth during the later part of pregnancy depends on prolactin and growth hormone of hypophysial origin as well as on estrogen and progesterone. The highest levels of the pituitary hormones are recorded for the last days before parturition.

The maintenance of secretion is dependent on corticotropin, thyroid-stimulating hormone, and somatotropin being present in normal amounts. Regular milking is also necessary if milk production is to be maintained. The act of milking stimulates the release of prolactin, corticotropin, and oxytocin; thus, within limits, more frequent milking increases the yield in consequence of the formation of more glandular tissue. Milk production can be enhanced artificially by administration of somatotropin.

The mammary gland is composed of tubuloalveolar secretory units grouped to form lobules defined by connective tissue septa (Plate 30/*G*). The secretory alveoli are lined by a simple epithelium that changes markedly in height during the cycle of activity. The cells demonstrate maximal activity in those alveoli prepared to release milk when stimulated by suckling (or milking). Following this the alveolar lumina are collapsed and irregular (Plate 30/*F*), and the epithelium is much reduced in height. All lobules within one gland do not necessarily exhibit the same stage

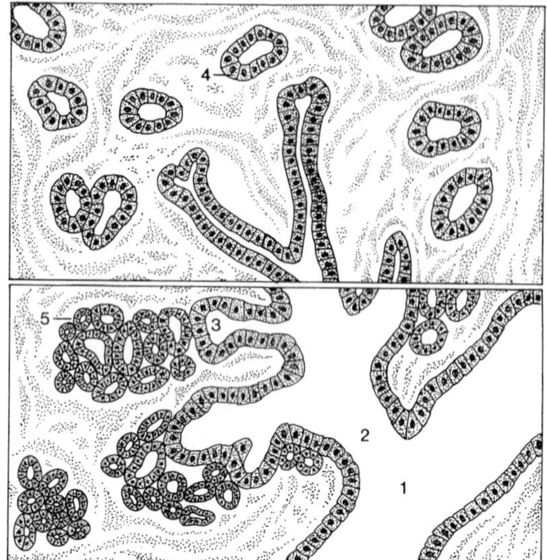


**Figure 31–10.** Two stages in the development of the mammary glandular tissue. The histology of the "dry" udder *(top)* and the lactating udder *(bottom)* is illustrated.

1, Lactiferous duct; 2, lesser lactiferous duct; 3, interlobular ducts; 4, inactive alveolus; 5, active alveolus.

of the secretory cycle and both active and nonactive lobules may be present concurrently. The milk is forced from the secretory units into the duct system by contraction of surrounding myoepithelial cells. The inter- and intralobular connective tissue provides important structural support and conveys blood, lymph vessels, and nerves.

In dairy cows the period of lactation is artificially prolonged by regular milking beginning a few days after calving. The majority of these cows are pregnant during most of the lactation period since they are bred again from about 60 days after calving. Milking is stopped about 2 months before the next calf is due and the cow is "dried up." The partial involution that then occurs is soon reversed, and the udder again enlarges shortly before the next calf is born (Fig. 31–10 and Plate 30/*F,G*). Thus, dairy cows that conceive following the first insemination lactate for about 10 months and are dry for about 2 months each year. A productive dairy cow produces some 7000 L of milk in the course of a lactation, a quantity far in excess of that required to raise a calf.

Permanent regressive changes are seen in senile cows, in which connective tissue increasingly replaces the gland parenchyma. A large proportion (25% in some surveys) of apparently normal cows exhibit induration of one or more quarters following inflammation of the gland tissue (mastitis).

## THE UDDER OF THE SMALL RUMINANTS

The udder of the small ruminants is situated in the inguinal region. It comprises only two glands that are more (goats) or less (sheep) distinctly demarcated externally. The gross appearance varies considerably. In milk goats the udder is relatively large in relation to body size and is deep and rather conical (Fig. 31–11); in ewes it is relatively smaller and more hemispherical, although sometimes inclining toward the caprine form in those breeds that are milked for cheese production. The teats also show considerable variation; they are cylindrical in the young, but in older animals, especially in goats of high productivity, they tend to become conical with wide bases that blend smoothly with the contours of the gland (Fig. 31–12). Accessory teats are not uncommon in goats.

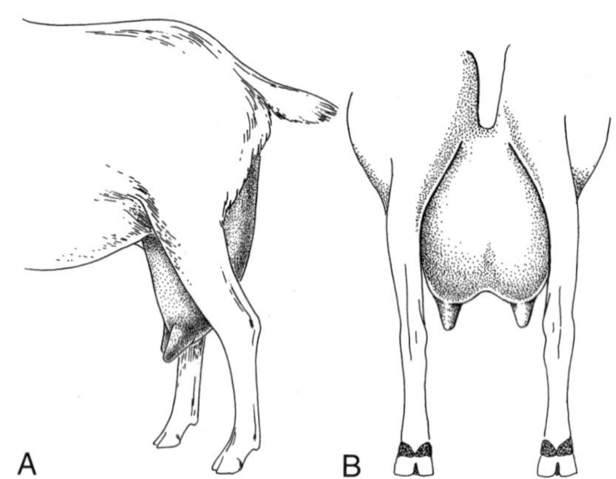


**Figure 31–11.** Lateral *(A)* and caudal *(B)* views of the goat's udder.

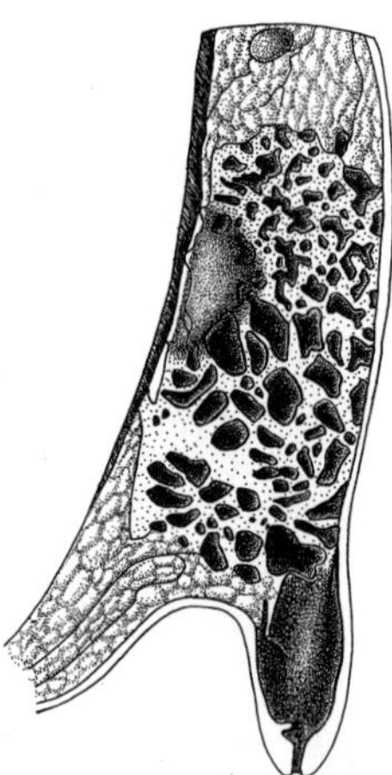

**Figure 31–12.** Sagittal section of a young goat's udder and teat. As in the cow, the superficial inguinal (mammary) lymph node lies, embedded in fat, above the glandular tissue.

In goats the skin over the udder is finely haired and pigmented according to the general pattern of the coat. In sheep the upper part may be covered by the fleece, but the part that is exposed is generally lightly pigmented and commonly dirtied by the secretion of the glands within the inguinal skin pouches interposed between the udder and the inner aspects of the thighs.

The structure, suspension, and vascular arrangements correspond with those of the bovine udder in most respects. However, the teats are not wholly naked in sheep or in goats, while closure of the teat orifice is achieved without the presence of a sphincter muscle in sheep. A milk vein develops in parous animals but is generally less conspicuous than in cows.

## Selected Bibliography


Adams, E.W., and C.B. Richard: The antistreptococcic activity of bovine teat canal keratin. Am. J. Vet. Res. 24:122–135, 1963.

Anderson, R.R.: Development and structure of the mammary gland. Endocrinological control. *In* Larson, B.L., and V.R. Smith (eds.): Lactation. Vol. I. The Mammary Gland/ Development and Maintenance. New York, Academic Press, 1974.

Ashdown, R.R., and S. Done: Color Atlas of Veterinary Anatomy: The Ruminants. Baltimore, University Park Press: and London, Gower Medical Publishing Ltd., 1984.

Baldwin, R.L.: Mammary growth and lactation. *In* Cupps, P.T. (ed.): Reproduction in Domestic Animals. 4th ed. New York, Academic Press, 1991.

Bristol, D.G.: Teat and udder surgery in dairy cattle—Part I. Compend. Contin. Educ. 11:868–873, 1989.

Bristol, D.G.: Teat and udder surgery in dairy cattle—Part II. Compend. Contin. Educ. 11:983–988, 1989.

Cartee, R.E., A.K. Ibrahim, and D. McLeary: B-mode ultrasonography of the bovine udder and teat. JAVMA 188:1284–1287, 1986.

Ducharme, N.G., M. Arighi, F.D. Horney, et al: Invasive teat surgery in dairy cattle. Can. Vet. J. 28:757–767, 1987.

González-Romano, N., A. Arencibia, A. Espinosa de los Monteros, et al.: Anatomical evaluation of the caprine mammary gland by computed tomography radiology and histology. Anat. Histol. Embryol. 29:25–30, 2000.

Heath, T.J., and R.L. Kerlin: Lymph drainage from the mammary gland in sheep. J. Anat. 144:61–70, 1986.

Hull, B.L.: Teat and udder surgery. Vet. Clin. North Am. 11:1–17, 1995.

Jalakas, M., P. Saks, and M. Klaassen: Suspensory apparatus of the bovine udder in the Estonian black and white Holstein breed: Increased milk production (udder mass) induced changes in the pelvic structure. Anat. Histol. Embryol. 29:51–61, 2000.

Kirk, J.H., F. deGraves, and J. Tyler: Recent progress in treatment and control of mastitis in cattle. JAVMA 204: 1152–1158, 1994.

Linzell, L.J.: Mammary blood flow and methods of identifying and measuring precursors of milk. *In* Larson, B.L., and V.R. Smith (eds.): Lactation. Vol. I. New York, Academic Press, 1974.

Makady, F.M., H.L. Whitmore, D.R. Nelson, and J. Simon: Effect of tissue adhesives and suture patterns on experimentally induced teat lacerations in lactating dairy cattle. JAVMA 198:1932–1934, 1991.

Miller, G.Y., P.C. Bartlett, S.E. Lance, et al: Costs of clinical mastitis and mastitis prevention in dairy herds. JAVMA 202:1230–1236, 1993.

Nickerson, S.C.: Resistance mechanisms of the bovine udder: New implications for mastitis control at the teat end. JAVMA 191:1484–1488, 1987.

Nickerson, S.C., and J.W. Pankey: Cytologic observations of the bovine teat end. Am. J. Vet. Res. 44:1433–1441, 1983.

Pavaux, C.: A Color Atlas of Bovine Visceral Anatomy. London, Wolfe Publishing, 1983.

Shinde, Y.: Role of milking in initiation and maintenance of lactation in the dairy animals. *In* Yokoyama, A., H. Mizuno, and H. Nagasawa (eds.): Physiology of the Mammary Gland. Tokyo, Japan Scientific Societies Press, 1978.

Sinha, Y.N., and H.A. Tucker: Mammary development and pituitary prolactin level of heifers from birth through puberty and during the estrous cycle. J. Dairy Sci. 52:507–512, 1969.

Turner, A.S., and C.W. McIlwraith: Repair of teat lacerations. *In* Techniques in Large Animal Surgery, 2nd ed. Philadelphia, Lea & Febiger, 1989.

Weber, A.F.: The bovine mammary gland. Structure and function. JAVMA 170:1133–1136, 1977.

# CHAPTER 32

# The Forelimb of the Ruminants

Cattle generally lead less energetic lives than horses and are consequently less exposed to injury of the more proximal segments of the limbs. Though cattle are prone to trauma and infection of the feet, the latter misfortunes being shared by sheep, it must be recognized that economic circumstances frequently argue against prolonged or costly clinical intervention. These circumstances suggest that bovine practitioners have less need of detailed knowledge of much of the anatomy of the limbs than their equine counterparts; therefore, rather cursory treatment is given to many topics in this and in the following chapter.

## THE SHOULDER AND ARM

The scapula, humerus, and associated muscles are enclosed within the skin of the trunk and generally fit closely against the thoracic wall, their caudal limit being indicated by a slight depression behind the triceps. Some cows (especially Jerseys) stand with their shoulders and elbows slightly abducted, which causes the humerus to angle away from the ribs. This defect in conformation, which appears to arise from an inherited weakness in certain girdle muscles, looks awkward but is of little consequence (Fig. 32–1). "Flying scapula," on the other hand, is a serious myopathy observed in cattle after they have been turned out to pasture in the spring. Muscle tissue actually deteriorates, allowing the dorsal borders of the scapulas to rise above the withers.

The position and slope of the scapula can be determined by palpation of its cranial and caudal angles and spine. The dorsal border of the bone is surmounted by a wide, semicircular plate of cartilage that lies opposite the spinous processes of the second to sixth thoracic vertebrae where it may be palpated in thin subjects. The ventral angle of the bone (and thus the shoulder joint) projects upon the middle of the first two ribs (see Fig. 26–1). The prominent spine, which ends in a sharp acromion, runs near the cranial border, dividing very unequal supra- and infraspinous fossae. The *humerus* is stout, especially its proximal end where the massive greater tubercle rises well above the head and extends onto the cranial surface, forming the point of the shoulder. The orientation of this bone is confirmed by the position of the more distal and readily palpable deltoid tuberosity. Movement at the capacious *shoulder joint* is largely confined to flexion and extension. The joint may be punctured at the cranial border of the infraspinatus tendon, just proximal to the salient greater tubercle.

Very few features of the shoulder and arm musculature can claim practical importance, and little benefit would accrue from descriptions that largely replicate the general accounts provided in Chapter 2. Only certain muscles are mentioned here, and only those features of the muscles that have a practical bearing. The *brachiocephalicus* forms the dorsal border of the jugular groove and is joined along its upper margin to the *omotransversarius* extending between the acromion and wing of the atlas. The latter muscle covers but does not prevent palpation of the large superficial cervical lymph node. The pectoral group is distinguished by the very rudimentary development of the *subclavius,* which explains the abrupt transition from the narrow neck to the greater width between the shoulder joints—a marked difference in the conformation of cattle and horses. The *rhomboideus* rarely attracts attention in cattle of European origin but makes the major contribution to the hump in zebu stock. The hump varies in size, position (cervicothoracic or thoracic), and structure in animals of different breeds and strains; in some it consists essentially of a thickening of the muscle, in others of a replacement of flesh by adipose tissue. The serratus ventralis, the principal supporter of the trunk, is adapted to this role by the inclusion of many tendinous strands and the stout aponeurotic covering. Despite these adaptations it is occasionally ruptured, a disaster of the first order that is made very evident by the projection of the scapular cartilage above the dorsal contour of the sunken thorax.

The muscles that operate at shoulder level are also generally unremarkable. The *infraspinatus*

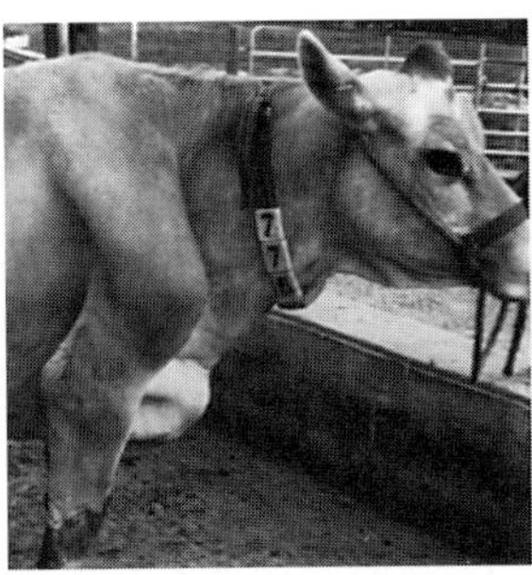
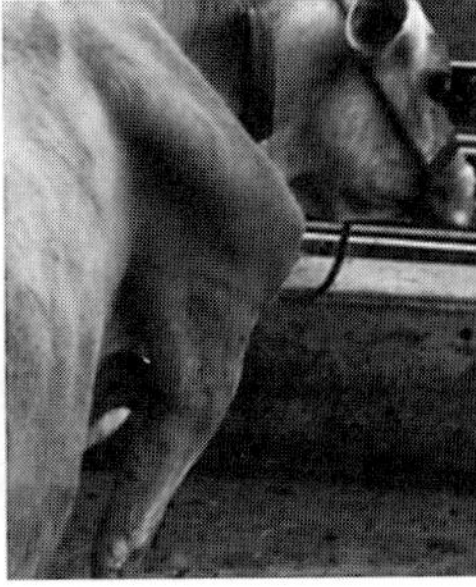

**Figure 32–1.** "Wing shoulder" in a 6-year-old Jersey cow.

tendon divides into the usual superficial and deep branches, the former protected by a synovial bursa interposed between the tendon and the humerus. The bursa is sometimes the seat of painful inflammation, which may be alleviated, and made obvious, by adduction of the arm. In cattle the tendon of origin of the *biceps* is also protected by a synovial (intertubercular) bursa on its deep face; in sheep and goats the corresponding protection is afforded by a pouch of the shoulder joint capsule that extends into the intertubercular groove. In the lower part of the arm, the covering aponeurosis of the biceps detaches a lacertus fibrosus that descends cranial to the elbow to blend with the covering of the extensor carpi radialis. The lacertus is much weaker than that found in the horse but has a similar function; it is palpable. The other muscles whose chief actions are on the shoulder or elbow joints are in no way remarkable. Synovial bursae are associated with the triceps tendon; one between the tendon and the olecranon just before the insertion, the other, inconstant, between the tendon and skin over the point of the elbow.

## THE ELBOW, FOREARM, AND CARPUS

The *elbow joint* is located opposite the ventral end of the fourth and fifth ribs. It presents no unusual features. The olecranon, the medial and lateral epicondyles of the humerus, and the robust collateral ligaments are all easily palpable and provide the necessary orientation for joint puncture. This is performed from the lateral aspect with the needle directed between the lateral epicondyle and the olecranon to enter a considerable pouch of the joint capsule within the deep olecranon fossa.

The ulna, although complete, is slender, and it is the massive radius that is the principal weight bearer. The *radius* is compressed from front to back along its length and is expanded medially and laterally at both ends. The entire medial border is subcutaneous and palpable and makes the usual division between the cranial extensor and caudal flexor muscle masses. The *ulna* is fused to the radius and is palpable only at its extremities—the olecranon and styloid process. The styloid process furnishes attachment to the lateral collateral ligament of the carpal joint. In most subjects the forearm inclines mediodistally to the expanded carpus while the foot angles laterally, producing a "knock-kneed" stance. Although straight limbs are preferred, this inward bulging at the carpus does not appear to interfere with function.

The proximal row of the *carpal skeleton* comprises radial, intermediate, and ulnar carpal bones extended caudolaterally by an accessory carpal (see Fig. 2–46). Since the rectangular accessory bone articulates only with the ulnar carpal its upper and lower margins provide rough guides to the levels of the antebrachiocarpal and midcarpal joints. The distal row consists of only two bones—fused second and third, and fourth carpals. Although movement is possible at three levels, most takes place between the forearm and carpus; a moderate amount is allowed at the midcarpal joint but very little at the flat carpometacarpal joint. Movements other than flexion and extension are largely prevented by the many ligaments, of which the collateral pair are most important. Irregularities on the palmar aspect of the carpal skeleton are covered and smoothed by the thick fibrous layer of the joint capsule (palmar carpal ligament), which combines with the accessory carpal bone and the flexor retinaculum to enclose the carpal canal. The pull of muscles attaching on the accessory carpal is transmitted to the lower carpus and metacarpus by several short ligaments. The fibrous layer of the joint capsule blends dorsally with the thick deep fascia (extensor retinaculum) that holds the extensor tendons in place. An inconstant bursa between the retinaculum and skin occasionally enlarges (hygroma) to form an unsightly, though painless, blemish. The capsules of the two distal joints communicate; occasionally, the antebrachiocarpal capsule communicates with the two distal joints as well. Puncture from the dorsal aspect is possible at the antebrachiocarpal and midcarpal levels; it is most easily performed when the joint is flexed.

Although most muscles of the *forearm* (extensor carpi radialis, ulnaris lateralis, extensor carpi obliquus, flexor carpi radialis, and flexor carpi ulnaris) resemble those of other species, significant differences affecting the digital extensor and flexor muscles are associated with the number of functional digits. The *common digital extensor* has two parts (Fig. 32–2/10). The insertion tendon of the larger medial belly ends on the middle phalanx of the medial digit and may therefore be regarded as the proper extensor of this digit—as it is indeed sometimes named. The tendon of the slighter lateral belly accompanies the medial tendon over the carpus, where they share a common sheath. The lateral tendon then splits into two branches that find insertion on the distal phalanges of both digits. The tendon of the *lateral digital extensor* (/11) descends over the lateral surface of the carpus, where it also receives protection from a synovial sheath, continues through the metacarpus with the common extensor tendons, and ends on the middle phalanx of the lateral digit (of which it is the proper extensor).

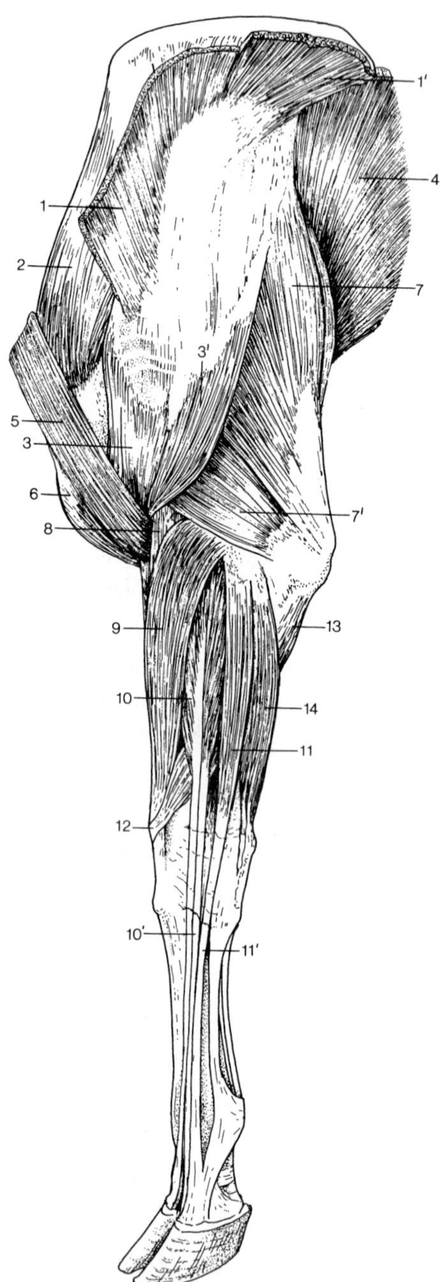


**Figure 32–2.** Muscles of the bovine forelimb, lateral view.

1, 1′, Trapezius; 2, supraspinatus; 3, 3′, deltoideus; 4, latissimus dorsi; 5, brachiocephalicus; 6, biceps; 7, 7′, long and lateral heads of triceps; 8, brachialis; 9, extensor carpi radialis; 10, common digital extensor; 10′, tendon of lateral belly; 11, 11′, lateral digital extensor; 12, extensor carpi obliquus; 13, ulnar head of deep digital flexor; 14, ulnaris lateralis.

The *superficial digital flexor* splits into two bellies. The tendon of the deep belly passes through the carpal canal, that of the superficial belly remains outside the flexor retinaculum; both are protected at carpal level by elongated carpal bursae that follow the tendons into the cannon where they merge. The resulting common cord bifurcates at the fetlock, and the divisions unite with branches of the interosseus to form sleeves around the branches of the deep flexor. The three heads of the *deep digital flexor* share a thick common tendon that passes through the carpal canal, where it is given the necessary protection by yet another carpal bursa. This tendon also splits in the metacarpus: its two branches proceed to insertion on the distal phalanges after limited connection with the middle phalanges.

The distal portions of the digital tendons, and the associated structures, are considered more fully in the next section.

## THE DISTAL PART OF THE LIMB

The distal part of the limb is commonly known as the foot, the digits as the toes. The foot (in this loose sense) consists of the expanded lower end of the metacarpus, the two principal toes, and the dewclaws. The toes are enclosed in a common envelope of skin that extends to the coronets so that the hoofs alone are separated by the interdigital cleft. The dewclaws project behind the fetlock and do not normally come into contact with firm ground.

In sheep the interdigital space contains a long (≈2 to 4 cm) blind pouch (sinus interdigitalis) that opens on the dorsal skin a little above the hoofs (see Fig. 10–24). The secretion of the apocrine glands in the wall of the pouch is said to be a territorial marker.

### The Skeleton and Joints

The skeleton is reduced to the bones of the principal digits (III and IV) together with vestiges of those of the flanking ones (II and V) (Fig. 32–5).

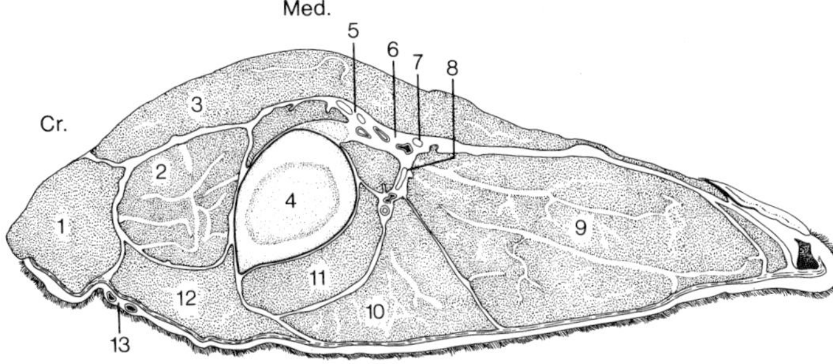


**Figure 32–3.** Transverse section of the middle of the bovine left arm.

1, Pectoralis descendens; 2, biceps; 3, pectoralis profundus; 4, humerus; 5, median nerve; 6, brachial vessels; 7, ulnar nerve; 8, radial nerve; 9, 10, long and lateral heads of triceps; 11, brachialis; 12, brachiocephalicus; 13, cephalic vein.

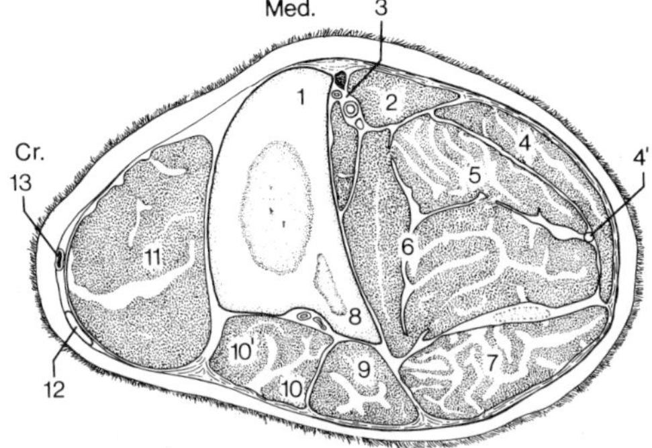


**Figure 32–4.** Transverse section of the middle of the bovine left forearm.

1, Radius; 2, flexor carpi radialis; 3, median vessels and nerve; 4, flexor carpi ulnaris; 4′, ulnar nerve; 5, superficial digital flexor; 6, deep digital flexor; 7, ulnaris lateralis; 8, ulna; 9, lateral digital extensor; 10, 10′, common digital extensor; 11, extensor carpi radialis; 12, superficial branch of radial nerve; 13, cephalic vein.

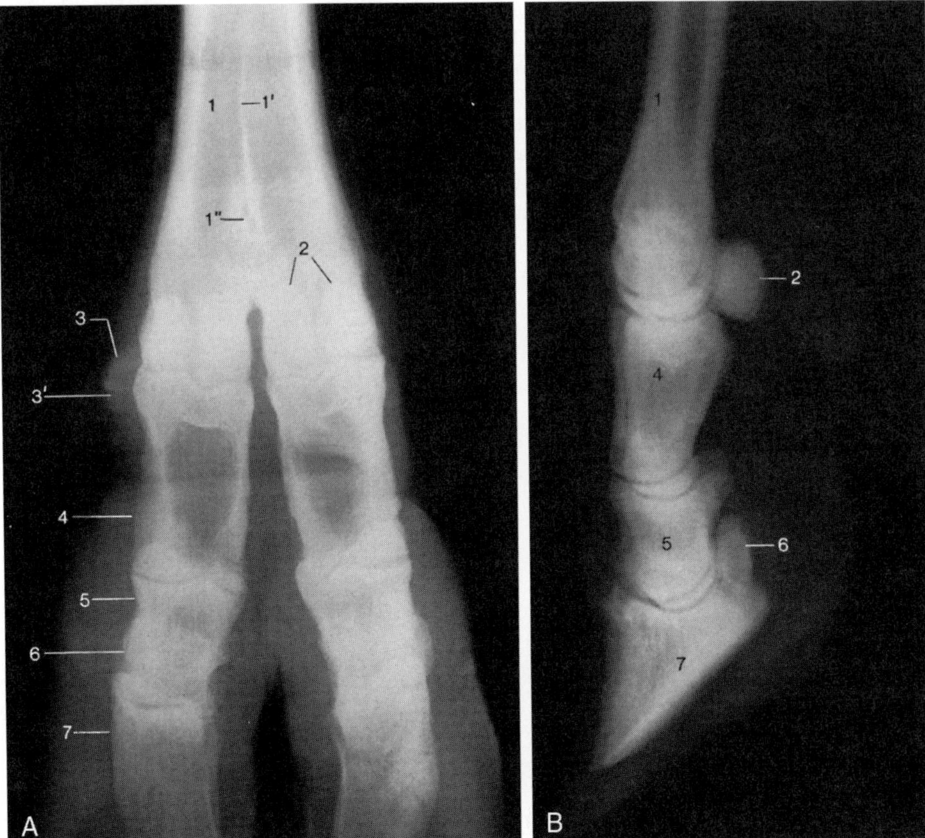


**Figure 32–5.** Dorsopalmar *(A)* and lateromedial *(B)* radiographs of the bovine foot.

1, Metacarpal bone; 1′, median septum; 1″, distal metacarpal canal; 2, proximal sesamoid bones; 3, dewclaw; 3′, rudimentary phalanx within dewclaw; 4, proximal phalanx; 5, middle phalanx; 6, navicular bone; 7, distal phalanx.

Although the principal metacarpal elements are fused to form a single cannon bone, this divides at its lower end into separate articular trochleae for the two proximal phalanges. All more distal bones are duplicated. Vestigial structures include the short, rodlike fifth metacarpal bone in articulation with the upper end of the cannon bone (see Fig. 2–46) and phalangeal rudiments isolated within the dewclaws.

The cannon bone is compressed from front to back and expanded to the sides at each end. A dorsal axial groove (presenting a vascular foramen at each end) and an incomplete internal septum (visible in radiographs) attest to the composite origin of the bone (Fig. 32–10/*B*,4). The proximal and middle phalanges are broadly alike, although the former are about twice the length of the latter. All four of these bones present proximopalmar tubercles, paired on the proximal phalanges, single and abaxial on the middle ones. Each has a distal surface that is grooved sagittally to fit the bifaceted surface of the bone with which it articulates. The distal phalanx is shaped like the hoof in which it is lodged and presents articular, axial, abaxial, and sole surfaces (Fig. 32–6). The extensor process is the highest point, and from it a crest runs to the apex of the bone, dividing the axial and abaxial surfaces. These surfaces are separated caudally by a thick transverse tubercle (/4) to which the deep flexor tendon attaches. Apart from the articular surface, the exterior displays numerous vascular foramina most conspicuously on the axial aspect of the extensor process and at the palmar end of the abaxial surface. (The proximal and distal sesamoid bones are described with the joints.)

As in the horse, the articulations linking the metacarpal and digital bones are commonly known as the fetlock, pastern, and coffin joints. The *fetlock joint,* the first duplicated joint of the limb, is slightly overextended when the animal stands at rest (Fig. 32–7/3). Its movements are confined to flexion and extension by reciprocally keeled and grooved articular surfaces and by strong collateral ligaments. The axial (interdigital) collateral ligaments of both joints have a common origin in the intertrochlear notch of the metacarpal bone (Fig. 32–5). The phalangeal articular surfaces are complemented on their palmar aspect by a row of four (proximal) sesamoid bones embedded within a continuous fibrocartilaginous bridge and joined by the interosseous muscle. These sesamoids are

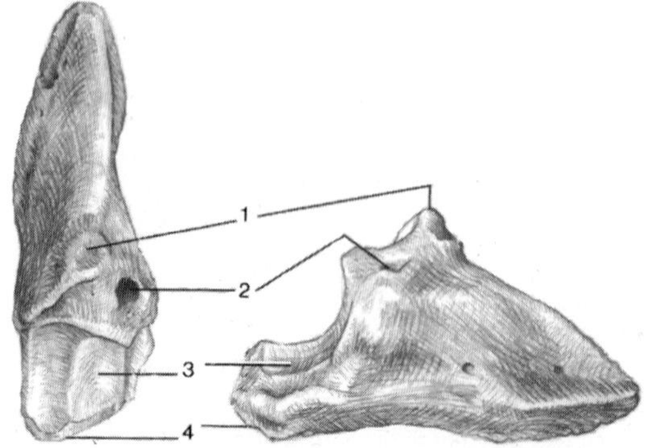


**Figure 32–6.** The distal phalanx of cattle looking distally *(left)* and axial surface *(right)*.

1, Extensor process; 2, axial foramen for the principal artery to the hoof; 3, articular surface; 4, tubercle on which the deep digital flexor attaches.

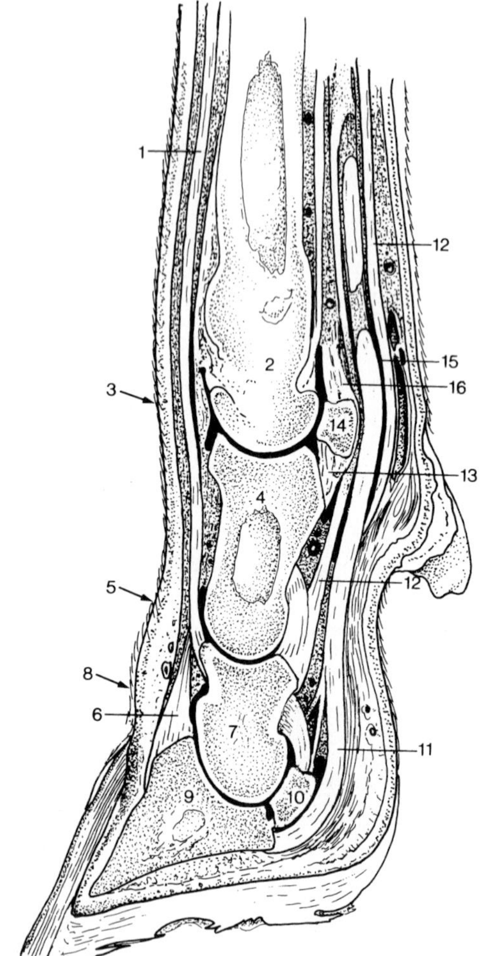


**Figure 32–7.** Sagittal section of the bovine foot, splitting the lateral digit.

1, Lateral digital extensor; 2, metacarpal bone; 3, fetlock joint; 4, proximal phalanx; 5, pastern joint; 6, common digital extensor; 7, middle phalanx; 8, coffin joint; 9, distal phalanx; 10, navicular bone; 11, deep digital flexor; 12, superficial flexor; 13, distal sesamoidean ligaments; 14, proximal sesamoid bone; 15, digital sheath; 16, interosseus.

additionally secured by collateral and distal sesamoidean ligaments. The collateral sesamoidean ligaments connect each abaxial sesamoid to the metacarpal bone and proximal phalanx. The ligaments that arise from the distal surfaces pass to the prominent tubercles on the proximopalmar aspect of the related phalanges, crossing in passage to their destinations (cruciate sesamoidean ligaments); fibers of the axial pair also cross the interdigital space (interdigital phalangosesamoidean ligaments; Fig. 32–8/10). Since the joints enjoy great mobility, the capsules are large; each extends proximally as a dorsal pouch between the metacarpal bone and extensor tendons and as a palmar pouch between the bone and the interosseous muscle (Fig. 32–10/9,9′). Although both may be punctured, the larger palmar pouch is reached more easily, entry being made from the side, about 2 or 3 cm proximal to the joint space. Communication between the paired capsules allows infection or injected material to travel from one joint to the other.

The less mobile *pastern joints* that link the proximal and middle phalanges also allow only flexion and extension. Each joint is supported by a pair of collateral ligaments, the axial one being better developed, presumably to resist excessive splaying of the toes under the body weight. An additional strong axial ligament extends from the proximal to the distal phalanx, bridging both pastern and coffin joints; its presence is given the same interpretation. The pastern joint obtains further support from a fibrocartilage that extends the palmar border of the articular surface of the middle phalanx, and from three palmar ligaments that resist overextension (Fig. 32–11/12). The most abaxial of these attaches on the prominent tubercle on the proximopalmar aspect of the middle phalanx. The capsules of the two pastern joints are separate. Each forms dorsal and palmar pouches

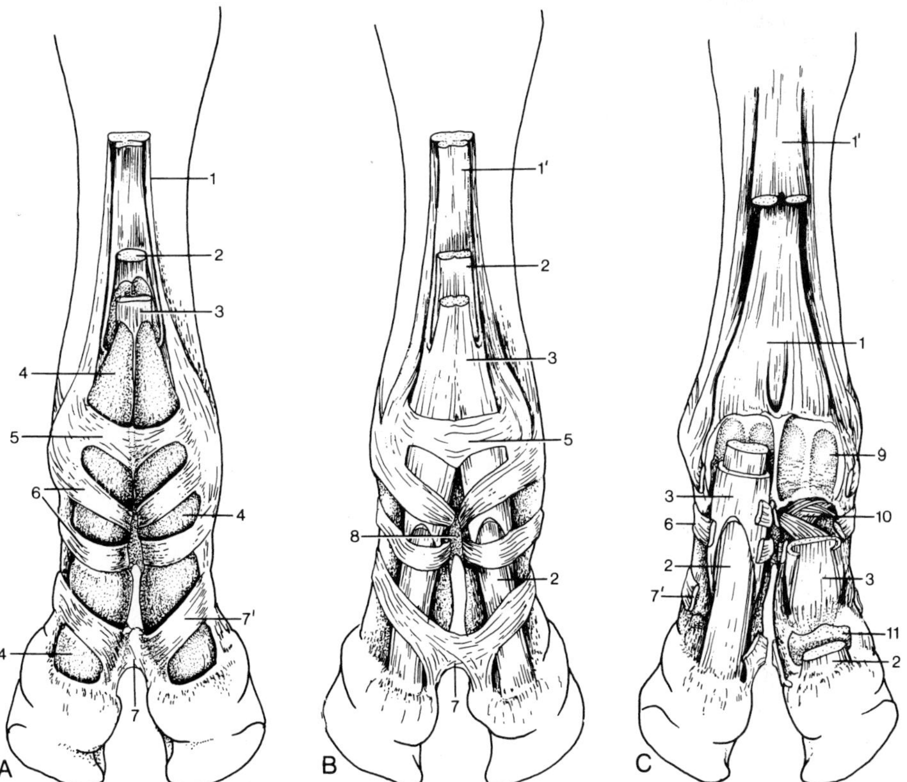


**Figure 32–8.** Palmar view of the bovine forefoot. *A,* Superficial dissection. *B,* Tissues of the digital sheath have been removed. *C,* Parts of the superficial and deep flexors have been removed.

1, Interosseus; 1′, band of interosseus to superficial flexor; 2, deep digital flexor; 3, superficial digital flexor; 4, digital sheath; 5, annular ligament of fetlock joint; 6, digital annular ligaments; 7, distal interdigital ligament, deep part; 7′, superficial part; 8, proximal interdigital ligament; 9, proximal sesamoid bones; 10, cruciate sesamoidean and interdigital phalangosesamoidean ligaments; 11, navicular bone.

on the proximal phalanx; the dorsal one is said to be accessible to puncture from the side.

The *coffin joint* resembles the pastern joint in conformation and in the possession of collateral ligaments. It is entirely within the hoof and, since the small dorsal and palmar pouches reach only to or a little beyond the coronet, injection is difficult (Fig. 32–7/8). The distal articular surface is enlarged by the navicular bone (distal sesamoid) placed at a depth of about 2 cm within the hoof (measured abaxially); its other end is above the lower axial wall of the hoof. This bone is mainly related to the middle phalanx and is held in place by a complex set of collateral and distal ligaments that pass to the middle and distal phalanges. These restrict overextension. An elastic ligament spanning the axial surface of the joint resembles that which retracts the cat's claw but has no obvious comparable function.

*Interdigital ligaments* prevent splaying of the toes. One connects the axial surfaces of the proximal phalanges (Fig. 32–8/8). A second (/7) crosses the interdigital space at the level of the navicular bones; its deep fibers, which connect the axial ends of these bones and adjacent areas of the phalanges, are related distally to the interdigital bridge of skin. The superficial (palmar) fibers pass obliquely over the palmar aspects of the deep flexor tendons to end on the abaxial surfaces of the middle phalanges.

## The Tendons

The *interosseus muscle** on the palmar surface of the metacarpal bone is important in supporting the fetlock. This flat muscle is fleshy in the young but becomes increasingly fibrous as the animal matures and gains weight. In the adult it forms a strong, almost wholly tendinous band that continues distally from the capsule of the carpal joint (Fig. 32–10/8). In midmetacarpus it gives rise to five principal branches; four of these—all but the central one—appear to terminate on the proximal sesamoid bones but obtain a functional continuation from the distal (sesamoidean) ligaments that attach on the proximal phalanges. The arrangement forms a "sling" that is tensed when the foot bears weight and the fetlock joint is overextended. Thin slips from the interosseus join the extensor tendons. Two of these split from the abaxial branches already mentioned and wind round the abaxial surfaces of the proximal phalanges to merge with the proper extensor tendons. Two more are provided by the bifurcation of the fifth (central) branch. They pass through the interdigital space, wind round the axial surfaces of the phalanges and merge in the same tendons. In midmetacarpus the interosseus also releases from its palmar surface a strong band (Fig. 32–10/*A*,7) that divides to join the branches of the superficial digital flexor tendon above the fetlock. (The band may be regarded as a check ligament of the superficial digital flexor.)

The three *extensor tendons* can be palpated where they lie side by side on the dorsal surface of the metacarpal bone. The middle tendon (from the lateral belly of the common digital extensor) bifurcates at the fetlock; the thin branches, each surrounded by an independent synovial sheath (Fig. 32–9/2′), follow the dorsal surface of the

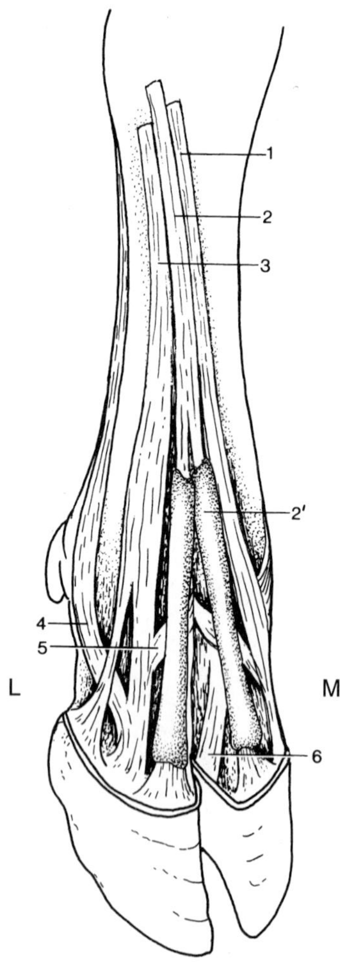


**Figure 32–9.** Dorsal view of the bovine right forefoot.

1, Medial tendon of common digital extensor to the medial digit; 2, common digital extensor; 2′, its sheaths; 3, lateral digital extensor; 4, 5, abaxial and axial extensor branches of the interosseus to the lateral digital extensor; 6, common axial collateral ligament.

*Morphologically a compound formation, it is nonetheless usual to speak of it in the singular.

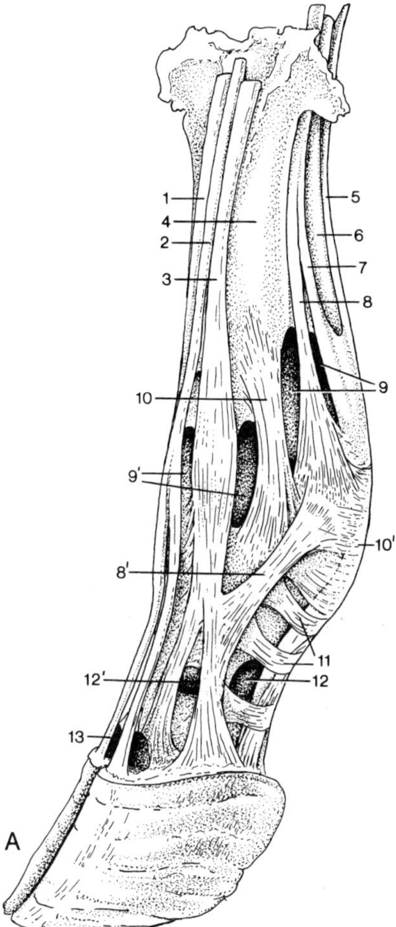


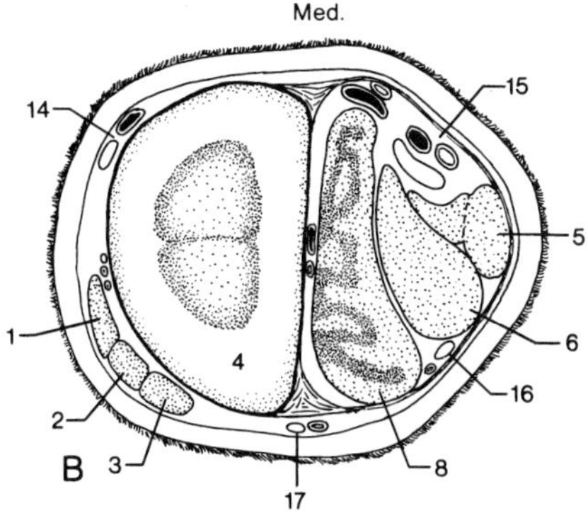


**Figure 32–10.** *A,* Bovine left forefoot, lateral view. *B,* Transverse section of the left metacarpus.

1, 2, Medial and lateral tendons of common digital extensor; 3, lateral digital extensor; 4, metacarpal bone; 5, superficial digital flexor; 6, deep digital flexor; 7, band from interosseus to superficial flexor; 8, interosseus, its extensor branch at 8′; 9, 9′, palmar and dorsal pouches of fetlock joint; 10, 10′, lateral collateral and annular ligaments of fetlock joint; 11, digital annular ligaments; 12, 12′, palmar and dorsal pouches of pastern joint; 13, dorsal pouch of medial coffin joint; 14, dorsal common digital vein III and superficial radial nerve; 15, median vessels and nerve; 16, palmar branch of ulnar nerve; 17, dorsal branch of ulnar nerve.

digits to insert on the extensor processes of the distal phalanges. The medial tendon (from the medial belly) widens as it passes over the dorsal pouch of the fetlock joint where a subtendinous bursa facilitates its passage. This tendon receives the extensor branches from the interosseus before it inserts on the proximal end of the middle phalanx (but with a secondary connection to the distal phalanx). The lateral tendon (lateral digital extensor; /3) comports itself identically in relation to the lateral digit.

The *superficial* and *deep flexor tendons* are separated from the metacarpal bone by the interosseus (Fig. 32–10). Together they can be palpated as they emerge from the carpus medial to the accessory carpal bone and they become individually distinguishable in the distal half of the cannon where the deep fascia is thin. They are never so easily identified as the sharp edged interosseus lying against the bone. The tendons are difficult to palpate in the digits.

The superficial flexor tendon splits above the fetlock joints (Fig. 32–8/*B*). Each branch receives a band from the interosseus with which it forms a sleeve about the corresponding branch of the deep flexor when level with the proximal sesamoid bones. These bones provide bearing surfaces around which the combined tendons bend, secured in place by annular ligaments (/9,5). The palmar wall of the sleeve ends at the middle of the proximal phalanx, exposing the deep tendon that has now exchanged relative position with the superficial flexor. The dorsal wall of the sleeve continues the superficial flexor tendon and terminates on the proximal end and complementary cartilage of the middle phalanx. Two narrower (digital) annular ligaments strap the tendons to the proximal phalanx. The deep flexor tendon widens after leaving the confines of the sleeve and continues over the insertion of the superficial flexor tendon, which provides it with another bearing surface. It then passes over the palmar surface of the navicular bone, where the interposed navicular bursa reduces friction, to end in a wide insertion on the hind end of the distal phalanx. The distal interdigital ligament binds the deep tendon down at the middle phalanx. The attachments of the superficial flexor tendon enable it to assist the interosseus in preventing overextension of the fetlock joint.

A complex sheath (digital sheath; /4) surrounds the two flexor tendons from the distal third of the metacarpus almost to the navicular bone. It facilitates their passage against each other and against the various bearing surfaces and annular ligaments. The sheaths of the medial and lateral branches of the tendons touch locally and occasionally communicate. They are independent of the digital joint capsules and navicular bursae. Distention of an infected sheath is possible where it is unsupported, namely at its proximal end and between the annular ligaments below the fetlock. The sheath may be punctured from the side at the dorsal border of the flexor tendons, about 5 cm proximal to the dewclaw.

The following skeletal features may be palpated at the fetlock (Fig. 32–5): the dorsal and abaxial surfaces of the metacarpal trochleae, the corresponding parts of the proximal phalanges, the abaxial sesamoid bones, the abaxial tubercles of the proximal phalanges, and the gaps between the proximal phalanges and the neighboring sesamoids, which mark the level of the joint spaces (opposite the dewclaws). Except for its palmar surface, most of the proximal phalanx is easily appreciated, but its distal end and the pastern joint space are obscure even though the level is marked by the insertion of the flat extensor tendon (3 cm above the coronet) and the prominent abaxial tubercle of the middle phalanx; the joint space itself lies about 2 cm above the coronet. The narrow branches of the common extensor are more easily appreciated than the wide but flat tendons of the proper extensors. The flexor tendons form a firm mass behind the bones. The dewclaws are attached to thickened deep fascia that forms two ligaments extending to the abaxial ends of the navicular bones; these ligaments become palpable when the dewclaws are raised.

## The Hoofs

The hoofs of the principal digits curve toward each other at both ends, making contact behind and occasionally also at their apices (Fig. 32–12). The lateral hoof carries the greater share of weight and is larger than the medial one (although this is not always so in the hind foot). Each hoof consists of periople, wall, sole, and bulb. The ground surface is formed by the distal border of the wall, the sole, and the dorsal part of the bulb (/1,3,4′); the parts visible in the standing animal are the wall to the sides and the bulb at the back of the hoof. The coronary border of the hoof is higher on the abaxial than on the axial side. The apical two thirds or so of the hoof are occupied by the distal phalanx and deep flexor tendon; the space behind is taken up by the digital cushion, the springy pad of fatty-fibrous tissue that also extends under the larger "half" of the bone (Fig. 32–11/8).

The *periople* provides a narrow (≈1 cm) strip along the coronary border that widens at the back where it grades into the bulb and merges with the periople of the other hoof. It is partly hidden by hair. In consistency it is intermediate between the epidermis of the skin and the hard horn of the wall (Fig. 32–13/6).

The *wall,* sharply flexed on itself, forms the greater part of both axial and abaxial surfaces (Fig. 32–12); the flexure produces a crest at the front that curves distally toward the tip or "toe" of the hoof. Both surfaces are bounded caudally by more

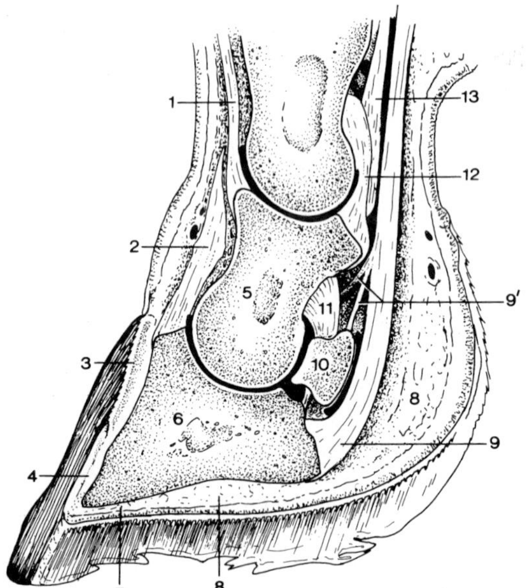


**Figure 32–11.** Sagittal section of the medial digit of the bovine forefoot.

1, Proper (medial) digital extensor; 2, common digital extensor; 3, coronary dermis; 4, laminar dermis; 5, middle phalanx; 6, distal phalanx; 7, sole dermis covered by sole; 8, digital cushion; 9, deep digital flexor; 9′, fibers of deep digital flexor to the middle phalanx and navicular bone; 10, navicular bone; 11, collateral navicular ligament; 12, palmar ligaments of pastern joint; 13, superficial digital flexor.

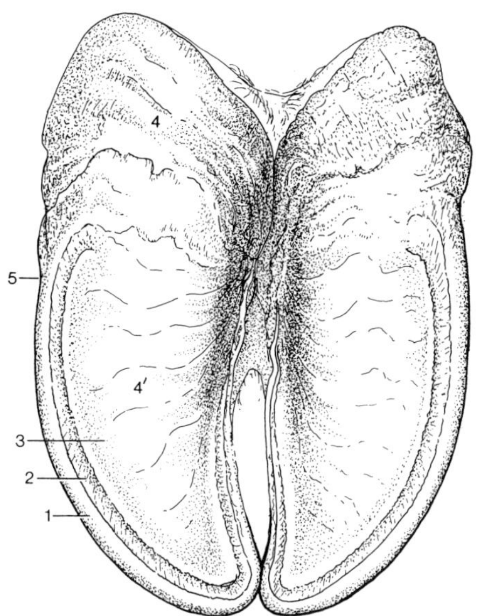


**Figure 32–12.** Ground surface of the hoofs of the bovine forefoot.

1, Wall; 2, white line; 3, sole; 4, bulb; 4′, dorsal part of bulb; 5, abaxial groove on the wall, dividing wall from bulb.

or less distinct grooves (/5) that extend from the coronary border to the ground surface; the horn caudal to the grooves belongs to the bulb. The axial groove is more cranial and provides an area of weakness that is sometimes penetrated; infection may then easily extend to the coffin joint only a few millimeters away. The wall is marked by prominent ridges that run parallel with the coronary border; they are caused by uneven production of horn that may be due to a local or more general disturbance. Although the distal border normally makes contact with the ground along the whole length of the abaxial wall, it does so only toward the toe on the axial side; because of its slight concavity, the greater part of this margin bears weight only on softer ground. The wall is not uniformly strong but is thicker near the apex and toward the ground, especially abaxially. It consists of both tubular and intertubular horn and is produced over the wide, flat coronary dermis. The coronary "groove," which is visible on the detached hoof, is molded to this dermis; it is therefore much wider and shallower (indeed, almost flat) than in the equine hoof. The horny laminae are short and low and form a weaker union with the laminar dermis than in the horse. This may be correlated with the greater extent of the weight-bearing surface, which includes the sole and bulb in ruminants.

The *sole* (/3) is a relatively smooth area confined within the inflected angle of the wall from which it is separated by the softer so-called white line. This line is actually little lighter than the generally unpigmented horn to each side; it is only a few millimeters wide and comprises the alternation of the distal ends of the horny laminae with the slightly darker horn produced over the terminal papillae of the sensitive laminae. Centrally, the sole blends imperceptibly with the apex of the bulb. The junction between the two depends on the extent of the digital cushion, which underlies the bulb (Fig. 32–11/8,7).

The *bulb* provides both the caudal aspect and a considerable portion of the ground surface where its apex inserts into the V-shaped sole. It is the chief weight-bearing part. A large proportion of intertubular horn makes it relatively soft, but its considerable thickness may compensate. Bulbar horn tends to flake when allowed to build up (as in animals stood on fouled bedding), and the resulting fissures provide access to infection; resulting abscesses may destroy the dermis and deeper structures.

The hoof capsule of the dissection subject may generally be removed intact, revealing that it is molded on a dermis attached to underlying structures by a modified subcutis. The subcutis is best developed where it forms the digital cushion. The dermis presents several segments that correspond to the parts of the hoof (Fig. 32–13). The horn of the wall is produced over the coronary dermis (/2) and slides distally over and between the dermal laminae where sufficient horn is produced to maintain adhesion. The covering of the terminal papillae at the distal ends of the dermal laminae (/3′) produces the horn that plugs the spaces between the horny laminae exposed in the white line.

The horn of other parts of the hoof grows away from the dermis at a rate of about 5 mm per month, a little faster in calves. In cattle allowed free range, wear of the ground surface equals growth, and at the toe the angle with the ground is maintained at about 50 degrees. On soft surfaces, growth exceeds wear, and the hoofs must be trimmed periodically if the toe is not to grow forward at a lesser angle. When this occurs the coffin joint is gradually overextended, the deep flexor tensed, and greater weight placed on the (caudal) part of the hoof over the insertion of the deep flexor and navicular bone. This causes pain and therefore lameness. In late fetal life the distal parts of the hoof are covered with soft horn, which is said to prevent injury to the fetal membranes and the birth canal. This soft cushion soon dries when exposed to air, revealing

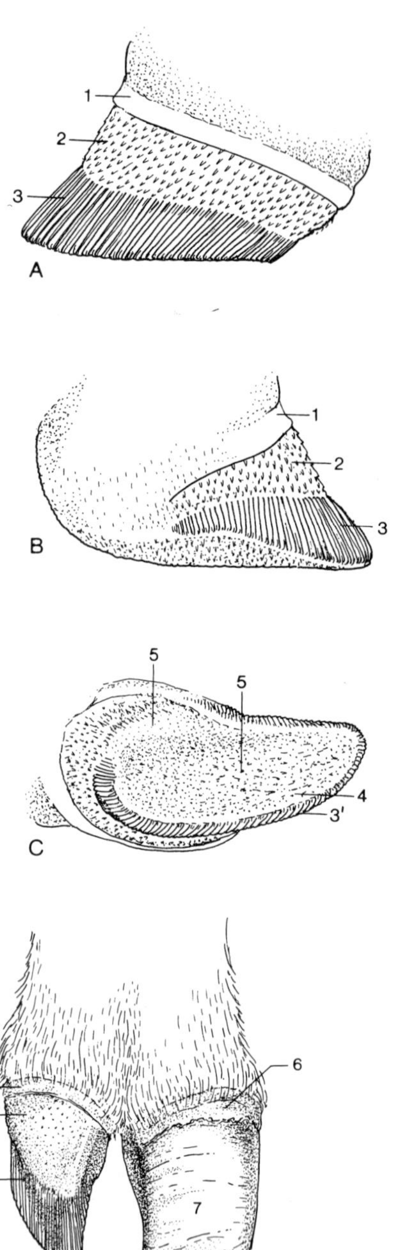


**Figure 32–13.** Dermis over which the horny bovine hoof is produced. *A* to *C*, Abaxial, axial, and ground surface. *D*, Dorsal surface of dermis and hoof.

1, Perioplic dermis; 2, coronary dermis; 3, laminar dermis; 3′, terminal papillae at the distal ends of the laminae; 4, sole dermis; 5, dermis of the bulb; 6, periople; 7, wall of hoof.

the harder hoof structures on which the calf supports itself within minutes of birth (see Fig. 23–37).

The dewclaws, miniatures of the principal hoofs, consist mainly of wall and bulb; they have no practical importance.

# THE BLOOD VESSELS AND LYMPHATIC STRUCTURES OF THE FORELIMB

The *axillary artery,* the main supply to the limb, is used occasionally as a source of arterial blood; it may be located on deep palpation where it winds around the first rib. The courses and branches of the arteries in the proximal segments follow the general pattern sufficiently closely to make description unnecessary. The account may be resumed where the *median artery* follows the medial border of the radius deep to the flexor carpi radialis (Fig. 32–4/3,2) before accompanying the deep digital flexor tendon through the carpal canal. It runs with a satellite vein and the median nerve within the metacarpus where it lies on the medial surface of the flexor tendons under cover of a thick deep fascia (Fig. 32–10/*B*,15). Throughout its course the trunk has many side branches that are linked by anastomoses sufficient to maintain an adequate collateral circulation should it be blocked. Branching is particularly profuse near the carpus, and several minor arteries that arise here descend to take part in the vascularization of the digits.

The median artery becomes superficial and vulnerable at the fetlock joint where its course takes it over the palmar surface of the medial branches of the flexor tendons. It is renamed the *palmar common digital artery III* when it dives into the interdigital space. The artery and satellite vein bulge visibly at this point in thin-skinned cows, and the artery can be palpated, although a pulse cannot usually be perceived (Fig. 32–14/9).

Within the interdigital space, the palmar common digital artery gives branches to the dewclaws and digital cushions; it also sends an anastomosis below the proximal interdigital ligament to the small dorsal common digital artery III that descends in the groove on the dorsal surface of the metacarpal bone. The common digital artery then splits into axial palmar digital arteries; each of these passes distally on the digit, slips under the axial common collateral ligament, and enters the distal phalanx through the large foramen by the extensor process. Lesser palmar digital arteries on the abaxial aspect of the digits are derived from palmar metacarpal continuations of the interosseous and radial arteries; each enters the distal phalanx at the palmar end of its abaxial surface. The palmar digital arteries anastomose inside the bone, forming a terminal arch from which numerous branches are released to the dermis. Small *dorsal* digital arteries are of lesser importance. The digital arteries are necessarily severed when a digit is amputated; the stump of the axial palmar digital artery, the largest of the set, bleeds most profusely and must be ligated.

The *veins* of the forelimb are divided between a deep system, satellite to the arteries, and a quasi-independent superficial system. The two are connected by prominent anastomoses at the elbow, above the carpus, and in the foot.

The superficial system comprises the cephalic and accessory cephalic veins and the tributaries of the latter in the foot (Fig. 32–15). Most can be palpated and form visible surface features in young, thin-skinned subjects. The *cephalic vein* (/2) arises from the radial vein, which ascends over the medial aspect of the carpus outside the flexor retinaculum. It crosses the medial surface of the radius (where it is joined by the accessory cephalic) and then climbs over the extensor carpi radialis (Fig. 32–4/13) to the elbow; at this level it is connected to the brachial vein by a long median cubital vein. The cephalic vein then ascends in the groove between the brachiocephalicus and pectoralis descendens to open into the external jugular vein at the base of the neck. The *accessory cephalic vein* continues the dorsal common digital vein III (Fig. 32–10/*B*,14), which ascends with the superficial branch of the radial nerve on the dorsal aspect of the cannon, having received blood from the dorsal surfaces of the digits; an interdigital anastomosis connects with the deep system at that level.

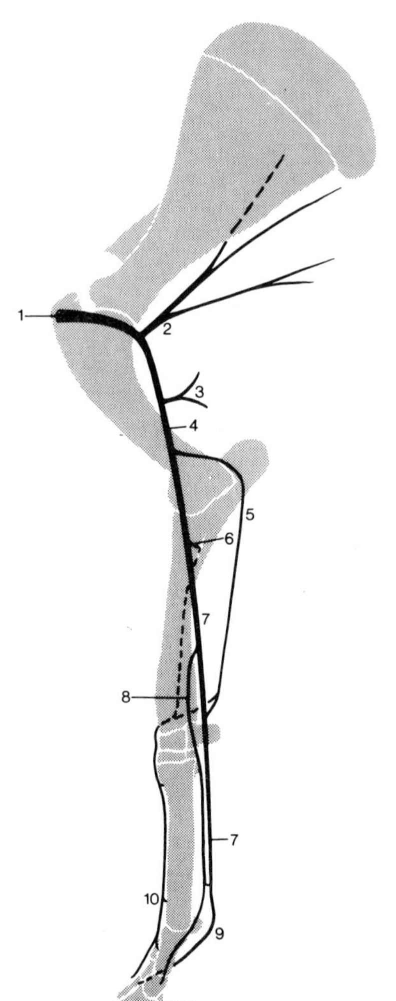


**Figure 32–14.** The principal arteries on the bovine right forelimb; medial view.

1, Axillary a.; 2, subscapular a.; 3, deep brachial a.; 4, brachial a.; 5, collateral ulnar a.; 6, common interosseous a.; 7, median a.; 8, radial a.; 9, palmar common digital artery III; 10, dorsal common digital artery III.

The larger superficial veins of the fore- and hindfeet are used for retrograde intravenous local anesthesia after being raised for puncture by application of a tourniquet distal to the carpus or hock. Those that best lend themselves to this procedure are shown in Figures 32–15, 33–9, and 33–10. The technique is simpler and more reliable than the alternative method (p. 747) that requires accurately placed deposits over several nerves.

The *lymph nodes* of the forelimb comprise the large proper axillary node, which lies against the chest wall caudal to the shoulder joint, and a few small accessory nodes (lnn. axillares primae costae) placed over the first rib and adjoining intercostal space. The axillary node receives lymph from the bones, joints, and muscles of the upper segments of the limb including the ventral girdle muscles. Its efferent vessels pass first to the accessory nodes and then either to the caudal deep cervical nodes or directly to one or other vein at the thoracic inlet. The node may be inspected through a medial incision in the middle of the first intercostal space of the split hanging carcass. The dorsal girdle muscles; the skin and subcutaneous fascia of the shoulder, arm, and forearm; and all distal structures drain directly into the superficial cervical node, which may be palpated in front of the shoulder.

# THE NERVES OF THE FORELIMB

## The Branches of the Brachial Plexus

The brachial plexus is formed by the last three cervical and first two thoracic nerves. Its branches generally conform to the common pattern, but a few points require brief description because of their clinical importance.

The *suprascapular* (C6–7) *nerve* winds around the cranial border of the scapula to reach the

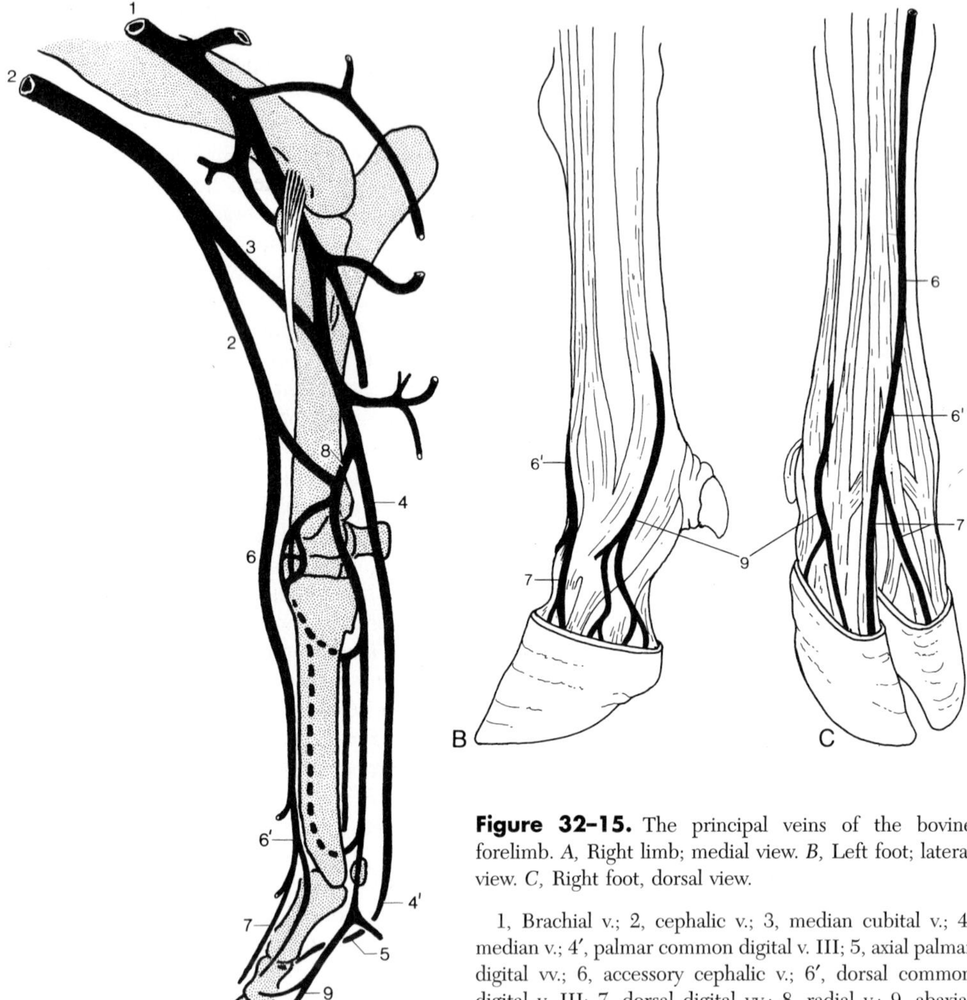


**Figure 32–15.** The principal veins of the bovine forelimb. *A,* Right limb; medial view. *B,* Left foot; lateral view. *C,* Right foot, dorsal view.

1, Brachial v.; 2, cephalic v.; 3, median cubital v.; 4, median v.; 4′, palmar common digital v. III; 5, axial palmar digital vv.; 6, accessory cephalic v.; 6′, dorsal common digital v. III; 7, dorsal digital vv.; 8, radial v.; 9, abaxial palmar digital vv.

supraspinatus and infraspinatus muscles (Fig. 32–16/4). Destruction* has little effect on the standing posture beyond producing occasional slight abduction of the arm. Walking is more severely affected, and the limb is advanced with a stiff, circumducted stride with the shoulder abducted most obviously in the support phase. In chronic paralysis the muscles atrophy and the scapular spine becomes sharply defined.

The *axillary nerve* (C7–8) supplies the skin over the craniolateral surface of the arm and craniomedial surface of the upper forearm.

*The descriptions of this and other nerve paralyses are based on experimental investigations. They do not always match the clinical accounts, presumably because injuries of accidental occurrence tend to be complicated by damage to other structures and do not always involve total severance of the nerve.

The *musculocutaneous nerve* (chiefly C6–8) after temporary embodiment within the median, breaks free in mid-arm and descends subcutaneously beside the cephalic vein. It then runs medial to the accessory cephalic vein before joining the superficial branch of the radial nerve (which runs lateral to the vein) at the carpus. It occasionally continues into the metacarpus independently. With the radial nerve it innervates an extensive skin area on the dorsal and medial surfaces of the limb. Paralysis of either of the axillary or musculocutaneous nerves has minimal effect on stance or gait.

The large *median nerve* (C8–T2) runs down the medial aspect of the arm, crosses the elbow joint (where it is palpable in front of the brachial artery; Fig. 32–3/5,6) and dips under the flexor muscles to which it sends branches. The much-reduced trunk then follows the median artery under cover of the flexor carpi radialis (Fig. 32–4/3) into the carpal canal before dividing in midmetacarpus into several branches that supply most of the palmar aspect of the foot; these are described later.

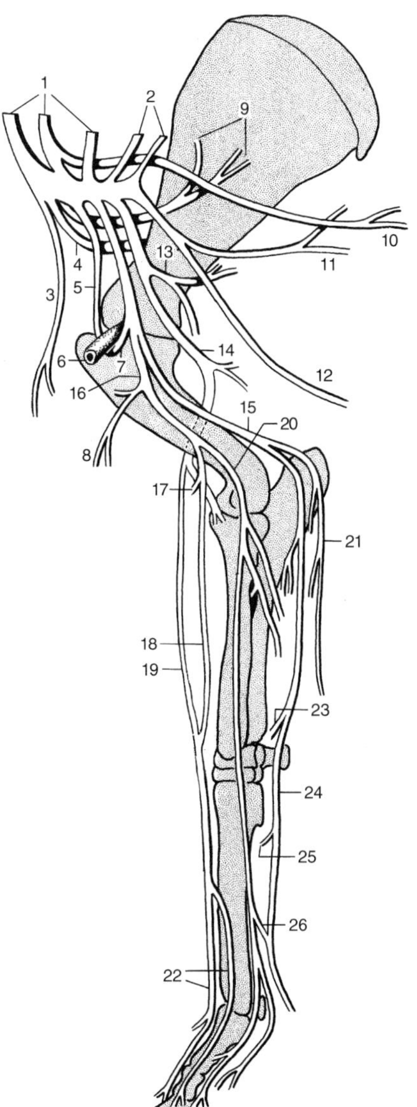


**Figure 32–16.** Nerves of the bovine forelimb; medial view.

1, 2, Roots of brachial plexus; 3, cranial pectoral n.; 4, suprascapular n.; 5, musculocutaneous n.; 6, axillary a.; 7, loop of musculocutaneous n. before joining median n.; 8, proximal branch of musculocutaneous n.; 9, subscapular n.; 10, long thoracic n.; 11, thoracodorsal n.; 12, lateral thoracic n.; 13, axillary n.; 14, radial n.; 15, ulnar n.; 16, combined musculocutaneous and median nn.; 17, distal branch of musculocutaneous n.; 18, medial cutaneous antebrachial n.; 19, superficial branch of radial n.; 20, median n.; 21, caudal cutaneous antebrachial n.; 22, dorsal common digital nn. III and II; 23, dorsal branch of ulnar n.; 24, palmar branch of ulnar n.; 25, deep branch of ulnar n. (to interosseous muscles); 26, communicating branch.

The *ulnar nerve* (C8–T2) arises with the median nerve but diverges from this in mid-arm (Fig. 32–16/15). After releasing a branch to the skin, it passes toward the olecranon where it dips between the origins of the flexor muscles. It detaches branches to these before continuing among the muscles in the caudal part of the forearm as a mainly sensory nerve (Fig. 32–4/4′), which divides a short distance above the accessory carpal bone. The palmar branch runs through the carpal canal lateral to the flexor tendons; the dorsal branch becomes superficial and may be palpated where it descends over the lateral aspect of the accessory carpal bone. Both branches are considered below.

Since the median and ulnar nerves share in the supply of the carpal and digital flexors, destruction of either one has little effect on posture or gait. Even when both are sectioned no immediate change in the appearance of the standing animal occurs, although overextension of the carpus develops later. Walking is affected by the double neurectomy and is performed with an exaggerated "goose-stepping" action in which the carpal and lower joints are overextended; but the stride is not shortened and the foot remains able to support weight.

The *radial nerve* (C7–T1) lies more caudally in the arm. It dives between the heads of the triceps (Fig. 32–3/8) before following the brachialis to reach the cranial surface of the elbow; it furnishes muscular branches en route. The trunk is vulnerable as it passes over the sharp epicondyloid crest of the humerus deep to the lateral head of the triceps. In this position it divides into several branches that innervate the extensor muscles of the carpus and digits, and a cutaneous branch that accompanies the cephalic and, more distally, the accessory cephalic vein. This sizable superficial branch is joined by the cutaneous branch of the musculocutaneous nerve before crossing the dorsomedial aspect of the carpus (Fig. 32–16/19,18). Its distribution to the dorsal surface of the foot is described later. The radial nerve is the exclusive supply to the extensors of all joints distal to the shoulder, and the effects of injury in the proximal part of its course are correspondingly severe. The elbow is "dropped" and the limb appears to be abnormally long. The animal moves with difficulty, dragging the toes and taking no weight on the affected limb. It is unable to place the sole of the hoof on the ground and rests on the dorsal surfaces of the digits. If the damage is more distal, the animal can usually learn to compensate for the loss of carpal and digital extensor muscle function.

## Innervation of the Forefoot

The following account has its main significance in relation to nerve-blocking techniques for the procurement of local anesthesia. Those who prefer the retrograde intravenous injection method are spared the necessity of mastering the details. The nerves traced across the carpus are the median, the palmar and dorsal branches of the ulnar, and the superficial branch of the radial (which incorporates the contribution from the musculocutaneous). Blockage of all (in midmetacarpus) completely desensitizes the digits.

The *median nerve* is accompanied by large satellite vessels in its descent medial to the flexor tendons. It divides into four branches above the fetlock (Fig. 32–17/*A*,1). The first (/2) runs distally in the groove between the flexor tendons and the interosseus and supplies the palmar and abaxial surfaces of the medial digit. Two axial nerves, often initially combined (/3), together with the palmar common digital artery and vein III, pass over the flexor tendons going to the medial digit and enter the interdigital space to supply the axial surfaces of the digits. The fourth, a communicating branch (/4), crosses the superficial flexor tendon to join the palmar branch of the ulnar nerve, which descends lateral to the flexor tendons.

The *palmar branch of the ulnar nerve* (/5), which receives the communicating branch from the median, runs distally in the groove between the flexor tendons and the interosseus, and supplies the palmar and abaxial surfaces of the lateral digit.

The *dorsal branch of the ulnar nerve* (/6) was seen to pass over the lateral aspect of the carpus and to continue in the groove between the

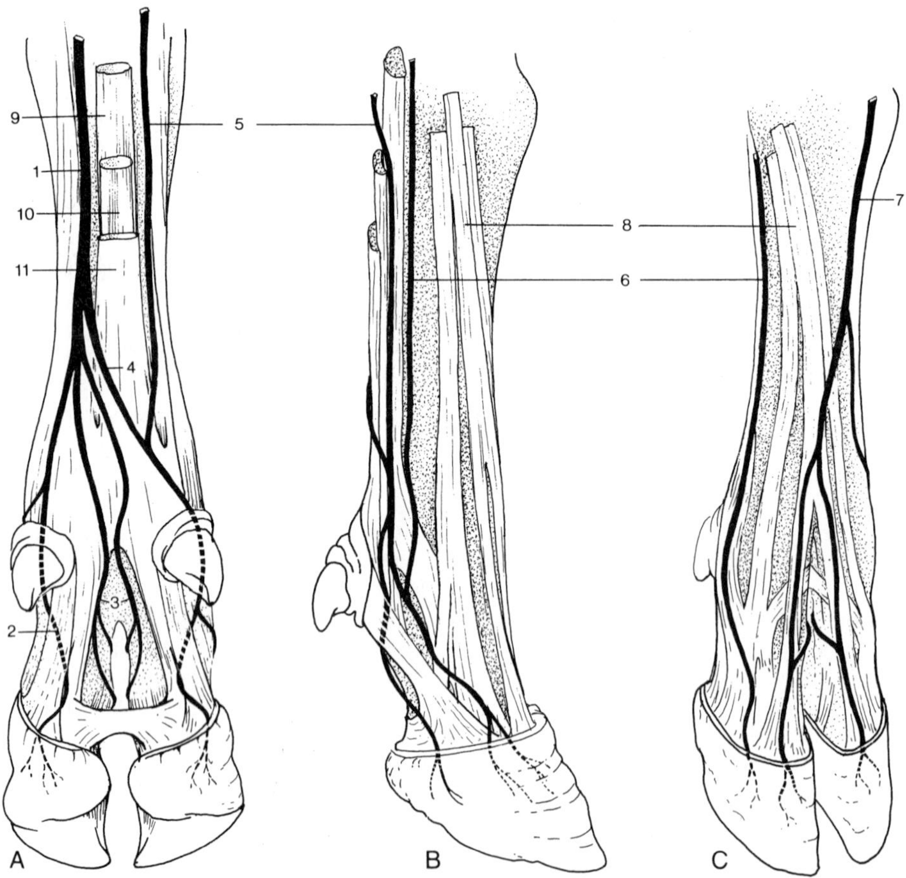


**Figure 32–17.** The principal nerves of the bovine right forefoot in palmar *(A)*, lateral *(B)*, and dorsal *(C)* views.

1, Median nerve; 2, palmar abaxial digital n.; 3, palmar axial digital nn.; 4, communicating branch; 5, palmar branch of ulnar n.; 6, dorsal branch of ulnar n.; 7, superficial branch of radial n.; 8, digital extensor tendons; 9, interosseus; 10, deep flexor tendon; 11, superficial flexor tendon.

interosseus and the metacarpal bone (where it is palpable) toward the fetlock. It crosses the fetlock dorsal to the interosseus and supplies the dorsoabaxial surface of the lateral digit.

The *superficial branch of the radial nerve* (/7) crosses the dorsomedial surface of the carpus. It then inclines laterally, reaches the extensor tendons in midmetacarpus, and comes to lie between them and the covering skin. This nerve and the accompanying accessory cephalic vein can be palpated most easily where they climb over the margins of the tendons. The first important branch, detached near this point, incorporates fibers obtained from the musculocutaneous nerve and returns to the medial side of the foot to supply the dorsoabaxial region of the medial digit. (The cutaneous branch of the musculocutaneous nerve occasionally continues independently to supply this digit.) The depleted radial branch splits at the fetlock joint to furnish axial dorsal nerves to both digits. These descend with the common digital extensor tendons and are connected with respective axial palmar nerves in the interdigital space.

In summary, the median nerve supplies most of the palmar aspect of the foot, the radial nerve most of the dorsal aspect, and the ulnar nerve the lateral margin. As a general guide it is useful to remember that the palmar nerves encroach on the territories of the dorsal nerves, and more medial nerves on the territories of those more lateral.

When blocking the foregoing nerves for surgery, it is necessary to bear in mind both their exact locations and their depths below the skin. One technique requires injection at four sites (Fig. 32–10/*B*): (1) over the median nerve (/15) between the medial border of the deep flexor tendon and interosseus, just above midmetacarpus where the nerve lies under the stout deep fascia; (2) over the palmar branch of the ulnar nerve (/16) between the lateral border of the deep flexor tendon and interosseus at the same depth and level; (3) over the dorsal branch of the ulnar nerve (/17) where it is subcutaneous and palpable in the groove between the interosseus and the metacarpal bone; and (4) over the superficial branch of the radial nerve (/14) in midmetacarpus where it is subcutaneous and palpable in relation to the extensor tendons.

## Selected Bibliography


Anderson, D.E., G. St Jean, D.E. Morin, et al.: Traumatic flexor tendon injuries in 27 cattle. Vet. Surg. 25:320–326, 1996.

Ashdown, R.R., and S. Done: Color Atlas of Veterinary Anatomy: The Ruminants. Baltimore, University Park Press; and London, Gower Medical Publishing Ltd. 1984.

Baxter, G.M., T.A. Broome, and J. Lakritz: Alternatives to digital amputation in cattle. Comp. Contin. Educ. Pract. Vet. 13:1022–1035, 1991.

Budras, K.D., C. Mülling, and A. Horowitz: Rate of keratinization of the wall segment of the hoof and its relation to width and structure of the zona alba (white line) with respect to claw disease in cattle. Am. J. Vet. Res. 57:444–455, 1996.

Copelan, R.W., and L.R. Bramlage: Surgery of the fetlock joint. Vet. Clin. North Am. L.A. Pract. 5:221–231, 1983.

deLahunta, A., and R.E. Habel: Applied Veterinary Anatomy. Philadelphia, W.B. Saunders Company, 1986.

Desrocher, A., G. St Jean, and D.E. Anderson: Use of facilitated ankylosis in the treatment of septic arthritis of the distal interphalangeal joint in cattle: 12 cases (1987–1992). JAVMA 206:1923–1927, 1995.

Desrocher, A., G. St Jean, W.C. Cash, et al.: Characterization of anatomic communications among the antebrachiocarpal, middle carpal, and carpometacarpal joints in cattle, using intra-articular latex, positive-contrast arthrography, and fluoroscopy. Am. J. Vet. Res. 58(1):7–10, 1997.

Desrocher, A., G. St Jean, W.C. Cash, et al.: Characterization of anatomic communications of the fetlock in cattle, using intra-articular latex injection and positive-contrast arthrography. Am. J. Vet. Res. 58(7):710–712, 1997.

Ebeid, M., and A. Steiner: Guidelines for taking and interpreting radiographs of the bovine foot. Vet. Med. 91:268–272, 1996.

Gogi, S.N., J.M. Nigam, and A.P. Singh: Angiographic evaluation of bovine foot abnormalities. Vet. Radiol. 23:171–174, 1982.

Greenough, P.R., F.J. MacCallum and A.D. Weaver: Lameness in Cattle, 2nd ed. Philadelphia, J.B. Lippincott, 1981.

Gunning, R.F., and R.J.W. Walters: Short communications: "Flying scapulas," a post turnout myopathy in cattle. Vet. Rec. 135:433–434, 1994.

Habel, R.E.: Guide to the Dissection of the Domestic Ruminants, 4th ed. Ithaca, 1989. [Published by the author.]

Hannam, D.A.R., L.R. Holden, M. Jeffrey, and N. Twiddy: Flying scapula of cattle. Vet. Rec. 134:356, 1994.

Jann, H.W., and R.R. Steckel: Treatment of lacerated flexor tendons in a dairy cow, using specialized farriery. JAVMA 195:772–774, 1989.

Kempson, S.A., and D.N. Logue: Ultrastructural observations of hoof horn from dairy cows: The structure of the white line. Vet. Rec. 132:499–502, 1993.

Knight, A.P.: Intravenous regional anesthesia of the bovine foot. Bovine Pract. 1:11–15, 1981.

Mascarello, F., and A. Rowlerson: Natural involution of the proximal sesamoidean ligament in sheep. J. Anat. 186:75–86, 1995.

Mills, M.L., G. St. Jean, and W. Cash: Clinical application of bovine distal limb anatomy. Agri. Prac. 17:14–19, 1996.

Nelson, D.R., and G.C. Petersen: Foot diseases in cattle, Part I: Examination and special procedures. Compend. Contin. Educ. 6/9:S543–S549, 1984.

Nuss, K., and M.P. Weaver: Resection of the distal interphalangeal joint in cattle: An alternative to amputation. Vet. Rec. 128:540–543, 1991.

Pejsa, T.G., G. St. Jean, G.F. Hoffsis, and J.M.B. Musser: Digit amputation in cattle: 85 cases (1971–1990) JAVMA 202: 981–984, 1993.

Petersen, G.C., and D.R. Nelson: Foot diseases in cattle, Part II: Diagnosis and treatment. Compend. Contin. Educ. 6/10: S565–S574, 1984.

Rakestraw, P.C., A.J. Nixon, R.E. Kaderly, and N.G. Ducharme: Cranial approach to the humerus for repair of fractures in horses and cattle. Vet. Surg. 20:1–8, 1991.

Rebhun, W.C., and E.G. Pearson: Clinical management of bovine foot problems. JAVMA 181:572–577, 1982.

Redding, W.R.: Ultrasonographic imaging of the structures of the digital flexor tendon sheath. Compend. Contin. Educ. 13:1824–1832, 1991.

Saber, A.S., A.E. Bolbol, and B. Schenk-Saber: A radiographic study of the development of the sheep carpus from birth to 18 months of age. Vet. Radiol. 30:189–192, 1989.

Sack, W.O., and W. Cottrell: Puncture of shoulder, elbow and carpal joints in goats and sheep. JAVMA 185:63–65, 1984.

Semevolos, S.A., A.J. Nixon, L.R. Goodrich, and N.G. Ducharme: Shoulder joint luxation in large animals: 14 cases (1976–1997). JAVMA 213:1608–1611, 1998.

Singh, S.S., W.R. Ward, and R.D. Murray: An angiographic evaluation of vascular changes in sole lesions in the hooves of cattle. Br. Vet. J. 150:41–52, 1994.

Tulleners, E.P.: Metcarpal and metatarsal fractures in dairy cattle. JAVMA 189:463–468, 1986.

Vaughan, L.C.: Peripheral nerve injuries: An experimental study in cattle. Vet. Rec. 76:1293–1300, 1964.

Weaver, A.D.: The bovine interdigital space. Vet. Rec. 93:132, 1973.

Weaver, A.D.: Performing amputation of the bovine digit. Vet. Med. 86:1230–1233, 1993.

Wegener, K.M., N.I. Heje, F.M. Aarestrup, et al: The morphology of synovial grooves *(Fossae synoviales)* in joints of cattle of different age groups. J. Vet. Med. A. 40:359–370, 1993.

West, D.M.: Anatomical considerations of the distal interphalangeal joint of sheep. N.Z. Vet. J. 31:58–60, 1983.

CHAPTER 33

# The Hindlimb of the Ruminants

The angular appearance of the hindquarters of cattle is due in part to the robust formation of the *pelvic girdle,* much of which is outlined below the skin, and in part to the weak development of the muscles of the *croup.* The sacral tuber is palpable to the side of the lumbosacral space even though it fails to reach the height of the sacral crest. (Its occasional elevation above the crest prompts suspicion of sacroiliac dislocation.) This tuber is joined to the much more prominent coxal tuber ("hook bone") by the iliac crest, which is only thinly—and incompletely—covered by the gluteus medius (Figs. 33–1 and 33–2). The triangular ischial tuber ("pin bone") is raised considerably above the pelvic floor and projects largely or wholly above the vulva. Its subcutaneous dorsal angle is joined by the sacrosciatic ligament; since the edge of this ligament is not covered by muscle it is readily palpable (Fig. 33–3/1′ and Plate 30/*H,I*), a convenience when checking for the softening that indicates impending parturition.

The line connecting coxal and ischial tubers reveals the slope of the pelvis measured against the horizon. An angle larger than usual is associated with a more upright pelvic inlet; a smaller angle (flattened rump) requires the femur to be carried more vertically, a conformation thought to predispose to concussive trauma of the hip joint. Neither inspection nor palpation directly reveals the position of this joint, which must be deduced by reference to the palpable greater trochanter; this is situated lateral and slightly caudal to the femoral head, below the intertuberal line (Fig. 33–3/2). Disturbance of this relationship suggests fracture of the neck or dislocation of the head of the femur. Dislocation may occur in several directions and is thought to be facilitated by the relative weakness, occasional absence, of the sole intra-articular ligament (lig. capitis). Most commonly the trochanter is displaced dorsocranially to project above the intertuberal line. Although nominally a ball-and-socket joint, the extension of the femoral articular surface onto the semicylindrical neck makes it evident that flexion and extension must be the principal movements. However, the degree of outward rotation of the thigh that accompanies flexion ensures that the stifle is carried free of the abdomen. The cavity of the joint may be reached by entering a needle directly in front of the trochanter and advancing it medially and slightly cranially. The deep location and contractions of the muscle pierced en route makes the procedure difficult to accomplish successfully.

The angle between the pelvic and vertebral axes is much reduced in sheep and goats. Other differences, though considerable, are of little practical importance.

The most striking features of the regional muscles are the relative weakness of the gluteal group and the absence of vertebral origins of the semitendinosus and semimembranosus. The gluteus superficialis is wholly incorporated within the biceps to form the combination sometimes known as gluteobiceps. The gluteus medius possesses a well-defined deep division (gluteus accessorius) with its own insertion tendon that enjoys the protection of a synovial bursa where it passes lateral to the greater trochanter. This bursa is occasionally inflamed. The biceps fills the caudolateral part of the thigh and has a wide insertion spread between the fascia lata, patella, lateral patellar ligament, and, via the crural fascia, the tibia and calcaneus. A large bicipital bursa intervenes between the lateral epicondyle of the femur and the part of the insertion proceeding to the patellar ligament. The bursa, which may communicate with the stifle joint cavity is sometimes the site of a painful inflammation, most often encountered in cattle required to rest on bare concrete. The insertions of the semitendinosus and semimembranosus follow the usual pattern and the three hamstring muscles principally act by extending the hip, stifle, and hock joints during the support phase of the stride, so providing the main propulsive force.

The adductor muscles of the medial thigh, the deep group about the hip joint, and the quadriceps femoris require no special notice (Fig. 33–4). The tensor fasciae latae at the cranial margin of the

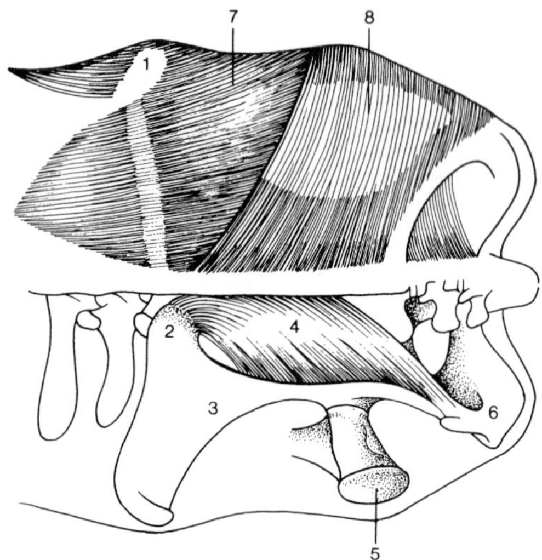


**Figure 33–1.** Dorsal view of the bovine croup; the muscles on the left side have been removed.

1, Coxal tuber; 2, sacral tuber; 3, ilium; 4, sacrosciatic ligament; 5, greater trochanter of femur; 6, ischial tuber; 7, gluteus medius; 8, biceps.

thigh is a guide to the location of the subiliac lymph node.

## THE STIFLE, LEG, AND HOCK

The stifle joint resembles that of the horse in possessing three patellar ligaments and an asymmetrical trochlea (Fig. 33–5/*B*). The patella, patellar ligaments, and tibial tuberosity can be palpated on its cranial surface; two palpable "dimples" at the proximal end of the tuberosity separate and conveniently identify the three ligaments. The prominent femoral epicondyle, collateral ligament (and its attachment to the rudimentary fibula; /*A*,9), and, more cranially, the common origin of the long digital extensor and peroneus tertius (/5) are palpable on the lateral aspect. As in the horse, the intermediate patellar ligament, the patella, a medial fibrocartilage, and the medial patellar ligament combine to form a loop that passes over the expanded proximal end of the medial ridge (/*B*,11) of the femoral trochlea. Although relatively little muscular effort keeps the loop in place, preventing flexion of the stifle, the mechanism is by no means as efficient as that of the horse, in which the stifle can be fully locked. Lateral and medial luxations of the patella are occasionally reported. Dorsal dislocation—better described as fixation—is more common, indeed relatively prevalent among working bullocks of the Indian subcontinent. The condition is usually intermittent and if not relieved spontaneously may be treated by section of the medial patellar ligament.

The femoropatellar and medial femorotibial joint cavities always communicate, but the lateral

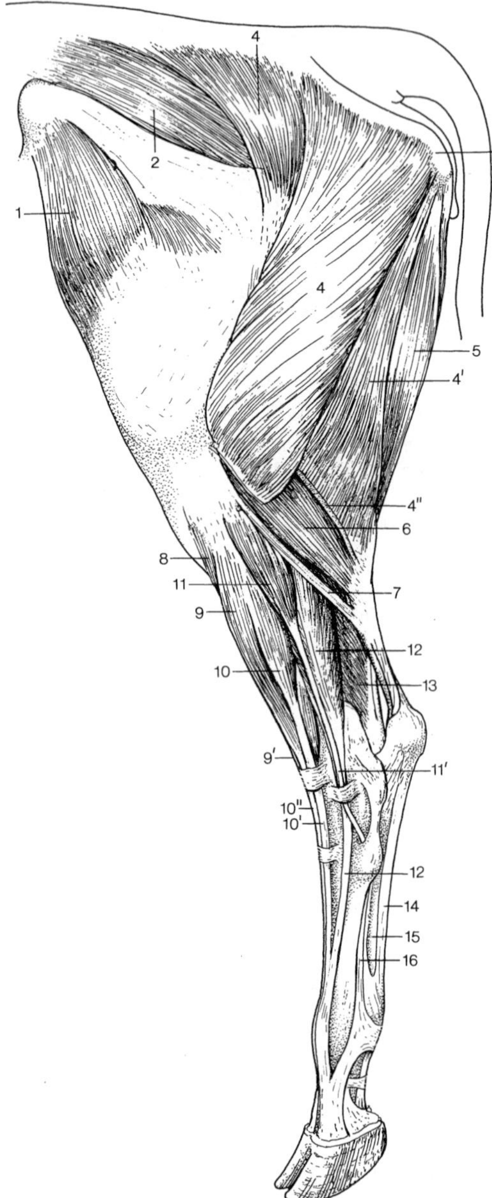


**Figure 33–2.** Muscles of the bovine left hindlimb; lateral view.

1, Tensor fasciae latae; 2, gluteus medius; 3, ischial tuber; 4, 4′, 4″, biceps, transected at 4″; 5, semitendinosus; 6, lateral head of gastrocnemius; 7, rudimentary soleus; 8, tibialis cranialis; 9, 9′, peroneus tertius; 10, 10′, 10″, long digital extensor; 11, 11′, peroneus longus; 12, lateral digital extensor; 13, lateral digital flexor; 14, tendon of superficial digital flexor; 15, combined tendon of deep digital flexors; 16, interosseus.

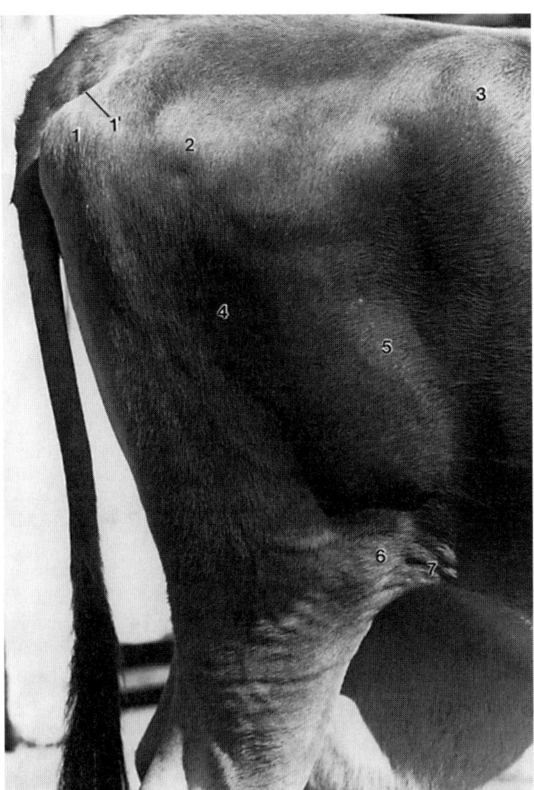


**Figure 33–3.** Right bovine thigh.

1, Ischial tuber; 1′, sacrotuberous part of sacrosciatic ligament; 2, greater trochanter of femur; 3, coxal tuber; 4, biceps; 5, lateral vastus; 6, patella; 7, flank fold.

femorotibial joint does not communicate with either of the other two. Two puncture sites are therefore in use. One, between the medial and intermediate patellar ligaments a short distance proximal to the tibia, gives access to the femoropatellar space; the other, in the extensor groove of the tibia cranial to the common tendon of the long digital extensor and peroneus tertius, provides access to the lateral femorotibial compartment.

The *tibia* is the only weight-bearing bone of the leg (crus). Its medial surface, including the prominent medial malleolus, is subcutaneous; the remaining surfaces are covered by muscle (Fig. 33–7). The distal articular surface (cochlea) presents two sagittal grooves separated by a ridge; each groove is bounded externally by the corresponding malleolus. The *fibula* is much reduced. A proximal rudiment, generally drawn into a distal point, is fused with the lateral condyle of the tibia and receives the lateral collateral ligament of the stifle. The distal rudiment is a separate (and palpable) quadrilateral bone (lateral malleolus; Fig. 33–6/2) that articulates securely with the tibia by means of an interlocking spike and groove. It also takes part in the formation of the hock joint.

The tarsal skeleton is formed by the following elements: calcaneus and talus in the proximal row; fused central and fourth bones in the intermediate row; and fused second and third bones, and a small independent first bone, in the distal row (see Fig. 2–58). In marked contrast to that of the horse, the *talus* carries a trochlea at each end (as in artiodactyls generally; Fig. 33–6/4′,4″). The proximal trochlea articulates with the tibial cochlea and malleolar bone, forming the tarsocrural joint; the distal trochlea articulates with the calcaneus behind and the fused central and fourth tarsal bones distally, forming the proximal intertarsal joint. Both joints allow flexion and extension, the principal movements at the hock, the proximal joint having the greater excursions. The *calcaneus,* more slender than the equine bone, has an additional articulation with the lateral malleolus. The tuber calcanei (point of hock) is slightly expanded. The combined central and fourth tarsals (/5) spans the breadth of the hock. The part provided by the fourth tarsal extends into the distal row and articulates with the metatarsal bone. It is related to the fused second and third bones on its medial side. The small first tarsal lies on the plantar aspect of the joint. The surfaces of the distal elements that concur in the formation of the

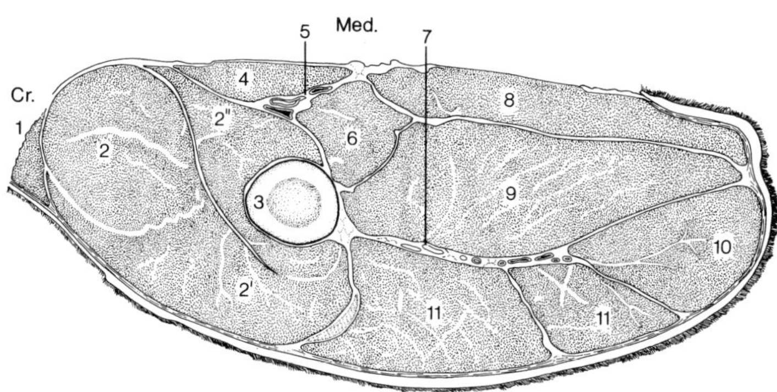


**Figure 33–4.** Transverse section of the bovine left thigh.

1, Tensor fasciae latae; 2, rectus femoris; 2′, 2″, vastus lateralis and medialis; 3, femur; 4, sartorius; 5, femoral vessels; 6, pectineus and adductor; 7, sciatic nerve (branching into tibial and peroneal nerves); 8, gracilis; 9, semimembranosus; 10, semitendinosus; 11, biceps.

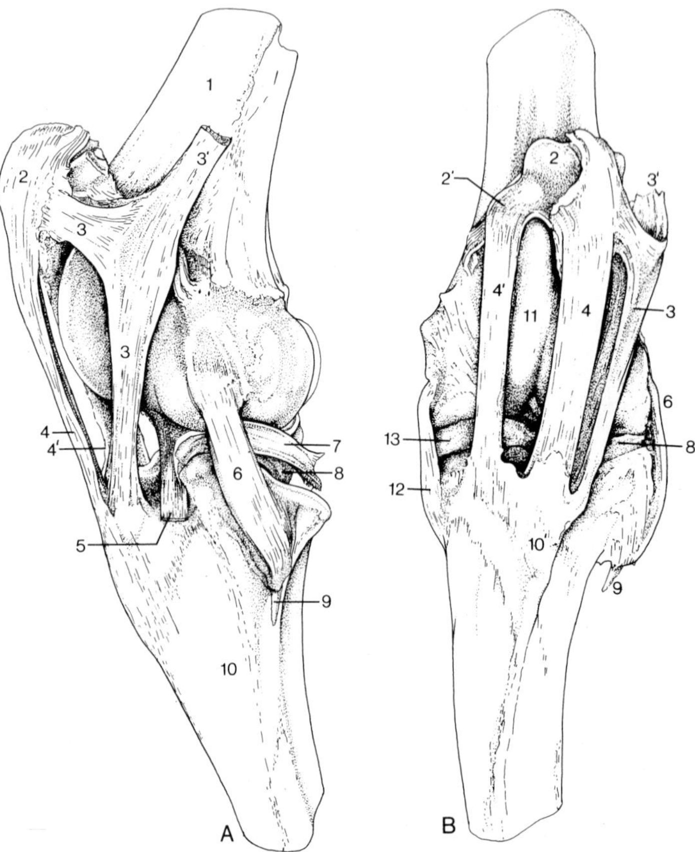


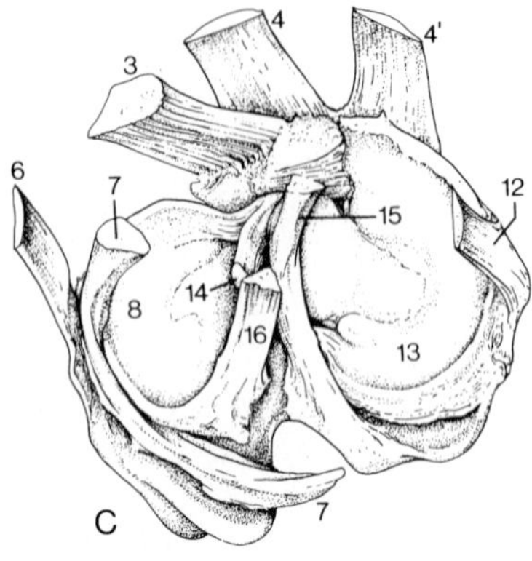


**Figure 33–5.** The left bovine stifle joint. *A*, Lateral view. *B*, Cranial view. *C*, The menisci and ligaments attaching on the proximal end of the left tibia.

1, Femur; 2, patella; 2′, fibrocartilage of patella; 3, lateral patellar ligament; 3′, attachment of biceps; 4, intermediate patellar ligament; 4′, medial patellar ligament; 5, combined tendon of long digital extensor and peroneus tertius; 6, lateral collateral ligament; 7, tendon of popliteus; 8, lateral meniscus; 9, fibula; 10, tibia; 10′, tibial tuberosity; 11, medial ridge of femoral trochlea; 12, medial collateral ligament; 13, medial meniscus; 14, cranial cruciate ligament; 15, caudal cruciate ligament; 16, meniscofemoral ligament.

distal intertarsal and tarsometatarsal joints are relatively flat and permit minimal movement. A small discoid sesamoid bone on the plantar surface of the metatarsal bone is embedded in the proximal part of the interosseus (/7).

Few of the many ligaments are individually important. The joint is supported on each side by collateral ligaments whose long components may be palpated in their full extents from the respective malleolus to the metatarsus. The long plantar ligament (palpable on the plantaromedial aspect) follows the plantar border of the calcaneus and extends beyond this to the metatarsus; it unites the bones on the plantar aspect that would otherwise be pulled apart by the powerful muscles attaching on the point of the hock.

The tarsocrural and proximal intertarsal articulations share a common and relatively capacious cavity. When enlarged, the capsule pouches noticeably on the dorsomedial aspect of the hock, medial to the tibialis cranialis tendon and directly distal to the medial malleolus. It can be punctured more safely than in the horse since the pouch is not overlain by a vein. The other joints are rarely of clinical concern.

The conformation of the hindlimb, particularly the hock, is important in the selection of animals for breeding. The points of the hock should be vertically below the ischial tubers in both lateral and caudal views. If they are too close the animal is said to be "cow-hocked" and its feet assume a wide stance. An adaptation to an overlarge udder is one cause of an exaggerated approximation of the points of the hocks. (The opposite bowlegged conformation brings the feet close together.) The normal angle of the hock joint (viewed from the side) is about 140 degrees, which gives the metatarsus a slightly forward inclination. When the angle is noticeably smaller, the hock sinks and the animal is said to be "sickle-hocked"; when it exceeds the normal, the animal is said to be "straight-hocked," a defect that may lead to "weak pasterns" because of the reduced angle at the fetlock joint. Abnormal postures of the hock cause faulty footing and risk damage to the tendons and synovial structures of the digits.

The *muscles of the leg* are divided into the usual craniolateral and caudal groups. Among the former, the tibialis cranialis and peroneus tertius broadly resemble those of the horse (Fig. 33–2/8,9); the peroneus tertius, though largely tendinous, is yet significantly fleshier than its equine equivalent. The long digital extensor resembles the common extensor of the forelimb in possessing two bellies, one that supplies the tendon proper to the medial digit and a second, smaller one whose tendon splits to reach both digits. A lateral extensor (/12), proper to the lateral digit, completes the group (as in the forelimb). All extensor tendons are of necessity held in place by (two) stout, palpable retention bands where they descend over the flexor surface of the hock; equally necessarily, they are protected here by synovial sheaths. The proximal retinaculum is easily palpated even in heavy, thick-skinned cows. The group is completed by a peroneus longus muscle (/11) that arises near the lateral collateral ligament of the stifle and descends on the lateral side of the leg. It then crosses over the tendon of the lateral digital extensor to wind around to the plantar aspect of the hock where it inserts. Some inward rotation of the foot is produced by its contraction.

The *gastrocnemius* (/6) arises by twin heads from the caudal surface of the femur and forms a muscular swelling at the upper end of the leg before narrowing abruptly to the strong tendon that inserts on the point of the hock.

The *superficial digital flexor,* though more muscular than that of the horse, is very tendinous and relatively inextensible (Fig. 33–7/14). It arises between the heads of the gastrocnemius, winds around the medial surface of that muscle's tendon, and spreads to cap the point of the hock. The edges of the cap attach here, but the bulk of the tendon continues down the plantar surface into the foot. The crural segment, acting in concert with the peroneus tertius, links the movements of the stifle and hock joints. (This needs to be kept in mind when attempting to correct the relatively common breech position of a fetus that presents the tail and flexed hocks.) An extensive subtendinous (calcanean) bursa protects the tendon both where it wraps around the gastrocnemius and again over the point of the hock. Occasionally a

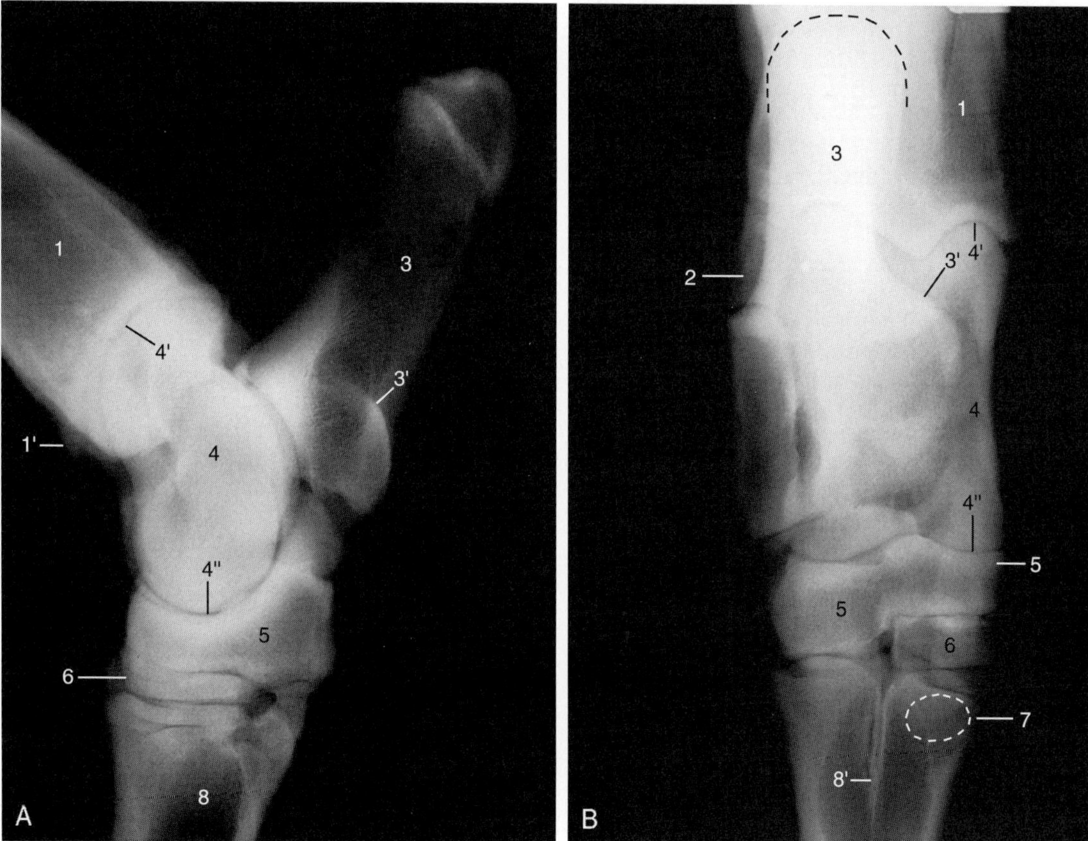


**Figure 33–6.** Lateral *(A)* and dorsoplantar *(B)* radiographs of the bovine hock.

1, Tibia; 1′, medial malleolus; 2, lateral malleolus (distal end of fibula); 3, calcaneus; 3′, sustentaculum tali; 4, talus; 4′, 4″, proximal and distal trochlea of talus; 5, fused central and 4th tarsal bones; 6, fused 2nd and 3rd tarsal bones, in *B* superimposed on small 1st tarsal bone (not labeled); 7, position of sesamoid bone in interosseus; 8, metatarsal bone; 8′, median septum.

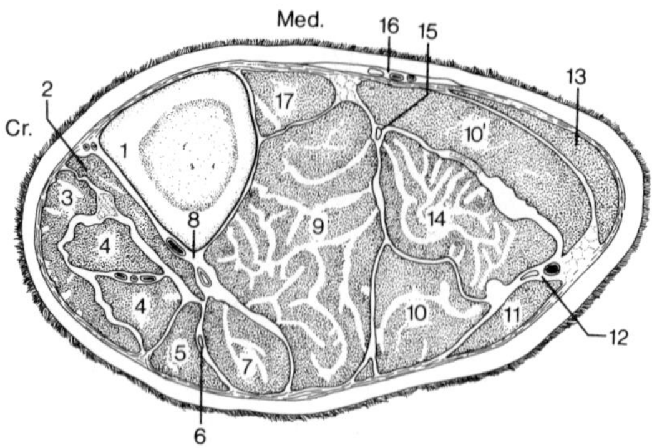


**Figure 33–7.** Transverse section of the left bovine leg.

1, Tibia; 2, tibialis cranialis; 3, peroneus tertius; 4, long digital extensor; 5, peroneus longus; 6, peroneal nerve; 7, lateral digital extensor; 8, cranial tibial vessels; 9, deep digital flexors; 10, 10′, lateral and medial heads of gastrocnemius; 11, biceps; 12, caudal cutaneous sural nerve and lateral saphenous vein; 13, semitendinosus; 14, superficial digital flexor; 15, tibial nerve; 16, saphenous vessels and nerve; 17, popliteus.

subcutaneous bursa (hygroma) develops over the tendon here.

Gastrocnemius and superficial flexor are in a continuous (reflex) state of contraction in calves with "spastic paresis." In these animals the hock and stifle are maximally extended, and the affected limb is used stiffly with only the toes of the hoofs touching the ground (Plate 27/*F*). Section of the tendons (or of the [tibial] nerve branches to the gastrocnemius) gives relief. Although there is no proof of inheritance, it is generally agreed that it is unwise to breed from affected animals even after surgical "cure."

The deep digital flexor (/9) has three heads. Two come together in the leg to form a thick tendon that passes over the plantar surface of the hock medial to the calcaneus, protected by the tarsal synovial sheath. The tendon is here bound down by the flexor retinaculum and other deep fasciae so that when distended the sheath bulges only at its ends, proximal and distal to the joint. The thin tendon of the third head tunnels through the dense medial tarsal fascia, within its own synovial investment, to join the major tendon in the metatarsus. The *popliteus* has no special features.

Most locomotor and cutaneous structures of the hindfoot are very similar to their forelimb counterparts and need not be described. However, the metatarsal bone is noticeably longer than the metacarpal and is quadrilateral in transverse section, giving the hind cannon a deeper appearance in lateral view (Fig. 33–13). The higher incidence of disease in the digits of the hindlimb, especially the lateral one, has not been fully explained.

# THE BLOOD VESSELS AND LYMPHATIC STRUCTURES OF THE HINDLIMB

The femoral artery continues the *external iliac artery* beyond the vascular lacuna. It passes between the medial muscles of the thigh to reach the flexor surface of the stifle where it is renamed the *popliteal artery.* This soon divides into cranial and caudal tibial arteries (Fig. 33–8/10,11). One branch of the femoral, the *saphenous artery* (/7), runs on the surface of the gracilis and is often used for taking the pulse of cows; it is most easily found

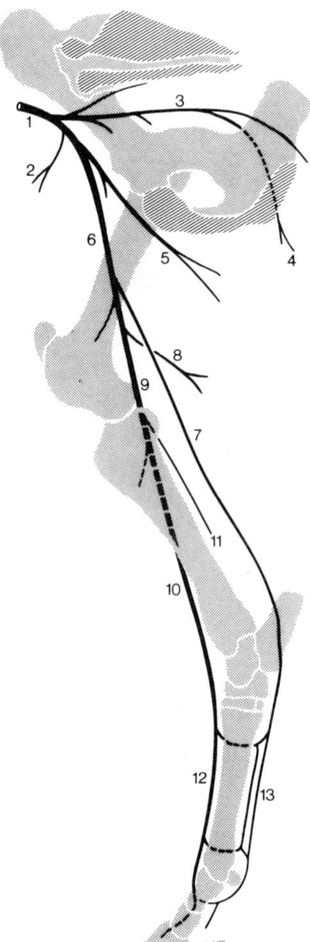


**Figure 33–8.** The principal arteries of the bovine right hindlimb; medial view.

1, External iliac a.; 2, deep circumflex iliac a.; 3, internal iliac a.; 4, caudal gluteal a.; 5, deep femoral a.; 6, femoral a.; 7, saphenous a.; 8, caudal femoral a.; 9, popliteal a.; 10, cranial tibial a.; 11, caudal tibial a.; 12, dorsal metatarsal aa.; 13, medial and lateral plantar, and metatarsal (closer to the bone) aa.

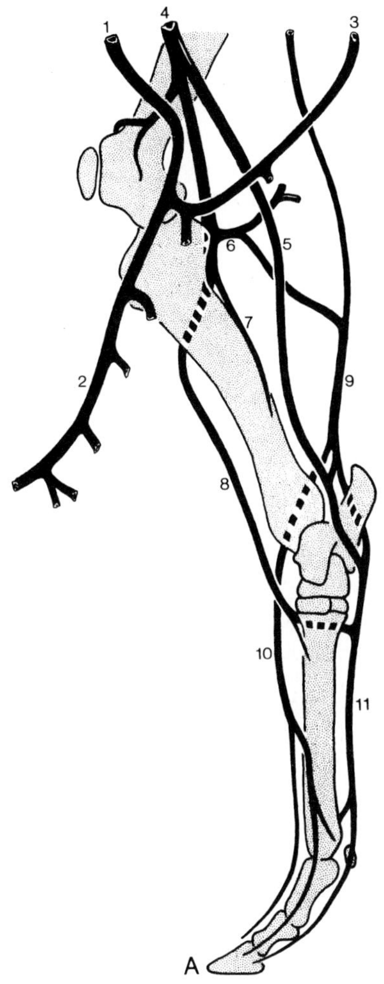


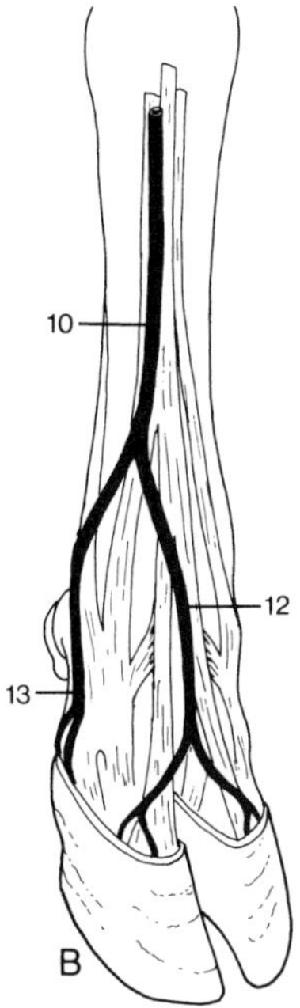


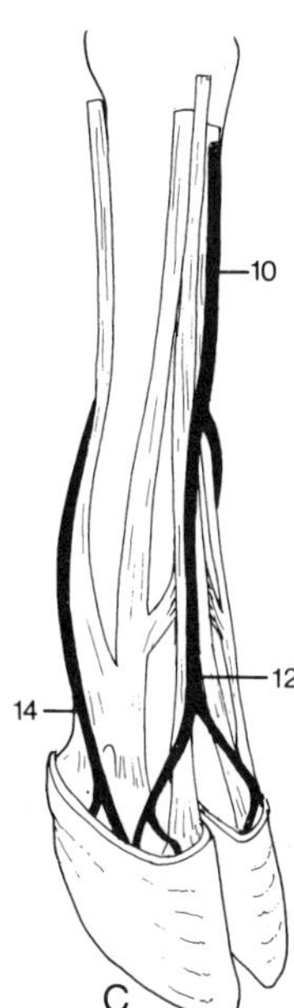


**Figure 33–9.** The major veins of the bovine hindlimb. *A*, Right limb; medial view: *B*, Right hindfoot; dorsolateral view: *C*, Left hindfoot; dorsomedial view.

1, External pudendal v.; 2, cranial mammary v.; 3, ventral labial v.; 4, femoral v.; 5, medial saphenous v.; 6, caudal femoral v.; 7, caudal tibial v.; 8, cranial tibial v.; 9, lateral saphenous v.; 10, cranial tributary of lateral saphenous v.; 11, medial and lateral plantar vv.; 12, dorsal common digital v. III; 13, plantar v. of lateral digit; 14, plantar v. of medial digits.

by sliding the hand from behind, between the udder and thigh. This vessel is responsible for the vascularization of the caudal part of the leg and follows the common calcanean tendon to the hock where it gives rise to medial and lateral plantar arteries.

The *cranial tibial artery* (Fig. 33–7/8), which may be regarded as the continuation of the femoral trunk, runs embedded between the crural muscles to reach the flexor (dorsal) surface of the hock joint under cover of the long digital extensor tendon. The caudal tibial artery is of minor local significance.

Renamed the *dorsal metatarsal artery* (Fig. 33–8/12), the main trunk now sends a perforating artery through the upper part of the metatarsal bone before continuing in the dorsal groove of this bone. A second perforating artery is released toward the fetlock. The perforating branches join the plantar arteries and are also connected by small deeper vessels. The plantar arteries resemble the corresponding forelimb vessels. One branch of the medial plantar artery crosses the plantar surface of the medial tendon of the superficial flexor proximal to the fetlock, and is here liable to injury. This branch continues into the interdigital space where it anastomoses with the main trunk. The anastomosis is substantial and winds around below the proximal interdigital ligament where it is encountered in amputation of a digit. The axial surfaces of the digits are supplied by branches arising from the anastomosis, the abaxial surfaces by direct continuations of the plantar arteries.

The very number and frequent anastomoses of other side branches deprive them of individual significance.

The *veins* are divided between a deep system satellite to the arteries and a few superficial vessels that follow independent courses (Fig. 33–9). The superficial vessels comprise the medial and lateral saphenous veins and their tributaries. The larger *lateral saphenous vein* (/9) arises from two tributaries; one ascends with the extensor tendons and superficial peroneal nerve and crosses on the dorsolateral aspect of the hock; the other ascends with the lateral plantar artery from a subcutaneous origin on the lateral digit and follows the flexor tendons under cover of the deep fascia to cross the joint plantarolaterally. The lateral saphenous vein (Fig. 33–10/1) raises a ridge below the skin as it crosses to the caudal border of the leg and then follows the curvature of the gastrocnemius, eventually to open into the femoral vein. The *medial saphenous vein* (Fig. 33–9/5) is also formed by two tributaries. The more important caudal one takes its origin from the abaxial aspect of the medial digit, ascends with the medial plantar artery, and passes the hock plantaromedially. The medial saphenous vein ascends together with the palpable saphenous artery on the medial aspect of the leg; above the stifle it dips between the gracilis and sartorius muscles to join the femoral vein.

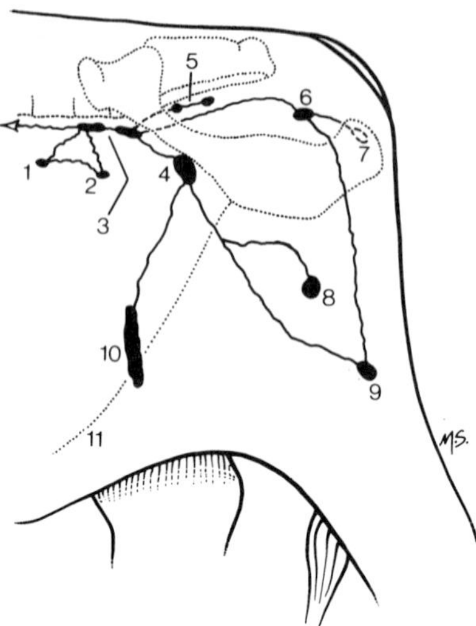


**Figure 33–11.** The lymph nodes of the bovine pelvis and hindlimb.

1, Lateral iliac l.n.; 2, coxal l.n.; 3, medial iliac and sacral l.nn.; 4, deep inguinal l.n.; 5, gluteal l.n.; 6, ischial l.n.; 7, tuberal l.n.; 8, superficial inguinal (mammary) l.n.; 9, popliteal l.n.; 10, subiliac l.n.; 11, linea alba.

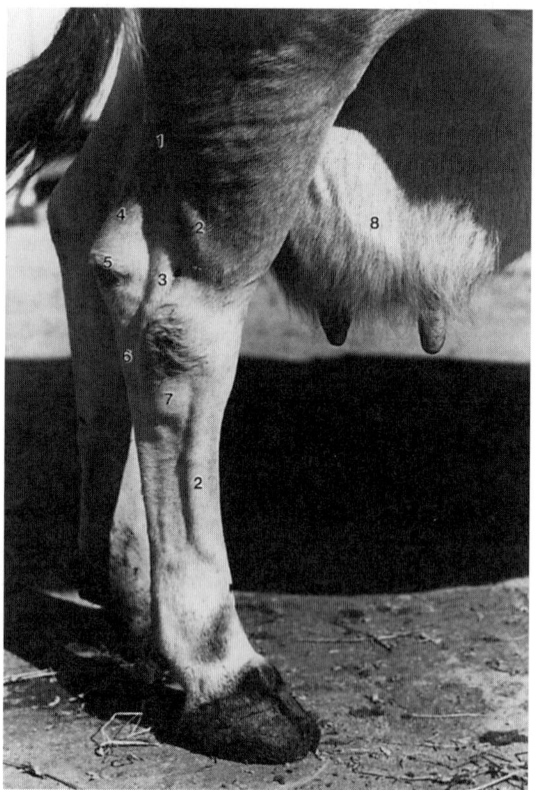


**Figure 33–10.** Right bovine hindfoot, lateral view.

1, Lateral saphenous vein (in shadow; compare with Fig. 33–9/9); 2, cranial tributary of lateral saphenous vein; 3, caudal tributary of lateral saphenous vein; 4, common calcanean tendon; 5, calcanean tuber; 6, superficial digital flexor tendon; 7, fused central and 4th tarsal bones; 8, udder.

The superficial veins (/B,C) may be raised by application of a tourniquet below the hock for injection of local anesthetic in order to desensitize the digits.

The *lymph nodes* include the popliteal node within the popliteal fossa and the very large subiliac node described with the abdominal wall (Fig. 33–11/9,10). A small coxal node ventral to the coxal tuber and a group of gluteal nodes on the lateral surface of the sacrosciatic ligament are also commonly present (/2,5). An ischial node (/6) that lies on the ligament just dorsal to the lesser sciatic foramen can be inspected in the split carcass by incising the ligament from within the pelvis. A tuberal node (/7) lies medial to the ischial tuber within the ischiorectal fossa.

The *popliteal node* collects from the distal part of the limb, including most of the leg, and sends its efferent vessels along two routes: one follows the sciatic nerve to the ischial node, while the second accompanies the femoral vessels to the large, deep inguinal node (/4) at the side of the pelvic inlet. The *subiliac node* drains the skin over the thigh and stifle in addition to the flank; its efferents also go chiefly to the deep inguinal node. The smaller nodes are only of local significance.

# THE NERVES OF THE HINDLIMB

## The Branches of the Lumbosacral Plexus

The lumbosacral plexus is formed from the nerves L4–S2.

The *obturator nerve* (L4–6) crosses the ventral surface of the sacroiliac joint, runs medial to the shaft of the ilium, and penetrates the obturator foramen to reach the medial muscles of the thigh (Fig. 33–12/1). It is vulnerable where it lies against bone, and the most common cause of obturator paralysis is compression during parturition. Conduction is rarely completely interrupted in this injury; cows can still stand and, on rough ground, walk even when both nerves have been damaged. However, they are unable to prevent their feet from sliding sideways on smooth floors and, once down, are often unable to rise (Plate 27/*G*). It is possible that the role of obturator nerve injury in postparturient paralysis (the "downer cow" syndrome) has been exaggerated, with insufficient attention directed toward traumatic or ischemic injury to the muscles ventral to the pelvis (the adductors in the broad sense) as alternative or aggravating causes. These muscles may suffer from compression, directly or through constriction of the arterial supply (deep and caudal femoral arteries), when recumbency is prolonged.

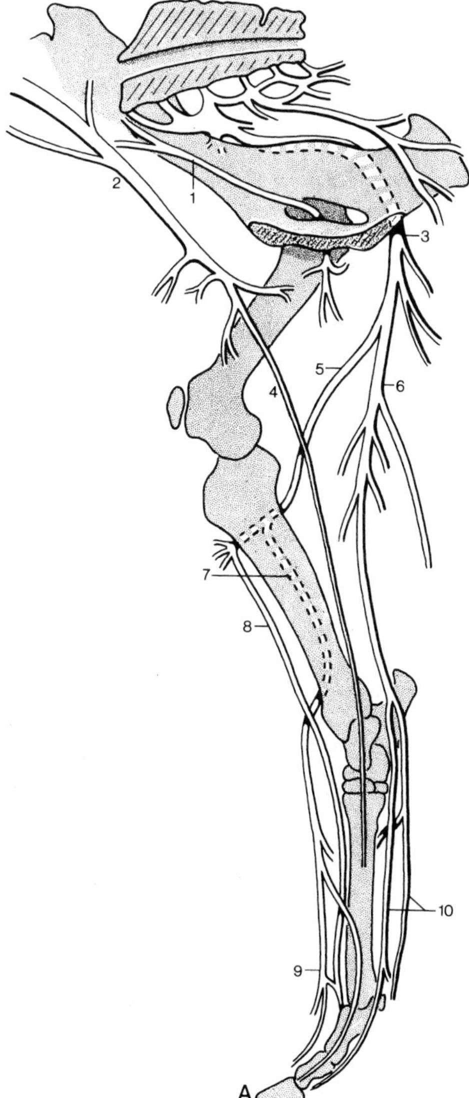


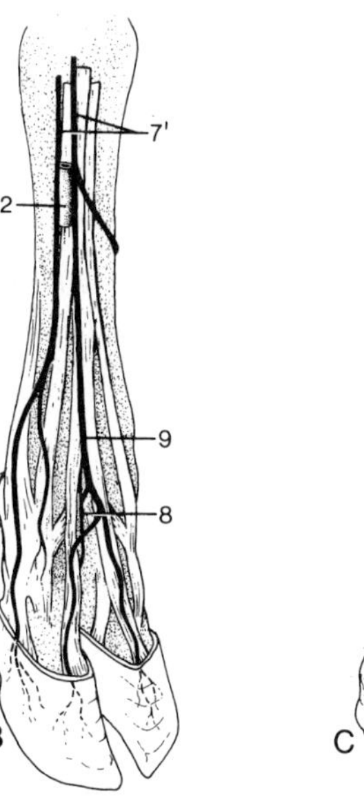


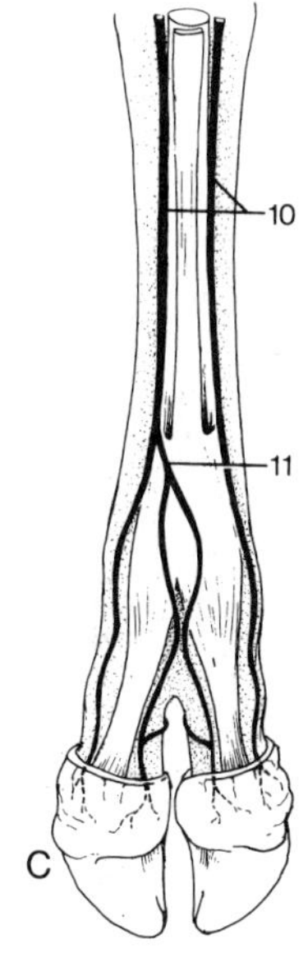


**Figure 33–12.** Nerves of the right bovine hindlimb. *A*, Medial view. *B*, Right hindfoot; dorsolateral view. *C*, Right hindfoot; plantar view.

1, Obturator n.; 2, femoral n.; 3, sciatic n.; 4, saphenous n.; 5, common peroneal n.; 6, tibial n.; 7, superficial peroneal n.; 7′, lateral and middle branches of superficial peroneal n.; 8, deep peroneal n.; 9, dorsal common digital n. III; 10, medial and lateral plantar nn.; 11, plantar common digital n. III; 12, cranial tributary of lateral saphenous vein.

The *femoral nerve* (also L4–6) (Fig. 33–12/2) has a very short course within the thigh; it ramifies within the quadriceps after detaching the saphenous branch. This supplies the skin over the medial surface of the limb (from mid-thigh to midmetatarsus). Damage to the femoral nerve is occasionally recognized in newborn calves delivered by strong traction on the hindlimbs. The affected limb is unable to bear weight; the diagnosis is confirmed by the loss of sensation in the appropriate area of skin.

On leaving the pelvis, the *sciatic nerve* (L6–S2) passes around the dorsal and caudal aspects of the hip joint before supplying the caudal thigh muscles. Its course between the biceps and semimembranosus, a few centimeters caudal to the femur, exposes it to risk of damage from intramuscular injection (Fig. 33–4/7). It divides into the tibial and common peroneal nerves before reaching the gastrocnemius. These share the responsibility for the innervation of all structures distal to the stifle (excepting only the medial skin). The sciatic nerve may also be injured during parturition of a large or ill-positioned fetus. When the lesion is severe, the affected limb hangs loose with the stifle and hock joints extended, the digital joints flexed, and the foot knuckled. Cutaneous sensation is lost over the entire extremity except in the area supplied by the saphenous nerve.

The *tibial nerve* (L6–S2) passes between the heads of the gastrocnemius a short distance cranial to the popliteal lymph node. It immediately detaches branches to the caudal crural muscles (Fig. 33–12/6); certain of these are severed in the treatment of spastic paresis (see earlier). The main trunk, now purely sensory continues toward the hock: it can be palpated in front of the common calcanean tendon (and blocked here). It divides opposite the point of the hock into medial and lateral plantar nerves, which accompany the deep flexor tendon distally. Their distribution within the foot is described later. Severe lesions of the tibial nerve manifest themselves by a pronounced overflexion of the hock and extension of the fetlock, producing a vertical pastern. As the innervation of the digital extensors remains intact, the hoofs are correctly set down when the animal walks and they continue to carry their share of the weight. The anomalous position of the joints becomes exaggerated at the walk.

The *common peroneal nerve* (L6–S2) (/5) crosses the lateral surface of the gastrocnemius under cover of the biceps before becoming superficial and palpable (and vulnerable) as it passes caudal to the lateral collateral ligament of the stifle. It then dives between the peroneus longus and lateral digital extensor muscles before dividing into superficial and deep branches (Fig. 33–7/6). The *superficial peroneal nerve,* the larger of the two, crosses the deep surface of the peroneus longus to re-emerge lateral to the long digital extensor tendon. It reaches the foot by crossing the dorsal aspect of the hock accompanied by the extensor tendons and the (palpable) cranial tributary of the lateral saphenous vein. The *deep peroneal nerve* (Fig. 33–12/8) supplies the cranial crural muscles among which it is embedded. It continues along the lateral edge of the tibialis cranialis, enters the foot deep to the long digital extensor tendon, and gains the groove on the dorsal surface of the cannon bone. The accounts of the two peroneal nerves are continued later. Paralysis of the peroneal nerve is betrayed by hyperextension of the hock and hyperflexion of the fetlock and digital joints (Plate 27/*C*). Unless passively placed in the correct position the limb rests on the dorsal surface of the flexed digits. The animal eventually learns to correct this by flicking the foot forward when walking.

## The Innervation of the Hindfoot

The superficial and deep branches of the peroneal and the medial and lateral plantar branches of the tibial all continue beyond the hock (Fig. 33–12/*B,C*). The branching pattern resembles that of the forefoot in that the dorsal aspect of the digits is the province of the peroneal nerve while, with some overlapping to the sides, the plantar aspect is that of the tibial.

The *superficial peroneal nerve* gives rise to three branches that in midmetatarsus lie dorsolateral to the three extensor tendons. The medial branch inclines to the side and enters the medial digit between the metatarsal bone and the interosseus. The larger middle branch (/*B*,9) splits at the fetlock to supply the axial parts of both digits. The lateral branch follows a similar course into the lateral digit as that adopted medially.

The smaller *deep peroneal nerve* shares the groove on the dorsal surface of the metatarsal bone with the principal artery to the foot; both are protected by the covering extensor tendons (/*B*,8). The nerve turns into the interdigital space and, after accepting a communication from the middle branch of the superficial nerve, divides into two branches that join the axial plantar nerves (see further on).

The *medial and lateral plantar nerves* (/*C*,10) course in the grooves between the deep flexor tendon and interosseus under cover of the thick metatarsal fascia. The smaller lateral nerve simply continues into the lateral digit. The medial nerve

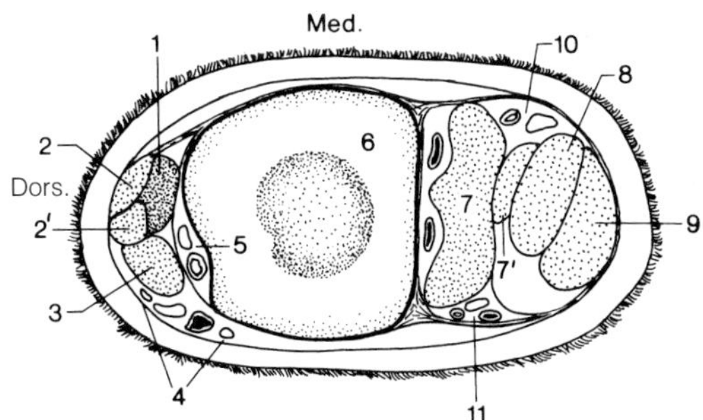


**Figure 33–13.** Transverse section of the bovine left cannon.

1, Extensor brevis; 2, 2′, long digital extensor; 3, lateral digital extensor; 4, branches of superficial peroneal nerve and cranial tributary of lateral saphenous vein; 5, deep peroneal nerve and dorsal metatarsal artery (continuation of cranial tibial); 6, metatarsal bone; 7, interosseus; 7′, band from interosseus to superficial digital flexor; 8, deep digital flexor; 9, superficial digital flexor; 10, 11, medial and lateral plantar nerves and vessels.

divides above the fetlock into a small branch for the medial digit and a common trunk (/11) for the two axial nerves. These are joined by the interdigital branches from the deep peroneal nerve.

Satisfactory anesthesia of the hind digits can be obtained by injecting at four sites. First, lateral and middle branches of the superficial peroneal nerve are reached dorsolaterally, in the upper half of the metatarsus where they are subcutaneous to each side of the cranial tributary of the lateral saphenous vein; the middle branch may be palpated against the extensor tendons (Fig. 33–13/4). Secondly, the deep peroneal nerve (/5) can also be reached here by passing the needle between the extensor tendons and the metatarsal bone to reach the dorsal groove. (Alternatively, the needle may be inserted into the interdigital space, just distal to the fetlock to a depth of 1 cm.) Thirdly and fourthly, medial and lateral plantar nerves are reached in the upper half of the metatarsus in the grooves between the deep flexor tendon and interosseus, deep to the heavy fascia (/10,11).

## Selected Bibliography

Allen, M.J., J.E.F. Houlton, S.B. Adams, and N. Rushton: The surgical anatomy of the stifle joint in sheep. Vet. Surg. 27:596–605, 1998.

Arighi, M., N.G. Ducharme, F.D. Horney, and P.W. Pennock: Proximal intertarsal subluxation in three Holstein-Friesian heifers. Can. Vet. J. 28:710–712, 1987.

Aron, D.N., and P.T. Purinton: Collateral ligaments of the tarsocrural joint—an anatomic and functional study. Vet. Surg. 14:173–177, 1985.

Ashdown, R.R., and S. Done: Color Atlas of Veterinary Anatomy: The Ruminants. Baltimore, University Park Press; and London, Gower Medical Publishing Ltd., 1984.

Baird, A.N., K.L. Angel, H.D. Moll, et al: Upward fixation of the patella in cattle: 38 cases (1984–1990). JAVMA 202:434–436, 1993.

Bartels, J.E.: Femoral-tibial osteoarthrosis in the Bull: I. Clinical survey and radiologic interpretation. J. Am. Vet. Rad. Soc. 16:151–159, 1975.

Bartels, J.E.: Femoral-tibial osteoarthrosis in the Bull: II. A correlation of the radiographic and pathologic findings of the torn meniscus and ruptured cranial cruciate ligament. J. Am. Vet. Rad. Soc. 16:159–174, 1975.

Baxter, G.M., T.A. Broome, and J. Lakritz: Alternatives to digital amputation in cattle. Comp. Contin. Educ. Pract. Vet. 13:1022–1035, 1991.

Bijleveld, K., and W. Hartman: Electromyographic studies in calves with spastic paralysis. Neth. J. Vet. Sci. 101:805–808, 1976.

Burt, J.K., V.S. Meyers, D.J. Hillman, and R. Getty: The radiographic locations of epiphyseal lines in bovine limbs. JAVMA 152:168–174, 1968.

deLahunta, A., and R.E. Habel: Applied Veterinary Anatomy. Philadelphia, W.B. Saunders Company, 1986.

De Ley, G., and A. De Moor: Bovine spastic paralysis: Results of surgical desafferentation of gastrocnemius muscle by means of spinal dorsal root section. Am. J. Vet. Res. 38:1899–1900, 1977.

Desrochers, A., G. St. Jean, W.C. Cash, et al.: Characterization of anatomic communications between the femoropatellar joint and lateral and medial femorotibial joints in cattle, using intra-articular latex, positive contrast arthrography, and fluoroscopy. Am. J. Vet. Res. 57(6):798–802, 1996.

Ducharme, N.G., M.E. Stanton, and G.R. Ducharme: Stifle lameness in cattle at two veterinary teaching hospitals: A retrospective study of forty-two cases: Can. Vet. J. 26:212–217, 1985.

Ducharme, N.G.: Stifle injuries in cattle. Vet. Clin. of North Am.: Food Animal Pract. 12:59–84, 1996.

Estill, C.T.: Intravenous local anesthesia of the bovine lower leg. Vet. Med. [SAC] 72:1499–1502, 1977.

Gibson, K.T., and C.W. McIlwraith: Identifying and managing stifle disorders that cause hind limb lameness. Vet. Med. 85:188–196, 1990.

Greenough, P.R.: The conformation of cattle. Bovine Pract. 1:20–34, 1980.

Greenough, P.R., F.J. MacCallum, and A.D. Weaver: Lameness in Cattle, 2nd ed. Philadelphia, J.B. Lippincott, 1981.

Habel, R.E.: Guide to the Dissection of the Domestic Ruminants, 4th ed. Ithaca, 1989. [Published by the author.]

Halata, Z., C. Wagner, and K.I. Baumann: Sensory nerve endings in the anterior cruciate ligament (lig. cruciatum anterius) of sheep. Anat. Rec. 254:13–21, 1999.

Knight, A.P.: Intravenous regional anesthesia of the bovine foot. Bovine Pract. 1:11–15, 1980.

Lopez, M.J., D. Wilson, M. Markel: Ligament injury in the bovine stifle. Compend. Contin. Educ. 18:S189–S198, 1996.

Larcombe, M.T., and J. Malmo: Dislocation of the coxofemoral joint in dairy cows. Austral. Vet. J. 66:351–354, 1989.

Madison, J.B., E.P. Tulleners, N.G. Ducharme, et al.: Idiopathic gonitis in heifers: 34 cases (1976–1986). JAVMA 194:273–277, 1989.

McIlwraith, C.W.: Surgery of the hock, stifle, and shoulder. Vet. Clin of. North Am.: LA Pract. 5:333–362, 1983.

Mgasa, M.N., and J. Arnbjerg: Radiographic study of postnatal development of the tarsus in West African Dwarf Goats. Anat. Histol. Embryol. 22:16–25, 1993.

Nelson, D.R., J.C. Huhn, and S.K. Kneller: Peripheral detachment of the medial meniscus with injury to the medial collateral ligament in 50 cattle. Vet. Rec. 85:59–60, 1990.

Nelson, D.R., J.C. Huhn, and S.K. Kneller: Surgical repair of peripheral detachment of the medial meniscus in 34 cattle. Vet. Rec. 85:571–573, 1990.

Paulsen, D.B., J.L. Noordsy, and H.W. Leipold: Femoral nerve paralysis in cattle. Bovine Pract. 2:14–26, 1981.

Pavaux, C., G. Arnault, M. Braussier, and M. Dumont: Triple tenectomy (Götze) as treatment of spastic paresis in cattle. Point Vet. 20:41–50, 1988.

Pavaux, C., J. Sautet, and Y. Lignereux: Anatomy of the bovine gastrocnemius muscle as application to the surgical correction of spastic paresis. Vlaams Diergeneesk. Tijdscrift. 54:296–312, 1985.

Pejsa, T.G., G. St. Jean, G.F. Hoffsis, and J.M.B. Musser: Digit amputation in cattle: 85 cases (1971–1990). JAVMA 202:981–984, 1993.

Ruberte, J., and C. Pavaux: Arterial blood supply of the bovine common calcanean tendon. Revue Méd. Vét. 138:33–44, 1987.

Smallwood, J.E., and M.J. Shively: Radiographic and xeroradiographic anatomy of the bovine tarsus. Bovine Pract. 2:28–45, 1981.

Tryphonas, L., G.F. Hamilton, and C.S. Rhodes: Perinatal femoral nerve degeneration and neurogenic atrophy of quadriceps femoris muscle in calves. JAVMA 164:801–807, 1974.

Tulleners, E.P.: Management of bovine orthopedic problems. Part II. Coxofemoral luxations, soft tissue problems, sepsis, and miscellaneous skull problems. Compend. Cont. Educ. 8:S117–S126, 1986.

Tulleners, E.P.: Metacarpal and metatarsal fractures in dairy cattle. JAVMA 189:463–468, 1986.

Tulleners, E.P., D.M. Nunamaker, and D.W. Richardson: Coxofemoral luxations in cattle: 22 cases (1980–1985). JAVMA 191:569–574, 1987.

Van Pelt, R.W.: Intra-articular treatment of tarsal degenerative joint disease in cattle. JAVMA 166:239–246, 1975.

Vermunt, J.J., and D.H. Leach: A scanning electron microscopic study of the vascular system of the bovine hind limb claw. New Zealand Vet. J. 40:146–154, 1992.

Weaver, A.D.: Performing amputation of the bovine digit. Vet. Med. 86:1230–1233, 1993.

Wegener, K.M., N.I. Heje, F.M. Aarestrup, et al: The morphology of synovial grooves (Fossae synoviales) in joints of cattle of different age groups. J. Vet. Med. A 40:359–370, 1993.

Weisbrode, S.E., D.R. Monke, S.T. Dodaro, and B.L. Hull: Osteochondrosis, degenerative joint disease, and vertebral osteophytosis in middle-aged bulls. JAVMA 181:700–705, 1982.

CHAPTER 34

# The Head and Neck of the Pig

Despite its imposing economic importance, the pig occupies a subordinate position in veterinary anatomical instruction. The reasons for this are to be found in the restriction of surgical procedures to a few regions of the body, in the nature of the animal itself, and in the way that most pigs are kept today. Physical examination is made difficult by a generally unfriendly disposition; young pigs react vociferously to the mildest restraint, while attempts to restrain older ones can be hazardous to the inexperienced. Furthermore, a thick layer of subcutaneous fat provides a formidable barrier to palpation and auscultation.

During the last few decades, the domestic pig has been relegated to a position similar to that of domestic fowl; large herds are kept under intensive husbandry, with the individual animal becoming less and less important and a healthy herd and high production being the overriding goals. Moreover, the pig's short life span (from birth to slaughter in 5 to 6 months) and the limitation of human interference generally protect it from much harm. Veterinary attention is mainly directed toward infectious diseases, reproductive problems, congenital anomalies, and inspection of the carcass after slaughter.

Significant structural and nutritional similarities to the human species have, in recent years, led the pig (including the "mini" variety) to become the subject of much biomedical research. Even so, the detailed anatomy required by the researcher is available for only some areas of the body; such information must be sought in the larger reference texts.*

*Barone, R.: Anatomie comparée des mammiferes domestiques; vols. 1–3. Lyon, Laboratoire d'Anatomie, Ecole Nationale Vétérinaire, 1966–1978; Ellenberger, W., and H. Baum: Handbuch der vergleichenden Anatomie der Haustiere, 18th ed. Berlin, Springer-Verlag, 1943; Getty, R.: Sisson and Grossman's Anatomy of the Domestic Animals. 5th ed., vol. 2. Philadelphia, W.B. Saunders Company, 1975; Montané, L., E. Bourdelle, and C. Bressou: Anatomie régionale des animaux domestiques. Vol. 3, Le Porc, 2nd ed. Paris, J.S. Baillière et Fils, 1964.

## THE SKULL

The skull of the pig varies greatly. It is more or less pyramidal in primitive breeds but sweeps sharply to a great height above the brain in some improved breeds (Figs. 34–1 and 34–2). The high nuchal surface is bounded by thick nuchal crests. The dorsal surface of the cranium is sharply demarcated from the temporal fossa by a prominent temporal line that continues into the zygomatic process of the frontal bone. This process is relatively short and fails to complete the orbital margin. The orbit is small. The zygomatic arch is extremely sturdy and deep, helping to bound the temporal fossa laterally. The articular surface is wide and flat. The fossa (/6) rostral to the orbit defines the origin of the levator labii superioris.

On the basal surface, the cranial and choanal regions are dorsal to the plane of the palate. The cranial region is most remarkable for the very long paracondylar processes (/23) and large tympanic bullae. The choanae are short but wide, particularly well enclosed, and placed far caudally.

The stout, rather rectilinear mandible is solid, the symphysis ossifying about 1 year after birth. Its chin region is cut away as an adaptation to the rooting habit. The coronoid process is short, the condylar process low and triangular.

## EXTERNAL FEATURES AND SUPERFICIAL STRUCTURES

The head and neck of the pig form a cone whose base blends with the trunk at the level of the forelimbs. The dorsal surface of the head is always concave, slightly so in breeds with long skulls, more markedly in those whose skulls are short. This gives the high caudal part of the skull unusual prominence. From here to the shoulders, the head-neck cone has a lesser slope, and in certain breeds it is almost cylindrical but with some lateral compression. The flabby lateroventral parts of the neck,

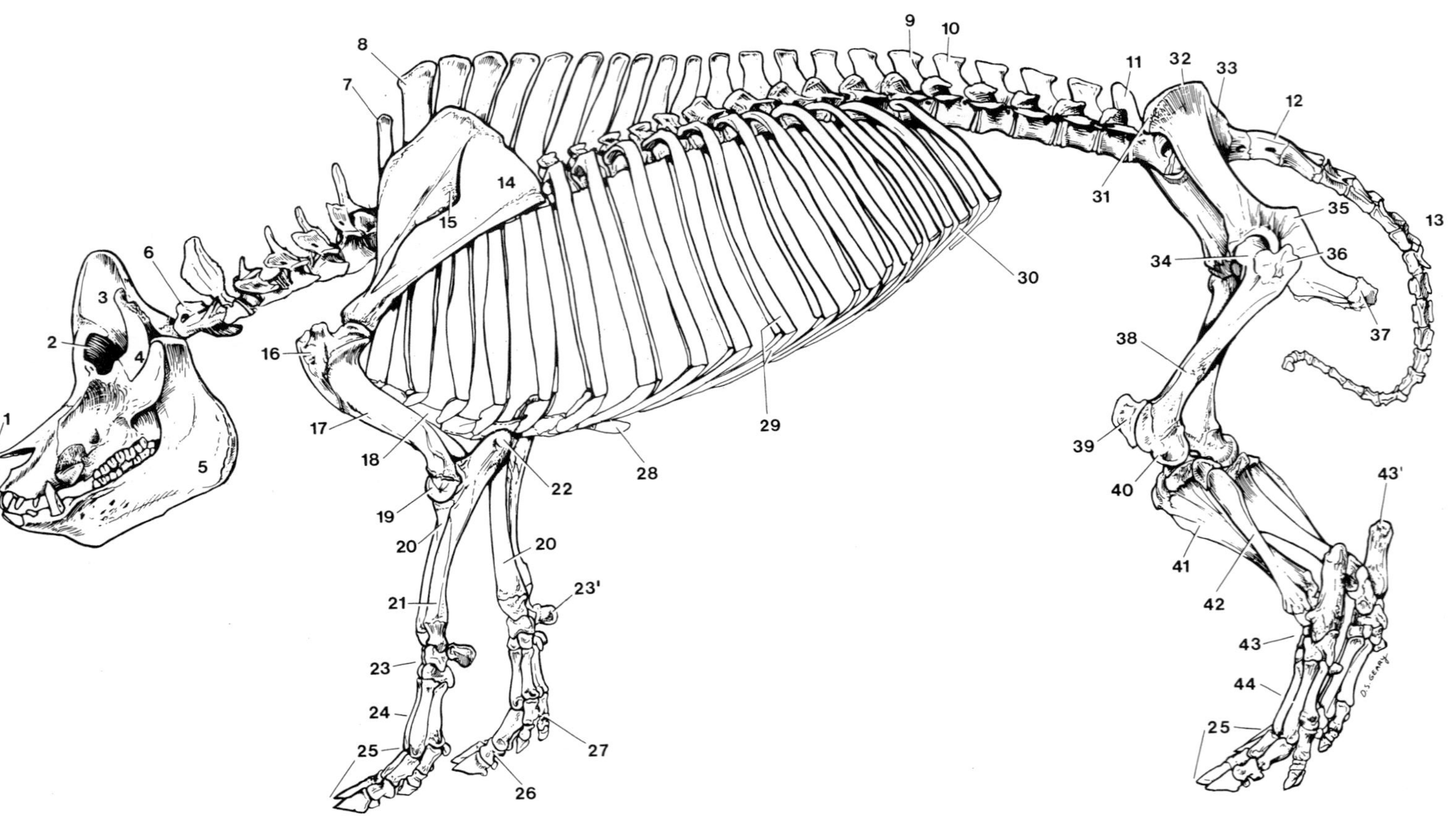


**Figure 34–1.** Skeleton of a boar.

1, Rostral bone; 2, orbit; 3, temporal fossa; 4, zygomatic arch; 5, mandible; 6, first cervical vertebra; 7, last cervical vertebra (C7); 8, first thoracic vertebra; 9, last thoracic vertebra (T16); 10, first lumbar vertebra; 11, last lumbar vertebra (L5); 12, sacrum; 13, caudal vertebrae; 14, scapula; 15, spine of scapula; 16, greater tubercle of humerus; 17, humerus; 18, sternum; 19, condyle of humerus; 20, radius; 21, ulna; 22, olecranon; 23, carpal bones; 23′, accessory carpal bone; 24, metacarpal bones; 25, phalanges; 26, phalanges of principal digit; 27, phalanges of accessory digit; 28, xiphoid cartilage; 29, 10th pair of ribs; 30, costal arch; 31, coxal tuber; 32, iliac crest; 33, sacral tuber; 34, head of femur in acetabulum; 35, ischial spine; 36, greater trochanter; 37, ischial tuber; 38, femur; 39, patella; 40, lateral condyle of femur; 41, tibia; 42, fibula; 43, tarsal bones; 43′, calcaneus; 44, metatarsal bones.

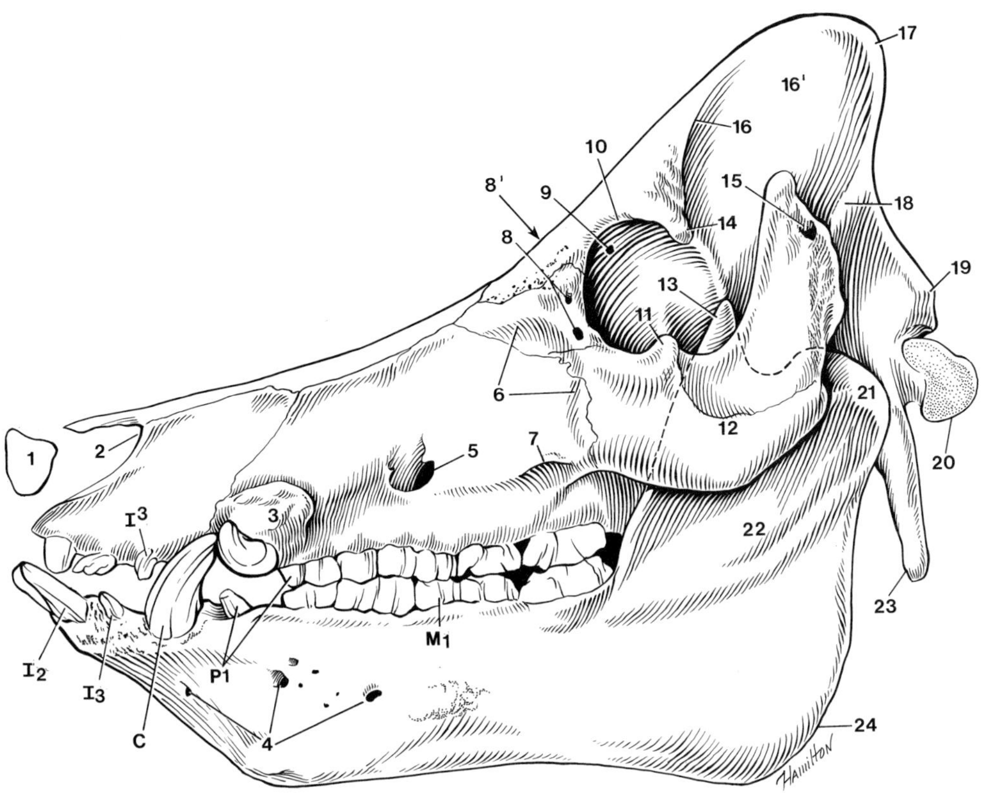


**Figure 34–2.** Skull of a boar.

1, Rostral bone; 2, nasoincisive notch; 3, canine eminence; 4, lateral mental foramina; 5, infraorbital foramen; 6, fossa canina; 7, facial crest; 8, lacrimal foramina; 8′, location of supraorbital foramen on dorsal surface; 9, orbital end of supraorbital canal; 10, orbital rim; 11, frontal process of zygomatic bone; 12, zygomatic arch; 13, coronoid process of mandible; 14, zygomatic process of frontal bone; 15, external acoustic meatus; 16, temporal line; 16′, temporal fossa; 17, nuchal crest; 18, temporal crest; 19, nuchal tubercle; 20, occipital condyle; 21, condylar process of mandible; 22, ramus of mandible; 23, paracondylar process; 24, angle of mandible; $I_2$, I3, incisors; C, canine teeth (tusks); P1, first premolars; $M_1$, first molar.

known as the jowls, are commonly the seat of abscesses. The neck is remarkably short, and this places the angle of the mandible close to the shoulder joint, an arrangement that prevents the pig from turning its head to any great degree (Fig. 34–1).

The most remarkable feature of the head is the rostrum, or *snout,* the disclike movable tip of the muzzle that incorporates the central part of the upper lip (Fig. 34–3). The snout is supported by the rostral bone (not present in other domestic species), which is set against the rostral end of the nasal septum; it gives attachment to the nasal cartilages and to the levator labii superioris, the principal mover of the snout. To prevent rooting, pigs with access to the soil are "ringed" through the dorsal border of the snout, not through the nostrils as in bulls. The lips are short and firm; the upper one is deeply notched to accommodate the projecting upper canine tooth (tusk), even when the tooth is small (Fig. 34–5).

The *eyes* are deeply placed and appear small, especially in fat adults. They lack a tapetum lucidum and thus do not reflect light as do the eyes of the other domestic mammals. A further difference is a large *deep* (lacrimal) gland of the third eyelid in the ventral part of the orbit (see Fig. 9–15/*B*,4′). The retrobulbar muscles are surrounded by an (orbital) venous sinus that is widest medioventral to the globe where it also engulfs the deep gland of the third eyelid. The sinus is said to be involved in the vascular thermoregulation of the brain by conveying cool blood, particularly from the nasal cavity, to the cavernous sinus surrounding the rete mirabile. It may be punctured through the medial angle of the eye by directing a needle medially and slightly ventrally between the globe and the third eyelid.

The *ears* are oval with a fairly wide base attached to the sides of the high caudal part of the head. They have a pointed tip and hang down over the face in some (lop-eared) domestic breeds but stand erect (prick ear) in others and in the wild species. The subcutaneous veins, often visible through the skin on the convex outer surface, are the only veins convenient for intravenous injection. The lateral auricular vein is preferred; it runs along the lateral border of the ear to an anastomosis at the tip with a similar vein that follows the medial border (Fig. 34–4/1,2). Compression (by rubber band) near the ear base raises the vein, which is often farther from the lateral border than is shown in Figure 34–4. The ears of young pigs are notched by most raisers for purposes of identification. Ear chewing is a vice of weanlings and young hogs; some come to slaughter with an ear lacking as a result of the aggressive behavior of their penmates.

A site just caudal to the base of the ear is convenient for subcutaneous injection; the parotid gland ventral to the ear must be avoided. The same site is used for deeper injection into the mass of muscle attaching to the caudal surface of the skull (Fig. 34–5).

Figure 34–5 shows the structures that lie deep to the cutaneous and certain other muscles of the face. The buccal branches (/20,19) of the facial nerve (VII) that supply the rostral muscles of facial expression are arranged as in cattle (the dorsal branch crossing the masseter, the ventral branch accompanying the parotid duct around the ventral border of the mandible). The facial vein runs with the ventral branch after draining the lips and crossing the face. It originates from the union of dorsal nasal and frontal veins, of which the latter, again as in cattle, passes through the prominent supraorbital foramen dorsomedial to the orbit. The facial artery is short; the blood supply of the dorsal half of the face is derived from a large infraorbital artery that emerges with the like-named nerve from the infraorbital foramen. The infraorbital nerve, which is relatively large since it supplies the sensitive snout, is well covered by muscle.

The large parotid gland lies caudal to the ramus of the mandible, extending almost to the shoulder joint (/15). The mandibular gland (Fig. 34–15/18) and the important lymph nodes of the head, of which the mandibular (/1) is routinely incised in meat inspection, lie deep to it.

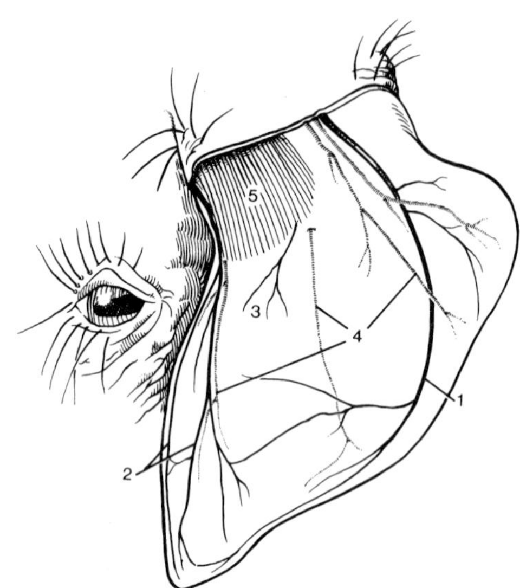


**Figure 34–4.** The left ear showing blood vessels.

1, Lateral auricular vein (for venipuncture); 2, medial auricular vein; 3, intermediate auricular vein; 4, medial, intermediate, and lateral auricular arterial branches; 5, parietoauricularis.

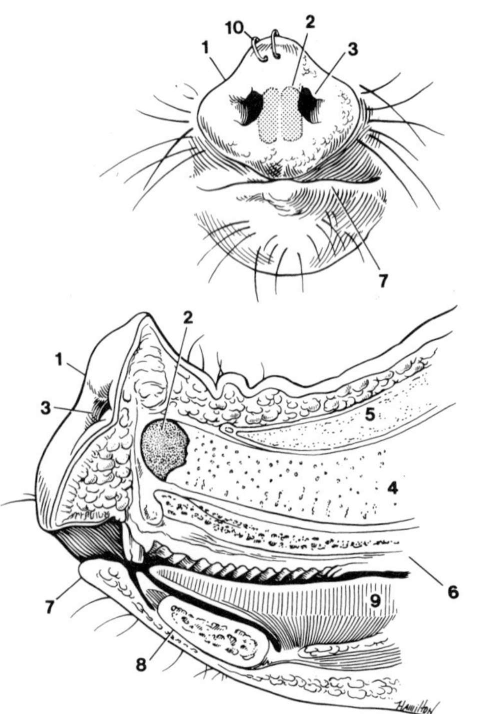


**Figure 34–3.** The snout from the front and in median section.

1, Rostral plate; 2, rostral bone; 3, nostril; 4, nasal septum; 5, nasal bone; 6, hard palate; 7, lower lip; 8, mandible with $I_1$; 9, tongue; 10, nose rings to discourage rooting.

## THE NASAL CAVITIES AND PARANASAL SINUSES

The nasal cavities are long and narrow and reach well behind the level of the orbits (Fig. 34–6/5,8).

Despite the widening face, they remain narrow, being separated from the lateral surface of the head by the thick muscles of facial expression and fat, not by extensive maxillary sinuses as in cattle and horses (Fig. 34–7/*A*). The round nostrils lead into the nasal cavities, which are divided by two conchae into three meatuses. The dorsal meatus leads to the ethmoidal conchae in the fundus of the cavity, while the middle and ventral meatuses conduct air through the choana into the nasopharynx. The fundus lies dorsal to the nasopharynx and, although dorsoventrally compressed, is very extensive (Fig. 34–6/5). It is filled with small ethmoidal conchae that carry the olfactory mucosa. The pig's sense of smell is very acute, an attribute exploited in France where pigs are used to locate truffles, which grow a few centimeters under the ground.

The dorsal nasal concha is a thick plate projecting ventrally from the dorsolateral wall of the nasal cavity (Fig. 34–7/2). The ventral nasal concha, although shorter, is much deeper and consists of upper and lower scrolls attached laterally by a common plate. The normal configuration of the nasal conchae must be known if their deformity in atrophic rhinitis, a common debilitating disease of young pigs, is to be assessed (/*B*).

The pig has maxillary, frontal, lacrimal, sphenoid, and conchal *sinuses* (see Fig. 4–7). Only the frontal is of more than passing interest. The

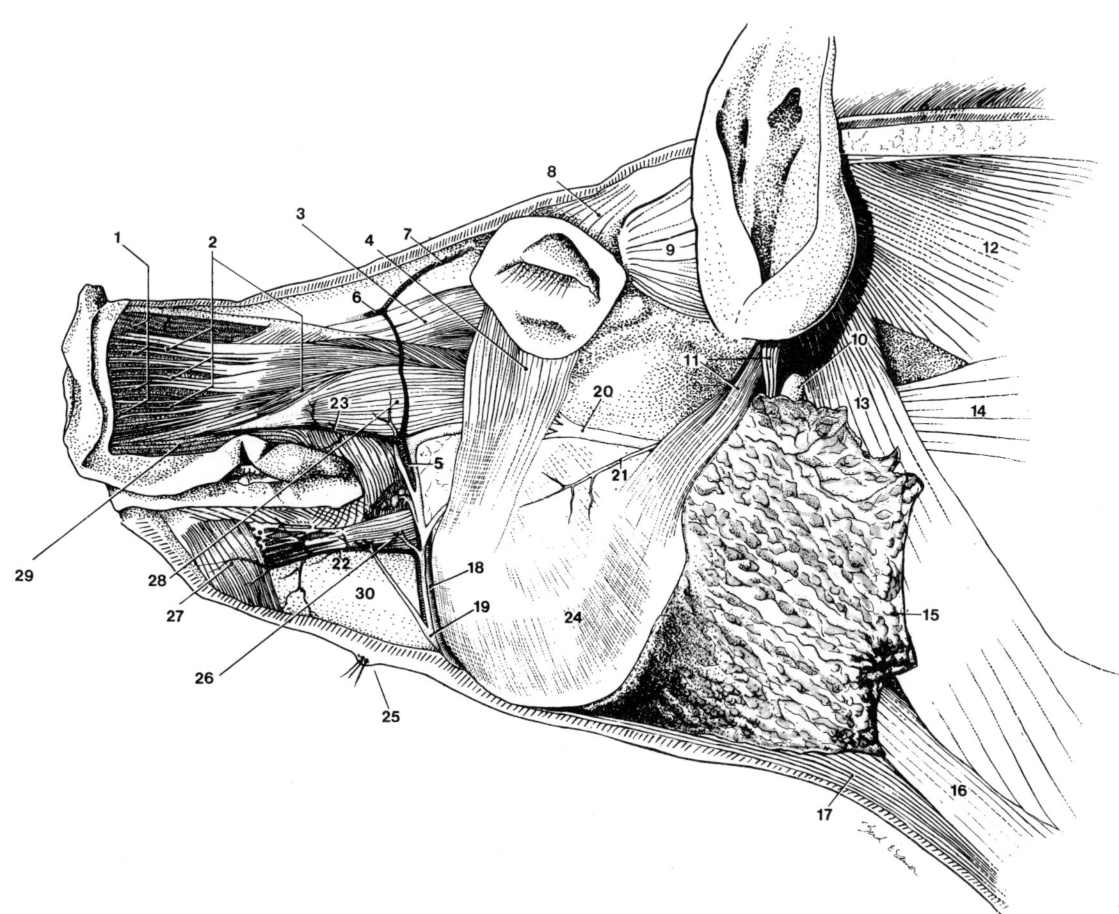


**Figure 34–5.** Head, superficial dissection.

1, Cut fasciculi of levator nasolabialis; 2, caninus; 3, levator labii superioris; 4, malaris; 5, facial vein; 6, dorsal nasal vein; 7, frontal vein; 8, levator anguli oculi; 9, frontoscutularis; 10, lateral retropharyneal lymph node; 11, parotidoauricularis; 12, trapezius; 13, cleido-occipitalis; 14, omotransversarius; 15, parotid gland; 16, sternocephalicus; 17, sternohyoideus; 18, parotid duct; 19, 20, ventral and dorsal buccal branches of facial nerve; 21, transverse facial nerve; 22, inferior labial vein; 23, superior labial vein; 24, masseter; 25, mental hairs and gland; 26, depressor labii inferioris; 27, mentalis; 28, depressor labii superioris; 29, orbicularis oris; 30, mandible.

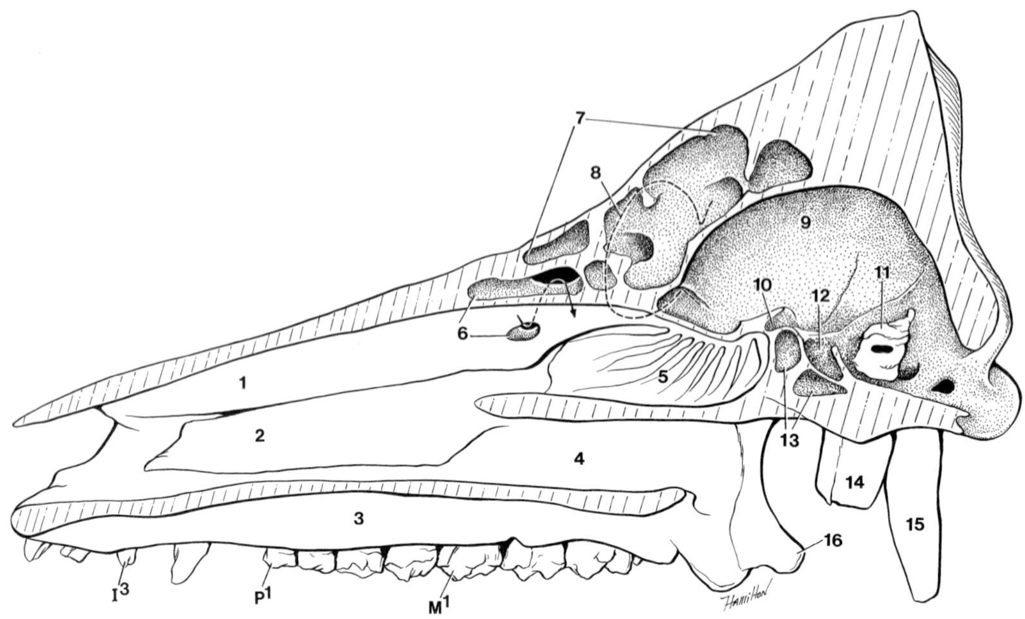


**Figure 34–6.** Paramedian section of the skull.

1, Dorsal turbinate bone, fenestrated at 6 to show conchal sinus; 2, ventral turbinate bone; 3, hard palate; 4, choana; 5, ethmoturbinates in fundus of nasal cavity; 6, conchal sinus; 7, portion of frontal sinus exposed by paramedian saw cut; 8, position of orbit; 9, cranial cavity; 10, optic canal; 11, petrous temporal bone; 12, fossa for hypophysis; 13, sphenoid sinus; 14, tympanic bulla; 15, paracondylar process; 16, hamulus of pterygoid bone.

restriction of the maxillary sinus (/4) to the level of the orbit has already been noted (p. 765). This sinus lies in the base of the wide zygomatic arch into which it extends some distance. The frontal sinuses

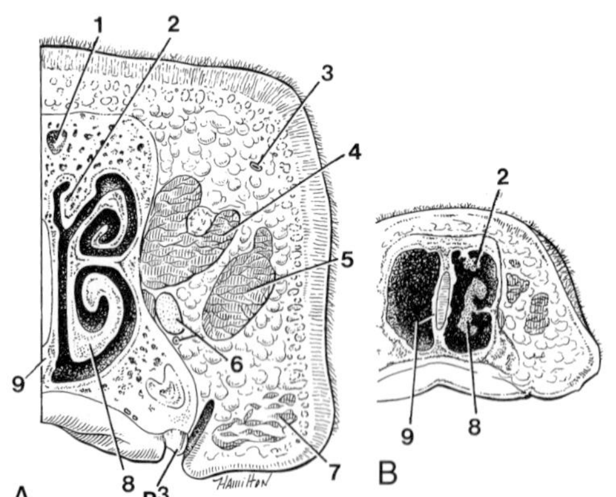


**Figure 34–7.** *A*, Transverse section of adult pig's nose level with p3. *B*, Transverse section of young pig's nose with advanced atrophic rhinitis (note complete absence of conchae in one nasal cavity); compare the nasal conchae with the normal ones in *A*.

1, Rostral extent of frontal sinus; 2, dorsal nasal concha; 3, dorsal nasal vein; 4, levator labii superioris; 5, caninus; 6, infraorbital nerve and artery; 7, orbicularis oris; 8, ventral nasal concha; 9, nasal septum.

(/1,2) of the mature pig excavate the entire dorsal surface of the skull caudal to the nasal bones. They spread the external and internal plates of the frontal and parietal bones so widely apart that all correspondence between the external form of the skull and the cranial cavity is lost. The brain is thus about 5 cm below the overlying skin and well protected by two plates of bone (Fig. 34–6/7). The origin of this and of other special features of the pig's skull is unclear, but it may be speculated that they are connected with the habits of rooting and fighting by sharp upward thrusts with the tusks.

The deep location of the brain has consequences at slaughter since pigs cannot be stunned reliably, hence humanely, by mechanical means (hammer or captive bolt). Electrocution or carbon dioxide gas is used for this purpose in most slaughterhouses today. When it is necessary to slaughter by shooting, the point of entry must be accurately determined lest the bullet miss the brain and cause unnecessary suffering. For most pigs the target point is the intersection of lines connecting the eye and the middle of the base of the opposite ear. In pigs of medium size this is about 5 cm caudal to the level of the eyes (Fig. 34–8). In particularly large animals, mainly boars, a more satisfactory alternative is shooting through the occipital bone from behind, because too much bone would have to be penetrated by the bullet in the method depicted.

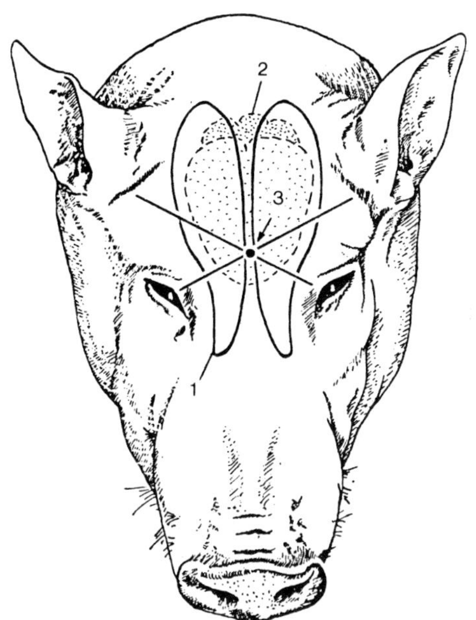


**Figure 34–8.** Head of a 9-month-old pig.

1, Outline of frontal sinuses; 2, position of brain; 3, point at which pig is best shot for stunning at slaughter.

## THE MOUTH AND THE DENTITION

Although the lips extend quite far caudally on the side of the face, pigs cannot open their mouth as widely as, for example, dogs and cats. In consequence, and apart from the difficulty with restraint, the caudal parts of the long and narrow oral cavity generally escape inspection. The roof of the cavity is marked by many prominent palatine ridges (Fig. 34–9/3) that end abruptly at the beginning of the soft palate where they are succeeded by two discrete patches, the *tonsils of the soft palate* (/5), which are the principal tonsils in the pig. Tonsils corresponding to those embedded in the lateral walls of the oropharynx of the other species are absent (see Fig. 3–26).

The floor of the oral cavity is occupied by the pointed tongue. In the newborn, the tongue is fringed with lacelike marginal papillae (Fig. 34–9/7) that persist for the first 15 to 18 days of life, and are thought to assist in sucking from the teat. They have been observed to swell preparatory to actual contact with the teat. They must be avoided when clipping the needle teeth (see further on).

Pigs have the most complete *dentition* of the domestic mammals (see Fig. 3–20). The formula for the permanent teeth is

$$\frac{3\text{-}1\text{-}4\text{-}3}{3\text{-}1\text{-}4\text{-}3}$$

The lower *incisors* are straight and project forward to meet the curved upper incisors in a grasping action (Fig. 34–2). The curved canine teeth, or *tusks,* are deeply anchored in the jaws; in boars their embedded proximal ends remain open, and the tusks grow throughout the animal's life. The lower ones are kept sharp by friction against the upper ones, providing boars with imposing weapons that must be treated with respect. The tusks can be sawn off under anesthesia, but herdsmen, disregarding the pain felt by the boar, often cut them off with heavy clippers using no more restraint than a snubbing rope. The tusks of the sow are smaller and except for their tips do not project from the mouth. They remain open for about 2 years, after which a root develops and growth ceases.

The crowns of the *cheek teeth* increase in both length and breadth from front to back. The occlusal surface of the massive molars is made irregular by numerous tubercles and is ideal for crushing food.

The pig is born with eight teeth: the deciduous upper and lower third incisors and the canines; these are commonly known as "needle teeth" (Fig. 34–9). They project almost laterally from the gums and may injure the teat of the sow or a littermate competing for the same teat. For these reasons they are usually nipped off by the breeder within hours of birth.

Upper and lower first incisors and third premolars erupt 1 to 3 weeks after birth, and the upper and lower fourth premolars follow a few days later. The upper and lower second premolars erupt at about 2 months, and the second incisors follow at about 3 months. This completes the deciduous dentition for which the formula is

$$\frac{3\text{-}1\text{-}3}{3\text{-}1\text{-}3}$$

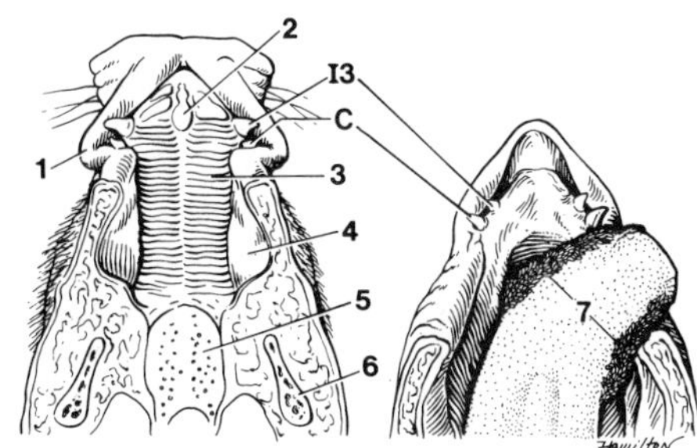


**Figure 34–9.** Upper *(left)* and lower *(right)* jaws of a newborn pig.

1, Permanent notch in upper lip opposite tusk; 2, incisive papilla; 3, hard palate with palatine ridges; 4, unerupted premolars 3 and 4 bulging the gums; 5, tonsils of the soft palate; 6, ramus of mandible; 7, marginal papillae on tongue; I3, deciduous third incisors; C, deciduous canine teeth.

**Table 34–1.** Eruption Dates of Porcine Teeth

| | Temporary Tooth | Permanent Tooth |
|---|---|---|
| Incisor 1 | 1–3 wk | 11–18 mo |
| Incisor 2 | 8–12 wk | 14–18 mo |
| Incisor 3 | Before birth | 8–12 mo |
| Canine | Before birth | 8–12 mo |
| Premolar 1 | 4–8 mo | |
| Premolar 2 | 6–12 wk | 12–16 mo |
| Premolar 3 | 1–3 wk | 12–16 mo |
| Premolar 4 | 2–5 wk | 12–16 mo |
| Molar 1 | | 4–8 mo |
| Molar 2 | | 7–13 mo |
| Molar 3 | | 17–22 mo |

By market age (roughly 6 months), the first permanent teeth, the upper and lower first molars, have erupted, but replacement of the deciduous teeth has yet to begin. A pig is at least 1½ years old before it acquires the full permanent dentition. Although criteria for the aging of pigs by their teeth exist (Table 34–1), they are rarely employed.

## THE PHARYNX AND LARYNX

Neither of these structures would warrant description were it not for one peculiar feature, the *pharyngeal diverticulum,* which arises from the pharyngeal wall dorsal to the entrance to the esophagus (Fig. 34–10/13). It is about 1 cm long in the piglet (3 to 4 cm in the adult) and burrows caudally into the pharyngeal muscles. Its significance lies in the risk of injury when pigs are dosed with a syringe. The nozzle of the syringe, if inserted too deeply, may enter and perforate the diverticulum and cause serious injury if the medication is deposited into the tissues of the neck. In the 4-week-old piglet the pharyngeal diverticulum is at the level of the cranial part of the base of the ear. Medication should be deposited in the oropharynx, which in the 4-week-old is level with the lateral angle of the eye. The difference between the two levels is only 2.5 cm, an indication of the care required.

The larynx has lateral ventricles and forms an obtuse angle with the trachea (/12,17). Both the ventricles and the angle have been cited as impediments to intubation for inhalation anesthesia.

Rostrolateral to the base of the epiglottis is the paraepiglottic tonsil (Fig. 34–11/8′). The other tonsils are the already mentioned tonsil of the soft palate (/8), the pharyngeal tonsil in the roof of the nasopharynx, and the tubal tonsil associated with the pharyngeal opening of the auditory tube. On occasion the paraepiglottic tonsil and that of the soft palate must be examined after slaughter, the former on the pluck (larynx, trachea, esophagus, heart, and lungs), and the latter on the cut surface of the head.

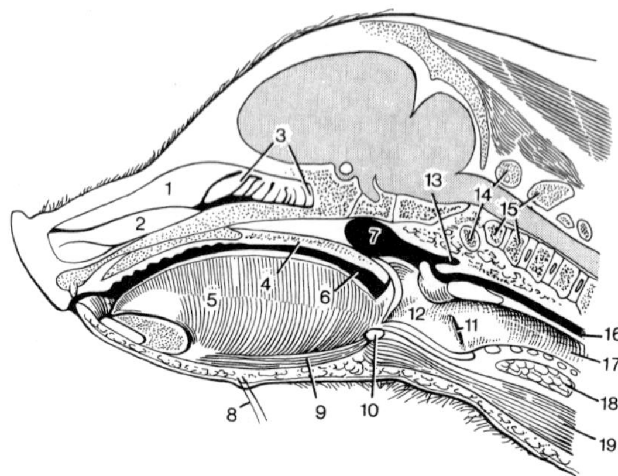


**Figure 34–10.** Median section of the head of a 4-week-old pig; the nasal septum has been removed.

1, Dorsal nasal concha; 2, ventral nasal concha; 3, ethmoidal conchae; 4, soft palate; 5, tongue; 6, oropharynx; 7, nasopharynx; 8, mental hairs; 9, geniohyoideus; 10, basihyoid; 11, laryngeal ventricle; 12, larynx; 13, pharyngeal diverticulum; 14, atlas; 15, axis; 16, esophagus; 17, trachea; 18, thyroid gland; 19, sternohyoideus.

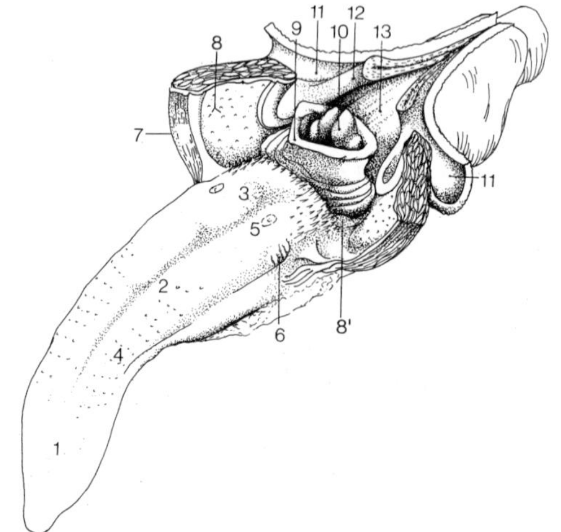


**Figure 34–11.** Tongue and pharynx. The soft palate and the dorsal wall of the esophagus have been split in the midline.

1–3, Apex, body, and root of tongue; 4, fungiform papillae; 5, vallate papillae; 6, foliate papillae; 7, palatoglossal arch; 8, tonsil of the soft palate; 8′, paraepiglottic tonsil; 9, epiglottis; 10, corniculate processes of the arytenoid cartilages; 11, dorsal wall of nasopharynx; 12, palatopharyngeal arch; 13, entrance to esophagus.

## THE VENTRAL PART OF THE NECK

The shortness and limited mobility of the neck have already been mentioned. A ligamentum nuchae is not present. The visceral compartment of the neck is relatively small; it houses the same structures as in the other species, including a fully functional internal jugular vein in the carotid sheath, and a well-developed cervical thymus to the side of the trachea.

Removal of the skin exposes the pale cutaneous muscles of which the cutaneus colli and platysma are best developed. The cutaneus colli arises from the manubrium sterni, where it is thick, and fans out over the ventral surface of the neck to blend with the cutaneous muscles of the face and lips.

The cutaneus colli at its origin overlies the depression between the palpable manubrium and the point of the shoulder, the site for cranial vena cava venipuncture (see further on). Removal of the muscle exposes the long ventral extremity of the large parotid gland (Fig. 34–12/1), which has the following relations: medially, the sternocephalicus, brachiocephalicus, and mandibular gland; cranially, the mandible; and ventrally, the fused sternohyoidei. The larynx is caudal to the intermandibular space; its (laryngeal) prominence is palpable in the middle of the neck. The thyroid gland, whose two lobes are broadly joined ventral to the trachea, lies close to the thoracic inlet (see Fig. 6–4/*D*). The triangular mandibular gland (Fig. 34–12/2), ventrolateral to the larynx, is covered laterally by the parotid gland and related craniolaterally to the angle of the mandible. The important mandibular lymph nodes (/19), which must be distinguished from the mandibular salivary gland in meat inspection, lie rostral, lateral, and slightly ventral to this gland (Fig. 34–15/1,18).

Removal of the parotid and mandibular glands exposes the brachiocephalicus, the sternocephalicus, the external jugular vein, and the omohyoideus. The brachiocephalicus (Fig. 34–12/12) is the most lateral muscle; it is wide and flat and passes from the distal part of the body of the humerus to the temporal and occipital bones at the back of the skull. The sternocephalicus (/14) extends from the sternum to the temporal bone and passes between the external and internal jugular veins. Although larger in diameter than its internal counterpart, the external jugular vein is not as easily punctured as in the other domestic species because it is nowhere subcutaneous. The omohyoideus (/15) extends between the fascia medial to the shoulder joint and the basihyoid; it crosses the medial aspects of the mandibular gland and sternocephalicus.

The thymus (/3) lies lateral to the larynx and trachea close to the carotid sheath. It is particularly well developed and attains its greatest size at about 9 months (should the pig survive so long); at about 1 year it begins to recede. Its cranial end is bulbous and contains on its surface the minute (1 to 4 mm) external parathyroid gland (III). (The internal parathyroid [IV] has not been located in the adult pig; it is thought to disappear in the embryo.)

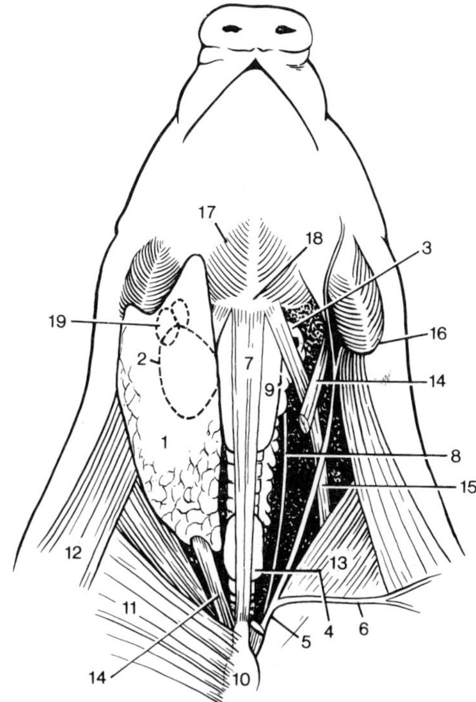


**Figure 34–12.** Ventral view of the neck. Deep dissection to the right; superficial dissection, from which the cutaneus colli has been removed, to the left; semischematic.

1, Parotid gland; 2, mandibular gland; 3, thymus—dot on cranial end indicates the position of the external parathyroid (III); 4, thyroid; 5, external jugular vein; 6, cephalic vein; 7, sternohyoideus (drawn narrower than actual width); 8, internal jugular vein; 9, larynx; 10, manubrium sterni; 11, superficial pectoral muscle; 12, brachiocephalicus; 13, subclavius; 14, sternocephalicus; 15, omohyoideus; 16, angle of mandible; 17, mylohyoideus; 18, basihyoid; 19, mandibular lymph nodes.

The most common clinical procedure involving the neck is *cranial vena cava venipuncture,* which may be performed in the standing animal restrained by a snubbing rope or in one held down on its back (Fig. 34–13/*C*). The needle, inserted in the depression between the palpable manubrium sterni and the point of the right shoulder, is advanced in the direction of the dorsal end of the left scapula, in an attempt to puncture any of the large veins between or just in front of the first pair of ribs. The needle passes through the cutaneus colli and then along the wedge-shaped space between the bra-

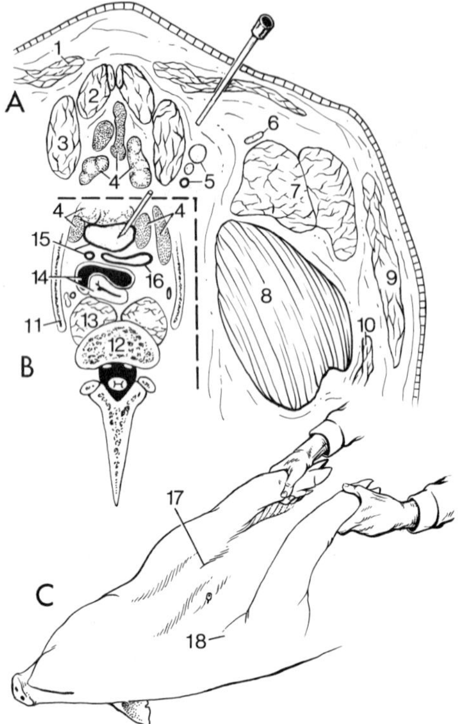


**Figure 34–13.** *A,* Transverse section of the ventral neck slightly cranial to the manubrium sterni. *B,* The area within the broken line represents the topography at the slightly more caudal level of the first ribs. *C,* Pig held on its back for cranial vena cava venipuncture; see needle in position.

1, Cutaneus colli; 2, sternohyoideus; 3, sternocephalicus; 4, lymph nodes and thymus; 5, common carotid artery and external and internal jugular veins; 6, cephalic vein; 7, brachiocephalicus; 8, subclavius; 9, platysma; 10, omotransversarius; 11, first rib; 12, body of C7; 13, longus colli; 14, trachea and esophagus; 15, cranial vena cava and left subclavian artery; 16, bicarotid trunk and right subclavian artery; 17, palpable manubrium sterni; 18, shoulder joint.

chiocephalicus and subclavius laterally, and the sternocephalicus and sternohyoideus medially. The right side is preferred because the left phrenic nerve occupies a more vulnerable position, while the unpaired thoracic duct is also more to the left. Blood may also be obtained from the external jugular vein one third the distance from the sternum to the jaw.

## THE LYMPH NODES OF THE HEAD AND NECK

These can be grouped into five lymph centers, all located in the ventrolateral part of the neck (Fig. 34–14). Most lymph from the head and neck passes through the regional nodes before being carried to the veins at the thoracic inlet by the tracheal trunks; some reaches its destination directly from the dorsal superficial cervical nodes into which several more cranial nodes drain.

The mandibular lymph center consists of up to six mandibular and four accessory mandibular nodes. The *mandibular lymph nodes* (Fig. 34–15/1) lie between the caudoventral border of the mandible and the cranial part of the sternohyoideus (/9) and are related caudally to the mandibular gland. The facial vein (/19) crosses their lateral surface. They drain the ventral half of the head, including the palate and larynx; their efferents go to the accessory mandibular and the ventral and dorsal superficial cervical nodes. The accessory mandibular lymph nodes (/2) are located near the caudoventral border of the mandibular gland and are covered by the parotid gland. They drain the same parts of the head as the mandibular nodes but also the ventral part of the neck; their efferents go to the ventral and dorsal superficial cervical nodes.

The parotid lymph center consists of a single group of *parotid lymph nodes* (/3) that lie ventral to the temporomandibular joint on the caudal border of the mandible, covered by the parotid gland. They drain the part of the head dorsal to the palate; their efferents go to the lateral retropharyngeal nodes.

The retropharyngeal lymph center consists of two lateral nodes and one medial node. The *lateral retropharyngeal lymph nodes* (/4) are found level with the temporomandibular joint between the parotid gland laterally and the cleidomastoideus medially, a few centimeters caudomedial to the parotid nodes. They drain the superficial parts of the head-neck junction; their efferents go to the dorsal superficial cervical nodes. The *medial retropharyngeal lymph node* (/5) is related ven-

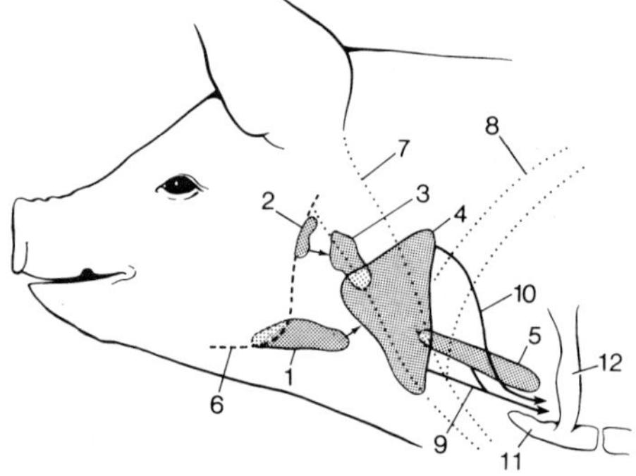


**Figure 34–14.** The lymph centers of the head and neck, schematic. The arrows indicate lymph flow.

1, Mandibular lymph center; 2, parotid lymph center; 3, retropharyngeal lymph center; 4, superficial cervical lymph center; 5, deep cervical lymph center; 6, mandible; 7, brachiocephalicus; 8, subclavius; 9, tracheal lymph trunk; 10, lymph from dorsal superficial cervical nodes; 11, manubrium sterni; 12, first rib.

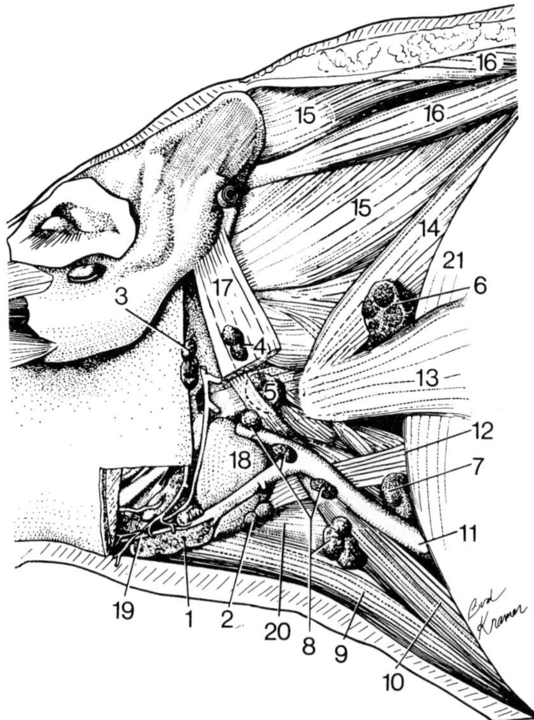


**Figure 34–15.** Dissection of the neck to show the lymph nodes, left lateral view.

1, Mandibular lymph nodes; 2, accessory mandibular lymph nodes; 3, parotid lymph nodes; 4, lateral retropharyngeal lymph nodes; 5, medial retropharyngeal lymph nodes; 6–8, dorsal, middle, and ventral superficial cervical lymph nodes; 9, sternohyoideus; 10, sternocephalicus; 11, external jugular vein; 12, omohyoideus; 13, omotransversarius; 14, serratus ventralis cervicis; 15, splenius; 16, rhomboideus cervicis et capitis; 17, cleidomastoideus; 18, mandibular gland; 19, facial vein; 20, thyrohyoideus; 21, subclavius.

trally to the muscles of the pharynx, and to the common carotid artery and internal jugular vein, medially to the sternocephalicus tendon. It drains the deep parts of the head-neck junction; its efferents join to form the tracheal trunk.

The superficial cervical lymph center consists of about 10 nodes widely spread in a triangular area cranial to the shoulder joint (Fig. 34–14/4). They are divided into dorsal, middle, and ventral nodes, and together they correspond to the single group of superficial cervical nodes found medial to the omotransversarius in the other species. The *dorsal superficial cervical lymph nodes* (Fig. 34–15/6) lie craniodorsal to the shoulder joint, partly under cover of the omotransversarius. They drain the neck, the cranial part of the thoracic wall, and parts of the forelimbs. They receive many efferents from other nodes of the head and neck (except the medial retropharyngeal) and, as already mentioned, convey through their own efferents a large portion of the lymph from the head and neck to the veins at the thoracic inlet. The *middle superficial cervical lymph nodes* (/7) are related ventrally to the external jugular vein and are covered laterally by the brachiocephalicus. They drain the superficial parts of the shoulder region; their efferents join or accompany those of the dorsal superficial cervical nodes. The *ventral superficial cervical lymph nodes* (/8) form a chain along the ventral border of the brachiocephalicus under cover of the parotid gland. They drain the superficial parts of the ventral neck, forelimb, and ventral thoracic wall (including the cranial mammary glands) and receive lymph from the mandibular and lateral retropharyngeal nodes.

The deep cervical lymph center (Fig. 34–14/5) consists of a large number of small nodes. These are supposedly divided into cranial, middle, and caudal groups, but the first two groups may be absent, while the caudal one may consist of only a few nodes. The deep cervical nodes follow the course of the internal jugular vein and trachea to the thoracic inlet. They drain adjacent structures, principally trachea, thyroid gland, and carotid sheath; their efferents pass variously to the large veins at the thoracic inlet.

## Selected Bibliography

Belz, G.T., and T.J. Heath: Lymphatic drainage from the tonsil of the soft palate in pigs. J. Anat. 187:491–495, 1995.

Brown, C.M.: A method for collecting blood from hogs using the thoracic inlet. Vet. Med. [SAC] 74:361–363, 1979.

Cox, J.E.: Immobilization and anesthesia of the pig. Vet. Rec. 92:143–146, 1973.

Davies, A.S.: Postnatal development of the lower canine and cheek teeth of the pig. Anat. Histol. Embryol. 19:269–275, 1990.

Ghoshal, N.G., and W.A. Khamas: Blood supply of the nasal cavity of the normal pig. Anat. Histol. Embryol. 15:14–22, 1986.

Huhn, R.G., G.D. Osweiler, and W.P. Switzer: Application of the orbital sinus bleeding technique to swine. Lab. Anim. Care 19:403–405, 1969.

Lawhorn, B.: A new approach for obtaining blood samples from pigs. JAVMA 192:781–782, 1988.

Pond, W.G., and K.A. Houpt: The Biology of the Pig. Ithaca, N.Y., Cornell University Press, 1978.

Sack, W.O. (ed.): Horowitz/Kramer Atlas of the Musculoskeletal Anatomy of the Pig. Ithaca, N.Y., Veterinary Textbooks, 1982.

Sankari, S.: A practical method of taking blood samples from the pig. Acta Vet. Scand. 24:133–134, 1983.

Schlotthauer, C.F., and G.M. Higgins: The parathyroid glands in swine. Mayo Clin. Proc. 9:374–376, 1934.

Schwartz, W.L., and J.E. Smallwood: Collection of blood from swine. Tex. Vet. Med. J. 39:6–7, 1977.

Simoens, P.: Morphologic Study of the Vasculature in the Orbit and Eyeball of the Pig [thesis]. Ghent, State University of Ghent, Faculty of Veterinary Medicine, 1985.

W.A.A.: Pharyngeal perforation in pigs. JAVMA 125:69, 1954.

Watson, S.A.J., and G.P.M. Moore: Postnatal development of the hair cycle in the domestic pig. J. Anat. 170:1–9, 1990.

CHAPTER 35

# The Vertebral Column, Back, and Thorax of the Pig

## THE VERTEBRAL COLUMN

The vertebral formula is C7, T14–15, L6–7, S4, Cd20–23. The seven cervical vertebrae are short and traverse the neck close to its center (Fig. 35–1). They exhibit the following species-specific features: C2 has a tall, relatively thin spinous process; C3 to C6 have bilateral, platelike processes that arise from the transverse processes and increase in size from C3 to C6; C7 has a tall spinous process (see Fig. 34–1).

Since the neck is nearly as deep dorsoventrally as the cranial part of the thorax, the first thoracic vertebra is also located near the midpoint of the dorsoventral diameter of the trunk. The vertebrae caudal to this gradually rise, and those of the caudal thoracic and lumbar regions lie nearer and almost parallel to the dorsal surface of the back.

The numbers of the thoracic and lumbar vertebrae vary considerably. Most pigs have either 14 or 15 thoracic and 6 lumbar vertebrae, giving a total of 20 or 21, but the full range observed is 19 to 23. Whether this variability is related to the practice of selectively breeding for longer-bodied animals is not known. Long-bodied pigs are desirable because they yield longer loins, which, aside from the hams, are the most valuable parts of the carcass (Fig. 35–1/14,22).

The sacrum consists of four partially fused units that lack spinous processes. Thus, an abrupt drop in the height of the vertebral column occurs at the lumbosacral junction, and the iliac crests, which flank the spinous process of L6, are the highest skeletal parts in the area (see Fig. 34–1/32). The *lumbosacral space* is used for the epidural administration of anesthetics: it measures about 2 cm craniocaudally and 3 cm transversely, is closed by an interarcuate ligament, and is situated 2 to 5 cm caudal to a line connecting the coxal tubers. In young hogs the spinal cord ends within the sacrum and is thus within range of the needle; in older animals it has ascended, ends cranial to L6, and is not at risk (see Fig. 8–56/*C*).

The pig has about 20 caudal vertebrae, of which the last 15 or so form the curly *tail.* The median caudal vessels on the ventral surface of the tail may be used for collecting blood. The artery and the two accompanying veins lie under the skin and are punctured at the tailhead (Cd4 or Cd5); the blood obtained may be arterial, venous, or mixed. Tail biting, a form of cannibalism among weanlings, is a problem when many animals are kept crowded together. The mutilation of the tail may be complicated by ascending infection via a direct venous route, circumventing the local lymphatics and resulting in pyemia; this may result in condemnation of all or part of the carcass. Trichinosis also can be transmitted through cannibalism. Excessive exploratory behavior is believed to be the underlying cause of tail biting and ear chewing. Removal of tails when piglets are 2 to 3 days old avoids the first risk.

## THE BACK

The contour of the back depends on breed and condition. In old, fat animals it is usually straight (parallel to the ground) but in most modern meat hogs the back is uniformly arched. In those of top quality, it is also broad from side to side. Pig breeders generally select animals with wide bodies and wide stance, as this promises good muscling in the trunk, and thick hams.

A thick layer of fat separates the skin from the muscles of the back and withers (Fig. 35–2). This is a segment of the panniculus adiposus, the well-developed fat deposit present nearly everywhere in the pig's subcutis. The panniculus is especially well formed and firm (back fat) over the "loin" and, since it has to be trimmed, represents a substantial loss to the producer. Some of the fat is rendered into lard, and some is cured to become

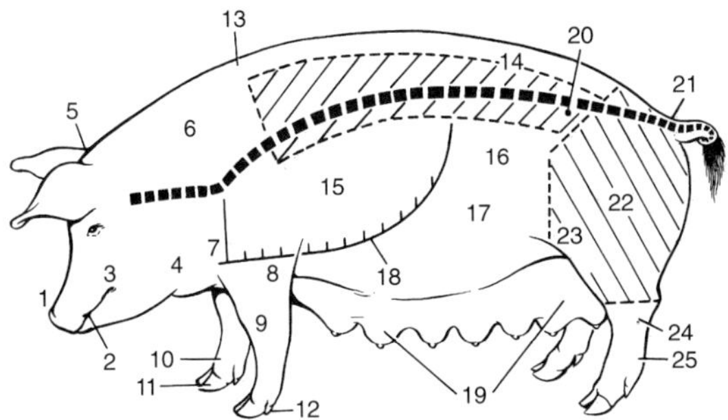


**Figure 35–1.** Parts of the pig. The position of the vertebral column is indicated. The hatched areas show ham and loin of the meat trade.

1, Snout; 2, mouth; 3, cheek; 4, jowls; 5, poll; 6, neck; 7, shoulder joint; 8, elbow joint; 9, carpus; 10, fetlock joint; 11, hoof; 12, accessory digit; 13, withers; 14, loin (lumbar area); 15, thorax; 16, flank; 17, abdomen; 18, ventral extent of bony thorax; 19, mammary glands; 20, position of coxal tuber; 21, tailhead; 22, thigh; 23, stifle joint; 24, hock joint; 25, metatarsus.

the "pork" in the popular canned food "pork and beans." Selective breeding has markedly reduced the thickness of the back fat to about 3 cm or less; it must be taken into account in injection into the back muscles.

The muscles of the back conform to the general pattern. They comprise (from lateral to medial) the iliocostalis, longissimus, and transversospinalis columns, which lie dorsal to the ribs and the lumbar transverse processes (/9,6,5). The longissimus (/6) has the largest diameter and is known as the "loin eye" in the meat trade. The psoas major and minor (filet mignon), the most desirable parts of the carcass, are found ventral to the lumbar transverse processes.

Ultrasound is used on the back of pigs to measure depth of subcutaneous fat and underlying muscle to predict carcass quality for the purpose of selective breeding; or on carcasses after slaughter, using the measurements for carcass evaluation.

## THE THORAX

The pig's body does not widen appreciably where the neck joins the trunk. The width of the neck and the subcutaneous fat allow the upper forelimb to blend in less obtrusively than in the other species; only the lateroventral depression between the flabby jowls and the shoulder joint marks the junction. A similar depression occurs between the elbow joint and the thoracic wall. The points of the shoulder and elbow are palpable, the latter opposite the ventral end of rib 5 in the standing animal (Fig. 35–3/3). The manubrium sterni is at the transverse level of the shoulder joint; it too is easily palpated.

Most pigs have 14 or 15 pairs of ribs, but the number varies between 13 and 17. Asymmetry in number is not rare (about 6.5%). The first seven ribs are sternal.

The bony thorax of the mature pig is considerably smaller than the external dimensions of the cranial part of the trunk would lead one to suspect (Fig. 35–1). It is compressed laterally in front to accommodate the scapula and arm within the trunk and attains its full height more caudally because of the upward sweep of the thoracic vertebrae.

The thoracic cavity is relatively long. The line of pleural reflection follows the dorsal half of the last rib and then descends in a gentle curve to the

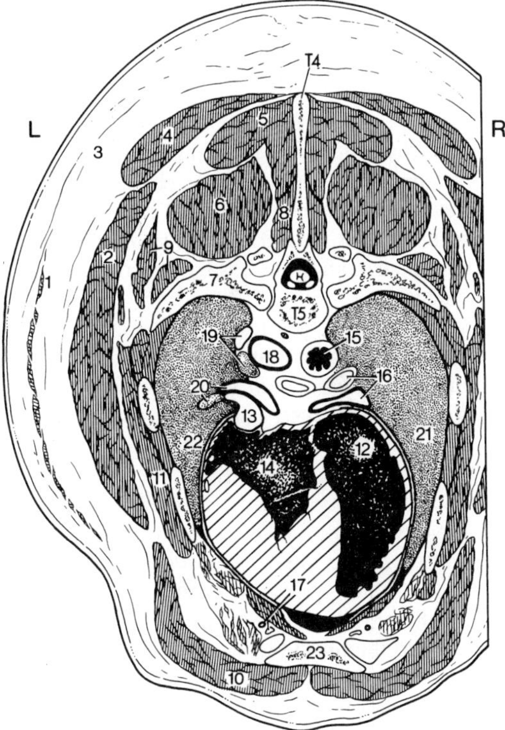


**Figure 35–2.** Transverse section of the thorax at T5; the ventral end of the section is slightly cranial to the dorsal. This pig was suspended by the hindlimbs before being frozen for sectioning; scapula and arm have fallen cranially.

1, Cutaneus trunci; 2, latissimus dorsi; 3, panniculus adiposus; 4, trapezius; 5, spinalis thoracis; 6, longissimus dorsi; 7, rib; 8, multifidus; 9, iliocostalis; 10, pectoralis ascendens; 11, serratus ventralis; 12, right atrium; 13, a pulmonary vein; 14, left atrium; 15, esophagus; 16, right principal bronchus *(above)*, right pulmonary artery; 17, internal thoracic artery and vein; 18, aorta; 19, left azygous vein, tracheobronchial lymph node; 20, left pulmonary artery, tracheobronchial lymph node; 21, cranial lobe of right lung; 22, cranial part of cranial lobe of left lung; 23, sternum.

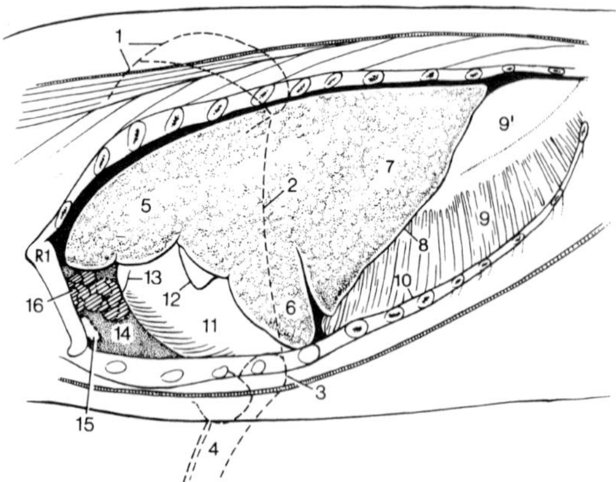


**Figure 35–3.** The thoracic viscera in situ, semischematic.

1, Scapula; 2, caudal border of triceps; 3, olecranon; 4, radius and ulna; 5, 6, cranial and caudal parts of cranial lobe of lung; 7, caudal lobe of lung; 8, basal border of lung; 9, 9′, muscular and tendinous parts of diaphragm; 10, line of pleural reflection; 11, heart; 12, 13, left and right auricles; 14, cranial mediastinum; 15, sternal lymph node; 16, thymus.

seventh costochondral junction (Fig. 35–3/10). The cranial mediastinum (/14), like that of the ruminants, lies against the ventral ends of the first one or two ribs of the left side, while more dorsally it is separated from these ribs by the cranial lobe of the left lung.

The *heart* of the pig is small in relation to the body, especially in fat animals. Its small size (0.3% of body weight compared with ca. 1.0% in horse and dog) has been cited as a predisposing factor in the relatively common and costly "sudden death syndrome" in pigs. Heart size apparently has not kept pace with body weight as ever–faster-growing pigs have been selected for breeding. (In the year 1800 it took 2 to 3 years for a domesticated pig to reach 40 kg; in 1850 pigs reached 70 kg in that span of time. Today, pigs reach an average of 100 kg in 5 to 6 months!)

The heart extends from the second to the fifth ribs and occupies slightly more than the ventral half of the available thoracic space (Figs. 35–2 and 35–4; see also Plate 11/*A–D*). It is covered by the arm and the triceps in the standing animal but can be made accessible by drawing the limb forward. The left cardiac notch, being larger than the right, allows the heart greater contact with the thoracic wall of that side.

Paracentesis is possible through the left fifth and the right fourth intercostal spaces; the needle is inserted about 5 cm dorsal to the level of the olecranon and directed medially.

The *lungs* have the following lobation. The right lung consists of cranial, middle, caudal, and accessory lobes, with the cardiac notch separating the first two (Fig. 35–5 and Plate 3/*D*). The left lung has a divided cranial lobe and a caudal lobe; the cardiac notch causes the division of the cranial lobe. The cranial lobe of the right lung is ventilated separately by a tracheal bronchus (/8; see Fig. 4–25/4) that arises a short distance cranial to the tracheal bifurcation. Lobulation, although not so distinct as in cattle, is visible over the entire surface.

The projection of the lungs onto the thoracic wall is relatively small. The left basal border extends from the sixth costochondral junction to the dorsal end of the rib third to last (Fig. 35–3/8).

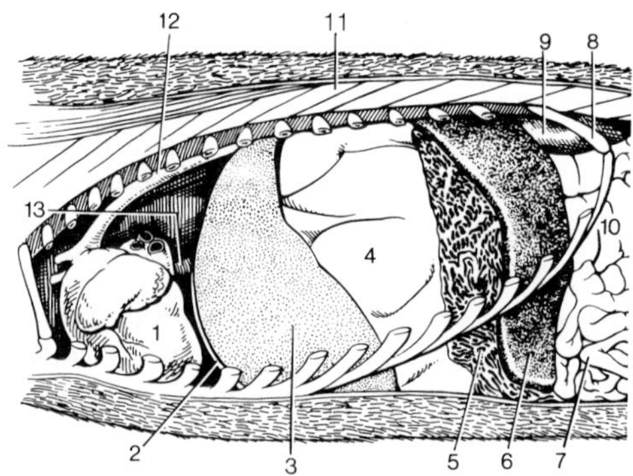


**Figure 35–4.** The heart in situ.

1, Heart; 2, diaphragm; 3, left lobe of liver; 4, stomach, greatly dilated; 5, greater omentum, gastrosplenic ligament; 6, spleen; 7, jejunum; 8, last rib; 9, left kidney; 10, ascending colon; 11, back muscles; 12, aorta; 13, caudal vena cava.

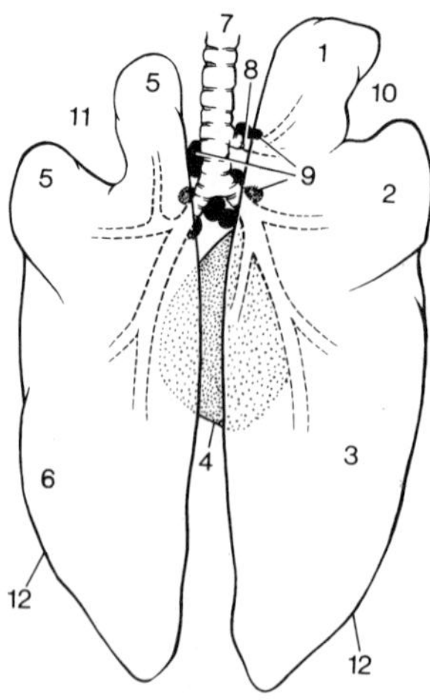


**Figure 35–5.** The lungs, dorsal view (see also Fig. 4–25).

1, Right cranial lobe; 2, right middle lobe; 3, right caudal lobe; 4, accessory lobe of right lung; 5, divided left cranial lobe; 6, left caudal lobe; 7, trachea; 8, tracheal bronchus; 9, tracheobronchial lymph nodes; 10, right cardiac notch; 11, left cardiac notch; 12, basal border.

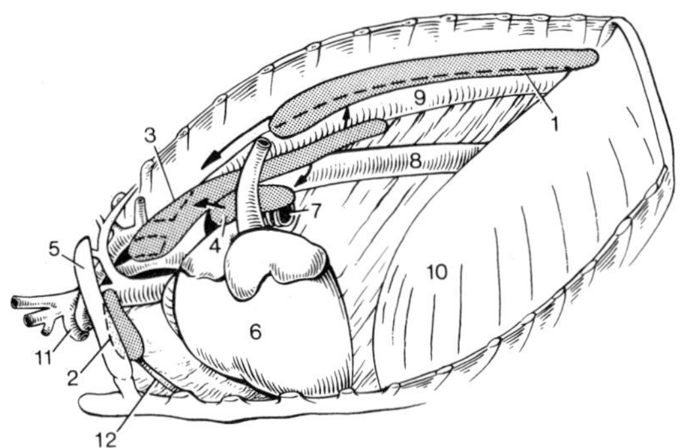


**Figure 35–6.** The lymph centers of the thorax, left lateral view.

1, Dorsal thoracic lymph center; 2, ventral thoracic lymph center; 3, mediastinal lymph center; 4, tracheobronchial lymph center; 5, first rib; 6, heart; 7, left bronchus; 8, esophagus; 9, aorta; 10, diaphragm; 11, axillary vein and artery; 12, internal thoracic artery.

On the right, the basal border is less steep and extends to the dorsal end of the rib second to last. Auscultation and percussion of the lungs are usually confined to young pigs of cooperative disposition.

## The Lymph Nodes of the Thorax

The lymph nodes of the thorax can be grouped into four lymph centers that are positioned as shown in Figure 35–6. They collect lymph from the thoracic organs, thoracic wall, and adjacent muscles and channel it into the thoracic duct or, where the more cranial nodes are concerned, directly into the veins at the thoracic inlet.

The dorsal thoracic lymph center (/1) is composed of 2 to 10 small *thoracic aortic lymph nodes* accompanying the aorta and left azygous vein caudal to the sixth thoracic vertebra. They drain muscles associated with the dorsal half of the thoracic wall, the mediastinum, and some caudal mediastinal nodes; their efferents join the thoracic duct.

The ventral thoracic lymph center (/2) consists of one to four fairly large *sternal lymph nodes* found at the level of the first intercostal space, between the right and left internal thoracic vessels. Only the most ventral are associated with the sternum. They drain lymph from the muscles related to the ventral half of the thoracic wall, the mediastinum, and the first three pairs of mammary glands; their efferents enter large lymphatics or veins at the thoracic inlet.

The mediastinal lymph center (/3) comprises two to eight cranial and, but inconstantly, one to three caudal mediastinal nodes that form a long chain across the base of the heart. The *cranial mediastinal lymph nodes* lie in the cranial mediastinum and are related to the trachea, the esophagus, and the great blood vessels. They drain dorsal muscles of neck and thorax, the organs in the cranial mediastinum, and some tracheobronchial nodes; their efferents go to the thoracic duct or to lymphatics and large veins at the thoracic inlet. *Caudal mediastinal lymph nodes* are occasionally found along the esophagus caudal to the tracheal bifurcation. They drain neighboring structures and send efferents to the nearby tracheobronchial or thoracic aortic nodes.

The bronchial lymph center (/4) consists of 9 to 15 *tracheobronchial lymph nodes,* grouped about the bifurcation of the trachea, and a more cranial group of one to five nodes associated with the tracheal bronchus (Fig. 35–5/9). They drain the lungs, heart, and pericardium; their efferents go to the cranial mediastinal nodes or to the thoracic duct.

When the thoracic viscera are removed at slaughter, only the thoracic aortic and the ventral-most sternal nodes remain within the carcass.

## Selected Bibliography

Fraser, A.F.: Farm Animal Behavior, 2nd ed. London, Baillière-Tindall, 1980, p. 181.

Fredeen, H.T., and J.A. Newman: Rib and vertebral numbers in swine. Can. J. Anim. Sci. 42:232–239, 1962.

Getty, R., and N.G. Goshal: Applied anatomy of the sacrococcygeal region of the pig as related to tail bleeding. Vet. Med. [SAC] 62:361–367, 1967.

Hanbury, R.D., P.B. Doby, H.O. Miller, and K.D. Murrell: Trichinosis in a herd of swine: Cannibalism as a major mode of transmission. JAVMA 188:1155–1158, 1986.

Huisman, G.H.: The circulation of blood in pigs [in Dutch]. Tijdschr. Diergeneeskd. 94:1428–1436, 1969.

Mickwitz, G.W., and U. Feider: Auscultation of the lung in the pig [in German]. Dtsch. Tierarztl. Wochenschr. 79:231–235, 1972.

Nakakuki, S.: Bronchial tree, lobular division and blood vessels of the pig lung. J. Vet. Med. Sci. 56:685–689, 1994.

Penny, R. H.C., and F.W. Hill: Observations of some conditions in pigs at an abattoir with particular reference to tail biting. Vet. Rec. 94:174–180, 1974.

Skarda, R.T.: Techniques of local analgesia in ruminants and swine. Vet. Clin. North Am. Food Anim. Pract. 2:621–663, 1986.

Winkler, G.C., and N.F. Cheville: Morphometry of postnatal development in the porcine lung. Anat. Rec. 211:427–433, 1985.

Wissdorf, H.: The blood vessels of the porcine vertebral column [in German]. Zbl. Veterinarmed. A 12(Suppl.):1–104, 1970.

Wood, A.K.W.: Radiological observations of the thorax and abdomen of the piglet. Anat. Histol. Embryol. 14:193–214, 1985.

Yujun, L., and J.R. Stouffer: Pork carcass evaluation with an automated and computerized ultrasonic system. J. Anim. Sci. 73:29–38, 1995.

# CHAPTER 36

# The Abdomen of the Pig

The abdomen continues evenly from the bony thorax to the pelvis, giving the trunk the shape of a cylinder with some lateral compression. In fat or pregnant animals an expansion may occur caudal to the costal arch, especially ventrally, but it is never so marked as in ruminants. The more cranial abdominal organs are intrathoracic and covered laterally by the ribs. Similarly, the caudal end of the abdomen is covered by the thighs (Fig. 36–3/*B*,18).

## THE ABDOMINAL WALL

From a clinical standpoint the ventrolateral part of the abdominal wall is the most important since it is incised in the operation for cesarean section, the most common condition requiring surgical entry in this species. The preferred incision follows the dorsal edge of the abdominal mammary glands. Inguinal (and scrotal) hernia are common in male weanlings and also require surgical correction; although not actually penetrating the abdominal wall, the surgeon works at the superficial inguinal ring, the cleft in the outermost abdominal muscle.

The abdominal wall of the pig consists of the usual layers: skin, superficial fascia and cutaneus trunci, deep fascia, muscular layer, transverse fascia, and peritoneum. Generous amounts of fat separate certain layers, and for better exposure of deeper structures some may be removed during surgery. The fleshy parts of the abdominal muscles of the pig do not hold sutures well, and many surgeons place their incisions in the aponeuroses and fasciae. Nevertheless, it is important to know which muscles are encountered in incisions of any part of the abdominal wall.

The *cutaneus trunci* covers the side of the trunk and extends dorsally to about the level of the vertebral column; the dorsal half is thin and of no consequence. The muscle is thicker ventrally, particularly where it ends in the fold of the flank. The fibers of this part begin at the ventral midline and pursue a caudodorsal course, leaving the prepuce, and the floor of the abdomen caudal to the prepuce, uncovered. An isolated detachment of the cutaneus provides the cranial preputial muscle, which arises near the xiphoid cartilage and passes to the side of the prepuce, below which it unites with its contralateral fellow. A weak caudal preputial muscle is sometimes present.

The underlying deep fascia closely adheres to the ventral part of the external abdominal oblique. It contains some elastic fibers but not enough to tinge it yellow or to give it the supportive elasticity for which it is noted in horses and cattle. The layer gives rise caudally to the thick external spermatic fascia that covers the entire extra-abdominal vaginal tunic in males.

The *external abdominal oblique muscle* arises from the lateral surface of the ribs and from the lumbodorsal fascia (Fig. 36–1/1). The fleshy part of the muscle (which covers much of the flank) is succeeded by a small aponeurotic part along a line that sweeps from the coxal tuber toward the costal arch, the curved junction being entirely covered by the cutaneus trunci. The aponeurotic part is inserted in the linea alba and attaches to the prepubic tendon and the coxal tuber. Between these attachments the aponeurosis ends by fusing with the fascia covering the iliopsoas, the fusion line often being referred to as the inguinal ligament. The superficial inguinal ring, the large cleft in the aponeurosis, is directed laterally and slightly cranioventrally from the prepubic attachment.

The fleshy part of the *internal abdominal oblique muscle* is not so large as that of the external oblique. It arises from the lumbodorsal fascia and by a narrow aponeurosis from the coxal tuber and the lateral half of the "inguinal ligament." The fibers pass cranioventrally toward the linea alba and costal arch where the most cranial fascicles attach directly. The remainder of the fleshy part is succeeded by an extensive aponeurosis that passes external to the rectus and fuses with that of the external oblique to form the external sheath (of the rectus) through which the two muscles attach to the linea alba. The internal oblique, arising only from the lateral part of the inguinal ligament and attaching via the linea alba to the cranial end of the pelvic symphysis, thus has a curved free border (Fig. 36–2/12). The border fuses with the triangular insertion tendon of the rectus (/10′), and together they form the cranial boundary of the deep inguinal ring (/17).

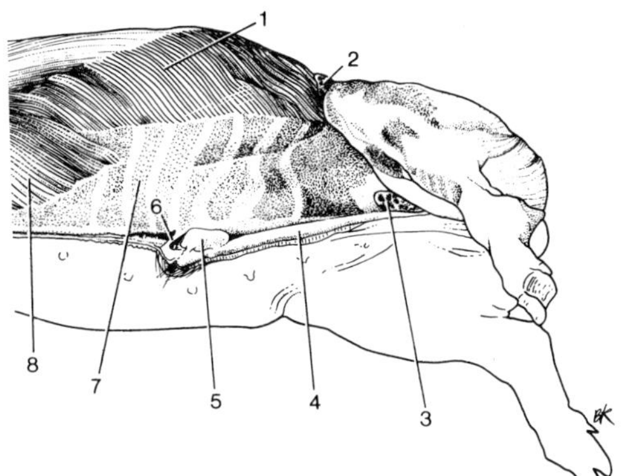


**Figure 36–1.** Ventrolateral view of the right abdominal wall. The cutaneus trunci has been removed.

1, External abdominal oblique; 2, subiliac lymph nodes; 3, superficial inguinal lymph nodes; 4, penis; 5, preputial diverticulum; 6, fibrous cord to umbilicus; 7, rectus abdominis with tendinous intersections shining through superficial lamina of rectus sheath; 8, pectoralis ascendens.

The *rectus abdominis* (/10) originates from the ventral surface of the sternum and costal arch and ends by a flat, triangular tendon cranioventral to the pelvic symphysis. The muscle is relatively narrow in its middle part and so does not extend onto the lateral surface of the abdominal wall as in the large species. It is thickest caudally.

The *transversus abdominis* continues without interruption from the transversus thoracis, which lies dorsal to the sternum and costal cartilages. It has an extensive fleshy part that covers the entire flank except for a narrow vertical strip at the thigh. Its fibers run dorsoventrally from the deep surface of the costal arch, the last rib, and the lumbar transverse processes, to be succeeded by an aponeurosis; the transition extends from the xiphoid cartilage and gradually moves laterally on the deep surface of the rectus before finally rising sharply to just in front of the coxal tuber. The aponeurosis lies deep to the rectus, and with the transverse fascia it forms the internal rectus sheath.

The abdominal wall is thus largely aponeurotic over a strip along the lateral border of the rectus that is about 10 cm long and up to 5 cm wide. The strip is deep to the base of the flank fold and covered by the cutaneus trunci, which is about 1 cm thick here. The *linea alba,* a narrow seam cranial to the prepuce, widens to about 2 cm above the prepuce before gradually narrowing again (/18). The umbilicus of the male is only a few centimeters cranial to the prepuce (Fig. 37–10/8). The prepuce impedes the surgical repair of an umbilical hernia and must be reflected to allow the edges of the hernia ring to be overlapped and sutured.

In principle, the *inguinal canal* of the pig conforms to the description given for other species. It is a potential space between the external and internal abdominal oblique muscles with deep and superficial openings (rings); the former leads from the canal into the abdominal cavity, the latter from the canal into the subcutaneous tissues of the groin (in the male into the blind sleeve formed by the external spermatic fascia). The deep ring is formed by the caudal free border of the internal oblique and the inguinal ligament. The superficial ring is a split in the aponeurosis of the external oblique situated near the pecten pubis and directed laterally, cranially, and slightly ventrally. Certain features warrant additional description.

At the deep inguinal ring the caudal free border of the internal oblique muscles does not reach very far caudally, with the result that the deep ring is large and the superficial ring is close to the caudal border of the internal oblique (Fig. 36–2/17,16,12). Thus, the inguinal canal is short. In addition, the insertion tendon of the rectus muscle (/10′) is wide enough to fuse with the medial half of the caudal border of the internal oblique, involving it in the formation of the deep inguinal ring whose borders

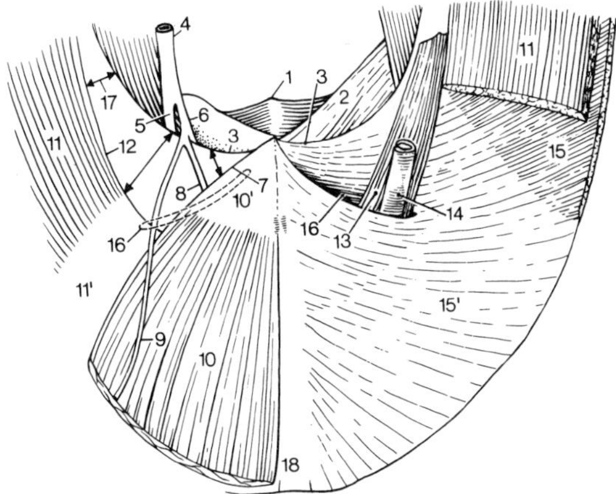


**Figure 36–2.** Inguinal canal of the male made visible on the interior (deep) surface of the caudal abdominal wall; semischematic, cranial view.

1, Pelvic symphysis; 2, prepubic tendon; 3, caudal border of external oblique aponeurosis (“inguinal ligament”); 4, external iliac artery; 5, femoral artery; 6, deep femoral artery; 7, lateral border of rectus tendon; 8, external pudendal artery; 9, caudal epigastric artery; 10, rectus abdominis; 10′, rectus tendon; 11, muscular part of internal abdominal oblique; 11′, aponeurotic part of internal abdominal oblique; 12, caudal free border of internal abdominal oblique; 13, cremaster; 14, tunica vaginalis and spermatic cord; 15, muscular part of external abdominal oblique; 15′, aponeurotic part of external abdominal oblique; 16, superficial inguinal ring; 17, deep inguinal ring (*arrows*); 18, linea alba.

are thus: cranially, the caudal free border of the internal oblique and the lateral border of the rectus tendon (/12,10′); caudally, the inguinal ligament (/3). The vaginal ring lies over the deep inguinal ring near the caudal free border of the internal oblique. Although normally much smaller than the deep inguinal ring, it has the potential to widen if a loop of bowel forces its way into it (indirect inguinal hernia).

The superficial inguinal ring is not a simple split in the external oblique aponeurosis; the medial crus is drawn dorsally, the lateral crus ventrally, so creating a flat passage with overlapping walls. Thus, the superficial inguinal ring itself has considerable depth; the subcutaneous end of the passage is more caudal than the abdominal end.

The two inguinal rings are quite large and partly superimposed; this predisposes the young male pig to inguinal hernia when an abnormal outgrowth reaction of the gubernaculum is present. Herniation involves the passage of a loop of intestine through the vaginal ring into the tubular tunica vaginalis, producing a subcutaneous swelling between the thighs. The inclusion of intestine within the tunica vaginalis makes castration of these animals hazardous.

The lamina femoralis, which continues the lateral crus of the superficial inguinal ring onto the medial surface of the thigh, is well developed.

The *blood supply* of the flank and ventrolateral abdominal wall is derived from two dorsal and two ventral arteries. The dorsal arteries are the cranial abdominal and deep circumflex iliac, and the ventral ones are the cranial and caudal epigastric arteries; all anastomose with each other. The cranial abdominal arises from the aorta and with two long branches supplies the abdominal muscles near the last rib. The deep circumflex iliac artery arises from the external iliac and with its cranial branch supplies the remainder of the flank. The cranial and caudal epigastric arteries arise from the internal thoracic and pudendoepigastric trunk, respectively; they pass toward each other on the deep surface of the rectus, which they supply. Lateral branches from the cranial epigastric supply the abdominal muscles adjacent to the rectus; they also supply the middle mammary glands (the caudal glands are supplied by branches of the caudal superficial epigastric).

The superficial inguinal lymph center comprising the subiliac and superficial inguinal nodes drains much of the abdominal wall. The *subiliac lymph nodes* form a small group on the cranial border of the thigh above the fold of the flank (Fig. 36–1/2). They drain the skin over a wide area of trunk and pelvis, the cutaneus trunci, and the cranial part of the thigh; their efferents usually go to the lateral iliac nodes but may go directly to the medial iliac nodes. The *superficial inguinal lymph nodes* (/3) form an elongated group in the groin, lateral to the penis or dorsolateral to the last pair of mammary glands. They drain much of the more superficial caudoventral parts of the animal, including the prepuce, the mammary glands (as far forward as the third pair), and the skin between the thighs; the perineum; and the distal parts of the hindlimbs. Their efferents pass through the inguinal canal to the medial iliac nodes.

### The Mammary Glands

Most sows have seven pairs of mammary glands forming the ventral contour of the trunk and extending from the axilla to the stifle (see Fig. 35–1). The glands are suspended by medial and lateral fibrous laminae derived from the deep abdominal fascia. The teats are long and perforated at the tip by two orifices through which the milk is withdrawn from the same number of duct systems within each gland. The blood supply is derived from the external thoracic and the cranial and caudal superficial epigastric arteries; satellite veins return the blood. Lymph drainage is via the ventral superficial cervical and sternal nodes for the first two pairs of glands and via the superficial inguinal nodes for the five caudal pairs.

In lactating multiparous sows the caudal glands are more pendulous than the cranial ones and their teats point somewhat laterally; despite their greater prominence they are said to be less productive. During nursing in lateral recumbency, the teats on the lower side may point toward the ground and be inaccessible to the litter. Although the sow has 14 glands, the average nursing litter does not exceed 8 or 10 piglets. For the first few days of the piglet's life the milk produced by one gland suffices. Several glands are, therefore, underused and begin to atrophy, with the result that in any lactation the number of functional glands more or less corresponds to the number in the litter. Later, when the piglet requires more milk than one gland can supply, its diet must be supplemented; the glands that have regressed remain quiescent until the next lactation.

## THE ABDOMINAL ORGANS

Except for a greatly elongated ascending colon and large cecum the abdominal organs resemble those of the dog in shape and position although these two species are not closely related. The description that follows includes the stomach, spleen, intestines,

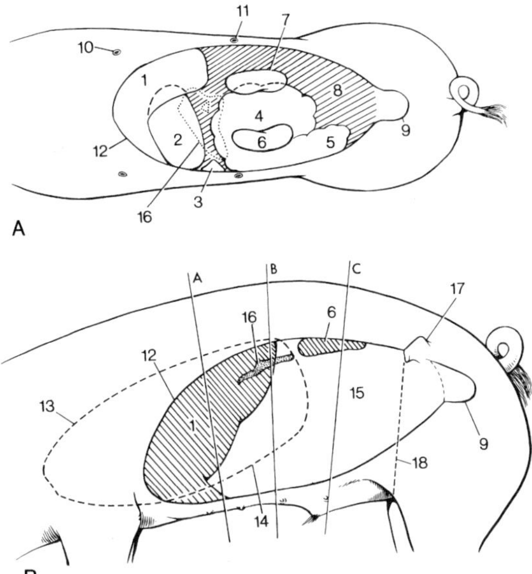


**Figure 36–3.** *A,* Dorsal projection of the abdominal cavity showing the approximate position of the major abdominal organs, schematic. *B,* Lateral projection with the relatively constant positions of liver, pancreas, and kidneys; the approximate levels of the three transverse sections in Figure 36–10 are indicated by A, B, and C.

1, Liver; 2, stomach; 3, spleen; 4, mass of ascending colon; 5, cecum; 6, left kidney; 7, right kidney; 8, space for small intestine; 9, pelvic cavity; 10, position of fifth rib; 11, position of last rib; 12, position of diaphragm; 13, cranial extent of thoracic cavity; 14, costal arch; 15, space for abdominal organs less constant in position (intestines, stomach, spleen); 16, pancreas; 17, wing of ilium; 18, cranial extent of thigh.

liver, pancreas, and kidneys. The other urinary and the reproductive organs that share the same space are described with the pelvis (p. 786).

The intestines, stomach, and spleen are loosely anchored to the abdominal wall and can expand or change their positions with food intake, pregnancy, or respiration. The more firmly attached liver, pancreas, and kidneys are less likely to shift. The latter group of organs occupies the craniodorsal part of the abdomen, while the more mobile ones fill the larger caudoventral part. The cecum and the ascending part of the colon form a distinct mass that, although attached dorsally, moves freely on the floor of the cavity. A general impression of the topography may be gained from the dorsal and lateral views in Figure 36–3.

## The Stomach and Spleen

The pig has a simple *stomach* distinguished from other simple stomachs by the presence of a diverticulum surmounting the fundus. The diverticulum points caudoventrally (Fig. 36–4/2); it is largely lined with glandular mucosa, and its interior is set off from the fundus by a spiral fold.

Except for a narrow strip near the cardia, the stomach is lined with glandular mucosa. The nonglandular area is whitish and easily recognized by its resemblance to the lining of the esophagus. It surrounds the cardiac opening and extends to the diverticulum, of which it lines a small part (/4). The mucosa of the fundus, diverticulum, and upper part of the body, a large third of the whole lining, contains cardiac glands, giving the pig by far the largest cardiac gland region (/6). The region of the proper gastric glands (/7) is more ventral and lines the remainder of the body except for the lesser curvature. The pyloric gland region (/9) lines the rest of the lesser curvature and the pyloric part. These regions, more readily distinguishable by their different hues in the pig than in the other domestic species, are not as sharply defined as Figure 36–4 suggests. The pylorus, like that of the ruminants, is accentuated by a fleshy protuberance (torus pyloricus; /10) that consists of muscle and adipose tissue; its function is still uncertain.

The median plane divides the moderately filled stomach so that fundus and body are to the left, the relatively small pyloric part to the right; the left parts are slanted cranioventrally.

The cranial relations of the stomach are the liver and the diaphragm. Caudally, the stomach is in contact with the spleen to the left, the intestines (usually the mass of ascending colon) ventrally,

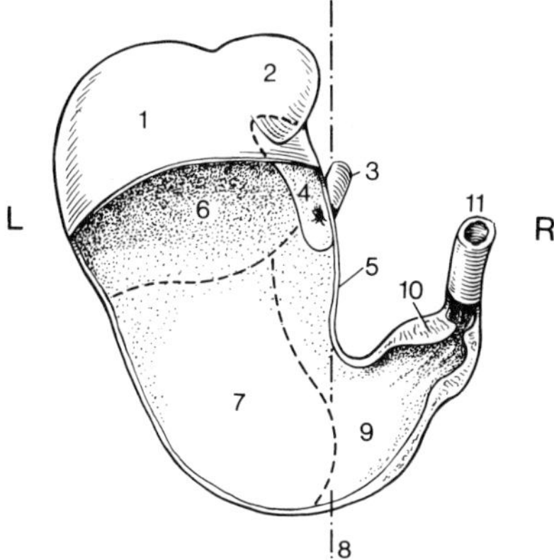


**Figure 36–4.** Stomach partially opened, caudoventral view, semischematic.

1, Fundus; 2, diverticulum; 3, esophagus; 4, nonglandular mucosa; 5, lesser curvature; 6, cardiac gland region; 7, region of proper gastric glands; 8, approximate position of median plane; 9, pyloric gland region; 10, torus pyloricus; 11, duodenum.

and the pancreas dorsally. Depending on the position of the colic mass, the visceral surface of the stomach may also relate to the jejunum. The stomach does not reach the floor of the abdominal cavity when moderately filled; if greatly distended it expands caudally and ventrally, displacing the spleen and ascending colon caudally (Fig. 36–5/6). The size of the stomach is then such that its pyloric part may reach the floor of the abdomen by the right costal arch.

The greater and lesser omenta are disposed as in the dog, but the caudal recess of the greater omentum is much shorter and does not cover the ventral surface of the intestines; it is therefore not the first structure encountered on incision of the abdominal wall.

The *spleen* can be recognized by its bright-red color, its elongated shape, and the surface marbling produced by the prominence of the splenic corpuscles. It is loosely attached to the greater curvature of the stomach by a rather wide gastrosplenic ligament and has a more or less dorsoventral orientation (/8). Its dorsal end fits between the fundus of the stomach, the cranial pole of the left kidney, and the left lobe of the pancreas; these relationships are not immediate as fat invariably intervenes. Its middle portion is in contact with the stomach and the intestine. When the stomach is moderately full the spleen lies opposite the last three or four ribs, and its ventral end crosses the costal arch or even the median plane. When the stomach is greatly dilated the spleen is pushed to the vicinity of the last rib.

## The Intestines

The small intestine is similar to that of the dog. The *duodenum* leaves the pylorus to the right of the median plane and passes caudodorsally, ventral to the right lobe of the liver and the right kidney. As it turns around the caudal aspect of the root of the mesentery, it passes between this and the descending colon before dipping ventrally to be continued by the jejunum. The bile duct enters the duodenum about 3 cm, and the single pancreatic duct (ductus pancreaticus accessorius) about 12 cm, from the pylorus on papillae visible with the unaided eye in hogs of slaughter size.

The *jejunum* is unremarkable. Its coils, only loosely tethered by a long mesentery, occupy the caudoventral portion of the abdominal cavity, which they share with the mass of the ascending colon (/11,9). Since the latter is to the left of the mesentery, the jejunum lies largely to the right, but portions may be found in contact with the left abdominal wall both cranial and caudal to the ascending colon (Fig. 36–3/*A*,8).

The *ileum* near the left flank rises to join the cecum, to which it is connected by the ileocecal fold. Its end raises within the cecum a distinct papilla, which is provided with a sphincter thought to prevent reflux of ingesta.

A better understanding of the pig's *large intestine* may be gained by reference to the simple arrangement in the dog. The transverse and descending colons are similar in both species—they hook around the cranial and left aspects of the

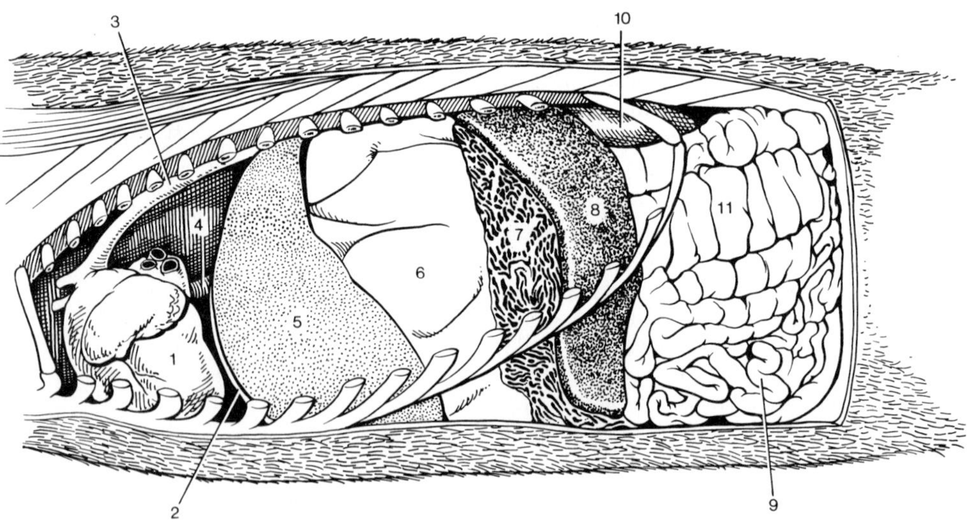


**Figure 36–5.** Heart and abdominal viscera, left lateral view.

1, Heart; 2, diaphragm, cut; 3, aorta; 4, caudal vena cava; 5, left lateral lobe of liver; 6, greatly distended stomach; 7, greater omentum (gastrosplenic ligament); 8, spleen; 9, jejunum; 10, left kidney; 11, mass of ascending colon.

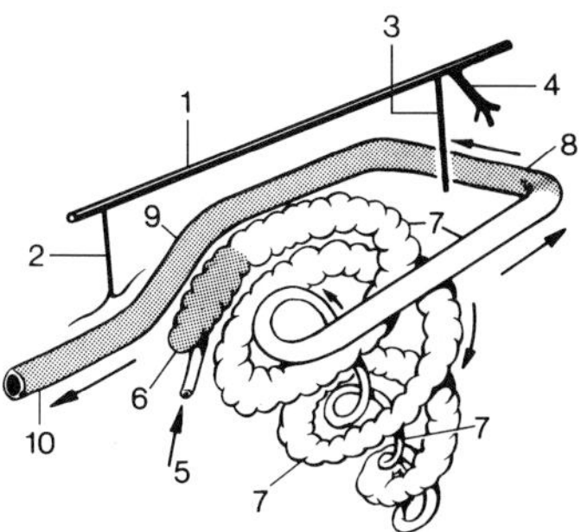


**Figure 36–6.** The large intestine, schematic.

1, Aorta; 2, caudal mesenteric artery; 3, cranial mesenteric artery; 4, celiac artery; 5, ileum; 6, cecum; 7, ascending colon; 8, transverse colon; 9, descending colon; 10, rectum.

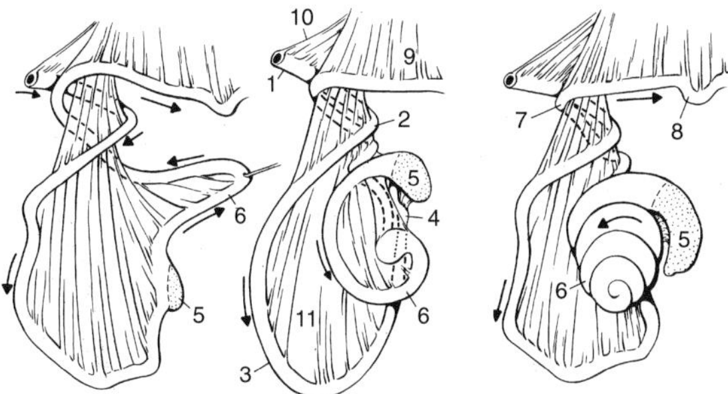


**Figure 36–7.** The development of the ascending colon, left lateral view.

1, Descending duodenum; 2, caudal flexure of duodenum; 3, jejunum; 4, ileum; 5, cecum; 6, ascending colon; 7, transverse colon; 8, descending colon; 9, descending mesocolon; 10, mesoduodenum; 11, mesentery.

root of the mesentery (Fig. 36–6/9,8). The ascending colon is greatly elongated in the pig and is coiled to form a cone-shaped mass. During development, the initial loop of the ascending colon (Fig. 36–7/6) falls to the left of the mesentery that suspends jejunum and ileum. The proximal limb proceeding from the cecum crosses the distal limb and as it elongates spirals around this. Thus, the proximal limb of the initial loop gives rise to the centripetal turns located on the outside of the cone, while the distal limb gives rise to the concealed centrifugal turns. The base of the cone is dorsal and is attached to the roof of the abdominal cavity in the vicinity of the left kidney and pancreas; the apex of the cone is ventral. Beginning at the cecum, which in this extraordinary arrangement comes to lie near the left (!) flank, the centripetal turns pass clockwise (when seen from above) to the apex of the cone. They then reverse and return to the base in tight counterclockwise turns (Fig. 36–6). The turn arriving at the base passes cranially to the right of the root of the mesentery and, becoming the transverse colon, begins to hook around the root. The axis of the cone is dorsoventral, but its ventral end enjoys considerable freedom to move along the abdominal floor. The outer centripetal turns of the cone are sacculated by the presence of two bands; the inner turns are smooth.

Jejunum and ileum contain numerous prominent patches of aggregate lymph nodules. One is extremely long and extends through the ileal papilla into the ascending colon.

The *rectum* conforms in structure and position to that of the other species. It is slightly dilated before the narrow anal canal begins. For the anus and surrounding structures see page 786.

## The Liver and Pancreas

The relatively large *liver* resembles that of the dog in lobation and position. It exhibits deep fissures that divide it into left lateral and medial, and right lateral and medial lobes (Fig. 36–8 and Plate 2/*C*). Additionally, the short quadrate lobe and the caudate process are present centrally; the latter generally fails to make contact with the right kidney. The gallbladder lies between the quadrate and right medial lobes. The high content of interlobular fibrous tissues outlines minute liver lobules on the surface (Plate 2/*D*); it results in pork

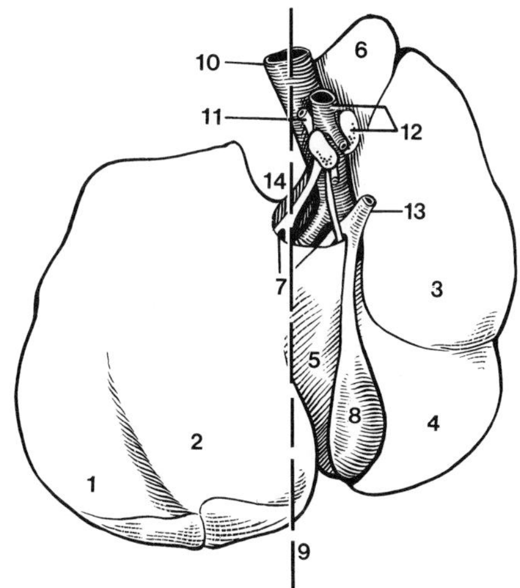


**Figure 36–8.** Visceral surface of the liver.

1, Left lateral lobe; 2, left medial lobe; 3, right lateral lobe; 4, right medial lobe; 5, quadrate lobe; 6, caudate process; 7, porta; 8, gallbladder; 9, approximate position of median plane; 10, caudal vena cava; 11, hepatic artery; 12, portal vein and hepatic lymph nodes; 13, bile duct; 14, esophageal notch.

liver being less palatable and considerably cheaper than bovine liver, which contains less connective tissue. The surface markings caused by the fibrous tissue identify the isolated pig liver. The fibrous tissue is so abundant that aspiration biopsy, as used in ruminants, for example, is unsuccessful. Surgical biopsy can be performed, however, through the ventral midline just caudal to the sternum where the liver lies broadly on the abdominal floor (Fig. 36–9/8).

Except ventrally, the liver is covered by the ribs. Despite the initial impression, more lies on the right side than on the left (Fig. 36–10*A*,7). The axis of the liver inclines in a left cranial and ventral direction from its most caudal part high on the right side. The liver has extensive cranial contact with the diaphragm, to which it is attached by left triangular and coronary ligaments that closely surround the caudal vena cava as this passes over the thick dorsal border (/4). The relations of the deeply concave visceral surface include the stomach to the left and the pancreas centrally; the remaining parts of the visceral surface are related to the duodenum, jejunum, and, at times, the ascending colon. When the stomach is distended, its contact with the liver increases ventrally and to the right, displacing the intestines.

The *pancreas* is applied to the roof of the abdominal cavity, which slopes so that the cranial portion of the gland is a little more ventral than the caudal. About two thirds lie to the left of the median plane where relationships with the fundus of the stomach, the spleen, and the cranial pole of the left kidney are established (Fig. 36–3/16). The right border follows the descending duodenum; it makes contact with the liver cranially and may reach the cranial pole of the right kidney caudally. The portal vein passes through the pancreas at an acute angle on its way from the root of the mesentery to the liver. The pancreas is surrounded by fat and may be covered by serosa in the vicinity of the duodenum.

## The Kidneys

The dorsoventrally flattened kidneys lie flat against the psoas muscles (embedded in generous amounts of fat), the cranial pole ventral to the last rib, and the caudal pole below the fourth lumbar vertebra. They are thus positioned more or less symmetrically in contrast to the arrangement in other species. The left kidney is related ventrally to the ascending colon, the base of the cecum, and the pancreas (Fig. 36–5/10). The right kidney is related ventrally to the descending duodenum, the jejunum, and possibly the pancreas, but does not make contact with the liver as in other domestic species (Fig. 36–9/5).

The hilus is situated in the medial border. The long renal pelvis consists of a central cavity and two large recesses (major calices) that are directed toward the poles (Fig. 36–11 and Plate 4/*C,D*). About 10 cup-shaped minor calices embrace an equal number of renal papillae through whose tips urine oozes into the pelvis. As a result of fusion of

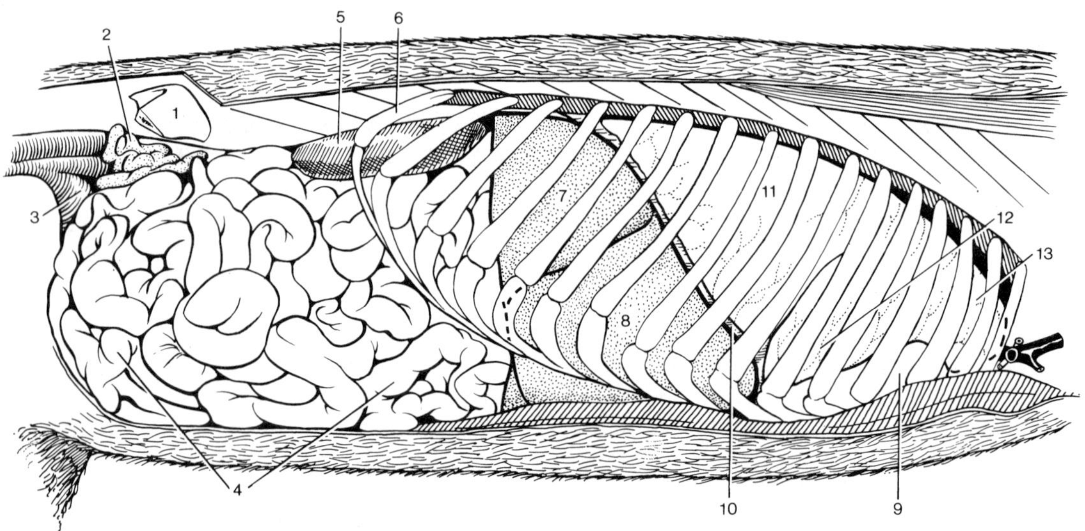


**Figure 36–9.** Abdominal and thoracic viscera, right lateral view.

1, Wing of ilium; 2, uterine horns; 3, bladder; 4, jejunum; 5, right kidney; 6, last rib; 7, 8, right lateral and medial lobes of liver; 9, heart in pericardium; 10, diaphragm, cut; 11–13, caudal, middle, and cranial lobes of right lung.

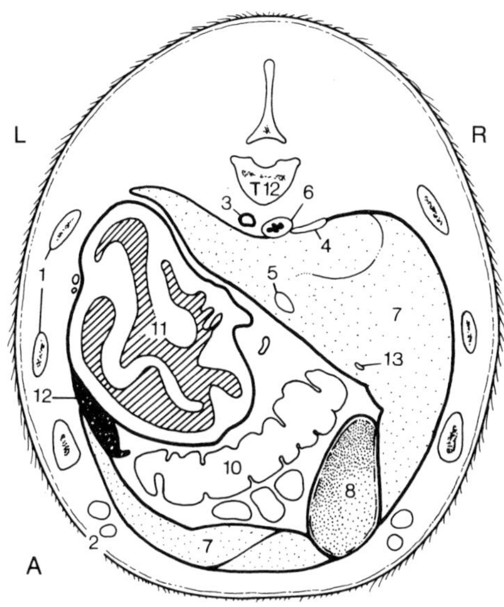


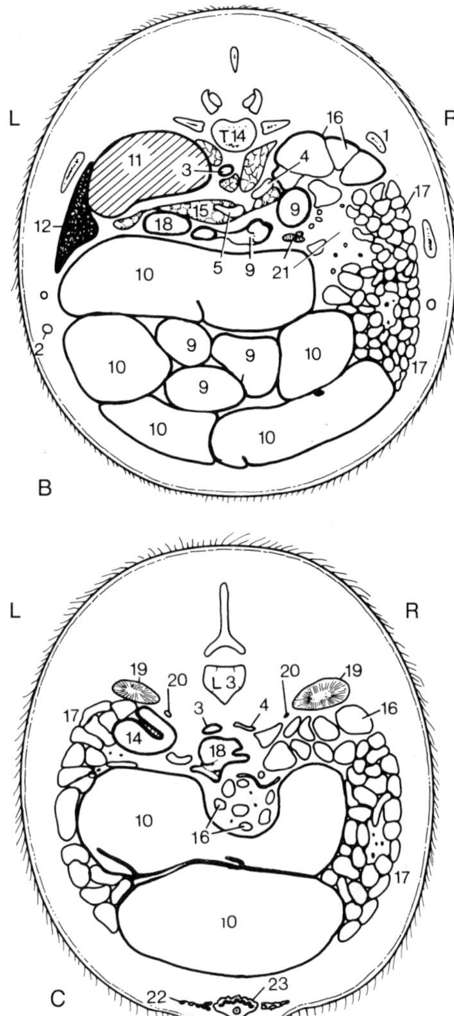


**Figure 36–10.** Schematic transverse sections of the abdomen at the levels of T12 *(A)*, T14 *(B)*, and L3 *(C)*; see Figure 36–3/*B*.

1, Ribs; 2, costal arch; 3, aorta, in *B* passing between crura of diaphragm; 4, caudal vena cava; 5, portal vein, in *B* passing through pancreas; 6, esophagus; 7, liver; 8, gallbladder; 9, centrifugal turns of ascending colon; 10, centripetal turns of ascending colon; 11, stomach (almost empty), fundus in *B;* 12, spleen; 13, hepatic ducts; 14, cecum; 15, pancreas; 16, gas-filled small intestines; 17, jejunum; 18, ascending colon; 19, caudal poles of kidneys; 20, ureters; 21, jejunal lymph nodes and mesentery; 22, cranial preputial muscle; 23, prepuce and preputial diverticulum.

neighboring renal pyramids during development, some papillae are larger than others. The interior of the pig's kidney is thus similar to that of the human organ.

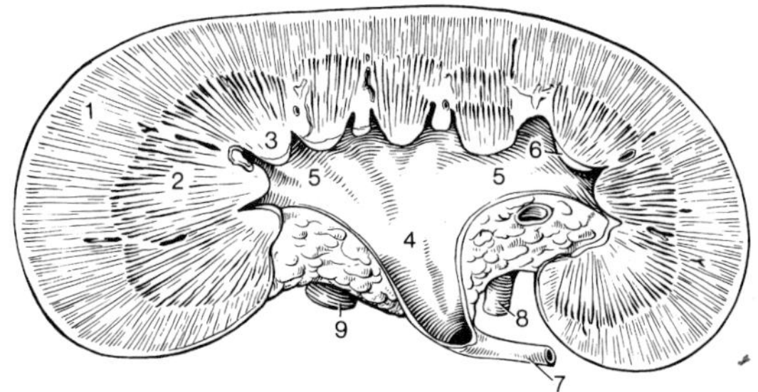


**Figure 36–11.** Kidney sectioned through poles and hilus.

1, Cortex; 2, medulla; 3, papilla; 4, pelvis; 5, major calices; 6, minor calyx; 7, ureter; 8, renal artery; 9, renal vein.

## THE LYMPHATIC STRUCTURES OF THE ABDOMINAL CAVITY

These can be divided into three groups that are associated with the dorsal abdominal wall and kidneys, the organs supplied by the celiac artery, and the organs supplied by the cranial and caudal mesenteric arteries.

The first group consists of the lumbar aortic, renal, and iliac nodes (Fig. 36–12/6,7,18,13). The *lumbar aortic lymph nodes* accompany the abdominal aorta and continue the thoracic aortic nodes. They drain the dorsal and lateral abdominal wall, perirenal fat, kidneys, and testes (or ovaries); their efferents combine to form lumbar trunks that empty into the cisterna chyli. Some are exposed in the slaughterhouse by the saw cut that splits the carcass.

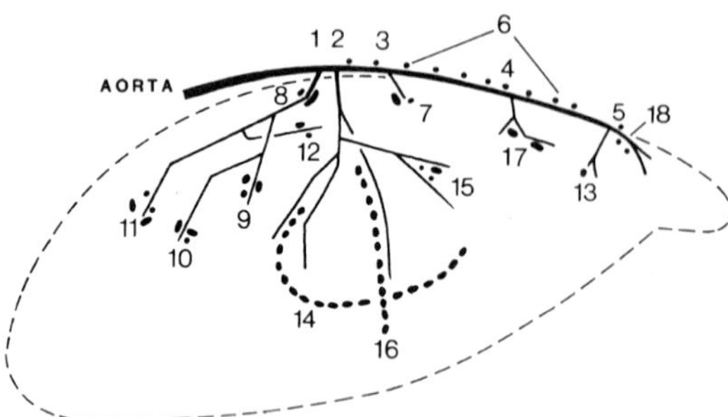


**Figure 36–12.** Schema of the major abdominal arteries and lymph nodes.

1, Celiac artery; 2, cranial mesenteric artery; 3, renal artery; 4, caudal mesenteric artery; 5, deep circumflex iliac artery; 6, lumbar aortic nodes; 7, renal nodes; 8, celiac nodes; 9, splenic nodes; 10, gastric nodes; 11, hepatic nodes; 12, pancreaticoduodenal nodes; 13, lateral iliac nodes; 14, jejunal nodes; 15, ileocolic nodes; 16, colic nodes; 17, caudal mesenteric nodes; 18, medial iliac nodes.

The two to four *renal lymph nodes* are located near the hilus of the kidney. They drain the kidney and adjacent territory; their efferents enter the lumbar trunks or the cisterna chyli.

Inconstant *phrenicoabdominal* and *testicular nodes* may be found on the lateral border of the psoas major and at the origin of the testicular artery (even in the spermatic cord), respectively.

The large group of *medial iliac lymph nodes* surround the terminal branches of the aorta and follow the external iliac vessels (Fig. 36–13/10). They drain the adjacent muscles, hindlimb, bladder, and genital organs and receive efferents from the nodes of the pelvis and hindlimb. The efferent vessels join the lumbar trunks in which the lymph reaches the cisterna chyli.

One to three small, inconstant *lateral iliac lymph nodes* (/11) lie at the bifurcation of the deep circumflex iliac vessels. They drain the caudodorsal abdominal wall and the superficial inguinal nodes; their efferents pass to the medial iliac nodes.

The group associated with the organs supplied by the celiac artery consists of the celiac, splenic, gastric, hepatic, and pancreaticoduodenal nodes (Fig. 36–12/8–12). Most are usually found close to the entry of the arteries to the various organs. A small group of *celiac lymph nodes* lie on the celiac artery itself; they refilter the lymph from the splenic, gastric, hepatic, and pancreaticoduodenal nodes and also drain the caudal parts of the lungs, mediastinum, and diaphragm. The efferents pass to the cisterna chyli.

The *splenic lymph nodes* are found at the dorsal end of the hilus of the spleen. They drain that organ and adjacent parts of the greater omentum, stomach, and pancreas; their efferents pass to the celiac nodes.

The *gastric lymph nodes* lie near the cardia and lesser curvature of the stomach. They drain the stomach and (in part) the caudal end of the esophagus, diaphragm, and pancreas; their efferents pass to the celiac nodes.

The two to seven *hepatic lymph nodes* lie at the porta of the liver (Fig. 36–8/12). They drain the liver, the pancreas (in part), and the pancreaticoduodenal nodes; their efferents pass to the celiac nodes.

The *pancreaticoduodenal lymph nodes* are distributed along the duodenum; some are embedded in the pancreas. They drain the pancreas, duodenum, and part of the stomach and omentum; the efferents of the more cranial nodes go to the celiac nodes, those from more caudal ones go to the colic nodes in the group associated with the cranial mesenteric artery.

The group associated with the organs supplied

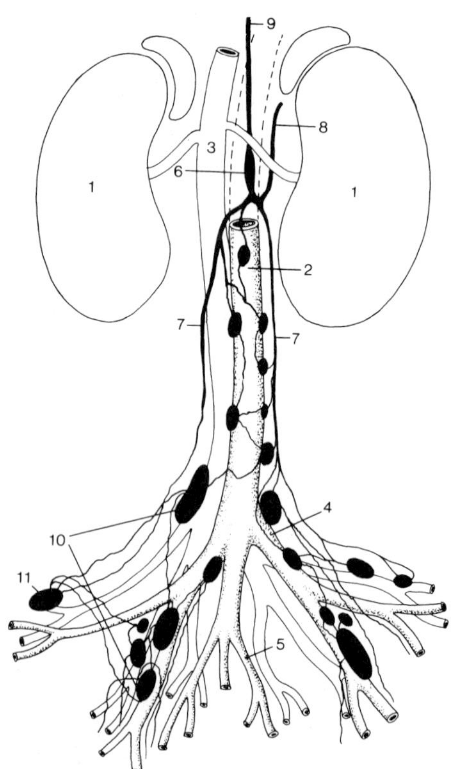


**Figure 36–13.** The lymph nodes of the sublumbar area, ventral view.

1, Kidneys; 2, aorta; 3, caudal vena cava; 4, external iliac artery; 5, internal iliac artery; 6, cisterna chyli; 7, lumbar trunks and lumbar aortic nodes; 8, intestinal trunk; 9, thoracic duct; 10, medial iliac nodes; 11, lateral iliac node.

by the mesenteric arteries drain the bulk of the small and large intestines and include the jejunal, ileocolic, colic, and caudal mesenteric nodes (Fig. 36–12/14–17). The most important of these (and of the entire abdominal cavity) are the *jejunal lymph nodes.* They form a long, raised band in the mesentery midway between the root and the attachment to the small intestine. They drain jejunum and ileum; their efferents form the large jejunal lymph trunk that joins the colic trunk in the root of the mesentery. The jejunal lymph nodes are regularly examined after slaughter because they reveal evidence of enteric diseases (also of tuberculosis) that often necessitate condemnation of the entire carcass.

The small group of *ileocolic lymph nodes* is located by the ileocolic junction and drain both cecum and ileum. The efferents pass to the trunk that arises from the colic nodes.

The numerous *colic lymph nodes* form a long chain in the center of the cone-shaped mass of the ascending colon and are therefore inaccessible to routine inspection. They drain the entire ascending colon, the transverse colon, and parts of the cecum and descending colon. Their efferents combine to form the colic trunk, which together with the jejunal trunk gives rise to the intestinal trunk that conveys lymph to the cisterna chyli.

A group of small *caudal mesenteric lymph nodes* lies in the mesocolon and drains the descending colon and also the nearby pancreas. The efferents go to the lumbar aortic nodes.

## Selected Bibliography


Ashdown, R.R.: The anatomy of the inguinal canal in the domesticated mammals. Vet. Rec. 75:1345–1351, 1963.

Becker, H.N.: Castration, inguinal hernia repair and vasectomy in boars. *In* Morrow, D.A. (ed.): Current Therapy in Theriogenology. Philadelphia, W.B. Saunders Company, 1986.

de Kruijf, J.M.: Liver biopsy in the pig [in German]. Dtsch. Tierarztl. Wochenschr. 81:10, 1974.

Prado, I.M.M., M.A. Niglino, and L.J.A. DiDio: Morphology of the swine ileum terminale. Ann. Anat. 179:475–479, 1997.

Runnels, L.J.: Obstetrics and cesarean section in swine. *In* Morrow, D.A. (ed.): Current Therapy in Theriogenology. Philadelphia, W.B. Saunders Company, 1986.

Sack, W.O. (ed.): Horowitz/Kramer Atlas of Musculoskeletal Anatomy of the Pig. Ithaca, N.Y., Veterinary Textbooks, 1982.

Snook, C.S.: Use of the subcutaneous abdominal vein for blood sampling and intravenous catheterization in potbellied pigs. JAVMA 219:809–810, 2001.

Wood, A.K.W.: Radiological observations of the thorax and abdomen of the piglet. Anat. Histol. Embryol. 14:193–214, 1985.

Zahner, M, and K.-H. Wille: The blood vascular system of the terminal position of the porcine gut [in German]. Anat. Histol. Embryol. 25:55–63, 1996.

CHAPTER 37

# The Pelvis and Reproductive Organs of the Pig

## THE PELVIS

The pelvic part of the trunk continues the back and abdomen without producing noticeable landmarks; ventrally it blends smoothly with the thighs. A slight vertical indentation above the fold of the flank marks the junction between abdomen and thigh. Because of the thick layer of fat on the dorsal and lateral surfaces and the muscling of the thighs, the bony pelvis appears proportionately rather small. Even so, coxal and ischial tubers can be palpated, the latter through the vertebral heads of biceps and semitendinosus. This tuber (Fig. 37–1/3) does not fuse with the body of the ischium for several years; it is therefore subject to detachment and ventral displacement by the pull of the strong hamstring muscles attaching to it. Pigs so afflicted, most commonly young sows, are in great pain and cannot rise; they die or must be slaughtered.

On lateral view, the bony pelvis appears much less angulated than that of most domestic mammals. The angle formed between the pelvic floor and the *conjugata* (the line connecting the cranial end of the symphysis with the promontory) is large and approaches 180 degrees (/10); this results in a long conjugata and a large, oval pelvic inlet so oblique that it is almost in the dorsal plane. The floor of the pelvis in the standing pig (particularly that with an arched back) slopes toward the ground caudally.

The conjugata of the sow is 12 to 15 cm, the transverse diameter of the inlet only 7 to 10 cm; the *vertical diameter* of the pelvis, the actual height of the birth canal, measures 8 to 10 cm. The vertical diameter strikes the caudal segment of the sacrum, which remains movable for some years so that some adjustment for the passage of the fetus is possible. The transverse diameter at this level is less accommodating and is diminished by the inward bend of the ischial spines (/2,14). The bony birth canal, therefore, has a diameter of about 8 or 9 cm in all directions. The actual passage is, of course, reduced by the vaginal wall, rectum, urethra, internal obturator, and fat, preventing veterinarians—unless they have small hands—from giving assistance per vaginam in cases of dystocia.

The space between sacrum and ischial spine is closed by the sacrosciatic ligament (/9), which relaxes at farrowing time, increasing the vertical diameter of the pelvis and its outlet. Simultaneous loosening of the symphysis and sacroiliac joints may help, but the transverse diameter is probably not affected.

The determination of the sex of a dressed, split carcass is assisted by recognition of the short stump (pizzle eye) of the crus penis beside the caudal end of the pelvic symphysis of the male. The name refers to the appearance of a transected crus, a red center (corpus cavernosum) inside a white ring of tunica albuginea, of the "pizzle."

### The Bladder, the Anus, and Surrounding Structures

The *urinary bladder* varies greatly in topography and appearance according to the volume of urine it contains. The recently voided organ is small, ovoid, and firm and placed over the pubic pecten. The grossly distended organ is more or less spherical and lies almost entirely within the abdomen, resting on the abdominal floor (Fig. 37–3/*A*,5). A small suburethral diverticulum is associated with the opening of the female urethra into the vestibule. It may impede the progress of a catheter (/6).

Congenital absence of the anus (atresia ani) is frequent in piglets and often is traceable to a particular boar. It is remarkable that such piglets often survive 3 to 4 weeks untreated. If the blind end of the rectum is not too distant from the skin, a passage to the exterior may be created by

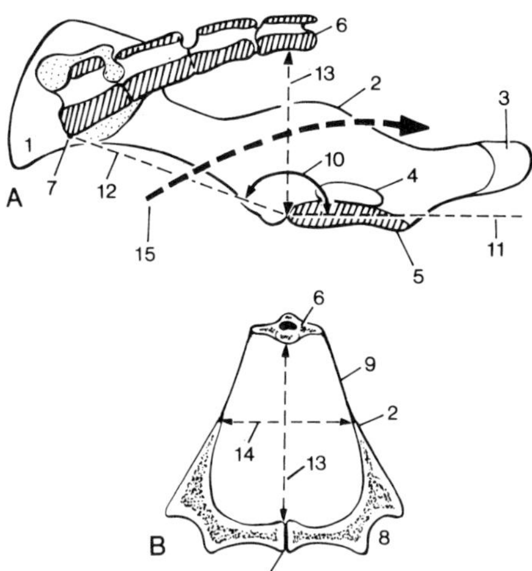


**Figure 37–1.** *A*, Median section of the sow's pelvis. *B*, Transverse section of the pelvis near the level of the vertical diameter.

1, Coxal tuber; 2, ischial spine; 3, ischial tuber; 4, obturator foramen; 5, pelvic symphysis; 6, S4; 7, promontory; 8, acetabulum; 9, sacrosciatic ligament; 10, angle between pelvic floor and conjugata; 11, plane of pelvic floor; 12, conjugata; 13, vertical diameter; 14, transverse diameter; 15, pelvic axis.

relatively simple surgery. Prolapse of the rectum, a condition that is encountered in pigs over 50 pounds (22.5 kg) in weight, requires more sophisticated surgery, especially when the everted rectum has been mutilated by penmates, as often happens.

Although little attention is paid, generally, to the structures surrounding the anus when correcting rectal prolapse, an understanding of the muscles associated with the rectum and anal canal is essential for the more complicated case. The outer longitudinal muscle layer of the rectum is gathered to the dorsal surface and, as the rectococcygeus, passes caudally to attach to the first few caudal vertebrae. The inner circular muscle layer thickens to form the internal anal sphincter. The external anal sphincter is anchored to the fascia of the tail above and to the muscles associated with the genital tract below. The levator ani is inserted into the lateral surface of the anal canal, having arisen from the sacrosciatic ligament a few centimeters craniolateral to the anus. The retractor penis (clitoridis) arises from the ventral surface of the sacrum and passes lateral to the rectum on its way to the penis (clitoris); its rectal part is independent, arises from the tail vertebrae, and forms a thin loop around the ventral aspect of the rectum.

*Rectal palpation* is possible in sows weighing over 330 pounds (150 kg) without great difficulty or ill effects on the animals. It seems that the small diameter and short suspension of the descending colon are a greater impediment than the narrowness of the pelvis. With ample lubrication and sufficient cooperation, the arm can be introduced almost to the elbow. The forearm becomes wedged solidly in the pelvic canal so that the internal range depends entirely on the length and mobility of the hand. The procedure allows examination of the pelvic inlet and bladder and, more important, the ovaries, cervix, and uterine arteries for pregnancy diagnosis. The right kidney and the spiral colon (recognized by its coarse, granular contents) may also be palpated. Examination of the more confined pelvic cavity of boars is unsuccessful, as the hand causes the animals obvious pain.

### The Lymph Nodes of the Pelvis

The *medial iliac lymph nodes,* grouped around the terminal branches of the aorta, have been described (p. 784). They are continued into the pelvic cavity by the *sacral lymph nodes,* which lie against the ventral surface of the sacrum; inconstant *anorectal lymph nodes* may continue the chain between the tailhead and rectum. The last-named drain the anus, rectum, and tail; their efferents pass to the medial iliac nodes. The *ischial* and the *gluteal lymph nodes* are found lateral to the sacrosciatic ligament (see Fig. 38–3/4,4′). The latter drain the gluteal region, the former the perineum, the bony pelvis, and the caudal thigh muscles and also receive lymph from the popliteal nodes. Their efferents pass through the gluteal nodes to the medial iliac nodes.

## THE FEMALE REPRODUCTIVE ORGANS

The rather mobile *ovaries* are about 5 cm long and characteristically irregular with many follicles and corpora lutea protruding from the surface (see Figs. 5–43/1 and 37–2/1 and Plate 7/*E*). They are suspended among the intestines by long mesovaria, usually a few centimeters lateroventral to the pelvic inlet. Both may lie near one flank and removal through a single flank incision is therefore possible. The ovaries sink with the horns as pregnancy advances and eventually become inaccessible on rectal exploration.

The *uterine tube* is about 20 cm long and begins within the ovarian bursa; its large orifice faces the ovary. It courses over the cone-shaped mesosalpinx to join the horn of the uterus without a noticeable constriction (/4). Obstruction of the tube (producing hydrosalpinx) is the most common cause of infertility in sows.

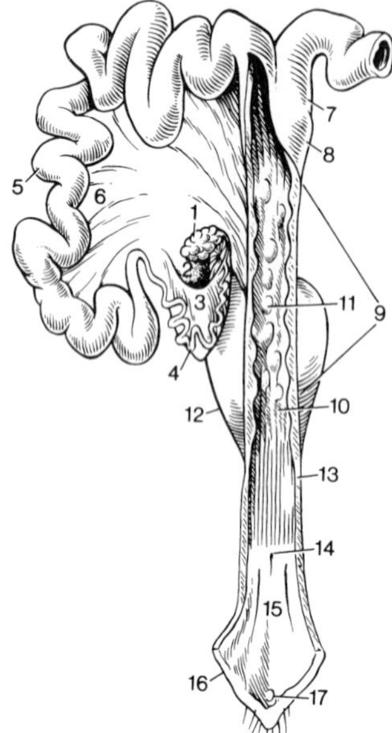


**Figure 37–2.** The reproductive tract of the sow opened dorsally in part; the right uterine horn and ovary are not shown.

1, Left ovary; 2, ovarian bursa; 3, mesosalpinx; 4, uterine tube; 5, uterine horn; 6, broad ligament; 7, parallel segments of uterine horns; 8, body of uterus; 9, cervix; 10, external uterine orifice; 11, mucosal prominences; 12, bladder; 13, vagina; 14, external urethral orifice; 15, vestibule; 16, vulva; 17, glans of clitoris.

The body of the *uterus* is short. The horns continue forward for a few centimeters within a common investment of longitudinal muscle, creating the impression that the uterine body is longer than it actually is. The deeper circular muscle at the junction of body and horns forms a complex sphincter that operates in such a way that when the entrance of one horn is closed that of the other is open. This arrangement comes into play at farrowing when it regulates the presentation of fetuses at the pelvic inlet and prevents the collision that otherwise might occur should both horns contract together. The sphincter effect is such that a hand introduced into the tract does not detect the bifurcation of the uterus. The mechanism does not prevent transuterine migration of embryos in early pregnancy. It also does not function in the atonic organ, as at cesarean section it is often possible to remove fetuses from one horn through an incision in the other.

The uterine horns are remarkable for their length. In the nongravid state, each is about 1 m long; at the height of pregnancy this may easily be doubled as occasionally it must accommodate eight fetuses. The nongravid horns and, for that matter, the ovaries are so mobile that they cannot be assigned exact positions in the abdominal cavity. The horns lie cranial to the pelvic inlet midway between roof and floor and are suspended by extensive broad ligaments (Fig. 37–3/4). They are related to the spiral colon, small intestine, and possibly the bladder. Their length and flexuous nature cause them to resemble coils of small

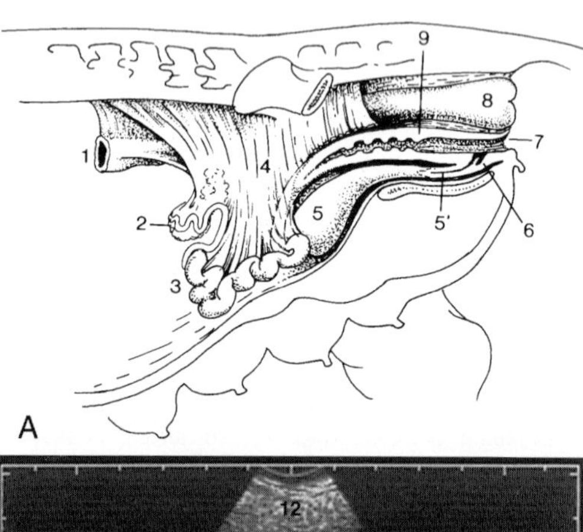


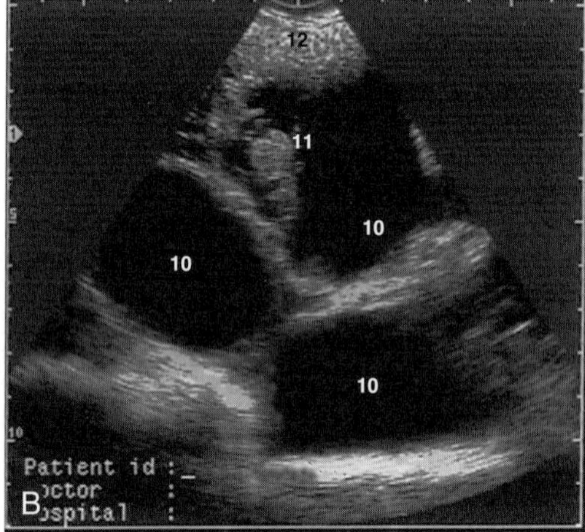


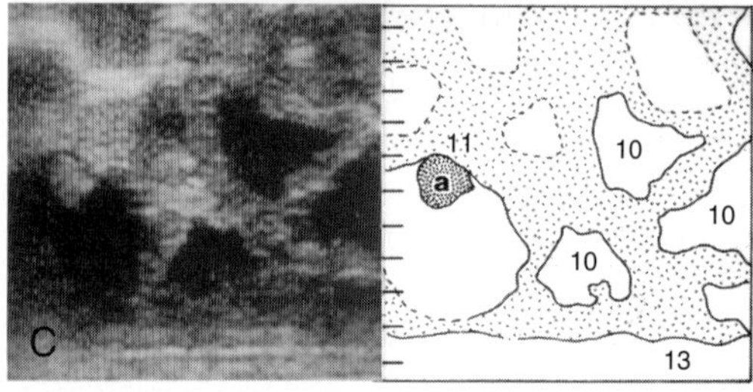


**Figure 37–3.** *A*, The reproductive organs of the sow in situ. (The presence of the intestines in the intact animal causes the ovaries and uterine horns to lie more dorsal than shown here.) Transrectal *(B)* and transabdominal *(C)* ultrasonic images of 30-day gravid porcine uteruses. (Scales in cm.)

1, Descending colon; 2, ovary; 3, uterine horns; 4, broad ligament; 5, bladder; 5′, urethra; 6, suburethral diverticulum; 7, vulva; 8, rectum; 9, cervix; 10, allantoic fluid-filled spaces; 11, (a), embryo; 12, rectal wall; 13, abdominal wall.

intestine. The broad ligaments, which contain much smooth muscle, enlarge considerably during pregnancy, allowing the horns to sink to the abdominal floor where the fetuses become inaccessible on rectal exploration; pregnancy diagnosis per rectum therefore depends almost entirely on palpating the cervix and the uterine artery. The gravid uterus may be visualized by transrectal or transabdominal ultrasound (/*B, C*). Toward the end of pregnancy the uterine horns almost fill the ventral half of the abdomen; they push the intestines craniodorsally and reach the stomach and the liver.

Table 37–1 lists criteria by which pig fetuses may be aged.

The uterine artery (Fig. 37–4/6), a substantial vessel, is the principal supply to the uterus, which also receives blood from branches of the ovarian and vaginal arteries (/2,7). The uterine artery arises from the umbilical and crosses the medial surface of the external iliac artery where it can be palpated rectally during pregnancy; close to term it may be as large as the iliac. "Fremitus," a reliable indicator of advanced pregnancy, can be felt, as in the cow.

The ovarian vein, which drains most of the uterus in addition to the ovary and uterine tube, consists of two or three interconnected channels. The ovarian artery combines with branches from the uterine artery to form a dense plexus around the venous channels, enabling luteolytic prostaglandins from the uterine horn to reach the ipsilateral ovary.

The fetuses are attached to the endometrium of the uterine horns by a *diffuse placenta* (Plate 8/*A,B*); except at its tips, which become necrotic, the fusiform sac grows chorionic folds that maintain extensive contact with the maternal tissues. This contact is not destructive, and the chorion can be peeled from the endometrium without difficulty; retained fetal membranes are consequently rare. The fetuses leave their placentas behind when they begin their journey toward the outside. The ruptured chorionic and amniotic sacs create a continuous, mucus-lubricated tube through which the fetuses move freely until they are propelled by a peristaltic contraction toward the birth canal. During this time, they remain connected to their placentas by umbilical cords that are so extensible that the fetuses can pass each other. The structure of the placenta may explain the lack of antibody transfer in utero and the newborn's need of colostrum to repair this deficiency.

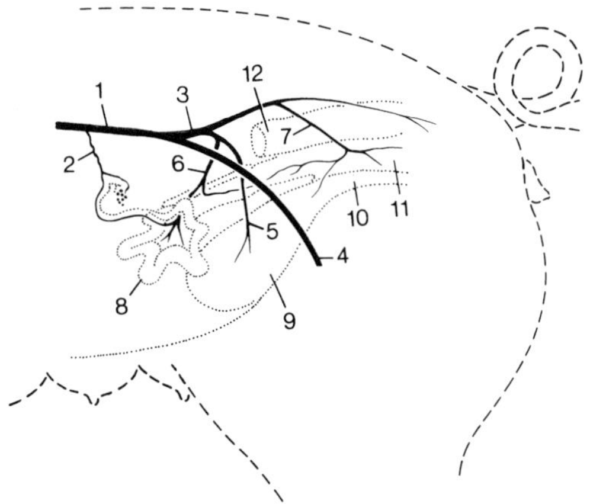


**Figure 37–4.** The principal arteries supplying the left side of the female reproductive tract, schematic.

1, Aorta; 2, ovarian a. with cranial uterine branch; 3, internal iliac a.; 4, external iliac a. continued by femoral into left thigh; 5, umbilical a.; 6, left uterine a. crossing medial surface of external iliac; 7, vaginal a. with caudal uterine branch; 8, left uterine horn; 9, bladder; 10, urethra; 11, vagina; 12, rectum.

The *cervix* (which lies half within the pelvic cavity, half within the abdomen) is peculiar for its length (up to 25 cm). It presents rows of mucosal prominences that project into the lumen, interdigitate, and occlude the canal (Fig. 37–2/11). The ends are ill-defined; the cervical canal simply

**Table 37–1.** Guide to the Aging of Pig Fetuses

| Weeks | Crown–Rump Length (cm) | External Features |
|---|---|---|
| 2.5 | ≈1 | Limb buds forming |
| 4 | ≈2 | Tactile hair follicles appear; mammary primordia present |
| 5 | ≈3.5 | Palate fused; facial clefts closed |
| 6 | ≈6.5 | Prepuce and scrotum, or labia and clitoris present |
| 7 | ≈9 | Eyelids fused; intestines returned to abdomen |
| 13 | ≈24 | Eyelids separated |
| Full term | | On average 114 days |

From Evans H.E., and W.O. Sack: Prenatal development of domestic and laboratory animals. Growth curves, external features, and selected references. Anat. Histol. Embryol. 2:11–45, 1973.

widens at each end to continue into the uterus and the vagina. On rectal palpation the cervix feels hard and distinct during diestrus and pregnancy; during estrus and prior to farrowing it becomes strikingly large and edematous, the mucosal prominences then being soft and indistinct.

The vagina is unremarkable.

The *vestibule* (/15) is relatively long since the urethra enters the genital tract rather far cranially. Correlated with this is the wholly abdominal position of the bladder, which, when full, can reach as far forward as the umbilicus. The bladder is entirely invested with peritoneum that ventrally extends between the urethra and the pubis.

The *vulva* is somewhat conical and slopes so that the cleft faces dorsocaudally. In some gilts the cone is more upturned, making the cleft inaccessible to the boar. Gilts with an infantile vulva are relatively common and equally undesirable as breeding stock since the defect suggests poor development of the reproductive tract with a considerable chance of infertility. The clitoris of the normal sow, although approximately 6 cm long, is barely visible. The enlarged clitoris that is commonly encountered is associated with intersexuality (female pseudohermaphroditism).

## THE MALE REPRODUCTIVE ORGANS

The reproductive organs of the boar are characterized by a perineal position of the scrotum, large vesicular and bulbourethral glands, and a thin penis with a sigmoid flexure (Fig. 37–5).

The palpable tail of the epididymis and the associated pole of the *testis* point caudodorsally, producing a prominent landmark close to the anus. The free border of the testis faces caudoventrally, while the attached border is applied against the caudal surface of the thigh (Fig. 37–6/5).

Male pigs that are not retained for breeding are commonly castrated when 2 to 4 weeks old to ensure that only untainted meat reaches the market. In some countries, the necessity for routine castration is questioned since most pigs are slaughtered before the taint develops. The rapid "open method" of castration is used; the skin incision exposes the testis within the vaginal cavity, and the operation is completed by its removal together with part of the spermatic cord (Fig. 37–7). The ligament (/9) that attaches the tail of the epididymis to the tunica vaginalis parietalis is cut or torn to free the testis and to cut the spermatic cord (/5). Essentially the same procedure is employed for castrating older boars. In the alternative "closed method" the skin incision spares the tunica vaginalis parietalis. The unopened tunic (and surrounding spermatic fascia) is bluntly separated from the scrotal wall and after ligation is transected close to the external inguinal ring.

The long spermatic cords flank the penis in the subcutaneous space between the thighs. The vaginal tunics and the cremasters adhering to their medial surfaces are enclosed by thick spermatic fascia that blends with the medial fascia of the thighs.

The descent of the testis begins at about 60 days of gestation. The extra-abdominal part of the gubernaculum, the part distal to the inguinal canal, enlarges and gradually pulls the testis toward the inguinal canal. At about 90 days, regression of the extra-abdominal gubernaculum sets in, creating space for the testis external to the inguinal canal. For several days before term the testis may slide back and forth through the canal. By birth, the gubernaculum has regressed sufficiently for the testis to take up a scrotal position (see p. 173). Retention of the testis (cryptorchidism) is common.

An abnormally large or malpositioned gubernaculum, possibly combined with delayed regression, expands the inguinal canal more than usual. This may cause insufficient descent or, if the testis has passed through the inguinal canal, may permit a

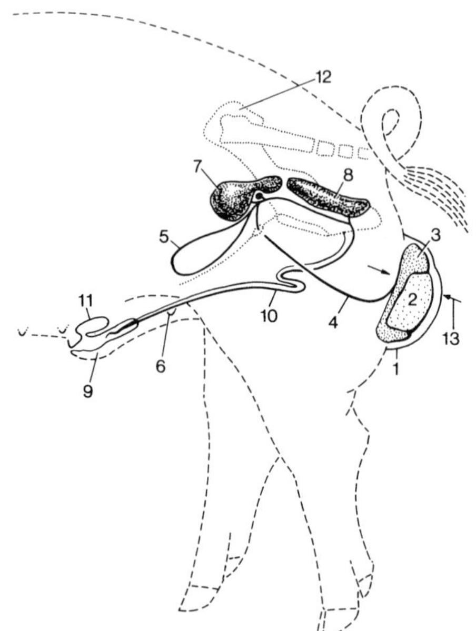


**Figure 37–5.** Schema of the boar's reproductive organs.

1, Scrotum; 2, left testis; 3, tail of epididymis; 4, deferent duct; 5, bladder; 6, rudimentary teat; 7, vesicular gland covering the small body of the prostate; 8, bulbourethral gland; 9, prepuce; 10, penis; 11, preputial diverticulum; 12, right hip bone; 13, level of section shown in Figure 37–6.

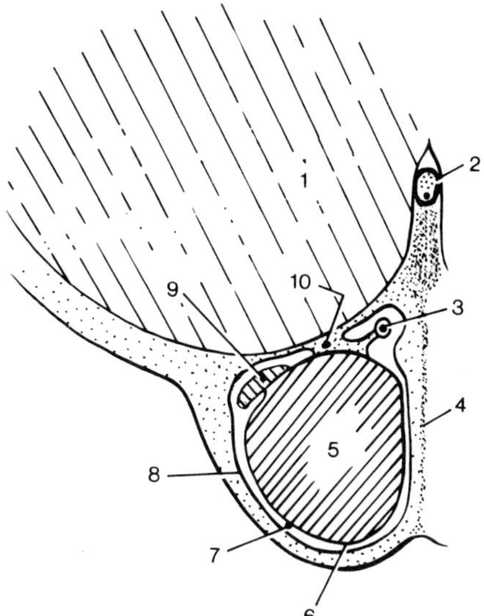


**Figure 37–6.** Transverse section of left testis in situ, dorsal surface. See Figure 37–5/13 for the level of this section.

1, Left thigh; 2, penis; 3, deferent duct; 4, scrotal septum; 5, testis; 6, tunica albuginea covered by tunica vaginalis visceralis; 7, vaginal cavity; 8, tunica vaginalis parietalis; 9, body of epididymis; 10, mesorchium.

loop of intestine to enter the vaginal cavity later (indirect inguinal—scrotal, if the loop of intestine is long enough to reach the testis—hernia). Surgical correction of this defect is combined with a closed castration; the freed vaginal tunic (and surrounding spermatic fascia) is twisted from the testicular end forward to push the herniated jejunum back into the abdominal cavity. The vaginal tunic with its contents of spermatic cord and testis is then ligated and removed, and the superficial inguinal ring is sutured to prevent another loop of bowel from entering the stump. The inguinal hernias occasionally seen in young females are associated with grossly abnormal genital tracts resembling those of bovine freemartins (Plate 5/*G*,*H*).

On entering the abdominal cavity, the *deferent duct* turns sharply dorsomedially to disappear between the bladder and the large vesicular gland (Fig. 37–8). Without enlarging to form ampullae, the right and left ducts converge dorsal to the urethra, penetrate the body of the prostate (/8), and open into the pelvic urethra on a low elevation.

The ducts of the *vesicular glands* (/7) enter the urethra beside the deferent ducts. These glands are so large that only their caudal ends are in the pelvic cavity, the bulk projecting into the abdominal cavity beyond the neck of the bladder where they are enclosed in the genital fold. The glands conceal the small, irregular body of the prostate. The bulk of the boar's prostate is disseminated within the wall of the pelvic urethra; it secretes through numerous small openings.

The *bulbourethral glands* (/11) are compound tubular glands lined with secretory columnar epithelium with occasional basal cells. The passages draining the secretion ultimately unite to form a single—sometimes replicated—duct. The glands are remarkable for their shape and size. They lie dorsolateral to the pelvic urethra into which they discharge their secretion near the ischial arch (Fig. 37–8/*A*). The glands are long and cranially touch the vesicular glands (see Fig. 5–40/*C*). They are covered dorsally by the bulboglandularis muscles whose contraction promotes their evacuation. The caudal ends are identified without difficulty on rectal examination. In the entire male their mutual contact prevents the finger from touching the urethra. In males without palpable testes, inability to touch the urethra suggests that the animal is a cryptorchid. The accessory glands of juveniles and castrates are naturally small (Fig. 37–8/*B*).

The size of the accessory genital glands is related to the large ejaculate, which averages about 200 mL (but may be as large as a liter). However,

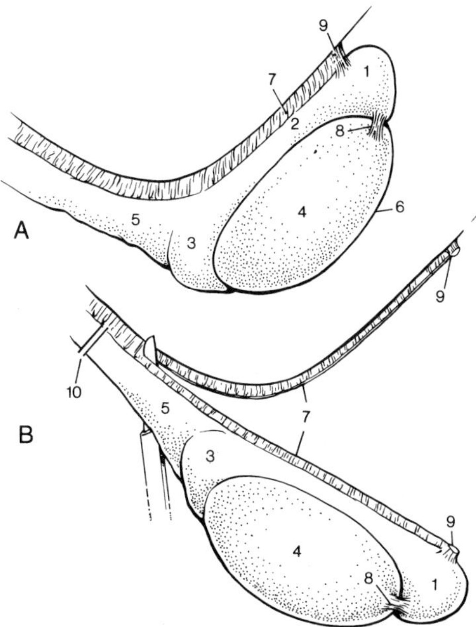


**Figure 37–7.** *A*, Left testis of a boar in situ, lateral view. *B*, The testis is detached from the body, as in one method of open castration, by cutting the ligament of the tail of the epididymis and the mesorchium.

1, Tail of epididymis; 2, body of epididymis; 3, head of epididymis; 4, testis; 5, spermatic cord; 6, free border of testis; 7, mesorchium; 8, proper ligament of testis; 9, ligament of tail of epididymis; 10, ligation and section of spermatic cord to remove testis.

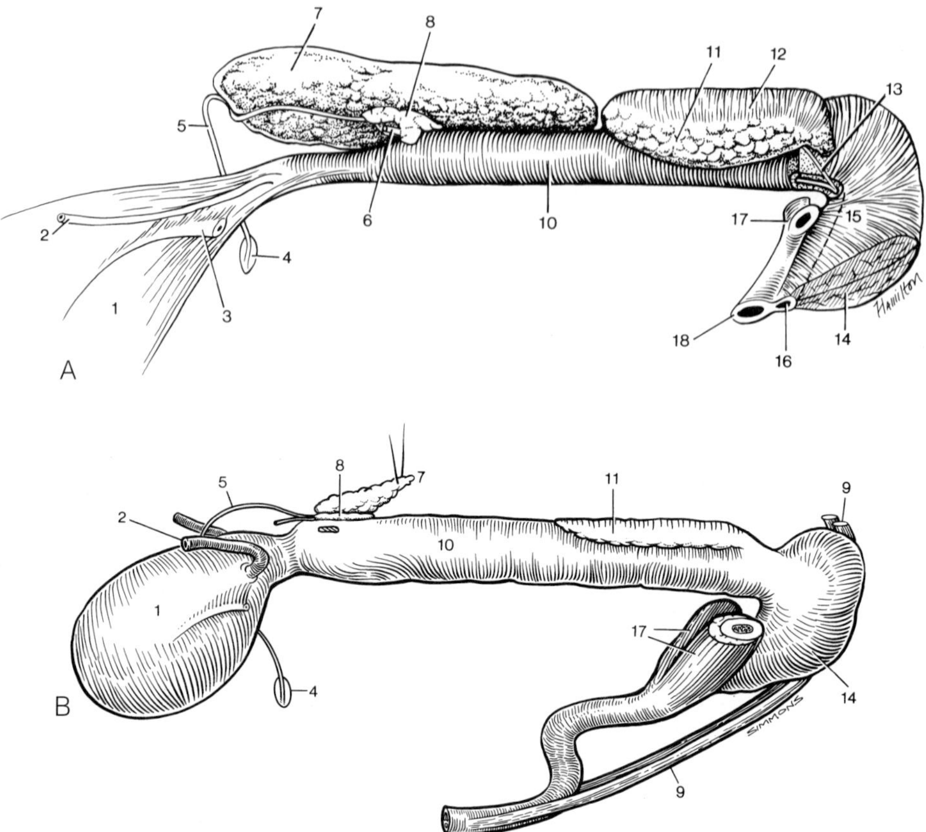


**Figure 37–8.** Pelvic urethra and associated organs of an 8-month-old boar *(A)* and of a 6-month-old castrate *(B)*, left lateral views. The left vesicular gland has been removed to expose the prostate.

1, Bladder; 2, left ureter; 3, left umbilical artery; 4, right vaginal ring; 5, right deferent duct; 6, left deferent duct, cut at prostate; 7, right vesicular gland; 8, body of prostate; 9, retractor penis; 10, pelvic urethra, surrounded by urethralis; 11, left bulbourethral gland; 12, bulboglandularis covering dorsal half of bulbourethral gland; 13, excretory duct of left bulbourethral gland; 14, bulbospongiosus; 15, bulb of penis; 16, urethra and corpus spongiosum; 17, right and left crura, cut; 18, corpus cavernosum.

the exceptionally large vesicular and bulbourethral glands produce only 15% to 20% and 10% to 25% of the ejaculate, respectively; the bulk of the seminal fluid (55% to 75%) is produced by the prostate and urethral glands. The seminal component of the ejaculate is only 2% to 5%.

As the urethra passes around the ischial arch to become incorporated in the *penis,* its lumen increases in diameter and the associated corpus spongiosum enlarges to form a swelling on its caudal surface. The swelling is covered caudally by the thick bulbospongiosus and forms the palpable bulb of the penis (*/A,*15). The urethra presents a small diverticulum as it leaves the pelvis; this is bounded ventrally by a membranous thickening enclosing the ducts of the bulbourethral glands. The two crura (/17) of the penis arise from the ischial arch cranial to the bulb and, surrounded by ischiocavernosus muscles, converge to form the shaft of the penis. The bulbospongiosus and ischiocavernosus muscles end a few centimeters proximal to the sigmoid flexure. A transverse section at this level is shown in Figure 37–9/*A*.

The penis is broadly similar to that of the bull (Fig. 37–5). It is relatively thin, about 60 cm long in the flaccid state, and has a thick tunica albuginea enclosing both corpus cavernosum and corpus spongiosum. The latter at first lies on the flat ventral surface of the corpus cavernosum, but more distally it occupies a deep urethral groove, bringing the urethra toward the center of the penis (Fig. 37–9/*B,*5). Apart from the sigmoid flexure, the shaft of the penis is twisted on its longitudinal axis by about one full turn counterclockwise when looking distally. The direction of this twist is the same as that of the shorter corkscrew spiral of the free part (/*C*).

During erection the blood pressure in the cavernous spaces rises sharply, and this straightens the sigmoid flexure, increasing the length of the penis by about 25%. The diameter of the shaft enlarges by about 20%. The longitudinal twist increases to six turns while the corkscrew spiral of the free part also becomes more pronounced.

During coitus, a slow process that may last up to 30 minutes, the boar is said to "soak" because of the absence of obvious activity on his part. However, forward and backward twisting movements of the penis do occur and are produced by the alternating contraction and relaxation of the retractor penis, which attaches asymmetrically distal to the sigmoid flexure. The assumption that the mucosal prominences in the cervix are arranged to form a canal with a "left-hand thread" adapted to the spiraled end of the penis has no basis. However, the end of the penis is believed to enter the uterus.

The *prepuce* is relatively long and houses the free part of the penis in its narrow caudal half (Fig. 37–10/*A*). The cranial half is wider and communicates dorsally with a preputial diverticulum (/5), a pouch containing a foul-smelling fluid made up of cell debris soaked with urine. The diverticulum is covered by the cranial preputial muscle (/1), which empties it prior to copulation, and this fluid is said to lubricate the penis. Apart from producing the odor that surrounds a boar, the fluid contains a pheromone that encourages sows in estrus to assume the immobile mating stance. This substance is also elaborated in the salivary glands and is found on the breath of the boar. An infected diverticulum can be opened for drainage and irrigation by a dorsolateral incision that includes the preputial muscle. If the contents of the diverticulum accumulate, the cranial end of the prepuce enlarges and may mimic an umbilical hernia (since the umbilicus [/8] is only a few centimeters cranial to the preputial orifice). The diverticulum is often removed in boars used in artificial insemination to decrease contamination of the semen and to eliminate the foul smell

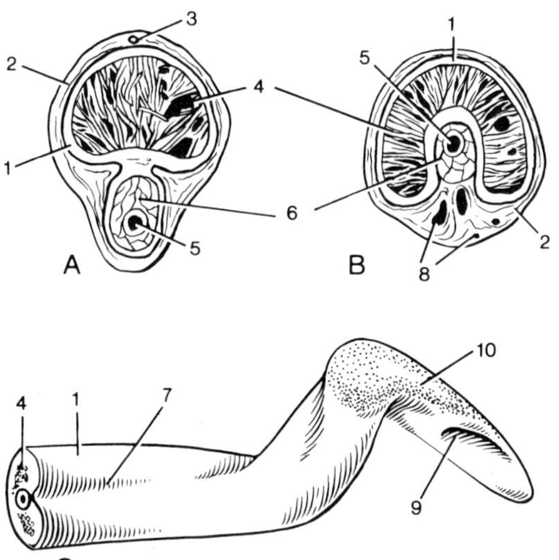


**Figure 37–9.** Transverse sections of the penis. *A*, Proximal to the sigmoid flexure. *B*, Distal to the sigmoid flexure. *C*, Free end of penis.

1, Tunica albuginea; 2, connective tissue surrounding penis; 3, dorsal artery of penis; 4, corpus cavernosum; 5, urethra; 6, corpus spongiosum; 7, urethral groove; 8, blood vessels; 9, external urethral orifice; 10, thin glans penis.

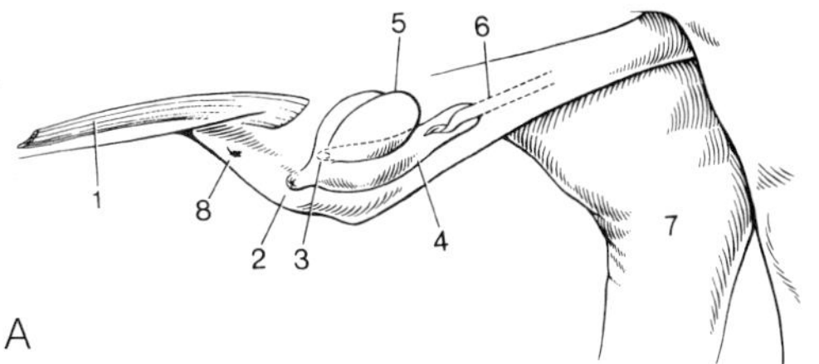


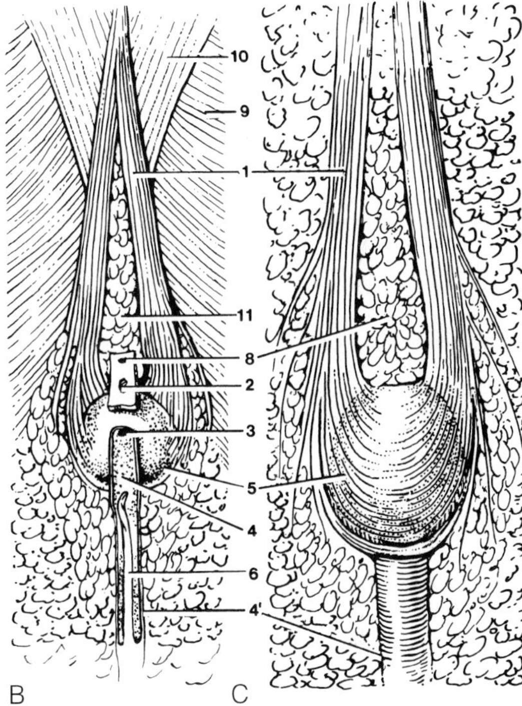


**Figure 37–10.** Prepuce and preputial diverticulum. *A*, In situ, schematic, craniolateral view. *B*, Ventral view. *C*, Dorsal view.

1, Cranial preputial muscle, in *A* cut at both ends; 2, preputial orifice; 3, orifice between prepuce and diverticulum; 4, 4′, wide cranial and narrow caudal parts of preputial cavity; 5, preputial diverticulum; 6, penis; 7, medial surface of right hock; 8, umbilicus; 9, cutaneous trunci; 10, pectoralis profundus; 11, preputial fat.

attending collection. Occasionally, a boar cannot protrude the penis because its tip has entered the preputial diverticulum; the penis can be freed with a finger passed through the preputial orifice. The diverticulum is small in castrates.

## Selected Bibliography

Balke, J.M.E., and R.G. Elmore: Pregnancy diagnosis in swine: A comparison of the technique of rectal palpation and ultrasound. Theriogenology 17:231–236, 1982.

Barone, R.: Anatomie Compafee des Mammifères Domestiques. Vol. 3, Part 2. Lyon, Laboratoire d'Anatomie, Ecole Nationale Vétérinaire, 1978.

Cameron, R.D.A.: Pregnancy diagnosis in the sow by rectal examination. Aust. Vet. J. 53:432–435, 1977.

Cartee, R.E., T.A. Powe, B.W. Gray, et al.: Ultrasonographic evaluation of normal boar testicles. Am. J. Vet. Res. 47:2543–2548, 1985.

Colenbrander, B., and C.J.G. Wensing: Studies on phenotypically female pigs with hernia inguinalis and ovarian aplasia. Proc. K. Ned. Akad. Wet. C 78:33–46, 1975.

Dhindsa, D.S., P.J. Dzuik, and H.W. Norton: Time of transuterine migration and distribution of embryos in the pig. Anat. Rec. 159:325–330, 1967.

Done, S.H., M.J. Meredith, and R.R. Ashdown: Detachment of ischial tuberosity in sows. Vet. Rec. 105:520–523, 1979.

Dutton, D.M., B. Lawhorn, and R.N. Hooper: Ablation of the cranial portion of the preputial cavity in a pig. JAVMA 211:598–599, 1997.

Dzuik, P.J.: Reproduction in pigs. *In* Cupps, P.T. (ed.): Reproduction in Domestic Animals. San Diego, Academic Press, 1991.

el Campo, C.H., and O.J. Ginther: Vascular anatomy of the uterus and ovaries and the unilateral luteolytic effect of the uterus: Horses, sheep, and swine. Am. J. Vet. Res. 34:305–316, 1973.

Garrett, P.D.: Urethral recess in male goats, sheep, cattle, and swine. JAVMA 191:689–691, 1987.

Ginther, O.J.: Internal regulation of physiological processes through local venoarterial pathways. A review. J. Anim. Sci. 39:550–564, 1974.

Glover, T.D.: The semen of the pig. Vet. Rec. 67:36–40, 1955.

Hansen, L.H., and I.J. Christiansen: The accuracy of porcine pregnancy diagnosis by a newly developed ultrasonic A-scan tester. Br. Vet. J. 132:66–67, 1976.

Lawhorn, B., P.D. Jarrett, G.F. Lackey, et al.: Removal of the preputial diverticulum in swine. JAVMA 205:92–96, 1994.

McGlone, J.J., R.I. Nicholson, J.M. Hellman, and D.N. Herzog: The development of pain in young pigs associated with castration and attempts to prevent castration-induced behavioral changes. J. Anim. Sci. 71:1441–1446, 1993.

Meredith, M.J.: Pregnancy diagnosis in the sow by examination of the uterine arteries. *In* Proceedings of the International Pig Veterinary Society Congress, Ames, Iowa, 1976, D5:1–2.

Meredith, M.J.: Clinical examination of the ovaries and cervix of the sow. Vet. Rec. 101:70–74, 1977.

Morton, D.B., and J.E.F. Rankin: The histology of the vaginal epithelium of the sow in oestrus and its use in pregnancy diagnosis. Vet. Rec. 84:658–662, 1969.

Perry, J.S.: Parturition in the pig. Vet. Rec. 66:706–709, 1954.

Roberts, S.J.: Veterinary Obstetrics and Genital Diseases (Theriogenology). Woodstock, Vt., 1986. Published by the author.

van Alstine, W.G., and C.G. Toben: Detachment of the tuber ischiadicum in swine. Compend. Contin. Educ. Food Anim. 11:874–879, 1989.

Wensing, C.J.G.: Testicular descent in some domestic mammals. I. Anatomical aspect of testicular descent. Proc. K. Ned. Akad. Wet. 71:423–434, 1968.

Wensing, C.J.G.: Testicular descent in some domestic mammals. II. The nature of the gubernacular change during the process of testicular descent in the pig. Proc. K. Ned. Akad. Wet. C 76:190–195, 1973.

Wensing, C.J.G.: Abnormalities of testicular descent. Proc. K. Ned. Akad. Wet. C 76:373–381, 1973.

Wensing, C.J.G., and B. Colenbrander: Cryptorchidism and inguinal hernia. Proc. K. Ned. Akad. Wet. C 76:489–494, 1973.

Wrobel, K.H., and B. Brandl: The autonomous innervation of the porcine testis in the period from birth to adulthood. Ann Anat 180:145–156, 1998.

# CHAPTER 38

# The Limbs of the Pig

Generally speaking, the limbs of the pig receive little veterinary attention. The features that principally distinguish the limb skeleton are the well-developed and weight-bearing ulnae and fibulae and the pairs of principal and accessory digits (see Fig. 34–1). The accessory digits ("dewclaws") are caudal to the principal ones and have a full complement of bones—quite unlike the rudimentary dewclaws of cattle (see Fig. 10–23).

The *hoofs* are similar to those of cattle but are straight (not bent inward at the tips) and have a soft digital pad (bulb) that is well set off from the wall and sole (Fig. 38–1). Those of the accessory digits are miniatures of the principal ones but bear weight only on soft ground. A short life span, and the common practice of running pigs on concrete, make hoof trimming rarely necessary.

Recently, joint disease has been found to be surprisingly common. The cause is unknown, although evidence exists that the practice of selecting for rapid weight gain may be contributory. As already mentioned, pigs now reach a weight of over 220 pounds (100 kg) within 5 to 6 months, long before their skeletons have finished growing, a process requiring 5 to 6 years. Even breeding stock nowadays rarely attain skeletal maturity since sows are culled when about 4 years old and boars before they are 2, to minimize inbreeding. The immature skeleton cannot support these loads; breakdown of articular cartilage and bone deformity result. The increase in joint disease has given impetus to studies of the structure of the joints and of procedures for their injection.

## THE FORELIMB

The following skeletal features may be palpated: the cranial and caudal angles, and the prominent tubercle on the spine, of the scapula (see Fig. 34–1); the caudal part of the greater tubercle of the humerus on the lateral aspect of the shoulder joint; the olecranon and the medial and lateral epicondyles of the humerus (especially their caudal borders) at the elbow; and, about 15 to 20 cm farther distally, the accessory carpal, which reveals the level of the proximal row of carpal bones. The cephalic vein on the cranial aspect of the arm may be punctured in some pigs, in which its position is visible through the skin.

**Shoulder Joint.** The larger cranial part of the greater tubercle deflects the intertubercular groove (and the biceps tendon) medially. Although smaller, it is the caudal part that is palpable as is the infraspinatus tendon related to it. Intra-articular injection is made across the cranial border of this tendon just proximal to its passage over the tubercle.

**Elbow Joint.** The lateral epicondyle of the humerus is accentuated by a crest, readily palpable, that follows its caudal border. In intra-articular injection the needle is inserted just caudal to this border, between it and the ulna (Fig. 34–1/19). A second method uses the same crest as a landmark but enters the needle 2 to 3 cm proximal to the preceding site; the needle is passed mediodistally, caudal to the crest, to enter the olecranon fossa.

**Carpal Joint.** This is exceptionally movable, permitting flexion of nearly 180 degrees. The midcarpal and carpometacarpal compartments communicate so that an injection into one reaches the other. The injections are made from the dorsal surface, medial and lateral to the extensor carpi radialis tendon, into the antebrachiocarpal and midcarpal spaces.

The *principal arterial trunk* (brachial artery) lies medial to the humerus and crosses the elbow joint a little in front of the medial epicondyle. From here it passes distally under cover of the flexor carpi radialis on the medial surface of the forearm (as the median artery). The median artery accompanies the flexor tendons through the carpal canal and lies on their caudomedial aspect in the metacarpus. At all levels in the limb branches exist that are capable of maintaining the circulation should the principal trunk be occluded.

**Lymphatic Structures.** Lymph originating from the superficial parts of the arm and forearm drains into the ventral superficial cervical nodes. Lymph from deeper structures, and from the entire distal part of the limb, passes through the *axillary lymph nodes of the first rib.* These lie cranial to the

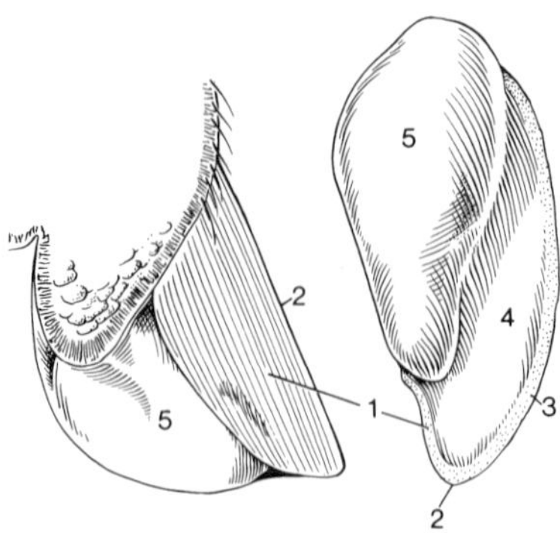


**Figure 38–1.** Axial and ground surfaces of the hoof.

1, Axial surface of wall (the lines indicate the direction of the horn tubules); 2, dorsal border of wall; 3, abaxial surface of wall; 4, sole; 5, digital pad (bulb) of hoof.

first rib and ventral to the axillary vessels. They also receive lymph from structures of the ventral part of the neck (including the thymus and thyroid glands) and brisket; their efferents go to the veins at the thoracic inlet.

So-called *carpal glands* are present on the caudomedial aspect of the carpus (Fig. 38–2). They consist of flat packages of glands adherent to the undersurface of the skin and open by three to four small but visible orifices; they are thought to function as territorial markers.

## THE HINDLIMB

Palpable landmarks include the coxal tuber (the slight enlargement on the ventral end of the iliac crest) (see Fig. 34–1/31) and the ischial tuber (/37), which is lateral to the vulva in the female. The greater trochanter of the femur is a less definite firmness slightly ventral to the line connecting these landmarks. The subiliac lymph nodes on the cranial border of the thigh are normally not palpable (see Fig. 36–1/2). The caudal muscles of the thigh (biceps, semitendinosus, semimembranosus) are used for intramuscular injection, although apart from possible injury to the sciatic nerve, this may affect the quality of the ham. The tibial crest, the single patellar ligament, the patella, the extensor groove of the tibia, and the collateral ligaments are palpable landmarks at the level of the stifle. The medial surface of the tibia can be followed from the stifle to its distal end (medial malleolus). Distally, the calcanean tendon leads to the calcaneus, the only fully palpable bone in the tarsus. However, both medial and lateral malleoli and the distal fourth of the prominent fibula can be palpated. As a result of insufficient bedding and subsequent trauma many pigs suffer from acquired bursitis on the lateral surface of the hock and over the tuber calcanei (capped hock).

**Hip Joint.** Because of the hip joint's deep location, the landmarks for injection are distant from the joint. A line is imagined connecting the coxal with the lateral part of the ischial tuber. Depending on the size of the pig, the trochanter major is palpated 2 to 4 cm ventral to this line. The needle is inserted on the line 2 to 4 cm cranial to the trochanter and advanced at right angles to the surface to pass through the gluteal muscles to the dorsal part of the joint capsule. The thick fibrous tissue of the capsule and of the gluteus profundus may be felt as an obstruction.

**Stifle Joint.** The femoropatellar joint communicates with both medial and lateral femorotibial joints at the distal end of the trochlea; the medial and lateral femorotibial joints also communicate across the intercondylar space. Therefore, one injection serves all three. The puncture is made lateral to the patellar ligament about one third of the way from the patella to the tibial tuberosity.

**Hock Joint.** The tarsometatarsal joint has two independent joint capsules, one proximal to metatarsals II and III and the other proximal to metatarsals IV and V; the distal intertarsal joint

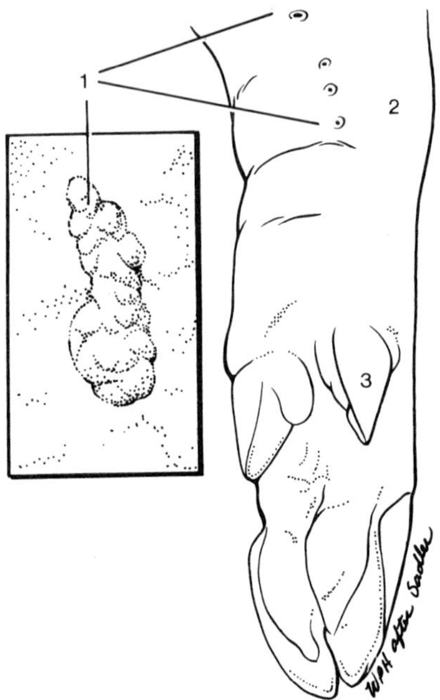


**Figure 38–2.** Left forefoot, caudomedial view. The inset shows the carpal glands on the undersurface of the skin, enlarged.

1, Carpal glands; 2, medial surface of carpus; 3, hoof of medial dewclaw.

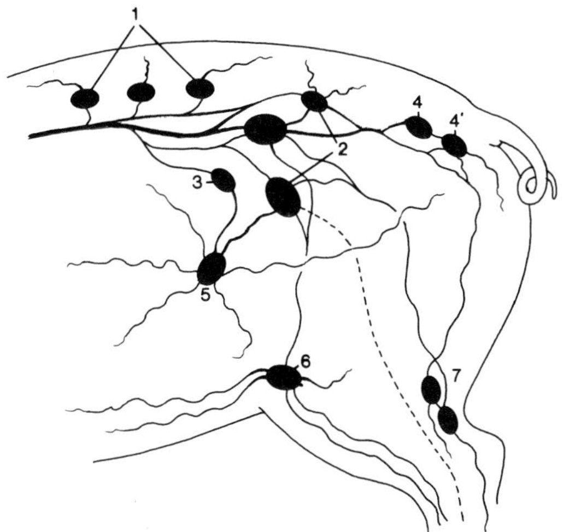


**Figure 38–3.** Lymph flow of the hindlimb, lateral view.

1, Lumbar aortic nodes; 2, medial iliac nodes; 3, lateral iliac node; 4, ischial node; 4′, gluteal nodes; 5, subiliac nodes; 6, superficial inguinal nodes; 7, popliteal nodes.

communicates with the former. No communication occurs between the tarsocrural and the proximal intertarsal joints, which are the only joints accessible to injection. Two sites, both lateral, may be used for the tarsocrural joint; one is dorsal, the other plantar to the collateral ligament. The proximal intertarsal joint is injected from the medial surface, plantar to the collateral ligament.

The femoral is the *principal artery* supplying the thigh and leg. It crosses the medial surface of the femur and, after passing the stifle (where it is known as the popliteal), it divides into cranial and caudal tibial arteries. The largest artery of the distal half of the limb is the saphenous, a branch of the femoral. It passes the stifle on the medial surface and is subcutaneous midway between the tibia and the calcanean tendon. It then passes the caudomedial aspect of the hock with the deep flexor tendon and lies between the flexor tendons and the skin in the metatarsus; it is the principal supply to the digits.

**Lymphatic Structures.** Lymph originating from the superficial parts of the thigh and leg is drained into the superficial inguinal and subiliac nodes (Fig. 38–3/6,5). Lymph originating from the deep parts travels centrally in lymphatics accompanying the popliteal and femoral arteries to reach the medial iliac nodes (/2). The deep structures of the distal half of the limb are drained by the *popliteal lymph nodes* (/7), which in most pigs are palpable between the distal ends of the biceps and semitendinosus; sometimes they are too deep to be palpated. Their efferents go to the gluteal and ischial nodes on the lateral surface of the sacrosciatic ligament or join the lymphatics that run to the medial iliac nodes.

## Selected Bibliography

Ham, G.W., I. MacDonald, and S.W.H. Elsley: A radiographic study of the development of the skeleton of the fetal pig. J. Agric. Sci. 72:123–130, 1969.

Klug-Simon, C., J. Dimigen, H. Wissdorf, and H. Wilkens: Possibility of injecting the porcine shoulder joint [in German]. Dtsch. Tierarztl. Wochenschr. 77:603–606, 1970.

Skarda, R.T.: Local and regional anesthesia in ruminants and swine. Vet. Clin. North Am. Food Anim. Pract. 12:579–625, 1996.

Van Alstine, W., and J.A. Dietrich: Porcine sciatic nerve damage after intramuscular injection. Compend. Contin. Educ. Food Anim. 10:1329–1332, 1988.

Van Alstine, W.G., and C.G. Toben: Detachment of the tuber ischiadicum in swine. Compend. Contin. Educ. Food Anim. Pract. 11:874–879, 1989.

Wissdorf, H.: Anatomical basis for the injection of the porcine stifle joint [in German]. Dtsch. Tierarztl. Wochenschr. 72:289–294, 1965.

Wissdorf, H.: Anatomical basis for the injection of the porcine elbow joint [in German]. Dtsch. Tierarztl. Wochenschr. 72:569–570, 1965.

Wissdorf, H.: Anatomical basis for the injection of the porcine hock joint [in German]. Zentralbl. Veterinarmed. [A] 13:369–383, 1966.

Wissdorf, H., and K. Neurand: Anatomical basis for the injection of the porcine carpal joint [in German]. Dtsch. Tierarztl. Wochenschr. 73:401–404, 1966.

Wissdorf, H., C. Simon, and J. Dimigen: Anatomical basis for the injection of the porcine hip joint [in German]. Dtsch. Tierarztl. Wochenschr. 77:107–109, 1970. (in German)

# CHAPTER 39

# Avian Anatomy

Two significant branches of avian medicine exist, one concerned with disease control in commercial flocks of the half-dozen species of domestic poultry, the other with the treatment, frequently on an individual basis, of the much larger variety of cage, aviary, and menagerie birds. In addition, rehabilitation of wild species (notably waterfowl and raptors) is rapidly increasing. This chapter seeks to supply practitioners of the first branch with a basic knowledge sufficient for the understanding of the special features of the physiology and pathology of birds and for the conduct of routine postmortem examinations. It is based on the chicken; all measurements and, with a few exceptions, all illustrations refer to that species. The comparative detail relevant to the growing number of veterinarians concerned with the examination and treatment of more exotic birds is beyond the scope of this book. Interested readers are referred to a number of titles listed at the end of the chapter.

The extreme evolutionary success of birds (approximately 8600 species compared with about 5000 species of mammals) relates largely to flight. The flight-awarded ability to disperse so ubiquitously has enabled birds to adapt to more niches than any other class of vertebrate. Nonetheless, the anatomical restrictions of flight are so rigid that morphology among all bird species presents less variation than is seen among the 300 species of mammalian carnivores. Flight is so highly demanding metabolically that anatomical or physiological modifications, or both, are present in nearly every body system. These adaptations increase energy output and stability, and decrease body weight and wind resistance. They range from the grossly visible, as in the loss of heavy teeth and mastication musculature, to the microscopic, as in the airways of the lung and the arrangement of conduction fibers in the heart. Together, these specializations render birds at once singularly uniform and strikingly diverse.

## EXTERNAL FEATURES AND INTEGUMENT

Feathers provide the principal characteristic that distinguishes birds from mammals. They streamline the body and assist in transforming the forelimbs into wings. The feathers are among the features (others are mentioned later) that lighten birds relative to their size and thus enhance their efficiency in the air.

The *skin* is thin and loose and tears easily, but since it is poorly supplied with blood vessels and nerves, wounds do not bleed as much as in mammals, and birds seem insensitive to manipulation of their skin. The skin is yellowish over the body but may be more deeply pigmented on the shanks and feet. It is paler in productive laying hens, in which the pigment is withdrawn and incorporated in the yolk. The dorsal surface of the neck-trunk junction is recommended for subcutaneous injections. In most species of bird, including the domestic chicken, localized changes in the skin occur during the brooding period for the more efficient incubation of the eggs. The brooding (incubation) patches that develop on the breast are characterized by feather loss and by thickening and increased vascularity of the skin.

The *comb, wattles,* and *ear lobes* (and the snood of turkeys) are soft ornamental outgrowths of the skin about the head (Fig. 39–1/*A,B* and Plate 31/*A,E*). Their dermis is thick and vascular, but the covering epidermis is thin. They are thus easily injured and potential portals for infection. In nearly all commercially reared chicks the comb (and snood) are snipped off (dubbing, desnooding) to prevent their traumatization in the confined spaces in which these birds are held. The edges of the wattles are used for intradermal injections.

The *beak* (bill) is the functional counterpart of the lips and teeth of mammals. It is a derivative of the skin and provides a horny cover for the rostral parts of both upper and lower jaws that grows continuously to compensate for natural wear. The beak varies tremendously in form among species, according to diet (Plate 31/*A–D,F*). A rich innervation causes the beak to be quite sensitive. Most commercially raised chickens and turkeys are debeaked when young (cutting off the upper beak in front of the nostrils) to prevent cannibalism. In psittacines (parrot-like birds), pigeons, and raptors, the base of the beak is covered by a fleshy membrane (cere) that may enclose the nostrils (Plate 31/*C,D*). It is a prominent feature of

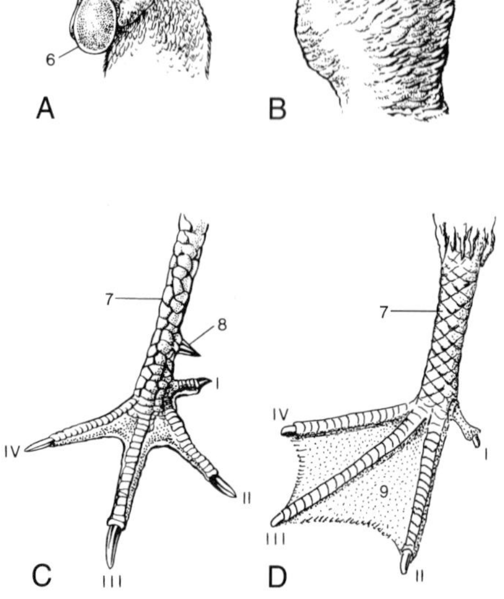


**Figure 39–1.** Head of the chicken *(A)* and the turkey *(B)*; right foot of a cockerel *(C)*; right foot of a goose *(D)*.

1, Nostril; 2, comb; 3, ear opening; 4, ear lobe; 5, snood; 6, wattles; 7, shank (metatarsus); 8, spur; 9, web between toes; I–IV, toes.

budgerigars, useful as a guide to their sex; the cere of the cock is blue, that of the hen light brown.

The scales on the shanks and feet are cornified epidermal patches similar to those of reptiles (Fig. 39–1/*C,D*). In waterfowl the three forward-pointing toes are connected by skin (webbed) to make more efficient sculls. The *spur* (/8) developed on the caudomedial surface of the rooster's shank is used as a weapon; it has an osseous core within a cone of horn. The length of the spur and the growth rings at its base may be used for determining age. Removal of the spur papilla in the chick inhibits its growth, much as the removal of the horn bud prevents horn growth in ruminants.

The sebaceous *uropygial gland* (oil gland; Fig. 39–2/1) is the only skin gland present apart from those in the external ear and at the vent; neither sebaceous nor sweat glands are present. The uropygial gland is bilobed, about 2 cm in diameter, and located dorsal to the caudal vertebrae that form the short tail. Its fatty secretion emerges from paired openings atop a small cutaneous papilla (/2). The secretion is carried to the body and wing feathers during preening. In waterfowl the secretion is important for waterproofing the feathers and insulating the submerged part of the body. The uropygial gland is prominent in the budgerigar; it is absent in some species.

## The Feathers

Feathers are highly specialized epidermal structures that have evolved from the scales of reptiles. Although light in relation to their size, they are of sturdy construction. Six types are recognized, but only the contour and down feathers are described here. The former are the externally visible feathers that modify the body contours, the wings and the tail. They conceal the down feathers, which create an effective dead air space that insulates the body. Feathers are concentrated in tracts (pterylae), leaving bare areas (apteria) that are preferred surgical sites. They also hide emaciation.

The exposed portion of a typical *contour feather* consists of a main shaft extended on each side by the vane (Fig. 39–3/*A*). The vane consists of numerous closely ranked branches (barbs; /2) that leave the shaft at angles of about 45 degrees. Adjacent barbs are connected by large numbers of minute barbules to form the level surfaces of the vane. This connection is effected by microscopic hooks on the distal ranks of barbules that loosely engage the proximal barbules crossing under them (/3′). Neighboring barbs are easily disconnected but reattach if brought together, as in preening or grooming the feathers.

The main shaft on the undersurface of the feather presents a longitudinal groove that ends in a depression (distal umbilicus; /*B*,8) opposite the fluffy proximal part of the vane. A small downy afterfeather (/9) may emerge from the umbilicus and contribute to the fluffiness.

The embedded part (quill, calamus) of the feather occupies the feather follicle, a tubular oblique invagination of the skin (/5′). The small

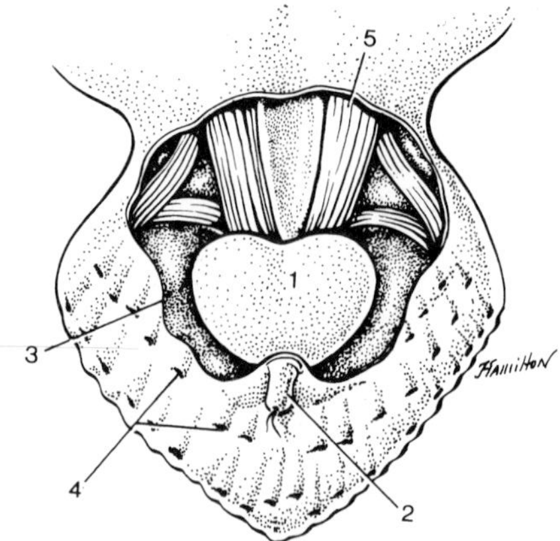


**Figure 39–2.** Uropygial (preen) gland; dorsal view.

1, Uropygial gland; 2, papilla of uropygial gland through which the secretion is extruded; 3, cut edge of skin; 4, feather follicles; 5, caudal vertebrae and associated muscles.

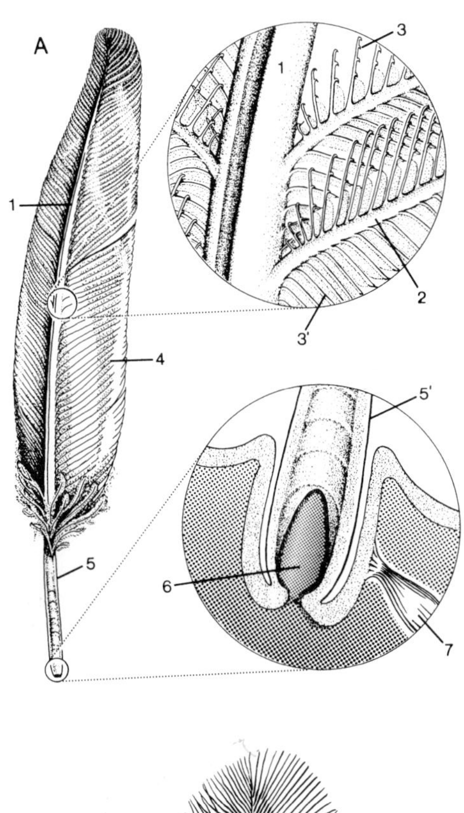


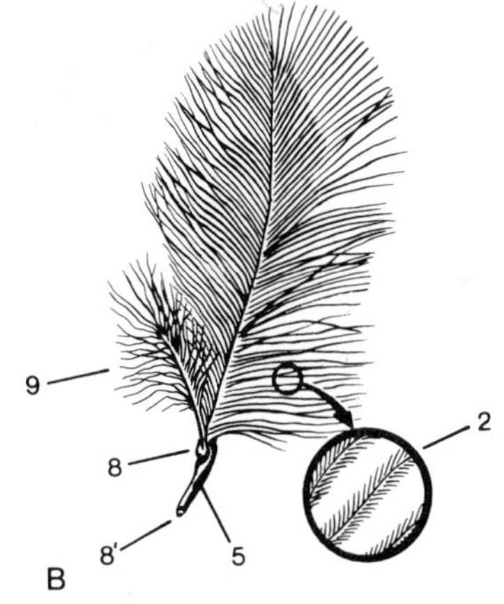


**Figure 39–3.** *A*, Contour feather. *B*, Down feather; with enlargements.

1, Main shaft; 2, barb with barbules; 3, distal barbule with microscopic hooks; 3′, proximal barbule; 4, vane formed by the barbs; 5, quill; 5′, quill in feather follicle; 6, dermal papilla; 7, feather muscle; 8, distal umbilicus; 8′, proximal umbilicus; 9, afterfeather.

dermal papilla at the bottom of the follicle extends into the opening (proximal umbilicus) at the proximal end of the quill. The quill itself is hollow and contains air and cellular debris (pulp caps) derived from the papilla. Feather muscles (/7), similar to the mammalian arrector pili muscles, attach to the sides of the follicles; they often form extensive networks that elevate or lower whole groups of feathers.

The barbs of the *down feathers* do not unite to form a closed vane. Their haphazard arrangement gives the feather its fluffy appearance.

At set times birds replace their feathers (molt) to discard worn ones or to change their plumage for display or camouflage. This occurs usually once a year following the breeding season and is set in motion by hormonal changes related mainly to length of day and temperature. During molt, which is a slow and gradual process, birds should not be stressed; they require rest and a diet rich in protein and minerals to support the high metabolic demands made by the rapid epidermal proliferation. Birds in poor condition often produce misshapen feathers. In most species, replacement of the large contour (flight) feathers is sequential and symmetrical so that flight always remains possible. Ducks and geese, however, lose these feathers at once, leaving them temporarily flightless. The old feather is pushed out by epidermal growth at the base of the follicle and as it vacates the follicle its replacement begins to grow. The loss of a feather by plucking initiates a similar sequence of events. Therefore, when feathers are clipped, it should be remembered that this is unlikely to disable birds for flight permanently.

In many species the sex is indicated by the shape and color of certain feathers or feather tracts.

## THE MUSCULOSKELETAL SYSTEM

The *skeleton* is light, compact, and strong with a greater content of calcium phosphate than in mammalian bone. It is characterized by fusion of vertebrae, a prominent sternum, and a pelvis that is open ventrally (Fig. 39–4). A peculiar avian feature is the pneumatization of bones by air sacs, extensions of the lungs; the sacs are principally found in the body cavity where they mingle with the viscera. Diverticula of the sacs extend through pneumatic foramina into the medullary cavities of neighboring bones, filling a considerable part of the skeleton with air. Pneumatization is gradual and is achieved at the expense of the bone marrow. The process is most advanced in the best fliers, which obtain a skeleton that is large and strong without being correspondingly heavy. Much of the adult skull is also pneumatized with spaces that connect to the airways in the head and not to the air sac system. Another peculiarity is the appearance prior to the laying season of (trabecular) medullary bone, thought to be a calcium store; on radiographs the extra bone may be mistaken for pathological processes.

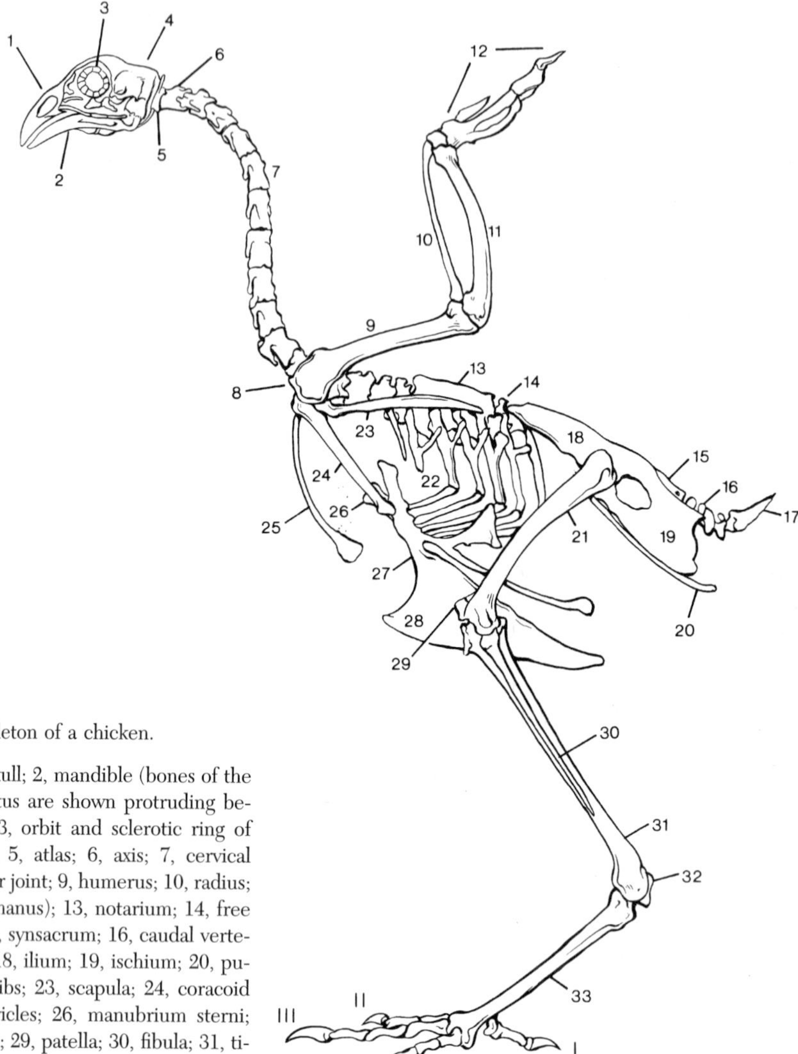


**Figure 39–4.** Skeleton of a chicken.

1, Facial part of skull; 2, mandible (bones of the hyobranchial apparatus are shown protruding below the mandible); 3, orbit and sclerotic ring of eyeball; 4, cranium; 5, atlas; 6, axis; 7, cervical vertebrae; 8, shoulder joint; 9, humerus; 10, radius; 11, ulna; 12, hand (manus); 13, notarium; 14, free thoracic vertebra; 15, synsacrum; 16, caudal vertebrae; 17, pygostyle; 18, ilium; 19, ischium; 20, pubis; 21, femur; 22, ribs; 23, scapula; 24, coracoid bone; 25, fused clavicles; 26, manubrium sterni; 27, sternum; 28, keel; 29, patella; 30, fibula; 31, tibiotarsus; 32, sesamoid bone (ossified tibial cartilage) in hock joint; 33, tarsometatarsus; I–IV, digits.

## The Skull

The salient features of the skull are the large orbits placed between the bulbous cranium and the pyramidal face (Fig. 39–5). The mandible is flat and adds only marginally to the height of the head. The enormous eyes have displaced the bones found between the orbits in most mammalian skulls and have reduced others to a thin median plate (interorbital septum; ./11). Several cranial bones consist of two plates separated by spongy bone; they are thus thicker than would be supposed and give the impression that the cranial cavity is greater than it is. The occipital bone encloses the foramen magnum. A single occipital condyle immediately ventral to this articulates with the atlas, forming a joint that enables birds to rotate the head on the vertebral column to a much greater extent than is allowed to mammals. The semispherical depression in the lower part of the lateral cranial wall is the tympanic cavity (/19). Its rim bounds the external acoustic meatus, which is closed by the tympanic membrane in life. Cochlear and vestibular windows in the depth of the depression lead into the inner ear.

Euthanasia (by injection into the brain) may be performed through the foramen magnum after flexion of the atlanto-occipital joint (Fig. 39–26/arrow).

The *facial part of the skull* is formed principally by the nasal and premaxillary bones that surround the large nasal aperture (Fig. 39–5/2). The nasal bone is dorsal, and in many birds, the psittacine species, for example, it makes a flexible cartilaginous connection with the frontal bone, permitting the upper jaw to be raised as the mandible is depressed. The maxilla below the nasal aperture is small and is connected to the mandibular joint by the long and thin jugal arch (/4), the homologue of the mammalian zygomatic arch. The palatine bones (/6) are caudally directed rods connecting the premaxillae with the pterygoid bones ventral to the orbits. Thus the osseous partition between the nasal and oral cavities exists only rostrally where it is formed by the palatine processes of the premaxillae.

The *mandible* (/5) consists of two thin bones fused rostrally where they are covered by the lower beak. Caudally, the mandible is connected to the skull, between the orbit and the external acoustic meatus, by the articular and quadrate bones (/21,15), elements that correspond to the mammalian middle ear ossicles, the malleus and incus. The quadrate bone is connected to the jugal arch, and, by interposition of the pyterygoid, to the rodlike palatine bone. In birds with a craniofacial hinge (e.g., budgerigar, parrot), depression of the lower jaw rotates the quadrate bone, which pushes the jugal arch and palatine bone rostrally, so elevating the upper jaw (craniokinesis).

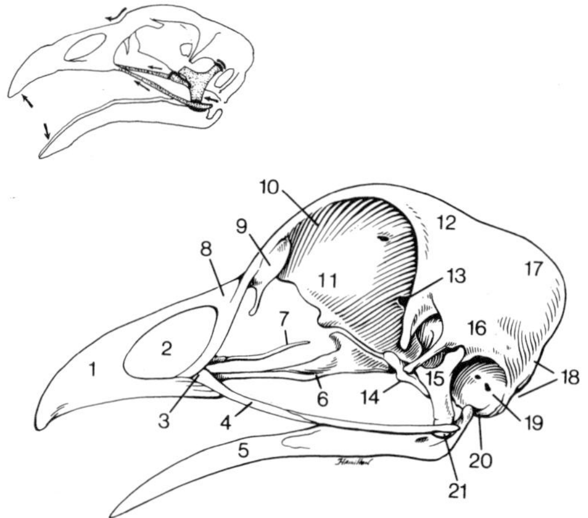


**Figure 39–5.** Skull; the inset shows how the upper jaw is raised by depression of the lower jaw in birds with a craniofacial hinge. (The hyobranchial apparatus and the sclerotic ring of the eyeball are not shown.)

1, Premaxilla; 2, nasal aperture; 3, maxilla; 4, jugal arch; 5, mandible; 6, palatine bone; 7, vomer; 8, nasal bone; 9, lacrimal bone; 10, orbit; 11, interorbital septum; 12, frontal bone; 13, optic foramen; 14, pterygoid bone; 15, quadrate bone; 16, temporal bone; 17, parietal bone; 18, occipital bone; 19, tympanic cavity with cochlear and vestibular windows; 20, sphenoid bone; 21, articular bone.

## The Axial Skeleton

This strictly comprises the vertebral column, ribs, and sternum, but the pelvis may be included since it is firmly attached to the synsacrum formed of fused lumbar, sacral, and caudal vertebrae (Fig. 39–4/15).

Division of the *vertebral column* into definite numbers of cervical, thoracic, lumbar, sacral, and caudal vertebrae is made difficult by the extensive fusion and the uncertainty of the location of the junction between the cervical and thoracic elements.

The number of *cervical vertebrae* varies with the length of the neck. Small birds may have only 8, while swans have as many as 25; in the chicken the number ranges from 14 to 17. The atlas (/5) is a small ring that articulates by a depression in its ventral arch with the single occipital condyle. Caudally, this arch has a facet for the dens of the axis. Except for the presence of the dens and short cranial articular processes, the axis differs little from the remaining cervical vertebrae, which are uniformly cylindrical with prominent articular processes and rudimentary caudally directed (cervical) ribs.

Usually seven *thoracic vertebrae* are present, most carrying complete ribs for connection with the sternum. Four fuse to form a single bone (notarium; /13),which is followed by a single free thoracic vertebra, the only mobile vertebra of the trunk. This vertebra articulates cranially and caudally by synovial joints in which both the articular processes and the bodies participate. It is the weak link in the column; its cranial end may be displaced ventrally, impinging on the spinal cord (kinky back in broilers). The last one or two thoracic vertebrae fuse with the lumbar, sacral, and first caudal vertebrae to form the *synsacrum* (/15). Synsacrum and notarium render the dorsal part of the trunk rigid, a rigidity that is extended laterally and caudally by the fusion of the synsacrum with the long hip bones. The synsacrum is followed by five or six free caudal vertebrae that allow movement to the tail. The most caudal segment (pygostyle; /17) consists of several fused rudiments and gives support to the flight feathers of the tail.

As in mammals, the bony *pelvis* consists of right and left hip bones and the (syn)sacrum. It is deeply concave ventrally and relatively long, bracing as much as half the trunk, an arrangement thought to be related to the bipedal posture. The broad dorsal and lateral surfaces of the hip bones are formed by the ilium and ischium, respectively (/18,19). The pubis is a thin rod attached to the ventral border of the ischium (/20). Ilium and ischium join to form the perforated acetabulum. Caudodorsal to this, a blunt process (antitrochanter) articulates with the trochanter of the femur and limits abduction. The hip bones do not meet in a ventral symphysis; the wide clearance favors the passage of the egg.

Five or six pairs of *ribs* connect the extensive sternum to the throacic vertebrae. Each complete rib consists of dorsal and ventral (vertebral and sternal) parts that meet at a cartilaginous joint. The vertebral rib corresponds to the osseous, the sternal rib to the cartilaginous part of the mammalian rib. Most vertebral ribs present a caudodorsally directed (uncinate) process that overlaps the next rib. These processes give attachment to muscles and ligaments and strengthen the thoracic wall. Floating (vertebral) ribs from the last few cervical vertebrae precede the complete ribs.

The *sternum* is a large unsegmented bone, which with its long processes forms a considerable part of the ventral body wall (Fig. 39–4/27). It gives attachment to the large flight muscles (see further on). It has a prominent keel (carina) in many good fliers, while in other species the keel is low but compensated by greater sternal width. The sternum of the chicken is relatively long and narrow and, although the chicken is a poor flier, it has a deep keel (/28). The subcutaneous position of the keel is ideal for bone marrow sampling in large cage birds but exposes it to injury when perching (twisted or bruised keels are an important factor in grading poultry). The manubrium (/26), a median process on the cranial end of the sternum, is flanked by large facets that receive the massive coracoid bones from above. Long processes, cranial and caudal to the articulations with the sternal ribs, enlarge the support provided to the lateral and ventral body wall. Pneumatic foramina on the concave dorsal surface of the sternum connect with the clavicular air sac. The caudal end of the sternum is cartilaginous in the young but later ossifies; its flexibility is thus an indicator of age.

## The Appendicular Skeleton

The appendicular skeleton is greatly modified by the conversion of the forelimbs to wings and by the hindlimbs assuming sole responsibility for locomotion on the ground, perching, and withstanding the stresses of landing. Avian long bones have thin, brittle cortices, unsuitable for bone plating or pinning that might be contemplated for fracture repair in large cage birds. The bones of the forelimbs are braced against the axial skeleton, notably the sternum, by a well-developed shoulder girdle; the distal bones of the wing have undergone reduction. The skeleton of the hindlimb is strong and distally simplified by fusion and loss.

### Forelimb

The *scapula* (Fig. 39–4/23) is a flat rod lying lateral and parallel to the vertebral column and extending caudally to the pelvis. It is joined to the axial skeleton by muscles and ligaments, while cranially it is connected to the clavicle and coracoid; with the latter it forms the articular surface that receives the head of the humerus (shoulder joint). The strong *coracoid bone* (/24) extends from the shoulder joint to a firm articulation with the cranial end of the sternum; it acts as a brace against the vigorous up-and-down strokes of the wing. The right and left *clavicles* unite to form the furcula (wishbone; /25) whose borders and median ventral expansion are tethered to the cranial end of the sternum and coracoids by tough membrane. The furcula connects the shoulder joints in springlike fashion and helps to brace the girdle against the axial skeleton. A foramen (canalis triosseus) at the junction of scapula,

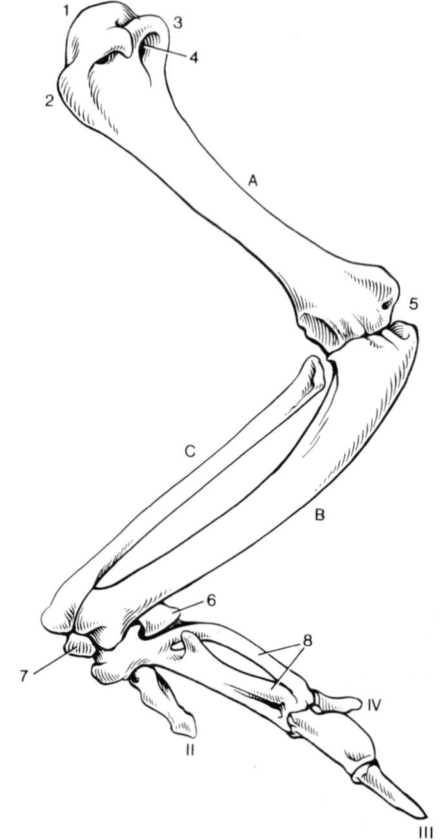


**Figure 39–6.** Skeleton of the left wing, partially extended laterally; dorsal surface. A, Humerus; B, ulna; C, radius.

1, Head; 2, dorsal tubercle; 3, ventral tubercle; 4, pneumatic foramen; 5, elbow joint; 6, ulnar carpal; 7, radial carpal; 8, carpometacarpals; II–IV, digits.

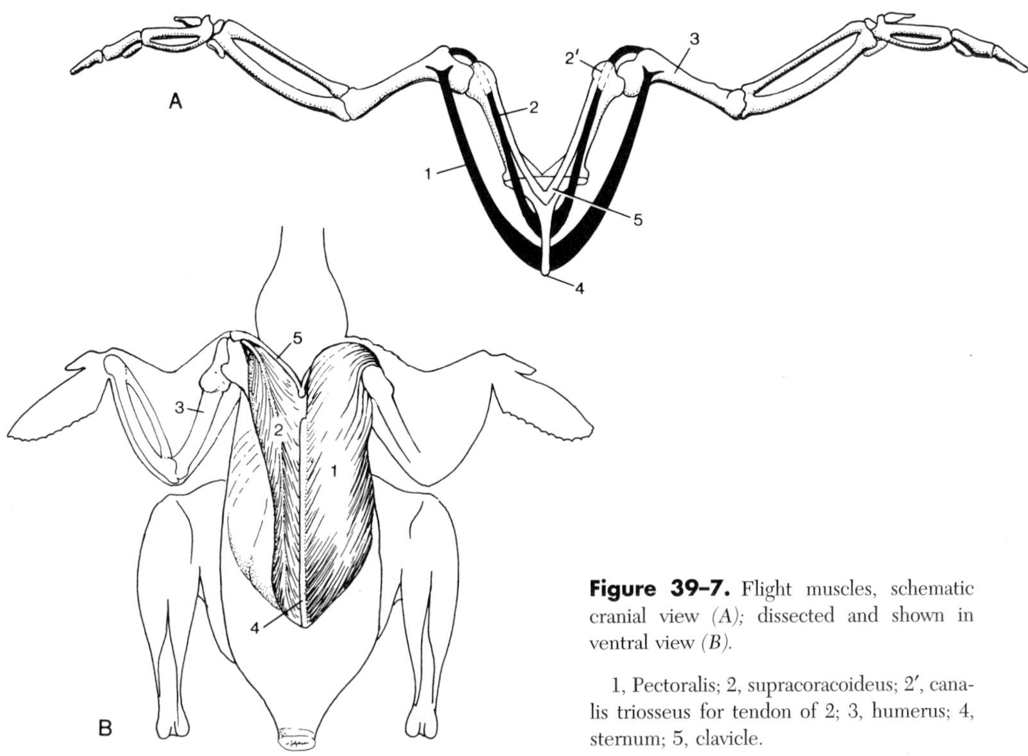


**Figure 39–7.** Flight muscles, schematic cranial view *(A);* dissected and shown in ventral view *(B).*

1, Pectoralis; 2, supracoracoideus; 2′, canalis triosseus for tendon of 2; 3, humerus; 4, sternum; 5, clavicle.

coracoid, and clavicle transmits the tendon of one of the flight muscles (see further on).

The stout *humerus* (/9) is flat at both ends. The proximal extremity carries dorsal and ventral tubercles (Fig. 39–6/2,3). A pneumatic foramen (/4) is present close to the ventral tubercle. The ulna is thicker and longer than the radius (*/B,C*). The proximal row of carpal bones is reduced by fusion to only two separate bones (radial and ulnar; /7,6); the distal row has fused with the metacarpus. The number of metacarpal bones and corresponding digits is reduced to three.

The *breast muscles* that move the wing are well developed and in some species represent as much as 20% of the body weight. The pectoralis (Fig. 39–7/1), the superficial muscle, arises from the keel of the sternum and the clavicle and passes directly to the ventral surface of the dorsal tubercle of the humerus. Its contraction produces the powerful downbeat of the wing. The smaller *supracoracoideus* (/2) also arises from sternum and clavicle. Its tendon is directed dorsally through the canalis triosseus and then across the head of the humerus to end close to its antagonist. The breast muscles are routinely palpated for an indication of the general health of the bird. They are also used for intramuscular injection when care must be taken not to enter the body cavity (Fig. 39–16/2,2′). The cranial portion of the muscles should be avoided for this purpose, as the larger vessels enter here and, if injured, may give rise to fatal hemorrhage.

Section of the tendon of the extensor carpi radialis at carpal level renders a bird unable to fly (pinioning). This prominent muscle lies dorsal to the radius in the laterally extended wing; its short tendon passes subcutaneously over the craniodorsal surface of the carpal joint and ends on the proximal end of the carpometacarpal bone (Fig. 39–8/5′).

## Hindlimb

The *femur* (Fig. 39–4/21) resembles the mammalian bone in its general form. Its palpable proximal end may be used for sampling bone marrow. A patella is present. The *tibia* of birds fuses with tarsal elements, forming a *tibiotarsus* (/31) that is much longer than the femur and carries a feebly developed fibula on its lateral aspect. The fibula is robust proximally where it articulates with the femur (unlike in mammals) as well as the tibiotarsus, but is incomplete distally tapering to a needle-sharp point about three quarters of the length down the tibiotarsus. This part of the limb is popularly known as the "drumstick." The distal tarsal elements merge with the metatarsal bone (itself a fusion of metatarsals II, III, and IV) to form the *tarsometatarsus* (/33). With no free tarsal bones present, the hock is an intertarsal joint that unites the tibiotarsus with the tarsometatarsus.

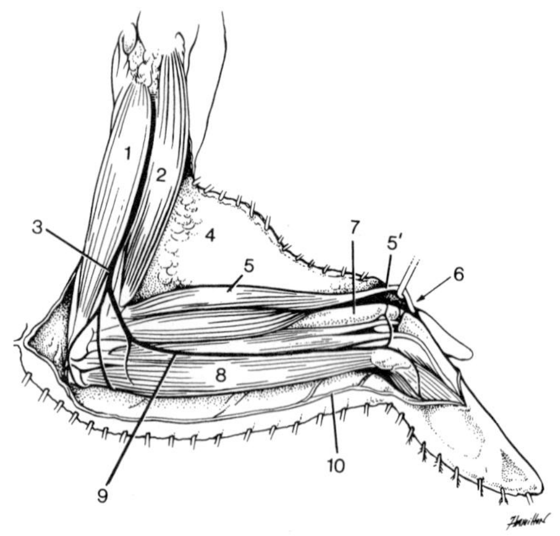


**Figure 39–8.** Superficial dissection of laterally extended left wing, ventral surface.

1, Triceps; 2, biceps; 3, brachial vein; 4, skin fold (propatagium); 5, extensor carpi radialis; 5′, tendon of 5; 6, carpal joint; 7, subcutaneous part of radius; 8, flexor carpi ulnaris; 9, cutaneous ulnar (wing) vein; 10, reflected skin.

The latter extends to the ground where it gives rise to the four digits whose bones are shown in Figure 39–4.

On the caudal surface of the intertarsal joint is a (tibial) cartilage through which the tendons of the digital flexors pass. The palpable gastrocnemius tendon passes through a sleeve connected to the caudal surface of the cartilage and ends on the plantar aspect of the tarsometatarsus. In case of dietary insufficiency (perosis), which disfigures the cartilage, the tendons may slip off the hock, causing severe lameness and deformity. The digital flexors are arranged so that perching is possible with a minimum of muscular energy; the bird in lowering its body flexes knee and hock joints, which passively tenses those tendons that clamp the digits about the perch. Conversely, when trying to undo the grip of a *large* bird, its legs should be extended first to release the tension on the flexor tendons. Budgerigars perch with digits II and III to the front, I and IV to the back (compare with Fig. 39–4). Tendons of limb muscles generally ossify in large birds, which makes them radiographically visible.

Red and white muscles (dark and white meat) are very clearly distinguished in birds. *Red muscles* contain larger amounts of myoglobin, are more heavily vascularized, and have more mitochondria and lipid globules within their fibers. They use fat rather than glycogen (carbohydrate) as a source of energy. Since fat supplies more energy than does carbohydrate per unit weight, muscles containing a predominance of red fibers are more suited to sustained effort. *White muscles* are more powerful but have less endurance. The breast muscles of birds with well-developed capacity for flight are red, those of the chicken and turkey are white, reflective of the galliform's preference for running. Selective breeding of farm-raised turkeys has greatly increased their weight and produced massive breast muscles.

## THE DIGESTIVE APPARATUS

The digestive apparatus consists of oropharynx, esophagus, stomach, duodenum, jejunum, ileum, paired ceca, and colon; the last ends at the cloaca, which also serves the urogenital system. As in the mammal, the liver and pancreas discharge their secretions into the gut and form part of the system. Several parts, including the beak, show considerable modifications and adaptations to diet.

### The Oropharynx

Birds lack a soft palate and obvious constriction separating the mouth from the pharynx. "Oropharynx" thus denotes the combined cavity that extends from the beak to the esophagus. The roof of this dorsoventrally flattened cavity is formed by the palate, its floor by the mandible, tongue, and laryngeal mound (Fig. 39–9). Lips and teeth are absent, their functions being met by the edges of the beak and the ventriculus (see further on). The *palate* presents a long median cleft (choana) that connects with the nasal cavity. A shorter, more caudal (infundibular) cleft (/4 and Plate 31/*E*) is the common opening of the auditory tubes. Choana and infundibular cleft open together in the budgerigar. Numerous "mechanical" *papillae* populate the oropharyngeal wall, either scattered singly or arranged in transverse rows; they are directed caudally and aid in moving the bolus toward the esophagus. Generous amounts of saliva, discharged through the barely visible openings (Fig. 39–9/2) of several sets of salivary glands, moisten the food. The triangular *tongue* (/5,6 and Plate 31/*E*) is supported by a delicate hyoid apparatus and is nonprotrusible. It moves the bolus within the oropharynx and, on swallowing, propels it into the esophagus while the choanal cleft closes. Ducks and geese have tongues fringed with papillae that fit loosely into grooves in the edges of the beak, providing a means of sifting food particles from water (Plate 31/*F*). The *laryngeal mound* (Fig. 39–9/8) rises caudal to the base of the tongue. It presents a median slit (glottis), which is not guarded by an epiglottis. A row of papillae marks the level of origin of the esophagus. The larynx modifies vocalization (unlike in mammals) but is not its actual source.

## The Esophagus

The esophagus at first lies between the trachea and the cervical muscles but soon deviates to the right, a position it maintains throughout the remainder of the neck, although both it and the trachea are quite movable (Fig. 39–10). At the thoracic inlet its ventral wall is greatly expanded to form the *crop* (/8 and Plate 31/*H*), which bulges yet farther to the right and lies against the breast muscles. (In ducks and geese, as in most birds, the crop is merely a fusiform enlargement of the esophagus.) Both cervical esophagus and crop are subcutaneous and palpable, ideally placed for surgery (foreign bodies, impaction) but vulnerable to laceration. The crop stores food for short periods when the muscular stomach is full. Within the body cavity the esophagus passes over the bifurcation of the trachea, below the ventral surface of the lungs, and over the base of the heart (Fig. 39–11 and Plate 31/*G*); it merges into the proventriculus (see further on) directly to the left of the median plane. Much lymphoid tissue (esophageal tonsil) is present in the caudal segment of the duck's esophagus.

The esophagus is capable of great distention; its lamina propria contains mucous glands whose secretion lubricates the passage of the bolus. During brooding, the large symmetrical crop of both male and female pigeons elaborates a crumbly material (crop milk) consisting of desquamated lipid-laden cells; mixed with ingested food, it is regurgitated and fed to the nestlings.

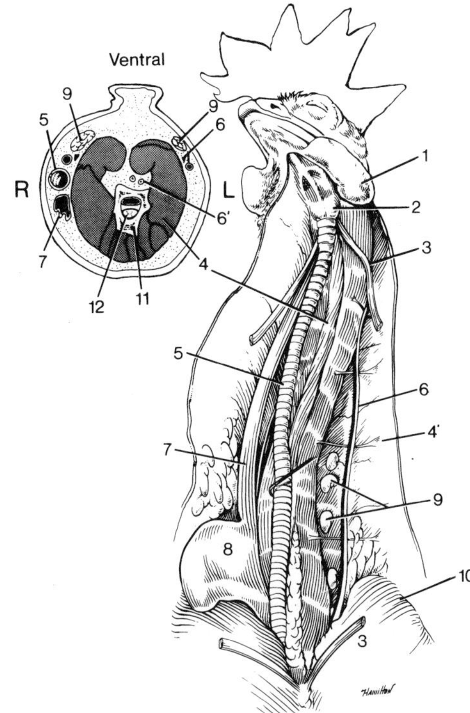


**Figure 39–10.** Ventral view of the dissected neck. The inset shows a transverse section through the middle of the neck.

1, Wattle; 2, larynx; 3, sternothyroideus, cut; 4, cervical muscles; 4′, cervical nerve; 5, trachea; 6, jugular vein and vagus; 6′, internal carotid arteries; 7, esophagus; 8, crop; 9, thymus; 10, pectoralis; 11, vertebra; 12, spinal cord.

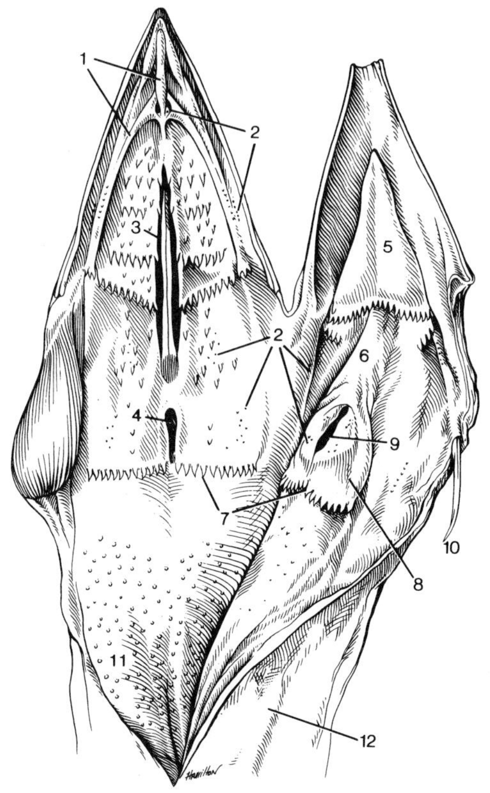


**Figure 39–9.** Oropharynx opened by the reflection of the lower jaw.

1, Median and lateral palatine ridges; 2, openings of salivary glands; 3, choana; 4, infundibular cleft; 5, body of tongue; 6, root of tongue; 7, "mechanical" papillae; 8, laryngeal mound; 9, glottis; 10, branchial cornu of hyobranchial apparatus; 11, esophagus; 12, position of trachea.

## The Stomach

Species variation in the gastrointestinal tract, much less extensive among birds than among mammals,

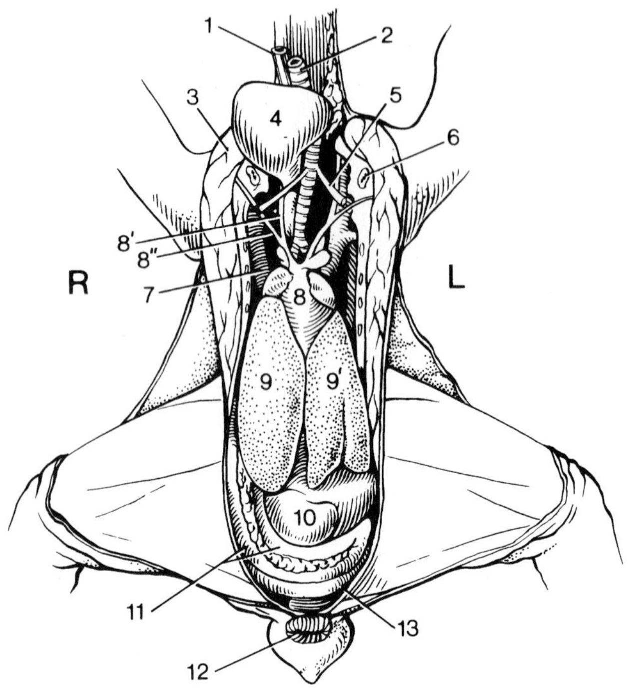


**Figure 39–11.** Viscera after removal of ventral body wall, ventral view.

1, Esophagus; 2, trachea; 3, pectoralis, cut; 4, crop; 5, sternotrachealis; 6, coracoid bone, cut; 7, right cranial vena cava; 8, heart; 8′, common carotid artery; 8″, subclavian artery; 9, 9′, right and left lobes of liver; 10, gizzard (its caudal blind sac); 11, duodenal loop, enclosing pancreas; 12, vent; 13, one of the ceca.

is most marked where the stomach is concerned. The stomach of fish- and flesh-eating species (raptors: hawks, eagles, owls, and vultures) is primarily a storage organ appropriate to the chemical digestion of a soft diet. In contrast, the stomach of species dependent on a vegetable diet is adapted to the mechanical reduction of tougher material through powerful muscular development. Domestic poultry, galliform and anseriform (chicken- and gooselike) birds, possess stomachs that all belong to the second category and exhibit only minor interspecific variation.

The stomach of domestic poultry is divided by a constriction into a predominantly glandular proventriculus and a predominantly muscular ventriculus (gizzard) placed one behind the other and found close to the median plane. The proventriculus is in contact ventrally with the left lobe of the liver; the larger, more caudal gizzard also touches the liver but has more extensive contact with the sternum and the lower part of the left lateral abdominal wall; it is thus exposed when the sternum and abdominal muscles are removed during necropsy (Fig. 39–11/10 and Plate 31/*H*).

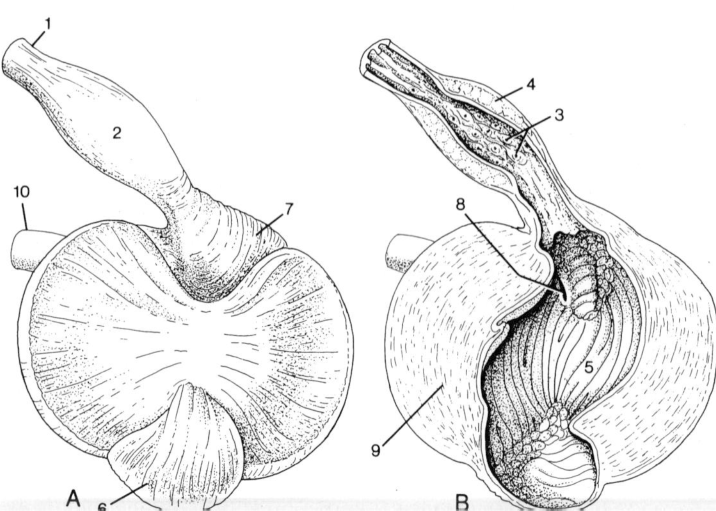


**Figure 39–12.** Stomach, ventral surface *(A)*, and opened ventrally *(B)*.

1, Esophagus; 2, proventriculus; 3, papillae; 4, deep proventricular glands, visible on cut surface; 5, lumen of gizzard; 6, caudal blind sac; 7, cranial blind sac; 8, pyloric orifice; 9, cranioventral muscle mass; 10, duodenum.

The *proventriculus* is spindle-shaped and about 4 cm long. Its whitish mucosa is lined with a mucus-secreting, columnar epithelium that is clearly demarcated from the more reddish lining of the esophagus (Fig. 39–12 and Plates 31/*H* and 32/*A,B*). It presents numerous macroscopic elevations (papillae) through which pass the collecting ducts from a thick bed of glands. These produce hydrochloric acid and pepsin and are readily seen on the cut surface of the wall, deep to the thin tunica muscularis (Fig. 39–12/4). The papillae are so prominent that they may be mistaken for parasitic lesions.

The *ventriculus* or *gizzard* is lens-shaped and is positioned with its convex surfaces facing more or less to right and left. Its interior is elongated and enlarged by cranial and caudal blind sacs, of which the former connects with the proventriculus (/7,6). The pylorus and the origin of the duodenum are on the right surface, adjacent to the cranial blind sac (Fig. 39–14/4). The bulk of the organ consists of two thick masses of muscle that insert on glistening tendinous centers, one on each surface. Two thinner muscles cover the blind sacs. The mucous membrane is thin but very tough; bounded on the surface by a cuboidal epithelium, it largely consists of tubular glands. The secretion of the glands solidifies on the surface and forms a hard *cuticle* of koilin, a carbohydrate-protein complex. The cuticle, rough and plicated, is replenished from the glands below as it is worn on the surface. In seed-eating birds powerful contractions of the gizzard crush the food with the aid of ingested grit, inviting comparison with the masticatory function performed by teeth in mammals. Grit therefore should be provided for such species; it is radiodense and identifies the gizzard in radiographs.

## The Intestines

The intestines occupy the caudal part of the body cavity, making extensive contact with the gizzard and reproductive organs (Plate 31/*H*). They consist of duodenum, jejunum, ileum, and a short colon that lies ventral to the synsacrum and opens into the cloaca. Two ceca arise from the ileocolic junction and accompany the ileum in retrograde fashion (Fig. 39–13/9).

The *duodenum* passes caudally from the right surface of the gizzard. It forms a tight U-shaped loop that returns the duodenojejunal junction to the vicinity of the stomach. Most of the loop lies on the abdominal floor and follows the caudal curvature of the gizzard (Fig. 39–11/11). The pancreas lies between the limbs and empties into

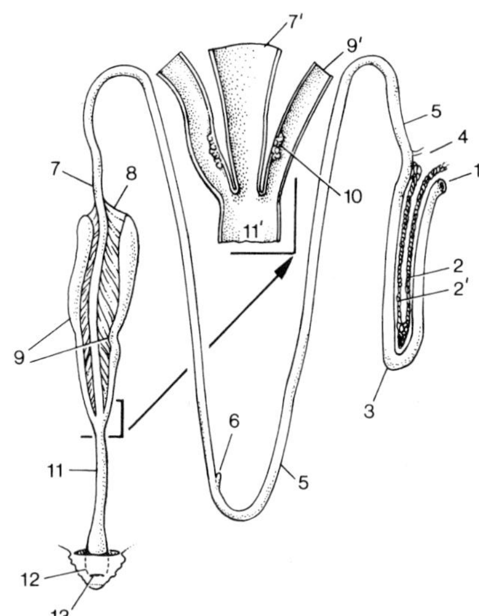


**Figure 39–13.** Isolated intestinal tract with detail of ileocolic junction.

1, Pylorus; 2, 2′, dorsal and ventral lobes of pancreas; 3, duodenal loop; 4, bile and pancreatic ducts entering duodenum; 5, jejunum; 6, vitelline diverticulum; 7, ileum; 7′, ileum opened; 8, ileocecal fold; 9, ceca; 9′, cecum opened; 10, cecal tonsil; 11, colon; 11′, colon opened; 12, cloaca; 13, vent.

the distal end of the duodenum; the bile ducts enter close by (Fig. 39–13/4).

The *jejunum* forms loose coils along the edge of the mesentery and is so thin-walled that its content causes it to appear greenish (Fig. 39–14/7). A small outgrowth (vitelline diverticulum; /8) marks the former connection with the yolk sac. (The yolk sac persists within the body cavity to nourish the hatchling for a few days.) Patches of aggregate lymph nodules are present. In the duck and goose, the jejunum is arranged in several U-shaped loops; in the pigeon, it forms a cone-shaped mass with outer centripetal and inner centrifugal turns.

The *ileum* continues from the jejunum without demarcation. It is variably described as beginning at the vitelline diverticulum or opposite the apices of the ceca (Fig. 39–13/7).

The large intestine comprises ceca and colon (/9,11). The *ceca,* relatively long in the chicken and the turkey, arise at the ileocolic junction and pursue retrograde courses beside the ileum to which they are attached by ileocecal folds. They pass cranially at first, then double back so that their blind ends usually lie near the cloaca (Fig. 39–11/13). The proximal segment has a heavy muscle coat (cecal sphincter) and contains much lymphoid tissue (the so-called cecal tonsil; Fig. 39–13/10). The thin-walled middle part appears greenish because of its content. The blind ends are

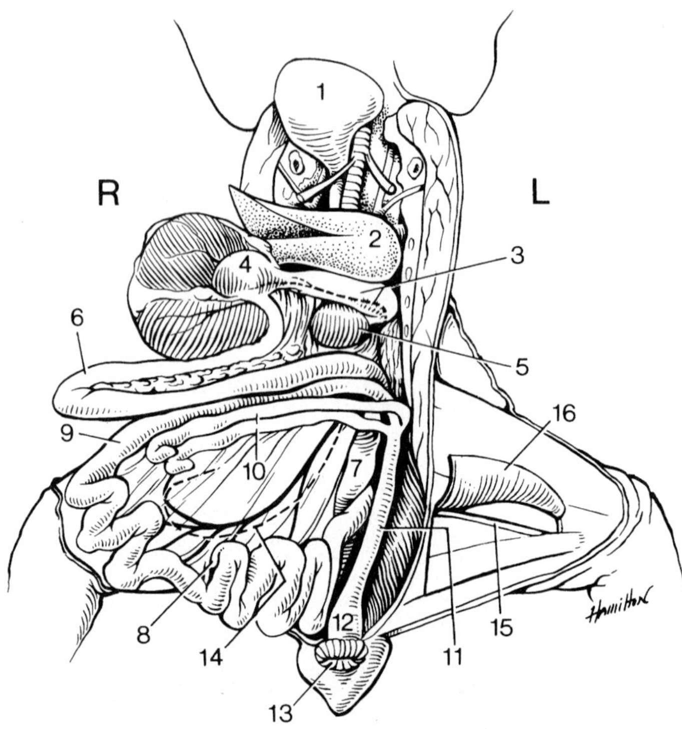


**Figure 39–14.** Gastrointestinal tract after reflection of liver, stomach, and small intestine craniodextrally, ventral view.

1, Crop; 2, left lobe of liver; 3, proventriculus with vagus on dorsal surface; 4, cranial blind sac on right side of reflected gizzard; 5, spleen; 6, duodenal loop enclosing pancreas; 7, jejunum; 8, vitelline diverticulum; 9, ileum; 10, ceca; 11, colon; 12, cloaca; 13, vent; 14, cranial mesenteric vessels and intestinal nerve in mesentery; 15, sciatic nerve and ischial artery; 16, gracilis and adductor.

thicker-walled and bulbous. Bacterial breakdown of cellulose occurs in the ceca. Passerine birds (generally known as song birds) and pigeons have very short ceca; psittacines have none.

The *colon* is about 10 cm long and ends by a slight enlargement at the cloaca.

## The Cloaca

The cloaca, common to the digestive and urogenital systems, opens to the exterior at the *vent* (Fig. 39–15/5). Colon, ureters, and deferent ducts (or the left oviduct) enter it at various levels. The cloaca is

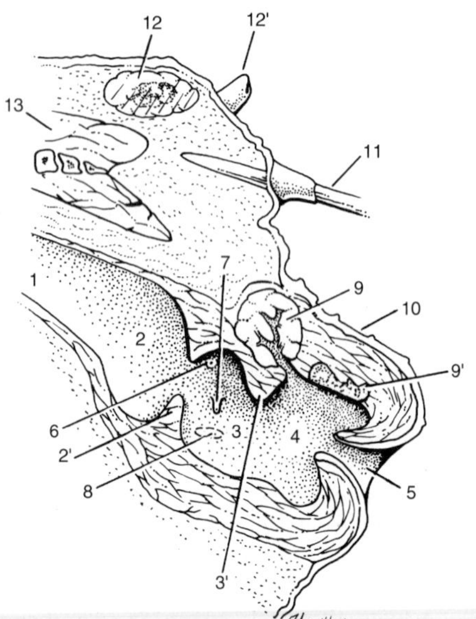


**Figure 39–15.** Median section of the cloaca, semischematic.

1, Colon; 2, coprodeum; 2′, coprourodeal fold; 3, urodeum; 3′, uroproctodeal fold; 4, proctodeum; 5, vent; 6, ureteric orifice; 7, papilla of deferent duct; 8, position of oviduct orifice (only on left side); 9, cloacal bursa; 9′, dorsal proctodeal gland; 10, skin; 11, tail feather; 12, uropygial gland; 12′, papilla of uropygial gland; 13, muscles surrounding caudal vertebrae.

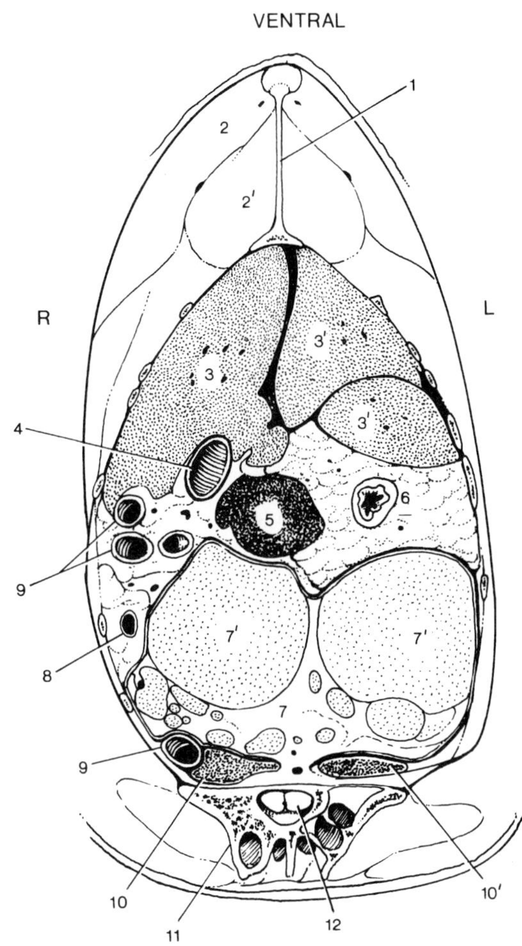


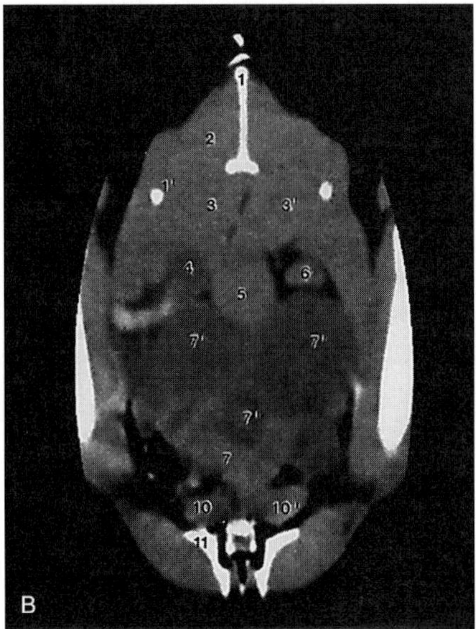


**Figure 39–16.** *A*, Transverse section of the trunk at the cranial end of the ilium. *B*, Corresponding CT image to illustrate the ability of computed tomography to produce transverse images of birds on which structures of different densities can be distinguished.

1, Keel of sternum, its sternocoracoidal processes at 1′; 2, pectoralis (pectoral muscles in *B*); 2′, supracoracoideus; 3, 3′, right and left lobes of liver; 4, gallbladder; 5, spleen; 6, constriction between proventriculus and gizzard; 7, ovary; 7′, follicle; 8, cranial mesenteric vein in mesenteric fat; 9, small intestine; 10, 10′, right and left kidneys; 11, ilium; 12, spinal cord.

divided sequentially into coprodeum, urodeum, and proctodeum by two more or less complete annular folds.

The *coprodeum* is the ampulliform continuation of the colon in which feces are stored (/2). It is bounded caudally by the coprourodeal fold (/2′), which may be stretched by the pressure of the feces so that its central opening is everted through the vent. Urodeum and proctodeum (/3,4) are described with the urogenital system (p. 817).

## The Liver and Pancreas

The avian *liver* is dark brown except in the first two weeks after hatching when it obtains a yellow color from yolk pigments, which continue to be absorbed from the intestine before the yolk sac finally regresses. The liver consists of right and left lobes, connected cranially by a bridge dorsal to the heart (Fig. 39–11). In striking contrast to mammals, birds lack a diaphragm; thus, the lobes of the liver, rather than the lungs, embrace the caudal portion of the heart. The larger right lobe carries the gallbladder in its visceral surface and is perforated by the caudal vena cava; the left lobe is divided (Fig. 39–16/3′). The parietal surface is convex and lies against the sternal ribs and sternum; it is thus exposed when the breast muscles and sternum are removed in postmortem examination. The visceral surface is concave and makes contact with the spleen, proventriculus, gizzard, duodenum, jejunum, and ovary (or right testis). Two bile ducts, one from each lobe, enter the distal end of the duodenum close to the pancreatic ducts; only the duct from the right lobe is connected to the gallbladder. Except near the hilus, the hepatic lobules are indistinct because of the lack of perilobular connective tissue. The pigeon and budgerigar lack a gallbladder.

The elongated *pancreas* lies between the limbs of the duodenal loop (Fig. 39–13/2,2′). It consists of dorsal and ventral lobes that are connected distally. Two or three ducts convey pancreatic juice into the distal end of the duodenum.

## The Spleen

The spleen (see also p. 822) is mentioned here because of its relationship to the stomach and liver (Plates 31/*H* and 32/*A*). It is a brownish-red sphere, about 2 cm in diameter, that lies in the median plane beside the proventriculus; it contacts the liver cranioventrally (Fig. 39–16/5). It is best exposed during postmortem examination by reflecting the right lobe of the liver and the gizzard, duodenum, and jejunum craniodextrally (Fig. 39–14/5). The spleen is triangular in the duck and goose, oval in the pigeon, and elongated in the budgerigar.

# THE RESPIRATORY SYSTEM

The indoor flocks of the modern poultry industry are particularly prone to respiratory infections, which may be very costly. The respiratory apparatus, which differs considerably from that of mammals, has a corresponding importance to the veterinarian.

## The Nasal Cavity

The *nostrils* (Fig. 39–1/1 and Plate 31/*B–D*) at the base of the beak are overhung by a horny flap (operculum). They lead into the nasal cavity, which is divided, as in the mammal, by a median septum and is in wide communication with the oropharynx through the choana (Fig. 39–9/3).

The nasal cavities are laterally compressed and extend to the large orbits. Rostral, middle, and caudal *conchae* that arise from the lateral wall encroach on the space (Fig. 39–26/2,2′,2″). The rostral and middle conchae enclose recesses that communicate with the nasal cavity; the caudal one encloses a diverticulum of the *infraorbital sinus.* This sinus lies lateral to the nasal cavity into which it opens by a narrow duct so placed that natural drainage is impeded. The sinus wall is thin and directly subcutaneous rostral and ventral to the eye where it may be identified by its yielding on palpation; it may be opened and the exudate, which accumulates within the sinus in several diseases, flushed out. The relatively wide nasolacrimal duct opens into the nasal cavity ventral to the middle concha. The elongated *nasal gland* extends forward from the dorsal part of the orbit in the lateral wall of the nasal cavity. Its duct opens into the cavity at the level of the rostral concha. The gland is widely known as the salt gland; however, it secretes sodium only in marine (and a few other) species.

## The Larynx, Trachea, and Syrinx

The *larynx* occupies a mound on the floor of the oropharynx (Fig. 39–9/8). It is supported by cricoid and paired arytenoid cartilages that differ markedly from their mammalian counterparts but occupy similar positions. The arytenoids articulate with the rostrodorsal part of the annular cricoid. The glottis, formed by the arytenoids, closes the entrance to the larynx by reflex muscular action, preventing food particles and other foreign matter from reaching the lower air passages. Despite the narrowness of the glottis it is possible to intubate the trachea in larger cage birds. There are no vocal folds; voice production occurs in the syrinx, a specialization at the tracheal bifurcation.

The *trachea,* composed of tightly stacked, complete, and overlapping cartilaginous rings, accompanies the esophagus through the neck; it can be palpated on the right side (Fig. 39–10/5). In a long-necked species, for example, trumpeter swans, it is much longer than the neck and forms a loop that is accommodated in an excavation of the sternum at the thoracic inlet. The trachea bifurcates into two primary bronchi dorsal to the base of the heart. These enter the ventral surface of the lungs after a short course.

The *syrinx* is formed by the terminal part of the trachea and the beginning of the primary bronchi (Fig. 39–17). The tracheal cartilages of the syrinx are sturdy, whereas the bronchial cartilages are largely lacking, although a short vertical bar (pessulus; /3) separates the bronchial openings. The lateral and medial walls of the initial segments of the bronchi are membranous and produce the voice when caused to flutter (/2,2′). A small paired muscle, sternotrachealis (Fig. 39–11/5), pulls the trachea toward the syrinx and aids in vocalization. The male duck and swan have an osseous bulla (believed to be a resonator) on the left side of the syrinx. An elaborate set of syringeal muscles is present in songbirds.

## The Lungs

The lungs are relatively small, unlobed, bright pink, and nonexpansile. Though firmer than mammalian lungs due to containing far more cartilage, fresh avian lungs are soft and velvety to the touch.

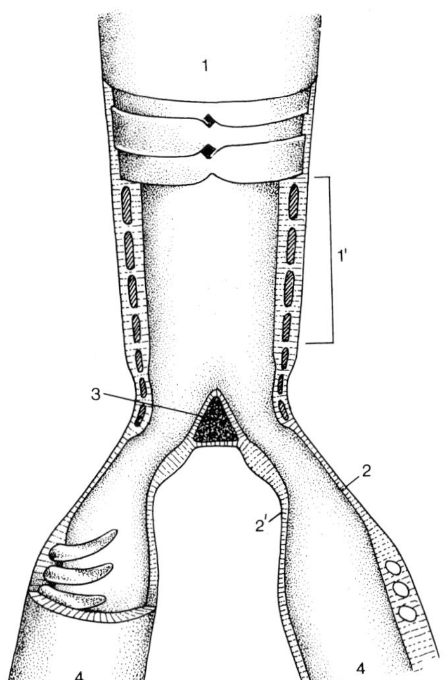


**Figure 39–17.** Semischematic representation of the opened syrinx.

1, Trachea; 1′, tympanum; 2, 2′, lateral and medial tympaniform membranes; 3, pessulus; 4, primary bronchi.

The lungs are confined to the craniodorsal part of the body cavity, lying against, and deeply indented by, the thoracic vertebrae and vertebral ribs. They fail to cover the lateral surfaces of the heart as they do in mammals. The convex dorsal surface is shaped to the curvature of the ribs; the concave ventral (septal) surface lies against the horizontal septum (see further on) and faces the esophagus, heart, and liver (Fig. 39–18). The lungs are lightly attached to the body wall and to the horizontal septum that confines them from below. No pleural cavity corresponding to that of mammals is necessary, since the capacity for expansion is negligible. The nonexpansile nature of the lungs, their abundant cartilage, and their confinement high within the body cavity surrounded by bone also renders them largely incompressible. This calls into question whether euthanasia by thoracic compression in birds is indeed humane.

The *primary bronchus* (Fig. 39–19/1) enters the ventral surface, passes diagonally through the lung, narrowing as it goes, and at the caudal border becomes continuous with the abdominal air sac (/13; see later). In the chicken it gives off 40 to 50 *secondary bronchi* classified as medioventral, mediodorsal, lateroventral, and laterodorsal according to the general areas of the lung they supply (Figs. 39–18/a–d and 39–19/2–5). Various connections of these groups of secondary bronchi exist with various air sacs. These communications are essential to passage of air through the lungs.

The secondary bronchi give off 400 to 500 *parabronchi* in whose relatively thick walls are contained the sites where gas exchange takes place. The parabronchi arising from the medioventral and mediodorsal bronchi connect with each other end to end to form loops of various lengths (/6). These loops, which are tightly packed and parallel, constitute about three quarters of the lung tissue, forming the functional division known as the paleopulmo. The parabronchi from the smaller

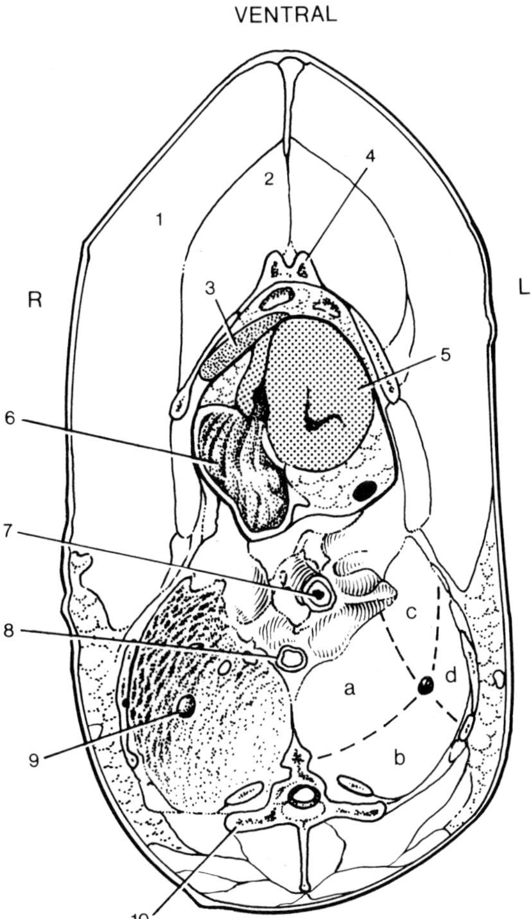


**Figure 39–18.** Transverse section of the trunk at the level of the heart and lungs.

1, Pectoralis; 2, supracoracoideus; 3, liver; 4, sternum; 5, left ventricle; 6, right atrium; 7, esophagus; 8, descending aorta; 9, primary bronchus in right lung; 10, thoracic vertebra (notarium).

a, b, c, d, Left lung showing areas supplied by medioventral, mediodorsal, lateroventral, and laterodorsal secondary bronchi, respectively.

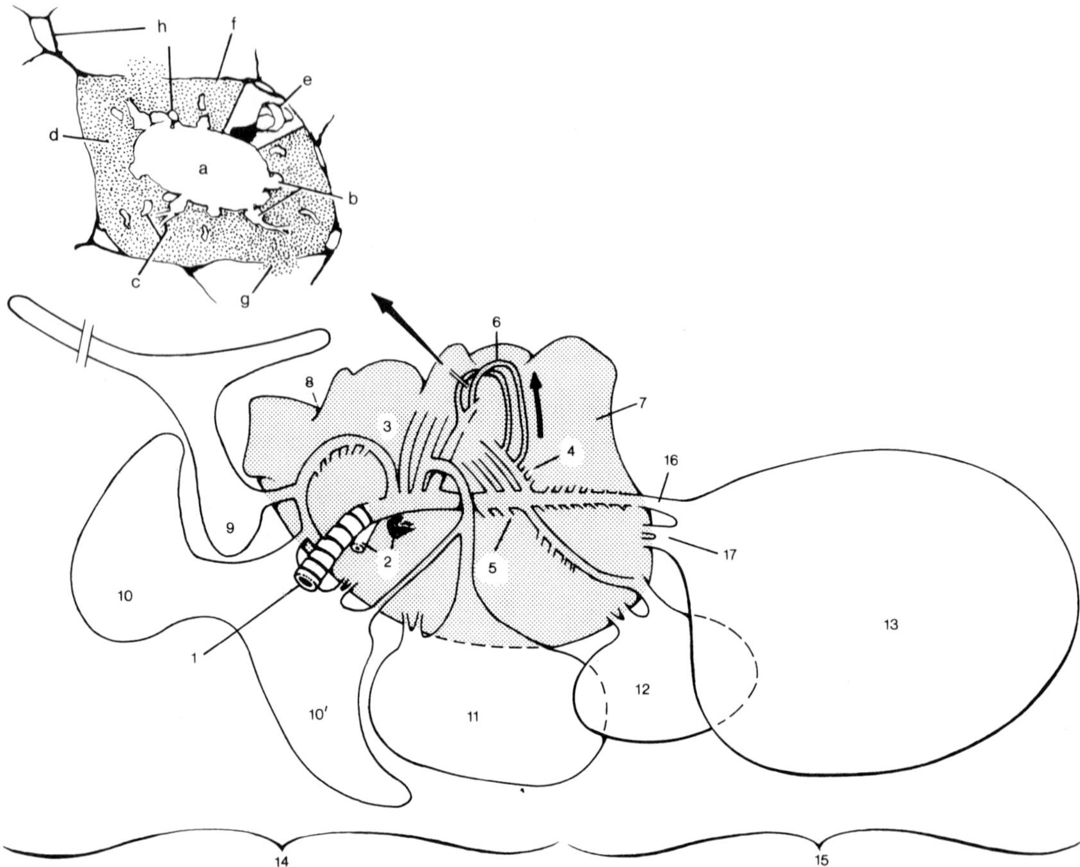


**Figure 39–19.** Right lung (medioventral view) and related air sacs, schematic. The intrapulmonic structures have been simplified. The inset shows a transverse section of a parabronchus.

1, Primary bronchus; 2, pulmonary vessels at hilus; 3, medioventral bronchi; 4, mediodorsal bronchi; 5, lateroventral bronchi; 6, loops of parabronchi; 7, lung; 8, indentations caused by ribs; 9, cervical air sac; 10, 10′ extra- and intrathoracic parts of clavicular air sac; 11, cranial thoracic air sac; 12, caudal thoracic air sac; 13, abdominal air sac; 14, cranial air sacs, functionally related to paleopulmonic parabronchi; 15, caudal air sacs, functionally related to neopulmonic parabronchi; 16, direct (saccobronchial) connection; 17, indirect (recurrent bronchial) connection of air sac to lung.

a, Lumen; b, atria; c, infundibula; d, network of air and blood capillaries; e, solidly drawn atrium and schematic air capillaries to show their continuity; f, interparabronchial septum; g, gas exchange tissue anastomosing through gap in interparabronchial septum; h, blood vessels.

lateroventral and laterodorsal bronchi form a less regular and more caudal functional division, known as the neopulmo.

The internal and external diameters of the parabronchi measure about 1 mm and 2 mm, respectively. The parabronchi anastomose with neighboring ones from which they are separated by fenestrated septa (/f). Numerous extensions (atria) of the parabronchial lumen give rise to the *air capillaries.* These form a dense network of interconnected loops (/e) that spread into the interparabronchial septa. Anastomoses with air capillaries of adjacent parabronchi are found where the septa are deficient (/g). The air capillaries are closely intertwined with blood capillaries, the two networks constituting the bulk of the parabronchial wall. The arrangement of flow in the blood capillaries is crosscurrent, a feature contributing to the super efficiency of the avian lung. The air capillaries, about 5 μm in diameter, are lined by a single layer of epithelial cells resting on a basement membrane. The capillary endothelium is applied to the other side of the basement membrane. Gas exchange takes place across the barrier. The air capillaries are therefore homologous with the alveoli of the mammalian lung. An essential difference is that the air capillaries are not terminations of the respiratory tree but continuous channels that can receive oxygen-rich air from either direction.

The *air sacs* are blind, thin-walled enlargements of the bronchial system that extend beyond the lung in close relationship to the thoracic and abdominal viscera. Diverticula from these sacs enter various bones and even extend between skeletal muscles.

The chicken has eight air sacs: single cervical and clavicular, and paired cranial thoracic, caudal thoracic, and abdominal sacs. The *cervical sac* (Fig. 39–19/9) consists of a small central chamber ventral to the lungs from which long diverticula extend into and alongside the cervical and thoracic vertebrae. The much larger *clavicular sac* lies in the thoracic inlet. Its thoracic part (/10′) fills the space cranial to and around the heart, and extends into the sternum. Its extrathoracic diverticula (/10) pass between the muscles and bones of the shoulder girdle to pneumatize the humerus. Compound fractures of the humerus may therefore introduce infection to the air sacs and lungs. The paired *cranial thoracic sacs* (/11) lie ventral to the lungs between the sternal ribs and the heart and liver. The paired *caudal thoracic sacs* (/12) lie more caudally between the body wall and the abdominal sacs. The paired *abdominal sacs* (/13) are the largest. They occupy the caudodorsal parts of the abdominal cavity where they are in broad contact with the intestines, gizzard, genital organs, and kidneys. Their diverticula enter recesses of the synsacrum and the acetabulum.

The air sacs function primarily in respiration, although their poorly vascularized walls deny them a role in gas exchange. Nonetheless, healthy air sacs are requisite to normal lung function. Indeed, their general arrangement is such that, in stark contrast to mammalian lungs, fresh air is moved through the lung on expiration as well as inspiration. This feature is an obvious contribution to the remarkable efficiency of the avian lung and the truly prodigious athletic capabilities it supports. The air sacs also lighten the body and, being broadly dorsal in position, lower the center of gravity, presumably for improved stability in flight. Those in the body cavity sharply delineate certain organs in radiographs.

The cervical, clavicular, and cranial thoracic sacs form one (cranial) functional group, and the caudal thoracic and abdominal sacs form a second (caudal) group. The cranial air sacs are related to the paleopulmo, the caudal to the neopulmo, the functional divisions of the lung already noted. Respiration in birds is complex, and the account given here is greatly simplified. Inspiratory movements (in which the ribs are drawn forward and the sternum lowered) draw air through the lungs into the air sacs; the caudal sacs (/15) receiving relatively fresh air, the cranial sacs (/14) receiving air that has already lost much oxygen by passing through the paleopulmonic parabronchi. During expiration the air sacs are compressed; most air from the caudal sacs now passes through the neopulmonic parabronchi, while most of that from the cranial ones leaves through the trachea. The air sacs thus act like bellows, moving the air through a largely passive lung. Air flow in them is tidal (as in the mammalian lung). Air flow in the lung, however, is circular; that is, air passes through the loops of paleopulmonic parabronchi always in the same direction. Thus, oxygen-rich air moves through the paleopulmo on both inspiration and expiration, a feature unique among vertebrates. How this is achieved is not yet fully understood.

## THE UROGENITAL APPARATUS

### The Kidneys and Ureters

The *kidneys* are brown and elongated (Fig. 39–20/*A–C* and Plate 32/*E*). They fill the recesses in the ventral surfaces of the hip bones and lie against the synsacrum, reaching almost to its caudal limit; cranially, they are in contact with the lungs. The abdominal air sacs that lie against their ventral surfaces extend diverticula that reach the dorsal renal surfaces. Several vessels and nerves pass through the kidneys, making it impossible to remove them uninjured. Birds suffering from renal gout (not uncommon in commercial flocks) may therefore have lameness as the presenting sign.

Each kidney is arbitrarily divided into cranial, middle, and caudal divisions by the external iliac and ischial arteries (Fig. 39–20/12,18), branches of the abdominal aorta. In some other species, but not the chicken, the right and left caudal divisions are fused.

The *ureter* (/20) arises in the cranial division by the confluence of several primary branches and passes over the medioventral surface of the kidney, receiving further branches from the middle and caudal divisions in its passage; no renal pelvis exists. The ureter then continues caudally alongside the genital duct to end in the urodeum (see later). It obtains a whitish tinge from the concentrated urine within it. Neither bladder nor urethra is present.

The primary branches of the ureter (/8) result from the confluence of several secondary branches that each receive urine from a small group (five or six) of cone-shaped *renal lobules,* each 1 to 2 mm in diameter. Those near the surface bulge slightly, providing a visible pattern. Each lobule is composed of nephrons and the vascular networks responsible for the extraction of urine from the

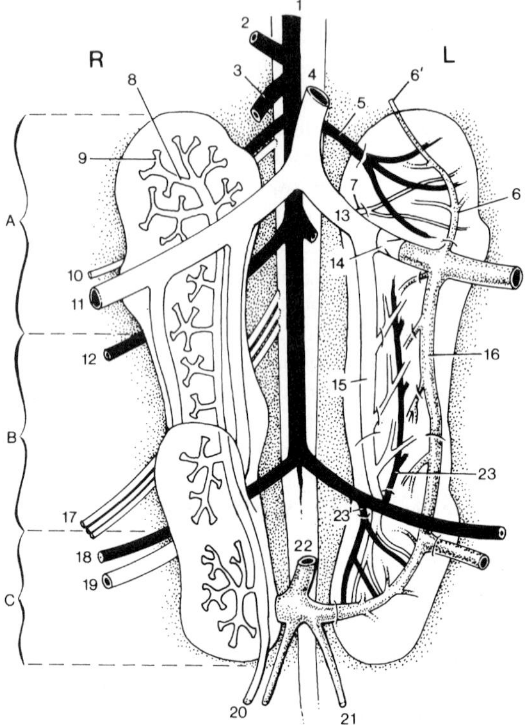


**Figure 39–20.** Ventral view of the kidneys, and vessels and nerves in their vicinity, schematic. The right kidney shows the branches of the ureter; the left, the renal vessels. Cranial (A), middle (B), and caudal (C) divisions of kidney.

1, Aorta; 2, celiac a.; 3, cranial mesenteric a.; 4, caudal vena cava; 5, cranial renal a.; 6, cranial renal portal v.; 6′, anastomosis with vertebral venous sinus; 7, cranial renal v.; 8, primary branch of ureter; 9, secondary branch of ureter; 10, femoral n.; 11, external iliac v.; 12, external iliac a.; 13, common iliac v.; 14, portal valve; 15, caudal renal v.; 16, caudal renal portal v.; 17, sciatic n.; 18, ischial a.; 19, ischial v.; 20, ureter; 21, internal iliac v.; 22, caudal mesenteric v.; 23, 23′, middle and caudal renal aa.

blood. The collecting tubules lie in the periphery of the cone and become confluent at the apex.

### *The Blood Vessels of the Kidneys*

The kidney is supplied by cranial, middle, and caudal *renal arteries,* one to each division (Fig. 39–20/5,23,23′). The cranial artery arises from the aorta, the others from the ischial artery. After repeated division, each gives rise to microscopic intralobular arteries that typically occupy the center of the renal lobules. The interlobular arteries supply the renal corpuscles and tubules. The smaller veins are satellite to the arteries, but the several *renal veins* (/7,15) leaving the organ join the common iliac vein (/13), and through it, the caudal vena cava. Superimposed on this is a renal portal system composed of cranial and caudal *renal portal veins* (/6,16). The portal veins receive blood from the caudal parts of the body and channel it to the intralobular capillary beds that receive arterial blood from the renal arteries. Thus, blood that has already passed one capillary bed in the hindlimb or the pelvis enters the kidney to pass through a second bed. A *portal valve* (/14) regulates the amount of venous blood entering the kidney; when narrowed, more blood enters the kidneys, although some always escapes via connections with the vertebral sinuses and caudal mesenteric vein (/6′,22) at the cranial and caudal ends of the system. Most blood in the caudal mesenteric vein passes through the right hepatic portal vein and through the liver before arriving at the heart. (It has been suggested that antibiotics should not be injected into the muscles of the hindlimb, as some of the drug would be excreted by the kidney before reaching the heart for general distribution.)

## The Male Reproductive Organs

These consist of paired testes, epididymides, deferent ducts, and a single phallus, which is the copulatory organ. The testes remain at their sites of origin; spermatic cord, tunica vaginalis, and scrotum are lacking. Furthermore, no accessory reproductive glands and no urethra exist.

### *The Testis*

The bean-shaped testes are relatively large (about 5 cm long) and white during the breeding season (Plate 32/*E*); in the quiescent period (during molt) they shrink to about half that size and become yellowish. Attached by short mesorchia, they are placed symmetrically against the cranial ends of the kidneys, related ventrally to the abdominal sacs, proventriculus, liver, and intestines (Fig. 39–21/3). Removal of the testes (caponizing) to induce fattening may be performed through an incision near the last rib. Prior to the advent of simpler and safer blood testing to determine the sex of a bird, sexing of larger cage birds could be performed by introducing an endoscope through a small incision—a bird whose sex is known has a greatly increased value.

The serosa covers a thin tunica albuginea from which a scanty stroma is derived; no mediastinum testis exists. Dark pigmentation on and in the testis is not uncommon in some species. The seminiferous tubules pass to the dorsomedial wall where they open into the rete testis. The *epididymis* is not divided into head, body, and tail and appears as a slight bulge on the testis. It is formed by tightly packed efferent ductules that join to form the epididymal duct through which the spermatozoa reach the *deferent duct* (/7 and Plate 32/*E*). This arises from the caudal end of the epididymis and is tightly coiled; it accompanies the ureter to the cloaca where it opens on a low papilla on the lateral wall of the urodeum (Fig. 39–15/7). The duct shows a slight terminal enlargement (receptacle). During the reproductive period the duct is packed with spermatozoa, which cause it to be white. The ejaculate of the cockerel is generally not quite 1 mL. The seminal fluid is elaborated in the testes and by the epithelial cells lining the extratesticular ducts.

## The Cloaca and Phallus

The *coprodeum,* the most cranial division of the cloaca, has already been described (p. 810). The *urodeum* (Fig. 39–15/3), caudal to the coprourodeal fold, is indistinctly demarcated from the proctodeum by a shallow, ventrally incomplete uroproctodeal fold (/3′). The ureteric orifice is in the dorsolateral wall, above the papilla of the deferent duct. In the female, the slitlike opening of the oviduct (/8) occupies a similar position on the left side (see further on). A small patch of vascular tissue (paracloacal vascular body; Fig. 39–21/15′) in the lateral wall of the urodeum is thought to supply the lymph for the tumescence of the phallus.

The *proctodeum,* the short, most caudal segment of the cloaca, ends at the vent. A small opening in its dorsal wall leads to the cloacal bursa (Fig. 39–15/9), an accumulation of lymphatic tissue that is the differentiation site of B-lymphocytes. The cloacal bursa is thus an immunological organ similar to the thymus (see p. 258). A small (dorsal proctodeal) gland is found caudal to the bursa (/9′).

The vent is a horizontal slit. The ventral lip is of interest because in the male it bears the nonprotrusible *phallus,* the analogue of the mammalian penis, on its internal surface. The phallus consists of a small median tubercle flanked by a pair of larger lateral phallic bodies (Fig. 39–21/13,14). These enlarge in the tumescent state and together form a groove that receives the ejaculate from the deferent ducts (/*C*). During insemination, the vent is everted and the phallus pressed against the cloacal mucosa of the female (cloacal "kiss"). The phallus of the tom turkey has a similar appearance. The gander and the drake have a protrusible

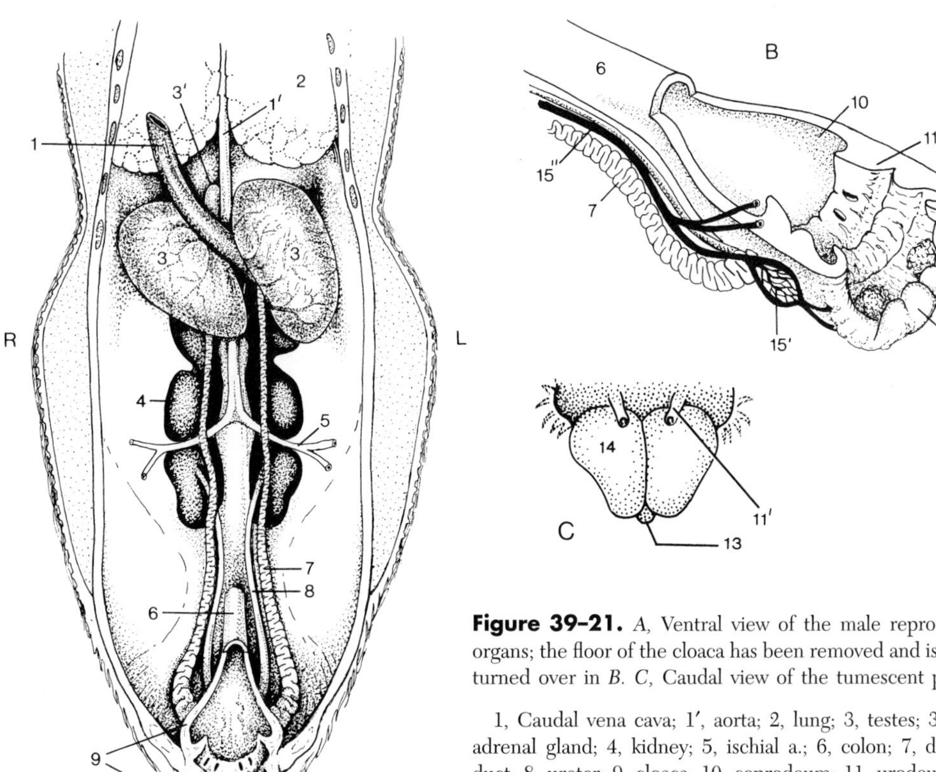


**Figure 39–21.** *A,* Ventral view of the male reproductive organs; the floor of the cloaca has been removed and is shown turned over in *B. C,* Caudal view of the tumescent phallus.

1, Caudal vena cava; 1′, aorta; 2, lung; 3, testes; 3′, right adrenal gland; 4, kidney; 5, ischial a.; 6, colon; 7, deferent duct; 8, ureter; 9, cloaca; 10, coprodeum; 11, urodeum; 11′, papilla of right deferent duct; 12, proctodeum; 13, median phallic tubercle; 14, lateral phallic body; 15, lymphatic folds; 15′, paracloacal vascular body; 15″, pudendal artery.

phallus, several centimeters long and capable of intromission. It is shaped like a thin cone and exhibits a spiral groove that conveys the semen to the tip (Fig. 39–22/8).

Day-old chicks of both sexes present a minute genital protuberance at the future location of the phallus. A barely visible difference in form (which is rounded in males and conical in females) enables almost all male chicks to be discarded when a laying flock is selected.

## The Female Reproductive Organs

These consist of ovary and oviduct. In birds generally, only the left organs are functional; the right set is formed but later regress. The avian oviduct, in contrast to its nominal counterpart in mammals (uterine tube), represents the entire genital tract and extends from the ovary to the cloaca.

Remarkably, both the gonad(s) and tubular tract(s) of both male and female undergo extreme involution outside the breeding season. The organs fill much of the body cavity while productive, but regress to such an extent that they may be difficult to locate.

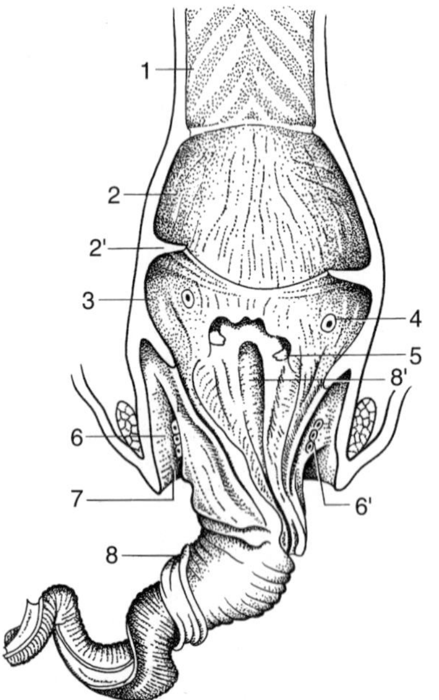


**Figure 39–22.** Cloaca of a drake with protruded phallus whose tip has been cut off, dorsal view.

1, Colon; 2, coprodeum; 2′, coprourodeal fold; 3, urodeum; 4, ureteric orifice; 5, papilla of deferent duct; 6, proctodeum; 6′, proctodeal glands; 7, lip of vent; 8, spiral groove of phallus; 8′, beginning of spiral groove.

### The Ovary

In the first 5 months after hatching, the ovary gradually develops from a small irregular structure with a finely granular surface to one in which individual *follicles* can be observed. These then rapidly increase in number and size until some are several centimeters in diameter (the size of an egg yolk; Fig. 39–16/7 and Plate 32/*C,D*). The mature ovary resembles a bunch of irregular grapes and is broadly attached to the cranial division of the left kidney. It contains several thousand follicles—far more than the number of eggs (about 1500) that even the most productive hen will lay. The larger follicles are pendulous and make contact with the stomach, spleen, and intestines. Each consists of a large, yolk-filled oocyte surrounded by a highly vascular follicular wall. Shortly before ovulation, a devascularized white band (stigma) appears opposite the stalk, indicating where the wall will rupture at ovulation (Fig. 39–23/2 and Plate 32/*C*). The empty follicle (calix) regresses following ovulation and disappears in a few days. No corpus luteum is required since there is no embryo to maintain as there is in mammals.

### The Oviduct

The oviduct is of much greater functional significance than its name implies. It not only conducts the fertilized ovum to the cloaca but also adds substantial amounts of nutrients (including the albumen) and, by enclosing the ovum with membranes and a shell, provides protection for the embryo. It conveys spermatozoa to the ovum for immediate fertilization and stores them for future use—one insemination is sufficient to fertilize the ova released during the following 10 days or so.

The oviduct (Fig. 39–23/3–7 and Plate 32/*C,D*) may be divided into infundibulum, magnum, isthmus, uterus, and vagina according to the function of its parts; the uterus and vagina are, of course, not analogous to the like-named organs of mammals. The oviduct occupies the left dorsal part of the body cavity where it is related to the kidney, intestines, and gizzard. It is a massive coil, approximately 60 cm long (i.e., about twice the body length) when fully functional. It is much reduced in juveniles and during the nonlaying period. It is suspended from the roof of the body cavity by a peritoneal fold (mesoviductus), and some coils are connected by a ventral continuation that forms the prominent muscular ventral ligament (/12). The wall of the oviduct consists of the usual layers—serosa, tunica muscularis (consisting of outer spiral and inner circular layers), a scanty submucosa, and a tunica mucosa containing many glands.

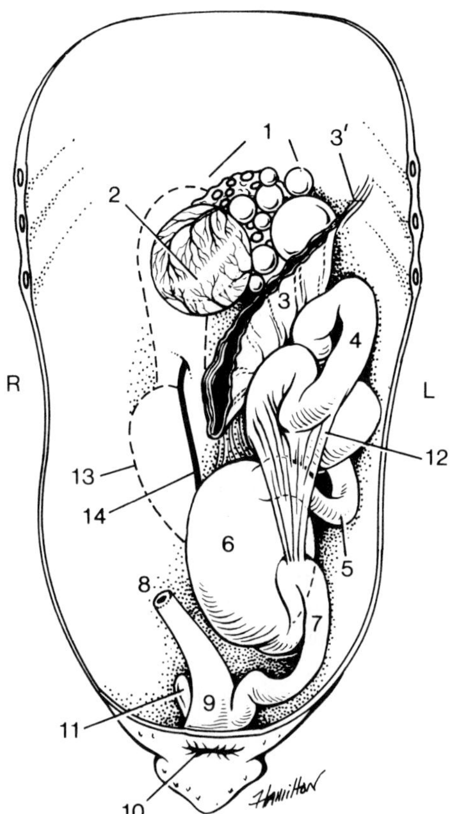


**Figure 39–23.** Ventral view of the reproductive organs of a laying hen, semischematic.

1, Ovary; 2, stigma on mature follicle; 3, infundibulum; 3′, attachment of infundibulum to body wall; 4, magnum; 5, isthmus; 6, uterus containing egg; 7, vagina; 8, colon; 9, cloaca; 10, vent; 11, vestigial right oviduct; 12, free border of ventral ligament of oviduct; 13, outline of right kidney; 14, right ureter.

The cranial end is formed by the 7-cm-long *infundibulum* (/3) consisting of fluted and tubular parts. The fluted part is thin-walled and stretched to form a slit (infundibular ostium) several centimeters long; its lateral end is attached to the body wall near the last rib. The ostium is positioned by the left abdominal air sac in such a way that it can grasp the newly released oocyte. The oocyte passes through the infundibulum in about 15 minutes but during this time infundibular glands provide it with its chalaziferous layer, the thin coating of dense albumen around the yolk. The chalazae, the coiled strands that suspend the yolk and allow it to rotate so that the germinal disc remains uppermost, although part of this layer, develop farther along the genital duct (Fig. 39–24/3′).

The highly coiled *magnum* (Fig. 39–23/4 and Plate 32/*C,D*) measures about 30 cm and is the longest segment of the duct. Its walls carry massive mucosal folds and are thickened by the glands that add about half the total albumen to the egg. In the distal end of the magnum the mucosal folds are lower and the secretion more mucous. The egg takes about 3 hours to pass through this part.

The *isthmus* (/5), about 8 cm long, is demarcated from the magnum by a narrow aglandular (translucent) zone. It is thinner and has lower mucosal folds than the magnum. Its glands secrete more albumen and also a material that rapidly congeals to form the two homogeneous membranes found between the albumen and the shell. The egg takes upward of 1 hour to traverse the isthmus.

The *uterus* (shell gland; /6) is a thinner-walled, slightly enlarged chamber, about 8 cm long. Its mucosa bears many low folds and ridges that flatten themselves against the egg, which remains here for about 20 hours. Some watery albumen is added here to plump out the egg by passing through the permeable membranes. This is followed by the deposition of the shell and shell pigments and a glazelike outer layer (cuticle).

Finally, the *vagina* (/7) is a muscular, S-shaped tube through which the completed egg passes in seconds when it is expelled. Its junction with the uterus is marked by a sphincter. Glandular crypts in the region of the sphincter have been found to store sperm. The vagina ends at a slitlike opening in the lateral wall of the urodeum. When the egg is laid (blunt end first) the vaginal opening protrudes through the vent, minimizing contact with the feces.

A remnant of the right oviduct (/11) is found on the right side of the cloaca; it may be cystic and enlarged.

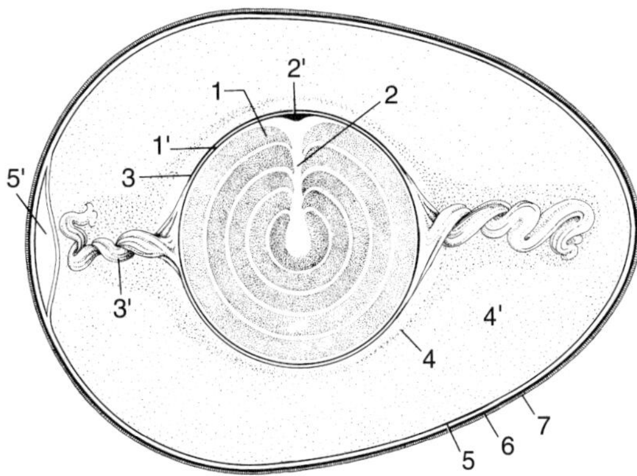


**Figure 39–24.** A semischematic section of a fertilized egg.

1, Yolk; 1′, yolk membrane; 2, latebra; 2′, germinal disc; 3, chalaziferous layer; 3′, chalaza; 4, 4′, thin and dense albumen; 5, internal and external shell membranes; 5′, air cell; 6, shell; 7, cuticle.

## THE BODY CAVITY

Now that the organs and air sacs have been described, a brief account of how the body cavity is subdivided may be helpful. In birds no diaphragm separates thoracic from abdominal organs. However, the body cavity is divided into three parts by horizontal and oblique septa in the cranial portion of the cavity. These septa are thin and translucent, although they contain some fibrous tissue and, where the horizontal septum is concerned, some muscle toward the periphery. The oblique septum is usually destroyed when the viscera are moved during dissection.

The *horizontal septum* is attached laterally to the ribs and medially to the bodies of the thoracic vertebrae; caudally it makes contact with the oblique septum. It forms the ventral surface of paired cavities that are bounded laterally and dorsally by the ribs and thoracic vertebrae. These spaces contain the lungs.

The larger *oblique septum* is attached to the sternum ventrally, the sixth and seventh ribs laterally, and the horizontal septum and thoracic vertebrae dorsally. It forms the caudoventral surface of the paired cavities that are bounded dorsally by the horizontal septum and laterally by the thoracic and abdominal wall. This part of the body cavity contains the thoracic air sacs and the thoracic parts of the cervical and clavicular air sacs.

The largest of the three parts is caudal to the oblique septum. It is bounded dorsally by the pelvis, dorsocranially by the oblique septum, and ventrally by the caudal portion of the sternum and abdominal muscles. It contains the heart, liver, spleen, gastrointestinal and urogenital tracts, and abdominal air sacs. It is further divided by mesenteries and peritoneal folds, resulting in a complex set of compartments whose description is beyond the scope of this book.

## THE ENDOCRINE GLANDS

The paired *thyroid glands* (Fig. 39–25/5) of the chicken are reddish brown, oval, and about 10 mm long and 5 mm wide. In the budgerigar, in which thyroid disease is a major problem, they are pale and only 2 to 3 mm long and 1 to 2 mm wide. The thyroid glands are located in the thoracic inlet, caudal to the crop and closely related to the common carotid artery, jugular vein, and vagus nerve (which accompanies the vein)—indeed they lie just cranial to where these vessels are joined by the subclavian vessels (/16). Their color distinguishes them from the neighboring rather similar but beige thymic lobes.

The *parathyroid glands* (/7), two or three on each side, are minute (1 to 3 mm) yellowish-brown structures immediately caudal to the thyroid gland; one may be attached to that gland.

The even more minute pink *ultimobranchial glands* (/8) lie next to the parathyroids.

The *adrenal glands* (Fig. 39–21/3′) are yellowish brown, oval or triangular and about 13 mm long and 8 mm wide. Each lies at the cranial pole of the corresponding kidney, related ventrally to the ovary (or epididymis).

The *hypophysis* (Fig. 39–26/7) is attached below the diencephalon and occupies the hypophysial fossa in the base of the skull. It resembles that of mammals in its division—adeno- and neurohypophysis—and formation.

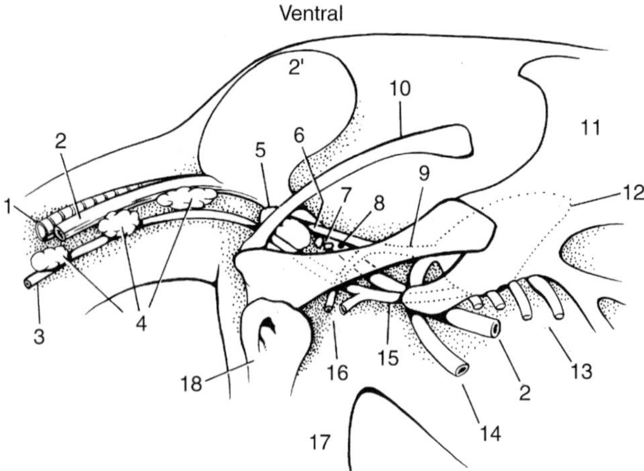


**Figure 39–25.** Junction of neck and trunk as viewed from the right, semischematic. Cranial is to the left.

1, Trachea; 2, esophagus; 2′, crop; 3, right jugular v.; 4, thymus; 5, thyroid gland; 6, right common carotid a.; 7, parathyroid glands; 8, ultimobranchial gland; 9, right brachiocephalic a.; 10, clavicle; 11, sternum; 12, position of heart; 13, sternal ribs; 14, descending aorta; 15, right cranial vena cava; 16, subclavian a. and v.; 17, wing; 18, humerus.

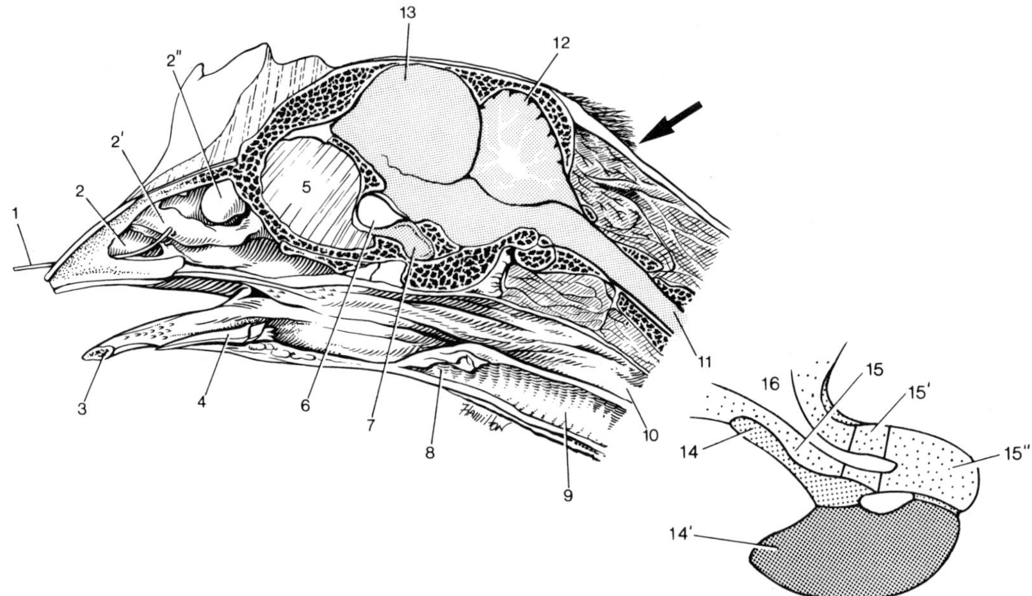


**Figure 39–26.** Median section of the head with an enlargement of the hypophysis *(inset)*. The arrow indicates the approach to the foramen magnum through which euthanasia may be performed by injection into the brain.

1, Wire in nostril; 2, 2′, 2″, rostral, middle, and caudal nasal conchae; 3, mandible; 4, tongue; 5, interorbital septum; 6, optic chiasm; 7, hypophysis (see also *inset*); 8, larynx; 9, trachea; 10, esophagus; 11, spinal cord; 12, cerebellum; 13, cerebrum; 14, 14′, pars tuberalis and pars distalis of the adenohypophysis; 15, 15′, 15″, median eminence, infundibulum, and neural lobe of the neurohypophysis; 16, third ventricle.

# THE CIRCULATORY SYSTEM

## The Heart

The avian heart is four-chambered and similar to that of mammals except for some minor features. It is, however, relatively much larger, and its rate of contraction is much greater—up to 1000 times per minute in certain small birds! In shape it is conical, with the apex formed solely by the left ventricle. The heart lies within the thorax both between and in front of the lobes of the liver (Fig. 39–11/8 and Plate 31/*G*). It is attached to the sternum by the fibrous pericardium.

The right atrium receives paired cranial venae cavae and a single caudal vena cava. The right atrioventricular valve is formed by a single muscular flap unprovided with chordae tendineae. The thin-walled right ventricle lays itself around the left ventricle so that its lumen on cross section is shaped like a crescent. The pulmonary veins combine to form a single trunk before entering the left atrium at an entrance provided with a valve to prevent reflux. The left atrioventricular valve has three cusps attached to chordae tendineae. The thick-walled left ventricle (Fig. 39–18/5) is shaped like a pointed cylinder. Muscular bars on its interior give the cross section a rosette-like appearance. Cardiac puncture, performed for blood sampling, is dangerous in small birds.

## Arteries

While still concealed by the heart, the aorta gives rise to right and left coronary arteries and a brachiocephalic trunk. The trunk immediately divides into right and left brachiocephalic arteries that send common carotid arteries forward into the neck, and subclavian arteries toward the wings (Fig. 39–11/8′,8″). In the thoracic inlet, the common carotids continue as internal carotids lying side by side on the ventral surface of the cervical vertebrae (Fig. 39–10/6′). The subclavian artery gives off a large pectoral trunk for the breast muscles and sternum before accompanying the humerus into the wing. In its descent along the vertebral column, the aorta gives rise to the following major branches: celiac (stomach, spleen, liver, intestine [Fig. 39–20/2]), cranial mesenteric (intestines [/3]), cranial renal (kidney, gonad [/5]), external iliac (thigh [/12]), ischial (kidney, oviduct, hindlimb [/18]), and caudal mesenteric (intestine, cloaca). It ends by supplying the end of the oviduct, pelvic structures, and tail.

### Veins

The two *cranial venae cavae* (Fig. 39–11/7; only one in mammals) are satellite to the brachiocephalic arteries and receive tributaries (jugular and subclavian veins) from the neck and head and the breast and wing. The right jugular vein, always larger than the left, is visible through the skin. This feature renders it useful for venipuncture (Fig. 39–10/6). Many small cage birds lack a left jugular. The cutaneous ulnar vein (wing vein), subcutaneous on the ventral surface of the extended wing, may also be used for the administration of fluids or collection of very small volumes of blood (Fig. 39–8/9). For a small amount of blood a claw may be clipped short or the comb incised.

The *caudal vena cava* drains the liver, kidney, gonads, and oviduct. It forms ventral to the kidneys from the union of the common iliac veins that drain the pelvis and hindlimb (Fig. 39–20/13). As described on page 816, some blood from the pelvis and hindlimb passes through the kidney (renal portal system) before reaching the caudal vena cava. Blood from the gastrointestinal tract reaches the liver by separate (again unlike mammals) right and left *hepatic portal veins* that enter the respective lobes. The left vein drains the left and ventral parts of the stomach. The much larger right vein drains the right and dorsal parts of the stomach, the spleen, and the remainder of the tract through cranial and caudal mesenteric veins. The caudal mesenteric vein, connected to the caudal end of the renal portal system (/22), also conveys a considerable amount of blood toward the kidney. Thus, blood from the gastrointestinal tract may return to the heart without passing through the liver.

### Lymphatic Structures

Only the goose and duck have lymphoid tissue encapsulated as true lymph nodes—a pair of cervicothoracic nodes in the thoracic inlet and a pair of lumbar nodes close to the kidneys. Lymphatic tissue is indeed present in all birds, but in most species exists as relatively unorganized aggregates of lymphoid tissue.

*Lymphatics* are less numerous than in mammals. They accompany the blood vessels, are valved, and contain microscopic lymph nodules scattered at intervals in their walls. They conduct the lymph to the thoracic inlet where it is discharged into the cranial venae cavae.

Although true lymph nodes are absent, much lymphatic tissue occurs in various organs (liver, pancreas, lung, and kidney) in the form of *solitary lymph nodules* and in the oropharynx and intestine as patches of *aggregate lymph nodules.* Cecal patches (cecal tonsils; Fig. 39–13/10 and p. 809) are particularly prominent.

The *thymus* consists of several separate lobes that accompany the jugular veins (Fig. 39–10/9). The lobes are divided into lobules, each of which consists of a dark cortex and a pale medulla. The thymus, best developed in the young, regresses with the onset of sexual maturity.

The location of the *cloacal bursa* has been described (p. 817; Fig. 39–15/9). Like the thymus, the bursa is a lymphoepithelial organ; it consists of a thin wall made uneven by the lobules it encloses, and surrounds an irregular lumen. In the second week of embryonic development in the chicken, lymphoid precursor cells migrate into the developing organ (Plate 32/*F*), and longitudinal plicae form that protrude into the lumen. Nodular epithelial formations, originating from the plicae, now begin to penetrate the lamina propria, while lymphoid cells invade these buds from the lamina propria; lymphopoiesis is now initiated. By day 18 these buds have considerably increased in size due to active proliferation of lymphoid cells (Plate 32/G). The bursa reaches its greatest size approximately 6 weeks after hatching, when the plicae are completely filled by large epithelial accumulations (or bursa follicles), resulting in the histology of the organ showing many similarities with that of the thymus (Plate 32/H). The main function of the bursa as a primary lymphatic organ is thought to be the antigen-independent differentiation of B-lymphocytes. The bursa gradually regresses from the age of 2 to 3 months, but a small nodule remains in the adult.

The location and shape of the *spleen* have been described (p. 812; Fig. 39–16/5). Its structure resembles that of the mammal, although the distinction between the red and white pulp is less marked.

## THE NERVOUS SYSTEM AND SENSE ORGANS

### The Brain and Spinal Cord

The brain is small, indeed barely larger than one of the eyes (Fig. 39–26). The *cerebral hemispheres* are pear-shaped; their pointed rostral ends (olfactory bulbs) are wedged between the large orbits. Compared with their mammalian counterparts, the hemispheres are small and relatively smooth. The right and left hemispheres are separated by a median fissure, and from the cerebellum by a transverse fissure. The tip of the epiphysis can be seen at the intersection of those fissures. The *optic lobes,* homologous to the rostral colliculi of the mammal, are found caudoventral to the hemispheres. They are exceedingly large—corresponding to the development of the eyes—and are visible from both dorsal and ventral aspects. The optic chiasm (/6) is also correspondingly large. (The small olfactory bulbs point to an underdeveloped sense of smell.) The *cerebellum* (/12), also relatively large, consists essentially of a central body (homologous to the mammalian vermis) with small lateral appendages (flocculi).

A peculiarity of the *spinal cord* is a glycogen-rich gelatinous body in the dorsal surface of the lumbosacral enlargement; it is 3 to 5 mm in size and should not be mistaken for a lesion.

## Some Peripheral Nerves

The normal peripheral nerve is white, has faint cross striations, and is of uniform width. Marek's disease (neural lymphomatosis) alters the appearance of nerves, especially those to the limbs. The following nerves are usually examined post mortem.

The *cervical nerves* emerge from the cervical muscles and pass to the skin at right angles to the neck (Fig. 39–10/4′). The *vagus nerve* (/6) accompanies the jugular vein. The cervical sympathetic trunk lies deep to the muscles. The vagus is seen again on the dorsal surface of the proventriculus (Fig. 39–14/3). The *brachial plexus* is exposed on each side of the cervical muscles when the esophagus, trachea, and major vessels cranial to the heart are reflected. Most branches pass into the wing ventral to the scapula and caudal to the humerus. The *intercostal nerves* are exposed by the removal of the lungs. The *intestinal nerve* (/14) accompanies the cranial mesenteric vessels in the mesentery. Nerves of the *lumbar* and *synsacral plexuses* pass through the kidney, which must be removed to expose them (Fig. 39–20/10,17). Finally, the *sciatic nerve* can be examined on the medial surface of the thigh by reflecting two thin muscles (Fig. 39–14/15).

## The Eye

Although the shape of the eyeball differs somewhat from the globular mammalian one, the general structure is the same (Fig. 39–27). The eyeball almost fills the orbit and thus has little room for movement; the long neck and mobile occipitoatlantal joint compensate for this.

The lower lid is the larger and more movable. The third eyelid has a stiffened edge; being translucent it does not seem to impair vision when drawn across the cornea. The secretions of the lacrimal gland and of the deep gland of the third eyelid leave the conjunctival sac through two puncta that lead to a spacious nasolacrimal duct. The upper punctum is surprisingly large.

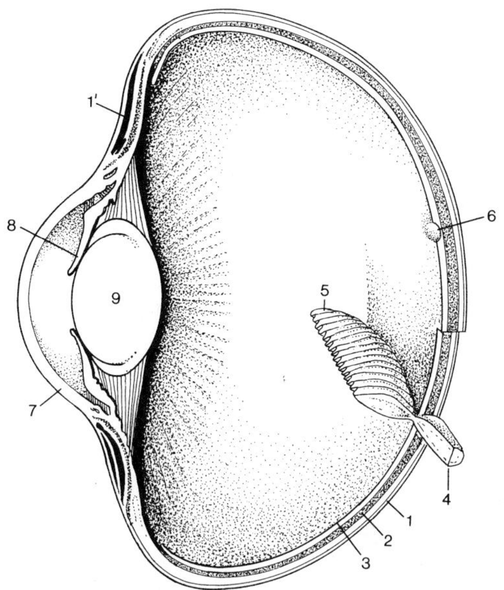


**Figure 39–27.** Section through the eyeball, schematic.

1, Sclera; 1′, ring of scleral ossicles; 2, choroid; 3, retina; 4, optic nerve; 5, pecten; 6, fovea centralis; 7, cornea; 8, iris; 9, lens.

The *cornea* is thin and strongly curved. Its small diameter belies the enormous eyeball to which it belongs. The *sclera* is reinforced by a layer of cartilage transformed to a ring of ossicles near the cornea (/1′). No tapetum lucidum is present. The *iris* of the chicken is yellow-brown but turns slightly paler during the laying period. It surrounds a round pupil that can rapidly change in size through the action of the *striated* sphincter and dilator muscles. Even so, the avian iris is surprisingly unresponsive to light. The *retina* is devoid of blood vessels. It displays a remarkable outgrowth (pecten; /5) over the optic disc. This is a black, pleated ridge that projects into the vitreous; it is rich in blood vessels and is thought to play a role in the nutrition of the retina. The extraocular muscles are similar to those of mammals, but a retractor bulbi is lacking.

## The Ear

No auricle is present. The *external ear* consists only of the external acoustic meatus, which opens on the side of the head under cover of a patch of small feathers. The meatus is short and straight so that the relatively large tympanic membrane can be easily examined (and as easily injured). A lobe, similar in structure to comb and wattle, is present ventral to the opening (Fig. 39–1/4). Among domestic chickens, the color of the ear lobe matches the color of the eggshell the hen lays.

The *middle ear* resembles that of mammals. The tympanic membrane is connected by the columella and associated cartilages to the vestibular window; these transmit the vibrations of the membrane to the perilymph in the inner ear. The columella, the homologue of the mammalian stapes, is a tiny osseous rod expanded at each end; the medial expansion (foot plate) occludes the vestibular window.

The structure and subdivision of the *inner ear* follow the mammalian pattern, although the cochlea does not form a spiral; it is only slightly curved and is significantly shorter than its mammalian counterpart. A relatively thick layer of sensory cells seems to compensate for the shortness of the duct.

## Selected Bibliography


Akester, A.R.: Renal portal shunts in the kidney of the domestic fowl. J. Anat. 101:569–594, 1967.

Altman, R.B., S. Clubb, G. Dorrestein, K. Quesenberry (eds.): Avian Medicine and Surgery. Philadelphia, W.B. Saunders Company, 1997.

Baumel, J.J. (ed.): Handbook of Avian Anatomy: Nomina Anatomica Avium, 2nd. ed. Cambridge, Mass., Nuttall Ornithological Club, Harvard University, 1993.

Canfield, T.H.: Sex determination of day-old chicks. Poult. Sci. 19:235–238, 1940.

Fedde, M.R.: Respiration in birds. *In* Swenson, M.J. (ed.): Duke's Physiology of Domestic Animals, 11th ed. Ithaca, N.Y., Cornell University Press, 1993.

Harrison, G.J.: Endoscopic examination of avian gonadal tissues. Vet. Med. [SAC] 73:479–484, 1978.

Harrison, G.J. and L.R. Harrison (eds.): Clinical Avian Medicine and Surgery, Including Aviculture. Philadelphia, W.B. Saunders Company, 1986.

King, A.S.: The urogenital system. *In* Getty, R. (ed.): Sisson and Grossman's The Anatomy of the Domestic Animals, 5th ed. Philadelphia, W.B. Saunders Company, 1975.

King, A.S., and J. McLelland: Birds—Their Structure and Function, 2nd ed. London, Baillière Tindall, 1984.

King, A.S., and J. McLelland: Form and Function in Birds, Vols. 1–3. London, Academic Press, 1979–1985.

King, A.S., and V. Molony: The anatomy of respiration. *In* Bell, D.J., and B.M. Freemon (eds.): The Physiology and Biochemistry of the Domestic Fowl, vol. 1. New York, Academic Press, 1971, p. 109.

Krautwald, M.E., B. Tellhelm, G. Hummel, V. Kostka, and E.F. Kaleta: Atlas of Radiographic Anatomy and Diagnosis of Cage Birds. Berlin, Paul Parey Verlag, 1992.

Lowenstine, L.J.: Avian anatomy and its relation to disease processes. *In* Proceedings of the Meeting of the Association of Avian Veterinarians, San Diego, June 1983.

Lucas, A.M., and P.R. Stettenheim: Avian Anatomy: Integument, Parts I and II. Agriculture Handbook 362. Washington, D.C., U.S. Government Printing Office, 1972.

Ludders, J.W.: Is euthanasia in birds by thoracic compression humane? (Letter to the editor.) JAVMA 218:1721, 2001.

Lumeij, J.T. (ed.): Raptor Biomedicine III. Lake Worth, Fla., Zoological Education Network, 2000.

McKibben, J.S., and G.J. Harrison: Clinical anatomy with emphasis on the Amazon parrot. *In* Harrison, G.J., and L.R. Harrison (eds.): Clinical Avian Medicine and Surgery, Including Aviculture. Philadelphia, W.B. Saunders Company, 1986, pp. 31–66.

McLelland, J.: A Color Atlas of Avian Anatomy. Philadelphia, W.B. Saunders Company, 1991.

Olsen, G.H., and S.E. Orosz: Manual of Avian Medicine. St. Louis, Mosby–Year Book, 2000.

Orosz, S.E., P.K. Ensley, and C.J. Haynes: Avian Surgical Anatomy: Thoracic and Pelvic Limb. Philadelphia, W.B. Saunders Company, 1992.

Redig, P.: Raptor Biomedicine. Minneapolis, University of Minnesota Press, 1993.

Ritchie, B.W., G.J. Harrison, and L.R. Harrison: Avian Medicine—Principles and Applications. Lake Worth, Fla., Wingers Publishing, 1994.

Rübel, G.A., Isenbügel, E., and Wolvekamp, P.: Atlas of Diagnostic Radiology of Exotic Pets: Small Mammals, Birds, Reptiles and Amphibians. Philadelphia, W.B. Saunders Company, 1991.

Satterfield, W.C., and R.B. Altman: Avian sex determination by endoscopy. *In* Proceedings of the American Association of Zoological Veterinarians, Honolulu, 1977, pp. 45–48.

Schultz, D.J.: Avian Physiology and Its Effect on Therapy. Proc. No. 55: Refresher Course for Veterinarians on Aviary and Caged Birds. Sydney, University of Sydney, 1981, p. 475.

Smith, B.J., and Smith, S.A.: Atlas of Avian Radiographic Anatomy. Philadelphia, W.B. Saunders Company, 1992.

Smith, B.J., S.A. Smith, K. Flammer, et al.: The normal xeroradiographic and radiographic anatomy of the orange-winged Amazon Parrot *(Amazona amazonica amazonica).* Vet. Radiol. 31:114–124, 1990.

# INDEX

The entries for structures in certain categories have been grouped under generic heads: Artery(ies); Ligament(s); Lymphatic System; Muscle(s); Nerve(s); and Vein(s).

Compound terms (in English) are ordered according to their adjectival components but disregarding, for this purpose, adjectives indicating relative size and position, e.g., major, lateral, superficial. Terms conventionally retained in Latin appear in their official (N.A.V.) forms.

Page references for the first ten (systematic) chapters, which are predominantly based upon the anatomy of the dog, are given without prefix. References to the remaining (topographical) chapters are prefixed by an appropriate initial: C, carnivore; H, horse; R, ruminant; P, pig; and A, avian anatomy. References to secondary features that *manifestly* pertain to a major indexed structure are commonly not separately listed. References to structures considered in the systematic chapters may not be repeated for species when the specific account does not substantially strengthen, modify, or add relevance to the initial description.

Page references followed by the letter f refer to figures, and those followed by t refer to tables.

## A

## D

## N

## R



## S

## T



## U



## V

## W



## X



## Y



## Z

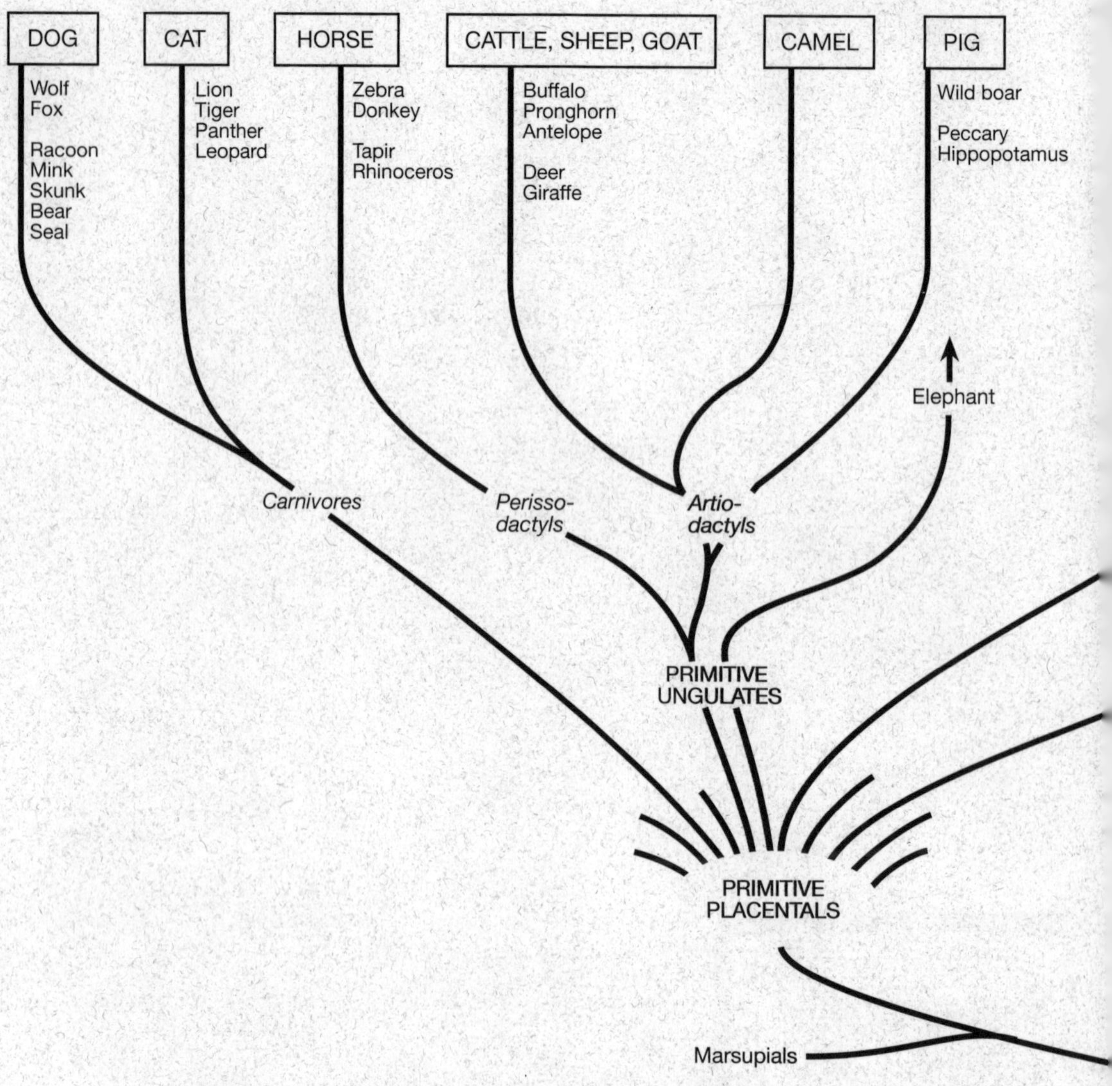


# THE ORIGIN OF THE DOMESTIC AND LABORATORY MAMMALS AND THEIR BETTER KNOWN RELATIVES

UNIVERSITY OF LINCOLN

KT-440-347

# International Cuisine

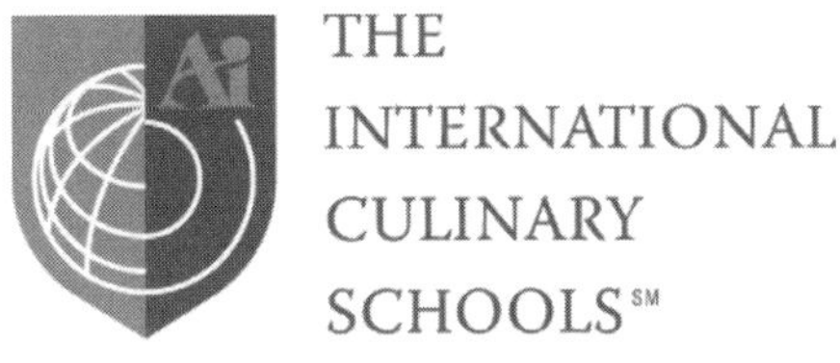


Michael F. Nenes, CEC, CCE

*Photography by Joe Robbins*

NORWICH CITY COLLEGE LIBRARY
Stock No. 217465
Class 641.59 NEN
Cat. Proc. 1WL

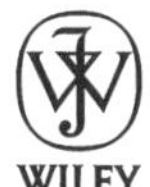


JOHN WILEY & SONS, INC.

This book is printed on acid-free paper.♾

Copyright © 2009 by Education Management Corporation. All rights reserved.

Published by John Wiley & Sons, Inc., Hoboken, New Jersey.

Published simultaneously in Canada.

No part of this publication may be reproduced, stored in a retrieval system, or transmitted in any form or by any means, electronic, mechanical, photocopying, recording, scanning, or otherwise, except as permitted under Section 107 or 108 of the 1976 United States Copyright Act, without either the prior written permission of the Publisher, or authorization through payment of the appropriate per-copy fee to the Copyright Clearance Center, Inc., 222 Rosewood Drive, Danvers, MA 01923, 978-750-8400, fax 978-646-8600, or on the web at www.copyright.com. Requests to the Publisher for permission should be addressed to the Permissions Department, John Wiley & Sons, Inc., 111 River Street, Hoboken, NJ 07030, 201-748-6011, fax 201-748-6008, or online at http://www.wiley.com/go/permissions.

Limit of Liability/Disclaimer of Warranty: While the publisher and author have used their best efforts in preparing this book, they make no representations or warranties with respect to the accuracy or completeness of the contents of this book and specifically disclaim any implied warranties of merchantability or fitness for a particular purpose. No warranty may be created or extended by sales representatives or written sales materials. The advice and strategies contained herein may not be suitable for your situation. You should consult with a professional where appropriate. Neither the publisher nor author shall be liable for any loss of profit or any other commercial damages, including but not limited to special, incidental, consequential, or other damages.

For general information on our other products and services, or technical support, please contact our Customer Care Department within the United States at 800-762-2974, outside the United States at 317-572-3993 or fax 317-572-4002.

Wiley also publishes its books in a variety of electronic formats. Some content that appears in print may not be available in electronic books.

For more information about Wiley products, visit our Web site at http://www.wiley.com.

Library of Congress Cataloging-in-Publication Data:

Nenes, Michael F.
International cuisine / Michael F. Nenes; photography by Joe Robbins.
p. cm.
Includes index.
ISBN 978-0-470-05240-2 (cloth)
ISBN 978-0-470-41076-9 (custom)
1. Cookery, International. I. Title.
TX725.A1N46 2009
641.59–dc22

2008009580

Printed in the United States of America
10 9 8 7 6 5 4 3 2 1

# Contents

# Foreword

Despite my training in classical French cooking techniques, I have long valued the cuisines of countries from all over the world and found great inspiration in them. As a young apprentice, I was fortunate to have trained in France's most famous kitchens including those of Paul Bocuse, Roger Vergé, and Paul Haeberlin, and then spent a number of years on cruise ships that exposed me to the excitement of world cuisines. Later, after a two-year stint in Brazil, I settled in San Francisco, a city with a food community that has always deeply appreciated a wide variety of international cuisines. At Fleur de Lys and more recently at our Burger Bar restaurants, I have created dishes which are sometimes directly—sometimes subtly—enhanced with flavors and cooking techniques found outside my original French classical training, and I have seen how these international influences have drawn enthusiasm from my diners.

I am delighted that The International Culinary Schools at The Art Institutes have put together this comprehensive book of world cuisines that is certain to become a treasured resource for anyone who cooks, both professionally and at home. It has everything needed to truly understand and master a wide array of international cuisines, especially Asian cuisines, which are now such an important part of the American dining landscape. The detailed and vivid descriptions of the history of the food culture for each cuisine are not only fascinating, but also give the reader an understanding of how each cuisine evolved. The comprehensive ingredient lists are a tremendous resource for anyone wishing to recreate the recipes. It is also extremely interesting to read about the cooking utensils from each cuisine along with the detailed descriptions of the cooking techniques. Finally, the book contains a treasure of authentic recipes that not only look delicious, but truly and accurately reflect the featured cuisine.

I know that ***International Cuisine*** is certain to have a prominent place in my culinary library and I hope yours as well.

Hubert Keller
Chef-Owner
Fleur de Lys, San Francisco and Las Vegas
Burger Bar, Las Vegas, San Francisco, and St. Louis
SLeeK Steakhouse, St. Louis

# Acknowledgments

The International Culinary Schools at The Art Institutes wish to thank the following contributors for their efforts on behalf of *International Cuisine*:

Author Michael F. Nenes, MBA, CEC, CCE. This first edition of ***International Cuisine*** is the result of intensive cooperative and collaborative effort by many individuals. Thanks to Lois Nenes, M.Ed., for her tremendous amount of research, writing, editing, and support. Every effort was made to find information that could be supported by at least two documented sources. Lois was a supportive colleague and we both enjoyed the tremendous amount of exploring and learning needed to complete this project.

Photographer Joe Robbins of Joe Robbins Photography, Houston, Texas. Joe taught at The Art Institute of Houston for over 15 years, helping to shape the careers of students in the visual arts. His collaboration and outstanding photography contribute to the effectiveness of this book.

Certified Master Chef Klaus Friedenreich, Chef Hugh Chang, and Chef Scott Fernandez worked with culinary students at The Art Institute of Houston, testing recipes to prepare and plate the food photographed for the book. This was a tremendous task made possible by hard work, organization, and culinary passion.

Thank you to the following Art Institutes' instructors, staff, and students for their efforts on behalf of *International Cuisine*: Staff members Jose Ferreira and Waldemar "Wally" Marbach; Instructors Soren Fakstrop; Joseph Bonaparte, CCE, CCC, MHM; Mark Matin, MBA; Michael Edrington, CCC, MHM; Nathan Hashmonay; Shannon Hayashi, CEC, M.Ed; Anita Bouffard, MBA, CWA, CWS; Jeff Kennedy, CHE; Scott Maxwell, M.Ed; Stephan Kleinman, CEC, CCE, AAC; Matthew J. Bennett, M.Ed, CEC, CCE, CWPC, CFBE; Ricardo Castro; Simon Vaz, MBA, Ed.S. CHE; Eyad Joseph, CEC, CCE, CCA; Mark Mattern, MBA, CEC; Hugh Chang; and Scott Fernandez; and students Claudia Turcios; Bryce Smith; Ian Caughey; Camilla Guerrero; Amber Bush; and Elizabeth Sanchez.

# Introduction

The idea for ***International Cuisine*** seemed natural and obvious in light of the importance of increased globalization. At the same time, The International Culinary School at The Art Institutes went through an extensive review process that emphasizes an international focus. The most compelling concept, explored with industry professionals, current students, our faculty, and prospective students, centered on teaching students about a wide variety of countries and regions, cultures, and ingredients and the crucial role they play in a variety of cuisines. Industry professionals acknowledge that while fundamental skills are still most critical, it is important for culinary students to have exposure to a wide range of cultural, sociological, and geographical information because the marketplace is demanding it. Due to changing demographics and evolving tastes of consumers, restaurateurs are under increasing pressure to offer more diverse and/or creative menus. Culinary students who have had a broader exposure to a variety of international cuisines will be more versatile and creative culinarians. We believe students who develop a good palate, expand their range of taste, and develop the techniques gain a better understanding of the culinary arts.

The intent of ***International Cuisine*** is to serve as a window for students to explore the different cultures and cuisines of the world. Culinary programs have always taught some type of international cuisine course, but while there are numerous good books centered on a particular country (such as Italy) or region (such as Latin America), there has been no one book that adequately brings together the world's regions. ***International Cuisine*** does just that, teaching the wide range of regions around the world and how history, geography, and religion—not to mention the ingredients—influence the different cuisines.

***International Cuisine*** is unique. Many of a cuisine's culinary traits result from conditions that naturally exist in the region or country—factors such as geography, climate, agriculture, as well as historical, cultural and religious influences from settlers, invaders, and neighboring countries. Each chapter is divided into the geography of the area (including a map of the country or countries being discussed), the history, the people and their contributions, and the foods particular to the region. Some chapters are countries discussed individually, others include two or more countries, and several discuss an entire continent. The effort was to choose countries that are culinary representatives of the world. Following this introduction of each country or countries, each chapter contains a glossary of ingredients and dishes as well as a selection of menus and recipes characteristic of the cuisine and its heritage.

Each menu and recipe in ***International Cuisine*** was selected and tested for its representation of the cuisine, to insure a variety of culinary techniques, a variety of ingredients, and availability of ingredients. However, many of the recipes have been influenced by local customs, ingredient availability, and the inspiration of international chefs, so they have been reformulated to conform to current practices. Methods of preparation are clearly broken down into straightforward steps, and follow a logical progression for completion of the recipe.

Here are some important tips for using ***International Cuisine***:

- It is important to understand that to yield a superior dish, you must start with high-quality ingredients. Good results cannot be obtained with substandard ingredients.
- Some ingredients are highly specific to a region and may be difficult to obtain elsewhere. The goal was to keep the unusual ingredients to a minimum so that the recipes can be prepared in areas that do not have large ethnic communities. These recipes are followed by Chef Tips, which indicate suitable substitutions.
- All herbs called for in recipes should be fresh unless specified as dried.
- All butter called for in recipes should be unsalted unless specified otherwise.
- It is recommended that the olive oil produced by each country be used for that country's recipes. For countries that do not produce olive oil but the ingredient is used in its recipes, use a good quality olive oil.
- It is recommended that both white and black pepper be ground fresh to the level of coarseness called for in the recipes. Ground pepper loses strength over time, making it difficult to judge the quantity needed.
- When citrus juice is called for in the recipes, it should be squeezed from fresh fruit rather than reconstituted from concentrate.
- Many of the cooking times indicated in the recipes are approximations. The altitude, type of cookware used, and amount of heat applied are all variables that affect cooking time. Professional cooks use these times as a guide but determine doneness by appropriate means.

One of the wonderful outcomes of our exploration turned out to be the discovery that most of these cuisines are based on sustainable food choices. Sustainable production enables the resources from which it was made to continue to be available for future generations. We support the positive shift in America and world-wide toward local, small-scale sustainable farming.

An ***Instructor's Manual*** (978-0-470-25406-6) is also available to qualified adopters of this book. It contains chapter objectives, the skills and techniques required to prepare the recipes, suggestions for mise en place demonstrations, additional information on each menu, expanded and detailed chef's tips, and a chapter test. For an electronic version of this ***Instructor's Manual***, please visit www.wiley.com/college and click on Culinary Arts.

# Mexico

## The Land

Long and narrow, Mexico forms what looks like a curved horn between the United States to the north and Guatemala and Belize to the south. To the west is the Pacific Ocean. The Gulf of Mexico and the Caribbean Sea lie to the east. Two huge mountain ranges, the Sierra Madre Occidental to the west, and the Sierra Madre Oriental to the east, run the length of the country, forming a giant V. Between these mountain ranges lie a series of plateaus. The plateau in the north is largely desert land, while the long central plateau father south is more fertile. Near the tip of the horn, the Yucatan Peninsula juts into the Atlantic Ocean. A long, narrow peninsula called Baja dangles from California's southern border. The southern coasts are home to tropical rain forests and jungles.

With most of its eastern and western borders being on the coast, some Mexican cuisine is based on seafood. There are good grazing areas in the north, with some fertile agricultural land to the south; however, between arid conditions and challenging terrain, only 12 percent of the country gets enough rain for crops.

## History

Mexico is a country of great contrasts. Within its borders, there are scorching deserts, snow-capped volcanoes, and lush tropical rain forests. Mexico is also one of the twenty richest nations in the world but, as in nearby Central American countries, there are big differences between standards of living of the rich and the poor. Long before the first European explorers arrived in 1519, Mexico was the home of some of the world's greatest civilizations.

A thousand years ago, Mexico was inhabited by groups of Mayan Indians, who had developed a very advanced civilization. They built large cities out of stone, developed systems of writing and arithmetic, and created beautiful works of art. Mayan settlements were situated close to *cenotes*, natural water holes that allowed for survival in an inhospitable tropical climate. The basis of the culture was farming, which included the cultivation of corn, beans, squash, and chile peppers. Chiles, both fresh and dried, are used more for flavor than heat and popular varieties include jalapeño, poblano, serrano, guajillo, chipotle, pasilla, habanero, ancho, mulatto, and cascabel. Squash, including pumpkins, and zucchini are used as vegetables; their blossoms are stuffed or incorporated in soups and sauces; and squash seeds are dried, ground, and used in sauces. Tomatoes were cultivated and became an essential ingredient along with tomatillos, small green tomatoes encased in papery husks.

It was the conquest of Mexico by Spain in 1521 that had the most influence on Mexican cuisine. Not only did the conquistadors introduce new types of livestock to the area, such as pigs, cows, and sheep, but they also introduced dairy products such as cheese and the fat from the cattle. The Spanish, themselves heavily influenced by the Arabic Moors of western Africa, introduced the most distinctive features of their cuisine to Mexico. Perhaps most characteristic is the combination in one dish of various finely chopped ingredients. Highly seasoned and spiced meat casseroles, hot pots of meats and vegetables, fruit syrups, and pasta and rice pilaf are Arab in origin. The Spanish brought many herbs as well as an abundance of Far Eastern spices like cinnamon and cloves. Wheat, an essential staple of the Spanish diet, was introduced to the region. Citrus fruits, peaches, melons, figs, and cherries as well as garlic, carrots, turnips, and eggplants became regular items in the diet.

Sugarcane was cultivated and became an important trade item, and with this widely available sweet Mexicans developed many deserts and sweets. Many Spanish-style "convent" desserts were developed by the nuns and priests who came to cook for the viceroys (royal officials that governed the provinces). For many years convents all over Mexico have supported themselves by making marzipan-like candies, with almonds and *pepitas* (pumpkin seeds). This period also saw the assimilation of many other cultures, cuisines, and ingredients, including French, Portuguese, Caribbean (particularly in the Veracruz area in the southeast), West African, and South American.

Today, almost 80 percent of contemporary Mexicans are descendants of both native and Spanish cultures and are called *mestizo.* There are more than fifty native groups, including the Nahua, Zapotec, Mixtec, Maya, Purepecha, Trahumara, Huastec, Mayo, Yaqui, and Otomi Indians, who account for fewer than 10 percent of the population. The remaining 10 percent comprises others of European descent. The Roman Catholic Church plays an important part in the everyday life of most Mexicans and religious festivals and celebrations take place in towns and cities across the country throughout the year.

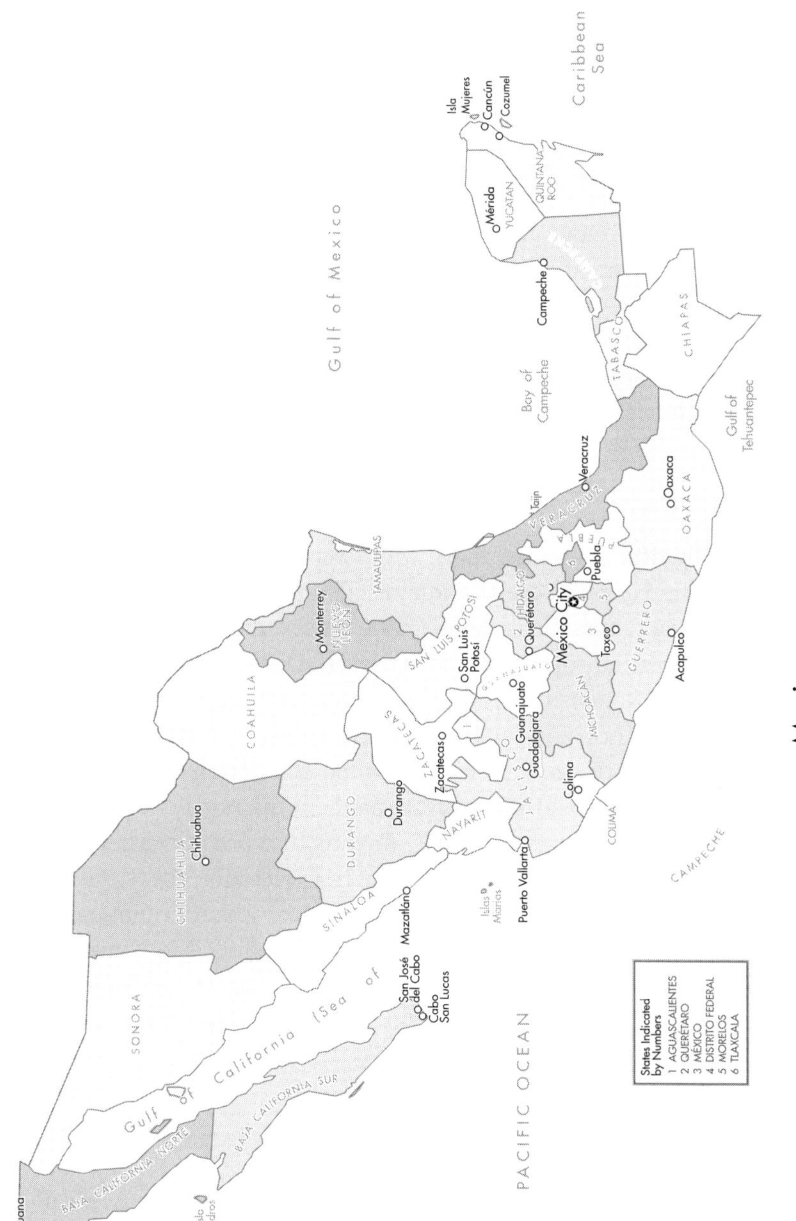

Gulf of Mexico
Caribbean Sea
Bay of Campeche
Gulf of Tehuantepec
PACIFIC OCEAN
Gulf of California (Sea of
Isla Mujeres
Cancún
Cozumel
Mérida
YUCATAN
QUINTANA ROO
Campeche
TABASCO
CHIAPAS
Veracruz
VERACRUZ
Tajín
Oaxaca
OAXACA
Puebla
Mexico City
Taxco
GUERRERO
Acapulco
Querétaro
HIDALGO
TAMAULIPAS
Monterrey
NUEVO LEÓN
SAN LUIS POTOSÍ
San Luis Potosí
COAHUILA
GUANAJUATO
Guanajuato
Guadalajara
MICHOACÁN
JALISCO
Colima
COLIMA
CAMPECHE
Zacatecas
ZACATECAS
Durango
DURANGO
NAYARIT
Puerto Vallarta
Islas Marías
Chihuahua
CHIHUAHUA
SINALOA
Mazatlán
San José del Cabo
Cabo San Lucas
SONORA
BAJA CALIFORNIA SUR
BAJA CALIFORNIA NORTE
Tijuana
Isla Cedros
States Indicated by Numbers
1 AGUASCALIENTES
2 QUERÉTARO
3 MÉXICO
4 DISTRITO FEDERAL
5 MORELOS
6 TLAXCALA


Mexico

# The Food

Although it is very diverse among the various Mexican regions, Mexican food is rich in color and flavor. Areas along the ocean are famous for their abundant *mariscos* (seafood dishes). Inland and highland mountain areas are famous for stews, intricate sauces, and corn-based recipes. Desert areas have cultivated delicacies of different sorts. In some desert regions, for example, there are numerous dishes containing varieties of cactus plants. While Mexico is made up of thirty-one states and one federal district, the country can be divided into six regions: northern Mexico, central Mexico, southern Mexico and the Gulf of Mexico, the Yucatan Peninsula, the Pacific Coast, and the Baja Peninsula.

## NORTHERN MEXICO

The north is mostly desert—a vast, high, windswept plateau flanked by the Occidental and Oriental chains of the Sierra Madre Mountains. The states of Chihuahua, Coajuila, Durango, Nuevo Leon, Sonora, Tamaulipas, and Zacatecas are part of this region. The cooking of northern Mexico gets its strongest influence from the ranching culture, predominately cattle, goats, pigs, and sheep. Ranch-style food is prepared with indigenous ingredients and cooked over an open fire. Cabrito is roast kid goat, a specialty of the city of Monterrey and its state of Nuevo Leon. Flour tortillas were created when the Spanish brought wheat to the New World; however, they are considered a bread staple in the northern states only. In the valleys of the eastern states farmers raise peaches, melons, nuts, and more than thirty varieties of apples. Queso Chihuahua or Chihuahua cheese is a soft white cow's milk cheese available in braids, balls or rounds. The cheese is named after its place of origin and is also called *queso menonita* after the Mennonite communities that first produced it. In the 1920s the Mexican government wanted to settle the barren northern areas of the country with industrious farmers. At the invitation of the then-president, 20,000 Mennonites left Canada and settled in the state of Chihuahua where the community still flourishes.

## CENTRAL MEXICO

The Distrito Federal, or Mexico City as it is called in English, is the Mexican capital in every sense of the word. With over 20 million people, it is not only many times larger than any other city in Mexico, but is also the second most populous city in the world, just behind Tokyo. There has been a capital here since before the arrival of the Spanish, although then it was the Aztec capital of Tenoctitlan. Unfortunately, almost all this old city was destroyed by the Spanish in their zeal to convert the Indians to Christianity. One impressive remain, however, still survives. El Templo Mayor is what's left of the Great Temple of the Aztecs. The ruin sits off the northeast corner of the Zocalo, the city's massive main square. In Mexico City, there is a full range of national cuisine. Because it is the capital, cooking from every region is available here.

The state of Michoacán derives its name from the Náhuatl terms *michin* (fish), *hua* (those who have), and *can* (place), which roughly translates into "place of the fisherman." Today there are national fishing tournaments and annual international sport fishing competitions focusing upon catching sailfish, marlin, and mahi-mahi. This state, along with the states of Morelas, Puebla, Queretaro, and Tlaxcala, are known as "the Central Breadbasket," and are one of Mexico's most important agricultural regions. Sugarcane fields, rice fields, coffee plantations, and macadamia trees are cultivated. Michoaca is the largest producer of avocados in the country. The area also produces large quantities of corn, beans, chickpeas, and potatoes. Fruit crops such as mangoes, strawberries, papaya, bananas, lemons, and limes are grown as well.

The food in this region is based heavily on corn. The early Indian tribes served it as a kind of porridge, called *atoll*. Corn kernels were also softened in water and lime and then ground into a fine meal known as *masa*. The *masa* is then shaped into flat, round cakes called tortillas, which are cooked on a *comal*, or griddle. Specialties include *corundas*, a triangular puffy tamale made with white corn and unfilled. *Huitacoche*, a small, dark fungus that grows on a cornstalk, is considered a particular delicacy. One of the other important crops is agave (also known as maguey), used to produce syrup, vinegar, and *pulque*, an alcoholic beverage. *Pulque* was the historical predecessor of mescal and tequila, which wielded a heavy sociological influence during both pre-Hispanic and Colonial periods of Mexican history. There are more than 400 species of agave native to North America and Mexico. It was one of the most sacred and important plants in ancient Mexico and had a privileged place in mythology, religious rituals, and the economy. *Pulque* is still made and drunk in limited quantities in parts of Mexico today. However, because it cannot easily be stored or preserved, it is not well known outside the country. Mezcal (or mescal) is the name given to a double-distilled spirit that comes from the maguey plant. Tequila is made exclusively from the agave azul that grows in semiarid soils and takes from eight to twelve years to mature.

The state of Puebla has been considered the gastronomic capital of Mexico. Its location between the coastal city of Veracruz and Mexico City gives it ample access to fresh seafood. The state produces fresh fruits and vegetables year-round, and raises some of the best beef and pork in the world. It cultivates cinnamon and nuts, as well as different types of hot peppers. *Mole* (the word means stew, or "concoctions") is a dish regarded with national pride and a culinary touchstone of Mexican cooking. It is a rich dark sauce with chocolate, chiles, spices, herbs, groundnuts, seeds, and a variety of other ingredients. Every Mexican household has its version of a *mole*, most of which are named for the color given by the variety of chiles used. Without a doubt the most famous type of *mole* is *mole poblano* (made from any fresh or dried chiles from the poblano pepper family). Other commonly prepared *moles* include *mole verde* (uses green chiles), *mole rojo* (uses red chiles) and *mole pipian* (uses pumpkin seeds).

The cities in this region all have their own enchiladas, from the Enchiladas Potosinas of San Luis Potosí (cheese and onion, with red chile ground into the masa tortillas) to the Enchiladas Mineras (miners' enchiladas) of Guanajuato (cheese or chicken filling topped with potatoes and carrots in a *guajillo* salsa). The *zacahuil*, a three-foot-long tamale that may weigh as much as 150 pounds, is perhaps the most famous food of the region. Stuffed with pork and a variety of ingredients including potatoes, hard-boiled eggs, and vegetables, the *zacahuil* requires nearly all the leaves of a banana tree to wrap it.

## SOUTHERN MEXICO AND THE GULF OF MEXICO

This region lies between two major bodies of water—the Gulf and Mexico and the Pacific Ocean—and includes the states of Veracruz, Chiapas, and Tabasco. Veracruz is located on the eastern shore of Mexico known as the Gulf Lowlands as it stretches along the Gulf Coast. Veracruz is the busiest port in Mexico and home to one of the most fertile fishing banks in the world. This is where the European conquest started and where the Spanish first settled, so there are significant Mediterranean influences. *Red Snapper Veracruz* is considered representative of the area. Traditionally, the whole fish is covered in a sauce of tomatoes, onions, capers, Spanish olives, olive oil, and pickled jalapeños. Veracruz is one of the few places in Mexico where people cook with olive oil, and ingredients like green olives and capers and raisins have been incorporated into the cuisine. In the city of Pampantla, vanilla pods are harvested from an orchid-type plant called *tlixochitl.*

During the first years after the Spanish arrived, diseases brought by the Europeans and unknown to the indigenous people decimated the population. Sugarcane production made heavy demands on labor, and African slaves were brought to work in the plantations. These slaves were some of the many thousands to bring their culinary influence with them. The peanut, an important ingredient in West African cooking, was added to meat, fish, and vegetable dishes and ground with spices as part of a paste-like condiment. Plantains, yucca, and sweet potatoes, all important elements of West African cooking, also became part of this region's cuisine.

More than half of Mexico's coffee beans are grown in Chiapas, and this state is one of the largest producers of cacao, used to make chocolate. The ancient Maya were the first to cultivate the cacao tree, native to the Central American rainforest. They found that by first fermenting the pulpy seeds, then drying, roasting, and crushing them, they could make a potent and delicious drink that they called *xocoatl* or *chocoatl.* When the Aztecs conquered the Maya in Central America, they demanded cacao seeds as tribute, and in their empire the seeds became a kind of currency. The Aztecs, like the Maya before them, used the chocoatl in religious ceremonies and considered the seeds a gift from the gods.

Here the tamales are made of fresh corn and pork wrapped in the large leaf of the *hoja santa* herb. When heated, the leaves produce a sweet, musky anise steam that flavors the tamale.

## THE YUCATAN PENINSULA

This region comprises the states of Campeche, Yucatan, and Quintana Rol. The Yucatan was once an isolated region of Mexico due to the mountainous terrain surrounding it. The Mayan civilization originated in the Yucatan near 2500 B.C. The Toltec culture arrived in A.D. 987, followed by the Spanish in the 1500s. Game meats such as venison and wild turkey, and vegetables like squash, cucumbers, chiles, and tomatoes are from the Mayans. Black beans, rather than pinto beans or kidney beans, are used in this area. Cooking methods like the *pib*, a hand-dug pit lined with stones and coals in which meats wrapped in banana leaves are cooked, are typical of Mayan cooking. The Spanish introduced pork, beef, and chicken. The Mayans had never fried foods before, but with the pig came lard, and with lard came frying. This produced one of the most significant changes in Mexican cooking.

Seville oranges came from Spain and are a key ingredient in this region's cuisine along with herbs and spices such as garlic, oregano, cinnamon, and cumin. Northern Europeans have a legacy in this region as well, especially the Dutch. Holland was an active trading partner in the nineteenth century and Edam cheese continues to be a regional staple. Ground spice pastes used for marinades are called *recado*. The red version (*rojo*) contains annatto, Mexican oregano, cumin, clove, cinnamon, black pepper, allspice, garlic, and salt. The annatto seeds dye the mixture red, which gives the meat or vegetables cooked with it a distinctive red hue. There are hundreds of variations and each *recado* is for a different dish.

## THE PACIFIC COAST

Many of the traditions considered characteristically "Mexican" were created in Guadalajara in the state of Jalisco. It is the country's second-largest city and has large mountain ranges, volcanoes, valleys, and plateaus. Guadalajara is the origin for traditions such as mariachi music, the Mexican hat dance, broad-brimmed sombrero hats, the Mexican rodeo, and tequila. The most important crops in this region include peanuts, sugarcane, and agave (for the production of tequila). In the mountainous regions ranch cooking dominates. *Pozole*, Mexico's pork and hominy stew, originated here, as did *birria*, mutton or goat prepared in an adobo sauce and served in a rich tomato and meat broth.

The state of Oaxaca is one of the most mountainous states in Mexico. Most of the people today are farmers and the most common crops are mangoes and coffee. A festival every December celebrates the radish, which was introduced to Mexico by the Spanish in the late 1500s. Specially grown radishes, some reaching over seven pounds, are carved into works of art. Sometimes called the "land of seven moles," Oaxaca is best known for its seven major varieties of mole. From the most elaborate to the simplest, the seven types are *mole negro* (black mole, the one that uses cocoa), *mole amarillo* (yellow), *mole coloradito* (little red), *mole almendrado* (with almonds), *mole chichilo* (a local name without translation), *mole verde* (green), and *mole colorado* (red). In the way of wine tasting, *mole* tasting is also practiced in several regions of Mexico.

*Chocolate con leche*, or more commonly *chocolate con agua* (hot chocolate prepared with milk or with water) is one of the most famous products of Oaxaca. The drink is prepared with fresh paste or tablets of cocoa, which in some stores are custom made with a mix of fresh cocoa, sugar, and cinnamon. The paste or tablets are dissolved in either water or milk. The hot liquid is mixed with a special wooden shaker (*molinillo*), which has loose rings that help produce foam. In many places it is served inside a large bowl accompanied with traditional bread made with egg and anise (*pan de huevo*).

The states of Colima, Nayarit, and Sinoloa border the Pacific Ocean. Sinaloa is one of Mexico's largest agricultural states, and also has one of the largest fishing fleets. The coast provides deep-sea fish such as marlin, swordfish, tuna, and sea bass as well as shallow-water fish and shellfish. All three states are important for their coconut, coffee, and banana plantations and orchards of avocado, limes, mango, mamey, and tamarind. Nayarit is famous for its chile sauce, called *Salsa Huichol.* This sauce is made from a variety of chiles, spices, vinegar, and salt and is used like American Tabasco.

### THE BAJA CALIFORNIA PENINSULA

This territory is divided into two states, Baja California and Baja California Sur. In Baja California, Tijuana is one of the most visited border cities in the world. The fertile valleys of Guadalupe, San Antonio, Santo Tomas, and San Vicente make up part of Mexico's famous wine-producing region. The state also hosts many food festivals throughout the year, including the Paella and Wine Fair, the Seafood and Fish Festival, the Tequila Festival, and the Caesar Salad Festival (the caesar salad was created in this state). The food in this region tends to be influenced by the north with the use of flour tortillas, burritos, tacos, red meat, and *machaca* (the Mexican equivalent of beef jerky). Baja California Sur only became a state in 1974, when tourist resorts such as Cabo San Lucas and San José del Cabo were developed. In the coastal waters off Baja California and Baja California Sur the seafood harvested includes sole, tuna, sardines, mackerel, clams, shrimp, and lobster.

## Glossary

**Achiote** Small, hard red seeds of the annatto tree, known as achiote, which are used to give color and flavor. Achiote seeds are widely available in Caribbean and Latin groceries. The seeds should have a healthy, earthy-red color; avoid seeds that have a dull brown color. The seeds alone have a slightly musky flavor, but they are most often combined with other herbs and seasoning to make achiote paste, which is popular in the Yucatan for marinades and sauces. In Mexico, the whole seeds are ground and used. Achiote should always be cooked in fat to remove any chalkiness.

**Avocado** The avocado tree, a member of the laurel family, is native of the tropical Americas. The pear-shaped fruit is sometimes known as the alligator pear. The word "avocado" is derived from the Nahuatl word *ahuacatl,* meaning "testicle." The medicinal properties of the avocado have been lauded since the Spanish conquest.

**Avocado Leaves** Fresh or dried; used for their flavor in Mexican cooking, particularly in the states of Morelos, Puebla, and Oaxaca. Avocado leaves should be stored dried in an airtight container away from light.

**Banana Leaves** Available year-round, fresh or frozen, in most Latin American markets. Banana leaves are popular in the southern and Gulf coast Mexican states for wrapping fish, tamales, pork, and chicken. Items wrapped with banana leaves stay moist during the cooking process, plus they pick up a fruity flavor.

**Beans** Two beans are typically associated with Mexican cooking: black beans and larger mottled pink pintos. Small black beans, eaten extensively in Latin regions of the world including Mexico, are small and quite hard, requiring a longer cooking time than other dried beans such as the pinto. Beans and rice are normally served at every meal and are a complete protein.

**Cactus Paddles (Nopales)** The prickly pear cactus is the most common type of cactus eaten in Mexico. *Nopal* means cactus in Spanish and *nopales* is the term for "cactus stem." *Nopalitos* refers to the pads once they are cut up and prepared for eating. Nopales are usually sold already cleaned (needles removed); look for bright green and firm pads. They are typically eaten grilled or boiled.

**Chayote** The chayote, or vegetable pear, is a native of Mexico, and its name is derived from the Nahuatl word *chayutli.* Chayote was one of the principal foods of the Aztec and Mayan people. This pear-shaped squash has the mild taste of zucchini. The flesh is quite crisp, something like a water chestnut. Chayotes come in both smooth and prickly varieties (covered in spines).

**Cheeses**

**Fresh Cheeses**

**Queso Blanco** A creamy white cheese made from skimmed cow's milk. It is described as being a cross between salty cottage cheese and mozzarella. It is traditionally coagulated with lemon juice, giving it a fresh, distinctive lemon flavor, although today it is often commercially made with rennet.

**Queso Fresco** A pale cream-colored, moist, crumbly, soft cheese made in round cakes of different sizes. It has a slight acidity but with a creamy flavor. It is sometimes called *queso* *de metate* because the curds are pressed out on the *metate* (grinding stone) until compact enough to be packed into the small wooden hoops that give them shape. It is usually made with a combination of cow's milk and goat's milk.

**Panela** The most popular fresh cheese in Mexico, also called *queso de canasta* because it carries the imprint of the basket in which it is molded. It is a white, spongy, salty, semi-soft cheese mild in flavor. It absorbs other flavors easily.

**Requesón** A loose, ricotta-like cheese used to fill *enchiladas* and to make cheese spreads. It is typically sold in the markets wrapped in fresh corn husks. *Requesón* has a very mild and semisweet flavor. Its color is white and its texture is soft, moist, and grainy.

**Soft Cheeses**

**Oaxaca** Also referred to as Asadero or Queso Oaxaca cheese. It is a semi-soft, white, string-type cheese. It is stretched, kneaded, then formed into a ball shape, which is plunged in brine for several minutes. The flavor ranges from mild to sweet and buttery.

**Semi-Soft Cheeses**

**Asadero** The literal translation of this cheese's name is "broiler" or "roaster"; the cheese itself is made by the same method as the braided Oaxaca cheese. The cheese melts easily when heated and strings appropriately.

**Chihuahua** Also called *queso menonita*, after the Mennonite communities of northern Mexico that first produced it. This is a mild, spongy, pale-yellow cheese. Unlike most Mexican cheeses, it is pale yellow rather than white, and can vary in taste from mild to a nearly cheddar-like sharpness.

**Queso Jalapeño** A smooth, soft white cow's milk cheese with bits of jalapeño chile in it.

**Queso Quesadilla** This cheese is smooth, soft, mild, and white. It melts easily to make dishes rich and creamy.

**Semi-Firm Cheeses**

**Queso Criollo** This pale yellow cheese is a specialty of the region around Taxco, Guerrero, and is similar to Munster.

**Edam** Although not considered a Mexican cheese, edam has become an intrinsic part of Yucatan regional cooking.

**Manchego** This cheese has a black, gray, or buff-colored rind with a crosshatch pattern. The interior ranges from stark white to yellowish, depending on age. It has a number of holes and a mild, slightly briny, nutty flavor.

**Firm Cheeses**

**Añejo** An aged cheese, white and crumbly, often very dry and salty, rather resembling a dry feta. This cheese is not as strongly flavored as cotija, but can be easily shredded or grated.

**Cotija** This is a sharp, crumbly goat cheese. This cheese is strongly flavored, firm and perfect for grating. It was originally made with goat's milk but today cow's milk is preferred.

**Chicharrón** Crispy fried pig skin used in salads, fillings, and as a snack.

**Chiles, Canned** Many Mexican recipes call for chiles serranos or jalapeños *en escabeche*, which means that they are canned in a souse, or pickled. Traditionally this includes vinegar, oil, herbs, garlic, onion, and slices of carrot. Canned *chiles chipotles en vinagre* or *adobo* are also widely used.

**Chiles** The most prominent feature of Mexican cooking is the emphasis it places on chiles, with more than seventy varieties.

**Dried Chiles**

Each chile has its own characteristics, flavor, and quality; you should not interchange chiles within a recipe unless it is indicated in the recipe.

**Ancho Chile** A ripened and dried *chile poblano*, one of the most commonly used throughout Mexico. Chile Ancho has a deep, reddish-brown color—brick red when soaked in water—and a wrinkled, fairly shiny skin. It is triangular in shape, and measures about 3 inches at its widest point and 5 inches in length. The ancho has a pleasant, sweet flavor, similar to a bell pepper. It may be stuffed; however, it is mostly soaked and ground for cooked sauces. It rates between 1,000 and 2,000 Scoville units on the heat index.

**Árbol Chile** The name means "tree chile." It is long and skinny, $2\frac{1}{2}$ by $\frac{1}{2}$ inches on average, and has a brilliant red, thin, smooth, shiny skin. This chile has a vicious bite, and should be treated with caution. It has a tannic, smoky, and grassy flavor, and a searing, acidic heat on the tip of the tongue. It rates between 15,000 and 30,000 Scoville units on the heat index.

**Cascabel Chile** Small and round, it is so named because it sounds like a rattle when it is shaken (cascabel means "jingle bells" in Spanish). It has a smooth, brownish-red skin, and usually measures 1 inch in diameter. Cascabel adds a deep smoky, nutty flavor to dishes. It is typically toasted and ground for sauce. The cascabel rates between 1,500 and 2,500 Scoville units on the heat index.

**Chipotle Chile** This is chile jalapeño, ripened, dried, and then smoked. Its light brown, wrinkled skin smells distinctly of smoke and its name means "smoked chile." It measures

# Where's the Chile's Heat?

Chiles get their "heat"—or "pungency"—from a group of chemical compounds called capsaicinoids, the best known of which is capsaicin. According to the Chile Pepper Institute, a research and education center housed at New Mexico State University, capsaicin is produced in the whitish pith (also called membranes or ribs), not by the seeds.

## HEAT SCALE

The pungency of chile peppers is measured in multiples of 100 units. It ranges from the sweet bell peppers at zero Scoville units to the habanero at 300,000-plus Scoville units! One part of chile "heat" per 1,000,000 drops of water is rated at only 1.5 Scoville Units. The substance that makes a chile so hot is called capsaicin. Pure capsaicin rates between 15,000,000 and 16,000,000 Scoville units! Today a more scientific and accurate method called liquid chromatography is used to determine capsaicin levels.

## GENERAL NOTES

- Smaller peppers are usually hotter than larger peppers.
- Peppers often become hotter as they ripen, and hotter still when they're dried. Dried peppers tend to have a richer, more concentrated flavor.
- The majority of the chile's heat is concentrated in the seeds and ribs. To tone down the heat of a pepper, remove some or all of the seeds and the white ribs.
- When working with peppers, wear rubber gloves or coat your hands with vegetable oil. Wash your hands carefully afterward.
- Chiles don't freeze well.

## TIPS FOR WORKING WITH FRESH CHILES

- It is advisable to wear gloves when handling fresh or dried chiles.
- Never bring your hands near your eyes during or after working with fresh chiles.
- Keep some vinegar or bleach on hand to neutralize the capsaicin, if it comes in contact with your skin.
- Be very careful of the hotter chiles like the habanero. It has been known to create first-degree burns.
- Gently wash your hands and arms after working with the chiles. The chile oils will need soap to break them up. Scrub fingertips, especially under the nails, and then soak them for a few minutes in strongly salted water, if necessary.

approximately 2 to 4 inches in length and about an inch wide. As much as one-fifth of the Mexican jalapeño crop is processed into chipotles. It rates between 5,000 and 8,000 Scoville units on the heat index.

**Guajillo Chile** A long, slender, pointed chile whose brownish-red skin is smooth, shiny, and tough, the *guajillo* averages $4\frac{1}{2}$ inches in length and $1\frac{1}{4}$ inches in width. Sweet and mild, this chile is a base for rich chile con carne and classic Tex-Mex cuisine. The *guajillo* is used in table and cooked sauces. The skin is extra tough, so it needs longer time for cooking. It rates between 2,000 and 4,500 Scoville units on the heat index.

**Mora Chile** This is a smoked and dried large red jalapeño pepper. Blackish red in color, it has a wrinkled, tough skin, with a round tip. A typical size is 2 inches long and $\frac{3}{4}$ inch wide. Like the *chipotle*, it has a smoky flavor and is very *picante* (hot and spicy). It rates between 5,000 and 8,000 Scoville units on the heat index.

**Morita Chile** A small, mulberry-red chile, triangular in shape and about 1 inch long and $\frac{1}{2}$ inch wide, with a slightly smoky flavor. This smoked and dried small red jalapeño pepper is very hot and spicy. It rates between 5,500 and 8,500 Scoville units on the heat index.

**Mulato Chile** This very popular chile looks like the ancho, only slightly larger with tougher and smoother skin and a brownish black hue. It's fairly mild and has an earthy flavor; when soaked in water it has a sweetish, almost chocolaty flavor. This chile is normally used soaked and ground in cooked sauces, the classic example being *mole poblano.* It rates between 900 and 1,500 Scoville units on the heat index.

**Pasilla Chile** This is a long, slender chile with a rounded tip. The skin is wrinkled with a blackish tone. It is a standard ingredient in mole sauces. The average size is 6 inches long and $\frac{3}{4}$ to 1 inch wide. The seeds and veins clustered at the top by the stem are very hot; however, the flesh is generally mild and has a slight "tobaccoish" flavor. It is toasted and ground for table sauces and soaked and ground for cooked sauces. It rates between 1,000 and 1,500 Scoville units on the heat index.

**Chile de la Tierra, Colorado Chile** This is the *chile verde,* or Anaheim, ripened and dried. When dried it has a tough, dark, reddish brown matte skin. It is very mild and does not have much flavor. It rates between 700 and 1,000 Scoville units on the heat index.

### Fresh Chiles

**Güero Chile** A pale yellow chile that varies in size, averaging 4 to 5 inches long and 1 inch wide. It is pointed at the end, with a smooth, small-ridged, undulated surface. This chile can be very hot and has a delicious and distinctive flavor. It rates between 2,000 and 6,500 Scoville units on the heat index.

**Habanero Chile** This chile is shaped like a small lantern, about 1 inch across as its widest part and a bit over 2 inches long. This extremely hot chile has a distinctive fruity flavor. It is a light green color and as it ripens it turns to one of various colors including red, orange, salmon, white, and chocolate, depending on the variety. It rates 200,000 to 300,000 Scoville units.

**Jalapeños Chile** The most well known of Mexico's chiles. It is a mid- to dark-green chile with a smooth surface and more often rounded at the tip than pointed. It averages $2\frac{1}{2}$ inches long and $\frac{3}{4}$ inch at its widest part. It has a unique rich fresh flavor and is hot. *Jalapeños*, like *serranos*, are used in various ways: fresh in a relish, cut and cooked, boiled and blended. It rates between 2,500 and 8,000 Scoville units on the heat index.

**Poblano Chile** The poblano can vary in shape, color, size, and flavor, depending on where it was grown, the time of year, and so forth. Typically, they are mild, large, heart-shaped peppers with very thick walls, 5 inches long and about 3 inches wide at the top, tapering to the apex. They are great for stuffing. They can be fairly mild to hot. With minor exceptions they are always charred and peeled. It rates between 1,200 and 2,500 Scoville units on the heat index.

**Serrano Chile** A small, smooth, mid-green chile, mostly rounded but sometimes pointed at the end. It averages $1\frac{1}{2}$ inch long and about $\frac{1}{2}$ inch wide. The flesh has a strong, fresh flavor, and the seeds and veins are very hot and spicy. It has thin walls, so it doesn't need to be charred, steamed, and peeled before using. It rates between 8,000 and 22,000 Scoville units on the heat index.

**Chile Verde, Anaheim Chile** A light green chile with a rounded tip, averaging 1 inch wide and 6 inches long. Anaheim chiles range from mild to hot. They have a tough skin that is typically charred and peeled before being used. When mature and red, an Anaheim is called a *chile colorado.* It rates between 1,000 and 2,000 Scoville units on the heat index.

**Chorizos** Brought to Mexico by Spanish explorers, this pork sausage is made all over Mexico, and each region has its own balance of spices, chiles, and herbs. Many cooks believe that lean pork is *the* important factor when making chorizos. The pork for Mexican *chorizos* is chopped (not ground), seasoned, and stuffed into casings made from pigs' small intestine.

**Cilantro** The fresh green leaves and tender stems of coriander, or Chinese parsley. The dried seed is occasionally used, but the two are not interchangeable. There is no substitute for its crisp and pungent flavor. Thick stems should be discarded and only thin stems and leaves used.

**Cinnamon** The light brown cinnamon bark originally from Ceylon is used extensively in Mexican cooking. Mexican cinnamon has a softer and more delicate flavor, and flavors both savories and sweets.

**Corn Husks** The dried outer sheath that surrounds each ear of corn. They are the traditional wrappers for tamales, but they can be used to wrap other foods for steaming or grilling. In addition to protecting foods as they cook, they also impart a mild corn essence. Cornhusks are used fresh as well as dried.

**Cumin** The flavor of cumin plays a major role in Mexican cuisine. Cumin is the dried seed of the herb *Cuminum cyminum*, a member of the parsley family. The cumin plant grows to about 1 to 2 feet tall and is harvested by hand. Cumin is a key component in both chile powder and curry powder. Always develop the flavor by cooking it first in fat.

**Epazote** A weed that grows all over North America. It is a strong-tasting herb; the flavor is dominant and should be used alone, not in combination with other herbs. It is quite pungent and some say it smells like gasoline or kerosene. It is most commonly used in black bean recipes to ward off some of the "negative" side affects of eating beans.

**Huitlacoche** An exotic fungus that grows naturally on ears of corn. The kernels are swollen and deformed, black and juicy inside and covered with a crisp, slivery-gray skin. The texture and inky flavor is unique. The earthy and somewhat smoky fungus is used to flavor quesadillas, tamales, soups, and other specialty dishes.

**Jicama** Like potatoes, jicama grows underground as a tuber. It is a round brown-skinned vegetable that yields crisp white flesh that looks like an apple or raw potato. Raw jicama is sweet and juicy. Always remove the fibrous brown skin. Cooked lightly it becomes milder but retains its crispness, like a water chestnut. Jicama is primarily a texture food since its flavor is rather bland.

**Lime** Mexican cooks use the yellow-skinned key lime, because it tastes sweeter than other limes. If key limes are unavailable, use half lemon juice and half lime juice. Mexican cuisine uses limes for marinating fish and chicken, in salsas, soups, and best of all balancing margaritas.

**Masa, Masa Harina** Masa means "dough" in Spanish, but in Mexico it is generally understood as "corn dough." It is made by boiling corn kernels in powdered lime (calcium oxide), washing them, and then grinding; water is mixed in to make dough. Smoother, soft masa is required for tortillas, and coarser, stiff masa is used for tamales. Masa harina is factory-made powdered masa. It can be used to make anything that calls for masa. Ordinary yellow cornmeal for making cornbread is not a substitute.

**Oregano** Mexican oregano has a more assertive flavor than the Mediterranean oregano. Thirteen varieties of oregano grow throughout Mexico. However, Mexican cooks normally use dried oregano.

**Pepitas or Pumpkin Seeds** These seeds have been used in Mexican cuisine since pre-Columbian times. Toasted in their hulls or hulled but unroasted and unsalted, they are used in moles, sauces, salads, and snack foods.

**Plantains** Plantains are popular in Latin American, Asian, and African cuisines, and are prepared and eaten in a number of ways. Unlike their common sweet banana cousin, plantains have to be cooked. They are starchy, only slightly sweet, and are no more appealing to eat raw than a potato. They can be pink, green, red, blackish-brown, and yellow with black spots. In Mexican cooking they must be very ripe, almost juicy, and sweet.

**Sesame Seeds** Widely used as a topping for breads and pastries or as a thickener for sauces.

**Seville or Sour Oranges** Small, brilliantly orange, thin-skinned oranges. There is no real substitute for the sharp, fragrant juice.

**Tamarind Seeds and Paste** Widely grown in Mexico since the sixteenth century, this is a 3- to 8-inch-long, brown, irregularly curved pod, which produces a juicy brown to reddish brown acidulous pulp. When fully ripe, the shells are brittle and easily broken. The pulp dehydrates to a sticky paste enclosed by a few coarse stands of fiber. The pods may contain from one to twelve large, flat, glossy brown seeds embedded in the brown, edible pulp. The pulp has a pleasing sweet-sour flavor and is high in both acid and sugar.

**Tomatillos (Tomates Verdes, Mexican Green Tomatoes)** The *tomatillo* is of Mexican origin; however, it now grows everywhere in the Western Hemisphere. It is a pale green fruit enclosed in a green, papery husk that ripens to yellow. It is not an ordinary unripe tomato. In central Mexico it is called *tomate verde*, and in the northeast *fresadilla*; elsewhere it is *tomatillo*, *tomate de cascara*, or *tomate de bolsa*. Generally used when they are green rather than yellow, *tomatillos*, vary in acidity and have a very tart flavor. When working with *tomatillos* always remove the husks and wash the fruit.

**Tomatoes** Tomatoes are indigenous to Mexico and South America, and are grown year round. The Italian plum tomato, called *jitomato guaje* ("gourd" tomato) or *guajillo*, like the chile, is also grown extensively. However, the skin of the plum tomato is much tougher than an ordinary tomato.

**Tortillas** Indispensable in Mexican cuisine, made with either corn or wheat flour. Available both fresh and frozen.

## KITCHEN TOOLS

**Cazuela** An earthenware casserole used to make moles. Its great advantage is that it heats evenly, eliminating that nemesis of all cooks, the dreaded "hot spot."

**Coffee/Spice Grinder** A necessity for many Mexican dishes that call for ground *achiote*, pumpkin or sesame seeds, or spices.

**Comal** A round plate, usually made of unglazed earthenware, cast iron, or tin, about $\frac{1}{2}$ inch thick. It is a Mexican griddle used for cooking tortillas, toasting chiles, garlic, and the like.

**Molcajete y Tejolote** This mortar and pestle combination, made of basalt, is used for grinding. The tejolote is a heavy, oval shaped rock used to grind spices, onions, peppers, and tomatoes into thick purees in a molcajete.

**Molinillo** Found in every Mexican kitchen, this wooden implement will, when twirled between the palms of both hands, give hot chocolate a spectacular collar of froth.

**Tortilla Press** An absolute must if you plan to make your own tortillas, the wooden variety of tortilla presses have largely been replaced by the cast-iron variety. There is also an aluminum model that is decidedly less popular.

## COOKING METHODS

**Charring, Peeling, and Cleaning Fresh Chiles and Bell Peppers** In Mexican peasant cooking this is done by charring peppers right on the charcoal or wood fire, which also serves to enhance the flavor. They can also be put directly over a gas flame, grill, or on a tray under the broiler. Char the pepper, turning it frequently, until the skin is blackened. The entire chile will not be completely black, but it should be charred about 60 percent. They will char evenly and in all the little irregular surfaces if they are first lightly coated with oil. After charring, place the pepper immediately into a plastic bag to "sweat" for about 15 minutes. Remove from the bag and when cool enough to work with, remove the blackened skin. You can use your hands, continually dipping them in water to remove the blackened bits, or use a paper towel. Use a knife to remove any skin that sticks. Do not peel roasted peppers under running water because this will wash away juices and flavor.

**Guisar (Braising or Stewing)** This is the most common way of cooking meat and poultry (with the possible exception of northern Mexico, where much of it is grilled). The meat, poultry, and in some cases vegetables are prepared separately from the sauce in the making of *mole, pipian,* and other complex dishes. A heavy-bottomed Dutch oven is a good substitute for a *cazuela* when doing this long, slow type of cooking.

**Moler (Grinding)** This is traditionally done in a *molcajete* but today a blender is more frequently used. The *molcajete* allows more control over the final texture of a *salsa;* however, if the sauce is a smooth one, a blender does quite well. The process of grinding chiles, herbs, spices, and tomatoes in a *molcajete* is labor-intensive, and an alternative is to grind dry ingredients in a spice or coffee mill before combining them with other ingredients. Whether using a *molcajete,* blender, or food processor, garlic and salt should be ground together before adding the remaining ingredients.

**Poner a Sudar (Sweating)** This refers to the method used for removing the skins from fresh chiles, especially poblanos, which are usually cooked without skins, either for stuffing or for making *rajas,* strips of chiles that are used in a great number of dishes.

**Sofreir (Soft-Frying/Sautéing)** Not much deep-frying is done in Mexican cooking, with the exception of some street snacks. A far more common technique is "soft-frying" or sautéing, which is done to soften ingredients and intensify their flavor. Dried chiles, for example, are sometimes soft-fried in combination with dry-roasting. Tortillas usually need to be soft-fried before being covered with sauce, as with *enchiladas.*

**Tostar/Asar** Toasting or dry-roasting. This is commonly done on the *comal,* but any well-seasoned griddle or dry skillet will work. It is a quick process, done over high heat and involving no liquid or oil. Toasting ingredients adds a distinctive flavor to the dish in which they are cooked.

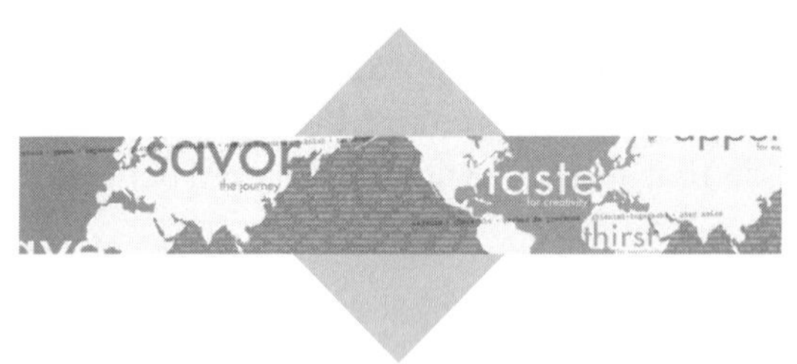

# Menus and Recipes from Mexico

MENU ONE

***Sopa de Lima con Pollo y Elote:* Chicken, Corn, and Lime Soup**

***Arroz Blanco con Verduras:* White Rice with Vegetables**

***Mole Verde con Hierbas:* Pork Herbed Green Mole**

**Corn Tortillas**

***Flan de Naranja:* Orange Flan**

MENU TWO

***Sopa de Ajo:* Garlic Soup**

***Nopales en Chipotle Adobado:* Nopales in Chipotle Sauce**

***Pavo con Salsa de Achiote a la Yucataneca:* Yucatán-Style Steamed Turkey in Achiote Sauce**

**Pickled Red Onions**

***Frijoles Refritos:* Well-Fried Beans**

***Arroz Blanco:* White Rice**

***Salsa de Jitomate Cocida:* Cooked Tomato Sauce**

**Churros**

**Mexican Hot Chocolate**

**Pico de Gallo**

MENU THREE

***Guacamole:* Avocado Dip**

***Sopa de Fideos Aguada:* Noodles in Tomato Broth**

***Chiles en Nogada:* Chiles in Walnut Sauce**

***Frijoles de Olla:* "Pot" Beans**

**Corn Tortillas**

***Arroz con Leche:* Mexican Rice Pudding**

OTHER RECIPES

***Mole Negro Oaxaqueño:* Oaxacan Black Mole**

***Pozole Blanco:* White Pozole**

***Arroz à la Mexicana:* Mexican Rice**

***Pescado à la Veracruzana:* Fish Veracruz Style**

**Jicama Salad**

# Sopa de Lima con Pollo y Elote

## Chicken, Corn, and Lime Soup

SERVES 4–6

| AMOUNT | MEASURE | INGREDIENT |
|---|---|---|
| **1 tablespoon** | **$\frac{1}{2}$ ounce, 14 ml** | **Vegetable oil** |
| **1 cup** | **4 ounces, 112 g** | **White onion, $\frac{1}{4}$ inch (.6 cm) dice** |
| **2** | | **Garlic cloves, minced** |
| **3 cups** | **18 ounces, 504 ml** | **Chicken stock** |
| **1$\frac{1}{2}$ cups** | **9 ounces, 252 g** | **Roma tomatoes, peeled, seeded, $\frac{1}{4}$ inch (.6 cm) dice** |
| **1$\frac{1}{2}$ cups** | **8 ounces, 224 g** | **Corn kernels** |
| **2** | | **Jalapeño chiles, seeded, minced** |
| **1 teaspoon** | | **Cumin, ground** |
| **1 cup** | **6 ounces, 168 g** | **Chicken thigh meat, fat trimmed, thinly sliced** |
| **3 tablespoons** | **8 g** | **Cilantro, chopped** |
| **1$\frac{1}{2}$ tablespoons** | **$\frac{3}{4}$ ounce, 21 ml** | **Fresh lime juice** |
| **To taste** | | **Salt and pepper** |

### PROCEDURE

1. Heat oil over medium heat, add onion and garlic, cook 8–10 minutes or until very soft.
2. Add chicken stock, tomatoes, corn, chiles, and cumin, bring to boil, reduce to simmer, and cook 5–8 minutes to blend flavors.
3. Add chicken and simmer about 3 minutes to cook meat.
4. Stir in cilantro and lime juice.
5. Correct seasoning.

# Arroz Blanco con Verduras

## White Rice with Vegetables

SERVES 4

**Chef Tip** **For all Mexican rice dishes, the grains are soaked, drained, and sautéed before steaming, then cooked with onion and garlic, as one would make a pilaf. This method produces fluffy, separate grains and a nutty, full flavor.**

| AMOUNT | MEASURE | INGREDIENT |
|---|---|---|
| 1 cup | 7 ounces, 198 g | Long-grain, unconverted white rice |
| 2 tablespoons | 1 ounce, 28 g | Corn oil |
| $\frac{1}{4}$ cup | 1 ounce, 28 g | White onion, $\frac{1}{4}$ inch (.6 cm) dice |
| $\frac{1}{2}$ cup | 1 ounce, 28 g | Green onions and tops, finely chopped |
| 2 | | Garlic cloves, minced |
| 1 cup | $2\frac{1}{2}$ ounces, 70 g | White mushrooms, $\frac{1}{4}$ inch (.6 cm) slices |
| 1 | | Serrano chile, seeds and veins removed, minced |
| $1\frac{1}{2}$ cups | 12 ounces, 353 ml | Chicken stock |
| $\frac{1}{2}$ cup | 2 ounces, 56 g | Corn kernels |
| 1 cup | 4 ounces, 113 g | Queso fresco, grated |
| 2 tablespoons | $\frac{1}{4}$ ounce, 7 g | Cilantro, chopped |
| To taste | | Salt and pepper |

**PROCEDURE**

1. Cover the rice with hot water and let stand for 20 minutes. Drain and rinse well under cold water. Let drain for 10 minutes.
2. Heat the oil until it smokes and add the rice; stir until all the grains are well coated.
3. Cook until the rice just begins to take on a color.
4. Add the onions, garlic, mushrooms, and chile; cook over high heat for 10 minutes, until white onion and garlic are translucent, stirring constantly.
5. Add chicken stock and corn; cook uncovered over medium heat—do not stir again—until the liquid has been absorbed and small air holes appear in the rice.
6. Remove from heat and let stand, covered, for 10 to 15 minutes.
7. Add the cheese and cilantro, and stir into the rice with a fork.

# Mole Verde con Hierbas

## Pork Herbed Green Mole

SERVES 4

**Green mole is most commonly found in the states of Puebla, Tlaxcala, and Oaxaca, where it is one of *los siete moles*—the seven famous moles, each with a distinctive color, flavor, and aroma. Unlike the other moles, which nearly always contain nuts and seeds, this recipe gets its characteristic flavor and bright green color from fresh herbs. If you prefer chicken, it may be substituted for pork in this recipe**

| AMOUNT | MEASURE | INGREDIENT |
|---|---|---|
| $1\frac{1}{2}$ pounds | 24 ounces, 672 g | Pork stew meat, $1\frac{1}{2}$ inch (3.8 cm) cube |
| $\frac{1}{2}$ teaspoon | 1 g | Black peppercorns, bruised |
| 1 cup | 4 ounces, 112 g | White onion, cut $1\frac{1}{2}$ inch (3.8 cm) cube |
| 10 | | Garlic cloves, peeled and split lengthwise |
| 8 | | Cloves, whole, or $\frac{1}{4}$ teaspoon ground |
| 1 teaspoon | 2 g | Cumin seeds |
| 2 | | Jalapeño chiles, seeds removed |
| 1 pound | 16 ounces, 448 g | Tomatillos, husks removed |
| 2 | | Thyme sprigs, fresh |
| 2 | | Marjoram sprigs, fresh |
| 1 cup | 8 ounces, 224 g | Masa, either fresh or reconstituted by mixing 6 tablespoons masa harina to a smooth paste with 1 cup water |
| $\frac{1}{2}$ cup | 1 ounce, 28 g | Italian parsley, chopped |
| $\frac{1}{2}$ cup | 1 ounce, 28 g | Cilantro leaves, chopped |
| $\frac{1}{4}$ cup | $\frac{1}{2}$ ounce, 14 g | Epazote, fresh or $\frac{1}{8}$ cup dried, crumbled |
| $\frac{1}{4}$ cup | $\frac{1}{2}$ ounce, 14 g | Hoja santa leaves, fresh, or 3 dried leaves (Also called hierba santa or root beer plant, it has a distinctive anise flavor that's hard to duplicate.) |
| 2 cups | 14 ounces, 392 g | White beans, cooked |
| To taste | | Salt and pepper |

**PROCEDURE**

1. Combine pork stew meat, peppercorns, $\frac{1}{2}$ cup white onions, and 5 garlic cloves, cover by 1 inch with cold water. Bring to a boil, cover, and reduce to simmer. Cook until just tender, 30–45 minutes. Remove meat and strain stock, reserve.
2. Grind the cloves and cumin seeds with a spice grinder or a mortar and pestle.
3. In a blender combine ground spices, jalapeño, tomatillos, thyme, marjoram, remaining garlic cloves and onions and $\frac{1}{2}$ cup stock from the cooked pork. Blend until smooth.

4 Combine reserved pork stock and tomatillo mixture; simmer, uncovered, 3 minutes.

5 Whisk masa into pork and tomatillo liquid; whisking constantly, return to simmer.

6 Cook, uncovered, over low heat 10 minutes, whisking occasionally. If lumps form, pass through a medium-mesh sieve and return to heat. Mixture should thicken to the consistency of whipping cream; if necessary, reduce to correct consistency or thin with more stock.

7 Combine parsley, cilantro, *epazote*, and *hoja santa* in a blender or food processor. If necessary, add a few tablespoons of liquid; process to a smooth puree.

8 Add beans, cooked pork, and pureed herbs to the *masa*-thickened sauce and let return to a simmer. Correct seasoning and serve.

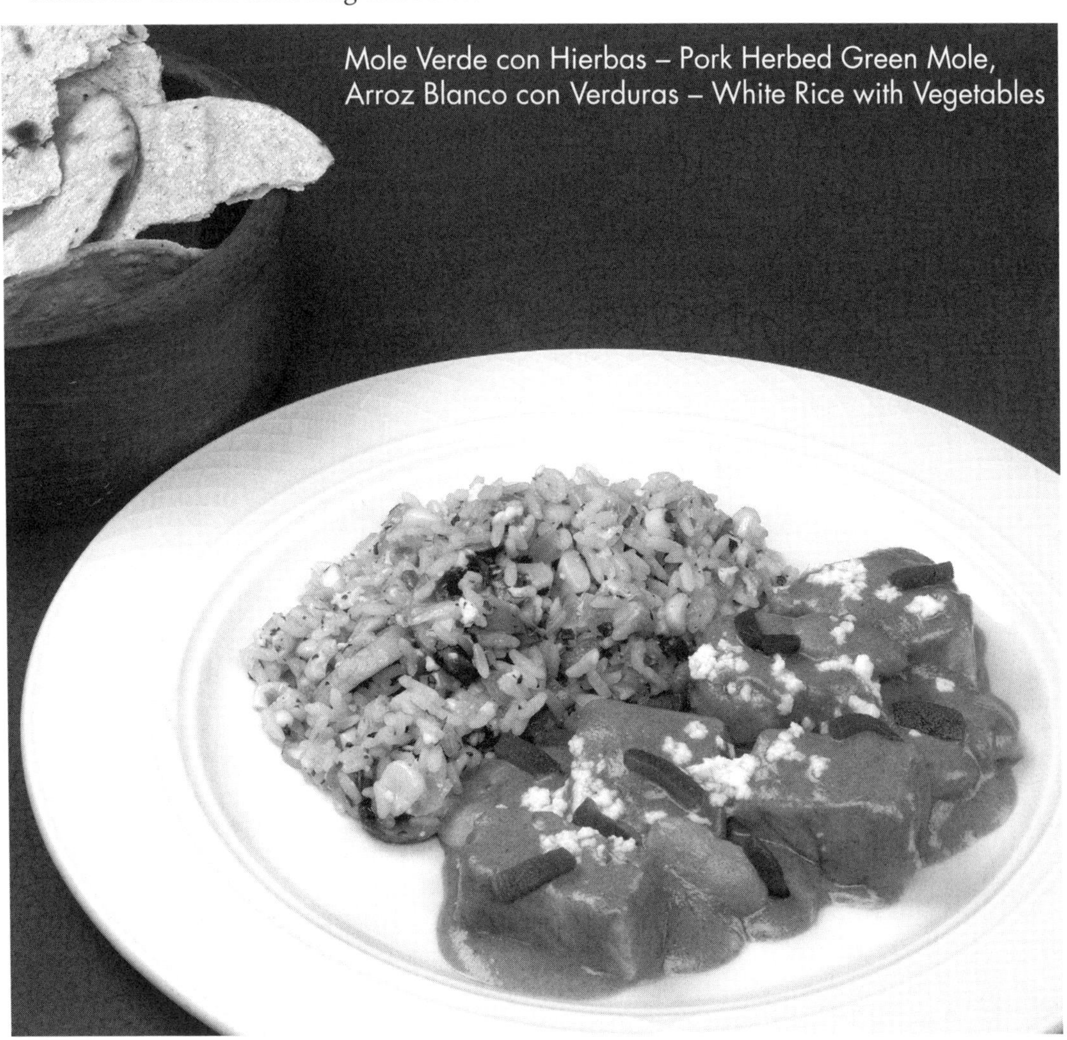

Mole Verde con Hierbas – Pork Herbed Green Mole, Arroz Blanco con Verduras – White Rice with Vegetables

# Corn Tortillas

YIELD: 1 POUND

| AMOUNT | MEASURE | INGREDIENT |
|---|---|---|
| **2 cups** | **10 ounces, 280 grams** | **Prepared masa harina** |
| **$1\frac{1}{3}$ cups** | **21 ounces, 588 ml** | **Warm water, approximately** |
| **1 teaspoon** | | **Salt** |

**PROCEDURE**

1. Dissolve the salt in the warm water. To the masa harina, add the water all at once (this keeps lumps from forming) and mix quickly, just until the ingredients are combined.
2. Let rest 5 minutes. Masa will dry out quickly, so keep covered with plastic wrap or a damp cloth.
3. Pinch off golf-ball-sized pieces and roll into balls.
4. Flatten the balls and roll out to $\frac{1}{8}$ inch (.3 cm) thick or use a tortilla press. If using a tortilla press, line both sides with plastic.
5. Gently place the tortilla on a hot skillet or griddle. It should make a soft sizzling sound. Cook for 30–40 seconds or until the tortilla starts to bubble on top. Turn tortilla over and cook an additional 20–30 seconds.
6. Remove the tortilla from pan and keep warm.
7. To reheat, bake covered in a 350°F (176°C) oven for 10–12 minutes.

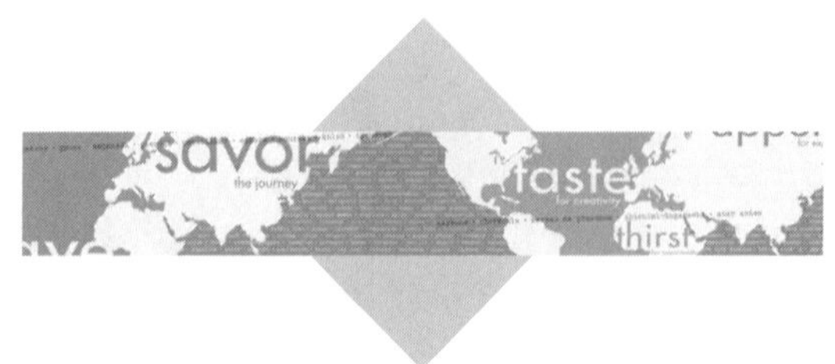

# Flan de Naranja Orange Flan

SERVES 4

| AMOUNT | MEASURE | INGREDIENT |
|---|---|---|
| $\frac{1}{2}$ cup | $3\frac{1}{2}$ ounces, 98 g | Sugar, granulated |
| 1 tablespoon | $\frac{1}{2}$ ounce, 15 ml | Water |
| $\frac{1}{4}$ teaspoon | | Lemon juice |
| Pinch | | Cayenne pepper |
| $\frac{1}{2}$ cup | 2 ounces, 56 g | Blanched almonds |
| $\frac{1}{4}$ cup | $1\frac{3}{4}$ ounces, 50 g | Sugar |
| | | Finely grated zest of 1 orange |
| 4 | | Eggs |
| $\frac{1}{4}$ cup | 2 ounces, 60 ml | Heavy cream |
| $\frac{3}{4}$ cup | 6 ounces, 180 ml | Orange juice |

PROCEDURE

1. Preheat oven to 350°F (176°C).
2. Make caramel by melting $\frac{1}{2}$ cup sugar ($3\frac{1}{2}$ ounces, 98 g), water, lemon juice (lemon juice keeps the mixture from hardening or crystallizing), and cayenne over low heat and cook for 8 to 10 minutes, without stirring. Gently tilt the pan off the heat to distribute color evenly as sugar caramelizes. When sugar reaches a uniform golden brown (light amber) color, immediately remove from heat.
3. Pour caramel into 4 individual custard cups; tip the molds side to side until there is an even coating of caramel over the bottom and halfway up the sides. Set aside.
4. Grind the almonds in a food processor.
5. Add the remaining sugar, orange zest, and the eggs, process until smooth.
6. Add cream and orange juice, process to mix.
7. Let the froth subside before pouring into custard cup.
8. Bake in a water bath, covered, until the flan is set. Test by inserting the blade of a knife into the center of the custard. If the blade comes out clean, cooking is done.
9. Set aside to cool before unmolding.

# Sopa de Ajo Garlic Soup

SERVES 4

| AMOUNT | MEASURE | INGREDIENT |
|---|---|---|
| $\frac{1}{4}$ cup | 2 ounces, 56 ml | Vegetable oil |
| 1 cup | 4 ounces, 112 g | Leeks, white and light green parts, cleaned, thinly sliced |
| $\frac{1}{3}$ cup | 2 ounces, 56 g | Garlic cloves, peeled, thinly sliced |
| 1 | | Chile morita or arbol, seeded and soaked in hot water until soft |
| 1 cup | 6 ounces, 168 g | Roma tomatoes, roasted and peeled, rough chopped |
| 3 cups | 24 ounces, 672 ml | Chicken stock |
| 3 | | Eggs, lightly beaten with 1 tablespoon oil |
| 2 tablespoons | 6 g | Parsley, chopped |
| To taste | | Salt |
| 4 | | 2-inch round croutons |
| 2 tablespoons | 1 ounce, 56 g | Panela or queso fresco cheese, crumbled |

PROCEDURE

1. Heat oil over medium high heat; add leeks and garlic and sauté until soft but not brown.
2. Puree the chile and tomatoes and add to the leek mixture.
3. Cook over medium high heat until mixture is thick.
4. Add chicken stock and bring to boil; return to simmer and cook 10–12 minutes.
5. Add beaten eggs, stirring constantly in a circular motion. Add parsley and simmer until eggs are set.
6. Correct seasoning.
7. Serve with a crouton in each bowl and sprinkle with cheese.

# Nopales en Chipotle Adobado

## Nopales in Chipotle Sauce

SERVES 4

**The mild flavor of nopales makes them ideal for combining with strong-flavored ingredients.**

**Chef Tip** **Nopal means cactus in Spanish and nopales is the term for "cactus stem." The term nopalitos refers to the pads once they are cut and prepared for eating. Nopales can be eaten grilled or boiled. Overcooking may give them a slightly slimy texture.**

| AMOUNT | MEASURE | INGREDIENT |
|---|---|---|
| 2 cups | 12 ounces, 336 g | Nopales paddles, cleaned and $\frac{1}{2}$ inch (1.27 cm) dice |
| 1 $\frac{1}{2}$ pounds | 672 g | Tomatillos, husked and roasted on a dry griddle or comal until soft |
| 2 | | Garlic cloves, peeled and chopped |
| 2 | | Chipotles in adobo sauce |
| 1 tablespoon | $\frac{1}{2}$ ounce, 14 ml | Vegetable oil |
| 1 cup | 4 ounces, 112 g | White onion, sliced very thin |
| To taste | | Salt |
| 2 cups | | Arroz blanco |

### PROCEDURE

1. To prepare the nopales remove the thorns and the "eyes" with a vegetable peeler or small paring knife. Wash the pads well with cool water and peel or trim off any blemished or discolored areas.
2. Combine nopales with enough salted water to cover. Bring to a boil and cook 10 minutes. Drain and set aside.
3. Combine tomatillos, garlic, and chipotles in a blender and blend until smooth.
4. Heat oil and sauté onions over low heat until transparent.
5. Add puree and nopales, stir and cook over low heat 10–15 minutes. Season to taste.
6. Serve hot with rice and warm tortillas

# Pavo con Salsa de Achiote a la Yucataneca Yucatán-Style Steamed Turkey in Achiote Sauce

SERVES 4

| AMOUNT | MEASURE | INGREDIENT |
|---|---|---|
| $\frac{1}{2}$ cup | 4 ounces, 112 g | Achiote paste (recipe follows) |
| 3 cups | 18 ounces, 504 ml | Seville or sour orange juice |
| $\frac{1}{4}$ cup | 2 ounces, 46 ml | Honey |
| 1 tablespoon | $\frac{1}{4}$ ounce, 6 grams | Cumin seeds, toasted and ground |
| 1 teaspoon | 1 g | Oregano, dried |
| 1 | 47 ounces, 1.33 kg | Turkey breast, bone in, skin on |
| $\frac{1}{4}$ cup | 2 ounces, 46 g | Butter, softened, or lard |
| 3 | | Banana leaves or enough fresh corn husks to line the roasting pan and cover the turkey |
| 2 tablespoons | 1 ounce, 28 ml | Vegetable oil |
| $1\frac{1}{2}$ cups | 12 ounces, 336 ml | Beer |
| 1 cup | 8 ounces, 113 g | Pickled red onion, thinly sliced (recipe follows) |
| 1 | 8 ounces, 224 g | Avocado, sliced |
| 8 | | Corn tortillas, 8 inches (20 cm), warmed |
| | | Pico de Gallo (see p. 34) |
| | | Salsa de Jitomate Cocida (see p. 32) |

**PROCEDURE**

1 Combine achiote paste, juice, honey, cumin, and oregano.

2 Lift the turkey skin and rub softened butter over meat.

3 Spread the achiote mixture evenly over turkey; let marinate at room temperature for 45 minutes or under refrigeration 3–4 hours.

4 Line a pan with half the banana leaves or corn husks. Place the turkey on a rack on top of the banana leaves and cover with excess marinade.

5 Add beer to pan, cover turkey with remaining banana leaves or cornhusks.

6 Wrap pan with foil or use an airtight lid.

7 Steam until turkey reaches an internal temperature of 165°F (74°C). Steaming may be done in a preheated 350°F (176°C) oven. Check liquid level and add more beer or water if necessary. (Some Mexican cooks place a coin at the bottom of the steamer; when the coin begins to rattle, they add more water.)

8 When cooked, remove from pan and let cool. Shred as for tacos, combining meat with any sauce left in steamer. Turkey can also be placed on a platter, whole or in pieces, with any remaining sauce poured over it.

9 Serve turkey with pickled onion, avocado, tortillas, salsa (Pico de Gallo) and Salsa de Jitomate Cocida (p. 32; cooked tomato sauce).

## Achiote Paste

MAKES $\frac{1}{4}$ CUP

| AMOUNT | MEASURE | INGREDIENT |
|---|---|---|
| **4 tablespoons** | | **Achiote seeds** |
| **15** | | **Peppercorns** |
| **1 tablespoon** | | **Oregano** |
| **1 tablespoon** | | **Cumin seeds** |
| **2** | | **Whole cloves** |
| **1 tablespoon** | | **Coriander seeds** |
| **6** | | **Garlic cloves** |
| **4 tablespoons** | | **White wine vinegar** |

**PROCEDURE**

1 Grind all but the garlic and vinegar in a coffee grinder. Crush the garlic in a mortar; gradually add the vinegar. Add the ground spices to the crushed garlic and mix well.

# Pickled Red Onions

SERVES

| AMOUNT | MEASURE | INGREDIENT |
|---|---|---|
| 1 pound | 16 ounces, 448 g | Red onions, $\frac{1}{4}$ inch slices |
| 1 tablespoon | 18 g | Kosher salt |
| 1 tablespoon | 2 g | Oregano |
| 1 teaspoon | 1 g | Cumin seeds |
| $1\frac{1}{4}$ cup | 10 ounces, 280 ml | Vinegar |
| 5–6 tablespoons | $1\frac{3}{4}$ ounces, 49 g | Granulated sugar |
| 1 teaspoon | 2 g | Black pepper |

**PROCEDURE**

1. Separate the onion rings, toss with the salt until coated, and let stand 30 minutes.
2. Rinse the onions under cold water, drain very well, and pat dry with paper towels.
3. Combine well the oregano, cumin seeds, vinegar, sugar, and black pepper; pour over the rings in the bowl; toss to coat well. Chill for at least 2 hours before serving.

# Frijoles Refritos Well-Fried Beans

SERVES 4

| AMOUNT | MEASURE | INGREDIENT |
|---|---|---|
| 3 tablespoons | $1\frac{1}{2}$ ounce, 42 g | Pork lard or vegetable oil |
| $\frac{1}{4}$ cup | 1 ounce, 28 g | White onion, $\frac{1}{4}$ inch (.6 cm) dice |
| 2 cups | 9 ounces, 252 g | Black, pink, or pinot beans, cooked, with cooking liquid |
| To taste | | Salt and pepper |

**PROCEDURE**

1. In a heavy pan, heat the lard or oil over medium-high heat.
2. Sauté the onions until brown, 3–4 minutes.
3. Increase heat to high and add half the beans and all the cooking liquid; mash well.
4. Gradually add the remaining beans and mash to a coarse puree.
5. Cook additional 10–12 minutes or until the beans begin to dry out and sizzle at the edges.

# Arroz Blanco White Rice

SERVES 4

| AMOUNT | MEASURE | INGREDIENT |
|---|---|---|
| | | Hot water to cover |
| 1 cup | $6\frac{1}{2}$ ounces, 184 g | Long-grain rice |
| $\frac{1}{4}$ cup | 2 ounces, 56 ml | Vegetable oil |
| $\frac{1}{4}$ cup | 1 ounce, 28 g | Carrots, $\frac{1}{4}$ inch (.6 cm) dice |
| $\frac{1}{4}$ cup | 1 ounce, 28 g | Onions, thinly sliced |
| 1 | | Garlic clove, minced |
| 2 cups | 16 ounces, 470 ml | Chicken stock |
| 2 tablespoons | $\frac{1}{2}$ ounce, 14 g | Green peas, cooked |

**PROCEDURE**

1 Soak rice in hot water for 20 minutes.

2 Drain and rinse well in cold water, let drain 10 minutes.

3 Heat oil to smoke point, add rice and stir to cover well with oil.

4 Cook, stirring, until rice is just turning color.

5 Add carrots, onions, and garlic; cook until onions are translucent, stirring constantly. Allow about 10 minutes over high heat to color rice and cook vegetables.

6 Add chicken stock and cook uncovered over medium heat—do not stir—until the liquid has been absorbed and small air holes appear.

7 Cover rice with a tight lid or aluminum foil, to prevent steam from escaping. Let set for 25 minutes.

8 Remove cover; stir in peas.

# Salsa de Jitomate Cocida

## Cooked Tomato Sauce

**YIELD: $1\frac{1}{2}$ CUPS**

| AMOUNT | MEASURE | INGREDIENT |
|---|---|---|
| 1 | | Poblano chile, charred, peeled, seeded, and $\frac{1}{4}$ inch (.6 cm) dice (see step 1) |
| 8 ounces | 224 g | Tomatoes, charred, seeded, and chopped (see step 1) |
| 1 tablespoon | $\frac{1}{2}$ ounce, 14 ml | Vegetable oil |
| $\frac{1}{2}$ cup | 3 ounces, 84 g | Red onion, $\frac{1}{4}$ inch (.6 cm) dice |
| 2 | | Garlic cloves, minced |
| 1 teaspoon | 3 g | Oregano, fresh, or $\frac{1}{2}$ teaspoon dried |
| 1 teaspoon | 3 g | Basil, fresh, or $\frac{1}{2}$ teaspoon dried |
| $\frac{1}{2}$ cup | 4 ounces, 112 g | Tomato sauce |
| 1 teaspoon | 5 g | Fresh lime juice |
| To taste | | Salt and pepper |

**PROCEDURE**

1. Char poblano and tomatoes, turning frequently, until lightly charred on all sides, 3 to 5 minutes for chiles, 6 to 8 minutes for tomatoes (flesh should be soft).
2. Heat oil over medium heat and sauté onion and garlic until translucent, about 5 minutes.
3. Puree charred tomato and poblano.
4. Combine all ingredients except lime juice and salt and pepper, and cook over medium heat until slightly thickened and flavors are blended, about 5 minutes.
5. Add lime juice and correct seasoning.

# Churros

SERVES 4

***Churros* are fried strips of dough typically served hot and sprinkled with powdered sugar or cinnamon and sugar, or dipped in chocolate. While the churro is actually an import from Spain, the dessert became very popular in Mexico. It is customary to serve churros with Mexican hot chocolate (see p. 34) or Cafe de Olla.**

| AMOUNT | MEASURE | INGREDIENT |
|---|---|---|
| 1 $\frac{1}{2}$ cups | 6 ounces, 168 g | All-purpose flour |
| 1 teaspoon | 2 g | Baking powder |
| 1 $\frac{1}{4}$ cups | 10 ounces, 280 ml | Water |
| $\frac{1}{4}$ teaspoon | 1 g | Salt |
| 1 $\frac{1}{2}$ tablespoons | 21 g | Brown sugar |
| 1 | | Egg yolk |
| | | Oil for deep frying |
| 1 | | Lime, cut into wedges |
| | | Powdered sugar for dusting |

PROCEDURE

1. Sift the flour and baking powder together; set aside.
2. Bring water to a boil, add salt and brown sugar, stirring constantly, until both have dissolved.
3. Remove from heat, add the flour and baking powder mixture, and beat continuously until smooth.
4. Beat in the egg yolk until the mixture is smooth and glossy. Set the batter aside to cool. Have ready a churro maker or a piping bag fitted with a large star nozzle, which will give the churros their traditional shape.
5. Heat to the oil to 375°F (190°C) or until a cube of dried bread floats and turns golden after 1 minute.
6. Spoon the batter into a churros maker or a piping bag. Pipe five or six 4-inch lengths of the mixture into the hot oil, using a knife to slice off each length as it emerges from the nozzle.
7. Fry for 3–4 minutes or until golden brown.
8. Drain the churros on paper towels while cooking successive batches. Arrange on a plate with lime wedges, dust with powdered sugar, and serve warm.

# Mexican Hot Chocolate

SERVES 4

**Mexican chocolate is a grainy chocolate disk flavored with sugar, cinnamon, almonds, and vanilla. It is used to prepare hot chocolate and mole sauces. For 1 ounce Mexican chocolate, substitute 1 ounce semisweet chocolate, $\frac{1}{2}$ teaspoon ground cinnamon, and 1 drop almond extract.**

| AMOUNT | MEASURE | INGREDIENT |
|---|---|---|
| 1 quart | 32 ounces, 896 ml | Milk |
| 1 pound | 16 ounces, 448 g | Mexican chocolate or dark bitter chocolate |
| 2 | | Vanilla beans, split lengthwise |

**PROCEDURE**

1 Warm milk and chocolate.

2 Scrape seeds from the vanilla bean and add the seeds and beans to milk.

3 Stir with a *molinillo* or whisk until the chocolate is melted and the mixture begins to boil. Remove the vanilla beans. Remove from the heat and froth the chocolate with the *molinillo* or the whisk. Serve immediately in ample mugs.

# Pico de Gallo

SERVES 4

| AMOUNT | MEASURE | INGREDIENT |
|---|---|---|
| 1 tablespoon | $\frac{1}{2}$ ounce, 0.015 l | Olive oil |
| 1 cup | 4 ounces, 113 g | Yellow onion, $\frac{1}{4}$ inch (.6 cm) dice |
| 1 | | Serrano pepper, minced |
| 1 | | Garlic clove, minced |
| 1$\frac{1}{2}$ tablespoons | | Cilantro, minced |
| 1 cup | 6 ounces, 170 g | Tomatoes, peeled, seeded, $\frac{1}{4}$ inch (.6 cm) dice |
| 1 tablespoon | $\frac{1}{2}$ ounce, 0.015 l | Fresh lime juice |
| To taste | | Salt and black pepper |

**PROCEDURE**

1 Heat oil over medium heat. Add onions, serrano pepper, garlic, and cilantro. Toss and remove from heat. Let cool.

2 Combine onion mixture with tomatoes and lime juice and correct seasoning.

3 Serve warm or at room temperature.

# Guacamole Avocado Dip

**The word *guacamole* comes from the Nahuatl words for avocado (*ahuacatl*) and "mixture" or "concoction" (*molli*). It should be made in the *molcajete*, never in a blender or food processor. Guacamole can contain a seemingly infinite variety of ingredients; however, it is best when kept simple: avocados, chiles, onions, cilantro, and seasoning. Even tomatoes may cause problems if they are too watery.**

**Guacamole is usually eaten in Mexico at the beginning of a meal with a pile of hot, freshly made tortillas, crisp pork skins (*chicharron*), or little pieces of crispy pork (*carnitas*).**

YIELD: 2 CUPS

| AMOUNT | MEASURE | INGREDIENT |
|---|---|---|
| $\frac{1}{2}$ cup | 2 ounces, 56 g | White onion, $\frac{1}{8}$ inch (.3 cm) dice |
| 2 | | Jalapeño chiles, stemmed, seeded, and $\frac{1}{8}$ inch (.3 cm.) dice |
| $\frac{1}{4}$ cup | 1 ounce, 28 g | Cilantro, chopped fine |
| 2 tablespoons | 1 ounce, 28 ml | Fresh lime juice |
| To taste | | Salt |
| 3 | | Hass avocados, ripe |
| Optional | | |
| $\frac{3}{4}$ cup | 5 ounces, 140 g | Tomatoes, $\frac{1}{4}$ inch (.6 cm) dice |
| Garnish | | |
| $\frac{1}{4}$ cup | 1 ounce, 28 g | White onion, $\frac{1}{8}$ inch (.3 cm) dice |
| 1 tablespoon | 2 g | Cilantro, chopped fine |
| As needed | | Tortilla chips |

PROCEDURE

1. In a *molcajete* or with a regular mortar and pestle, grind together the onion, chiles, cilantro, lime juice, and salt until smooth.
2. Cut the avocadoes in half. Remove the pits, scoop out the flesh, and mash roughly into the chile mixture in the *molcajete.* Mix well to incorporate flavors.
3. Stir in tomatoes, if desired.
4. Adjust the salt.
5. Sprinkle with garnish and serve immediately with warm tortilla chips.

# Sopa de Fideos Aguada

## Noodles in Tomato Broth

SERVES 4

| AMOUNT | MEASURE | INGREDIENT |
|---|---|---|
| 2 tablespoons | 1 ounce, 28 g | Chicken fat or vegetable oil |
| | 3 ounces, 84 g | Mexican fideos, angelhair pasta, or vermicelli |
| $1\frac{1}{2}$ cups | 9 ounces, 252 g | Roma tomatoes, roasted and peeled |
| 1 | | Garlic clove, chopped |
| $\frac{1}{4}$ cup | 1 ounce, 28 g | White onion, roughly chopped |
| $5\frac{1}{4}$ cups | 42 ounces, 1.24 liter | Chicken stock, heated |
| 1 tablespoon | 3 g | Italian parsley, roughly chopped |
| To taste | | Salt |

PROCEDURE

1. Heat fat or oil until it begins to smoke; add the whole bundles of noodles without breaking them up.
2. Sauté, stirring constantly to prevent scorching, until they are just golden brown.
3. Drain off excess fat; reserve 2 tablespoon in pan.
4. In a blender, combine tomatoes, garlic, and onions; blend until smooth.
5. Add mixture to the browned noodles; stir to coat noodles.
6. Add hot chicken stock and parsley; bring to a boil.
7. Reduce heat and simmer until pasta is cooked (soft).
8. Adjust seasoning.

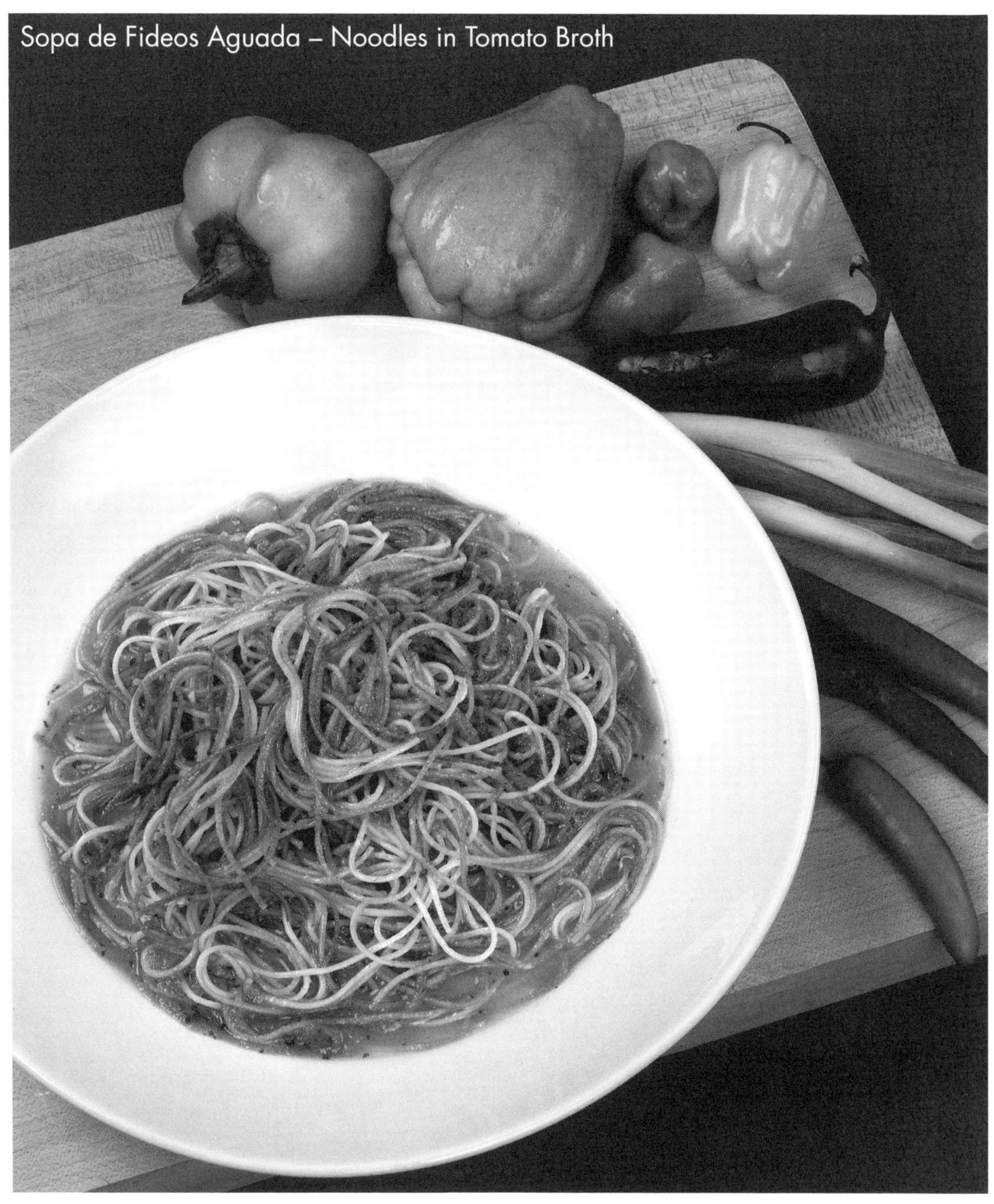
Sopa de Fideos Aguada – Noodles in Tomato Broth

# Chiles en Nogada

## Chiles in Walnut Sauce

SERVES 4

**This is one of the famous dishes of Mexico: large, dark green chiles poblanos stuffed with a pork meat picadillo and covered with a walnut sauce. It is decorated with red pomegranate seeds and large-leafed Italian parsley. The recipe is said to have been concocted by the grateful people of Puebla, for a banquet in honor of Don Agustin de Iturbide's saint's day, August 28, in 1821. He and his followers had led the final revolt against Spanish domination; as self-proclaimed emperor he had just signed the Treaty of Cordoba. All the dishes at the banquet were made with ingredients the colors of the Mexican flag: in this dish green chiles, white sauce, and red pomegranate seeds.**

| AMOUNT | MEASURE | INGREDIENT |
|---|---|---|
| 4 | | Chiles poblano, large and smooth |
| 1 tablespoon | $\frac{1}{2}$ ounce, 14 ml | Vegetable oil |
| 1$\frac{1}{2}$ cups | 12 ounces, 336 g | Pork, chopped fine |
| $\frac{1}{2}$ cup | 2 ounces, 56 g | White onion, $\frac{1}{4}$-inch (.6 cm) dice |
| 1 | | Garlic clove, minced |
| 1 cup | 6 ounces, 170 g | Tomato, peeled, seeded, $\frac{1}{4}$-inch (.6) dice |
| 1 | | Apple, sweet or tart, $\frac{1}{4}$-inch (.6 cm) dice |
| $\frac{1}{2}$ cup | 2 ounces, 56 g | Peaches, $\frac{1}{4}$-inch (.6 cm) dice |
| $\frac{1}{4}$ cup | 1 ounce, 28 g | Plantain, $\frac{1}{4}$-inch (.6 cm) dice |
| $\frac{1}{4}$ cup | 1 ounce, 28 g | Raisins |
| $\frac{1}{4}$ cup | 1 ounce, 28 g | Almond slivers |
| 2 teaspoons | $\frac{1}{2}$ ounce, 14 g | Pine nuts |
| 1 tablespoon | $\frac{1}{3}$ ounce, 10 g | Lemon zest |
| $\frac{1}{4}$ cup | 2 ounces, 56 ml | Chicken stock |
| $\frac{1}{2}$ teaspoon | 1 g | Coriander seeds |
| To taste | | Salt and black pepper |
| 3 | | Eggs, separated |
| As needed | | Flour |
| As needed | | Oil |
| 2 cups | 16 ounces, 448 ml | Walnut sauce (recipe follows) |
| Garnish | | Seeds of two pomegranates |

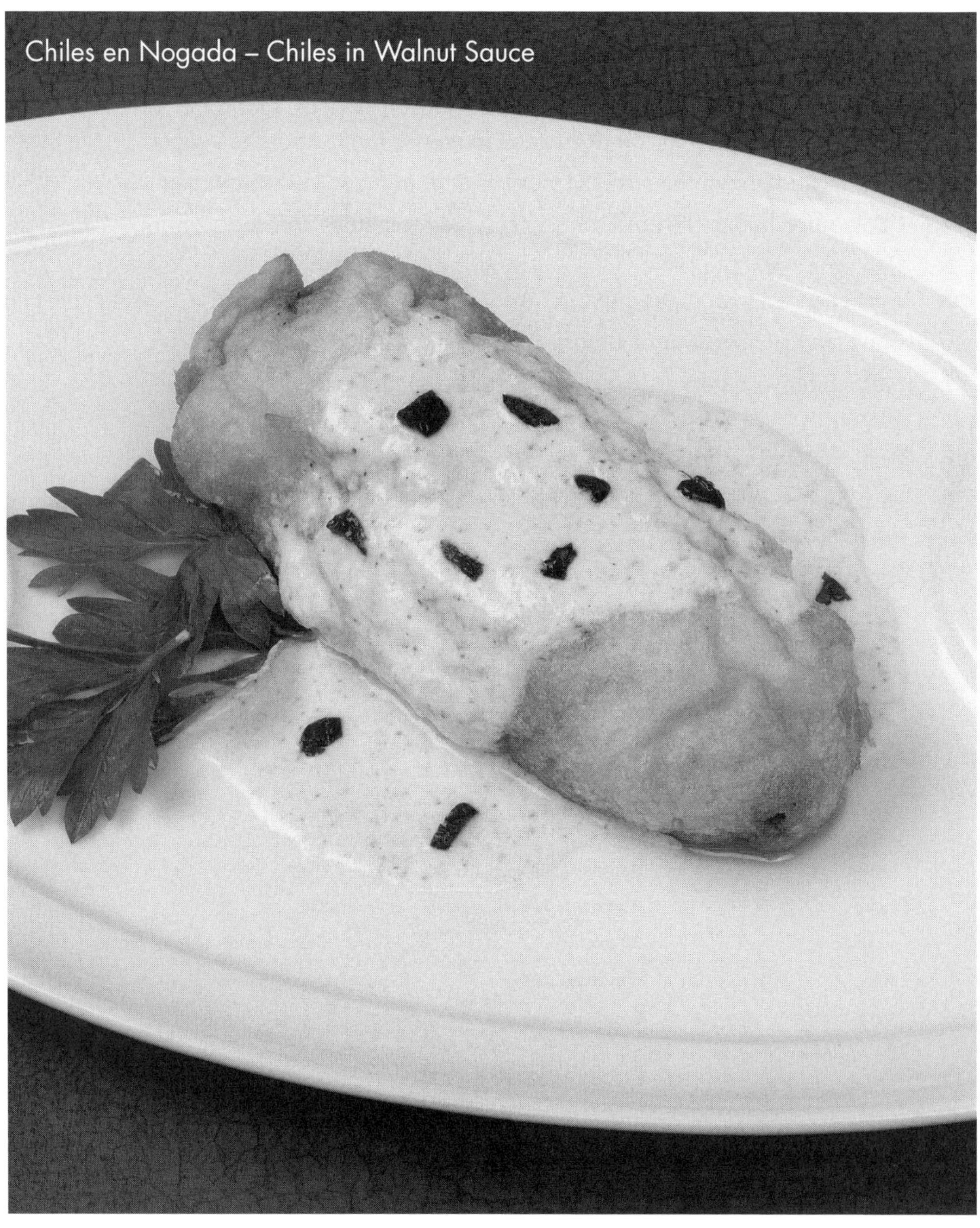
Chiles en Nogada – Chiles in Walnut Sauce

**PROCEDURE**

1 Roast (char) the chiles, steam, and peel off outer skin without removing the stem.
2 Make a lengthwise slit in each chile and remove the veins. Optional: Soak in a salt water and vinegar solution for up to 2 hours to reduce the heat of the pepper.
3 Heat oil and brown the pork. Remove and drain meat; leave fat in pan.
4 Cook onion and garlic until translucent. Add tomatoes and cook 2 minutes.
5 Combine pork, apples, peaches, plantain, raisins, almonds, pine nuts, lemon zest, and chicken stock with onion mixture. Add coriander and season with salt and pepper.
6 Cook over slow heat until almost dry. Allow to cool.
7 Stuff chiles with pork mixture. Reshape and secure openings with a toothpicks; chill for 30 minutes.
8 Beat egg whites until stiff peaks form. Lightly beat the egg yolk and mix into whites.
9 Heat oil to 350°F (175°C) in a deep fryer or pan fry using enough oil so it comes up half the thickness of the chiles.
10 Dip the stuffed chiles in flour and then in the egg batter, and fry until golden brown on each side. Drain on paper towels and remove toothpicks.
11 Just before serving, coat with warm walnut sauce and garnish with pomegranate seeds.

## Walnut Sauce

| AMOUNT | MEASURE | INGREDIENT |
|---|---|---|
| 1 cup | 4 ounces, 112 g | Walnut halves |
| 1 cup | 8 ounces, 240 ml | Milk |
| 1 ounce | 28 grams | Sliced bread, torn in pieces |
| 1 cup | 8 ounces, 224 g | Queso fresco or whole-milk ricotta cheese |
| 1 cup | 8 ounces, 240 g | Heavy cream |
| $\frac{1}{2}$ teaspoon | 2 g | Sugar |

**PROCEDURE**

1 Soak walnuts in half the milk for 1 hour. Strain and reserve the milk. Rub walnuts in a clean towel to remove the skin.
2 Soak the bread in remaining milk for at least 30 minutes.
3 Combine all ingredients in a blender and process until smooth.

# Frijoles de Olla "Pot" Beans SERVES 4

**This is traditionally served in a small earthenware bowl.**

| AMOUNT | MEASURE | INGREDIENT |
|---|---|---|
| 2 cups | 15 ounces, 420 g | Dried beans, black, pink, or pinto |
| $\frac{1}{2}$ cup | 2 ounces, 56 g | White onion, $\frac{1}{4}$ inch (.6) dice |
| 2 tablespoon | 1 ounce, 28 g | Pork lard or vegetable oil |
| 1 tablespoon | 15 g | Salt |
| To taste | | Salt and pepper |

PROCEDURE

1. Rinse beans in cold water and check for and remove small stones.
2. Cover beans with hot water, add onion and lard, and bring to boil.
3. Reduce to simmer; cover and cook until they are just soft and the skins are breaking open, $1\frac{1}{2}$–2 hours.
4. Add salt and continue to cook until the beans are soft and the liquid is somewhat thick.
5. Correct seasoning.

# Arroz con Leche Mexican Rice Pudding

SERVES 4

| AMOUNT | MEASURE | INGREDIENT |
|---|---|---|
| 2 cups | 16 ounces, 480 ml | Milk |
| 1 | | Cinnamon stick |
| 1 cup | $6\frac{1}{2}$ ounces, 184 g | Long-grain rice |
| $\frac{1}{2}$ cup | $3\frac{1}{2}$ ounces, 98 g | Granulated sugar |
| $\frac{1}{2}$ cup | 4 ounces, 112 ml | Sweetened condensed milk |
| $1\frac{1}{2}$ teaspoons | 8 ml | Vanilla extract |

PROCEDURE

1. Combine milk and cinnamon; bring to boil.
2. Add rice, reduce to a simmer, cover, and cook 15 minutes.
3. Combine sugar, condensed milk, and vanilla; stir to dissolve. Stir into rice and simmer 5 minutes. Remove from heat and serve warm.

# Mole Negro Oaxaqueño

## Oaxacan Black Mole SERVES 4–6

**The most famous of *Oaxaca's* many moles, traditionally served with pork, chicken, or particularly turkey, this is the choice for festive occasions. In Mexico, the ingredients for large batches of mole are usually taken to a *molino*-mill to eliminate the laborious process of grinding with the *metate* (stone mortar and pestle).**

| AMOUNT | MEASURE | INGREDIENT |
|---|---|---|
| | 5 ounces, 140 g | Mulato chiles |
| | 4 ounces, 112 g | Ancho chiles |
| | 2 ounces, 56 g | Pasilla chiles |
| | 4 ounces, 114 g | Chile negro |
| 2 cups | 16 ounces, 448 ml | Chicken stock |
| 1 | | Dried avocado leaves |
| $\frac{1}{4}$ cup | 1 ounces, 56 g | Sesame seeds |
| 1 | 2 ounces, 56 g | Corn tortilla, finely chopped |
| | 2 ounces, 56 g | Bolillo or French roll, crumbled |
| $\frac{1}{4}$ cup | 2 ounces, 56 ml | Lard or vegetable oil |
| $\frac{1}{2}$ cup | 2 ounces, 56 g | Almonds, sliced |
| $\frac{1}{2}$ cup | 2 ounces, 56 g | Peanuts, shelled and skinned |
| $\frac{1}{4}$ cup | 2 ounces, 56 g | Raisins |
| $\frac{1}{4}$ cup | 2 ounces, 56 g | Prunes, pitted and chopped |
| $\frac{1}{2}$ cup | 3 ounces, 84 g | Plantain, peeled and chopped |
| 1 teaspoon | 2 g | Black pepper |
| 2 | | Allspice, whole |
| $\frac{1}{8}$ teaspoon | | Marjoram |
| $\frac{1}{8}$ teaspoon | | Thyme |
| $\frac{1}{8}$ teaspoon | | Oregano |
| 1 | | Cinnamon stick, 2 inches |

*(Continued)*

| AMOUNT | MEASURE | INGREDIENT |
|---|---|---|
| **Pinch** | | **Anise** |
| **$\frac{1}{2}$ teaspoon** | **3 g** | **Cumin, ground** |
| **$\frac{1}{4}$ cup** | **1 ounce, 28 g** | **Garlic clove, minced** |
| **1 cup** | **4 ounces, 112 g** | **White onion, chopped** |
| **$\frac{1}{2}$ cup** | **2 ounces, 56 g** | **Tomatillos, husked** |
| **$\frac{1}{2}$ cup** | **2 ounces, 56 g** | **Tomato** |
| **$\frac{1}{2}$ cup** | **4 ounces, 112 ml** | **Vegetable oil** |
| | **2 ounce, 56 g** | **Mexican chocolate** |
| **To taste** | | **Sugar and salt** |

**PROCEDURE**

1 Roast chiles and remove the veins and seeds; soak in chicken stock for 20 minutes. Puree chiles in a blender or food processor with stock. Reserve.

2 Dry-toast the avocado leaves, sesame seeds, tortillas, and *bolillo* until browned, set aside.

3 Heat the lard and fry the almonds, peanuts, raisins, prunes, plantain, herbs, spices, garlic, and onions until the onion begin to soften. Add more oil if needed.

4 Roast the *tomatillos* and tomatoes on the *comal* or on a sheet pan under the broiler.

5 Blend all ingredients in a food processor, blender, or mortar except chile puree, vegetable oil, and chocolate; puree until smooth, adding enough water or stock to allow the blades to move. May be done in batches.

6 Heat the vegetable oil over medium heat.

7 Add blended ingredients and cook over low heat for 35 minutes.

8 Add chile puree and continue to cook 30 minutes or until thickened.

9 Add chocolate; stir until melted.

10 Adjust seasoning with sugar and salt.

# Pozole Blanco White Pozole

SERVES 4–6

**Pozole, a Mexican soup, is made with a special type of corn that has been slaked (soaked) in a solution of lime. The traditional corn used is *maiz blanco* or *cacahuazintle* [kaw-kaw-WAH-SEEN-til]. This is a very large-kerneled white corn grown in Mexico.**

| AMOUNT | MEASURE | INGREDIENT |
|---|---|---|
| | | Water to cover |
| 2 cups | 13 ounces, 364 g | Hominy |
| 1 pound | 16 ounces, 448 g | Pork stew meat, $\frac{1}{2}$ inch (1.2 cm) cubes |
| 1 pound | 16 ounces, 448 g | Pork neck bones |
| 1 | | Pork trotters (optional), cut in 4 pieces |
| 1 cup | 4 ounces, 112 g | White onion, $\frac{1}{2}$ inch (1.2 cm) dice |
| $\frac{1}{4}$ cup | 1 ounce, 28 g | Garlic cloves, minced |
| To taste | | Salt and pepper |
| Garnish | | |
| 2 | | Limes, quartered |
| 2 cups | 4 ounces, 112 g | Lettuce or cabbage, shredded |
| $\frac{1}{2}$ cup | 2 ounces, 56 g | Radishes, washed, sliced thin |
| 1 tablespoon | | Dried oregano |
| 1 tablespoon | | Crumbled chiles piquin or other small, dried hot red chiles |
| 1 cup | 4 ounces, 112 g | White onion, $\frac{1}{4}$ inch (.6) dice |
| 8 | | Corn tortillas, 4 inch, fried crisp |

PROCEDURE

1. Add water to hominy to cover by $\frac{1}{2}$ inch (1.2 cm).
2. Bring to boil and cook until corn kernels start to blossom or "flower" (they will open out at one end).
3. Add all pork items, first quantity of onion, and garlic; cook until pork is tender, adjusting water as needed.
4. Correct seasoning.
5. Arrange lime wedges, shredded lettuce or cabbage, radishes, oregano, chiles, and onions in bowls.
6. Ladle soup over garnish.
7. Serve with fried tortillas.

# Arroz à la Mexicana

## Mexican Rice

SERVES 4–6

| AMOUNT | MEASURE | INGREDIENT |
|---|---|---|
| | | Hot water to cover |
| 1 cup | $6\frac{1}{2}$ ounces, 184 g | Long-grain rice |
| $\frac{1}{4}$ cup | 2 ounces, 56 ml | Vegetable oil |
| 1 cup | 6 ounces, 168 g | Tomato, $\frac{1}{4}$ inch (.6 cm) dice |
| $\frac{1}{4}$ cup | 1 ounce, 28 g | Onions, thinly sliced |
| 1 | | Garlic clove, minced |
| $\frac{1}{4}$ cup | 1 ounce, 28 g | Carrots, $\frac{1}{4}$ inch (.6 cm) dice |
| 2 cups | 16 ounces 470 ml | Chicken stock |
| 2 tablespoons | $\frac{1}{2}$ ounce, 14 g | Green peas, cooked |

PROCEDURE

1. Add hot water to cover rice and soak for 20 minutes.
2. Drain and rinse well in cold water; let drain 10 minutes.
3. Heat oil until smoke point; add rice and stir to cover well with oil.
4. Cook, stirring, until rice is light golden, stirring and turning so the rice cooks evenly. This process should take about 8 minutes and should be done over high heat or the rice will become mushy in its final cooking stage.
5. Blend the tomato, onion, and garlic until smooth; add to the fried rice.
6. Cook until the mixture is dry.
7. Add carrots and chicken stock; cook uncovered over medium heat—do not stir—until the liquid has been absorbed and small air holes appear.
8. Cover rice with a tight lid or aluminum foil to prevent steam from escaping. Let set for 25 minutes.
9. Remove cover; stir in peas.

# Pescado à la Veracruzana

## Fish Veracruz Style

SERVES 4

*Pescado à la Veracruzana* is one of the most famous dishes of Veracruz, which lies on the Caribbean coast of eastern Mexico. This dish shows a strong influence of Spanish cuisine.

**Chef Tip** Be careful with how much salt you add to this dish. The olives and capers will add their own salt to the sauce.

Red snapper is the fish most commonly associated with this dish, but any firm white fish fillet may be used.

| AMOUNT | MEASURE | INGREDIENT |
|---|---|---|
| 4 | 4–6 ounces, 113–1170 g | Fish fillets, boneless white firm flesh |
| 1 tablespoon | $\frac{1}{2}$ ounce, 14 ml | Fresh lime juice |
| 1 teaspoon | 8 g | Salt |
| 2 tablespoons | 1 ounce, 28 ml | Vegetable oil |
| 1 cup | 4 ounces, 112 g | White onion, sliced thin |
| 2 | | Garlic cloves, minced |
| 3 cups | 18 ounces, 508 ml | Tomatoes, peeled, seeded, $\frac{1}{4}$ inch (.6 cm) dice |
| 1 cup | 8 ounces, 224 ml | Fish stock or water |
| $\frac{1}{3}$ cup | 2 ounces, 56 g | Green olives, pitted, sliced thin |
| 2 tablespoon | 6 g | Parsley, minced |
| 1 teaspoon | 1 g | Oregano, dried |
| 1 | | Bay leaf |
| 1 tablespoon | $\frac{1}{2}$ ounce, 14 g | Capers, rinsed, drained |
| 2 | | Jalapeños, seeds and veins removed, sliced thin |
| 1 | | Cinnamon stick |
| 2 | | Whole cloves |
| To taste | | Salt and pepper |
| | | Rice, for serving |

**PROCEDURE**

1. Marinate the fish in the lime juice and salt, 30 minutes to 1 hour.
2. Heat oil over medium heat; add onion and cook until translucent.
3. Add garlic and cook 1 minute.
4. Add remaining ingredients, bring to simmer, and cook 15 minutes until almost sauce consistency.
5. Add fish to tomato sauce, cover with sauce; cover and simmer until fish is cooked.
6. Serve with rice.

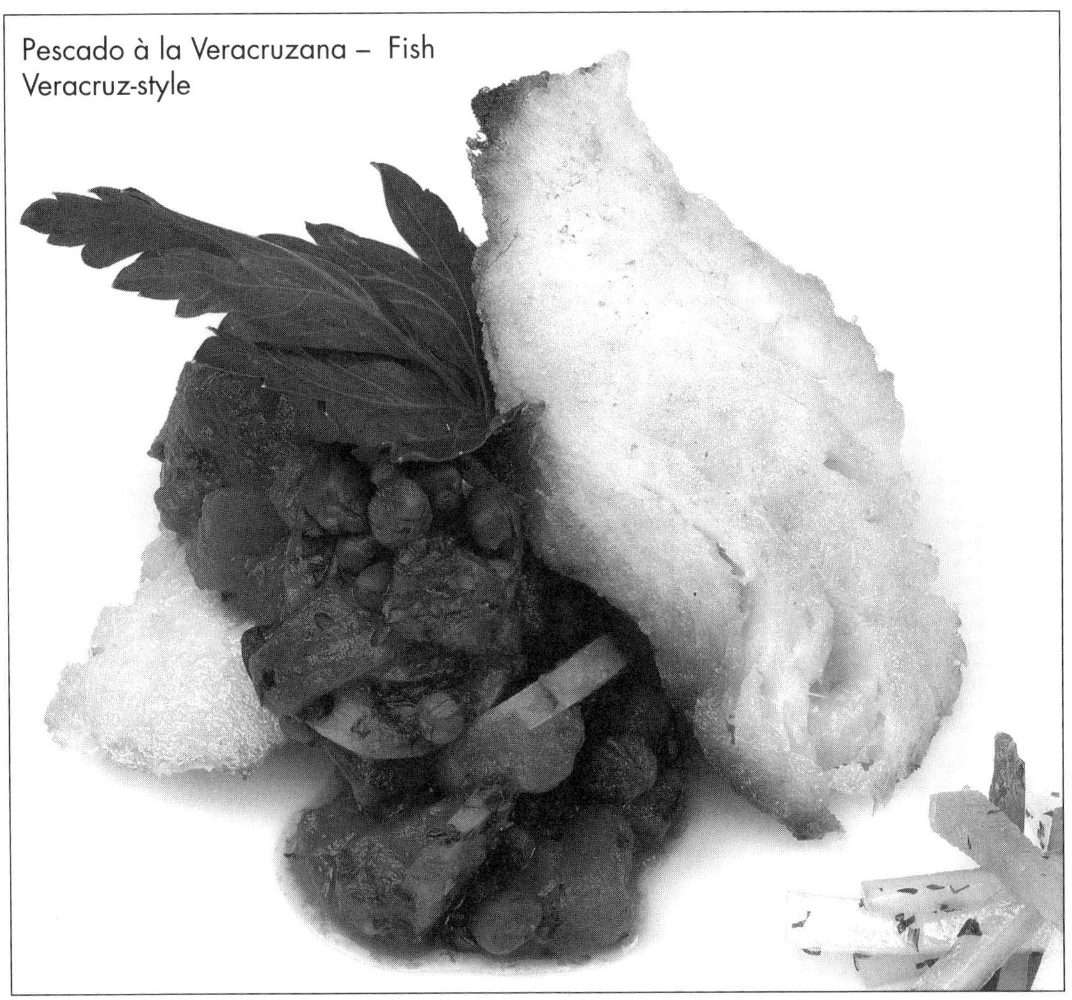
Pescado à la Veracruzana – Fish Veracruz-style

# Jicama Salad

SERVES 4

| AMOUNT | MEASURE | INGREDIENT |
|---|---|---|
| $\frac{1}{2}$ cup | 2 ounces, 56 g | Red bell pepper, julienned |
| $\frac{1}{2}$ cup | 2 ounces, 56 g | Green bell pepper, julienned |
| $\frac{1}{2}$ cup | 2 ounces, 56 g | Yellow bell pepper, julienned |
| $\frac{1}{2}$ cup | 2 ounces, 56 g | Carrot, julienned |
| 2 cups | 8 ounces, 224 g | Jicama, peeled, julienned |
| $\frac{1}{2}$ cup | 3 ounces, 84 g | Cucumber, peeled, seeded, julienned |
| 1 tablespoon | 3 g | Fresh cilantro, minced |
| 1 teaspoon | | Fresh parsley, minced |
| 1 teaspoon | | Fresh chives, minced |
| 2 | | Shallot, minced |
| 1 | | Garlic clove, minced |
| 2 tablespoons | 1 ounce, 28 ml | Vinegar or sherry wine vinegar |
| $\frac{1}{4}$ cup | 2 ounce, 56 ml | Olive oil |
| To taste | | Salt and pepper |

PROCEDURE

1. Combine the first six ingredients.
2. Combine the remaining ingredients and whisk mixture until well incorporated.
3. Toss vegetables with dressing; refrigerate until ready to serve.

# South America

## The Land

South America, the fourth largest continent, contains the world's highest waterfall, Angel Falls; the largest river (by volume), the Amazon River; the longest mountain range, the Andes; the driest desert, Atacama; the largest rain forest, the Amazon rain forest; the highest capital city, La Paz, Bolivia; and the world's southernmost city, Ushuaia, Argentina.

In the high reaches of the Andes Mountains, along the border between Bolivia and Peru, lies one of the highest regions inhabited by people anywhere in the world. Here in the altiplano farmers raise sheep, llamas, and alpacas, as they have for thousands of years. But unlike most farmlands, the altiplano is surrounded by jagged mountains, volcanic peaks that drop steeply down to deserts in some places, to rain forests in others, and on the western side, to the deep trench of the Pacific Ocean. South America is home to some of the planet's largest volcanoes, and in the far south along the coast of Chile, large ice sheets are commonplace.

The Amazon River Basin is roughly the size of the forty-eight contiguous United States and covers some 40 percent of the South American continent. Reflecting environmental conditions as well as past human influence, the Amazon is made up of ecosystems and vegetation types that include rain forests, seasonal forests, deciduous forests, flooded forests, and savannas.

The Eastern Highlands of South America belong to the older geologic period (almost of the same time as that of North America's Appalachian Mountains). The northern section of the Eastern Highlands is known as Guiana Highlands, which consists of a vast plateau marked by deep gorges and tropical rain forests, and is home to Angel Falls. The southern section is known as the Brazilian Highlands and includes several mountain ranges.

Venezuela's rugged Llanos are one of the world's richest tropical grasslands. This large, very fertile plain is located in central and southern Venezuela and eastern and central Colombia. It is drained by the Orinoco River and its many tributaries. This mostly flat, grassy country is teeming with wildlife, including more than 100 species of mammals and over 300 species of birds. Here, a catfish known as the *lau-lau* weighs up to 330 pounds and is considered a culinary delicacy.

*Pampas* is a word of Quechua origin that means "a plain without trees." This flat land is Argentina's agricultural heartland, home of the gaucho (cowboy) and is famed for its many cattle ranches.

Patagonia is the area between the Andes Mountains and the Atlantic Ocean. It stretches south from the Rio Negro River in southern Argentina to Tierra del Fuego and the Strait of Magellan and is one of the less populated regions in the world. Its mostly rugged, barren land is not suitable for extensive farming, but is compatible with sheep raising.

# History

In the sixteenth century, Spanish explorers in the Americas encountered two great civilizations, one in Mesoamerica (the territory controlled by the Aztecs and the Mayas at the time of the conquest) and the other in South America (the territory in the central Andean region under Inca rule). The people of these regions included many tribes and nations, with achievements that included art, cities, and strong foundations of economic, political, and social organization.

The Inca empire, with its capital at Cuzco (in modern-day Peru), covered a large portion of South America in the fifteenth century and the first quarter of the sixteenth century. The empire stretched nearly 2,500 miles down the west coast of South America, and covered coastal desert, high mountains, and low-lying jungle. It covered most of modern-day Peru, part of Ecuador, and Bolivia, northwest Argentina, and the greater part of Chile. To control such a huge area, the Incas built roads, including both mountainous and coastal routes. This road system was key to farming success since it allowed distribution of foodstuffs over long distances. Agriculture was an important part of Incan life and farmers used sophisticated methods of cultivation. By the time of the Spanish conquest, the ancient Americans were some of the greatest plant cultivators in the world. Maize from Mesoamerica and potatoes from the Andes were some of their contributions to the European diet. To get the highest yield from their crops, the Incas used terracing and irrigation methods on hillsides in the highlands. Building terraces meant that they could use more land for cultivation, and it also helped to resist erosion of the land by wind and rain.

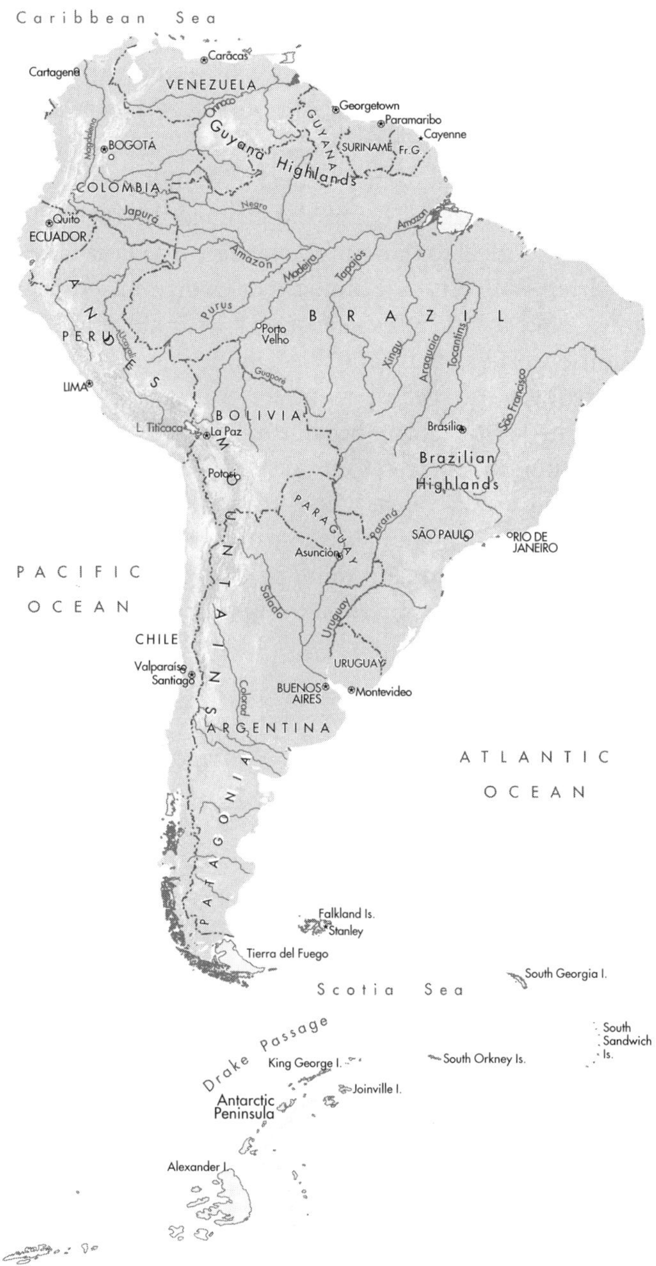


South America

By the sixteenth century, rumors of gold and other riches attracted the Spanish to the area. Spanish conquistadors, led by Francisco Pizarro, explored south from Panama, reaching Inca territory. It was clear that they had reached a wealthy land with prospects of great treasure, and after one more expedition in 1529, Pizarro traveled to Spain and received royal approval to conquer the region and be its viceroy.

Pedros Alvares Cabral set sail from Portugal in 1500 to sail to the eastern side of South America. He arrived on the coast of Brazil and claimed the region for Portugal. Finding the warm climate and rich soil ideal for planting sugarcane, the Portuguese built large plantations and brought slaves from West Africa. Shiploads of Euorpean settlers poured in to make their fortune. Many grew coffee in the rich soil around São Paulo, and Brazil became the foremost coffee producer in the world at that time. Gold mines flourished in the interior, and a new industry to produce rubber emerged up along the Amazon. Cattle ranches sprang up to feed developing mining centers. Brazil soon began exporting coffee, rubber, cocoa, and cattle.

Today these are countries of great contrasts. In each one, there are wealthy and cosmopolitan cities, but there are also areas where many people live in conditions of great poverty. Significant ecological and environmental issues, such as the destruction of the rain forest, loss of plant and animal species, and air and water pollution, are being addressed. Rich in natural resources with growing economies, there is great potential for the future.

## The Food

The inhabitants of the Andean region developed more than half the agricultural products that the world eats today. Among these are more than 20 varieties of corn, 240 varieties of potato, as well as one or more varieties of squash, beans, peppers, peanuts, and cassava (a starchy root). Quinoa (which in the language of Incans means "mother of cereals") is a cereal grain crop domesticated in the high plains area around Lake Titicaca (on the border of Peru and Bolivia).

By far the most important of the crops was the potato. The Incas planted the potato, which is able to withstand heavy frosts, in elevations as high as 15,000 feet. At these heights the Incas could use the freezing night temperatures and the heat of the day to alternately freeze and dry harvested potatoes until all the moisture had been removed. The Incas then reduced the potato to a light flour. Corn could also be grown up to an altitude of 13,500 feet; it was consumed fresh, dried, or popped. They also made it into an alcoholic beverage known as *saraiaka* or *chicha.*

The manioc tuber, or cassava root, was another important staple of the natives. This carbohydrate-rich food was easy to propagate but difficult to process, at least for the bitter variety, which is poisonous when raw. To detoxify manioc, the tubers had to be peeled and grated and the pulp put into long, supple cylinders—called *tipitis*—made of woven plant fibers. Each tube was then hung with a heavy weight at the bottom, which compressed the pulp and expressed the poisonous juice. The pulp could then be removed, washed, and roasted, rendering it safe to eat. The product was toasted into coarse meal or flour known as *farinha de mandioc.* Starch settling out from the extracted juice was heated on a flat surface, causing individual starch grains to pop open and clump together into small, round granules called tapioca. The extracted juice, boiled down to remove the poison, was used as the basis of the sauce known as *tucupi.*

Manioc meal became many things in the hands of the Indian women. Pulverized meal was mixed with ground fish to produce a concoction called *paçoka,* or *paçoca.* For the children, small, sun-dried cakes called *carimã* were prepared. There was a porridge or paste known as *mingau,* and thin, crisp snacks called *beijus,* made of either tapioca flour or dough from a nonpoisonous, or sweet variety of manioc known as *macaxeira* or *aipim.* These sweet manioc tubers, which are somewhat fibrous but considerably easier to prepare, were also pared, boiled for several hours to soften them, and eaten like potatoes.

Soups are an indispensable part of the main meal and frequently are a meal in themselves. Most South American soups originated in European kitchens; a few date back to pre-Hispanic times. In the Andean countries there are the *mazamorroas* or *coladoas,* creamlike soups made with ground dried corn and ground dried beans, quinoa, amaranth, or squash. Variations of this type of soup, called *sangos,* are probably the oldest Indian food. *Sango* was the sacred dish of the Incas. The Spaniards introduced *potajes* (hearty soups), *pucheros* (*pot-au-feu*-type soups), and *cocidos* (meat and vegetables soups) that are popular in the southern countries of South America. Chile, Argentina, Uruguay, Bolivia, and Paraguay have *locros*—thick soups made with hominy, beans, squash, and sweet potatoes. *Chupes,* popular in Bolivia, Chile, Peru, and Ecuador, are stewlike soups prepared with fish, chicken, or other meat along with potatoes, cheese, vegetables, and may include eggs.

## VENEZUELA

Venezuela is located on the northern edge of South America, bordered by Guyana, Brazil, Colombia, and the southern waters of the Caribbean Sea. The explorer Christopher Columbus, on his third voyage sailing from Spain, landed on its coast in 1498. Venezuela declared itself independent of Spain in 1811 but retains a strong Spanish influence.

The country is one of the world's top ten producers of oil, which has helped it to develop its economy. Due to the diversity in the landscape, Venezuela has an ability to grow a wide variety of crops. Its main crop is sugarcane, followed by fruits such as bananas, oranges, pineapple, papayas, strawberries, passion fruit, watermelons, limes, and avocados. Because of its long Caribbean coastline Venezuela is as much a Caribbean country as it is a South American one. Venezuela has a strong fishing industry, famous for sardines, shrimp, clams, mussels, crabs, and tuna.

*Arepas*, thick, flattened balls of fried or baked corn or wheat flour, are the main staple of Venezuelan cuisine. These flatbreads can be filled with meats, cheeses, jelly, or vegetables. Favorite fillings include tuna or chicken salad, shredded beef, or ham and cheese. *Arepas* usually accompany Venezuela's national dish, *pabellon criollo*. This is a hearty dish that includes black beans and shredded beef seasoned with onions, garlic, green peppers, tomatoes, and cilantro. This is served atop a mound of rice alongside a fried egg and strips of fried plantain. White cheese is grated over the top. *Hallaca* is a special dish served only during the holidays. A packet of cornmeal dough is steamed in a wrapping of palm leaves with a filling of pork, chicken, and beef, and mixed with olives, capers, raisins, tomatoes, peppers, nuts, and spices. *Hallaca* were first made by servants trying to use up leftovers from their plantation master's tables. Among the unusual foods in this country are *logarto sancocho* (lizard soup) and fried ants, considered a special treat.

## BRAZIL

Brazil covers nearly half of South America and both the equator and the Tropic of Capricorn run through the country. Brazil is bordered by Argentina, Paraguay, Uruguay, Bolivia, Peru, Colombia, Venezuela, Guyana, Suriname, and French Guiana, as well as the Atlantic Ocean. The country's main regions are the Amazon Basin, the dry northeast where farmers raise cattle, and the southeast, Brazil's most populated region.

Brazil's population is the largest in Latin America and constitutes about half the population of South America. With nearly all of the people living in cities and towns, Brazil is one of the most urbanized and industrialized countries in Latin America. São Paulo and Rio de Janeiro are among the ten largest cities in the world. Yet parts of Brazil's Amazon region, which has some of the world's most extensive wilderness areas, are sparsely inhabited by indigenous peoples who rarely come into contact with the modern world.

Until 1822 the country was a Portuguese colony and even today its official language is Portuguese. The Portuguese and Spanish brought African slaves to South America, and nowhere is their influence stronger than in Brazil. Dendê (palm oil), peppers, okra, and coconut milk, staples of West African cooking, are firmly established on the Brazilian palate. Brazil's national dish, *feijoada* (literally "big bean" stew), is said to have originated during slave times. Originally *feijoada* contained inexpensive and less desirable cuts of meat such as tripe and pigs feet, as slaves had only the leftovers of the master's table for themselves. Today *feijoada* consists of a variety of meats slowly cooked with black beans and condiments. A *feijoada completa*, or "complete feijoada," is accompanied by rice, fresh orange slices, a side dish of peppery onion sauce, chopped greens such as collards, and *farinha* (toasted manioc flour).

The Portuguese influence shows in the rich, sweet egg breads that are served at nearly every meal, and in the seafood dishes that blend assorted seafoods with coconut and other native fruits and vegetables. Seafood stews predominate in the north, while the south is the land of *churrascos*. *Churrasco* is a Brazilian word that means "to barbecue" and stems from the pampas of Brazil, where ranchers cook large portions of marinated meats on long skewers over an open fire pit. The range of barbecued meats includes pork, beef, chicken, goat, and the very special *galinha do coracao*, or chicken hearts. The meats are cut straight from the skewer with large butcher knives directly onto the plate. They make great use of their rich assortment of tubers, squash, and beans. Manioc is at the heart of Brazilian vegetable consumption. It is the "flour" of the region, and is eaten in one form or another at nearly every meal. Brazilian food, unlike the cuisines of many of the surrounding countries, favors the sweet rather than the hot.

## THE GUIANAS

Guyana (formerly British Guiana), Suriname (formerly Dutch Guiana), and French Guiana (an overseas department of France) are situated in northeastern South America. Together they are called the Guianas and the influences are varied.

The Dutch were among the first to settle in Guyana. With the Dutch, many Germans and Austrians also settled in the area, which added to the cuisine of this region. Peas, rice, and bread are staples in the diet of many Guyanese. Locally grown vegetables such as manioc, plantains, and breadfruit are widely consumed, but are available only in season. A popular festive food is *cook-up*, which is any kind of meat prepared in coconut milk and served with rice and beans. There are influences from India and many traditional dishes are very spicy, made with curries and habanero peppers, or Scotch bonnet, which is native to the region.

Suriname is more prosperous than Guyana and has a diversity of ethnic influences. The Indonesian population has contributed a number of spicy meat and vegetable side dishes, including *nasi goring* (fried rice) and *bami goring* (fried noodles). From the Creole population has come *pom* (ground tayer roots, which are a relative of the cassava, mixed with poultry), and *pastei* (chicken pie with vegetables). The African influence is found in the popular peanut soup.

French Guiana is the only remaining nonindependent country on the South American mainland. The French used it as a penal colony between 1852 and 1939, and it is the location of the infamous Devil's Island. In 1947 it became an overseas department of France. It is governed by French law and the French constitution, and enjoys French customs, currency, and holidays. Most of the food here is imported and people in French Guiana enjoy an international cuisine, including Chinese, Vietnamese, and Indonesian dishes.

## COLOMBIA

Located in the northwest corner of South America, Columbia is the only country in South America with both Caribbean and Pacific coastlines. Colombia also shares its borders with Panama, Venezuela, Brazil, Peru, and Ecuador. Coffee is Colombia's leading agricultural crop. With its two coastlines, seafood makes a major impact on the cuisine, along with chicken, pork, potatoes, rice, beans, and soup. Columbia's cuisine also has a strong Spanish influence. Interesting regional dishes include *ajiaco*, a specialty from Bogota that is a potato-based soup accompanied by chicken and maize and served with cream, capers, and chunks of avocado; the famous *hormiga culona*, a large ant that is fried and eaten; and *lechona*, a whole suckling pig, spit-roasted and stuffed with rice, which is a specialty of Tolima.

### ECUADOR

This county's name comes from the Spanish word meaning "equator" as it sits directly on the equator. It is bordered by Colombia, Peru, and the Pacific Ocean and includes the Galápagos Islands. Ecuador is renowned for its *ceviche*, made with bitter orange juice and chilies. Afro-Ecuadorians along the northern coast enjoy seafood seasoned with coconut milk. Peanuts and bananas are found on the lower-coastal regions. Corn and potato pancakes and soups, as well as grilled *cuy* (guinea pig), are popular further inland along the Andes. Ecuador is also known for its fabulous exotic fruits that include cherimoya (custard apple), physalis (cape gooseberry), tamarillo (tree tomato), babaco (mountain papaya), granadilla (passion fruit), baby bananas, and red bananas. There is also high-quality fish and seafood, and the countless varieties of Andean potatoes. Across the country national and regional dishes include lemon-marinated shrimp, toasted corn, and pastries stuffed with spiced meats. The core of the Ecuadorian diet is rice, potatoes, and meat (beef and chicken throughout the country and pork in the Sierra region). Foods are cooked in *achiote* oil or lard. *Refrito*, a fried mixture containing chopped onions, green peppers, tomato, *achiote*, and salt and/or garlic, is added to many cooked dishes. Meats are often seasoned with a spicy *aji* sauce. The *aji* sauce (made from a spicy red pepper) is a national delicacy and is found on most tables. Ecuador's specialties are fresh soups such as *Locro* soup (cheese, avocado, and potato). *Fanesca* is a soup made of many ingredients including twelve different grains and salted cod served during Lent. Other popular dishes include *lomo salteado* (thin sliced steak, covered with onions and tomatoes) and *chocio* (grilled Andean corn) sold by street vendors.

### PERU

Peru, just south of the equator, is located on the western coast of South America. It is bordered by Ecuador, Colombia, Brazil, Bolivia, Chile, and the Pacific Ocean. East of the dry coastal plain of Peru lie the Andes Mountains, which contain active volcanoes and high plateaus between the ranges. East of the Andes are plains covered by rain forests.

This "land of the Incas" is the world's potato capital, with more than three hundred varieties and colors (including purple, blue, yellow, and shades of brown to pink), as well as various sizes, textures, and flavors. This tuber, in addition to rice, chicken, pork, lamb, and fish, comprise the basic ingredient from which most Peruvian dishes originate. Most corn and beans cannot grow in the Andes Mountains because of the cold and the short growing season; thus, the potato was the main staple grown by the Incas and Indians. The Indians also grew quinoa and the grain *kiwicha,* which grows at high altitudes and produces small seeds that are very rich in protein. These were used by the Incas to supplement their diet. The areas surrounding the Pacific Ocean, the Amazon River, and Lake Titicaca have abundant seafood and turtles. *Ceviche* comes in many variations, and is typically served with boiled potato, sweet potato, or *cancha* (toasted corn kernels). Meats are served in a variety of ways. *Butifarras* is a sandwich with Peruvian ham and spicy sauce. *Carapulcra* is a stew made with pork, chicken, yellow potatoes, chiles, peanuts, and cumin. *Aji de gallina* is a peppery chicken served in a creamy, yellow, spicy nut-based sauce. *Seco de cabrito* is goat marinated with *chichi de jora* (a fermented maize drink) or beer, cilantro, and garlic. *Chaiona* is cured lamb, alpaca, or llama. Grilled or fried guinea pig (*cuy*) is a favorite in the highlands. The cuisine's flavor is spicy and sweet and it varies by region. Some Peruvian chile peppers are not spicy but give color to sauces. In Peru rice production is significant and today rice often accompanies Peruvian dishes rather than potatoes.

### BOLIVIA

The landlocked country of Bolivia is located in west-central South America and is bordered by Peru, Brazil, Paraguay, Argentina, and Chile. Due to the number of mountains with elevations of 18,000 to 20,000 feet, many people refer to the country as the "Tibet of the Americas." The portion of the Andes Mountains that runs through Bolivia includes some of the highest peaks and most remote regions found anywhere in South America. Lake Titicaca and surrounding streams and rivers offer fresh trout and other fishes. Bolivia is known for its *saltenas* and *empanadas,* which are meat or vegetable pies. Other traditional dishes include *majao,* a rice dish with eggs, beef, and fried banana; *silpancho,* meat served with rice and potatoes; and *pacumutu,* a rice dish with grilled beef, fried yuca, and cheese. Spicy sauces and condiments made with ajis are served with stews and soups such as *chairo* (with cured lamb or alpaca), *chuno* (freeze-dried potatoes), or *saice* (meat soup with onions and tomatoes). Bolivian beer is popular, but the most favored local drink is *chicha cochabambina,* a very potent alcohol made from corn.

### PARAGUAY

Although landlocked, Paraguay is bordered and crisscrossed by navigable rivers. Corn and manioc are the cornerstones of the cuisine in Paraguay. Other principal food crops include beans, peanuts, sorghum, sweet potatoes, and rice. Many types of beans are grown in Paraguay, including lima beans, French beans, and peas. The most popular dishes are based on corn, meat, milk, and cheese. *Yerba mate* is a national drink made from the green dried leaves and stemlets of the tree *Ilex paraguarensis* and is an important ritualistic process among the people of Paraguay and Argentina. It is served in a hollow gourd that is filled two-thirds of the way with the moistened mate herb. Hot water is then poured into the gourd. The person sucks the *mate* water out of the gourd with a *bombilla* (a metal filter straw with a strainer at the end, which can range from the functional to the elaborately crafted). When the water is gone, the gourd is refilled by the server with hot water and passed to the next person in the group. When that person finishes, the gourd is handed back to the server for another refill and this rotating process of sharing is what makes the act of mate drinking a moment of intimacy for those present. *Yerba mate* is supposed to have powers that include mental stimulation, fatigue reduction, and stress reduction. Another local drink preferred by Paraguayans is locally produced dark rum made from sugarcane.

## CHILE

More than 2600 miles long and only 110 miles at its widest point, the terrain of Chile ranges from the desert in the north to the Antarctic in the south. Chile is located on the western coast of South America and bordered by Argentina, Bolivia, and Peru, as well as the Pacific Ocean. Chile's agriculture is well established in North American and European supermarkets, with major exports of fruit and wine. Spanish priests first introduced vines to Chile in the sixteenth century because they needed wine for religious celebrations. Vines were planted in the central valley around Santiago and grew well. In the 1850s, the Spanish vines were replaced by French varieties and winemaking became a serious industry. Historically, Chile has grown mostly the Cabernet Sauvignon grape, but recent successes with Merlot, Carmenere, and Syrah grapes make a wider range of wines available. Muscatel grapes are grown in the northern region, but mainly for the production of *pisco*, the national drink. During the nineteenth century, the newly independent government sought to stimulate European immigration. Beginning in 1845, it had some success in attracting primarily German migrants to the Chilean south, principally to the lake district. For this reason, that area of the country still shows a German influence in its architecture and cuisine, and German (peppered with archaic expressions and intonations) is still spoken by some descendants of these migrants.

Because of its location in the Southern Hemisphere, the fruits grown there are ready for export in the Northern Hemisphere's winter season. Fruits exported to the United States include apples, avocados, peaches, nectarines, kiwifruits, plums, pears, blueberries, and cherries, and the main vegetables are garlic, asparagus, and onions.

A typical Chilean dish is *cazuela de ave*, a thick stew of chicken, potatoes, rice, green peppers, and, occasionally, onions. *Humitas* are a national favorite, and they come from the Amerindians who are native to Chile. Humitas are made with grated fresh corn, mixed into a paste with fried onions, basil, salt, and pepper. The mixture is then wrapped in corn husks and cooked in boiling water.

Chile's long coastline makes it a natural for seafood such as abalone, eel, scallops, turbot, king crab, sea urchin, and algae. The Juan Fernadez Islands are known for their huge lobsters. Seafood is an ingredient prepared in almost every technique, including stews, *ceviches*, *escabeches*, or snacks with potatoes, corn, squash, and other vegetables. Many of Chile's lamb dishes, such as lamb ribs or lamb shish kebabs, as well as baked deer dishes and cakes, stem from Welsh influence. Chile's most distinctive desserts trace their origins to the southern lake region, where German immigrants left a legacy of *kuchen*—a delicious pastry loaded with fresh fruits like raspberries and apricots. A more common Chilean pastry is the *alfajor*, which consists of *dulce de leche* (caramelized milk) sandwiched between thin pastries and rolled in powdered sugar. Another favorite is *macedonia*, diced fruit with a fruit syrup topping. There is also *arroz con leche*, or chilled rice with milk, sugar, and cinnamon. *Semola con leche* is a flan made of sweet corn flour topped with caramel.

## ARGENTINA

Argentina, which means "land of silver," is a rich and vast land—the second largest country (after Brazil) in South America and eighth largest in the world. Located in southern South America, it is bordered by Chile, Bolivia, Paraguay, Brazil, Uruguay, and the Atlantic Ocean.

Argentina's heartland is a broad grassy plain known as the Pampas. The cuisine has been influenced by waves of European immigration. Italian immigrants have had considerable influence, and Italian standards like lasagna, pizza, pasta, and ravioli are commonly seen on the Argentine table, at least in the country's major cities.

Argentina is the beef capital of the world. The rich grassland of the Pampas are home to cattle and sheep, raised by gauchos (Argentine cowboys). The national dish is *matambre*, made from thin flank steak rolled with fillings that include spinach, whole hard-boiled eggs, other vegetables, herbs, and spices. The steak is then tied with a string and either poached in broth or baked. Its name is derived from *mata hambre*, which means "kill your hunger." Probably the most famous Argentine dish is the *parrillada*, a mixed grill plate of different meats and sausages (chorizos). The meat is cooked on a very large grill called a *parilla*. Spit roasting is also very popular. For this the meat to be roasted is placed on spits that look like swords and are placed tip down into and around hot coals. Classic Argentinean cuisine includes *chimichurri* sauce (a cross between Mexican salsa and Italian vinaigrette) and the empanada. Here tortillas are made with potato dough, in contrast to the traditional Mexican corn or flour tortilla.

Argentina is the world's fifth largest producer of wine. The grape varieties are almost entirely of European derivation: Chardonnay, Riesling, Cabernet Sauvignon, Merlot, and Malbec are only a few of some 60 different varieties cultivated. Almost 75 percent of the total wine production originates in the province of Mendoza found in the Andean foothills. Mendoza cultivates its vines on desert flatlands made fertile by irrigated water, which descends from the Andes. Although made from European grapes, Argentine wines have their own flavor because of the climate and soil conditions and irrigation methods. There are two varieties that can be considered exclusively Argentinean in quality if not in origin. The first is Malbec, a grape not considered particularly distinguished in France, but considered by many in Argentina to make fine red wine. The second is the Torrontes, a grape of Spanish origin, which makes a full, fruity, rich white wine.

### URUGUAY

Uruguay is located on the southeastern coast of South America, bordered by Brazil, Argentina, and the Atlantic Ocean. It is a land of grassy plains and hills. Sheep and cattle ranches make up 80 percent of the land. Uruguayan cuisine is the result of many influences, including gaucho, Spanish, and Italian. In Uruguay, food and meat are almost synonymous. Most restaurants in Uruguay are *parrillada* (grill-rooms), which specialize in *asado* (barbecued beef), the country's most famous dish. Besides beef, pork, sausage, and grilled chicken are popular. *Chivito* (a sandwich filled with slices of meat, lettuce, and egg) and *puchero* (beef with vegetables, bacon, beans, and sausages) are local favorites. With the arrival of large numbers of Italian immigrants in the twentieth century, many businesses opened by Italians were pasta-making factories. They also imported Parmesan cheese and prosciutto ham into Uruguay and these foods have made their way into the national cuisine.

## Glossary

**Aji (a'hee)** Spicy chili or seasoning: very hot Andean chili pepper, malagueta.

**Aji Caco de Cabra** Fresh red pepper, long, thin, and very hot, used to make Chile hot pepper sauce.

**Ají de Gallina** Shredded chicken in a piquant cream sauce (Peru).

**Aji Mirasol, aji Amarillo** A common pepper in Peruvian and Bolivian cuisine, bright yellow and hot.

**Aji Verde** Milder variety of *aji caco de cabra*, with a thicker flesh and a waxy, lime green skin. Used in Chile to make condiments.

**Alfajores** Wafer-thin spirals of shortbread dusted with icing sugar, served with *manjar blanco* (a caramel sauce) (Peru).

**Amaranth** Tiny ancient seeds cultivated in the Americas for several millennia. One of the staple grains of the Incas and other pre-Columbian Indians. They are rich in protein and calcium, and have a pleasant, peppery flavor. Substitutes: millet, quinoa, buckwheat groats.

**Anticuchos** Strips of beef or fish marinated in vinegar and spices, then barbecued on skewers (Peru).

**Arepa Flour** A precooked corn flour used to make *arepas* and tamales in Colombia and Venezuela. It has a grainy texture. It should not be confused with Mexican *masa harina*.

**Arepas** The native bread made from primitive ground corn, water, and salt (Venezuela).

**Arroz Brasileiro or *Arroz Simples*** Rice, Brazilian style. Long-grained rice briefly sautéed in garlic and oil before the addition of boiling water. In addition to garlic, some Brazilian cooks add small amounts of onion, diced tomato, or sliced black olives for additional flavor. Properly done, each grain is fluffy and separate from others.

**Asada (Asado)** Spanish for roasted or broiled. A roast cooked on an open fire or grill. Often served with chimichurri sauce.

**Asador** A Spanish word for a wire-mesh stovetop grill that can be used to roast vegetables over an outdoor fire or on the stovetop.

**Babaco** A member of the papaya family. Looks like a papaya but is smaller in diameter and has a tougher skin. The fruit has a delicate white flesh and seeds that are like those of passion fruit.

**Bacalao** Dried, salted codfish. Introduced by Spanish and Portuguese settlers, it is very popular in Latin America. The whiter *bacalao* is the better quality.

**Batida** These tropical fruits cocktails are a mixture of fresh fruit juice and *cachaça*, the potent sugarcane liquor from Brazil. Sometimes the recipe will also call for *leite condensado* (sweetened condensed milk) and/or other liquor. They are usually prepared in a blender and served with crushed ice in tiny glasses.

**Bedidas Calientes** Hot beverages. Hot drinks are as common as cold ones in South America.

**Bouillon d'Aoura** A dish of smoked fish, crab, prawns, vegetables, and chicken served with aoura (the fruit of Savana trees) (French Guiana).

**Breadfruit** Resembling a melon with bumpy green scales, breadfruit weighs 2 to 4 pounds. When green, it tastes like a raw potato. When partially ripened, it resembles eggplant and has the sticky consistency of a ripe plantain. When fully ripe it has the texture of soft Brie cheese. It is cooked like potatoes and is never eaten raw.

**Café** Coffee.

**Café con Leche** Coffee with warm milk, the preferred South American style.

**Camarao Seco** Dried shrimp. In various sizes, dried shrimp are utilized in many dishes. Before use they are covered with cold water and soaked overnight. The water is discarded before the shrimp are used. The residual salt is usually enough that more is not added to a recipe.

**Carbonada** An Argentine stew with meats, vegetables, and fruits.

**Cassava** People in Hispanic countries use cassavas much like Americans use potatoes. There are sweet and bitter varieties of cassava. The sweet can be eaten raw, but the bitter variety requires cooking to destroy the harmful prussic acid it contains. Cassava played a major role in the expansion by Spanish and Portuguese explorers. Cassava could be prepared in large quantities, it was cheap, and it kept well. Explorers also exported cassava to Africa, the Philippines, and Southeast Asia, where it has become a significant ingredient in those regions' cuisines. It's often best to buy frozen cassava, since the fresh kind is hard to peel. Look for it in Hispanic markets. Unprepared cassava doesn't store well, so use it within a day or two of purchase. Malanga, dasheen, or potato (not as gluey) can be used as substitutes.

**Cau Cau** Tripe cooked with potato, peppers, and parsley (Peru).

**Cazuela** A stew made with beef, chicken, or seafood along with various vegetables.

**Ceviche** Marinated foods, also spelled *seviche* or *cebiche.*

**Cheese (Quesos)**

**Queso Blanco or Queso Fresco** (white cheese) The primary cheese used in South America. A fresh, moist, lightly salted, unripened cheese made from cow's milk.

**Quesillo** A cheese used the same day it is made or within a few days. *Quesillo* is refreshing, similar to ricotta cheese, but it is molded and can be cut into slices. For crumbling use *queso fresco.*

**Queso Blanco** Also called *queso de mesa.* A firmer cheese because it is pressed and left to mature for weeks. In areas of South American, *queso blanco* comes in various degrees of maturation, from ricotta type to hard cheese.

**Queso de Cabra** Goat cheese.

**Cherimoya** A species of *Annona* native to the Andean-highland valleys of Peru, Ecuador, Colombia, and Bolivia. The fruit is fleshy, soft and sweet, white in color, with a custard-like texture, which gives it its secondary name, custard apple. Some characterize the flavor as a blend of pineapple, mango, and strawberry. Similar in size to a grapefruit, it has large, glossy, dark seeds that are easily removed. The seeds are poisonous if crushed open; one should also avoid eating the skin. It is green when ripe and gives slightly to pressure, similar to the avocado.

**Chichas** Beerlike drink made from many types of seeds, roots, or fruits, such as quinoa, peanuts, grapes, oca, yuca, corn, rice, and the berries of the mulli tree (pink peppercorns).

**Chimichurri Sauce** Vinegar-based mixture of herbs, vegetables, and spices, traditionally used as the marinade or main sauce with grilled meats (Argentina).

**Chocolate** A preparation made from cocoa seeds that have been roasted, husked, and ground. Chocolate today is often sweetened and flavored with vanilla. Aztec king Montezuma drank 50 goblets a day in the belief that it was an aphrodisiac.

# Ceviche, Seviche, or Cebiche

## MARINATED FOODS

*Ceviche* is seafood prepared in a centuries-old method of cooking by contact with the acidic juice of citrus juice instead of heat. *Ceviche* dates back to the Incas, who seasoned fish with sea salt and *aji* (chile peppers) and cured it in the acidic juice of *tumbo*, a tart tropical fruit. Ceviche's origin is somewhat disputed—either the invention of the pre-Columbians who, food historians tell us, ate their raw fish laced with dried chiles, salt, and foraged herbs; or ceviche as we know it was the creation of Moorish cooks who were brought to South America as Spanish slaves, and who, it is believed, were responsible for the addition of citrus juice to the earlier cooks' traditional salt/spice/herb mix. Traditionally, the citrus marinade was made with *naranja agria* (sour or bitter orange); however, today lemon, lime, and orange juices are used to prepare most ceviche. It can be eaten as a first course or main dish, depending on what is served with it.

Every Latin American country has given ceviche its own touch of individuality by adding particular garnishes. In Peru, it is served on lettuce leaves, without the marinade, garnished with slices of cold sweet potatoes, corn-on-the-cob, slices of hard-cooked egg and cheese, with a bowl of *cancaha* (toasted dried corn) on the side. Peruvians also prefer ceviche spicy. In Ecuador, the hot sauce is normally served on the side, the marinade is served in small bowl, and the ceviche is accompanied by popcorn, French bread, or *cancaha* (toasted dried corn). In Mexico, ceviche is accompanied by slices of raw onions and served on toasted tortillas.

The most famous ceviche comes from Ecuador and Peru, and Ecuadorian ceviche may enjoy the reputation of being the best in South America. In Peru and Ecuador, ceviches are popular snack foods. Ceviche can be made with just about any type of seafood: fish, shrimp, scallops, clams, mussels, squid, langostinos, or lobster. The common denominators among the countries are the lemon and lime juices used as the basis for the marinade. The acid in the marinade "cooks" the fish. Depending on the type of fish and the thickness of the pieces, this "cooking" takes anywhere from three to six hours. Shellfish is usually cooked or blanched first before adding to the marinade.

Colombian ceviches use citrus juices and tomato sauce for the marinade and are served on lettuce leaves, as in Peru. Colombians also have a unique ceviche made with coconut milk, an African contribution.

**Chuchoca** Corn that is boiled and sun-dried for two to three days.

**Chupe de Camarones** Chowder-type soup made with shrimp, milk, eggs, potatoes, and peppers (Peru).

**Churrascaria** A Brazilian or Portuguese steakhouse.

**Cochayuyo** Seaweed found along the coast of Chile; very important in the Chilean diet.

**Cocoa** The fruit of the cocoa plant. These beans are fermented, dried, roasted, cracked, and ground. After extracting half the fat, it is again dried into unsweetened cocoa. Dutch cocoa is treated with alkali to neutralize acidity.

**Coconut Cream** Made by combining one part water and four parts shredded fresh or desiccated coconut meat and simmering until foamy. The coconut is then discarded. It is particularly used in curry dishes.

**Coconut Milk** Made by combining equal parts water and shredded fresh or desiccated coconut meat and simmering until foamy. The coconut is then discarded. It is particularly used in curry dishes.

**Coconut Water** The opaque white liquid in the unripe coconut that serves as a beverage for those living near the coconut palm.

**Corvina** Sea bass.

**Creole** Style of cooking melding Incan and Spanish culinary techniques and ingredients.

**Dendê Oil (Palm Oil)** A form of edible vegetable oil obtained from the fruit of the oil palm tree.

**Dulce de Leche** Caramel-like candy popular in Argentina, Brazil, Chile, Paraguay, Peru, Uruguay, and other parts of the Americas. Its most basic recipe mixes boiled milk and sugar, or it may also be prepared with sweetened condensed milk cooked for several hours.

**Empanada Salteña** A Bolivian national specialty that is a mixture of diced meat, chicken, chives, raisins, diced potatoes, hot sauce, and pepper baked in dough.

**Ensaladas** Salads. The most popular salads are cooked vegetable salads and those that include fresh beans. A common characteristic of South American salads is the sparse use of dressing.

Tossed salad (*ensalada mixta*) is generally made with lettuce and tomatoes, thinly sliced onions, shredded carrots, radishes, or watercress and usually tossed with oil and vinegar. South American cuisines also include main course salads, seasoned with a vinaigrette or a mayonnaise dressing (popular in the southern countries, especially during hot months). Potato and rice salads, simple or complex, can be found throughout South America.

**Escabeches** Escabeches is a very popular technique of pickling food used throughout South America. The technique is of Arab origin introduced by Spanish explorers and traders, adopted as a way of preserving foods, such as fish, poultry, meat, and vegetables.

**Fritada** Called *chicharron* in the areas around the Andes, usually made with different cuts of pork. In Argentina it is made with beef. This dish requires the meat to be cooked in beer until tender and then browned in its own fat.

**Guinea Pigs** Called *cuy* or *curi* in the Andean regions, these vegetarian rodents are raised for food in native Indian homes.

**Hallaca** Cornmeal combined with beef, pork, ham, and green peppers, wrapped in individual pieces of banana leaves and cooked in boiling water. Traditionally eaten at Christmas and New Year's (Colombia and Venezuela).

**Hearts of Palm** Tender, ivory-colored buds of a particular palm tree. They can be used in salads, soups, as a vegetable, or with *ceviche.*

**Ilajhua** A hot sauce consisting of tomatoes and pepper pods, used to add spice and flavor (Bolivia).

**Jugos** Fruit juice drinks that can be made from any fruit mixed with water and sugar.

**Kaniwa** A nutritious grain that grows at high altitudes, thriving in places where quinoa cannot survive. A prominent early grain used by the Indians of Bolivia and the Peruvian altiplano.

**Lingüica** Brazilian garlic pork sausage of Portuguese origin. Polish sausage may be substituted.

**Llapingachos** Pancakes stuffed with mashed potato and cheese (Ecuador).

**Lomo Montado** Fried tenderloin steak with two fried eggs on top, rice, and fried banana (Bolivia).

**Malagueta** Small green, yellow, or red pepper from Brazil. This pepper is extremely hot and an essential ingredient in the kitchen. They come preserved in jars or as a table sauce. They are pickled in a 2:1 oil to grain alcohol ratio and then rested for one month before using. Tabasco sauce can be used as a substitute.

**Manioc (see Cassava)**

**Manioc Flour** Widely used in Brazil as a breading for chicken. Manioc is not a grain; it comes from the tropical cassava root. When seasoned with spices, roasted manioc flour has a texture and flavor similar to a cornflake crumb breading.

**Matambre** Rolled stuffed flank steak (Argentina).

# Empanadas

**In Spain, Portugal, the Caribbean, Latin America, and the Philippines, an empanada (Portuguese empada) is basically a stuffed pastry. The name comes from the Spanish verb *empanar*, meaning to wrap or coat in bread. Empanadas are also known by a wide variety of regional names.**

**It is likely that the Latin American empanadas were originally from Galicia, Spain, where an empanada is prepared similar to a pie that is cut in pieces, making it a portable and hearty meal for working people. The Galician empanada is usually prepared with codfish or chicken. The addition of the empanada to the cuisine may be due to the influence of the Moors, who occupied Spain for eight hundred years. Middle Eastern cuisine to this day has similar foods, like simbusak (a fried, chickpea-filled "empanada") from Iraq.**

**Varieties by Country**

| | |
|---|---|
| **Argentina** | **The filling is ground beef, perhaps spiced with cumin and with onion, green olive, chopped boiled egg, and even raisins. While empanadas are usually baked, they can also be fried. They may also contain cheese, ham and cheese, chicken, tuna, *humita* (sweet corn with bechamel sauce) or spinach; a fruit filling is used to create a dessert empanada. Empanadas of the interior can be spiced with peppers. In restaurants where several types are served, a *repulgue*, or pattern, is added to the pastry fold. These patterns, which can be quite elaborate, distinguish the filling.** |
| **Bolivia** | **Widely known as *salteÃas* (after an Argentine province bordering the country to the south), they are made with beef or chicken and usually contain potatoes, peas, and carrots. They are customarily seamed along the top of the pastry and are generally sweeter than the Chilean variety.** |
| **Brazil** | **Empanadas are a common ready-to-go lunch item available at fast-food counters. A wide variety of different fillings and combinations are available, with the most common being chicken, beef, shrimp, cheese, olives, and palmito (heart of palm).** |
| **Chile** | **The dough for these empanadas is wheat flour based, but the meat filling is slightly different and often contains more onion. There are two types of Chilean empanadas: baked and fried. The baked empanadas are much larger than the fried variety. There are three main types of fillings: *pino*, cheese, and seafood. *Pino* contain chopped (or sometimes minced) meat, onion, chopped boiled egg, olives, and raisins. Fried empanadas containing shrimp and cheese are prevalent along the coastal areas. Seafood empanadas are essentially the same as *pino*, but with seafood instead of meat. Sweet empanadas, sugarcoated and filled with jam, are popular during September 18 Independence Day celebrations.** |
| **Colombia** | **Empanadas are either baked or fried. Fillings can vary according to the region, but they usually contain ingredients such as salt, rice, beef or ground beef, boiled potatoes, hard-boiled eggs, and peas. However, variations can also be found (cheese empanadas, chicken-only empanadas, and even *trucha*—trout—empanadas). The pastry is mostly corn based, although potato flour is commonly used. They are usually served with *aji* (*picante*), a sauce made of cilantro, green onions, vinegar, salt, lemon juice, and bottled hot sauces.** |

| | |
|---|---|
| **Cuba** | **These empanadas are typically filled with seasoned meats (usually ground beef or chicken) folded into dough and deep-fried. These are not to be confused with Cuban *pastelitos*, which are very similar but use lighter pastry dough and may or may not be fried. Cubans eat empanadas at any meal, but usually during lunch or as a snack.** |
| **Dominican Republic** | **Very similar in preparation and consumption as Cuban empanadas, but modern versions, promoted by some specialty food chains, include stuffing like pepperoni and cheese, conch, Danish cheese, and chicken. A variety in which the dough is made from cassava flour is called *catibías*.** |
| **Iraq** | **Iraq has a traditional "ancestor" to the empanada called *simbusak* or *sambusac*, prepared with a basic bread dough and a variety of fillings, baked or fried. The most traditional simbusak is filled with garbanzo beans, onions, and parsley, and shallow fried. Others have meat or cheese (*jibun*) as a filling.** |
| **Mexico** | **Mexican empanadas are most commonly a dessert or a breakfast item. Sweetened fillings include pumpkin, yams, sweet potato, and cream, as well as a wide variety of fruit fillings. Meat, cheese, and vegetable fillings are not as popular. Particular regions such as Hidalgo are famous for their empanadas.** |
| **Peru** | **Peruvian empanadas are similar to Argentine empanadas, but slightly smaller and eaten with lime juice.** |
| **Philippines** | **Filipino empanadas usually contain a filling flavored with soy sauce and consisting of ground beef or chicken, chopped onion, and raisins in a wheat flour dough. Empanadas in the northern Ilocos region are made of a savory filling of green papaya and, upon request, chopped Ilocano sausage (*longganisa*) and/or an egg. Rather than the soft, sweet dough favored in the Tagalog region, the dough is thin and crisp, mostly because Ilocano empanada is deep-fried rather than baked.** |
| **Portugal** | **In Portugal, empanadas are a common option for a small meal, found universally in patisseries. They are normally smaller than others, about the size of a golf ball; size and shape vary depending on establishment. The most common fillings are chicken, beef, tuna, codfish, or mushrooms, and vegetables. They are usually served hot.** |
| **Puerto Rico and the Dominican Republic** | **Puerto Rican empanadas, called *pastelillos*, are made of flour dough and fried. Fillings are typically ground beef, chicken, guava, cheese, or both guava and cheese.** |
| **Venezuela** | **Venezuelan empanadas use cornstarch-based dough and are deep-fried. Stuffing varies according to region; most common are cheese and ground beef. Other types use fish, *caraotas negras* (black beans), oysters, clams, and other types of seafood popular in the coastal areas, especially in Margarita Island.** |

**Milanesas** Breaded cutlets brought to South America by Italian immigrants. They are especially popular in Argentina and Uruguay.

**Morcilla Dulce** Sweet black sausage made from blood, orange peel, and walnuts.

**Pabellón Criollo** Hash made with shredded meat and served with fried plantains and black beans on rice (Venezuela).

**Pachamanca** Typical dish from the desert. It consists of lamb, pork, potatoes, sweet potatoes, and tamales. The food is placed inside a sack and buried in hot rocks to cook. It has to be repeatedly checked to see when it is done because the temperature is unstable. An important part of Peruvian cuisine.

**Parrillada** A selection of meat grilled over hot coals, often including delicacies such as intestines, udders, and blood sausages (Argentina and Chile).

**Postres y Dulces (Desserts and Sweets)** Before the arrival of the Portuguese in 1502, South America Indians did not have sugar. They did have honey and a few fruit and vegetable sweeteners. Most early sweets or desserts were fresh fruit, and fruit-based sweets remain the South Americans' favorite desserts.

**Quimbolitos** Sweet tamales of Ecuador, served for dessert or as a snack with coffee.

**Quinoa** This ancient seed was a staple of the Incas. It cooks quickly, has a mild flavor, and a slightly crunchy texture. High in the amino acid lysine, it provides a more complete protein than many other cereal grains. It comes in different colors, ranging from pale yellow to red to black. Rinse quinoa before using to remove its bitter natural coating. Couscous, rice, bulgur, millet, buckwheat groats, or amaranth can be substituted.

**Refrescos (Refreshments)** A term used for all cold nonalcoholic beverages, including *jugos*, sorbets, *licuados*, and *batidos*, all of which are generally made with milk and sometimes ice cream.

**Rocoto** Cultivated pepper in the Andes, with a thick flesh similar to bell pepper. It is a hotter pepper than other *ajies*. The Mexican *manzano* pepper, though much hotter, is a good substitute.

**Rose Water** A flavoring used in the preparation of desserts. Brought over by the Spaniards, it is the extract of roses mixed with distilled water.

**Shrimp, Dried** Tiny shrimp that have been salted and dried, used extensively in Bahian cooking and some Peruvian specialties. They come in two varieties, head and shell on or peeled. Normally, dried shrimp are ground before using.

**Tacacá** A thick yellow soup with shrimp and garlic (Brazil).

**Tamales** An important food that has sustained cultures in Central and South America, as well as the southwestern region of North America for millennia.

**Tostones** Twice-fried slices of plantain that are pounded thin before the second frying.

## Tamales

The word *tamale* comes from *tamalli* in Nahuatl, the language of the Aztecs. The word for corn tamale in the Inca language (Quechua) is *choclotanda*, which means "cornbread." We have no record of which culture actually created it, but the tamale is recorded as early as 5000 B.C., possibly 7000 B.C. in pre-Columbian history. Initially, women were taken along in battle as army cooks to make the masa for the tortillas and the meats, stews, and drinks. As the warring tribes of the Aztec, Mayan, and Incan cultures grew, the demand of readying the *nixtamal* (corn) itself became so overwhelming a process, a need arose to have a more portable sustaining foodstuff, creating the tamale.

No history of the tamale would be complete without discussing the process of "nixtamalization," which is the processing of field corn with wood ashes (pre-Colombian) or now with *cal*, or slaked lime. This processing softens the corn for easier grinding and also aids in digestibility and increases the nutrients absorbed by the human body. Nixtamalization dates back to around 1200–1500 B.C. on the southern coast of Guatemala, where kitchens were found equipped with the necessities of nixtamal making.

In South America, tamales are found in Andean countries where there is a concentrated Indian population. The Amazonian Indians also make tamales with corn, yuca, or plantains. Each of the Andean countries has a variety of tamales both savory and sweet. They also go by different names depending not only on the country but also on the region. In Venezuela, they are called *ayacas* or *hallacas*, *bolos*, and *cachapas*; in Colombia *tamales*, *envueltos*, *hallacas*, and *bolos*; and in Ecuador *humitas*, *tamales*, *quimobolitos*, *hallacas*, and *chiguiles*. Peruvians have *tamales*, *humitas*, *juanes*, and *chapanas*; Bolivians *humintas* and *tamales*; Chileans and Argentines *humitas*; and Brazilians *pamonhas*.

In pre-Columbian times tamales were made only from corn and quinoa. Now they are made from potatoes, yuca, plantains, rice, squash, eggplant, sweet potatoes, and a variety of flours. Fillings usually include cheese, chicken, pork, beef, or fish. Raisins, prunes, hard-cooked eggs, hot peppers, almonds, and olives are the traditional garnish. The wrappings were corn husks, banana leaves, fabric, avocado leaves, soft tree bark, and other edible, nontoxic leaves. Tamales were steamed, grilled on the *comal* (grill) over the fire, or put directly on top of the coals to warm, or they were eaten cold.

Superstition has it that a chef must be in a good mood when cooking tamales or they will come out raw.

**Vatapá** A rich puree that can be made with fish, dried shrimp, cod, or chicken. Thought to have been brought from the Iberian peninsula and modified by African slaves, who added *dendê* (palm oil) and coconut milk. It can be thickened with bread, the Portuguese way of thickening stews, or with rice flour or manioc meal. Groundnuts, peanuts, almonds, or cashews, as well as dried shrimp, are essential to the dish. *Dendê* gives the *Vatapá* its characteristic taste and color. Cooks all have their own preparation of this dish (Brazil).

**Yuca Root** Although there are many varieties of yuca root, there are only two main categories: bitter and sweet. Used as a thickener in the making of tapioca. Bitter yuca root must be cooked to be edible.

**Yuca Flour** Made from the bitter cassava (yuca). Once grated and sun-dried, it is also called yuca root meal. It has a texture similar to that of cornstarch and is used to make breads, cookies, cakes, and tapioca.

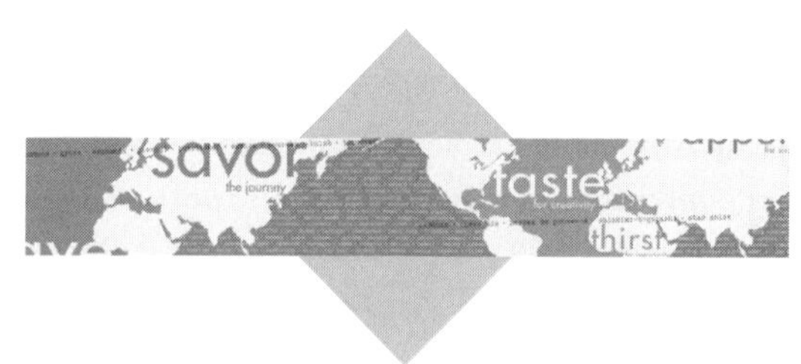

# Menus and Recipes from South America

MENU ONE

*Sopa de Palmito:* **Hearts of Palm Soup (Brazil)**

*Ceviche de Champiñones:* **Mushroom Ceviche (Peru)**

*Vatapá de Galinha:* **Chicken in Nut and Dried Shrimp Sauce (Brazil)**

*Pirão de Arroz:* **Rice Flour Pudding (Brazil)**

*Couve à Mineira:* **Shredded Kale**

*Ensalada de Tomate y Cebolla:* **Tomato and Onion Salad (Chile)**

*Crepas con Salsa de Dulce de Leche:* **Crepes with Dulce de Leche Sauce**

MENU TWO

*Ceviche de Pescado:* **Fish Ceviche (Peru)**

*Tamales de Espinaca con Queso:* **Spinach and Cheese Tamales (Argentina)**

*Chifles:* **Green Plantain Chips**

*Pabellón Criollo:* **Shredded Beef with Beans, Rice, and Plantains (Venezuela)**

MENU THREE

*Chupe de Quinua:* **Quinoa Chowder (Bolivia)**

*Salada de Chuchu:* **Chayote Salad (Brazil)**

*Patata y Carne de vaca Empanadas:* **Potato and Beef Empanadas with Chimichurri Sauce (Argentina)**

*Ceviche Mixto:* **Shellfish Ceviche (Ecuador)**

*Feijoada:* **Bean Stew with Beef and Pork (Brazil)**

*Cuscuz de Tapioca Molho de Chocolate:* **Tapioca and Coconut Cake with Chocolate Sauce**

OTHER RECIPES

*Truchs à la Parrilla:* **Grilled Trout (Argentina)**

*Bobó de Camarão:* **Shrimp with Yuca Sauce**

*Cuñapès:* **Yuca Flour Rolls**

*Escabeche de Pescado:* **Pickled Fish (Bolivia)**

*Ají Colombiano:* **Colombian Sauce**

*Humitas Ecuatorianas:* **Ecuadorian Humitas**

# Sopa de Palmito

## Hearts of Palm Soup (Brazi) SERVES 4

| AMOUNT | MEASURE | INGREDIENT |
|---|---|---|
| 2 tablespoons | 1 ounce, 28 ml | Butter |
| 1 cup | 4 ounces, 112 g | Leeks, thinly sliced, white parts and 1 inch (2.5 cm) green, washed well |
| 1 tablespoon | 7 g | All-purpose flour |
| 1 tablespoon | 7 g | Cornstarch |
| $\frac{1}{4}$ teaspoon | 1 g | White pepper |
| | 14 ounces, 392 g | Hearts of palm |
| 2 cups | 16 ounces, 470 ml | Chicken stock |
| 1 cup | 8 ounces 235 ml | Milk |
| To taste | | Salt and pepper |
| For garnish | | Sweet paprika or cayenne pepper |

### PROCEDURE

1. Heat butter over low to medium heat; sauté leeks 3 minutes; do not color.
2. Add flour, cornstarch, and white pepper; toss to coat.
3. Add hearts of palm and stock; bring to simmer and cook 25 minutes or until hearts of palm are tender.
4. Puree mixture until smooth.
5. Strain using a small-hole china cap and return to a clean pan.
6. Add milk and bring to boil; reduce to simmer and cook 3 minutes.
7. Correct seasoning and serve with a sprinkling of paprika or cayenne on top.

# Ceviche de Champiñones

## Mushroom Ceviche (Peru) SERVES 4

| AMOUNT | MEASURE | INGREDIENT |
|---|---|---|
| 3 cups | 12 ounces, 336 g | Fresh, firm cremini or white button mushrooms, cleaned, dry, quartered or sliced ($\frac{1}{4}$ inch, .6 cm) |
| 1/3 cup | $\frac{1}{2}$ ounce, 42 g | Celery, $\frac{1}{4}$ inch (.6 cm) dice |
| 1/3 cup | $\frac{1}{2}$ ounce, 42 g | Red onion, 1 inch (2.4 cm) dice, soaked in hot water for 5 minutes and drained |
| 2 | | Garlic cloves, minced |
| $\frac{1}{2}$ teaspoon | 2 g | Salt |
| $\frac{1}{4}$ teaspoon | 1 g | White pepper |
| $\frac{1}{2}$ teaspoon | 2 ml | Hot pepper sauce |
| $\frac{1}{2}$ teaspoon | 2 g | Dried oregano |
| $\frac{1}{2}$ cup | 4 ounces, 118 ml | Fresh lime or lemon juice |
| 1 tablespoon | $\frac{1}{2}$ ounce, 14 ml | Olive oil |
| $\frac{1}{4}$ cup | 1 ounce, 28 g | Red bell pepper, julienned |
| $\frac{1}{4}$ cup | 1 ounce, 28 g | Green bell pepper, julienned |
| 1 | | Jalapeño, seeded, minced |
| For garnish | | Alfonso or kalamata olives |

**PROCEDURE**

1. Blanch mushrooms in boiling water for 30 seconds and drain well.
2. Combine celery, onion, and blanched mushrooms.
3. Puree, garlic, salt, pepper, hot sauce, oregano, lime juice, and olive oil until well mixed.
4. Toss with mushroom mixture.
5. Adjust salt and pepper to taste. Refrigerate for 2 hours.
6. Drain well and toss with bell peppers and jalapeño.
7. Garnish with black olives.

# Vatapá de Galinha

## Chicken in Nut and Dried Shrimp Sauce (Brazil)

SERVES 4

**This classic Bahia dish is considered to be one of the best representations of Afro-Brazilian cuisine. The Portuguese thicken their soups and stews with bread, rice flour, or manioc meal. Groundnuts, dried shrimp, and *dendê* give the *vatapá* its characteristic taste and color. Vatapá can be made with fish, shrimp, dried cod, or chicken.**

| AMOUNT | MEASURE | INGREDIENT |
|---|---|---|
| 1 cup | 4 ounces, 112 g | Onion, $\frac{1}{4}$ inch (.6 cm) dice |
| 2 | | Garlic cloves, minced |
| 1 tablespoon | 1 ounce, 28 g | Fresh ginger, peeled, minced |
| 1 tablespoon | $\frac{1}{2}$ ounce, 14 g | Serrano pepper or to taste |
| 2 cups | 12 ounces, 336 g | Tomato, peeled, chopped, seeded, $\frac{1}{4}$ inch (.6 cm) dice |
| $\frac{1}{2}$ cup | 2 ounces, 56 g | Green bell pepper, deveined and seeded, $\frac{1}{4}$ inch (.6 cm) dice |
| $\frac{1}{2}$ cup | 1 ounce, 28 g | Cilantro, leaves only, chopped |
| 3 tablespoons | $\frac{1}{2}$ ounce, 45 ml | Dendê oil |
| 1 | $2\frac{1}{2}$ pounds, 1.13 kg | Chicken, cut into eight pieces, skinned and patted dry |
| 1 teaspoon | 5 g | Salt |
| $\frac{1}{2}$ teaspoon | 3 g | Freshly ground black pepper |
| $\frac{1}{2}$ cup | $\frac{1}{2}$ ounce, 14 g | Bread, day-old, $\frac{1}{2}$ inch (1.2 cm) cubes |
| $\frac{1}{2}$ cup | 4 ounces, 120 ml | Water |
| $\frac{1}{4}$ cup | $\frac{1}{2}$ ounce, 14 g | Dried peeled shrimp, ground |
| $\frac{1}{2}$ cup | $\frac{1}{2}$ ounces, 42 g | Peanuts, almonds, or cashews, toasted and ground |
| 1 tablespoon | $\frac{1}{2}$ ounce, 15 ml | Fresh lime juice |
| $\frac{3}{4}$ cup | 14 ounces, 420 ml | Unsweetened coconut milk |
| To taste | | Salt and black pepper |

### PROCEDURE

1. Puree first seven ingredients until smooth.
2. Heat dendê oil over medium heat, add puree and cook, stirring occasionally, 10 minutes.
3. Season chicken pieces with salt and pepper.
4. Add to sauce and toss to coat; bring to simmer.

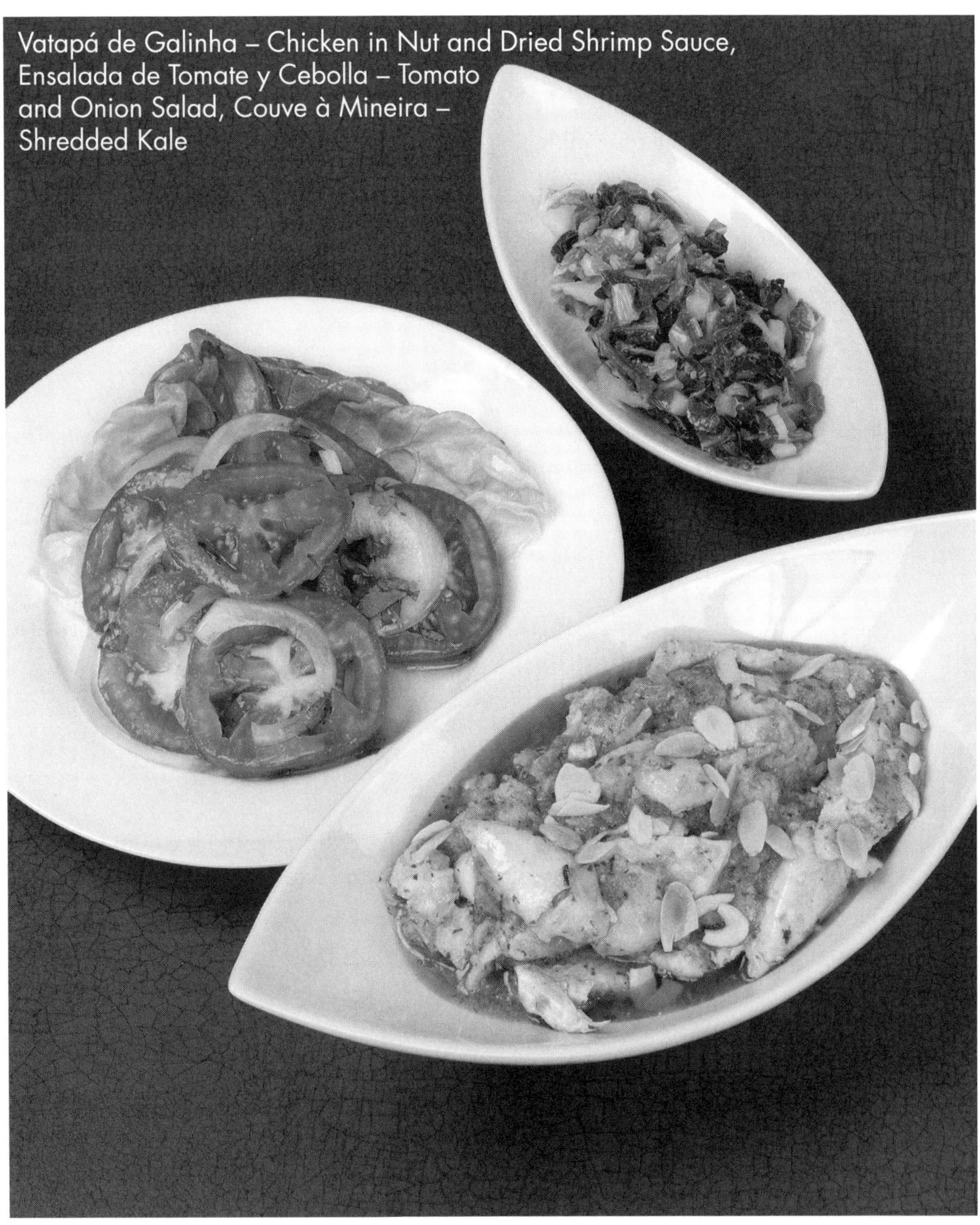

Vatapá de Galinha – Chicken in Nut and Dried Shrimp Sauce, Ensalada de Tomate y Cebolla – Tomato and Onion Salad, Couve à Mineira – Shredded Kale

5 Cover and cook, 15 to 20 minutes.
6 Remove chicken, cut meat into ½ inch (1.2 cm) wide by 1½ inch (3.8 cm) long boneless pieces.
7 Return to sauce with all remaining ingredients; simmer until sauce thickens.
8 Correct seasoning and serve with Pirão de Arroz (recipe follows).

# Pirão de Arroz

## Rice Flour Pudding (Brazil) SERVES 4–6

**Pirãos are very thick, savory porridges or mushes, like polenta but of African origin. They may be served either hot or at room temperature.**

| AMOUNT | MEASURE | INGREDIENT |
|---|---|---|
| ¾ cup | 3⅓ ounces, 95 g | Rice flour |
| 1 teaspoon | | Salt |
| 4 cups | 32 ounces, 1 liter | Unsweetened coconut milk |

### PROCEDURE

1 Scald 3 cups (24 ounces, 720 ml) coconut milk over medium heat.
2 Mix remaining milk with the rice flour and salt.
3 Add flour mixture and stir until mixture is smooth, reduce heat to medium low and cook stirring often until mixture is very thick and smooth, 15 to 20 minutes.
4 Fill lightly oiled molds, let cool to room temperature.
5 Refrigerate until firm, 2 to 3 hours, unmold, and serve.

# Couve à Mineira

## Shredded Kale SERVES 4

| AMOUNT | MEASURE | INGREDIENT |
|---|---|---|
| **2 pounds** | **907 g** | **Fresh kale,** |
| **$\frac{1}{4}$ cup** | **2 ounces, 60 ml** | **Olive oil or bacon fat** |
| **$\frac{1}{2}$ cup** | **2 ounces, 56 g** | **Onions, $\frac{1}{4}$ inch (.6 cm) dice** |
| **1** | | **Garlic clove, minced** |
| **To taste** | | **Salt and pepper** |

**PROCEDURE**

1. Trim blemishes and tough stems from kale leaves. Rinse thoroughly under running water.
2. Layer leaves on top of each other, and slice crosswise into very thin strips.
3. Heat oil over medium high heat; add onion and garlic and cook 3 to 5 minutes until softened.
4. Add kale and cook about 5 to 7 minutes, stirring often, until kale is softened but not discolored or browned. Season to taste.

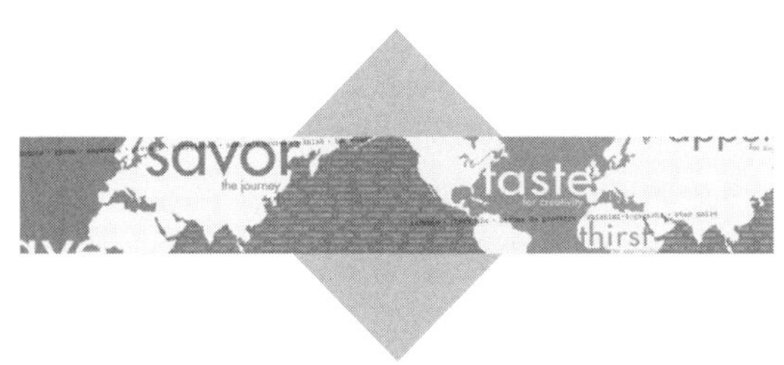

# Ensalada de Tomate y Cebolla

## Tomato and Onion Salad (Chile)

SERVES 4

| AMOUNT | MEASURE | INGREDIENT |
|---|---|---|
| **1 cup** | **4 ounces, 112 g** | **Sweet onion, julienned** |
| **1 pound** | **16 ounces, 448 g** | **Tomatoes, firm, peeled, sliced $\frac{1}{4}$ inch (.6 cm) thick** |
| **1 tablespoon** | **3 g** | **Fresh cilantro, chopped** |
| **1 tablespoon** | **$\frac{1}{2}$ ounce, 15 ml** | **Fresh lemon juice** |
| **2 tablespoons** | **1 ounce, 30 ml** | **Olive oil** |
| **To taste** | | **Salt and pepper** |

**PROCEDURE**

1. Soak onion in cold water to cover 20 minutes; drain and rinse well.
2. Drain and rinse the onions, squeeze, and drain well again.
3. Combine all ingredients, toss, and correct seasoning.

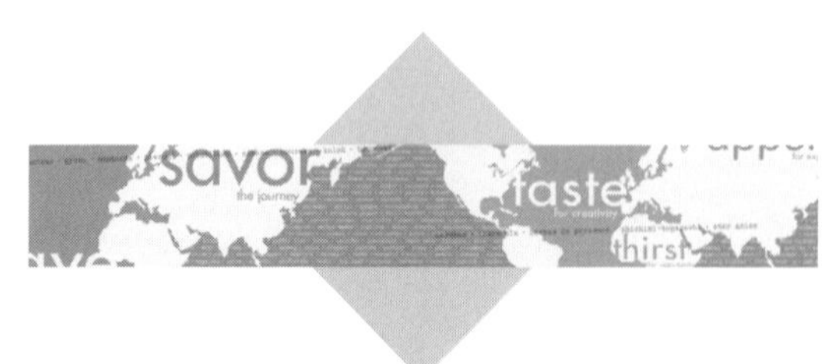

# Crepas con Salsa de Dulce de Leche Crepes with Dulce De Leche Sauce

SERVES 4

| AMOUNT | MEASURE | INGREDIENT |
|---|---|---|
| **1 cup** | **8 ounces, 240 ml** | **Dulce de leche sauce** |
| **1 cup** | **8 ounces, 240 ml** | **Heavy cream** |
| **$\frac{1}{4}$ cup** | **2 ounces, 60 ml** | **Rum** |
| **8** | | **Crepes, cooked** |
| **$\frac{1}{2}$ cup** | **2 ounces, 56 g** | **Pistachios, chopped** |
| **2 tablespoons** | **1 ounce, 28 g** | **Butter** |

**PROCEDURE**

1. Add heavy cream to sauce and return to simmer; stir in rum.
2. Place crepe brown-side down, spread 1 tablespoon ($\frac{1}{2}$ ounce, 15 ml) sauce over half, and sprinkle with 1 teaspoon pistachios.
3. Fold in half, then fold in half again; set aside. Repeat with remaining crepes.
4. Arrange crepes in a lightly buttered ovenproof pan and cover. Bake for 10 minutes in a 375°F (190°C) oven.
5. Serve two crepes; top with additional sauce and chopped nuts.

## Dulce de Leche Sauce

YIELD: 1 CUP (8 OUNCES, 240 ML)

| AMOUNT | MEASURE | INGREDIENT |
|---|---|---|
| **1 quart** | **32 ounces, 960 ml** | **Milk** |
| **$\frac{1}{4}$ cups** | **9 ounces, 252 g** | **Granulated sugar** |
| **$\frac{1}{4}$ teaspoon** | | **Baking soda** |
| **1 teaspoon** | | **Vanilla extract** |

**PROCEDURE**

1. Over medium high heat, combine milk, sugar, and baking soda. Bring to a boil.
2. Reduce heat to low and simmer, stirring occasionally. As it begins to thicken, stir periodically and cook until caramel-colored and very thick (caramel sauce), about 1 hour.
3. Stir in vanilla extract.

# Ceviche de Pescado

## Fish Ceviche SERVES 4

**Fish must be extremely fresh. The classic fish for this dish is corvina in Ecuador and tuna in Peru, but any white-fleshed fish, such as sea bass, flounder, red snapper, tilapia, or sole, may be used.**

| AMOUNT | MEASURE | INGREDIENT |
|---|---|---|
| 12 ounces | 336 g | White-fleshed lean fish fillets, cut $\frac{1}{4}$ inch (.6 cm) thick and 1 inch (2.4 cm) long |
| Marinade | | |
| $\frac{1}{2}$ cup | 4 ounces, 118 ml | Fresh lemon juice |
| $\frac{1}{4}$ cup | 2 ounces, 59 ml | Fresh lime juice |
| $\frac{1}{2}$ cup | 4 ounces, 118 ml | Fresh orange juice |
| 1 tablespoon | $\frac{1}{2}$ ounce, 14 ml | Olive oil |
| $\frac{1}{2}$ teaspoon | 3 g | Salt |
| 1 | | Garlic clove, minced |
| 1 | | Ali Amarillo (yellow Peruvian chile), seeded and minced, or canned aji or serrano chile |
| To taste | | Hot pepper sauce |
| 1 teaspoon | 1 g | Parsley, chopped |
| 1 teaspoon | 1 g | Cilantro, chopped |
| $\frac{1}{3}$ cup | $1\frac{1}{2}$ ounces, 42 g | Green onions (white part and 1 inch of green), minced |
| Garnish | | |
| 4 | | Bib, romaine, or green leaf lettuce leaves |
| 2 | | Corn ears, cut into 2 inch (4.8 cm) pieces |
| 8 ounces | 224 g | Sweet potatoes, roasted in the skin, peeled, $\frac{1}{2}$ inch (1.2 cm) thick rounds |
| 8 ounces | 224 g | Yuca, peeled, cut into batonnets, boiled soft, cooled |

**PROCEDURE**

1. Soak the fish for 1 hour in lightly salted water; drain and rise well.
2. Combine the citrus juices, salt, garlic, chile, and fish; mix well, cover, and let marinate in refrigerator until it is "cooked" (milky white throughout), 3 to 6 hours. Start checking at 3 hours.
3. Add all remaining marinade ingredients and correct seasoning.
4. To serve, line serving platter with lettuce. Place ceviche in center and display garnish around.

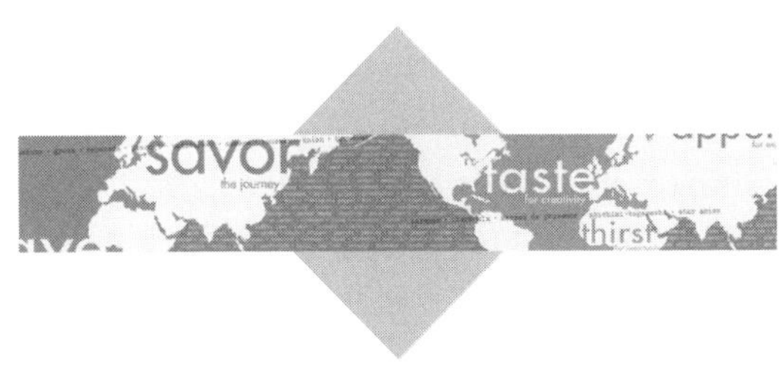

# Tamales de Espinaca con Queso Spinach and Cheese Tamales

YIELD: ABOUT 12, DEPENDING ON SIZE OF CORN HUSKS

## Basic Tamales

| AMOUNT | MEASURE | INGREDIENT |
|---|---|---|
| 12 | | Dried corn husks |
| 1 cup | 8 ounces, 224 g | Lard or vegetable shortening |
| 2/3 cup | 6 ounces, 176 ml | Chicken stock or water |
| 3 cups | 18 ounces, 504 g | Masa harina or fresh masa (1 $\frac{1}{2}$ pounds) |
| 2 teaspoons | 10 g | Salt |
| 1 teaspoon | 4 g | Baking powder |

**PROCEDURE**

1. Place corn husks in warm water to cover and soak 2 hours. Remove, drain, and pat dry.
2. Beat the lard by hand or in mixer until soft and light.
3. Gradually add stock to the masa harina and knead until the dough is no longer sticky. Add salt and baking powder.
4. Move masa harina mixture to mixer and beat lard into the dough, a little at a time, until the dough is light and fluffy. Test for lightness by pinching off a small piece and dropping into a glass of cold water. It should float when ready; if not, continue to beat and test again. The lighter the dough, the better; it results in moist and fluffy tamales. It is impossible to overmix this dough.

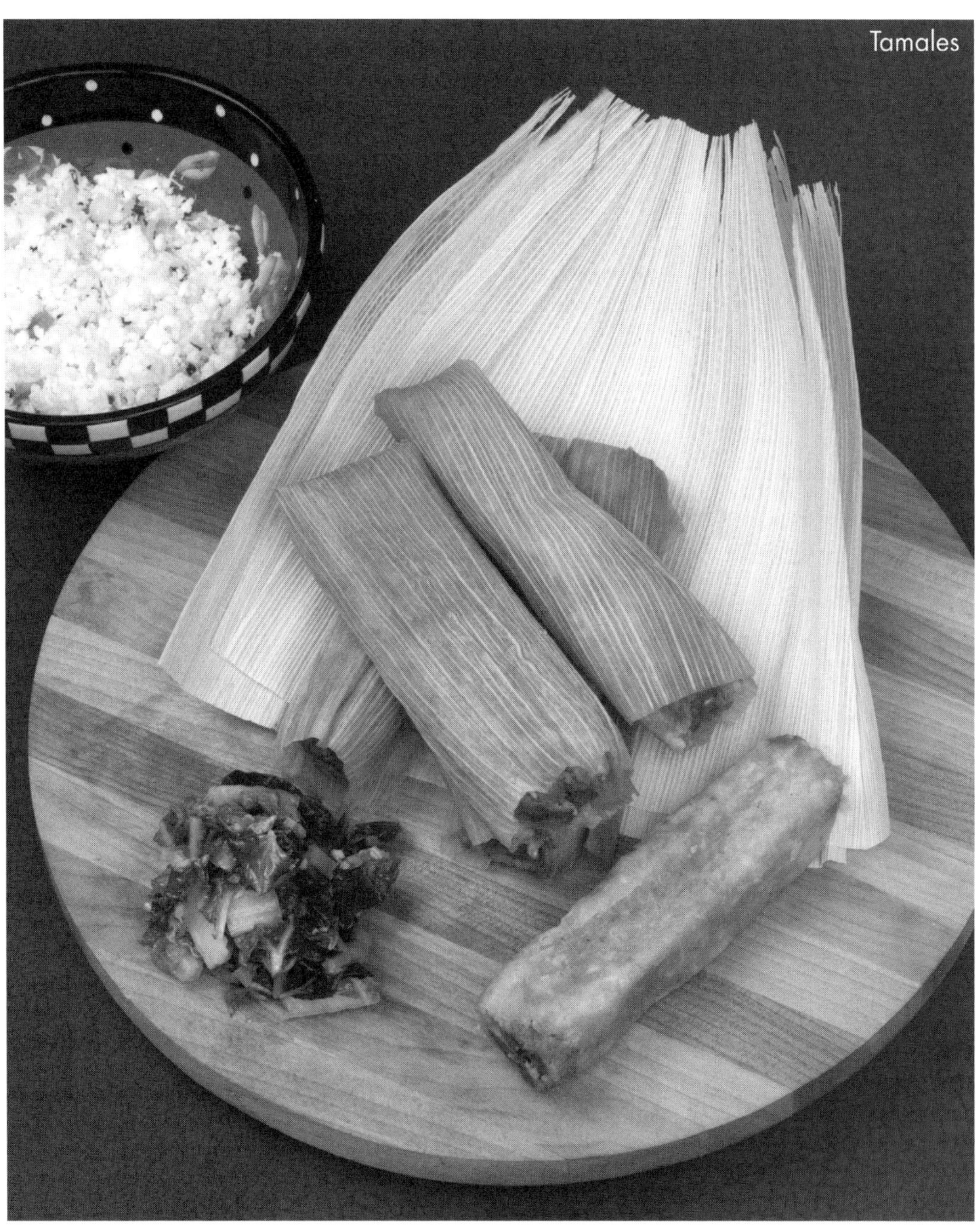
Tamales

# Spinach and Cheese Filling

**YIELD: ABOUT 12, DEPENDING ON SIZE OF CORN HUSKS**

| AMOUNT | MEASURE | INGREDIENT |
|---|---|---|
| $\frac{1}{2}$ tablespoon | $\frac{3}{4}$ ounce, 21 ml | Vegetable oil |
| $\frac{1}{2}$ cup | 2 ounces, 56 g | Onion, $\frac{1}{4}$ inch (.6 cm) dice |
| $\frac{1}{2}$ cup | 3 ounces, 84 g | Tomato, peeled, seeded, $\frac{1}{4}$ inch (.6 cm) dice |
| 4 cups | 8 ounces, 224 g | Fresh spinach, or 8 ounces frozen chopped |
| 1 cup | 4 ounces, 112 g | Adobera, Asadero, or Monterey Jack cheese, shredded |
| To taste | | Salt and pepper |

**PROCEDURE**

1. Heat oil and sauté onions until translucent. Add tomatoes and cook until almost dry.
2. Add spinach and wilt.
3. Let cool and mix well with cheese.
4. Adjust seasoning.
5. Combine spinach and cheese filling with Basic Tamales (masa harina mixture); mix well and check seasoning again.

**TO MAKE TAMALES**

1. Place an unbroken corn husk on a work surface in front of you with the small tapering end of the husk facing you.
2. Using a spatula or masa spreader, spread approximately $\frac{1}{4}$ cup of dough onto the husk, leaving a border of at least $1\frac{1}{2}$ inches of husk at the tapered end.
3. Fold the two long sides of the corn husk in over the corn mixture.
4. Fold the tapered end up, leaving the top open.
5. Secure the tamale by tying with a strip of husk or a string.
6. Line the steamer with husks. Stand the tamales up in a row around the edge of the steamer.
7. Cover and steam, checking water level frequently and replenishing with boiling water as needed, until tamales easily come free from husks, about 1 hour for tamales made with fresh masa or $1\frac{1}{4}$ to $1\frac{1}{2}$ hours if made with masa harina mixture.

# Chifles Green Plantain Chips

SERVES 4

| AMOUNT | MEASURE | INGREDIENT |
|---|---|---|
| **2** | | **Green plantains** |
| **As needed** | | **Peanut oil for frying** |
| **To taste** | | **Salt** |

**PROCEDURE**

1 Peel plantains by trimming both ends with a sharp knife, cutting incisions along the natural ridges and then pulling away the skin. Cut into very thin slices and place in ice-cold water for 15 minutes (this helps keep them crisp). Drain well and dry on paper towels.

2 Heat oil to 375°F (190°C) or until a cube of dried bread added to the oil floats and turns golden after 1 minute.

3 Fry in batches, until golden, about 2 minutes. Drain well on paper towels.

4 Season with salt and serve when cool.

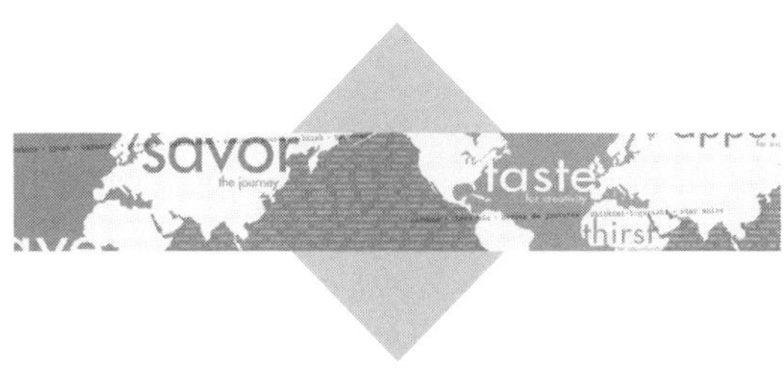

# Pabellón Criollo

## Shredded Beef with Beans, Rice, and Plantains (Venezuela) SERVES 4

**Pabellón means "flag," and the finished dish resembles a Venezuelan flag.**

| AMOUNT | MEASURE | INGREDIENT |
|---|---|---|
| $1\frac{1}{2}$ pounds | 672 g | Flank steak; cut in 3 or 4 pieces |
| 1 | | Bay leaf |
| 1 quart | 32 ounces, 960 ml | Beef stock; to cover |
| 2 tablespoons | 1 ounces, 30 ml | Olive oil |
| 1 cup | 4 ounces, 112 | Onion, $\frac{1}{4}$ inch (.6 cm) dice |
| 2 | | Garlic cloves; minced |
| $1\frac{1}{2}$ cups | 9 ounces, 252 g | Tomatoes, peeled, seeded, $\frac{1}{4}$ inch (.6 cm) dice |
| $\frac{1}{2}$ teaspoon | | Cumin seeds; crushed |
| 1 teaspoon | | Oregano |
| To taste | | Salt and pepper |
| 2 tablespoons | 1 ounce, 40 ml | Vegetable oil |
| 4 cups | | Arroz blanco (see recipe on page 31) |
| 4 cups | | Caraotas negras (see recipe on page 41 for Frijoles de Olla; use black beans) |
| 1 | | Plantain (use ripe plantains with black skins for this dish; green plantains will be too dry). Cut into 2 inch (5 cm), pieces |
| As needed | | Vegetable oil for frying plantain |

PROCEDURE

1. Combine flank steak, bay leaf, and stock, bring to simmer, and cook 1 to $1\frac{1}{2}$ hours until very tender.
2. Cool in stock. When cool, shred meat and set aside.
3. Heat olive oil over medium high heat; add onions and cook until translucent.
4. Add garlic, tomatoes, cumin, oregano, salt, and pepper; cook until almost dry.
5. Add shredded beef; cook 5 minutes and correct seasoning.

6 Heat vegetable oil over medium heat and sauté plantains until they are browned all over. Drain on paper towels.

7 To assemble the "flag," arrange beef, rice, and beans on a rectangular platter in three rows with the rice in the center. Garnish with chifles.

In some recipes, fried eggs are placed on top of the meat—one per person.

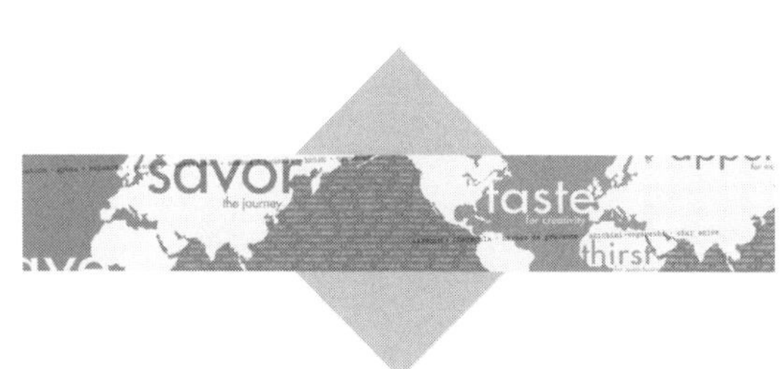

# Chupe de Quinua Quinoa Chowder

SERVES 4

| AMOUNT | MEASURE | INGREDIENT |
|---|---|---|
| 2 tablespoons | 1 ounce, 60 ml | Butter |
| 1 cup | 4 ounces, 112 g | Onion, $\frac{1}{4}$ inch (.6 cm) dice |
| 2 | | Garlic cloves, chopped |
| 1 teaspoon | 5 g | Salt |
| $\frac{1}{2}$ teaspoon | 2 g | Pepper, freshly ground |
| $\frac{1}{2}$ teaspoon | 2 g | Cumin, ground |
| $\frac{1}{2}$ teaspoon | 2 g | Sweet paprika |
| 3 cups | 24 ounces, 720 ml | Hot chicken or vegetable stock |
| $\frac{1}{2}$ cup | 9 ounces, 252 g | Quinoa, cooked |
| 1 cup | 6 ounces, 168 g | All-purpose potatoes, peeled, cooked, 1-inch (2.5 cm) cubes |
| $\frac{3}{4}$ cup | 6 ounces, 180 ml | Milk |
| $\frac{1}{2}$ cup | 2 ounces, 56 g | Fresh or frozen corn kernels |
| $\frac{1}{2}$ cup | 3 ounces, 84 g | Fava beans or peas, blanched and peeled |
| $\frac{1}{2}$ cup | 2 ounces, 56 g | Manchego: or Cheddar cheese, shredded |
| 2 | | Large eggs, beaten |
| To taste | | Salt and pepper |
| 1 tablespoon | 3 g | Fresh mint, chopped |
| 1 tablespoon | 3 g | Fresh cilantro, chopped |
| $\frac{1}{2}$ cup | 2 ounces, 56 g | Avocado, peeled, pitted $\frac{1}{4}$ inch (.6 cm) dice |

PROCEDURE

1. Heat butter over low heat, add onions, and cook for 10 minutes without coloring.
2. Make a paste with garlic, salt, and pepper.
3. Add garlic paste, cumin, and paprika to onions; cook 1 minute.
4. Add stock, quinoa, and potatoes; simmer 15 minutes or until potatoes are tender.
5. Add milk, corn, and beans; simmer until tender, 5 minutes. Do not boil after adding the milk. Adjust the consistency with more hot stock if necessary.
6. Add cheese and eggs, stirring constantly, until cheese has melted and eggs have set.
7. Correct seasoning and serve hot, garnished with mint, cilantro, and avocado.

# Salada de Chuchu

## Chayote Salad (Brazil) SERVES 4

| AMOUNT | MEASURE | INGREDIENT |
|---|---|---|
| 2 | | Preserved malagueta peppers, minced, or 1 teaspoon Tabasco sauce |
| 1 teaspoon | 3 g | Salt |
| $\frac{1}{2}$ cup | 2 ounces | White onions, minced |
| 1 | | Garlic clove, minced |
| 1 tablespoon | $\frac{1}{2}$ ounce, 15 ml | Lemon juice, fresh |
| To taste | | Salt and pepper |
| 2 tablespoons | 1 ounce, 30 ml | Olive oil |
| 2 cups | 12 ounces, 336 g | Chayote, peeled, seeded, $\frac{1}{4}$ inch (.6 cm) slices |
| 4 | | Romaine or green leaf lettuce leaves |

PROCEDURE

1 In a mortar and pestle, blender, or food processor, combine the peppers and salt; process to a paste.

2 Gradually add onions and garlic and process to a paste.

3 Add lemon juice and oil to make dressing, correct seasoning.

4 Cook chayote in boiling salted water until just tender.

5 Drain and toss with half the dressing, cool.

6 Arrange on lettuce leaf and drizzle with remaining dressing.

# Patata y Carne de vaca Empanadas

## Potato and Beef Empanadas with Chimichurri Sauce (Argentina)

SERVES 4–6

### Dough

YIELD: 20–24 ROUNDS

| AMOUNT | MEASURE | INGREDIENT |
|---|---|---|
| 2 teaspoons | 6 g | Salt |
| $\frac{3}{4}$ cup | 6 ounces, 180 ml | Warm water |
| $4\frac{1}{2}$ cups | 18 ounces, 510 g | All purpose flour |
| $\frac{1}{4}$ teaspoon | | Paprika |
| $\frac{3}{4}$ cup | 6 ounces, 170 g | Lard or vegetable shortening |

PROCEDURE

1. Dissolve salt in warm water.
2. Sift together flour and paprika. Add lard or vegetable shortening, blend fat and flour to a fine meal.
3. Add salted water until mixture forms a ball. Add more flour a tablespoon at a time if the dough is too sticky.
4. Shape dough into a ball; knead vigorously for 10 minutes on a lightly floured surface or until smooth and elastic. Reshape into a ball, refrigerate to let rest covered for at least 30 minutes (preferably 2 hours).
5. Roll dough to 1/8 inch (.3 cm) thickness on lightly floured surface and cut into 5-inch (12 cm) rounds. Stack rounds and cover to prevent drying.

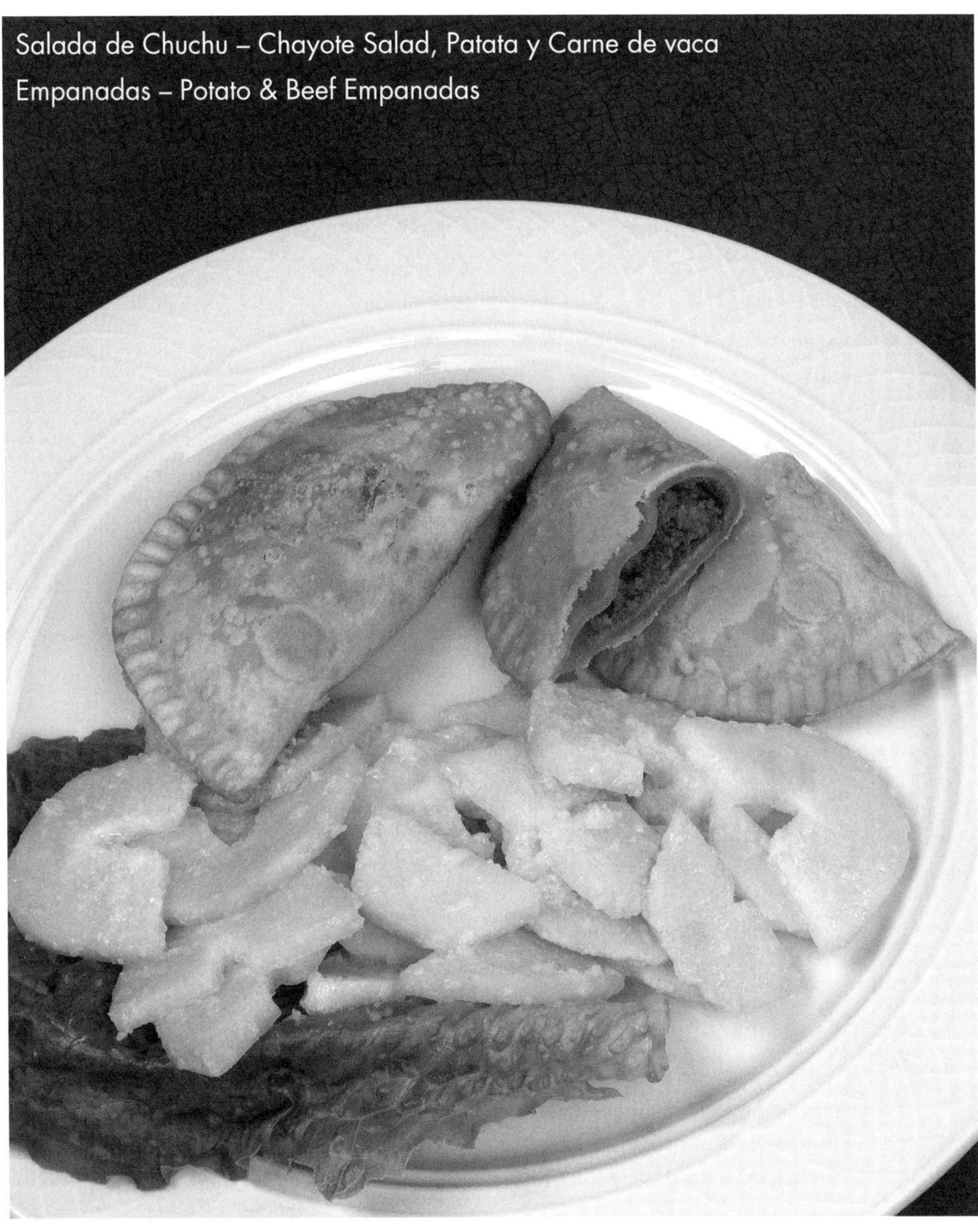

Salada de Chuchu – Chayote Salad, Patata y Carne de vaca Empanadas – Potato & Beef Empanadas

## Filling

| AMOUNT | MEASURE | INGREDIENT |
|---|---|---|
| 3 tablespoons | $1\frac{1}{2}$ ounce, 45 ml | Olive oil |
| 1 cup | 4 ounces, 112 g | Onion, minced |
| $\frac{1}{2}$ cup | 2 ounces, 56 g | Red bell pepper, cored, seeded, $\frac{1}{4}$ inch (.6 cm) dice |
| $\frac{1}{2}$ teaspoon | 2 g | Red pepper flakes |
| $\frac{1}{2}$ teaspoon | 2 g | Paprika |
| $\frac{1}{2}$ teaspoon | 2 g | White pepper |
| $\frac{1}{2}$ teaspoon | 2 g | Ground cumin |
| 1 cup | 6 ounces, 168 g | Beef shoulder, minced |
| To taste | | Salt and pepper |
| $\frac{1}{2}$ cup | 2 ounces, 56 g | Potato, russet, peeled, $\frac{1}{4}$ inch (.6 cm) dice, boiled, drained, and cooled |
| $\frac{1}{4}$ cup | 1 ounce, 28 g | Raisins |
| $\frac{1}{4}$ cup | 2 ounces, 56 g | Green Spanish olives, pitted, $\frac{1}{4}$ inch (.6 cm) dice |
| $\frac{1}{4}$ cup | 1 ounce, 28 g | Green onions, white part and 1 inch green, finely chopped |
| 1 | | Hard-boiled egg, peeled and chopped |

**PROCEDURE**

1. Heat oil over medium heat and add onion, bell pepper, red pepper flakes, paprika, white pepper, and cumin, cook 6 to 7 minutes or until onions are soft.
2. Add beef and cook, stirring, until meat is brown and cooked.
3. Correct seasoning; set aside to cool.
4. To cooled meat mixture, add cooked potatoes, raisins, olives, green onions, and egg; combine well.
5. Correct seasoning.
6. Preheat oven to 400°F (204°C).
7. To assemble empanadas, place about 3 tablespoons of filling in the center of each dough circle. Fold over and press the edges firmly to seal, starting from the middle and working out to the edges. Curve the ends of the empanada to form a crescent. To make the "rope"

around edge, pinch $\frac{1}{2}$ inch of one corner edge between your thumb and index finger and fold edge over onto itself. Pinch and pull another $\frac{1}{2}$ inch of the edge and fold again, making a rough triangle over the first fold. Repeat this folding around edge, pressing each fold tight.

8 Bake until golden brown, 15 to 20 minutes.

9 Serve warm with chimichurri sauce.

## Chimichurri Sauce

SERVES 4–6

| AMOUNT | MEASURE | INGREDIENT |
|---|---|---|
| $\frac{1}{2}$ cup | 4 ounces, 120 ml | Olive oil |
| $\frac{1}{4}$ cup | 2 ounces, 60 ml | Lemon juice, fresh |
| $\frac{1}{4}$ cup | 2 ounces, 60 ml | Sherry or red wine vinegar |
| $\frac{1}{2}$ cup | 2 ounces, 56 g | Onion; finely minced |
| 1 tablespoon | 6 g | Garlic, finely minced |
| $\frac{1}{2}$ cup | 1 ounce, 28 g | Flat-leaf parsley; chopped |
| 1 tablespoon | 3 g | Fresh oregano leaves, chopped |
| $\frac{1}{2}$ teaspoon | | Dried red chile pepper |
| $1\frac{1}{2}$ teaspoons | | Salt |
| 1 teaspoon | | Black pepper, freshly ground |

PROCEDURE

1 Combine all ingredients; rest for at least 2 hours. This is best if prepared overnight. The parsley may be added just before serving to preserve the color.

# Ceviche Mixto
## Shellfish Ceviche SERVES 4

| AMOUNT | MEASURE | INGREDIENT |
|---|---|---|
| 1 quart | 32 ounces, 938 ml | Water |
| 1 | | Green onion, white part and 1 inch green, sliced |
| 12 ounces | 340 g | Shrimp (16–20 count), peeled and deveined |
| 6 ounces | 168 g | Scallops, rinsed |
| $\frac{1}{4}$ cup | 2 ounces, 60 ml | Dry white wine |
| 12 ounces | 340 g | Mussels, scrubbed and debearded |
| 12 | | Baby clams |
| | | Marinade (recipe follows) |
| | | Garnishes (recipe follows) |

PROCEDURE

1 Bring water and green onion to boil; let simmer 5 minutes. Add shrimp, remove from heat, and let stand 1 minute or until shrimp are just cooked. Remove from hot water (reserving the cooking liquid) and cool shrimp so they do not become rubbery.

2 Return cooking liquid to boil, add scallops, remove from heat, and let stand for 3 minutes, depending on size. Cut a scallop in half to see if it is cooked through (it should be milky white in the center). Drain and rinse under cold running water.

3 Bring wine, mussels, and clams to a boil over high heat. Cover and let cook until the shells are open, 3 to 5 minutes. Discard any clams or mussels that do not open. Remove clams and mussels from shells and discard shells. Cool shellfish.

4 Combine cooked shellfish with marinade and refrigerate for at least 2 hours.

5 Before serving, check seasoning for salt, sugar, and hot pepper sauce.

6 Divide seafood equally between four serving containers. Garnish each in the center with 1 teaspoon each chopped tomato, bell pepper, onion, cilantro, and parsley.

7 Serve with the side dishes.

# Marinade

| AMOUNT | MEASURE | INGREDIENT |
|---|---|---|
| $\frac{1}{4}$ cup | 2 ounces, 60 ml | Fresh lemon juice |
| $\frac{1}{4}$ cup | 2 ounces, 60 ml | Fresh lime juice |
| $\frac{1}{2}$ cup | 4 ounces, 120 ml | Fresh orange juice |
| $\frac{1}{2}$ cup | 4 ounces, 120 ml | Fish or chicken stock |
| 1 tablespoon | $\frac{1}{2}$ ounce, 14 ml | Olive oil |
| $\frac{1}{2}$ teaspoon | 3 g | Sugar |
| $\frac{1}{2}$ teaspoon | 3 g | Salt |
| $\frac{1}{4}$ teaspoon | 2 g | Black pepper, freshly ground |
| To taste | | Hot pepper sauce |

**PROCEDURE**

1 Combine all ingredients and mix well.

# Garnishes

| AMOUNT | MEASURE | INGREDIENT |
|---|---|---|
| $\frac{1}{2}$ cup | 3 ounces, 84 g | Tomato, peeled, seeded, $\frac{1}{4}$ inch (.6 cm) dice |
| $\frac{1}{2}$ cup | 2 ounces, 56 g | Green bell pepper, seeded, $\frac{1}{8}$ inch (.3 cm) dice |
| $\frac{1}{2}$ cup | 2 ounces, 56 g | White onion, $\frac{1}{8}$ inch (.3 cm) dice, rinsed with hot water, and drained |
| 2 tablespoons | 6 g | Cilantro, leaves only, minced |
| 2 tablespoons | 6 g | Parsley, minced |

**SIDE DISHES**

Popcorn

Tostado (corn nuts)

# Feijoada Bean Stew with Beef and Pork (Brazil)

SERVES 4–6

**Reputedly introduced in Brazil by black slaves as early as the sixteenth century, *feijoada*—a bean potpourri type dish—is the Brazilian equivalent of American "soul food." It is considered the Brazilian national dish. In *uma feijoada legitima*, the real *feijoada*, every part of the pig is used: ears, tail, and snout.**

| AMOUNT | MEASURE | INGREDIENT |
|---|---|---|
| 1 cup | 7 ounces, 196 g | Dried black beans, washed and sorted, soaked overnight, or 2 cups cooked black beans |
| 1 piece | 5 ounces, 140 g | Ham hock, smoked, 1 inch (2.4 cm) dice |
| 1 | | Pork foot, ear, tail, tongue (optional) |
| 1 cup | 5 ounces, 140 g | Chorizo, pepperoni, or Brazilian *lingüica*, $\frac{1}{2}$ inch (1.2 cm) dice |
| $\frac{1}{2}$ cup | 3 ounces, 84 g | Lean Canadian bacon or Brazilian *carne seca*, cut $\frac{1}{2}$ inch (1.2 cm) dice |
| 4 ounces | 112 g | Smoked pork or beef ribs |
| $\frac{1}{2}$ cup | 3 ounces, 84 g | Lean pork, 1 inch (2.4 cm) dice |
| $\frac{1}{2}$ cup | 3 ounces, 84 g | Lean beef, 1 inch (2.4 cm) dice |
| 1 tablespoon | $\frac{1}{2}$ ounce, 15 ml | Olive oil |
| 1 ounce | 56 g | Smoked bacon, $\frac{1}{2}$ inch (1.2 cm) dice |
| 1 cup | 4 ounces, 112 g | Onion, $\frac{1}{2}$ inch (1.2 cm) dice |
| 2 | | Garlic cloves, minced |
| 1 tablespoon | $\frac{1}{2}$ ounce, 15 ml | Sherry vinegar |
| 1 | | Bay leaf |
| To taste | | Salt and pepper |
| To taste | | Hot sauce |
| 4 cups | | Arroz blanco (see recipe on page 31) |
| 2 cups | | Couve à Mineira (see recipe on page 77) |

**PROCEDURE**

1. Place the beans in a large saucepot and cover with cold water. Bring to a boil and turn the heat down to simmer. Simmer until soft.
2. Combine ham hock, pork parts, chorizo, Canadian bacon, ribs, lean pork, and beef in saucepot; Add cold water just to cover; bring to a boil and cook 10 minutes or until meat is cooked.
3. Strain meat and retain liquid.
4. Heat oil over medium high heat and render diced bacon.
5. Add onion, garlic, and vinegar; cook until onions are caramelized.
6. Add $\frac{1}{2}$ cup cooked black beans to onion mixture and mash together.
7. Add bay leaf and fry for two minutes remove bay leaf.
8. Combine cooked beans, onion mixture, and cooked meats.
9. Add one cup or more retained liquid from meat.
10. Cook meat and beans together, adding liquid as needed, until meat is tender.
11. Correct seasoning and hot sauce.
12. Serve over rice with Couve à Mineira.

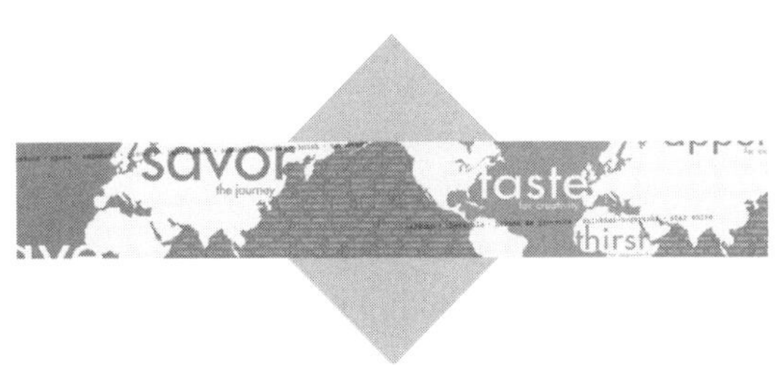

# Cuscuz de Tapioca Molho de Chocolate Tapioca and Coconut Cake with Chocolate Sauce

SERVES 4

| AMOUNT | MEASURE | INGREDIENT |
|---|---|---|
| 1 cup | 8 ounces, 240 ml | Unsweetened coconut milk |
| 1 cup | 8 ounces, 240 ml | Milk |
| ½ cup | 3½ ounces, 98 g | Sugar |
| ½ teaspoon | | Salt |
| 1 cup | 2½ ounces, 42 g | Coconut, grated |
| 1 cup | 5½ ounces, 154 g | Quick-cooking tapioca |

PROCEDURE

1. Over medium-high heat, combine coconut milk, milk, sugar, and salt.
2. Stir to dissolve sugar and bring to a boil.
3. Combine tapioca and coconut.
4. Add tapioca mixture to milk mixture and simmer until tapioca is clear, 2 minutes.
5. Pour into molds or serving containers; let set up.
6. Serve with chocolate sauce.

## Chocolate Sauce

| AMOUNT | MEASURE | INGREDIENT |
|---|---|---|
| 1¾ cups | 14 ounce, 420 ml | Sweetened condensed milk |
| 2 tablespoons | ¾ ounce, 21 g | Unsweetened cocoa powder |
| 1 tablespoon | ½ ounce, 15 ml | Unsalted butter |
| 1 tablespoon | ½ ounce, 15 ml | Water |
| Pinch | | Salt |

PROCEDURE

1. Combine all ingredients over low heat; cook, stirring, until smooth and hot.
2. Let cool to room temperature.

# Truchas à la Parrilla

## Grilled Trout

SERVES 4

| AMOUNT | MEASURE | INGREDIENT |
|---|---|---|
| 4 | 8 ounce, 224 g | Pan-dressed trout |
| 2 tablespoons | 1 ounce, 30 ml | Fresh lemon juice |
| 2 tablespoons | 1 ounce, 30 ml | Fresh lime juice |
| 2 teaspoons | 6 g | Salt |
| 1 teaspoon | 3 g | Black pepper, freshly ground |
| 1 teaspoon | 3 g | Ground cumin |
| 2 | | Garlic cloves, minced |
| 1 cup | 8 ounces, 240 ml | Unsalted butter, melted |

**PROCEDURE**

1. Make 3 deep incisions in both sides of each trout.
2. Combine lemon juice, lime juice, salt, pepper, cumin, and garlic and coat the trout with it, making sure it gets into the incisions. Cover and refrigerate for at least 1 hour.
3. Grill trout on a oiled perforated grill rack over low heat, basting frequently with melted butter, until just cooked through, about 5 minutes per side.
4. Serve with rice and a salad.

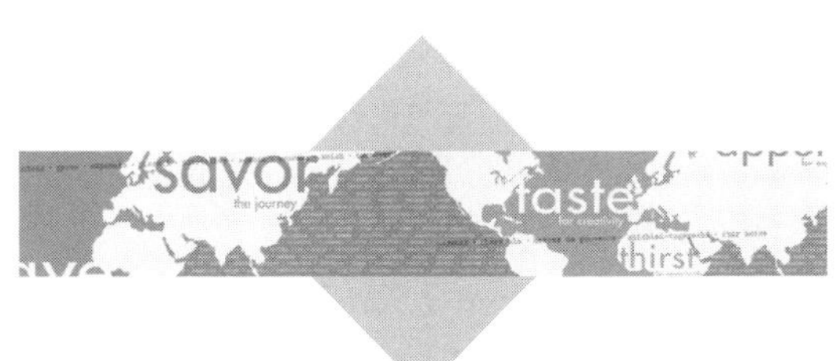

# Bobó de Camarão

## Shrimp with Yuca Sauce

SERVES 4

| AMOUNT | MEASURE | INGREDIENT |
|---|---|---|
| 1 pound | 448 g | 16–20 ct shrimp, unpeeled |
| 2 tablespoons | 1 ounce, 30 ml | Fresh lime juice |
| 1 $\frac{1}{2}$ cups | 9 ounces, 252 g | Yuca, fresh or frozen, peeled, cut $\frac{1}{2}$ inch (1.2 cm) dice |
| 2 cups | 16 ounces, 480 ml | Water |
| 1 tablespoon | $\frac{1}{2}$ ounce, 15 ml | Olive oil |
| 2 tablespoons | 1 ounce, 30 ml | Dendê or palm oil |
| 1 cup | 4 ounces, 112 g | Onions, $\frac{1}{4}$ inch (.6 cm) dice |
| 3 | | Garlic cloves, minced |
| $\frac{1}{2}$ cup | 2 ounces, 56 g | Green bell pepper, seeded, $\frac{1}{4}$ inch (.6 cm) dice |
| $\frac{1}{2}$ cup | 2 ounces, 56 g | Red bell pepper, seeded, $\frac{1}{4}$ inch (.6 cm) dice |
| 1 cup | 6 ounces, 168 g | Tomatoes, peeled, seeded, $\frac{1}{4}$ inch (.6 cm) dice |
| 2 tablespoons | 6 g | Parsley, chopped |
| 2 tablespoons | 6 g | Cilantro, chopped |
| 2 tablespoons | $\frac{1}{2}$ ounce, 14 g | Fresh ginger, peeled, grated |
| $\frac{1}{2}$ teaspoon | 2 g | Salt |
| $\frac{1}{2}$ teaspoon | 2 g | White pepper |
| 1 cup | 8 ounces, 240 ml | Unsweetened coconut milk, |
| To taste | | Salt, pepper, and hot pepper sauce |

PROCEDURE

1. Peel and devein shrimp, reserving the shells; rinse and toss with lime juice.
2. Add water just to cover shrimp shells. Bring to boil, reduce heat, and simmer 10 minutes. Strain the broth and discard the shells.
3. Bring shrimp stock to boil and add yuca, and if necessary enough boiling water to cover. Cook over low heat until tender, about 20 minutes.
4. Drain and reserve liquid.
5. Mash yuca with potato masher or fork, add enough cooking liquid to make a coarse puree (it should not be smooth).
6. Heat oil and dendê over medium heat; add onion and cook, stirring, until softened, 5 minutes.

7 Add garlic, green and red bell peppers, tomatoes, parsley, cilantro, ginger, salt, and pepper. Cover and cook to reduce to a saucelike consistency, 10 minutes.

8 Add coconut milk and cook 5 minutes.

9 Add shrimp and cook 1 minute.

10 Add yuca puree; cook 1 minute.

11 Correct seasoning with salt, pepper, and hot sauce.

12 Add cooking liquid as needed to reach the consistency of heavy cream.

13 Serve with white rice.

## Cuñapès Yuca Flour Rolls

YIELD: 24 ROLLS

| AMOUNT | MEASURE | INGREDIENT |
|---|---|---|
| $\frac{3}{4}$ cup, more if necessary | 5 ounces, 140 g | Yuca flour |
| $\frac{3}{4}$ teaspoon | 2 g | Baking powder |
| 2 | | Medium eggs |
| $1\frac{1}{2}$ cups | 6 ounces, 170 g | Queso fresco, crumbled |
| As needed | | Milk |

PROCEDURE

1 Sift flour and baking powder until well mixed.

2 Add eggs and cheese; mix—preferably with a food processor—until a dough is formed.

3 If dough is too dry, add a little milk.

4 Shape dough and let rest for 30 minutes.

5 Preheat oven to 375°F (190°C).

6 Bake rolls until lightly colored, about 20 minutes. Serve warm.

# Escabeche de Pescado

## Pickled Fish SERVES 4

**The most commonly used fish for escabeche is tuna, corvina, red snapper, trout, and catfish. This escabeche can be served warm or at room temperature.**

| AMOUNT | MEASURE | INGREDIENT |
|---|---|---|
| 1 pound | 448 g | Firm white-fish fillets, lean flesh, skinless, all bones removed |
| 1 tablespoon | $\frac{1}{2}$ ounce, 14 ml | Fresh lemon juice |
| $\frac{1}{2}$ teaspoon | 2 g | Salt |
| $\frac{1}{4}$ teaspoon | 1 g | Black pepper, freshly ground |
| $\frac{1}{4}$ cup | 2 ounces, 60 ml | Olive oil |
| $\frac{1}{2}$ cup | 2 ounces, 56 g | Red onions, julienne |
| $\frac{1}{4}$ cup | 1 ounce, 28 g | Red bell pepper, julienne |
| $\frac{1}{4}$ cup | 1 ounce, 28 g | Green bell pepper, julienne |
| | | Garlic cloves, minced |
| 1 tablespoon | $\frac{1}{2}$ ounce, 14 g | Capers, washed and drained |
| 1 | | Bouquet garni (1 sprig fresh thyme, 2 sprigs fresh parsley, 1 bay leaf, $\frac{1}{4}$ teaspoon black peppercorns, tied up in cheesecloth) |
| $\frac{1}{4}$ cup | 2 ounces, 60 ml | Dry white wine |
| $\frac{1}{4}$ cup | 2 ounces, 60 ml | Sherry vinegar |
| $\frac{1}{4}$ cup | 2 ounces, 60 ml | Fish or chicken stock |
| | | Lettuce leaves for garnish |

### PROCEDURE

1. Rub fish with lemon juice and half the salt and black pepper. Let marinate in refrigerator for 1 hour. Cut into 1 inch (2.4 cm) by 2 inch (4.8 cm) pieces and set aside.
2. Heat oil over medium heat; sauté onion, bell peppers, and garlic for 5 minutes or until soft.
3. Add capers and remaining salt and pepper, bouquet garni, wine, vinegar, and stock; bring to simmer.
4. Add fish, baste with sauce, cover, and simmer until opaque in center, 2 to 4 minutes or less. Do not overcook.

5 Discard bouquet garni and correct seasoning.
6 Transfer fish to clean container; pour sauce over and let cool.
7 Before serving, refrigerate 1 to 2 hours or overnight.
8 Arrange on lettuce leaves to serve.

# Ají Colombiano

## Colombian Sauce

YIELD: 2 CUPS

***Ají* is as important to Colombians as *chimichurri* is to Argentines**

| AMOUNT | MEASURE | INGREDIENT |
|---|---|---|
| $\frac{1}{2}$ cup | 2 ounces, 56 g | Green onions, white and light green parts, thinly sliced |
| $\frac{1}{2}$ cup | 3 ounces, 84 g | Tomatoes, peeled, seeded, $\frac{1}{4}$ inch (.6 cm) dice |
| $\frac{1}{2}$ cup | 2 ounces, 56 g | Red onion, $\frac{1}{4}$ inch (.6 cm) dice |
| $\frac{1}{4}$ cup | $\frac{1}{2}$ ounce, 14 g | Cilantro, stemmed, chopped |
| 3 | | Hard-cooked egg whites, chopped |
| 1 tablespoons | 3 g | Fresh chives, chopped |
| $\frac{1}{2}$ cup | 4 ounces, 120 ml | Olive oil |
| 1 teaspoon | | Tabasco sauce |
| $\frac{1}{4}$ cup | 2 ounces, 60 ml | White wine vinegar |
| 1 tablespoon | $\frac{1}{2}$ ounce, 15 ml | Fresh lime juice |
| To taste | | Kosher salt and freshly ground pepper |

### PROCEDURE

1 Combine green onions, tomatoes, and red onions. Stir to blend.
2 Add the cilantro, egg whites, and chives. Stir to blend. Gradually stir in the olive oil.
3 Add the Tabasco, vinegar, lime juice, salt, and pepper. Stir to blend.

# Humitas Ecuatorianas

## Ecuadorian Humitas

YIELD: ABOUT 12, DEPENDING ON SIZE OF CORN HUSKS

**_Humitas_ are the South American cousin of tamale. Made with grated tender corn, the dough is wrapped and tied in corn husks, which are then steamed. _Humitas_ can be found throughout the Andes from Ecuador down to Argentina. Each country has its own version.**

Chef Tip **Ecuadorian cooks place a coin in the bottom of the pot before adding the steamer filled with _humitas_. The coin vibrates noisily on the bottom of the pot as the water simmers. The coin stops making noise when all the water has evaporated. This tells the cook that additional boiling water is needed.**

| AMOUNT | MEASURE | INGREDIENT |
|---|---|---|
| 12 | | Corn husks |
| 4 cups | 20 ounces, 560 g | Corn kernels |
| $\frac{1}{4}$ cup | 1 ounce, 28 g | Onion, $\frac{1}{4}$ inch (.6 cm) dice |
| $\frac{1}{2}$ cup | 4 ounces, 112 g | Butter, melted or vegetable oil |
| 3 | | Large eggs, separated |
| $\frac{1}{2}$ cup (approximately) | 3 ounces, 84 g | Cornmeal |
| 1 teaspoon | 4 g | Baking powder |
| 1 teaspoon | 8 g | Salt |
| 1 teaspoon | 8 g | Sugar |
| 1$\frac{1}{2}$ cups | 6 ounces, 168 g | Chihuahua, mozzarella, or Muenster cheese, shredded |
| | | Kitchen twine, cut into twelve 15 inch lengths |
| 2 cups | 16 ounces, 469 ml | Water |
| | | Aji Criollo (recipe follows) |

PROCEDURE

1. If using dried corn husks, soak them in water for at least 2 hours. Separate them one by one and stack them ready for use. If using fresh, blanch in boiling water for 2 to 3 minutes to make pliable; remove, drain, and cool.
2. Puree corn kernels and onion until finely ground.

3 Add butter, egg yolks, cornmeal, baking powder, salt, sugar, and cheese to corn and onion mixture. Pulse until well incorporated and smooth. The mixture should not be runny; add more cornmeal if necessary.

4 Whip egg whites to soft peaks and fold into mixture.

5 ASSEMBLY: Dry corn husks and place 2 overlapping; place $\frac{1}{2}$ cup (3 ounces, 84 g) corn batter on the lower half of the husks. Fold the two long sides of the corn husk in over the corn mixture. Fold the tapered end up, leaving the top open. Secure the tamale by tying with a strip of husk or a string.

6 Set up a steamer in a large saucepot with an elevated bottom and tight-fitting lid. Add water to reach just under the elevated bottom. Place *humitas* on the elevated bottom, standing up or laying down. Cover with any leftover husks and place the cover on the steamer. Steam until the *humitas* feel firm to the touch, about 30 minutes if small, 45 minutes if large. Add more water if needed.

7 To serve, remove the twine and place on a plate with the husks open to expose the *humitas*. Serve *aji criollo* on the side.

## Aji Criollo Creole Hot Pepper Salsa

YIELD: 3/4 CUP

| AMOUNT | MEASURE | INGREDIENT |
|---|---|---|
| **4** | | **Red or green serranos, or jalapeños peppers, seeded and minced (1/8 inch, 3 cm)** |
| **6 tablespoons** | **3 ounces, 90 ml** | **Water** |
| **$\frac{1}{2}$ teaspoon** | **3 g** | **Salt** |
| **$\frac{1}{4}$ cup** | **1 ounce, 28 g** | **Green onion, white part only, minced** |
| **2 tablespoons** | **6 g** | **Cilantro or parsley leaves, minced** |

PROCEDURE

1 Combine peppers, 2 tablespoons water, and salt. Puree in blender.

2 Combine puree with green onion, cilantro and remaining water and mix well. This is best served the same day it's made.

# The Caribbean

## The Land

The West Indian archipelago forms a massive breakwater 2,000 miles long consisting of thousands of islands and reefs that protect the Caribbean Sea against the Atlantic Ocean. This barrier provides the Caribbean its calm and clear waters.

This area is known by a variety of names. The earliest name, and the one most frequently used, is West Indies. Christopher Columbus gave the region that name erroneously when he arrived in 1492. He thought that he had circumnavigated the earth and that the islands were off the coast of India.

Spain and France called the islands the Antilles, after the mythological Atlantic island of Antilia. The larger islands (Cuba, Jamaica, Hispaniola, and Puerto Rico) came to be known as the Greater Antilles, while the remaining smaller islands were called the Lesser Antilles. Today the area is broken into four island chains: the Bahamas, the Greater Antilles, and the eastern and southern islands of the Lesser Antilles. Together, these islands cover more than 91,000 square miles of land area.

The northernmost island chain is the Bahamas, which include 29 inhabited islands and nearly 3,000 islets stretching southeastward from Florida. Most of them are flat islands formed from coral and limestone.

The Greater Antilles is the largest and westernmost chain. It includes Cuba, Hispaniola, Jamaica, and Puerto Rico. The four main islands comprise nine-tenths of the entire land area of the West Indies. Cuba alone has almost half this area. The main island of Cuba covers 40,543 square miles. Much of the landmass of the Greater Antilles is formed by a partially submerged mountain range, which forms the Sierra Maestras and Sierra de Nipe on Cuba, the Blue Mountains on Jamaica, the Cordillera Central on Hispaniola, and the mountainous core of Puerto Rico farther to the east. The western three-fourths of the island is a vast limestone platform similar to the limestone platforms of Florida and Mexico's Yucatán Peninsula.

The third island chain includes the eastern islands of the Lesser Antilles, which curve north from the coast of Venezuela toward Puerto Rico. The islands along this arc fall into two distinct geographic groups. Some islands formed as a result of volcanic activity, while others emerged from the ocean as low-lying coral islands. Saint Vincent, Saint Lucia, Martinique, Dominica, the western half of Guadeloupe, Montserrat, Nevis, Saint Kitts, and the Virgin Islands are mountainous with rims of coastal plain. There are many active volcanoes in the West Indies, including Montagne Pelée on Martinique and Soufrière on Saint Vincent. The Soufrière Hills volcano on Montserrat erupted during the mid-1990s, destroying the island's capital of Plymouth. The islands of Barbados, Antigua, Barbuda, Anguilla, and the eastern half of Guadeloupe generally have low elevations and more level terrain.

The fourth island chain, the southern islands of the Lesser Antilles, follows the coast of Venezuela, from Lake Maracaibo to the mouth of the Orinoco River. These islands are extreme northeastern extensions of the Andes Mountains and have complex geologic structures. They include Aruba, Bonaire, Curaçao, Margarita, and Trinidad and Tobago. One of the smallest inhabited islands is Saba, part of the Netherlands Antilles. A volcanic cone, Saba towers 2,854 feet above the ocean. Its capital, the Bottom, is built at the bottom of the extinct crater—the only patch of level land on the island. Many smaller uninhabited coral islets are found in the region.

# History

The English word *Caribbean*, its Spanish equivalent *Caribe*, and its French version *Caraïbe* comes from the name of an Indian tribe that, in pre-Columbian time, inhabited the northwest portion of South America, Central America, and the southeast islands of the region now known as the Caribbean Basin. The Carib people left their name behind as a symbol of the region they inhabited. On land, they lived in small settlements, farmed and fished, and hunted game with blowguns and bows and arrows and were noted for their ferocity. However the most dominant culture was that of the Tainos or Arawack. These people practiced a highly productive form of agriculture and had an advanced social and material culture.

The arrival of Christopher Columbus was the beginning of the end of the indigenous people of the Caribbean and beginning of the European conquest and domination. The

Caribbean became the most precious jewel in the crown of Spain. They began to settle the Greater Antilles soon after Christopher Columbus landed in the Bahamas in 1492. For the Arawak/Tainos, the Spanish conquest was disaster. Aside of the pressure exerted on them through the destruction of social structures and the disruption of their food supply the Arawaks had to face European diseases for which they were not immunologically prepared.

Spanish control of the region was not undisputed, and other European colonial powers constantly challenged it. The British, French, and Dutch encouraged and at times even licensed their citizens to attack Spanish merchant ships, fleets, and ports. They harassed the Spaniards with some success for nearly two hundred years, most intensively between the mid-1500s and mid-1600s.

The history of the years of massive colonial prosperity of the West Indies, especially in Jamaica (English rule) and St. Domingue (French rule, today Haiti) is centered around the economics of sugarcane production. When the Arawak population disappeared, the lack of manpower resulted in the introduction of African slaves. The flow of slaves to the West Indies was at first a trickle but became a flood in the eighteenth century. At that time, an increase of the demand for sugar in Europe triggered the astronomic growth of production by the West Indian sugar plantations. According to some historians the estimated number of people uprooted from Africa varies between sixty and one hundred million. Though many died during the Middle Passage, many also survived. And, after nearly three hundred years of struggle, the people of African descent became the inheritors of the lands of the Caribbean.

Politically the islands of the West Indies are made up of thirteen independent nations and a number of colonial dependencies, territories, and possessions. The Republic of Cuba, consisting of the island of Cuba and several nearby islands, is the largest West Indian nation. Haiti and the Dominican Republic, two other independent nations, occupy Hispaniola, the second largest island in the archipelago. Jamaica, Barbados, the Bahamas, Trinidad and Tobago, Dominica, Grenada, the Federation of Saint Kitts and Nevis, Saint Lucia, Saint Vincent and the Grenadines, and Antigua and Barbuda are the other sovereign nations.

Rule over nearly all the other West Indies islands is distributed among the United States, France, the Netherlands, Venezuela, and the United Kingdom. Puerto Rico, the fourth largest island of the archipelago, is a U.S. commonwealth and several of the Virgin Islands are United States territories. The French West Indies includes Martinique, Guadeloupe, and a number of smaller dependencies of Guadeloupe. Martinique and Guadeloupe and its dependencies are overseas departments of France. The Dutch possessions consist of the Netherlands Antilles (Curaçao and Bonaire), Aruba, and smaller Lesser Antilles islands. Venezuela controls about seventy Lesser Antilles islands, including Margarita Island. Dependencies of the United Kingdom are Anguilla, the Cayman Islands, Montserrat, Turks and Caicos Islands, and some of the Virgin Islands.

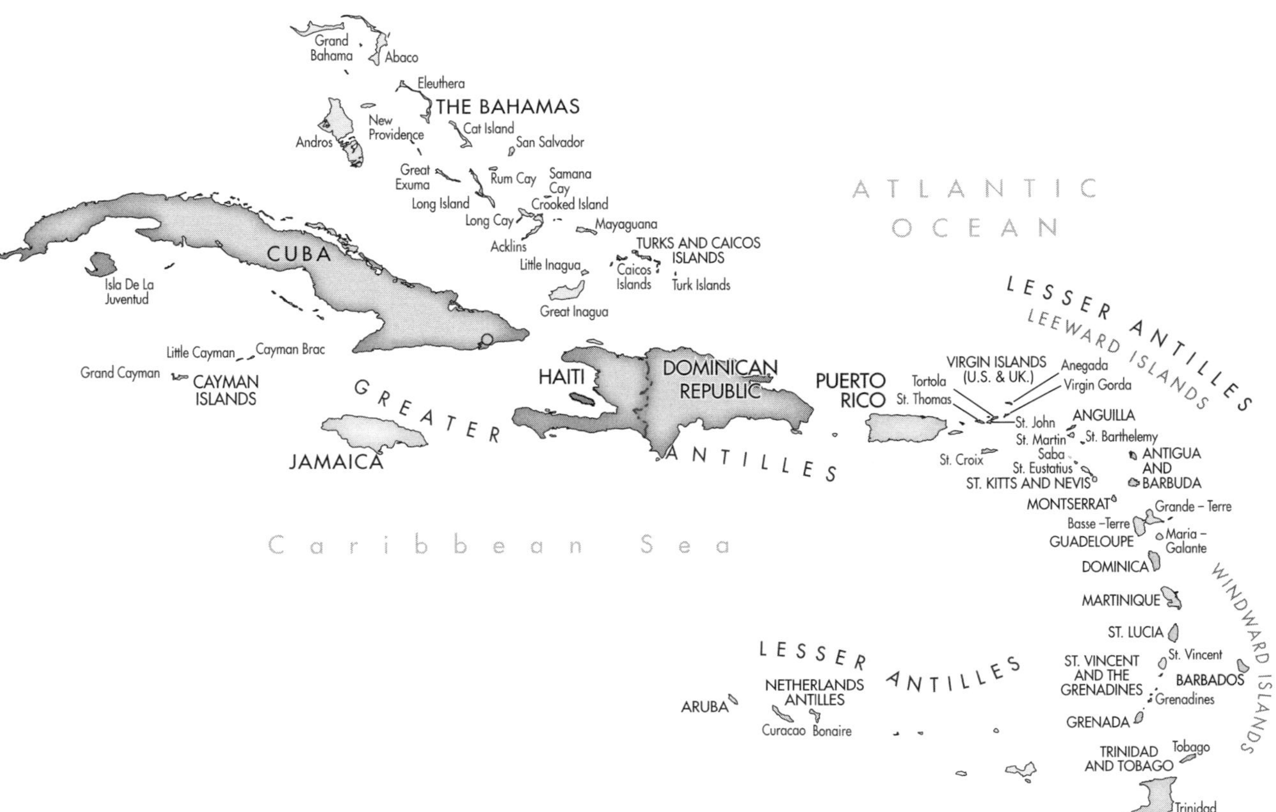


The Caribbean

# The People

The roots of the vast majority of Caribbean island people can be traced to Europe, Africa, and Asia. During the seventeenth century the English, Dutch, and French joined the Spanish in settling and exploring the Caribbean islands. At first, the English and French met their needs for labor by bringing Europeans to the islands as indentured servants, individuals who agreed to work for a specific number of years in exchange for passage to the colonies, food, and shelter. Eventually, all the colonizing countries imported slaves from Africa to provide labor. The number of slaves increased dramatically after the sugar plantations were established in the seventeenth century, making slavery the dominant economic institution on many islands.

The African people soon became the majority on most of the islands. Their culture and customs influence much of the religious worship, artistic expression, rhythmic dancing, singing, and even ways of thinking in the Caribbean. Spiritual practices such as Junkanoo in the Bahamas, Santeria in Cuba, Voodun in Haiti, and Rastafari in Jamaica are African-influenced movements that have Caribbean origin and a worldwide following. Reggae music and jerk cooking are also Africa-inspired contributions to the world from the Caribbean.

After the abolition of slave trade in the British West Indies during the early nineteenth century, Asian workers arrived in Cuba and Jamaica and indentured workers from India came to the Lesser Antilles.

Today, an estimated 70 percent of the people of the region are of African descent or *mulatto* (mixed African and European descent), 25 percent European descent, and 5 percent Asian descent. The racial composition of individual islands, however, differs widely. Most of the Caucasians live in Cuba, the Dominican Republic, and Puerto Rico. Most of the Asians live in Trinidad. The inhabitants of the other islands and the third of Hispaniola occupied by Haiti are overwhelmingly of African descent. Jamaica is typical of the older plantation islands, with 76 percent of its population of African descent, 15 percent mulatto, 1 percent of European descent, and 8 percent of Chinese, Indian, or other heritage.

# The Food

The islands originally inhabited by the Arawak and Carib Indian tribes had established a varied combination of foodstuffs and cooking techniques. The Caribs were cannibalistic but are credited by food historians to be the people who began ritually spicing their food with chile peppers. The Arawaks, on the other hand, devised a method of slow-cooking their meat by placing it over an open fire on a makeshift grate or grill made out of thin green sticks. They called this a *barbacoa*, which gave rise in both method and name to what is known today as a barbecue.

After Christopher Columbus arrived in the area in 1492, other Europeans followed Spain in colonizing the islands and brought with them their culinary trademarks. Some of the ingredients the Spanish and Europeans introduced included not only sugarcane, but varieties of coconut, chickpeas, cilantro, eggplant, onions, garlic, oranges, limes, mangoes, rice, and coffee.

The Caribbean's close proximity to Mexico and South America encouraged trade between the early settlers. Mexico traded papaya, avocado, chayote, and cocoa. Potatoes and passion fruit came from South America. Later breadfruit was introduced by Polynesians and corn, beans, and chile by Americans. Beginning in the early 1600s the slave trade brought foods from West Africa to the islands. The Africans brought crops of okra, callaloo, and *ackee*. Cuisine is similar from island to island, but each island has its specialties.

Typical Cuban foods include black beans, white rice, yellow rice, citrus marinades, garlic, and fried sliced banana (plantain). Olive oil and garlic marinades are often used as sauces. Popular spices include cumin, cayenne, and cilantro. Meat is often prepared roasted and in a *creola* style marinade. Two things not often seen in Cuban food are cream and milk products and cheeses in heavy sauces. These products, popular in Europe and North America, are expensive to purchase and often difficult to store. Pork and chicken are relatively plentiful, fresh and inexpensive. *Ajiaco*, a thick soup made with pork along with different kinds of edible vegetable roots and stems, is the national dish of Cuba. The taste depends on the vegetables and the seasonings chosen by the cook. Other typical Cuban dishes include *moros y cristianos* (white rice and black beans), *congrí* (a combination of rice and red kidney beans), and *picadillo à la habanera* (a mincemeat dish, Havana style).

Jamaica's national dish is said to be *ackee and saltfish*, usually served at breakfast, but can also be a main dish. *Ackee* is a fruit whose color and flavor when cooked are said to resemble scrambled eggs. A "closed" ackee is unripe and poisonous and is only safe to consume when it ripens and is thus "open." Saltfish is fish (usually cod) that has been heavily immersed in salt for preservation, drying, and curing purposes. Saltfish is usually soaked overnight in cold water to remove most of the salt before eating. Jamaica's saltfish (or codfish) fritters, called *Stamp and Go*, an island form of fast food, are made from a batter of soaked, cooked, skinned, and flaked saltfish, with scallions, chiles, and tomato, fried in coconut oil until golden brown. The long lasting Oriental and Indian influences in Caribbean cooking are represented by curries and rice. Curried goat is a favorite, usually reserved for special occasions. Jamaican *jerk* is another signature dish of the island. It can be either a dry seasoning mixture that is rubbed directly into the meat or it can be combined with water to create a marinade. *Jerk* recipes have passed through generations but the basic ingredients involve allspice, hot chiles (scotch bonnet), salt, and a mixture of up to thirty or more herbs and spices that blend to create one of the hottest and spiciest foods known. The Blue Mountains of Jamaica lend their name to the famous Blue Mountain Coffee, renowned for being smooth and full flavored. Coffee beans were first introduced to Jamaica in 1728 from the country of Martinique. The climatic conditions of the island ensured that the seedlings flourished, which triggered the cultivation of coffee bean crops in the region.

From Puerto Rico come *adobo* and *sofrito*—blends of herbs and spices that give many of the native foods their distinctive taste and color. *Adobo*, made by crushing together peppercorns, oregano, garlic, salt, olive oil, and lime juice or vinegar, is rubbed into meats before they are roasted. *Sofrito*, a potpourri of onions, garlic, and peppers browned in either olive oil or lard and colored with achiote (annatto seeds), imparts the bright yellow color to the island's rice, soups and stews. Soups include *sopón de pollo con arroz* (chicken soup with rice), which tastes different across the island's regions; *sopón de pescado* (fish soup), which is prepared with the head and tail intact; and *sopón de garbanzos con patas de cerdo* (chickpea soup with pig's feet), which is made with pumpkin, chorizo (Spanish sausage), salt pork, chile peppers, cabbage, potatoes, tomatoes, and fresh cilantro. The most traditional Puerto Rican dish is *asopao*, a hearty gumbo made with either chicken or shellfish. One well-known and low-budget version is *asopao de gandules* (pigeon peas). Another is *asopao de pollo* (chicken), which adds a whole chicken flavored with oregano, garlic, and paprika to a rich gumbo of salt pork, cured ham, green peppers, chile peppers, onions, cilantro, olives, tomatoes, chorizo, and pimientos. Stews, which are usually cooked in heavy kettles called *calderas*, are a large part of the Puerto Rican diet. A popular one is *carne guisada puertorriqueña* (Puerto Rican beef stew). The ingredients that flavor the beef vary but might include green peppers, sweet chile peppers, onions, garlic, cilantro, potatoes, pimento-stuffed olives, capers, and raisins. *Pastelón de carne*, or meat pie filled with salt pork, ham, and spices, is a staple of many Puerto Rican dinners. Other typical dishes include *carne frita con cebolla* (fried beefsteak with onions), *ternera a la parmesana* (veal parmesan) and roast leg of pork, fresh ham, lamb, or veal, which are prepared Creole style and flavored with adobo. Exotic fare, such as *Cabrito en Fricasé* (goat meat fricasse,) *Carne Mechada* (larded pork or beef loin with chorizo sausage,) and *Cuajito* and *Mollejas Guisadas* (stews popular during Christmas season) are also enjoyed by locals.

A festive island dish is *lechón asado* (barbecued pig). A recipe dating back to the Taino Indians, it is traditional for picnics and outdoor parties. The pig is basted with *jugo de naranja agria* (sour orange juice) and achiote coloring. Green plantains are peeled and roasted over hot stones, then served as a side dish. The traditional dressing served with the pig is *aji -li-mojili*, a sour garlic sauce consisting of garlic, whole black peppercorns, and sweet seeded chile peppers, flavored further with vinegar, lime juice, salt, and olive oil. Chicken is a Puerto Rican staple, *arroz con pollo* (chicken with rice) being the most common dish. Other preparations include *pollo al Jérez* (chicken in sherry), *pollo agridulce* (sweet-and-sour chicken) and *pollitos asados a la parrilla* (broiled chicken). Fish specialties include *mojo isleño*, fried fish in a typical sauce of olives, olive oil, onions, pimientos, capers, tomato sauce, vinegar, garlic, and bay leaves. Puerto Ricans often cook *camarones en cerveza* (shrimp in beer) and *jueyes hervidos* (boiled crab). Rice and plantains are prepared in dozens of ways and accompany nearly every meal. Rice (*arroz*) is simmered slowly with sofrito and generally served with *habichuelas* (beans) or *gandules* (pigeon peas). Another typical rice specialty is *pegao*, which is rice that is prepared so that it sticks to the bottom of the pan and gets crispy. Plantains also are served in many forms. *Amarillos* are ripe plantains fried with sugar to enhance their sweetness. Green plantains are either mashed into discs and deep fried to make *tostones* or mashed into balls of *mofongo* and mixed with pork or seafood and spices.

In St. Vincent the national dish is roasted breadfruit and jackfish. Seafood is abundant, including lobster, crab, conch (pronounced conk), shrimp, whelk, and mahimahi. A favorite delicacy is *tri tri*, a tiny fish seasoned with spices and curry powder and fried into cakes. Other popular dishes include callaloo stew, *souse* (a soupy stew made with pigs feet), pumpkin soup, *roti*, and *buljol* (salted fish, tomatoes, sweet peppers, and onions served with roasted breadfruit). A favorite dessert, *duckanoo*, originally from Africa, is made with cornmeal, coconut, spices, and brown sugar. The ingredients are tied up in a banana leaf (hence its other name, *Tie-a-Leaf*), and slowly cooked in boiling water.

Native cooking in the Dominican Republic combines Spanish influences with local produce. Beef is expensive (Dominicans raise fine cattle, but mostly for export) and local favorites are pork and goat meat. Breakfast typically calls for a serving of *mangu*, a mix of plantains, cheese, and bacon. *Mangu* has been called "mashed potatoes" of the Dominican Republic. A foundation of the native diet, '*La Bandera Dominicana*, or the Dominican flag meal, is eaten by nearly everyone at lunchtime. The most important meal of the day, *La Bandera* consists of rice, beans, meat, vegetables, and fried plantains. Another popular dish is *Sancocho*, a Spanish-style stew usually served with rice. Ingredients include various roots, green plantains, avocado, and typically chicken or beef, although it sometimes includes a combination of seven different types of meat (*Sancocho prieto*). Goat meat, a staple in many Dominican homes, may also be used in this recipe. It offers a unique addition to the character of any dish since these animals graze on wild oregano. *Locrio*, or Dominican rice, varies. An adaptation of the Spanish paella, *locrio* is made with achiote (a colored dye produced from the seeds of the achiote plant), because saffron spice is unavailable. *Casabe* (a round flat cassava bread) and *catibias* (cassava flour fritters filled with meat) are the only culinary legacy of the Taino Indians. Desserts here are very sweet, made with sugar and condensed milk in various flavors (coconut, papaya, banana, pineapple, soursop, ginger), prepared as flans, puddings, and creams. Tropical fruits are abundant and are used in desserts throughout the year, but many different varieties are found depending on the altitude (for example, cherries, plums, and strawberries grow in the central regions).

Barbados is distinguished for its *flying fish/coo-coo* dinners. Sleek, silver-blue fish with fins that resemble dragonfly wings, flying fish are able to propel themselves in the air at speeds up to thirty miles an hour to escape predators. *Coo-coo* is a polenta-like porridge made from yellow cornmeal, water, salt, pepper, butter, and okra. Other specialties include *conkies*, from Ghana, which are steamed sweet or savory preparations with mixtures of cornmeal, coconut, pumpkin, raisins, sweet potato, and spices, in preboiled banana leaf pieces. *Eddo*, sometimes called *coco*, is a hairy root vegetable with the size and flavor of a potato that is used in soups.

Peas and rice, or pigeon peas are a mainstay of the diet. The peas are cooked with rice and flavored with coconut. The peas are also known as *congo* or *gongo* peas on other islands. *Jug-jug* is a stew made from corned beef, pork, pigeon peas, and guinea corn. Lamb in Barbados is from a breed of black-bellied sheep that look like goats.

Antigua's national dish is *fungi and pepperpot,* a thick vegetable stew with salted meat. *Ducana* (sweet potato dumpling) is served with saltfish and *chop up* (mashed eggplant, okra and seasoning). *Black pineapples* from Antigua are famous throughout the East Caribbean for their unique, extra-sweet flavor.

The signature dish of Curaçao is *keshi yená,* or "stuffed cheese." This dish is traditionally made with chicken, vegetables, seasonings, and raisins, which are stuffed into a scooped-out Edam or Gouda cheese shell. The "top" of the cheese is replaced and the whole is baked for at least an hour. In Colonial times, the Dutch masters would eat the cheese and "generously" donate the shell to their workers. Having to make due with what they had, the poor people of the island came up with this specialty. Two very popular dishes are *funchi* and *tutu.* Both based on cornmeal, they are commonly served as side dishes or appetizers. Taken directly from African cuisine, these two dishes are still cooked in the traditional manner. Funchi is much like polenta, in that cornmeal is poured into boiling water seasoned with butter and salt. It is stirred with a spoonlike utensil called a *mealie* or *funchi stick.* It is most often left mushy and served in a mound, although sometimes it is allowed to stiffen and then shaped into dumplings, much like hushpuppies. Some fancy eateries will shape the *funchi* into ramekins or other molds. *Tutu* is like *funchi* but with the addition of mashed black-eyed peas and is mixed with a *lélé* (a stick with three points, used like a whisk.) *Bitterbal,* another popular Dutch-inspired dish, is sausage meat formed into balls, coated in bread crumbs and fried. It is eaten for breakfast, lunch, and snacks.

*Rotis* in Trinidad are as common as hamburgers in the United States. This unofficial national dish consists of a curry meal wrapped in thin pastry; its prototype was brought to the Caribbean by Indian immigrants some decades ago. The little packets of food have turned into a top seller for a quick snack.

# Glossary

**Ackee** The fruit of a West African tree, named in honor of Captain Bligh, who introduced it to Jamaica. The ackee fruit is bright red. When ripe it bursts open to reveal three large black seeds and bright yellow flesh. It is popular as a breakfast food throughout Jamaica. Ackee is poisonous if eaten before it is fully mature and because of its toxicity, it is subject to import restrictions and may be hard to obtain in some countries. Never open an ackee pod; it will open itself when it ceases to be deadly. The edible part is the aril, sometimes called Vegetable

Brains; it looks like a small brain or scrambled eggs, with a delicate flavor. It is best known in the Jamaican dish saltfish and ackee.

**Allspice, Pimienta** Dark-brown berry, similar to peppercorns, that combines the flavors of cinnamon, clove, and nutmeg.

**Annatto** This slightly musky-flavored reddish yellow spice, ground from the seeds of a flowering tree, is native to the West Indies and the Latin tropics. Islanders store their annatto seeds in oil, giving the oil a beautiful color. Saffron or turmeric can be substituted. The Spanish name *achiote* is sometimes referred to as achote. Available in Latin American and some Oriental markets.

**Bay Rum** The bay rum tree is related to the evergreen that produces allspice and the West African tree that produces melgueta pepper. Used to flavor soups, stews, and, particularly, *blaff.*

**Beans, Peas** Interchangeable terms for beans. Kidney beans in Jamaica are called peas. In Trinidad pigeon peas are referred to as peas. The French islands use the term *pois* for kidney beans. Cuba calls beans *frijoles.* Puerto Rico uses the term *habichuelas,* and in the Dominican Republic both terms are used. Often combined with rice, used in soups and stews, or pulped and made into fritters.

**Bitter or Seville Orange** Also called sour and bigarade orange. It is large, with a rough, reddish-orange skin. The pulp is too acid to be eaten raw, but the juice is used in meat and poultry dishes. The oranges are also used to make marmalade. A mixture of lime or lemon juice and sweet orange juice can be used as a substitute.

**Blaff** A broth infused with whole Scotch bonnet peppers and bay rum leaves in which whole or filleted fish is poached.

**Boniato** Tropical sweet potato.

**Boudin, Black Pudding** Sausage that may include pig's blood, thyme, and Scotch bonnet peppers. Frequently served with souse, a pork dish that can include any part of the pig.

**Breadfruit** Large green fruits, usually about 10 inches in diameter, with a potato-like flesh. It was introduced to Jamaica from its native Tahiti in 1793 by Captain Bligh. Breadfruit is not edible until cooked; when cooked the flesh is yellowish-white, like a dense potato. Breadfruit is picked and eaten before it ripens and is typically served like squash: baked, grilled, fried, boiled, or roasted after being stuffed with meat, or in place of any starch vegetable, rice, or pasta. It makes an excellent soup.

**Calabaza** A squash, also called West Indian or green pumpkin. It comes in a variety of sizes and shapes. The best substitutes are Hubbard or butternut squash.

**Callaloo** The principal ingredient in the most famous of all the island soups. The term applies to the leaves of two distinct types of plant that are used interchangeably. The first are the elephant-ear leaves of the taro plant. The other is Chinese spinach, a leafy vegetable typically prepared as one would prepare turnip or collard greens.

**Carambola, Star Fruit** Tart or acidy-sweet star-shaped fruit used in desserts, as a garnish for drinks, tossed into salads, or cooked together with seafood.

**Cassareep** The boiled down juice of grated cassava root, flavored with cinnamon, cloves, and sugar. It is the essential ingredient in pepperpot, the Caribbean island stew. It may be purchased bottled in West Indian markets.

**Cassava** This tuber, also known as manioc and yuca, is a rather large root vegetable, 6–12 inches length and 2–3 inches in diameter. Cassava has a tough brown skin with a very firm white flesh. Tapioca and cassareep are both made from cassava. There are two varieties of the plant: sweet and bitter. Sweet cassava is boiled and eaten as a starch vegetable. Bitter cassava contains a poisonous acid that can be deadly and must be processed before it can be eaten. This is done by boiling the root in water for at least 45 minutes; discard the water. Alternatively, grate the cassava and place it in a muslin cloth, then squeeze out as much of the acid as possible before cooking. Bitter cassava is used commercially but is not sold unprocessed in some countries.

**Chayote, Christophine, Cho-cho, Mirliton** A small pear-shaped vegetable, light green or cream colored, and often covered with a prickly skin. Bland, similar in texture to squash, and used primarily in Island cuisine as a side dish or in gratins and soufflés. Like pawpaw (papaya), it is also a meat tenderizer.

**Cherimoya** Pale-green fruit with white sweet flesh that has the texture of flan. Used for mousse and fruit sauces, the fruit is best when fully ripe, well chilled and eaten with a spoon.

**Chorizo** Spanish sausage that combines pork, hot peppers, and garlic.

**Coo-coo (or cou-cou)** The Caribbean equivalent of polenta or grits. Once based on cassava or manioc meal it is now made almost exclusively with cornmeal. Coo-coo can be baked, fried, or rolled into little balls and poached in soups or stews.

**Conch** Also known as *lambi* or *concha.* These large mollusks from the gastropod family are up to a foot long, with a heavy spiral shell with yellow that shades to pink inside. When preparing conch soup, conch salad or conch fritters, the tough conch flesh must be tenderized by pounding.

**Crapaud** Very large frogs, known as mountain chicken, found on the islands of Dominica and Monserrat. Fried or stewed legs are considered a national delicacy.

**Creole, Criolla** Creole refers to the cooking of the French-speaking West Indies, as well as to southern Louisiana and the U.S. Gulf states. Criolla refers to the cuisine of Spanish-speaking islands. Both terms encompass a melding of ingredients and cooking methods from France, Spain, Africa, the Caribbean, and the Americas.

**Dhal** Hindu name for legumes; in the Caribbean, it refers only to split peas or lentils.

**Darne** The Caribbean name for kingfish.

**Dasheen** Also known a coco, taro, and tannia, dasheen is a starchy tuber usually served boiled or cut up and used as a thickener in hearty soups. They are considered by some to have a texture and flavor superior to that of a Jerusalem artichoke or potato, but potatoes can often be used as a substitute for dasheen in recipes. Dasheen is often called coco, but coco is actually a slightly smaller relative of dasheen.

**Escabeche** The Spanish word for "pickled." It usually refers to fresh fish (and sometimes poultry) that is cooked in oil and vinegar, or cooked and then pickled in an oil and vinegar marinade.

**Guava, Guayaba** Tropical fruit that has over one hundred species. It is pear-shaped, yellow to green skinned, with creamy yellow, pink, or red granular flesh and rows of small hard seeds. Ripe guava have a perfume-like scent. Guava is used green or ripe in punches, syrups, jams, chutneys, and ice creams.

**Hearts of Palm** Ivory-colored core of some varieties of palm trees. They are used fresh or canned in salads and as a vegetable.

**Hibiscus** Also known as sorrel, rosell, or flor de Jamaica, this tropical flower is used for drinks, jams, and sauces. The flower blooms in December, after which it is dried and used to make a bright red drink that has a slightly tart taste and is the color of cranberry juice. It should not be confused with the American hibiscus found in the garden.

**Jack** A fish family of over two hundred species, these colorful saltwater fish are also known as yellowtail, greenback, burnfin, black, and amber jack. These delicately flavored fish tend to be large, weighing as much as 150 pounds, and readily available in waters around the world. Tuna and swordfish may be substituted.

**Lobster** Caribbean rock lobster. Unlike the Maine variety, this lobster has no claws.

**Malanga, Yautia** A relative of dasheen or taro, this tuber is prevalent throughout the Caribbean.

**Mamey Apple** The large tropical fruit, native to the New World, yields edible pulp that is tangerine in color. The flavor is similar to a peach.

**Mango** A native of India, this fruit is known as "the fruit of the tropics." Green mangoes are used in hot sauces and condiments, while ripe mangoes appear in desserts, candies, and drinks.

**Name** This giant tuber is called by a variety of different names. The Spanish translation of the word *ñame* is *yam*. The outer skin is brown and coarsely textured, while the inside is porous and very moist. The ñame grows to enormous size and is considered to be the "king" of tubers.

**Otaheite Apple** This pear-shaped apple ranges from pink to ruby red in color. This fruit is usually eaten fresh, but also poached in wine, or juiced and served as a beverage.

**Papaya** Also known as "pawpaw" in Jamaica. Green papaya is often used as an ingredient in chutney or relishes and as a main dish when stuffed. When ripe, it is yellow or orange and eaten as a melon, or served in fruit salad.

**Passion Fruit, Maracudja, Granadilla** Oval-shaped fruit that has a tough shell and a color range from yellow-purple to eggplant to deep chocolate. The golden-yellow pulp is sweet and it must be strained to remove the seeds. Used in juices, desserts, drinks, and sauces.

**Picadillo** Spicy Cuban hash, made of ground beef and cooked with olives and raisins.

**Pickapeppa Sauce** This sauce, manufactured in Jamaica at Shooters Hill near Mandeville, is a secret combination of tamarind, onions, tomatoes, sugar, cane vinegar, mangoes, raisins, and spices. Since 1921 the company has produced this savory sauce, which has won many awards and is distributed throughout North America. The sauce is aged in oak barrels for a minimum of one year.

**Saltfish** Saltfish is any fried, salted fish, but most often cod. With the increasing availability of fresh fish all over Jamaica, some cooks are moving away from this preserved fish, which originated in the days before refrigeration. Still, Jamaicans have a soft place in their hearts for the taste of this salted cod (sold around the world in Italian, Spanish, and Portuguese markets under some variant of the name *bacalao*). Ackee and saltfish is the preferred breakfast of Jamaicans. When imported saltfish is unavailable, Jamaicans have been known to make their own from fresh fish.

**Sofrito** A seasoning staple, there are many variations. Most contain pork, lard, green peppers, tomatoes, onions, and coriander. Typically they are prepared in advance and stored under refrigeration. The word comes from a Spanish verb that means "to fry lightly."

**Soursop, Corossol, Guanabana** Elongated, spike-covered fruit, slightly tart and delicately flavored. It is used mainly in drinks, punches, sherbets, and ice cream.

**Stamp and Go, Accra, or Baclaitos** Spicy-hot fritters popular throughout the Caribbean. Methods, ingredients, and names vary from island to island.

**Star Apple** The local fruit is the main ingredient in a popular holiday dish called matrimony, a mix of star apple and oranges. It is similar to an orange but is made up of clear segments. The eight-pointed star that gives the name can be seen when the fruit is sliced.

**Stinking Toe** A pod that resembles a human toe, this fruit possesses a foul smelling rough exterior. The sugary power inside is eaten, or used in custards or beverages.

**Sugar Apple, Sweetsop** The flesh of the sweetsop is actually black seeds surrounded by sweet white pulp. The sweetsop is native to the tropical Americas.

**Tamarind** A large, decorative tree that produces brown pods containing a sweet and tangy pulp used for flavoring curries, sauces, and even beverages.

**Yam** Similar in size and color to the potato, but nuttier in flavor, it is not to be confused with the Southern sweet yam or sweet potato. Caribbean yams are served boiled, mashed, or baked.

**Yautía** A member of the taro root family, the yautía is the size of a potato, but more pear-shaped. It has a brown fuzzy outer skin. The flesh is white and slimy and is custard-like when cooked. It is one of the most natural thickeners, used to thicken soups, stews, and bean dishes. There is also a purple yautía, also called *mora.*

**Yuca** Root vegetable similar in length and shape to a turnip, with scaly yam-like skin. Universally made into flour for breads and cakes, and used as a base for tapioca.

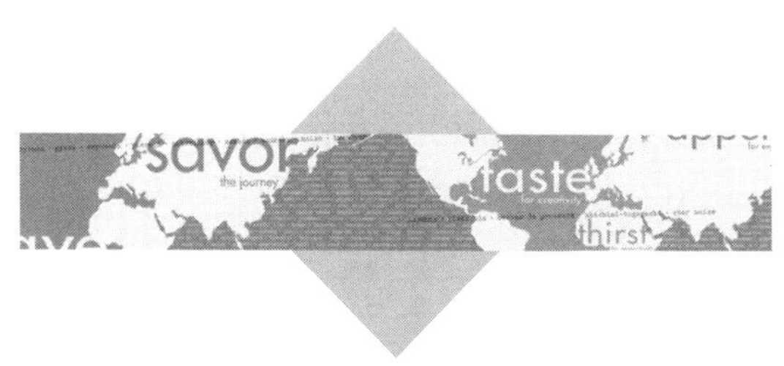

# Menus and Recipes from the Caribbean

MENU ONE

*Buljol:* Flaked Saltfish (Trinidad)

*Yuca Mufongo* with Cilantro Aioli Sauce (Puerto Rico)

Jamaican Jerk Beef Steak or Jamaican Jerk Chicken

*Arroz Mamposteao:* Rice and Beans (Puerto Rico)

*Mojo de Amarilos:* Ripe Plantain Chutney (Puerto Rico)

*Coo-Coo* (Barbados)

*Coco Quemado:* Coconut Pudding (Cuba)

MENU TWO

Run Down (Jamaica)

*Ensalada de Aguacate y Piña:* Avocado and Pineapple Salad (Cuba)

*Arroz con Pollo:* Chicken and Rice (Puerto Rico)

Pepperpot Soup (Jamaica)

Sweet Potato Cake (Martinique)

MENU THREE

*Camarones Sofrito:* Shrimp in Green Sofrito (Dominican Republic)

*Sopa de Frijol Negro:* Black Bean Soup (Cuba)

Salad of Hearts of Palm with Passion Fruit Vinaigrette (Puerto Rico)

Curried Kid or Lamb (Trinidad)

Fried Ripe Plantains (All Islands)

Tamarind Balls (Jamaica)

Stuffed Dates (Curacao)

ADDITIONAL RECIPES

*Tostones:* Twice-Fried Plantains (All Islands)

Roasted Breadfruit (Barbados)

Stewed Conch (Cayman Islands)

# Buljol

## Flaked Saltfish (Trinidad) SERVES 4

**The name is from the French *brule gueule*, meaning "to burn your mouth."**

| AMOUNT | MEASURE | INGREDIENT |
|---|---|---|
| ½ pound | 8 ounce, 224 g | Saltfish, boneless |
| 2 tablespoons | 1 ounce, 30 ml | Fresh lime juice |
| 1 cup | 6 ounces, 168 g | Cucumber, peeled and seeded, ¼ inch (.6 cm) dice |
| 1 cup | 4 ounces, 112 g | Onion, ¼ inch dice (.6 cm) |
| 2 teaspoons | | Garlic, minced |
| 1 cup | 6 ounces, 168 g | Tomato, peeled, seeded, ¼ inch (.6 cm) dice |
| 2 tablespoons | | Green onion, tops, minced |
| ½ | | Scotch bonnet chile, seeded, minced |
| 3 tablespoons | 1½ ounce, 45 ml | Olive oil |
| 1 | | Avocado, peeled and cut into 12 slices |

**PROCEDURE**

1. Desalt the salt fish: cover with boiling water and allow to cool in the water. Drain. Remove any skin and bones. Shred the fish and cover again with boiling water, let cool. Drain and press out all the water.
2. Combine all the other ingredients except the avocado and mix well.
3. Add fish and toss well, refrigerate for at least two hours.
4. Serve with sliced avocado.

# Yuca Mufongo with Cilantro Aioli Sauce (Puerto Rico)

SERVES 4

**Yuca is also known as manioc or cassava.**

| AMOUNT | MEASURE | INGREDIENT |
|---|---|---|
| 1 pound | 448 g | Fresh yuca |
| $\frac{1}{2}$ cup | $2\frac{1}{2}$ ounces, 70 g | Bacon, $\frac{1}{4}$ inch (.6 cm) dice |
| $\frac{1}{3}$ cup | $1\frac{1}{2}$ ounces, 42 g | Onion, $\frac{1}{4}$ inch (.6 cm) dice |
| 1 | | Garlic clove, minced |
| 1 teaspoon | | Oregano, dried ground |
| 1 tablespoon | | Cilantro, minced |
| 2 | | Eggs, beaten |
| 1 teaspoon | | Adobo |
| To taste | | Salt and pepper |
| As needed | | All purpose flour |
| As needed | | Oil for frying |

**PROCEDURE**

1. Trim ends from fresh yuca and peel remainder, removing all waxy brown skin and pinkish layer underneath. Cut yuca into 3 inch thick pieces. Cover with salted water by 2 inches and boil until soft, but firm and almost translucent. Drain. Carefully halve hot yuca pieces lengthwise and remove thin woody cores. Mash until smooth.
2. Over medium heat, render the bacon until crisp.
3. Add the onions and garlic to bacon and cook 2 to 3 minutes or until soft.
4. Add mashed yuca, oregano, cilantro, and eggs; mix well.
5. Season with adobo, salt and pepper to taste.
6. Chill for 1 hour or until firm.
7. Preheat deep fat fryer to 350°F (175°C).
8. Shape two tablespoons of the mixture into balls. Roll in flour, shake off excess, and fry until golden brown. Drain on paper towels.
9. Serve hot or warm with Cilantro Aioli Sauce.

# Adobo Spice Mix 1

YIELD: 2 OUNCES

| AMOUNT | MEASURE | INGREDIENT |
|---|---|---|
| 1 teaspoon | 4 g | Coriander seeds, toasted and ground |
| 1 teaspoon | | Ground ginger |
| 1½ teaspoons | | Red pepper flakes, crushed |
| 1 teaspoon | | Turmeric, ground |
| 1 tablespoon | | Dry mustard |
| 1 teaspoon | | Nutmeg, freshly grated |
| 1½ teaspoons | | Cayenne pepper |
| 1 teaspoon | | Black pepper, freshly ground |
| 1½ tablespoons | | Kosher salt |
| 1 tablespoon | | Paprika |
| 1 tablespoon | | Sugar |

PROCEDURE

1 Mix all ingredients together.

# Adobo Spice Mix 2

YIELD: 2 OUNCES

| AMOUNT | MEASURE | INGREDIENT |
|---|---|---|
| 1 tablespoon | 6 g | Garlic powder |
| 1 tablespoon | | Onion powder |
| 1 tablespoon | | Dried oregano, ground |
| ½ teaspoon | | Ground cumin |
| ½ tablespoon | | Salt |
| 1 teaspoon | | White pepper, freshly ground |

PROCEDURE

1 Mix all ingredients together.

# Cilantro Aioli Sauce

SERVES 4

| AMOUNT | MEASURE | INGREDIENT |
|---|---|---|
| 4 | | Garlic cloves, chopped |
| $\frac{1}{4}$ teaspoon | | Salt |
| 1 cup | 8 ounces, 240 ml | Mayonnaise, commercial or made with pasteurized eggs |
| 2 tablespoons | 1 ounces, 30 ml | Fresh lime juice |
| 2 tablespoons | | Cilantro, leaves only, minced |
| To taste | | Salt and pepper |

**PROCEDURE**

1. Combine garlic and $\frac{1}{4}$ teaspoon salt; mash to a paste.
2. Combine garlic, mayonnaise, lime juice, and cilantro. Adjust seasoning.
3. Chill for 1 hour to blend flavors.

# Jamaican Jerk Beef Steak

SERVES 4

| AMOUNT | MEASURE | INGREDIENT |
|---|---|---|
| 1 $\frac{1}{2}$ pounds | 24 ounces, 672 g | Skirt or flank steak |
| To taste | | Salt and black pepper, freshly ground |
| 2 tablespoons | | Adobo spice mix 1 |
| 1 tablespoon | | Fresh thyme, fresh, chopped |
| 2 tablespoons | 1 ounce, 30 ml | White vinegar |
| $\frac{1}{4}$ cup | 2 ounces, 60 ml | Olive oil |

**PROCEDURE**

1. Season the meat with salt and pepper to taste.
2. Combine the adobo spice, thyme, vinegar and oil; whisk to combine well. Add meat and marinate 1 hour at room temperate or 2 to 3 hours under refrigeration.
3. Grill over high heat to desired temperature.
4. Slice and serve hot with *arroz mamposteao* and *mojo de amarilos*.

# Jamaican Jerk Chicken

SERVES 4

| AMOUNT | MEASURE | INGREDIENT |
|---|---|---|
| $\frac{1}{4}$ cup | 2 ounces, 60 ml | Fresh lime juice |
| $\frac{1}{4}$ cup | 2 ounces, 60 ml | Water |
| $3\frac{1}{2}$ pounds | | Whole chicken, cut in half |
| 2 | | Garlic cloves, minced |
| Jerk Marinade | | |
| 2 teaspoons | | Jamaican pimiento, ground |
| $\frac{1}{2}$ teaspoon | | Nutmeg, grated |
| $\frac{1}{2}$ teaspoon | | Mace, ground |
| 1 teaspoon | | Salt |
| 1 teaspoon | | Sugar |
| 2 teaspoons | | Dried thyme |
| 1 teaspoon | | Black pepper |
| 1 cup | 4 ounces, 112 g | Green onions, chopped |
| 1 cup | 4 ounces, 112 g | Yellow onion, chopped |
| 1 | | Whole Scotch bonnet |
| 2 tablespoons | 1 ounce, 30 ml | Vegetable oil |

PROCEDURE

1. Preheat grill.
2. Combine lime juice and water and use to rinse chicken. Pat dry and rub with garlic.
3. Combine remaining ingredients in a blender, mortar, or food processor. Process ingredients to almost smooth and pour over chicken; marinate in refrigerator for at least 2 hours.
4. Remove chicken from marinade.
5. Grill, turning often, until fully cooked. Cut chicken into 8 to 12 pieces.

# Arroz Mamposteao

## Rice and Beans (Puerto Rico)

SERVES 4

| AMOUNT | MEASURE | INGREDIENT |
|---|---|---|
| **Green Sofrito Mix** | | |
| 1 cup | 4 ounces, 112 g | Onion, $\frac{1}{2}$ inch (1.2 cm) dice |
| 1 cup | 4 ounces, 112 g | Cubanelle pepper (Italian), $\frac{1}{2}$ inch (1.2 cm) dice |
| 1 cup | 4 ounce, 112 g | Green bell pepper, $\frac{1}{2}$ inch (1.2 cm) dice |
| 6 | | Garlic cloves, chopped |
| $\frac{1}{2}$ cup | 1 ounce, 28 g | Fresh cilantro, leaves only |
| 2 tablespoons | 1 ounce, 30 ml | Water |

PROCEDURE

1 Using a food processor, blender, or mortar and pestle, process all ingredients into a loose puree paste. Add additional water if necessary.

| **Bean Stew** | | |
|---|---|---|
| 1 cup | 6 ounces, 168 g | Pink beans or red kidney beans (dried) |
| 1 cups | 6 ounces, 168 g | Corned pork or smoked ham, 1 inch (2.4 cm) cubes |
| 3 cups | 24 ounces, 720 ml | Water |

PROCEDURE

1 Soak the beans overnight in water. Drain.

2 Combine beans, pork, and water; bring to a boil, cover, and simmer gently until the beans are just tender, about 1 hour.

3 Drain, retaining beans and pork.

| **Garnish for Bean Stew** | | |
|---|---|---|
| 2 tablespoons | 1 ounce, 30 ml | Oil |
| $\frac{1}{2}$ cup | 2 ounces, 56 g | Onion, $\frac{1}{4}$ inch (.6 cm) dice |
| 2 | | Garlic cloves, minced |
| 1 | | Small hot red or green pepper, seeded, minced |

| | | |
|---|---|---|
| 3 tablespoons | ½ ounce, 45 ml | Green sofrito |
| ¼ cup | 6 ounces, 180 ml | Tomato sauce |
| 1 cup | 8 ounces, 240 ml | Water |
| 1 cup | 6 ounces, 168 g | West Indian pumpkin (calabaza) or Hubbard squash |
| 2 teaspoons | | Adobo spice mix (1 or 2) |

**PROCEDURE**

1. Heat the oil over medium heat, sauté onion and garlic until soft but not brown, 2 to 3 minutes.
2. Add pepper and sofrito; cook 2 minutes.
3. Add tomato sauce; cook 2 minutes.
4. Add cooked beans and pork mixture, water, squash, and adobo spice mix. Cook, uncovered, 15 to 20 minutes or until squash is cooked and sauce has thickened. Remove from heat and reserve.

**Mamposteao Rice**

| | | |
|---|---|---|
| 2 tablespoons | 1 ounce, 30 ml | Corn oil |
| ¼ cup | 2 ounces, 56 g | Chorizo, chopped |
| ½ cup | 2 ounces, 56 g | Bacon, chopped fine |
| ⅓ cup | 2 ounces, 56 g | Onion, ¼ inch (.6 cm) dice |
| 2 | | Garlic cloves, minced |
| 1 tablespoon | | Cilantro, minced |
| 2 tablespoons | | Green bell pepper, ⅛ inch (.3 cm) dice |
| 2 tablespoons | | Red bell pepper, ⅛ inch (.3 cm) dice |
| 1 cup | 6 ounces, 180 ml | Bean stew |
| 2 cups | 8 ounces, 224 g | Cooked rice |

**PROCEDURE**

1. Heat oil over medium heat; sauté chorizo and bacon for 2 to 3 minutes, until cooked.
2. Add onion and garlic; sauté for 3 minute or until soft.
3. Add cilantro and peppers; sauté for 3 minutes or until soft.
4. Add bean stew; cook 2 minutes.
5. Add rice, stirring constantly; cook 4 minutes until the consistency of a wet risotto.

# Mojo de Amarilos

## Ripe Plantain Chutney (Puerto Rico) SERVES 4

**Chef Tip** **When peeling plantains (plátanos), moisten your hands and rub with salt to prevent the juices from sticking to your hands.**

| AMOUNT | MEASURE | INGREDIENT |
|---|---|---|
| 2 tablespoons | 1 ounce, 30 ml | Vegetable oil |
| 1 cup | 6 ounces, 168 g | Very ripe plantain, very yellow, almost orange, with black spots, peeled, $\frac{1}{2}$ inch (1.2 cm) dice |
| 10 | | Cherry tomato cut in half |
| $\frac{1}{4}$ cup | 1 ounce, 28 g | Red onion, 1 inch (2.4 cm) julienne |
| $\frac{1}{4}$ cup | 1 ounce, 28 g | Red bell pepper, 1 inch (2.4 cm) julienne |
| $\frac{1}{4}$ cup | 1 ounce, 28 g | Yellow bell pepper, 1 inch (2.4 cm) julienne |
| 1 | | Garlic clove, thinly sliced |
| 2 teaspoons | | Golden raisins |
| $\frac{1}{4}$ cup | 2 ounces, 60 ml | Olive oil |
| 2 tablespoons | | Fresh cilantro, leaves only |
| To taste | | Salt and pepper |

### PROCEDURE

1. Heat oil over medium heat and sauté plantain until tender and brown.
2. Combine remaining ingredients except cilantro, salt, and pepper; simmer together for 5 to 6 minutes.
3. Add cilantro and correct seasoning. Serve warm to hot about 160°F (71°C).

# Coo-Coo (Barbados) SERVES 4

| AMOUNT | MEASURE | INGREDIENT |
|---|---|---|
| **3 cups** | **24 ounces, 720 ml** | **Water** |
| **To taste** | | **Salt** |
| **1 cup** | **4 ounces, 112 g** | **Young okras, cut $\frac{1}{4}$ inch (.6 cm) thick** |
| **1 cup** | **$6\frac{1}{4}$ ounces, 175 g** | **Yellow cornmeal** |
| **2 tablespoons** | **1 ounce, 30 ml** | **Butter** |

**PROCEDURE**

1. Bring water and salt to a boil. Add okras and simmer, covered for 10 minutes.
2. Add cornmeal in a slow, steady stream, stirring constantly with a wooden spoon.
3. Cook over medium heat until mixture is thick and smooth, stirring constantly, 5 minutes.
4. Remove from heat and let stand 3 to 5 minutes.
5. Place on serving dish and spread butter on top.

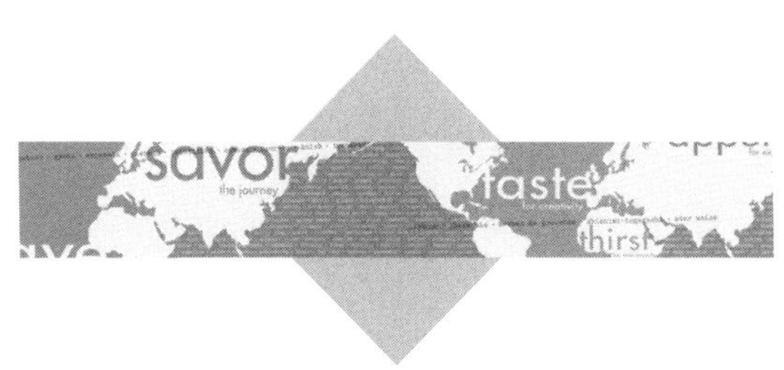

# Coco Quemado

## Coconut Pudding (Cuba)

SERVES 4

| AMOUNT | MEASURE | INGREDIENT |
| --- | --- | --- |
| 1 $\frac{1}{2}$ cups | 12 ounces, 336 g | Granulated sugar |
| $\frac{3}{4}$ cup | 6 ounces, 180 ml | Water |
| 3 cups | 9 ounces, 252 g | Grated coconut |
| 3 | | Egg yolks, lightly beaten |
| 1 teaspoon | | Ground cinnamon |
| 6 tablespoons | 3 ounces, 180 ml | Dry sherry |

**PROCEDURE**

1. Cook the sugar and water to syrup at the thread stage. When sugar syrup reaches this stage, a drop of boiling syrup forms a soft 2-inch thread when immersed in cold water. On a candy thermometer, the thread stage is between 230–234°F (110–112°C).
2. Add coconut, and then stir in egg yolks, cinnamon and sherry. Cook over low heat, stirring constantly until mixture is thick.
3. Pour into serving dish and brown the top under a broiler or with a torch.
4. Serve warm or chilled.

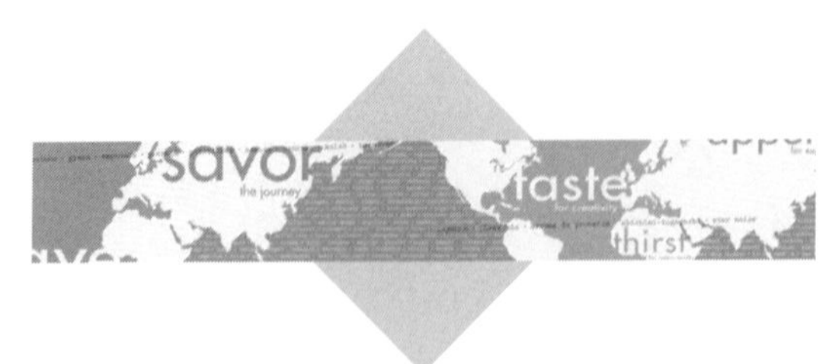

# Run Down (Jamaica) SERVES 4

| AMOUNT | MEASURE | INGREDIENT |
|---|---|---|
| 1 pound | 16 ounces, 448 g | Mackerel or shad fillets, or other oily fish, such as bluefish, mullet or pompano |
| $\frac{1}{4}$ cup | 2 ounces, 60 ml | Fresh lime juice |
| $1\frac{1}{2}$ cups | 12 ounces, 360 ml | Coconut milk |
| $\frac{1}{2}$ cup | 2 ounces, 56 g | Onion, minced |
| $\frac{1}{2}$, or to taste | | Scotch bonnet chile, seeded and minced |
| 2 | | Garlic cloves, minced |
| 1 cup | 6 ounces, 168 g | Tomato, peeled, seeded, $\frac{1}{2}$ inch (.6 cm) dice |
| 2 teaspoons | 10 ml | Apple-cider vinegar |
| 1 teaspoon | | Fresh thyme leaves |
| To taste | | Salt and black pepper |

**PROCEDURE**

1. Marinate fish in the lime juice for 15 minutes.
2. Cook coconut milk over medium heat for 5 to 8 minutes or until it begins to turn oily.
3. Add onion, chile and garlic, cook 5 minutes or until onions are soft.
4. Add tomatoes, vinegar, and thyme and season with salt and pepper.
5. Drain the fish and add to the mixture. Cover and cook over low heat 8 to 10 minutes or until the fish flakes easily.
6. Serve hot with boiled bananas or roasted breadfruit.

# Ensalada de Aguacate y Piña

## Avocado and Pineapple Salad (Cuba)

SERVES 4

| AMOUNT | MEASURE | INGREDIENT |
|---|---|---|
| $\frac{1}{4}$ cup | 2 ounces, 60 ml | Olive oil |
| $\frac{1}{4}$ cup | 2 ounces, 60 ml | Cider vinegar |
| $\frac{1}{4}$ cup | 2 ounces, 60 ml | Fresh orange juice |
| $\frac{1}{4}$ cup | 2 ounces, 56 g | Granulated sugar |
| To taste | | Salt and pepper |
| 4 cups | 8 ounces, 224 g | Iceberg or Boston lettuce, shredded |
| 1 cup | 6 ounces, 168 g | Fresh pineapple, $\frac{1}{2}$ inch (1.2 cm) cubes |
| 1 cup | 4 ounces, 112 g | Sweet red onions, thinly sliced |
| 1 | | Avocado, peeled, sliced $\frac{1}{4}$ inch (.6 cm) thick |
| 4 | | Fresh lime wedges |

PROCEDURE

1 Combine olive oil, vinegar, orange juice, and sugar in a blender until smooth. Season with salt and pepper.

2 Lightly toss together the lettuce, pineapple, and red onions. Dress with oil and vinegar mixture; adjust the amount used to taste.

3 Garnish individual salads with several avocado slices lightly seasoned with salt and pepper and a squeeze of lime juice. Serve with lime wedges.

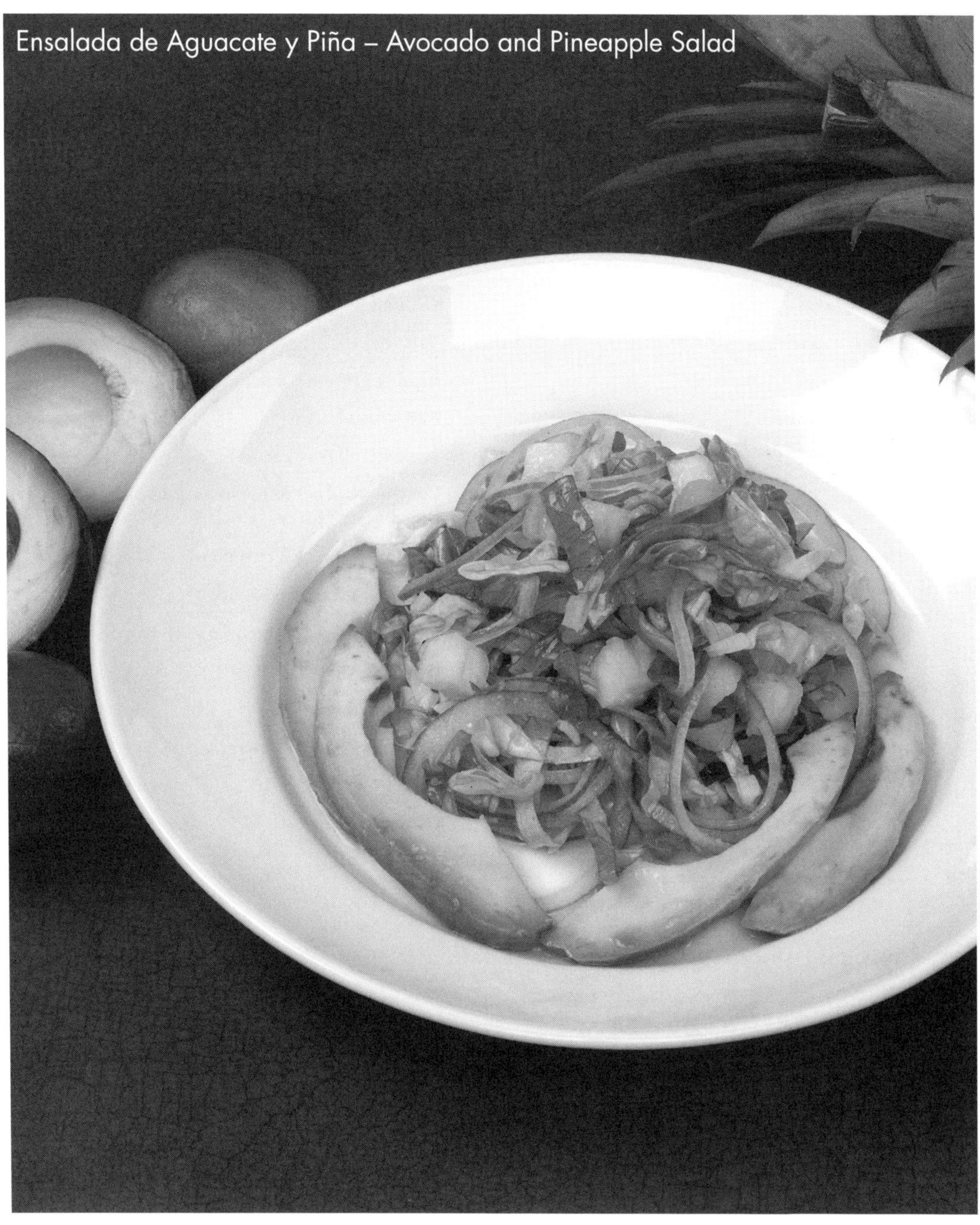

Ensalada de Aguacate y Piña – Avocado and Pineapple Salad

# Arroz con Pollo

## Chicken and Rice (Puerto Rico) SERVES 4

| AMOUNT | MEASURE | INGREDIENT |
|---|---|---|
| 1 $2\frac{1}{2}$ to 3 pound | 1 1.12 to 1.34 kg | Chicken, cut into 8 pieces |
| 2 | | Garlic cloves, minced |
| $\frac{1}{2}$ teaspoon | | Ground oregano |
| 2 teaspoons | | Salt |
| $\frac{3}{4}$ teaspoon | | Freshly ground black pepper |
| 2 tablespoons | 1 ounce, 30 ml | Red wine vinegar |
| 2 tablespoons | 1 ounce, 30 ml | Annatto oil (see recipe) |
| $\frac{1}{2}$ cup | 3 ounces, 84 g | Longaniza (Puerto Rican pork or sausage) or ham, sliced $\frac{1}{4}$ inch (.6 cm) thick |
| $\frac{1}{2}$ cup | 3 ounces, 84 g | Bacon, $\frac{1}{2}$ inch (1.2 cm) dice |
| 1 cup | 4 ounces, 112 g | Onion, $\frac{3}{4}$ inch (.6 cm) dice |
| 1 cup | 4 ounces, 112 g | Red bell pepper, $\frac{3}{4}$ inch (.6 cm) dice |
| 2 tablespoons | 1 ounce, 30 ml | Green sofrito |
| $\frac{1}{2}$ cup | 4 ounces, 120 ml | Tomato sauce |
| 1 cup | 4 ounces, 112 g | Banana peppers, $\frac{3}{4}$ inch (.6 cm) dice |
| 2 cups | 14 ounces, 392 g | Long grain rice |
| 2 tablespoons | $\frac{1}{2}$ ounce, 15 ml | Capers, rinsed |
| $4\frac{1}{2}$ cups | 36 ounces, 1.08 l | Chicken stock |

### PROCEDURE

1. Wash the chicken and pat dry.
2. Mix together the garlic, oregano, salt, pepper, and vinegar; rub into the chicken pieces. Let stand 45 minutes.
3. Brown the chicken in the annatto oil until golden; remove and set aside.
4. Brown the longaniza and bacon. Drain off all but approximately 3 tablespoons ($1\frac{1}{2}$ ounces, 45 ml) fat.
5. Add onions and cook until soft, 3 minutes. Add red pepper sofrito, tomato sauce, and banana peppers; stir well and cook 2 minutes.
6. Add rice and stir to coat; cook stirring 2 minutes.

7 Add chicken pieces, capers, stock, and salt to taste. Bring to a boil. Lower heat to a simmer; cover and cook for 20 minutes or until the liquid has been absorbed and the rice and chicken are tender. Serve hot.

**Annatto Oil**

| | | |
|---|---|---|
| **1 cup** | **8 ounces, 240 ml** | **Vegetable oil** |
| **$\frac{1}{2}$ cup** | **2 ounces, 56 g** | **Achiote seeds** |

**PROCEDURE**

1 Heat the oil over low heat, add seeds, and cook for 5 minutes, stirring occasionally, until a rich orange color. Cool, strain, and store, covered, in the refrigerator.

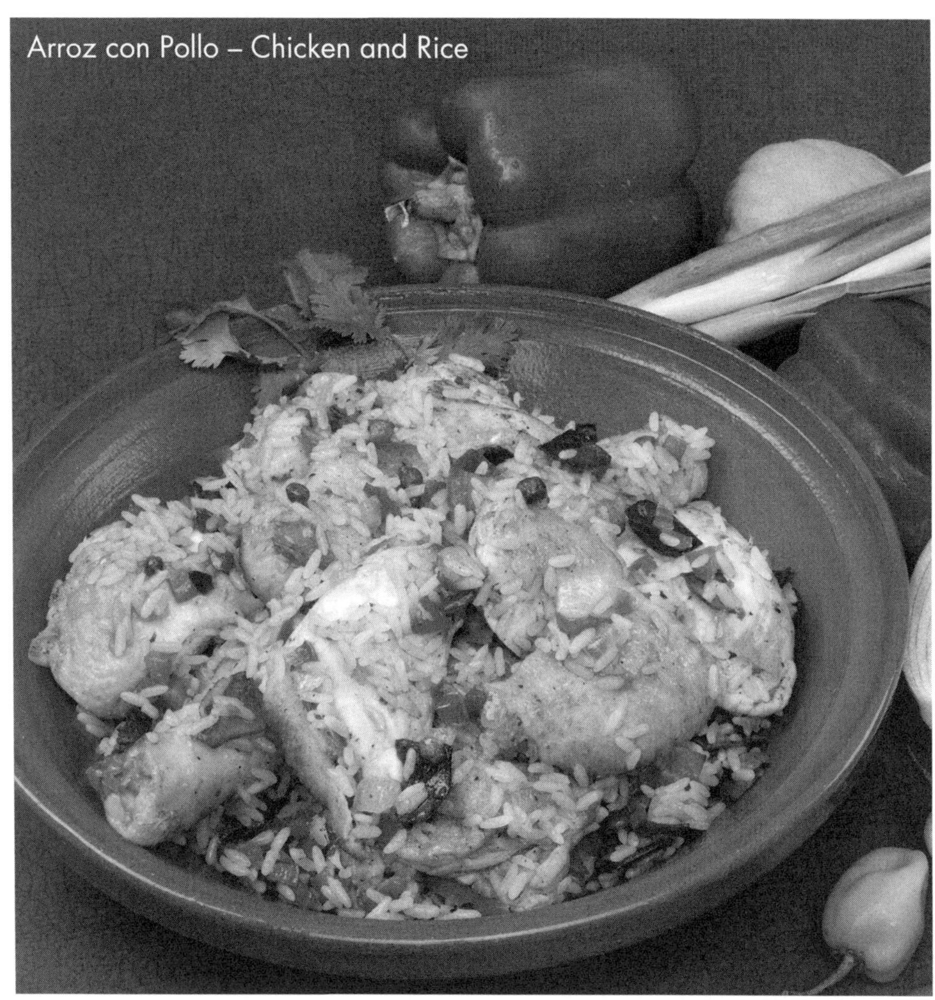

Arroz con Pollo – Chicken and Rice

# Pepperpot Soup

## (Jamaica) SERVES 4

| AMOUNT | MEASURE | INGREDIENT |
|---|---|---|
| 1 $\frac{1}{4}$ cup | 8 ounces, 224 g | Lean beef stew meat, $\frac{1}{2}$ inch (1.2 cm) dice |
| $\frac{1}{2}$ cup | 3 ounces, 84 g | Corned beef or salt pork, $\frac{1}{2}$ inch (1.2 cm) dice |
| 1 quart | 32 ounces, 960 ml | Water |
| 4 cups | 8 ounces, 224 g | Kale or collard greens, chopped |
| 4 cups | 8 ounces, 224 g | Callaloo or spinach, chopped |
| $\frac{1}{2}$ cup | 2 ounces, 56 g | Onion, $\frac{1}{4}$ inch (.6 cm) dice |
| 1 | | Garlic clove, minced |
| $\frac{1}{2}$ cup | 2 ounces, 56 g | Green onions, white and green parts, minced |
| 1 teaspoon | | Fresh thyme leaves |
| 1 | | Green hot pepper, seedless, minced |
| 1 cup | 4 ounces, 112 g | Yam, peeled, $\frac{1}{2}$ inch (1.2 cm) dice |
| $\frac{1}{2}$ cup | 2 ounces, 56 g | Taro root, peeled, $\frac{1}{2}$ inch (1.2 cm) dice |
| To taste | | Salt and pepper |
| 1 tablespoon | $\frac{1}{2}$ ounce, 15 ml | Butter |
| 1 cup | 4 ounces, 112 ml | Okra, sliced $\frac{3}{4}$ inch (.6 cm) thick |
| $\frac{1}{2}$ cup | 2 ounces, 56 g | Small cooked shrimp |
| $\frac{1}{2}$ cup | 4 ounces, 120 ml | Coconut milk |

**PROCEDURE**

1. Combine meat and water; simmer, covered for 1 hour.
2. Combine kale and callaloo with 2 cups (16 ounces, 480 ml) water in a separate pan and cook until tender, about 30 minutes. Puree kale, callallo and liquid, add to the cooked meat.
3. Add onion, garlic, green onions, thyme, pepper, yam, and taro root and season with salt and pepper. Cover and simmer until meats are tender and yam and taro are cooked, 30 to 45 minutes.
4. Heat butter over medium heat and sauté okra until lightly brown. Add to soup.
5. Add shrimp and coconut milk and simmer 3 to 5 minutes. Correct seasoning.

# Sweet Potato Cake

## (Martinique) SERVES 4

| AMOUNT | MEASURE | INGREDIENT |
|---|---|---|
| 2 pounds | 896 g | Sweet potatoes, peeled, thickly sliced |
| 2 tablespoons | 1 ounce, 30 ml | Butter |
| $\frac{3}{4}$ cup | 6 ounces, 168 g | Brown sugar |
| $\frac{1}{4}$ cup | 2 ounces, 60 ml | Dark rum |
| 4 | | Eggs |
| $\frac{1}{2}$ cup | 4 ounces, 120 ml | Milk |
| 2 teaspoons | | Lime rind, grated |
| 1 tablespoon | $\frac{1}{2}$ ounce, 15 ml | Lime juice |
| $\frac{1}{2}$ teaspoon | | Ground cinnamon |
| $\frac{1}{2}$ teaspoon | | Ground nutmeg |
| $\frac{1}{2}$ teaspoon | | Salt |
| 2 teaspoons | | Baking powder |

**PROCEDURE**

1. Preheat oven at 350°F (176°C)
2. Cook sweet potatoes in just enough water to cover until tender, 20 to 25 minutes. Drain and mash.
3. While still warm mix in butter, sugar, and rum.
4. Beat in eggs, one at a time.
5. Add milk, grated rind, and lime juice.
6. Sift together cinnamon, nutmeg, salt, and baking powder. Add to sweet potatoes and mix thoroughly.
7. Pour into a greased 9 × 5-inch (22.5 × 12.5 cm) loaf pan.
8. Bake at 350°F (176°C) 1 hour or until a cake tester comes out clean.
9. Let cool 5 minutes, then turn onto a rack to cool.

# Camarones Sofrito Shrimp in Green Sofrito (Dominican Republic)

SERVES 4

| AMOUNT | MEASURE | INGREDIENT |
|---|---|---|
| $\frac{1}{4}$ cup | 2 ounces, 60 ml | Butter |
| 1 cup | 4 ounces, 112 g | Onion, $\frac{1}{4}$ inch (.6 cm) dice |
| 1 | | Garlic clove, minced |
| 1, or to taste | | Scotch bonnet chile, seeded and minced |
| $\frac{1}{2}$ cup | 2 ounces, 56 g | Celery, $\frac{1}{4}$ inch (.6 cm) dice |
| 1 cup | 6 ounces, 168 g | Tomato, peeled, seeded, $\frac{1}{4}$ inch (.6 cm) dice |
| To Taste | | Salt and pepper |
| $\frac{1}{2}$ teaspoon | | Sugar |
| 1 tablespoon | $\frac{1}{2}$ ounce, 15 ml | Lime juice |
| 1 | | Bay leaf |
| 1 tablespoon | | Parsley, minced |
| $\frac{1}{2}$ cup | 4 ounces, 120 ml | Green Sofrito (see *Arroz Mamposteao*) |
| 1 pound | 448 g | Shrimp, 16–20 ct, shelled and deveined |

**PROCEDURE**

1. Heat butter over medium heat, add the onion and garlic, and cook 2 minutes. Add chile and celery, cook 3 minutes, until celery is soft.
2. Add tomatoes, salt, pepper, sugar, lime juice, bay leaf, and parsley; simmer uncovered, until sauce is well blended and slightly reduced, 10 to 15 minutes.
3. In a separate pan heat the sofrito and stir in the shrimp; cook until the shrimp lose their translucency, about 3 minutes.
4. Serve shrimp on top of tomato sauce.

# Sopa de Frijol Negro
## Black Bean Soup (Cuba) SERVES 4

| AMOUNT | MEASURE | INGREDIENT |
|---|---|---|
| **Sofrito** | | |
| $\frac{1}{2}$ cup | 2 ounces, 56 g | Green bell pepper, seeded, chopped |
| $\frac{1}{2}$ cup | 3 ounces, 56 g | Tomatoes, peeled, seeded, chopped |
| $\frac{1}{2}$ cup | 2 ounces, 56 g | Onion, chopped |
| 2 | | Garlic cloves, chopped |
| 2 tablespoons | | Fresh cilantro leaves, chopped |
| 1 tablespoon | | Fresh parsley, chopped |
| 1$\frac{1}{2}$ tablespoons | $\frac{3}{4}$ ounce, 23 ml | Annatto oil |
| **Soup** | | |
| 2 ounces | 56 g | Salt pork, minced |
| 2 ounces | 56 g | Lean Virginia ham, trimmed, minced |
| 1 teaspoon | | Dried oregano, crushed |
| 1$\frac{1}{2}$ cup | 9 ounces, 252 g | Dried black beans, picked over and soaked |
| 1 teaspoon | | Ground cumin |
| 3$\frac{1}{2}$ cups | 28 ounces, 840 ml | Chicken or beef stock |
| To taste | | Salt and pepper |
| **Garnish** | | |
| $\frac{1}{4}$ cup | | White onions, minced |

### PROCEDURE

1. Pound or process peppers, tomatoes, onions, garlic, cilantro and parsley to a paste.
2. Heat annatto oil and render the salt pork until crisp. Drain, reserve the oil and salt pork.
3. Return fat to medium-low heat, add the vegetable paste, and sauté 2 to 3 minutes, until vegetables are cooked but not brown. Add ham and cook 1 minute.
4. Drain and rinse beans. Add to sofrito along with the oregano, cumin, stock and seasoning. Stock should cover beans by 1 to 2 inches (2.4 to 4.8 cm).
5. Bring to a boil, lower heat, cover and simmer for 1$\frac{1}{2}$ to 2 hours, until beans are very tender. Add additional stock if necessary.
6. Puree half the soup, combine and simmer 5 minutes.
7. Correct seasoning and serve with minced white onions.

# Salad of Hearts of Palm with Passion Fruit Vinaigrette (Puerto Rico)

SERVES 4

**Fresh hearts of palm are available in Cryovac bags and will last up to two weeks in a refrigerator. Canned hearts of palm may be substituted for fresh.**

| AMOUNT | MEASURE | INGREDIENT |
|---|---|---|
| 1 tablespoon | $\frac{1}{2}$ ounce, 15 ml | Passion fruit puree |
| $\frac{1}{4}$ cup | 2 ounces, 60 ml | Red wine vinegar |
| $\frac{1}{8}$ teaspoon | | Dijon-style mustard |
| $\frac{1}{2}$ cup | 4 ounces, 120 ml | Olive oil |
| To taste | | Salt and pepper |

**PROCEDURE**

1 Combine puree, vinegar, and Dijon mustard. Gradually add olive oil, whisking continuously. Correct seasoning.

| AMOUNT | MEASURE | INGREDIENT |
|---|---|---|
| 12 | | Tomato wedges, peeled |
| 2 cups | 12 ounces, 336 g | Fresh hearts of palm, $\frac{1}{2}$ inch (1.2 cm) dice |
| $\frac{1}{2}$ cup | 2 ounces, 56 g | Red bell pepper, $\frac{1}{4}$ inch (.6 cm) dice |
| $\frac{1}{2}$ cup | 2 ounces, 56 g | Green bell pepper, $\frac{1}{4}$ inch (.6 cm) dice |
| 3 cups | 6 ounces, 168 g | Boston lettuce leaves, washed, dried, torn |
| $\frac{1}{2}$ cup | 2 ounces, 56 g | Red onion, cut into very thin rings, soaked in ice water for 30 minutes, drained, and patted dry |
| $\frac{1}{3}$ cup | 2 ounces, 56 g | Queso fresco |

**PROCEDURE**

1 Toss tomato wedges with 2 tablespoons of vinaigrette and let stand at least 30 minutes.

2 When ready to assemble salad, combine hearts of palm and red and green bell pepper; toss with a little vinaigrette.

3 Toss lettuce with dressing and place on salad plate. Arrange 3 tomato wedges on each plate. Top lettuce with hearts of palm mixture. Arrange a few sliced onions over salad and sprinkle with queso fresco.

# Tamarind Balls (Jamaica) SERVES 4

**Tamarind is one of the legacies brought to the Caribbean region by the indentured Indian servants, who replaced the enslaved Africans.**

| AMOUNT | MEASURE | INGREDIENT |
|---|---|---|
| $\frac{1}{2}$ cup | 4 ounces, 120 ml | Tamarind paste with seeds |
| $3\frac{1}{4}$ cups | 23 ounces, 644 g | Granulated sugar |

**PROCEDURE**

1. Combine the tamarind paste and 1 pound ($2\frac{1}{4}$ cups, 448 g) sugar on a worktable and knead to together until the mixture is light in color and the majority of the sugar is absorbed.
2. Roll 1 tablespoon ($\frac{1}{2}$ ounce, 15 ml) of the mixture into a ball around one or two of the tamarind seeds (if using). Proceed until all the paste has been used.
3. Spread the remaining sugar on the worktable and roll each ball in sugar until coated.
4. Store in an airtight container.

# Stuffed Dates (Curacao) SERVES 4

| AMOUNT | MEASURE | INGREDIENT |
|---|---|---|
| $\frac{1}{2}$ cup | $2\frac{1}{2}$ ounces, 70 g | Walnuts, chopped fine |
| $\frac{1}{2}$ cup | 3 ounces, 84 g | Dried apricots, minced |
| 1 to 2 tablespoons | $\frac{1}{2}$ to 1 ounce, 15 to 30 ml | Water |
| 24 | | Dates (Medjool), pitted |

**PROCEDURE**

1. Mix together the walnuts, apricots, and water and spoon 1 teaspoon of the mixture into each date. Do not overfill.
2. Serve at room temperature.

# Curried Kid or Lamb

## (Trinidad) SERVES 4

| AMOUNT | MEASURE | INGREDIENT |
|---|---|---|
| 1 tablespoon | $\frac{1}{2}$ ounce, 15 ml | Lime juice |
| 1 | | Lime, cut into quarters |
| 1 tablespoon | | Coarse salt |
| 1 $\frac{1}{2}$ pounds | 24 ounces, 672 g | Boneless lean lamb or goat, 1 $\frac{1}{2}$ inch (3.6 cm) cubes |
| 2 tablespoons | 1 ounce, 30 ml | Vegetable oil |
| 1 cup | 4 ounces, 112 g | Onion, $\frac{3}{4}$ inch (.6 cm) dice |
| 2 | | Garlic cloves, minced |
| 2 teaspoons | 10 ml | Tarmarind pulp |
| 1 cup | 4 ounces, 112 g | Green mango, peeled, $\frac{1}{2}$ inch (1.2 cm) dice (optional) |
| 1 tablespoon | | Curry powder |
| 1 or $\frac{1}{2}$, to taste | | Habanera pepper, seeded and minced |
| 1 cup | 6 ounces, 168 g | Tomatoes peeled, seeded, $\frac{1}{2}$ inch (1.2 cm) dice |
| 1 cup | 8 ounces, 240 ml | Vegetable or chicken stock |
| 1 cup | 6 ounces, 168 g | Potatoes, peeled, $\frac{1}{2}$ inch (1.2 cm) dice |
| 1 cup | 6 ounces, 168 g | West Indian pumpkin (calabaza) or Hubbard squash, peeled, $\frac{1}{2}$ inch (1.2 cm) dice |
| $\frac{1}{2}$ cup | 3 ounces, 84 g | Chayote, peeled, $\frac{1}{2}$ inch (1.2 cm) dice |
| 1 tablespoon | | Fresh thyme, chopped |
| 1 teaspoon | | Lime juice |
| To taste | | Salt and pepper |
| As needed | | White rice, cooked |
| As needed | | Fried ripe plantains (recipe follows) |

**PROCEDURE**

1 Combine the 1 tablespoon lime juice, lime quarters, coarse salt, and meat with 1 cup of water. Cover and allow to stand for 30 minutes. Drain and pat dry.

2 Heat oil over medium-high heat and brown the meat on all sides. Remove meat.

3 Add onions; cook 3 to 4 minutes until golden brown. Add garlic, tamarind pulp, mango, curry powder, and habanera pepper. Cook, stirring, for 3 to 4 minutes. Add tomatoes and

cook 2 minutes. Return meat to mixture; cook 2 to 3 minutes to make sure the meat is coated with spice mixture. Add the stock.

4 Bring to a boil, reduce to a simmer, cover, and cook 30 minutes.

5 Add potatoes, calabaza, and chayote; correct salt. Cover and simmer 30 minutes or until meat and vegetables are tender. Stir in the fresh thyme, 1 teaspoon lime juice and correct seasoning.

6 Serve hot with rice and fried ripe plantains.

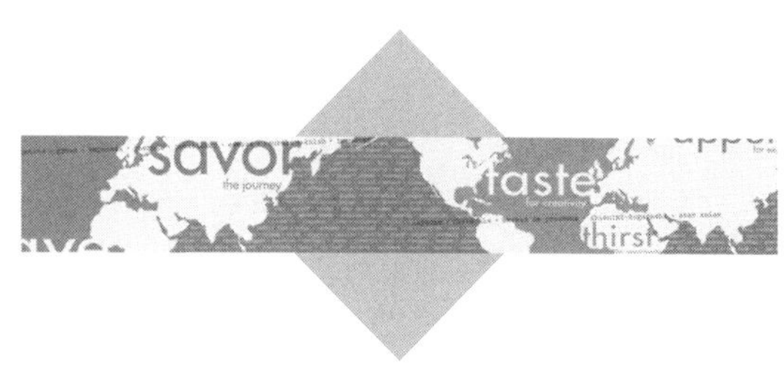

# Fried Ripe Plantains
## (All Islands) SERVES 4

**Ripe plantain skins are quite black. If bananas are used as a substitute, use ripe but still firm bananas and be sure the skins are yellow, not black.**

| AMOUNT | MEASURE | INGREDIENT |
|---|---|---|
| 2 large | | Ripe plantains |
| As needed | | Butter or oil |

**PROCEDURE**

1. Cut off ends of the plantains, peel, and halve lengthwise.
2. Slice in half crosswise, yielding 8 slices.
3. Heat butter or oil over medium heat. Add slices and sauté until browned on both sides. Drain on paper towels and serve hot.

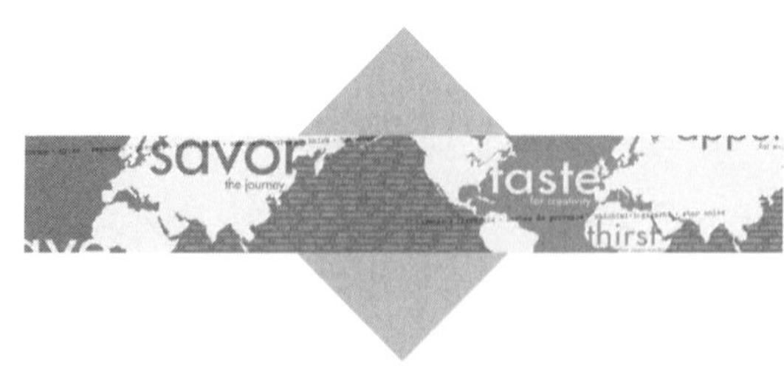

# Tostones Twice-Fried Plantains (All Islands)

YIELD: 12 TO 16 TOSTONES

| AMOUNT | MEASURE | INGREDIENT |
|---|---|---|
| 2 | | Large green plantains |
| As needed | | Salted water |
| As needed | | Oil for frying |
| To taste | | Kosher salt and freshly ground black pepper |

**PROCEDURE**

1 Cut off about 1 inch (2.4 cm) from both ends of plantains. Make 2 lengthwise cuts at opposite ends.

2 Cover with very hot water for 5 to 10 minutes to help loosen the peel. Drain.

3 Hold the plantain steady with one hand and use the other hand to slide the tip of the knife under the skin and begin to pull it away, going from top to bottom.

4 Cut into diagonal slices 1 to $1\frac{1}{2}$ inch (2.4 to 4.8 cm) thick. Soak the slices in salted water for 30 minutes. Drain and pat dry.

5 Heat 2 inches (4.8 cm) oil over medium heat to 350°F (176°C) and sauté the pieces until tender, 3 to 4 minutes; do not let them get crusty on the outside. Drain on absorbent paper.

6 While they are still warm, lay a sheet of parchment paper, waxed paper, or a clean towel over the slices and flatten until half as thick.

7 When ready to serve, refry at 375°F (190°C) until golden. Drain on absorbent paper, season, and serve.

# Roasted Breadfruit

## (Barbados) SERVES 4

**Chef Tip** **Breadfruit is cooked and handled like a potato.**

| AMOUNT | MEASURE | INGREDIENT |
|---|---|---|
| **1 medium** | | **Breadfruit** |

**PROCEDURE**

1. Roast breadfruit over charcoal grill or directly over a gas burner.
2. Turn the fruit as it begins to char. Cook on all sides till brownish black. This process can take up to 1 hour.
3. When steam starts to escape from the stem end, the breadfruit is done. Or use skewer to check if cooked.
4. Remove from grill and peel off skin.
5. Cut in half.
6. Cut out the "heart" (inedible portion in the middle).
7. Cut breadfruit into appropriate size pieces. Serve hot.
8. To bake, place breadfruit in a baking pan, with water covering the pan bottom. Bake at 350°F (176°C) one hour or until tender.

# Stewed Conch
## (Cayman Islands) SERVES 4

| AMOUNT | MEASURE | INGREDIENT |
| --- | --- | --- |
| 1 pound | 448 g | Conch meat, fresh or frozen |
| $\frac{3}{4}$ cup | 2 ounces, 60 ml | Lime juice |
| To taste | | Salt and pepper |
| 8 ounces | 224 g | Salt pork, $\frac{1}{2}$ inch (1.2 cm) cubes |
| 3 cups | 24 ounces, 720 ml | Coconut milk |
| 1 cup | 6 ounces, 168 g | Green plantain, peeled, sliced $\frac{1}{2}$ inch (1.2 cm) slices |
| 1 cup | 6 ounces, 168 g | Yuca, peeled, 1 inch (2.4 cm) cubes |
| 1 cup | 6 ounces, 168 g | Yam, peeled, 1 inch (2.4 cm) cubes |
| 1 cup | 6 ounces, 168 g | Sweet potato, peeled, $\frac{1}{2}$ inch (1.2 cm) cubes |
| $\frac{1}{2}$ cup | 3 ounces, 112 84 | Breadfruit, peeled, 1 inch (2.4 cm) cubes (optional) |
| 1 tablespoon | | Fresh thyme, minced |
| 2 teaspoons | | Fresh basil, minced |

**PROCEDURE**

1. Marinate conch in the lime juice for 30 minutes. Drain, rinse, and then tenderize the conch meat by pounding it with a meat mallet. Cover with water, season with salt and pepper, and simmer for 10 minutes. Drain and cut into 1 to $1\frac{1}{2}$-inch (2.4 to 3.6 cm) pieces.
2. In a separate pan, cook salt pork in water to cover for 20 minutes to remove the salt.
3. Combine conch, salt pork, and coconut milk over medium heat; bring to a boil, then lower to a simmer.
4. Add plantain, yuca, yam, and sweet potato; cook 25 minutes. Add breadfruit, adjust seasoning, and cook until everything is tender, about 20 minutes.
5. Add thyme and basil, stir, and adjust seasonings. Serve hot.

# Japan

## The Land

Japan is a small nation of more than 3,000 scattered islands off the eastern coast of mainland Asia. The Japanese call it *Nippon,* which means "source of the sun"; others call it "Land of the Rising Sun." It is an archipelago, or chain of islands, including four major islands—Hokkaido, Honshu, Shikoku, and Kyusha—and thousands of smaller ones that lie scattered along a southwest to northeast axis of nearly 3,000 miles. Historically, its location isolated the country from the rest of the world. Considering the country's physical geography, its history, and its huge population, Japan has had to overcome many obstacles to achieve its present-day place among major world nations.

Japan is located in a region of geologic instability known as the Pacific Ring of Fire. This region includes approximately 100 active volcanoes and as a result it averages about 1,500 earthquakes each year. Japan is also subject to floods, blizzards, and typhoons that sweep over the islands each year. And volcanic events occurring on the ocean floor can cause devastating tsunamis. Although no longer active, the most recognized of Japan's volcanoes is Mount Fuji. This cone-shaped peak rises 12,388 feet above the Kanto Plain, about 70 miles southwest of Tokyo.

The small valleys of flat land and narrow coastal plains support much of Japan's population and economy. Japan's population is over 127 million people, all of whom occupy an area slightly smaller than the state of California.

# History

In 1543, Portuguese traders arrived at one of the small islands of Japan and offered to exchange "what they had for what they did not have." The Japanese were eager for trade and soon Portuguese traders and Jesuit missionaries arrived in increasing numbers, followed by the Dutch and the English. During this time the Shogun (the emperor's commander in chief) Tokugawa Ieyaso, with the aid of the English sailor Will Adams as naval advisor, worked to unify the country.

More than a hundred years later, the Shogun, fearing too much Western influence, closed Japan to "foreigners." During this time Japan was able to develop in its own way. Two hundred years later, when Commodore Matthew Perry of the U.S. Navy demanded reopening of trade in 1853, Japan was again ready to face the West.

Under the modern thinking of Emperor Meiji, Japan soon became a power in the Far East, defeating imperial China and Russia in the late nineteenth and early twentieth centuries. Then an expanding need for raw materials not available set Japan on a course of conquest of Asia and the islands of the Pacific, ultimately leading to their role in World War II. In 1945, Japan was defeated by the United States and its Allies, and occupying American troops helped rebuild its cities and industries.

Today, Japan has one of the most successful economies of any non-Western nation.

# The People

Few places in the world are as crowded as Japanese cities. Over 98 percent of the country's inhabitants are ethnic Japanese. Koreans make up the largest group of immigrants and there are small numbers of Chinese, Brazilians, Filipinos, and Americans living in the country.

Religious beliefs and practices in Japan primarily revolve around two faiths: Shintoism and Buddism. Originating in ancient times, Shinto is the polytheistic (believing in many gods) religion of Japan. Followers of Shinto worship their ancestors, offer prayers, and observe various rituals. They believe that *kami* (the many gods of Shinto) control the forces of nature and the human condition, including creativity, sickness, and healing. Because the followers of Shinto believe that the *kami* live in shrines, they erect places of worship in their homes as well as in public places. These structures are often quite extensive, involving several buildings and gardens, to which people make pilgrimages. Buddism, which originated in India and reached Japan from Korea in the sixth century A.D., focuses on enlightenment and meditation.

Chanoyu has been referred to as the "Japanese Tea Ceremony" for many years but the word literally means hot water for tea. The simple art of Chanoyu is really a synthesis of many Japanese arts with the focus of preparing and serving a bowl of tea with a pure heart. Tea was first introduced to Japan from China with Buddhism in the sixth century. It wasn't until 1191 that tea really took hold in Japan with the return from China of the Zen priest Eisai (1141–1215). Eisai, the founder of the Rinzai sect of Zen Buddhism in Japan, introduced powdered tea and tea seeds that he brought back with him from China. The tea seeds were planted at the Kozanji temple in the hills northwest of Kyoto. The tea master Sen Rikyu developed *wabicha,* or the style of tea that reflects a simple and quiet taste. It is this simple style of tea that is practiced and taught in Japan and throughout the world today. The principles of *Wa Kei Sei Jaku* (harmony, respect, purity, and tranquility) are the principles that practitioners of Chanoyu integrate into their study of tea and into their daily lives. The tea ceremony varies according to the seasons, with tea bowls, types of tea, flowers, and scrolls carefully chosen.

## The Food

Rice is Japan's most important crop and has been cultivated by the Japanese for over 2000 years. Japanese rice is short grain rice that becomes sticky when cooked. Most rice is sold as *hakumai* ("white rice"), with the outer portion of the grains (*nuka*) polished away. Unpolished rice (*gemmai*) is considered less desirable. A second major rice variety used in Japan is *mochi* rice. Cooked mochi rice is more sticky than conventional Japanese rice, and it is commonly used for *sekihan* (cooked mochi rice with red beans) or pounded into rice cakes. The rice cakes are traditionally eaten on New Year's day and are usually grilled and then served in a soup or wrapped in nori seaweed. Rice flour is used in various Japanese sweets (*wagashi*) and rice crackers (*sembei*). Daifuku is sweetened red bean paste wrapped in rice flour dough, and *kushi-dango* are rice flour dumplings on skewers. Rice is also used to produce vinegar. Rice wine is commonly known as sake which is the general term for "alcohol" in Japanese.

The importance of rice in the daily diet is revealed in the word *gohan,* which means both "cooked rice" and "meal." This word is extended to *asagohan* (breakfast), *hirugohan* (lunch), and *bangohan* (dinner). A traditional Japanese breakfast is a bowl of rice, *miso* (fermented soy paste) soup, a plain omelet, some dried fish, and pickled vegetables. Lunches are light, often consisting of noodles (*soba* made from buckwheat or *udon* made from wheat), *domburi mono* (a bowl of rice with vegetables, meat, or eggs on top), or a *bento box.* Dinner is a bowl of rice, *miso* or *dashi* soup (a stock made from kelp and dried bonito flakes), a small portion of protein, vegetables, pickled vegetables, and a dessert (usually a seasonal fruit).

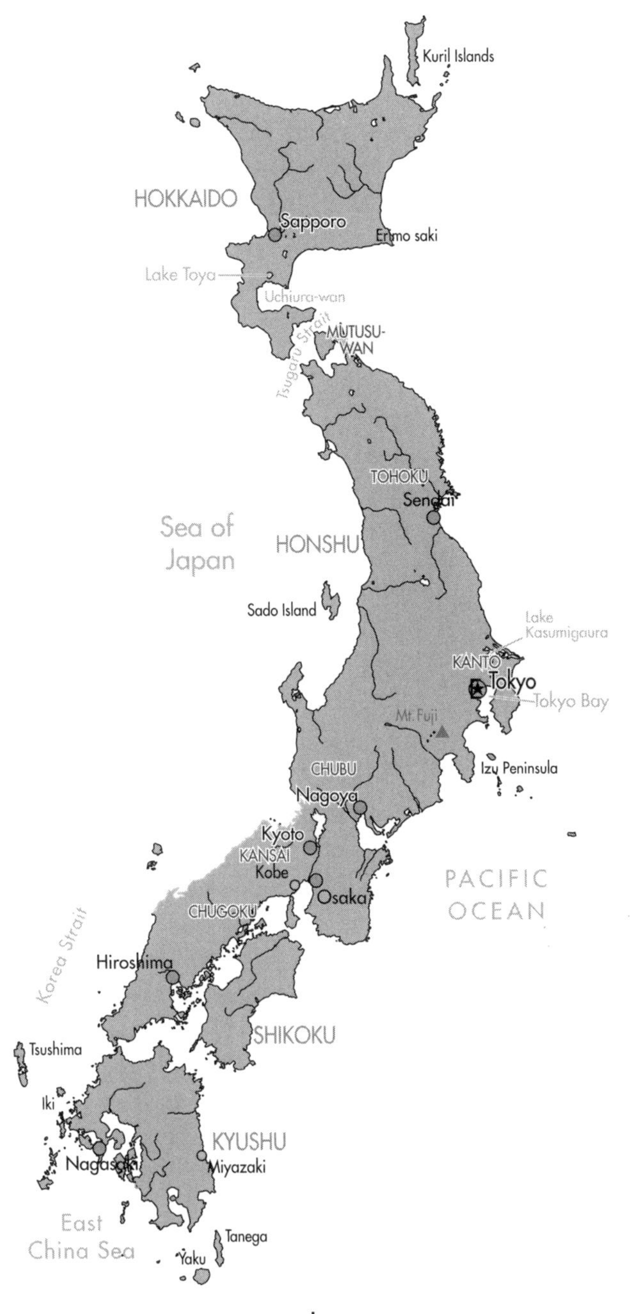
Kuril Islands
HOKKAIDO
Sapporo
Erimo saki
Lake Toya
Uchiura-wan
Tsugaru Strait
MUTUSU-
WAN
TOHOKU
Sendai
Sea of
Japan
HONSHU
Sado Island
Lake
Kasumigaura
KANTO
Tokyo
Tokyo Bay
Mt. Fuji
Izu Peninsula
CHUBU
Nagoya
Kyoto
KANSAI
Kobe
Osaka
PACIFIC
OCEAN
CHUGOKU
Korea Strait
Hiroshima
SHIKOKU
Tsushima
Iki
KYUSHU
Nagasaki
Miyazaki
East
China Sea
Tanega
Yaku

Japan

So close to the sea where warm (*kurosio*) currents meet with cold (*oyashio*), the area is home to some of the world's richest fishing grounds. Fish is a main element in the Japanese diet and is eaten in a variety of preparations: steamed, fried, boiled, broiled, and raw.

Preserving fish also became popular and sushi originated as a means of preserving fish by fermenting it in boiled rice. Salted fish was placed in rice and preserved by lactic acid fermentation, which prevents growth of the bacteria that bring about putrefaction. This older type of sushi is still produced in the areas surrounding Lake Biwa in western Japan, and similar types are also known in Korea, southwestern China, and Southeast Asia. A unique fifteenth-century development shortened the fermentation period of sushi to one or two weeks and made both the fish and the rice edible. As a result, sushi became a popular snack food. Sushi without fermentation appeared during the 1600s, and sushi was finally united with sashimi at the end of the eighteenth century, when the hand-rolled type, *nigiri-sushi,* was devised.

In the thirteenth century, Zen monks from China popularized a form of vegetarian cuisine known in Japan as *shojin ryori.* The practice of preparing meals with seasonal vegetables and wild plants from the mountains, served with seaweed, fresh soybean curd (or dehydrated forms), and seeds (such as walnuts, pine nuts and peanuts) is a tradition that is still alive at Zen temples today. Stemming from the Buddhist precept that it is wrong to kill animals, including fish, *shojin ryori* is completely vegetarian. Buddhism prescribes partaking of a simple diet every day and abstaining from drinking alcohol or eating meat. Such a lifestyle, it is thought, together with physical training, clears the mind of confusion and leads to understanding.

In the sixteenth century the Portuguese traders, followed by the Dutch, began to introduce foods such as sugar and corn that were adopted by the Japanese. The use of fried foods such as tempura might seem to be unusual since a scarcity of meat and dairy products in the Japanese diet meant that oil was not commonly used for cooking. However, tempura was enjoyed by many people and is now used for a wide variety of seafood, meats, and vegetables.

Buddhist influences and cultural factors caused Japanese emperors to ban consumption of beef and meat from other hoofed animals in Japan for more than a thousand years until the Meiji Restoration in 1868. It is thought that before this time, Japanese soldiers, involved in many armed conflicts over the years, were fed beef to strengthen them for battle. When the soldiers came home from war, they brought their appetite for beef with them. Village elders believed that consuming beef inside the house was a sacrilege, a desecration of the house, and an insult to their ancestors. Thus young men were forced to cook their beef outside on plowshares (this process became known as *sukiyaki,* which literally means *plow cooking*) until the Meijii Restoration finally relaxed the restriction against eating beef. During the Meiji Restoration the new emperor went as far as staging a New Year's feast in 1872 designed to embrace the Western world. It had a European emphasis and for the first time in over a thousand years, people publicly ate meat.

Kobe beef is a legendary delicacy of Japan that comes from the capital city of Kobe in the Hyogo prefecture (province) of Japan. Cattle were first introduced into Japan around the second century, brought in from the Asian mainland via the Korean Peninsula. The cattle provided a much-needed source of agricultural power, power to pull the plows for the cultivation of rice, power for the growth of a nation. The Shikoku region received the first imports, but because of rugged terrain and difficult traveling in the region, further migration of the cattle was slow. The cattle were in isolated areas, each essentially a closed population. These herds were developed with an emphasis on quality.

Very protective of the breed, Japan went so far as to have the Wagyu classified as a national treasure. Wagyu produce consistently marbled, low-cholesterol carcasses, recognized as the world's finest, unmatched for flavor, tenderness, and overall eating quality. Wagyu is the Japanese breed of cattle used to produce Kobe, Matzukya, and Hokkido beef and is similar to the Hereford, Holstein, and Angus breeds. In order to earn the designation "Kobe beef," the Wagyu beef must come from the Hyogo province and meet strict production standards imposed by the industry. In Japan, Kobe beef is occasionally eaten as sushi, but is more frequently eaten as sukiyaki or steak. To cook a Kobe steak properly one should use high heat to sear the steak for a short amount of time. Since the fat is what gives Kobe beef its exquisite flavor, it is important to cook the steak only to medium rare (at most), since anything more would cause all of the fat to melt away. Most recipes recommend cooking a Kobe steak on the grill or a cast-iron pan, and seasoning only with salt and pepper.

*Nabemono* dishes are a hearty wintertime specialty, prepared from fish, seafood, chicken, meat and/or vegetables in a bubbling cauldron at the table. Serving trays piled high with raw ingredients arrive at the table, then everyone begins cooking, finally eating together out of the communal pot. There are many different types of nabemono, depending on the ingredients used. Oysters, scallops, cod, salmon, and chicken are all popular. *Chanko-nabe*, a variety made with chicken, seafood, potatoes, and other vegetables, is the staple diet of Japan's sumo wrestlers. Another special type of nabemono is beef sukiyaki.

Grilled *unagi* (eel) is a delicacy in Japan. The cooking process is what makes the eel both crisp and tender: the eels are first grilled over hot charcoal, then steamed to remove excess fat, then seasoned with a sweetish sauce and grilled a second time. The ingredients in the sweet basting sauce differs depending on the family or restaurant. Fancy unagi restaurants keep tanks full of live eels.

*Yakitori* itself means broiled chicken. Various cuts of chicken, including heart, liver, and cartilage are cooked on skewers over a charcoal grill. Also cooked this way are an assortment of vegetables such as green peppers (*piman*), garlic cloves (*ninniku*) and onions (*negi*). They are flavored using either a tangy sauce (*tare*) or salt (*shio*).

*Okonomiyaki* restaurants serve large, savory pancakes made with diced seafood, meat, and vegetables. It is topped with a special sauce and mayonnaise and sprinkled with nori and dried fish flakes (*katsuobushi*). Variations include adding a fried egg or soba. The okonomiyaki style of cooking originated in Osaka and is very popular around the country,

*Oden* is a very simple stew made by simmering fish dumplings, fried tofu, eggs, and vegetables in a kelp based stock for several hours. Sides include daikon (white radish), potatoes, kelp, transparent cakes made from *kon'nyaku* (devil's tongue starch) and *fukuro* (fried tofu pouches stuffed with chopped mushrooms and noodles). There is also a selection of fish cakes such as *chijuwaw*—made by molding fish paste into a tubular shape, steaming it, and finally grilling it. The fish cakes are made from fish that are not popular on their own, such as shark, flying fish, and pollack. *Kaiseki ryouri* is Japanese formal cuisine. Today it is considered an art form that celebrates the harmony between food and nature, with an emphasis on flavors, textures, and colors. A traditional *kaiseki* meal consists of a set sequence of courses based on preparation techniques. One meal can consist of as many as 15 different courses featuring sashimi, tempura, fish and meat dishes, and tofu prepared in diverse traditional style and designed to please all of the senses. Everything, down to the timing of each course and the choice of ceramics is planned to perfection. An example of this meal would be: *sakitsuke* (hors d'ouvre), *zensai* (appetizer), *suimono* (clear soup), *sashimi* (slices of raw fish), *nimono* (stewed seafood and vegetables*), yakimono* (broiled fish), agemono (deep-fried seafood and vegetables), *sunomono* (vinegared seafood and vegetables) *gohan* (cooked rice), *tomewan* (miso soup), konomono (pickled vegetables) and *kudamono* or *mizugashi* (fruit). *Senscha* (green tea) is served before the meal. During and after the meal *hojicha* (roasted tea) is served. Dishes focus on seasonal ingredients, and *kaiseki* chefs give zealous attention to presentation.

*Shippoku ryouri,* the specialty cuisine of the city of Nagasaki, combines European, Chinese, and Japanese tastes. Although *shippoku* benefited from Chinese, Dutch, and Portuguese culinary influences, it was the original creation of the Chinese living in Nagasaki's Chinese quarters. While it was intended to entertain Japanese and Western visitors, it spread to common households and evolved into a feast that is presented in traditional Japanese restaurants even today. The primary characteristic of Shippoku cuisine is *jikabashi,* the seating of the diners around a lacquered round table on which the food is served in one dish, with all diners serving themselves. This creates an atmosphere of *omoyai* (sharing) and contributes to a harmonious atmosphere. In addition, even before the toast, it is customary for the host to signal the start of the meal with one phrase: "Please help yourself to the *ohire* broth." Varying according to the season, the menu includes *ohire* (clear fish soup); *sashimi* (raw fish); vinegared, cooked, fried, and boiled vegetables and meat; and at the end *umewan* (sweet red bean soup with a salted cherry blossom).

# Glossary

**Aburage** Deep-fried tofu pouch. Before being deep-fried, the tofu is cut into thin sheets.

**Akatogarashi** Japanese dried red chile pepper, one of the hottest chile varieties in the world. It is sold in a powdered form, called *ichimi togarashi.*

## The Bento Box

**A *bento* box is a compact container designed to hold a single serving of rice and several side dishes. The earliest records of packed lunches in Japan date back to around the fifth century, when people going out to hunt, farm, or wage war took food along with them. They typically carried dried rice, which was eaten either in its dried state or after being rehydrated with cold or hot water, or rice balls.**

**Traditionally, people working outdoors—whether in the fields, in the mountains, on fishing boats, or in town—carried their lunches with them because they did not have time to go home for meals. These box lunches were built around such staples as white rice, rice mixed with millet, or potatoes, depending on the region.**

**During the Edo period (1603–1868), people considered *bento* an essential accompaniment to any outdoor excursions, including the theater. The *makunouchi bento,* which typically contains small rice balls sprinkled with sesame seeds and a rich assortment of side dishes, made its first appearance during this era. *Makunouchi* refers to the interval between the acts of a play, and the *bento* is said to have gotten its name from the fact that spectators ate it during intermission.**

**In the Meiji period (1868–1912), with the introduction of Japan's railway system, the *ekiben* ("station *bento,*" or box lunches sold at train stations) appeared. The first *ekiben*—rice balls with pickled apricots inside—was reportedly sold in 1885. *Ekiben* are still sold at Japanese train stations today in vast quantities.**

**Aji-no-moto** Monosodium glutamate (MSG).

**Atsuage** Regular or firm tofu, deep-fried until the outside is crisp and golden brown; the inside remains white.

**Azuki beans** Tiny, reddish, purplish dried beans, cooked to a sweetened paste and used in a variety of ways; often used in Japanese sweets.

**Beni shoga** Red pickled ginger.

**Bonito** Tuna, also known as skipjack tuna.

**Buta** Pork.

**Chutoro** The belly area of the tuna.

**Daikon** A large white radish, crisp, juicy, and refreshing. Available year-round, daikon becomes sweeter during the cold season. The flavor differs slightly depending on the part of the root used. The upper part is sweeter and without bitterness, typically used for *daikon oroshi* (peeled and grated daikon), which accompanies deep-fried foods such as tempura and grilled oily fish and meat. The top part is also used in salads. The bottom half of the root has a mild and pleasant bitter taste. It is usually simmered until soft enough to be broken with chopsticks. Simmered daikon (*furofuki daikon*) is served very hot, with a flavored *miso* sauce.

**Dashi** Basic Japanese stock made with *kombu* and *katsuoboshi.*

**Ebi** Cooked shrimp. *Ami Ebi* shrimp is prepared by "curing" the shrimp in a mixture of citrus juices.

**Edamame** Green soybeans.

**Fugu** Puffer fish, considered a delicacy, though its innards and blood contain the extremely poisonous neurotoxin *tetrodotoxin*. In Japan only licensed fugu chefs are allowed to prepare fugu.

**Futo-Maki** Big, oversized sushi rolls.

**Gari** Pickled ginger (pink or white) served with sushi.

**Ginnan** Gingko nuts. Asian cooks like to use ginnan in desserts and stir-fries. They're available fresh (in the fall), canned, or dried in Asian markets. To prepare fresh nuts, remove the soft pale yellow nutmeat from the hard shell. Simmer the nuts in salted boiling water. The meat will turn a bright green color. Drain and peel off the skins; refresh under cold water. Ginnan are used in stir-fry, deep-fried, or added to simmered or steamed dishes or soups. Canned nuts have already been shelled, skinned, and boiled, but they're mealier than fresh nuts. Rinse them before using. Substitute blanched almonds or pine nuts.

**Goma** Sesame seeds, found in two colors: white and black. White sesame seeds contain more oil than black seeds and are used to produce sesame oil. Black sesame seeds have a stronger, nuttier flavor than the white variety. Sesame seeds are sold untoasted, toasted, toasted and roughly ground, and toasted and ground to a smooth paste, with a little oil from the seeds floating on top. Japanese sesame paste is similar to Middle Eastern *tahini.*

**Goma Abura** Sesame oil. Introduced to Japan by China during the eighth century. There are two types of sesame oil, one made with toasted seeds and the other with raw seeds. Sesame oil made with toasted seeds has a golden brown color and a rich, nutty flavor. It is the preferred type used in Japan. Sesame oil made with raw seeds is clear and milder in flavor. Japanese have also adopted a chile-flavored sesame oil, called *rayu.*

**Hakusai** Chinese cabbage, about ten inches in length and six inches across the base. The lower parts of the leaves are white and quite thick. The upper parts are light green, thin and wrinkled. Hakusai does not have a strong flavor, making it a very good match with rich flavored stocks. When cooked for only a short amount of time it has a crisp texture.

**Hamachi** Young yellowtail tuna, or amberjack.

**Hanakatsuo** Dried bonito, shaved or flaked.

**Ichiban Dashi** "First fish stock." This stock extracts the best flavor and nutrients from the *kombu* (kelp) and *katsuobushi* (bonito flake). A very short cooking time prevents the stock from becoming strongly flavored or yellowish.

**Japan Green Teas** First brought to Japan from China in the ninth century by Buddhist Monks, tea has become the beverage of choice in all of Japan. Tea may be divided into three groups, according to how the leaves are processed: unfermented, partially fermented, or fully fermented. Japanese tea is an unfermented type, also called green tea. In Japan, fresh-picked tea leaves are steamed, quickly cooled, and rolled by hand or machine while hot air blows them dry. This process helps to preserve the leaves' maximum flavor, to be released only when the tea is brewed.

**Kabocha** A winter squash shaped like a pumpkin, six to seven inches in diameter, with a thick, tough, dark green skin. It has a deep orange flesh; when cooked it becomes very sweet and creamy. As with other winter squash it is a versatile vegetable. Substitute pumpkin or butter nut squash.

**Kaiware (Daikon Sprouts)** These have a pleasantly bitter, refreshing taste and are eaten raw. Used in salads, rolled sushi, or as a condiment for sashimi or noodle dishes.

**Kaki** Persimmon, native to China and cultivated in Japan for centuries. Both sweet and astringent varieties are grown in Japan. Sweet *kaki* contains chemicals called tannins that produce the astringency in unripe persimmons. The ripening process inactivates the tannins, so the astringency disappears. These sweet varieties have a round and slightly flattened shape. Astringent *kaki,* which is shaped like an acorn, becomes less astringent when the fruit becomes very soft and mushy.

**Kamaboko** Imitation crab meat, used in California rolls and other *maki.*

**Kanten (Agar-Agar)** When *kanten* is cooked with liquid and cooled, it forms a gel that is very stable at relatively high temperatures.

**Karashi** General word for mustard; *wa-garashi* is the expression for Japanese mustard, which is hotter than Western mustard. *Wa-garashi* has a dark yellow color and a pleasant bitter flavor. Colman's English mustard can be a substitute.

**Katsuobushi** Dried bonito fish flakes. Bonito is a type of tuna, which is a member of the mackerel family, and one of the most important fish in Japanese cuisine. To make *katsuobushi* the tuna is filleted, boned, boiled, smoked, and dried in the sun to make a hard, woodlike block with a concentrated, rich, and smoky flavor. A special tool is used to flake the extremely hard chunks. Bonito shavings form the base for many Japanese sauces and stocks (such as dashi, made with bonito and seaweed). The flakes are frequently sprinkled over boiled or steamed vegetables and into soups.

**Kinoko** Mushrooms, literally meaning "child of a tree." Various mushrooms are used in Japanese cuisine. Some of the most popular ones are introduced below.

**Bunashimeji.** A firm-textured cultivated mushroom that is suitable for Japanese, Chinese, and Western-style cooking

**Enokitake.** Pale yellow mushrooms with long, slender stems and tiny caps, both of which are edible. Enokitake mushrooms have a faint but distinctive flavor: raw they have a pleasant, crisp bite; blanched they have a chewy texture.

**Hiratake** The Japanese name for oyster mushrooms. This mushroom looks, smells, and tastes like oysters,

**Maitake** Mushrooms popular in Japanese cuisine. They have a wonderful taste, crisp texture, and excellent aroma. Appearing to be a clump of small suspicious-looking fronds or petals, the *maitake* mushroom is firm and fleshy. Its aroma is somewhat similar to that of the oyster mushroom. Entirely edible, the flavor is mild and deliciously pleasant.

**Matsutake** Highly priced gourmet mushrooms that grow only in red pine forests. The mushrooms have a firm, chewy texture, and a spicy, clean smell and taste.

**Shiitake** Large meaty mushrooms with a distinctive, appealing "woody-fruity" flavor and a spongy, chewy texture, which allows it to partner with stronger flavors like beef, pork, and soy sauce.

**Kombu** A dark green long thick sea vegetable from the kelp family. Used frequently in Japanese cooking, it is an essential ingredient of *dashi.* Never wash or rinse before using. The speckled surface of the kelp is just natural salts and minerals, resulting in great flavor. *Kombu* contains significant amounts of glutamic acid, the basis of monosodium glutamate (MSG).

**Kome** Rice. More than 300 varieties of rice are grown in Japan. Japanese cuisine typically uses short-grain types that, when cooked, are faintly sweet and slightly sticky. Rice is the most important crop and has been cultivated by the Japanese for over 2000 years and it was once used as a currency. The Japanese word for cooked rice *(gohan)* also has the general meaning of "meal" and the literal meaning of breakfast (*asagohan*) is "morning rice."

There are three major types of *kome* typically used in Japanese cuisine:

**Genmai** Unpolished brown rice.

**Haigamai** Partially polished white rice.

**Seihakumai** Highly polished white rice, the most common type.

In addition to ordinary table rice, short-grain *mochigome,* glutinous rice or sweet rice, is popular.

**Komezu** Rice vinegar. A light and mild-tasting Japanese vinegar. An essential ingredient for making sushi rice and *sunomono* (vinegary salads). It has a lower acid level than Western vinegars. Vinegar is also known for its antibacterial properties and this is one reason komezu is often used in Japanese dishes that include raw fish, seafood, or meat.

**Kyuri** Japanese cucumber. This is a slender and long cucumber, about 8 inches, with a bumpy skin that is thick and dark green. Kyuri is very crispy to the bite, with very few seeds.

**Menrui** Japanese noodles, made from wheat and buckwheat flours, and mung-bean and potato starch. In Japan, rice flour is not used to make noodles.

**Mirin** A golden yellow, sweet, rich-textured rice wine with an alcohol content of about 14 percent. When used in cooking, it is frequently heated to cook off the alcohol before other flavoring ingredients are added. This technique is called *nikirimirin. Mirin* contributes a rich flavor and an attractive, glossy brown appearance.

**Miso** A fermented soybean paste made from a starter culture that includes either steamed rice or barley mixed with cooked beans and salt. When the beans ferment the taste is somewhat meaty or mushroom-like, with a texture of nut butters, but is not oily. Miso is used in a variety of ways: to flavor soups or stews, in marinades, and spread on items before cooking. The different types of grains used in production process yield three different kinds of *miso*: *komemiso* is made of rice and soybeans, *mugimiso* of barley and soybeans, and *mamemiso* nearly entirely of soybeans. The lighter-colored misos, called "white miso"(*shiro miso*), are made from soybeans. They are sweeter, milder, and more delicate than the darker misos. The darker-colored misos (*aka miso*) are made from red adzuki beans (*aka* means "red" in Japanese). It has a richer, saltier taste because it is allowed to ferment longer. *Aka miso* is a specialty of Hokkaido, the northern island of Japan. *Kuro miso* is a dark, almost black miso that is strong tasting and usually aged the longest. *Hinsu miso* is yellow miso that is readily available. *Mugi miso* is made with all barley and no soybeans, usually a medium brown color. All miso is nutrient dense and high in protein, containing live enzymes that aid in digestion.

**Mitsuba** Literally, "three leaves," often translated as "trefoil." This member of the parsley family has a flavor somewhere between sorrel and celery. Used in soups, eggs, custards, hot stews, and salads.

**Mizuna** A member of the mustard family, it grows in bunches of thin, snow-white stalks with light green leaves. Each leaf is about the size of an arugula leaf, but is deeply serrated. One of the few indigenous vegetables of Japan, *mizuna* means "water greens" because it is grown in fields that are shallowly flooded with water. May be pickled, eaten raw in salads, stir-fried, simmered, and used in hot-pot dishes.

**Moyashi** Bean sprouts. Sprouts grown from many different kinds of legume seeds—soybeans, mung beans, azuki beans, alfalfa, peas, and lentils—are generally known as moyashi. Japanese cuisine predominantly uses soybean sprouts, which have yellow heads and thick, snow-white stems. Mung bean sprouts have small green heads and thinner, longer stems and have become more commonplace. Neither soybean nor mung bean sprouts have a distinctive flavor; they are used more for their crisp texture. Bean sprouts are used in soups, stir-fries, and simmered preparations. Generally they are added at the very last preparation step.

**Naganegi** Literally, "long onion." These are nonbulbing onions 12–16 inches long and 1 inch at the base. Both the white and green parts are used in cooking. The white stem has a strong onion flavor when eaten raw, but becomes very mild and sweet when cooked. It is typically grilled or used in simmered dishes.

**Nasu** Japanese eggplant. A distinctive eggplant variety, it is short—about 4–5 inches–and slender. Less seedy than other eggplant varieties, it becomes very creamy when cooked. Eggplant is pickled, stir-fried, deep-fried, steamed, grilled, or simmered.

**Niban Dashi** A "second fish stock" prepared by simmering the kelp and dried bonito flakes used in preparing ichiban *dashi* in the same volume of fresh water. It will have a less refined flavor and a cloudy appearance, but is still good in everyday miso soups and simmered dishes where strong-flavored condiments or ingredients are incorporated.

**Nira** Chinese chives, also called garlic chives, for their mixed flavor of garlic and chives. These chives have long (up to 16 inches), flat, thin, dark green leaves. When quickly stir-fried, they become bright green and crisp in texture, with a garlicky flavor.

**Nori** Dried or roasted seaweed. Nori seaweed grows around bamboo stakes placed under water. When harvested it is washed, laid out in thin sheets, and dried. The best quality nori seaweed is glossy black-purple. It is typically toasted before using, which improves flavor and texture. To toast, simply pass the sheet of nori several inches over the heat until it turns from dark green to an even darker green. It only takes a few seconds to toast both sides. In Japan it is eaten for breakfast with a little soup and rice. Nori has two sides: one shinier than the other. When using to make *makizushi* (sushi rolls), roll them with the shiny side facing out.

**Panko** Japanese bread crumbs that are extremely crunchy.

**Okara** A by-product of the tofu making process, It is like a moist, white, crumbly sawdust. It is used in soups, stews, or as a side dish.

**Renkon** This is the root of the lotus or water lily plant, *hasu.* The root grows in sausage-like links and has longitudinal tubular channels, usually ten. When cut crosswise, the root has an attractive flowerlike pattern. Mild flavored when raw; when briefly cooked, it has a pleasant crunchy texture.

**Sake** Rice wine. The premiere Japanese alcoholic drink. Sake is often used in marinades for meat and fish to soften them as well as to mask their smell. In cooking, it is often used to add body and flavor to various *dashi* (soup stocks) and sauces, or to make *nimono* (simmered dishes) and *yakimono* (grilled dishes).

**Sashimi** Raw fish fillets.

**Sato-Imo** Taro is the root of a perennial plant that is found everywhere in tropical Asia. The shape varies from small and round to long and sticklike, with a snow-white flesh. It has no distinctive flavor, but has a pleasant, soft texture. Taro is traditionally simmered in a flavored broth, stewed with proteins, or added to soups. Taro will absorb the flavor it is cooked with. Taro must be washed, peeled, and parboiled before final preparation.

**Satsuma-Imo** Sweet potato. Originally from Central and South America, sweet potatoes were introduced by Spanish conquistadors to the Philippines; from there they reached China. They were introduced to Japan from China in the seventeenth century. The Japanese produce a very sweet and creamy sweet potato, with a bright, reddish purple skin. The meat is creamy white when uncooked and a bright yellow when cooked. North American sweet potatoes are less sweet and creamy; when cooked they are more watery. Yams may be the best substitute.

**Shichimi-Tōgarashi** A Japanese spice mixture made from seven spices. *Shichimi* means "seven flavors." It is not the same as Chinese five-spice mixture. The ingredients and proportions used will vary but usually include red pepper flakes, ground roasted orange or mandarin peel, yellow (aka white) sesame seed, black sesame seed or black hemp seeds or poppy seeds, sansho (Japanese pepper also known as Szechuan peppercorns), dark green dried seaweed flakes (nori), rapeseed, or chipi (dried mikan peel).

**Shishitogarashi** Small green pepper, literally "Chinese lion pepper." A 3-inch-long pepper resembling a miniature Chinese lion head. This pepper has been hybridized to remove most of the heat; it is a uniquely Japanese pepper variety. Shishitogarashi peppers are best when stir-fried or deep-fried. When not available, substitute green bell peppers.

**Shiso** Herb, a member of the mint family, tasting of cumin and cinnamon. The leaves are used to wrap sushi and as a garnish for sashimi.

**Shoga** Ginger. One of the oldest seasonings in Japan. It has a pleasant, sharp bite and fragrant bouquet, said to stimulate the appetite. Ginger suppresses undesirable odors from other foods. It is an important condiment for sashimi and sushi because of its antiseptic properties.

**Shoyu (see Soy Sauce)**

**Shungiku** Chrysanthemum leaves. These leaves are cultivated to be edible. They are slightly bitter and can be used raw or cooked. Substitute spinach, turnip greens, or mustard greens.

**Soba** These noodles, which were first called *sobakiri,* are now simply called soba. They are linguine-sized noodles that are hearty, healthy, and served both hot and cold. The quality of the soba noodle is dependent on how much other starchy material, such as wheat flour or yam flour, has been added to the buckwheat flour. Buckwheat, which is not a grain, lacks the gluten needed to form dough. A 100-percent buckwheat flour noodle would lack the "bite" of good pasta. Soba noodles are a regional food. The cooler the climate, the more fragrant and rich-tasting the buckwheat.

**Chukasoba** Literally, "Chinese-style soba noodles." They are a type of wheat noodle that contains no buckwheat flour, mixed with water and a naturally obtained alkaline agent called *kansui.* The *kansui* provides the noodles with their distinctive elasticity. These noodles are creamy yellow (although they contain no eggs), curly, and resilient in texture. They are served hot, with a richly flavored broth made from chicken and pork bones. The most famous dish made from these noodles and broth is *ramen.*

**Harusame** Potato starch noodles, slender and transparent, as thin and straight as angel-hair pasta.

**Kishimen** Flat wheat noodles similar to fettuccini, with a distinctive chewy bite. They are also served both hot and cold.

**Ryokuto Harusame** Mung bean noodles, clear, thin, wrinkled starch noodles.

**Somen and Hiyamugi** Thin wheat noodles. *Somen* are as thin as vermicelli, and *hiyamugi* are slightly thicker than *somen.* Both are summertime noodles, usually served cold, with a dipping sauce.

**Udon** The most popular of the wheat noodles. They are a thick, long, cream-colored, noodle that may be served hot or cold.

**Soy Sauce** Three types of soy sauce are used in Japanese cooking, which differ in color, flavor, and degree of saltiness.

**Koikuchi shoyu,** or simply *shoyu,* means brewed with wheat. It has a dark brown color, rich flavor, and complex aroma, with a salt content around 17 to 18 percent. Used in all types of preparations, it gives foods a dark brown color and rich flavor.

**Tamari** is made nearly entirely from soybeans, and only a small amount of water is added to the fermenting mixture. Tamari is thicker, with a dark brown color, rich in bean flavor and about as salty as regular *shoyu.* Tamari is preferred as a condiment or flavor enhancer rather than a basic cooking ingredient. Follow these key points when cooking with *shoyu:* cook it only for a short time. Brief cooking preserves its natural fragrance, flavor, and color. Because of its high salt content, it should be added toward the end of the cooking process. In stir-frying, *shoyu* is added at the end of the cooking.

**Usukuchi shoyu,** light-colored soy sauce, is produced by not roasting the wheat as much, and more salt is added to slow the fermentation. The resulting *shoyu* is lighter in color, less flavorful, and has a slightly higher salt content, about 19 percent. *Usukuchi shoyu* is used in recipes where a refined color and weak flavor are required.

**Sushi** The term is actually sweetened, pickled rice. Raw fish (*sashimi*) wrapped together with a portion of sushi rice is sold as *"sushi." Sushi* is the term for the special rice; in Japanese it is modified to *zushi* when coupled with modifiers that describe the different styles.

**Takenoko** Bamboo shoots. It is a member of the grass family. Bamboo shoots are young, new canes that are harvested for food before they are two weeks old or one-foot tall. Bamboo shoots are crisp and tender, comparable to asparagus, with a flavor similar to corn. However, fresh bamboo shoots are very difficult to find. Fresh shoots need to be peeled and cooked before using. Raw shoots are bitter tasting and hard to digest.

**Tofu** Soybean curd. This soft, cheeselike food is made by curdling fresh hot soy milk with a coagulant. Traditionally, the curdling agent used to make tofu is *nigari,* a compound found in natural ocean water, or calcium sulfate, a naturally occurring mineral. The curds then are generally pressed into a solid block.

**Firm tofu** is dense and solid and holds up well in stir-fry dishes, soups, or on the grill—anywhere you want the tofu to maintain its shape. Firm tofu also is higher in protein, fat, and calcium than other forms of tofu.

**Kōya-dofu** is freeze-dried tofu, which comes in flat, creamy white squares. When soaked in warm water it absorbs a large amount of liquid and takes on a slightly spongy texture. It has a mild but distinctive flavor. Reconstituted dried tofu has no resemblance to fresh tofu.

**Silken tofu** is a Japanese-style tofu, with a mild, light, delicate taste. Unlike other types of tofu, the water is not pressed out of it, nor is it strained. A slightly different process that results in a creamy, custardlike product makes silken tofu higher in water content, so it does not hold its shape as well as firm tofu. Silken tofu works well in pureed or blended dishes and soups. In Japan, silken tofu is enjoyed "as is," with a touch of soy sauce and topped with chopped scallions.

**Yaki-dofu** is tofu that has been grilled on both sides over charcoal, producing a firm texture.

**Umami** The elusive fifth flavor, translated from Japanese as "delicious," "savory," or "brothy." It refers to a synergy of intricate, balanced flavors. Umami is a taste that occurs when foods with glutamate (like MSG) are eaten.

**Ume** Japanese green plum. Typically pickled, ume is used as a base for preserves, or for *umeshu* (plum wine).

**Wakame** One of the most popular sea vegetables in the Japanese diet.

**Wasabi** Japanese horseradish, pale green in color with a delicate aroma; milder tasting than Western horseradish. *Wasabi* is similar to horseradish in its taste and culinary function but is unrelated. Wasabi grows in the water while horseradish grows in soil. Like ginger, wasabi has antiseptic properties, so it has traditionally been served with sushi and sashimi dishes. Wasabi also helps to promote digestion. Fresh wasabi root should be grated just before consumption; however, fresh is hard to obtain outside of Japan. Powdered or paste *wasabi* is more pungent than freshly grated root, and it is also less fragrant and flavorful. The paste form of wasabi, *neriwasabi,* comes in a tube ready to serve. Powdered wasabi, *konawasabi,* is a mixture of wasabi and horseradish powder; frequently mustard powder is added to increase the pungency and an artificial green color is added to simulate real wasabi.

**Yuzu** A tangerine-size variety of citron (citrus fruit), with a thick, bumpy rind. Like a lemon, yuzu is valued for both its juice and its rind, which has a pleasant tart and bitter flavor. Substitute lime or lemon rind and equal parts lime, orange, and grapefruit juice for *yuzu* juice.

## KITCHEN TOOLS

**Deba bocho** A heavy-duty knife, similar to the chef's knife, with a thicker blade and a pointed tip. Used to chop fish heads and chicken bones.

**Donabe** Earthenware pot with lid, used directly for stovetop cooking (on a gas stove) or at the dinner table with a portable stove. It should not be used in an oven. Often used for *sukiyaki, oden,* and *shabu shabu.*

**Fukin** A thin, rectangular cotton cloth, 12 to 16 inches in length and 10 inches in width. Like cheesecloth, a *fukin* is used for a variety of purposes, including wrapping and forming cooked rice into shapes, lining a colander to strain stock, and squeezing excess water from tofu. A larger version of this is *daifukin.*

**Hangiri** Wooden sushi tub usually made of cypress wood, in the shape of a large circular plate with high sides. The large surface area cools the rice quickly, and the wood absorbs excess moisture. Used to mix rice with sugar and vinegar to make sushi rice.

**Hocho** Japanese knives. Most Japanese knives are made for cutting fish and green leafy vegetables only. They are thin-bladed knives not intended to cut root vegetables, winter squash, carrots, or anything else that might chip the blade. Except for *nakkiri bocho* and *bunka bocho,* only one side of the Japanese blade is ground to form the cutting edge, which is straight, not curved. These characteristics give Japanese knives a cleaner, quicker cut.

**Burka bocho** All-purpose knives.

**Deba bocho** A heavy knife with a sharp tip, used for fish.

**Nakkiri bocho** Knives specifically for vegetables. The name derives from its function: *na* refers to "vegetable" and *giri* means "cut."

**Ryuba** Used to cut fish. *Ryuba* means "willow blade cutting edge."

**Sashimi bocho** Long, thin blade a bit more than an inch wide. Used to cut filleted fish for sushi and sashimi.

**Takobiki** Very long and thin blunt-tipped knife, traditional tool of the sushi chef, perfect for accurate slicing.

**Usuba bocho** A light and efficient knife designed for cutting vegetables, it resembles a basic cleaver, with a slightly rounded end. The straight blade edge is suitable for cutting all the way to the cutting board without the need for a horizontal pull or push.

**Kushi** Bamboo skewers used for preparing certain grilled Japanese dishes, such as *yakitori.* The cook continually turns the skewers so that the meat is evenly cooked and basted. For this reason, bamboo skewers are essential; steel skewers would become too hot to handle. The skewers are soaked in water for 30 minutes before use so they won't burn during cooking.

**Makisu** Bamboo rolling mats, made from thin pieces of bamboo tied together. Makisu are used to make sushi rolls (*makizushi*).

**Oroshigane** A steel grater with very fine spikes, used to grate *wasabi,* ginger, and *daikon* radish.

**Oroshiki** Porcelain grater, considered better than the metal grater (*oroshigane*), because it does not impart any metallic flavor to the food and is safer on the hands.

**Oshizushi no kata** Wooden sushi mold. Used when making pressed sushi, such as *oshizushi.* The rice and toppings placed in an *oshizushi no kata* are pressed, resulting in a pressed "cake."

**Otoshibuta** Literally "drop lid"—a lightweight round lid used to keep foods submerged. It ensures heat is evenly distributed and reduces the tendency of liquid to boil with large bubbles, thus preventing fragile ingredients from losing their original shape. Typically made from wood.

**Ryoribashi** Cooking chopsticks, typically 14 inches long. Normally, *ryoribashi* have a string at the top to tie the chopsticks together.

**Shamoji** A paddle made from wood or plastic, used to serve rice. Also used to stir sushi rice after adding sweetened vinegar and cooling. Nowadays, *shamoji* are usually made from plastic, since they are much easier to clean than their wooden counterparts.

**Suribachi** A bowl with a corrugated pattern on the inside, used as a mortar along with the *surikogi* (pestle) to grind sesame seeds into a paste. It is glazed ceramic on the outside and unglazed on the inside, often brown and beige in color.

**Surikogi** A wooden pestle, often made from cypress wood, shaped like a big cucumber. The grinder part to *suribachi* (bowl), which makes up the Japanese version of the mortar and pestle.

**Wok** For stir-frying. Japanese cuisine uses the traditional, round-bottomed Chinese wok.

**Zaru** A shallow bamboo basket used to drain, rinse, or dry foods. In the summer, cold soba noodles are served in a *zaru,* accompanied by a small bowl filled with dipping sauce, called *zaru soba.*

## COOKING TERMS

**Agemono** Fish or vegetables fried in vegetable oil. The first cooking oil used in Japan was probably sesame oil, goma abura, introduced by the Chinese during the eighth century. However, the majority of deep-frying is now accomplished using refined, flavorless vegetables oils such as canola, soybean, cottonseed, or corn oils, or a combination of these.

There are two styles of deep-frying: tempura and *kara-age.* Tempura is batter frying, while kara-age uses no batter. Instead, ingredients are breaded or dusted with cornstarch and fried. The word *kara* refers to China, meaning that this method originated in Chinese cooking (*age* means deep-fried).

**Daikon Oroshi** Grated daikon. Many fried dishes, including tempura and grilled or broiled oily fish, are almost always served with grated daikon. Choose a radish that is heavy for its size, so it will be juicy. Grate only the top part, which is sweeter than the lower part.

**Hana Ninjin** Floral-cut carrots.

**Hiya-Gohan** Day-old rice, used in stir-frying or rice soup.

**Itameru** Stir-frying.

**Katsura Muki** A technique used with daikon, cucumber, and carrots to cut a continuous paper-thin sheet of flesh.

**Mizukiri** The process of removing excess water from tofu before it is used.

**Momiji Oroshi** Spicy grated daikon. *Momiji* means "autumn leaf color." To prepare *momiji oroshi,* make two deep holes on the cut surface of a disk of daikon, Insert one *skatog arashi* (Japanese dried red chile) into each hole. Grate the daikon and chile together, producing a slightly red, spicy *oroshi.*

**Nabemono** One-pot cooking, a specific style of Japanese preparation, with ingredients added in succession to a pot to cook and ultimately to be served from the cooking pot. The term is also used for simmered dishes. The technique is often applied to vegetables, chicken, and fish. Foods are typically cut into manageable pieces with chopsticks before they are simmered. The basic liquids used include *dashi* (fish stock), *kombu dashi* (kelp stock), water, or sake (rice wine). *Otoshibuta,* or "drop-lid," is frequently used in simmering.

**Shiraga Negi** Literally, "gray-hair long onion," the white part of Japanese long onion *(naganegi),* cut into very thin strips. These thin strips are soaked in ice water so they are crisp and curly. Used as a garnish.

**Tamagoyaki** Egg omelet, sweet and light. In Japan it is the trademark of each sushi chef.

**Yakimono** Foods (usually meat) that are grilled, broiled, or pan-fried. The ingredients are generally marinated in sauce or salted then skewered so they retain their shape and grilled over a hot fire so the skin (if any) is very crisp while the meat stays tender and juicy. *Yakitori* is a type of *yakimono.*

## SUSHI TERMS

**Chirashi-zushi** Translates as "scattered sushi." A bowl or box of sushi rice topped with a variety of sashimi (usually nine, which is considered a lucky number).

**Gunkam-maki** Battleship roll. The maki is rolled to form a container for the liquid of an item, such as oysters, *uni,* quail eggs, *ikora,* and *tobiko.*

**Inari-zushi** *Aburage* (simmered with sweet sake, shoyu, and water), then stuffed with sushi rice.

**Kaiten-zushi** A sushi restaurant where the plates with the sushi are placed on a rotating conveyor belt that winds through the restaurant and moves past every table and counter seat. Customers may place special orders, but most simply pick their selections from a steady stream of fresh sushi moving along the conveyor belt. The final bill is calculated based on the number and type of plates of the consumed sushi. Besides conveyor belts, some restaurants use a fancier form of presentation such as miniature wooden "sushi boats" traveling small canals, or miniature locomotive cars.

**Maki-zushi** Rice and seaweed rolls with fish and/or vegetables made with a makisu mat made from thin pieces of bamboo that facilitates the rolling process. Most rolls are made with the rice inside the *nori,* a few—like the California roll—place the rice on the outside of the *nori.*

**Ana-kyu Maki** Conger eel and cucumber rolls.

**Chutoro Maki** Marbled tuna roll.

**Futo Maki** Large rolls with nori on the outside.

**Hosomaki** Thin rolls, similar to *futomaki* but about half the size in diameter.

**Kaiware Maki** Daikon sprout roll.

**Kanpyo Maki** Pickled gourd rolls.

**Kappa Maki** Cucumber-filled *maki zuchi.*

**Maguro Temaki** Tuna *temaki.*

**Maki Mono** Vinegared rice and fish (or other ingredient) rolled in nori.

**Natto Maki** Sticky, strong-tasting fermented soybean rolls.

**Negitoro Maki** Scallion and tuna roll.

**Nori Maki** Same as *kanpyo maki;* in Osada, same as *futo maki.*

**Oshinko Maki** Pickled daikon rolls.

**Otoro Maki** Fatty tuna roll.

**Tekka Maki** Tuna filled *maki zushi.*

**Tekkappa Maki** Selection of both tuna and cucumber rolls.

**Temaki** Hand-rolled cones made from nori.

**Uramaki** Inside-out rolls; the rice is on the outside with the nori and filling inside.

**Neta** The piece of fish that is placed on top of the sushi rice for *nigiri.*

**Nigiri-zushi** The little fingers of rice topped with wasabi and a filet of raw or cooked fish or shellfish. This is the most common form of sushi.

**Oshinko** Japanese pickles.

**Oshi-zushi** Sushi made from rice pressed in a box or mold.

**Sashimi** Raw fish without rice.

**Tamaki-zushi** Hand-rolled cones of sushi rice, fish, and vegetables wrapped in seaweed.

# Menus and Recipes from Japan

MENU ONE

***Gyoza:* Japanese Pot-Stickers**
***Miso-Shiru:* Miso Soup**
***Dashi:* Japanese Basic Stock**
***Kyuri No Sunome:* Japanese Cucumber Salad**
***Sashimi:* Sliced Raw Fish**
***Sushi:* Basic Vinegared Rice**
***Nigiri-Zushi***
***Yakitori:* Grilled Chicken**
***Hiyashi Chukasoba:* Summertime Chilled Chukasoba**
**Thin Omelet**

MENU TWO

***Asari no Ushio-jiru:* Asari Clam Soup**
***Maki Sushi: Futomaki:* Seasoned Vegetables**
***Horenso Goma-ae:* Spinach with Sesame Dressing**
***Chawan Mushi:* Savory Custard**
***Buta Teriyaki:* Pork on Skewers**
***Nasu No Karashi:* Mustard-Pickled Eggplant**
***Kamonanban Soba:* Soba with Duck and Long Onions**
***Kakejiru:* Broth for Hot Noodles**
**Tempura**
***Goma-anko Manju:* Steamed Dumplings with Sweet Azuki Paste and Sesame Seeds**
***Anko:* Sweet Azuki Bean Paste**

# Gyoza
## Japanese Pot-Stickers

YIELD: 4 SERVINGS OR 40 SMALL DUMPLINGS

**The primary difference between packaged gyoza skins and packaged wonton skins is the shape (round for gyoza skins, square for wonton skins) this is a matter of preference. The dough can be made but it is a time-consuming process and the dough must be rolled quite thin.**

| AMOUNT | MEASURE | INGREDIENT |
|---|---|---|
| 2 cups | 9 ounces, 252 g | All-purpose flour, plus extra for dusting |
| 1 teaspoon | | Salt |
| $1\frac{1}{2}$ cups | 12 ounces, 360 ml | Boiling water |
| $2\frac{1}{2}$ cups | 7 ounces, 196 g | Chinese cabbage, upper leafy parts only, or bib lettuce, minced |
| 1 cup | 8 ounces, 224 g | Ground pork, or $\frac{1}{2}$ cup (4 ounces, 112 g) ground pork and $\frac{1}{2}$ cup (4 ounces, 112 g) ground shrimp |
| 2 teaspoons | 10 ml | Shoyu |
| 1 teaspoon | 5 ml | Grated ginger |
| 1 | | Garlic clove |
| 1 tablespoon | | Green onions, green part only, minced |
| Pinch | | Sugar |
| $\frac{1}{2}$ teaspoon | | Black pepper, fresh ground |
| 40 | | Gyoza or Wonton skins |
| 3 tablespoons | $1\frac{1}{2}$ ounces, 45 ml | Sesame oil mixed with vegetable oil |
| 3 tablespoons | $1\frac{1}{2}$ ounces, 45 ml | Vegetable oil |
| 1 cup | 8 ounces, 240 ml | Boiling water |
| As needed | | Hot mustard paste |
| As needed | | Shoyu |

PROCEDURE

1 Sift flour and $\frac{1}{2}$ teaspoon salt together.

2 Add $1\frac{1}{2}$ cups boiling water to flour little by little, stirring with chopsticks, until mixture is shaped into a ball. Cover and let stand 1 hour.

3. On floured work surface, knead the dough for 6 minutes or until smooth. Form the dough into a long log, and cut the log crosswise into 40 disks. Dust each cut side with additional flour to prevent the surfaces from drying out.
4. Roll each piece of dough into a 3-inch disk, making the rim thinner than the center. Dust liberally with additional flour; stack and wrap in plastic. Set aside.
5. Toss Chinese cabbage with remaining salt. Let stand for 10 minutes. Squeeze the cabbage to remove excess water.
6. Combine ground pork with shoyu and mix until the pork is sticky. Mix in the cabbage, ginger, garlic, green onion, sugar, and black pepper.
7. Have a small bowl of water at hand. Place a wrapper in one hand, wet half the rim of the wrapper with water, and place a little stuffing in the center of the wrapper. Fold the wrapper in half by placing the dry edge over the wet edge. While sealing the dumpling, make six to eight pleats in the top, dry edge, starting at one side and continuing around the rim.
8. Over medium heat, heat a pan large enough to hold 20 dumplings; add 2 tablespoons (1 ounce, 30 ml) oil. When hot, add dumplings to the skillet, pleated sides up, and cook until the bottoms are golden and crisp.
9. Combine 1 cup boiling water and 2 tablespoons (1 ounce, 30 ml) oil. When dumplings are golden, add enough of the liquid mixture to reach to $\frac{1}{4}$ the height of the dumplings. Immediately cover and steam dumplings over medium to low heat for 4 to 5 minutes.
10. Remove lid, turn heat up to high, and cook away any remaining liquid.
11. Remove dumplings from the pan and keep warm. Repeat with remaining dumplings.
12. Serve hot with mustard paste and shoyu.

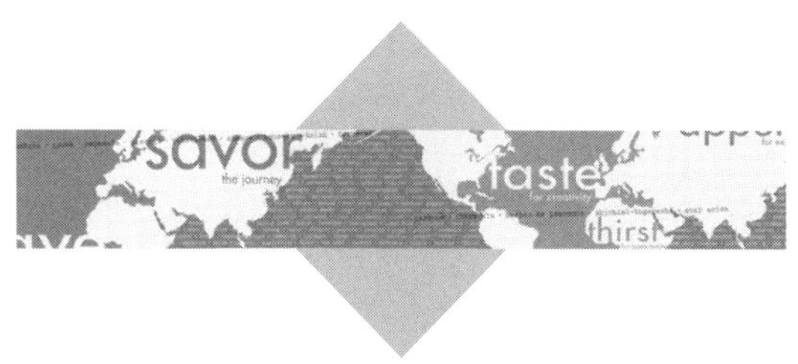

# Miso-Shiru

## Miso Soup SERVES 4

**This is a traditional soup, which can be served at any meal.**

| AMOUNT | MEASURE | INGREDIENT |
|---|---|---|
| 4 cups | 32 ounces, 950 ml | Ichiban dashi (recipe follows) |
| $\frac{1}{2}$ cup | $1\frac{1}{3}$ ounces, 37 g | Wakeme seaweed or shiitake mushrooms, thinly sliced |
| 3 tablespoons | $1\frac{1}{2}$ ounces, 45 ml | Shiro miso (sweet white miso) |
| 1 cup ($\frac{1}{2}$ block) | 7 ounces, 196 g | Firm or soft tofu, $\frac{1}{2}$ inch (1.27 cm) dice |
| 3 tablespoons | $\frac{1}{2}$ ounce, 14 g | Green onion, green and white parts, $\frac{1}{8}$ inch (.3 cm) thin diagonal cut |

**PROCEDURE**

1 Combine dashi and mushrooms; simmer over medium heat 3 minutes.

2 Soften the miso with a little stock and stir into the dashi until miso is dissolved. Do not boil: miso's flavor changes when boiled. Add the tofu and heat 30 seconds.

3 Divide the green onion, mushrooms, and tofu equally among serving bowls.

4 Ladle in dashi. Serve immediately, as hot as possible.

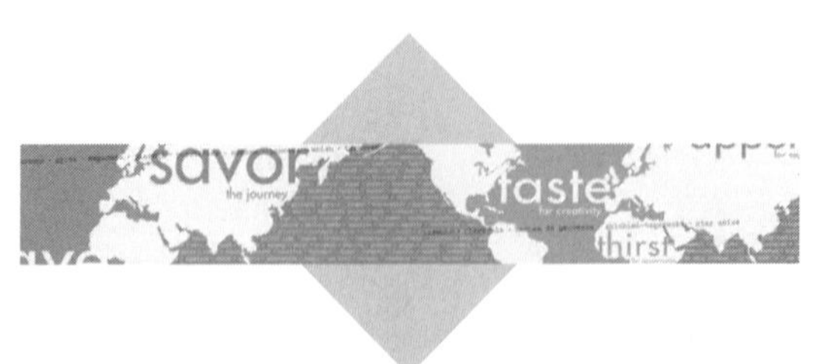

# Dashi
## Japanese Basic Stock

***Dashi* is indispensable in Japanese cooking. Although chicken stock can be a suitable substitute, to cook truly "Japanese," *dashi* should always be used when a recipe calls for stock or broth.**

## Ichiban Dashi (First Fish Stock)

YIELD: 1 QUART

| AMOUNT | MEASURE | INGREDIENT |
|---|---|---|
| **1 quart** | **32 ounces, 1 liter** | **Water** |
| **1** | **1 x 4 inch (10 cm)** | **Kombu (kelp), wiped clean** |
| **$\frac{1}{2}$ cup** | **$\frac{1}{2}$ ounce, 14 g** | **Katsuobushi (bonito fish flakes), tightly packed** |

PROCEDURE

1. Combine water with *kombu* over medium heat; bring almost to a boil but do not let the *kombu* boil or the stock will become stronger than desired.
2. Immediately remove *kombu*; save.
3. Bring back to boiling point; remove from heat and stir in bonito flakes. Let sit for 1 to 2 minutes; flakes will settle to the bottom.
4. Strain the stock through a cheesecloth-lined strainer. Store in an airtight container for up to 4 days.

# Kyuri No Sunome

## Japanese Cucumber Salad

SERVES 4

| AMOUNT | MEASURE | INGREDIENT |
|---|---|---|
| 2 cups | 8 ounces, 224 g | Cucumber, peeled, seeded, cut lengthwise in half and sliced very thin |
| $\frac{1}{2}$ cup | 1 ounce, 28g | Green onions, chopped $\frac{1}{4}$ inch (.6 cm) |
| 2 tablespoons | 1 ounce, 30 ml | Shoyu |
| 1 tablespoon | $\frac{1}{2}$ ounce, 15 ml | Sesame oil |
| 1 tablespoon | $\frac{1}{2}$ ounce, 14 g | Granulated sugar |
| 4 tablespoons | 2 ounces, 120 ml | Rice vinegar |
| To taste | | Salt |
| 2 teaspoons | | Mixture of black and white sesame seeds, toasted |

**PROCEDURE**

1. Combine all ingredients except sesame seeds and let stand for 1 hour.
2. Sprinkle with toasted sesame seeds.

# Sashimi

## Sliced Raw Fish

SERVES 4

| AMOUNT | MEASURE | INGREDIENT |
|---|---|---|
| **1$\frac{1}{2}$ pounds** | **672 g** | **Impeccably fresh sea bass, tuna, or other saltwater fish, filleted** |
| **2 cups** | **6 ounces, 168 g** | **Daikon, shredded** |
| **$\frac{1}{2}$ cup** | **1 ounce, 28 g** | **Carrot, shredded** |
| **$\frac{1}{2}$ cup** | **2 ounces, 56 g** | **Green onion, white and green parts, minced** |
| **1 tablespoon** | **$\frac{1}{2}$ ounce, 14 g** | **Wasabi** |
| **To taste** | | **Shoyu** |
| **1 tablespoon** | **$\frac{1}{2}$ ounce, 14 g** | **Ginger, grated** |

**PROCEDURE**

1. Remove any skin, blood, and dark sections from the fish.
2. Cut diagonally into slices 1 inch (2.5 cm) long and $\frac{1}{4}$ inch (5 mm) thick.
3. Arrange shredded *daikon,* carrot, and green onion in mounds on a serving platter.
4. Arrange raw fish slices on platter.
5. Mix wasabi to a thick paste with a little water and place on platter.
6. To serve, pour shoyu into individual bowls, then allow diners to add wasabi and ginger to their own bowls.
7. Serve with rice, if desired. Dip fish and vegetables into sauce before eating.

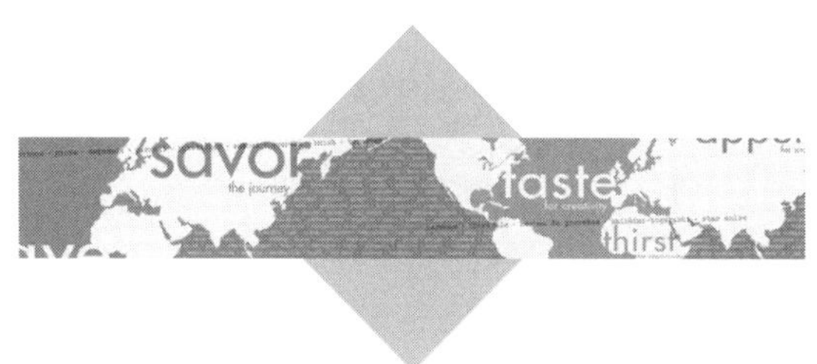

# Sushi

## Basic Vinegared Rice

**Chef Tip** **Keys to success: Use white short-grain Japanese rice or medium-grain California rice.**

**Wash rice thoroughly under cold running water, rubbing it well between the palms of the hands. Drain and repeat the process 3 times until the water is clear. Drain and set in a colander to air dry for 30 minutes, tossing once or twice for even air circulation, before cooking. This produces firmly cooked rice, perfect for tossing with vinegar dressing. Rice for sushi should not be soaked.**

**Use good-quality rice vinegar.**

**Mix cooked rice and vinegar dressing in a *hangiri* tub. Because the wood absorbs moisture and retains heat, the rice doesn't become watery, nor does it cool too quickly. An unfinished wooden salad bowl is a good substitute for a *hangiri*. Soak wood bowls and spatula in cold water for at least 20 minutes so the rice will not stick.**

**Never refrigerate sushi rice; it will become unpleasantly firm.**

## Gohan (Rice)

YIELD: 8–9 CUPS

| AMOUNT | MEASURE | INGREDIENT |
|---|---|---|
| 3 cups | 19 ounces, 532 g | Rice |
| 4 cups | 32 ounces, 960 ml | Water |
| 2 tablespoons | 1 ounce, 30 ml | Sake |
| 1 | 2 inch (4.8 cm) square | Kombu |
| Vinegar Dressing | | |
| 3 tablespoons | $1\frac{1}{2}$ ounces, 42 g | Sugar |
| 2 teaspoons | $\frac{1}{2}$ ounce, 14 g | Salt |
| $\frac{1}{2}$ cup | 4 ounces, 120 ml | Rice vinegar |

PROCEDURE

1. Prepare rice for cooking.
2. Combine rice, water, and sake in correct-size pot (three times deeper than water level). Place the *kombu* on top, bring to a boil, and then immediately remove the *kombu*.

3 Cook, uncovered, until the water level is almost level with the rice.

4 Reduce heat to low and cover with a tight-fitting lid. Cook for another 10 to 15 minutes.

5 Remove from heat and let stand, covered, for 10 minutes. This resting makes the rice easier to toss.

6 Dissolve the sugar and salt in the vinegar. Do not allow to boil vigorously or the flavor of the vinegar will be compromised. Cool slightly.

7 Transfer the hot rice to a *hangiri,* wooden bowl, or sheet pan. Spread into a thin layer.

8 Pour the vinegar dressing over the cooling rice and cut into the rice with a wooden spatula, while fanning the rice to cool it. Do not use all the dressing right away or the rice may get mushy. Keep fanning, stirring, and adding vinegar dressing until the rice is at room temperature. Taste as you go; you may not need all the dressing.

9 The rice is ready to make sushi when it has cooled to room temperature.

Chef Tip **To prevent cooked sushi rice from becoming sticky when handling, keep your hands damp with *tezu* ("hand-vinegar"), which is a combination of water and vinegar that can be used to dip your fingers into while making sushi. To create *tezu,* combine 1 tablespoon sushi dressing with 3 tablespoons cold water.**

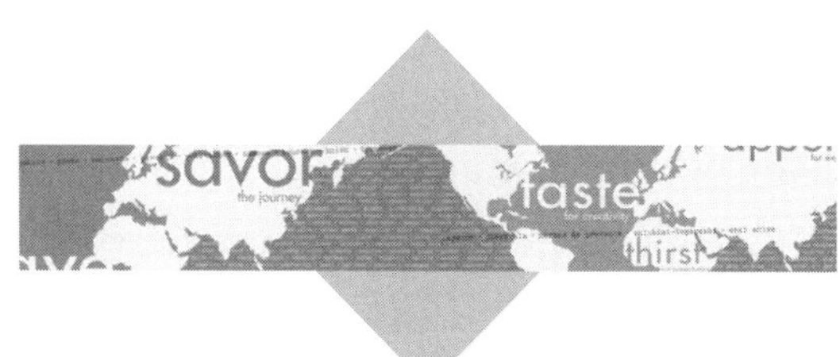

# Nigiri-Zushi

YIELD: 24 PIECES

| AMOUNT | MEASURE | INGREDIENT |
|---|---|---|
| **Tezu** | | |
| $\frac{3}{4}$ cup | 6 ounces, 180 ml | Water |
| 1 $\frac{1}{2}$ tablespoons | $\frac{3}{4}$ ounce, 23 ml | Rice vinegar |
| 1 tablespoon | | Wasabi powder |
| 1 tablespoon | $\frac{1}{2}$ ounce, 15 ml | Warm water |
| 2 cups | 14 ounces, 418 g | Cooked sushi rice |
| 12 ounces | 336 g | 24 assorted pieces raw fish cut for sushi—1 $\frac{1}{2}$ inches (3.6 cm) long by 2 inches (4.8 cm) wide by $\frac{1}{4}$ inch (.6 cm) thick |
| As needed | | Pickled ginger |
| As needed | | Shoyu |

PROCEDURE

1. Make the tezu by stirring together the water and rice vinegar.
2. Mix wasabi powder with the warm water to make a paste; set aside to rest for 30 minutes.
3. Dip fingers in the tezu and clasp your hands together to dampen palms. Take about 1$\frac{1}{2}$ tablespoons of rice in your fingers and gently compress into the shape of a finger, about $\frac{3}{4}$ inch (1.8 cm) wide, 1$\frac{1}{2}$ inches (3.6 cm) long, and $\frac{3}{4}$ inch (1.8 cm) high.
4. Smear a bit of wasabi paste down the center of one flat side of a piece of fish. Holding the rice in one hand and the fish in the other, press the two together. The fish should completely cover the top of the rice.
5. Repeat with remaining rice and fish and place on a serving platter.
6. Mound a small amount of wasabi on the platter and serve with shoyu and pickled ginger.

# Yakitori

## Grilled Chicken

SERVES 4

| AMOUNT | MEASURE | INGREDIENT |
| --- | --- | --- |
| **4** | **16 ounces, 448 g** | **Chicken thighs, skinned, boned, and cut into 1 inch (2.4 cm) by $1\frac{1}{4}$ inch (3 cm) pieces** |
| **2** | | **Green onion, cut diagonally to match the size of chicken** |
| **8** | | **Bamboo skewers, soaked in water for 1 hour** |
| **As needed** | | **Salt** |
| **As needed** | | **Yakitori Basting Sauce (recipe follows)** |

**PROCEDURE**

1. Preheat broiler or grill.
2. Thread chicken and green onions alternately onto skewers. Salt chicken and green onions.
3. Cook the skewered chicken and onions for 4 minutes, turning the skewers several times. Remove from heat and baste with *tare* (basting sauce).
4. Return to heat and cook 2 minutes, turning several times. Remove from heat and baste.
5. Return to heat and cook 2 minutes, turning once. Remove from heat and baste once more. Serve hot.

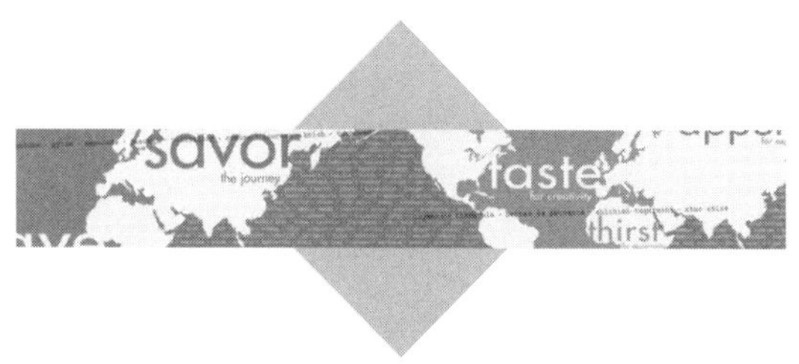

# Yakitori Tare
## Yakitori Basting Sauce

YIELD: $\frac{1}{2}$ CUP, 4 OUNCES, 120 ML

| AMOUNT | MEASURE | INGREDIENT |
|---|---|---|
| **8** | | **Chicken wings** |
| **$\frac{3}{4}$ cup** | **6 ounces, 180 ml** | **Sake** |
| **1 $\frac{1}{3}$ cups** | **10 $\frac{1}{2}$ ounces, 315 ml** | **Mirin** |
| **3 tablespoons** | **1 $\frac{1}{2}$ ounces, 42 g** | **Granulated sugar** |
| **1 $\frac{1}{3}$ cups** | **10 $\frac{1}{2}$ ounces, 315 ml** | **Shoyu** |

**PROCEDURE**

1. Char chicken wings over about half their surfaces.
2. Over medium heat, bring sake and mirin to boil; add sugar and cook to dissolve. Add shoyu and chicken wings; bring to a boil and reduce heat to low.
3. Cook over low heat for 30 minutes, until sauce is thick and glossy.
4. Strain through cheesecloth; serve warm to hot.

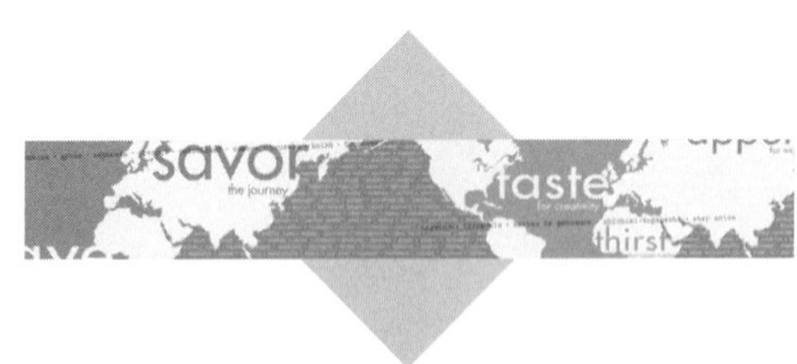

# Hiyashi Chukasoba

## Summertime Chilled Chukasoba

SERVES: 4

**Chef Tip** **To make ginger juice, peel and grate ginger. Wrap grated ginger in cheesecloth and squeeze the juice through the cheesecloth.**

### Sauce

| AMOUNT | MEASURE | INGREDIENT |
|---|---|---|
| $\frac{1}{4}$ cup | 2 ounces, 60 ml | Mirin |
| 1 tablespoon | $\frac{1}{2}$ ounce, 14 g | Granulated sugar |
| $1\frac{1}{2}$ cups | 12 ounces, 360 ml | Chicken stock or ramen stock |
| $\frac{1}{2}$ cup | 4 ounces, 120 ml | Shoyu |
| 3 tablespoons | $1\frac{1}{2}$ ounces, 45 ml | Rice vinegar |
| 1 tablespoon | $\frac{1}{2}$ ounce, 15 ml | Sesame oil |
| 1–2 teaspoons | | Ginger juice, to taste |

**PROCEDURE**

1. Over high heat bring mirin to a boil; add sugar and chicken stock and return to a boil.
2. Add shoyu, return to boil, remove from heat, and transfer to a clean, cooled container.
3. Add rice vinegar, sesame oil, and ginger juice. Let cool and refrigerate for at least 1 hour.

### Toppings

| AMOUNT | MEASURE | INGREDIENT |
|---|---|---|
| 3 cups | 12 ounces, 336 g | Soybean or mung bean sprouts |
| 2 ounces | 48 g | Mung bean noodles, soaked in boiling water for 6 minutes |

**PROCEDURE**

1. Blanch sprouts in boiling water for 30 seconds. Drain and set aside.
2. Drain soaked mung-bean noodles, cool under cold running water, and cut into 6-inch (14.4 cm) lengths.

# Thin Omelet

| AMOUNT | MEASURE | INGREDIENT |
|---|---|---|
| Pinch | | Salt |
| 1 teaspoon | 5 g | Granulated sugar |
| 4 | | Eggs, lightly beaten |
| $1\frac{1}{2}$ tablespoons | $\frac{3}{4}$ ounce, 23 ml | Vegetable oil |
| **Noodles** | | |
| 13 ounces | | Dried chukasoba noodles |
| 2 teaspoons | 10 ml | Sesame oil |
| **Plating** | | |
| 1 cup | 6 ounces, 168 g | Japanese or salad cucumber, julienned in $2\frac{1}{2}$ inch (6 cm) lengths |
| 8 | | Cherry tomatoes, cut in half |
| 8 | | Shrimp (16–20 count), cooked, peeled, and cut in half |
| **Garnish** | | |
| 2 tablespoons | | White or black sesame seeds, toasted |
| To taste | | Hot mustard paste or smooth French-style mustard |

**PROCEDURE**

1. Combine salt, sugar, and eggs.
2. Use oil and eggs to make 8 small very thin omelets. Cut into 2-inch (4.8 cm) julienne strips.
3. Cook noodles in large amount of boiling water until al dente, 3 to 5 minutes or as instructed on package.
4. Drain and rinse under cold running water. Drain again, toss with sesame oil.
5. Divide the noodles among 4 individual shallow bowls. Top noodles with cucumber, tomatoes, shrimp, sprouts, mung bean noodles, and omelets strips. In traditional presentations, the items are placed in separate mounds like the colorful spokes of a wheel. Pour some of the sauce over each dish, garnish with sesame seeds on top, and place a dab of mustard on the rim of the bowl.

# Asari no Ushio-jiru

## Asari Clam Soup

YIELD: 16 PIECES

| AMOUNT | MEASURE | INGREDIENT |
|---|---|---|
| **12** | **24 ounces, 672 g** | **Asari clams, or littleneck or New Zealand cockles** |
| **4 cups** | **32 ounces, 960 ml** | **Water** |
| **1** | **3 inch (7.2 cm)** | **Square kombu (kelp)** |
| **1 tablespoon** | **$\frac{1}{2}$ ounce, 15 ml** | **Sake** |
| **To taste** | **$\frac{1}{2}$ ounce, 15 ml** | **Light soy sauce** |
| **To taste** | | **Salt** |
| **To taste** | | **Lemon juice** |
| **To taste** | | **Sugar** |
| **Garnish** | | |
| **$\frac{1}{2}$ cup** | **2 ounces, 48 g** | **Daikon sprouts, roots removed, or watercress leaves** |
| **$\frac{1}{4}$** | | **Yuzu citron or lemon rind, julienned** |

PROCEDURE

1. Place clams into a colander, and place the colander in a large bowl of salted cold water (1 tablespoon salt to 1 quart water). Let clams stand in a cool place for 2 hours to expel any sand, then rub and rinse under cold running water.
2. Combine clams, water, and *kombu* and bring almost to a boil over medium heat, skimming any foam. Remove and discard the *kombu.*
3. Add the sake and cook clams, covered, until they open, 3 to 4 minutes. Discard any unopened clams.
4. Strain soup through a sieve lined with cheesecloth. Reserve clams, and return both clams and soup broth to pot. Season to taste with soy sauce, salt, lemon juice, and sugar.
5. Serve each portion with equal amounts of clams and broth.
6. Top each serving with daikon sprouts and julienned lemon rind.

# Maki Sushi

## *Futomaki:* Seasoned Vegetables

YIELD: 16 PIECES

| AMOUNT | MEASURE | INGREDIENT |
|---|---|---|
| 1 tablespoon | | Wasabi powder |
| 1 tablespoon | $\frac{1}{2}$ ounce, 15 ml | Warm water |
| 1 cup | 6 ounces, 168 g | Vegetables, julienned—(suitable vegetables include bamboo shoots, carrot, celery, daikon, spinach (squeeze especially well), green beans, asparagus, snow peas) |
| 1 cup | 8 ounces, 240 ml | Dashi |
| 1 $\frac{1}{2}$ tablespoons | | Sugar |
| 1 $\frac{1}{2}$ tablespoons | $\frac{3}{4}$ ounce, 22.5 ml | Mirin |
| 1 $\frac{1}{2}$ tablespoons | $\frac{3}{4}$ ounce, 22.5 ml | Soy sauce |
| $\frac{3}{4}$ cup | 6 ounces, 180 ml | Water |
| 2 tablespoons | 1 ounce, 30 ml | Rice vinegar |
| 2 | | Full sheet nori, toasted |
| 3 cups | 21 ounces, 588 g | Cooked sushi rice |
| As needed | | Soy sauce |
| As needed | | Pickled ginger |

PROCEDURE

1. Mix wasabi with warm water to make a paste and set aside to rest for 30 minutes.
2. Combine vegetables, dashi, sugar, mirin, and 1$\frac{1}{2}$ tablespoons soy sauce. Simmer over medium heat until the vegetables are just tender.
3. Remove from heat, cool, and squeeze to remove excess liquid.
4. Make the tezu by stirring together the water and rice vinegar.
5. Place the rolling mat in front so the bamboo pieces are horizontal. Cover with film, if desired.
6. Place the nori shiny side down (textured side up) on top of the mat, with the shorter edge near you. Align the edge of the nori with the edge of the rolling mat so that the nori is squared off.

7. Dip fingers in to tezu and spread the rice over the nori, covering the surface from edge to edge but leaving a 1-inch (2.4 cm) portion of nori bare at the top. The rice should be about $\frac{1}{4}$ inch (.6 cm) thick.
8. Use your finger to make a shallow indentation in the center of the rice that runs horizontally across.
9. Smear wasabi in the indentation and add half the vegetables down the center line.
10. Place your fingers on top of the filling to help keep it in place and use your thumbs to lift the bamboo mat up and over, rolling it forward. Bring the bottom edge of the nori and rice up and over the filling to meet the end of the rice.
11. Squeeze your fingers back toward you, tucking under the bottom and far side of the roll. Doing so compresses the filling and rice to make a tight roll.
12. Remove the mat and gently squeeze the roll to firm it and round out its shape.
13. Moisten the blade of a thin, sharp knife and slice each roll into 8 × $\frac{3}{4}$ inch (19.2 × 1.8 cm) pieces. Wipe the blade with a clean, warm cloth between slices.
14. Arrange on a serving plate; serve with soy sauce, wasabi, and pickled ginger on the side.

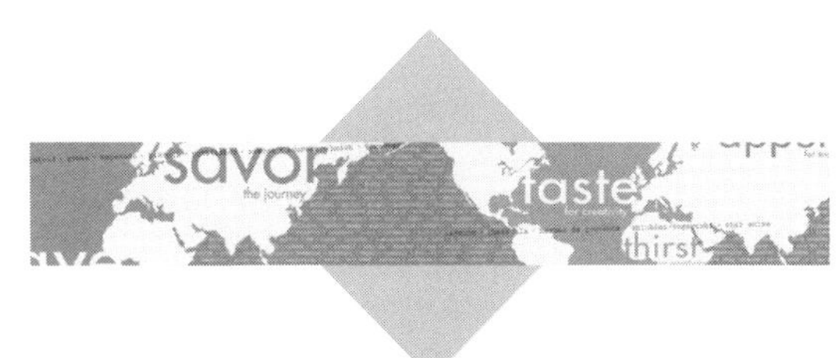

# Horenso Goma-ae

## Spinach with Sesame Dressing

SERVES 4

| AMOUNT | MEASURE | INGREDIENT |
|---|---|---|
| **5 tablespoons** | **$1\frac{1}{4}$ ounces, 35 g** | **Sesame seeds, toasted** |
| **1 tablespoon** | **$\frac{1}{3}$ ounce, 10 g** | **Granulated sugar** |
| **2 tablespoons** | **1 ounce, 30 ml** | **Dashi** |
| **$\frac{1}{2}$ teaspoon** | | **Tamari** |
| **$3\frac{1}{4}$ cups** | **7 ounces, 196 g** | **Spinach, washed** |
| **As needed** | | **Yuzu citron or lime rind** |

**PROCEDURE**

1. Grind toasted sesame seeds with a mortar and pestle until an oily paste. Add sugar, blending thoroughly. Add dashi a little at a time, mixing until smooth. Use additional dashi, if necessary, to make a smooth paste. Blend in tamari. (A food processor or blender can also be used to make the dressing.)
2. Cook spinach in salted boiling water for 45 seconds.
3. Drain spinach and cool under running water. Squeeze tightly to remove excess water.
4. Cut spinach into $1\frac{1}{2}$ inch (3.6 cm) lengths.
5. Just before serving, toss the spinach with sesame dressing and garnish with yuzu citron or lime rind.

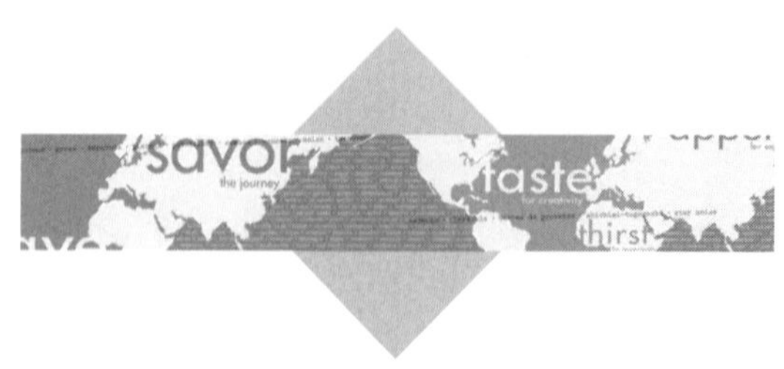

# Chawan Mushi Savory Custard

SERVES 4 (6 OUNCES EACH)

| AMOUNT | MEASURE | INGREDIENT |
|---|---|---|
| $\frac{1}{2}$ cup | 2 ounces, 56 g | Chicken breast fillet |
| As needed | | Salt |
| 4 | 4 ounces, 112 g | Shrimp, headed, peeled, deveined, cut in $\frac{1}{4}$ inch (.6 cm) pieces |
| 2 | 2 ounces, 56 g | Shiitake mushrooms, stems removed, quartered |
| 2 teaspoons | 7 ml | Light soy sauce |
| 4 | | Large eggs |
| $1\frac{1}{2}$ cups | 12 ounces, 360 ml | Dashi |
| Pinch | | Salt |
| 1 teaspoon | 5 ml | Mirin |
| 8 | | Watercress leaves, stems removed |
| Garnish | | Yuzu citron or lemon rind, julienned |

PROCEDURE

1. Remove any sinew from the chicken breast, lightly salt, and let stand 15 minutes.
2. Wipe chicken with a paper towel to remove the salt and exuded juice.
3. Cut the fillet in half diagonally, then halve the two pieces crosswise into $\frac{1}{2}$-inch (1.2 cm) pieces.
4. Blanch chicken and shrimp in salted boiling water for about 10 seconds. Drain and wipe dry.
5. Toss shrimp, chicken, and mushrooms with $1\frac{1}{2}$ teaspoon soy sauce. Let stand 15 minutes.
6. Wipe dry with paper towel and divide equally among four custard cups or ramekins.
7. Beat eggs lightly, add remaining soy sauce, dashi, salt, and mirin, and mix again.
8. Strain egg mixture through a fine sieve; divide among ramekins.
9. Wrap the ramekins with film and steam custard for 2 minutes over high heat; reduce heat to medium and continue to steam for 13 minutes or until clear liquid runs out when a wooden skewer is inserted. It is important that the steam temperature is not too high; the custard should be silky and smooth, similar to soft tofu.
10. Remove film and place a watercress leaf on top of each ramekin; steam for 30 seconds. Remove from steamer and cover with a lid to keep warm.
11. Serve the custard with a spoon. Garnish with yuzu or lemon rind.

# Buta Teriyaki

## Pork on Skewers

SERVES 4

| AMOUNT | MEASURE | INGREDIENT |
|---|---|---|
| $\frac{1}{2}$ cup | 4 ounces, 120 ml | Mirin |
| $\frac{1}{4}$ cup | 2 ounces, 60 ml | Sake |
| $\frac{1}{4}$ cup | 2 ounces, 60 ml | Shoyu |
| 2 tablespoons | 1 ounce, 28 g | Granulated sugar |
| 2 pounds | 896 g | Pork tenderloin, cleaned and thinly sliced $\frac{1}{4}$ inch (.6 cm) thick |
| 1 teaspoon | 5 g | Fresh ginger root, grated |
| 1 cup | 4 ounces, 112 g | Onion, minced |

**PROCEDURE**

1. To make teriyaki sauce, over medium heat, combine the mirin and sake for 5 minutes. Add shoyu and sugar; stir to dissolve the sugar.
2. Cook over low heat for 25 minutes; cool before using.
3. Combine remaining ingredients with teriyaki sauce and marinate for 1 hour.
4. Thread the pork on 4 skewers, reserving marinade.
5. Grill (broil) for 3 minutes on each side, basting frequently with the marinade. Serve immediately with plain white rice.

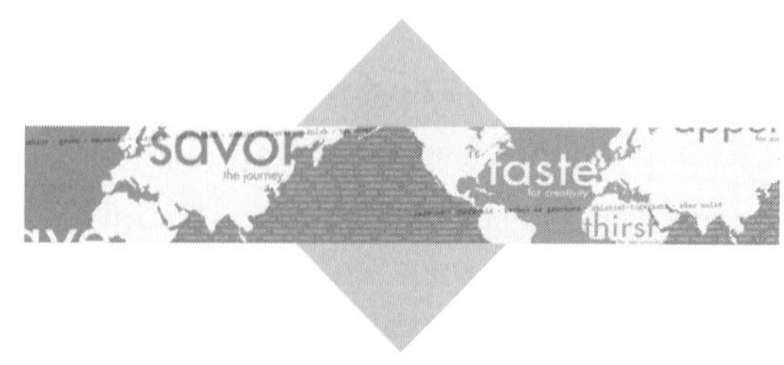

# Nasu No Karashi

## Mustard-Pickled Eggplant

SERVES 4

| AMOUNT | MEASURE | INGREDIENT |
|---|---|---|
| **6** | | **Small Japanese elongated eggplants** |
| **3 cups** | **24 ounces, 720 ml** | **Water** |
| **1 tablespoon** | **$\frac{1}{2}$ ounce, 15 g** | **Salt** |
| **Dressing** | | |
| **$1\frac{1}{2}$ teaspoons** | **7 g** | **Dry mustard or wasabi** |
| **3 tablespoons** | **$1\frac{1}{2}$ ounces, 45 ml** | **Shoyu** |
| **4 tablespoons** | **2 ounces, 60 ml** | **Mirin** |
| **2 tablespoons** | **1 ounce, 28 g** | **Granulated sugar** |

**PROCEDURE**

1. Cut eggplant crossways into slices about $\frac{1}{8}$ inch (2.5 mm) thick, then cut into quarters.
2. Combine water and salt; add eggplant and soak for 1 hour.
3. Drain eggplant and pat dry.
4. Combine remaining ingredients to make the dressing, mix well.
5. Combine eggplant and dressing. Chill for 2 hours or longer to combine flavors before serving.

# Kamonanban Soba

## Soba with Duck and Long Onions

SERVES 4

| AMOUNT | MEASURE | INGREDIENT |
|---|---|---|
| **2** | **8 ounces, 224 g** | **Duck breast, excess fat removed and reserved** |
| **14 ounces** | **392 g** | **Dried soba noodles** |
| **1** | | **Naganegi long onion, or 4 thick scallions** |
| **$\frac{1}{4}$ cup** | **2 ounces, 60 ml** | **Sake** |
| **6 cups** | **48 ounces, 1440 ml** | **Kakejiru, warm to hot (recipe follows)** |
| **1 cup** | **2 ounces, 56 g** | **Watercress leaves** |
| **As needed** | | **Seven-spice powder** |

**PROCEDURE**

1. Slice duck breast diagonally into $\frac{1}{4}$ inch (.6 cm) thick slices.
2. Cook noodles al dente; drain and rinse under cold running water, rubbing them between your hands until they are cold and no longer starchy. Drain well.
3. Heat reserved duck fat over medium heat; cook until fat covers the bottom of the pan. Remove the solid duck fat.
4. Add duck and long onion or scallion; cover and cook until the surface of the duck turns whitish and the bottom is slightly golden.
5. Turn the duck and long onion, sprinkle with sake, cover, and continue to cook 2 more minutes.
6. Add duck and onions to the *kakejiru.*
7. Add noodles and reheat for 1 to 2 minutes.
8. Divide noodles among the serving bowls and pour over hot broth.
9. Serve noodles topped with duck, onion, and watercress.
10. Sprinkle with seven-spice powder.

# Kakejiru
## Broth for Hot Noodles

**YIELD: 1 QUART, 32 OUNCES, 960 ML**

| AMOUNT | MEASURE | INGREDIENT |
|---|---|---|
| 1 quart | 32 ounces, 960 ml | Ichiban dashi |
| $1\frac{1}{2}$ tablespoons | $\frac{3}{4}$ ounce, 21 g | Granulated sugar |
| $1\frac{1}{2}$ teaspoons | 10 g | Salt |
| 1 tablespoon | $\frac{1}{2}$ ounce, 15 ml | Shoyu |
| $1\frac{1}{2}$ teaspoons | 8 ml | Light soy sauce |

**PROCEDURE**

1 Bring all ingredients to a slow boil over low heat.

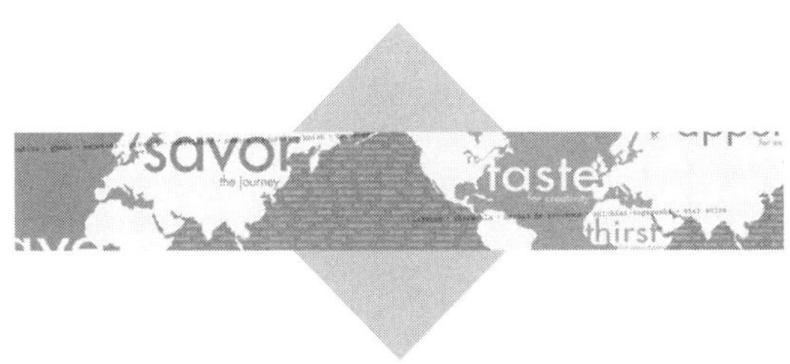

# Tempura

**Portuguese missionaries first brought tempura to Japan in the sixteenth century, but there are many legends about its origins. One is that it was named after the Buddhist curator who, centuries ago, invented the dish to please his noble lord. Another explanation is that the word *tempura* is broken down into three *kanji,* or picture characters: *tem,* signifying heaven; *pu,* signifying woman; and *ra,* meaning silken gauze; the combination means something like "woman veiled in silken gauze, giving a glimpse of heaven."**

***Tempura* refers to vegetables or seafood that have been battered and deep-fried. Tempura reflects many qualities of the Japanese cuisine; absolutely fresh ingredients, artful presentation, and the perfection of a technique. When correctly executed, tempura results in a fried food that is light and fresh tasting, a triumph of Japanese cooking.**

**The secret to tempura's crispiness is in its batter coating, or more precisely, the lumps, which are apt to form in the tenuous mixture of egg, ice water, and flour. Because these ingredients remain unmixed, each morsel dipped to the bottom of the batter is coated in an egg-water-flour sequence. The batter must be made in small batches and not left to stand. If the batter is overmixed, the result will be armorlike pancake casing, rather than the crispy coating the Japanese call a *koromo,* or "cloak." The Japanese claim that they can tell the difference between tempura made by a five-year "novice" and a twenty-year veteran, so subtle is the chemistry at work in the tempura chef's powdery-ringed batter bowl.**

## Traditional Tempura Batter

YIELD: 4

| AMOUNT | MEASURE | INGREDIENT |
|---|---|---|
| 1 | | Large egg |
| ½ cup | 4 ounces, 120 ml | Ice cold club soda or water |
| 1 cup | 4 ounces, 112 g | Rice flour |

PROCEDURE

1. Combine egg and club soda or water.
2. Add the flour to the liquid and stir together with chopsticks. Do not overmix; the batter should be a bit lumpy.
3. Let rest at least 15 minutes but no more than 1 hour before using.
4. If too thick, add water to achieve the consistency of whipping cream; stir with chopsticks.

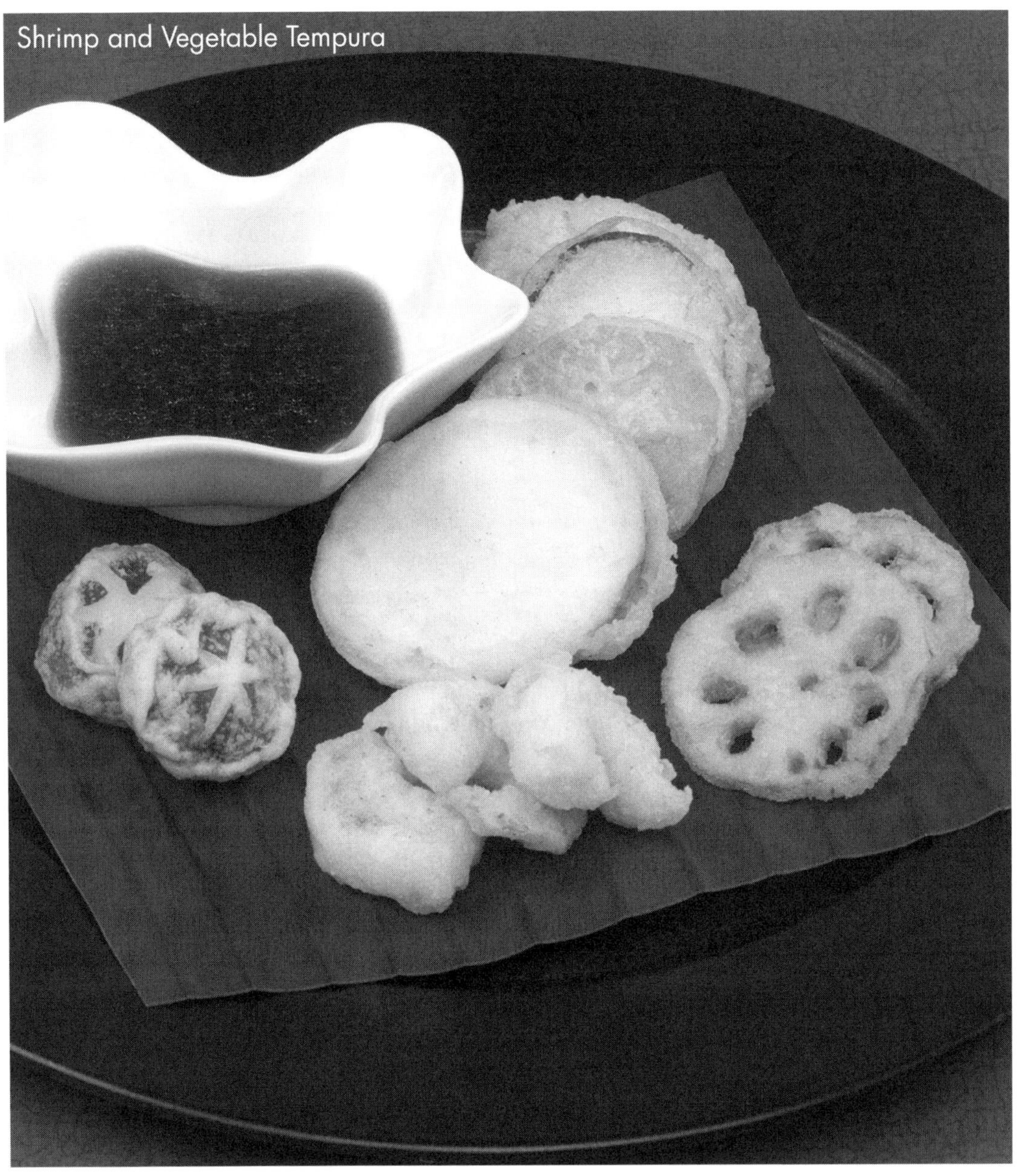
Shrimp and Vegetable Tempura

# Shrimp and Vegetables

| AMOUNT | MEASURE | INGREDIENT |
|---|---|---|
| **8** | **8 ounces, 224 g** | **Shrimp (16–20 count)** |
| **As needed** | | **All-purpose flour** |
| **Oil for frying** | | **80/20 blend of vegetable oil and sesame oil, minimum 2 inches deep, heated to 350°F (180°C)** |
| **8** | | **Small button mushrooms, stems removed** |
| **1** | **8 ounces, 224 g** | **Zucchini, cut diagonally into 8 slices, $\frac{1}{3}$ inch (.8 cm) thick** |
| **8 slices** | | **Lotus root, cut into $\frac{1}{4}$ inch (.6 cm) rings** |
| **8 ounces** | **224 g** | **Sweet potato, peeled, cut diagonally into eight slices $\frac{1}{4}$ inch (.6 cm) thick** |
| **As needed** | | **Tentsuyu (dipping sauce; recipe follows)** |
| **Garnish** | | |
| **$\frac{1}{2}$ cup** | **3 ounces, 84 g** | **Daikon, grated** |
| **2 tablespoons** | **1 ounce, 28 g** | **Fresh ginger root, grated** |

**PROCEDURE**

1. Peel shrimp, being careful to retain the tails for handling. Cut the back of the shrimp along the vein and wash in cold water to remove.
2. Spread the shrimp out flat with the tail end toward you.
3. Make two shallow vertical cuts the length of each half. This cuts the muscles to prevent curling during frying.
4. Using the side of your hand tap shrimp, cut side up, gently pushing out and away with lengthwise strokes from tail to blunt end of the shrimp, being careful not to destroy the shrimp. The object is to spread it to $1\frac{1}{2}$–2 times its original size.
5. Dip shrimp in flour and let set for 5 to 10 minutes to assure a good adhesion of batter to shrimp in frying.
6. Prepare oil for frying; be sure to maintain heat while frying.
7. Have all the vegetables and shrimp ingredients ready: coat with batter, and cook similar ingredients together for even cooking, frying until light golden. Fry in small batches, turning frequently with clean chopsticks. The pieces should move freely.

8 Remove from oil and drain on paper towels. Serve immediately. Between batches, skim off the small bits of batter (*tenkasu*) that float in the oil. The Japanese save these bits of *tenkasu* to use as croutons in soup or over rice.

9 Serve with dipping sauce and garnish. Diners should mix together dipping sauce and garnish according to taste.

## Tentsuyu

***Tentsuyu* is a dipping sauce served with fresh hot fried foods, such as tempura. Dipping hot foods in *tentsuyu* cools them a little and provides additional flavor. The sauce is served warm or at room temperature.**

| AMOUNT | MEASURE | INGREDIENT |
|---|---|---|
| **1 cup** | **8 ounces, 240 ml** | **Ichiban dashi** |
| **3 tablespoons** | **$1\frac{1}{2}$ ounces, 458 ml** | **Light soy sauce** |
| **1 teaspoon** | **5 ml** | **Shoyu** |
| **2 tablespoons** | **1 ounce, 30 ml** | **Mirin** |

**PROCEDURE**

1 Combine all and bring to a boil. Remove from heat.

2 Serve in individual serving bowls, warm or at room temperature.

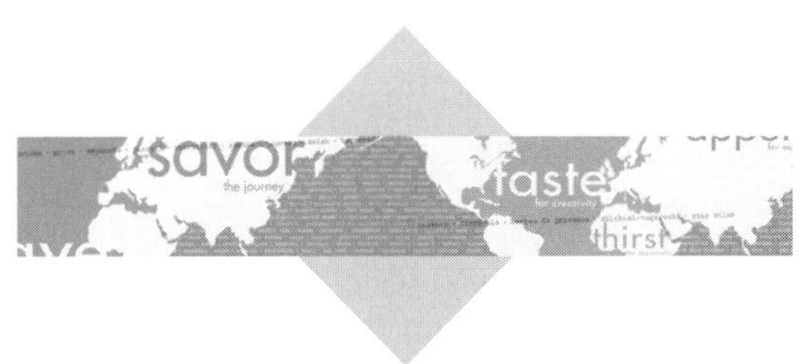

# Goma-anko Manju

## Steamed Dumplings with Sweet Azuki Paste and Sesame Seeds

YIELD: 12 DUMPLINGS

| AMOUNT | MEASURE | INGREDIENT |
|---|---|---|
| $\frac{1}{2}$ cup | $4\frac{1}{2}$ ounces, 135 ml | Anko (sweet azuki bean paste; recipe follows) |
| 2 tablespoons | 2 ounces, 60 ml | Water |
| 1 teaspoon | | Black sesame seeds, toasted |
| $\frac{3}{4}$ cup plus 2 tsp | 3 ounces, 84 g | Cake flour |
| $\frac{1}{2}$ teaspoon | | Baking powder |
| 5 tablespoons | $2\frac{1}{2}$ ounces, 70 ml | Water |
| $4\frac{1}{2}$ tablespoons | $2\frac{1}{4}$ ounces, 63 g | Granulated sugar |

PROCEDURE

1. Combine anko and 2 tablespoons water. Cook over medium heat, stirring, until thoroughly mixed. Add sesame seeds and stir to mix. Cool to room temperature. Divide into 12 portions.
2. Sift together flour and baking powder.
3. Combine 5 tablespoons water and the sugar; cook mixture to dissolve sugar; cool to room temperature.
4. Combine flour and sugar water to form a ball. Let stand, covered, for 30 minutes.
5. Line a bamboo or metal steamer basket with parchment paper and place steamer on boiling water.
6. On a floured counter, knead the dough briefly, 10 to 20 times. The dough should be somewhat soft. Roll the dough into a long, thin log, and cut the log into 12 equal pieces. Flatten dough with palms into a 1-inch (2.4 cm) disk, $\frac{1}{8}$ inch (.3 cm) thick.
7. Wrap the dough around each portion of bean paste (about 1 teaspoon), so you have 12 dumplings (shao mai style). To fill each dumpling, place a wrapper on the palm of your hand and cup it loosely. Place one filling in the cup. Then, with the other hand, gather the sides of the wrapper around the filling, letting the wrapper pleat naturally. Squeeze the middle gently to make sure the wrapper fits firmly against the filling, and to give the cylinder a wasp-waisted look. Tap the dumpling to flatten the bottom so it can stand upright.
8. Transfer to steamer and cook over high steam for 8 to 10 minutes. Serve with green tea.

# Anko

## Sweet Azuki Bean Paste

YIELD: 19 OUNCES

**Sweet bean paste is available at most Asian markets.**

| AMOUNT | MEASURE | INGREDIENT |
|---|---|---|
| **1 cup** | **7 ounces, 196 g** | **Dried azuki beans** |
| **1 cup** | **7 ounces, 196 g** | **Granulated sugar** |

**PROCEDURE**

1 Over medium heat, combine dried beans and 4 cups (32 ounces, 960 ml) water. Bring to a boil, drain, and discard the water.

2 Repeat with 4 cups (32 ounces, 960 ml) water and bring to boil over medium heat. Reduce heat to low and cook, uncovered, until tender, 60 minutes. Add more water, if necessary; at the end of the cooking time the beans should barely be covered with liquid.

3 In a food processor or blender, blend the beans with some of the cooking liquid to a smooth puree. Press the puree through a fine sieve; yield should be about $2\frac{1}{4}$ cups.

4 Transfer pureed beans to cheesecloth, make a sachet, close the ends, and grip tightly.

5 Plunge the cloth into a bowl of cold water, enough to completely cover and rinse the beans by squeezing the cloth in the water.

6 Discard the water and rinse again using fresh cold water. Remove and squeeze the cloth to remove excess water.

7 Combine pureed beans, sugar, and $\frac{1}{3}$ cup (80 ml) water over medium-low heat; bring to boil and reduce heat to low.

8 Cook until the mixture resembles soft peanut butter, about 20 minutes. cool quickly. Use a shallow pan to spread the mixture out and expose maximum surface, or use and ice bath (place the bean spread over in a container into an ice bath and stir frequently to avoid hot spots and to enhance cooling.

# China

## The Land

China shares its border with twelve countries. To the north is Mongolia, the east North Korea, and the northeast and northwest, Russia. Afghanistan, Pakistan, India, Nepal, Sikkim, and Bhutan are to the west and southwest, and to the south are Myanmar, Laos, and Vietnam. China's coastline is bounded by the Bohai, Yellow, East, and South China seas. With a population of 1.3 billion and a land area of 3.7 million square miles, China dominates not only Asia, but the entire world. It has about 22 percent of the total world population, but only some 6.5 percent of the world's land area.

The diversity of China is best recognized in the features of the landscape. China is a rugged country, with mountains, hills, and plateaus occupying about 65 percent of the total land area. The highest peak in the world, Mount Everest, stands on the border between China and Nepal. Moving north, the terrain drops to between 3,280 and 6,560 feet above sea level. Here are the famous grasslands of Mongolia, important to cattle breeding, and the Gobi Desert. In the northwest is the largest desert in China, the Taklamakan Desert, through which the ancient Silk Road passed. Nearby, bordered by the Tian Mountains, is the Turfan Depression; known as the Oasis of Fire, its temperatures can reach 120°F. In central China is the Yang Zi river delta, an important agricultural area, heavily populated. Further south, the geography changes more dramatically, with unusually shaped cliffs, gorges, and waterfalls.

The growth of civilization in China has centered on three great river systems, all of which flow from west to east. The northern quarter is drained by the Huang He (Yellow River); the middle half of the country is drained by the Chang Jiang (Yangtze River, the third longest in the world); and the southern quarter of China is dominated by the Xi Jiang (West River). The two noted cities of Guangzhou (formerly Canton) and Hong Kong are situated at the mouth of the West River. These river systems were the cheapest and most practical form of transportation, and were an important source for irrigation and energy. The river valleys also provided fertile soils for the surrounding level land. As a result, much of China's population is concentrated along these rivers and reaches its highest and most extensive density at their mouths.

# History

China has one of the world's oldest continuous civilizations. It is thought that some form of organized society began around 2000 B.C., and throughout the centuries, China has made significant world contributions in philosophy, religion, science, math, politics, agriculture, writing, and the arts. Confucius, whose teachings and writing still influence Chinese thought, lived during the Zhou Dynasty, about 2,500 years ago. The Confucian classics were the guide for Chinese civilization, highlighting education and family as the foundation of society. Taoists believed that people should renounce worldly ambitions and turn to nature and the Tao, the eternal force that permeates everything in nature. Buddhism has become a very powerful belief system for the Chinese. It provided a refuge in the political chaos that followed the fall of the Han Dynasty (206 B.C.–A.D. 220). By the fifth century A.D., Buddhism was widely embraced throughout China. Over the centuries, openness to new ideas fostered the emergence of many Chinese inventions and discoveries.

The ancient Silk Road was established over 2,000 years ago. It started at the Han capital of Changan (today's Xian) and stretched west for 4,350 miles. Crossing mountains and deserts, it branched into two routes, one going through central and western Asia to the eastern shore of the Mediterranean, the other crossing the Aral and Caspian Seas to Constantinople (Turkey). From here, silk was carried on to Rome and Venice. Chinese silk and the four great Chinese inventions—paper, printing, gunpowder, and the compass—made their way to the rest of Asia and to Europe along this route. In return, merchants brought religion, and the art and culture of these foreign regions to China. Trade along the route brought and enriched the northern provinces with herbs, fruits, vegetables, and spices. Coriander, sesame seeds, grapes, walnuts, peas, and garlic were imported from the west and became a hallmark of much of northern Chinese cooking.

The Chinese government has always been characterized by some form of central authority, dating as far back as the Xia Dynasty of 2200 B.C. Subsequent dynasties reinforced cultural unity and continuity for the Chinese civilization. One dynasty succeeded another through warfare, but with only occasional intrusion by forces outside of China. The lack of outside contacts allowed the Chinese to develop one culture across many regions with a strong sense of national identity. A series of emperors served as political leaders supported by well-equipped armies. The Chinese people believed their emperors ruled by "Mandate of Heaven." These dynasties continued over the centuries until the opening of China to the West in the 1800s.

The twentieth century saw dynamic forces change the political landscape of China. Shortly after the century began, the ages-old imperial dynastic system was swept away. Along the way, the country survived occupation by foreign troops, a short-lived republican government, a failed attempt at monarchical restoration, a war against Japan, and five years of civil war. The People's Republic of China emerged on October 1, 1949, a Communist government under the authoritarian Chairman Mao Zedong. By century's end, global realities forced China to experiment with forms of capitalism. Over the last half century, there has been major land and social reform, the Great Leap Forward Campaign, the Cultural Revolution, famine, the market reforms of Deng Xiaoping, and the move to put China on the world political and economic map. Through it all, Chinese culture has endured and even thrived. A strong sense of unity has held the Chinese nation together through 4,000 years. Its stable territorial boundaries, borders that defy easy penetration, culture, language, rich philosophy, and political institutions have allowed China to remain unified through dynastic changes and periodic social upheavals. The country has proved resilient and enduring.

# The People

China is a united multi-ethnic nation of 56 ethnic groups. According to the fourth national census, taken in 1990, the Han people made up 92 percent of the country's total population, and the other 55 ethnic groups, 8 percent. China's ethnic groups include Zhuang, Uygurs, Mongols, Tibetans, and others scattered over vast areas, mainly in the border regions.

The peasants of China make up 80 percent of the population and are the backbone of the economy. They alone make up one-third of all the farmers in the world. *Feng shui*, or "wind and water," is about living in harmony with the natural environment and tapping the goodness of nature for good fortune and health. It was first practiced in ancient China by farmers, to whom wind and water were the important natural forces that could either destroy or nurture their crops. Feng shui has developed into an art of locating buildings and other man-made structures (for example, fountains and bridges) to harmonize with and benefit from the surrounding physical environment.

*Yin and yang* is a concept in Chinese philosophy that consists of two opposing yet complementary forces. Yin is the female, passive, cool force. Yang is the male, active, hot force. These forces are engaged in an endless cycle of movement and change. This is best illustrated

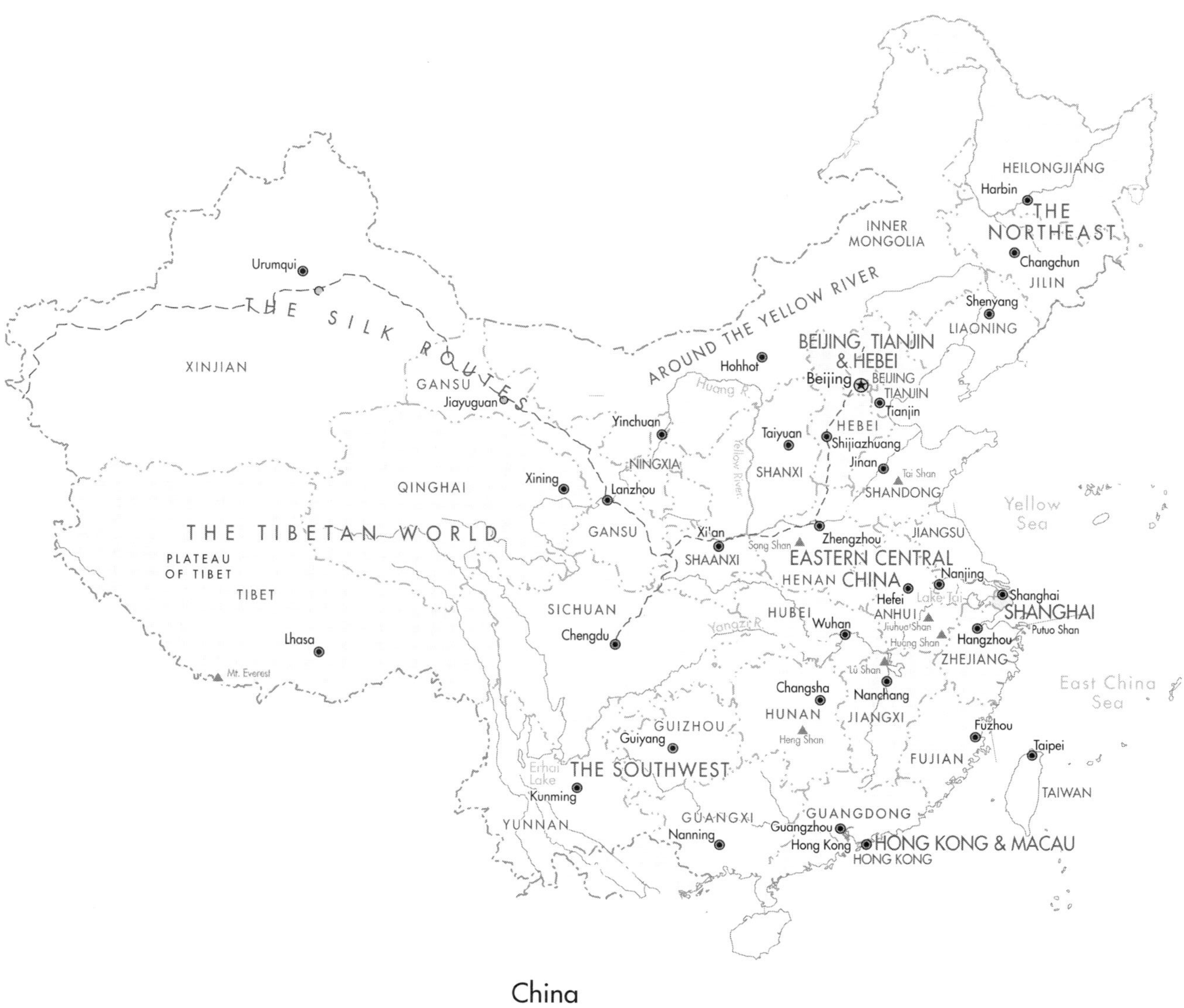
HEILONGJIANG
Harbin
THE NORTHEAST
Changchun
JILIN
INNER MONGOLIA
Shenyang
LIAONING
Urumqui
THE SILK ROUTES
AROUND THE YELLOW RIVER
XINJIAN
GANSU
Jiayuguan
Hohhot
BEIJING, TIANJIN & HEBEI
Beijing
BEIJING
TIANJIN
Tianjin
Huang R.
Yinchuan
Taiyuan
HEBEI
Shijiazhuang
Jinan
Tai Shan
SHANDONG
NINGXIA
Yellow River
SHANXI
Yellow Sea
QINGHAI
Xining
Lanzhou
THE TIBETAN WORLD
GANSU
Xi'an
Zhengzhou
JIANGSU
Song Shan
EASTERN CENTRAL CHINA
SHAANXI
PLATEAU OF TIBET
HENAN
Nanjing
TIBET
Hefei
Lake Tai
Shanghai
SICHUAN
HUBEI
ANHUI
SHANGHAI
Jiuhua Shan
Wuhan
Yangzi R.
Putuo Shan
Hangzhou
Huang Shan
Chengdu
Lhasa
ZHEJIANG
Mt. Everest
Lu Shan
Changsha
Nanchang
East China Sea
HUNAN
JIANGXI
GUIZHOU
Guiyang
Heng Shan
Fuzhou
Taipei
FUJIAN
Erhai Lake
THE SOUTHWEST
Kunming
TAIWAN
GUANGXI
GUANGDONG
YUNNAN
Guangzhou
Nanning
Hong Kong
HONG KONG & MACAU
HONG KONG

China

by the *taiji*, a symbol that shows a light patch and a dark patch winding around each other. This symbol illustrates how each of the two forces contains some of the opposing force. As yang reaches its peak, it changes into yin. As the cycle continues and yin peaks, it changes into yang. This never-ending cycle of peaks and valley expresses the Chinese view of life, history, and everything else in the world.

# The Food

Not surprisingly, given China's size, there are a number of distinct regional cooking styles that can be divided into four major traditions: the northern plains, including Beijing; the fertile east, watered by the Yangtze River; the south, famous for the Cantonese cooking of the Guangdong Province; and the luxuriant west of Szechwan and Hunan Provinces. Some observers characterize those regional cuisines as salty in north, sweet in south, hot in east, and sour in west.

## NORTH CHINA

Severe winters, a short growing season, and arid climate shape the hearty cuisine of China's north. The staples are wheat, barley, millet, potatoes, and soybeans, as opposed to rice, which characterizes the other regions. Noodles such as cellophane noodles (made from mung bean flour), rice ribbon noodles (made from rice flour), and breads such as steamed wheat buns, pancakes, and dumplings are the base of the meal. Soy milk is extracted from soybean paste and used to make bean curd, commonly known as tofu. Tofu is used in a variety of ways because it absorbs the flavor of sauces and seasonings, readily resulting in very tasty dishes. The most commonly eaten vegetable is Chinese cabbage, or bok choy. Salted and pickled vegetables such as turnips and white radish are common. The food is flavored with onions, garlic, and dark soy sauce. Soybean paste is the basis of many other pastes like hoisin (also known as Chinese barbeque sauce or plum sauce) and yellow bean, usually used to thicken sauces or as a marinade or seasoning. The northern portion of China also has a distinct Mongolian influence, characterized by the nomadic simplicity of the fire pot. Fuel being scarce in this region, the Mongols would huddle around the fire pot warming their hands while a tureen of broth was heating. Paper-thin slices of lamb or beef were dipped into the boiling broth until cooked and then dipped in spicy sauces. After the meal, the then richly seasoned broth was poured into bowls and served as soup. Northern cooking is known also as *Mandarin* or *Beijing* cooking and was influenced by the imperial court, where royal haute cuisine was developed. Peking duck is a traditional delicacy where thin slices of barbecued duck skin, wrapped in thin pancakes, are eaten with hoisin sauce. Beijing is known for *jiaozi*, the traditional Chinese dumpling filled with pork and vegetables, but variations may include sweet fruits or chestnuts during the holidays.

## CENTRAL CHINA

The central coast provinces are known as "The Land of Fish and Rice" and produce the eastern style of cooking, based on fresh seafood and river fish. Wheat, barley, rice, corn, sweet potatoes, and soybeans are the major staple crops. Sugar cane is grown in the humid valleys. Numerous varieties of bamboo shoots, beans, melons, gourds, squashes, and leafy vegetables are found here, and peaches, plums, and grapes flourish. Based around the cities of Shanghai, Zhejiang, and Fujian, as well as the Yangtze River, eastern Chinese cuisine includes careful preparation and fine knife skills, delicate forms, and light, fresh, sweet flavors based on the use of stocks and slow cooking. Stir-fried dishes and steaming are also common cooking methods. Dried and salted meats and preserved vegetables are commonly used to flavor dishes. It was in this region that Chinese vegetarian cuisine was elevated to sophisticated heights, as a result of the wealth of ingredients and the expertise of the regional chefs.

One of the most striking features in eastern cooking is the quantity of sugar included in both vegetable and meat cooking. Sugar combined with a dark soy sauce creates perhaps the most fundamental eastern flavor. Rice wine appears in regional specialties such as Drunken Chicken, Drunken Spare Ribs, and Drunken Prawns. Regional specialties include soy-braised duck and goose and Beggar's Chicken, a dish wrapped in lotus leaves, covered in clay, and oven baked. Century egg is also known as a preserved egg, or thousand-year egg. It is made by preserving duck, chicken, or quail egg in clay, ash, salt, or lime, for several weeks or months. The yolk of the egg turns pale and dark green, while the egg white turns dark brown and translucent. The egg white has a gelatinous texture, similar to that of a cooked egg, but has very little taste. *Wuxi* spare ribs features the common eastern technique of "red cooking," in a stock of soy sauce and rice wine to produce a flavorful stew. Hangzhou and the West Lake area boast the delicate ham known as *jinhua*, a type of cured ham known for its smoky flavor and scarlet color, and the world-famous Dragon Tea Well, for which only the top three leaves of each branch are considered worthy. Shanghai is known for its unusual "soup inject" dishes (*xiao long bao, or xiao long tang bao*), which are meatballs, dumplings, or buns filled with a gelatin and stock mixture and cooked until the inside is soupy.

## WESTERN CHINA

Western China is known for Sichuan, or Szechuan, cooking. A basin in the southwestern part of the country, Sichuan is one of the most agriculturally productive areas in China. Broken by small hills, the countryside is cut into squares, each an irrigated paddy field. Rice is grown during the summer, and after it has been harvested in the late autumn, wheat is planted in its place to be harvested six months later. The government, which controls all the supplies of grain in China, uses the surplus to help feed the big cities further east. On the lower slopes of the hills are an abundance of citrus fruit orchards (tangerines in particular) and bamboo groves, while on the higher forested mountainsides the people collect various kinds of edible fungi, such as *muer* (wood-ears) and silver fungi. The western half of Sichuan is very mountainous and sparsely populated. The people, mainly of Tibetan origin, keep sheep, cows, and horses.

The tea plant has long been of great agricultural importance for China. Its origins trace to the second century A.D., when it was grown in plantations in the uplands of central China and the ranges of the coastal provinces. Tea is also important in the interior Sichuan province. Green tea accounts for 45 percent of tea production. Black and brick tea comprise another 45 percent, and *wulung*, chrysanthemum, and jasmine tea are other varieties. Yunnan grows magnificent teas, especially the exotic *pu-erh*, that is sometimes aged for up to a hundred years before being served at banquets. Another well-known product is Yunnan ham (similar to Spanish serrano). China's west also grows some of the world's hottest chile peppers, which have given Sichuan a reputation for heat. There are several thoughts behind this; one is that the fire will stimulate the palate to distinguish the flavors beneath; another is that the heat induces perspiration and helps people to keep cool; and some say the spices are used to mask the taste of foods that rot quickly in the heat.

The texture of different ingredients in a dish is important to western Chinese cooking and care is taken to produce "chewy" and "crunchy" results. Unlike dishes in eastern China, many western dishes are accompanied by only the minimum of sauce to convey the seasonings; the sauce itself is not an important feature in the dish. The resulting dishes are drier. Similar to the southern regional cuisine, it is usual to find garlic, chiles, vinegar, sugar, and soy sauce in one dish. Because of the region's humidity, the preservation of food takes top priority. Salting, drying, pickling, and smoking are traditionally all employed. Pungent vegetables like onions, garlic, and ginger are used, as well as aromatic sesame, peanuts, soybean products, fermented black soybeans, orange peel, aniseed, ginger, and spring onions. Also known as pepper flower, Chinese pepper, and *fagara*, Szechuan pepper is not a pepper at all. Instead, the reddish-brown fruit, one of the ingredients in five-spice power, is a berry that comes from the prickly ash tree. While not as hot as chile pepper, it has a unique flavor, famous for its numbing effect on the tongue. Some notable Szechuan dishes include *kung pao chicken*, tea-smoked duck, *chengdu chicken* (chicken cubes with hot bean paste), and *mapo tofu*, a snow-white bean curd with fried, minced beef and green garlic shoots flavored with crushed peppercorns.

## SOUTH CHINA

Hunan (south of the river) cuisine is less well known and descriptions of Chinese cuisine often lump the two together. Hunan cuisine is often even hotter than Szechuan cooking.

While Szechuan recipes often call for chile paste, Hunan dishes frequently use fresh chile peppers, including the seeds and membranes, where most of the heat is contained. Simmering, steaming, stewing, and frying are popular cooking techniques in Hunan Province. Hunan cooks have a great variety of ingredients to work with and they tend to have several steps in preparation. For example, a classic Hunan dish is orange beef, where the beef is marinated overnight, then washed and marinated again with a mixture including egg white, wine, and white pepper. In braised soy sauce beef, the meat is simmered in an aromatic mixture including star anise, sugar, ginger, soy sauce, and sherry. Another popular dish is crispy duck, where the duck is seasoned with peppercorns, star anise, fennel, and other spices, then steamed and finally deep fried.

China's southernmost province, Guangdong (formerly Canton), is the home of the most famous of the Chinese regional cuisines. Though densely populated, this is very fertile land with mild winters. Rice is the main staple, but the farmers grow a profusion of fruit and green vegetables throughout the year. The subtropical climate is perfect for fruits such as pineapple, lychee, oranges, and bananas. Subtler than other Chinese cuisines, Cantonese is best known for its freshness and emphasis on natural flavors. As an example of the high standard for freshness in Cantonese meals, cows and pigs used for meat are usually killed earlier the same day. Chickens are often killed just hours beforehand, and fish are displayed in tanks for customers to choose for immediate preparation. The spices used in Cantonese cooking tend to be light and natural: ginger, salt, soy sauce, white pepper, spring onion, and rice wine or fresh citrus. Fish is quickly steamed with minimal touches of ginger and soy sauce; soups are slow-cooked; pork and duck are barbecued or roasted; and virtually everything that walks, crawls, or flies with "its back to heaven" (as the Cantonese saying goes) is quickly stir-fried in blazing-hot woks. The people of this region are known to eat nearly everything: fish maw, snake liver, dog, and guinea pig are some of the more unusual ingredients.

Guangdong is also praised for its perfected tradition of presentation. Cantonese cooks often make artistic and colorful presentational accents, such as radish roses or scallion flowers. Seafood flavors are incorporated into meat cookery, such as oyster sauce, made from a distillation of the oysters grown in the shallow waters of the Pear River, or shrimp sauce. Salted black beans are used to impart a highly savory taste; ginger is used to counteract fishiness; and garlic is used as an aromatic. Barbecue-roasted duck, chicken, and pork dishes are important here. Fruit is often included in Cantonese cooking, especially lemon, plum, tangerine, and orange, which are evident in the tangy, sweet-and-sour sauces. The tradition of *dim sum* ("touching the heart" or "little eats") originated here. It is usually eaten in the mornings and early afternoons. Popular dim sum items are *ha gau* (shrimp dumpling), *siu mai* (prawn and pork dumpling), *pai gwat* (steamed spareribs), *chun guen* (spring rolls), *cha siu pau* (steamed barbecued pork buns), and *cheung fun* (steamed rice flour rolls with barbecue pork, beef, or shrimp). Other well-known Cantonese dishes include shark's fin soup, roasted suckling pig, barbecued pork or *char siu*, lo mein, and the omelets known as *fu young.*

# Glossary

**Agar-Agar** A Japanese seaweed product sold in the form of 8-inch long bars with 1-inch-square cross section or thin sticks $\frac{1}{8}$ inch in diameter. Usually colorless but sometimes dyed a deep red, it is used much like clear gelatin, but has a different texture. While gelatin gels are resilient, gels made of agar-agar liquid break cleanly on the bite. For best results, pass the boiled agar-agar liquid through a sieve to remove the undissolved particles before gelling. Agar-agar sticks, cut into 2-inch lengths, are often mixed with fresh cucumber shreds and soy sauce in a northern Chinese salad. A favorite agar-agar dessert is almond bean curd, which is agar-agar gel flavored with milk, sugar, and almond essence, but no bean curd.

**Amaranth** Young leaves and stems of this decorative plant are a common vegetable (*xiancai*) in east and south China. Salt-preserved amaranth stems, thick as a thumb, is an east China specialty.

**Aniseeds** Seeds from the anise plant, similar to fennel in both taste and appearance.

**Bacon, Chinese** Meat from the belly of the pig, with lean and fat layers interlaced and skin attached, is called five-flower meat in China, and is used extensively, especially in braised dishes in which $\frac{1}{4}$-inch-thick slices are separated by slices of starchy vegetables, such as taro. Winter-preserved meat (laro), often called Chinese bacon, also uses this cut, and is marinated first, then dried in the winter sun.

**Bamboo Fungi** Often mistakenly thought to be the lining of the hollow bamboo stem, these are a relative of the North American stinkhorn. The unique crisp texture is similar to bamboo shoots. This is one of the most expensive edible fungi in China, often three times more the price of French truffles.

**Bamboo Shoots** Bamboo plants propagate by issuing shoots from below the ground. The texture of the shoots changes with the seasons. Winter shoots, stubby and firm, have a meatlike chewiness; spring shoots are slender and tender; most commonly available are summer shoots, looser in texture, succulent, though inclined to be bitter. In North America fresh shoots are a rarity and the quality of canned shoots varies greatly with the brand. Winter and spring shoots are so specified on cans; unspecified ones are summer shoots, which should be ivory-white rather than yellow, and firm rather than mushy.

**Bean Cheese** Also called fermented bean cake, or *furu.* A fermented soybean product in the form of tiny yellow bricks, it is soft, salty, and pungent. It is used to accompany congee and oil-strips for breakfast. Subtle-tasting red bean cheese (*nanru*) is used extensively to flavor pork dishes and Cantonese snacks.

**Bean Curd** The process of making bean curd from soybeans has much in common with making cheese. Known as *doufu* in China and *tofu* in Japan and commonly called "meat without bones," it is extremely high in protein. Although quite bland in taste, it absorbs the flavors of the food it is cooked with and is used in a number of dishes, from soups and sauces to stir-fries. It is offered in three texture grades; **Soft**—Soft and smooth, used mostly for soups and steamed dishes; **Semi-soft**; and **Hard**—More substantial, used mostly for cutting into slices and cubes, or pressed and then shredded.

**Bean Sprouts** Sprouts from both soybeans and mung beans are used extensively in Chinese cooking. Mung bean sprouts have a fresh taste and a crisp, almost crystalline texture. This is true also of the stems of soybean sprouts. However, the large, yellow head of the latter is chewy and meatlike.

**Bird Chiles** Tiny chiles, extremely hot.

**Bird's Nest** Nests formed on sheer cliffs made of dried swallow saliva, found in Malaysia, Thailand, and Indonesia. The best ones are crystalline white, sometimes tinged with pink. Lower grades may be gray with adhered swallow down. Very expensive and getting rarer every year.

**Bitter Melon or Foo Gwa** Also known as balsam pear, this is a very strange-looking gourd, shaped something like a cucumber with a rough, pockmarked skin. The flavor is unusual as well; like cilantro, it's an acquired taste.

**Black Beans, Fermented** These beans come already cooked, fermented, and seasoned with salt and ginger. They are widely used in stir-frying and steaming in country cooking all over south China.

**Blackfish Roe** Dried roe of the blackfish (*wu* fish); thin slices are roasted and consumed as a snack in Fujian and Taiwan.

**Broad Beans (Fava Beans)** A very common vegetable, especially in north China. The pods are poisonous and must be removed. Served as a vegetable in stir-fries, in soups, as a paste, or as a snack.

**Brown Sugar** Chinese brown sugar comes in slabs like an elongated domino. Each slab looks like a sandwich, brown and solid top and bottom, and lightly yellow and powdery in between. Common brown sugar serves the same purpose except for the appearance.

**Cassia Blossoms, Preserved (Guihua)** Tiny yellow flowers of the osmanthus preserved in sugar or salt. They are used extensively in east and north China for their sweet fragrance in dumplings, pastries, and sauces.

**Caul or Lace Fat (Wangyou, "Net-fat")** This is a net of stringy fat that forms a casing, used for wrapping food before cooking for a self-braising effect, to improve external appearance, and to add special chewiness.

**Cellophane Noodles (Fensi, Flour Threads, Bean Threads)** Dried white threads made of the flour of the mung bean, they turn translucent and resilient when cooked, and are important in country cooking. A related product is *fenpi* (flour skin), which is a platter-size sheet of the same material.

**Chestnuts** Considered one of the best companions to chicken, available fresh or dried. The Chinese chestnut is easy to peel and has a smooth surface. Dried chestnuts should be soaked for hours before use. Chestnut paste is used commonly in North China for cakes and fillings of pastries or puddings.

**Chile Pepper Products** Chile pepper oil is red and very hot. It is a common table condiment and comes in two types: those made of ground chiles are orange red, somewhat like Tabasco sauce, but are thicker in consistency and are not vinegary; those made of crushed chiles often contain added ingredients such as ginger, fermented black beans, and shallots. Dried chile peppers are used liberally in Sichuan and Hunan cooking. Chile pepper powder is not found in Cantonese kitchens.

**Chinese Almonds** Not really almonds at all, Chinese almonds are seeds of the apricot, and come in two varieties. Southern almonds are mild, interchangeable in taste with American almonds; northern almonds are more bitter. A soup recipe may call for both types. American almonds are known to the herbist as flatpeach seed.

**Chinese Cabbage (Sui Choy) or Napa Cabbage** Several types of Chinese cabbage exist. The variety most commonly associated with Chinese cabbage is Napa cabbage, the large-headed cabbage with firmly packed, pale green leaves. It is also known as Peking cabbage and celery cabbage. Lining a bamboo steamer with cabbage helps prevent food from sticking to the bottom.

**Chinese Sausage or Lop Cheong** Smaller (up to 6 inches in length) and thinner than western sausages, these are usually made from pork or liver. The taste varies somewhat depending on the ingredients used, but they generally have a sweet-salty flavor.

**Chinese White Radish or Lo Bak** Also known simply as white radish and in Japan as daikon, this popular Asian vegetable has no resemblance to the round red radishes. Chinese cooks use it for soups and stir-fries.

**Chives, Chinese and Yellow** Chinese chives, often called Chinese leeks, have the shape of chives and the odor of leeks. They are used for stir-frying, for making egg pancakes, and for stuffing dumplings in north China cuisine. Yellow chives are grown in the dark; they are pale yellow and tender. Both Chinese chives and yellow chives are available in large Western Chinatowns.

**Chrysanthemums** Fresh white chrysanthemum petals are edible. They are used as a garnish for a number of banquet dishes or dried and used for tea. Chrysanthemum tea is popular with

Cantonese people when eating dim sum and it is often sweetened with rock sugar. As with all edible flowers, they should not be exposed to pesticides.

**Cilantro or Chinese Parsley** An aromatic herb with flat leaves, cilantro is the leaf of the coriander plant. Featured prominently in Asian and Latin cuisines, Chinese cooks use cilantro in soups, stir-fries, and frequently as a garnish. Although a member of the parsley family, cilantro has a much stronger flavor, which its detractors have described as "soapy."

**Cloud Ear, Black** Ruffle-edged, thin, black mushrooms. Cloud ears are similar in appearance to wood ears except wood ears are black with a brownish-tan inner color, whereas cloud ears are black with a slightly lighter shade of black as their inner color. Cloud ears have a more delicate, milder flavor and are much smaller than wood ears. Cloud ears reconstitute to a puffy, soft, smooth texture and delicate flavor.

**Congee** Boiled rice porridge. Plain congee with oil-strips, bean cheese, and pickles is a standard breakfast for many Chinese. Common in South China is congee with meat, chicken, roast duck, animal organs, and/or peanuts.

**Cornstarch (Cornflour)** A powdery "flour," nearly all starch, obtained from the endosperm of corn. Mixed with water to form a paste, it is often added to stir-fries as a thickening agent near the final cooking stages, as overcooked cornstarch loses its power as a thickener. If necessary, cornstarch can be used as a substitute for tapioca starch.

## CUTTING TECHNIQUES

**Slicing** Hold the knife vertical or horizontal to the cutting board and cut straight across the ingredient.

**Julienne and Shredding** To get narrow strips, slice the ingredient into pieces of roughly $\frac{1}{8}$-inch (.3 cm) thickness, stack two or three of these pieces, and cut them again into $\frac{1}{8}$-inch (.3 cm) sticks.

**Dicing** Make the julienne sticks above, line the sticks up perpendicular to the knife blade, and cut straight down to get the size cubes called for in your recipe, usually $\frac{1}{4}$- to $\frac{1}{2}$-inch (.6 to 1.2 cm).

**Mincing** Slice or dice the ingredient into small pieces, then using the tip of the knife as a pivot, move only the lower blade in a chopping motion, from side to side across the ingredient until it is finely minced.

**Roll-cutting** For carrots, zucchini, and other cylindrical vegetables, hold the knife perpendicular to the board and slice down on a diagonal angle, then roll the vegetable a quarter turn and slice at the same angle; keep rolling and slicing a quarter turn at a time.

**Crushing** A fast, easy way to smash ginger, garlic, and lemongrass, place the knife flat on the ingredient with the blade facing away and press down hard on the blade with the palm of your hand.

**Dates, Chinese Red** Also called jujube dates, these are sold in dried form. They are used in soups, steamed chicken as garnish, and also as a filling for pastries.

**Dragon Well Tea** This is the most well-known green tea, grown in Hangzhou Province near Dragon Well Spring, the water of which is almost as famous.

**Dried Bean Curd Sticks** Made from soybeans and water, bean curd sticks resemble long yellowish icicles. They feel like thin plastic and break apart quite easily. They must be soaked overnight in cold water before use, or boiled for 20 minutes, or soaked in warm water for 1–2 hours.

**Dried Lily Buds** Also known as golden needles and tiger lilies, dried lily buds are the unopened flowers of day lilies. Dried lily buds are yellow-gold in color, with a musky or earthy taste. Before using, cut off about $\frac{1}{4}$ inch at the bottom to get rid of the woody stem. Like many other "woodsy" Chinese vegetables, lily buds must be soaked in warm water before use, for about 30 minutes.

**Dried Shrimps** Made from small shrimp tails, usually sun-dried.

**Dried Tangerine Peel** Soak the tangerine peel in warm water to soften it before using.

**Duck, Preserved (Laya, Winter-Preserved Duck)** A salted whole duck, flattened into a roughly circular disc and dried. The best ones come from Nanan in Jiangxi Province, just north of the border with Guangdong. Preserved duck from Nanking is called *banya* (board duck).

**Eggs, Thousand-Year-Old** Duck eggs that have been preserved in potash, they acquire a blue-black yolk and a translucent brown egg white.

**Fennel** An important ingredient in five-spice powder and in *lu*, the south China simmering sauce. Aniseed is often substituted.

**Fish Lips and Fish Maws** Fish lips are the meaty part of the shark near the mouth and fins. Fish maws are dried, deep-fried bladders of a large fish, usually cod.

**Fish Sauce** Fish sauce is a thin, salty liquid used in place of salt as a seasoning in many Asian recipes. It is also used as a dipping sauce. Chinese brands are often labeled "fish gravy" or "fish sauce," while it is called *nuoc mam* in Vietnam and *nam pla* in Thailand. However, they are all basically the same product, although the Thai and Vietnamese brands are considered superior.

**Five-Spice Powder** A common ingredient in Chinese cooking, this delicious mixture of five ground spices usually consists of equal parts of cinnamon, cloves, fennel seed, star anise, and Szechwan peppercorns.

**Fuzzy Melon (Mo Gwa)** Looks like a zucchini covered with fuzz. While zucchini is a type of squash, fuzzy melon is a gourd, related to winter melon. Peel off the skin or scrub well to remove the fuzz before using.

**Gingko Nuts or White Nuts** Typically used in desserts and stir-fries. Substitute blanched almonds or pine nuts.

**Ginger** The roots of the ginger plant, an indispensable ingredient in Chinese cuisine. Valued for its clean, sharp flavor, ginger is used in soups, stir-fries, and marinades. It is especially good with seafood, as it can cover up strong fish odors.

**Green Onion, Spring Onion, or Scallion** An immature onion with a white base (not yet a bulb) and long green leaves. Both parts are edible.

**Hair Vegetable (Facai)** Freshwater algae, with the appearance of course, dull, black human hair. Valued in vegetarian cuisine.

**Hoisin Sauce** A thick sauce valued for its unique combination of sweet and spicy flavors. It is made from soybean paste and flavored with garlic, sugar, chiles, and other spices and ingredients.

**Hot Mustard** A popular condiment served with Chinese appetizers; you'll also often find it added to sauces in Japanese dishes. It is made by mixing dry mustard powder with water, causing a chemical reaction that produces a sharp, hot taste.

**Hua Diao ("Flower-Engraved")** The best yellow wine from Xiaoxing Province.

**Lo Mein** In this dish, boiled and drained noodles are added to the other ingredients and stir-fried briefly during the final stages of cooking. This gives the noodles more flavor than is the case with chow mein, where the meat and vegetables are served over noodles that have been cooked separately.

**Lotus root** Grows underwater. It is starchy when cooked, but crispy and refreshing when raw. Slices of the lotus root have a beautiful pattern. Substitute water chestnuts or jicama.

**Lychee** Also called litchi, lichee, lichi, leeched, and laichee. Popular Chinese fruit about the size of a walnut, with a bumpy red shell encasing white translucent pulp that's similar in texture to a grape. The flavor is sweet, exotic, and very juicy.

**Lychee Nuts** Also called litchi nut, lichee nut, lichi nut, and leechee nut. These are sun-dried litchis. The outer shells are brown and the meat inside looks like a large raisin.

**Marinade** In Chinese cooking the primary reason meat is marinated before cooking is to improve flavor. The amount of marinade should be just sufficient to coat the meat or fish. Red meat is typically marinated with a little oil to prevent them from becoming dry and sticking together during the cooking process. Dark meat is marinated with whole egg and white meat and fish with egg white.

**Monosodium Glutamate (MSG)** A white crystalline compound used to enhance flavor. Note that MSG may not be suitable for everyone.

**Mushrooms, Chinese Black** Dried mushrooms. The name is a bit of a misnomer, since Chinese black mushrooms can be light brown, dark brown, and even gray. They are frequently speckled. Chinese black mushrooms (also known as shiitake mushrooms) range in price from moderate to quite expensive. The more costly are often called flower mushrooms because they have a thick cap and a nice curl. The drying process gives them a stronger flavor. Before use, soak them in warm water for 20 to 30 minutes, and remove the stems.

**Mushroom Soy Sauce** Soy sauce that has been infused with the flavor of straw mushrooms.

**Oil (Dipping) Poaching** A technique used to give the meat a more tender texture, oil poaching (also called velveting) seals the meat.

**Oyster Sauce** A rich sauce made from boiled oysters and seasonings, it does not have a fishy taste. Its savory flavor is used in meat and vegetable dishes, and is an important ingredient in Cantonese cooking.

**Red Cooking** Similar to Western braising, the cooking liquid is a soy sauce–based liquid.

**Rice Vinegar** Chinese rice vinegars are milder and less acidic than regular vinegar (as are Japanese vinegars). There are three basic types—black, red, and white—as well as sweetened black vinegars. The black variety is somewhat similar to balsamic vinegar, while red vinegar has both a sweet and tart taste. White vinegar is the closest in acidity and flavor to cider vinegar. There are no hard and fast rules, but black vinegar is generally recommended for braised dishes and as a dipping sauce; red vinegar for soups, noodle, and seafood dishes; and white for sweet and sour dishes and for pickling. In recipes, rice vinegar is sometimes also called rice wine vinegar.

**Rice Wine** Known colloquially as yellow wine, rice wine is a rich-flavored liquid made from fermented glutinous rice or millet and has a relatively low alcohol content. Aged for ten years or more, rice wine is used both in drinking and cooking. Pale dry sherry is the most acceptable substitute.

**Sesame Oil** Amber-colored, aromatic oil, made from pressed and toasted sesame seeds. Not for use as a cooking oil. Has an intense flavor and very low smoke point.

**Sesame Seed Paste** Roasted sesame seeds ground to a thick aromatic paste.

**Shark's Fin** The pale yellow, translucent ligaments within the fins of the shark.

**Snow Peas** Also known as *mangetout*, French for "eat it all." The French name comes from the fact that the whole pea including the pod is eaten.

**Snow Pea Shoots** The tips of the vines and the top set of leaves of the pea plant are an Oriental delicacy. They can be served raw in salads, quickly cooked in stir-fries, or blanched and used in soups.

**Soy Sauce** Invented by the Chinese approximately 3,000 years ago, soy sauce is made from fermented soybeans, wheat flour, water, and salt. The two main types of soy sauce are light and dark. As the name implies, light soy sauce is lighter in color, and also sweeter than dark soy sauce. Aged for a longer period of time, dark soy sauce is thicker and blacker in color. It is also less salty than light soy. It is used in certain recipes to add color, and as a dipping sauce.

**Star Anise** Whole star anise looks like an eight-pointed star about 1 inch (2.5 cm) across. It gives a licorice flavor to savory dishes, particularly those with pork and poultry.

**Straw Mushrooms** Delicate meaty texture and fine flavor, used for many soups and vegetable dishes.

**Sugar, Rock** Comes in chunks that look like crystals, has a subtle taste, and is used in most braised or "red-cooked" dishes.

**Szechuan (Sichuan) Peppercorn** Also called anise pepper, brown peppercorn, Chinese aromatic pepper, Chinese pepper, flower pepper, sancho, Japanese pepper, Japan pepper, wild pepper, and fagara pepper. Reddish-brown peppercorns, native to Szechuan Province. Much stronger and more fragrant than black peppercorns. These aren't true peppercorns, but rather dried flower buds.

**Tapioca** Made from the starch of the cassava root, tapioca comes in several forms, including granules and flour, as well as the pellets that are called pearl tapioca. Tapioca starch is often used to make dumpling dough, or as a thickening agent.

**Water Chestnuts** A knobby vegetable with papery brown skin, it is an aquatic vegetable that grows in marshes. Indigenous to Southeast Asia, the water chestnut is valued both for its sweetness and its ability to maintain a crisp texture when cooked.

**White-Cooking** A typical Cantonese technique to cook a whole fowl or fish by immersing it in boiling water. The heat is then turned off and the pot is covered until the item is done. The word for "white" in Chinese means "plain."

**Winter Melon (Dong Gua)** Resembles a large watermelon with dark green skin. The flesh inside is white, looking much like it has been lightly covered with snow, and the seeds are white as well. Winter melon has a very mild, sweet taste. It is used in soups and stir-fries, where it absorbs the flavors of the ingredients it is cooked with.

**Wok** The most important piece of Chinese cooking equipment, a wok can be used for stir-frying, deep-frying, steaming, and roasting. While a frying pan can be used in place of a wok for stir-frying (cast iron is particularly good), a wok has numerous advantages in shape, design, and material. It distributes heat more evenly, and requires less oil to cook with. There are two instruments traditionally used for cooking with a wok: a long-handled spoon and a long-handled perforated scoop with a slightly rounded edge.

**Wonton Wrappers** Made of flour, water, salt, and eggs; sold fresh or frozen. The dough is cut in $3\frac{1}{2}$ inch (8.75 cm) squares.

**Wood Ear Mushroom** A distant relative of the cloud ear fungus. Larger and somewhat tougher, they lack the delicate taste of cloud ears. They can be soaked in cold instead of warm water.

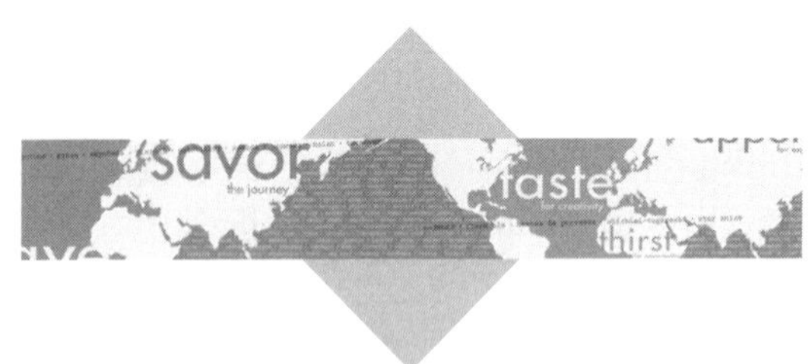

# Menus and Recipes from China

MENU ONE (NORTH)

**Pungent and Hot Soup (Hot and Sour Soup)**

**Mandarin Pancakes**

***Jiao Zi or Guo-tieh:* Pot-Stickers**

**Chinese Egg Noodles**

**Stir-Fried Bok Choy**

**Vinegar-Slipped Fish Chunks**

**Mo Shu, Moshu, Moo shu, or Mu Shu Pork ('Wood Shavings Pork')**

**Fortune Cookies**

**Lamb on Rice Sticks**

MENU TWO (EAST)

**Wonton Soup**

**Jellyfish and White Radish Salad**

**Pearl Balls (Porcupine Meatballs)**

**Emerald Shrimp**

**Red-Cooked Duck**

***Yangchow (Yangzhou)* Fried Rice**

**Shanghai Sweet-and-Sour Spareribs**

**Bean Curd in Oyster Sauce**

MENU THREE (WEST)

**Tea and Spice Smoked Quail with Sweet and Sour Cucumbers**

***Ma-Puo (Mapo) Doufu***

**Sichuan Stuffed Eggplant**

**Kung Pao Chicken**

**Stir-Fried Long Beans**

***Dan Dan Mian:* Spicy Noodles**

**Fish-Flavored Pork Shreds**

**Sichuan Spicy Fired Beef Shreds**

MENU FOUR (SOUTH)

**Spinach Velvet Soup**

***Char Siu:* Cantonese Roast Pork**

***Char Sui Bau:* Steamed Pork Buns**

**Stir-Fried Squid with Fermented Black Bean Paste**

**Buddha's Delight**

**Fried Chicken, Hong Kong Style**

**Steamed Whole Fish**

**Tea Leaf Eggs**

# Pungent and Hot Soup

## Hot and Sour Soup

SERVES 4

**Different versions of this soup are found in northern, eastern, central, and even southern China. This northern version has the lightest color.**

**Chinese black mushrooms are the dried mushrooms sold in Asian grocery stores. The name is a bit of a misnomer, since Chinese black mushrooms can be light brown, dark brown, and even gray. They are frequently speckled.**

| AMOUNT | MEASURE | INGREDIENT |
|---|---|---|
| **Seasoning** | | |
| 1 teaspoon | | Tapioca powder or cornstarch |
| 1 $\frac{1}{2}$ teaspoons | | Soy sauce |
| $\frac{1}{4}$ teaspoon | | Sugar |
| $\frac{1}{2}$ cup | 3 ounces, 84 g | Pork, lean boneless, julienned $\frac{1}{8}$ x $\frac{1}{8}$ x 2 inches (.3 x .3 x 5 cm) |
| **Hot and Sour Mixture** | | |
| 1 $\frac{1}{2}$ teaspoons | 7 ml | Sesame oil |
| 1 tablespoon | $\frac{1}{2}$ ounce, 15 ml | Soy sauce |
| $\frac{1}{2}$ teaspoon | | White pepper |
| 1 tablespoon | $\frac{1}{2}$ ounce, 15 ml | Black or rice vinegar |
| $\frac{1}{2}$ teaspoon | | Sugar |
| 3 cups | | Chicken stock |
| 3 | | Medium dried black mushrooms, soaked in hot water 5 minutes, or until soft, rinsed thoroughly, tough ends trimmed; cut into $\frac{1}{8}$ x $\frac{1}{8}$ x 2 inch (.3 x .3 x 5 cm) pieces |
| | $\frac{1}{4}$ ounce, 4 g | Dried black cloud ears, soaked in hot water 20 minutes, cut into $\frac{1}{8}$ x $\frac{1}{8}$ x 2 inch (.3 x .3 x 5 cm) pieces |
| $\frac{1}{2}$ cup | 3 ounces, 84 g | Bamboo shoots, $\frac{1}{8}$ x $\frac{1}{8}$ x 2 inches (.3 x .3 x 5 cm) |
| 1 $\frac{1}{2}$ tablespoons | | Tapioca powder or cornstarch |
| 1 tablespoon | $\frac{1}{2}$ ounce, 15 ml | Water |
| 1 cup | 6 ounces, 168 g | Soft bean curd, $\frac{1}{8}$ x $\frac{1}{8}$ x 2 inches (.3 x .3 x 5 cm) |
| 1 | | Egg, lightly beaten |
| 1 tablespoon | | Green onion, minced |
| 2 tablespoon | | Cilantro leaves and short stems, 2 inches (5 cm) |

**PROCEDURE**

1. Mix seasoning ingredients and combine with julienne pork; mix well.
2. Combine hot and sour mixture ingredients.
3. Bring chicken stock to a boil; add mushrooms, bamboo shoots, and pork shreds. Bring back to a boil; reduce heat to medium. Stir to separate pork shreds and cook for 5 minutes.
4. Reduce heat to low. Mix $1\frac{1}{2}$ tablespoons tapioca powder with the water and add gradually to soup, stirring constantly until thickened. Add bean curd.
5. Add hot and sour mixture to soup. Stir, correct seasoning.
6. Return to a boil, using a ladle float the eggs in very thin petals. Immediately remove from heat. Allow soup to set for 15 seconds. Garnish with green onion and cilantro.

# Mandarin Pancakes

SERVES 4

**Chef Tip** **Cooking pancakes in pairs makes the inside moist and assures a paper-thin pancake.**

| AMOUNT | MEASURE | INGREDIENT |
|---|---|---|
| 2 cups | 8 ounces, 224 g | All-purpose flour |
| $\frac{3}{4}$ cup | 6 ounces, 180 ml | Boiling water |
| As needed | | Sesame oil |

PROCEDURE

1. Place the flour in a mixing bowl, making a well in the center. Add water to the flour, incorporating the flour by stirring it into the water with a wooden spoon or chopsticks. Let the dough cool slightly and turn onto a floured surface.
2. Knead for about 10 to 12 minutes or until smooth. Cover the dough and allow it to rest for 30 minutes. Knead an additional 1 to 2 minutes.
3. Roll the dough into a sausage shape, about $1\frac{1}{2}$ inches (3.6 cm) in diameter. Measure the cylinder and cut into 16 equal size pieces. Roll each piece into a smooth ball. Grease an area of the kneading board about 10 inches (24 cm) square with oil to prevent sticking. Moisten fingers with a bit of sesame oil. Flatten each ball into a 2-inch (4.8 cm) round and brush evenly with sesame oil on the surface. Place another round on top, forming a 2-layered round. Using a rolling pin, roll out this double-layered disk into a circle about 6 inches (14.4 cm) in diameter and $\frac{1}{8}$ inch (.3 cm) thick. Grease the board with more oil if needed.
4. Roll 2 pancakes, then proceed with the cooking. Continue to roll and cook, 2 pancakes at a time, until all the dough is used up.
5. To cook, heat a griddle or heavy pan over medium heat until hot. Cook the pancake on an ungreased surface for 1 minute or until the surface puffs up and brown spots appear on the bottom side. Turn to brown on the other side for about 30 seconds to 1 minute.
6. Transfer pancakes to a clean plate and cover with foil or a lightly dampened cloth to keep moist and warm.
7. Separate the two layers carefully; fold into quarters, with the cooked side on the inside. Serve warm.

# Jiao Zi or Guo-tieh

## Pot-Stickers

YIELD: 25 TO 30 POT-STICKERS

**Chef Tip** **The additional chicken stock is to insure a moist filling, and adds intensity.**

**Dough**

| AMOUNT | MEASURE | INGREDIENT |
|---|---|---|
| 2 cups | 8 ounces, 224 g | All-purpose flour |
| $\frac{1}{8}$ teaspoon | | Salt |
| $\frac{1}{2}$ cup | 4 ounces, 120 ml | Boiling water |
| 2 tablespoons | 1 ounce, 30 ml | Cold water |

PROCEDURE

1. Sift together the flour and salt. Make a well in the center add the boiling water. Mix together with a wood spoon or spatula.
2. Cover and let set for 5 minutes, and then add the cold water and mix to combine. Cover and let set for 15 minutes.
3. Turn out onto a floured board and knead until smooth, sprinkling additional flour as needed, for about 15 minutes.
4. Divide dough into two parts and roll each out 1 inch (2.4 cm) in diameter and about 12 inches (29 cm) long. Cut the rolls into $\frac{1}{2}$-inch (1.2 cm) slices. Lightly flour, then flatten and roll out each piece to a 3-inch (7.2 cm) diameter circle, $\frac{1}{8}$ inch (.3 cm) thick. The wrappers can be dusted with tapioca powder and stacked.

# Chinese Egg Noodle

**This dough may also be used for wonton and egg-roll wrappers.**

**Dough (optional dough)**

| AMOUNT | MEASURE | INGREDIENT |
|---|---|---|
| $1\frac{3}{4}$ cups | $9\frac{1}{4}$ ounces, 260 g | All-purpose flour |
| 4 tablespoons | $1\frac{1}{3}$ ounce, 37 g | Bread flour |
| $\frac{1}{2}$ teaspoon | | Salt |
| 1 | | Egg |
| 7 tablespoons | | Water |
| $\frac{1}{8}$ teaspoon | $3\frac{1}{2}$ ounces, 105 ml | Sesame oil |
| $\frac{1}{3}$ cup | $1\frac{1}{2}$ ounces, 42 g | Cornstarch |

**PROCEDURE**

1. In a food processor fitted with a metal blade, process the flours and salt together.
2. Beat the egg with 5 tablespoons ($2\frac{1}{2}$ ounces, 75 ml) water and sesame oil. Gradually add egg mixture, processing just until the dough begins to form a ball; add additional water if necessary. Process 10 seconds if using a pasta machine; process 30 seconds longer if rolling by hand.
3. Turn the dough, which should be barely sticky, onto a lightly floured board, and knead for 1 minute. Dough should be satiny and not stick to the palm of the hand. Cover and let rest 30 minutes to 1 hour.
4. To roll out with a pasta machine, roll the dough into a sausage shape $1\frac{1}{2}$ inch (3.6 cm) in diameter and cut into thirds. Flatten each piece to a rectangle about $\frac{1}{4}$ inches (.6 cm) thick and lightly coat both sides with cornstarch. Pass the dough through the thickest setting. Then fold the dough into thirds, flatten, dust with cornstarch, and run it through the rollers again, feeding in the unfolded end first. Repeat the procedure three times. Turn the machine to the next thinnest setting, dust the dough, and roll it though unfolded. Repeat this procedure with each setting until it is $\frac{1}{16}$ inch (.15 cm) thick for pot-stickers.
5. Cut the dough, allow the cut pieces to dry about 10 minutes, then dust them with cornstarch and stack them.

**Filling**

| AMOUNT | MEASURE | INGREDIENT |
|---|---|---|
| 2 cups | 8 ounces, 224 g | Napa cabbage, $\frac{1}{4}$ inch (.6 cm) dice |
| 1 teaspoon | | Salt |
| 1 cup | 8 ounces, 224 g | Ground pork |
| $\frac{1}{4}$ cup | 1 ounce, 28 g | Green onion, minced |
| 2 teaspoons | | Ginger, grated |
| 1 tablespoon | | Garlic clove, minced |
| 1 tablespoon | $\frac{1}{2}$ ounce, 15 ml | Soy sauce |
| 1 tablespoon | $\frac{1}{2}$ ounce, 15 ml | Dry sherry |
| 2 tablespoons | 1 ounce, 30 ml | Sesame oil |
| 2 teaspoons | | Rice vinegar |
| $\frac{1}{2}$ cup | 4 ounces, 120 ml | Chicken Stock, depending on the moisture content of the mixture |
| 2 teaspoons | | Tapioca or cornstarch powder |
| **For Frying** | | |
| 3 tablespoons | $\frac{3}{4}$ ounce, 20 ml | Vegetable oil |
| $\frac{1}{2}$ cup | 4 ounces, 120 ml | Water |
| 1 teaspoon | | Vinegar |
| **Ginger and Vinegar Sauce** | | |
| 2 tablespoons | 1 ounce, 28 ml | Ginger, finely shredded |
| $\frac{1}{4}$ cup | 2 ounces, 60 ml | Chinese black (Chinkiang) or rice vinegar |
| 1 tablespoon | $\frac{1}{2}$ ounce, 15 ml | Sesame oil |

**PROCEDURE**

1. Mix cabbage with the 1 teaspoon salt. Allow to sit for 30 minutes, then wrap in cheesecloth and squeeze to remove as much moisture as possible.
2. Combine cabbage with remaining filling ingredients. It should bind together; if not, add a little more cornstarch.
3. To assemble the dumplings, place about 1 tablespoon filling in the center of each wrapper and shape the filling into a strip.
4. Fold the wrapper over to make a half-moon shape and pinch the edges together at the center of the arc, leaving the two ends open.
5. With your fingers, make about 3 to 4 pleats in one side of the opening at each end. Pinch all along the edges to seal.

6 Remove the finished pot-sticker to a tray dusted with flour or cornstarch; keep covered with a cloth.

7 To cook, heat a heavy 10-inch (24 cm) skillet over high heat until drops of water sprinkled into it sizzle and dry up. Add oil to coat the bottom evenly.

8 Add enough pot-stickers to fill the pan, arranging them closely together with pleated sides up. Pan-fry over medium heat for 2 minutes, or until the bottoms are lightly browned.

9 Mix water with vinegar and add to skillet. Cover the skillet and cook for 6 to 8 minutes or until the liquid is evaporated.

10 Remove cover and continue to pan-fry until they can be moved around easily. Remove from the heat and transfer to a serving platter, brown side up.

11 Combine sauce ingredients. Serve pot-stickers hot with ginger and vinegar sauce on the side.

**Chef Tip** **Boiled dumplings (*jiaozi*) are made with the same filling. However, the dough is made with only cold water. Assembly of the *jiaozi* is made simple by pinching the edges together instead of pleating. They are then boiled in salted water in the following manner: bring water to a boil and add the dumplings and stir immediately. When the water returns to the boil, add cold water to reduce the temperature. Cook for 5 minutes or until the *jiaozi* float to the top.**

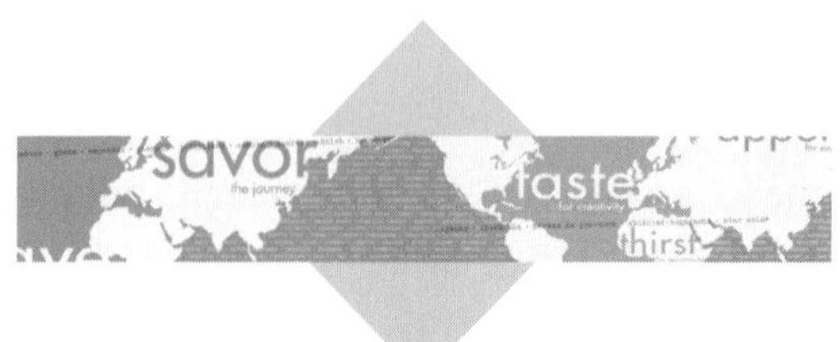

# Stir-Fried Bok Choy

SERVES 4

| AMOUNT | MEASURE | INGREDIENT |
|---|---|---|
| **Sauce** | | |
| I teaspoon | | Cornstarch |
| 2 tablespoons | I ounce, 30 ml | Chicken stock. |
| $\frac{1}{4}$ teaspoon | | Sesame oil |
| 3 tablespoons | I $\frac{1}{2}$ ounces, 45 ml | Oil |
| To taste | | Salt and white pepper |
| **Bok Choy** | | |
| 3 tablespoons | I $\frac{1}{2}$ ounces, 45 ml | Vegetable oil |
| 2 slices | | Ginger root |
| I cup | 4 ounces,I I2 g | Onions, thinly sliced |
| 2 cups | 4 ounces, I I2 g | Mushrooms, washed, $\frac{1}{2}$ inch (I.2 cm) sliced |
| 2 cups | I2 ounces, 336 g | Bok choy, washed, $\frac{1}{2}$ inch (I.2 cm) sliced on the bias |
| 2 tablespoons | I ounce, 30 ml | Chicken stock |

PROCEDURE

1. Combine the sauce ingredients.
2. Set a wok over high heat until the bottom turns a dull red. Add 3 tablespoons (1 $\frac{1}{2}$ ounces, 45 ml) oil. When oil is hot and smoky, add ginger briefly to flavor oil, and then discard when brown.
3. Add onions, stirring and turning, for 30 seconds. Add mushrooms, stirring and turning, for 30 seconds.
4. And bok choy, stirring and turning until each piece is well coated with oil.
5. Whirl in stock along edge of wok and cover immediately. Cook for two minutes.
6. Add the sauce; stir until thickened, season with salt and white pepper to taste, cover.
7. Keep wok covered for one minute. Serve immediately.

# Vinegar-Slipped Fish Chunks

SERVES 4

**Made from the starch of the cassava root, tapioca powder thickens at a lower temperature than cornstarch, remains stable when frozen, and imparts a glossy sheen. With the exception of dumpling dough, in most cases cornstarch can be used as a substitute.**

**Chef Tip** **Ginger juice is often used as a seasoning, along with wine. The best process to maximize the ginger is to grate as much ginger as needed into a small bowl, and then add the wine and mix well. Pour the mixture through a small strainer and squeeze the grated ginger against the wall of the strainer to extract all the juice. A normal-size slice of gingerroot is the size and thickness of an American quarter.**

| AMOUNT | MEASURE | INGREDIENT |
|---|---|---|
| 1 pound | 16 ounces, 448 g | Boneless, skinless fish fillet (cod, red snapper, or sole) |
| 2 | | Green onions, white and green parts, separated |
| 3 cups | 24 ounces, 720 ml | Oil |
| 1 | | Garlic clove, crushed |
| 1 tablespoon | ½ ounce, 15 ml | Dry sherry |
| 2 teaspoons | | Sesame oil |
| Marinade | | |
| 2 | | Egg whites |
| 2 tablespoons | | Tapioca powder or cornstarch |
| 1 tablespoon | ½ ounce, 15 ml | Dry sherry |
| ½ teaspoon | | Salt |
| 2 slices | | Ginger juice (see Chef Tip) |

| AMOUNT | MEASURE | INGREDIENT |
|---|---|---|
| **Vinegar Sauce** | | |
| **$\frac{3}{4}$ cup** | **6 ounces, 180 ml** | **Chicken stock** |
| **2 tablespoons** | **1 ounce, 30 ml** | **Red rice vinegar** |
| **2 tablespoons** | **1 ounce, 28 g** | **Sugar, granulated** |
| **2 teaspoons** | | **Tapioca powder or cornstarch** |
| **$\frac{1}{4}$ teaspoon** | | **Salt** |

**PROCEDURE**

1. Cut fillets lengthwise into strips 1 inch (2.4 cm) wide. Cut each strip into chunks about 1 × 1$\frac{1}{2}$ inches (2.4 cm × 3.6 cm).
2. Mix ingredients for marinade and add to the fish. Mix well, using your fingers or chopsticks.
3. Cut white parts of green onion into 4-inch (9.6 cm) lengths, then flatten with a cleaver. Add them to the marinating fish.
4. Chop the green onion greens very fine and set aside.
5. Mix ingredients for sauce and set aside.
6. When ready to cook, remove green onion whites and chop fine. Combine with green parts.

**To Cook**

1. Set wok over medium heat. When hot, add the oil. Wait 2 to 3 minutes, heat to 325°F (163°C) or until a piece of green onion dropped in oil bubbles, sizzles, and moves around.
2. Add the fish chunks to the oil. Lightly stir in a spading manner to separate (30 seconds). Cook fish 2 minutes, then turn heat up and continue to cook 1 minute longer, at 375°F (190°C). Drain fish and oil into a colander or strainer-lined container. Leave about 1 tablespoon ($\frac{1}{2}$ ounce, 15 ml) oil in wok.
3. Return wok to high heat. When very hot add the garlic, stirring 10 seconds. Sizzle in the wine along the sides of the wok, and then add the sauce mixture. Turn heat to low; stir sauce until thickened.
4. Glaze sauce with sesame oil, and then slip in the fish chunks. Add the chopped green onions and mix together. Correct seasoning and serve.

# Mo Shu, Moshu, Moo Shu, or Mu Shu Pork

## Wood Shavings Pork

SERVES 4

**Chef Tip** **Nappa cabbage may have a high moisture content, green cabbage has a lower moisture content.**

| AMOUNT | MEASURE | INGREDIENT |
|---|---|---|
| | | **Mandarin pancakes** **(see p. 218)** |
| **6 tablespoons** | **3 ounces, 90 ml** | **Vegetable oil** |
| **2** | | **Eggs** |

**PROCEDURE**

1 Prepare mandarin pancakes. Cover finished pancakes with a clean cloth to prevent condensation from dropping onto the surface. Cover and keep warm until ready to serve.

2 Set a wok over high heat. Add one tablespoon ($\frac{1}{2}$ ounce, 15 ml) oil, swirl around wok.

3 Beat eggs lightly. When oil is hot, pour in eggs, and tilt the wok so that the whole surface is covered with a thin coat of eggs. Flip the egg sheet over and cook for a few seconds. Transfer to plate; when cool, shred into narrow strips 2 inches (4.8 cm) long.

| AMOUNT | MEASURE | INGREDIENT |
|---|---|---|
| **$\frac{1}{2}$ pound** | | **Lean pork** |
| **Marinade** | | |
| **To taste** | | **Freshly ground pepper** |
| **$\frac{1}{4}$ teaspoon** | | **Fresh ginger, minced** |
| **2 teaspoons** | | **Cornstarch** |
| **1 teaspoon** | | **Dry sherry** |
| **1 tablespoon** | **$\frac{1}{2}$ ounce, 15 ml** | **Soy sauce** |

**PROCEDURE**

1 Shred pork by slicing it $\frac{1}{8}$ inch (.3 cm) thick across the grain, then cut the slices into strips about $\frac{1}{8}$ inch × $\frac{1}{8}$ inch × 2 inches (.3 cm × .3 cm × 4.8 cm).

2 Combine marinade ingredients; mix with shredded pork. Toss to coat thoroughly; let stand at least 30 minutes.

| AMOUNT | MEASURE | INGREDIENT |
|---|---|---|
| 6 | | Chinese dried mushrooms |
| ¼ cup | | Dried black cloud ears |
| 25 | | Dried tiger lily buds |
| 1 cup | 4 ounces, 112 g | Cabbage, ⅛ x ⅛ x 2 inches (.3 x .3 x 5 cm) |

**PROCEDURE**

1 Soak mushrooms and black cloud ears in 2 cups (16 ounces, 480 ml) hot water for 20 minutes. Discard the water. Remove stems; shred mushrooms into thin strips.

2 Soak tiger lily buds in 1 cup (8 ounces, 240 ml) hot water for 10 minutes. Discard the water. Snap off hard ends of the buds. Rinse and cut each bud in half. Combine with mushrooms and black cloud ears.

| AMOUNT | MEASURE | INGREDIENT |
|---|---|---|
| Sauce | | |
| 1 teaspoon | | Tapioca powder or cornstarch |
| 1 tablespoon | ½ ounce, 15 ml | Light soy sauce |
| 4 tablespoons | 2 ounces, 60 ml | Chicken stock or water |
| ½ teaspoon | | Sesame oil |

**PROCEDURE**

1 Mix all ingredients to combine.

| AMOUNT | MEASURE | INGREDIENT |
|---|---|---|
| 2 | | Garlic cloves, crushed |
| 1 teaspoon | | Garlic cloves, minced |
| ½ teaspoon | | Salt |
| 2 | | Green onions, minced |

**PROCEDURE**

1 Return wok to high heat. When very hot, add 2 tablespoons (1 ounce, 30 ml) of oil. Flavor the oil with crushed garlic and discard the garlic when browned. Add the tiger lilies, wood ears black mushrooms, and cabbage, stirring for 3 to 4 minutes. Toss and season. Remove from wok.

2 Rinse wok and reset over high heat. When very hot, add two (1 ounce, 30 ml) tablespoons oil. Flavor with minced garlic for 10 seconds, then add the meat and green onions, stirring continuously until the shreds separate.

3 Push ingredients to the side of wok and restir sauce mixture. Add sauce mixture to the center of the wok, stirring sauce until it thickens. Return the tiger lilies, mushrooms, bean sprouts, and eggs to wok; mix well and remove.

4 Serve with steamed mandarin pancakes as wrappers. Serve with Hoisin dipping sauce to be spread on the pancakes before wrapping filling.

## Hoisin Dipping Sauce

| AMOUNT | MEASURE | INGREDIENT |
|---|---|---|
| **$\frac{1}{4}$ cup** | **2 ounce, 60 ml** | **Hoisin sauce** |
| **2 tablespoons** | **1 ounce, 30 ml** | **Water** |

**PROCEDURE**

1 Combine to a smooth sauce.

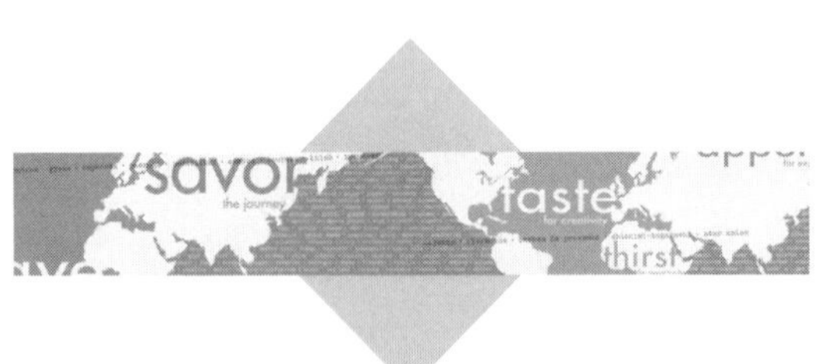

# Fortune Cookies

SERVES 4

**Before making the cookies, prepare the fortunes on small slips of paper.**

| AMOUNT | MEASURE | INGREDIENT |
|---|---|---|
| 3 | | Eggs |
| $\frac{3}{4}$ cup | 6 ounces, 168 g | Sugar |
| $\frac{1}{2}$ cup | 4 ounces, 112 g | Butter, melted |
| $\frac{1}{4}$ teaspoon | | Vanilla extract |
| 1 cup | 4 ounces, 112 g | All-purpose flour |
| 2 tablespoon | 1 ounce, 30 ml | Water |

**PROCEDURE**

1. Preheat oven to 350°F (176°C).
2. Combine ingredients in order listed, mixing well after each addition.
3. Chill for 20 minutes.
4. On a nonstick baking pad or parchment paper, fill a 3-inch (7.2 cm) circle mold with cookie butter and spread to $\frac{1}{8}$-inch (.3 cm) thickness. Bake two cookies at a time
5. Bake 4 to 5 minutes, until edges are lightly browned.
6. Working quickly, place a fortune paper slip in the center of each cookie. Fold cookie in half, enclosing the fortune slip and forming a semicircle.
7. Grasp the rounded edges of the semicircle between thumb and forefinger with both hands. Push the fortune cookie down over a dowel, making certain the solid sides of cookie puff out.
8. Place each cookie in small muffin tin, open end up, until cookies are set.
9. Return to oven to finish baking until golden brown, about 1 to 2 minutes.

# Lamb on Rice Sticks

SERVES 4

**Lamb is a tradition in Peking.**

**When marinating meats be sure to add oil or the meat will stick together when cooking.**

| AMOUNT | MEASURE | INGREDIENT |
|---|---|---|
| | 12 ounces | Lamb, trimmed of all visible fat and all gristle removed, cut $\frac{1}{8}$ x $\frac{1}{8}$ x 1$\frac{1}{2}$ inch (.3 x .3 x 3.6 cm) shreds |
| 1 teaspoon | | Ginger juice |
| $\frac{1}{2}$ cup | 3 ounces, 84 g | Bamboo shoots |
| 2 cups plus 1 tablespoon | 16.5 ounces, 495 ml | Vegetable oil |
| 1 ounce | | Rice sticks |
| 2 cups | 8 ounces, 224 g | Leeks, white part only, washed well, $\frac{1}{8}$ x $\frac{1}{8}$ x 1$\frac{1}{2}$ inch (.3 x .3 x 3.6 cm) shreds |
| 4 medium | | Black mushrooms, soaked in warm water until soft, stems trimmed; squeeze to extract moisture, $\frac{1}{8}$ x $\frac{1}{8}$ x 1$\frac{1}{2}$ inch (.3 x .3 x 3.6 cm) shreds |
| 1 | | Garlic clove, minced |
| 1 cup | 4 ounces, 112 g | Carrots, peeled, $\frac{1}{8}$ x $\frac{1}{8}$ x 1$\frac{1}{2}$ inch (.3 x .3 x 3.6 cm) shreds |
| 3, or to taste | | Hot chiles, seeds and pulp removed, shredded finely |
| $\frac{1}{2}$ teaspoon | | Salt |
| 1 teaspoon | | Granulated sugar |
| 1 tablespoon | $\frac{1}{2}$ ounce, 15 ml | Dry sherry |
| 1 teaspoon | | Tapioca powder or cornstarch mixed with 1 tablespoon ($\frac{1}{2}$ ounce, 15 ml) chicken stock |
| 1 teaspoon | | Sesame oil |
| Marinade | | |
| 1 | | Egg |
| 1 tablespoon | | Tapioca powder or cornstarch |
| 1 tablespoon | $\frac{1}{2}$ ounce, 15 ml | Soy sauce |
| 1 tablespoon | | Ginger juice |
| $\frac{1}{4}$ teaspoon | | Salt |
| $\frac{1}{8}$ teaspoon | | White pepper |
| 1 tablespoon | $\frac{1}{2}$ ounce, 15 ml | Vegetable oil |

**PROCEDURE**

1. Combine all marinade ingredients and add to lamb. Mix until well blended; refrigerate 30 minutes.
2. Blanch bamboo shoots in boiling water 1 minute; rinse with cold water. Shred finely, $\frac{1}{8} \times \frac{1}{8} \times 1\frac{1}{2}$ inch (.3 × .3 × 3.6 cm) shreds; drain and pat dry with paper towels.
3. Set wok over high heat. When very hot, add 2 cups (16 ounces, 480 ml) oil and heat to 400°F (204°C). Test temperature by dropping a few inches of rice stick into the oil. If it puffs up immediately, the oil is hot enough.
4. Add the rice sticks, turning over quickly when puffed up. Deep-fry for 5 more seconds and remove; drain on paper towels. The rice sticks should be creamy white in color.
5. Remove wok from heat, strain sediments from oil, and return to 400°F (204°C). Add the lamb shreds to the wok, stirring to separate. Cook 1 to 2 minutes, then pour oil and lamb into a strainer-lined container to drain.
6. Return wok and two tablespoons (1 ounce, 30 ml) oil to high heat. When hot, add the leeks and garlic to the oil, stir-fry until limp. Add mushrooms, carrots, bamboo shoots, and chiles, in that order, stirring after each is added. Season with salt.
7. Return lamb to wok. Stir and sizzle in the sherry along the edge. Push all the ingredients to the side, restir thicking mixture, and add to center of wok. Stir until thickened, then add sesame oil. Mix all ingredients.
8. Line a serving platter with rice sticks, pressing down to break sticks into smaller pieces. Place the lamb shreds on top. Serve hot.

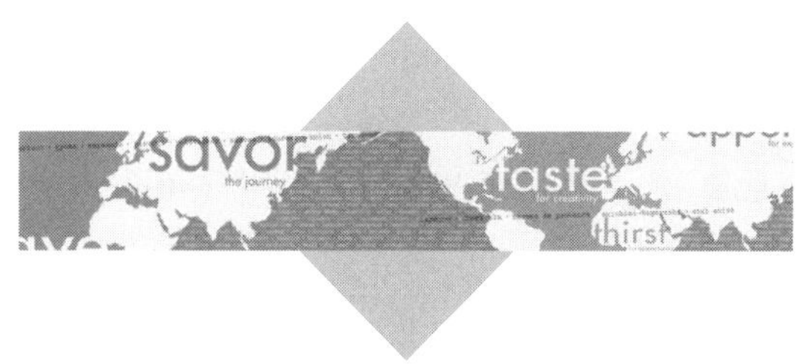

# Wonton Soup

SERVES 4

| AMOUNT | MEASURE | INGREDIENT |
|---|---|---|
| 40 | | Wonton Wrappers, packaged |
| Filling | | |
| $\frac{1}{2}$ pound | 8 ounces, 224 g | Ground pork, chicken or shrimp |
| 2 tablespoons | 1 ounce, 30 ml | Soy Sauce |
| 1 tablespoon | $\frac{1}{2}$ ounce, 15 ml | Rice wine or dry sherry |
| $\frac{1}{2}$ teaspoon | | Salt |
| 1 | | Egg |
| 2 tablespoons | 1 ounce, 30 ml | Sesame oil |
| $\frac{1}{4}$ cup | 1 ounce, 28 g | Green onions, minced |
| $\frac{1}{2}$ cup | 3 ounces, 84 g | Chinese cabbage or bamboo shoots, minced |
| Dash | | White pepper |
| Soup | | |
| 6 cups | 48 ounces, 1.4 L | Chicken or beef stock |
| 2 tablespoons | 1 ounce, 30 ml | Soy sauce |
| To taste | | Salt |
| 2 tablespoons | | Green onions, minced |

## PROCEDURE

1. Mix filling ingredients, chill until needed.
2. Place 1 teaspoon filling in the center of each wrapper.
3. Fold over at the center, wet the edges with water and press to seal.
4. Fold in half lengthwise at the open side, bring the two ends over the other and press together with a little water.
5. Bring 3 quarts (96 ounces, 2.8 L) of water to a boil. Add wontons, stir. Cover and return to boil.
6. Add 1 cup (8 ounces, 240 ml) of cold water, cover and return to boil. When cooked the wontons will float.
7. Drain and rinse with cold water to stop cooking.
8. Combine stock, soy sauce and salt, bring to a boil.
9. Add wontons and return to a boil. Add minced green onions, serve hot.

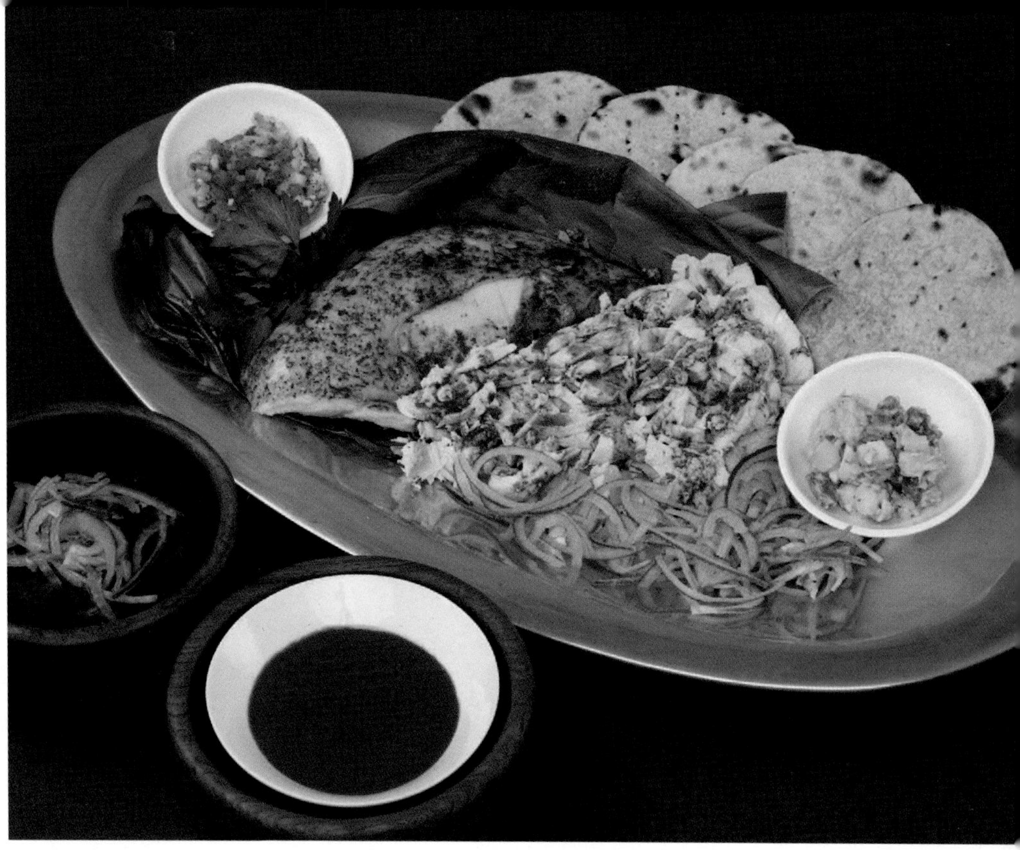

**Pavo con Salsa de Achiote a la Yucataneca—Yucatán-Style Steamed Turkey in Achiote Sauce (Mexico)**

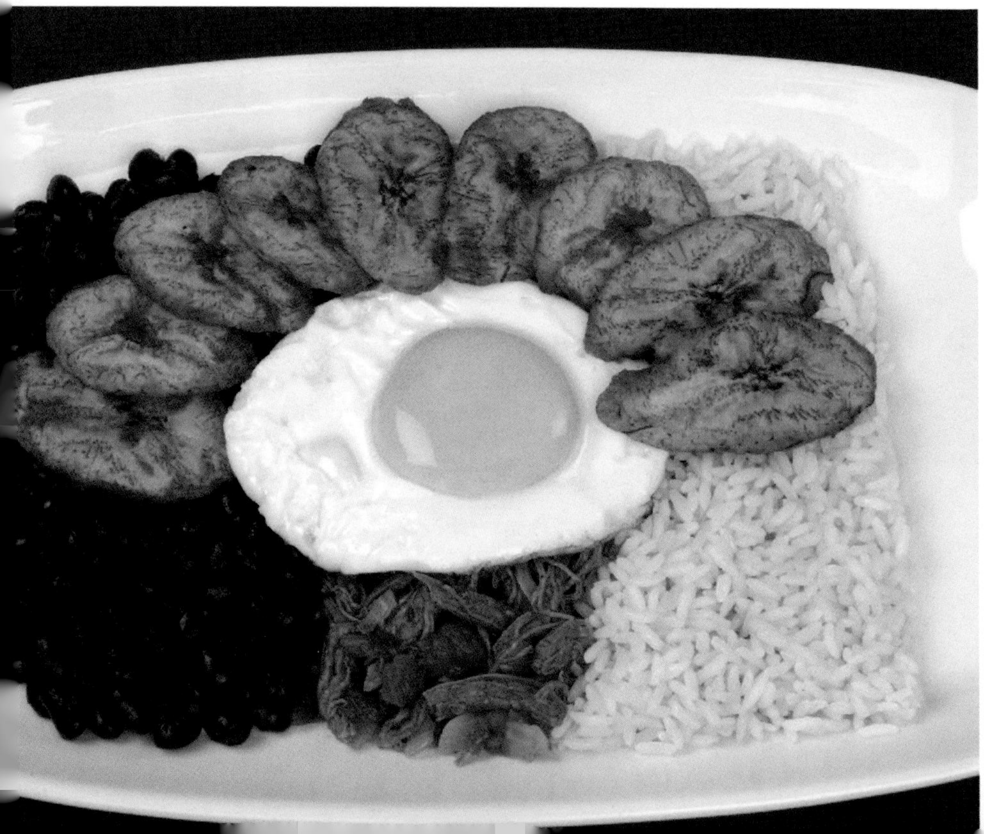

**Pabellón Criollo—Venezuelan Shredded Beef with Beans, Rice and Plantains (South America)**

**Ceviche de Pescado—Fish Ceviche (South America)**

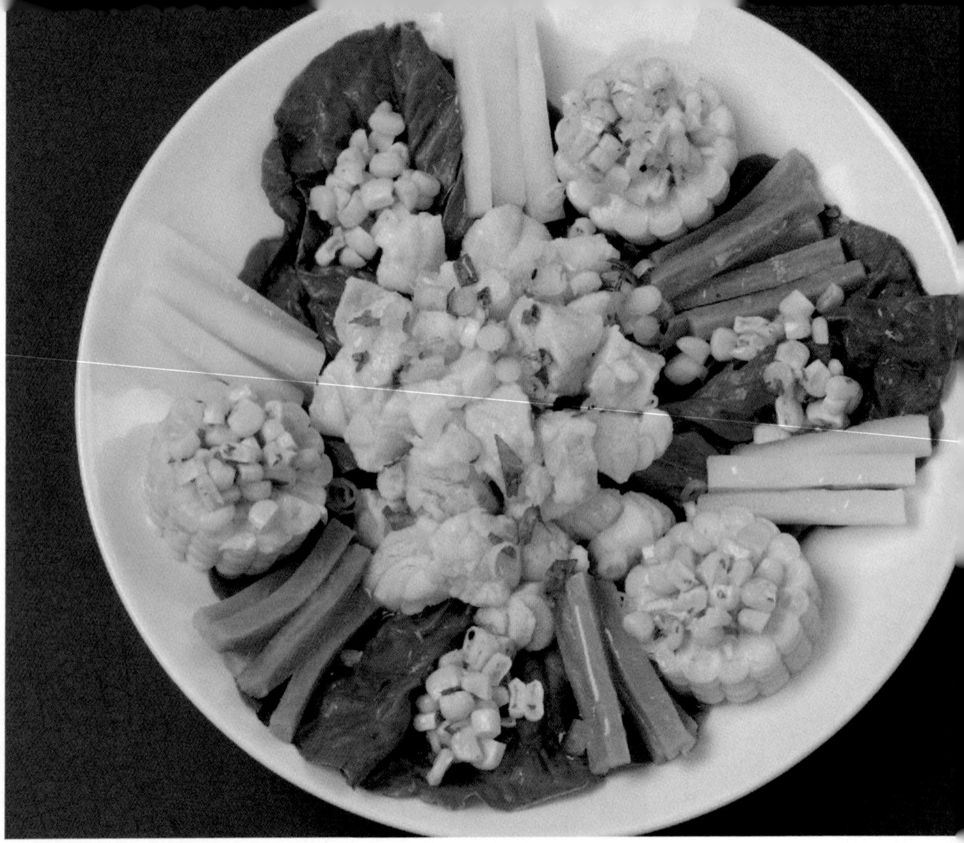

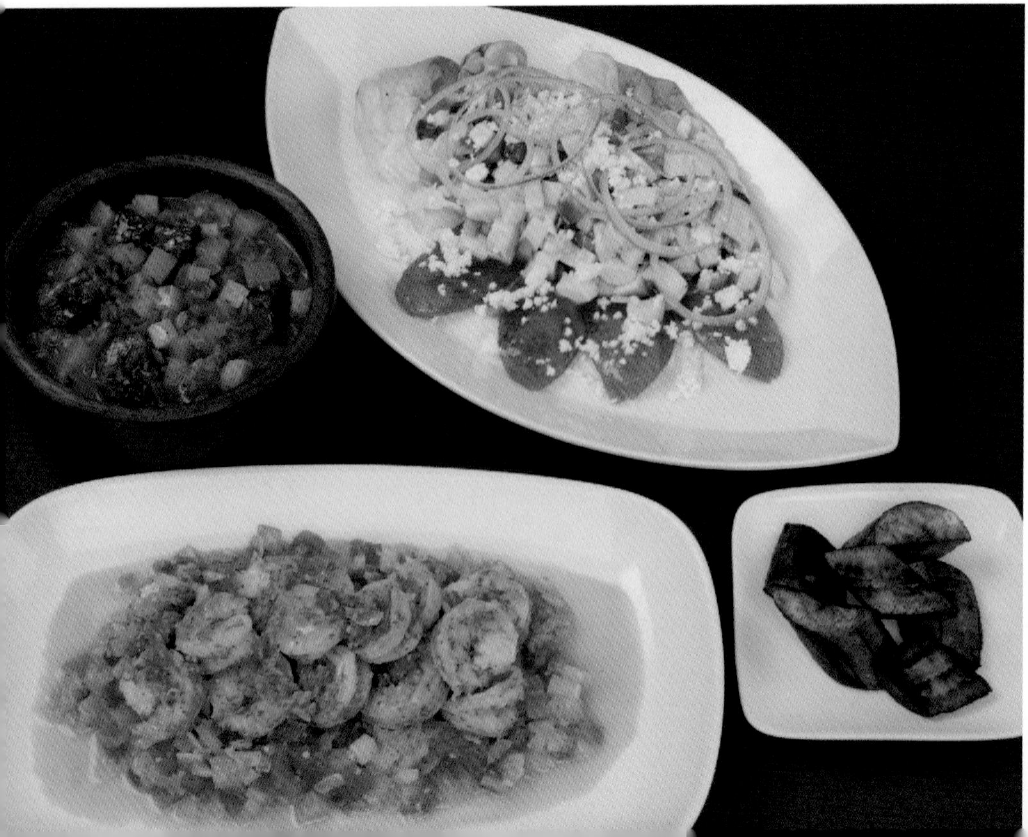

**(Bottom left) Camarones Sofrito—Shrimp in Green Sofrito (Dominican Republic); (Top right) Curried Lamb, Salad of Hearts of Palm, with Passion Fruit Vinaigrette and Fried Ripe Plantains (Caribbean)**

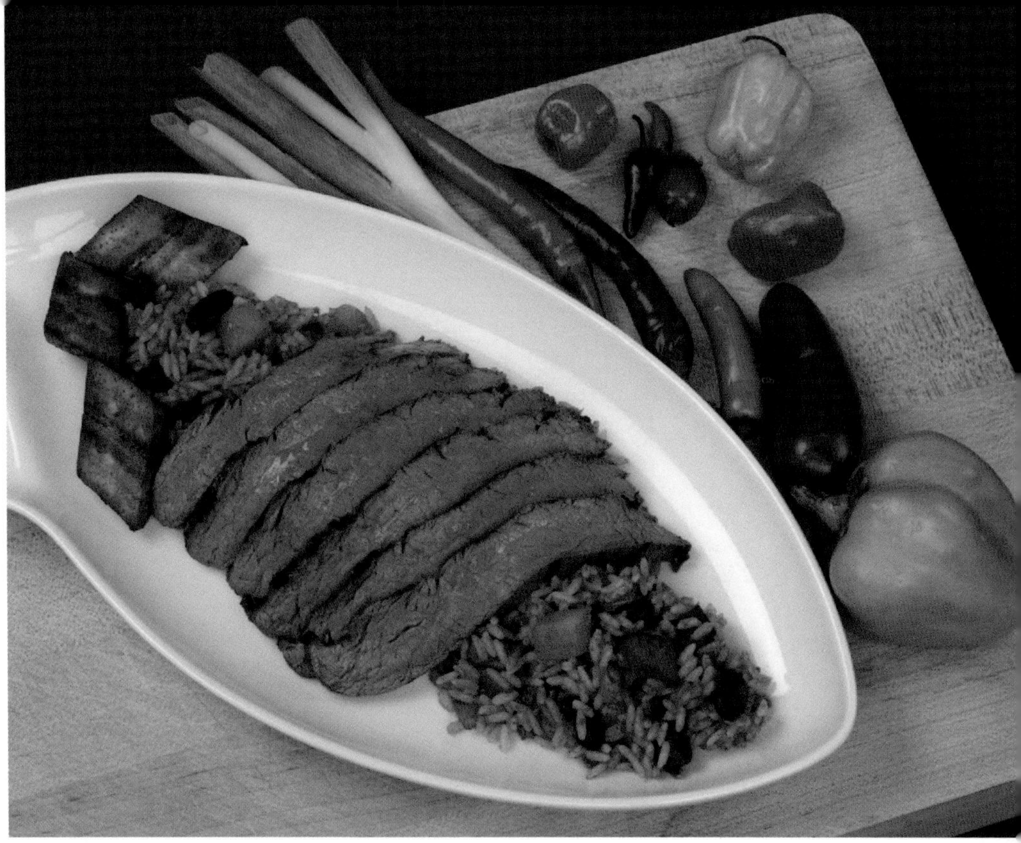

**Jamaican Jerk Beef Steak on Arroz Mamposteao—Rice and Beans**

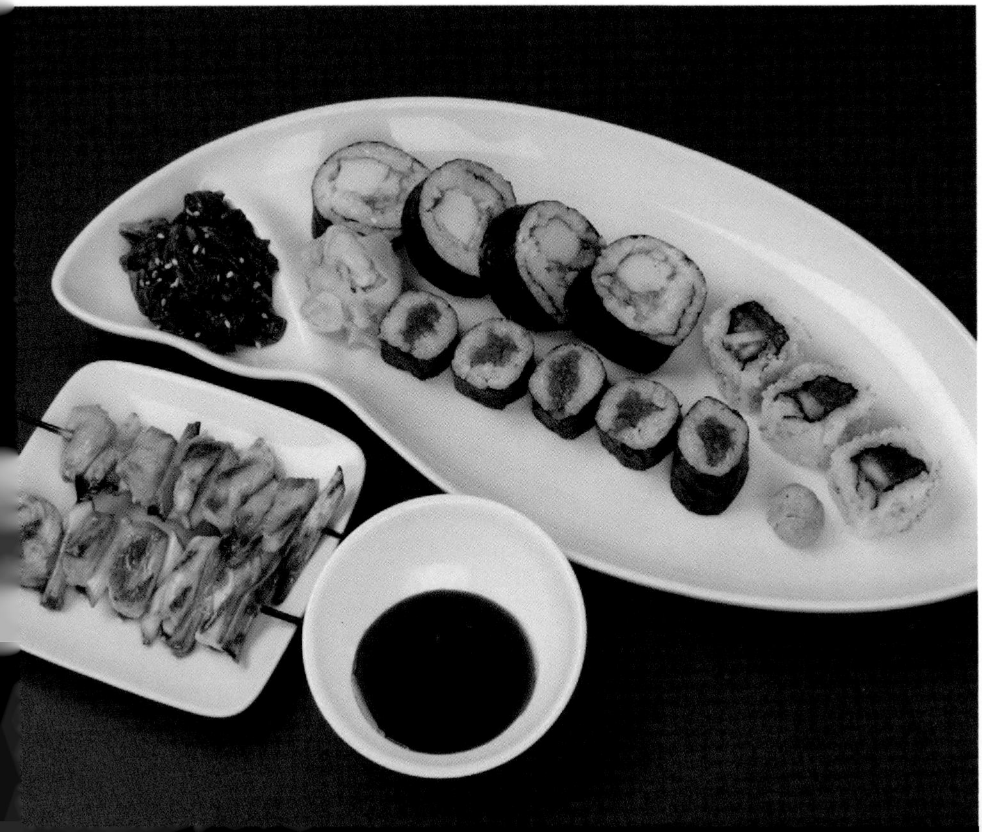

**Yakitori—Grilled Chicken, Maki Sushi, Horenso Goma-ae—Spinach in Sesame Dressing (Japan)**

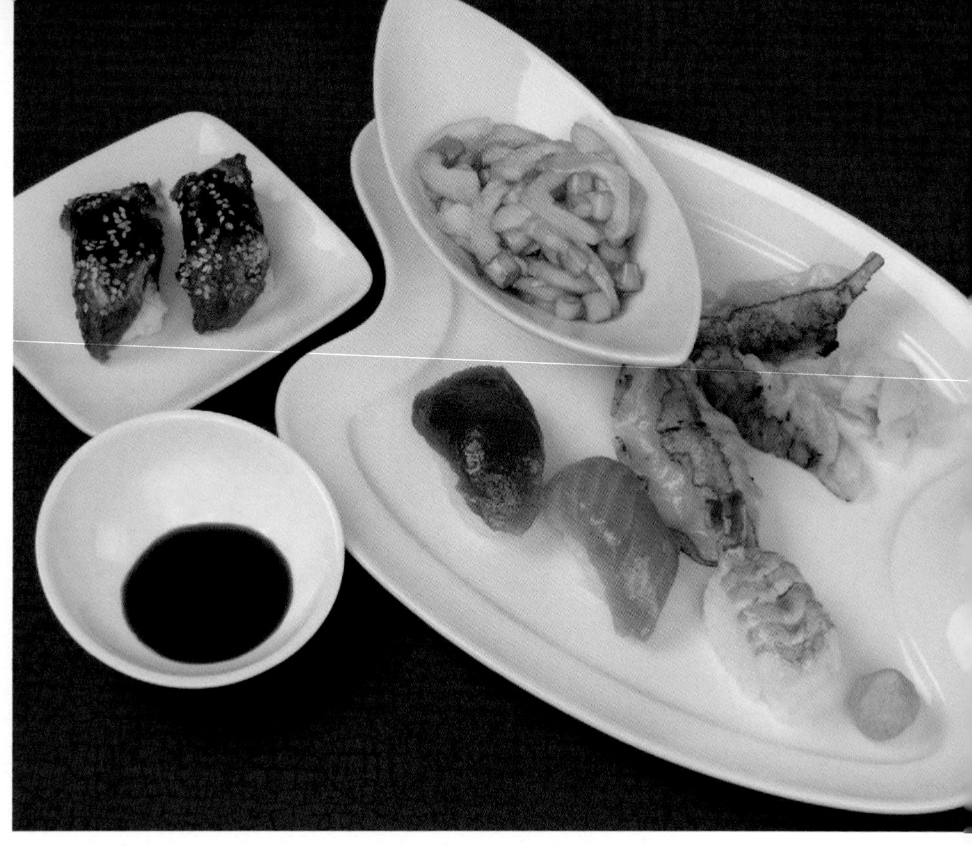

**Gyoza—Japanese Pot-Stickers, Kyuri No Sunome—Japanese Cucumber Salad, and Nigiri-Zushi (Japan)**

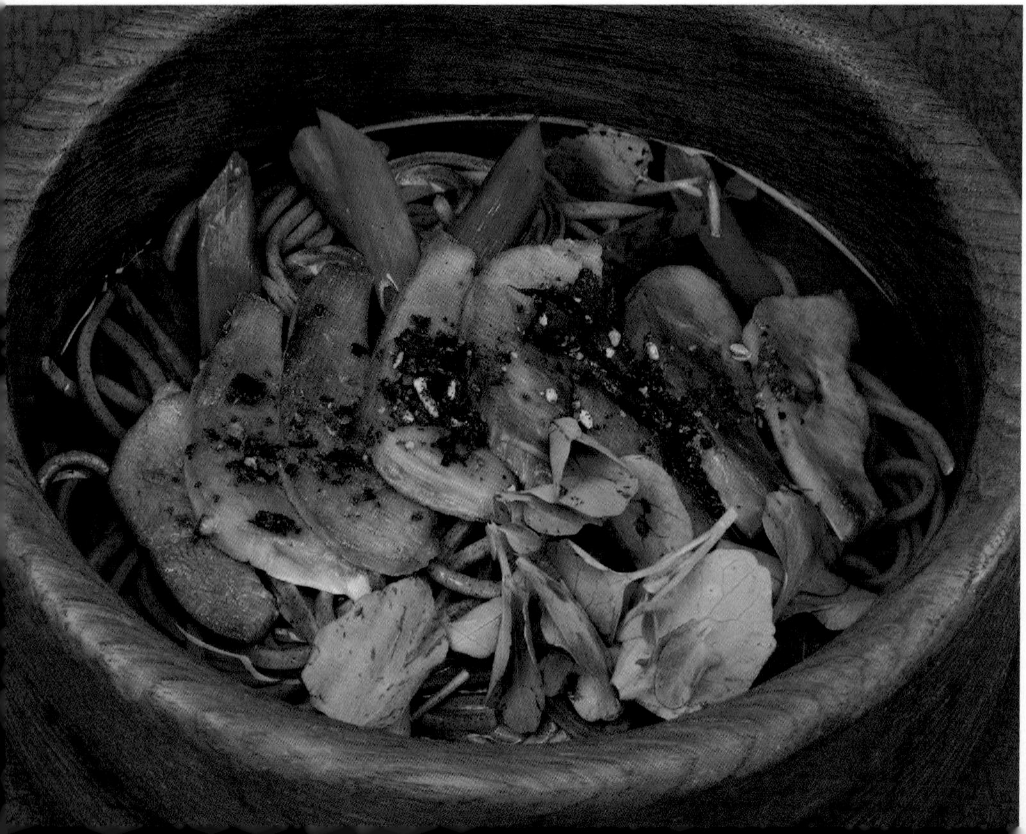

**Kamonanban Soba—Soba with Duck and Long Onions (Japan)**

**Emerald Shrimp and Shanghai Sweet and Sour Spareribs (China)**

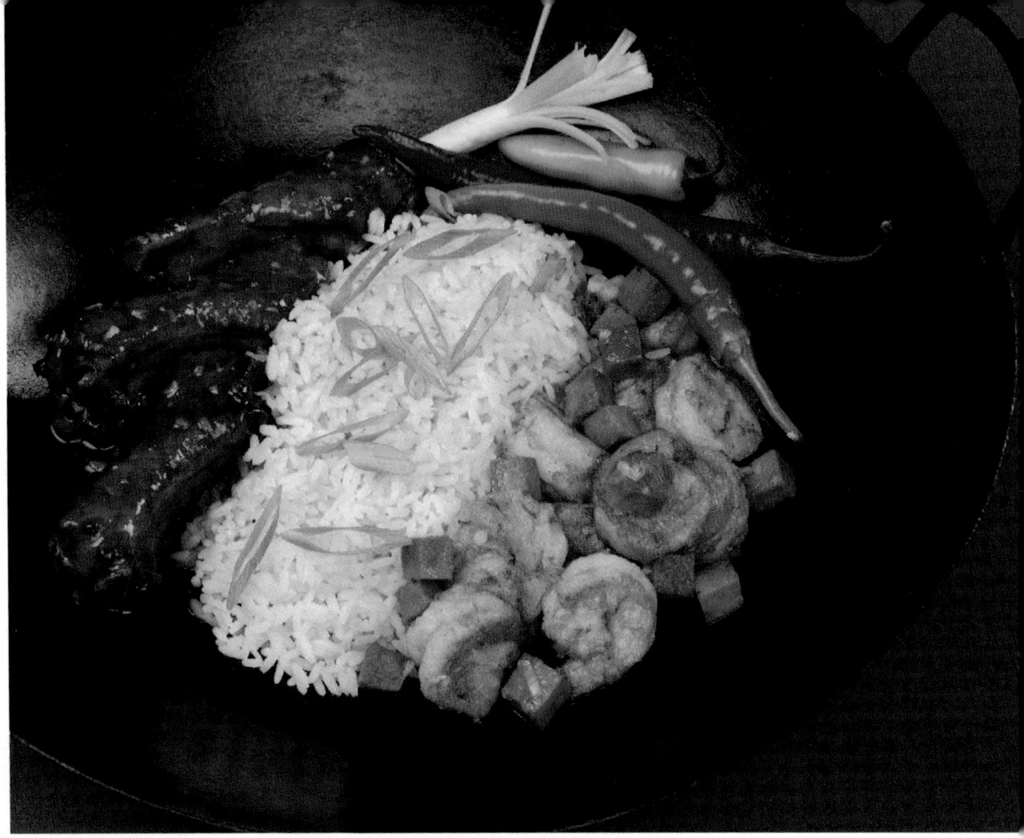

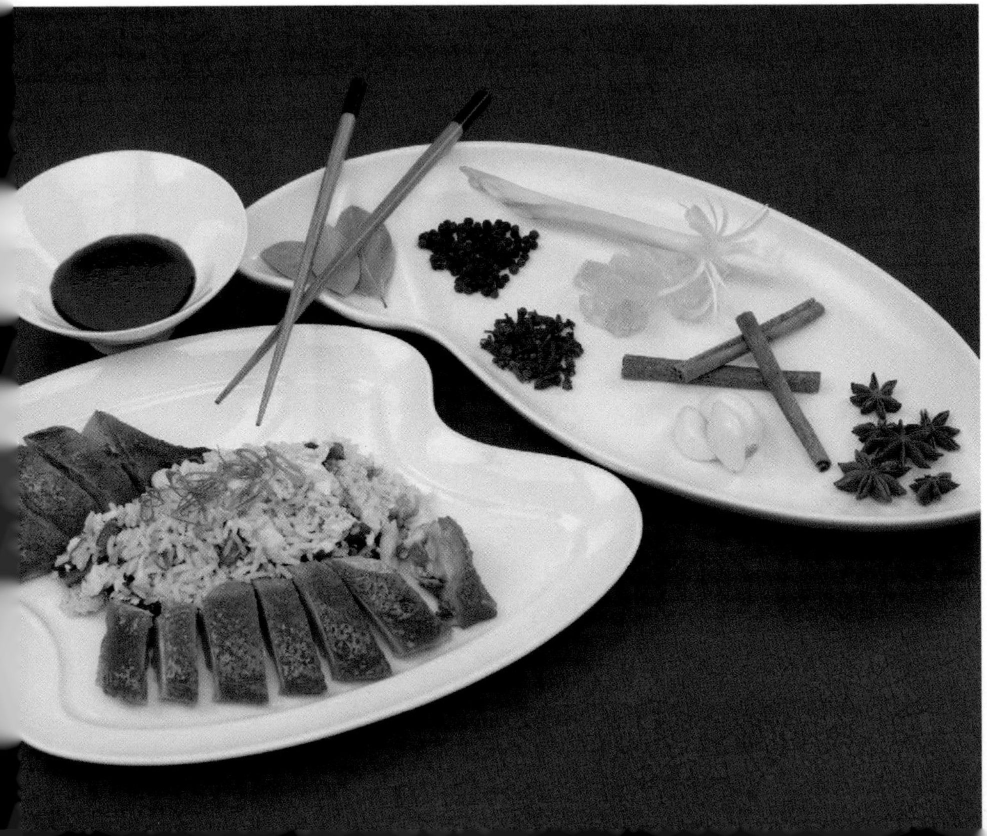

**Red Cooked Duck and Yangchow (Yangzhou) Fried Rice (China)**

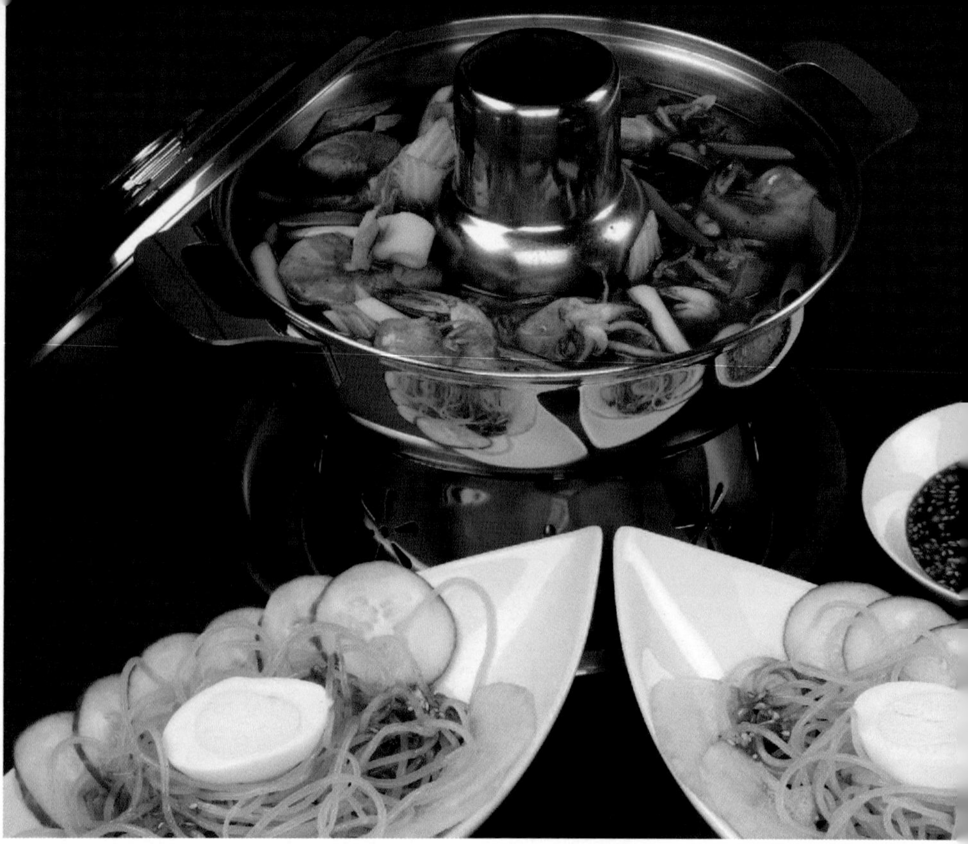

**Hacmul Jungol—Seafood Hot Pot and Bibim Naeng Myun—Garden's Cold Mixed Noodles (Korea)**

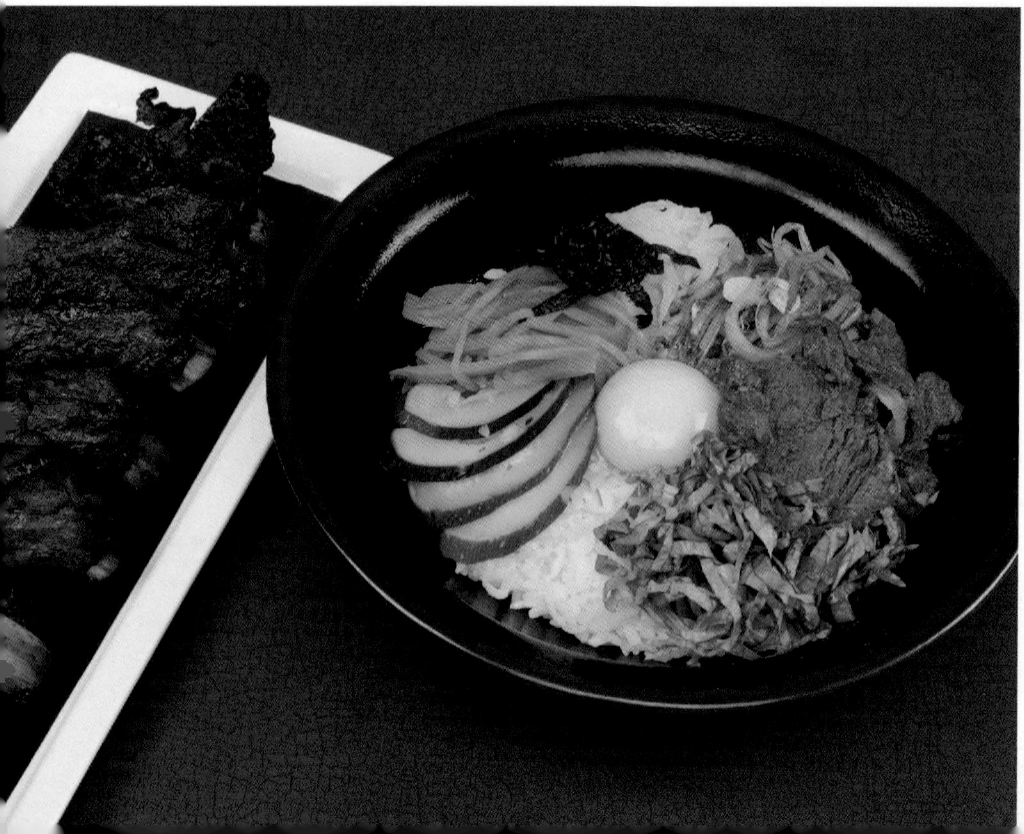

**Dwaeji Galbi—Spicy Pork Ribs and Bibimbap – Garnished Rice (Korea)**

ssorted spices and erbs—Bottom platter, lockwise from bottom left: ine nuts, ground cayenne, enugreek, walnut pieces, araway seeds, white ardamom. Between the latters, clockwise from the ottom: Green onions, emon grass, red chile de rbol, mint leaf, lime, hallots, curry leaf, kaffir me leaves, habanero, garlic oves, ginger, red onion; op platter, clockwise from ottom left: cloves, chives, antaka chile, dried red chili akes, árbol, chile basil, umpkin seeds, cinnamon icks (Southeast Asia)

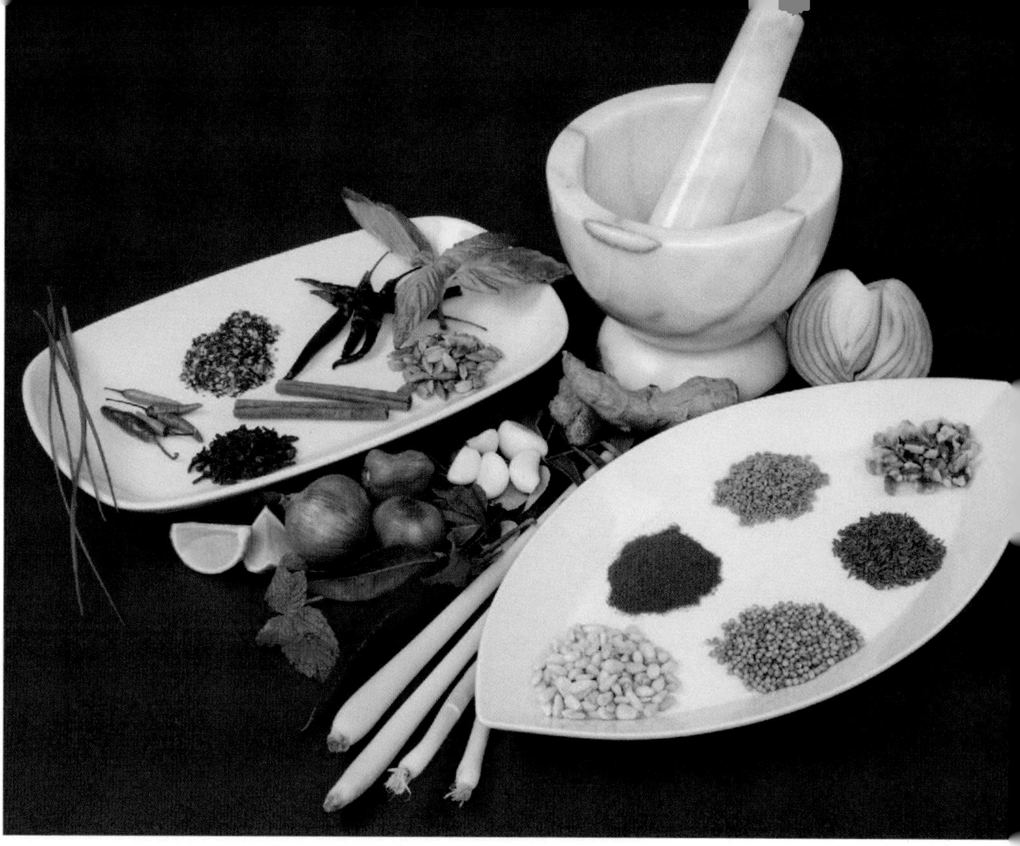

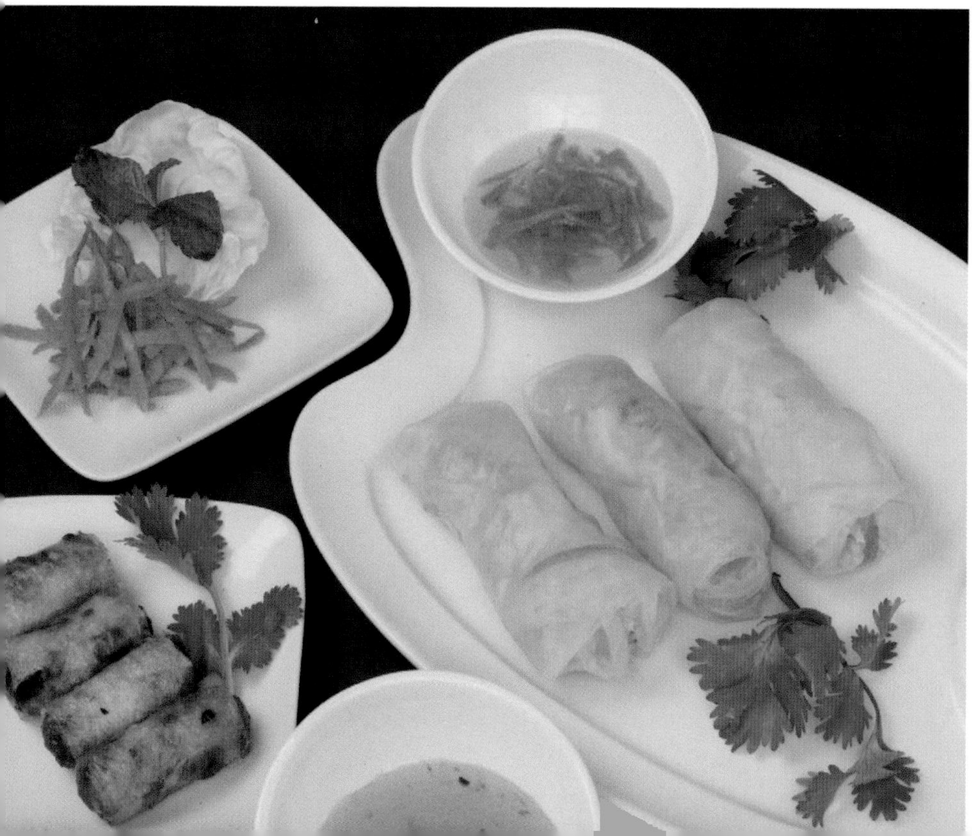

**Goi Cuon—Fresh Spring Rolls and Cha Gio—Fried Spring Rolls (Vietnam, Southeast Asia)**

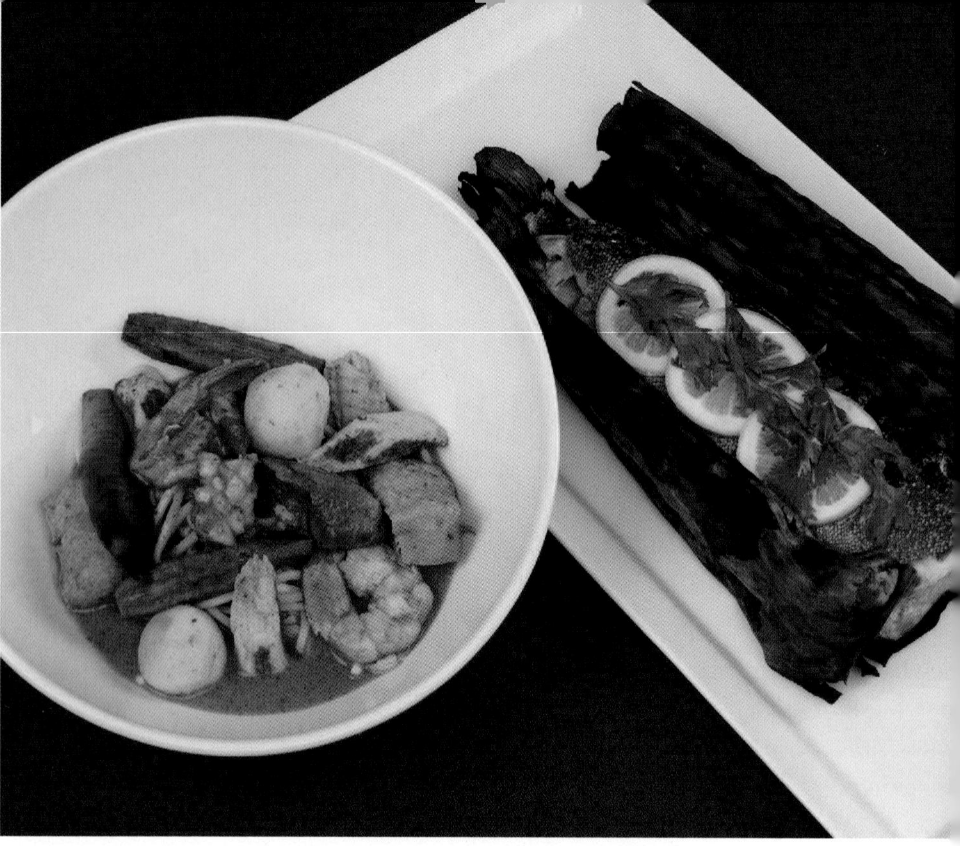

**Laksa Lemak—Chicken, Shrimp and Rice Noodles in Coconut Sauce; Pepes Ikan—Grilled Fish in Banana Leaf (Indonesia, Southeast Asia)**

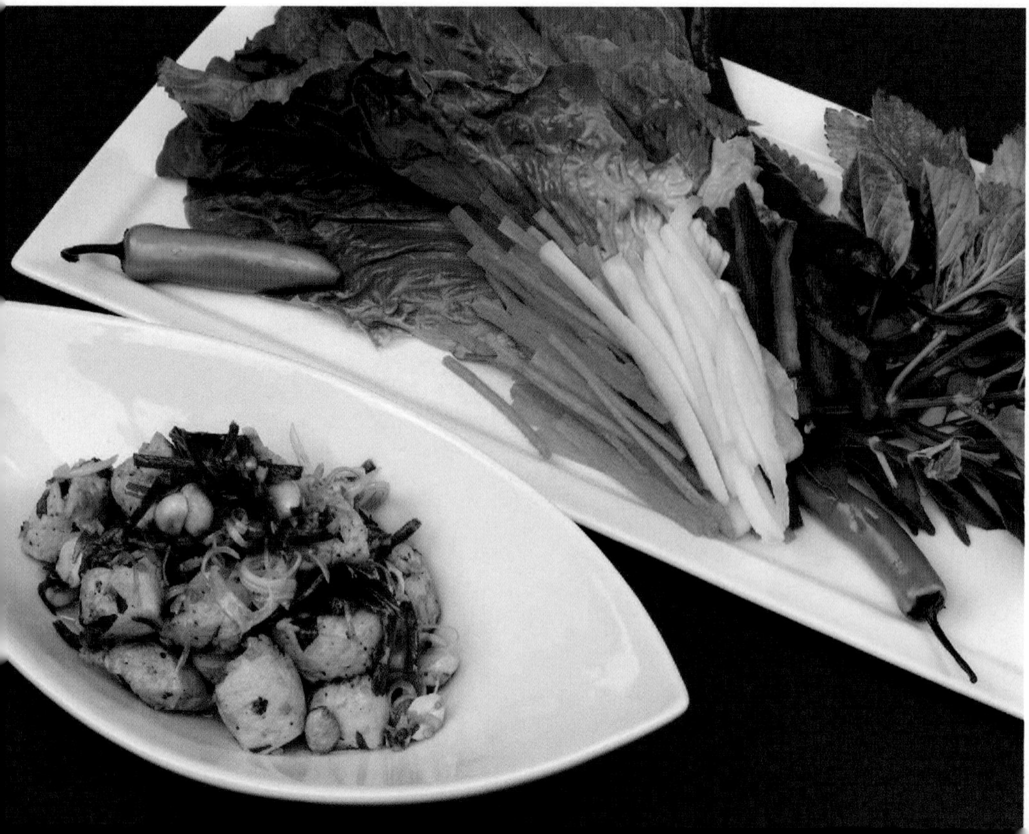

**Dia Rau Song—Vegetable Platter; Ga Xao Sa Ot—Lemon Grass Chicken (Vietnam, Southeast Asia)**

# Jellyfish and White Radish Salad

SERVES 4

**Chef Tip** **It is best to soak the jellyfish overnight. Keep it as dry as possible so the dressing will not be diluted.**

| AMOUNT | MEASURE | INGREDIENT |
|---|---|---|
| | 4 ounces, 112 g | Precut jellyfish shreds, soaked overnight |
| $1\frac{1}{2}$ cup | 8 ounces, 224 g | Chinese white radish (daikon), peeled, $\frac{1}{8} \times \frac{1}{8} \times 1\frac{1}{2}$ inch (.3 x .3 x 3.6 cm) shreds |
| | | Salt |
| $\frac{1}{2}$ cup | 2 ounces, 56 | Carrot, peeled, $\frac{1}{8} \times \frac{1}{8} \times 1\frac{1}{2}$ inch (.3 x .3 x 3.6 cm) shreds |
| 1 | | Green onion, trimmed, white part and 2-in. (4.8 cm) green part, minced |
| 2 | | Chinese parsley (cilantro) sprigs, cut into 2-in. (4.8 cm) pieces |
| Dressing | | |
| 2 teaspoons | | Rice vinegar |
| 2 teaspoons | | Sesame oil |
| 2 tablespoons | 1 ounce, 30 ml | Peanut oil |
| 2 teaspoons | | Granulated sugar |
| To taste | | White pepper and cayenne |

PROCEDURE

1. Rinse jellyfish with cold water, squeezing and rubbing to remove salt. Cover in cold water and soak, preferably overnight, then rinse thoroughly. Drain in colander for 1 hour, or until most moisture is gone. Pat dry and wrap with a towel. Chill and refrigerate.
2. Rub radish with 1 tablespoon salt and let stand at room temperature for 2–3 hours or until limp. Rinse radish with cold water to remove salt, then squeeze shreds by hand to remove excess moisture. Repeat until all shreds are squeezed dry.
3. Process carrot in the same manner as radish.
4. One hour before serving, mix dressing, and combine with all ingredients. Toss well. Serve chilled.

# Pearl Balls

## Porcupine Meatballs

SERVES 4 AS AN APPETIZER

**Chef Tip** **Make sure the egg is well incorporated, it is a binding agent. If rice is not sticking to the pearl balls, wet with a little cold water.**

| AMOUNT | MEASURE | INGREDIENT |
|---|---|---|
| ½ cup | 3½ ounces, 98 g | Glutinous rice |
| 1 cup | 8 ounces, 224 g | Lean ground pork |
| ¼ teaspoon | | Salt |
| 1 tablespoon | ½ ounce, 15 ml | Light soy sauce |
| 1 | | Egg |
| 2 teaspoons | | Dry sherry |
| ¼ teaspoon | | Granulated sugar |
| 1 teaspoon | | Ginger, grated |
| 2 teaspoons | | Sesame oil |
| 2 teaspoons | | Tapioca powder or cornstarch |
| To taste | | White pepper |
| ½ cup | 3 ounces, 84 g | Bamboo shoots |
| 2 tablespoons | | Green onion, white parts only, minced |
| ¼ cup | 2 ounces, 60 ml | Rice vinegar |
| 1 tablespoon | | Ginger, minced |

### PROCEDURE

1. Rinse the rice and soak in cold water for a least 1 hour. Drain thoroughly and spread in one layer on pan lined with paper towels. Make sure the rice is dry before using.
2. Combine pork, salt, and soy sauce. Mix with your fingers and scoop up pork mixture by the hand, beating it back into the bowl several times until firm. Add the egg, sherry, sugar, ginger, sesame oil, tapioca powder and pepper to the meat, scooping and beating several more times.
3. Blanch the bamboo shoots in boiling water for two minutes. Run cold water over to stop the cooking process; shred into bite sized bits. Squeeze out as much moisture as possible.

4 Add the green onion to the pork together with bamboo shoots. Mix well; chill for at least 2 hours or until ready to use.

5 Scoop up a handful of pork mixture and squeeze out through the fist until it reaches the size of a walnut (1 tablespoon is 1 ounce). Scrape off with a wet spoon.

6 Drop pork balls onto the rice, rolling around until the surface is evenly covered with the rice. Place on a greased container that can be used in a steamer; or on a lettuce leaf (banana leaf, bamboo leaf, napa cabbage) allow $\frac{1}{2}$ inch (1.2 cm) separation between each pearly ball.

7 Place the meatballs in a steamer; steam over high heat 25 to 30 minutes or until the rice is cooked and turns shiny and translucent.

8 Combine vinegar and ginger to make sauce. Serve meatballs hot or warm with sauce.

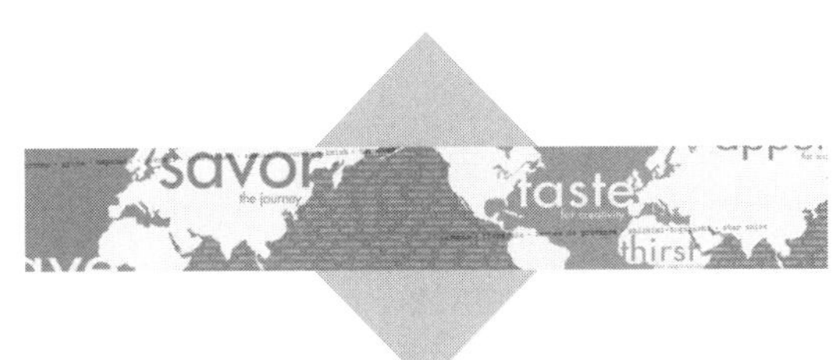

# Emerald Shrimp

SERVES 4

| AMOUNT | MEASURE | INGREDIENT |
|---|---|---|
| 12 ounces | | Shrimp (16–20 count), shelled, deveined, and cut down the middle from the back |
| 4 cups | 8 ounces, 224 g | Flat leaf spinach, washed well, stems removed, coarsely chopped |
| 2 tablespoons | | Green onion, white part only, roll-cut in ½ inch (1.2 cm) cuts |
| | ½ ounce, 14 g | Smithfield ham, ½ inch (1.2 cm) dice |
| 2 cups | 16 ounces, 480 ml | Water |
| 1½ cup | 12 ounces, 360 ml | Vegetable oil |
| 1 | | Garlic clove |
| 2 teaspoons | | Mirin |
| Marinade | | |
| 1 | | Egg white |
| ½ teaspoon | | Salt |
| 2 teaspoons | | Tapioca powder or cornstarch |
| ¼ teaspoon | | Sesame oil |
| ¼ teaspoon | | Sugar |
| Dash | | White pepper |

PROCEDURE

1. Arrange the shrimp in one layer on double paper towels. Roll up like a jelly roll and chill for at least two hours. The shrimp need to be very dry.
2. In a blender, combine 1 cup (8 ounces, 240 ml) water with the spinach. Process until reduced to a puree. Pour the puree into a very fine-mesh strainer; press the pureed spinach to extract liquid. Reserve strained liquid and spinach.
3. Transfer spinach puree to a bowl and thin with remaining water. Pour it through the strainer again to combine liquid with the previously extracted spinach juice.
4. Heat the spinach juice over high heat until small bubbles start to appear gradually along the sides of the pan and the liquid begins to foam. Remove immediately from heat.

5 Set a coffee filter into a cone and skim the spinach foam from the pan into the filter. Let it drain thoroughly and squeeze to extract all the liquid; there should be about 1 tablespoon of very fine spinach paste. Cover and chill until ready to use. Discard the juice in the pan.

6 Pat shrimp with paper towel; they must be very dry for the green spinach coloring to adhere. Combine shrimp and 1 teaspoon spinach paste, mixing it well by hand. Continue to add $\frac{1}{2}$ teaspoon at a time, mixing well after each addition until shrimp is tinted evenly with green coloring. You need at least 2 teaspoons of spinach paste; avoid over-coloring.

7 Mix marinade with wire whisk until smooth. Add to the green shrimp, mixing well by hand until evenly coated. Chill for 1 to 2 hours.

8 Set a wok over high heat. When very hot, add about $\frac{1}{4}$ cup (2 ounces, 60 ml) oil, swish around the wok to grease the surface, and remove that oil from the wok. Add remaining oil, heat to 325°F (163°C) or until a piece of green onion dropped in oil bubbles, sizzles, and moves around.

9 Stir shrimp mixture, and then add the whole batch to the oil at once. Stir to separate shrimp quickly, about 20 seconds. Pour shrimp and oil into a strainer-lined container to drain oil, leaving about 1 tablespoon ($\frac{1}{2}$ ounce, 15 ml) of oil in wok.

10 Return wok to high heat. Add garlic. Remove wok quickly from heat, let garlic cook in hot oil for 10 seconds, then discard. (This ensures the oil in wok is clear.)

11 Reset wok on high heat. Return the shrimp to wok and stir-fry 15 to 20 seconds. Sizzle in the mirin, then add green onions and ham. Stir 20 seconds and serve immediately.

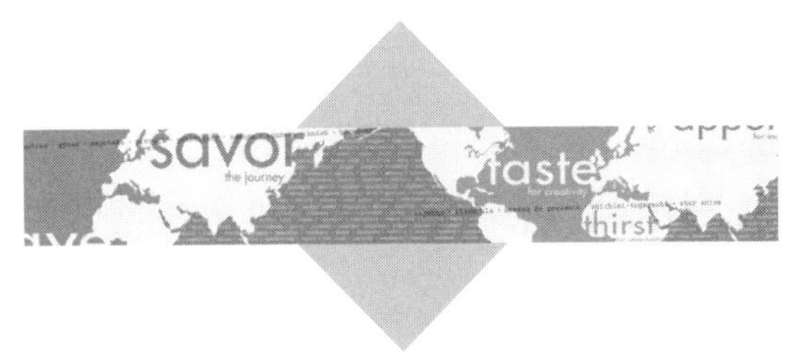

# Red-Cooked Duck

SERVES 4

**Chef Tip** Cold Red-Cooked Duck is outstanding, should be served garnished with cilantro.

| AMOUNT | MEASURE | INGREDIENT |
|---|---|---|
| $3\frac{1}{2}$ pound | 1.5 kg | Young duck, cut in quarters |
| 2 tablespoons | 1 ounce, 30 ml | Vegetable oil |
| 1 | | Garlic clove, flattened |
| 2 | | Green onions, $\frac{1}{4}$ inch (.6 cm) lengths |
| 1 | | Star anise |
| 2 teaspoons | | Tapioca powder or cornstarch |
| 1 tablespoon | $\frac{1}{2}$ ounce, 15 ml | Water |
| 1 teaspoon | | Sesame oil |
| To taste | | Salt |
| Marinade | | |
| 2 teaspoons | | Ginger juice |
| 2 tablespoons | 1 ounce, 30 ml | Dry sherry |
| 2 tablespoons | 1 ounce, 30 ml | Dark soy sauce |
| $\frac{1}{2}$ teaspoon | | Salt |
| Braising Mixture | | |
| 2 cups | 16 ounces, 480 ml | Chicken stock |
| 1 tablespoon | $\frac{1}{2}$ ounce, 15 ml | Oyster sauce |
| 1 tablespoon | $\frac{1}{2}$ ounce, 14 g | Rock sugar or granulated sugar |
| 1 | | Thai bird chile (small red) |

PROCEDURE

1 Remove excess loose fat from duck, then flatten the duck. Rinse and pat dry. Prick the skin.

2 Combine marinade ingredients, mix well, and rub evenly on the skin and cavity. Let marinate at room temperature for at least 1 hour, turning occasionally.

3 Drain duck, reserving excess marinade. Set wok over high heat; when hot, add 2 (1 ounce, 30 ml) tablespoons oil. Swish oil around and then place duck in wok. Turn heat to medium and brown the duck slowly and evenly on all sides.

4 Mix together the braising mixture and bring to boil over high heat, then add the duck. Return to a boil; add reserved marinade, garlic, green onion, and star anise. Cover and reduce to a simmer; cook 1 to $1\frac{1}{2}$ hours or until a chopstick pierces through the thigh easily. Remove duck and chile; degrease the sauce.

5 Return braising liquid to a boil, add duck to reheat, remove, drain, cut into serving pieces, and place on serving platter.

6 Mix tapioca powder with the water and add to the liquid in the wok, stirring constantly until thickened. Correct seasoning, then glaze sauce with sesame oil. Pour over duck. Serve hot or cold.

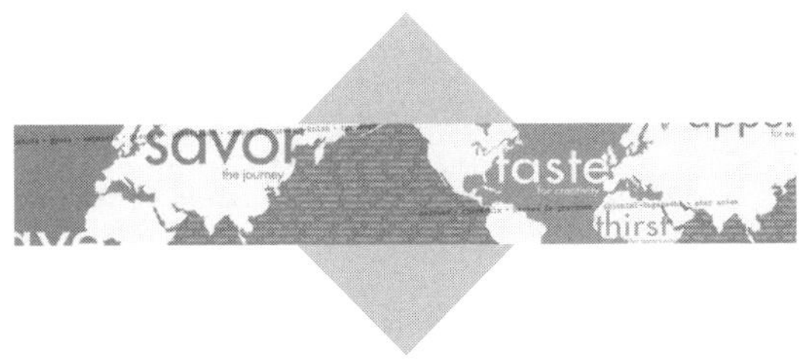

# Yangchow (Yangzhou) Fried Rice

SERVES 4

**This colorful fried rice may have started in Yangzhou, a city famous for Eastern cuisine, but many versions are found all over China. The original version was said to have at least eight ingredients and each grain of rice coated with egg!**

**Chef Tip** **Always marinate dark meat with whole egg.**

| AMOUNT | MEASURE | INGREDIENT |
|---|---|---|
| 1 cup | 6 ounces, 168 g | Boneless, skinless chicken thigh meat, cut $\frac{1}{2}$ inch (1.2 cm) dice |
| 9 tablespoons | $3\frac{1}{2}$ ounces, 105 ml | Vegetable oil |
| $\frac{3}{4}$ cup | 4 ounces, 112 g | Shrimp, raw, dice $\frac{1}{2}$ inch (1.2 cm). |
| $\frac{3}{4}$ cup | 4 ounces, 112 g | Cantonese roast pork (*char siu*), dice $\frac{1}{2}$ inch (1.2 cm). |
| $\frac{3}{4}$ cup | 4 ounces, 112 g | Chinese Ham |
| 3 | | Black mushrooms, soaked in hot water until soft. Trim stems and squeeze to extract moisture, dice $\frac{1}{2}$ inch (1.2 cm). |
| 2 | | Eggs and 1 egg yolk, beaten with a pinch of salt |
| 2 tablespoons | 1 ounce, 28 g | Carrots, $\frac{1}{2}$ inch (1.2 cm) dice, blanched |
| $\frac{1}{4}$ cup | 2 ounces, 56 g | Green peas, cooked |
| 3 cups | 12 ounces, 336 g | Cold cooked rice, grains separated |
| 4 | | Green onions, $\frac{1}{4}$ inch (.6 cm) lengths |
| Marinade for Chicken | | |
| 2 tablespoons | 1 ounce, 30 ml | Water |
| $\frac{1}{2}$ teaspoon | | Salt |
| 1 | | Egg whole |
| 1 tablespoon | $\frac{1}{2}$ ounce, 15 ml | Dry, sherry |
| To taste | | White pepper |
| 1 tablespoon | | Tapioca powder or cornstarch |
| 1 tablespoon | | Oil |
| 1 teaspoon | | Sesame oil |

| AMOUNT | MEASURE | INGREDIENT |
|---|---|---|
| **Marinade for Shrimp** | | |
| **2 tablespoons** | **1 ounce, 30 ml** | **Water** |
| **$\frac{1}{2}$ teaspoon** | | **Salt** |
| **1** | | **Egg white** |
| **1 tablespoon** | **$\frac{1}{2}$ ounce, 15 ml** | **Sherry, dry** |
| **1 tablespoon** | **$\frac{1}{2}$ ounce, 15 ml** | **Vegetable oil** |
| **1 tablespoon** | **$\frac{1}{2}$ ounce, 15 ml** | **Sesame oil** |
| **To taste** | | **White pepper** |
| **1 tablespoon** | | **Tapioca powder or cornstarch** |
| **1 tablespoon** | | **Oil** |

**PROCEDURE**

1. In separate containers, combine the ingredients for the chicken marinade and shrimp marinade; mix well. Add the diced chicken thigh meat to the chicken marinade; toss to coat, chill for 30 minutes. Add the shrimp to the shrimp marinade; toss to coat, chill 30 minutes.
2. Set wok over high heat. When very hot, add two tablespoons (1 ounce, 30 ml) oil. Add chicken, stirring constantly until separated and just cooked (no longer pink). Remove and reserve.
3. Heat one tablespoon oil in wok, over high heat. When oil is hot, add the pork and mushrooms. Stir 1 minute, add ham, stir 30 seconds. Add green peas and carrots, stir-fry 15 seconds. Remove and reserve with chicken and shrimp.
4. Rinse wok and wipe dry. Set over high heat; when wok is hot, add remaining oil. Scramble the eggs until set, and turn heat to medium. Break the scrambled eggs in the wok into small pieces; about the same size as the chicken. Add the rice and sprinkle with salt. Stir-fry the rice, about 5 to 7 minutes.
5. Return all cooked items to the wok and stir-fry to mix with rice.
6. Add green onions, and correct seasoning with $\frac{1}{4}$ teaspoon sesame oil, white pepper and salt.

# Shanghai Sweet-and-Sour Spareribs

SERVES 4

| AMOUNT | MEASURE | INGREDIENT |
|---|---|---|
| $\frac{1}{2}$ teaspoon | | Salt |
| 1 tablespoon | $\frac{1}{2}$ ounce, 15 ml | Dry sherry or rice wine |
| 1 teaspoon | | Tapioca powder or cornstarch |
| 1 pound | 448 g | Pork spareribs cut $\frac{1}{2}$ inch wide by 1 inch in length (1.2 cm x 2.4 cm), silver skin removed (or substitute pork chops) |
| $\frac{1}{4}$ cup | 2 ounces, 60 ml | Vegetable oil |
| Sauce | | |
| $\frac{1}{3}$ cup | 2.3 ounces, 64 g | Granulated sugar |
| 3 tablespoons | 1$\frac{1}{2}$ ounces, 45 ml | Rice wine vinegar |
| 2 tablespoons | 1 ounce, 30 ml | Soy sauce |
| 1 tablespoon | $\frac{1}{2}$ ounce, 15 ml | Tomato catsup |
| 1 teaspoon | | Tapioca powder or cornstarch |

PROCEDURE

1. Combine salt, sherry, and tapioca powder, and mix well. Add sparerib pieces, toss to coat, and marinate for minimum of 30 minutes.
2. Heat oil in a wok over medium heat to about 350°F (176°C) or until a piece of green onion dropped in oil bubbles, sizzles, and moves around.
3. Add the spareribs and deep-fry until crisp, stirring to keep them from sticking together, 5 to 7 minutes. Remove from oil and drain on paper towels.
4. Reset empty wok on medium high heat. Stir sauce ingredients to blend, pour into wok, and cook, stirring, until thickened. Return pork to wok and stir well until each piece is coated with sauce. Serve hot.

# Bean Curd in Oyster Sauce

SERVES 4

| AMOUNT | MEASURE | INGREDIENT |
|---|---|---|
| 2 tablespoons | 1 ounce, 30 ml | Oil |
| 2 | | Green onion, white and greens separated, minced |
| 1 1/4 cups | 8 ounces, 224 | Semi-firm bean curd (tofu), soaked in hot water 15 minutes, drained, dried, cut into 1 inch (2.4 cm) cubes |
| Sauce | | |
| 1 tablespoon | 1/2 ounce, 15 ml | Oyster sauce |
| 1/2 tablespoon | 1/4 ounce, 8 ml | Soy sauce |
| 1 tablespoon | 1/2 ounce, 15 ml | Dry sherry |
| To taste | | Salt |
| 2 tablespoons | 1 ounce, 30 ml | Chicken stock |

PROCEDURE

1. Combine sauce ingredients.
2. Heat wok over high heat; when hot add oil and swirl. When the oil is just below the smoke point, add the white parts of the green onions; stir-fry 10 seconds.
3. Add the tofu and stir-fry 1 minute, turning gently to coat with oil and onions.
4. Add sauce ingredients; Bring to boil, reduce to simmer and cook 2 minutes.
5. Add green onions tops; toss and serve.

# Tea and Spice Smoked Quail with Sweet-and-Sour Cucumbers

SERVES 4

| AMOUNT | MEASURE | INGREDIENT |
|---|---|---|
| 2 | | Quail, semi-boneless |
| | | Sweet-and-sour cucumbers (recipe follows) |
| **Seasoning Salt** | | |
| 1 tablespoon | 10 g | Sea salt |
| ½ teaspoon | 2 g | Toasted Sechuan pepper, ground |
| 1½ teaspoons | 5 g | Five-spice powder |
| 1 cup | 8 ounces, 240 ml | Vegetable oil |
| **Smoking Mixture** | | |
| ½ cup | 3½ ounces, 98 g | Long-grain rice |
| 3 pieces | | Dry mandarin peel |
| 1 piece | | Cassia bark |
| 1 ounce | 28 g | Jasmine tea leaves |
| 1½ ounces | 42 g | Brown sugar |
| 3 | | Star anise |

## PROCEDURE

1. Combine seasoning salt ingredients and rub on quail; marinate 30 minutes.
2. Combine smoking mixture ingredients. Line bottom of a wok with foil. Place smoking mixture on foil and place over high heat.
3. Place a rack in the wok and cover until it begins to smoke. Reduce heat and place quail on rack. Cover and smoke quail, 2–3 minutes. Watch to ensure quail is cooked only to rare. Remove quail and hold until ready to serve.
4. Set wok over high heat. Heat oil to 350°F (176°C°). Deep-fry quail until golden brown and crispy, 3–4 minutes. Serve with sweet-and-sour cucumbers.

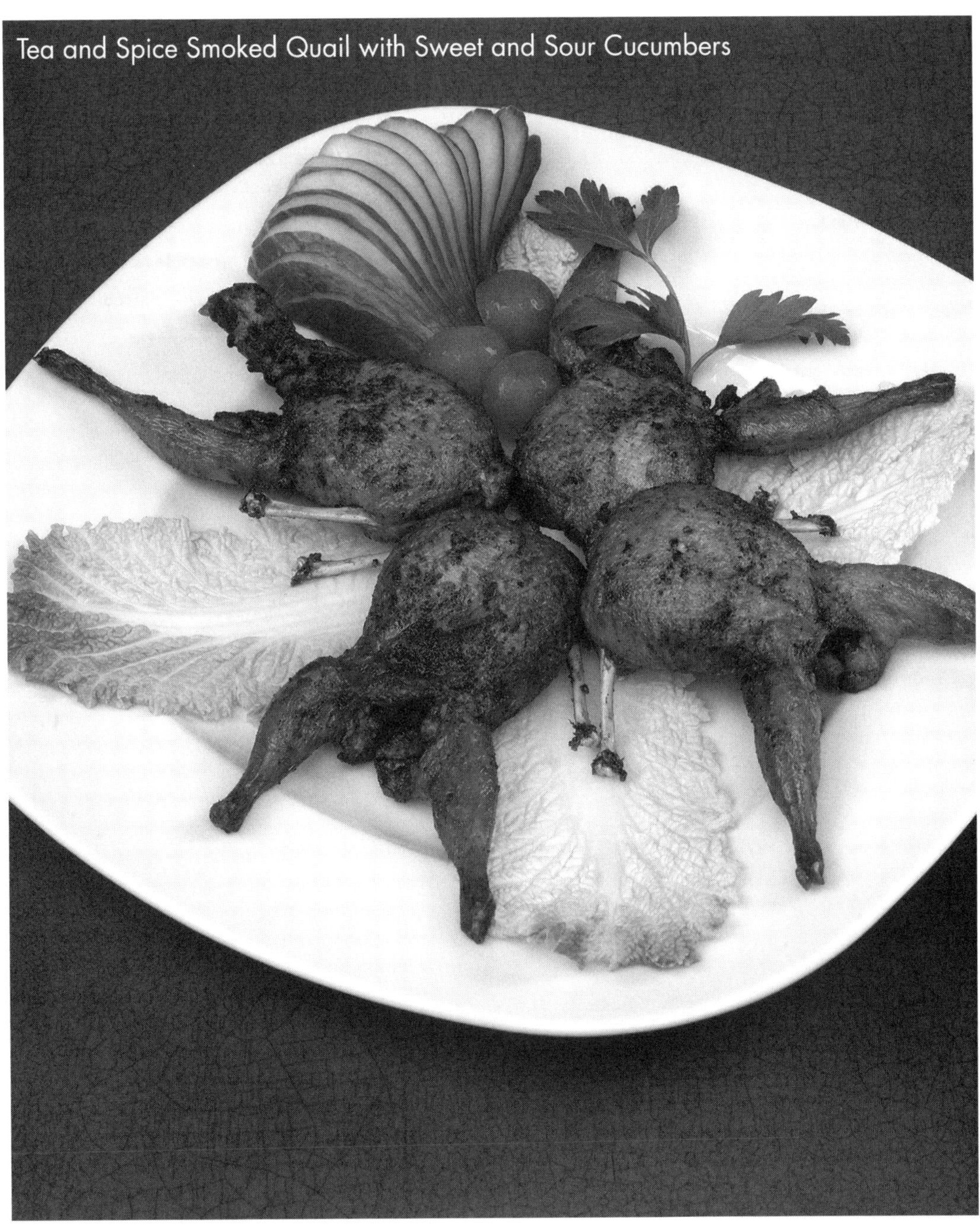

Tea and Spice Smoked Quail with Sweet and Sour Cucumbers

# Sweet-and-Sour Cucumbers

**SERVES 4**

| AMOUNT | MEASURE | INGREDIENT |
|---|---|---|
| 2 cups | 12 ounces, 336 g | English cucumber, julienned |
| Dressing | | |
| 2 | | Thai bird chile (small red), finely slice |
| 2 | | Garlic clove, minced |
| 3 tablespoons | $1\frac{1}{2}$ ounces, 45 ml | Rice wine vinegar |
| 4 teaspoons | 40 ml | Water |
| 2 teaspoons | 20 g | Granulated sugar |
| $\frac{1}{2}$ teaspoon | | Salt |

**PROCEDURE**

1 Combine all dressing ingredients; mix well to dissolve sugar. Toss cucumbers with dressing; let sit 30 minutes before serving.

# Ma-Puo (Mapo) Doufu

SERVES 4

| AMOUNT | MEASURE | INGREDIENT |
|---|---|---|
| 2 tablespoons | 1 ounce, 30 ml | Dark soy sauce |
| 2 tablespoons | 1 ounce, 30 ml | Shaoxing wine or dry sherry |
| 2 tablespoons | 1 ounce, 30 ml | Fermented chile bean paste |
| 1 cup | 8 ounces, 224 g | Pork, lean ground |
| $1\frac{1}{4}$ cups | 10 ounces, 300 ml | Chicken stock |
| 4 tablespoons | 2 ounces, 60 ml | Vegetable oil |
| 2 tablespoons | | Ginger, grated |
| 2 | | Garlic cloves, minced |
| 2 | | Green onions, white part, sliced thinly |
| 1 pound | 448 g | Tofu, semi-firm, blanch in hot water for 3 minutes, then cut $\frac{1}{2}$ inch (1.2 cm) cubes |
| 1 teaspoon | | Sichuan peppercorns, toasted and cracked finely, or 1 teaspoon ground in spice mill |
| 2 tablespoons | 1 ounce, 30 ml | Water |
| 1 tablespoon | | Tapioca powder or cornstarch |
| 1 teaspon | | Sesame oil |
| 1 tablespoon | | Cilantro, chopped |

PROCEDURE

1. Combine half the soy sauce, half the wine, bean paste, and pork. Mix well.
2. Combine remaining soy sauce and wine with chicken stock.
3. Set wok over high heat; when very hot, add oil. Add pork mixture; cook, stirring, to separate the grains of meat, about 30 seconds. Add ginger, garlic, and green onion; stir-fry 1 minute. Add chicken stock; cook 1 minute.
4. Add bean curd. Stir mixture gently; the bean curd breaks easily. Cook just to heat through, about 1 minute. Sprinkle Sichuan peppercorns over the mixture.
5. Blend water and tapioca powder and add, stirring gently to thicken. When dish is thickened, add sesame oil and transfer to serving dish and garnish with cilantro.

# Sichuan Stuffed Eggplant

SERVES 4

**Chef tip** The cornstarch between the eggplant slices helps to maintain the positioning of the ground pork.

| AMOUNT | MEASURE | INGREDIENT |
|---|---|---|
| ½ cup | 4 ounces, 112 g | Lean ground pork |
| 1 tablespoon | ½ ounce, 15 ml | Soy sauce |
| As needed for coating | | Cornstarch |
| 2 | | Eggs |
| ⅛ teaspoon | | White pepper |
| 3 | | Japanese eggplant, 6 ounces (168 g) each |
| 2 | | Eggs |
| ⅛ teaspoon | | Salt |
| 4 cups plus 1 tablespoon | 32½ ounces, 975 ml | Vegetable oil |
| 1 teaspoon | | Sesame oil |
| Seasoning | | |
| 1 tablespoon | ½ ounce, 15 ml | Soy sauce |
| 1 teaspoon | | Dry sherry |
| ¼ teaspoon | | Granulated sugar |
| 2 tablespoons | | Ginger, grated |
| 1 tablespoon | | Garlic, minced |
| 2 teaspoons | | Tapioca powder or cornstarch |
| 2 tablespoons | | Green onion, white part, minced |
| 1 teaspoon | | Sesame oil |
| Sauce for glazing | | |
| ½ cup | 4 ounces, 120 ml | Chicken stock |
| 1 tablespoon | ½ ounce, 15 ml | Sichuan hot bean paste |
| 2 teaspoons | 10 ml | Dark soy sauce |
| 1 tablespoon | ½ ounce, 15 ml | Rice vinegar |
| 1 tablespoon | ½ ounce, 15 ml | Brown sugar |

**PROCEDURE**

1. Combine pork with the soy sauce from the seasoning. Mix with your fingers, scooping up pork mixture with your hand and beating it back into the bowl several times until firm. Add the remaining seasoning and mix well.
2. Cut eggplant into $\frac{3}{4}$- to 1-inch (1.8 cm to 2.4 cm) pieces using a vertical slope-cut. Make a slit down the center of each slice and cut two thirds of the way down, forming double-layer slices with skin side not cut all the way through. Gently open up the double layer and brush the inside surface lightly with cornstarch. Slice and brush the remaining pieces the same way, noting that they are not uniform in size but in thickness only.
3. Stuff about one tablespoon of pork mixture into each piece of eggplant. Then dip the back of a spoon in a little water and smooth the pork mixture.
4. Mix the glazing sauce ingredients; set aside.
5. About 10 minutes before cooking, beat eggs with $\frac{1}{8}$ teaspoon salt until smooth. Dip each piece of stuffed eggplant into the egg mixture, then coat with cornstarch. Shake off excess cornstarch.
6. Set a wok over high heat. When hot, add 4 cups oil. Heat oil to 375°F (190°C), or until a piece of green onion or ginger sizzles noisily and quickly turns brown.
7. Add the eggplant pieces in succession to the oil; deep-fry until the coating is set, then remove. Reheat oil to very hot 400°F (204°C) and return all eggplant pieces to the oil. Deep-fry until golden, then remove and drain on paper towels.
8. Set in a separate wok or pan over high heat. When hot, add remaining tablespoon oil. Stir the glazing sauce and add it to the wok. Bring to a boil, glaze sauce with sesame oil.
9. Plate hot eggplant and glaze with sauce. Eggplant should be glazed within a minute or two after frying.

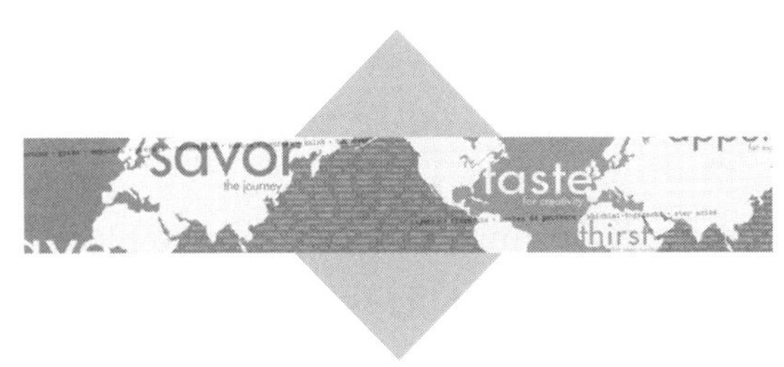

# Kung Pao Chicken

SERVES 4

| AMOUNT | MEASURE | INGREDIENT |
|---|---|---|
| **Marinade** | | |
| 1 tablespoon | $\frac{1}{2}$ ounce, 15 ml | Soy sauce |
| 1 teaspoon | | Chinese rice wine or dry sherry |
| 2 teaspoons | | Cold water |
| 1 | | Egg |
| 1 tablespoon | $\frac{1}{2}$ ounce, 15 ml | Vegetable oil |
| 2 teaspoons | | Tapioca powder or cornstarch |
| **Sauce** | | |
| 1 tablespoon | $\frac{1}{2}$ ounce, 15 ml | Dark soy sauce |
| 2 teaspoons | | Light soy sauce |
| 1 tablespoon | $\frac{1}{2}$ ounce, 15 ml | Rice vinegar |
| 1 tablespoon | $\frac{1}{2}$ ounce, 15 ml | Chicken stock |
| 1 tablespoon | $\frac{1}{2}$ ounce, 14 g | Granulated sugar |
| $\frac{1}{2}$ teaspoon | | Salt |
| $\frac{1}{2}$ teaspoon | | Sesame oil |
| 1 teaspoon | | Tapioca powder or cornstarch |
| **Other ingredients** | | |
| 2 cups | 12 ounces, 336 g | Chicken thigh meat, cut $\frac{1}{2}$ inch (1.2 cm) cubes |
| 3 cups | 24 ounces, 720 ml | Vegetable oil |
| 12 | | Dried red chile peppers, whole |
| 2 | | Garlic cloves, minced |
| $\frac{1}{8}$ teaspoon | | Sichuan peppercorns, ground |
| $\frac{1}{2}$ cup | $2\frac{1}{2}$ ounces, 70 g | Unsalted peanuts |

PROCEDURE

1 Combine marinade ingredients; mix well. Add chicken pieces and marinate 30 minutes.

2 Combine all sauce ingredients, whisking in tapioca powder last.

3 Set a wok over high heat. Heat the 3 cups oil to 350°F (176°C) or until a piece of green onion dropped in oil bubbles, sizzles, and moves around. Carefully slide the chicken into the wok; fry for 3–4 minute, until the cubes separate and turn white. Remove and drain on paper towels. Remove all but one tablespoons ($\frac{1}{2}$ ounce, 315 ml) of oil from the wok.

4 Heat oil, add chiles, and stir-fry until the skin starts turn dark red and chilies plump. Add garlic; stir-fry until you smell the garlic aroma, 10 seconds, add Sichuan peppercorn.

5 Return chicken to wok; stir-fry 30 seconds. Stir the sauce, and pour into the center. Toss with chicken, cook until sauce thickens, add the peanuts, and mix well. Serve hot.

# Stir-Fried Long Beans

SERVES 4

| AMOUNT | MEASURE | INGREDIENT |
|---|---|---|
| **1 pound** | **16 ounces, 448 g** | **Long beans, cut 2 inch (5 cm) pieces** |
| **4 tablespoons** | **2 ounces, 60 ml** | **Vegetable oil** |
| **1 tablespoon** | | **Garlic, minced** |
| **1 tablespoon** | | **Ginger, grated** |
| **$\frac{1}{2}$ teaspoon** | | **Sesame oil** |
| **$\frac{1}{2}$ teaspoon** | | **Rice vinegar** |
| **To taste** | | **Salt and white pepper** |

PROCEDURE

1 Wash beans, trim the ends, and cut diagonally into 2 inch (2 cm) pieces.

2 Blanch the beans in boiling salted water, remove, shock in ice water, drain, and set aside.

3 Set wok over high heat; when very hot, add oil. Swirl around wok, add garlic and ginger, and stir-fry 30 seconds.

4 Add long beans and stir-fry 1 to 2 minutes. Glaze with sesame oil, add vinegar, and correct seasoning.

# Dan Dan Mian Spicy Noodles

**SERVES 4**

| AMOUNT | MEASURE | INGREDIENT |
|---|---|---|
| 1 tablespoon | $\frac{1}{2}$ ounce, 14 g | Dried shrimp |
| $\frac{3}{4}$ cup | 6 ounces, 180 ml | Hot water |
| $\frac{1}{4}$ cup | 2 ounces, 56 g | Sichuan preserved vegetables |
| 6 tablespoons | 3 ounces, 90 ml | Vegetable oil |
| 4 cups | 32 ounces, 960 ml | Chicken stock |
| 1 pound | | Asian noodles, or 12 ounces dried Asian noodles (width between linguine and fettuccine), or 12 ounces linguine |
| 4 | | Green onions, whole |
| 1 tablespoon | | Sesame seeds |
| Dan Dan Sauce | | |
| 2 tablespoons | 1 ounce, 30 ml | Dark soy sauce |
| 2 tablespoons | 1 ounce, 30 ml | Light soy sauce |
| 1 tablespoon | $\frac{1}{2}$ ounce, 15 ml | Rice vinegar |
| 2 tablespoons | 1 ounce, 30 ml | Sesame paste |
| 1 tablespoon | $\frac{1}{2}$ ounce, 15 ml | Chile oil |
| 2 tablespoons | 1 ounce, 30 ml | Sesame oil |
| 1 tablespoon | $\frac{1}{2}$ ounce, 14 g | Granulated sugar |

**PROCEDURE**

1. Soak shrimp in hot water 20 minutes. Chop finely and reserve soaking liquid.
2. Rinse chile and spices off the preserved vegetables; chop finely.
3. Toast the sesame seeds until golden; set aside.
4. Mix ingredients for the dan dan sauce until smooth.
5. Set wok or heavy saucepan over medium high heat. When very hot, add one tablespoon ($\frac{1}{2}$ ounce, 15 ml) oil. Add shrimp; stir for 2 minutes or until oil is well flavored. Add the preserved vegetables; stir-fry 1 minute. Remove from heat.
6. Combine the dan dan sauce ingredients, the shrimp mixture, and 2 tablespoons (1 ounce, 30 ml) oil. Set aside.
7. Heat chicken stock and shrimp soaking liquid over very low heat.

8 Cook noodles following directions. Strain, shake the colander to drain excess water, and toss with remaining oil.

9 Serve the dan dan sauce in 4 separate bowls and place $\frac{1}{4}$ of the hot noodles on sauce. Sprinkle chopped green onions and sesame seeds on top. Serve with chicken/shrimp stock in separate bowls.

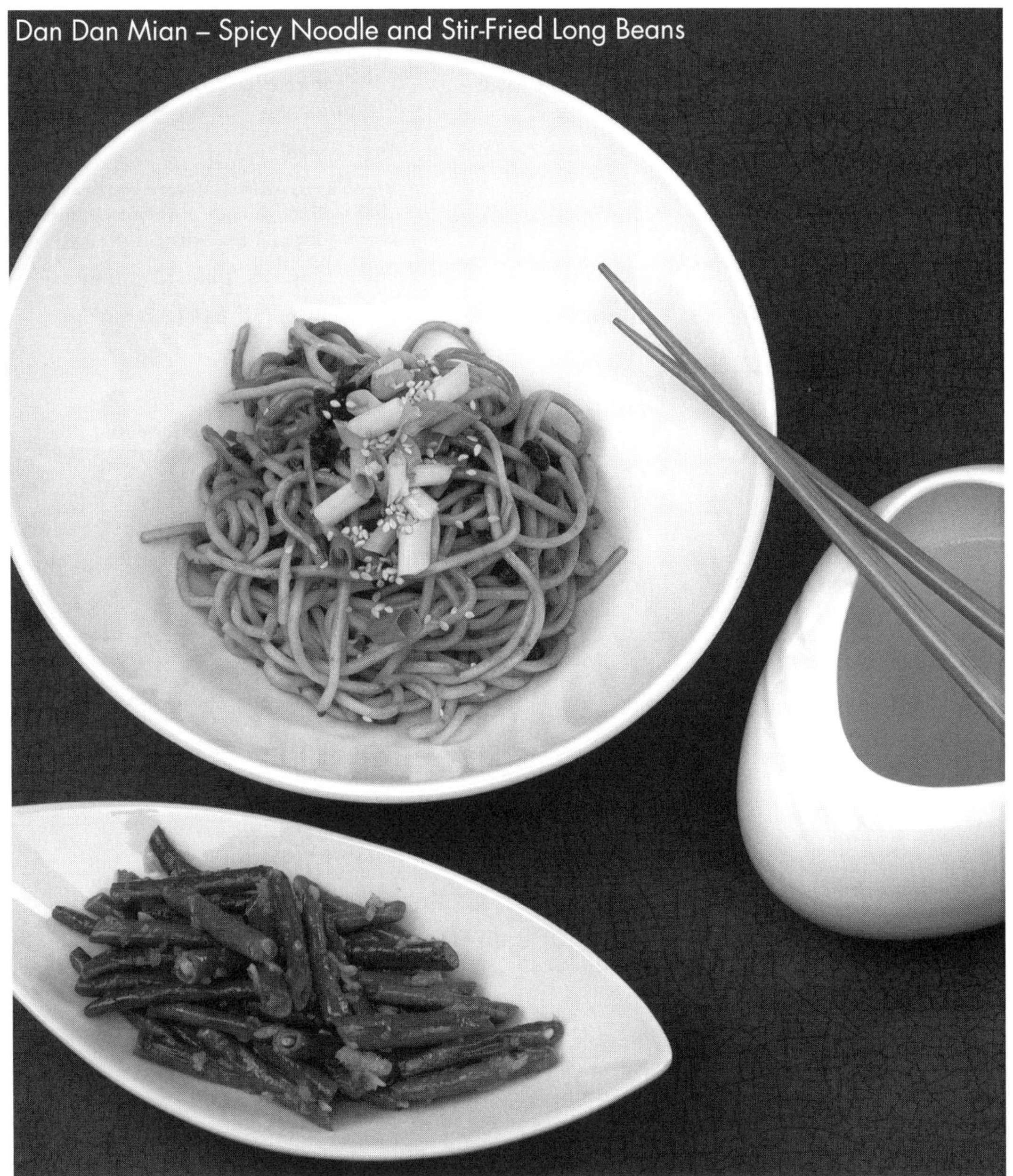
Dan Dan Mian – Spicy Noodle and Stir-Fried Long Beans

# Fish-Flavored Pork Shreds

SERVES 4

**There is no fish in this dish from fish-starved Sichuan. The flavor is adapted from the sauce used in braising fish.**

| AMOUNT | MEASURE | INGREDIENT |
|---|---|---|
| 1 $\frac{1}{2}$ cups | 12 ounces, 336 g | Pork, cut from loin, trimmed of excess fat, $\frac{1}{8}$ × $\frac{1}{8}$ × 2 inch (.3 × .3 × 4.8 cm) shreds |
| 2 cups plus 2 tablespoons | 17 ounces, 510 ml | Vegetable oil |
| 8 medium | | Wood ears, soaked in warm water 30 minutes until soft, tough ends trimmed; cut into strips, about $\frac{1}{8}$ inch (.3 cm) wide |
| $\frac{1}{4}$ cup | 2 ounces, 56 g | Water chestnuts, $\frac{1}{8}$ inch (.3 cm) strips |
| $\frac{1}{4}$ cup | 2 ounces, 56 g | Bamboo shoots, $\frac{1}{8}$ inch (.3 cm) strip |
| 1 tablespoon | | Carrots, $\frac{1}{8}$ inch (.3 cm) strips |
| To taste | | Salt |
| 2 tablespoons | | Green onions, white part, minced |
| 1 tablespoon | | Ginger, grated |
| 1 tablespoon | | Garlic clove, minced |
| 1 tablespoon | $\frac{1}{2}$ ounce, 15 ml | Dry sherry |
| 2 teaspoons | | Sesame oil |
| Seasoning | | |
| 2 tablespoons | 1 ounce, 30 ml | Dark soy sauce |
| 1 tablespoon | | Tapioca powder or cornstarch |
| Sauce mixture | | |
| 1 tablespoon | $\frac{1}{2}$ ounce, 15 ml | Sichuan hot bean paste |
| 1 tablespoon | $\frac{1}{2}$ ounce, 15 ml | Rice vinegar |
| 1 tablespoon | $\frac{1}{2}$ ounce, 15 ml | Dark soy sauce |
| 2 teaspoons | 10 ml | Granulated sugar |
| 1 teaspoon | | Tapioca powder or cornstarch |

PROCEDURE

1 Mix ingredients for sauce mixture; set aside. Mix seasoning ingredients and combine with pork.

2 Set wok over high heat; when very hot, add 2 cups (16 ounces, 360 ml) oil. Heat oil to 375°F (190°C), or until a piece of green onion or ginger sizzles noisily and quickly turns brown. Add the pork shreds, stirring to separate; stir-fry 1 minute. Pour both meat and oil into strainer-lined bowl to drain, leaving about 1 tablespoon ($\frac{1}{2}$ ounce, 15 ml) oil in wok.

3 Place wok over medium high heat and add the wood ears, water chestnuts, bamboo shoots and carrots stirring for 1 minute. Season with salt, stir, and remove.

4 Add remaining two tablespoons (1 ounce, 30 ml) oil to the wok. When the oil is hot, add green onions, ginger, and garlic. Stir for 10 seconds, then return pork to wok. Sizzle in the sherry along the edge of the wok, stirring constantly. Add wood ears, water chestnuts, bamboo shoots, and carrots.

5 Stir sauce mixture and add to the center of the wok, stirring until thickened. Glaze sauce with sesame oil, mix well, and serve.

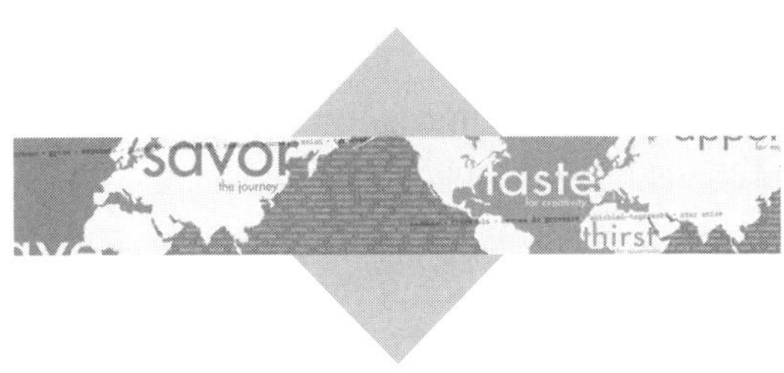

# Sichuan Spicy Fired Beef Shreds

SERVES 4

| AMOUNT | MEASURE | INGREDIENT |
|---|---|---|
| 1 pound | 16 ounces, 448 g | Flank steak, $\frac{1}{8} \times \frac{1}{8} \times 1\frac{1}{2}$ inch (.3 x .3 x 3.6 cm) shreds |
| $\frac{1}{2}$ cup/1 tablespoon | $4\frac{1}{2}$ ounces, 135 ml | Vegetable oil |
| 2 | | Garlic cloves, flattened |
| 3 | | Dried hot chiles, seeds removed |
| 1 cup | 4 ounces, 112 g | Celery, $\frac{1}{8} \times \frac{1}{8} \times 1\frac{1}{2}$ inch (.3 x .3 x 3.6 cm) shreds |
| $\frac{1}{2}$ cup | 2 ounces, 56 g | Carrot, peeled, $\frac{1}{8} \times \frac{1}{8} \times 1\frac{1}{2}$ inch (.3 x .3 x 3.6 cm) shreds |
| 3 | | Fresh hot chiles, $\frac{1}{8} \times \frac{1}{8} \times 1\frac{1}{2}$ inch (.3 x .3 x 3.6 cm) shreds |
| To taste | | Salt |
| 1 tablespoon | | Sesame oil |
| Marinade | | |
| 4 tablespoons | 2 ounces, 60 ml | Dark soy sauce |
| | | Juice of 3 slices gingerroot |
| 1 tablespoon | $\frac{1}{2}$ ounce, 15 ml | Dry sherry |
| 2 teaspoons | 10 g | Granulated sugar |

PROCEDURE

1 Mix marinade ingredients, add the meat, and toss. Let sit at room temperature for at least 30 minutes. Turn the meat occasionally.

2 Set wok over high heat; when very hot add $\frac{1}{2}$ cup (4 ounces, 120 ml) oil. Flavor the oil with the garlic; remove the garlic when it turns brown.

3 Add meat; stir-fry 1 to 2 minutes, or until strips separate. Turn heat to medium low; continue to stir-fry until strips turn brown, 1 to 2 minutes; remove from wok.

4 Rinse wok and wipe dry. Set on medium high heat; when hot, add sesame oil. Flavor oil with dried chile until brown. Add celery, carrots, and fresh chiles, stirring 30 seconds to 1 minute; season with salt.

5 Return meat and mix with vegetables. Glaze the meat with sesame oil and serve with rice.

# Spinach Velvet Soup

SERVES 4

**This soup does not reheat well. Do not prepare too far in advance or it will lose its beautiful bright green color.**

| AMOUNT | MEASURE | INGREDIENT |
|---|---|---|
| 3 cups | 6 ounces, 180 g | Spinach, leaves loosely packed |
| 2 teaspoons | | Granulated sugar |
| 2 | | Egg whites |
| 1 tablespoon | $\frac{1}{2}$ ounce, 15 ml | Water |
| 3 tablespoons | | Tapioca powder or cornstarch |
| $3\frac{1}{2}$ cups | 28 ounces, 840 ml | Chicken stock |
| 1 tablespoon | | Ginger juice |
| 2 tablespoons | | Smithfield ham, $\frac{1}{4}$ inch (.6 cm) dice |
| 1 teaspoon | | Sesame oil |
| $1\frac{1}{2}$ tablespoons | $\frac{3}{4}$ ounce, 20 ml | Vegetable oil |
| To taste | | Salt and white pepper |

PROCEDURE

1. Remove stems from spinach, rinse thoroughly, and drain.
2. Heat 2 quarts (1.9 l) water to a boil; add sugar and spinach, stirring until water boils again. Immediately drain in a colander, running cold water over the spinach to stop the cooking process.
3. Squeeze spinach leaves to extract as much water as possible. Julienne finely; do not use a blender.
4. Beat egg whites with water until smooth but not foamy.
5. Mix tapioca powder and $\frac{1}{4}$ cup (2 ounces, 60 ml) stock.
6. Heat remaining stock over high heat, bring to a boil, and reduce heat to medium. Add half the ham and ginger juice and cook 4 minutes. Turn heat to high and add the spinach, stirring until it returns to a boil.
7. Season soup and add the tapioca powder mixture. Stir until the soup thickens (creamy).
8. Remove from heat and whirl in the egg whites. Do not stir for 30 seconds, then stir to mix. Add sesame oil and vegetable oil.
9. Pour soup into bowls and garnish with remaining ham. Adjust seasoning. Serve immediately.

# Char Siu Cantonese Roast Pork

SERVES 4

| AMOUNT | MEASURE | INGREDIENT |
|---|---|---|
| 1 ½ pounds | 672 g | Lean pork butt (trimmed weight) |
| 1 | | Carrot, cut into 2 inch (4.8 cm) lengths, then cut in half vertically |
| ¼ cup | 2 ounces, 60 ml | Honey |
| 2 tablespoon | 1 ounce, 30 | Mirin wine |
| 1 tablespoon | ½ ounce, 15 ml | Sesame oil |
| Marinade | | |
| ¼ cup | 2 ounces, 60 ml | Dry sherry |
| 2 | | Garlic cloves, crushed |
| 3 tablespoons | 1 ½ ounces, 45 ml | Light soy sauce |
| 1 tablespoon | ½ ounce, 15 ml | Sesame paste |
| 1 tablespoon | 1 ounce, 30 ml | Brown bean paste |
| 2 tablespoons | 1 ounce, 30 ml | Hoisin sauce |
| 1 teaspoon | | Salt |
| ½ teaspoon | | Five-spice powder |
| ¼ cup | 2 ounces, 56 g | Granulated sugar |

PROCEDURE

1. Trim fat from meat and cut into 1 × 1 × 8 inch strips (2.4 × 2.4 × 20 cm).
2. Combine all marinade, ingredients; mix well. Add pork and toss to cover with marinade. Cover and set at room temperature for at least 1 hour or refrigerate 3 hours or overnight. Turn every 30 minutes or so.
3. Thread pieces of pork lengthwise on skewers, using pieces of carrots as the end pieces to keep the pork from sliding off.
4. Preheat oven to 375°F (190°C). Fill a shallow roasting pan with 1 inch (2.4 cm) boiling water to catch dripping and to prevent smoking. Place pan on the lowest rack in the oven and hook skewers to the highest rack, each 2 inches (4.8 cm) apart. Roast meat for 40 minutes.
5. Turn oven to 450°F (232°C). Mix the honey and mirin. Remove skewers from oven and brush with honey mixture, then sesame oil.
6. Empty the water from the roasting pan and return to the oven. Hang the skewers as before and roast 10 minutes. Remove.

# Char Sui Bau Steamed Pork Buns

YIELD: 12 BUNS (DOUGH FOR UP TO 24 BUNS)

| AMOUNT | MEASURE | INGREDIENT |
|---|---|---|
| 1 cup | 8 ounces, 224 g | Char sui, $\frac{1}{4}$ inch (.6 cm) dice |
| **Seasoning** | | |
| 1 tablespoon | $\frac{1}{2}$ ounce, 15 ml | Oyster sauce |
| 2 tablespoons | 1 ounce, 28 g | Granulated sugar |
| 1$\frac{1}{2}$ tablespoons | 1$\frac{1}{2}$ ounce, 45 ml | Peanut oil |
| 1 teaspoon | | Sesame oil |
| **Bun Dough** | | |
| 1 tablespoon | $\frac{1}{2}$ ounce, 14 g | Granulated sugar |
| $\frac{1}{4}$ cup | 2 ounces, 60 ml | Warm water (105°F, 40.5°C) |
| 2$\frac{1}{4}$ teaspoons | $\frac{1}{4}$ ounce, 7 g | Active dry yeast |
| 4 cups | 16 ounces, 448 g | All-purpose flour |
| 2 tablespoons | 1 ounce, 28 g | Lard or shortening |
| $\frac{1}{2}$ cup | 4 ounces, 112 g | Extra-fine granulated sugar |
| 1 cup | 8 ounces, 240 ml | Milk, warm (105°F, 40.5°C) |
| 1 tablespoon | $\frac{1}{2}$ ounce, 15 ml | Oil |
| 1 tablespoon | | Baking powder mixed with 1$\frac{1}{2}$ tablespoons ($\frac{3}{4}$ ounce, 23 ml) water |
| **Filling Base** | | |
| 2 tablespoons | 1 ounce, 30 ml | Peanut oil |
| 2 teaspoons | | Shallots, minced |
| 1$\frac{1}{2}$ tablespoons | | All-purpose flour |
| 6 tablespoons | 3 ounces, 90 ml | Chicken stock |
| 1 tablespoon | $\frac{1}{2}$ ounce, 15 ml | Dark soy sauce |

PROCEDURE

**Filling**

1 Heat the oil over medium heat and sauté the shallots 2 minutes or until light brown. Add the flour, stir to combine, and cook 1 minute.

2 Add the chicken stock, stir well, and cook 2 minutes. Add soy sauce and cook one minute.

3 Remove from heat and stir in cut pork and seasoning ingredients. Chill until very firm.

**Dough**

1. Dissolve sugar in warm water, sprinkle yeast over; let stand for 2 to 3 minutes, and then stir to mix well. Let set until it starts of foam, 10 minutes.
2. Sift flour and make a well in the center. Combine lard, extra-fine sugar, yeast mixture, and milk; mix well. Combine liquid mixture with the flour; gradually incorporate the flour with the liquid to make dough.
3. Knead the dough for 10 minutes, sprinkling with flour as necessary.
4. Use the oil to grease the dough; cover and let rest in a warm area $1\frac{1}{2}$ hours or until double in size.
5. Punch dough down and flatten out to about $\frac{3}{4}$ inch (1.8 cm) thick. Spread the baking powder mixture evenly on the dough (this acts as a stabilizer). Roll dough up and knead about 15 minutes, or until smooth and satiny. The dough should be firmer than regular white bread dough.
6. Cover and let rest 30 minutes.

**Dough Breaking**

1. Divide dough into four equal parts. Roll one part by hand to form a rope approximately 9 (22.5 cm) inches long and $1\frac{1}{4}$ inchs in (3.12 cm) diameter.
2. Mark into 6 equal parts, $1\frac{1}{2}$-inch (3.75 cm) long.
3. Holding the dough with one hand, grip at the first mark with the thumb and index finger of the other hand and tear away briskly to break off a small dough piece. Continue breaking off until you have 12 pieces.

**Dough Rolling**

1. Flatten each piece of dough with your palm.
2. Using a rolling pin, roll each into a round disc, making a quarter turn with each roll.
3. Roll to leave the center thick; thinner edges are easier to pleat.

**Assembling**

1. Place about $1\frac{1}{2}$ tablespoons ($\frac{3}{4}$ ounce, 21 g) of filling at the center of each dough round, flat side up.
2. Gather the edges by first pleating counterclockwise, then twisting to seal securely.
3. Let rest, covered, for at least 30 minutes.

**Cooking**

1. Steam on high heat for 8 to 10 minutes. Do not uncover the steamer any time during the steaming. If a flat-lid steamer is used, wrap the lid with a kitchen towel to prevent condensed steam from dripping on the buns.

**Chef Tip** **Dough breaking instead of cutting is a traditional Cantonese practice in dim sum restaurants. The breaking leaves no sharp cutting edges, which would require longer time for the dough to round out.**

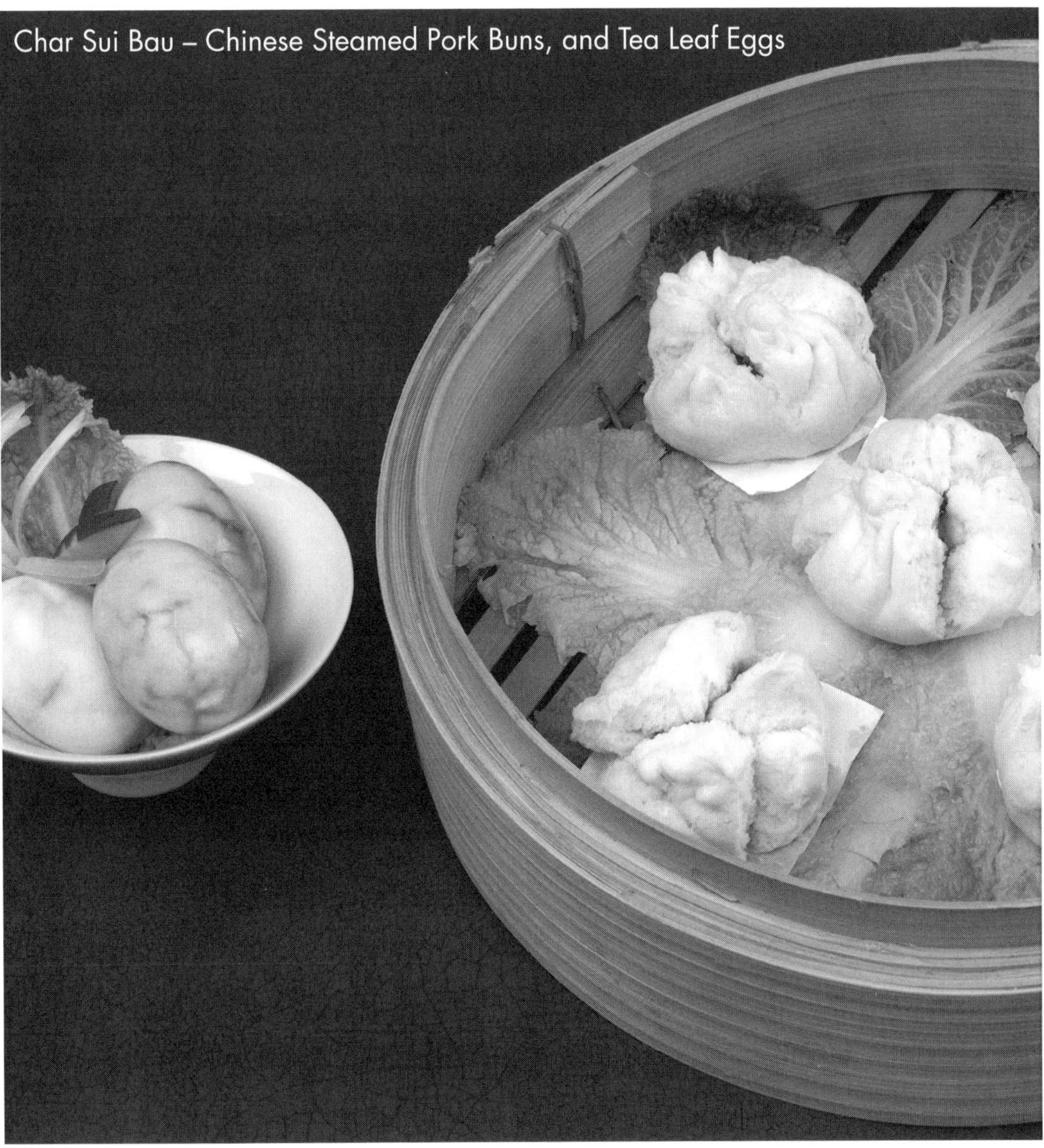

Char Sui Bau – Chinese Steamed Pork Buns, and Tea Leaf Eggs

# Stir-Fried Squid with Fermented Black Bean Paste

SERVES 4

**Chef Tip** Squid is cut (scored) because as it cooks it rolls up, and the crosshatching cuts will catch and hold the sauce.

| AMOUNT | MEASURE | INGREDIENT |
|---|---|---|
| 14 ounces | 392 g | Squid body meat, scored and cut into 1 inch (2.4 cm × 2.4 cm) cubes |
| 1 tablespoon | | Salt |
| 2 tablespoons | | Vegetable oil |
| 1 tablespoon | | Ginger, grated |
| 1 tablespoon | | Garlic clove, minced |
| 1 | | Red chile (hot) seeded, sliced thinly |
| 3 tablespoons | $1\frac{1}{2}$ ounces, 45 ml | Fermented black bean paste |
| 1 cup | 4 ounces, 112 g | Red bell peppers, seeded, 1 inch (2.4 cm) cubes |
| 1 cup | 4 ounces, 112 g | Onion, 1 inch (2.4 cm) cubes |
| 1 cup | 4 ounces, 112 g | Green bell peppers, seeded, 1 inch (2.4 cm) cubes |
| 2 tablespoons | 1 ounce, 30 ml | Shaoxing wine or dry sherry |
| 2 teaspoons | | Sesame oil |
| 1 tablespoon | | Cilantro, chopped |
| Sauce | | |
| 2 tablespoons | 1 ounce, 30 ml | Chicken stock |
| 2 teaspoons | | Tapioca powder or cornstarch |
| 1 tablespoon | $\frac{1}{2}$ ounce, 15 ml | Light soy sauce |

**PROCEDURE**

1 To clean squid, grip the head in one hand and the body in the other. Gently pull the head away from the body. The ink sac will come out at the same time. Pull out the yellow jelly pouch and the translucent center bone inside the body.

2 Reserve only the body for this recipe and discard the rest or keep the tentacles for some other use. Open up the body cavity and under running water rub the purplish outer skin with fingers, peeling it off. On larger squid, the skin tends to be tough when cooked.

3 Rub and squeeze the squid with salt; rinse and drain well.

4 Turn the inner side of a piece of squid up, scoring gently on the diagonal at $\frac{1}{4}$ inch (.6 cm) intervals, forming a diamond pattern.

5 Bring 6 cups (1.4 l) water to a boil. Remove from the heat and add the squid immediately. Stir once and pour into a colander to drain. Arrange in a single layer on paper towels and pat dry.

6 Prepare ingredients for sauce and set aside.

7 Set wok over high heat; when very hot; add the oil. Add the ginger, garlic, and chile; stir-fry for 10 seconds. Add the bean paste and cook 10 seconds. Add the bell peppers and onions; stir-fry 1 minute.

8 Add squid and stir-fry 45 seconds. Push squid and vegetables to the side, restir the sauce mixture, and add to the center of the wok, stirring until thickened. Sizzle in the wine along the edges, stir to mix all ingredients, and glaze with sesame oil.

9 Sprinkle with chopped cilantro, mix well, and serve.

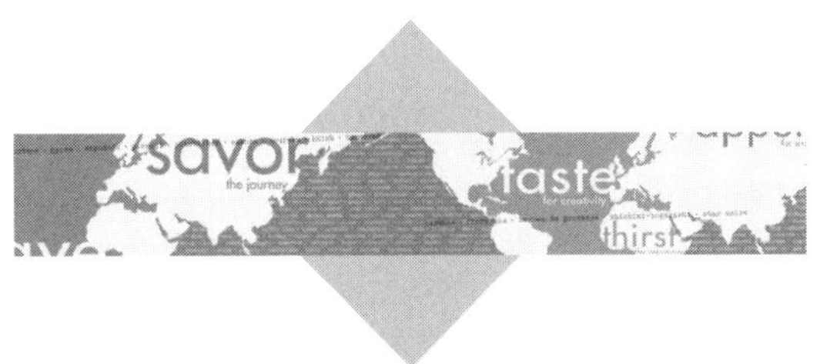

# Buddha's Delight

SERVES 4

**Adapted from *Louhan Zhai*, the vegetarian dish for the five hundred disciples sworn to protect the Buddhist way.**

| AMOUNT | MEASURE | INGREDIENT |
|---|---|---|
| 8 | | Medium dried shiitake mushrooms or fresh |
| $\frac{1}{2}$ cup | 3 ounces, 84 g | Bamboo shoots |
| $\frac{1}{2}$ cup | 2.5 ounces, 70 g | Firm tofu, 1 inch (2.4 cm) cubes |
| 1 slice | | Ginger |
| $\frac{1}{2}$ cup | 2 ounces, 56 g | Snow peas or sugar snap beans, strings removed, rinsed |
| $\frac{1}{2}$ cup | 2 ounces, 56 g | Carrots, julienned |
| $\frac{1}{4}$ cup | 2 ounces, 56 g | Water chestnuts, sliced thin |
| 1 cup | 4 ounces, 112 g | Napa cabbage, julienned |
| $\frac{1}{2}$ cup | 3 ounces, 84 g | Baby corn |
| $\frac{1}{2}$ cup | 2 ounces, 56 g | Red pepper, diamond cut |
| $\frac{1}{4}$ cup | 2 ounces, 56 g | Gingko nuts, drained and rinsed |
| 1 teaspoon | | Sesame oil |
| Seasoning | | |
| $1\frac{1}{2}$ teaspoons | | Granulated sugar |
| $\frac{1}{2}$ cup | 4 ounces, 120 ml | Chicken stock, vegetable stock, or water |
| $\frac{1}{2}$ teaspoon | | White pepper |
| 1 teaspoon | | Salt |
| Slurry | | |
| 2 tablespoons | 1 ounce, 30 ml | Water |
| 1 tablespoon | | Cornstarch |

**PROCEDURE**

1 If using dried mushrooms, soak them in $\frac{1}{2}$ cup (4 ounce, 120 ml) of warm water for about 15 minutes or until soft. Trim the stems and tough ends. Squeeze to extract moisture from shiitake. Reserve mushroom liquid; strain through cheesecloth.

2 Blanch all the vegetables individually in boiling water, rinse with cold water and reserve.

3 Cut the bamboo shoots finely into $\frac{1}{8} \times \frac{1}{8} \times 1\frac{1}{2}$ inch (.3 × .3 × 3.6 cm) shreds. Drain and pat dry with paper towel.

4 Set wok or heavy-bottomed pot over medium high heat. When hot, add 2 tablespoons (1 ounce, 30 ml) oil. Flavor oil with 1 garlic clove; remove garlic when brown. Add the shiitake, stirring for 1 minute.

5 Add remaining blanched vegetables, stir fry for 3 to 4 minutes

6 Add mushroom liquid and all seasoning and bring to boil.

7 Make a slurry by mixing water and cornstarch and add 1 to 2 tablespoons to vegetable mixture.

8 Add sesame oil and serve hot.

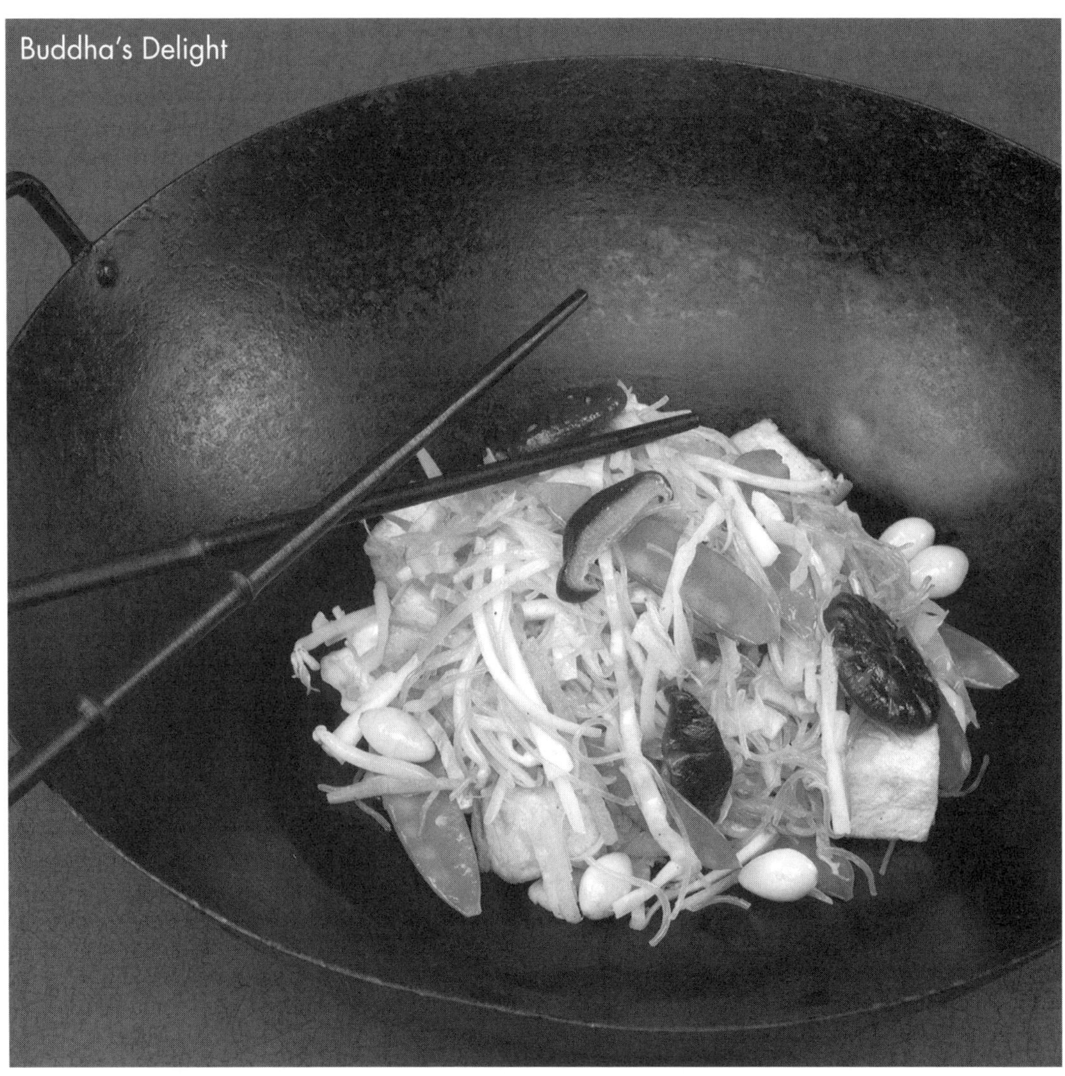
Buddha's Delight

# Fried Chicken Hong Kong Style

SERVES 4

| AMOUNT | MEASURE | INGREDIENT |
|---|---|---|
| 1 pound | 16 ounces, 448 g | Boneless, skinless chicken thighs |
| 6 cups plus 2 tablespoons | 49 ounces, 1.47 l | Vegetable oil |
| 1 | | Egg, lightly beaten |
| As needed | | Cornstarch and all-purpose flour mixed in 50:50 ratio |
| 1 cup | 4 ounces, 112 g | Onions, julienned |
| 1 tablespoon | | Garlic clove, minced |
| Marinade | | |
| 2 tablespoons | 1 ounce, 30 ml | Light soy sauce |
| 1 tablespoon | ½ ounce, 15 ml | Dry sherry |
| 1 teaspoon | | Ginger juice |
| Sauce | | |
| ½ cup | 4 ounces, 120 ml | Chicken stock |
| 2 tablespoons | 1 ounce, 30 ml | Tomato catsup |
| 2 tablespoons | 1 ounce, 30 ml | Worcestershire sauce |
| 1 tablespoon | ½ ounce, 15 ml | Lemon juice |
| 1 teaspoon | | Lemon zest |
| 1 tablespoon | | Tapioca powder or cornstarch |
| ¼ teaspoon | | Salt |
| 2 tablespoons | 1 ounce, 28 g | Brown sugar |

PROCEDURE

1. Remove any yellow film on chicken thighs; rinse and pat dry. Prick with a fork so marinade can penetrate.
2. Mix marinade ingredients, combine with chicken, and allow to rest at room temperature for 30 minutes or in refrigerator 2 to 3 hours. Drain and reserve marinade.
3. Combine marinade with sauce ingredients and set aside.
4. Heat 6 cups (48 ounces, 1.4 l) oil to 375°F (190°C), or until a piece of green onion or ginger sizzles noisily and quickly turns brown. While waiting on the oil, dip the chicken in egg and dredge in cornstarch-flour mixture. Shake off excess.

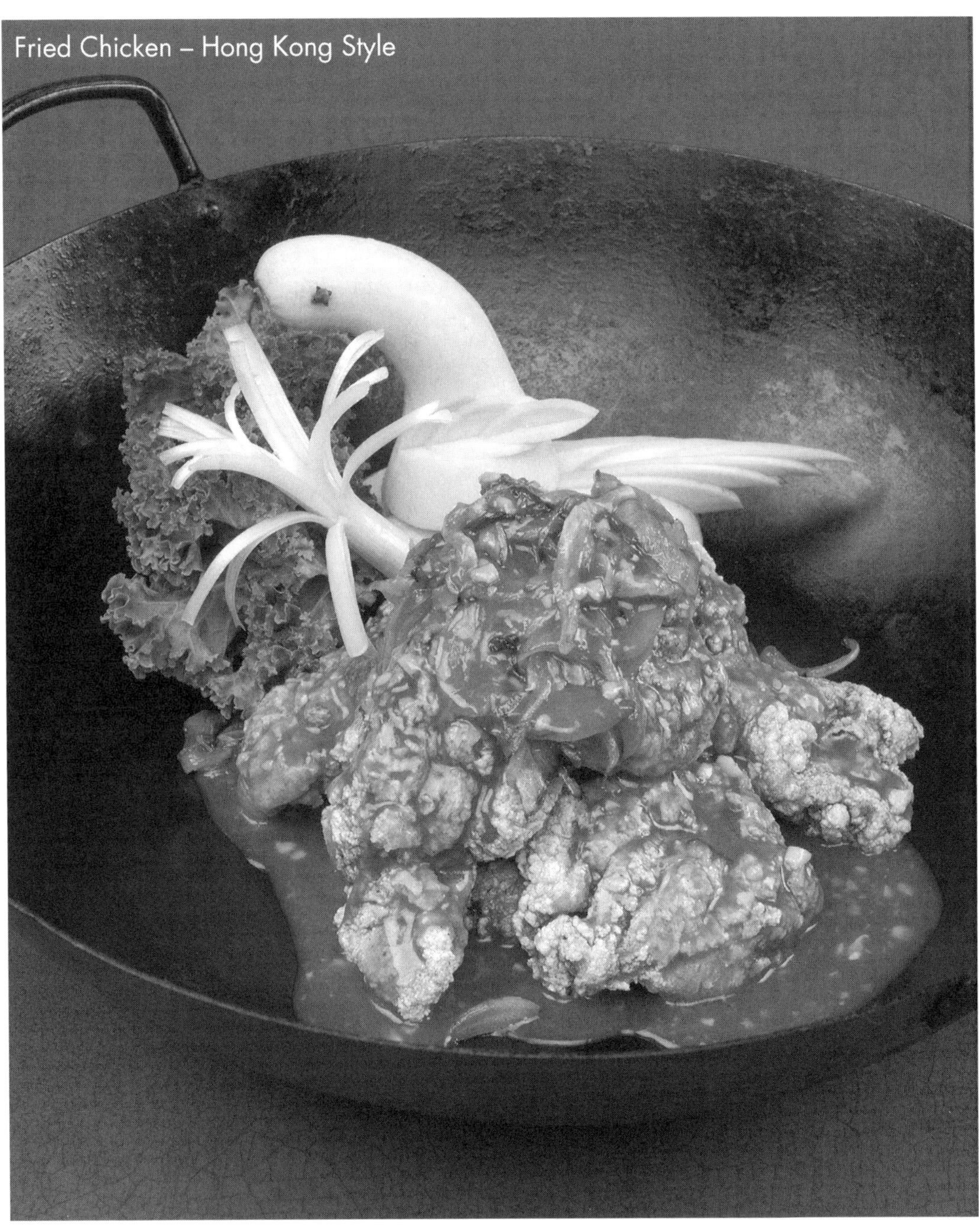

Fried Chicken – Hong Kong Style

5. Add chicken to hot oil and deep fry until the coating sets and is lightly browned. Remove and drain.
6. Use a fine-mesh strainer to remove sediment from the oil. Reheat oil 400°F (204°C). Return chicken pieces and deep-fry until golden brown; remove and drain on paper towels.
7. Using a basket, add onions to hot oil. Fry onions 1 minute, until soft and translucent. Remove onions. Pour out oil and wipe wok clean.
8. Set wok over high heat and add 1 tablespoon ($\frac{1}{2}$ ounce, 15 ml) oil. Flavor oil with garlic; stir-fry 10 seconds. Mix sauce ingredients again and add to wok, stirring constantly until thickened. Turn heat to low, glaze the sauce with remaining oil, and turn off heat.
9. Arrange thighs in single layer on serving platter, top with fried onions, pour sauce over, and serve immediately.

# Steamed Whole Fish

SERVES 4

| AMOUNT | MEASURE | INGREDIENT |
|---|---|---|
| **1 each $1\frac{1}{2}$ pound** | **673 g** | **Whole firm fish, head and tail on (any firm, white fish such as rock cod, striped bass, snapper, perch, sole, or tilapia)** |
| **2** | | **Whole green onions** |
| **$\frac{1}{8}$ teaspoon** | | **White pepper** |
| **$\frac{1}{4}$ teaspoon** | | **Salt** |
| **1 tablespoon** | | **Ginger, grated** |
| **2** | | **Green onions, thinly sliced** |
| **$\frac{1}{4}$ cup** | **2 ounces, 60 ml** | **Vegetable oil** |
| **2 teaspoons** | | **Sesame oil** |
| **3 tablespoons** | **$1\frac{1}{2}$ ounces, 45 ml** | **Light soy sauce** |
| **2** | | **Cilantro sprigs, 2 inch lengths** |

**PROCEDURE**

1. Clean and scale the fish; rinse well and pat dry.
2. Arrange green onions lengthwise on a heatproof fish platter; the platter should be large enough to hold the fish and be placed in the steamer. Place the fish on the green onions, so the steam will flow under and over the fish.
3. Steam fish for approximately 10 minutes or until a chopstick can go easily into the thickest part of the fish. Remove from steamer; drain excess liquid. Discard green onions.
4. Sprinkle the white pepper and salt over the fish. Spread ginger and green onions on top of the fish.
5. Heat the oil and sesame oil to very hot and pour over the fish. Add the soy sauce to the bottom of the serving platter. Garnish with cilantro sprigs and serve.

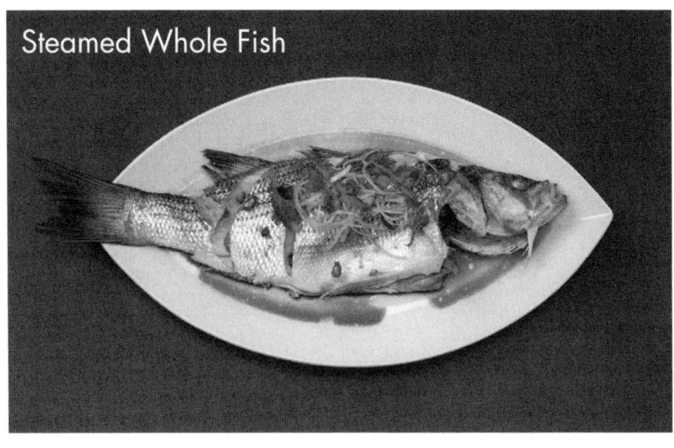
Steamed Whole Fish

# Tea Leaf Eggs

SERVES 4

| AMOUNT | MEASURE | INGREDIENT |
|---|---|---|
| **4** | | **Large eggs** |
| **Tea Leaf Mixture** | | |
| **3 cups** | **24 ounces, 720 ml** | **Water** |
| **1 tablespoon** | **$\frac{1}{2}$ ounce, 15 ml** | **Dark soy sauce** |
| **1** | | **Star anise, whole** |
| **2 teaspoon** | | **Salt** |
| **2 tablespoons** | | **Green tea leaves** |
| **1 tablespoon** | **$\frac{1}{2}$ ounce, 15 ml** | **Rock sugar** |

PROCEDURE

1. Combine eggs and enough cold water to cover. Bring to a boil and cook 10 minutes.
2. Remove eggs and immerse in ice water until cool.
3. Using a tablespoon, tap the shells gently to make fine cracks.
4. Combine tea-leaf ingredients and bring to a boil. Add the cracked eggs and bring back to a boil. Turn heat to low and simmer for 30 minutes.
5. Remove pan from heat and let eggs cool to room temperature.
6. Shell the eggs and serve cold.

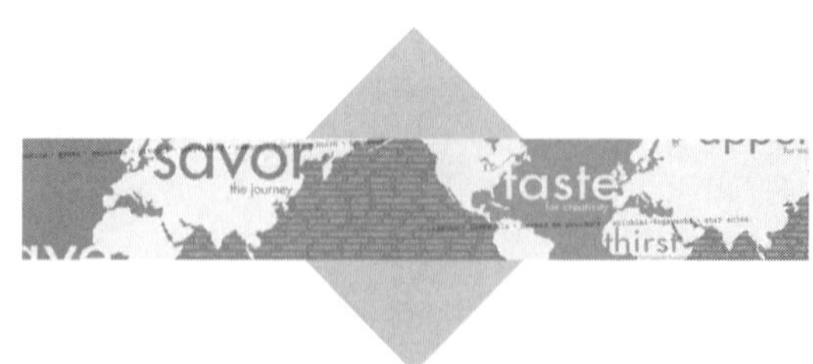

# Korea

## The Land

Korea is a rugged peninsula lying between China on the west and north and Japan to the east. It shares a very small border with Russia to the extreme northeast. Korea is surrounded by water on three sides: the Korea Bay and the Yellow Sea to the west, the Korea Strait to the south, and the East Sea (also known as the Sea of Japan) to the east. There are more than 3,400 islands along the coast. Mountains and hills make up about 70 percent of the country. The Korean peninsula is divided by two political states: the Democratic People's Republic of Korea (North Korea) and the Republic of Korea (South Korea). The counties are separated by a line 38 degrees north of the equator. North Korea occupies about 55 percent of the peninsula's 84,402 square miles of land. To the west and south of the peninsula are broad coastal plains where the larger cities are located and where most of the agricultural land is found. With a combined population of nearly 72 million Koreans, in a country the size of Great Britain or New Zealand, the land is well used. The land gently slopes from the south and western coastal plains toward the mountains and drops steeply from the mountains to the East Sea.

# History

The Korean Peninsula's first inhabitants migrated from the northwestern regions of Asia. Some of these peoples also populated parts of northeast China (Manchuria); Koreans and Manchurians still show physical similarities.

According to legend, the god-king Tangun founded the Korean nation in 2333 B.C. By the first century A.D., the Korean peninsula was divided into the kingdoms of Silla, Koguryo, and Paekche. In A.D. 668, the Silla kingdom unified the peninsula. The Koryo dynasty—from which Portuguese missionaries in the sixteenth century derived the Western name *Korea*—succeeded the Silla kingdom in 935. The Choson dynasty, ruled by members of the Yi clan, replaced Koryo in 1392 and lasted until the Japanese annexed Korea in 1910.

Throughout most of its history, Korea has been invaded, influenced, and fought over by its larger neighbors. Korea was under Mongolian occupation from 1231 until the early fourteenth century and was plundered by Japanese pirates in 1359 and 1361. The unifier of Japan, Hideyoshi, launched major invasions of Korea in 1592 and 1597. When Western powers focused "gunboat" diplomacy on Korea in the mid-nineteenth century, Korea's rulers adopted a closed-door policy, earning Korea the title of "Hermit Kingdom."

Though the Choson dynasty paid loyalty to the Chinese court and recognized China's control in East Asia, Korea was independent until the late nineteenth century. At that time, China sought to block growing Japanese influence on the Korean peninsula and Russian pressure for commercial gains there. This competition resulted in the Sino-Japanese War of 1894–95 and the Russo-Japanese War of 1904–05. Japan emerged victorious from both wars and in 1910 annexed Korea as part of its growing empire.

Japanese colonial administration was characterized by tight control from Tokyo and ruthless efforts to supplant Korean language and culture. Organized Korean resistance during this era—such as the March 1, 1919, Independence Movement—was unsuccessful, and Japan remained firmly in control until the end of World War II in 1945.

Japan surrendered to the Allied Forces in August 1945, and Korea was liberated. However, the unexpectedly early surrender of Japan led to the immediate division of Korea into two occupation zones, with the United States administering the southern half of the peninsula and the U.S.S.R taking over the area to the north of the 38th parallel. This division was meant to be temporary and to facilitate the Japanese surrender until the U.S., Britain, the Soviet Union, and China could arrange a trusteeship administration.

At a meeting in Cairo, it was agreed that Korea would be free "in due course." At a later meeting in Yalta, it was agreed to establish a four-power trusteeship over Korea. In December 1945, a conference convened in Moscow to discuss the future of Korea. A five-year trusteeship was discussed, and a joint Soviet-American commission was established. The commission met intermittently in Seoul but deadlocked over the issue of establishing a national government.

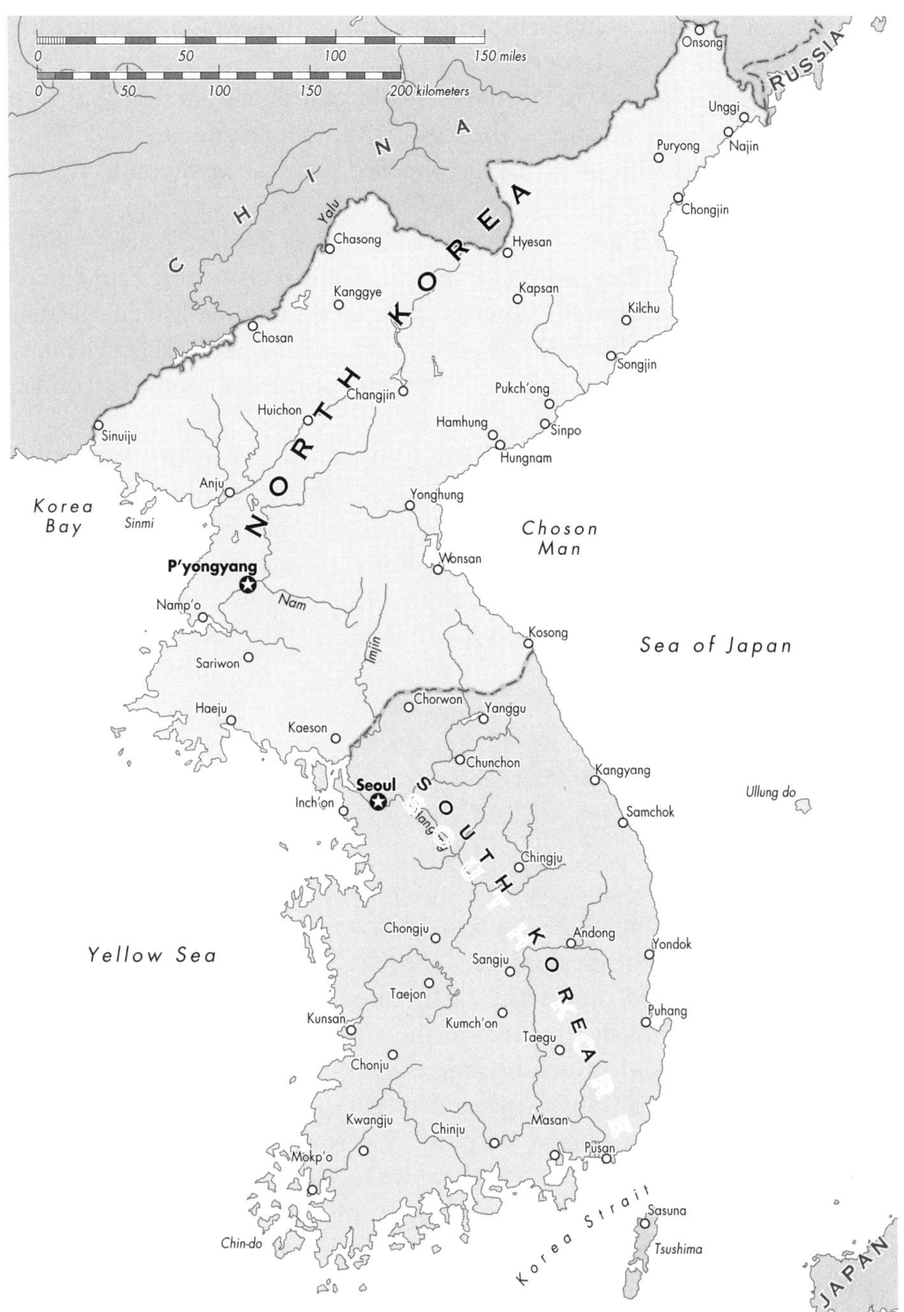


North and South Korea

In September 1947, with no solution in sight, the United States submitted the Korean question to the United Nations (U.N.) General Assembly.

Initial hopes for a unified, independent Korea quickly evaporated as the politics of the Cold War and domestic opposition to the trusteeship plan resulted in the 1948 establishment of two separate nations with diametrically opposed political, economic, and social systems. War broke out in 1950.

North Korea invaded South Korea on June 25, 1950. The U.N. sent military assistance. The Korean War lasted three years and inflicted terrible damage to Korea before a cease-fire ended the war in 1953. The four-kilometer-wide area along the Military Demarcation Line that divides North and South Korea has become known as the DMZ, or Demilitarized Zone. In the forty-five years since the Korean War there have been continual conflicts along the DMZ.

In 1993, Kim Young Sam became South Korea's first civilian president following thirty-two years of military rule. South Korea today is a fully functioning modern democracy. By contrast, North Korea is a communist government and one of the most isolated countries in the world. In June 2000, a historic first North-South summit took place between the South's President Kim Tae-chung and the North's leader Kim Jong Il.

Efforts continue to unify North and South Korea.

# The People

Korea's markets, its fishing and farming villages, modern though the buildings might be, remain very much the same as in the past. And its artisans—celadon pottery makers, for example—have re-created the great works of the past. All are traditional expressions of Korean culture, which is still based on certain six-hundred-year-old Confucian principles. Unlike a religion, Confucianism does not involve the worship of a higher being. But like some religions, it attempts to guide human relationships and improve social and ethical conduct. The fundamental thrust of Confucianism is to maintain peace and order. It has rules for familial relationships that emphasize harmony. It stresses the importance of education and respect for authority.

The Korean family structure is part of a larger kinship structure that is defined by specific obligations. Multigenerational households are quite common in rural areas and in a Korean home, the head of the family—usually the oldest male—holds the position of authority and every family member is expected to do as he says. Large families have been prized and over many centuries families intermarried within the regions of Korea to form large clans. Family names reflect this. A dozen family names predominate, especially Kim, Park, Lee, Kang, and Cho. But Kims from the city of Pusan in the south are not the Kims from Seoul and all the Kims know exactly to which group they belong. Custom forbids people marrying within their own clan, no matter how distant the cousin might be. In order to know who is who, families and clans keep detailed genealogical records that might go back many hundreds of years. Even in today's Westernized Korea, many people can still recite the history of their clans and take pride in it.

The oldest religious ideas in Korea are called shamanism. These are beliefs that the natural world is filled with spirits, both helpful and harmful, that can be addressed by people with special powers called shamans. Herbal medicines, dances, chants, and other ceremonies mark the work of shamans, most of whom are women. Though few people believe in the religious teachings today, they do accept old ideas about the natural world and use many ancient herbal remedies. Buddhism is one of the most popular religions in South Korea. The religion is based on the teachings of the Buddha; the basic idea is that salvation can come from giving up worldly desires and living in moderation. By living according to the Buddha's teachings, a Buddhist believes that he or she can reach the state of nirvana—ultimate peace—wherein a person experiences no pain or worry.

Taoism came from China and is similar to shamanism in its worship of many equally important gods. Taoism's main principle is to create harmony between humans and nature. The many gods are used as ideals toward which humans can strive and Taoists believe that spiritual perfections can be attained in this life through patience, purity, and peace.

Christianity was brought to Korea in the sixteenth century by Confucian intellectuals who learned about it in the Chinese capital of Peking. The first half of the nineteenth century was a difficult time for Korean Christians; thousands were persecuted and many were killed. Today South Korea is second in Asia only to the Philippines in its percentage of Christians.

# The Food

The climate of the Korean peninsula resembles the north central region of the United States: cold winters, warm summers, and long, pleasant autumns. Because the land is made up mostly of mountains and extends from the North Asian landmass into warmer seas in the south, Korea has many microenvironments. In the mountainous northeastern part of the country the most famous dishes have wild ferns, mushrooms, and native roots in them. *Namul* (raw or cooked vegetable or wild green dishes) is one of the most basic side dishes in the Korean diet. In the rice-growing valleys of the south, in the region of Chonju city, the best known dish, *pibimpap* (*bibimpap*), is a large bowl of rice covered in a variety of finely sliced vegetables, meats, and a fiery red pepper sauce. The basic flavors of Korean food include garlic, ginger, black pepper, spring onions, soy sauce, sesame oil, and toasted sesame seed. The chile, a native to Central and South America, was spread across the world by Portuguese and Spanish merchants. Chiles and chile paste has become an important part of all Korean tables and many food preparations.

Its peninsular location gives Koreans three different seas from which to gather fish: the Yellow Sea, the East Sea, and the unique microenvironment where the two seas come together at the south end of the peninsula, the Korea Strait. Fish from the Yellow Sea differ from those of the Eastern Sea (Sea of Japan) and those of the south coast differ from the others. Koreans are seafood connoisseurs and seek out the specialties of each region. But three types of seafood are served all the time. One kind is a small dried sardine, used not as a main dish but as condiments to be eaten with others and bowls of these appear at every meal, including breakfast. Another is dried cuttlefish (similar to squid or octopus), which is the most popular snack food. All along the road and streets near fishing ports are lines of these cephalopods hanging out to dry. Seaweed and seaweed products are known for numerous health benefits and are prepared to keep well in a climate that endures long winters. Pregnant women, new mothers, and babies are fed seaweed soups. *Miyeok guk* is a brown seaweed soup known as birthday soup.

Koreans eat many preserved foods, prepared to keep over wintertime. *Kimchi* is Korea's signature dish of spicy, pickled vegetables and is served every day at every meal. *Kimchi* is characterized by its sour, sweet, and carbonated taste, yet is very different from sauerkraut, which is a popular fermented vegetable product in the West. The first written description of making *kimchi* dates to about A.D. 1250. Many different recipes were published and fermentation methods "invented" for making *kimchi*, so it is not surprising that the tastes are quite different from one another. Despite the uniqueness of every *kimchi*, the basic taste is derived from salt, lactic acid fermentation of vegetables, spices (including hot red pepper, garlic, ginger, and green onion), and pickled fish or fresh seafood. There are about 170 different varieties and two or three kinds are served with meals. It is also used as a seasoning in soups and stews. In summer, *kimchi* is prepared weekly, since the vegetables are in season. But when winter sets in, no crops can be produced until late spring. The approach of winter marks the start of a long *kimchee*-making time called *gimjang*. During *gimjang*, Koreans gather in groups to cut, wash, and salt hundreds of pounds of the vegetables. After it is prepared, it is stored in the yard in large earthenware crocks. In the countryside, the crocks are buried up to their necks to keep the pickled vegetables from freezing.

*Bulgogi* is one of Korea's most famous grilled dishes. It is made from sirloin or another prime cut of beef (such as top round), cut into thin strips. For an outside barbecue, the meat is marinated in a mixture of sesame oil, soy sauce, black pepper, garlic, sugar, onions, ginger, and wine for at least four hours to enhance the flavor and to tenderize it. The marinated beef is cooked on a metal dish over the burner. Whole cloves of garlic, sliced onions, and chopped green peppers are often grilled at the same time. To eat, a piece of cooked beef is wrapped in lettuce with rice, *kimchi*, and shredded vegetables.

There are no real "courses" in a Korean meal. Generally, all food is laid out on the table at the same time and eaten in any order. Dessert is not a Korean tradition; seasonal fruit is normally served with hot tea or coffee.

# Glossary

**An-ju** Appetizers or bar snacks, like tapas, usually savory, pungent, and strong-flavored foods intended to promote thirst.

**Baechu (Napa Cabbage)** The most popular vegetable used in traditional kimchi.

**Bap (pab)-or (Ssal)** Rice; Koreans eat short-grain rice.

**Bokeum** Stir-fried or sautéed dish.

**Boo** Long white radish resembling a parsnip in appearance, with a mild flavor. Tender white turnips can be substituted.

**Buchu** Korean chives, resembling a bundle of long grass rather than ordinary chives. They are highly perishable.

**Bulgogi** Grilled, marinated beef or other meat.

**Busut** Mushrooms.

**Cellophane Noodles** See Mung Bean Threads.

**Chang Gilum** A strongly flavored sesame oil used for seasoning; made from roasted sesame seeds.

**Chongol (Jongol)** Korean one-pot stew, similar to Japanese sukiyaki.

**Dalaji** White bellflower roots. Crunchy with a slightly sweet flavor, used both fresh and dried.

**Dang-myun** Sweet potato noodles that are distinctly Korean. Made from potato and sweet potato starch, they must be soaked in boiling water for 10 minutes before using.

**Dubu** Tofu or soybean curd.

**Dwenjang** Fermented soybean paste, brownish yellow in color and chunky in texture, different from the Japanese miso.

**Gam** Persimmons.

**Gochu** A chile pepper, introduced by Portuguese and Spanish traders in the seventeenth century.

**Gochu Galu** Korean chile powder made from sun-dried thin red peppers.

**Gooksu, Myon or Kuksu** Noodles.

**Gui** Barbecued or grilled food.

**Jajang-myeon** Korean noodle dish, black bean sauce, minced pork, and vegetables.

**Jjigae Jungol** Liquid-based hot-pot main courses for everyone to share.

**Jjim, Jolim** Simmered or stewed foods.

**Jook** Porridge.

**Jon, Jun, Buchingae** Batter-fried vegetables, meat, or fish.

**Kalbi** Short ribs, either barbecued or braised in soy sauce.

**Kimchi** Essentially the national dish of Korea, it combines countless varieties of pickled (fermented) vegetables. Most common kimchi consists of salted Korean cabbage, layered with garlic, ginger, chile paste, and salt or fermented fish, shrimp, or oysters.

**Kochujang (Gochujang)** Hot chile and bean curd paste, a staple of the Korean kitchen.

**Kochukaru (Gochu Galu)** Korean chile powder. Dried, powdered spicy red pepper.

**Kong-namul (Kohng Namool)** Soybean sprouts.

**Laver (Gim)** Edible seaweed.

**Mae un Tang** *Mae un* means spicy; *tang* is a meat-based soup boiled for a long time. It has been described as a "Korean bouillabaisse"—hot and spicy fish soup with chiles and kochujang.

**Malt Powder (Yut Gilum)** Beige-colored powder made from dried barley. Malt powder made from dried soybeans is called *meju galu.*

**Mandu** Korean dumplings, filled with ground pork, kimchi, spring onions, and bean curd, usually poached in a rich beef broth.

**Manul** Korea is number one in the world for garlic consumption per capita. Three major types of *manul* are grown in Korea: *soinpyun*, which has three or four large cloves; *dainpyun*, with many small cloves; and *jangsun*, grown mostly for its stems.

**Miwon** Pure MSG in white crystal form.

**Miyuk or Dashima** Kelp, sold dry. When soaked for about 10 minutes, it softens and expands, becoming slightly slimy and flowing.

**Mu** Radish, Asian or daikon.

**Mung Bean (Nokdu)** Dried mung beans are very small and green in color, yellow if the green husks have been removed. Dried split peas may be used as a substitute.

**Mung Bean Sprouts (Nokdu Namool) or Green Bean Sprouts (Sookju Namool)** Mung bean sprouts and green bean sprouts are interchangeable. Smaller than soybean sprouts, they do not have the large yellow bean head.

**Mung Bean Threads** Very fine dried noodles made from mung bean flour. Soak in water for 10 minutes before using.

**Myuichi** Anchovies. Dried anchovies are commonly used in Korean cooking; salted anchovies (paste) are also used. Korean brands are usually less salty and pungent than those of other Asian countries.

**Naeng myon** Literally, "cold noodle." Korean noodles made from buckwheat flour and potato starch. They are brownish in color with a translucent appearance, most often eaten cold.

**Naju Bae** An Asian pear that looks like a large brown apple with tough skin. It is very crispy and juicy, often peeled.

**Namool** Vegetables.

**Oi** Cucumbers; small pickling varieties are used in Korean cooking.

**Pa** Green onions.

**Panchan** Side dishes.

**Pibimbap** One-dish meal of rice, vegetables, meat, fried egg, and kochujang.

**Pindaettok** Mung bean pancake.

**Pokkum** Stir-fried or braised dish.

**Saengsonhoe** Raw fish.

**Saewu Jut** Salted shrimp; tiny salted shrimp (krill) is one of the major ingredients in making *kimchi*. Not to be confused with the more salty and pungent Southeast Asian shrimp paste.

**Sang-chi-sam** Lettuce-wrapped meal accompanied by many side dishes.

**Sesame Seeds (Ggae)** Used raw and toasted. There are two types, white and black.

**Shil Gochu** These chile pepper threads are a traditional garnish. The hair-thin threads, which resemble saffron, are machine-cut from dried red chile peppers.

**Shinsollo** Korean hot pot.

**Soybean Paste** Known as miso in Japan, a basic seasoning made from cooked soybeans, malt, and salt.

**Tang** Meat-based soup.

**Toen Jang** Miso-like fermented soybean paste used in soups and stews.

**Twoenjangtchigae** Pungent soybean paste soup, the soul of Korean cuisine.

**Wun Tun Skins** Called wonton skins in North America, paper-thin squares or circles of dough.

# Menus and Recipes from Korea

MENU ONE

***Pa Jon:* Korean-Style Pancake**

***Yangnyum Ganjang:* Seasoned Soy Sauce**

***Mu Sangchae:* Spicy Radish Salad**

***Buhsut Namool:* Seasoned Mushrooms**

***Twigim Mandu:* Fried Meat Dumplings**

***Bibim Naeng Myun:* Garden's Cold Mixed Noodles**

**Marinated Cucumbers**

***Hacmul Jungol:* Seafood Hot Pot**

***Kalbi-Kui:* Barbecue Beef Ribs**

***Kimchi:* Traditional Napa Cabbage**

***Soo Jeung Kwa:* Persimmon Punch**

MENU TWO

***Jahb Chae:* Mung Bean Noodles**

***Dak Chochu Jang Boekum:* Chicken in Hot Chile Sauce**

***Dubu Jolim:* Simmered Tofu**

***Dan Kim Kui:* Crispy Seaweed**

***Kohng Namool:* Seasoned Soybean Sprouts**

***Bulgogi (Boolgogi):* Fire Meat**

***Ojingo Pokum:* Squid with Vegetables in Chile Hot-Sweet Sauce**

MENU THREE

***Bibimbap:* Garnished Rice**

***Dwaeji Galbi:* Spicy Pork Ribs**

***Bibim Gooksu:* Spicy Summer Noodles**

***Maeum Tang:* Spiced Fish Soup**

***Kaji Namul:* Marinated Eggplant**

***Oi Bok Kum Namul:* Cooked Cucumbers**

***Seng Sun Bulgogi:* Barbecued Spiced Fish**

***Yak Sik:* Steamed Rice Pudding**

# Pa Jon Korean-Style Pancake

SERVES 4

**Chef Tip** **For crispy pancakes, use very cold water in the batter.**

| AMOUNT | MEASURE | INGREDIENT |
|---|---|---|
| 1 teaspoon | | Salt |
| $\frac{3}{4}$ cup | 3 ounces, 84 g | All-purpose flour |
| $\frac{1}{4}$ cup | 1 ounce, 28 g | Rice flour |
| $\frac{3}{4}$ cup | 6 ounces, 180 ml | Ice cold water |
| 1 cup | 4 ounces, 112 g | Green onions, $1\frac{1}{2}$ inch (3.75 cm) long, julienned |
| $\frac{1}{4}$ cup | 1 ounce, 28 g | Zucchini (skin on), seeded, julienned |
| $\frac{1}{4}$ cup | 1 ounce, 28 g | Red bell pepper, julienned |
| 4 tablespoons | 2 ounces, 60 ml | Vegetable oil |
| | | *Yangnyum Ganjang* or *Cho Ganjang* (recipes follow) |

PROCEDURE

1. Sift salt and flours together; add water a little at time, mixing until it is the consistency of thin pancake batter.
2. Add vegetables and mix.
3. Over medium-high heat, coat griddle or frying pan with just enough oil to thinly cover.
4. Cook batter in two batches, creating two large flat circles. Distribute the batter and vegetables evenly around the pan. Cook to golden brown, 3 minutes. Flip and cook other side, 2–3 minutes. Adjust heat if necessary to prevent burning; add oil as needed. Smaller pancakes are acceptable.
5. Cut pancake into 4 or 8 pieces and serve hot with *Yangnyum Ganjang* (seasoned soy sauce) or *Cho Ganjang* (vinegar soy sauce).

# Yangnyum Ganjang

## Seasoned Soy Sauce

YIELD: $\frac{1}{2}$ CUP (4 OUNCES, 120 ML)

| AMOUNT | MEASURE | INGREDIENT |
|---|---|---|
| **4 tablespoons** | **2 ounces, 60 ml** | **Soy sauce** |
| **$\frac{1}{4}$ cup** | **1 ounce, 28 g** | **Green onion, minced** |
| **1 tablespoon** | | **Toasted sesame seeds** |
| **1 tablespoon** | **$\frac{1}{2}$ ounce, 15 ml** | **Sesame oil** |
| **$\frac{1}{2}$ tablespoon** | | ***Kochukaru* (Korean chile powder)** |
| **$\frac{1}{2}$ teaspoon** | | **Black pepper** |

**PROCEDURE**

1 Combine all ingredients.

## Cho Ganjang Vinegar Soy Sauce

YIELD: $\frac{1}{2}$ CUP (4 OUNCES, 120 ML)

| AMOUNT | MEASURE | INGREDIENT |
|---|---|---|
| **4 tablespoons** | **2 ounces, 60 ml** | **Soy sauce** |
| **2 tablespoons** | **2 ounces, 60 ml** | **Rice vinegar** |
| **2 tablespoons** | **1 ounce, 30 ml** | **Sesame oil** |
| **1 tablespoon** | | **Toasted sesame seeds** |
| **1 teaspoon** | | **Black pepper** |

**PROCEDURE**

1 Combine all ingredients.

# Mu Sangchae

## Spicy Radish Salad SERVES 4–6

| AMOUNT | MEASURE | INGREDIENT |
|---|---|---|
| 1 teaspoon | | *Kochukaru* (Korean chile powder) |
| 2 tablespoons | 1 ounce, 30 ml | Rice or white vinegar |
| 1 tablespoon | | Sugar |
| 1 tablespoon | | Salt |
| 2 cups | 12 ounces, 336 | Daikon, peeled and julienned |

**PROCEDURE**

1 Combine chile powder vinegar, sugar, and salt, stir to dissolve completely. Mix vinegar with daikon, let marinate under refrigeration for 2 hours before serving.

2 Serve chilled.

# Buhsut Namool

## Seasoned Mushrooms SERVES 4

| AMOUNT | MEASURE | INGREDIENT |
|---|---|---|
| 1 tablespoon | $\frac{1}{2}$ ounce, 15 ml | Sesame oil |
| 1 | | Garlic clove, minced |
| 2 cups | 5 ounces, 140 g | Shiitake mushrooms, $\frac{1}{4}$ inch (.6 cm) slices |
| 1 teaspoon | | Soy sauce |
| 1 teaspoon | | Sesame seeds, toasted |

**PROCEDURE**

1 Heat sesame oil over medium-high heat; add garlic and mushrooms and stir-fry 2–3 minutes. Add soy sauce, toss, and remove from heat.

2 Serve warm or cold, sprinkled with toasted sesame seeds.

# Twigim Mandu
## Fried Meat Dumplings

YIELD: 24 DUMPLINGS

| AMOUNT | MEASURE | INGREDIENT |
|---|---|---|
| $\frac{1}{2}$ cup | 2 ounces, 56 g | Mung bean or green bean sprouts |
| | 4 ounces, 112 g | Ground pork |
| $\frac{1}{4}$ cup | 1 ounce, 28 g | Onion, minced |
| $\frac{1}{4}$ cup | 1 ounce, 28 g | Green onion, white and green top, minced |
| 2 | | Garlic cloves, minced |
| $\frac{1}{2}$ tablespoon | $\frac{1}{2}$ ounce, 14 g | Ginger, peeled and minced |
| 1 | | Small egg |
| $\frac{1}{2}$ teaspoon | | Sesame oil |
| $\frac{1}{4}$ teaspoon | | Salt |
| $\frac{1}{4}$ teaspoon | | White pepper |
| 24 | | Round or square dumpling (wonton) wrappers, fresh (recipe follows) or purchased |
| As needed | | Vegetable oil, for frying |

PROCEDURE

1. Blanch mung bean sprouts in boiling water, shock in ice water, and squeeze out all excess moisture. Chop fine.
2. Combine chopped sprouts and remaining ingredients except dumpling wrappers and vegetable oil; mix well.
3. To make each dumpling, place $1\frac{1}{2}$ teaspoons (7.5 ml) filling in the center of a wrapper. Fold the wrapper over the filling in a semicircle for a round wrapper or a triangle for a square wrapper. Seal the edges by moistening them with a little water and pinching them. (To form a hat-shaped *mandu*, moisten the corners for the semicircular dumplings and bring them together, pinching them so that the dumpling forms a sort of fat tortellini.) Keep both wonton skins and dumplings moist under plastic or damp towels as you work. Repeat until all filling or wrappers are used.
4. Over medium-high heat, added enough oil to a frying pan to cover the bottom surface. Place dumpling in hot pan, filling but not crowding; you don't want the dumplings to touch and stick together.

5 Fry until golden brown and crispy on one side. Flip (long wooden chopsticks work great), cooking on all sides until golden and crispy all over. Continue cooking, adding oil as needed.

6 Serve with warm *Cho Ganjang.*

## Mandu Pi Fresh Dumpling Skins

YIELD: 50 SKINS

| AMOUNT | MEASURE | INGREDIENT |
|---|---|---|
| **3 cups** | **12 ounces, 336 g** | **All-purpose flour** |
| **$\frac{1}{4}$ teaspoon** | | **Salt** |
| **$\frac{2}{3}$ cup** | **5.25 ounces, 158 ml** | **Water** |

**PROCEDURE**

1 Sift together flour and salt. Add water to a bowl; add flour a little at a time, mixing with each addition. Continue kneading until dough is well mixed and stiff. Cover and let rest 30 minutes.

2 Roll out on a floured surface or use a pasta machine. Pinch off small pieces and make them into round balls to roll out flat with a rolling pin. Alternately, roll the dough into small sausage-shaped rolls and slice them before rolling them into flat thin circles.

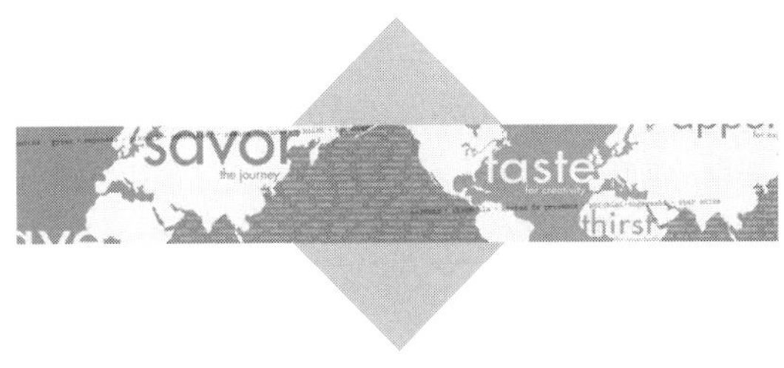

# Bibim Naeng Myun

## Garden's Cold Mixed Noodles SERVES 4

**After serving, the dish is eaten by stirring everything into the sauce with chopsticks. Note: the sauce is very hot and spicy.**

| AMOUNT | MEASURE | INGREDIENT |
|---|---|---|
| $\frac{1}{2}$ cup | 4 ounces, 120 ml | Red pepper paste (recipe follows) |
| $\frac{1}{3}$ cup | 2.66 ounces, 80 ml | Soy sauce |
| 2 tablespoons | | Granulated sugar |
| 1$\frac{1}{4}$ tablespoons | | Garlic, minced |
| 2$\frac{1}{4}$ tablespoons | | Green onions, minced, white part |
| 1 tablespoon | | Sesame seeds, toasted and crushed |
| $\frac{1}{4}$ cup | 2 ounces, 60 ml | Sesame oil |
| 3 tablespoons | 1$\frac{1}{2}$ ounces, 45 ml | Beef broth |
| 1$\frac{1}{2}$ pounds | | Fresh-frozen buckwheat noodles (*naeng myun*), or 12 ounces dried, or 9 ounces bean threads |
| 1 | | Asian pear or other hard pear, peel, cored, and sliced lengthwise, $\frac{1}{4}$ inch (.6 cm) |
| 1 cup | 8 ounces, 224 g | Marinated cucumbers (recipe follows) |
| 2 | | Hard-cooked eggs |

**PROCEDURE**

1. Combine red pepper paste, soy sauce, sugar, garlic, onion, sesame seeds, sesame oil, and broth. Mix or process until well blended and almost smooth.
2. Cook frozen noodles about 45 seconds in boiling water or until they are chewy but tender. Rinse with cold water, drain well, and chill. Or, if using dried noodles or bean threads, soak in water to cover 20 minutes, boil 1 minute; drain, rinse, and chill.
3. Divide the sauce among 4 bowls. Mound a fourth of the noodles in each bowl in the center of the sauce with a border of red sauce showing.
4. Arrange the pear slices and cucumbers on noodles.
5. Top with half a hard-cooked egg.

## Red Pepper Paste

| AMOUNT | MEASURE | INGREDIENT |
|---|---|---|
| $\frac{3}{4}$ cup plus 1 tablespoon | | Crushed red hot Korean peppers, or New Mexico or *Guajillo* chile peppers |
| $\frac{3}{4}$ cup plus 1 tablespoon | $6\frac{1}{2}$ ounces, 195 ml | Water |

**PROCEDURE**

1. Combine water and crushed peppers; let soak 30 minutes.
2. Process in a blender or food processor, or use a mortar and pestle to get a thick, slightly textured paste. Adjust thickness with water.

# Marinated Cucumbers

SERVES 4

| AMOUNT | MEASURE | INGREDIENT |
|---|---|---|
| 2 tablespoons | 1 ounce, 30 ml | Rice vinegar |
| 1 tablespoon | | Granulated sugar |
| $1\frac{1}{2}$ teaspoons | | Salt |
| $1\frac{1}{2}$ cups | 8 ounces, 224 g | European cucumber, unpeeled, sliced lengthwise $\frac{1}{8}$ inch (.3 cm) thick and $2\frac{1}{2}$ inches (6.25 cm) long |

**PROCEDURE**

1. Combine vinegar, sugar, and salt; stir to dissolve.
2. Add cucumbers; cover and marinate at least 2 hours at room temperature. Refrigerate until ready to use.

# Hacmul Jungol

## Seafood Hot Pot

SERVES 4

| AMOUNT | MEASURE | INGREDIENT |
|---|---|---|
| 1 cup | 5 ounces, 140 g | Onion, $\frac{1}{4}$ inch (.6 cm) slices |
| $\frac{1}{2}$ cup | 2 ounces, 56 g | Shiitake mushrooms, $\frac{1}{4}$ inch (.6 cm) slice |
| 2 cups | 8 ounces, 224 g | Napa cabbage, (5 cm) 2-inch-long strips |
| 1$\frac{1}{2}$ teaspoons | | Garlic, minced |
| 1$\frac{1}{2}$ teaspoons | | Ginger, minced |
| 3 cups | 24 ounces, 720 ml | Chicken broth (stock) |
| $\frac{3}{4}$ cup | 4 ounces, 112 g | Squid, cleaned, sliced into thin (5 cm) 2-inch-long strips |
| 4 ounces | 112 g | 16–20 shrimp |
| 4 ounces | 112 g | Fresh oysters, shelled, cleaned |
| 4 | | Medium clams, shelled, cleaned |
| 1 tablespoon | | Chile paste (red pepper paste) |
| 1 tablespoon | | Kochukaru (Korean chile powder) |
| $\frac{1}{2}$ cup | 2 ounces, 56 g | Green onion, cut on the diagonal, 2 inch (5 cm) long |
| 3 | | Chrysanthemum leaves (optional) |
| To taste | | Salt and pepper |

### PROCEDURE

1. Combine onion, mushroom, cabbage, garlic, and ginger with stock. Bring to boil and reduce to simmer.
2. Add seafood, chile paste, and chile powder to taste. Let cook until seafood is just done, 2 to 3 minutes.
3. Add green onions and chrysanthemum leaves; simmer 1 minute.
4. Correct seasoning.
5. Serve by placing the hot pot in middle of the table.

# Kalbi-Kui

## Barbecue Beef Ribs

SERVES 4

| AMOUNT | MEASURE | INGREDIENT |
|---|---|---|
| $\frac{1}{2}$ cup | 4 ounces, 120 ml | Soy sauce |
| 2 tablespoons | 1 ounce, 28 g | Granulated sugar |
| $\frac{1}{4}$ teaspoon | | Dry mustard |
| $\frac{1}{4}$ teaspoon | | Black pepper, freshly ground |
| 1 teaspoon | | Sesame seeds |
| 2 tablespoons | 1 ounce, 30 ml | Rice vinegar |
| 2 tablespoons | 1 ounce, 30 ml | Sesame oil |
| 1 teaspoon | | Ginger, minced |
| 4 | | Garlic cloves, minced |
| $\frac{1}{4}$ cup | 1 ounce, 28 g | Green onions, chopped |
| $2\frac{1}{2}$ pounds | 1.12 kg | Korean-style short ribs (beef chuck flanken), cut $\frac{1}{3}$ to $\frac{1}{2}$ inch (.83 cm to 1.2 cm) thick across the bones, about 8 to 10 pieces |

**PROCEDURE**

1. Combine all ingredients except short ribs; whisk well.
2. Trim the excess fat from the ribs. Score the meat deeply every $\frac{1}{2}$ inch (1.2 cm), almost to the bone.
3. Add short ribs to the marinade and coat evenly, turning the meat so the scored side is face-down in the marinade. Cover and let stand at least 3 hours, or refrigerate overnight, if possible.
4. Broil over charcoal, grill, or cook under a broiler. Look for outside to become crisp.

# Kimchi

## Traditional Napa Cabbage

YIELD: 1 GALLON

| AMOUNT | MEASURE | INGREDIENT |
|---|---|---|
| 1 cup plus 1 tablespoon | $8\frac{1}{2}$ ounces, 238 g | Salt |
| $\frac{1}{2}$ gallon | 64 ounces, 1.92 l | Water |
| 2 | | Napa cabbage heads, cut into 2 inch (5 cm) wedges |
| 1 | | Garlic head, cloves separated and peeled |
| 2 | 1-inch (2.4 cm) pieces | Ginger root |
| $\frac{1}{4}$ cup | 2 ounces, 60 ml | Fish sauce or Korean salted shrimp |
| 1 bunch | | Green onion, 1 inch (2.4 cm) pieces |
| $\frac{1}{2}$ cup | 4 ounces, 112 g | Korean ground chile |
| 1 teaspoon | | Granulated sugar |

### PROCEDURE

1. Dissolve 1 cup (8 ounces, 224 g) salt in water. Soak cabbage in salt water 3 to 4 hours.
2. Combine garlic, ginger, and fish sauce and process until almost smooth.
3. Combine green onions, garlic mixture, chile, 1 tablespoon ($\frac{1}{2}$ ounce, 14 g) salt, and sugar.
4. Drain cabbage and rinse thoroughly. Drain well in colander, squeezing as much water from the leaves as possible.
5. Spread green onion/chile mixture between cabbage leaves, making sure to fill each leaf adequately.
6. When all the cabbage has been stuffed, wrap a few of the larger leaves tightly around the rest of the cabbage, making tight bundles.
7. Divide cabbage among four 1-quart (960 ml) jars or one 1-gallon (1.28 l) jar, pressing down firmly to remove any air bubbles.
8. Let stand 2 to 3 days in the refrigerator to ferment.

# Soo Jeung Kwa

## Persimmon Punch

YIELD: 1 QUART

| AMOUNT | MEASURE | INGREDIENT |
| --- | --- | --- |
| 1 quart | 32 ounces, 960 ml | Cold water |
| $\frac{1}{4}$ cup | 1 ounce, 28 g | Ginger, peeled, sliced thin |
| 2 | | Cinnamon sticks |
| $\frac{1}{2}$ cup | 4 ounces, 112 g | Granulated sugar |
| 2 | | Dried persimmons, sliced, or 4 fresh or 10 dried apricots, 1 inch (2.5 cm) dice |
| $\frac{1}{4}$ cup | 1 ounce, 28 g | Pine nuts |

PROCEDURE

1 Simmer water, ginger, and cinnamon sticks for 30 minutes or until water turns slightly red.

2 Strain, add sugar and persimmons, and let cool.

3 Serve well chilled with a teaspoon of pine nuts floating in each cup.

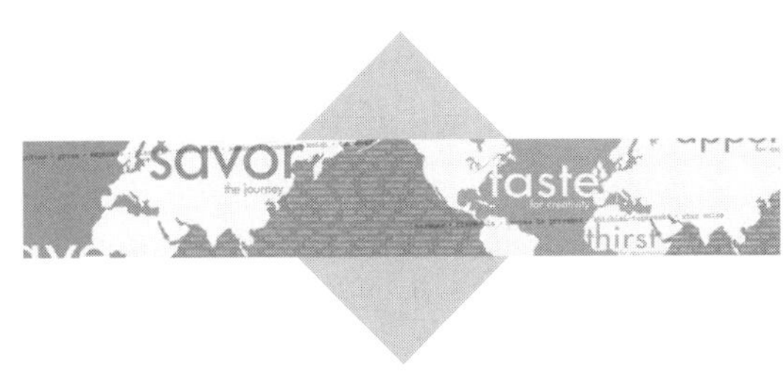

# Jahb Chae

## Mung Bean Noodles

SERVES 4

| AMOUNT | MEASURE | INGREDIENT |
|---|---|---|
| 3 cups | 6 ounces, 168 g | Spinach |
| 2 tablespoons | 1 ounce, 30 ml | Sesame oil |
| 1 tablespoon | | Minced garlic |
| As needed | | Salt |
| 1 cup | 4 ounces, 112 g | Onion, julienned |
| 1 cup | 4 ounces, 112 g | Green onions, bias cut into 2 inch (5 cm) pieces |
| $\frac{1}{2}$ cup | 2 ounces, 56 g | Carrots, peeled, julienned |
| 1 cup | 3 ounces, 84 g | Shiitake mushrooms, thinly sliced |
| As needed | | Soy sauce |
| As needed | | Granulated sugar |
| As needed | | Vegetable oil |
| 6 ounces | 168 g | *Dang myun* (Korean starch noodles), cover with boiling water, let stand 15 to 20 minutes or until softened, drained |
| As needed | | Pepper |
| As needed | | Sesame seeds, toasted |

PROCEDURE

1. Blanch spinach in boiling salted water; cool under cold running water. Squeeze out as much moisture as possible. Cut into 3 inch (7.2 cm) lengths.
2. Combine sesame oil, minced garlic, and a pinch of salt. Toss with spinach and set aside.
3. Over medium high heat sauté all the vegetables separately with vegetable oil. To use the same pan, start with light-colored vegetables: onions, green onions, carrots, then shiitake mushrooms. The vegetables do not need to take on color, they just need to be softened.
4. Toss the sautéed shiitake mushrooms with $\frac{1}{2}$ teaspoon (2.5 ml) soy sauce, 1 teaspoon (5 ml) sugar, and 1 teaspoon (5 ml) sesame oil mix together.
5. Combine $1\frac{1}{2}$ cups (12 ounces, 360 ml) water, $\frac{1}{4}$ cup (2 ounces, 56 g) sugar, 2 tablespoons (1 ounce, 30 ml) soy sauce, and $\frac{1}{4}$ cup (2 ounces, 60 ml) vegetable oil to make *dang myon* seasoning.

6 In correct size pan, combine *dang myon* seasoning and soaked noodles. Bring to a boil, stirring occasionally for a few minutes until liquid is absorbed, then stir constantly until noodles are soft and translucent. Remove from heat, let cool, and cut into manageable length.

7 Toss noodles and vegetables; correct seasoning with salt and pepper. Transfer to a shallow serving dish and serve warm or at room temperature. Sprinkle with sesame seeds.

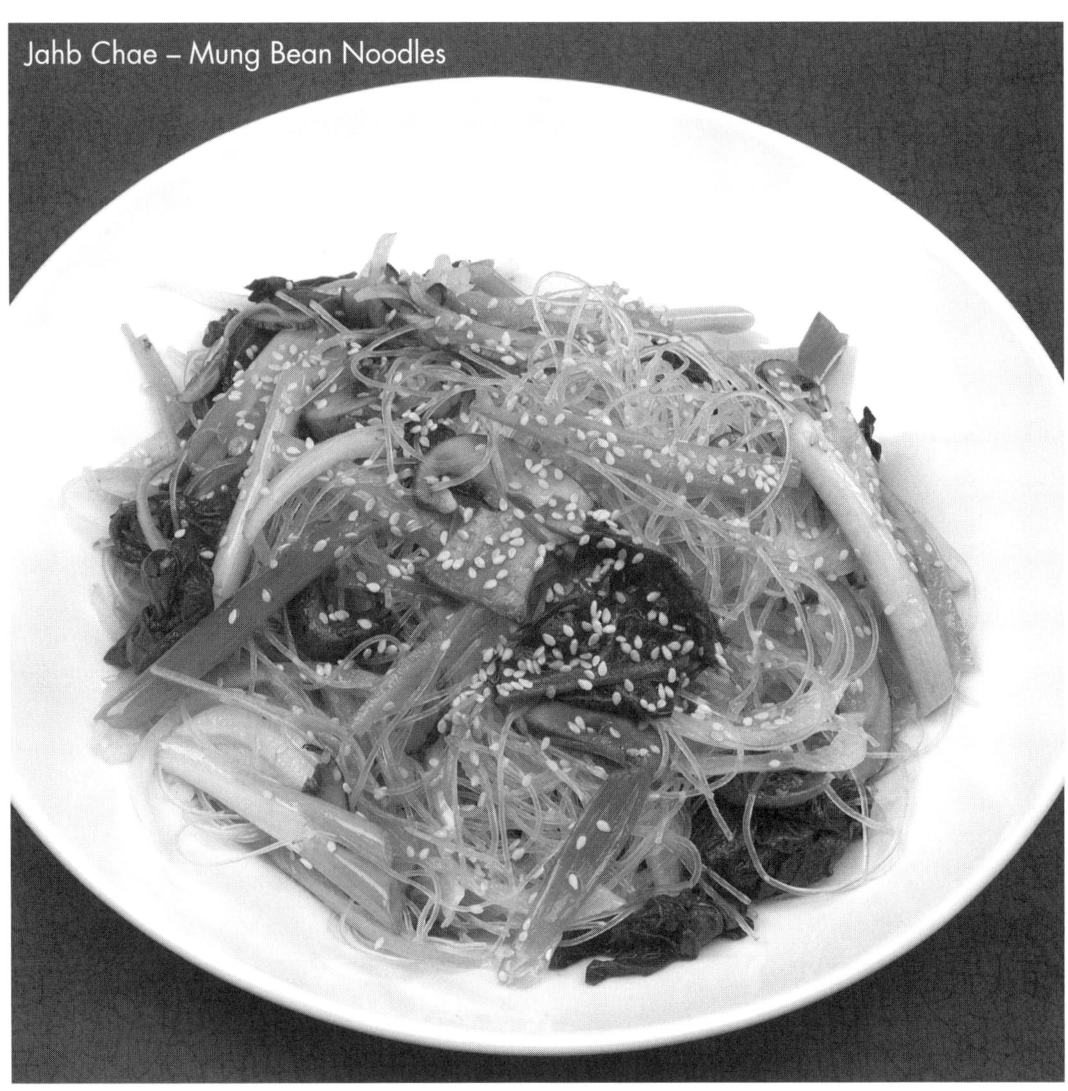
Jahb Chae – Mung Bean Noodles

# Dak Chochu Jang Boekum

## Chicken in Hot Chile Sauce

SERVES 4

| AMOUNT | MEASURE | INGREDIENT |
|---|---|---|
| 1 $\frac{1}{2}$ pounds | 672 g | Chicken, cut into 3 inch (7.2 cm) pieces |
| 4 tablespoons | 2 ounces, 56 g | Granulated sugar |
| 2 | | Garlic cloves, minced |
| $\frac{1}{4}$ cup | 1 ounce, 28 g | Green onions, chopped |
| 1 tablespoon | $\frac{1}{2}$ ounce, 15 ml | Fresh ginger, peeled, minced |
| 2 tablespoons | 1 ounce, 30 ml | Soy sauce |
| 4 tablespoons | 2 ounces, 60 ml | *Gochu jang* (Korean hot fermented chile paste) |
| 2 tablespoons | 1 ounce, 30 ml | Sesame oil |
| 2 tablespoons | $\frac{1}{3}$ ounce, 10 g | Sesame seeds, toasted |
| $\frac{1}{2}$ cup | 4 ounces, 120 ml | Water |

### PROCEDURE

1. Toss chicken pieces with sugar and let stand 1 hour.
2. Combine all other ingredients except water.
3. Toss chicken pieces with mixture and let stand 1 hour.
4. Bring water to a boil, add chicken and marinade, and bring to a simmer. Cover and simmer 30 minutes, or until chicken is cooked and most of the liquid has evaporated. Stir to prevent burning.

# Dubu Jolim Simmered Tofu

**SERVES 4**

| AMOUNT | MEASURE | INGREDIENT |
|---|---|---|
| **18 ounces** | **504 g** | **Firm tofu** |
| **2 tablespoons** | **1 ounce, 30 ml** | **Soy sauce** |
| **1** | | **Garlic clove, minced** |
| **$\frac{1}{2}$ cup** | **2 ounces, 56 g** | **Green onion, sliced thin** |
| **$\frac{1}{4}$ cup** | **1 ounce, 28 g** | **Red bell pepper, minced** |
| **1 tablespoon** | **$\frac{1}{2}$ ounce, 15 ml** | **Vegetable oil** |

**PROCEDURE**

1. Rinse tofu in cold water. Cut into $\frac{1}{2}$ inch (1.2 cm) cubes. Set aside to drain on paper towels.
2. Combine soy sauce, garlic, green onions, and red bell pepper. Set aside.
3. Heat oil over medium high heat and add tofu; make sure a flat side of each piece is in contact with the pan. The tofu will still have moisture, so be careful of splatters. Cook until first side is light brown, 2 to 4 minutes. Turn over and brown the opposite side, 2 to 4 minutes.
4. Reduce heat to medium; add soy mixture, spooning over the top. Cover and cook 2 to 3 minutes until infused with the seasoning.

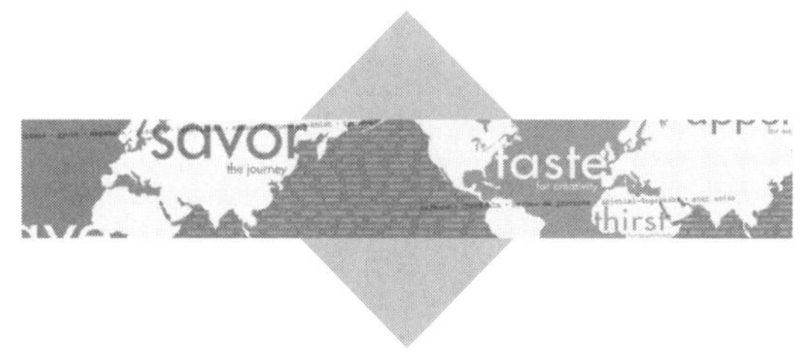

# Dan Kim Kui Crispy Seaweed

SERVES 4

| AMOUNT | MEASURE | INGREDIENT |
|---|---|---|
| As needed | | Sesame oil |
| 10 | | Nori (seaweed) sheets |
| As needed | | Salt |

PROCEDURE

1 Using a pastry brush, brush a thin layer of oil onto the seaweed. Sprinkle a little salt over the entire sheet. Turn over and repeat on the other side.

2 In a large fry pan over medium heat, toast the nori until they turn brownish dark green; flip and toast the other side.

3 Cut toasted nori sheets down the middle lengthwise, then cut twice crosswise to make 6 small pieces.

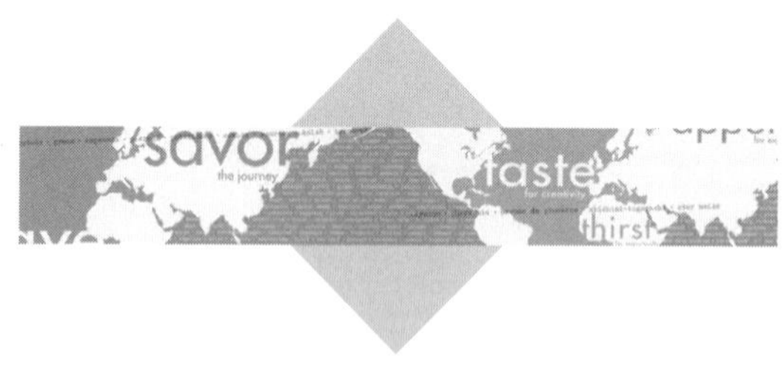

# Kohng Namool

## Seasoned Soybean Sprouts

SERVES 4

| AMOUNT | MEASURE | INGREDIENT |
|---|---|---|
| **4 cups** | **16 ounces, 448 g** | **Soybean sprouts** |
| **½ cup** | **2 ounces, 56 g** | **Green onions, thinly sliced** |
| **1½ tablespoons** | | **Garlic cloves, minced** |
| **1 tablespoon** | | **Toasted sesame seeds, crushed** |
| **1 tablespoon** | **½ ounce, 15 ml** | **Sesame oil** |
| **1 teaspoon** | | **White vinegar** |
| **1 teaspoon** | | **Salt** |
| **1 teaspoon** | | ***Kochukaru* (Korean chile powder)** |

**PROCEDURE**

1. Wash bean sprouts in cold water, removing any bean husks.
2. Combine sprouts and 1 cup (8 ounces, 240 ml) water in a pot with lid. Bring to a boil and cook 3 minutes. Do not lift lid. Remove from heat.
3. Rinse in cold water and drain.
4. Combine remaining ingredients, mix well, and toss with sprouts. Correct seasoning with salt and chile powder.

# Bulgogi (Boolgogi)

## Fire Meat SERVES 4

**While literally translated as "fire meat," *bulgogi* is a nonspicy dish. Traditionally, it is eaten wrapped in green lettuce with *gochujang* (bean-paste hot sauce), but it may also simply be placed over a bowl of rice.**

| AMOUNT | MEASURE | INGREDIENT |
|---|---|---|
| $\frac{1}{2}$ cup | 4 ounces, 112 g | Asian or hard pear, peeled, cored, and grated |
| 2 tablespoons | $\frac{1}{2}$ ounce, 14 g | Onion, minced |
| $\frac{1}{4}$ cup | 1 ounce, 28 g | Green onion, sliced thin |
| 2 tablespoons | 1 ounce, 30 ml | Sake |
| $\frac{1}{2}$ cup | 4 ounces, 120 ml | Water |
| 1 tablespoon | | Garlic, minced |
| 2 tablespoons | 1 ounce, 30 ml | Sesame oil |
| 2 teaspoons | | Sesame seeds |
| 1 teaspoon | | Black pepper, freshly ground |
| 2 tablespoons | 1 ounce, 28 g | Granulated sugar |
| 1 pound | 448 g | Beef top round, partially frozen, cut very thin into 2 inch (5 cm) squares. |
| As needed | | *Bulgogi* sauce (recipe follows) |

**PROCEDURE**

1 Combine all ingredients except the beef; stir well to dissolve.
2 Add beef to marinade and toss; marinate for at least 3 hours.
3 Drain meat, discarding marinade.
4 Cook beef on a *bulgogi* grill pan or grill over hot charcoal or stir-fry over high heat.
5 Dip broiled, grilled, or stir-fried meat slices in *bulgogi* sauce.

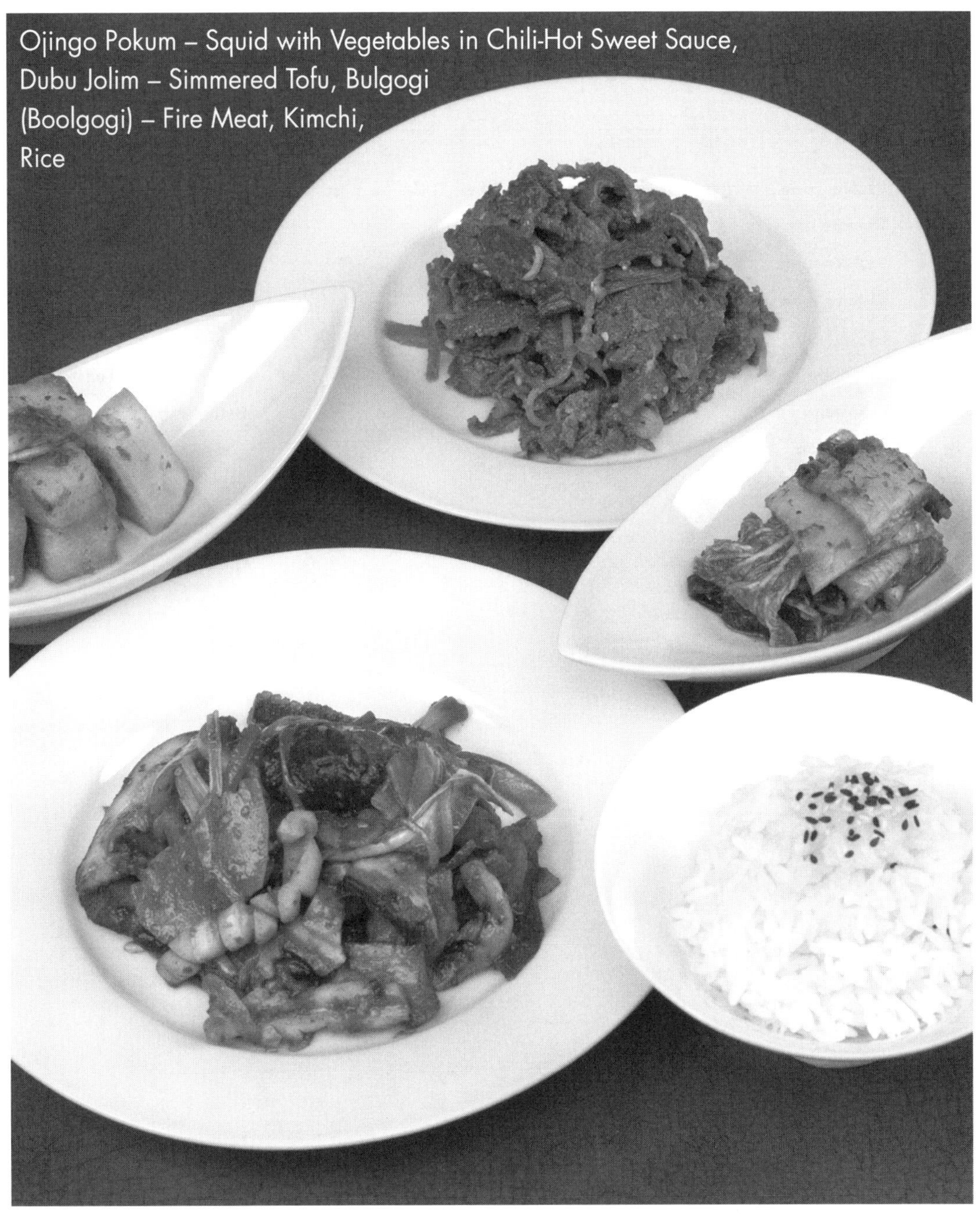

Ojingo Pokum – Squid with Vegetables in Chili-Hot Sweet Sauce, Dubu Jolim – Simmered Tofu, Bulgogi (Boolgogi) – Fire Meat, Kimchi, Rice

# Bulgogi Sauce

SERVES 4

| AMOUNT | MEASURE | INGREDIENT |
|---|---|---|
| 1 | | Garlic clove |
| 1 tablespoon | $\frac{1}{2}$ ounce, 14 g | Granulated sugar |
| To taste | | Salt |
| 3 tablespoons | $1\frac{1}{2}$ ounces, 45 ml | Dark soy sauce |
| 1 tablespoon | $\frac{1}{2}$ ounce, 15 ml | Sesame oil |
| 1 teaspoon | | Chinese bean paste |
| 1 teaspoon | | Sesame seeds, toasted |
| 2 tablespoons | 1 ounce, 30 ml | Sake or dry sherry |
| 1 teaspoon | | Green onion, white part, minced |
| 1 tablespoon | $\frac{1}{2}$ ounce, 15 ml | Oil |
| $\frac{1}{4}$ teaspoon | | Cayenne pepper |

**PROCEDURE**

1 Crush garlic with sugar and salt to make a smooth paste.

2 Combine remaining ingredients.

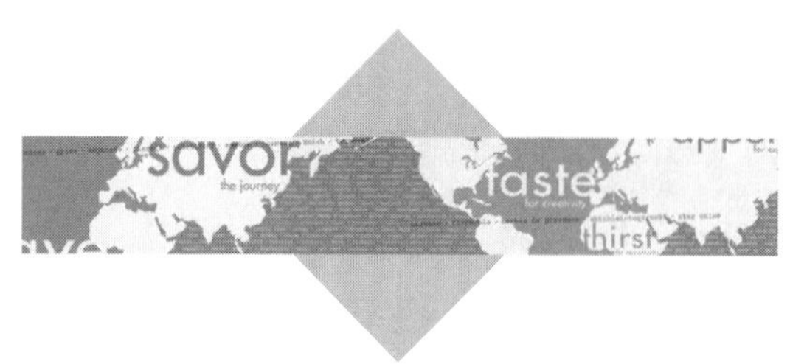

# Ojingo Pokum

## Squid with Vegetables in Chile Hot-Sweet Sauce SERVES 4

| AMOUNT | MEASURE | INGREDIENT |
|---|---|---|
| 2 tablespoons | 1 ounce, 30 ml | Vegetable oil |
| 1 cup | 4 ounces, 112 g | Green onions, cut into 1 inch (2.4 cm) lengths |
| 1 cup | 4 ounces, 112 g | Spicy Korean red peppers, or red bell peppers, julienned |
| 1 cup | 4 ounces, 112 g | Carrots, julienned |
| 1 cup | 4 ounces, 112 g | Onions, julienned |
| 1 cup | 4 ounces, 112 g | Mushrooms, sliced thin |
| 1 pound | 448 g | Squid, cleaned and cut into flat 1 × 2 inch (2.4 × 4.8 cm) inch pieces |
| 2 teaspoons | | Garlic, minced |
| 2 teaspoons | | Granulated sugar |
| 1 tablespoon | | Red pepper flakes or *kochukaru* (Korean chile powder) |

**PROCEDURE**

1. Heat the oil, add the vegetables, and stir-fry 2 minutes.
2. Remove from heat and add squid, garlic, and sugar. Stir-fry 2 minutes.
3. Add chile powder and cook over high heat 1 minute. Serve hot.

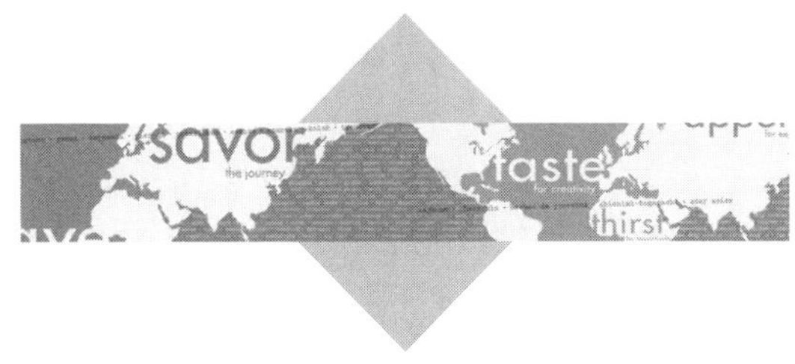

# Bibimbap Garnished Rice SERVES 4

**This is a one-dish meal with rice and an assortment of seasonal vegetables, and often a small bit of meat may be added. It is traditionally served in a heated stone pot, garnished with a raw egg yolk on top. When eaten, everything is mixed together, and the raw yolk is fully cooked by the heated stone.**

## Red Pepper Paste

| AMOUNT | MEASURE | INGREDIENT |
|---|---|---|
| 2 tablespoons | 1 ounce, 30 ml | Red pepper paste |
| 2 tablespoons | 1 ounce, 30 ml | Soy sauce |
| 1 tablespoon | | Garlic, minced |
| 2 tablespoons | $\frac{1}{2}$ ounce, 14 g | Green onion, white part, minced |
| 1 tablespoon | $\frac{1}{2}$ ounce, 14 g | Granulated sugar |
| 1 tablespoon | | Sesame seed, toasted |
| 2 tablespoons | 1 ounce, 30 ml | Sesame oil |

**PROCEDURE**

1 Combine all ingredients and simmer on low heat until thick.

## Seasoning Sauce

| AMOUNT | MEASURE | INGREDIENT |
|---|---|---|
| 4 tablespoons | 2 ounces, 60 ml | Soy sauce |
| 2 tablespoons | 1 ounce, 30 ml | Granulated sugar |
| 1 tablespoon | $\frac{1}{2}$ ounce, 15 ml | Rice wine |
| 1 tablespoon | | Green onion, minced |
| 1 tablespoon | | Garlic, minced |
| 1 tablespoon | $\frac{1}{2}$ ounce, 15 ml | Sesame oil |
| 1 tablespoon | | Sesame seeds, toasted |
| $\frac{1}{2}$ teaspoon | | Black pepper |

**PROCEDURE**

1 Combine all ingredients.

| AMOUNT | MEASURE | INGREDIENT |
|---|---|---|
| 3 cups | 18 ounces, 504 g | White rice, cooked |
| 1 cup | 4 ounces, 112 g | Carrots, julienned blanched |
| 1 teaspoon | | Soy sauce |
| 1 tablespoon | | Sesame seeds |
| Pinch | | Salt |

**PROCEDURE**

1 Stir-fry rice and carrots with 1 teaspoon (5 ml) soy sauce, $\frac{1}{2}$ teaspoon (2.5 ml) sesame oil, 1 tablespoon (5 ml) sesame seed, and a pinch of salt.

| AMOUNT | MEASURE | INGREDIENT |
|---|---|---|
| 1 cup | 6 ounces, 168 g | English cucumber, julienned |
| 2 teaspoons | | Salt |
| $\frac{1}{2}$ teaspoon | | Sesame oil |

**PROCEDURE**

1 Sprinkle cucumber with 1 teaspoon salt; toss and let stand 10 minutes. Squeeze out the moisture and stir-fry in 1 teaspoon salt and $\frac{1}{2}$ teaspoon sesame oil until hot.

| AMOUNT | MEASURE | INGREDIENT |
|---|---|---|
| 2 cups | 8 ounces, 224 g | Bean sprouts |
| $\frac{1}{2}$ cup | 4 ounces, 120 ml | Boiling water, salted |
| 1 teaspoon | | Salt |
| 1 teaspoon | | Sesame oil |
| 1 teaspoon | | Green onion |
| $\frac{1}{2}$ teaspoon | | Garlic |

**PROCEDURE**

1 Scald bean sprouts in boiling salted water. Drain and mix with remaining ingredients.

| AMOUNT | MEASURE | INGREDIENT |
|---|---|---|
| 1 cup | 6 ounces, 168 g | Spinach, blanched, moisture squeezed out |
| 1 teaspoon | | Soy sauce |
| $\frac{1}{2}$ teaspoon | | Sesame oil |
| $\frac{1}{2}$ teaspoon | | Sesame seeds |
| 1 teaspoon | | Green onion |
| $\frac{1}{2}$ teaspoon | | Garlic |
| To taste | | Black pepper |

**PROCEDURE**

1 Stir-fry spinach with soy sauce, sesame oil, sesame seed, green onion, garlic, and black pepper.

| AMOUNT | MEASURE | INGREDIENT |
|---|---|---|
| 4 | | Whole eggs |

**PROCEDURE**

1 Fry egg to taste.

**Serving**

1 Place $\frac{1}{4}$ of the rice in 4 warm bowls. Arrange vegetables in separate mounds around the rice. Top each serving with 1 egg. Serve with red pepper paste, which is normally mixed together with the rice and vegetables. Serve the seasoning sauce on the side.

# Dwaeji Galbi

## Spicy Pork Ribs

SERVES 4

| AMOUNT | MEASURE | INGREDIENT |
|---|---|---|
| 1 inch (2.4 cm) | | Ginger root, peeled, minced |
| 1 | | Garlic clove, minced |
| $\frac{1}{4}$ cup | 2 ounces, 60 ml | Chile paste |
| 2 tablespoons | 1 ounce, 30 ml | Korean malt syrup *(mool yut)* or corn syrup or honey |
| 2 tablespoons | 1 ounce, 28 g | Granulated sugar |
| 1 tablespoon | $\frac{1}{2}$ ounce, 15 ml | Soy sauce |
| 1 tablespoon | $\frac{1}{2}$ ounce, 15 ml | Sesame oil |
| $\frac{1}{2}$ teaspoon | | Black pepper |
| $1\frac{1}{4}$ pound | 560 g | Pork back ribs, trimmed and cut into serving pieces |

**PROCEDURE**

1. Preheat oven to 350°F (176°C)
2. Combine ginger, garlic, chile paste, malt syrup, sugar, soy sauce, sesame oil, and black pepper. Rub marinade generously over meat. Cover and refrigerate 2 hours or longer.
3. Arrange ribs, slightly overlapping in roasting pan. Cover with foil; bake 1 hour or until ribs are tender. Set aside and reserve roasting juices.
4. When ready to serve, heat grill to medium-high heat and grill 5 to 6 minutes per side. Baste with roasting juices.

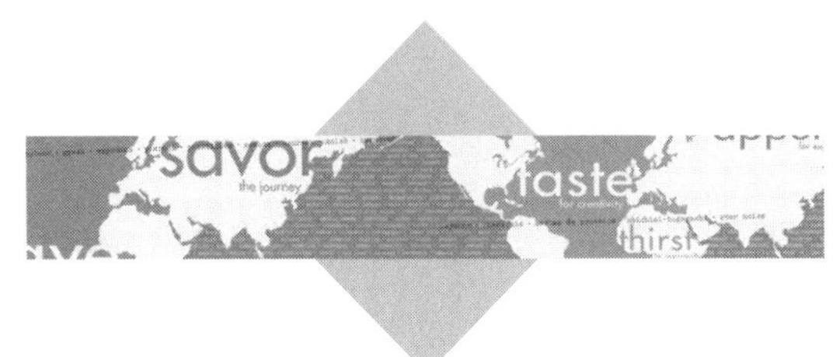

# Bibim Gooksu

## Spicy Summer Noodles

SERVES 4

| AMOUNT | MEASURE | INGREDIENT |
|---|---|---|
| **1 cup** | **8 ounces, 224 g** | **Kimchi, chopped** |
| **$1\frac{1}{2}$ cup** | **9 ounces, 252 g** | **Cucumber, peeled, seeded, julienned** |
| **1 tablespoon** | **$\frac{1}{2}$ ounce, 15 ml** | **Soy sauce** |
| **1 tablespoon** | **$\frac{1}{2}$ ounce, 15 ml** | **Sesame oil** |
| **1** | | **Garlic clove, minced** |
| **1 tablespoon** | **$\frac{1}{2}$ ounce, 15 ml** | **Rice vinegar** |
| **1 tablespoon** | **$\frac{1}{2}$ ounce, 14 g** | **Granulated sugar** |
| **10 ounces** | **280 g** | **Dried buckwheat noodles (*naeng myun*), cooked and cooled in ice water** |

PROCEDURE

1. Combine kimchi and cucumbers.
2. Combine soy sauce, sesame oil, garlic, vinegar, and sugar; stir to dissolve.
3. Toss dressing with vegetables.
4. Drain the noodles thoroughly and divide among four shallow bowls. Top each portion with the vegetable mixture and serve immediately.

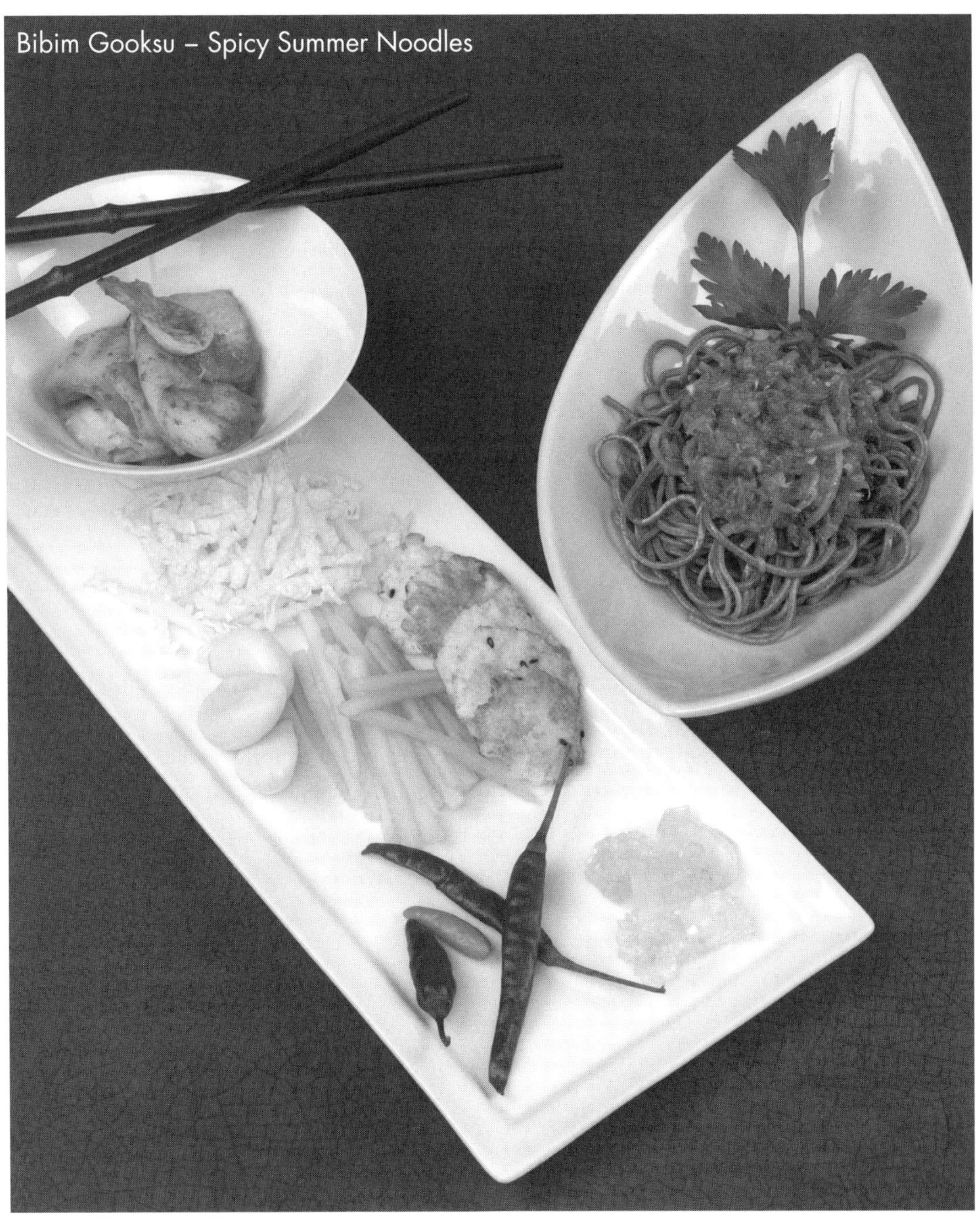
Bibim Gooksu – Spicy Summer Noodles

# Maeum Tang Spiced Fish Soup

SERVES 4

| AMOUNT | MEASURE | INGREDIENT |
|---|---|---|
| **1 pound** | **448 g** | **Cod fillets, skinned, boned, $1\frac{1}{2}$ inch (3.6 cm) cubes** |
| **$2\frac{1}{2}$ cups** | **20 ounces, 600 ml** | **Water or light fish stock** |
| **2 tablespoons** | **1 ounces, 30 ml** | **Vegetable oil** |
| **1 cup** | **4 ounces, 112 g** | **Onion, $\frac{1}{4}$ inch (.6 cm) dice** |
| **2 tablespoons** | **$\frac{1}{2}$ ounce, 14 g** | **Green onion, white part, minced** |
| **2** | | **Garlic cloves, minced** |
| **1 teaspoon** | | **Ginger, minced** |
| **2–4 teaspoons** | | **Chile powder, to taste** |
| **2 teaspoons** | | **Salt** |
| **1 cup** | **4 ounces, 112 g** | **Zucchini, halved lengthwise and sliced thin** |
| **$\frac{1}{2}$ cup** | **2 ounces, 56 g** | **Green pepper, julienne cut** |

PROCEDURE

1. Combine cod and water; bring to a simmer and cook 3–4 minutes or until just cooked. Remove from heat and set aside.
2. Heat oil over medium high heat; stir-fry onions, green onions, garlic, ginger, and chile powder for 1 minute. Add salt, zucchini, and green peppers; stir-fry one minute.
3. Combine vegetables with soup, bring back to simmer, and serve hot.

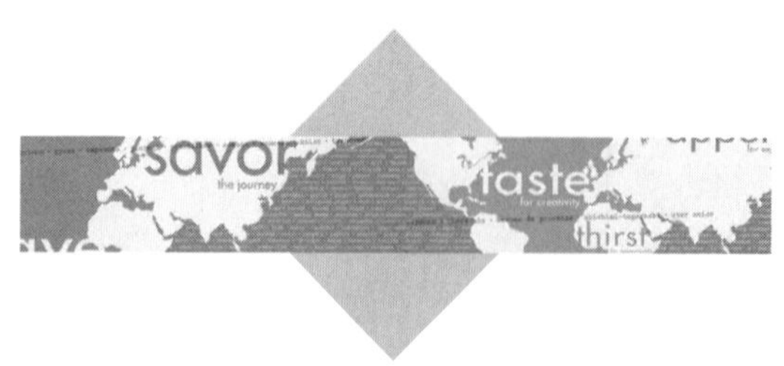

# Kaji Namul
## Marinated Eggplant

SERVES 4

| AMOUNT | MEASURE | INGREDIENT |
|---|---|---|
| 2 or 3 | 8 ounces, 224 g | Japanese eggplants, ends trimmed |
| $\frac{1}{2}$ cup | 2 ounces, 56 g | Green onions, green and white parts, minced |
| 2 tablespoons | 1 ounce, 30 ml | Soy sauce |
| 1 | | Garlic clove, minced |
| 1 teaspoon | | Sesame seeds |
| 2 teaspoon | | Sesame oil |
| 1 teaspoon | | Rice vinegar |

PROCEDURE

1 Steam eggplant in a Chinese-style steamer until tender, 8 to 10 minutes. Let cool and cut into 3-inch (7.2 cm) strips.

2 Combine remaining ingredients; whisk together. Toss dressing with eggplant and refrigerate until ready to serve. Serve at room temperature.

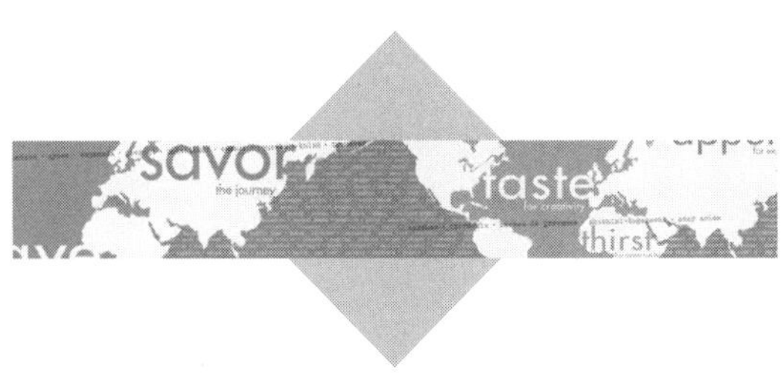

# Oi Bok Kum Namul

## Cooked Cucumbers

SERVES 4

| AMOUNT | MEASURE | INGREDIENT |
|---|---|---|
| 2 cups | 8 ounces, 224 g | Cucumber, peeled, seeded, cut $\frac{1}{4}$ x $\frac{1}{4}$ x 2$\frac{1}{2}$ inches (.6 cm x .6 cm x .6 cm) long |
| 1$\frac{1}{4}$ teaspoons | | Salt |
| 1$\frac{1}{2}$ tablespoons | $\frac{3}{4}$ ounce, 20 ml | Sesame seed oil |
| 2 tablespoons | $\frac{1}{2}$ ounce, 14 g | Green onions, minced |
| 2 tablespoons | 1 ounce, 30 ml | Soy sauce |
| 2 teaspoons | | Chile powder |
| 1$\frac{1}{2}$ teaspoon | | Granulated sugar |
| 1 tablespoon | | Sesame seeds, toasted |

### PROCEDURE

1. Toss cucumber with salt and let stand 10 minutes. Rinse and dry thoroughly.
2. Heat oil over medium heat and sauté cucumbers and green onions until they begin to soften, 2 to 3 minutes.
3. Add soy sauce, chile powder, and sugar; toss to distribute evenly. Transfer to serving dish and sprinkle with sesame seeds.
4. Serve warm or slightly chilled.

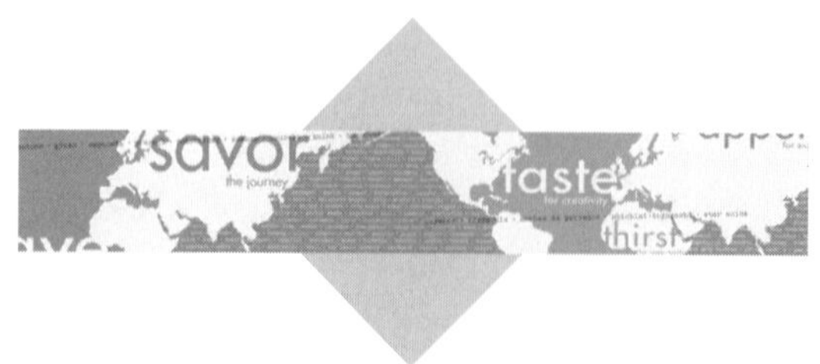

# Seng Sun Bulgogi
## Barbecued Spiced Fish
SERVES 4

| AMOUNT | MEASURE | INGREDIENT |
|---|---|---|
| 1 teaspoons | | Salt |
| 1 $\frac{1}{2}$ pounds | 5 ounces each, 140 g each | Fillet of fish, sea bass, red snapper, flounder, or similar fish, skin on |
| 2 teaspoons | | *Kochujang (Gochujang)* paste |
| 1 teaspoon | | Granulated sugar |
| $\frac{1}{2}$ teaspoon | | Black pepper |
| 1 teaspoon | | Toasted sesame seeds |
| 1 teaspoon | | Sesame oil |
| 1 teaspoon | | Rice wine |
| 2 tablespoons | | Green onions, minced |
| 1 | | Garlic clove, minced |
| 1 teaspoon | | Ginger root, minced |

PROCEDURE

1. Sprinkle salt over fish fillet and let stand under refrigeration for at least 3 hours, preferably overnight, to dry out. Turn the pieces over a few times.
2. Mix remaining ingredients to a paste. Rub paste into fish fillets. Let stand 30 minutes.
3. Grill or broil filets until just done, 3 to 5 minutes per side, according to thickness. Do not overcook. Serve hot or warm.

# Yak Sik Steamed Rice Pudding

SERVES 4

| AMOUNT | MEASURE | INGREDIENT |
|---|---|---|
| 1¾ cup | 12¼ ounces, 343 g | Glutinous rice |
| 2 tablespoons | 1 ounce, 30 ml | Sesame oil |
| ½ teaspoon | | Ground cinnamon |
| ½ cup | 2½ ounces, 70 g | Raisins |
| ½ cup | 3½ ounces, 98 g | Dates, pitted, cut in half |
| 1 cup | 7 ounces, 196 g | Packaged chestnuts, peeled, cut in half |
| ¼ cup | 2 ounces, 60 ml | Honey |
| 2 tablespoons | | Pine nuts |
| Seasoning Mix | | |
| 1½ tablespoons | ¾ ounce, 22.5 ml | Soy sauce |
| ¼ cup | 2 ounces, 56 g | Brown sugar |
| ¾ cup | 5¼ ounces, 147 g | Granulated sugar |

PROCEDURE

1. Wash rice and soak in cold water 4 hours, if possible. Drain and steam 30 minutes. Transfer hot cooked rice to a large bowl.
2. Combine seasoning mix ingredients and fold into the hot rice until well mixed. Add sesame oil and cinnamon and mix again. Gently add the raisins, dates, and chestnuts while stirring.
3. Return mixture to steamer and steam for one hour. Test one of the chestnuts to make sure everything is cooked. Sprinkle with honey and mix while steaming. Serve topped with pine nuts.
4. For an alternative serving presentation, press the hot steamed rice pudding into a form lined with film or foil. Make at least three layers, sprinkling pine nuts on each layer. Let cool enough to slice into squares. Serve warm or at room temperature.

# Southeast Asia

## The Land

Southeast Asia, a region of Asia of over 1,740,000 square miles, is bordered by the Indian subcontinent on the west, China on the north, and the Pacific Ocean on the east. The name "Southeast Asia" came into popular use after World War II and has replaced such phrases as "Further India," "East Indies," "Indo-China," and "Malay Peninsula," which formerly designated all or part of the region. Southeast Asia includes the Indochina Peninsula, which juts into the South China Sea, the Malay Peninsula, and the Indonesian and Philippine archipelagos. The region has ten independent countries: Brunei, Cambodia, Indonesia, Laos, Malaysia, Myanmar, the Philippines, Singapore, Thailand, and Vietnam.

Peninsular Southeast Asia is a rugged region traversed by many mountains and drained by great rivers such as the Thanlwin, Ayeyarwady, Chao Phraya, and Mekong. Insular Southeast Asia is made up of numerous volcanic and coral islands. Overall, the region has a generally tropical rainy climate, with the exception of the northwestern part, which has a humid subtropical climate. The wet monsoon winds are vital for the economic well-being of the region. Tropical forests cover most of the area. Rice is the chief crop of the region; rubber, tea, spices, and coconuts are also important. The region has a great variety of minerals and produces most of the world's tin.

# History

Throughout the early human history of Southeast Asia, one group after another was displaced and pushed southward by successive waves of immigrants from China and Tibet. Only the inhabitants of the highlands retained their traditional culture.

By the first century A.D., traders from India and China were vying for a foothold in the region, drawn there by its rich abundance of minerals, spices, and forest products. For the next thirteen or fourteen centuries, India's influence dominated, except in what is now Vietnam. Although there is some small Indian influence seen in the cuisine, China maintained a political foothold in Vietnam for a thousand years. Even after it lost control over the area during the 900s, Chinese migrants and merchants continued to make a strong impact on the region.

Throughout this long period, local kingdoms, such as the Khmer empire, rose and fell, but the peoples of the region were never unified culturally. Frequently, they were caught up in savage wars with one another. Even today, there is a legacy of distrust among groups of differing ancestries in Southeast Asia.

In the late fifteenth century Islamic influences grew strong but were overshadowed by the arrival of Europeans, who established their power throughout Southeast Asia; only Thailand remained free of colonial occupation. Because of Southeast Asia's strategic location between Japan and India, and the importance of shipping routes that traverse it, the region became the scene of battles between Allied and Japanese forces during World War II.

Since the war the countries of Southeast Asia have reemerged as independent nations. They have been plagued by political turmoil, weak economies, ethnic strife, and social inequities, although the situation for most Southeast Asian nations improved in the 1980s and 1990s. Throughout the 1960s and early 1970s, however, there were open conflicts between communist and non-Communist factions, especially in Vietnam, Laos, and Cambodia. In 1967 Indonesia, Malaysia, the Philippines, Singapore, and Thailand created the Association of Southeast Asian Nations (ASEAN), the objectives of which are to promote regional economic growth, political stability, social progress, and cultural developments. Since then, Brunei (1984), Vietnam (1995), Laos (1997), and Myanmar and Cambodia (1999) have joined ASEAN. In 1997 a monetary collapse in Thailand sparked a general economic crisis in several nations in the region; the results were most severe in Indonesia, which underwent economic, political, and social turmoil in the late 1990s.

Religion, ethnicity, and language are diverse throughout Southeast Asia. There are dozens of religions, including Buddhism, Confucianism, Hinduism, Islam, and Roman Catholicism. Hundreds of languages are spoken throughout.

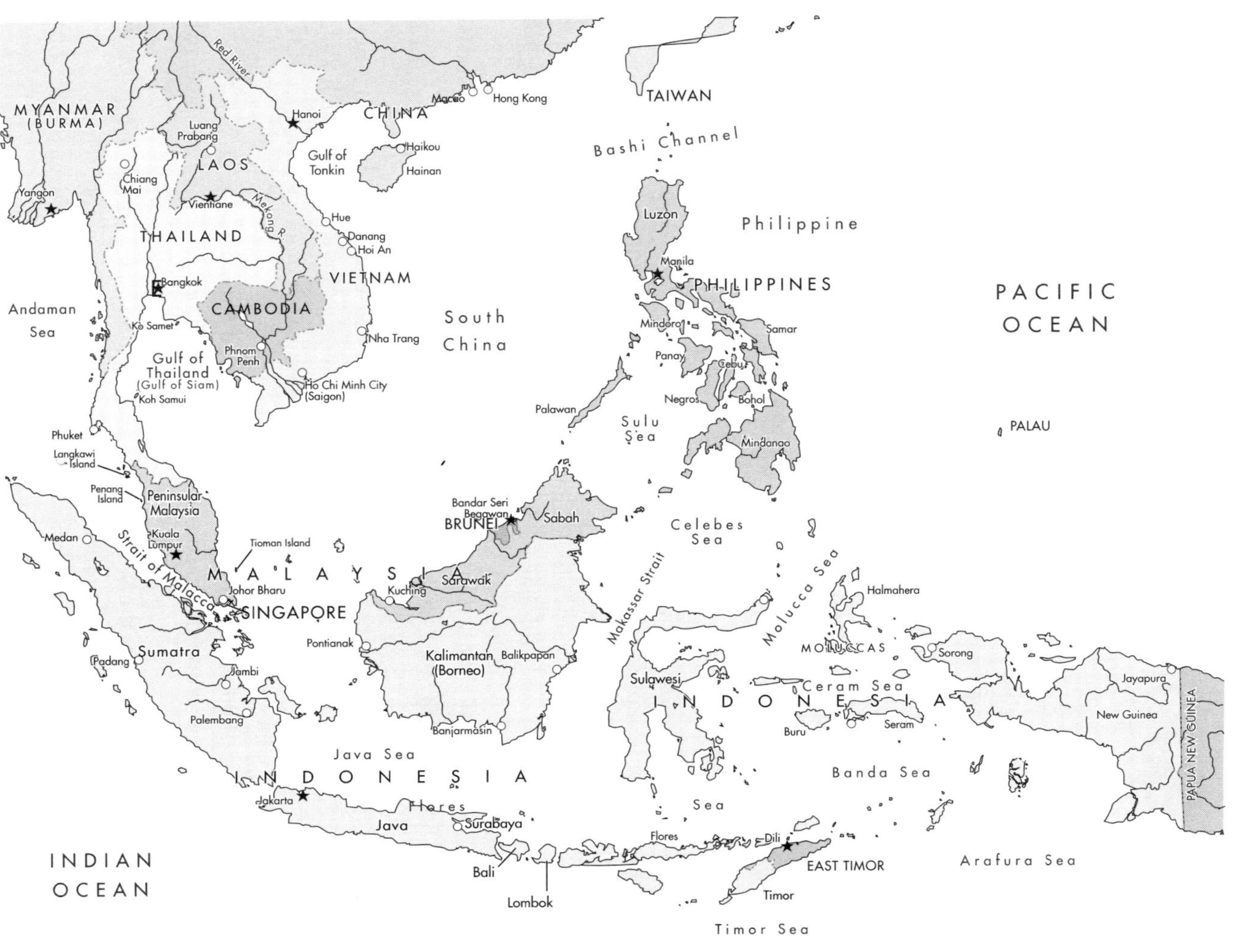


Southeast Asia

# The People

Southeast Asia is one of the world's great melting pots. Its diverse peoples moved into the region in search of a better life and greater security. The original inhabitants of Southeast Asia can be found in the highland regions of the Philippines, Indonesia, and Malaysia. Around 2500 B.C., the first major wave of migrating peoples entered the area. They were the Malays, or Indonesians, and it is their descendants who form the great majority of the populations of the Philippines and Indonesia today. The Malays formerly lived in what is now southern China, but pressure from the Chinese population in the north forced other peoples southward. These people in turn pressed upon the Malays, who moved through the mountain passes into mainland Southeast Asia, down the Malay Peninsula, and out into the Indonesian and Philippine islands. Skilled sailors, the Malays expanded eastward through these islands.

Others followed, principally the Cambodians, the Vietnamese, the Myanmar (Burmese), and the Thai moving south out of China, to settle in mainland Southeast Asia. The Thai were the last of the major groups to settle in here, establishing their first important kingdom during the 1200s.

These various groups brought with them their own customs, cultures, and living patterns, but they were to be strongly influenced by still other people. Traders from India brought Indian philosophies to Southeast Asia, especially the Hindu and Buddhist religions. Myanmar, Thailand, Laos, and Cambodia are today Buddhist countries as a result. Later, Muslim traders brought Islam to Malaysia and Indonesia, which are now predominantly Muslim. The culture and religion of Vietnam were influenced by China.

This process of infusion of both people and ideas has continued into modern times. The European powers began their colonization of the region (except for Thailand, which was never colonized) during the 1500s, bringing with them Western ideas of government, culture, and religion. The Philippines, colonized by Spain, became largely Roman Catholic. During the late 1700s and early 1800s large numbers of Chinese and Indians came to Southeast Asia to take advantage of the economic opportunities during the height of the European colonial period.

More than three-quarters of the Southeast Asia population is agriculture-based. Much fish is consumed in this region, reflecting the long coastlines and river environments of Southeast Asia. The staple food throughout the region is rice, which has been cultivated for thousands of years.

In Asia, there are different styles of eating food. In India and the Middle East, as well as Southeast Asia, people typically eat food with their hands. It is a very direct way to experience the texture of the food, and people wash their hands before and after each meal. Normally, only the right hand is used, so that one knows to keep it especially clean. Generally, the foods to be eaten are placed on plates in the center of the mat or table, and people take food in small portions as they eat. The exception to this pattern is Vietnam, where the influence of China was much stronger than anywhere else in Southeast Asia. Here, chopsticks are the utensil of choice, and food is served onto individual plates or into individual bowls. Today, the influence of Western cultures is found not only in the use of tables and chairs in many modern Southeast Asian households, but also in the use of spoons and forks. Knives are not necessary, since meat and vegetables are chopped into smaller portions before cooking or serving. A large spoon is held in the right hand, while the left hand is used to scoop food into the spoon.

# The Food

Due to the close proximity of the borders between countries in Southeast Asia, and to combined influences from India and China that have affected indigenous taste and cooking styles, the ingredients are similar throughout most of the region, while they are individualized by each culture to suit their palate and taste. Indian cooking has influenced much of Southeast Asia. However, Indian cooking traditions vary throughout the region and according to ethnic and religious preference. Muslims do not eat pork, and the month of Ramadan (the ninth month of the Muslim lunar calendar) is a time of fasting for Muslims all over the world, during which time they may neither eat nor drink during the daylight hours. Hindus, in contrast, believe that cows are sacred and the eating of beef is forbidden. Others from the south of India are vegetarians. Buddhists, too, are expected not to eat meat, as the killing of any animal is against Buddhist beliefs. However, many Buddhists do eat meat as well as fish, and this belief tends to be most closely observed by monks or ascetics rather than by ordinary people today. Curries originated in India, with the milk and butter from cows being included in the recipes. In Southeast Asia, coconut milk is substituted for cow's milk, which gives a very different taste to the curries. Noodles are popular throughout Southeast Asia, and reflect Chinese as well as Indian influence in the spices and methods of preparation.

Europeans have had their culinary influence in Southeast Asia. In the Philippines, for example, Spanish influence is clearly present not only in the languages of the country but in their love of such dishes as *pan de sal* (a type of bread), *kilawin* (marinated raw seafood with chile), *paella* (a seafood, meat, and rice stir fry dish), empanadas (turnovers), and a variety of other seasoned meat dishes. Conventional dishes in the Philippines reflect more influence from a blend of Chinese, Spanish, and indigenous Southeast Asian traditions than is found anywhere else in Southeast Asia.

Popular meals in Southeast Asia consist of rice, fish, vegetables, fruits, and spices. Curry, *satay* (spiced or marinated meat on a stick that is barbecued), *sour fish soup*, noodles, and soy products are popular. Common flavorings include ginger, pepper, chile peppers, onions, garlic, soy sauce, fish sauce, fermented fish paste, turmeric, candlenut, lemongrass, cloves, nutmeg, cinnamon, as well as tamarind and lime (for a sour taste). Coconut milk is often used to bind sharp flavors, while palm sugar is used to balance the spices. Unique combinations of sweet and sour, hot and sour, or hot and sweet are common in various regions. Fish paste and prawn paste is spicy-sour, and is popularly consumed with green mangoes, fresh fish, or in stews. Fish sauce is used in almost all Southeast Asian curries as well as in various forms of cooking fish and pork. Popular vegetables are sweet potatoes, maize, taro, tapioca, legumes, blossoms, and the leaves of many green plants. Popular fruits are pineapple, coconut, star fruit, jackfruit, papaya, bananas, rambutan, mangosteen, and the somewhat foul-smelling durian. Tea and coffee are abundant throughout the region, although the popular drink with a meal is water.

The islands of Indonesia support the fourth most populous nation in the world, a population that is 90 percent Muslim, with hundreds of tribes, subcultures, and languages. *Satay*—pieces of grilled meat, poultry, or seafood served with spicy peanut sauce—is Indonesia's best-known dish. One of the region's most unique foods is the vegetarian *tempeh* or *tempe*. This is made from soybeans and was originally produced to be a food similar to China's tofu. *Gado-gado*, a dish of mixed vegetables and salad with both tofu and tempeh, topped with a spicy peanut sauce, is one of the typical ways in which it is used. *Sambal*, a spicy sauce made from chiles, shrimp paste, and tomatoes, is available everywhere and is eaten with main dishes and snacks.

In Bali the cuisine and culture are distinctively different due to the predominance of the Hindu religion on the island. *Babi guling*, a dish of spit-roast suckling pig stuffed with herbs, is one of the most distinctive Balinese dishes, and often accompanied by the local version of black pudding. Along with rice, proximity to the Pacific Islands means other sources of starch; sago, cassava, and taro are popular staples. There is a large variety of fresh fish to choose from, including eels, squid, barracuda, crab, and shrimp.

Cambodian and Laotian dishes rely on the original ingredients for the core of the flavoring. The most frequent methods of cooking are steaming, grilling over a charcoal fire, or a quick stir-fry in a wok. One of the most popular flavorings is *tik marij*, a mixture of ground black pepper, salt, and lime juice. A main course in the Cambodian diet is simply cooked meat or fish with *tik marij*. Banana leaves are used for wrapping food during grilling or steaming. The leaves retain liquid while adding some flavor to a dish. A favorite Cambodian dessert consists of grilling sticky rice balls with coconut and jackfruit inside a banana leaf.

A combination of different Asian culinary tastes, Lao cuisine combines a love of sticky rice, raw greens, and spicy dipping sauce. Their national dish, *larb*, is a mixture of marinated meat or fish, sometimes served raw, and offered with a combination of vegetables, herbs, and spices. Another popular dish is *tam mak houng*, green papaya salad. Except for crisp green vegetables, Lao foods favor sour over sweet. Galangal, lemongrass, shallots, and garlic are also herbs and vegetables seen as a necessity.

Malaysia has been influenced by Chinese, Indian, and Arabic roots. A majority of Malays are Muslims who consume rice, but not pork or alcohol. However, similar to its Thai neighbors in the north, Malay cooking extensively uses chile peppers and thick coconut milk. East Asian spices contribute flavor to many of the sauces. Malaysian dishes are typically seasoned with curry, shallots, garlic, shrimp paste, tamarind, lemongrass, or coconut milk.

For almost four hundred years, the Spanish had control in the Philippines, leaving a lasting effect that is apparent in Filipino cooking today. Many dishes have Spanish names, regardless of a Spanish connection. A basic technique to start off many Filipino dishes was introduced by the Spaniards: sautéing tomatoes, garlic, and onions in olive oil. The Spaniards also introduced sausages and dishes using meat and dairy. Beef was initially brought to the Philippines by Spanish ships, so many beef entrees are of Spanish origin. In the Philippines, four meals a day are served: breakfast, lunch, *merienda* (snack), and dinner. *Pancit*, or noodles, is considered a *merienda* dish and is served with a sponge cake called *puto* and a glutinous rice cake called *cuchinta.* Lunch is the heaviest meal and consists of rice, a vegetable, a meat, and sometimes fish as well. Vegetables include *kangkung* (a local spinach), broccoli, Chinese broccoli, bitter melon, mung bean, bean sprouts, eggplant, and okra. Beef, pork, and chicken are eaten often, and water buffalo are eaten in the provinces. Other important foods include rice, corn, coconuts, sugarcane, bananas, coffee, mangoes, and pineapples.

In Singapore, cooking—known as Straits Chinese, Baba, or Peranakan cuisine, or Nonya cooking—is a mixture of Chinese and Malay traditions. Described as a fusion of Chinese techniques and tropical produce, Nonya cooking tends to be spicier and tangier than Chinese food but, unlike indigenous Malay cuisines, features the use of pork and noodles. The result is highly refined but also boldly flavored. *Laksa,* the rich coconut soup-noodle dish, is one of the best-known Nonya dishes. *Otak otak* is mashed fish with coconut milk and chile, wrapped in banana leaf and grilled over coals. Singapore is particularly famous for its crab dishes. *Chile crab* features pieces of shellfish smothered in tangy chile and tomato sauce, while black pepper crabs are seasoned in a thick black pepper and soy sauce. The European influence can be seen in curry puffs (pastry parcels filled with curried potato and chicken or lamb), which are similar to England's pasties, and *kaya,* which is a sweet preserve most likely based on Europe's imported jams, but made of coconut and egg. It is usually served with bread.

Thailand can be broken into four regions. The influences of neighboring Laos are reflected strongly in the northeastern region food, with glutinous rice being the staple food, eaten both as a base for a meal and also as a dessert, steamed with coconut milk and black beans. Herbs such as dill are widely used, and a popular regional dish is *Khanom Buang,* a thin crispy egg omelette stuffed with shrimp and bean sprouts. Northeastern food is highly spiced, with regional specialties like *lap,* spicy minced meat or chicken, or the famous *som tam* (papaya salad) and *kai yang* (barbecued chicken). Freshwater fish and shrimp are the main sources of protein in northeastern dishes, as meat is a scarce commodity.

The central plains area is considered to be the cultural and economic heart of Thailand due to the fertility of the land. A vast number of paddy fields have traditionally provided the country with its principal source of food, hence the Thai expression *kin khao* ("to eat"), which literally translates as "to eat rice." Unlike the north and northeast, the central plains use plain rice, traditionally steamed, but sometimes boiled or fried. The central region provided much of what is known as traditional Thai cuisine: rice, fish, and vegetables flavored with garlic, fish sauce, and black pepper, along with an abundance of fresh fruits. When Ayutthaya became the capital of Thailand, the increase in the use of chiles occurred, along with coriander, lime, and tomato. As well as freshwater fish from the river, the central plains have access to the nearby Gulf and so the cuisine features much seafood. A wide range of vegetables grows in the fertile soils, along with fruit such as mango, durian, custard apple, pomelos, and guavas. The north of Thailand is a region of wild, densely forested mountains and temple filled towns. Rice tends to be of the glutinous variety, eaten after being kneaded into small balls with the fingers and using it to scoop up more liquid dishes.

Northern curries are generally milder than elsewhere in Thailand, with the influence of neighboring countries such as Myanmar evident in dishes such as *kaeng hang le*, a pork curry with ginger, tamarind, and turmeric, and *khao soi*, a curry broth with egg noodles. Another northern specialty is a spicy pork sausage, called *name*. The south of Thailand has vast plantations of pineapple, coconut, and rubber, and due to the large Muslim influence along the Malaysian border, a distinctive culture. Southern food is characterized by local produce. Coconut has a prominent role in most dishes—its milk to cool the chiles in curries and soups, its flesh when grated to serve as a condiment, or its oil for frying. Fresh seafood is featured prominently. The cashew nuts from local plantations are used as starters or stir-fried—particularly with chicken and chiles—and an exotic, bitter flavor is provided by the pungent flat bean called *sato*. A variety of cultural influences can be seen in southern Thai cuisine; several Malaysian dishes such as fish curries are found. *Kaeng massaman* is a mild Indian-style curry with cardamom, cloves, and cinnamon; *satay*—originally an Indonesian dish—is widely eaten with a spicy peanut sauce. Probably most famous is the influence of the large Chinese community, who hold a ten-day vegetarian festival in Phuket every October.

Vietnamese cuisine can be divided into three regional varieties. In the cool, mountainous north, in the city of Hanoi, a history of Chinese rule is evident in Cantonese-style stir-fries and simple, brothy soups. The flat, arid central region serves up heartier, more refined dishes. In the hot, steamy south, including the city of Ho Chi Minh City (formerly Saigon), tropical abundance is the rule: seafood, pork, and numerous fruits and vegetables are found in bold and spicy dishes, including curries influenced from nearby India. And throughout the country, *banh mi* (a kind of Vietnamese po'boy with meat, pâté, hot peppers, and pickled vegetables) and strong, sweet coffee serve as reminders of Vietnam's French colonial past.

The presence of fresh herbs is one of the most distinctive elements in Vietnamese cooking. Collectively called *rau thom*, Vietnamese herbs include mint; purplish Thai basil (also called holy or Asian basil); aniselike red perilla (also known as shiso); lemony green perilla; floral, cilantro-like saw leaf herb; and spicy, sharp Vietnamese coriander. A table salad known as *rau song* includes a plateful of herbs, along with lettuces, cucumbers, mung bean sprouts, and sometimes pickled vegetables; it is served at every meal. It is also tucked inside leaves of lettuce and wrapped around grilled meats and fried spring rolls, lending a clean, crisp dimension to foods that might otherwise taste heavy in Vietnam's hot climate.

Vietnamese food does not include large amounts of meat and fish; instead, rice is supplemented with vegetables and eggs. Similar to Chinese cooking, Vietnamese cooking uses little fat or oil for frying. Instead of using soy sauce for seasoning, *nuoc mam* (fish sauce) is used as the main flavoring in almost every dish. *Pho* is a type of soup in which noodles, beef, chicken, or pork are added, and the soup is then garnished with basil, bean sprouts, and other seasonings. Vietnamese spring rolls are an alternative to Chinese egg rolls. These wraps are characterized by their rice paper packaging. *Bahn trang* are paper-thin, white crepes that have a criss-cross pattern from the trays on which they are dried. Rice flour is a crucial item in a Vietnamese kitchen. The flour is the main element of a Vietnamese pancake/crepe, bánh Xèo. These pancakes are stuffed with minced pork, shrimp, and bean sprouts. They are garnished with mint and served with a spicy, sweet dipping sauce. Fruits are an integral part of each meal—bananas, mangoes, papayas, oranges, coconuts, and pineapple are all popular. Vietnamese coffee is made with condensed milk to make the drink sweet. Hot green tea is very popular as well.

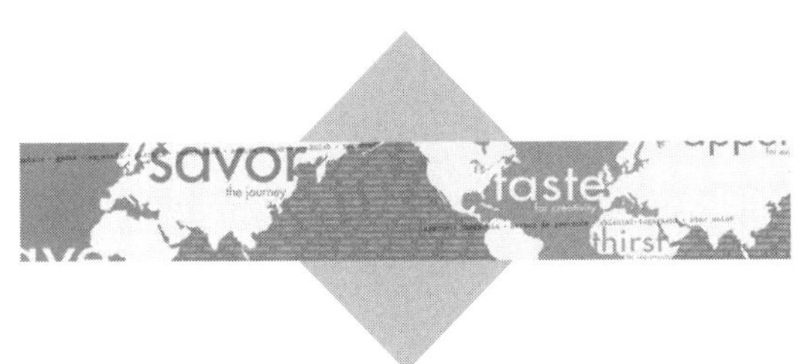

# Glossary

**Bac ha** Eaten as a vegetable, the long, strong, bright green stem of the giant taro plant looks like a smooth stalk of celery but does not have thick fibers. It is frequently used in Vietnamese sour soup.

**Banh Pho** Short, flat, white Vietnamese rice stick noodle about $\frac{1}{8}$ inch wide. They cook in minutes in boiling water or soup and should not be overdone. They are used in soup noodle dishes, particularly the Hanoi soup that goes by the common name of *pho*.

**Banh Trang** The Vietnamese equivalent of ravioli skins. It is round, semitransparent, thin, hard, and dry rice paper and is used as the wrapping on Vietnamese spring rolls and broiled meats, along with salad and herbs. It is made from a dough of finely ground rice, water, and salt, with tapioca (cassava) flour as a binding agent. The dough is passed through rollers and then cut into circles 7 to 14 inches in diameter. These are then put on bamboo mats to dry in the sun. Once dry, they will keep indefinitely. To use, they must be moistened by covering with a damp cloth until soft or by dipping quickly into warm water. To get a crisp, golden-brown color, the wrappers can be brushed lightly with a sugar-water solution before frying.

**Basil, Asian Basil, Thai Basil** This medium to dark green basil with purple flowers has a sharp anise taste that handles heat better than sweet basil. It has little taste or aroma when raw; the strong flavor emerges when it is cooked.

**Bean Curd** Made from dried soybeans soaked, pureed, and boiled with water. The resulting milky liquid is strained and then mixed with a coagulant or natural solidifier, which causes curds to form. These are then taken to wooden tubs lined with cloth and pressed until they form bean curd.

**Bean Sprouts** The tender young sprouts of the germinating mung bean are used in Asia as a vegetable and fried in cooked dishes. They are also often used raw in salads.

**Black Vinegar** A dark, mild, almost sweet vinegar that has only one equivalent: balsamic vinegar. It is usually made from glutinous rice or sorghum, which gives it its distinctive taste.

**Cabbage** There are many varieties of cabbages; the white or pale green cabbages are popular in South East Asia.

**Candlenut** A round, cream-colored nut with an oily consistency used to add texture and a faint flavor to many dishes. Substitute macadamia nuts or raw cashews.

**Chiles (Cabai Cabe, or Lombok)** There are several types of chile pepper used in Indonesia. The amount of heat of a chile pepper increases as the size of the chile pepper decreases. Green chiles are the unripe fruit, with a flavor different from red chiles. Fresh, finger-length red chiles are the most commonly used types in Southeast Asia. Dried chiles are also used in some dishes; they should be torn into pieces and soaked in hot water to soften before grinding or blending. Hottest of all chiles are the tiny fiery bird's-eye chiles (*cabe* or *rawit*). To reduce the heat of the dish while retaining the flavor, remove some or all the chile's seeds.

**Chile Sauce** Usually a fairly thick, hot sauce. Chile sauce is prepared from pulped peppers, flavored with garlic and vinegar, and thickened with cornstarch.

**Chinese Five-spice Powder** A blend of spices consisting of anise-pepper, star anise, cassia, cloves, and fennel seed. A licorice flavor predominates.

**Chinese Mushroom** Also called shiitake mushroom, these are the most widely used mushrooms in east Asian cooking and are grown in China and Japan on the wood of dead deciduous trees. Dried mushrooms should be soaked in warm water for 20 minutes before cooking.

**Coconut Milk and Coconut Cream** These are two of the most important ingredients in this region's cooking and are used in both curries and desserts, as well as beverages. Coconut milk is the liquid squeezed from the grated flesh of mature coconut after the flesh has been soaked in lukewarm water. Coconut cream is a richer version. Coconut milk uses 3 cups of grated coconut to 5 cups of water, whereas coconut cream uses just 2 cups of water. Both must be soaked for 15 minutes, mixed, and then poured through muslin lined strainer; all of the liquid must be squeezed out of the muslin.

**Cup Leaves (Daun Mangkok)** The shape of the leaf is like a cup. Also known as *tapak leman* (*Nothopanax scutellarium*), it is usually used to cook stew dishes. A good substitute is curly kale.

**Curry Paste** Red curry paste is the most common of all the curry pastes. It is a mixture of dried chile pepper, shallot, garlic, galangal, lemongrass, cilantro root, peppercorn, coriander, salt, shrimp paste, and kaffir lime zest. Green curry paste has the same ingredients as the red, except that fresh green pepper is substituted for the dried chile pepper. Yellow curry paste comes from southern Thailand and is similar to red or green curry, but it is made with yellow peppers and turmeric.

**Fermented Black Beans** Oxidized soybeans that are salt-dried, with a savory, salty, and slightly bitter flavor. They are used in stir-fries, marinades, and sauces. Before using, they should be soaked in water for 10 to 30 minutes to get rid of excess salt. When purchasing fermented black beans, look for shiny and firm beans, rather than dull and dry ones with salt spots. Once open, store in plastic in the refrigerator for up to one year.

# Noodles

**While noodles are known by an assortment of names, they are made from just four basic four groups: wheat, rice, mung bean, and buckwheat. Noodles also come in a variety of shapes and width, but are customarily served long and uncut. The noodle's length symbolized longevity in the Asian culture; according to this belief, the longer the noodle, the longer the life.**

- **Egg noodles, udon, kishimen, hiyanmugi, somen, and ramen noodles are all made from wheat flour. These noodles are similar to American noodles. Their sizes range from fine to coarse and they can be pale yellow in color, the result of an egg and wheat mixture, or white if made without eggs. Egg noodles are commonly used in chow mein, which translates to "fried noodles." Udon noodles are thick wheat noodles eaten in Japan. Usually round in shape and white in color, they are used in soups like *kake udon*, a hot broth topped with thin slices of green onions, and in dishes such as *yakiudon*, which is udon stir-fried in soy-based sauce. *Japanese* somen noodles are fine white noodles made from wheat flour, water, and a small bit of oil. Like soba noodles, they're often served cold with a dipping sauce. Ramen are curly, long, brick-shaped noodles often purchased as instant noodles. In the Philippines, *Filipino noodles*, or *pancit*, is made from wheat flour and coconut oil and is often used in soups and salads. Indonesians use noodles made from wheat flour and eggs in a local fried noodle dish called *bami goring*.**
- **Rice vermicelli, rice sticks, and bun noodles are made from rice flour. The noodles are named for their shape and thickness, which can range in diameter from 1 cm to almost threadlike. *Rice vermicelli* is fine, while *rice sticks* are thicker and can be round or flat. Rice noodles are opaque and the texture resembles that of rice.**
- **Cellophane noodles are made from mung beans. Also called glass noodles, bean threads, bean noodles, or cellophane vermicelli, these noodles are aptly named because of their transparent appearance when cooked. Cellophane noodles are long, slippery, and soft, and because they are flavorless on their own, will readily absorb the flavors of the ingredients they are prepared with. They do not need to be cooked, but merely heated and softened in warm water for best results.**
- **Buckwheat, or soba, noodles are made from buckwheat flour. These thin noodles are slightly brown in color. They are often served chilled with a dipping sauce or as a noodle soup.**

**Fermented Soya Beans (Tao Jiaw)** These are available whole and fermented from either yellow or black beans; in English they are most commonly known as black bean and yellow bean sauce. They are nutritious, strongly flavored, and salty, replacing salt completely in some Thai dishes.

**Fish Sauce** Fish sauce, called *nam pla* in Thai (the salt of Thai cuisine) or *nuoc mam* in Vietnamese, is used much like salt or soy sauce as a flavor enhancer. Made from the liquid drained from fermented anchovies, it is very is potent. It is usually combined with other ingredients when used as a dipping sauce. For cooking it can be used straight, but never add it to a dry pan or the smell will be overpowering. Like olive oil, there are several grades of fish sauce. High-quality fish sauce, which is the first to be drained off the fermented fish, is usually pale amber, like clear brewed tea, and used in dipping sauces. For cooking usually stronger-flavored, lower-grade brands, which are made from a secondary draining, are used.

**Galangal** A member of the ginger family, galangal is used in many countries as a substitute for ginger. It has a hot, peppery taste and is used mainly as flavoring and as a pungent ingredient in ground curry pastes. Galangal can be found in fresh root, frozen, dry, and powdered form in most Asian grocery stores. If using dried slices of galangal, soak them in warm water for at least 30 minutes. Substitute the fresh galangal with half the amount of dry galangal in the recipe.

**Ground Coriander** One of the essential ingredients in curry powders. The whole spice is ground when needed. To get the best out of the coriander seed, it is advisable to toast first in an oven and then finely grind it.

**Hoisin Sauce** The barbecue sauce of Vietnam. Made from red rice colored with a natural food dye, usually from annatto seeds, it is a sweet-tasting, thick, reddish brown sauce best used as a condiment for roast pork and poultry.

**Holy Basil, or Sacred Basil (Bai Gkaprow)** Often called hot basil because of its peppery taste, especially when very fresh, with a hint of mint and cloves. Since its exotic flavor becomes fully released with cooking, it is not eaten raw, but added in generous amounts to stir-fried dishes and some spicy soups. Holy basil is so called because it is a sacred herb in India where it is frequently planted around Hindu shrines.

**Kaffir Lime leaves, Makrut, Thai Lime Leaves** One of the signature flavors in Thai cooking, lemony and floral. If not available, substitute regular lime leaves and fruit. Kaffir limes, however, are used for their rind, since they are very dry inside. The zest is highly aromatic. Kaffir lime leaves may be frozen or dried for future use, or even kept green by standing leafy twigs in water on a sunny windowsill.

**Kangkon** Green, smooth-leafed vegetable native to the Philippines. It has a flavor that is milder than spinach and a texture similar to watercress.

## Rice

**Deriving originally from wild grasses, rice is a staple food in Asia. Historians believe that it was first domesticated in the area covering the foothills of the eastern Himalayas (northeastern India), and stretching through Burma, Thailand, Laos, Vietnam, and southern China. From here, it spread in all directions and human cultivation created numerous varieties. Different types of rice cross-breed easily. According to the International Rice Research Institute (IRRI), based in the Philippines, there are 120,000 varieties of rice worldwide. Over the centuries, three main types of rice developed in Asia, depending on the amylose content of the grain. They are *indica* (high in amylose and cooking to fluffy grains to be eaten with the fingers), *japonica* (low in amylase and cooking to sticky masses suitable for eating as clumps with chopsticks), and *javanica* (intermediate amylose content and stickiness). Rice is further divided into long-, medium-, and short-grained varieties, and in the subcontinent different populations grow and consume different varieties.**

**Rice grains are grown in a variety of colors and textures. Brown rice grains, unlike white, still have an outer coating of bran. This bran carries twice as much fiber and increased levels of vitamin E and magnesium as enriched white rice does. Usually produced as long or medium grains, brown rice takes more time to cook, tastes chewier, and retains a mild, nutty bran flavor.**

**Black sticky rice, often called forbidden rice, is a nutty, medium-grain rice. When cooked, the brown-black rice turns a shade of purple-black. It may also be labeled "black**

**Kare-Kare** Philippine meat-vegetable stew with oxtail, beef, or tripe; eggplant, banana buds, and other vegetables cooked in peanut sauce and ground toasted rice.

**Lemongrass** An essential ingredient in Southeast Asian cooking, it is a long, thin, pale green edible grass with bright lemon fragrance and taste. To use a lemongrass stalk, cut off the grassy top and root end. Peel and remove the large, tough outer leaves of the stalk until you reach a light purple color. Chop it very fine to use in salads and grind into curry pastes if eating them directly. Or cut into 2-inch portions and bruise them to extract the flavor before boiling with soup broth. Lemongrass can be found fresh in most grocery stores because it has a very long shelf life. Dry and frozen forms are also available in most Asian stores.

**Lumpia** Philippine egg rolls.

**Nuoc Mam** A fish sauce that is a powerfully flavored, pungent seasoning sauce, used extensively in Southeast Asia. It is made by layering fish and salt into large barrels and allowing the fish to ferment for three or more months before the accumulated liquid is siphoned off, filtered, and

**glutinous rice" or "black sweet rice." Cultivated in Indonesia and the Philippines, stickier varieties of black rice are often used for sweets such as rice pudding in countries throughout Southeast Asia including Thailand, Malaysia, and Singapore.**

**Thailand originated the planting of the aromatic jasmine rice. This fragrant long-grain rice has a soft texture due to a special water-milling process. When cooked, this rice comes out moist and tender like medium grains. Available in brown and white, jasmine rice is a staple of Thai cooking.**

**In medium-grain rice, the length of the grain is less than twice its width. High in starch, the cooked grains come out moist and tender with a bit of stickiness. Medium grains are harvested in Italy and Spain; they tend to grow in regions farther from the equator. This rice, known as arborio, is found in European dishes such as risotto and paella.**

**Short-grain rice also has a length that is less than twice its width. When cooked, the grains are softer and stickier than medium grain. In Japan, sushi is only as good as the short-grain sticky rice that is used. Sticky rice has numerous uses. While it is also used for desserts, it is an integral part of every meal in the regions of Laos, Cambodia, and Vietnam. In addition, sticky rice is a primary source for brewing rice-based alcohol like sake.**

**Another type of rice essential to this region is glutinous rice. Although it does not contain any gluten, this short-grain, starchy rice becomes quite sticky and dense when cooked. This rice is labeled as sticky, waxy, and sweet. Generally used for desserts, glutinous rice is used for making little cakes in Japan, Thailand, Malaysia, and Indonesia.**

bottled. In Vietnam *nuoc mam* is made into different dipping sauces by adding chiles, ground roasted peanuts, sugar, and other ingredients.

**Oyster Sauce** One of the most popular bottled sauces in Vietnam. Made from dried oysters, it is thick and richly flavored. The cheaper brands tend to be saltier. The original sauce was much thinner and contained fragments of fermented, dried oysters. It is mostly used in stir-fried dishes.

**Palm Sugar** An unrefined sweetener similar in flavor to brown sugar. Used in sweet and savory Asian dishes. Commonly available in podlike cakes, it is also sold in paste form at Asian markets. Store as you would other sugar.

**Paprika** Derived from bell peppers. In Vietnam it is used as a vegetable and as a spice. In its latter guise, it is dried and ground to a powder.

**Pomelo** A large fruit that resembles a grapefruit. It tapers slightly at the stem end and has a thick, sweet, slightly rough-textured skin, and a dry, semi-sweet flesh.

**Sambal** A spicy condiment used especially in Indonesia and Malaysia, made with chile peppers and other ingredients, such as sugar or coconut.

**Satay or Saté or Sateh** Pieces of meat or fish threaded onto skewers and grilled. Meat satay is typically served with a spicy peanut sauce.

**Shallots** Like the French, Vietnamese cooks use shallots rather than onions as a major flavoring ingredient, prizing their sweeter, more aromatic quality. Shallots, along with garlic and lemongrass, are among the few seasonings that are typically cooked, rather than added to dishes raw. Fried shallots, along with crushed, roasted peanuts, also appear on the Vietnamese table as a garnish for noodle dishes and soups.

**Shrimp Paste** Shrimp paste adds depth to noodle dishes, soups, and curries. It comes in bottled form and is available at most Asian grocery stores. As it is salty and highly concentrated, it is used sparingly.

**Sinigang** Sour soup dish of meat or fish with vegetables, seasoned with tomatoes, onions, and lemon juice.

**Soy Sauce** Made from fermented soybeans mixed with a roasted grain, normally wheat. It is infected with a yeast mold and after fermentation begins, salt is added. Yeast is added for further fermentation and the liquid is left in vats for several months and then filtered.

**Star Anise** The seedpods of one type of magnolia tree. The tan eight-pointed pods resemble stars, hence the name. When dried, a shiny, flat, light brown seed is revealed in each point.

**Straw Mushrooms** Grown on paddy straw, left over from harvested wheat, which gives them a distinctly earthy taste. Generally, they are packed in water and canned.

**Sugarcane** The sugarcane bought for cooking consists of the stem, the leaves being chopped off in the cane fields. The cane should be very carefully peeled with a strong, sharp knife. Reasonably easy to obtain from large grocers.

**Szechwan Peppercorns** Aromatic, small, red-brown seeds from the prickly ash tree known as fagara. The whole peppercorns can be kept for years without loss of flavor if stored in a tightly sealed jar.

**Tamarind** The dark brown pod of the tamarind tree contains a sour fleshy pulp, which adds a fruity sourness to many dishes. Packets of pulp usually contain the seeds and fibers. To make tamarind juice, measure the pulp and soak it in hot water for 5 minutes before squeezing it to extract the juice, discarding the seeds, fiber, and any skin.

**Tausi** Black soybeans, salted and fermented.

**Turmeric** A native of Southeast Asia, it belongs to the same family as ginger and galangal. It has a bright orange yellow flesh with a strong, earthy smell and a slightly bitter taste. The flesh is responsible for the yellow color we associate with curry powder and it overpowers all other spices.

**Wood Ear Fungus** Perhaps the most common is derived from its habitat of decayed wood. It is valued for its subtle, delicate flavor and slightly crunchy "bite."

**Yellow Bean Sauce** Made according to the ancient recipe for *jiang*, or pickled yellow soybeans in a salty liquid. It is normally bought in cans and jars but it is best transferred to a jar in which it can be stored in a refrigerator almost indefinitely.

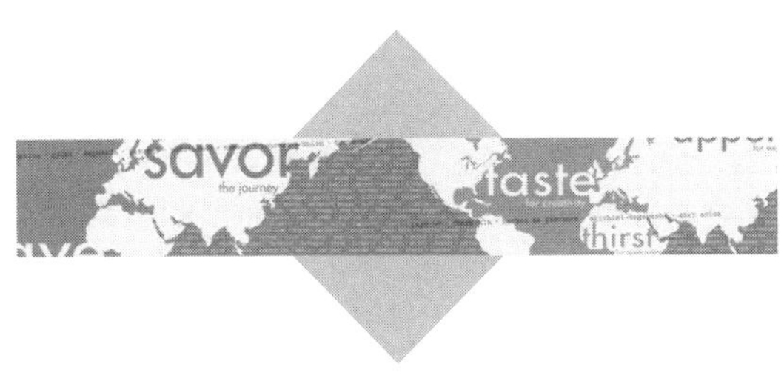

# Menus and Recipes from Southeast Asia

MENU ONE (INDONESIA)

***Krupuk Udang:* Shrimp Chips**

***Sambal Ulek:* Chile Sauce**

***Serundeng Kacang:* Toasted Spiced Coconut with Peanuts**

***Tahu Telur:* Spicy Tofu Omelet**

***Satay Babi:* Pork Satay**

***Satay Ayam:* Chicken Satay**

***Gado Gado:* Cooked Vegetable Salad, Sumatran Style**

***Laksa Lemak:* Chicken, Shrimp, and Rice Noodles in Coconut Sauce**

***Pepes Ikan:* Grilled Fish in Banana Leaf**

***Tumis Terong:* Sautéed Eggplant**

***Lapis Daging:* Stir-fried Beef**

MENU TWO (THAILAND)

***Ma Hor:* Galloping Horses**

***Tord Man Pla:* Fried Fish Cakes**

***Tom Yam Goong:* Hot and Spicy Shrimp Soup**

***Mun Tot:* Fried Sweet Potatoes**

***Yam Makeua Issaan:* Grilled Eggplant Salad**

***Khao Tang:* Crispy Rice Crackers**

***Pad Thai:* Thai Fried Noodles**

***Kaeng Kiew Warn Kai:* Green Curry with Chicken**

***Khao Niew Mam Uang:* Mangoes and Sticky Rice**

***Cha Yen:* Thai Iced Tea**

MENU THREE (VIETNAM)

***Banh Hoi Thit Nuong:* Shrimp Toast**

***Cha Gio:* Fried Spring Rolls**

***Cha Bo:* Grilled Beef Patties**

***Goi Cuon:* Fresh Spring Rolls**

***Dia Rau Song:* Vegetable Platter**

***Pho Bo:* Vietnamese Beef and Noodle Soup**

***Dua Chua:* Pickled Carrot and Daikon Salad**

***Ga Xao Sa Ot:* Lemongrass Chicken**

***Bo Nuong:* Grilled Beef**

***Suon Rang:* Glazed Spareribs**

# Krupuk Udang Shrimp Chips

SERVES 4

**Uncooked shrimp chips come in many shapes and sizes. Most are Indonesian, pale-pink in color with a distinct shrimp flavor. When deep-fried in hot oil, they become light, crisp, and crunchy, and swell to more than twice their size within seconds.**

| AMOUNT | MEASURE | INGREDIENT |
|---|---|---|
| As needed | | Oil for deep frying |
| 12 | | Dried shrimp chips |

PROCEDURE

1 Heat oil in a wok or deep-fat fryer to 360°F (182°C). Fry the chips, a few at a time, if the oil is hot enough; they will puff up within 2 to 3 seconds. Fry until lightly colored, approximately 15 seconds. Remove and drain on paper towels.

# Sambal Ulek Chile Sauce

YIELD: $\frac{3}{4}$ CUP (6 OUNCES, 180 ML)

**This is served during most meals to allow each person to season soup, meat, and fish dishes.**

| AMOUNT | MEASURE | INGREDIENT |
|---|---|---|
| $\frac{1}{2}$ teaspoon | | Salt |
| 10 | | Hot red chiles, thinly sliced |
| $\frac{1}{2}$ teaspoon | | Shrimp paste (*terasi*) |
| $\frac{1}{2}$ teaspoon | | Granulated sugar |
| $\frac{3}{4}$ cup | 5 ounces, 140 ml | Tomatoes, peeled, seeded, $\frac{1}{4}$ inch (.6 cm) dice |

PROCEDURE

1 Pound or process salt, chiles, shrimp paste, and sugar in a mortar or processor to form a coarse paste. Add tomatoes and crush slightly to blend flavors.

# Serundeng Kacang

## Toasted Spiced Coconut with Peanuts

YIELD: 1–1 $\frac{1}{2}$ CUPS

**Serve this sprinkled over practically any dish.**

| AMOUNT | MEASURE | INGREDIENT |
|---|---|---|
| 5 | | Shallots, chopped |
| 3 | | Garlic cloves, chopped |
| 2 tablespoons | 1 ounce, 30 ml | Vegetable oil |
| 1 teaspoon | | Coriander, ground |
| $\frac{1}{2}$ teaspoon | | Cumin, ground |
| $\frac{1}{2}$ teaspoon | | Galangal, ground |
| 1 tablespoon | $\frac{1}{2}$ ounce, 15 ml | Tamarind water |
| 1 teaspoon | | Brown sugar |
| $\frac{1}{2}$ teaspoon | | Salt |
| 1 cup | 6 ounces, 168 g | Coconut, freshly grated, or $\frac{1}{2}$ cup dried coconut flakes soaked 5 minutes in 1 cup (8 ounces, 240 ml) water |
| $\frac{1}{2}$ cup | 2$\frac{1}{2}$ ounces, 70 g | Unsalted peanuts, roasted |

### PROCEDURE

1. Pound or process shallots and garlic to a smooth paste; heat oil and stir-fry paste over medium heat for approximately 2 minutes or until translucent. Do not brown.
2. Add coriander, cumin, galangal, tamarind water, brown sugar, and salt. Stir-fry 1 minute on low heat to blend flavors.
3. Add coconut (if using rehydrated, let simmer until all the water has been soaked up by the coconut before stirring). Cook over low heat, stirring until coconut is nearly dry and medium brown in color, about 20 to 30 minutes.
4. Add peanuts and toast 5 minutes, stirring constantly until coconut is golden brown. Be careful not to let it burn.
5. Remove from heat and let cool before serving.

# Tahu Telur

## Spicy Tofu Omelet

SERVES 4

| AMOUNT | MEASURE | INGREDIENT |
|---|---|---|
| 1 cup | 2 ounces, 56 g | Fresh bean sprouts |
| 1 cup | 8 ounces, 224 g | Fresh tofu, drained, $\frac{1}{4}$ inch (.6 cm) dice |
| 4 | | Eggs, beaten with $\frac{1}{4}$ teaspoon salt |
| $\frac{1}{2}$ teaspoon | | Salt |
| 1 teaspoon | | Vegetable oil |
| 2 | | Green hot chiles, seeds removed, finely sliced |
| 2 tablespoons | 1 ounce, 30 ml | Sweet soy sauce (*kecap manis*) (recipe follows) |
| 1 tablespoon | $\frac{1}{2}$ ounce, 15 ml | White vinegar |
| 3 tablespoons | | Fried peanuts, crushed |
| 3 tablespoons | | Fried shallot flakes (recipe follows) |
| 1 tablespoon | | Parsley leaves |

PROCEDURE

1. Blanch bean sprouts in boiling water 30 seconds. Drain, refresh with cold water, and drain again.
2. Combine tofu, eggs, and salt.
3. Heat oil in a 10-inch omelet pan. Add half the egg mixture, tilting the pan to make a thin omelet. Cook over medium heat until set and lightly browned. Remove and keep warm. Repeat to make a second omelet.
4. Evenly spread bean sprouts and chiles over omelets.
5. Combine *kecap manis* and vinegar; drizzle over omelets.
6. Garnish with peanuts, fried shallot flakes, and parsley leaves.
7. To serve, cut in wedges.

## Kecap Manis Indonesian Sweet Soy Sauce

YIELD: $1\frac{1}{2}$ CUPS (12 OUNCES, 360 ML)

| AMOUNT | MEASURE | INGREDIENT |
|---|---|---|
| 1 cup | 8 ounces, 224 g | Dark brown sugar, packed |
| 1 cup | 8 ounces, 240 ml | Water |
| $\frac{3}{4}$ cup | 6 ounces, 180 ml | Soy sauce |
| 7 tablespoons | $3\frac{1}{2}$ ounces, 105 ml | Dark molasses |
| $\frac{1}{2}$ teaspoon | | Laos (galangal) ground |
| $\frac{1}{4}$ teaspoon | | Coriander, ground |
| $\frac{1}{4}$ teaspoon | | Black pepper, freshly ground |
| 1 | | Star anise |

PROCEDURE

1 Combine the sugar and water; simmer over low heat, stirring frequently, until the sugar dissolves. Bring to a boil and cook to 200°F (93°C) on a sugar thermometer, approximately 5 minutes. Reduce heat to low, add remaining ingredients, and simmer 5 minutes.

2 Remove from heat and let cool.

## Fried Shallot Flakes

| AMOUNT | MEASURE | INGREDIENT |
|---|---|---|
| 10 | | Shallots |
| 1 tablespoon | $\frac{1}{2}$ ounce, 15 ml | Vegetable oil |

PROCEDURE

1 Slice shallots very thin.

2 Lightly oil a small skillet. Heat pan over medium heat and add shallots.

3 Cook for approximately 5 to 7 minutes, shaking the pan so they brown slowly and evenly.

4 When golden brown, remove from the oil and drain on paper towels until cool. They will crisp and turn darker brown as they stand.

# Satay Babi Pork Satay SERVES 4

| AMOUNT | MEASURE | INGREDIENT |
|---|---|---|
| 1 pound | 448 g | Boneless, skinless pork tenderloin or loin |
| 1 tablespoon | $\frac{1}{2}$ ounce, 15 ml | Butter |
| 1 | | Garlic clove, crushed |
| 2 teaspoons | | Dark soy sauce |
| 2 teaspoons | | Fresh lemon juice |
| Marinade | | |
| 2 tablespoons | 1 ounce, 30 ml | Soy sauce |
| 2 | | Garlic clove, crushed |
| 1 teaspoon | | Ginger, ground |
| 1 teaspoon | | Five-spice powder |
| 1 tablespoon | $\frac{1}{2}$ ounce, 15 ml | Honey |
| $\frac{1}{2}$ teaspoon | | White pepper |
| As needed | | *Sambal Kecap* (recipe follows) |

PROCEDURE

1. Slice pork across the grain into thin slices, $\frac{1}{4}$ inch (.6 cm) wide by 3 to 4 inches (7.2 to 9.6 cm) long.
2. Combine marinade ingredients and mix well. Add pork, mix well, and let stand 2 hours.
3. Remove from marinade and thread onto skewers.
4. Melt butter and add remaining ingredients. Before placing on the grill, brush with this mixture.
5. Grill 2 to 3 minutes or until just done.
6. Serve hot or warm with Sambal Kecap (Chile and Soy Sauce).

## Sambal Kecap Chile and Soy Sauce SERVES 4

| AMOUNT | MEASURE | INGREDIENT |
|---|---|---|
| 6 tablespoons | 3 ounces, 90 ml | Dark soy sauce |
| 1 teaspoon | | Chile powder |
| 3 | | Serrano chiles, sliced very thin |
| ½ cup | 2 ounces, 56 g | Onions, minced |
| 2 tablespoons | 1 ounce, 30 ml | Fresh lime juice |
| 2 | | Garlic cloves, minced. |

**PROCEDURE**

1 Place all the ingredients in a small saucepan and cook over a medium to low heat for about 5 minutes, stirring constantly. Let cool.

## Satay Ayam Chicken Satay SERVES 4

| AMOUNT | MEASURE | INGREDIENT |
|---|---|---|
| 1 pound | 448 g | Chicken thigh meat, boneless, skinless |
| 1 stalk | | Lemongrass, finely minced |
| 2 | | Garlic cloves, minced |
| ½ teaspoon | | Turmeric, ground |
| ½ teaspoon | | Fennel, ground |
| ½ teaspoon | | Cumin, ground |
| 2 tablespoons | 1 ounce, 30 ml | Vegetable oil |
| To taste | | Salt |
| | | 12-inch bamboo skewers, soaked in water for 1 hour |

**PROCEDURE**

1 Slice chicken across the grain into thin slices ¼ inch (.6 cm) wide by 3 to 4 inches (7.2 to 9.6 cm) long.

2 Combine lemongrass, garlic, turmeric, fennel, cumin, and oil to a paste. Add chicken, mix well, and let stand 2 hours.

3 Remove from marinate and thread on to skewers. Season with salt before cooking.

4 Grill or broil, basting occasionally with oil.

5 Serve hot or warm with peanut sauce and cucumber salad.

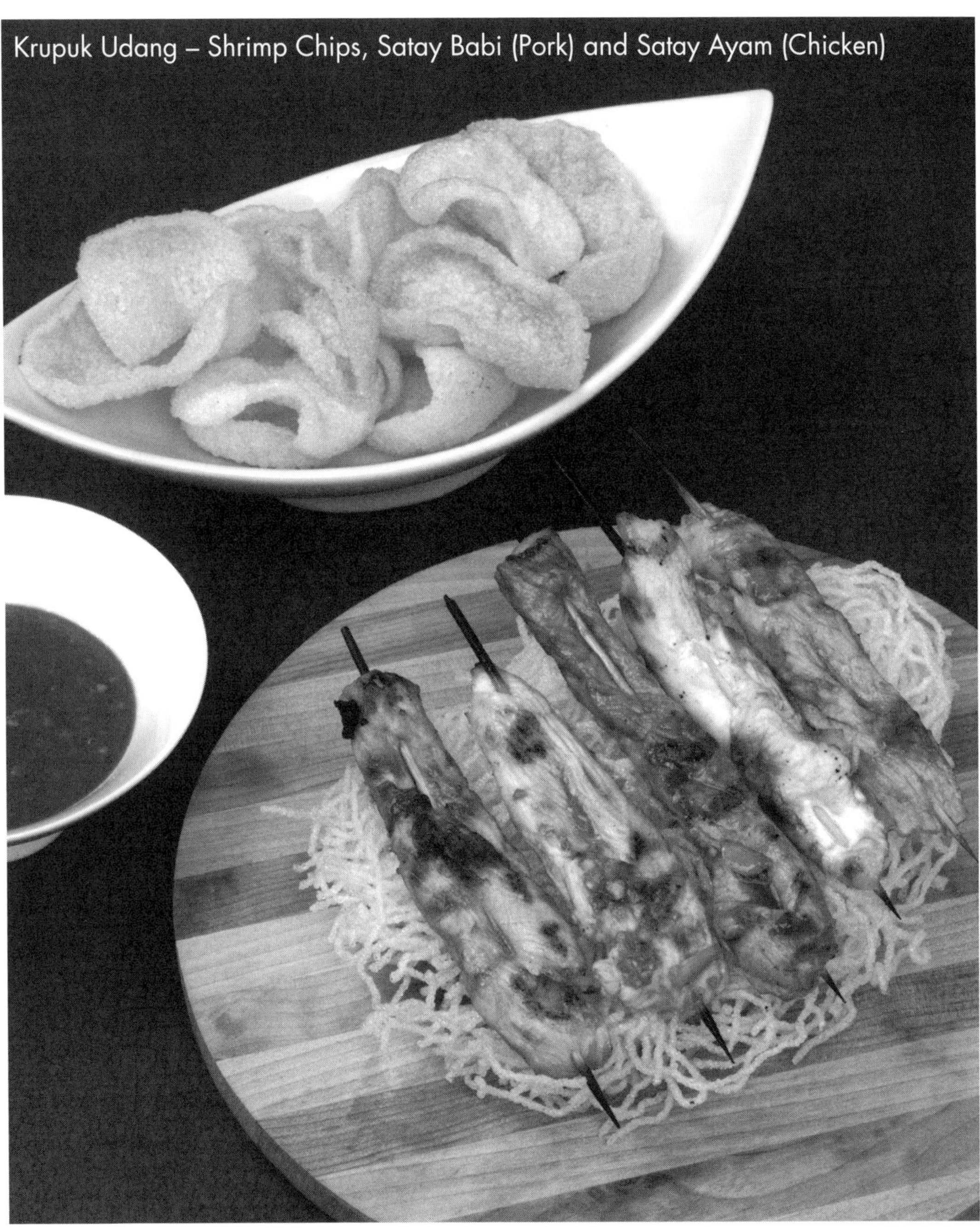

Krupuk Udang – Shrimp Chips, Satay Babi (Pork) and Satay Ayam (Chicken)

# Gado Gado

## Cooked Vegetable Salad, Sumatran Style

SERVES 4

| AMOUNT | MEASURE | INGREDIENT |
|---|---|---|
| 4 ounces | 112 g | Firm tofu |
| 1 teaspoon | | *Kecap manis* (Sweet soy sauce) |
| 3 tablespoons | $1\frac{1}{2}$ ounces, 45 ml | Vegetable oil |
| $\frac{1}{2}$ cup | $2\frac{1}{2}$ ounces, 70 g | Boiling potatoes, cooked, $\frac{1}{4}$ inch (.6 cm) slice |
| $\frac{1}{2}$ cup | 2 ounces, 56 g | Carrots, 2 inch (4.8 cm) julienne |
| $\frac{1}{2}$ cup | 2 ounces, 56 g | Green beans, 2 inch (4.8 cm) julienne |
| 1 cup | 4 ounces, 112 g | Cabbage, shredded, 2 inch (4.8 cm) |
| 1 cup | 4 ounces, 112 g | Bean sprouts |
| $\frac{1}{2}$ cup | 3 ounces, 84 g | Cucumber, peeled, halved, seeded, $\frac{1}{4}$ inch (.6 cm) slice |
| 2 | | Eggs, hard-boiled, sliced |
| Garnish | | |
| As needed | | *Sambal kacang* (peanut sauce) |
| $\frac{1}{4}$ cup | | Fried shallots flakes (see recipe on page 334) |
| As needed | | Shrimp chips |
| As needed | | Soy sauce |

PROCEDURE

1 Drain tofu. Rinse and cut into two pieces. Place on a plate. Top with another plate and put 1 to 2 pounds (448 to 896 g) on top (heavy canned goods work well as a weight). Let stand 30 minutes. Discard liquid. Pat tofu dry. Sprinkle with *kecap manis.*

2 Set wok over high heat. When hot, add the oil. When the oil is hot but not smoking, add the tofu. Stir-fry 3 to 4 minutes or until golden. Transfer to paper towels to drain. Cut the tofu into $\frac{1}{2}$ inch (1.2 cm) pieces. Heat oil in wok to 350°F (176°C). Return tofu and fry until golden brown and puffy, about 3 to 4 minutes. Remove and drain on paper towels.

3 Boil the potatoes; peel and cut into $\frac{1}{4}$ inch (.6 cm) slices.

4 Blanch carrots, green beans, and cabbage separately for 1 to 2 minutes. Drain and refresh with cold water; drain again.

5 Blanch bean sprouts in boiling water 30 seconds. Rinse under cold water; drain well.

6 Arrange vegetables and tofu in separate sections on a platter, with the egg in the center.

7 Serve with warm peanut sauce, spooning a little on the salad and the rest on the side.

8 Sprinkle with fried shallot flakes.
9 Serve at room temperature with shrimp chips and soy sauce.

## Sambal Kacang (Bumbu Sate) Peanut Sauce

YIELD: 1 CUP(8 OUNCES, 240 ML)

| AMOUNT | MEASURE | INGREDIENT |
|---|---|---|
| 2 teaspoons | | Coriander seed, toasted |
| 1 teaspoon | | Fennel seed, toasted |
| 1 teaspoon | | Cumin seed, toasted |
| 6 | | Dry red chiles, seeded and soaked |
| ½ teaspoon | | Shrimp paste |
| 5 | | Shallots, sliced thin |
| 2 | | Garlic clove, sliced thin |
| 1 tablespoon | ½ ounce, 15 ml | Vegetable oil |
| ½ cup | 2½ ounces, 75 g | Peanuts, roasted, roughly ground (crunchy peanut butter) |
| ¾ cup | 6 ounces, 180 ml | Coconut milk |
| 1 tablespoon | | Tamarind paste, dissolved in 4 tablespoons (2 ounces, 60 ml) water |
| 1 teaspoon | | Palm sugar |
| To taste | | Salt and pepper |

PROCEDURE

1 Grind the dry spices in a spice grinder or mortar and pestle.
2 Pound or process the chiles, shrimp paste, shallots, and garlic into a paste.
3 Over low heat, sauté the paste lightly until fragrant in oil, 1 minute. Add the dry spices and cook 1 minute. Be careful not to burn the paste after adding the dry spices.
4 Add the peanuts, coconut milk, tamarind, and sugar. Simmer about 10 minutes, adding water if the sauce thickens too fast.
5 Adjust seasoning and serve warm.

# Laksa Lemak Chicken, Shrimp, and Rice Noodles in Coconut Sauce

SERVES 4

| AMOUNT | MEASURE | INGREDIENT |
|---|---|---|
| **Paste** | | |
| 2 | | Garlic cloves, chopped |
| 1 tablespoon | | Ginger, grated |
| 4 | | Dried red chiles, soaked in hot water until softened, minced |
| 1 stalk | | Lemongrass, sliced, bottom 6 inches only, or thinly peeled rind of 1 lemon |
| 4 | | Shallots, peeled, chopped |
| 3 | | Candlenuts or macadamia nuts, minced |
| 2 teaspoons | | Turmeric, ground |
| 1 teaspoon | | Coriander, ground |
| 2 teaspoons | | Dried shrimp, soaked in hot water until soft, about 10 minutes |
| 4 tablespoons | 2 ounces, 60 ml | Vegetable oil |
| 1 cup | 6 ounces, 168 g | Shrimp, shelled, deveined |
| $1\frac{3}{4}$ cups | 14 ounces, 420 ml | Chicken stock |
| 1 cup | 6 ounces, 168 g | Chicken meat, cooked, skinless, boneless, $1\frac{1}{2}$ inch (3.6 cm) pieces |
| 10 ounces | 280 g | Dried rice noodles (rice vermicelli), soaked in hot water to soften, 15 minutes, drained |
| $\frac{3}{4}$ cup | 6 ounces, 180 ml | Coconut milk, thick |
| 1 cup | 4 ounces, 112 g | Bean sprouts (optional) |
| **Garnish** | | |
| 1 tablespoon | | Cilantro, chopped |
| $\frac{1}{4}$ cup | | Green or red hot chiles, sliced thin |
| $\frac{1}{4}$ cup | 1 ounce, 28 g | Green onions, chopped |
| 8 | | Lime wedges |

**PROCEDURE**

1. Pound or blend garlic, ginger, chiles, lemongrass, shallots, nuts, turmeric, and coriander to a fine paste.
2. Pound or blend dried shrimp separately until smooth; if necessary, add 1 to 2 tablespoons coconut milk.
3. Heat half the oil and add the dried shrimp paste; cook 1 minute. Add spice paste and cook 1 to 2 minutes.
4. Add remaining oil, heat, add raw shrimp, and stir-fry 1 minute.
5. Add chicken stock and chicken pieces; cook 5 minutes.
6. Add drained rice noodles and coconut milk; bring to a boil slowly, stirring gently to prevent milk from curdling.
7. Add bean sprouts and simmer 3 minutes or until hot. Sprinkle with cilantro.
8. Serve with separate bowls of chiles, green onions, and lime wedges.

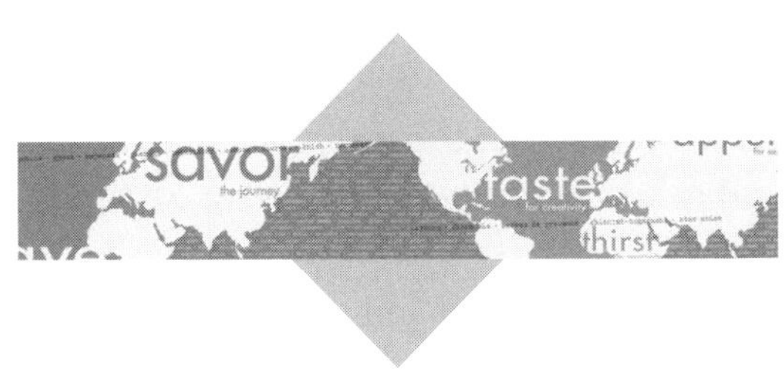

# Pepes Ikan

## Grilled Fish in Banana Leaf

SERVES 4

| AMOUNT | MEASURE | INGREDIENT |
|---|---|---|
| 6 | | Shallots, peeled and sliced |
| 3 | | Garlic cloves, chopped fine |
| 1 tablespoon | | Ginger, grated |
| 3 | | Red chiles fresh, seeded, sliced thin |
| $\frac{1}{4}$ cup | | Holy basil (hot basil) leaves, shredded |
| $\frac{1}{2}$ cup | | Green onion, green only, julienned on the bias |
| 2 | | Whole trout, cleaned, boned, head and tail removed |
| 1 tablespoon | $\frac{1}{2}$ ounce, 15 ml | Light soy sauce |
| 1 tablespoon | $\frac{1}{2}$ ounce, 15 ml | Fresh lime juice |
| As needed | | Banana leaf for wrapping |
| 12 slices | | Lemon, very thin |
| 6 | | Cilantro sprigs |

PROCEDURE

1. Pound or process shallots, garlic, ginger, chiles, basil, and green onion to a paste. Spread paste on the inside of the fish, sprinkle with soy sauce and lime juice, and marinate 30 minutes.
2. Cut the banana leaf in pieces to fit the width of the fish less the head and tail, and long enough to wrap the fish once. Pour boiling water over the banana leaf to soften and prevent splitting.
3. Place each fish in the middle of a leaf and wrap each fish in a leaf, making two packages. Place lemon slices and cilantro sprigs on top of fish. Wrap envelope style into a neat parcel, keeping seam side on top. Secure with a metal skewer, toothpick, or staples.
4. Grill over a very low grill until the leaf begins to brown; allow 10 minutes per inch thickness of fish.
5. Cut open the banana leaves. Serve fish in banana leaves with rice, and a sambal on the side.

# Tumis Terong

## Sautéed Eggplant

SERVES 4

| AMOUNT | MEASURE | INGREDIENT |
|---|---|---|
| 2 cups | 8 ounces, 240 g | Eggplant, 2 inch (4.8 cm) thick slices |
| 2 tablespoons | 1 ounce, 30 ml | Vegetable oil |
| 3 tablespoons | $1\frac{1}{2}$ ounces, 45 ml | Sweet soy sauce (kecap manis) (optional) |
| $\frac{1}{2}$ cup | 2 ounces, 56 g | Onions, sliced thin |
| 1 | | Garlic clove, minced |
| 1 teaspoon | | Shrimp paste |
| To taste | | Salt and pepper |

**PROCEDURE**

1. Heat deep fryer to 375°F (190°C). Deep-fry eggplant for 30 seconds; remove and drain.
2. Set a wok over high heat. When very hot, add the oil, onion, garlic, and shrimp paste. Stir-fry two minutes.
3. Add eggplant; pour in soy sauce, stir and cover pan. Simmer 10 minutes. If there is no juice from steaming the eggplant, add $\frac{1}{4}$ cup (2 ounces, 60 ml) water.
4. Correct seasoning and serve hot.

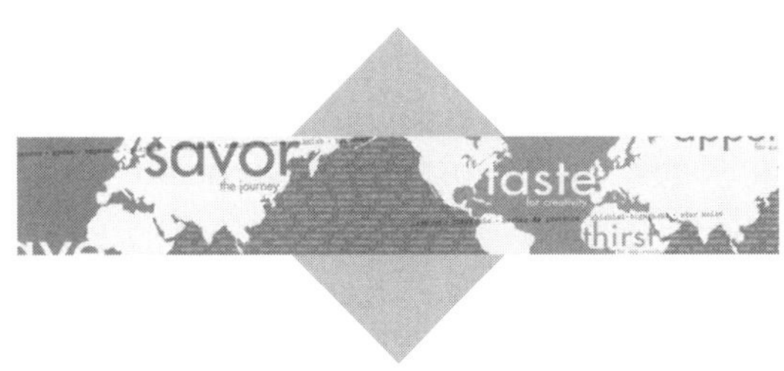

# Lapis Daging

## Stir-Fried Beef SERVES 4

| AMOUNT | MEASURE | INGREDIENT |
|---|---|---|
| $\frac{1}{2}$ teaspoon | | Nutmeg |
| 1 | | Egg, beaten |
| 8 ounces | 224 g | Flank steak, cut $\frac{1}{4}$ inch (.6 cm) wide and 2 to 3 inches (4.8 to 7.2 cm) in length |
| 1 tablespoon | $\frac{1}{2}$ ounce, 15 ml | Vegetable oil |
| $\frac{1}{4}$ cup | 1 ounce, 28 g | Onion, sliced thin |
| 1 | | Garlic clove, sliced thin |
| 1 tablespoon | $\frac{1}{2}$ ounce, 15 ml | Sweet soy sauce *(kecap manis)* |
| 1 | | Cinnamon stick, 1 inch (2.4 cm) long |
| 2 | | Whole cloves |
| To taste | | Pepper |
| $\frac{1}{2}$ cup | 3 ounces, 84 g | Tomato, peeled, seeded, chopped |
| As needed | | Fried shallot flakes (see recipe on page 334) |
| As needed | | Sambal tomat (recipe follows) |

PROCEDURE

1. Combine nutmeg and egg. Coat the steak slices with the egg mixture.
2. Heat the oil over medium heat and sauté the onion and garlic, 2 to 3 minutes or until soft.
3. Drain the egg from the meat and sauté until medium.
4. Combine sweet soy sauce, cinnamon, cloves, pepper, and tomato. Add to the cooked steak. Mix well and cook 3 to 5 minutes or until the sauce has thickened slightly. If necessary, add a little water.
5. Sprinkle with fried shallot flakes. Serve immediately with rice and sambal tomat.

## Sambal Tomat SERVES 4

| AMOUNT | MEASURE | INGREDIENT |
|---|---|---|
| 2 cups | 12 ounces, 336 g | Tomato, peeled, seeded, chopped |
| 3 | | Shallots, minced |
| 1 | | Red chile fresh, seeded, sliced |
| To taste | | Salt |
| 1 tablespoon | $\frac{1}{2}$ ounce, 15 ml | Fresh lime juice |
| 1 tablespoon | | Basil, shredded |

**PROCEDURE**

1 Combine tomato, shallots, and chile; season with salt and lime juice.
2 Let stand 1 hour, add basil, and serve.

## Naam Prik Chile Sauce YIELD: $\frac{3}{4}$ CUP

| AMOUNT | MEASURE | INGREDIENT |
|---|---|---|
| 4 tablespoons | 2 ounces, 30 ml | Palm sugar |
| 7 tablespoons | $3\frac{1}{2}$ ounces, 105 ml | Hot water |
| 2 tablespoons | 1 ounce, 30 ml | Fish sauce (*nam pla*) |
| | 100 ml | Water, hot |
| 2 tablespoons | | Fish sauce |
| 1 | | Red chile, fresh, thinly sliced |
| 2 tablespoons | 1 ounce, 30 ml | Fresh lime juice |

**PROCEDURE**

1 Dissolve the sugar in the hot water. Let cool.
2 Combine remaining ingredients.

# Ma Hor Galloping Horses SERVES 4

| AMOUNT | MEASURE | INGREDIENT |
|---|---|---|
| 1 tablespoon | $\frac{1}{2}$ ounce, 15 ml | Vegetable oil |
| 2 teaspoons | | Garlic, minced |
| 1 cup | 6 ounces, 168 g | Pork, ground |
| 1 tablespoon | $\frac{1}{2}$ ounce, 15 ml | Fish sauce (*nam pla*) |
| 2 tablespoons | 1 ounce, 28 g | Brown sugar |
| $\frac{1}{8}$ teaspoon | | Black pepper, freshly ground |
| $\frac{1}{4}$ cup | 1$\frac{1}{2}$ ounces, 42 g | Peanuts, roasted, coarsely chopped |
| 1 | | Butter lettuce, head, separated into leaves |
| 2 | | Tangerines, peeled, pith and white fibers removed, cut horizontally into $\frac{1}{3}$ inch (.8 cm) thick, or pineapple wedges |
| Garnish | | |
| $\frac{1}{4}$ cup | | Mint leaves |
| $\frac{1}{4}$ cup | | Cilantro leaves |
| 2 | | Red chiles, fresh, seeded, cut into thin shreds |

PROCEDURE

1. Heat wok over medium heat. When hot, add oil. Add garlic, and stir-fry 30 seconds.
2. Add pork, fish sauce, brown sugar, and black pepper. Stir-fry until pork is cooked.
3. Stir in peanuts; mix. Remove from heat and let cool.
4. Place lettuce leaves on serving platter. Arrange tangerine slices on lettuce. Put a heaping teaspoon of the cooked meat on each slice.
5. Garnish with mint and cilantro leaves.
6. Serve chilled or room temperature with chiles on the side.

# Tord Man Pla Fried Fish Cakes SERVES 4

| AMOUNT | MEASURE | INGREDIENT |
|---|---|---|
| $\frac{3}{4}$ pound | 12 ounces, 336 g | Catfish or any white-fleshed fish fillet |
| 1 $\frac{1}{2}$ tablespoons | $\frac{3}{4}$ ounce, 22 ml | Fish sauce (*nam pla*) |
| 1 tablespoon | $\frac{1}{2}$ ounce, 15 ml | Red curry paste |
| 1 tablespoon | | Galangal or ginger |
| 1 | | Egg, lightly beaten |
| 4 | | Kaffir lime leaves, stems removed, finely shredded |
| $\frac{1}{4}$ cup | 2 ounces, 60 ml | Vegetable oil |

**PROCEDURE**

1 Pound or process fish, fish sauce, curry paste, galangal, and egg to a smooth paste. Do not overprocess.

2 Add kaffir leaves and mix well. Moisten hands with water and shape mixture into small cakes, about 3 inches (7.2 cm) by $\frac{1}{4}$ inch (.6 cm) thick.

3 Heat oil to 350°F (176°C). Fry cakes until both sides are light brown, pressing down on the cakes. Drain on paper towels.

## Nam Prik Kaeng Ped Red Curry Paste

YIELD: 3 TABLESPOONS

| AMOUNT | MEASURE | INGREDIENT |
|---|---|---|
| 14 | | Red chiles, dried, seeded soaked in water 10 minutes to soften |
| 2 teaspoons | | Galangal, chopped |
| 1 | | Lemongrass stalk, bottom 6 inches (14.4 cm) only |
| 1 teaspoon | | Lime zest |
| 2 tablespoons | | Cilantro roots, chopped |
| 1 | | Shallot, chopped |
| 1 teaspoon | | Shrimp paste |
| 10 | | Peppercorns, black |
| 2 tablespoons | 1 ounce, 30 ml | Vegetable oil |

**PROCEDURE**

1 Pound or process all ingredients in a mortar, blender, or processor to a smooth paste. Add a little more oil if necessary.

# Tom Yam Goong

## Hot and Spicy Shrimp Soup

YIELD: SERVES 4

| AMOUNT | MEASURE | INGREDIENT |
|---|---|---|
| **1 pound** | **448 g** | **Shrimp, 30-count size** |
| **1 tablespoon** | **$\frac{1}{2}$ ounce, 15 ml** | **Vegetable oil** |
| **5 cups** | **40 ounces, 1.2 l** | **Chicken stock** |
| **2** | | **Lemongrass stalks** |
| **1$\frac{1}{2}$ tablespoons** | | **Cilantro stems, minced** |
| **2** | | **Garlic cloves, minced** |
| **2** | | **Green hot chiles, seeds removed, minced** |
| **4** | | **Kaffir lime leaves, chopped** |
| **$\frac{1}{2}$ teaspoon** | | **Lime zest** |
| **$\frac{1}{2}$ teaspoon** | | **White pepper** |
| **15 ounce** | **420 g** | **Straw mushrooms, drained** |
| **1 tablespoon** | **$\frac{1}{2}$ ounce, 15 ml** | **Fish sauce (*nam pla*)** |
| **2 tablespoons** | **1 ounce, 30 ml** | **Lime juice** |
| **2** | | **Red chiles, seeds removed, julienned** |
| **2 tablespoons** | | **Cilantro, leaves only, chopped** |
| **2 tablespoons** | | **Green onion, sliced on the thin on the bias** |

### PROCEDURE

1. Peel, wash, and devein shrimp; reserve the shells. Cut shrimp in half lengthwise.
2. Heat the oil and sauté the shrimp shells until they turn pink, 2 to 3 minutes.
3. Add chicken stock. Cut off the top of the lemongrass; reserve the bottom 5 inches (12 cm). Bruise the lemongrass stalks with the side of a cleaver or knife. Add to stock. Slice the remaining bottom inches into paper-thin slices.
4. Pound or process the sliced lemongrass, cilantro stems, garlic, green chiles, Kaffir leaves, lime zest, and white pepper to a paste.
5. Add the paste to the stock and stir to combine. Bring to a boil. Cover, reduce to a simmer, and cook 20 minutes. Strain.

6 Return stock to heat and bring back to a boil.
7 Add shrimp and mushrooms; cook 2 to 3 minutes, or until shrimp are just cooked.
8 Remove from heat; add fish sauce and lime juice, and correct seasoning.
9 Serve hot, with red chiles, cilantro leaves, and green onions on the side.

# Mun Tot

## Fried Sweet Potatoes

SERVES 4

| AMOUNT | MEASURE | INGREDIENT |
|---|---|---|
| $\frac{3}{4}$ cup | $5\frac{1}{4}$ ounces, 147 g | Rice Flour |
| $\frac{1}{4}$ cup | 1 ounce, 28 g | Unsweetened coconut, grated |
| $\frac{1}{4}$ cup | 2 ounces, 56 g | Granulated sugar |
| 1 teaspoon | | Red curry paste |
| 6 tablespoons | 3 ounces, 90 ml | Coconut cream, thick |
| 2 cups | 8 ounces, 224 g | Sweet potatoes, peeled, $\frac{1}{4}$ inch (.6 cm) pieces, rounds, bias cuts, or sticks |
| As needed | | Peanut sauce (see recipe on page 339) |

**PROCEDURE**

1 Combine all ingredients except sweet potatoes and stir to a paste. Do not overmix.
2 Heat deep fryer to 375°F (190°C).
3 Dip sweet potato pieces into batter and fry until golden. Drain on paper towels.
4 Serve with peanut sauce.

# Yam Makeua Issaan

## Grilled Eggplant Salad

SERVES 4

| AMOUNT | MEASURE | INGREDIENT |
|---|---|---|
| **1 pound** | **448 g** | **Eggplant** |
| **3** | | **Shallots, unpeeled** |
| **5** | | **Garlic cloves, unpeeled** |
| **2** | | **Anaheim or banana chiles** |
| **2** | | **Green onions, minced** |
| **½ cup** | | **Cilantro leaves, chopped** |
| **¼ cup** | | **Mint leaves, chopped** |
| **2 tablespoons** | **1 ounce, 30 ml** | **Fresh lime juice** |
| **3 tablespoons** | **1½ ounces, 45 ml** | **Fish sauce (*nam pla*)** |
| **2 tablespoons** | | **Sesame seeds, dry roasted** |
| **As needed** | | **Crispy rice crackers (recipe follows)** |

PROCEDURE

1. Prick the eggplant all over with a small knife or fork. Grill or broil until well softened and browned, 10 to 15 minutes, or oven-roast. Remove from heat and cool.
2. Broil or roast shallots, garlic, and chiles until soft and covered with a few black spots. Remove from heat and cool. Peel and coarsely chop.
3. Pound or process shallots, garlic, and chiles to a coarse paste.
4. Remove skin from the eggplants and coarsely chop. Mash to a lumpy mixture; add chile paste and mix.
5. Stir in the green onions, cilantro, mint, lime juice, and fish sauce.
6. Garnish with sesame seeds. Serve with Crispy Rice Crackers.

# Khao Tang

## Crispy Rice Crackers

**SERVES 4**

| AMOUNT | MEASURE | INGREDIENT |
|---|---|---|
| **2 cups** | **12 ounces, 336 g** | **Cooked jasmine rice, warm or hot** |
| **As needed** | | **Peanut or other oil** |

**PROCEDURE**

1 Preheat oven to 350°F (176°C).

2 With a rice paddle or wooden spoon, spread the rice onto a lightly oiled baking sheet to make a layer about $\frac{1}{2}$ inch (1.2 cm) thick. Press down to compact the rice so that it sticks together.

3 Place sheet pan into oven and turn down the temperature to 250°F (121°C). Let dry 3 to 4 hours; the bottom will be a light brown.

4 Heat 2 inches (4.8 cm) oil to 350°F (176°C) or use a deep fryer. To test the temperature, drop a small piece of dried rice cake into the oil. It should sink to the bottom and immediately float back to the surface without burning or crisping. Adjust the heat as necessary.

5 Break off rice cakes and fry in the hot oil. When the first side stops swelling, turn over and cook on the other side until well puffed and just starting to brown, 30 seconds. Remove and drain on a paper towels.

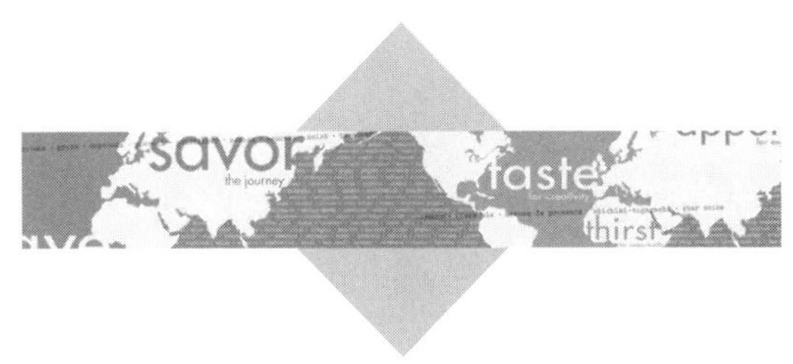

# Pad Thai Thai Fried Noodles SERVES 4

**Chef Tip** **Noodles for Pad Thai should be soaked with warm, not boiling, water. Noodles should be somewhat flexible and solid, not completely expanded and soft.**

| AMOUNT | MEASURE | INGREDIENT |
|---|---|---|
| 2 tablespoons | 1 ounce, 30 ml | Tamarind water or white vinegar |
| 2 tablespoons | 1 ounce, 28 g | Granulated sugar |
| 4 teaspoons | 20 ml | Fish sauce |
| ½ teaspoon | | Dried chile peppers |
| 1 tablespoon | ½ ounce, 15 ml | Preserved turnips (optional) |
| 2 tablespoons | 1 ounce, 30 ml | Peanut oil |
| 2 tablespoons | ¾ ounce, 20 g | Peanuts |
| 1 | | Shallot, minced |
| 3 | | Garlic cloves, minced |
| ¾ cup | 4 ounces, 112 g | Extra-firm tofu, 1 inch (2.4 cm) julienned |
| 5 ounces | 140 g | Thai rice noodles, soaked in lukewarm water for 5 to 10 minutes, drained |
| 1 | | Egg |
| ½ pound | 8 ounces, 224 g | Shrimp, peeled, washed, and deveined |
| ½ pound | 8 ounces, 224 g | Lean-cut pork, ¼ inch (.6 cm) wide and 2 to 3 inches (4.8 to 7.2 cm) long |
| 1 cup | 4 ounces, 112 g | Bean sprouts, washed and drained |
| 1 cup | 2 ounces, 56 g | Green onions, 2 inch (4.8 cm) pieces |
| 4 | | Lime wedges |

**PROCEDURE**

1. Mix together tamarind, sugar, fish sauce, chile peppers, and preserved turnip, set aside.
2. Heat wok over high heat; when hot, add oil. Fry the peanuts until toasted and remove from wok.
3. Add shallot, garlic, and tofu; stir-fry until they start to brown, 2 to 3 minutes.
4. Add drained noodles; they should be flexible but not expanded.
5. Stir-fry to prevent sticking. Add tamarind mixture; stir. If the wok is not hot enough you will see a lot of juice; if so, turn up the heat.

6 Move the ingredients to one side and crack the egg into the wok. Scramble until it is almost set. Fold the egg into the noodles.

7 Add shrimp and pork and stir-fry until cooked.

8 Add half the bean sprouts and chives. Stir and cook 30 seconds. The noodles should be soft and very tangled.

9 Serve sprinkled with peanuts, the remaining bean sprouts, and chives, and lime wedge on the side.

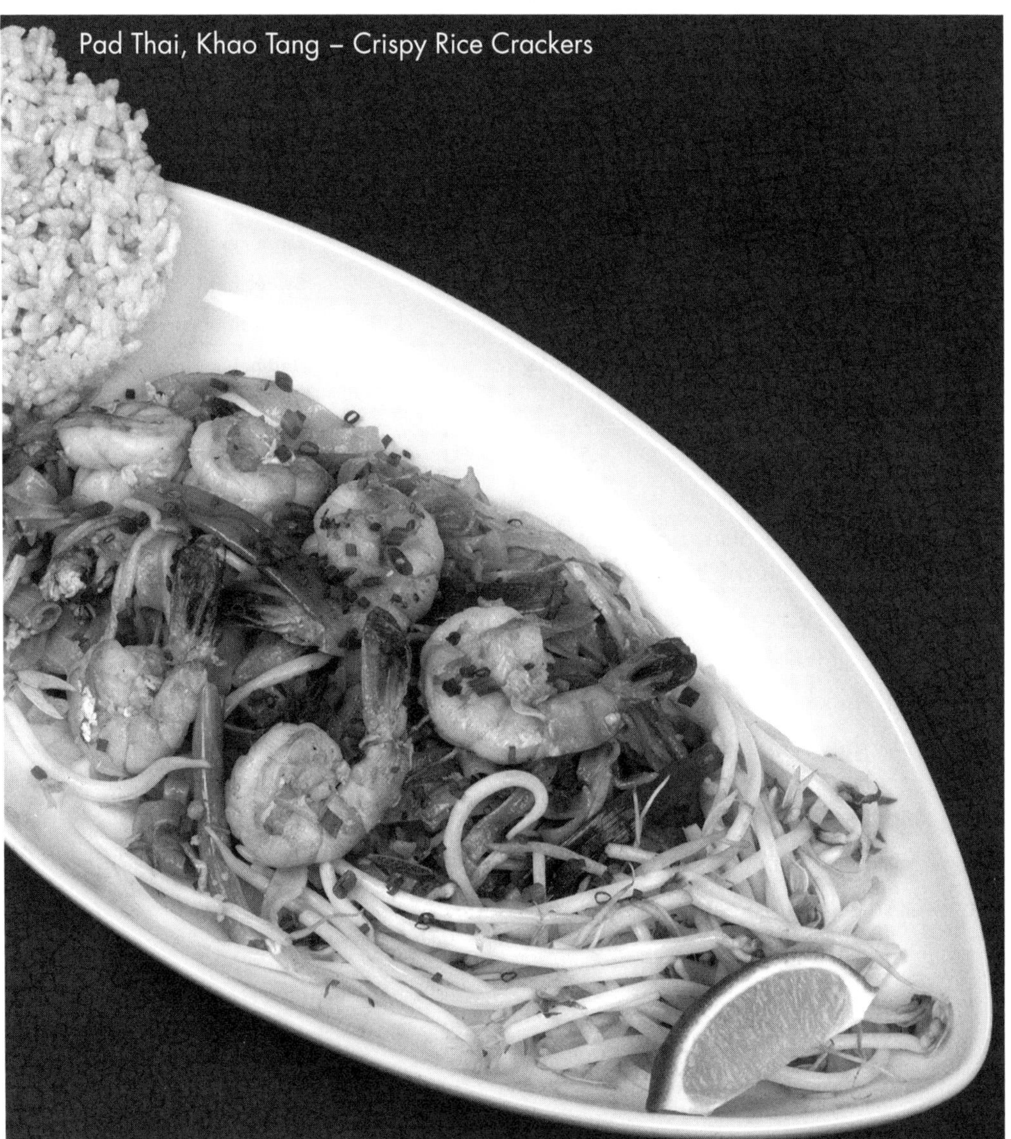
Pad Thai, Khao Tang – Crispy Rice Crackers

# Kaeng Kiew Warn Kai

## Green Curry with Chicken SERVES 4

| AMOUNT | MEASURE | INGREDIENT |
|---|---|---|
| $\frac{1}{2}$ cup | 4 ounces, 120 ml | Coconut milk, thick |
| $\frac{1}{4}$ cup | 2 ounces, 56 g | Green curry paste (recipe follows) |
| 3 cups | 24 ounces, 720 ml | Coconut milk |
| 1 | $2\frac{1}{2}$ pound, 1.12 kg each | Whole chicken, cut into 8 pieces |
| 1 | | Japanese eggplant, 1 inch (2.4 cm) sections |
| 2 tablespoons | 1 ounce, 30 ml | Fish sauce (*nam pla*) |
| 1 tablespoon | $\frac{1}{2}$ ounce, 14 g | Brown sugar |
| $\frac{1}{2}$ teaspoon | | Salt |
| 1 teaspoon | | Lime zest |
| $\frac{1}{2}$ cup | 1 ounce, 14 g | Sweet basil |
| 4 | | Kaffir lime leaves, shredded |
| $\frac{1}{2}$ cup | 2 ounces, 56 g | Red bell pepper, julienned |
| As needed | | Jasmine rice |

**PROCEDURE**

1. Over medium heat, bring the $\frac{1}{2}$ cup (4 ounces, 120 ml) thick coconut milk to a boil, stirring until it thickens and has an oily surface.
2. Add the curry paste. Continue cooking and stirring until the oil has separated from the curry, about 3 to 5 minutes. Be careful not to burn it.
3. Add the chicken and stir-fry until the chicken is firm, 3 to 5 minutes.
4. Add the 3 cups coconut milk; gradually stirring, return to a low boil. Reduce heat, add eggplant, fish sauce, brown sugar, salt, lime zest, half the basil leaves, and Kaffir lime; and simmer 5 to 10 minutes until the chicken and eggplant are tender.
5. Add red bell pepper and cook 1 minute.
6. Garnish with remaining basil leaves and serve with jasmine rice.

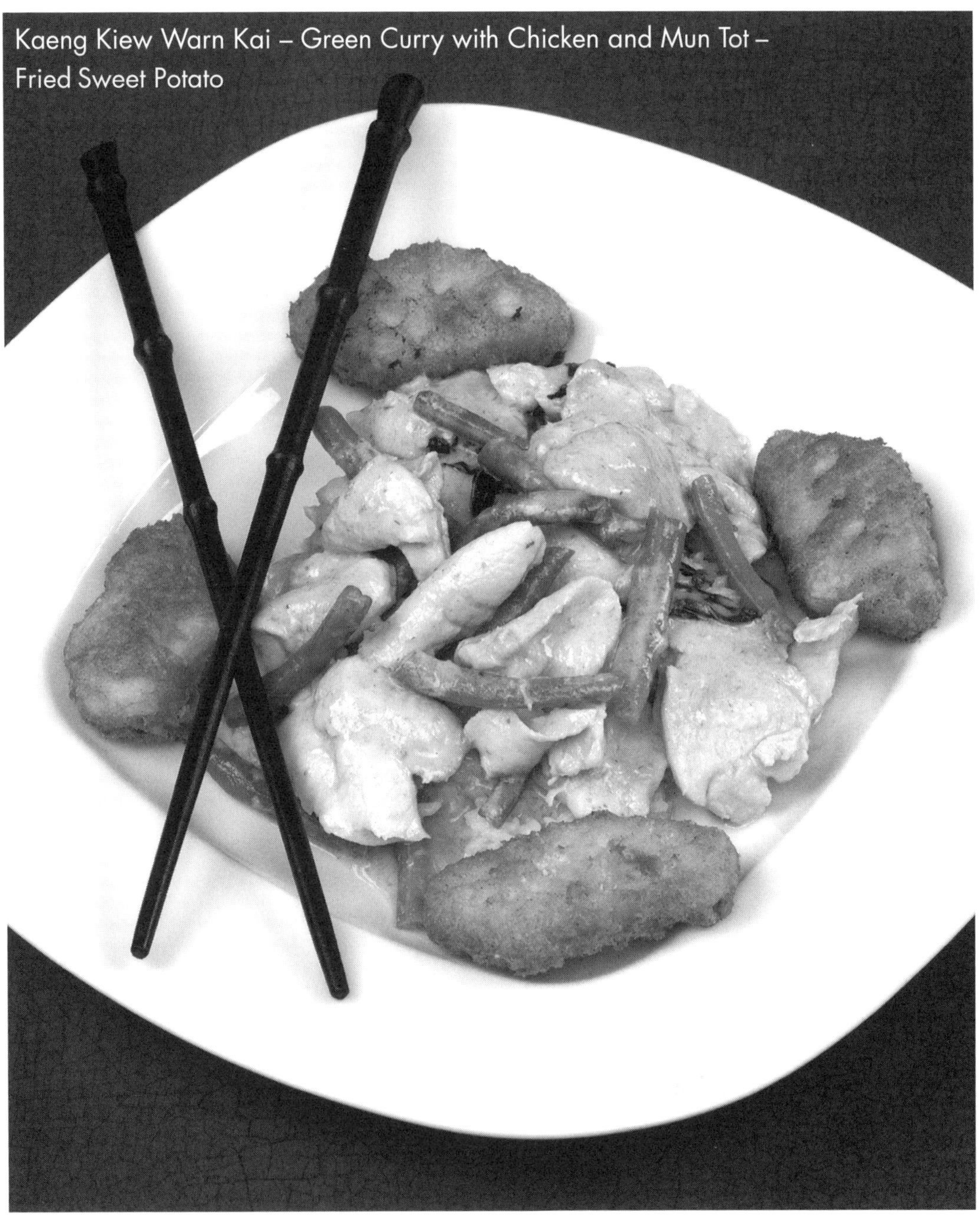

Kaeng Kiew Warn Kai – Green Curry with Chicken and Mun Tot – Fried Sweet Potato

# Green Curry Paste

| AMOUNT | MEASURE | INGREDIENT |
|---|---|---|
| 1 tablespoon | | Coriander seeds, dry roasted and ground |
| 2 teaspoons | | Cumin seeds, dry roasted and ground |
| 1 teaspoon | | Black peppercorns, ground |
| $\frac{1}{4}$ cup | | Cilantro stems, minced |
| $1\frac{1}{2}$ teaspoons | | Salt |
| $\frac{1}{2}$ cup | | Lemongrass, minced |
| $\frac{1}{4}$ cup | | Garlic, chopped |
| $\frac{1}{4}$ cup | | Shallots, chopped |
| 1 tablespoon | | Ginger, minced |
| 1 tablespoon | $\frac{1}{2}$ ounce, 15 ml | Fresh lime juice |
| 1 tablespoon | | Lime zest |
| $\frac{1}{2}$ cup | 1 ounce, 28 g | Green bird chiles, stemmed and coarsely chopped |
| 1 tablespoon | | Shrimp paste |

**PROCEDURE**

1 Combine coriander, cumin, and peppercorns.

2 Pound or process to reduce ingredients to a paste. Place cilantro stems in a mortar with a pinch of salt and pound until well soft and breaking down. Add the lemongrass and work to mash. Add garlic and another pinch of salt and continue to work. Once the garlic is mashed, add the shallots, then the ginger and lime juice mash. Add the lime zest and another pinch of salt; work to a coarse paste.

3 Add the spice blend and mash and pound until well combined. Add chopped chiles and remaining salt, work until broken down and somewhat smooth. Set aside.

4 Place the shrimp paste on a piece of aluminum foil about 8 × 4 9. (19.2 × 6 cm) inches. Spread it out in a thin layer; fold to a flat package. Place in a pan over high heat and cook 3 minutes on the first side, pressing it down. Turn over and repeat. You should smell the hot shrimp paste. Remove and work into the curry while hot.

# Khao Niew Mam Uang

## Mangoes and Sticky Rice

SERVES 4

| AMOUNT | MEASURE | INGREDIENT |
|---|---|---|
| 2 cups | 13 ounces, 364 g | Rice, glutinous (sticky or sweet rice), washed, soaked overnight (8 hours), and drained |
| $\frac{1}{2}$ cup | 4 ounces, 112 g | Granulated sugar |
| 1 teaspoon | | Salt |
| 1 cup | 8 ounces, 240 ml | Coconut milk, thick |
| Topping | | |
| 1 cup | 8 ounces, 230 ml | Coconut milk |
| $\frac{1}{2}$ teaspoon | | Salt |
| $\frac{1}{4}$ cup | 2 ounces, 56 g | Granulated sugar |
| 2 cups | 12 ounces, 336 g | Mangoes, peeled, halved, stone removed, $\frac{1}{2}$ inch (1.2 cm) thick slices |

**PROCEDURE**

1. Place the rice on cheesecloth and steam over water 20 to 25 minutes or until the rice is soft.
2. Dissolve the $\frac{1}{2}$ cup (4 ounces, 112 g) sugar, salt, and thick coconut milk together over medium heat. Bring to a slow boil and remove from heat immediately.
3. Add the rice to the hot milk; stir until completely mixed. Cover and let stand 30 minutes.
4. Bring the remaining coconut milk to a boil, add the salt and $\frac{1}{4}$ cup (4 ounces, 112 g) sugar. Stir to dissolve the sugar.
5. Serve the sliced mangoes with sticky rice and coconut topping.

# Cha Yen Thai Iced Tea SERVES 4

| AMOUNT | MEASURE | INGREDIENT |
|---|---|---|
| $\frac{1}{2}$ cup | 4 ounces, 120 ml | Thai tea |
| 3 cups | 24 ounces, 720 ml | Water |
| $1\frac{3}{4}$ cups | 14 ounces, 420 ml | Sweetened condensed milk |
| $1\frac{1}{2}$ cups | 12 ounces, 360 ml | Milk |

**PROCEDURE**

1 Place tea in a coffee filter in a drip cone set over a pot.

2 Bring water to a boil and pour over the tea. Allow tea to drip through. Repeat this procedure 5 times, until the tea is a deep reddish orange color and very strong.

3 Add the condensed milk to the tea and allow the mixture to come to room temperature.

4 To serve, fill tall glasses with ice; fill half full with the tea/condensed milk mixture, then fill the other half with milk. Stir.

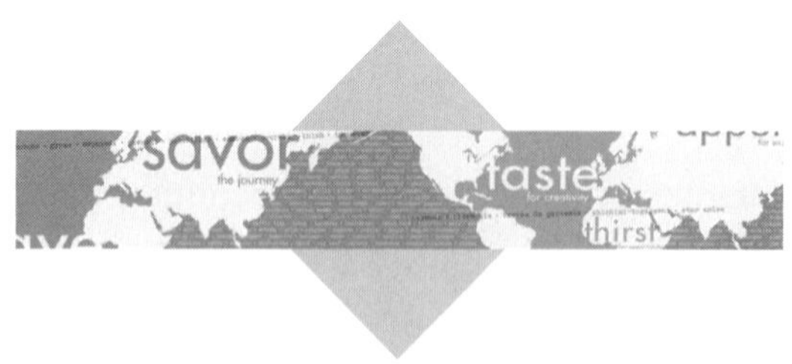

# Banh Hoi Thit Nuong

## Shrimp Toast

YIELD: 20 SHRIMP TOASTS

| AMOUNT | MEASURE | INGREDIENT |
|---|---|---|
| **8 ounces** | **224 g** | **Shrimp, peeled and deveined** |
| **4** | | **Garlic cloves, chopped** |
| **6** | | **Shallots, chopped** |
| **$\frac{1}{2}$ teaspoon** | | **Ginger, grated** |
| **$\frac{1}{2}$ teaspoon** | | **Salt** |
| **1 $\frac{1}{2}$ teaspoons** | | **Granulated sugar** |
| **1 tablespoon** | | **Cornstarch** |
| **To taste** | | **Black pepper, freshly ground** |
| **1 tablespoon** | **$\frac{1}{2}$ ounce, 15 ml** | **Vietnamese fish sauce (*Nuoc mam*)** |
| **1** | | **Baguette, $\frac{1}{2}$ inch (1.2 cm) thick slices** |
| **1 cup** | **2 ounces, 56 g** | **Fresh bread crumbs** |
| **As needed** | | **Oil for frying** |
| **As needed** | | **Nuoc cham (see recipe on page 369)** |

PROCEDURE

1 Pound or puree the shrimp, garlic, shallots, ginger, salt, sugar, cornstarch, and pepper. Process to a coarse paste. Add fish sauce and mix well.

2 Spread about 1 tablespoon of the shrimp paste on each slice of bread; round off the top. Dip the shrimp-coated side in the bread crumbs. Refrigerate.

3 Heat $\frac{1}{2}$ inch (.6 cm) of oil to 360°F (182°C) or until bubbles form around a dry wooden chopstick when inserted in the oil. Working in batches, add the shrimp toast, shrimp side down. Fry 1 minute or until golden brown. Turn over, bread side down, and fry 1 minute. Drain on paper towels.

4 Serve hot with *nuoc cham*.

# Cha Gio Fried Spring Rolls SERVES 4

| AMOUNT | MEASURE | INGREDIENT |
|---|---|---|
| 1 ounce | 28 g | Fine bean threads, soaked/cooked, drained, and cooled |
| 2 tablespoons | | Cloud ears or shiitake, dried, soaked in warm water 20 minutes to soften, drained, chopped into 2 inch (4.8 cm) strips |
| $\frac{1}{4}$ cup | 1 ounce, 28 g | Water chestnuts (or jicama), $\frac{1}{4}$ inch (.6 cm) dice |
| 1 cup | 6 ounces, 168 g | Chicken breast, raw, skinned, boned, minced |
| $\frac{1}{2}$ cup | 3 ounces, 84 g | Crabmeat, picked over and flaked |
| $\frac{1}{2}$ cup | 3 ounces, 84 g | Shrimp, raw, peeled, deveined, minced |
| 2 | | Garlic cloves, minced |
| 2 tablespoons | | Shallots, minced |
| $\frac{1}{4}$ cup | 1 ounce, 28 g | Red onions, minced |
| 1 tablespoon | $\frac{1}{2}$ ounce, 15 ml | Vietnamese fish sauce (*nuoc mam*) |
| 2 tablespoons | 1 ounce, 28 g | Granulated sugar |
| $\frac{1}{2}$ teaspoon | | Black pepper, freshly ground |
| 4 cups | 32 ounces, 960 ml | Water, warm (110°F, 43°C) |
| 4 tablespoons | 2 ounces, 56 g | Granulated sugar |
| 14 | | Rice paper, $6\frac{1}{2}$ inches (15.6 cm) (*banh trang*) |
| 2 | | Egg whites, beaten |
| As needed | | Oil for frying |
| Garnish | | |
| As needed | | *Dia rau song* (vegetable platter; see recipe on page 363) |

**PROCEDURE**

1 Combine bean threads, cloud ears, water chestnuts, chicken, crab, shrimp, garlic, shallots, onions, fish sauce, 2 tablespoons sugar, and pepper; mix well.

2 Combine warm water with 4 tablespoons sugar; stir to dissolve.

3 Dip 3 or 4 rice papers separately into the water for 3 to 4 seconds. Remove and place on a flat work surface. Allow rice paper to soften, 1 to 2 minutes, until soft and transparent.

4 Fold up the bottom third of each wrapper. Center 1 to 2 teaspoons (.5 to 1.0 ml) filling near curved end of the wrappers, leaving space on both ends. Press filling into a compact rectangle. Fold one side of the wrapper over the mixture, then the other. Roll from

bottom to top to completely enclose. Seal with egg white. Continue making packages until wrappers are filled.

5 Heat $1\frac{1}{2}$ to 2 inches (3.6 to 4.8 cm) oil to 325°F (163°C). Add rolls but do not crowd or let them touch; they will stick together. Fry over medium heat 10 to 12 minutes, turning often, until golden and crisp. Drain on paper towels. Keep warm while frying the remaining rolls.

6 To eat, each diner wraps a roll in a lettuce leaf along with a few strands of noodles and a variety of other ingredients from the vegetable platter before dipping it in the *nuoc cham.*

# Cha Bo Grilled Beef Patties SERVES 4

| AMOUNT | MEASURE | INGREDIENT |
|---|---|---|
| **2 tablespoons** | **$\frac{1}{3}$ ounce, 9 g** | **Peanuts, roasted, ground** |
| **$1\frac{1}{2}$ cups** | **9 ounces, 252 g** | **Lean ground beef** |
| **2 tablespoons** | | **Shallots, minced** |
| **2 teaspoons** | | **Vietnamese fish sauce (*nuoc mam*)** |
| **2 tablespoons** | **1 ounce, 30 ml** | **Coconut milk** |
| **$\frac{1}{2}$ teaspoon** | | **Cumin, ground** |
| **$\frac{1}{2}$ teaspoon** | | **Granulated sugar** |
| **To taste** | | **Salt and pepper** |
| **8** | | **Bamboo skewers, soaked in water 30 minutes** |

**PROCEDURE**

1 Combine all ingredients; mix well. Divide into 16 portions.

2 Shape into a ball and then flatten to form a $1\frac{1}{2}$ inch (3.6 cm) patty.

3 Thread 2 patties on each skewer.

4 Grill or broil over high heat until desired temperature, 4 to 5 minutes. Turn only once.

5 Serve immediately with *nuoc cham.*

# Goi Cuon Fresh Spring Rolls

YIELD: 4–8 ROLLS

| AMOUNT | MEASURE | INGREDIENT |
|---|---|---|
| 1 cup | 4 ounces, 112 g | Carrots, shredded |
| 1 teaspoon | | Granulated sugar |
| 8 | | Rice paper (*banh trang*), $8\frac{1}{2}$ inches (20.4 cm) in diameter |
| 4 | | Red leaf or Boston lettuce leaves, thick stem ends removed, cut in half |
| 2 ounces | 56 g | Rice vermicelli or Japanese alimentary paste noodles (*somen*), soaked/cooked, drained, and cooled |
| 12 ounces | 336 g | Pork loin, thinly sliced 1 x 2 inch (2.4 x 4.8 cm) pieces |
| 1 cup | 4 ounces, 112 g | Bean sprouts, washed and drained |
| $\frac{1}{2}$ cup | | Mint leaves |
| 8 | | Shrimp (16–20 ct), cooked, cooled, shelled, deveined, and cut lengthwise in half |
| $\frac{1}{2}$ cup | | Cilantro leaves |
| 1 tablespoon | | Peanuts, roasted, chopped |
| As needed | | Peanut sauce |
| As needed | | Nuoc cham with shredded carrot and daikon |

PROCEDURE

1 Combine shredded carrots and sugar; let stand 10 minutes to soften.

2 Fill a container of warm water (110°F, 43°C) large enough to hold the rice paper. Work with only 2 sheets of rice paper at a time; keep the remaining sheets covered with a damp cloth to prevent curling.

3 Immerse each sheet individually into the warm water, 5 seconds. Remove and spread out flat; do not let the sheets touch each other. Allow the rice paper to soften 2 to 3 minutes. When soft and transparent, assemble the rolls.

4 Lay one piece of lettuce over the bottom third of the rice paper. On the lettuce, place 1 tablespoon of noodles, 1 tablespoon (14 g) carrots, 2 to 3 pieces of pork, a few bean sprouts and several mint leaves. Roll up the paper halfway into a cylinder. Fold in the sides in an envelope pattern. Lay 2 shrimp halves, cut side down, along the crease. Place a few cilantro leaves next to the shrimp. Keep rolling the paper into a tight cylinder to seal. Repeat with remaining wrappers. Store with seam side down.

5 Sprinkle the chopped nuts over the dipping sauce and serve.

# Dia Rau Song

## Vegetable Platter

SERVES 4

| AMOUNT | MEASURE | INGREDIENT |
|---|---|---|
| 1 | | Head of Boston or other soft lettuce, separated into individual leaves (approximately 3 leaves per person) |
| 1 cup | 4 ounces, 112 g | Green onions, cut into 2-inch lengths |
| 1 cup | 2 ounces, 56 g | Cilantro leaves |
| 1 cup | 2 ounces, 56 g | Mint leaves |
| 1 cup | 2 ounces, 56 g | Basil leaves |
| $1\frac{1}{2}$ cups | 9 ounces, 252 g | Seedless cucumber, peeled in alternating strips, halved lengthwise, sliced thinly crosswise |
| 1 cup | 4 ounces, 112 g | Bean sprouts, washed, drained |
| $\frac{1}{2}$ cup | 2 ounces, 56 g | Carrots, julienned |
| As needed | | Lime slices |

PROCEDURE

1 Arrange ingredients in separate groups.

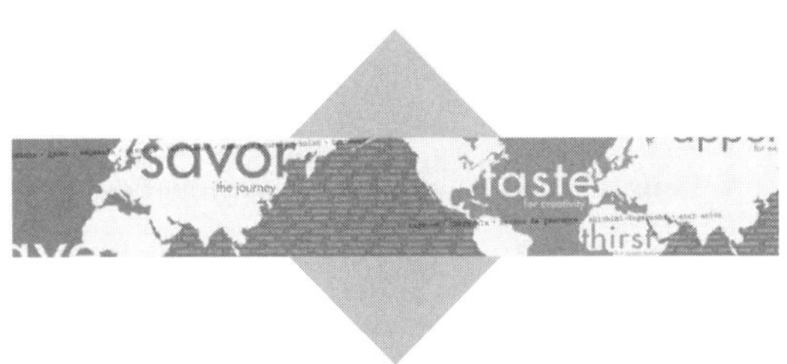

# Pho Bo

## Vietnamese Beef and Noodle Soup

YIELD: 3 TO 4 QUARTS

| AMOUNT | MEASURE | INGREDIENTS |
|---|---|---|
| 1 pound | 448 g | Oxtail, cut 3 inch (7.2 cm) pieces |
| 1 pound | 448 g | Beef bones |
| 2 quarts | 64 ounces, 1.92 l | Beef stock |
| 1 tablespoon | ½ ounce, 15 ml | Vegetable oil |
| 2 | | Onions, cut in ¼ inch (.6 cm) slices |
| 8 ounces | 224 g | Daikon, chopped |
| 1½ ounces | 42 g | Ginger, peeled, sliced |
| 3 | | Green onions, crushed |
| 3 | | Garlic cloves |
| 1 | | Cinnamon stick, 2 inch (4.8 cm) |
| 1 piece | | Star anise |
| 1 teaspoon | | Black pepper |
| Garnish | | |
| 4 ounces | 112 g | Dried rice sticks (*bahn pho*), soaked in hot water for 30 minutes, drained |
| 8 ounces | 224 g | Flank steak, cut very thin |
| 1 cup | 4 ounces, 112 g | Bean sprouts |
| 1 cup | 4 ounces, 112 g | Red onions, thinly sliced |
| 1 | | Green chili pepper (jalapeño), sliced thinly |
| ½ cup | 2 ounces, 56 g | Green onions, ½ inch pieces |
| ½ cup | 1 ounce, 28 g | Cilantro leaves, fresh |
| ½ cup | 1 ounce, 28 g | Mint leaves, fresh |
| ½ cup | 1 ounce, 28 g | Basil leaves, fresh |
| 2 tablespoons | 1 ounce, 30 ml | Vietnamese fish sauce (*nuoc mam*) |
| 8 | | Lime wedges |

**PROCEDURE**

1 Rinse the oxtail and beef bones. Cover with cold stock and additional water if necessary, bring to a slow boil. Reduce heat and simmer, skim as necessary for the first 30 minutes.

2 Heat oil and add sliced onions; cook, stirring until the onions are browned. Remove and drain the fat.

3 After the stock has stopped foaming add the browned onions, daikon, ginger, green onions, garlic, cinnamon, star anise and black pepper. Simmer and continue to skim for 2 hours. Strain the stock using two layers of cheese cloth. Remove oxtail and shred the meat; serve with the soup.

4 Blanch the bean sprouts in boiling water for 3 seconds. Drain, rinse with cold water and drain.

5 Arrange the sliced beef on a platter. Garnish with red onions, sliced chilies, lime wedges, mint leaves, and basil.

6 At serving time, cook rice sticks in boiling water to heat. Drain.

7 Divide rice sticks equally among 4 serving bowls.

8 Season hot beef stock with fish sauce and black pepper.

9 Each person adds cooked beef, raw flank steak and red onions to their noodles; ladle hot stock over the meat, stirring to cook the meat.

10 Add green chili, bean sprouts, cilantro, mint, basil, and lime to taste.

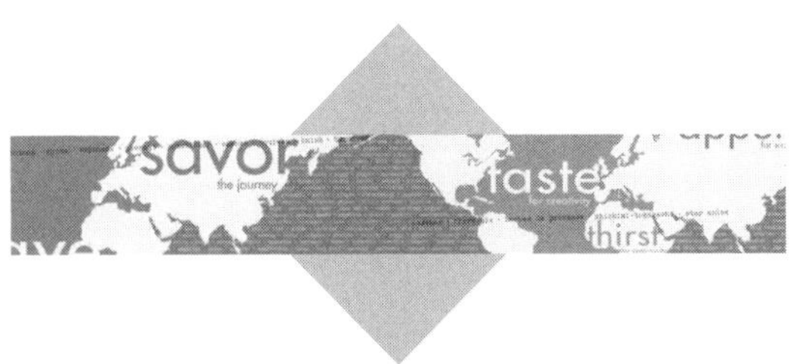

# Dua Chua
## Pickled Carrot and Daikon Salad

SERVES 4

| AMOUNT | MEASURE | INGREDIENTS |
|---|---|---|
| **2 cups** | **8 ounces, 224 g** | **Carrots, julienned** |
| **2 cups** | **8 ounces, 224 g** | **Daikon, julienned** |
| **1 teaspoon** | | **Salt** |
| **$\frac{1}{2}$ cup** | **4 ounces, 120 ml** | **Water** |
| **11 tablespoons** | **$5\frac{1}{2}$ ounces, 165 ml** | **Rice wine vinegar** |
| **$\frac{1}{4}$ cup** | **2 ounces, 56 g** | **Granulated sugar** |
| **$\frac{1}{2}$ teaspoon** | | **Vietnamese fish sauce (*nuoc mam*)** |
| **1 tablespoon** | | **Cilantro leaves, shredded** |
| **1 tablespoon** | | **Mint leaves, shredded** |
| **1 tablespoon** | | **Basil leaves, shredded** |

### PROCEDURE

1. Combine carrots, daikon, and salt; toss to coat. Place in a colander to drain for 30 minutes. Rinse and squeeze dry.
2. Combine water, vinegar, sugar, and fish sauce, bring to a boil, and cool to room temperature.
3. Add vegetables to cool vinegar mixture and let marinate 1 hour.
4. Just before serving, toss with herbs.

# Ga Xao Sa Ot

## Lemongrass Chicken SERVES 4

| AMOUNT | MEASURE | INGREDIENT |
|---|---|---|
| 2 | | Lemongrass stalks, bottom 6 inches, only, minced |
| 3 tablespoons | 1 $\frac{1}{2}$ ounces, 45 ml | Vietnamese fish sauce (*nuoc mam*) |
| $\frac{1}{4}$ teaspoon | | Black pepper, ground |
| 1 tablespoon | | Garlic, minced |
| 1 pound | 16 ounces, 448 g | Chicken thigh meat, boned, skinned, cut into 1-inch (2.4 cm) cubes |
| 1 tablespoon | $\frac{1}{2}$ ounce, 15 ml | Vegetable oil |
| 2 | | Red chile, fresh, seeded, shredded into 1 $\frac{1}{2}$ inch (3.6 cm) lengths |
| $\frac{1}{2}$ cup | 2 ounces, 56 g | Green onions, shredded into 1 $\frac{1}{2}$ inch (3.6 cm) lengths |
| 1 teaspoon | | Granulated sugar |
| 2 tablespoons | | Basil leaves |
| 1 tablespoon | | Mint leaves |
| Garnish | | |
| $\frac{1}{4}$ cup | 1 ounce, 28 g | Peanuts, unsalted roasted |
| | | *Dia Rau Song* (vegetable platter; see recipe on page 363) |

PROCEDURE

1 Combine lemongrass, 2 tablespoons (1 ounce, 30 ml) fish sauce, pepper, and garlic; mix well. Add chicken and toss to combine, let marinate for 1 hour.

2 Heat a wok over medium heat. Add oil; stir-fry chicken, 2 to 3 minutes, until chicken is no longer pink. Add a little water if mixture is too dry.

3 Add remaining fish sauce, chiles, green onions, and sugar. Stir for 30 seconds. Add basil and mint leaves; toss to combine.

4 Serve garnished with peanuts and vegetable platter or rice.

# Bo Nuong Grilled Beef SERVES 4

| AMOUNT | MEASURE | INGREDIENT |
|---|---|---|
| 2 | | Lemongrass stalks, bottom 6 inches only, sliced thin, or 2 tablespoons dried lemongrass, soaked in warm water 1 hour |
| $\frac{1}{4}$ cup | 1 ounce, 28 g | Shallots, sliced thin |
| 4 | | Garlic cloves, crushed |
| 1 tablespoon | $\frac{1}{2}$ ounce, 14 g | Granulated sugar |
| 1 | | Fresh red chile peppers, seeded |
| 2 tablespoons | 1 ounce, 30 ml | Vietnamese fish sauce (*nuoc mam*) |
| 1 tablespoon | $\frac{1}{2}$ ounce, 15 ml | Sesame oil |
| 1 tablespoon | $\frac{1}{2}$ ounce, 15 ml | Peanut oil |
| 2 tablespoons | | Sesame seeds |
| 1 pound | | Beef, sirloin or flat iron steak, very cold, cut into thin strips, 1$\frac{1}{2}$ (3.6 cm) inches by 4 to 5 (9.6 to 12 cm) long. |
| 24 | | Bamboo skewers, 8 inches (19.2 cm), soaked in water 30 minutes |
| Garnish | | |
| 4 ounces | 112 g | Rice vermicelli, thin, soaked/cooked, drained, and cooled |
| As needed | | *Dia Rau Song* (Vegetable Platter; see recipe on page 363) |
| As needed | | *Nuoc cham* with shredded carrots and daikon (recipe folllows) |

**PROCEDURE**

1. Combine lemongrass, shallots, garlic, sugar, and chiles in a mortar; pound to a fine paste. Move to a bowl and stir in fish sauce, sesame oil, peanut oil, and sesame seeds; blend well.
2. Add beef strips to the paste; toss to coat well. Let marinate for 30 minutes.
3. Weave a skewer through each strip of meat.
4. Grill or pan sear, 1 minute per side. Serve at room temperature with cooked noodles, vegetable platter, and *nuoc cham*.
5. Each diner fills a lettuce leaf with vegetables, noodles, and barbecued beef. The leaf is wrapped into a neat roll and dipped in individual bowls of *nuoc cham* and eaten by hand.

# Nuoc Cham with Shredded Carrots and Daikon

YIELD: 1 ½ CUP

| AMOUNT | MEASURE | INGREDIENT |
|---|---|---|
| **2 tablespoons** | **1 ounce, 30 ml** | **Rice vinegar** |
| **3 tablespoons** | **1 ½ ounces, 45 l** | **Fresh lime juice** |
| **¼ cup** | **2 ounces, 60 ml** | **Vietnamese fish sauce (*nuoc mam*)** |
| **¼ cup** | **2 ounces, 60 ml** | **Water** |
| **2 tablespoons** | **1 ounce, 28 g** | **Granulated sugar** |
| **1** | | **Garlic clove, minced** |
| **½ teaspoon** | | **Red pepper flakes** |
| **½ cup** | **2 ounces, 56 g** | **Carrot, shredded** |
| **½ cup** | **2 ounces, 56 g** | **Daikon or turnip, peeled, shredded** |
| **1 teaspoon** | | **Granulated sugar** |
| **As needed** | | ***Nuoc cham* (recipe follows)** |

PROCEDURE

1 Combine rice vinegar, lime juice, fish sauce, water, and sugar; stir to dissolve. Add garlic and red pepper flakes. Stir. Cover and let stand for at least 1 hour.

2 Toss the carrot and daikon shreds with the 1 teaspoon of sugar. Let stand 15 minutes to soften. Combine with the *nuoc cham*.

# Nuoc Cham

YIELD: 1 CUP

| AMOUNT | MEASURE | INGREDIENT |
|---|---|---|
| **2** | | **Garlic cloves, crushed** |
| **1** | | **Fresh red chile pepper, seeded, minced** |
| **2 tablespoons** | **1 ounce, 28 g** | **Granulated sugar** |
| **2 tablespoons** | **1 ounce, 30 ml** | **Fresh lime or lemon juice** |
| **¼ cup** | **2 ounces, 60 ml** | **Rice vinegar** |
| **¼ cup** | **2 ounces, 60 ml** | **Nuoc mam (Vietnamese fish sauce)** |
| **¼ cup** | **2 ounces, 60 ml** | **Water** |

PROCEDURE

1 Using a mortar, make a paste of the garlic, chile, and sugar. Add remaining ingredients; stir to blend.

# Suon Rang

## Glazed Spareribs SERVES 4

| AMOUNT | MEASURE | INGREDIENT |
|---|---|---|
| 1 tablespoon | ½ ounce, 15 ml | Vegetable oil |
| 2 pounds | 32 ounces, 896 g | Spareribs, lean, cut into 2 inch (4.8 cm) pieces |
| 2 tablespoons | 1 ounce, 28 g | Granulated sugar |
| 2 tablespoons | 1 ounce, 30 ml | Vietnamese fish sauce (*nuoc mam*) |
| 1 tablespoon | ½ ounce, 15 ml | Soy sauce |
| 6 | | Garlic cloves, mashed |
| 1½ cups | 6 ounces, 168 g | Onions, 1 inch (2.4 cm) cubes |
| 1½ cups | 6 ounces, 168 g | Red bell peppers, 1½ inch (3.6 cm) cubes |
| ½ cup | 2 ounces, 56 g | Green onions, 2 inch (4.8 cm) lengths |
| To taste | | Black pepper, freshly ground |
| As needed | | Cilantro sprigs |

PROCEDURE

1 Heat wok over medium heat; add oil. Add ribs and cook on both sides until browned, about 15 to 20 minutes.

2 Add sugar and stir. Cook 10 minutes.

3 Pour off all but 1 tablespoon (½ ounce, 15 ml) fat. Add fish sauce and soy sauce and stir-fry 3 to 4 minutes. Add garlic, onions, bell peppers, and green onions. Stir-fry 3 to 4 minutes or until onions are lightly browned and peppers are tender but firm. Transfer to serving dish.

4 Sprinkle with black pepper and garnish with cilantro sprigs. Serve with rice.

# Spain

## The Land

Spain is Europe's third largest nation and occupies most of the Iberian Peninsula at the southwestern edge of the continent. It borders France and Andorra in the north and Portugal in the west. Spain's rule once extended all over the world, but today it has been reduced to the mainland, the Balearic Islands in the Mediterranean Sea, the Canary Islands off the northwestern coast of Africa, the Spanish free ports of Ceuta and Melilla on the northern coast of Africa in Morocco, and several other small islands off the coast of Morocco. Spain's physical geography comprises a large peninsula protected by a ring of mountains on nearly all sides. These mountains make Spain the second highest country in Europe, after Switzerland. Continental Spain consists of the Meseta or central plateau, the largest plateau of its kind in Europe, which is surrounded by the Baetic, Andalusian, and Iberian Mountains to the south and southeast, and the Pyrenees to the north, as well as the Cordillera Cantabrica (Catabrian Mountains) to the northwest. The eastern and southern coasts of Spain border the Mediterranean Sea. The varied topography makes for diversity in both climate and natural resources.

## History

Around 1100 B.C., Phoenicians from the area that is now present-day Lebanon set up trading colonies along the Spanish coast. Greeks also traded along the northeastern coast. After the fall of Phoenecia it was occupied by Rome for six centuries, laying such important foundations as the Latin language, Roman law, the municipality structure, and the Christian religion.

After the Roman Empire fell, the Suevi, Vandals, and Alans came to Spain but were defeated by the Visigoths, who, by the end of the sixth century, had occupied most of the peninsula. The Arabs entered from the south at the beginning of the eighth century. They conquered the country quickly except for a small area in the north that would become the initial springboard for the reconquest that would occur eight centuries later. The era of Muslim rule is divided into three periods: the Emirate (711–756), the Caliphate (756–1031), and the Reinos de Taifas (small independent kingdoms, 1031–1492).

In 1469, two Catholic monarchs were married: Isabella of Castile and Ferdinand of Aragon. The marriage prepared the way for the two kingdoms to be united. This union marked the opening of a period of growing success for Spain. The year 1492 heralded the discovery of the Americas under the command of Christopher Columbus. During the sixteenth and seventeenth centuries the Spanish Empire became the world's foremost power, and a huge presence in European politics. In 1808 Joseph Bonaparte was installed on the Spanish throne, following the Napoleonic invasion. A fierce resistance followed and Spanish rule was restored with Fernando VII occupying the throne. The Spanish overseas empire finally dissolved in 1898 when, after a brief war with the United States, Spain lost Cuba, Puerto Rico, and the Philippines.

During elections in 1931, it became clear that the people no longer wanted the monarchy ruling over them. In all the large towns of Spain the candidates who supported the monarchy were defeated heavily. However, many smaller country towns supported the monarchy, and thus it was able to keep power. The cities held much power, however, and within them support for Republicans was enormous. Great crowds gathered in Madrid, and the king's most trusted friends advised him to leave. He did so, and the Republic was established on April 14, 1931. During the five-year lifetime of the Republic, it was riddled with political, economic, and social conflicts, which split opinion into two irreconcilable sides: those who still supported a republic and those who did not. The climate of violence grew and on July 18, 1936, a military uprising turned into a tragic three-year civil war.

On October 1, 1936, General Francisco Franco took over as head of state and commander-in-chief of the armed forces. Spain began a period of forty years' dictatorship. The early years were years of economic privation and political repression. Later in Franco's rule, steps toward modernizing Spain's economy began, and increased external influence began to be felt both from the burgeoning tourist trade and industrial investments in Spain.

Franco died in 1975, bringing to an end a significant period of modern Spanish history and opening the way to the restoration of the monarchy with the rise to the throne of Juan Carlos I. Once in power, the young king pushed for change to a western-style democracy. Adolfo Suarez, the prime minister of the second monarchy government, carried out the transition

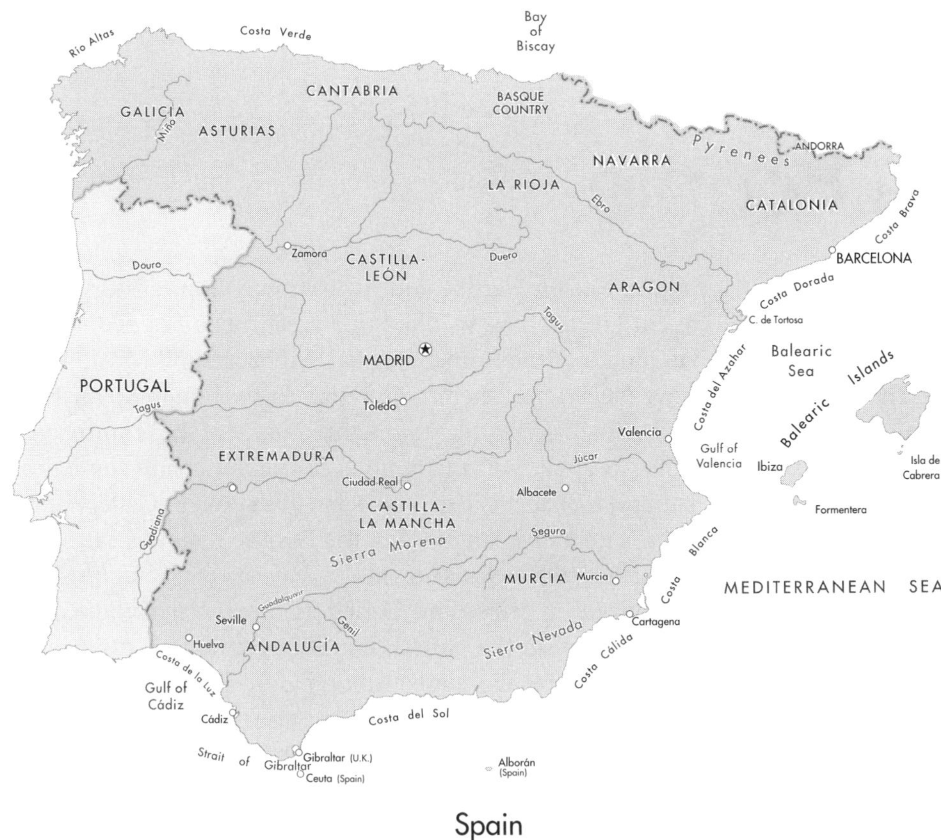


Spain

to democracy, which culminated in the first democratic parliamentary elections in forty-one years, on June 15, 1977. The years since have been years of rapid change, politically, economically, and socially. In 1982, Spain became a member of the North Atlantic Treaty Organization (NATO). In 1995, Spain joined the European Union. Spain's economy has grown at a rapid pace, and now has reached near parity with the northern European industrialized democracies. Socially, Spain also has moved toward the European mean, with the younger generation more urban and more cosmopolitan than generations before.

On March 11, 2004, Spain was the victim of a massive terrorist attack when Islamic extremists exploded a series of bombs on trains in the crowded Atocha train station in central Madrid. Nearly three hundred died, and hundreds more were injured. In an election a few days later, voters angry at a lack of transparency in the government's handling of the attack—and especially angry at apparently politically-motivated government attempts to link the bombings to Basque terrorists and denial of any Al Queda involvement—led to a surprise victory for the Socialists and their regional allies after eight years of right-wing Partido Popular rule.

# The People

Spain's land-bridge location between Europe and Africa and its long history of invasion and settlement by many different groups have resulted in a great mixing of peoples and cultures, particularly the strong influences of the Roman, Jewish, Moorish, and Muslim cultures.

The language of Spain reflects this inherent diversity. Even though Spanish is the official language, other languages in Spain are highly dominant in parts of the country and have been officially recognized. Catalan is spoken in the regions of Catalonia and the Balearic Islands. In Valencia both Castilian and a dialect called Valencian are spoken. Gallego, or Galician, is popular in northwest Spain. The native language of the Basque region is called Euskera. It is not a form of Spanish, and its origins are unknown.

Most Spaniards are baptized, married, and buried as members of the Roman Catholic Church. Under the 1978 constitution the church is no longer Spain's official faith, though financial support is still provided by the state. Among non-Catholic Spaniards, Muslims from Morocco form the largest community. Many other non-Catholics are Protestants, and Spain is also home to small Jewish and Eastern Orthodox congregations. One long-standing minority group is the Roma (Gypsies), who are known as Gitanos. Some of the Roma follow a traditional nomadic lifestyle, while others have assimilated into mainstream Spanish society. Some Basques also claim an ethnic or racial uniqueness from other Spaniards, in addition to a language difference. In the late twentieth century, Spain began receiving large numbers of immigrants for the first time since the sixteenth century. Most of the country's foreign populations are from Latin America, elsewhere in Europe, or North Africa.

The discussion of Spanish culture would not be complete without mentioning two of the most popular customs of Spain: flamenco and bullfighting. These customs are synonymous with Spain throughout the world and hence have become a part of its culture. They are an important part of any fiesta or carnival in Spain. Traditionally, flamenco is an intense artistic expression that originated in southern Spain. Song, dance, and guitar are blended into passionate rhythms that are often improvised and spontaneous. Bullfighting had its first mention as a sport during the Greek and Roman periods. Many northern Europeans are critical of bullfighting and condemn it as a cruel blood sport. Most Spaniards, however, do not see it this way. To them bullfighting is an exciting test of bravery, skill, and grace.

The Spanish are known for eating late. Breakfast often consists of rolls, butter or preserves, and coffee. Lunch, served between 2 and 3 p.m., is the main meal of the day. Dinner is eaten after 9 p.m., often as late as midnight, and is lighter.

# The Food

The Moors' occupation of Spain for 750 years greatly influenced Spanish culinary development. The Moorish invaders introduced the cultivation of rice; spices such as saffron, cumin, and anise; nuts (especially almonds); and fruit such as figs, citrus, and bananas. The Moors also introduced their own methods of food preparation. For example, the technique of marinating fish in a strong, vinegary sauce and the combination of sweet and spicy foods are of Arab origin. From the Spanish conquests in the New World in the sixteenth century came eggplant, tomatoes, potatoes, red and green peppers (both hot and sweet), and chocolate.

The Spanish mainland can be broadly divided into five distinct regions: Green Spain, Central Spain, the Pyrenees, Mediterranean Spain, and Andalusia.

Green Spain is located in the north and northwest and includes the regions of Galicia, Asturias, Cantabria, and the Basque provinces. Galicia is known for its abundance of seafood, especially scallops, hake, salmon, and trout. An elegant fan-shaped sea scallop that the Galacians call *vieira* has flavor and history. Travelers from the south kept the shells as proof of their journey through the rocky coastlines. The Asturias is known for its abundance of fish and vegetables. Known for contented cows and mountain ranges full of forests, Asturias and Cantabria are cheese and apple country. *Arroz con leche* is a simple rice pudding made with famous rich and creamy milk. The milk not used for bottling is used for some of the best cheeses in Spain. Cow, sheep, and goat's milk is used to make a soft creamy cheese known as Cabrales Blue that is wrapped in chestnut leaves and stored in humid caves. Light green-blue veins develop to intensify its taste and aroma. Also famous in this region is a blood sausage made with cow's blood, bacon, and onions.

Basque cuisine has agriculture, pastoral, and fishery influences. Peas, beans, green and red peppers, tomatoes, onions, and other mixed vegetables are the stars of many Basque dishes. The Basque district curves around the Bay of Biscay and these waters provide many varieties of fish and shellfish that include crab, hake, tuna, cod, mussels, oysters, lobsters, edible sea barnacles, and baby eels, or angulas. Octopus that inhabit the deep bay waters also find their way to the table as *pulpo gallega.* In Basque country the people enjoy *pintxos* (tapas) twice during the day. One is the *aperitivo* in the morning, and the other is the *txikiteo*, in the evening. Examples of pintxos include tiny rolls filled with ham, grilled eggplant, red peppers, various omelets, fish, sausage, fresh anchovies, as well as croquettes and towering creations of potato salad, egg, mayonnaise, and shrimp supported by a toothpick and topped by an olive. *Bacalao*, or dried salted cod, is a staple food that is affordable and can be stored for days. All salt cod needs to be refreshed in water to remove the salt that has preserved the cod. Cooks will first slap the fish against a hard surface to break down the fibers and then leave it to soak for at least 24 hours, changing the water frequently. It is then simmered, or cooked with vegetables, or pureed with cream, olive oil, and spices.

Central Spain is located on the vast Meseta plateau and includes the provinces of La Rioja, Castile-Leon, Castile-LaMancha, Extremadura, and the country's capital, Madrid. Food here is a blend of Jewish, Muslim, and Christian traditions producing a rustic style of cooking. Dishes range from simple broths such as warm garlic soup (*sopas de ajo*) to more complex winter dishes. *Cocido Madrileno*, or simply *cocido*, is one of Spain's notable dishes. Cocido is based on a large cauldron, which simmers all day. The meats used are chosen for their diversity; salt meat, fresh meat, and sausage are used, as well as meat bones and trotters to add richness to the stock. *Caldo* is a clear stock to which sherry is added. The pot also contains vegetables, the first being chickpeas, then onion, garlic, and leek, and finally fresh vegetables. The order and manner of serving is governed by family tradition. Some families like a large display, with everything served at the same time on different platters, or it may be served in courses. The region is also well known for its roasts; lamb, veal, suckling pig, young goat, and other meats are slowly cooked in wood ovens. The Manchegos have great meat roasting traditions and have produced numerous recipes for cooking game, such as the *gazpacho manchego* (a stew of partridge, hare, rabbit, and pheasant). This region produces some of the finest iberico pork and cheese products in Spain. The foods are reminiscent of those described in *Don Quixote*, prepared with saffron, honey, and manchego cheese. The Castile–La Mancha district produces a range of fine foods and drink, including Spain's best sheep cheese (manchego), excellent table wines (*Valdepenas*), honey, asparagus, strawberries, and saffron. The city of Toledo is renowned for its *yemas* (egg yolk sweets) and marzipans; Madrid is known for its *chocolate con churros*, *orejuelas* (honey fritters); and Ciudad Real for its *bizcochos, borrachos* or wine-soaked cakes. The cool Mediterranean climate, semi-arid conditions, and high altitude of central Spain provide the perfect environment for growing olive trees. In the slopes of the Sierras (Montes de Toledo, Sierra de Alcaraz, La Alcarria) the trees are protected from frost. The olive oils of this region have been appreciated for their quality and taste with the cultivation of the first olive trees dating back to the twelfth century. Central Spain is also where one of their most precious products is produced, saffron. The Moors brought with them the spice *az-zafaran* over a thousand years ago. Today over 70 percent of the world's saffron is grown on the high Castilian plateau known as La Mancha. Every October the crocus flowers open at night. The people from Toledo to Albacete rush to the fields at dawn, the opening of the crocus creating a purple blanket as far as the eye can see. All the saffron crocuses must be gathered before dusk; otherwise they lose their flavor. The La Vera region of Spain produces a particularly high quality smoked paprika. Over the centuries, the Yuste monks shared their secrets for growing and processing the chile with local farmers. But it was not until the mid-nineteenth century that the farmers began growing their pimientos on a large scale and processing them into pimentón. These days the pimenton is the region's main source of income. The pimientos are slowly dried over smoldering oak logs for ten to fifteen days and are hand-turned twenty-four hours a day before they are ready to be processed. The smoke-dried pods are then ground into powder and packed in bulk containers. The majority of the pimenton goes to the sausage factories to flavor chorizo. But it is also packed in tins for the consumer market. There are three varieties of pimenton—sweet (dulce), hot (picante), and bittersweet (agridulce).

The rugged mountain chain of the Pyrenees extends along the Spanish-French border from the Bay of Biscay to the Gulf of Valencia. Throughout this mountainous region there are upper meadows, pasture land, glacial lakes, and streams. At the foot of the mountains lie a series of valleys that turn to fertile orchards and vineyards at the Ebro river basin. The cuisine of this region is typically mountain cuisine. Trout and other fish from mountain streams are cooked *a la llosa:* on a slate slab over hot coals. Beef can also be prepared this way. Dishes made with rabbit, quail, partridge, venison, and duck are popular as well. Wild mushrooms are also a local delicacy.

Mediterranean Spain includes the regions of Catalonia, Valencia, and Murcia. The coastal or irrigated plains are home to citrus orchards and produce. Rice fields, vineyards, olive groves, almond, fig, and citrus orchards are characteristic of this area. Seafood and shellfish are abundant here. Catalan cuisine is the oldest, most well-known, most individual, and most traditional cuisine in Spain. It is made up of seven primary ingredients: olive oil, garlic, onions, tomatoes, nuts (almonds, hazelnuts, and pine nuts), dried fruits (raisins and prunes), and herbs (oregano, rosemary, thyme, and bay leaves). There are seventeen officially recognized varieties of chorizo in Catalonia. It is usually made from lean pork, garlic, paprika, red bell peppers and red chile pepper flakes. This region's cuisine is as varied as that of most Spanish regions, but it is a rice-growing land. The short-grain rice was mass-produced around the city of Valencia as a result of the sophisticated irrigation system introduced by the Moors. It was the poor peasant people of the Valencian region who first prepared *paella*, Spain's most famous dish. The original recipe combined homegrown vegetables (usually green and broad beans) with off-cuts of rabbit. Today paella has many variations, most commonly rice cooked with both seafood and chicken or rabbit and then scented and colored with saffron. Another variation is the *paella negra* (black paella), which is colored by the ink from the squid. The region of Valencia produces a wide variety of oranges, mandarins, and lemons. Valencia is also the birthplace of the soft drink *horchata*, made from something called a *chufa*, which translates as "tiger nut," grown all over eastern Spain. *Horchata* looks like an off-white milk, with a toffeelike aroma, and is served cold. Valencia is the home of the famous Spanish candy, *turron*, thought to have been introduced by the Moors. It is traditionally eaten at Christmas. Turron is made by roasting almonds and slow-cooking them with honey and egg white.

Andalusia in southern Spain is the largest of the country's provinces. Andalusia is the world's largest producer of olive oil and its flavor is the foundation of the region's cooking. Black and green olives are grown on the same tree; green olives are simply unripe black olives and are picked in October. Remaining olives ripen and turn black, ready for picking in January or February. In Spain black olives are hardly ever eaten, being used mostly for making oil. Green olives are harvested for eating as tapas or for use as cooking ingredients. Tapas, the age-old custom in Spain originated in Andalusia. The word *tapa* literally means "cover" or "lid" and it is said that the first tapas was simply a hunk of bread placed over the glass to keep out the fruit flies. As the tradition developed, tapas became more elaborate small portions of foods, both hot and cold, served in bars, bodegas, and tascas to accompany a *copa of fino* (dry Spanish sherry), or draught beer. Tapas recipes vary according to the taste and gastronomic traditions of each region. But the tapas most often served are usually those including the many varieties of olives: green, Manzanilla, *machacadas* (crushed), *goradales* (big), *rellenas* (stuffed), *aliñadas* (flavored), and *deshuesadas* (stoneless), dry nuts, as well as many kinds of cold cuts.

Andalusia's most famous contribution to world gastronomy is said to be gazpacho. Traditionally gazpacho is known as peasant food consisting of bread, olive oil, and crushed garlic. None of those forerunners of gazpacho contained tomatoes, as tomatoes were unknown in Spain until after the discovery of the New World. The Moorish influence is evident in some of the variations on the basic theme, such as *ajo blanco*, made with ground almonds. The mountainous province of Huelva in western Andalusia is famous for producing cured hams from pigs fed partially or entirely on a diet of acorns. The hams hang from the ceilings of most establishments, most with hooves still attached and a small container attached at the bottom to catch draining fluids. The hams are taken down and placed on special clamps and very thin slices are carved using a flexible and very sharp knife.

Sherry is a fortified wine, made in and around the town of Jerez. According to Spanish law, Sherry must come from the triangular area of the province of Cadiz, between Jerez, Sanlucar de Barrameda, and El Puerto de Santa Maria. In earlier times Sherry was known as sack, a rendering of the Spanish *saca*, meaning a removal (from the *solera*, or barrel). Sherry differs from other wines by how it is treated after fermentation. After fermentation is complete, it is fortified with brandy. Sherry vinegar can only be made from wines produced in the "sherry triangle." Not only must sherry vinegar be made from wines from this small area but it has to be aged in one of these sherry towns.

Spain is the world leader in the production of air-dried hams, about 190,000 tons per year, which represents some 30 million hams, produced by 1,700 companies. The hams spend a short period of time in salt and then at least three months curing in the mountain air. Most are produced from white pigs but the darker Iberian pigs produce the most expensive hams. All these hams are subject to stringent quality control and are awarded certain classes depending on their production methods. They are best eaten on their own, without bread. A significant amount of Spanish hams are exported each year, mainly to Germany and France.

# Glossary

**Aioli** Garlic flavored mayonnaise, typical of Catalonia and the Balearic Islands.

**Anisette** A digestive, the flavoring for many liqueurs (anisette or anise). Its flavor varies according to which seeds are used—aniseed or star anise.

**Bacalao** Preserved salt cod.

**Capaplanas** Traditional domed clam cookers from the Algarve region in southern Portugal.

**Chorizo** Brick-colored sausage prepared with light variations in various parts of Spain. Normally made with pork, fat, and pimentón, which gives it its characteristic color and smokiness. In Spain chorizo comes in three varieties. *Fully cured dry chorizo* has a texture similar to pepperoni. *Semi-cured, fully cooked soft chorizo* has a consistency similar to kielbasa. *Fresh chorizo* is raw, uncooked sausage.

**Churro** Choux pastry dough deep-fried in olive oil, spiral shaped, and similar to a doughnut. *Churros* are made from dough extruded into thin tubes; these have a star-shaped cross section and are several inches long. Traditionally eaten at breakfast with hot chocolate.

**Cocido** Stews, famous in northern and central Spain. More than just a stew, they are elaborate creations, an event, usually prepared to feed a large group of friends and family.

**Empanada** In Spanish the word *empanada* means "in dough" and describes pies with savory fillings enclosed in bread dough, short pastry, or puff pastry.

**Flan** Baked custard dessert, usually served with caramel sauce.

**Gazpacho** Cold vegetable soup, the best-known version of which is from the southern Spanish region of Andalusia. It is made of ripe tomatoes, bell peppers, cucumbers, garlic, and bread moistened with water that is blended with olive oil, vinegar, and ice water and is served cold.

**Jambon Serrano** Cured ham similar to the prosciutto of Italy, with a sweet-salty flavor.

**Paella** Traditional rice dish originating from Valencia, an authentic *paella valenciana* contains chicken, rabbit, sometimes duck, and the land snails called *vaquetes*, for which a rosemary sprig can be substituted. The only permissible vegetables are flat green beans, artichokes, and butter beans. The star of this dish is rice. Other authentic ingredients include a *sofrito* of tomatoes, garlic, saffron, and pimiento. The Valencian word *paella*, meaning "pan," comes from the Latin *patella*, which also means "pan."

**Paella Pan** Thin, round, shallow, flat-bottomed, two-handled pan. The wide, shallow shape allows the largest area of rice to come in contact with the bottom of the pan, where the flavor of the ingredients is concentrated. It also helps liquid evaporate rapidly.

**Pimentón** Smoked paprika. It differs from other European paprikas because of the characteristic smoked aroma that it gives off during processing from being dried by means of wood smoke.

**Piquillo Peppers** Spanish wood-roasted sweet peppers.

**Queso (Cheese) PDO Status** The governments in most European countries have instituted a government-controlled quality program known as PDO (Protected Designation of Origin) for

# About Olive Oil

Spain is the largest producer of olive oil in the world, followed closely by Italy. Greece is the third-largest producer, though it uses more olive oil per capita than any other country. No two olive oils are exactly alike. Just as with wine, each oil is distinct, a unique product of soil, climate, olive type (there are at least 60 varieties of olives), and processing method.

The olive tree is a hearty evergreen with silver-green leaves that thrives in the mild winters and long hot summers of the Mediterranean and does well in dry, arid climates. In many cases olive trees, which start bearing usable fruit after five to eight years, can be hundreds of years old and still produce fruit. Olive trees planted near the sea can produce up to 20 times more fruit than those planted inland. A mature olive tree will produce only 15 to 20 kilograms (33 to 44 pounds) of olives each year. Since it takes about 5 kilograms of olives to make a liter of oil, one tree is capable of producing only about 3 to 4 liters of oil per year.

Picked olives are taken to an olive oil mill, where they are pressed for their oil. This is done the same day, or at most a day later, before they start to oxidize and ferment. The actual fruit of the tree—the just-picked olives—is far too bitter and acrid to eat and it must be washed and soaked and then either brined or salted and allowed to age before it is edible.

Virgin olive oil is extracted without heat, additives, or solvents from the freshly picked bitter olives, and should have a lush, rich taste and velvety texture. The oil from olives is ready to use immediately after extraction.

Olive oil that is "cold-pressed" is made from olives that have been crushed with a traditional millstone or stainless steel grindstone. No heat or chemicals are added during the process, which produces a heavy olive paste. The paste is then spread over thick, round straw or plastic mats that are placed in a press. This press extracts the liquid from the paste—a combination of oil and water. The oil is separated from the water either by decanting or by centrifuge and then filtered to remove any large particles. The resulting oil is then graded and classified, according to standards established by the IOOC. The finest olive oils are those that have the lowest acidity, which is measured as a percentage per 100 grams of oil.

## TYPES OF OLIVE OIL

- Extra-Virgin Olive Oil: Any olive oil that is less than 1 percent acidity, produced by the first cold pressing of the olive fruit. Most olive oils today are extra virgin in name only, meeting only the minimum requirements. Extra virgin is a chemical requirement that does not indicate quality and taste.

- **Virgin Olive Oil:** It is made from olives that are slightly riper than those used for extra-virgin oil and is produced in exactly the same manner but has a slightly higher level of acidity ($1\frac{1}{2}$ percent).
- **Unfiltered Olive Oil:** This oil contains small particles of olive flesh. Some claim this adds additional flavor. Unfortunately, it causes a sediment to form at the bottom of the bottle, which can become rancid, negatively impacting flavor and shelf life. It is recommended that this oil not be used for cooking. Unfiltered oil should be carefully stored and used within three to six months of bottling.
- **Early Harvest (Fall Harvest Olive Oil):** Olives reach their full size in the fall but may not fully ripen from green to black until late winter. Green olives have slightly less oil and more bitterness and can be higher in polyphenols. The oil tends to be more expensive because it takes more olives to make a bottle of oil. This oil has a more peppery and bitter flavor.
- **Late Harvest (Winter Harvest Olive Oil):** The fruit is picked ripe and the olives have a little more oil. It has a light, mellow taste with little bitterness and more floral flavors.
- **Refined Olive Oil:** This olive oil is obtained from refining virgin olive oil that has defects (the result is an essentially tasteless olive oil). Among the defects are a natural acidity higher than 3.3 percent, poor flavor, and an unpleasant odor. This product is also known as "A" refined olive oil.
- **Refined Olive-Pomace Oil:** Oil obtained by treating olive pomace with solvents and refined using methods that do not lead to alterations in the initial glyceridic structure.
- **Olive-Pomace Oil:** Olive oil that consists of a blend of refined olive-pomace oil and virgin olive oil.
- **Light and Extra Light Olive Oil:** The olive oil advertised as "light" or as "extra light" olive oil contains the exact same number of calories as regular olive oil and is a mixture of refined olive oils that are derived from the lowest-quality olive oils available through chemical processing.
- **First Press:** This is no longer an official definition for olive oil. A century ago, oil was pressed in screw or hydraulic presses. The paste was subjected to increasingly high pressures with subsequent degradation in the flavor of the oil. Today the vast majority of oil is made in continuous centrifugal presses. There is no second pressing.

many agricultural and food products. Often called DO, this program means the government guarantees the origin, preparation methods, and production within a certain location in the country, and the quality of a product.

**Spanish DO Cheeses**

**Cabrales** One of the great blue cheeses of the world, produced from raw milk, mainly cow's milk. The rind is sticky and yellow, with an intense smell. The interior is compact but very open, with lots of holes and blue veins. The taste is strong, although not as strong as the smell, slightly piquant, acid, and creamy.

**Cantabria** Also called queso de nata or cantabrian cream cheese. Aged cheese from soft to semi-cured to cured, made from pasteurized cow's milk, it has a smooth flavor, ranging from sweet and slightly acidic to buttery.

**Ibores** Made with unpasteurized milk from the serrata goat breed of Verata and Retinta, using mixed coagulation (lactic and enzymatic) techniques. It is a semi-soft paste of medium aging. The rind is rubbed with olive oil or smoked paprika from Vera. Its flavor is creamy and very buttery, with aromas of unpasteurized milk.

**Idiazábal** Aged cheese, from semi-cured to cured, made exclusively from whole raw sheep's milk. Idiazábal is a robust and sharp cheese, made to be ripened for a long period, with a dry and crumbly paste.

**L'Alt Urgell y la Cerdanya** Made with pasteurized whole milk from frisona cows. It has a soft and creamy texture, with sweet aroma.

**L'Alt Urgell** A very aromatic soft cheese cured for a short time, with a buttery taste, although intense and persistent.

**La Serena** Cheese aged for at least eight weeks, from soft to semi-cured, made with unpasteurized whole milk, from merino sheep. The flavor is very buttery, thick, and creamy. It is full flavored with an underlying tart flavor and a spreadable texture. This is a cheese almost always made in an artisanal way, of a very small production, difficult to find and expensive.

**Mahón** Also known as Menorquín cheese. Fresh to much-cured cheese, depending on the state of aging, made from raw or pasteurized cow's milk. The taste is very particular, slightly acidic and salty, but not buttery. It can be milky and humid when fresh, and dry, strong, and piquant as it ages.

**Majorero** Also called queso de fuerteventura. Aged cheese, from aired to very cured. Made with goat's milk, it has a compact but open interior, and a slightly gummy texture. The taste of the little-cured variety is acidic, a little piquant, and buttery but not salty. Aged cheese is rubbed with oil, paprika, and gofio (a local sweet wheat flour) in order to avoid excessive drying.

**Manchego** Aged cheese, with a firm interior, compact and closed. The color is ivory to pale yellow. The taste is very characteristic, well developed but not too strong, buttery and slightly piquant, with a sheep's milk aftertaste. Semi-cured to cured cheese is made exclusively with raw or pasteurized sheep's milk and has a crumbly texture. The shape is cylindrical, with a flat top and bottom surfaces engraved with the typical "flower" left by the wooden presses. The sides show a zigzag pattern produced by the mat-weed (esparto) of the molds.

**Murcia al Vino** Aged cheese, from soft to semi-cured, made with pasteurized goat's milk, and aged by applying external washes with red wine. It has a mild aroma, and the flavor is pleasantly acid and a little salty.

**Picón** Also known as Queso de los Picos de Europa. Aged for at least three months, cured, made of a mixture of unpasteurized cow's, goat's, and sheep's milk. A type of blue cheese, it is robust and full flavored, cylindrical in shape. It is an artisanal cheese limited in production and aged in natural caves in the Picos de Europa in northern Spain.

**Quesucos de Liebana** Fresh cheese or aged and soft, produced mainly with cow's milk, although sometimes mixed with sheep's and goat's milk. Cylindrical in shape, smoked or with a natural rind, the unsmoked cheese has a smooth and buttery flavor, while the smoked variety has a more acidic and cured flavor.

**Roncal** Also queso del valle del roncal. Aged for at least four months, and cured, made from sheep's milk from Laxta or Aragonese breeds. Its flavor is well developed and structured, buttery with an aroma of straw, dried fruit, and mushrooms.

**Tetilla** Aged, from soft to semi-cured, made with cow's milk. The soft paste, thick and smooth with few air pockets, is very creamy on the palate. The flavor is clean and smooth. The word *tetilla*, meaning "nipple," clearly defines the traditional shape of this cheese: a flattened pear-shaped cone with a small nipple on the top.

**Zamorano** The rind is dark gray and oily. The inside is closed and compact, with tiny crystal-like dots spread evenly throughout. The cheese is compact, not easy to melt, and has a straw-yellow color. The taste is intense although not too strong, slightly piquant, and buttery.

**Saffron** The stigma of the purple crocus flower, intensely fragrant, slightly bitter in taste. By soaking saffron in warm water, the result is a bright yellow-orange solution.

**Sangria** Red wine mixed with fruit juices.

**Sherry** Sherry is a fortified wine from a small region of Spain, made from the Muscat, Palomino, and Pedro Ximenez grapes.

# Menus and Recipes from Spain

TAPAS MENU

*Aceitunas Verdes Rellenas de Pimiento y Anchoa:* **Green Olives Filled with Piquillo Peppers and Anchovy**

*Queso Idiazábal:* **Cheese with Fresh Herbs**

*Pan Con Tomate:* **Tomato Toast**

*Calamares Encebollados:* **Squid with Caramelized Onions**

*Garum:* **Black Olive, Anchovy, and Caper Spread**

*Croquetas de Jamón:* **Serrano Ham Fritters**

*Bacalad Al Ajo Arriero:* **Bacalao Hash**

*Tortilla de Patatas:* **Potato Omelet**

*Gambas Al Ajillo:* **Sizzling Garlic Shrimp**

MENU ONE

*Rape con Romesco:* **Monkfish with Romesco Sauce**

*Sopa De Ajo:* **Castilian Garlic Soup**

*Fabes con Almejas:* **Asturian Bean Stew with Clams**

*Paella Valenciana*

*Espinacas à la Catalana:* **Spinach, Catalan-Style**

*Pera Salsa de Caramelo al Café:* **Pears with Caramel-Coffee Sauce**

MENU TWO

*Gazpacho Sevillano:* **Classic Gazpacho**

*Pollo En Pepitoria:* **Chicken in Almond and Saffron Sauce**

*Ensalada con Higos, Cabrales, y Granada:* **Mesclun, Figs, Cabrales, and Pomegranate**

*Merluza en Salsa Verde:* **Hake in Green Sauce**

*Cerdo Cocido con la Fruta Seca:* **Braised Pork with Dried Fruit**

*Arroz con Leche:* **Rice and Milk**

# Aceitunas Verdes Rellenas de Pimiento y Anchoa

## Green Olives Filled with Piquillo Peppers and Anchovy

SERVES 4

| AMOUNT | MEASURE | INGREDIENT |
|---|---|---|
| 8 | | Extra-large green olives unpitted |
| 4 | | Anchovy fillets, oil-packed, cut in half lengthwise |
| 2 | | Piquillo pepper, cut into 8, $\frac{1}{2}$ inch (1.2 cm) wide strips |
| 1 | | Garlic clove, rough chopped |
| 3 tablespoons | 1 $\frac{1}{2}$ ounces, 45 ml | Spanish extra-virgin olive oil |
| 1 tablespoon | | Orange zest, grated |
| 1 tablespoon | $\frac{1}{2}$ ounce, 15 ml | Sherry vinegar |
| To taste | | Sea salt |

**PROCEDURE**

1. Using the flat side of a chef knife, press each olive until the pit pops out; do not split the olive in half.
2. Place one slice anchovy and pepper in each olive.
3. Combine garlic, olive oil, orange zest, and sherry vinegar to make a dressing.
4. Marinate stuffed olives in dressing for 30 minutes.
5. Serve sprinkled with sea salt.

# Queso Idiazábal

## Cheese with Fresh Herbs SERVES 4

**Chef Tip** **Any semi-hard cheese can be substituted.**

| AMOUNT | MEASURE | INGREDIENT |
|---|---|---|
| 3 | | Garlic cloves, split in half, crushed |
| 2 cups | 12 ounces, 336 g | Idiazábal cheese, cut into 1 inch (2.5 cm) cubes |
| 1 tablespoon | | Whole black peppercorns |
| 2 | | Fresh rosemary sprigs, rough chopped |
| 2 | | Fresh thyme sprigs, rough chopped |
| 1 cup | 8 ounces, 240 ml | Spanish extra-virgin olive oil |

**PROCEDURE**

1. Combine all ingredients and coat the cheese thoroughly.
2. Marinate at room temperature, for as long as overnight.

# Pan Con Tomate Tomato Toast SERVES 4

| AMOUNT | MEASURE | INGREDIENT |
|---|---|---|
| 4 | | Rustic bread, $\frac{1}{2}$ inch (1.2 cm) thick slices |
| 2 | | Ripe tomatoes, cut in half |
| $\frac{1}{2}$ cup | 4 ounces, 120 ml | Spanish extra-virgin olive oil |
| To taste | | Sea salt |
| Optional | | Garum (recipe follows) |
| Optional | | Jamón serrano (Spanish cured ham) |

**PROCEDURE**

1. Toast or grill bread.
2. Rub the open face of the tomato into one side of each piece of toast until all the flesh is grated. Discard skin.
3. Drizzle olive oil over tomato and season with salt.
4. Serve with garum, if desired, or a thin slice of jamón serrano.

# Calamares Encebollados

## Squid with Caramelized Onions

SERVES 4

| AMOUNT | MEASURE | INGREDIENT |
|---|---|---|
| $\frac{1}{4}$ cup | 2 ounces, 60 ml | Spanish extra-virgin olive oil |
| 1 | | Garlic clove |
| 2 cups | 8 ounces, 224 g | Spanish sweet onions, sliced thin |
| 1 | | Bay leaf |
| To taste | | Salt |
| 2 cups | 12 ounces, 336 g | Fresh squid, $\frac{1}{2}$ inch (1.2 cm) pieces |
| $\frac{1}{2}$ cup | 4 ounces, 120 ml | Dry white wine |
| 2 teaspoons | | Flat-leaf parsley, chopped |

### PROCEDURE

1. Heat the olive oil over medium heat in a medium sauté pan.
2. Add garlic and cook 2 minutes or until brown; remove.
3. Add onions and bay leaf; cook over medium-low heat until lightly brown, about 10 minutes.
4. Reduce heat to low and continue cooking until onions are soft and caramelized, about 20 minutes longer.
5. Remove onions from pan and set aside, leaving the oil in pan.
6. Return heat to high and sprinkle pan with salt. Add squid, making sure not to overcrowd the pan; there must be ample space so the squid does not boil. Sauté 15 to 20 seconds on each side. Remove from pan and repeat the process with remaining squid.
7. Return all the squid to the pan, add caramelized onions, and stir to mix. Add wine around sides and boil for 20 seconds.
8. Sprinkle with parsley and serve.

# Garum Black Olive, Anchovy, and Caper Spread

YIELD: $\frac{3}{4}$ CUP

**In ancient Rome, garum was a pungent all-purpose condiment made from fermented anchovies, similar to Asian fish sauce. This current version, from Catalonia, is closer to the French tapenade and works well with grilled meat, chicken, or fish. Try to find olives that are pungent, but not vinegary and briny.**

| AMOUNT | MEASURE | INGREDIENT |
|---|---|---|
| 1 cup | 6 ounces, 168 g | Pitted black olives, Niçoise |
| 2 | | Anchovy fillets, chopped and mashed to a paste |
| 1 tablespoon | $\frac{1}{2}$ ounce, 14 g | Capers, drained and rinsed |
| 1 | | Garlic clove, smashed |
| 1 | | Hard-cooked egg yolk, smashed |
| 1 tablespoon | $\frac{1}{2}$ ounce, 15 ml | Rum, brandy, or water |
| $\frac{1}{4}$ teaspoon | | Dijon mustard |
| 2 tablespoons | 1 ounce, 30 ml | Olive oil |

## PROCEDURE

1. Combine olives, anchovy, capers, garlic, egg yolk, rum, and mustard in a food processor or mortar; process to a medium-fine paste.
2. Gradually add olive oil.
3. Let stand 1 hour at room temperature to allow flavors to develop.
4. Serve with grilled bread or tomato toast.

# Croquetas de Jamón

## Serrano Ham Fritters

YIELD: 15 FRITTERS

| AMOUNT | MEASURE | INGREDIENT |
|---|---|---|
| 4 tablespoons | 2 ounces, 56 g | Butter |
| $\frac{1}{4}$ cup | 1 ounce, 28 g | Spanish onion, $\frac{1}{4}$ inch (.6 cm) diced |
| 1$\frac{1}{4}$ cups | 6 ounces, 168 g | All-purpose flour |
| 2 cups | 16 ounces, 480 ml | Milk |
| $\frac{1}{2}$ cup | 3 ounces, 84 g | Jamón serrano (Spanish cured ham), finely chopped |
| To taste | | Salt |
| Pinch | | Nutmeg |
| 1 | | Large egg, beaten with teaspoon of water |
| 1 cup | 1 ounce, 28 g | Dry bread crumbs |
| 2 cups | 16 ounces, 480 ml | Olive oil, for frying |

PROCEDURE

1. Heat butter over medium heat; add onion and sauté until translucent, 3 minutes.
2. Add 1 cup (4$\frac{1}{2}$ ounces, 126 g) flour and mix well. Cook to a blond roux, about 5 minutes.
3. Add milk gradually, stirring continuously; cook 3 to 4 minutes, until a thick béchamel.
4. Add ham, salt, and nutmeg; cook 2 minutes. The mixture should be thick enough to mold by hand. Test for correct consistency by carefully picking up a tablespoon-size bit and balling it with your hands. It should not be very sticky. If mixture sticks to your hands, return to heat and cook 2 more minutes; recheck.
5. Spread mixture out on a half sheet pan and cool to room temperature.
6. Form the mixture into small cylinders the size of a wine cork, using about a tablespoon of mixture for each.
7. Roll each fritter in remaining flour, the egg, and breadcrumbs.
8. Refrigerate for 30 minutes before frying.
9. Heat oil to 375°F (190°C).
10. Deep-fry fritters in small batches. Fry until golden color, about 1 minute; turn as needed.
11. Transfer to absorbent towels to drain. Repeat with all fritters and serve hot.

# Bacalad al Ajo Arriero

## Bacalao Hash SERVES 4

**Chef Tip** Cooked with care, desalted reconstituted bacalao is moist, plump, and falling apart in big, luxurious flakes. Depending on the grade of the fish and the salting method used, bacalao can take anywhere from 24 hours to 2 days to desalt properly. To desalt, cover with 2 inches of cold water and refrigerate, changing water every 4–5 hours if possible. Taste a small piece and if it is still too salty, soak longer, changing water as needed. It can also be cooked in milk instead of water to draw out some of the salt. It is important to cook salt cod very gently or it will become tough and rubbery; never boil it. The fish is cooked when it flakes easily with the point of a knife. There are small bones that need to be removed.

| AMOUNT | MEASURE | INGREDIENT |
|---|---|---|
| | 3 ounces, 84 g | Salt cod, soaked, cooked, drained |
| 2 tablespoons | 1 ounce, 30 ml | Olive oil |
| $\frac{1}{2}$ cup | 2 ounces, 56 g | Onion, $\frac{1}{4}$ inch (.6 cm) dice |
| 2 | | Garlic cloves, minced |
| $\frac{1}{4}$ cup | 1 ounce, 28 g | Green bell pepper, $\frac{1}{4}$ inch (.6 cm) dice |
| $\frac{1}{2}$ cup | 2 ounces | Piquillo peppers (from can or jar) or pimientos, or Red bell pepper, julienne cut |
| 1 cup | 6 ounces, 168 g | Boiling potatoes (Yukon gold), peeled, boiled, drained, $\frac{1}{4}$ inch (.6 cm) dice |
| $\frac{1}{4}$ teaspoon | | Sweet (not smoked) paprika |
| 2 tablespoons | 1 ounce, 30 ml | Tomato sauce |
| $\frac{1}{4}$ teaspoon | | White wine or sherry vinegar |
| To taste | | Coarse salt and freshly ground black pepper |
| 1 tablespoon | | Flat-leaf parsley, minced |
| For serving | | Sliced crusty baguette |

**PROCEDURE**

1. Flake salt cod finely, discard bones, skin, and any tough bits.
2. Heat olive over medium-low heat. Add onion and sauté until translucent, 3 minutes. Add garlic; cook 2 minutes.
3. Add green pepper and cook until pepper and onions are very soft, 5–6 minutes. Do not brown.
4. If pan looks dry add a little more oil, stir in cod, piquillo peppers, and potatoes; mix well, cover, and cook 5 minutes. Stir only 2–3 times.
5. Add paprika and stir for a few seconds. Add tomato sauce and wine, reduce heat to very low, re-cover, and simmer 7–8 minutes. Hash should still be moist; if not, add a little water and simmer 1 or 2 minutes.
6. Let hash cool to warm or room temperature; the flavor will develop as it cools.
7. Stir in parsley, adjust seasoning, and serve on or with bread.

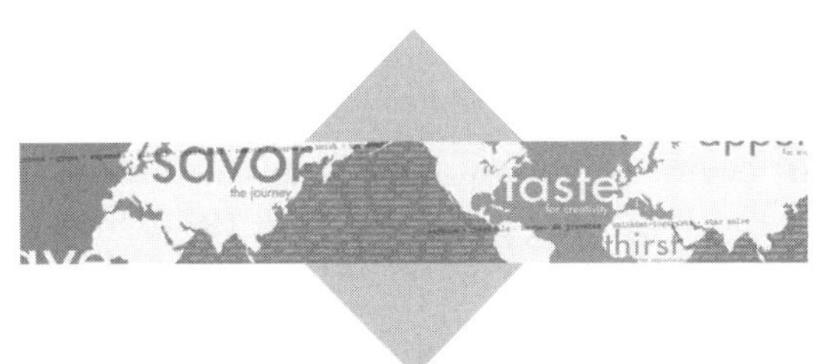

# Tortilla de Patatas

## Potato Omelet SERVES 4

| AMOUNT | MEASURE | INGREDIENT |
|---|---|---|
| $1\frac{1}{2}$ cups | 10 ounces, 300 ml | Olive oil |
| 2 cups | 8 ounces, 224 g | All-purpose potatoes, peeled, very thin slices |
| 1 teaspoon | 5 g | Salt |
| $\frac{1}{2}$ cup | 3 ounces, 84 g | Spanish onion thinly sliced |
| 4 | | Eggs, lightly beaten |

**PROCEDURE**

1. Heat olive oil over medium heat, until a piece of potato dropped in the oil jumps, 275°F (135°C).
2. Add potatoes to hot oil and cook until lightly browned and crispy around edges, 10 minutes. Remove from heat, strain potatoes from oil, and reserve oil.
3. Season potatoes with half the salt and set aside.
4. Reheat oil and add onions; cook over medium heat until golden brown, 8 minutes.
5. Strain onions, set aside, and reserve oil.
6. Combine egg, potatoes, and onions.
7. Add reserved oil to a 6-inch (15 cm) sauté pan over medium heat.
8. Heat oil until it just begins to smoke, add egg mixture. Shake pan 10 to 15 seconds, then cook 30 seconds without moving pan. Lower heat and cook 2 to 3 minutes until a crust has formed.
9. Flip tortilla when edges are cooked but the center is not completely set. Place a plate on top of the pan and gently flip tortilla onto the plate. Slide tortilla back into pan and continue cooking over low heat for 1 minute longer. Pan may need additional oil before returning tortilla.
10. Serve hot, at room temperature, or cold.

# Gambas al Ajillo
## Sizzling Garlic Shrimp
SERVES 4

| AMOUNT | MEASURE | INGREDIENT |
|---|---|---|
| 1 pound | 16 ounces, 448 g | Large shrimp (26 to 30 ct), in shell |
| To taste | | Coarse salt |
| 1 cup | 8 ounces, 240 ml | Olive oil |
| 5 | | Garlic cloves, finely chopped |
| $\frac{1}{2}$ | | Small dry red chile (arbol), crumbled |
| 2 tablespoons | | Flat-leaf parsley, minced |
| For serving | | Bread |

PROCEDURE

1 Pat shrimp dry and sprinkle with salt.

2 Combine olive oil and garlic over medium-low heat until oil is hot and garlic begins to sizzle gently. Cook until garlic is very fragrant but not colored, 2–3 minutes; reduce heat if necessary.

3 Add chile and stir for 30 seconds.

4 Add shrimp; cook, stirring, until shrimp are just cooked, about 3 minutes.

5 Season with salt to taste, stir in parsley, and cook 15 seconds.

6 Serve with bread.

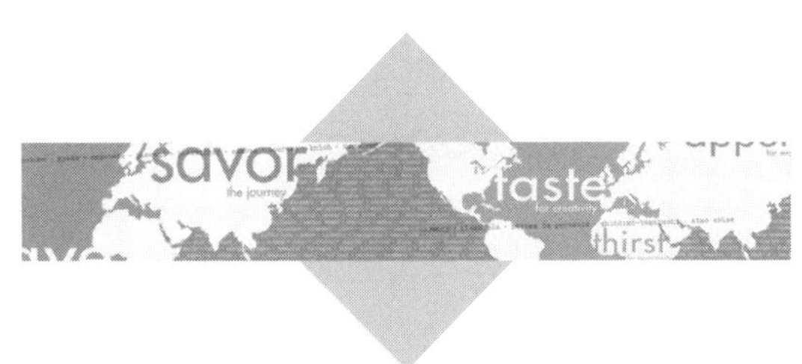

# Rape con Romesco

## Monkfish with Romesco Sauce

SERVES 4

| AMOUNT | MEASURE | INGREDIENT |
|---|---|---|
| | 12 ounces, 336 g | Monkfish fillet or any meaty fish |
| 5 | | Bay leaves, dry or fresh |
| 2 tablespoons | 1 ounce, 30 ml | Olive oil |
| To taste | | Salt and white pepper |
| 2 cups | 16 ounces, 480 ml | Romesco sauce (recipe follows) |

**PROCEDURE**

1. Clean fish of any membrane and cut 5 incisions about 1 inch apart in the fillet; do not cut all the way through.
2. Insert a bay leaf into each slot.
3. Heat oil over medium high heat and sauté fillet until lightly browned on each side, 3 to 4 minutes. Set fish aside to cool.
4. Remove bay leaves and discard. Slice fillet into 1-inch (2.5 cm) medallions; season with salt and white pepper.
5. Place medallions on romesco sauce and drizzle with olive oil to serve.

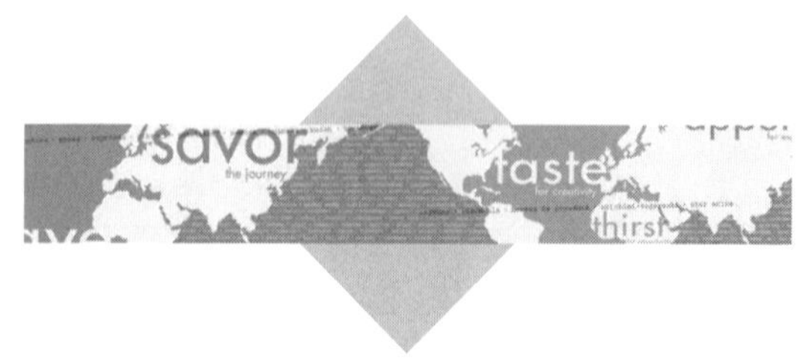

# Romesco Sauce

**Catalan roasted-vegetable sauce.**

YIELD: 2 CUPS

| AMOUNT | MEASURE | INGREDIENT |
|---|---|---|
| 1 | | Red bell pepper |
| 1 pound | 16 ounces, 448 g | Ripe plum tomatoes |
| 1 | | Garlic head, halved |
| 1 | 6 ounces, 180 g | Whole Spanish onion |
| $\frac{1}{2}$ cup plus 2 tablespoons | 5 ounces, 150 ml | Olive oil |
| 3 | | Ñora chile peppers or any dried sweet chili pepper |
| $\frac{1}{4}$ cup | 1 ounce, 28 g | Blanched almonds |
| $\frac{1}{2}$ cup | 1 ounce, 28 g | White bread, crust removed |
| 1 tablespoon | $\frac{1}{2}$ ounce, 15 ml | Sherry vinegar |
| 1 teaspoon | | Pimentón (Spanish sweet paprika) |
| To taste | | Salt |

PROCEDURE

1. Heat oven to 350°F (176°C).
2. Toss red bell pepper, tomatoes, garlic, and onion with 2 tablespoons (1 ounce, 30 ml) olive oil; place on baking sheet and roast until all are soft, 25 minutes. Let vegetables cool; peel and seed pepper; peel onion; seed tomatoes; peel garlic.
3. Cover ñora chile peppers with enough hot water to cover; soak 15 minutes. Strain and remove seeds.
4. Puree chiles until smooth. Pass the puree through a fine-mesh sieve and set aside.
5. Heat 1 tablespoon ($\frac{1}{2}$ ounce, 15 ml) oil over medium low heat, sauté almonds 1 minute or until lightly toasted; remove from pan to stop the cooking.
6. Toast the bread until it is a nice brown color.
7. Sauté the pureed ñora over medium heat 30 seconds; remove from heat
8. Place cooled peeled vegetables, almonds, toasted bread, pureed ñora, vinegar, pimentón, and remaining oil in a blender. Blend to a thick sauce; add salt.

# Sopa de Ajo

## Castilian Garlic Soup

SERVES 4

**Chef Tip** **Traditionally the eggs are poached right in the soup, but they can be poached ahead of time.**

| AMOUNT | MEASURE | INGREDIENT |
|---|---|---|
| 6 tablespoons | 3 ounces, 90 ml | Olive oil |
| 6 | | Garlic cloves, sliced thin |
| $\frac{1}{2}$ cup | 2 ounces, 56 g | Serrano ham or prosciutto, minced |
| 2 cups | 4 ounces, 112 g | Day-old country bread without crusts, 1 $\frac{1}{2}$ inch (3.75 cm) dice |
| 2 teaspoons | | Smoked sweet Spanish paprika |
| 5 cups | 40 ounces, 1.2 l | Chicken stock |
| To taste | | Salt and pepper |
| 4 | | Garlic cloves, smashed to a paste |
| 4 | | Poached eggs |
| 1 tablespoon | | Flat-leaf parsley, minced |

PROCEDURE

1. Heat olive oil over low heat; add garlic and ham. Cook, stirring, until garlic is very fragrant but not brown, 4 to 5 minutes.
2. Add bread, stirring to coat with oil; cook 2 to 3 minutes. Add more oil if the pan is dry.
3. Remove from heat and add paprika; toss the bread to coat evenly.
4. Return pan to heat and add stock. Increase heat to medium and simmer about 7 minutes or until bread swells but still holds its shape.
5. Season with salt and pepper, add garlic paste, and cook 1 minute.
6. Ladle soup into warm bowls, top each with a warm poached egg and parsley.
7. To eat, break the poached egg, stirring the yolk into the soup; the egg will cook slightly from the heat and thicken the broth.

# Fabes con Almejas

## Asturian Bean Stew with Clams

SERVES 4

| AMOUNT | MEASURE | INGREDIENT |
|---|---|---|
| 1 cup | 7 ounces, 196 g | Asturian beans or other large dried white beans such as cannellini, dried, sorted, soaked overnight |
| 1 $\frac{1}{2}$ quarts | 48 ounces, 1.44 l | Water |
| 1 | | Spanish onion, peeled |
| 1 | | Roma tomato |
| 2 inch (5 cm) | | Carrot piece, peeled |
| 3 | | Fresh parsley sprigs |
| 4 tablespoons | 2 ounces, 60 ml | Olive oil |
| To taste | | Salt |
| 16 | | Littleneck clams, cleaned |

**PROCEDURE**

1. Combine soaked beans and water; bring to a boil. Reduce heat to low and simmer 10 minutes, occasionally removing any foam that comes to the surface.
2. Add onion, tomato, carrot; and parsley; simmer 2 hours. Every 15 minutes, add $\frac{1}{4}$ cup (2 ounces, 60 ml) cold water to slow the simmering. Beans should always be covered with liquid. By the end of the cooking time the beans should be just covered with liquid.
3. Remove the vegetables and place in a food processor or blender with a $\frac{1}{2}$ cup (4 ounces) of beans that are split or broken and 1 tablespoon ($\frac{1}{2}$ ounce, 15 ml) cooking liquid. Blend until somewhat smooth, pass through a fine strainer, and return to the bean mixture.
4. Add 2 tablespoons (1 ounce, 30 ml) olive oil to beans and season with salt. Beans should be very soft and broth creamy and starchy. Return to a simmer.
5. Heat 1 quart of water to a boil. Add 4 clams at a time until they just open, 5 to 10 seconds. Remove from water. Repeat with remaining clams.
6. Working over a bowl to collect any clam juice, use a paring or clam knife to remove clams from shell.
7. Strain juices and add to the beans.
8. Serve beans topped with clams and drizzle clams with remaining olive oil.

# Paella Valenciana

SERVES 4

**Chef Tip According to Valencian traditionalists, this is the only legitimate paella. This dish evolved from a range of simpler rices prepared by laborers in the Levantine rice paddies and *huertas* (vegetable plots) with whatever could be hunted and gathered.**

**Paella is not a pilaf or risotto; the rice is never washed or the barley stirred. It should have a crispy, caramelized, toasted bottom (called socarrat).**

| AMOUNT | MEASURE | INGREDIENT |
|---|---|---|
| $1\frac{1}{2}$ cups | 10 ounces, 280 g | Skinless, boneless chicken thighs, $1\frac{1}{2}$ inch (3.75 cm) chunks |
| | 16 ounce, 448 g | Rabbit, bone-in, cut into small pieces |
| $1\frac{1}{2}$ teaspoons | | Smoked sweet Spanish paprika |
| To taste | | Salt and fresh black pepper |
| 6 | | Garlic cloves, minced or crushed with a garlic press |
| 4 cups | 32 ounces, 960 ml | Chicken stock |
| Pinch | | Saffron, pulverized in a mortar |
| 5 tablespoons | $2\frac{1}{2}$ ounces, 75 ml | Olive oil |
| 1 cup | 6 ounces, 168 g | Spanish chorizo, $1\frac{1}{2}$ inch (3.75 cm) pieces |
| $\frac{1}{4}$ cup | 2 ounces, 56 g | Green beans (Italian flat beans), trimmed, $1\frac{1}{2}$ inch (3.75 cm) lengths |
| $\frac{1}{2}$ cup | 3 ounces, 84 g | Cooked butter beans or baby lima beans |
| 1 cup | 6 ounces, 168 g | Frozen artichoke hearts, thawed, patted dry |
| $\frac{1}{2}$ cup | 3 ounces, 90 ml | Tomato, cut in half and grated on box grater, skin discarded |
| Pinch | | Cayenne |
| 2 cups | 14 ounces, 392 g | Short- to medium-grain rice |
| 12 large | | Snails (optional) |
| $\frac{1}{2}$ cup | 3 ounces, 84 g | Red bell pepper, roasted, peeled, julienned |

PROCEDURE

1 Preheat oven to 425°F (218°C).

2 Combine chicken, rabbit, $\frac{1}{2}$ teaspoon paprika, salt, pepper, and half the garlic; toss well and set aside for 15 minutes.

3 Bring chicken stock to a simmer. Add the saffron and continue to keep hot.

4 Using only one burner, place 4 tablespoons (2 ounces, 60 ml) olive oil in a 14-inch (53.6 cm) paella pan over medium heat until oil begins to smoke.

5 Add chicken and rabbit; brown, 6 to 7 minutes.

6 Add chorizo; cook 2 minutes.

7 Add green beans, butter beans, and artichokes; toss until vegetables begin to take on color, 5 minutes. Move all items to the edge of pan.

8 Add remaining oil to center of paella pan, add remaining garlic, and cook until fragrant, about 30 seconds.

9 Add tomatoes to center of the pan, reduce heat to low, and cook, stirring, until tomato is thickened and reduced, 5 to 6 minutes.

10 Toss tomato mixture with meat and vegetables, add remaining paprika and cayenne; stir to combine.

11 Add rice to pan and stir to coat. Add hot stock.

12 Place pan over two burners, stir in snails if using, and shake pan to distribute rice evenly. Cook over medium low heat until the cooking liquid is almost level with the rice, 6–8 minutes; rice will still be soupy. Move and rotate pan so the liquid cooks evenly. If liquid is absorbed too fast and the rice seems raw, add a little more stock.

13 Transfer paella pan to oven and bake until the rice is tender but still al dente, about 15 minutes. Check and sprinkle with more stock if necessary.

14 Remove paella from the oven, cover with aluminum foil, and let stand 5 minutes. Uncover and let stand 10 minutes; flavors will develop as it rests.

15 Garnish with roasted peppers and serve.

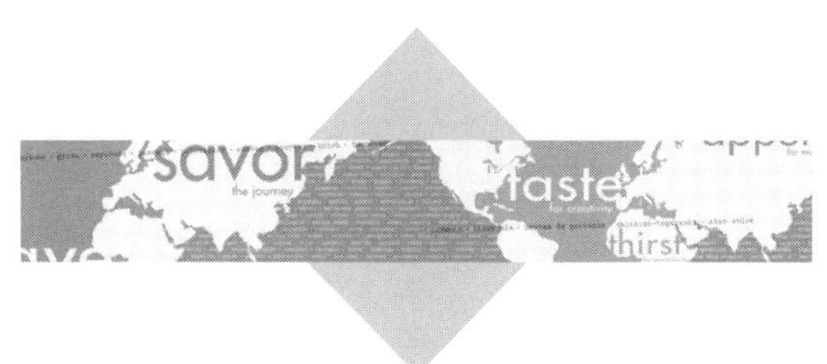

# Espinacas à la Catalana

## Spinach Catalan-Style

SERVES 4

**Catalans enjoy cooking with dried fruits.**

| AMOUNT | MEASURE | INGREDIENT |
|---|---|---|
| 2 tablespoons | 1 ounce, 30 ml | Olive oil |
| 1 cup | 4 ounces, 112 g | Sweet apple (golden delicious), peeled, $\frac{1}{4}$ inch (.6 cm) dice |
| $\frac{1}{4}$ cup | $\frac{1}{2}$ ounce, 14 g | Pine nuts |
| $\frac{1}{4}$ cup | 1 ounce, 28 g | Dark raisins |
| 5 cups | 10 ounces, 280 g | Baby spinach, washed |
| To taste | | Salt and white pepper |

PROCEDURE

1. Heat oil over high heat; add apples and brown lightly, about 1 minute.
2. Add pine nuts and cook until they are light brown, 30 seconds, stirring constantly. Add raisins.
3. Add spinach and toss; sauté until it begins to wilt, then remove from heat; it will continue to cook.
4. Correct seasoning and serve.

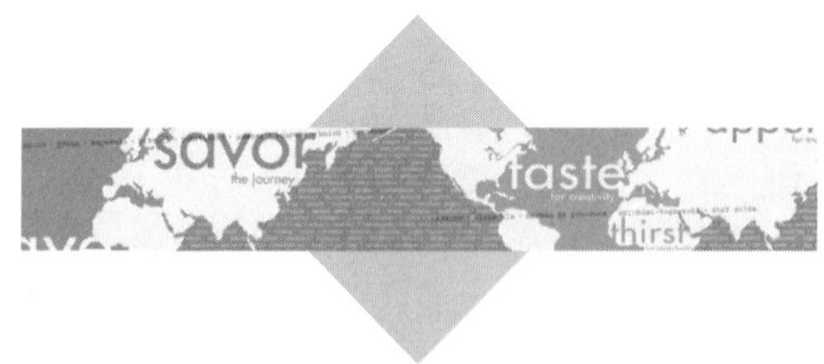

# Pera Salsa de Caramelo al Café

## Pears with Caramel-Coffee Sauce

SERVES 4

| AMOUNT | MEASURE | INGREDIENT |
|---|---|---|
| **4** | | **Anjou, Bosc, or Comice pears, medium, not too ripe** |
| **3 tablespoons** | | **Granulated sugar** |
| **2 tablespoons** | **1 ounce, 28 g** | **Butter, broken into bits** |
| **1 cup** | **8 ounces, 240 ml** | **Heavy cream** |
| **1 teaspoon** | | **Confectioner's sugar** |
| **1 tablespoon** | | **Coffee extract or strong espresso** |
| **$\frac{1}{8}$ teaspoon** | | **Vanilla extract** |

PROCEDURE

1. Preheat oven to 425°F (218°C).
2. Peel and split pears lengthwise, remove seeds, and core.
3. Place flat side down in a gratin dish; do not overlap. Sprinkle with sugar and top with butter.
4. Bake 35 minutes or until tender and sugar has caramelized. Check for tenderness by piercing with the point of a knife. If necessary, cook an additional 5–10 minutes.
5. Add $\frac{3}{4}$ cup (6 ounces, 180 ml) cream, coffee extract or espresso, and continue to cook for 10–15 minutes, basting every 5 minutes. The cream should have reduced to sauce consistency and taken on an ivory color. Remove from oven and cool to lukewarm.
6. Whip remaining cream with confectioner's sugar and vanilla extract.
7. Serve with sauce and whipped cream.

# Gazpacho Sevillano

## Classic Gazpacho SERVES 4

**Chef Tip** **The original mortar-pounded gazpachos were coarse in texture; modern Spanish cooks prefer a smooth soup.**

| AMOUNT | MEASURE | INGREDIENT |
|---|---|---|
| 1 cup | 1 ounce, 28 g | Day-old country bread, crust removed, 1 inch (2.5 cm) cubes |
| 1 | | Garlic clove, minced |
| Pinch | | Ground cumin |
| To taste | | Salt |
| 4 cups | 24 ounces, 672 g | Tomatoes, very ripe, peeled, seeded, $\frac{1}{2}$ inch (1.2 cm) dice |
| 1 cup | 5 ounces, 140 g | Kirby (pickling) cucumber, peeled, $\frac{1}{2}$ inch (1.2 cm) dice |
| $\frac{1}{2}$ cup | 2 ounces, 56 g | Italian frying pepper, Italianelles or cubanels (long, green peppers, sweet and tender with thin skin), $\frac{1}{4}$ inch (.6 cm) dice |
| $\frac{1}{2}$ cup | 2 ounces, 56 g | Red bell pepper, $\frac{1}{4}$ inch (.6 cm) dice |
| 2 tablespoons | $\frac{1}{2}$ ounce, 14 g | Spanish onion, $\frac{1}{4}$ inch (.6 cm) dice |
| $\frac{1}{4}$ cup | 2 ounces, 60 ml | Olive oil |
| $\frac{1}{4}$ cup, more if needed | 2 ounces, 60 ml | Water |
| $1\frac{1}{2}$ tablespoons, more to taste | $1\frac{1}{2}$ ounces, 45 ml | Aged sherry vinegar |
| To taste | | Freshly ground pepper |
| Garnishes | | |
| 2 tablespoons | $\frac{1}{2}$ ounce, 14 g | Cucumber, $\frac{1}{8}$ inch (.3 cm) dice |
| 2 tablespoons | $\frac{1}{2}$ ounce, 14 g | Granny Smith apple, $\frac{1}{8}$ inch (.3 cm) dice |
| 2 tablespoons | $\frac{3}{4}$ ounce, 21 g | Underripe tomato, peeled, seeded, $\frac{1}{8}$ inch (.3 cm) dice |
| 2 tablespoons | $\frac{1}{2}$ ounce, 14 g | Green bell pepper, $\frac{1}{8}$ inch (.3 cm) dice |
| 1 tablespoon | | Basil, chiffonade |

**PROCEDURE**

1 Cover bread with ice cold water; soak 10 minutes. Drain and squeeze out excess liquid.

2 Mash garlic, cumin, and $\frac{1}{2}$ teaspoon salt with a mortar and pestle.

3 Toss together tomatoes, cucumbers, Italian and red peppers, onion, soaked bread, and garlic paste. Let stand 15 minutes.

4 Using a food processor, process ingredients until smooth; add olive oil while processing.

5 Add water and vinegar, correct seasoning with salt, pepper, and additional vinegar.

6 Cover and chill, 1 hour or more.

7 Serve with garnishes.

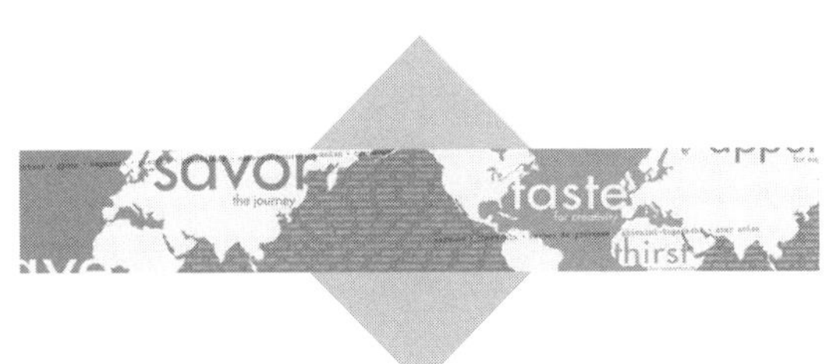

# Pollo En Pepitoria

## Chicken in Almond and Saffron Sauce

SERVES 4

| AMOUNT | MEASURE | INGREDIENT |
|---|---|---|
| 1 | | Chicken (about 2½ pounds; 1.3 kg), cut into 12 pieces, rinsed, patted dry, excess fat trimmed |
| To taste | | Coarse salt and freshly ground black pepper |
| ½ cup | 4 ounces, 120 ml | Olive oil |
| ¾ cup | 3 ounces, 84 g | Whole blanched almonds |
| 5 | | Garlic cloves |
| 6 | | Whole black peppercorns |
| ¼ cup | | Flat-leaf parsley, minced |
| 2 cups | 8 ounces, 228 | Onion, ¼ inch (.6 cm) dice |
| 1½ inch | 1 2.5–5 cm | Cinnamon stick |
| ¾ cup | 6 ounces, 180 ml | Dry white wine |
| 2¼ cup | 18 ounces, 540 ml | Chicken stock |
| 2 teaspoons | | Saffron, pulverized in a mortar and steeped in 3 tablespoons hot water |
| ¼ teaspoon | | Ground cloves |
| ⅓ cup | 1 ounce, 28 g | Lemon slices, paper thin, cut in half, seeds removed |
| 2 | | Eggs, hard-cooked, yolk and whites separate |
| ¼ cup | | Almonds, slivered, toasted |

### PROCEDURE

1. Season chicken and let stand 10 minutes.
2. Heat oil over medium heat; add whole almonds and cook 2 minutes until lightly colored.
3. Add garlic and cook with almonds until both are golden brown, 2 minutes. Remove from fat onto paper towels to drain, reserve oil.
4. In a mini food processor or mortar, grind almonds, garlic, peppercorns, and ⅔ of the parley to a paste, set aside.
5. Reheat oil over medium-high heat and brown chicken on all sides, 5–8 minutes. Remove and reserve.
6. Return only two tablespoons of oil to medium-low heat; add onion and cinnamon stick and cook slowly until onions are very soft, 10 minutes.

7. Return chicken to pan, add wine and stock, and bring to simmer over medium-high heat.
8. Add almond paste, saffron, and cloves; cover and reduce heat to medium low and simmer, covered, until chicken is tender, 30 minutes, turning pieces every 10 minutes. At the end of the 30 minutes, stir in lemon slices and cook 10 minutes. Check for tenderness and correct seasoning. Remove chicken pieces and keep hot.
9. Chop egg white for garnish.
10. Mash egg yolks and whisk 3 tablespoons ($1\frac{1}{2}$ ounces, 75 ml) cooking liquid.
11. Return cooking liquid to a boil and reduce to by $\frac{1}{3}$, 2–4 minutes.
12. Stir in mashed egg yolk and cook 3–4 minutes; sauce will thicken somewhat.
13. Return chicken pieces, coat with sauce, and reheat.
14. Serve chicken with sauce on top, garnish with slivered almonds, chopped egg white, and remaining parsley.

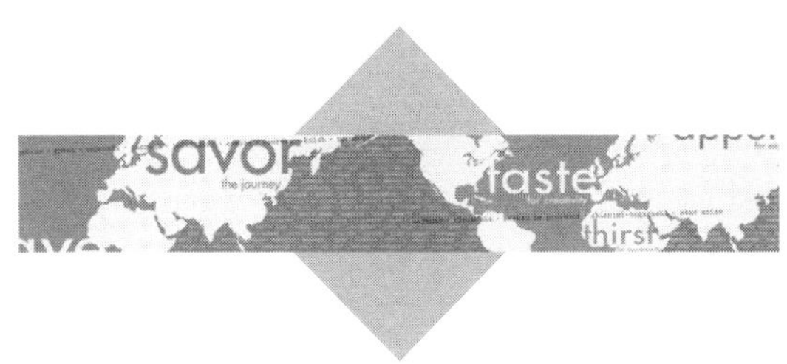

# Ensalada con Higos, Cabrales, y Granada

## Mesclun, Figs, Cabrales, and Pomegranate

SERVES 4

| AMOUNT | MEASURE | INGREDIENT |
|---|---|---|
| 1 | | Medium-size pomegranate |
| ½ teaspoon | | Honey |
| 4½ teaspoons | 1½ ounces, 45 ml | Fresh lemon juice |
| 4½ teaspoons | 1½ ounces, 45 ml | High-quality red wine vinegar |
| 2 tablespoons | ½ ounce, 14 g | Shallots, minced |
| ¼ cup | 2 ounces, 60 ml | Olive oil |
| 8 | | Purple figs, trimmed, quartered lengthwise |
| 4 cups | 6 ounces, 168 g | Mesclun, rinsed, dried, loosely packed |
| ¼ cup | 1 ounce, 28 g | Pine nuts, toasted |
| To taste | | Coarse salt and freshly ground black pepper |
| ⅓ cup | 2 ounces, 56 g | Cabrales or other blue cheese, crumbled |

PROCEDURE

1. Cut pomegranate into quarters. Remove seeds from 3 of the pieces and place in a bowl; pick out and discarding any membrane.
2. Working over a sieve, press the juice from the remaining pomegranate quarter into a separate bowl. Add honey, lemon juice, vinegar, and shallots; slowly whisk in the olive oil. Correct seasoning.
3. Broil fig quarters cut side up until they look caramelized and lightly charred, 4–5 minutes.
4. Combine figs, pomegranate seeds, mesclun, and toasted pine nuts, toss with dressing, and season with salt and pepper.
5. Toss in cheese and serve.

# Merluza en Salsa Verde

## Hake in Green Sauce SERVES 4

**If available, use a cazuela that just fits the fish. Cazuelas are terra cotta casserole dishes, and have been used in Spain for thousands of years.**

| AMOUNT | MEASURE | INGREDIENT |
|---|---|---|
| 8 | | Manila clams, medium size |
| 2 tablespoons | 1 ounce, 30 ml | Olive oil |
| 1 | | Garlic clove, minced |
| 1 teaspoon | | All-purpose flour |
| | 12 ounces, 336 g | Hake, skin on, cut into 4 pieces |
| To taste | | Salt |
| 1 tablespoon | | Flat-leaf parsley, minced |
| 1 $\frac{1}{2}$ tablespoons | $\frac{3}{4}$ ounce, 23 ml | Crisp dry white wine |

### PROCEDURE

1. Bring 1 quart (32 ounces, 960 ml) water to a boil. Add 4 clams at a time and cook 10–15 seconds or until they just open. Remove and repeat with the other four clams. Working over a bowl to collect juices, remove the clams from the shells and discard shells.
2. Heat oil over low heat, add garlic, and cook until it just begins to jump, 45 seconds; do not brown. Add flour.
3. Season fish with salt and place skin side down in pan. Add parsley.
4. Moving pan in a constant circular motion, cook 3 to 4 minutes. Turn fish over and repeat on second side, 3 to 4 minutes. Maintain a low temperature.
5. Add clams, clam juices, and white wine. Cook an additional 3 to 4 minutes; do not boil liquid.
6. The natural gelatins of the fish will emulsify with the oil, making a light green sauce. Correct seasoning and serve 1 piece of fish, 2 clams, and sauce for each portion.

# Cerdo Cocido con la Fruta Seca

## Braised Pork with Dried Fruit

SERVES 4

| AMOUNT | MEASURE | INGREDIENT |
|---|---|---|
| 2 pounds | 896 g | Boneless pork shoulder roast, trimmed of excess fat and tied |
| To taste | | Coarse salt and freshly ground black pepper |
| 2 | | Garlic cloves, chopped fine |
| 3 tablespoons | 1 ½ ounce, 45 ml | Olive oil |
| 1 cup | 4 ounces, 112 g | Onions, ¼ inch (.6 cm) dice |
| 1 cup | 4 ounces, 112 g | Carrot, ¼ inch (.6 cm) dice |
| 1 cup | 4 ounces, 112 g | Pearl onions, peeled |
| ¼ cup | 2 ounces, 60 ml | Kirsch or brandy |
| 1 ½ cups | 10 ounces, 300 ml | Full-bodied dry high-acidity red wine |
| 2 cups | 16 ounces, 480ml | Beef or chicken stock |
| ¾ cup | 3 ounces, 84 g | Pitted dried sour cherries |
| ½ cup | 2 ounces, 56 g | Dried apricots, quartered |
| 1 | | Bay leaf |
| 1 ½ inch | 1 2.5–5 cm | Cinnamon stick |
| 2 | | Fresh rosemary sprigs |
| As needed | | Saffron rice or boiled potatoes |

PROCEDURE

1. Preheat oven to 325°F (162.7°C).
2. Season pork roast with salt and pepper.
3. Heat 2 tablespoons (1 ounce, 30 ml) olive oil over medium-high heat until almost smoking.
4. Add pork and sear to a rich brown color, 8 minutes. Add remaining oil if needed. Transfer to a holding platter.
5. Add diced onions, garlic, carrots, and pearl onions; brown well, 6–7 minutes.
6. Add kirsch and reduce to almost dry, 1 minute.

7 Add wine, stock, cherries, apricots, bay leaf, cinnamon, and rosemary sprigs and bring to a simmer. Return pork to pan. Cover tightly and transfer to oven.

8 Cook until very tender, about 1 hour, turning every 30 minutes.

9 Remove pork from braising liquid; keep warm.

10 Remove and discard bay leaf, cinnamon stick, and rosemary sprigs; bring liquid back to boil and reduce to sauce consistency, 3 to 5 minutes. Correct seasoning.

11 Remove string, slice pork, and serve with the sauce and saffron rice or boiled potatoes.

# Arroz con Leche

## Rice and Milk SERVES 4

| AMOUNT | MEASURE | INGREDIENT |
|---|---|---|
| 10 cups | 80 ounces, 1.4 l | Milk |
| 1 inch | 2.5 cm | Lemon zest |
| $1\frac{1}{2}$ inch | 1 2.5–5 cm | Cinnamon stick |
| 1 cup | $6\frac{1}{4}$ ounces, 175 g | Arborio rice or any short-grain rice |
| 4 tablespoons | 2 ounces, 60 ml | Butter |
| 1 cup | 7 ounces, 196 g | Granulated sugar |

PROCEDURE

1 Combine milk, lemon zest, and cinnamon stick over medium-high heat and bring to a boil.

2 Stir in rice, reduce heat to low, and simmer 30 minutes, stirring constantly so rice does not stick to the bottom of the pan.

3 Add butter and simmer 5 minutes.

4 Add sugar and stir briskly. Remove from heat and spread rice out on a platter. Let rest; as it cools the milk will develop a thin skin on top. Fold back into the rice before serving.

5 Serve at room temperature or cold.

# The Middle East

## The Land

The Middle East is at the junction of trade routes connecting Europe and China, India and Africa, and all the cultures of the Mediterranean basin. Many of these routes have been documented from as early as five thousand years ago, and the presence of so many different people and products over the years has had a profound effect on the region's culture, politics, and economy. More specifically, the Middle East is a term used to describe the area covering sixteen countries and states: Bahrain, Egypt, Iran, Iraq, Israel, Jordan, Kuwait, Lebanon, Oman, Qatar, Saudi Arabia, Syria, Turkey, United Arab Emirates, West Bank/Gaza Strip, and Yemen. The Middle East region represents an area of over five million square miles.

The physical geography of the Middle East is varied. Vast deserts are common in the region. The Sahara Desert runs across North Africa, essentially limiting settlement to along the Mediterranean coastline and in Egypt along the Nile River. The desert of the Arabian Peninsula is so inhospitable that it has been given the name "Empty Quarter." In areas better served by rainfall and rivers (for example the Tigris-Euphrates river system, the Jordan River, and along the Mediterranean coast), rich agriculture is abundant. Mountain ranges exist throughout the Middle East, with some peaks rising as high as 19,000 feet.

Geography and natural resources have always influenced political power in this region. The Nile River and the rivers of the Mesopotamian region (now modern Iraq, and extending north into Syria and Turkey) can support a rich agricultural base, but only if the water supply is sustained and controlled through irrigation systems. Mesopotamian farmers used Persian Gulf seawater to irrigate for centuries, and, as a result, much of southern Iraq's soil is now too salty to grow crops. Agriculture in the region now relies on modern practices like fresh water irrigation, crop rotation, and technologically sophisticated dam projects.

Today, the wealth in Middle Eastern soil comes not from crops but from petroleum. This region contains about two-thirds of the world's known petroleum reserves. When the United States and Europe increased their consumption of oil drastically during World War II, the oil reserves in the Middle East became critically important to U.S. foreign policy, and have remained so ever since.

# History

The Middle East is the most ancient region of human civilization. The rich, fertile soil of the Middle East led early civilizations to settle, domesticate plants and animals, and thrive. The Fertile Crescent between the Tigris and Euphrates Rivers known as Mesopotamia was the home of the world's first urban culture, the Sumer, six thousand years ago. The Sumerians' Egyptian rivals took advantage of the annual flooding of the Nile for their regular harvest, later exporting a large portion of their produce to the Roman Empire. Some time later, the Hittites settled in the rolling hills of Anatolia (modern Turkey) and the Phoenicians off the eastern Mediterranean (modern-day Lebanon, Syria, and northern Israel). Over the years many different great civilizations and cultures developed from or invaded the area. The list of ancient empires includes the Egyptians (c. 2000–1000 B.C.); the Assyrians and Babylonians (c. 1000–500 B.C.); the Persians (c. 550–330 B.C.); and the Romans (c. 60 B.C.–140 A.D.).

During the first millennium B.C. through the middle of the second millennium A.D., a vast network of trade routes known as the Silk Road linked the people and traditions of Asia with those of Europe. These historic routes, covering over five thousand miles of land and sea, were a major conduit for the transport of knowledge, information, and material goods between East and West and resulted in the first global exchange of scientific and cultural traditions.

In modern times the Ottoman Empire (c. 1300–1923) became the largest political entity in Europe and western Asia. The Safavid Empire (1501–1736) dominated the area of modern Iran.

The Middle East has been the center of more than twenty major conflicts from the Persian-Greek Wars to the Crusades to the Iran-Iraq War. After World War I, the decline and disbursement of the Ottoman Empire marked the beginning of a new stage of conflict over territory centering around the lands of Palestine.

While today about 92 percent (292 million) of the people are Muslim, the Middle East is the geographic and emotional center of three of the world's most influential religions: Islam, Christianity, and Judaism.

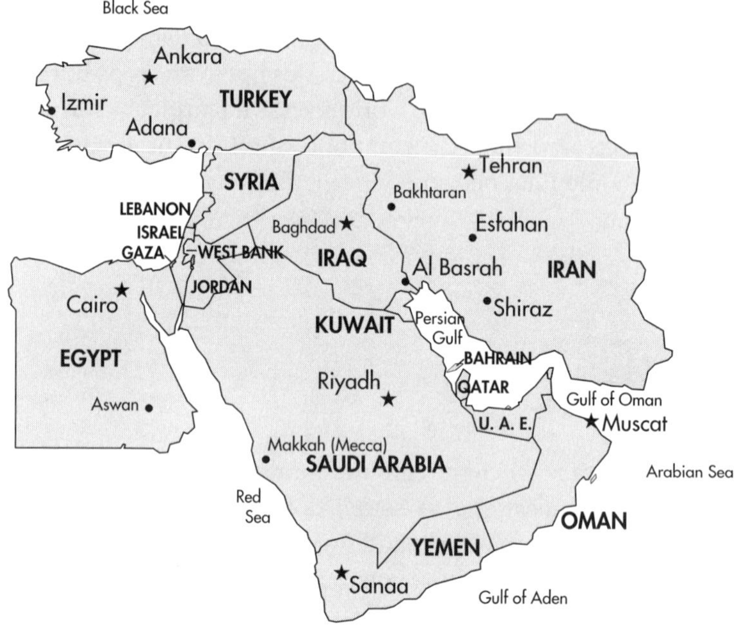


The Middle East

# The People

The people of the Middle East belong to various ethnic groups, which are based largely on culture, language, and history. Ethnically, more than three-fourths of the Middle Eastern people are Arabs. Although they live in different countries, Arabs share a common culture and a common language, Arabic. Iranians and Turks also form major ethnic groups in the region. Smaller groups in the Middle East include Armenians, Copts, Greeks, Jews, Kurds, and various black African groups.

# The Food

Originally, Arabic food was the food of the desert nomads—simple and portable. Nomads stopped in oases and settled farming areas to get some of their food, such as flour for bread, fruits, vegetables, and spices. They brought animals with them to provide meat and milk, and they cooked over campfires. During the early Middle Ages, Islamic empires spread from the Atlantic Ocean to India. The world of Islam would continue to expand to other areas of the world in later centuries. It was not uncommon for an exchange of foods from the various territories to occur. As the people settled in villages, towns, and large cities, the food was no longer only that of the desert nomads.

Flat bread was made along the caravan routes and in the nomads' camps. Made from wheat flour, water, and a little salt, the dough can be flattened and shaped by hand and put on a flat pan over a fire. Dates come from the date palm tree, which grows in the hottest desert oases, and are one of the most important foods of the Middle East. Sheep were the most important source of milk, used for cheese and yogurt, and mutton and lamb continue to be the most popular meat in Arabic cuisine. Goats were also raised for meat and milk. Beans and grains such as garbanzo beans, fava beans, and lentils were dried and carried on the nomads' travels. Other dried fruits such as grapes, dried apricots, figs, and nuts were an important part of the diet. Familiar spices and herbs like cinnamon, cloves, black pepper, hot red and green peppers, allspice, ginger, mint, parsley, bay leaves, basil, dill, rosemary, garlic, and onions were and still are used frequently.

It is a shared history, including that of two great world empires, which has brought unity to the kitchens of the Middle East. The spread of Islam and the establishment of an enormous Islamic state stretching across Asia, North Africa, and the Mediterranean was the most important factor in the development of a gastronomic tradition comparable to that of France and China. As the state grew, Arabs brought to each new region their own tastes as well as those of the countries they had already conquered. Cooking styles traveled with the massive migrations of people; large-scale transport brought into the cities, and even into distant parts of the Middle East, local produce from the desert, olive oil from Syria, dates from Iraq, and coffee from Arabia. Crops such as rice, sugar, hard wheat, eggplant, spinach, pomegranates, and even grapes are all part of the Arab heritage. The Ottoman Turks had significant influence in the Balkans, responsible for little cakes called turbans and puff pastry croissants found in the shape of the Turkish crescent. Certain cooking methods, like cooking skewered ingredients over charcoal or long, slow simmering in unglazed covered pots, are typical of the whole region. Skewering meats, chicken, or fish kebabs is believed to have been developed by the Turks on the field of battle.

All the countries have rice and wheat dishes, stuffed vegetables, pies wrapped in paper-thin pastry, meatballs, thick omelets, cold vegetables cooked in oil, scented rice puddings, nut-filled pastries, fritters soaked in syrup, and many other common elements. One of the most important parts of a meal in many parts of the region is the *mezeh,* which can be anything from half a dozen saucers of appetizers to a spread of fifty dishes, a veritable banquet. A basic selection will include raw carrot sticks, radishes, lettuce hearts, cucumber, and green pepper slices along with salted nuts, olives, crumbly goat's cheese, green onions, sprigs of mint and mountain thyme, pickled turnips and peppers, strained yogurt (*labneh*) topped with golden olive oil, and the national specialties: *hummus bi tahini, baba ghannouj*, and *tabbouleh*. In the center, in reach of all, will be a stack of the puffy hollow rounds of flat Arab bread or sheets of the paper-thin mountain bread. Bread is torn to make scoops for the dips and to wrap small pieces of meat and vegetables. It can also serve as a plate, tablecloth, and napkin. *Hummus bi tahini* is a paste of chickpeas flavored with sesame seed oil, lemon juice, and garlic. *Baba ghannouj* is a smoky dip of eggplant that has been charred over a flame and whipped with the same flavorings to a fluffy consistency. These dips are swirled into a saucer and garnished with whole chickpeas, pomegranate seeds, a sprinkling of paprika, or sprigs of cress or mint. *Tabbouleh* is a salad composed of chopped parsley, onions, tomatoes, and mint leaves mixed with softened cracked wheat kernels (bulgur) and dressed with lemon juice and a little oil.

Iranian cuisine is considered to be the most refined. Fragrance during cooking and at the table plays as important a role as taste. Iran was first to use many common herbs such as basil, mint, cumin, cloves, and coriander. The foods of the courts of ancient Persia (as Iran was called until the 1930s) included perfumed stews flavored with cinnamon, mint, and pomegranates; elaborate stuffed fruits and vegetables; and tender roasted meats. Many different foods originated in or were introduced by Iran, such as oranges, pistachios, spinach, saffron, sweet-and-sour sauces, kabobs, and almond pastries. The domesticated goat is believed to have originated in Persia since the goat's ability to subsist in sparse vegetation made it ideal for domestication by nomads. Wheat, barley, and rice are the most important Iranian crops. Long-grain rice, grown in moist areas bordering the Caspian Sea, has a place of honor, often prepared with a golden crust formed from clarified butter, saffron, and yogurt. Lamb and chicken are marinated and grilled as kebabs, or mixed into stews called *khoreshes* with fruit and sour ingredients such as lime juice. Pickles and flatbreads are served at every meal. Desserts feature rose water and pistachios, and refreshing drinks called *sharbats* are made from diluted fruit and herb syrups.

On the Mediterranean shore are the great network of rivers—the Euphrates, Tigris, Orontes, and Jordan—that irrigate the valleys and plains of Syria, Lebanon, Palestine, Jordan, and Iraq. Known as the Fertile Crescent, this region is a vegetarian's paradise, with a seasonal procession of fruits and vegetables, cereals, golden olive oil, and fragrant herbs. Syria, Lebanon, and Jordan have much the same style of cooking. Rice and cracked wheat are the primary grains. Syria's finest food is found in the city of Aleppo. Distinctly local foods are *muhammara*, a spicy paste eaten like *hummus* but made of the city's renowned hot pepper, pomegranate juice, and ground walnuts; a seasonal kebab in a sauce of stewed fresh cherries, called *kababbi-karaz*; and varieties of *kibbe* made with sumac and quince. Aleppo's famous pistachios are used in many sweets—rolled in doughs and smothered with syrup, or embedded in sweet gelatin.

There is a wide variety in the Jordanian style of cooking. The authentic Jordanian cuisine can range from grilling (*shish kababs, shish taouks*) to stuffing of vegetables (grape leaves, eggplants, and so on), meat, and poultry. Also common in the Jordanian style of cooking is roasting, and/or preparing foods with special sauces. Jordan's most distinctive dish is *mansaf*, a Bedouin dish often served for special occasions. *Mansaf* consists of Arabic rice, a rich broth made from dry sour milk (*jameed*), and either lamb or chicken. It is also considered the greatest symbol in Jordanian culture for generosity and the level of generosity is determined by the amount of lamb presented. Utensils are not commonly used when eating *mansaf.* Guests feast from the communal dish using their hands.

Lebanon is nestled along the eastern shore of the Mediterranean Sea at the very crook of the Fertile Crescent. Its contributions to Middle Eastern cuisine are unmistakable. The flavors that spice the foods of all the surrounding lands can be found here in abundance: olive oil, lemon, garlic, and mint. Lebanese cuisine features such staples as *kibbeh* (ground lamb with bulgur wheat) and *tabbouleh.* The food is simply prepared, with the flavors blending together into a complex medley of earthy, fruity tastes and scents.

With so much coastline and varying climatic conditions, Turkey has always had an abundance of fresh produce and fish, making for a varied diet. Turkey's geographical location made it a natural route for traders, travelers, and migrants, all of whom influenced Turkish cuisine. Since the Turkish sultan had complete control over the Spice Road, many spices and seasonings were adapted to flavor traditional dishes. The climatic and geographical differences within the country also heavily influence regional cooking, from desert-like heat in the southeast, where the food tends to be spicier and meat dishes such as kebabs are common, to temperate fertile zones to the west, where seafood and olive oil are frequently used ingredients. Then there is the eastern region, with its long cold winters where dairy, produce, honey, cereals, and meat are popular. Turkey is discussed in more detail in the next chapter.

The modern state of Israel is an ancient land that has been a formal nation only since 1948. Its citizens hail from over eighty countries. It is truly a culinary and ethnic melting pot. The majority of its population arrived from Eastern European countries such as Russia, Poland, and Hungary, and Middle Eastern and North African countries such as Morocco and Syria. There is also a sizable population originally from Greece. Jewish culinary traditions are ancient and strong. From the rituals of the Passover Seder to fasting at Yom Kippur, many of these observances date back to biblical times. Yet while Jews as a people have endured for over three thousand years, the modern state of Israel is still relatively young. That fact, and the uncertainty and instability associated with the Palestinian conflict, have made it difficult for a truly national Israeli cuisine to develop and flourish. Israeli cuisine was formed according to the availability (or lack) of certain foods. Fruits and vegetables are plentiful and are included in virtually every meal. Dairy products, including different types of yogurt and soured milks and creams, are also a major part of the Israeli diet. Red meat is rarely eaten, partly because the lack of quality grazing land for livestock produces a lower grade of meat. Turkey and chicken are a major part of the Israeli diet. *Cholent* is a traditional stew served on the Jewish Sabbath, which is observed from sundown on Friday to sundown on Saturday. Because the oven in a religious home cannot be lit after sundown on Friday, *cholent* simmers overnight in a warm oven turned on before the Sabbath begins. Various types of *cholent* reflect the traditional foods of the different Jewish ethnic groups. Moroccan Jews, for example, use beef, spices, chickpeas, and potatoes, while Sephardic Jews include beans, meat, potatoes, and eggs. *Kugel,* a noodle casserole that is a traditional food among Eastern European Jews, is also a Sabbath favorite because it can be left overnight in a warm oven and be ready for the meal on Saturday.

Another factor that plays a significant role in the Israeli menu is the dietary laws of the Jews and Muslims. Jewish kashrut dietary laws were developed during early times. Food prepared according to these rules is called kosher, or "proper." Jews are prohibited from eating pork, so lamb, mutton, and beef are the preferred meats. The consumption of blood is also forbidden, so meats must be butchered and prepared using a process of salting and curing, in order to remove all traces of blood. Meat and dairy are never mixed in the same dish or even, according to some interpretations, in the same meal. Orthodox homes maintain two separate sets of utensils and dishes, one for meat and one for dairy. The very wealthy may even have two separate kitchens. With regard to seafood, it is forbidden to eat anything without scales. That means no shrimp, shellfish, squid, or octopus. There are varying degrees of adherence to kashrut laws in modern Israel. While one finds strict fidelity among the Orthodox population, it is not uncommon to see only partial or no observation among secular Jews.

Throughout the Mediterranean Middle East, the cultures and people have intermingled, and carried with them their foods and traditions. In no other place in the world is there such a blending of cultures that has mingled so much, yet maintained their distinct, national flavors.

# Glossary

**Aleppo Pepper** Sweet and sharp chile from the Aleppo region of Syria, with moderate heat that doesn't overpower the fruity flavor of the pepper. As a substitute, combine an equal amount of crushed, hot red pepper with Spanish paprika.

**Arabic Bread (Khubz Arabi, Pita)** Flat, round bread, which can be easily split to make a sandwich, or broken apart and used as a utensil for scooping food.

**Ataif (Gatayef, Kataif)** Small pancakes stuffed with nuts or cheese and doused with syrup.

**Aysh abu Laham** Something like pizza, made from leavened dough, egg-rich and flavored with seeds of fennel, and black caraway. It is baked in the shape of a thick-bottomed pie shell, filled with fried mutton, chopped *kurrath,* or spring onion, and topped with a sauce made from tahina (Saudi Arabia).

**Baba Ghanoush (Baba Ganouj or Baba Gannoujh)** A puree of char-grilled eggplant, *tahina,* olive oil, lemon juice, and garlic, served as a dip.

**Baharat (Bjar)** Arabic mixed spices; in Egypt a mixture of ground cinnamon, allspice, and cloves often used with meat. In Morocco, a mixture of ground cinnamon and rosebuds.

**Baklawa (Baklava)** Dessert of layered pastry filled with nuts and steeped in honey-lemon syrup. Usually cut into triangular or diamond shapes.

**Bukhari Rice** Lamb and rice stir-fried with onion, lemon, carrot, and tomato paste.

**Bulgur** Also known as *bulghur, burghul, bulger, bulgar, wheat groats* (Arabic, Armenian, Turkish, British), kernels of whole wheat are steamed, dried, and then crushed to make bulgur. The process involved to make bulgur is what gives it a fine, nutty flavor. It requires no or little cooking; it is typically used in tabbouleh and mixed with lamb in kibbeh.

**Cardamom** Aromatic spice, used to flavor Arabic coffee, yogurt, and stews. Cardamom is an essential ingredient in that ubiquitous symbol of Arab hospitality, coffee. In the Arabian Peninsula, coffee is usually a straw-colored brew, made from lightly roasted beans, lavishly perfumed and flavored with crushed, large green cardamom pods, and served unsweetened in miniature handleless cups in a stream of generosity that ends only when the guest's thirst is satisfied. As it is one of the world's most expensive spices, cardamom's generous use is intended as an honor. In addition, coffee brewed from dark-roasted beans, and usually prepared with sugar, is drunk occasionally. That brew is sometimes spiced with a little ground cardamom seed as well. Cardamom is not limited to coffee; its pleasant, camphor-like flavor combines well with any food or beverage, hot or cold. The seedpods, slightly crushed, are a standard spice in the traditional Arabian dish *kabsah*, a lamb-and-rice stew, and it is a common ingredient in fruit desserts. Native to southern India, the spice traveled the short distance to the Arabian Peninsula along the Silk Road. The plant is a member of the ginger family, grows to a height of six to eight feet, and produces its aromatic seed pods on curly panicles at its base.

**Chai** Black tea brewed with selected spices and milk. Each ingredient adds subtle flavor changes and brewing methods vary widely.

**Chelo** Cooked (steamed) rice.

**Chelo Kebah** Rice, grilled marinated lamb, egg yolk, spices, and yogurt. National dish of Iran.

**Cheeses**

**Akawi or Akawieh** Made from sheep's milk, with complex flavor. It is a hard cheese used primarily as a table cheese.

**Baladi** Soft-white, smooth, creamy cheese with a mild flavor. Eaten for breakfast as well as snacks with fresh bread or crackers.

**Feta** Curd cheese that dates back thousands of years and is still made by shepherds in the Greek mountains with unpasteurized milk. Originally made with goat's or sheep's milk, but today much is often made commercially with pasteurized cow's milk. The milk, curdled with rennet, is separated and allowed to drain in a special mold or a cloth bag. It is cut into large slices (feta means "slice") that are salted and packed in barrels filled with whey or brine, for a week to several months. Feta cheese is white, usually formed into square cakes, and can range from soft to semi-hard, with a tangy, salty flavor that can range from mild to sharp. Its fat content can range from 30 to 60 percent; most is around 45 percent milk fat.

**Halloumi** A mild-flavored, creamy-tasting chewy textured cheese that is most often served cooked. Halloumi is usually made with sheep's milk and may be flavored with mint.

**Jibneh Arabieh** A simple cheese found all over the Middle East. It is particularly popular in Egypt and the Arabian Gulf area. The cheese has an open texture and a mild taste. The heritage of the product started with Bedouins, using goat's or sheep's milk; however, current practice is to use cow's milk to make the cheese. *Jibneh Arabieh* is used for cooking, or simply as a table cheese.

**Kenafa** An unsalted, very fresh, soft cheese that melts easily and freely. It is used to make the popular *knafe*. It can also be used as a base for other sweet cheese desserts.

**Labane** A cheese shaped into small balls, very popular in the Middle East. Made of sheep's or goat's milk and is eaten young, almost liquid in form.

**Labenah (Labneh)** Thick creamy cheese, made from sheep's or goat's milk, made by draining soured milk or yogurt. Soft texture and a tangy flavor, often spiced and used as a dip.

**Naboulsi** A salty, fresh, brined cheese popular in Syria, Lebanon, and Jordan. The cheese is packed in brine.

**Testouri** From Egypt shaped like an orange, made from sheep's or goat's milk, eaten fresh and lightly salted. This cheese was introduced into North Africa by the Ottomans after the fifteenth century.

**Tzfatit** A delicate, salty cheese. One of Israel's most popular cheeses, its flavor is especially delectable when served with slices of fresh vegetables, olive oil, and herbs such as zatar.

**Coriander (Cilantro)** Lacy, green-leaf relative of the parsley family with an extremely pungent flavor akin to a combination of lemon, sage, and caraway.

**Couscous** Small, grainlike semolina pasta.

**Dibbis** Date syrup, an Iraqi sweetening agent made by boiling dates and draining. Resembles thick brown molasses.

**Dried Limes** Lends a bright tang to stews, some varieties of *kabsah*, and fish dishes. The limes may be used whole and fished out of the dish before serving, or pounded to a fine powder. To make your own dried limes, boil the small round variety of lime vigorously for a few minutes, then dry them in a sunny or otherwise dry and warm place for several weeks until they turn brown and feel hollow.

**Falafel** Small deep-fried patties made of highly spiced ground chickpeas.

**Fatayer** Pastry pockets filled with spinach, meat, or cheese.

**Fattoush** A salad of toasted croutons, cucumbers, tomatoes, and mint.

**Fenugreek Leaves** Leaves with a pleasant bitter flavor, used fresh or dried, used in soups and stews (Iran; *shambabileh* in Persian).

**Fillo** Consists of thin sheets of unleavened flour dough. They are layered with butter and baked to make flaky pies and pastries. The layers of fillo dough can be as thin as paper or a millimeter or so thick. Fillo is used in many of the cuisines of the former Ottoman Empire. (*Phyllo* to the Greeks and *yufka* to the Turks.)

**Gyros (Sandwich)** Meat cooked on a rotisserie, sliced in thin shavings and served traditionally with tomatoes, onions, and tzatziki in pita or plain bread.

**Halwa (Halva)** Sesame paste; sweet, usually made in a slab and studded with fruit and nuts.

**Hamour** Red Sea fish from the grouper family.

**Hummus (Hommus)** Spreadable paste made of chickpeas, tahini, lemon juice, and garlic.

**Jarish** Crushed wheat and yogurt casserole.

**Kabsa** Classic Arabian dish of meat mixed with rice.

**Kamareddine** Apricot nectar used to break the fast during Ramadan.

**Kebab** Skewered chunks of meat or poultry cooked over charcoal or broiled.

**Khubz Marcook** Thin, dome-shaped Arabic bread.

**Kibbeh (Kibbe)** The national dish of Syria, Lebanon, and Jordan; there are countless versions, some widely known throughout the Middle East. It always involves a mixture of minced lamb, grated onion, and fine-ground bulgur pounded to a paste.

**Kibbeh Naye** Raw *kibbeh*, eaten like steak tartar.

**Kofta** Fingers, balls, or a flat cake of minced meat and spices. May be baked or charcoal-grilled on skewers. The word *kofta* is derived from the Persian word *kūfta*, meaning “meatball.”

**Kouzi** Whole lamb baked over rice so that the rice absorbs the juice of the meat.

**Kunafi (Kunafah)** Shoelace-like pastry dessert stuffed with sweet white cheese, nuts, and syrup.

**Lahma Bi Ajeen** Arabic pizza.

**Ma’amul** Date cookies shaped in a wooden mould called a *tabi*.

**Mahlab** Spice obtained from the dark kernels inside the pits of small wild black cherry trees. It has been used for centuries in the Middle East as a sweet/sour, nutty addition to breads, cookies, and pastries.

# Kosher and Halal

**Kosher and halal describe what is "fit and proper" to eat for two groups of people, Jews and Muslims, according to religious law. Although these terms are used to describe a wide array of foods and beverages that are acceptable to eat, the most significant laws refer to meat. Both of these food laws have their roots in Old Testament scripture, and Torah for kosher and the Quran for halal.**

| | KOSHER | HALAL |
|---|---|---|
| Blessing of animals | Blessing before entering slaughtering area, not of each animal | Blessing of each animal while slaughtering |
| Preparation of meat | Soaked and salted to drain all blood | No special preparation; blood drained during slaughtering |
| Gelatin | From kosher animals | From halal bones only |
| Dry bones | From kosher animals | From halal animals only |
| Fish | From kosher fish only | From any fish |
| Pork | Pork is forbidden | Pork is forbidden |
| Fish and other seafood | Permitted except fish that do not have fins and scales (e.g., catfish, eels, rays, sharks, swordfish) shellfish (e.g., oysters, clams), crustaceans (e.g., crab, lobster), and mollusks (e.g., scallops) not permitted | Permitted |
| Alcohol | Permitted, except for grape derivatives such as wine, brandy, or some liqueurs; alcohol must be certified kosher before permitted | Not permitted |
| Combining dairy and meat products | Not permitted | Permitted |
| Special occasions | Additional restrictions during Passover | Same rules apply all the time |

**Mastic** The resin exuded from the bark of a small evergreen shrub closely related to the pistachio tree; it is best known in the West today for its use in such products as varnish and paint, but cooks in Arabia continue their centuries-old custom of enjoying its unique, fresh, resinous aroma and flavor in meat soups and stews and in puddings. Mastic melts into the food rather than dissolving, so it is best to pulverize the translucent light-yellow lumps before adding them. Mastic is one of the many ingredients used in the popular *shawurma,* an elaborate construction of marinated meat, fat, and flavors, which rotates on a vertical spit placed close to a fire.

**Mehshi** Means *stuffed.* Eggplant, zucchini, vine leaves, or cabbage may be stuffed with a mixture of minced meat, rice, and onions.

**Melokhiyyah** Green spinachlike vegetable.

**Mezze (Mezza, Meze, Mezzah)** The Arabic word for appetizer (small plates).

**Mouhammara** A mixture of groundnuts, olive oil, cumin, and chiles, eaten with Arabic bread.

**Moutabe** Eggplant dip made with tahini, olive oil, and lemon juice.

**Mutabak** Sweet or savory pastry turnovers usually stuffed with cheese, banana, or meat.

**Nutmeg** The seed of a large evergreen tree native to the Spice Islands (the Moluccas) of what is now Indonesia. The fleshy yellow, peach-like fruit of this tree splits open when ripe, revealing the nutmeg encased in a dark-brown shell, which in turn is wrapped in a bright red net, or aril; this aril is the spice mace. Nutmeg has long been in popular use in Middle Eastern cuisine, as in the rest of the world, both as a flavoring and a medicine; however, its medicinal properties have caused it to be classified officially as a drug and it is therefore banned in Saudi Arabia today. Very large quantities of nutmeg can produce hallucinations followed by ferocious headaches, and an overdose can be lethal.

**Orange-Blossom Water *(Mai Qedda)*** Produced from the blossom of the sour-orange tree, it contributes a delicate perfume to syrups and pastries.

**Pomegranate Seeds** The juicy, shiny pink seeds of the fresh fruit, used as garnish.

**Pomegranate Syrup (Molasses or Concentrate)** Made from the juice of sour (not sweet) pomegranates boiled down to thick syrup. Prominent in Iranian and Syrian cooking.

**Rakwi** Long-handled coffee pot.

**Rose water *(Mai Ward)*** Distilled essence of rose petals, used to scent syrups and pastries. Rosewater is one of the earliest distilled products ever made, and its manufacture has been an important industry in the Middle East for about 1,200 years. Rosewater and orange-blossom water are added to food simply for the pleasure their fragrance gives, rather than for flavor.

**Saffron** The highly prized red saffron threads are the pistils of a particular purple crocus grown in Iran, Kashmir, and Spain. Saffron is used in a variety of ways in Persian and Moroccan cooking. This spice, the world's most expensive, is made up of the stigmas of an autumn-flowering crocus native to the Middle East. The stigmas and parts of their styles are dried to brittle red threads, which, when ground, yield a yellow powder. Each flower has only three tiny stigmas, and as many as 80,000 flowers are needed to produce a pound of spice. Most of the saffron in trade today comes from Spain, where it was introduced by the Arabs in the eighth or ninth century.

**Sahlab (Salep)** The root tuber of a type of orchid used in powder form to thicken milk and flavor hot drinks and ice cream. *Sahlab* is very expensive.

**Sambusek (Sambusak)** Triangular pies filled with meat, cheese, or spinach.

**Samneh (Ghee)** Ghee is the classic shortening of India and the Middle East. It is simple to make and it keeps forever even in the hot climate. In the Middle East it is called samneh. The solids are removed from butter.

**Seleek** Meat and rice dish in which the rice is cooked in milk rather than the juice of the meat.

**Sesame Seeds** The pale, small seeds of a tall herb grown in many parts of the Middle East are extremely important to the cuisine of the region. The seeds are pressed to extract a high-quality oil; lightly toasted; they add their nutty flavor to a large number of breads and pastries, or provide a tasty coating for sweet Medina dates stuffed with almonds. *Tahini,* a paste made from sesame, is mixed with mashed chickpeas, garlic, and lemon juice to make *hummus.* Sesame seeds mixed with honey are a nutritious, sweet snack. The seed pods of this plant (except for modern commercial varieties) burst open suddenly and forcefully when the seeds are ripe, scattering them widely.

**Shaour** Red Sea fish from the emperor family.

**Shawarma (Shawerma)** A cone of layered pressed lamb, chicken, or beef roasted on a vertical spit where the meat is shaved off from the outside as the spit keeps turning. Saudi Arabia's most popular sandwich is Arabic bread filled with *shawarma* meat, salad, hot sauce, and tahina.

**Shaybah** Also known as "old man's beard," a tree lichen found in the Arabian Peninsula whose complex, bitter, metallic flavor is popular in meat and vegetable stews. A small piece of curly black-and-silver lichen will flavor a large pot of stew.

**Shourba** Soup.

**Sumac (Sumac)** A dark, wine-colored spice with an astringent sour flavor, made from the coarsely ground dried berries of the sumac shrub. Iranians, Iraqis, Lebanese, and Syrians use it frequently. It is often sprinkled on kebabs, salads, and fish dishes. Powdered dark-red *sumac* berries provide a pleasant lemony spice that tastes especially good on meats such as shish kebabs. Although it is produced by a small Mediterranean/Persian tree related to the poisonous sumac of North America, and it is sometimes used in tanning leather, the acid of these berries is in no way harmful. Sumac was mentioned nearly two thousand years ago in the writing of Dioscorides, a Greek physician serving in the Roman army, as having healthful properties; Dioscorides says it was "sprinkled among sauces" and mixed with meat. Modern-day eaters find it excellent on pizza. Sumac is also generally considered an essential ingredient in the spice mixture *za'tar.*

**Tabbouleh** A salad of bulgur, tomato, mint, and parsley.

**Tahini** An oily paste made from ground sesame seeds. It is used raw, in dips and salads, and cooked, in sauces.

**Tahrini** A brass coffee grinder.

**Taklia** A spice consisting of ground coriander and garlic.

**Tamarind (Tamarhendi)** The name is derived from the Arabic for "Indian date." The pulp of the long brown seed pods of the tamarind tree yields an extremely viscous syrup with a distinctive sour flavor that is excellent in vegetables, meat, and fish dishes. Tamarind syrup makes a delicious and refreshing cold drink, prepared like lemonade with water and sugar. This spice is not as exotic in the West as it may seem at first; tamarind is an ingredient in Worcestershire sauce.

**Tamr** Dates.

**Taratour** A thick mayonnaise (water emulsified) of pureed pine nuts, garlic, and lemon, used as a sauce or dip.

**Turmeric** The rhizome or underground stem of a ginger-like plant, almost always available ground into a bright yellow, fine powder. Turmeric is used extensively in the East and Middle East as a condiment and culinary dye. It has an earthy and slightly acrid bouquet; its flavor is warm and aromatic with a bitter undertone.

**Tzatziki** Strained yogurt and cucumbers seasoned with onion and garlic.

**Um Ali** "Ali's mother" is a pastry pudding with raisins and coconut steeped in milk.

**Zattar (Zahtar)** Wild thyme. It is also the name of a mixture of this herb with sumac, salt, and toasted sesame seeds. It is made by combining 1 part ground dried thyme, 1 part lightly toasted sesame seeds, $\frac{1}{4}$ part sumac, and salt to taste.

**Zereshk** Called barberries in English, these are tart red berries used dried in Persian cooking.

# Menus and Recipes from the Middle East

MENU ONE

*Hummus Bi Tahini:* **Chickpea and Sesame Dip**

*Fatayer Sbanikh:* **Triangle Spinach Pies**

*Tabbouleh:* **Cracked Wheat and Herb Salad**

*Khobz:* **Whole Wheat Flat Bread**

*Kukuye Mohi:* **Fish Omelet**

*Bamia:* **Lamb and Okra Casserole**

*Muaddas:* **Rice with Lentils**

*Khoshaf:* **Dried Fruit Compote**

*Qahwah:* **Arabic Coffee**

MENU TWO

*Borani Chogondar:* **Beet and Yogurt Salad**

*Falafel:* **Dried Bean Croquettes**

*Khubz (Khoubiz):* **Arabic Flat Bread**

*Baba Ghannouj (Moutabal):* **Eggplant Dip**

*Morgh Polou:* **Chicken with Rice**

*Adas Bis Silq:* **Lentil and Swiss Chard Soup**

*Baklawa "Be'aj":* **Fillo and Nut Pastries**

MENU THREE

*Muhammara:* **Red Pepper and Walnut Dip**

*Besara:* **Broad Bean Puree**

*Samke Harrah al-Sahara:* **Baked Fish with Hot Chile Sauce**

*Shurabat al Kibbeh:* **Kibbeh Soup**

*Fattoush:* **Toasted Bread Salad**

*Nane Lavash (Taftoon):* **Flat Bread**

*Tapauch Ets Im Mits Tapuzim:* **Apples in Orange Juice**

*Tan:* **Yogurt Drink**

# Hummus Bi Tahini

## Chickpea and Sesame Dip

YIELD: 3 CUPS

| AMOUNT | MEASURE | INGREDIENT |
|---|---|---|
| 2 cups | 14 ounces, 392 g | Garbanzos (chickpeas), cooked, separated from their skins; drained and rinsed if canned |
| $\frac{1}{3}$ cup | 2.66 ounces, 80 ml | Tahini |
| $\frac{1}{2}$ cup | 4 ounces, 120 ml | Fresh lemon juice |
| 2 | | Garlic cloves, crushed |
| To taste | | Salt |
| For serving | | |
| 1 tablespoon | $\frac{1}{2}$ ounce, 15 ml | Olive oil |
| 1 teaspoon | | Parsley, chopped |
| Sprinkle | | Cayenne pepper or paprika |

**PROCEDURE**

1 Combine garbanzos (reserve 1 tablespoon), tahini, $\frac{1}{4}$ cup (2 ounces, 60 ml) lemon juice, and garlic in a food processor using a metal blade. Process until thick and smooth. Adjust flavor with lemon juice and salt. Adjust consistency with a little water.

2 Serve in a shallow dish, swirling with back of spoon to cover the dish. Pour olive oil in the center, garnish with reserved chickpeas, chopped parsley, and a sprinkling of paprika or cayenne.

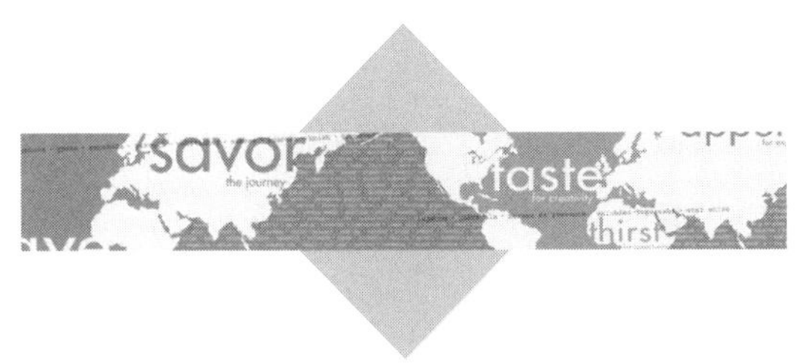

# Fatayer Sbanikh

## Triangle Spinach Pies

YIELD: ABOUT 15 TRIANGLES

| AMOUNT | MEASURE | INGREDIENT |
|---|---|---|
| **Dough** | | |
| 1 $\frac{1}{2}$ teaspoons | 8 g | Dry yeast |
| 1 cup | 8 ounces, 240 ml | Warm water |
| 1 teaspoon | 5 g | Salt |
| 4 cups | 16 ounces, 448 g | All-purpose flour |
| $\frac{1}{2}$ cup | 4 ounces, 120 ml | Olive oil |
| **Spinach Filling** | | |
| 6 cups | 12 ounces, 336 g | Fresh spinach, leaves and small stems, washed |
| 3 tablespoons | 1 $\frac{1}{2}$ ounces, 45 ml | Olive oil |
| $\frac{1}{2}$ cup | 2 ounces, 48 g | Onion, $\frac{1}{8}$ inch (.3 cm) dice |
| $\frac{1}{4}$ cup | 1 ounce, 28 g | Pine nuts or chopped walnuts |
| 1 tablespoon | 15 g | Sumac* |
| 2 tablespoons | 1 ounce, 30 ml | Fresh lemon juice |
| $\frac{1}{4}$ teaspoon | | Nutmeg |
| To taste | | Salt and freshly ground black pepper |

*If not using the sumac, increase lemon juice to taste.

### PROCEDURE

**Dough**

1 Soak yeast in warm water for 5 minutes.

2 Combine salt and flour.

3 Add oil to water and yeast mixture; stir to combine.

4 Make a well in the center of the flour mixture and gradually add yeast mixture, combining as you add the liquid.

5 Knead for 10 to 15 minutes until the dough is soft and not sticky.

6 Cover and let rise in a warm place 1 to 1$\frac{1}{2}$ hours or until double in size.

**Spinach Filling**

1 Chop spinach finely.

2 Cook spinach in a dry nonreactive deep pan, uncovered, until wilted and almost dry, about 4 minutes. Stir often.

3 When wilted, turn into a colander and press with the back of a spoon to remove as much moisture as possible.

4 Heat olive oil over medium heat and cook onion until transparent, 2 minutes.

5 Add spinach and cook 2 to 3 minutes longer.

6 Add pine nuts, lemon juice, and seasoning. Cook an additional 5 minutes or until moisture has evaporated. Cool.

7 Punch down dough and roll out on a lightly floured board until $\frac{1}{4}$ inch (.6 cm) thick. Cut into 4 inch (10.2 cm) squares; cover any unused dough.

8 Place a tablespoon of spinach filling in center of each square and fold corner to corner and pinch tightly. Press edges firmly with fingertips to seal pies completely.

9 Place close together on lightly oiled baking pans and brush each parcel with additional olive oil. Bake in a 350°F (180°C) preheated oven 10 to 15 minutes or until golden brown.

10 Serve hot or warm.

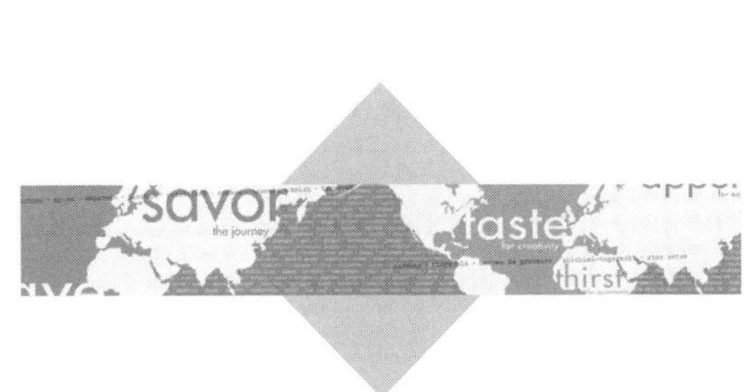

# Tabbouleh
## Cracked Wheat and Herb Salad

SERVES 4

| AMOUNT | MEASURE | INGREDIENT |
|---|---|---|
| $\frac{1}{2}$ cup | 3.5 ounces, 98 g | Bulgur wheat, fine |
| $1\frac{1}{4}$ cups | 10 ounces, 300 ml | Cold water |
| $1\frac{1}{4}$ cups | 2.25 ounces, 63 g | Flat-leaf parsley, coarsely chopped |
| $\frac{1}{2}$ cup | 2 ounces, 48 g | Green onions, coarsely chopped |
| $\frac{1}{4}$ cup | 1 ounce, 28 g | Mint, coarsely chopped |
| $2\frac{1}{2}$ tablespoons | 1.5 ounces, 45 ml | Olive oil |
| $1\frac{1}{2}$ tablespoons | $\frac{3}{4}$ ounce, 23 ml | Fresh lemon juice |
| 1 teaspoon | 5 g | Salt |
| $\frac{1}{2}$ teaspoon | 3 g | Black pepper, freshly ground |
| $\frac{1}{2}$ cup | 3 ounces, 84 g | Tomato, peeled, seeded $\frac{1}{4}$ inch (.6 cm) dice |
| 4 | | Romaine leaves |
| $\frac{1}{4}$ cup | 2 ounces, 60 ml | Fresh lemon juice |
| $\frac{1}{2}$ teaspoon | | Salt |

PROCEDURE

1. Cover bulgur with cold water; soak 30 minutes. Drain through a fine sieve, pressing with back of a spoon to extract moisture. Spread out on a lined pan to dry further.
2. Wash parsley, shake off excess, and remove thick stalks. Wrap in cheesecloth and refrigerate for 30 minutes to dry and crisp.
3. Combine dry bulgur and green onions; squeeze mixture so bulgur absorbs onion flavor.
4. Chop parsley, measure, and add to bulgur with mint.
5. Combine olive oil, $1\frac{1}{2}$ tablespoons ($\frac{3}{4}$ ounce, 23 ml) lemon juice, 1 teaspoon (5 g) salt, and black pepper; add to bulgur and toss well.
6. Gently stir in tomato; cover and chill 1 hour or more.
7. Serve with romaine. Combine remaining lemon juice and salt to serve on the side, to be added according to individual taste.

# Khobz

## Whole Wheat Flat Bread

YIELD: 6 ROUNDS

**Whole wheat: Whole grains that have been milled to a finer texture rather than leaving the grain intact become whole wheat. Whole wheat contains all the components of the grain, so whole wheat foods are also whole grain. Whole wheat bread and rye bread are typical examples of products made with whole wheat.**

| AMOUNT | MEASURE | INGREDIENT |
|---|---|---|
| 1 1/2 cups | 6 ounces, 168 g | Whole wheat flour |
| 1/2 teaspoon | 3 g | Salt |
| 1/2 cup | | Tepid water |
| As needed | | Oil |

**PROCEDURE**

1. Combine flour and salt.
2. Add water and work to a soft dough.
3. Knead for 10 minutes. Dough will feel slightly sticky at first but will become smooth as it is kneaded.
4. Cover and rest for at least 2 hours.
5. Divide dough into 6 even-sized balls the size of a large egg; roll out to 6-inch (15 cm) diameter rounds. Dough should be shaped without flour; dust lightly with white flour if needed.
6. Cover and rest rounds 20 minutes.
7. Heat a heavy frying pan or flat griddle. Cooking surface is hot enough when a little water sprinkled on bounces off the surface. Rub surface with a little oil.
8. Put in a round of dough and cook for about 1 minute, pressing top lightly with a folded cloth to encourage even bubbling of dough. When browned on the first side, turn and cook 1 minute or until bread looks cooked.
9. As breads are cooked, wrap in a cloth to keep soft and warm. Rub cooking surface occasionally with oil.

# Kukuye Mohi

## Fish Omelet SERVES 4

| AMOUNT | MEASURE | INGREDIENT |
|---|---|---|
| 12 ounces | 336 g | White fish fillets, skinless, boneless |
| 1 teaspoon | 5 g | Salt |
| $\frac{1}{4}$ cup | 2 ounces, 60 ml | Samneh (clarified butter) |
| $\frac{1}{2}$ cup | 3 ounces, 84 g | Onion, $\frac{1}{4}$ inch (.6 cm) dice |
| $\frac{1}{2}$ teaspoon | 3 g | Turmeric |
| 1 tablespoon | 5 g | Coriander leaves, finely chopped |
| 1 tablespoon | 15 g | All-purpose flour |
| 4 | | Large eggs |
| To taste | | Black pepper, freshly ground |

**PROCEDURE**

1. Preheat oven to 350°F (180°C).
2. Salt fish fillet and let sit 10 minutes.
3. Heat half the samneh over medium heat and sauté fish until cooked; fish does not have to brown. Remove, flake with a fork, and remove all bones.
4. In the same pan, add the onions and cook 3 minutes until transparent. Stir in turmeric and cook 2 minutes. Mix into fish with coriander and flour.
5. Beat eggs well with a pinch of salt. Add to fish mixture and season with pepper.
6. Heat remaining samneh in an 8-inch (20 cm) nonstick cake pan or casserole dish; swirl to coat base and sides.
7. Pour in egg mixture and bake in preheated oven for 30 minutes. Top should be slightly brown.
8. Unmold onto serving platter and serve hot or cold, cut into wedges.

# Bamia Lamb and Okra Casserole

SERVES 4

| AMOUNT | MEASURE | INGREDIENT |
|---|---|---|
| 2 tablespoons | 1 ounce, 30 ml | Samneh (clarified butter) |
| 12 ounces | 336 g | Boneless stewing lamb, 1 $\frac{1}{4}$ inch (3 cm) dice |
| $\frac{3}{4}$ cup | 4 ounces, 112 g | Onion, $\frac{1}{8}$ inch (.3 cm) dice |
| $\frac{1}{2}$ teaspoon | 2 g | Cumin, ground |
| $\frac{2}{3}$ cup | 4 ounces, 112 g | Tomato, peeled, seeded, $\frac{1}{4}$ inch (.6 cm) dice |
| 1 tablespoon | $\frac{1}{2}$ ounce, 14 g | Tomato paste |
| $\frac{1}{2}$ cup | 4 ounces, 120 ml | Lamb, beef, or chicken stock |
| To taste | | Salt and black pepper |
| $\frac{1}{2}$ teaspoon | 2 g | Granulated sugar |
| 12 ounces | 336 g | Fresh okra |
| 1 tablespoon | $\frac{1}{2}$ ounce, 15 ml | Samneh (clarified butter) |
| As needed | | Ta'leya I (recipe follows) |

PROCEDURE

1. Heat 2 tablespoons samneh over medium heat and brown meat on all sides. Transfer to another container as meat browns.
2. Reduce heat and add onions to the same pan the meat was browned in and cook 2 to 3 minutes until transparent. Add cumin, tomatoes, tomato paste, and cook 1 minute.
3. Add stock and stir well to collect browned sediment.
4. Return meat to pan, correct seasoning, and add sugar.
5. Cover and cook in a moderately slow oven or on top of stove for 1 $\frac{1}{2}$ hour or until meat is almost tender.
6. Prepare okra, remove stem, leave whole.
7. Heat remaining samneh (clarified butter) over medium heat and sauté okra 3 minutes, tossing as needed.
8. Arrange okra on top of meat; cover and cook until okra and meat are tender.
9. Prepare ta'leya and pour while hot over bamia. Serve at the table from the cooking dish.

# Muaddas Rice with Lentils SERVES 4

| AMOUNT | MEASURE | INGREDIENT |
|---|---|---|
| **1 cup** | **7 ounces, 196 g** | **Basmati (quality long-grain) rice** |
| **$\frac{1}{2}$ cup** | **3.5 ounces, 98 g** | **Brown or green lentils** |
| **2 tablespoons** | **1 ounce, 30 ml** | **Samneh (clarified butter)** |
| **$\frac{1}{2}$ cup** | **2 ounces, 56 g** | **Onion, $\frac{1}{4}$ inch (.6 cm) dice** |
| **2 cups** | **16 ounces, 480 ml** | **Boiling water** |
| **1 teaspoon** | **5 g** | **Salt** |

**PROCEDURE**

1 Pick over rice and wash in several changes of cold water until water runs clear. Drain well.

2 Pick over lentils to remove small stones and discolored seeds. Put in a bowl of water and remove any that float. Wash lentils well and drain thoroughly.

3 In a heavy, deep pan heat the samneh over medium high heat and sauté the onions until transparent and lightly browned.

4 Add rice and lentils; cook 3 to 4 minutes, stirring often.

5 Add boiling water and salt; return to a boil, stirring occasionally. Reduce heat to low, cover pan, and simmer gently 25 to 30 minutes.

6 Remove cover and cook 5 minutes longer. Fluff the rice with a fork and serve.

## Ta'leya I: Garlic Sauce

| AMOUNT | MEASURE | INGREDIENT |
|---|---|---|
| **4** | | **Garlic cloves** |
| **$\frac{1}{2}$ teaspoon** | **3 g** | **Salt** |
| **2 tablespoons** | **1 ounce, 30 ml** | **Samneh (clarified butter)** |
| **1 teaspoon** | | **Coriander, ground** |
| **Pinch** | | **Hot chile pepper** |

**PROCEDURE**

1 Crush garlic with salt in a mortar to make a garlic paste.

2 Heat samneh in a small pan and add garlic. Cook, stirring constantly, until golden brown; remove pan from heat and stir in coriander and pepper. Use while sizzling hot.

# Khoshaf Dried Fruit Compote

SERVES 4

| AMOUNT | MEASURE | INGREDIENT |
|---|---|---|
| $\frac{3}{4}$ cup | 3 ounces, 84 g | Prunes, pitted, coarse chopped |
| $\frac{3}{4}$ cup | 3 ounces, 84 g | Dried apricots, coarse chopped |
| $\frac{3}{4}$ cup | 3 ounces, 84 g | Sultanas (white raisins) |
| As needed | | Water to cover |
| $\frac{1}{3}$ cup | 2.3 ounces, 9.4 g | Granulated sugar |
| 1 | | Thin strip of lemon rind |
| 2 | | Cloves |
| $\frac{1}{4}$ teaspoon | | Allspice, ground |
| 2 tablespoons | $\frac{1}{2}$ ounce, 14 g | Walnuts, chopped |

PROCEDURE

1. Wash dried fruits well.
2. Place in a pan with cold water just to cover. Bring to boil, reduce to simmer, and cook over low heat 15 minutes.
3. Add sugar, lemon rind, and spices. Stir to dissolve and add water if necessary. Simmer gently, uncovered, until fruit is soft but not mushy, and syrup is thick. Remove lemon rind and whole spices.
4. Chill well before serving. Serve in dessert glasses sprinkled with chopped nuts.

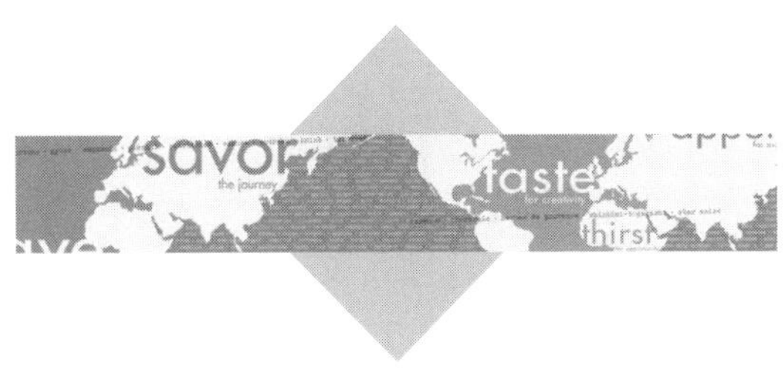

# Qahwah Arabic Coffee

SERVES 4

**Chef Tip** **Cardamom has a very strong flavor, and too much of it can cause a soapy taste.**

| AMOUNT | MEASURE | INGREDIENT |
|---|---|---|
| 1 | | Cardamom pods |
| 1 cup | 8 ounces, 240 ml | Water |
| $\frac{1}{4}$ cup | $\frac{1}{2}$ ounce, 14 g | Dark roast ground coffee beans |

PROCEDURE

1. Bruise cardamom pods.
2. Combine all ingredients and bring to boil.
3. Serve in Arabic coffee cups, half filled.

Traditionally a little silver urn of rose water or orange blossom water accompanies the coffee, so a few drops may be added to individual taste. Sugar is not generally served.

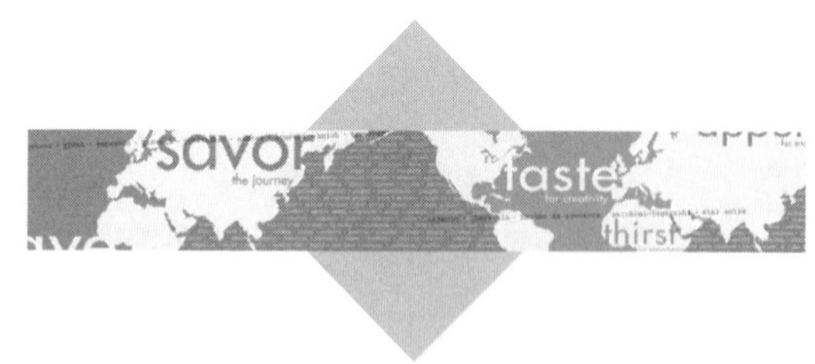

# Borani Chogondar

## Beet and Yogurt Salad

SERVES 4

**Chef Tip** **To make drained yogurt, place yogurt in cheesecloth, tie with string, and suspend from a fixed object over a receptacle to collect draining liquid. Hang for 2 to 4 hours, depending on initial thickness of yogurt. When drained, yogurt should have the consistency of softened cream cheese.**

| AMOUNT | MEASURE | INGREDIENT |
|---|---|---|
| 1 pound | 448 g | Beets, mixed red and golden, if available |
| $1\frac{1}{2}$ cups | 12 ounces, 360 ml | Drained yogurt |
| To taste | | Salt and pepper |
| To taste | | Vinegar or fresh lemon juice (optional) |
| 1 tablespoon | | Fresh mint, chopped |
| For garnish | | Fresh mint leaves |

PROCEDURE

1. Preheat oven to 400°F (205°C).
2. Rinse beets, leaving on roots and 1 inch (2.5 cm) of stems. Bake, covered, with $\frac{1}{4}$ inch (.6 cm) water, 25 to 40 minutes or until beets can be easily pierced with a knife. Cool.
3. When the beets are cool enough to handle, peel and dice $\frac{1}{2}$ inch (1.3 cm).
4. Reserve about $\frac{1}{4}$ cup (2 ounces, 60 ml) diced beets. Mix remainder into yogurt with salt and pepper to taste. Sharpen the flavor with vinegar or lemon if desired.
5. Blend in mint; cover and chill.
6. Serve garnished with reserved beets and mint leaves.

# Falafel Dried Bean Croquettes

YIELD: ABOUT 35 CROQUETTES

**Chef Tip** **Favas have a wonderful flavor, but if you can't find them, dried white beans, such as cannellini or navy, can be substituted.**

| AMOUNT | MEASURE | INGREDIENT |
|---|---|---|
| 1 cup | 6 ounces, 168 g | Fava beans (broad beans), dried and shelled, soaked overnight and drained |
| 1 cup | 6 ounces, 168 g | Garbanzo beans (chickpeas), dried, soaked overnight, and drained |
| $\frac{1}{2}$ cup | 2 ounces, 56 g | Onion, $\frac{1}{4}$ inch (.6 cm) dice |
| 2 | | Garlic cloves |
| $\frac{1}{2}$ cup | 1 ounce, 28 g | Flat-leaf parsley, finely chopped |
| 2 tablespoons | 6 g | Cilantro leaves, finely chopped |
| $\frac{1}{8}$ teaspoon | | Hot chile pepper, ground |
| 1 teaspoon | 4 g | Coriander, ground |
| $\frac{1}{2}$ teaspoon | 2 g | Cumin, ground |
| 1 teaspoon | 4 g | Baking soda |
| To taste | | Salt and freshly ground black pepper |
| | | Oil for deep-frying |
| As needed | | Taratour bi tahini (recipe follows) |
| As needed | | Khoubiz (Arabic flat bread; see recipe on page 438) |

PROCEDURE

1. Combine fava beans, chickpeas, onion, and garlic and grind twice in food grinder using a fine die, or process in food processor to form a coarse paste.
2. Combine with remaining ingredients except oil and tahini. Knead well and let rest for 30 minutes. Correct seasoning.
3. Shape a tablespoon of the mixture at a time into balls, then flatten into thick patties $1\frac{1}{2}$ inches (4 cm) in diameter. Let rest 30 minutes at room temperature.
4. Deep-fry in two inches of oil at 375°F (190°C), 6 to 8 at a time; cook 4 to 5 minutes, turning to brown evenly. Falafel should be toasty brown and crunchy on the outside. Remove and drain on a paper towel.
5. Serve hot as an appetizer with taratour bi tahini or in split khoubiz with the same sauce and salad vegetables.

## Taratour bi Tahini

YIELD: ABOUT 1 $\frac{1}{2}$ CUPS

| AMOUNT | MEASURE | INGREDIENT |
|---|---|---|
| 2 | | Garlic cloves, crushed with $\frac{1}{2}$ teaspoon salt |
| $\frac{1}{2}$ cup | 4 ounces, 120 ml | Tahini |
| $\frac{1}{4}$–$\frac{1}{2}$ cup | 2–4 ounces, 60–120 ml | Cold water |
| $\frac{1}{2}$ cup | 4 ounces, 120 ml | Fresh lemon juice |
| To taste | | Salt |

**PROCEDURE**

1. Using a food processor, combine garlic and tahini until smooth.
2. Beat in a little water and lemon juice alternately. The water thickens the mixture; lemon juice thins it.
3. Add all the lemon juice and enough water to give a thin or thick consistency, depending on the use. Correct seasoning; flavor should be tart.

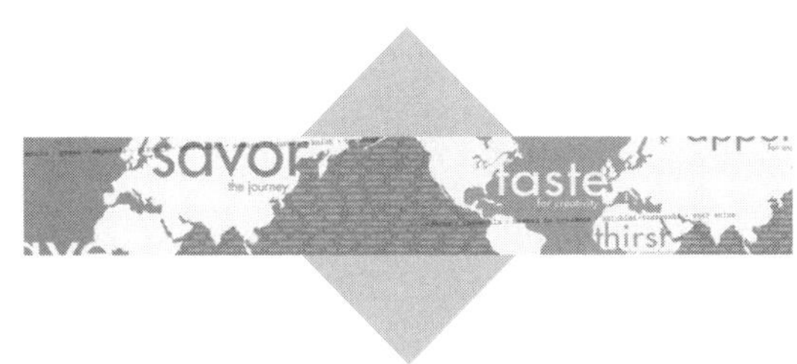

# Khubz (Khoubiz) Arabic Flat Bread

YIELD: ABOUT 10 6-INCH KHUBZ

**Chef Tip** **To cook in a sauté pan, preheat pan on highest heat with lid on. When heated, oil the base of the pan quickly and slide in the dough. Cover and cook 3 minutes, remove lid, turn bread over, re-cover, and cook 2 minutes.**

| AMOUNT | MEASURE | INGREDIENT |
|---|---|---|
| **½ cup** | **4 ounces, 120 ml** | **Warm water** |
| **2 teaspoons** | **8 g** | **Active dry yeast** |
| **4 cups** | **16 ounces, 448 g** | **Bread flour** |
| **1 teaspoon** | **5 g** | **Salt** |
| **1 cup** | **8 ounces, 240 ml** | **Warm milk** |
| **As needed** | | **Olive oil** |

PROCEDURE

1. Set a pizza stone on the bottom rack of a preheated 500°F (260°C) oven.
2. Combine warm water and yeast; let stand until foamy, about 10 minutes.
3. In a mixer, food processor, or by hand, combine flour and salt.
4. Add yeast mixture and then the warm milk; work to form dough.
5. On a lightly floured surface, knead one minute. Form the dough into a ball.
6. Lightly oil a bowl with olive oil. Transfer the dough to the bowl and turn to coat; cover and let rise in a warm place until doubled in bulk, about 1 hour.
7. Lightly dust a work surface with flour. Punch down dough and cut in half. Cut each half into 5 pieces, roll them into balls, then flatten into 6-inch rounds; cover. Let rise until puffy, 25 minutes.
8. Rub stone with oil and then slide dough rounds a few at a time onto it. Bake for 4 to 5 minutes until it puffs up like a balloon. To brown, turn quickly and leave for one minute. Remove bread and wrap in a cloth to keep warm and soft.

# Baba Ghannouj (Moutabal)

## Eggplant Dip

SERVES 4

| AMOUNT | MEASURE | INGREDIENT |
|---|---|---|
| 1 medium | 12 ounces, 336 g | Eggplant |
| $\frac{1}{4}$ cup | 2 ounces, 60 ml | Fresh lemon juice |
| $\frac{1}{4}$ cup | 2 ounces, 60 ml | Tahini |
| 2 | | Garlic cloves |
| 2 teaspoons or to taste | 10 g | Salt |
| 1 tablespoon | $\frac{1}{2}$ ounce, 15 ml | Olive oil |
| $\frac{1}{4}$ cup | $\frac{1}{2}$ ounce, 14 g | Flat-leaf parsley, chopped fine |
| As needed | | Khoubiz (Arabic flat bread; see recipe on page 438) |

**PROCEDURE**

1. Grill eggplant or roast in a hot oven, turning often; cook until soft.
2. Peel off skin while hot and remove stem and end if still firm.
3. Chop flesh and pound to a puree in a mortar with pestle, or puree in a blender or food processor.
4. Blend in $\frac{3}{4}$ of the lemon juice and gradually add the tahini.
5. Crush garlic to a paste with 1 teaspoon salt and add to eggplant. Beat well; adjust flavor with more lemon juice and salt.
6. Beat in olive oil and parsley. Do not puree the parsley.
7. Serve with khoubiz as an appetizer.

# Morgh Polou Chicken with Rice

SERVES 4

| AMOUNT | MEASURE | INGREDIENT |
|---|---|---|
| $2\frac{1}{2}$ to 3 pounds | 1.15–1.4 kg | Chicken, cut into 8 pieces |
| To taste | | Salt and black pepper |
| $\frac{1}{4}$ cup | 2 ounces, 60 ml | Samneh (clarified butter) |
| 1 cup | 4 ounces, 112 g | Onion, $\frac{1}{4}$ inch (.6 cm) dice |
| $\frac{1}{2}$ cup | 3 ounces, 84 g | Dried apricots, coarsely chopped |
| $\frac{1}{2}$ cup | 3 ounces, 84 g | Sultanas (white raisins) |
| $\frac{1}{2}$ teaspoon | | Cinnamon, ground |
| $\frac{1}{4}$ cup | 2 ounces, 60 ml | Water |
| 8 cups | 64 ounces, 1.89 liters | Water |
| 2 tablespoons | 1 ounce, 28 g | Salt |
| 2 cups | 14 ounces, 392 g | Basmati (quality-long grain) rice |
| $\frac{1}{4}$ cup | 2 ounces, 30 ml | Samneh (clarified butter) |
| $\frac{1}{4}$ cup | 2 ounces, 30 ml | Water |
| $\frac{1}{2}$ teaspoon | | Saffron threads |

**PROCEDURE**

1. Wipe chicken pieces dry with paper towels and season.
2. Heat half the first quantity of samneh and brown chicken well on all sides. Remove.
3. Add remaining samneh to same pan and sauté onion until transparent.
4. Add fruit and cook 5 minutes over low heat.
5. Stir in cinnamon and add $\frac{1}{4}$ cup (2 ounces, 60 ml) water to deglaze pan.
6. Wash rice until water runs clear; drain.
7. Bring 8 cups of water to a boil, add salt and rice, stir, and return to boil.
8. Boil for 5 minutes. Pour immediately into a large sieve or colander and drain.
9. Combine second quantity of samneh and $\frac{1}{4}$ cup water; bring to boil. Pour half into pan the rice was cooked in and swirl to coat base and sides.
10. Spread half the partly cooked rice in base of pan, and even out with back of spoon.
11. Place chicken pieces on top of rice. Spread apricot mixture over chicken and top with remaining rice and samneh mixture.

12 Cover top of pan with clean doubled tea towel or 2 paper towels, place lid on tightly, and cook over low heat (or in the oven) for 40 minutes or until chicken is tender. The cloth absorbs the steam and makes the rice fluffy and light.

13 While polou is cooking, boil 2 tablespoons (1 ounce, 30 ml) water and mix with saffron. Leave aside to steep.

14 Just before serving, sprinkle saffron liquid over rice and stir in gently. Serve piled on a platter.

# Adas Bis Silq

## Lentil and Swiss Chard Soup

SERVES 4

| AMOUNT | MEASURE | INGREDIENT |
| --- | --- | --- |
| 1 cup | 6 ounces, 168 g | Brown lentils |
| 4 cups | 32 ounces, 960 ml | Cold water |
| $\frac{1}{4}$ cup | 2 ounces, 60 ml | Olive oil |
| $\frac{1}{2}$ cup | 3 ounces, 84 g | Onion, $\frac{1}{4}$ inch (.6 cm) dice |
| 2 | | Garlic cloves, minced |
| 4 cups | 8 ounces, 224 g | Swiss chard leaves, washed, shredded coarsely |
| $\frac{1}{4}$ cup | $\frac{1}{2}$ ounce, 14 g | Cilantro leaves, coarsely chopped |
| To taste | | Salt and freshly ground black pepper |
| 3 tablespoons | 1$\frac{1}{2}$ ounces, 45 ml | Fresh lemon juice |

### PROCEDURE

1 Pick over lentils to remove small stones and discolored seeds. Put in a bowl of water and remove any that float. Wash lentils well and drain thoroughly.

2 Cover lentils with the cold water; bring to boil, skimming if necessary, then cover and simmer gently for 1 hour or until soft.

3 Heat oil over medium heat and sauté onions until transparent. Stir in garlic and cook for 15 seconds.

4 Add shredded Swiss chard to the onion mixture; cook, stirring often, until wilted.

5 Add onion mixture to cooked lentils, add remaining ingredients, and simmer gently, 15 to 20 minutes.

6 Serve with lemon wedges and khoubiz or other bread.

# Baklawa "Be'aj" Fillo and Nut Pastries

YIELD: ABOUT 20 PASTRIES

**Chef Tip** **The butter firms fairly quickly and it could be difficult to shape pastries if the buttered sheets are left for a long time. It is advisable to fill and shape in lots.**

| AMOUNT | MEASURE | INGREDIENT |
|---|---|---|
| $\frac{1}{2}$ pound | 8 ounces, 224 g | Fillo pastry |
| $\frac{1}{2}$ cup | 4 ounces, 120 ml | Samneh or unsalted butter, melted |
| Nut Filling | | |
| 1 | | Egg white |
| $\frac{1}{4}$ cup | 2 ounces, 56 g | Granulated sugar |
| 1 cup | 4 ounces, 112 g | Walnuts, coarsely ground |
| 1 cup | 4 ounces, 112 g | Almonds, coarsely ground |
| 1 teaspoon | 5 ml | Rose water |
| Atar Syrup | | |
| 1 cup | 7 ounces, 196 g | Granulated sugar |
| $\frac{3}{4}$ cup | 6 ounces, 180 ml | Water |
| $\frac{1}{2}$ teaspoon | | Fresh lemon juice |
| $\frac{1}{2}$ teaspoon | | Orange flower water |
| $\frac{1}{2}$ teaspoon | | Rose water |
| Garnish | | |
| $\frac{1}{2}$ cup | 2 ounces, 56 g | Pistachio nuts, peeled, chopped |

PROCEDURE

1. Stack 10 sheets fillo dough on a flat surface, keeping any reminder covered with a dry towel, then a damp towel on top.
2. Brush top sheet of stack with melted butter, lift sheet, and replace on stack, buttered side down. Brush top with butter, lift top two sheets, and turn over on stack. Repeat until all 10 sheets are buttered, lifting an extra sheet each time. Top and bottom of finished stack should remain unbuttered.
3. Cut stack into 4-inch (10 cm) squares. Stack and cover. Prepare any remaining sheets.

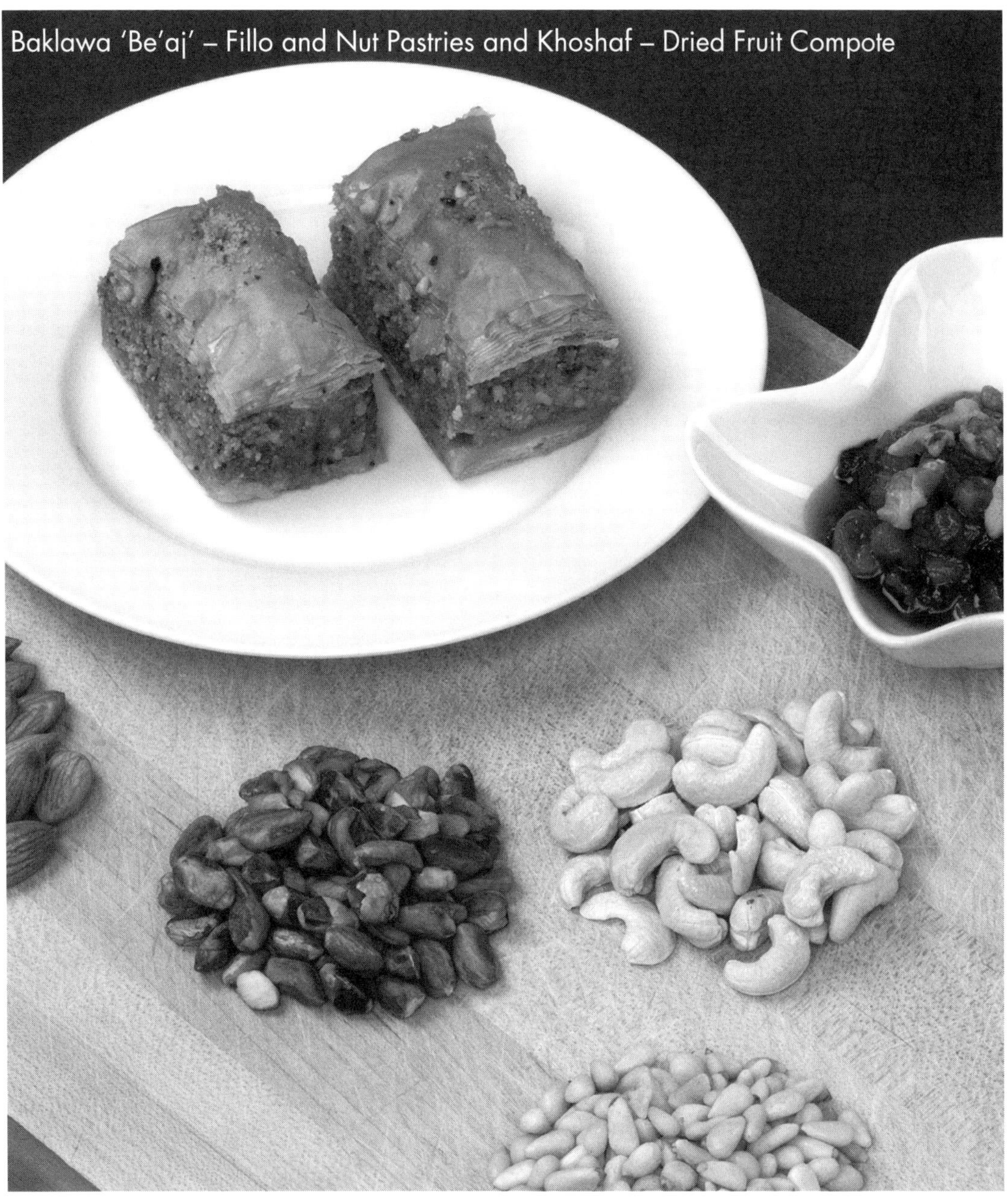

Baklawa 'Be'aj' – Fillo and Nut Pastries and Khoshaf – Dried Fruit Compote

4 Beat egg white until stiff and beat sugar in gradually. Fold in walnuts, almonds, and rose water.

5 Butter top of fillo square and place a tablespoon of nut mixture in the center. Gently squeeze into a lily shape, with four corners of square as petals and filling in center.

6 Place in a buttered baking pan close together.

7 Bake at 350°F (180°C) for 30 minutes; reduce to 300°F (150°C) and cook 15 minutes longer.

8 To make syrup, dissolve sugar in water over high heat, add lemon juice and orange flower water, and bring to boil. Boil 15 minutes, remove from heat, add rose water, and cool.

9 Spoon cool thick syrup over hot pastries. Leave until cool and sprinkle pistachio nuts in center.

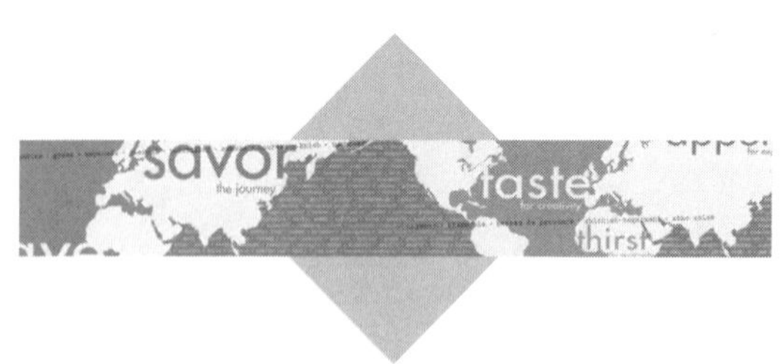

# Muhammara

## Red Pepper and Walnut Dip

SERVES 4

| AMOUNT | MEASURE | INGREDIENT |
|---|---|---|
| 1 pound | 448 g | Red bell peppers |
| $\frac{1}{2}$ cup | 2 ounces, 56 g | Walnuts, coarsely ground |
| 2 tablespoons | | Bread crumbs or sesame cracker crumbs |
| 1 tablespoon | $\frac{1}{2}$ ounce, 15 ml | Pomegranate molasses |
| 1 tablespoon | $\frac{1}{2}$ ounce, 15 ml | Fresh lemon juice |
| $\frac{1}{2}$ teaspoon, plus more for dusting | | Cumin, ground |
| $\frac{1}{2}$ teaspoon | | Aleppo pepper, or $\frac{1}{4}$ teaspoon crushed red pepper or red chile paste |
| To taste | | Salt and pepper |
| 1 tablespoon | $\frac{1}{2}$ ounce, 15 ml | Olive oil |

**PROCEDURE**

1. Roast bell peppers over gas flame or under broiler, turning until blackened and blistered. Wrap with film or place in a bag to steam 10 minutes to loosen the skin. Let cool slightly; remove skin, membranes, stems, and seeds. Allow to drain.
2. Combine walnuts and bread crumbs in a food processor and process until finely ground.
3. Add bell peppers, pomegranate molasses, lemon juice, cumin, and aleppo or crushed red pepper; blend until creamy. Adjust seasoning with salt, pepper, and aleppo or crushed peppers.
4. Chill at least two hours.
5. Serve with a dusting of ground cumin and a drizzle of olive oil.

# Besara Broad Bean Puree SERVES 4

| AMOUNT | MEASURE | INGREDIENT |
|---|---|---|
| 3 cups | 18 ounces, 504 g | Broad beans (fava), cooked, skin removed |
| To taste | | Salt and pepper |
| 2 teaspoons | | Dried mint |
| Garnish | | |
| | | Ta'leya II (recipe follows) |
| | | Olive oil |
| | | Chopped onion |
| | | Lemon wedges |

**PROCEDURE**

1. Pass the beans through a sieve or puree in a food processor.
2. Add enough hot water to give the beans a dip consistency.
3. Season to taste with salt and pepper and add mint; simmer 5 minutes.
4. Serve hot in small bowls, garnishing each with ta'leya.
5. Serve with a cruet of olive oil, chopped raw onion, and lemon wedges.

## Ta'leya II

| AMOUNT | MEASURE | INGREDIENT |
|---|---|---|
| $\frac{1}{4}$ cup | 2 ounces, 60 ml | Olive oil |
| 2 cups | 8 ounces, 224 g | Onions, thin semicircle cuts |
| 2 | | Garlic cloves, minced |

**PROCEDURE**

1. Heat oil over medium heat and sauté onions until golden brown.
2. Add garlic and cook 1 minute.

# Samke Harrah al-Sahara

## Baked Fish with Hot Chile Sauce SERVES 4

| AMOUNT | MEASURE | INGREDIENT |
|---|---|---|
| 1 | 4 pound, 1.81 kg | Snapper or other baking fish, cleaned, scaled, head on but eyes removed |
| As needed | | Salt |
| $\frac{1}{2}$ cup | 4 ounces, 120 ml | Olive oil, for frying |
| 4 | | Garlic cloves |
| 1 teaspoon | | Salt |
| $\frac{1}{4}$ cup | $\frac{1}{2}$ ounce, 14 g | Cilantro leaves, finely chopped |
| | | |
| $\frac{1}{2}$ cup | 4 ounces, 120 ml | Cold water |
| 1 cup | 8 ounces, 240 ml | Tahini |
| $\frac{1}{2}$ cup | 4 ounces, 120 ml | Fresh lemon juice |
| $\frac{1}{4}$–$\frac{1}{2}$ teaspoon | | Hot chile pepper |
| 1 tablespoon | | Pine nuts |
| For garnish | | Lemon wedges and coriander sprigs |

**PROCEDURE**

1. Preheat oven to 350°F (180°C).
2. Slash snapper in 2 places on each side. Sprinkle inside and out with salt; cover and refrigerate 1 hour. Pat dry before cooking.
3. Heat all but 1 tablespoon oil in large sauté pan and fry fish on high heat for 2 to 3 minutes on each side. Do not cook through. Remove from oil and place in baking dish.
4. Mash garlic with 1 teaspoon salt, and mix in cilantro.
5. Remove all but 2 tablespoons fat from sauté pan and reheat. Add garlic mixture; fry until mixture is crisp but not burnt. Cool.
6. Gradually add water to tahini, beating constantly. Mixture will thicken, then add lemon juice gradually and stir in garlic mixture and chile pepper to taste.
7. Pour sauce over fish, covering fish completely. Bake in preheated oven for 30 to 35 minutes or until fish is cooked through and sauce is bubbling.
8. Toast pine nuts in reserved tablespoon oil until golden brown.
9. Lift cooked fish onto platter and spoon sauce on top. Sprinkle with pine nuts and garnish with lemon wedges and coriander sprigs.

# Shurabat al Kibbeh

## Kibbeh Soup

SERVES: 4

**Kibbeh**

| AMOUNT | MEASURE | INGREDIENT |
|---|---|---|
| 1 cup | 4 ounces, 112 g | Bulgur wheat |
| 11 ounces | 308 g | Lean lamb |
| $\frac{1}{3}$ cup | 1.5 ounces, 42 g | Onion, chopped |
| 1 teaspoon | | Salt |
| $\frac{1}{2}$ teaspoon | | Black pepper |
| $\frac{1}{3}$ teaspoon | | Allspice |
| | | Ice water or ice chips |

**PROCEDURE**

1. Cover bulgur with cold water and let soak 10 minutes. Drain in a sieve and press with back of spoon to remove as much moisture as possible. Lay out flat and chill 1 hour.
2. Trim all fat and fine skin from lamb; cut into cubes. Chill 1 hour.
3. Pass meat through a food grinder twice, using fine die. Grind onion twice and combine with meat, bulgur, salt, pepper, and allspice.
4. Pass through grinder twice, adding a little ice water if necessary to keep mixture cold.
5. Knead to a smooth, light paste with hands, adding ice water when necessary. Cover and chill.

**Soup**

| AMOUNT | MEASURE | INGREDIENT |
|---|---|---|
| As needed | | Kibbeh mixture |
| $\frac{1}{4}$ cup | 1 ounce, 28 g | Pine nuts |
| $\frac{1}{4}$ cup | 2 ounces, 60 ml | Samneh (clarified butter) |
| 1 cup | 4 ounces, 112 g | Onion, $\frac{1}{4}$ inch (.6 cm) dice |
| 4 cups | 32 ounces, 960 ml | Water or stock |
| 1 small piece | | Cinnamon strck |
| To taste | | Salt and pepper |
| $\frac{1}{3}$ cup | 2 ounces, 56 g | Short-grain rice, washed |
| $\frac{1}{4}$ cup | $\frac{1}{2}$ ounce, 14 g | Parsley, chopped, for garnish |

**PROCEDURE**

1. Shape kibbeh into balls the size of a walnut. Make a hole in each, insert two pine nuts, and re-form into balls.
2. Heat samneh and brown kibbeh balls, shaking pan so they keep the round shape and brown evenly. Remove and leave fat in pan.
3. Add onion to pan and sauté until soft, 3 to 5 minutes.
4. Add 1 cup water or stock and bring to boil, scraping bottom of the pan to get all the drippings.
5. Remove to a soup pot and add remaining liquid, cinnamon, salt and pepper to taste, and rice.
6. Bring to boil, stirring occasionally; simmer, covered, 10 minutes.
7. Add kibbeh balls; cover and simmer 15 to 20 minutes.
8. Correct seasoning.
9. Serve with parsley sprinkled on top.

# Fattoush

## Toasted Bread Salad

SERVES 4

| AMOUNT | MEASURE | INGREDIENT |
|---|---|---|
| 1 6-inch | | Khoubiz, toasted golden brown, $\frac{1}{2}$ inch (1.2 cm) dice |
| 3 cups | 6 ounces, 168 g | Romaine, shredded or broken into small pieces |
| $\frac{3}{4}$ cup | 4 ounces, 112 g | Cucumber, peeled, $\frac{1}{2}$ inch (1.2 cm) dice |
| 1 cup | 6 ounces, 168 g | Tomato, peeled, seeded, $\frac{1}{2}$ inch (1.2 cm) dice |
| $\frac{1}{3}$ cup | 1 ounce, 28 g | Green onion, chopped |
| $\frac{1}{3}$ cup | $\frac{1}{2}$ ounce, 14 g | Flat-leaf parsley, chopped |
| 3 tablespoons | | Fresh mint, chopped |
| $\frac{3}{4}$ cup | 3 ounces, 84 g | Green bell pepper, $\frac{1}{2}$ inch (1.2 cm) dice |
| As needed | | Salad dressing (recipe follows) |

PROCEDURE

1 Combine all ingredients and toss with salad dressing.

## Salad Dressing

| AMOUNT | MEASURE | INGREDIENT |
|---|---|---|
| 1 | | Garlic clove |
| 1 teaspoon | | Salt |
| $\frac{1}{2}$ cup | 4 ounces, 120 ml | Fresh lemon juice |
| $\frac{1}{2}$ cup | 4 ounces, 120 ml | Olive oil |
| To taste | | Black pepper |

PROCEDURE

1 Mash garlic with salt and stir in remaining ingredients.

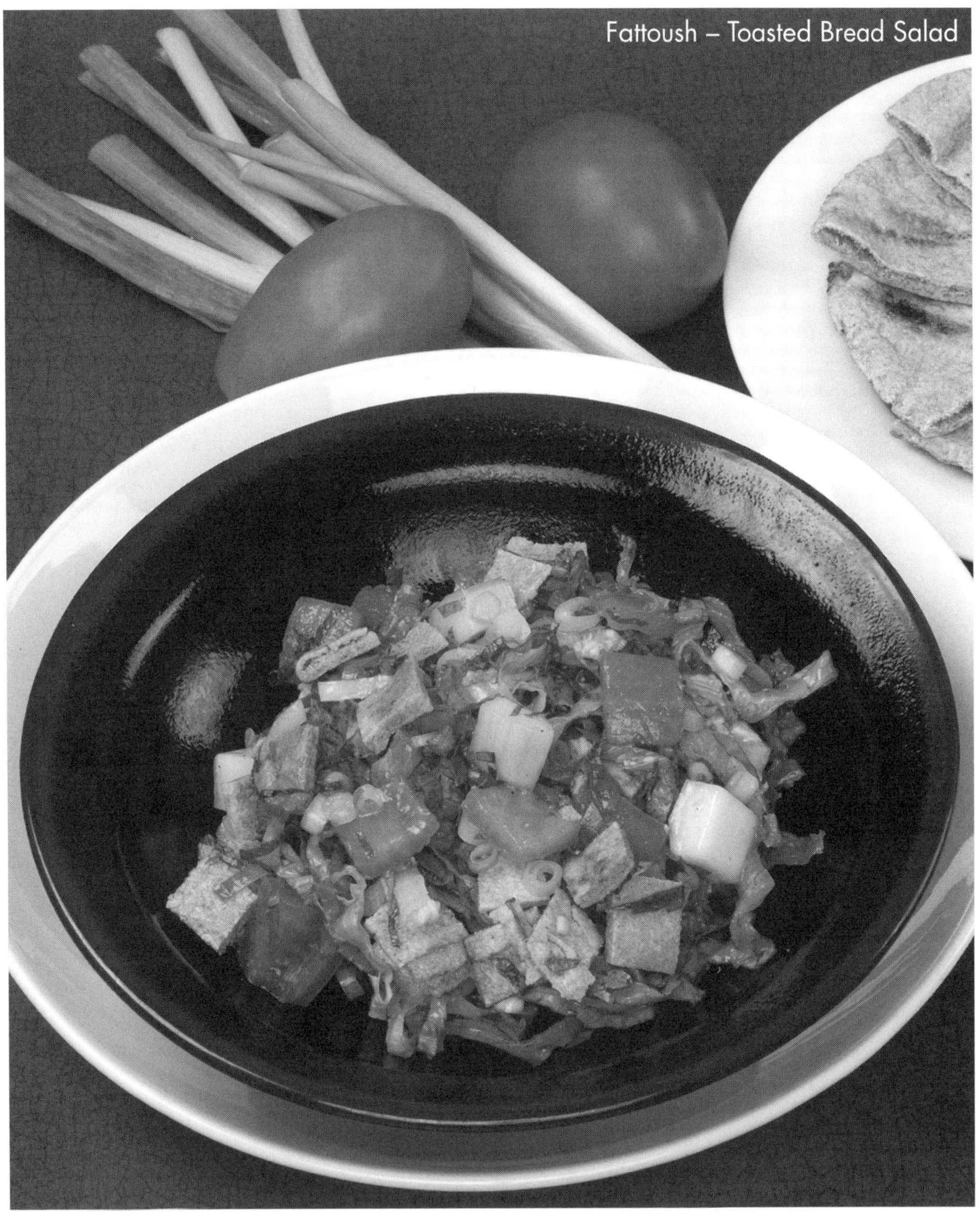

Fattoush – Toasted Bread Salad

# Nane Lavash (Taftoon)

## Flat Bread

YIELD: 4 ROUNDS

**The only difference between the breads is the size. Nane lavash is the better-known Persian bread, but it is very large. Taftoon is the same dough shaped in smaller rounds.**

| AMOUNT | MEASURE | INGREDIENT |
|---|---|---|
| $\frac{2}{3}$ cup | 3 ounces, 84 g | All-purpose flour |
| 2 cups | 8 ounces, 224 g | Whole wheat flour |
| 2 teaspoon | $\frac{1}{4}$ ounce, 7 g | Active dry yeast |
| 1$\frac{2}{3}$ cups | 13 ounces, 390 ml | Water |
| 1 teaspoon | 5 g | Salt |
| | | Oil for handling dough |

### PROCEDURE

1. Preheat oven to 500°F (260°C). Set a pizza stone or griddle on the center rack.
2. Sift flours together; discard any flakes left in sifter.
3. Dissolve yeast in $\frac{1}{4}$ cup (2 ounces, 60 ml) warm water. Combine warm water and yeast; let stand until foamy, about 10 minutes.
4. Add 1$\frac{1}{2}$ cups (12 ounces, 360 ml) of the remaining water and the salt.
5. Combine yeast with flour and mix using a dough hook on low speed for 15 to 20 minutes, gradually adding as much of the remaining $\frac{3}{4}$ cup (6 ounces, 180 ml) water as the dough will absorb. As the dough is worked, its ability to absorb water increases.
6. Oil your hands and divide dough into 4 equal-size pieces, shaping each into a ball.
7. Roll out one at a time as thin as possible with an oiled rolling pin. Prick well all over with a fork or pin wheel.
8. Take round and flip across the backs of your hands to stretch it.
9. Oil pizza stone or griddle and press dough on to it. Close oven and cook 1 minute; pat dough down again to prevent bread puffing up.
10. Bake until surface is bubbly, about 3 minutes; turn over and cook 2 minutes more. Remove and wrap in a cloth. Let oven regain heat and continue with remaining dough. Rolled-out dough should not rest before being baked.

# Tapauch Ets Im Mits Tapuzim

## Apples in Orange Juice

SERVES 4

| AMOUNT | MEASURE | INGREDIENT |
|---|---|---|
| 1 ½ cups | 12 ounces, 360 ml | Orange juice, fresh |
| 3 tablespoons | 1 ½ ounces, 42 g | Seedless raisins |
| 3 tablespoons | 1 ½ ounces, 42 g | Butter |
| 4 medium size | | Tart-eating apples |
| 2 teaspoons | | Cornstarch |
| 2 tablespoons | 1 ounce, 30 ml | Water |

PROCEDURE

1 Combine orange juice, raisins, and butter; bring to boil.
2 Peel, core, and cut the apples in half.
3 Add apples to orange juice; cover and simmer gently until tender and shape still holds.
4 Blend cornstarch with water and thicken liquid.
5 Serve warm with meal.

# Tan Yogurt Drink

***Tan* accompanies every Armenian meal.**

SERVES 4

| AMOUNT | MEASURE | INGREDIENT |
|---|---|---|
| 2 cups | 16 ounces, 480 ml | Plain yogurt |
| 1 cup | 8 ounces, 240 ml | Water |
| Salt | | Salt |

PROCEDURE

1 Process yogurt in blender until smooth.
2 Add water gradually, blending as you add, until mixture reaches a drink consistency. Add salt and chill well before serving.

# Turkey, Greece, and Crete

## The Land

### TURKEY

Turkey is located on two continents, Europe and Asia, and is close to where the three continents of Asia, Europe, and Africa come together. About 3 percent of the country lies within Europe and is called Eastern Thrace. The other 97 percent of Turkey is located in Asia and is called Anatolia, or Asia Minor. Unlike some of the lands that neighbor it, Turkey is not only a Middle Eastern country; it shares a lot of history with Europe and is considered to be one of the world's cradles of civilization. Over the centuries it has given birth to many civilizations, religions, empires, and states.

Turkey is shaped like a rectangle and is similar to a peninsula. To the north is the Black Sea; to the south is the Mediterranean Sea; and to the west is the Aegean Sea. The Bosporus Strait, the Sea of Marmara, and the Dardanelles Strait divide the continents of Europe and Asia from each other within Turkey. Turkey borders the countries of Greece, Bulgaria, Georgia, Armenia, Iran, Iraq, Azerbaijan, and Syria.

Geographically, Turkey can be divided into eight main regions, each with its own landscape and history. The small region of Eastern Thrace has rolling hills and fertile grasslands. This region produces maize, wine, and tobacco. Herds of sheep graze on the hilly slopes. The northern Black Sea region is cattle country and people on the western part of the coast mainly live in noncommercial fishing towns. The Marmara and the Aegean regions are important agricultural markets where groves of olives and other crops thrive. The Aegean coast is home to the historical sites of Troy and Pergamum and is important from an archaeological viewpoint. The Mediterranean region has some of the most beautiful scenery in the entire country with the Taurus Mountains and a rugged coastline in the east. Western Anatolia is covered with mountain ranges. Central Anatolia is considered to be Turkey's heartland because it is where the first Turkish tribes settled in the tenth century. Eastern Anatolia is far more isolated and underdeveloped; the land is barren and poverty is common. Southeastern Anatolia shares borders with Syria, Iraq, and Iran, so there is a Middle Eastern flair to its culture.

As of 1998, Turkey is the world's largest producer of hard-shell nuts, figs, and apricots, a leader in fresh vegetables, grape, and tobacco production, and seventh in the world in wheat and cotton production.

## GREECE

Like Turkey, Greece also lies at the crossroads of three continents. The country is located at the southeastern corner of Europe on the southern part of the Balkan Peninsula. Continental Asia lies to the east of Greece across the Aegean Sea, and Africa lies south across the Mediterranean Sea. Greece is famous for its jagged coastline bordered by the Aegean Sea on the east, the Mediterranean Sea on the south, and the Ionian Sea on the west. In the north, Greece shares a boundary with Albania, the former Yugoslav republic of Macedonia, and Bulgaria. Its territory includes more than 2,000 islands in the Aegean and Ionian seas, of which only 170 or so are inhabited.

The geography of Greece exercises an important influence upon the political destinies of its population. Greece is one of the most mountainous countries of Europe. Its surface is occupied by a number of small plains, either entirely surrounded by limestone mountains or open only to the sea. Arcadia was almost the only political division that did not possess some territory upon the coast. Each of the principal Grecian cities was founded in one of these small plains and, since the mountains that separated it from its neighbors were lofty and rugged, each city led solitary independence. Thus shut out from their neighbors by mountains, the Greeks were naturally attracted to the sea, and became a maritime people.

## CRETE

Crete is the largest of the Greek islands. A mountainous island, it lies south of the Aegean Sea, a link between Asia, Africa, and Europe. Its unique geographical position between the three continents determined its historical course both throughout antiquity and in modern times.

The island is an elongated shape. To the south it is bordered by the Libyan Sea, to the west the Myrtoon Sea, to the east the Karpathion Sea, and to the north the Sea of Crete. Its coastline, which consists of both sandy beaches and rocky shores, is framed by the small islets of Kouphonisi, Gaidouronisi, Dia, Aghioi Pantes, Spinalonga, and Gavdos in the Libyan Sea. Crete is the southernmost point of Europe.

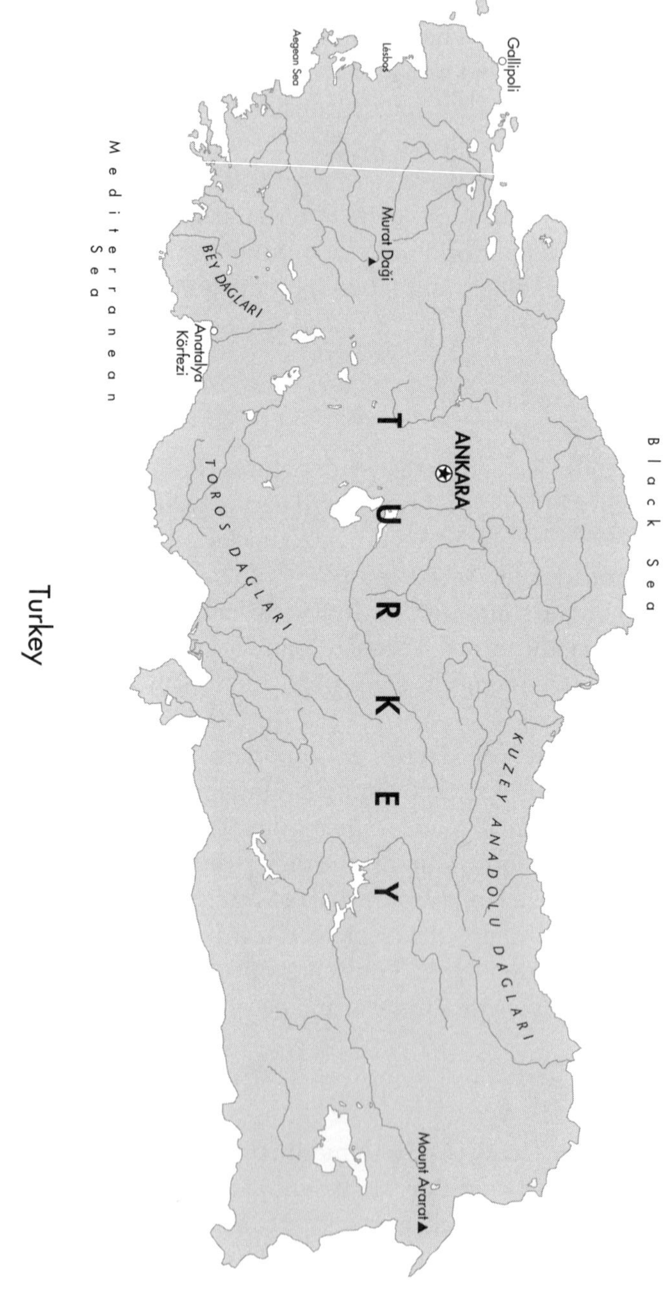
Gallipoli
Lésbos
Aegean Sea
Mediterranean Sea
Murat Daği
BEY DAGLARI
Anatalya Körfezi
ANKARA
TURKEY
Black Sea
TOROS DAGLARI
KUZEY ANADOLU DAGLARI
Mount Ararat

Turkey

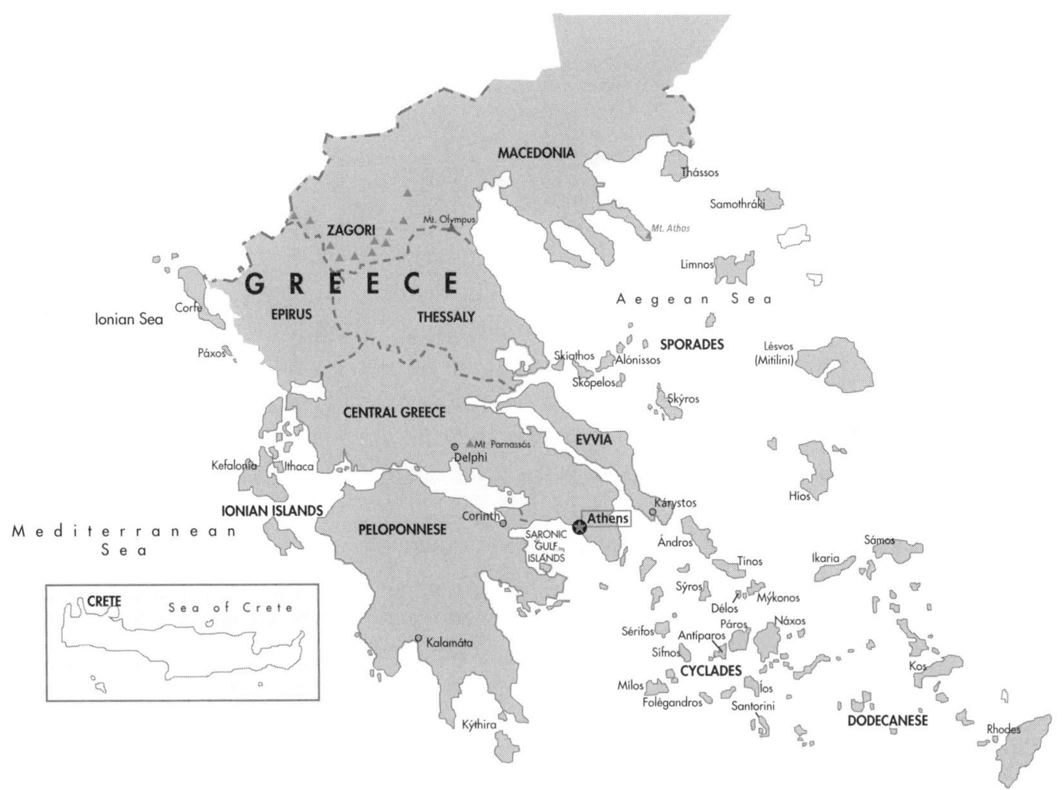


Greece and Crete

# History

## TURKEY

Archaeologists have found evidence of advanced societies living in this part of the world as early as 6000 B.C. As in many countries of the world, the years saw shifting power as one empire after another took control, and then others came along to challenge it. The first to dominate the region were the Hittites, the leading rulers of the Middle East in 1500 B.C. They were followed by the Greeks (eighth century B.C.), and the Persians (sixth century B.C.), and in A.D. 395 it became part of the Byzantine Empire. The area was conquered by the Ottoman Turks between the thirteenth and fifteenth centuries and remained the core of the Ottoman Empire. Its modern history dates to the rise of the Young Turks (after 1908) and the collapse of the empire in 1918. Under the leadership of Kemal Atatürk, a republic was proclaimed in 1923.

## GREECE

Greece is one of the cradles of European civilization, whose ancient scholars made great advances in philosophy, medicine, mathematics, and astronomy. Its city-states were pioneers in developing democratic forms of government. The historical and cultural heritage of Greece continues to resonate throughout the world in literature, art, philosophy, and politics.

The first settlement dated from the Paleolithic era (11,000–3,000 B.C.). During the second millennium B.C., Greece gave birth to the great civilizations of the Minoan, the Mycenaean, and the Cycladic on the Greek islands in the Aegean Sea. The classical period of Greek history (sixth to fourth centuries B.C.) was the golden age; during this period lived the great philosophers and mathematicians. Following that period, the history of Greece is a succession of various invasions and dominations; the Macedonians formed a strong empire, followed by the Romans and the Byzantine Empire, which ended with the invasion of the Turks. The Ottoman rule lasted for four hundred years and was a dark period for the inhabitants of Greece. Wanting to finally win their freedom, Greeks started to organize themselves and various revolts exploded against their Turkish oppressors.

The Independence War started in the Peloponnese peninsula in 1821 and ended in March 1831, with the establishment of the new and independent Greek state. Yet despite their illustrious history, the people of Greece are still striving to gain a role in world affairs. After enduring political and cultural oppression for centuries, their deep sense of cultural unity has preserved a rich society through occupation, wars, and political strife. In the last forty years Greece's main economic sectors have grown to include agriculture, tourism, construction, and shipping.

## CRETE

Crete's geography defined its historical course down through the ages. Situated between three continents, it was at the junction of the major cultural currents and at the crossroads of conflicting geopolitical interests and bloody clashes. On Cretan soil were hatched and developed features of civilization that mark the history of humankind. At the same time the island paid a heavy price because of its strategic position and was repeatedly invaded and periodically conquered, which contributed to the destruction of Crete's native civilization, the lowering of living standards, and the subsequent misery of the inhabitants. However, through successive restructuring new forms of social coexistence were forged, new intellectual values arose, and new material and cultural creations appeared that left their indelible mark on Crete and the historical role of the Cretans.

# The People

## TURKEY

The people of Turkey have changed along with their country. Their beginnings were primarily in Asia. About 85 percent of Turks are descended from people who migrated to Anatolia from central Asia during the tenth century A.D. The largest minority group in Turkey is the Kurds. About ten to twelve million Kurds live in the mountainous region of southeast Turkey as well as in the west. Many Kurds would like to form their own independent state, separate from Turkey. This issue has come into direct conflict with Turkey's plans for future development and is an ongoing battle that has yet to be solved. A small portion of the Turkish population consists of Arabs, Armenians, and Greeks. While there is no state religion and people have the freedom to choose, almost everyone who lives in Turkey is Muslim.

## GREECE

The Greek people are only partly descended from the ancient Greeks, having mingled through the ages with the numerous invaders of the Balkans. Modern vernacular Greek is the official language. There is a small Turkish-speaking minority, and many Greeks also speak English and French. The Greek Orthodox Church is the established church of the country, and it includes the great majority of the population.

In a country that traditionally has been poor agriculturally, making the most of meager produce has evolved from necessity to a national obsession with food. As necessity breeds innovation, Greek cuisine comprises a rich diversity of cooking styles, ingredients, and flavors. It also has a colorful history dating from antiquity and has incorporated outside elements from Italian, Turkish, and French cuisines. Vegetarianism has a long tradition in Greece and was espoused by Pythagoras, who abstained from meat for moral reasons. Even to this day, the ultra-religious abstain from meat and animal products on Wednesdays and Fridays as well as during the forty days of Lent.

## CRETE

The island of Crete has been inhabited since prehistoric times. There is evidence of organized habitation dating back to 8000 B.C., and twentieth-century excavations have revealed a splendid civilization that ruled the island and much of the Aegean region during the Bronze Age. The Minoan civilization is credited as the first civilization of Europe. It began around 2000 B.C. and it lasted for about two millennia before it was replaced on the island by the Mycenaean civilization circa 1375, and then by classical and Hellenistic Greeks, who in turn were replaced by the Romans. The Byzantine Empire and the Venetians controlled the island for a few hundred years before the Ottoman Empire invaded the island.

The Ottoman Empire ruled the island from 1645 until 1898 when the Greeks revolted and finally reunited the island with Greece in 1913.

# The Food

## TURKEY

In history, the Turks led a nomadic life, dependent on agriculture and on the breeding of domestic animals. The word "yogurt" is Turkish in origin and the fermenting process used in yogurt is thought to have originated among these nomadic tribes. Early Turks cultivated wheat and used it liberally, in several types of leavened and unleavened breads, which are baked in clay ovens, fried on a griddle, or buried in embers. Stuffing not only pastry but also all kinds of vegetables remains common practice, as evidenced by dozens of different types of "dolma." Skewering meat as another way of grilling, what we know as the kebab, was developed by the Turks. Turkish cuisine is full of vegetables, grains, fresh fish, and seemingly infinite varieties of lamb dishes. Fish and meat are typically served grilled or roasted, although often with inordinate amounts of *yag* (oil). The core group of seasonings is garlic, sage, oregano, cumin, mint, dill, lemon, and yogurt. The richness of Turkish cooking originated from Ottoman sultans. During their reign, many of the chefs were trying to create a new dish and taste to please the sultan in order to receive praise and reward. A sultan's palace kitchen might include hundreds of chefs and more than one thousand kitchen staff. As a result, a large variety of dish offerings from meat to many fresh vegetables were developed. The majority of these recipes, recorded in Arabic script, were regrettably lost in the language reforms. Some Ottoman favorites have continued, however, like *hünkar begendi* (the sultan was pleased), *imam bayaldi* (the priest fainted), and *hanim göbegi* (lady's navel), a syrupy dessert with a thumbprint in the middle.

The first meal of the day is breakfast. A typical Turkish breakfast is fresh tomatoes, white cheese, black olives, bread with honey and preserves, and sometimes an egg. Lunch often will include a rice or bulgar pilaf dish, lamb or chicken baked with peppers and eggplant, and fresh fish grilled with lemon. A popular lamb cut is *prizolla.* These are extra-thin-cut lamb chops seasoned with sumac (a tart red berry dried and coarsely ground, often referred to as a "souring agent") and thyme, and then quickly grilled. Other favorites include *sucuk,* a spicy sausage, and *pastirma,* a sun-dried cumin-fenugreek coated preserved beef. It is sliced thin much like pastrami.

Dinners will most commonly start with *mezeler* (singular, *mezze*), or appetizers. These often become a meal in themselves, accompanied by an ample serving of *raki* (a liquorlike anisette, licorice flavored; when diluted with water it assumes a milky color). Cold mezes include *patlican salatasi* (roasted eggplant puree flavored with garlic and lemon), *haydari* (a thick yogurt dip made with garlic and dill), *dolma, ezme* (a spicy paste of tomatoes, minced green pepper, onion, and parsley), *kizartma* (deep-fried eggplant, zucchini, or green pepper served with fresh yogurt), *cacik* (a garlicky cold yogurt "soup" with shredded cucumber, mint, or dill), *barbunya pilaki* (kidney beans, tomatoes, and onions cooked in olive oil), and *barbunya pilaki* (slow-roasted baby eggplant topped with olive oil-fried onions and tomatoes and seasoned with garlic). Hot appetizers, usually called *ara sicak,* include *börek* (a deep-fried or oven-baked pastry filled with cheese or meat), *kalamar* (deep-fried calamari served with a special sauce), and *midye tava* (deep-fried mussels). Fresh fish, often a main course, is commonly served grilled and drizzled with olive oil and lemon. Specialties include *alabalik* (trout), *barbunya* (red mullet), *kalkan* (turbot), *kefal* (gray mullet), *kiliç* (swordfish, sometimes served as a kebab), *levrek* (sea bass), *lüfer* (bluefish), and *palamut* (bonito). Grilled quail is most common inland; it's often marinated in tomatoes, yogurt, olive oil, and cinnamon. *Karisik izgara,* a mixed grill, usually combines chicken breast, beef, a lamb chop, and spicy lamb patties, all served with rice pilaf and vegetables.

Soups have traditional importance and are generally served as the first course or starter and can be eaten with any meal, even breakfast. They come in a wide variety and many are are based on meat stock. Lentil soup is the most common, but there are other preferred soups such as *yayla* (a yogurt-based soup), *tarhana* (cracked wheat or flour, yogurt, and vegetables fermented and then dried), *asiran* (made from bulgur wheat and yogurt), and *guli* (from greens, white beans, and lamb). The well-known "wedding soup" is made with lamb shanks in an egg broth.

One of the pillars of Turkish cooking is *pilavlar,* or pilaf. Generally made of rice, but sometimes with bulgur or *sehriye* (vermicelli), pilaf is one of the mainstays of the Turkish table. The rice should not be sticky but separate into individual grains. The pilaf may include eggplant, chickpeas, beans, or peas. Although pilaf is traditionally a course in its own right, it may also be used as a garnish with meat and chicken dishes.

*Börek* is a general Turkish term for filled pastries. The filling is often white sheep's milk cheese and a chopped vegetable such as parsley or spinach. Often the dough is paper-thin *yufka* (phyllo) layered, rolled, or folded around the ingredients, then baked, steamed, or fried.

Kebabs are dishes of plain or marinated meat either stewed or grilled. Although the ingredient of choice for Turks is lamb, some kebabs are made with beef, chicken, or fish, usually grilled with vegetables on a skewer. *Doner kebab* is a famous Turkish dish of a roll of lamb on a vertical skewer turning parallel to a hot grill. *Adana kebaps* are spicy ground-lamb patties arranged on a layer of sautéed pita bread, topped with a yogurt-and-garlic sauce. *Iskender kebaps,* also known as *bursa kebaps,* are sliced grilled lamb, smothered in tomato sauce, hot butter, and yogurt. *Sis kebaps* are the traditional skewered cubes of lamb, usually interspersed with peppers and onions. *Kofte* are meatballs, predominantly lamb, and there is a rich variety of kofte recipes within Turkey. Finely minced meat mixed with spices, onions, and other ingredients is shaped by hand, and grilled, fried, boiled, or baked. Some *koftes* are cooked in a sauce; as in the case of the *izmir kofte,* the *koftes* are first grilled and then cooked with green peppers, potato slices, and tomatoes in their own gravy. In southern and southeastern Turkey, bulgur wheat is an essential ingredient of many varieties of meatballs. The stuffed meatballs known as *içli kofte* have an outer shell of bulgur and minced meat and a filling of walnuts and spicy minced meat. Raw *kofte* are a specialty that requires top-quality meat without a trace of fat. This is then minced and kneaded with bulgur and the purplish hot pepper of the region.

*Dolmas* is family of stuffed vegetable dishes. This applies to tomatoes, peppers, eggplant, potatoes, onions, quince, and even apples; although stuffed mackerel and squid are also called *dolma. Dolmas* originated in Turkey, but are also found from the Balkans to Persia. Perhaps the best-known is the grape leaf *dolmas.* The stuffing may include meat or not. Meat *dolmas* are generally served warm, often with sauce; meatless ones are generally served cold.

Bread has major cultural significance in Turkey. It is usually baked twice a day, early in the morning and late in the afternoon. The freshly baked elongated loaf of bread, which looks like French bread, is the bread that most people eat during the day. Then there is flat bread, known as pita bread (*pide* in Turkish) which is good for wrapping; *lavash,* a wafer thin type of bread, is also good for wrapping; and *simit,* which is a round bread much like a bagel, covered with sesame seeds.

Many fresh and dried fruits are stewed into compotes in which the liquid is as important an element as is the fruit itself. Desserts made from apricots or figs are given a topping of fresh clotted cream and sometimes crushed walnuts. The same topping is used on *kabak tatlisi,* an unusual dessert made by cooking pieces of pumpkin in syrup. Milk-based desserts include a wide variety of puddings, some of which are baked. *Keskul* is a milk pudding made with coconut. *Gullac* is a confection of thin sheets of pastry in a milk sauce to which rosewater is added; and pastry-based desserts include baklava, as well as *kadayif* (made from shredded pastry baked in syrup, often filled with pistachio nuts, walnuts, or clotted cream), *revani* (a sweet made from semolina), *hanim göbegi,* and *sekerparee* (two kinds of small sweet cake). Turkish delight and helva are well-known candies. Turkish delight is made from cornstarch or gelatin, sugar, honey, and fruit juice or jelly, and is often tinted pink or green. Chopped almonds, pistachio nuts, pine nuts, or hazelnuts are frequently added. Once the candy becomes firm, it is cut into small squares and coated with confectioners' sugar. Helva is made by pan-sautéing flour or semolina and pine nuts in butter before adding sugar and milk or water, and briefly cooking until these are absorbed. The preparation of helva is conducive to communal cooking. People are invited for "helva conversations" to pass the long winter nights.

Tea (cay) is the national drink. It is served extremely hot and strong in tiny tulip-shaped glasses, accompanied by two sugar cubes. The size of the glass ensures that the tea gets consumed while hot. The coffee culture is a little less prevalent but no less "steeped" in tradition. Early clerics believed it to be an intoxicant and consequently had it banned. But the *kahvehane* (coffeehouse) refused to go away, and now the sharing of a cup of coffee is an excuse to prolong a discussion, plan, negotiate, or simply relax. Turkish coffee is ground to a fine dust, boiled directly in the correct quantity of water, and served as is. There are two national drinks, *raki* and *ayran. Raki* is an alcoholic drink distilled from raisins and then redistilled with aniseed. *Ayran* is a refreshing beverage made by diluting yogurt with water.

## GREECE

As in every culture of the world, local culinary traditions are the reflection of two interconnected factors, geography and history. The mainland cuisine of Greece is primarily a nomadic shepherd's cuisine. As recently as a generation ago, shepherds moved on foot with their flocks twice a year, in mid-fall and mid-spring, between the low-lying plains (where it was warmer) and the mountains, where they spent their summers. Foraging, not farming, was the norm. Butter and lard were the predominant fats, and cheese, yogurt, and myriad other dairy products played a dominant role in those diets, as did meat. Vegetables were typically wild greens, picked in and around nomadic settlements and often turned into pies, one of the backbones of mainland Greek cooking. For an itinerant shepherd, it was the most efficient food, a dish that could be easily prepared from accessible ingredients, baked in makeshift portable ovens, was satisfyingly filling, and could be carried with ease over long distances.

There are many pies in Greece that fall into several broad categories. *Tiropita* is a cheese pie. The filling is usually a simple combination of local cheese, usually feta, and eggs. Some pies are multilayered; others are very thin, almost like crepes filled with cheese. *Hortopita* is a category of pies, filled with seasonal, usually mild, greens. In some, a little cheese is added. *Kreatopita* translates as meat pie. Pork, lamb, and some beef appear in fillings from various regions. Chicken is also used as a filling for pies. These are called *kotopites.* There are also some unusual pies filled with eggplant (*thesalia*) and with pulses, such as lentils, which is a very old dish from Ipiros. *Bourekakia* are individual, hand-held pies that can be filled with cheese, vegetables, or meat. They are either fried or baked and shapes vary. *Glikes pites* are sweet pies. Baklava falls into this category. Other dessert pies include *galaktoboureko,* a custard-filled pie almost always prepared with commercial phyllo, not homemade and *galatopita,* or milk pie, which is a classic country dish in Roumeli, Thesalia, and Ipiros. Often, *trahana* or rice is added to the filling of milk pies to make it more substantial. There is also an unusual sweet Lenten pie found throughout Ipiros made with rice and raisins.

There are several subcategories of Greek cuisine: cooking large casseroles, stews, grilled meat and seafood specialties, and phyllo items (*pites*). Each type of cooking is represented by a specialty restaurant. *Tavernas* can be found all over Greece and specialize in preprepared casserole items (*moussaka, pastitsio,* vegetables stuffed with rice). *Psistaries* serve only grilled meats. *Pites,* phyllo pastry pies stuffed with greens, are generally considered as *laiko,* or village cuisine, made at home or purchased from either a bakery or a street vendor specializing in one type of pita.

Breakfast, or *proeeno,* is a light meal, usually eaten as early as 7 a.m. Many people have only Greek coffee, which is a strong, thick mixture of fine ground coffee, water, and sometimes sugar, boiled together. This may be accompanied by a roll with butter, honey, or jelly. Lunch, or *mesimeriano,* is the main meal, eaten at home at 2 or 3 p.m. Appetizers, meat or fish, salad, yogurt with honey, and fruit may be served at a typical midday meal. Dinner is *deipnon,* usually eaten in the late evening, as late as 10 p.m. Most Greeks have appetizers, or *mezedakia,* in the early evening, before dinner. The word *meze* describes a form of socializing as much as a group of dishes. Drinking without eating is frowned upon in Greece. People gather in *ouzeries* in the early evening not just for drinks, but also for *mezethes* to tide them over until dinner. *Meze* is eaten throughout the Eastern Mediterranean, and Greek *mezethes* share common flavors with the Turkish, Middle Eastern, and North African varieties (nearly four hundred years of Ottoman rule left a strong mark on the entire area). But this style of eating can be traced to ancient Greece; Plato's writings include descriptions of symposium spreads that would not be out of place in an *ouzerie* today. Greek *mezethes* generally have robust or spicy flavors to stand up to strong drinks. The hallmarks of Greek cuisine since antiquity—olives, fresh vegetables, spit-roasted or grilled meats, dried and fresh fruit, oregano, mint, yogurt, and honey—figure prominently. *Meze* in seaside areas includes dishes like wood-grilled squid and octopus, while the mountainous inland regions are known for pies stuffed with meat and cheese.

Feta cheese and yogurt are the backbone of the Greece's dairy industry. The country produces 150,000 tons of feta per year. Because of Greek emigrations, this brined cheese has become known worldwide.The European Union has granted this cheese a Protected Designation of Origin (PDO) and has prohibited other countries in its domain from using the name "feta." Derived from the milk of both sheep and goats (but never cows), its unique flavors result from these animals grazing on indigenous plants in rather dry pastures.

Whereas Greek mountain cooking is basically rooted in a pastoral tradition, the cuisine of the Peloponnese, the large peninsula joined to the rest of mainland Greece by a narrow strip of land (the Isthmus of Corinth), is rural, farm cuisine at its best. Here is Greece's most important olive grove—the tree grows virtually all over the Peloponnese—and olive oil figures prominently in the cuisine.

Perhaps no other symbol represents Greece as does the olive tree. The Greek poet Homer once described Greece's olive oil as "liquid gold" and for a long time olive groves were protected. Said to be given by the goddess of wisdom, Athena, to the city bearing her name, the olive tree provides two staples of Greek cuisine: table olives and olive oil. Today its production and sale plays a significant role in the economic life of twenty-first-century Greece. Greece is home to 120,000,000 olive trees, about twelve trees for every resident. About 120,000 tons of table olives each year are produced, which is the fifth largest total in the world. Two-thirds of the crop goes to export markets. Of the many varieties grown, three predominate: the *kalamata*, perhaps the best known; the *conservolia*; and the *halkidiki.* It is a point of pride that 80 percent of Greece's olive oil is rated extra virgin, making the country the world's largest producer in this category. Olive oil is used in virtually every method of cooking in Greece and is also used as a condiment, especially with the greener, more herbaceous varieties of oil. Common dishes like the green bean, eggplant, potato, or zucchini stew, cooked in lemon or tomato sauce, are called *ladera* (cooked in olive oil).

Other important elements in the cuisine of the Peloponnese are tomatoes, garlic, onions, spinach, artichokes, fennel, lettuce, cabbage, *horta* (wild greens), zucchini, eggplant, and peppers. Fruits are eaten either fresh, or preserved by drying. Popular varieties include apricots, grapes, dates, cherries, apples, pears, plums, and figs.

The excellent quality of Greek herbs and spices reflects the country's ample sunshine and the variability of its landscape. This special landscape makes Greek flora so rich that of the 7,500 different species of plants growing in Greece, 850 of them are found only there. Some of the best herbs grow there naturally: chamomile, mountain tea, *tilio* (lime blossom), sage, thyme, oregano, and basil are chosen above others by celebrity chefs across Europe. Spices from Greece include sesame, white sesame, *machlepi* (the kernel of a certain cherry; it has a pleasant, sweet and earthy aroma and is used to flavor certain holiday breads), and cumin. The most valuable and expensive spice, red saffron, is cultivated in Greece. There are certain defining flavors and combinations that make a dish unquestionably Greek. Among them are lemon and dill; lemon and olive oil; lemon, olive oil, oregano, and garlic; lemon and eggs (*avgolemono*); tomatoes and cinnamon (in sauces); tomatoes, honey, vinegar, and dill; garlic ground with mint (sometimes with the addition of walnuts); garlic and vinegar; anise (or *ouzo*) and pepper; and olives, orange, and fennel. Garlic is indispensable to Greek cooking and is used in stews and other savory dishes, but it most important in dipping sauces, such as *skordalia* and in yogurt-based dips, such as *tzatziki.* Greeks enjoy the taste of garlic and nuts, and there are several sauces that call for walnuts and garlic or almonds and garlic.

With documented production dating to sixth century B.C., honey has a special resonance in Greece. It's the basic sweetening ingredient in the Mediterranean diet and Greece is one of the primary providers of honey in Europe. The country defines its honey sources in two broad categories. Forest honey, most of which is pine honey, fir honey, and oak honey, accounts for 60 to 70 percent of all production. The balance is considered flower honey and includes sources such as orange, heather, chestnut, and aromatic plants like wild oregano, wild lavender, and salvia. Because Greece's vegetation is sparser than in some other parts of the world, bees must work harder. In Greece a beehive will average 10 kilos (about 22 pounds) production, while in the rest of Europe hives generate over 30 kilos (about 66 pounds). However, the Greek bees that struggle and collect nectar from a wider variety of plants produce a honey that is denser and richer in aromatic substances.

Wheat has been cultivated in Greece for thousands of years and is a staple of Greek cuisine. It's used to make a variety of breads including pita bread and crusty whole-grain peasant bread. Bulgur, which is made from cracked whole wheat, is eaten as an accompaniment to hearty stews or added to soups and salads. Pasta, introduced to the Greeks by the Italians, is also a popular wheat-based food. Another important grain food in the Greek diet is rice, which is used in pilafs and bakes, served with stews, or wrapped in grape leaves to make *dolmades.*

Legumes such as chickpeas, lima beans, split peas, and lentils are used in traditional Greek cooking. They are eaten either whole in stews, bakes, pilafs, soups, and salads, or pureed and used as a dip or spread such as hummus. The most popular dried beans are the *gigantes,* or giant beans, which resemble lima or butter beans but are bigger. These are made into casseroles, baked with tomatoes and other vegetables, and sometimes served up simply boiled with a little olive oil, lemon juice, and oregano. Greeks call the yellow split pea *fava.* The most common way to cook them is to simmer the yellow split peas until they become creamy and dense, like mashed potatoes. This is a classic Greek dish, usually topped with raw olive oil and raw onions. In Santorini, *fava* is "married," that is, it is served with a topping of either stewed capers, another local specialty, or stewed eggplants. Once the puree has been made, it can also sometimes be turned into fritters. Many types of nuts are used in cooking or eaten as snacks, particularly pine nuts, almonds, walnuts, and pistachios.

Meat, particularly large roasts, have been an important part of Greek culinary history. Today, Easter would be incomplete without lamb or kid on a spit, or its *kokoretsi* (innards sausage), skewered and grilled outdoors. On the everyday table, skewered meats are also prominent, in the form of *souvlaki,* sold all over the country. *Souvlaki*, like the kebab, is made by skewering small chunks of meat, usually pork or lamb, and grilling them over coals. *Souvlaki* may be made with or without slices of peppers, tomatoes, and onions on the skewer. A *souvlaki* pita is wrapped in grilled pita bread together with tomatoes, *tzatziki,* and onions. A *gyros* (also spelled *giros*) is like *souvlaki* pita, usually served wrapped in grilled pita bread with one difference: *gyros,* which means round, is made by stacking very thin slices of meat on a vertical skewer and grilling the resulting cone on a rotisserie for hours, until all the slices meld together. To serve it, the *gyro* maker slices off thin pieces and wraps them in pita bread with tomatoes, onions, and *tzatziki.* There are countless stews and stovetop meat preparations in the traditional Greek culinary repertoire. Meat is expensive and so used sparingly, most often in combination with other ingredients, such as vegetables, beans, and rice or pasta.

*Moussaka* is the best known of all Greek foods. It is a lamb and eggplant casserole covered with a thick layer of béchamel sauce that is baked until golden and crusty. It can be made with other ingredients besides lamb and eggplant, using beef, or vegetables such as zucchini or potatoes.

Greece is surrounded by the sea, so fish and shellfish are an important part of the diet. The most popular types of fish and shellfish include tuna, mullet, bass, halibut, swordfish, anchovies, sardines, shrimp, octopus, squid, and mussels. This fish and seafood is enjoyed in many ways, including grilled and seasoned with garlic and lemon juice, baked with yogurt and herbs, cooked in rich tomato sauce, added to soups, or served cold as a side dish.

Fresh and dried fruit are the usual dessert. Rich desserts and pastries, often sweetened with honey, are mostly reserved for special occasions or eaten in small amounts. Greek sweets made with fruits are a part of the Greek tradition and way of life since they represent a warm welcome for the visitor to the friendly environment of a Greek home. In the near past, these sweets were usually homemade according to the art and secrets of each housewife. They were called "spoon sweets" because the usual serving size was a well-filled teaspoon.

Most sweets were prepared at the time of year each fruit matured: apricots, prunes, grapes, quince, bergamot, citrus, wild cherries, and figs followed each other from early summer to late autumn. Other varieties such as pistachio, walnut, fig, and bitter orange used fruit that was not yet fully ripe. Sometimes spoon sweets were made by using vegetables (such as eggplants or tomatoes) or even flower petals. The Greek seamen and merchants traveling east to Mesopotamia particularly appreciated the Turkish dessert baklava. They brought the recipe to Athens. *Phyllo* was coined by Greeks and means "leaf" in the Greek language. In a relatively short time, in every kitchen of wealthy households in the region, trays of baklava were being baked for all kinds of special occasions from the third century B.C. onward.

Wine is consumed regularly in Greece, but mainly with food, and in moderation. Ouzo is Greece's national drink. Ouzo is made from a precise combination of pressed grapes, herbs, and berries including aniseed, licorice, mint, wintergreen, fennel, and hazelnut. It is usually served as an aperitif, but is also used in some mixed drinks and cocktails. When mixing Ouzo with water it will turn whitish and opaque.

### CRETE

Island cooking has always been shaped by the various rites of the Greek Orthodox Church. Christmas, Easter, and the feast of the Dormition of the Virgin Mary on August 15 (corresponding to the feast of the Assumption in the Roman Catholic Church) are the most colorful of the festivals. Easter is preceded by the forty days of Lent, during which people abstain from all foods derived from animals (meat, dairy products, and eggs), as they do every Wednesday and Friday throughout the year. This abstention has inspired cooks to develop a number of exquisite vegetarian dishes that substitute for the more familiar versions made with meat. Lenten grape leaves stuffed with rice; pasta with olive oil, onions, and spices; tomato and onion flatbread, and zucchini; and chickpea fritters are just a few of the flavorful examples. There is plenty of celebration food as well, like roast leg of lamb with potatoes, fragrant with garlic, oregano, and thyme, and baked chicken with orzo.

It is argued that the Cretan diet, based on olive oil, cereals, wine, and fish hasn't really changed since Minoan times. It has created the world's healthiest and long-lived people and is the basis of the famous Mediterranean diet. Research in the 1950s by the international scientific community concluded that Cretans were this healthy due to their diet. Today, it is generally agreed that following the traditional Cretan way of eating leads to less chance of suffering from heart disease compared to other Mediterranean countries. This seems to be due to the fact that Cretans eat twice as much fruit, a quarter less meat, and more pulses than other Europeans. Greek island cuisine is largely free from animal fats, an absence considered healthful. More than anywhere else in Greece, maybe more than anywhere else in the whole Mediterranean, the cooking of the Aegean islands is one in which the basic rule is that food be embellished as little as possible and altered as little as possible from its original state.

## Glossary

**Avgolemono** Egg-lemon sauce prepared by adding fresh lemon juice to whisked eggs.

**Baklava** Famed Mediterranean pastry whose origin is debatable. Made from many layers of butter-brushed, nut- and sugar-sprinkled layers of phyllo pastry.

**Barbouni** Red mullet, a favorite fish usually served grilled or fried. The cheeks and liver are considered special delicacies.

**Béchamel Sauce** By this name, the sauce's origin is attributed to Louis de Béchamel, of the court of King Louis XIV. However, it should be noted that this same sauce—a roux of fat and flour whisked with a liquid, usually milk or cream—was described by Athenaeus in A.D. 200 and widely used in Greek cuisine.

**Bourekakia** A Turkish name for all the tiny appetizer pastries made from phyllo pastry and filled with a variety of savory fillings, including vegetables, meats, and cheese. In Greece these appetizers commonly take their name from the filling.

**Greek Cheeses**

**Anthotiro** A variation of mizithra. It is buttery in texture and comes in two variations, soft and dry.

**Feta** The most popular and most ancient of the Greek cheeses, the traditional cheese of Greece. It is traditionally made from goat's or sheep's milk and is stored in barrels of brine. Most feta comes from mountainous areas. It is used in salads, baked in pies, crumbled on omelets, or even stuffed into fish. The most popular way to eat feta is to lay a thick slab on a plate, pour on some olive oil, and add a pinch of oregano on top.

**Graviera** Hard in texture, mild in taste, this cheese resembles Swiss or Gruyère in texture. It is served with meals or used for grating over spaghetti.

**Kapnisto Metsovone** One of the few smoked cheeses of Greece. It is made from cow's milk, but sometimes with the addition of a little sheep's or goat's milk.

**Kaser** *(Kasseri)* This mild- to sharp-tasting cheese (depending on variety) is faint yellow in color, oily in texture, and usually eaten on its own. It is made from sheep's milk and is good as a table cheese.

**Kefalograviera** A cross between Kefalotiri and Graviera, this cheese is made from cow's milk. It is a hard cheese, pale yellow in color with a sharp taste and smell, used as a table cheese and for grating or frying.

**Kefalotiri** This traditional Greek cheese is very hard in texture. It is made with a combination of sheep's and goat's milk. Salty and sharp tasting, it is similar to regato and Parmesan and is used for grating over spaghetti. It is primarily used for frying. It is ripened for at least three months and so acquires a sharp aroma and a rich, salty, tangy taste.

**Ladotyri** This is sheep's and goat's milk cheese. It is made in the shape of small spheres and so is sometimes called *kefalaki* (little head). Its proper name refers to olive oil, in which it is aged. It can be aged for as much as a year and emerge richer and tastier.

**Manouri** Like mizithra, ricotta, and cottage cheeses, manouri is soft in texture and unsalted. It is made from full-fat sheep's milk and is mainly used for sweet pies. In Athens and the islands it is the name of soft cream cheese.

**Mizithra** It is made from sheep's or goat's milk and comes in two forms. The fresh, ricotta-like mizithra is unsalted. The dried version is salted, aged until hard, and is good for grating and cooking. Mizithra is more often used for sweet pies.

**Telemes** A variation of feta cheese. The difference is that it is made from cow's milk.

**Touloumotiri** This sweet, moist, snow-white cheese is stored by hanging in goatskin or sheepskin bags.

**Dolmadakia** Any stuffed food, this term refers to tiny stuffed foods such as small rolls of cabbage, spinach, or vine leaves or tiny scooped-out vegetables. These are filled with savory mixtures such as béchamel sauce and cheese or rice with seasonings.

**Domates** Tomatoes.

**Fakki** Meatless brown lentil soup, a standby for busy days and a staple when meat is scarce.

**Fenugreek** Pleasantly bittersweet seed generally ground.

**Imam Bayaldi** Slowly baked eggplants stuffed with tomatoes and sliced onions and flavored with garlic. Literally, "the caliph fainted," so named because the dish was so delicious that the priest was said to have fainted (here the stories differ) either when he tasted it or when he was denied a taste.

**Kafes** Turkish coffee introduced to Greece, brewed in a long-handled pot called a *briki.* In Greece it is called Greek coffee, but it is still made in thirty-three variations, as is Turkish coffee.

**Kataifia** Sweetened very fine shreds of a wheat flour pastry rolled up with chopped nuts.

**Kefthedes or Keftethes** Tiny meatballs prepared with finely minced meat (any kind) blended with bread crumbs and eggs then seasoned with garlic, mint, oregano, and salt and pepper. The mixture is formed into tiny balls and fried in oil until brown.

**Kolokythia** Called baby marrows in England, courgettes in France, and zucchini in Italy. Greeks enjoy the flowers freshly picked, stuffed, and fried.

**Kouloura** A Greek bread.

**Kourabiedes** Rich buttery shortbread-type cookies baked in round balls, liberally sprinkled with rosewater or orange flower water, and dusted with powdered sugar.

**Mahlab** Used in dessert breads, the spice is actually the pit of a sour cherry.

**Mastica** Unique to Greek cooking, the powdered resin from a small evergreen grown mostly on the Greek isle of Chios. Like ginger and mahlab, mastic is used as a spice in desserts and sweets, as well as a way to sweeten main entrées. Used for flavoring yeast dough. There is also a liqueur by the same name.

**Melitzanosalata** A popular Mediterranean appetizer of pureed eggplant seasoned liberally with onion and vinegar and garnished with black olives and tomato wedges.

**Moussaka** Browned eggplant slices layered with tomatoes, cheese, onions, and ground meat finished with a béchamel sauce. Typically Greek, there is a faint taste of cinnamon.

**Nigella** Small black seed with a nutty, pepper flavor that looks like black sesame. Most often used to top breads and to flavor salads and vegetables.

**Ouzo** A Greek anise-flavored alcoholic beverage that turns opaque when mixed with water.

**Pastizzio** A baked layered casserole of cooked pasta sprinkled with cheese and a layer of seasoned minced meat. The casserole is finished with cheese and béchamel sauce.

**Phyllo or Fillo** This paper-thin pastry is usually made commercially of egg, flour, and water. The Greek word *phyllo* means "leaf."

**Saganaki or Tiraki** Any firm cheese cut in squares, dusted with flour, and quickly fried in hot oil and served as an appetizer.

**Skordalia or Skorthalia** A smooth, thick sauce made with oil, lemon juice, soft white bread, and garlic. There are many variations depending on the region and the family; many versions include potato.

**Souvlakia** Skewered cubes of lamb with onions, green peppers, and tomato wedges, all marinated then broiled.

**Spanakopita** A "pie" of buttery layers of phyllo with a center portion of chopped cooked spinach and feta mixed with béchamel.

**Stefado** A stew.

**Sumac** Deep red, slightly sour spice with citrus notes. Ground sumac is used in salads, on grilled meats, in soups, and in rice dishes.

**Taramosalata** Creamy dip made of roe, white bread or potato, garlic, oil, and lemon juice.

**Tzatziki** A tangy dip of plain yogurt, minced cucumber, garlic, salt, and pepper.

**Vasilopita** Sweet yeast bread flavored with grated orange rind, cinnamon, and mastic, made especially for Saint Basil's Day.

# Menus and Recipes from Greece and Turkey

MENU ONE

*Spanakopita Peloponniso:* **Peloponnese Spinach Rolls**

*Elliniki Salata:* **Greek Salad**

*Aginares me Avgolemono:* **Artichokes with Egg and Lemon Sauce**

*Fasoulatha:* **Bean Soup**

*Garithes Saganaki:* **Baked Shrimp**

*Afelia:* **Fried Pork with Coriander**

*Pourgouri Pilafi:* **Pilaf of Cracked Wheat**

**Fresh Fruit**

MENU TWO

*Dolmathakia me Rizi:* **Stuffed Grape Vine Leaves**

*Saganaki:* **Fried Cheese**

*Tzatziki:* **Garlic, Cucumber, and Yogurt Dip**

*Salata me Portokalia kai Elies:* **Orange and Olive Salad**

*Psari Savoro:* **Fried Fish with Rosemary and Vinegar**

*Fasolakia:* **Fresh Green Bean Ragout**

*Kataifi:* **Nut-stuffed Shredded Wheat Rolls**

*Moussaka:* **Eggplant Moussaka**

MENU THREE (TURKEY)

*Kabak Kizartmasi* **and** *Patlican Kizartmasi:* **Zucchini and Eggplant Fritters**

*Midye Dolmasi:* **Stuffed Mussels**

*Sis Kebap:* **Skewered Lamb and Vegetables**

*Balik Köftesi:* **Fish Balls**

*Domates Salatasi:* **Tomato Salad**

*Havuc Plakisi:* **Braised Carrots**

*Beyaz Pilave:* **Plain Pilaf**

*Íncír Compostu:* **Figs in Syrup**

# Spanakopita Peloponniso

## Peloponnese Spinach Rolls

SERVES 4

**Feta cheese comes packed in brine. Rinse it under cold water, let it drain on a paper towel for a few minutes, then crumble it into the bowl containing the spinach and onions.**

| AMOUNT | MEASURE | INGREDIENT |
|---|---|---|
| 8 cups | 16 ounces, 448 g | Spinach, washed, coarse stems removed, roughly chopped |
| $\frac{1}{4}$ cup | 2 ounces, 60 ml | Olive oil |
| $\frac{1}{2}$ cup | 2 ounces, 56 g | Onion, $\frac{1}{4}$ inch (.6 cm) dice |
| $\frac{1}{2}$ cup | 2 ounces, 56 g | Leek, white part only, $\frac{1}{4}$ inch (.6 cm) dice |
| $\frac{1}{2}$ cup | 2 ounces, 56 g | Green onion, $\frac{1}{4}$ inch (.6 cm) dice |
| $\frac{1}{4}$ cup | $\frac{1}{2}$ ounce, 14 g | Flat-leaf parsley, chopped fine |
| $1\frac{1}{2}$ teaspoons | | Fresh dill, chopped |
| $\frac{1}{8}$ teaspoon | | Nutmeg |
| $\frac{1}{2}$ cup | 2 ounces, 56 g | Feta cheese, crumbled |
| 1 | | Egg, beaten |
| To taste | | Salt and freshly ground black pepper |
| 4 | | Sheets phyllo pastry |
| As needed | | Olive oil or butter for assembling rolls |

### PROCEDURE

1. Preheat oven to 350°F (180°C).
2. Wilt spinach over medium heat and drain well in colander, pressing with spoon to remove all moisture.
3. Heat oil over medium heat and sauté onion for 5 minutes until soft. Add leeks and green onion, cook until soft, 5 minutes.
4. Combine the drained spinach, onion mixture, herbs, nutmeg, feta, and egg and season with salt and pepper. Cool.
5. Place a sheet of phyllo on work surface; brush lightly with olive oil or melted butter. Top with remaining sheets, brushing each with oil.
6. Brush top lightly with oil and place 2 ounces (56 g) spinach mixture along the length of the pastry toward one edge; leave $1\frac{1}{2}$ inches (4 cm) clear on each end.

7 Fold bottom edge of pastry over filling, roll once, fold in ends, then roll up. Place a hand at each end of roll and push it in gently, like an accordion.

8 Place roll on a parchment lined or oiled baking dish. Brush top with oil and bake at 350°F (180°C) for 30 minutes or until golden brown.

9 Serve hot, cut in portions.

# Elliniki Salata Greek Salad SERVES 4

| AMOUNT | MEASURE | INGREDIENT |
|---|---|---|
| 2 cups | 4 ounces, 112 g | Romaine lettuce, $\frac{1}{2}$ inch (1.27 cm) strips |
| $\frac{1}{4}$ cup | $\frac{1}{2}$ ounce, 14 g | Fresh dill |
| 1 cup | 6 ounces, 168 g | Tomatoes, peeled, seeded, $\frac{1}{2}$ inch (1.27 cm) dice |
| 1 cup | 6 ounces, 168 g | Cucumber, peeled, seeded, cut in half lengthwise, $\frac{1}{4}$ inch (.6 cm) slices |
| 1 cup | 4 ounces, 112 g | Red onion, cut into very thin rings |
| $\frac{1}{2}$ cup | 2 ounces, 56 g | Green Italian or green bell pepper, seeded, $\frac{1}{2}$ inch (1.27 cm) dice |
| $\frac{1}{2}$ cup | 3 ounces, 84 g | Kalamata olives, pitted |
| $\frac{1}{2}$ cup | 3 ounces, 84 g | Feta cheese, crumbled (optional) |
| Dressing | | |
| $\frac{1}{4}$ cup | 2 ounces, 60 ml | Olive oil |
| 1 tablespoon | $\frac{1}{2}$ ounce, 30 ml | Red wine vinegar |
| 1 tablespoon | $\frac{1}{2}$ ounce, 30 ml | Fresh lemon juice |
| 1 | | Garlic clove, mashed with $\frac{1}{2}$ teaspoon salt |
| 2 teaspoons | | Fresh oregano, or 1 teaspoon dried |
| To taste | | Salt and pepper |

PROCEDURE

1 Make dressing by whisking together all dressing ingredients.

2 Scatter lettuce on a platter; sprinkle with half the dill.

3 Combine remaining salad ingredients and dressing; toss well.

4 Distribute over lettuce and serve.

# Aginares me Avgolemono

## Artichokes with Egg and Lemon Sauce

SERVES 4

| AMOUNT | MEASURE | INGREDIENT |
|---|---|---|
| 4 | | Whole globe artichokes |
| 2 tablespoons | 1 ounce, 30 ml | Fresh lemon juice |
| 1 | | Lemon, sliced |
| 1 tablespoon | $\frac{1}{2}$ ounce, 15 ml | Olive oil |
| 1 $\frac{1}{4}$ cups | 10 ounces, 300 ml | Chicken stock, boiling |
| 1 $\frac{1}{2}$ teaspoons | | Cornstarch |
| 2 | | Eggs, separated |
| 1 tablespoon | $\frac{1}{2}$ ounce, 15 ml | Fresh lemon juice |
| To taste | | Salt and pepper |
| 1 tablespoon | | Dill and parsley, chopped fine for garnish |

**PROCEDURE**

1. Wash artichokes well and cut off stem close to base. Add 1 tablespoon (15 ml) lemon juice to enough cold water to cover artichokes.
2. Remove tough outer leaves and trim carefully. Cut off 1 $\frac{1}{4}$ inches (3 cm) from top and trim remaining leaf ends with scissors. Rub with lemon slices, to prevent discoloration.
3. Cook prepared artichokes in boiling salted water, 1 tablespoon (15 ml) lemon juice, and olive oil for 30 minutes or until tender. Test by pulling a leaf; if it comes away easily the artichokes are done.
4. Remove and invert to drain. Place in serving dish and keep warm.
5. Make avgolemono sauce using chicken stock or half stock and half artichoke water.
6. Mix cornstarch with enough cold water to make a paste and add to stock, stirring until thickened and bubbling. Let cook 1 minute.
7. Beat egg whites until stiff; add egg yolk and continue beating until light and fluffy. Add lemon juice gradually, beating constantly.
8. Gradually pour in thickened hot stock to egg, beating constantly.
9. Return sauce to heat and cook, stirring constantly, over low heat for 1 to 2 minutes to cook egg. Mixture should thicken enough to coat the back of a spoon. Do not boil.
10. Remove from heat and continue stirring; correct seasoning.
11. Serve immediately, pour over artichokes and sprinkle with chopped dill and parsley.

# Fasoulatha Bean Soup

SERVES 4 TO 6

| AMOUNT | MEASURE | INGREDIENT |
|---|---|---|
| 2 cups | 15 ounces, 420 g | Dried nave, cannellini, lima, or black-eyed beans |
| 8 cups | 64 ounces, 1.92 l | Water or stock |
| $\frac{1}{3}$ cup | $2\frac{1}{2}$ ounces, 75 ml | Olive oil |
| 1 cup | 4 ounces, 112 g | Onion, $\frac{1}{4}$ inch (.6 cm) dice |
| 1 cup | 4 ounces, 112 g | Celery, including leaves, $\frac{1}{4}$ inch (.6 cm) dice |
| 1 cup | 4 ounces, 112 g | Carrots, $\frac{1}{4}$ inch (.6 cm) dice |
| 1 tablespoon | $\frac{1}{2}$ ounce, 14 g | Garlic, minced |
| $1\frac{1}{2}$ cups | 9 ounces, 270 ml | Tomatoes, peeled, seeded, $\frac{1}{4}$ inch (.6 cm) dice |
| 2 tablespoons | 1 ounce, 28 g | Tomato paste |
| $\frac{1}{2}$ teaspoon | | Granulated sugar |
| To taste | | Salt and pepper |
| $\frac{1}{2}$ cup | 1 ounce, 28 g | Flat-leaf parsley, chopped |
| As needed | | Cayenne pepper |
| As needed | | Lemon juice |

PROCEDURE

1. Soak the beans in water overnight and drain.
2. Combine beans and water or stock; bring to boil.
3. Heat oil and sauté onions until transparent, 3 minutes.
4. Add celery and carrots and cook 3 to 4 minutes; add garlic and cook 1 minute.
5. Add tomatoes and tomato paste, cook 2 to 3 minutes.
6. Combine cooked vegetables with beans, bring to boil, reduce to simmer, and cook until beans are soft. Time depends on type of bean.
7. Add sugar and correct seasoning with salt and pepper.
8. To thicken the soup, mash some of the beans and vegetables against the side of the pot.
9. Stir in the chopped parsley and correct seasoning with toasted cayenne pepper and lemon juice if desired.

# Garithes Saganaki

## Baked Shrimp SERVES 4

| AMOUNT | MEASURE | INGREDIENT |
|---|---|---|
| | 1 pound, 448 g | 16–20 count uncooked shrimp, peeled and deveined |
| 2 tablespoons | 1 ounce, 30 ml | Fresh lemon juice |
| $\frac{1}{4}$ cup | 2 ounces, 60 ml | Olive oil |
| 1 cup | 4 ounces, 112 g | Onions, $\frac{1}{4}$ inch (.6 cm) dice |
| 2 tablespoons | 1 ounce, 28 g | Pepperoncini, minced |
| 2 | | Garlic cloves, minced |
| $\frac{1}{2}$ cup | 2 ounces, 56 g | Green onion, minced |
| 1 cup | 6 ounces, 240 ml | Tomatoes, peeled, seeded, $\frac{1}{4}$ inch (.6 cm) dice |
| $\frac{1}{4}$ cup | 2 ounces, 60 ml | Dry white wine |
| $\frac{1}{4}$ cup | $\frac{1}{2}$ ounce, 14 g | Parsley, chopped |
| $\frac{1}{2}$ teaspoon | | Oregano |
| To taste | | Salt and pepper |
| $\frac{1}{2}$ cup | 2 ounces, 56 g | Feta cheese, crumbled |

**PROCEDURE**

1. Sprinkle the cleaned shrimp with lemon juice and let stand until sauce is ready.
2. Heat oil over medium heat and sauté onions until transparent, 2 to 3 minutes. Add pepperoncini and garlic and cook 2 minutes; add green onion and cook 1 minute.
3. Add tomato to onion mixture and cook 5 minutes. Add shrimp, white wine, and half the parsley and oregano; cook 2 minutes. Correct seasoning.
4. Spoon half the tomato sauce into 4 individual oven dishes or 1 large dish. Add shrimp and spoon remaining sauce over shrimp; top with crumbled cheese.
5. Bake in a 450°F (232°C) oven for 6 to 7 minutes or until shrimp are firm (160°F, 71.1°C) and the feta is melted and lightly browned. Do not overcook or the shrimp will be tough.
6. Sprinkle with remaining parsley and serve with crusty bread.

# Afelia Fried Pork with Coriander

SERVES 4

| AMOUNT | MEASURE | INGREDIENT |
|---|---|---|
| **1 ½ pounds** | **680 g** | **Pork tenderloin, cut in ½ inch (1.2 cm) cubes** |
| **1 ½ cups** | **12 ounces, 360 ml** | **Good-quality dry red wine** |
| **1 teaspoon** | | **Salt** |
| **2 tablespoons** | | **Coriander seeds, coarsely crushed** |
| **1** | | **Cinnamon stick** |
| **To taste** | | **Black pepper, freshly ground** |
| **6 tablespoons** | **3 ounces, 180 ml** | **Olive oil** |
| **As needed** | | **Pourgouri pilafi (recipe follows)** |

PROCEDURE

1 Combine pork with red wine, salt, 1 tablespoon coriander seeds, cinnamon stick, and fresh pepper to taste (this dish requires lots of pepper). Marinate under refrigeration for at least 2 hours, turning pork occasionally.

2 Drain pork, reserving marinade, and pat dry. Do not discard the marinade.

3 Heat oil in pan over medium-high heat. Add pork; turn up heat to high and sauté, stirring frequently, until browned and just cooked through. Remove to serving plate.

4 Discard most of remaining fat, add remaining coriander seeds, and lightly toast until fragrant. Return marinade to pan, reduce until about ¼ cup (2 ounces, 60 ml) remains; should be sauce consistency. Discard cinnamon stick and correct seasoning.

5 Return pork, toss to coat, and reheat pork.

6 Serve immediately with pourgouri pilafi and yogurt.

# Pourgouri Pilafi

## Pilaf of Cracked Wheat

SERVES 4

| AMOUNT | MEASURE | INGREDIENT |
|---|---|---|
| 2 tablespoons | 1 ounce, 30 ml | Olive oil |
| 1 cup | 4 ounces, 112 g | Onion, $\frac{1}{4}$ inch (.6 cm) dice |
| $\frac{1}{2}$ cup | 1 ounce, 28 g | Vermicelli, crumbled |
| 2 cups | 16 ounces, 480 ml | Chicken stock |
| 1 cup | 7 ounces, 196 g | Pourgouri (coarse cracked wheat) |
| To taste | | Salt and pepper |

**PROCEDURE**

1. Heat oil over medium heat and sauté onion until transparent, 3 minutes.
2. Stir in vermicelli; sauté with onion until vermicelli begins to absorb the oil.
3. Add the stock and bring to a boil.
4. Wash the pourgouri under cold running water; add to liquid, and season to taste.
5. Stir until it boils again, reduce heat to a simmer, and cook 8 to 10 minutes or until all the stock is absorbed.
6. Let sit for 10 minutes before serving.

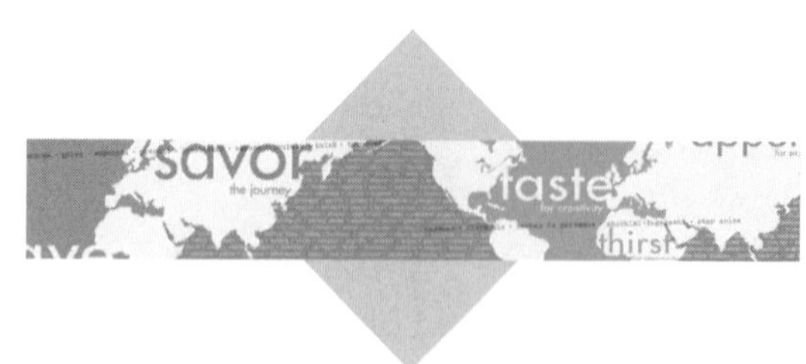

# Fresh Fruit

**Sweets are not the everyday desert in Greece but are rather reserved for special occasions, holidays, or between-meal treats. Serve fresh fruits such as grapes, figs, melons, pomegranates, or whatever is in season. In Greece, the fruits usually come in a large bowl of ice water. Dried fruits such as figs and raisins are standard winter fare. A bowl of nuts usually accompanies the fruits.**

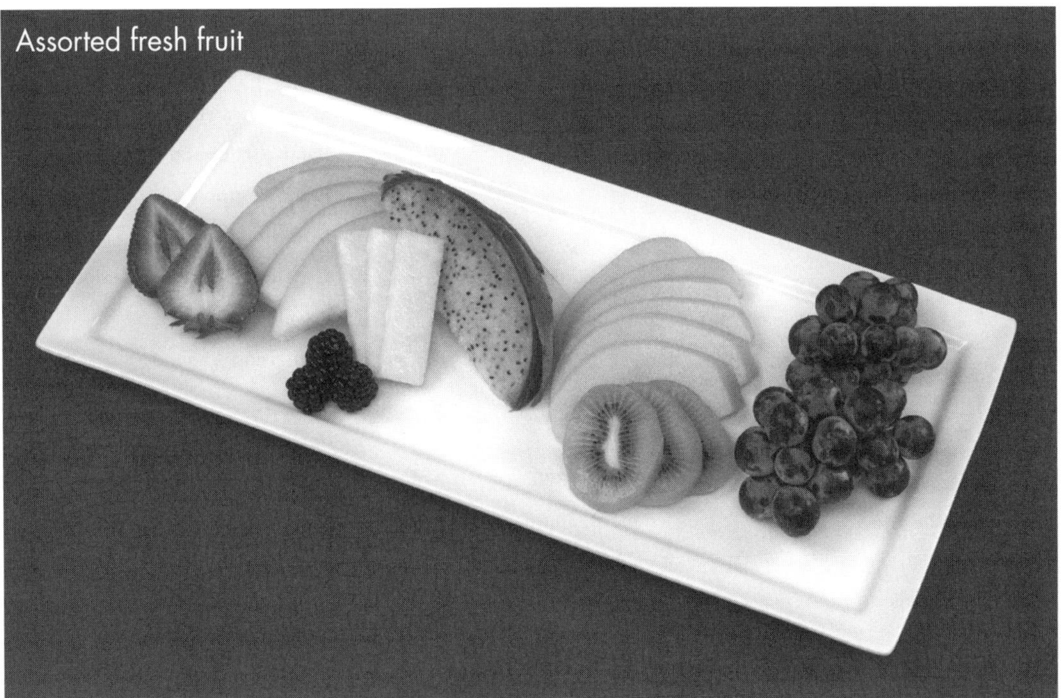
Assorted fresh fruit

# Dolmathakia me Rizi

## Stuffed Grape Vine Leaves

YIELD: ABOUT 30; SERVES 4–6

| AMOUNT | MEASURE | INGREDIENT |
|---|---|---|
| 8 ounces | 240 ml | Preserved vine leaves, or 40 fresh leaves |
| 2 tablespoons | $\frac{1}{2}$ ounce, 14 g | Pine nuts |
| $\frac{1}{4}$ cup | 2 ounces, 60 ml | Olive oil |
| 1 cup | 4 ounces, 112 g | Onions, $\frac{1}{8}$ inch (.3 cm) dice |
| $\frac{1}{2}$ cup | 3$\frac{1}{2}$ ounces, 98 g | Short-grain rice |
| $\frac{1}{4}$ cup | $\frac{1}{2}$ ounce, 14 g | Parsley, chopped |
| 1 teaspoon | | Mint, chopped |
| 1 tablespoon | | Dill, chopped |
| $\frac{1}{2}$ cup | 2 ounces, 56 g | Green onion, tops included, chopped |
| $\frac{1}{8}$ teaspoon | | Allspice, ground |
| $\frac{1}{8}$ teaspoon | | Cinnamon, ground |
| 1 teaspoon | | Salt |
| To taste | | Pepper, freshly ground |
| 1$\frac{1}{4}$ cups | 10 ounces, 300 ml | Vegetable or chicken stock |
| 2 tablespoons | 1 ounces, 30 ml | Lemon juice |
| 1 cup | 8 ounces, 240 ml | Olive oil |
| As needed | | *Tzatziki* (recipe follows) |

PROCEDURE

1 Drain brine from the grape leaves, rinse in cold water, and blanch in boiling water 1 minute. Transfer to a cold-water bath and drain in colander until needed. If using fresh leaves, blanch in boiling water for 3 to 4 minutes; shock and drain.

2 Toast pine nuts in oven until they just turn amber.

3 Heat oil over medium heat and sauté onions until transparent, 5 minutes.

4 Add rice; stir until completely coated with oil.

5 Add herbs, allspice, cinnamon, and season with salt and pepper. Add $\frac{1}{2}$ cup (4 ounces, 120 ml) stock.

6 Cover pan and simmer 5 minutes. Remove from heat and stir in pine nuts. Cool.

7. To shape dolma, place a vine leaf, shiny side down, on work surface. Snip off stem if necessary. Place about a tablespoon of mixture near stem end, fold end and sides over stuffing, and roll up firmly. (Do not roll too tightly because the rice will swell).
8. Line base of a shallow pan with vine leaves (use damaged ones) and place dolmas side by side in layers, seam side down and close together. Sprinkle with lemon juice; add 1 cup (8 ounces, 240 ml) olive oil and remaining stock (enough just to cover the dolmas). Cover top rolls with remaining grape vine leave.
9. Place a plate over dolma to prevent them from opening, cover and simmer over a low heat for about 35 to 40 minutes or until rice is completely cooked.
10. Uncover the dolmas so they can cool quickly. As soon as they can be handled, remove with a spatula and arrange on a platter. Serve warm or at room temperature with *tzatziki* and lemon wedges.

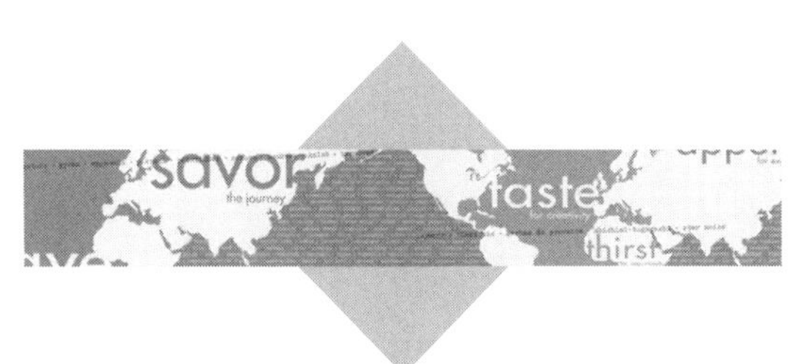

# Saganaki Fried Cheese SERVES 4

| AMOUNT | MEASURE | INGREDIENT |
| --- | --- | --- |
| | 12 ounces, 336 g | Kefalograviera, kasseri, or graviera cheese, or provolone |
| As needed | | Flour for dredging |
| $\frac{1}{2}$ cup | 4 ounces, 120 ml | Olive oil |
| 1 | | Lemon, cut in wedges |

**PROCEDURE**

1. Cut the cheese into strips 2 inches (4.9 cm) wide and $\frac{1}{2}$ inch (1.2 cm) thick.
2. Run strips under cold running water and dredge lightly with flour. Be sure to cover all surfaces of the cheese with flour.
3. Heat oil over medium-high heat and pan-fry cheese, turning once, until golden brown on both sides.
4. Remove, drain on paper towels, and serve immediately, accompanied by the lemon wedges. Or squeeze lemon juice to taste onto fried cheese, serve cheese in pan. Serve with additional lemon wedges and eat with crusty bread, which is dipped into the lemon-flavored oil in the pan.

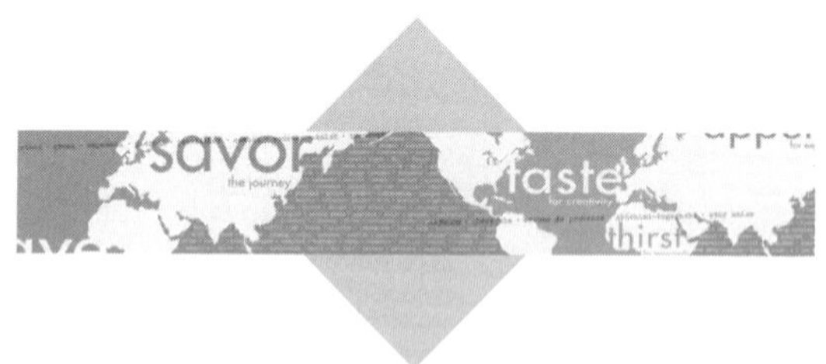

# Tzatziki

## Garlic, Cucumber, and Yogurt Dip

SERVES 4

| AMOUNT | MEASURE | INGREDIENT |
|---|---|---|
| 1 cup | 8 ounces, 240 ml | Plain yogurt |
| 1 cup | 6 ounces, 180 ml | Cucumber, peeled, seeded, and shredded |
| 3 | | Garlic cloves, minced |
| 2 tablespoons | 1 ounce, 30 ml | Olive oil |
| 1 tablespoon | $\frac{1}{2}$ ounce, 15 ml | Red wine vinegar or lemon juice |
| To taste | | Salt and black pepper |
| | | Mint leaves for garnish |

PROCEDURE

1. Drain the yogurt in a colander lined with cheesecloth for at least 1 hour. The yogurt will lose about a third of its volume and will be considerably creamier and thicker.
2. Press the shredded cucumbers in a colander with a dish on top of them to weigh them down, and let drain for one hour. Squeeze the cucumber to remove all excess moisture.
3. Combine yogurt, cucumbers, garlic, olive oil, vinegar, salt, and pepper; mix well. Refrigerate for 1 hour before serving.
4. Serve chilled with crusty bread, garnished with mint leaves.

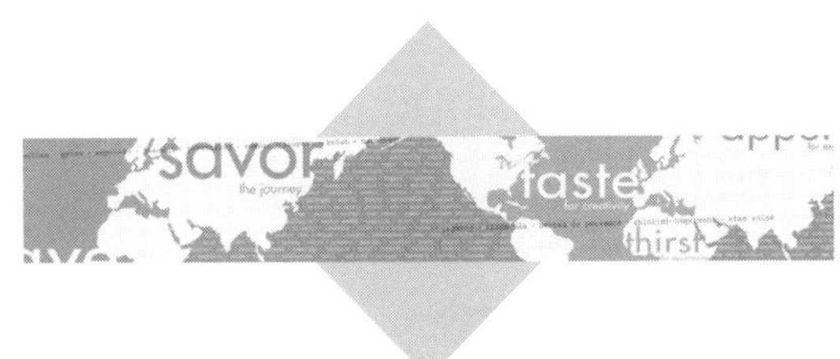

# Salata me Portokalia kai Elies

## Orange and Olive Salad

SERVES 4

| AMOUNT | MEASURE | INGREDIENT |
|---|---|---|
| 4 | | Navel oranges, peeled, pith removed, and sliced into $\frac{1}{4}$ inch (.6 cm) rounds |
| 1 cup | 4 ounces, 112 g | Red onion, cut into very thin rings |
| 1 cup | 4 ounces, 112 g | Kalamata olives, pitted, rinsed, and halved |
| 1 | | Garlic clove, smashed |
| $\frac{1}{2}$ teaspoon | | Dried thyme |
| $\frac{1}{2}$ teaspoon | | Black peppercorns |
| 2 tablespoons | 1 ounce, 30 ml | Orange juice, fresh strained |
| 2 teaspoons | 20 ml | Red wine vinegar |
| $\frac{1}{4}$ cup | 2 ounces, 60 ml | Extra virgin olive oil |
| 1 cup | 2 ounces, 56 g | Arugula leaves, washed, patted dry, and shredded |

PROCEDURE

1 Arrange the oranges, onions, and olives on a platter.

2 Using a mortar and pestle, crush together the garlic, thyme, and peppercorns. Combine spices with orange juice, vinegar, and olive oil; whisk well to combine.

3 Sprinkle the shredded arugula leaves over the oranges, onion slices, and drizzle with the dressing.

4 Serve immediately.

# Psari Savoro

## Fried Fish with Rosemary and Vinegar

SERVES 4

| AMOUNT | MEASURE | INGREDIENT |
|---|---|---|
| 4 | 4–5 ounce, 112–140 g | Fish fillets, boneless and skinned |
| 2 tablespoons | 1 ounce, 30 ml | Fresh lemon juice |
| As needed | | Salt |
| As needed | | Olive oil, for frying |
| As needed | | All-purpose flour |
| 2 | | Garlic cloves, minced |
| 1 teaspoon | | Rosemary leaves, fresh or dried |
| 3 tablespoons | $1\frac{1}{2}$ ounces, 45 ml | Sherry or red wine vinegar |
| 3 tablespoons | $1\frac{1}{2}$ ounces, 45 ml | White wine |
| To taste | | Salt and fresh pepper |

PROCEDURE

1 Sprinkle fish with lemon juice and salt; let sit 30 minutes.

2 Heat oil over medium heat.

3 Flour fish and pan-fry until golden brown on both sides and cooked completely. Drain and place on warm dish.

4 Pour off all but 2 tablespoons (1 ounce, 30 ml) oil. Add garlic and rosemary; cook 1 minute. Sprinkle in 2 teaspoons flour and stir over medium heat until lightly colored.

5 Add vinegar and white wine; cook 1 minute, stirring constantly. Correct seasoning and consistency (thin with water if too thick) and serve over fish.

# Fasolakia

## Fresh Green Bean Ragout

SERVES 4

| AMOUNT | MEASURE | INGREDIENT |
|---|---|---|
| $\frac{1}{4}$ cup | 2 ounces, 60 ml | Olive oil |
| 1 cup | 6 ounces, 168 g | Red onions, halved, thinly sliced |
| 3 | | Garlic cloves, minced |
| 1 pound | 16 ounces, 448 g | Green beans, trimmed |
| 2 cups | 10 ounces, 280 g | Potato, peeled, $\frac{1}{2}$ inch (1.2 cm) dice |
| 1 | | Fresh or dried chile pepper |
| 1 cup | 6 ounces, 168 g | Tomato, peeled, seeded, $\frac{1}{4}$ inch (.6 cm) dice |
| To taste | | Salt and pepper |
| $\frac{1}{2}$ cup | 1 ounce, 28 g | Parsley, chopped |
| 2 tablespoons | 1 ounce, 30 ml | Red wine vinegar |
| 1 cup | 6 ounces, 168 g | Feta cheese |

PROCEDURE

1. Heat olive oil over medium heat and sauté onions and garlic until soft, 7 minutes.
2. Add green beans and toss to coat. Cover pan, reduce heat, and steam green beans in the oil for 10 minutes.
3. Add potatoes and chile pepper, toss to coat, add tomatoes, and season with salt and pepper.
4. Add enough water just to cover vegetables. Cover pan and simmer until beans and potatoes are tender, 20 to 30 minutes.
5. Add parsley and vinegar, toss to coat, and cook 5 minutes.
6. Adjust seasoning. Serve warm or at room temperature, with feta cheese on the side.

# Kataifi Nut-Stuffed Shredded Wheat Rolls

YIELD: 12 ROLLS

| AMOUNT | MEASURE | INGREDIENT |
|---|---|---|
| 1 $\frac{1}{4}$ cups | 12 ounces, 360 ml | Butter, melted |
| $\frac{3}{4}$ cup | 3 ounces, 84 g | Walnuts, coarsely ground |
| $\frac{3}{4}$ cup | 3 ounces, 84 g | Almonds, coarsely ground |
| $\frac{1}{8}$ cup | 1 ounce, 28 g | Granulated sugar |
| $\frac{1}{2}$ teaspoon | | Cinnamon, ground |
| 1 | | Egg, beaten |
| 2 tablespoons | 1 ounce, 30 ml | Heavy cream |
| 8 ounces | | Kataifi pastry, thawed, room temperature |
| Galaktoboureko Syrup | | |
| 1 cup | 7 ounces, 196 g | Granulated sugar |
| 1 cup | 8 ounces, 240 ml | Water |
| 1 tablespoon | $\frac{1}{2}$ ounce, 15 ml | Fresh lemon juice |
| Pinch | | Cinnamon, ground |

PROCEDURE

1 Brush sheet pan with melted butter and set aside.

2 Combine nuts, sugar, and cinnamon; mix well.

3 Beat egg with cream and 3 tablespoons melted butter.

4 To prepare shredded wheat rolls, spread out a handful of the pastry to about 6 inches long. Brush generously with melted butter, place a tablespoon of nut filling on bottom, and roll up tightly, incorporating the loose ends inward as you go.

5 Place seam side down on buttered pan, and repeat with remaining pastry and filling.

6 Brush the tops of the pastries liberally with remaining butter.

7 Bake at 350°F (180°C), 1 hour.

8 Remove to a rack and let stand for 5 to 10 minutes.

9 Make syrup by combining sugar and water over medium heat; as soon as sugar dissolves, add lemon juice and cinnamon. Bring to a boil, reduce heat, and simmer 10 minutes.

10 Spoon hot syrup over rolls. Cover the pan with a clean towel and let stand 2 to 3 hours before serving, occasionally basting with syrup.

# Moussaka Eggplant Moussaka SERVES 4

| AMOUNT | MEASURE | INGREDIENT |
|---|---|---|
| 1 | 16 ounce, 448 g | Eggplant, skin on, cut into $\frac{1}{4}$ inch (.6 cm) slices |
| As needed | | Salt |
| **Meat Sauce** | | |
| 2 tablespoons | 1 ounce, 30 ml | Olive oil |
| 1 cup | 6 ounces, 168 g | Onion, $\frac{1}{4}$ inch (.6 cm) dice |
| 2 | | Garlic cloves, minced |
| 2 cups | 1 pound, 16 ounces, 448 g | Ground lamb or lean ground beef |
| 1 cup | 6 ounces, 180 ml | Tomato, peeled, seeded, $\frac{1}{4}$ inch (.6 cm) dice |
| 2 tablespoons | 1 ounce, 30 ml | Tomato paste |
| $\frac{1}{2}$ cup | 4 ounces, 120 ml | White wine |
| 2 tablespoons | | Chopped parsley |
| 1 teaspoon | | Sugar |
| $\frac{1}{4}$ teaspoon | | Cinnamon, ground |
| To taste | | Salt and pepper |
| **Cream Sauce** | | |
| $\frac{1}{4}$ cup | 2 ounces, 60 ml | Butter |
| $\frac{1}{3}$ cup | 2.33 ounces, 66 g | Flour, all-purpose |
| 2 cups | 16 ounces, 480 ml | Milk |
| $\frac{1}{8}$ teaspoon | | Nutmeg |
| $\frac{1}{4}$ cup | 1 ounce, 28 g | Kefalotiri or Parmesan cheese |
| To taste | | Salt and pepper |
| 1 | | Egg, lightly beaten |

## PROCEDURE

1 Sprinkle eggplant slices with salt and let sit 1 hour. Dry with paper towels.

### Meat Sauce

1 Heat oil over medium heat and sauté onion, 2 minutes. Add garlic; cook 2 minutes or until onions are soft.

2 Add lamb and brown over high heat, stirring well. Add remaining meat sauce ingredients; cover and cook 20 minutes. Correct seasoning.

**Cream Sauce**

1. Melt butter over medium heat and stir in flour; cook gently 2 minutes. Add milk, stir to combine, turn heat to high, and bring to a boil. Cook 2 minutes. Remove from heat.
2. Sir in nutmeg and 1 tablespoon cheese; correct seasoning.

**Assemble Moussaka**

1. Oil an 8 × 8 inch (20 × 20 cm) baking pan. Place a layer of eggplant slices in the base. Top with half the meat sauce, add another layer of eggplant, the remainder of meat sauce, and finish with eggplant.
2. Stir beaten egg into sauce and spread on top. Sprinkle with remaining cheese.
3. Bake at 350°F (180°C), 1 hour. Let stand 10 minutes before cutting into squares to serve.

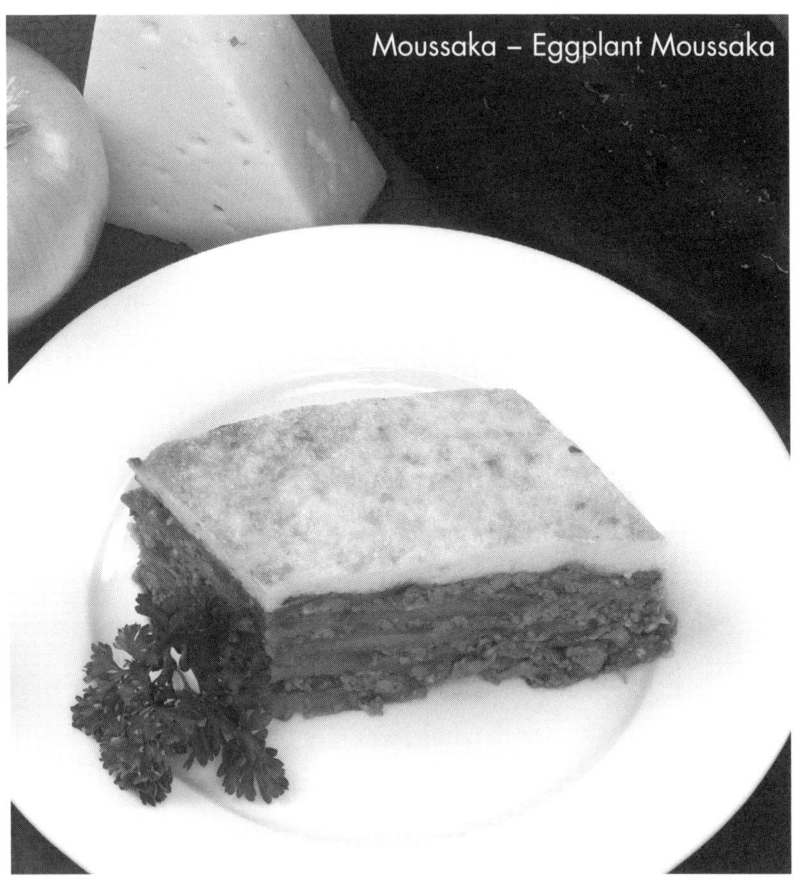

Moussaka – Eggplant Moussaka

# Kabak Kizartmasi and Patlican Kizartmasi

## Zucchini and Eggplant Fritters

SERVES 4

| AMOUNT | MEASURE | INGREDIENT |
|---|---|---|
| 2 cups | 10 ounces, 280 g | Long slender eggplant |
| 2 cups | 10 ounces, 280 g | Zucchini, $\frac{3}{4}$ inch (1.8 cm) slices lengthwise or diagonally |
| As needed | | Oil for pan-frying |
| 1 cup | 7 ounce, 196 g | All-purpose flour |
| 1 teaspoon | | Salt |
| $\frac{3}{4}$ cup | 6 ounces, 180 ml | Beer |
| 2 | | Garlic cloves |
| $\frac{1}{2}$ teaspoon | | Salt |
| 1 cup | 8 ounces, 240 ml | Yogurt |
| As needed | | Tarator (recipe follows) |

### PROCEDURE

1. Peel off lengthwise strips of eggplant to give a striped effect, then cut into $\frac{1}{4}$ inch (.6 cm) diagonal slices. Sprinkle liberally with salt and leave for 30 minutes. Wipe off salt and dry with paper towels.
2. Oil eggplant slices on both sides and broil or grill, turning, until brown on both sides. Alternatively, eggplant may be pan-fried. Remove from heat or oil and stack until needed.
3. To make batter, sift flour and salt together; add beer and mix to a smooth batter.
4. Dip eggplant and zucchini into batter and pan-fry until tender and golden brown on both sides, approximately 2 to 3 minutes. Drain on paper towels.
5. Serve hot with *yogurt salcasi* and *tarator.*

### *Yogurt Salacasi:* Yogurt Sauce

1. Mash 2 cloves garlic with salt to a fine paste. Combine with yogurt and chill.

## Tarator Hazelnut Sauce

YIELD: 2 CUPS

| AMOUNT | MEASURE | INGREDIENT |
|---|---|---|
| **1 cup** | **4 ounces, 112 g** | **Hazelnuts, whole and peeled** |
| **1 cup** | **3 ounces, 84 g** | **Fresh white breadcrumbs** |
| **2** | | **Garlic cloves, crushed** |
| **1 tablespoon** | **$\frac{1}{2}$ ounce, 15 ml** | **Water** |
| **1 cup** | **8 ounces, 240 ml** | **Olive oil** |
| **$\frac{1}{2}$ cup** | **4 ounces, 120 ml** | **White vinegar or fresh lemon juice** |
| **1 teaspoon** | | **Salt** |

**PROCEDURE**

1. Grind hazelnuts in a blender or food processor or pound in mortar. If using a mortar, place nuts in a bowl when pulverized.
2. Add breadcrumbs, garlic, and water; process while adding oil.
3. Gradually add vinegar, process until smooth, and add salt.
4. Chill and serve.

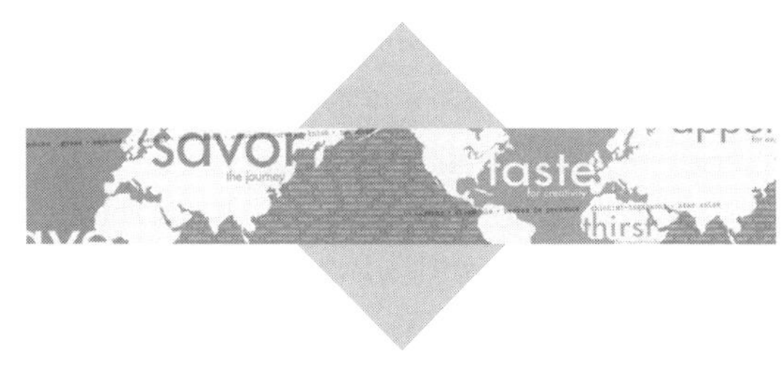

# Midye Dolmasi

## Stuffed Mussels SERVES 4

| AMOUNT | MEASURE | INGREDIENT |
|---|---|---|
| $\frac{1}{4}$ cup | 2 ounces, 60 ml | Olive oil |
| 1 cup | 4 ounces, 112 g | Onions, $\frac{1}{4}$ inch (.6 cm) dice |
| 1 tablespoon | | Pine nuts |
| $\frac{1}{2}$ cup | 4 ounces, 112 g | Long-grain rice, washed |
| 1 tablespoon | | Parsley, chopped |
| $\frac{1}{2}$ teaspoon | | Allspice, ground |
| $\frac{1}{2}$ cup | 3 ounces, 90 ml | Tomatoes, peeled, seeded, $\frac{1}{4}$ inch (.6 cm) dice |
| $\frac{1}{2}$ cup | 4 ounces, 120 ml | Fish stock or water |
| To taste | | Salt and fresh pepper |
| 20 large | | Mussels |
| $\frac{1}{2}$ cup | 4 ounces, 120 ml | Fish stock or water |
| 4 | | Lemon wedges, for serving |
| As needed | | Tarator (see recipe on page 491) |

**PROCEDURE**

1. Heat oil over medium heat; sauté onions until transparent, 5 minutes. Add pine nuts and cook 2 minutes. Stir in rice, parsley, allspice, tomatoes, and $\frac{1}{2}$ cup (4 ounces, 120 ml) stock; add salt and pepper. Cover and simmer on low 15 minutes until liquid is absorbed.
2. Prepare mussels. Scrub mussels well and tug beard toward pointed end of the mussel to remove. To open, place scrubbed mussels in warm salted water. As they open, insert point of knife between the shells and slice it toward pointed end to sever the closing mechanism. For stuffing do not separate shells.
3. Place 2 teaspoons of filling in each mussel and close the shell as much as possible. Arrange mussels in a even layer, and place a weight on top to keep them closed.
4. Add water or stock, bring to a simmer, cover pan, and simmer 15 to 20 minutes, until mussel meat is cooked. Turn off heat and cool in pan.
5. Carefully remove mussels and wipe shell with paper towel. Shells may be lightly oiled for a more attractive appearance.
6. Serve chilled or at room temperature with lemon wedges and tarator.

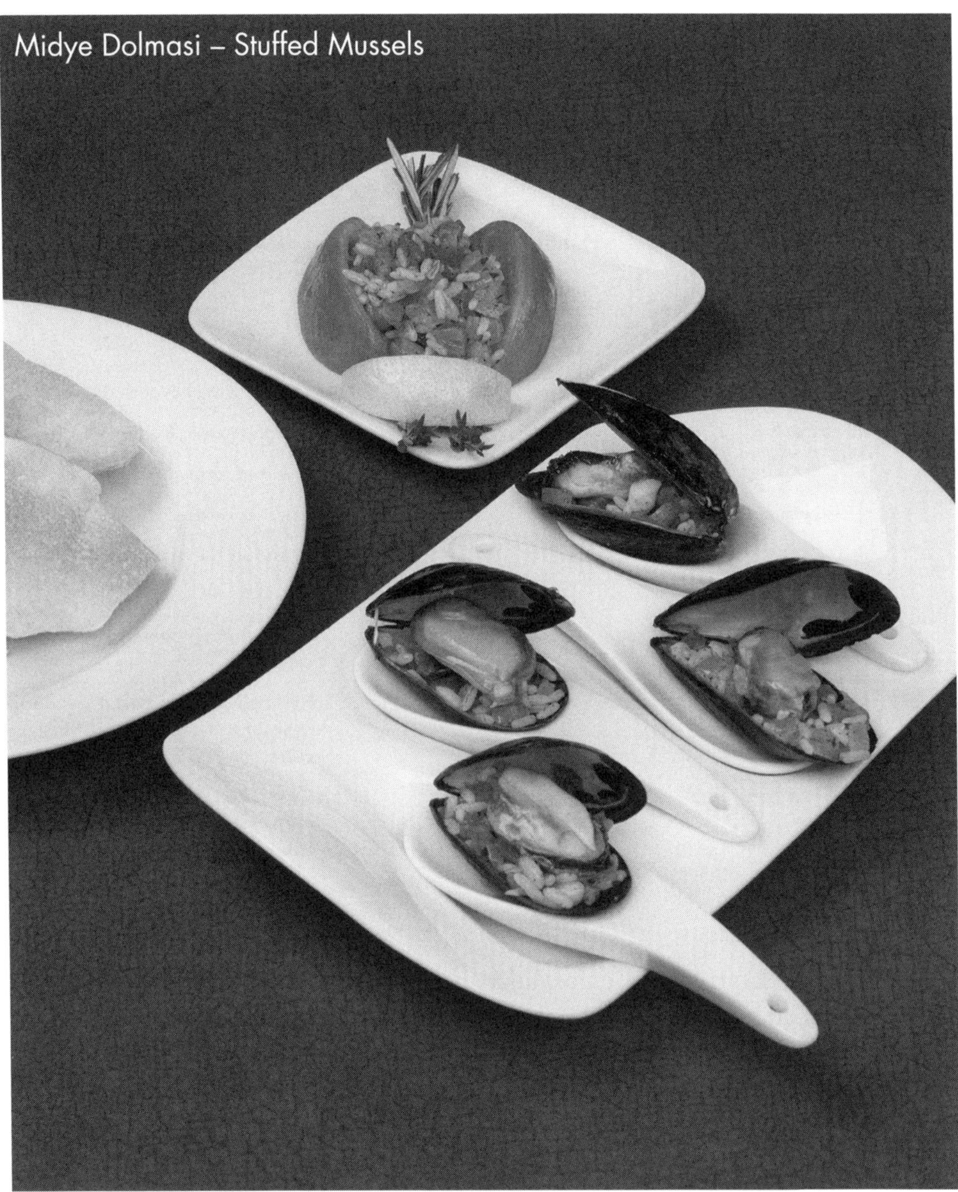
Midye Dolmasi – Stuffed Mussels

# Sis Kebap

## Skewered Lamb and Vegetables

SERVES 4

| AMOUNT | MEASURE | INGREDIENT |
|---|---|---|
| | 20 ounces, 560 g | Lamb meat, boneless from leg, $1\frac{1}{4}$ inch (3.18 cm) cubes |
| 2 tablespoons | 1 ounce, 30 ml | Fresh lemon juice |
| $\frac{1}{4}$ cup | 2 ounces, 60 ml | Olive oil |
| $\frac{3}{4}$ cup | 3 ounces, 84 g | Onion, thinly sliced |
| To taste | | Black pepper, freshly ground |
| 1 | | Bay leaf, crumbled |
| $\frac{1}{2}$ teaspoon | | Thyme, dried |
| 8 | | Wooden skewers, soaked in water 1 hour |
| Garnish | | |
| 8 | | Pearl onions, peeled and parboiled in salted water |
| 8 cubes | | Red bell pepper, cored, seeded, white membrane removed, cut in $1\frac{1}{4}$ inch (3.18 cm) cubes |
| 8 cubes | | Green bell pepper, cored, seeded, white membrane removed, cut in $1\frac{1}{4}$ inch (3.18 cm) cubes |

**PROCEDURE**

1. Combine lamb cubes, lemon juice, olive oil, onions, black pepper, bay leaf, and thyme. Do not add salt, it draws out the meat juices. Mix well and marinate at room temperature 1 hour or refrigerate 2 to 3 hours.
2. Blanch bell peppers in boiling salted water for 30 seconds; let cool.
3. To assemble skewers, remove meat from marinade and thread onto 8 skewers, alternating cubes of meat with onions and peppers.
4. Grill over medium high heat, turning frequently and brushing with marinade when required. After searing meat, move to lower heat to avoid burning vegetables.
5. Serve hot on a bed of Beyaz Pilav, colored with turmeric.

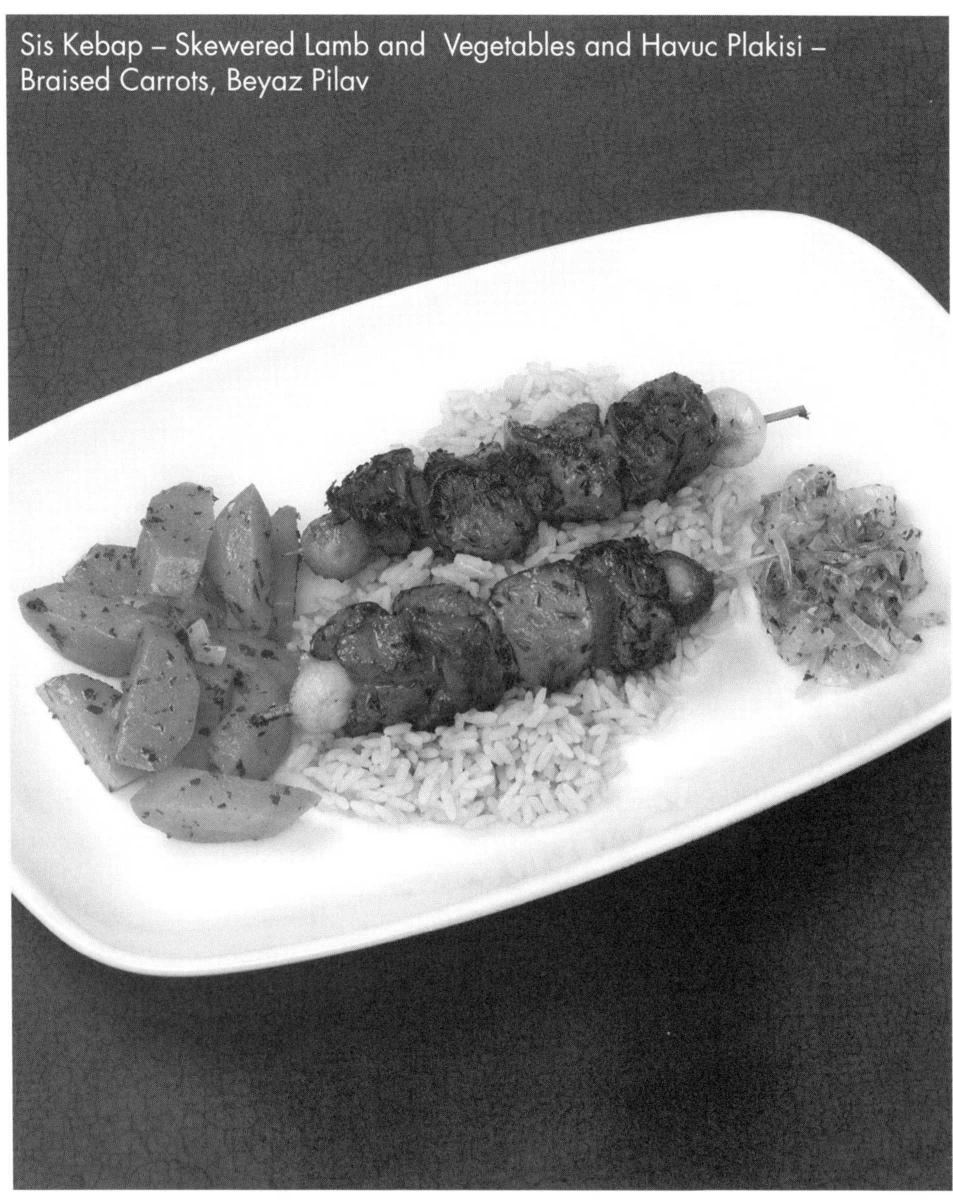

Sis Kebap – Skewered Lamb and Vegetables and Havuc Plakisi – Braised Carrots, Beyaz Pilav

# Balik Köftesi Fish Balls SERVES 4

| AMOUNT | MEASURE | INGREDIENT |
|---|---|---|
| | 12 ounces, 336 g | White fish fillets, skinless, boneless |
| $\frac{1}{4}$ cup | 1 ounce, 28 g | Green onion, white only, minced |
| 1 tablespoon | | Parsley, minced |
| 1 teaspoon | | Dill, minced |
| Pinch | | Hot red pepper |
| $\frac{3}{4}$ cup | 3 ounces, 84 g | Fresh white breadcrumbs |
| 1 | | Egg |
| To taste | | Salt and fresh pepper |
| As needed | | All-purpose flour |
| As needed | | Oil for deep-frying |
| 4 | | Lemon wedges, for serving |

**PROCEDURE**

1. In a food processor combine fish, onion, parsley, dill, and red pepper; process to a smooth paste.
2. Remove to a bowl and work in breadcrumbs and egg; work to a paste and correct seasoning. Do not overwork.
3. With moistened hands, shape into balls the size of walnuts. Chill until firm.
4. Coat with flour and deep-fry for 4 to 6 minutes at 370°F (188°C).
5. Drain on paper towels and serve hot with lemon wedges.

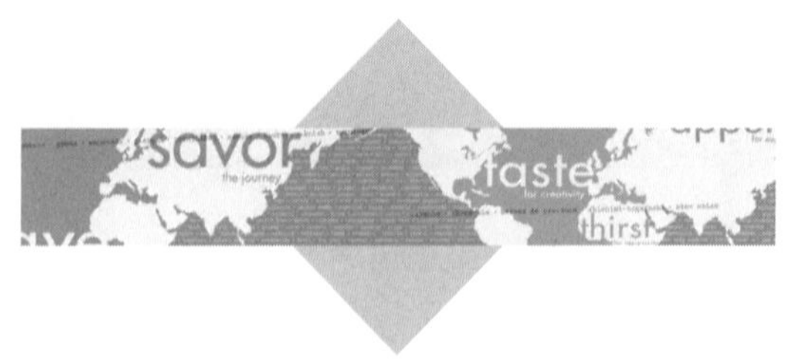

# Domates Salatasi

## Tomato Salad

SERVES 4

| AMOUNT | MEASURE | INGREDIENT |
|---|---|---|
| 2 | 10 ounces, 280 g | Tomatoes, firm |
| 1 | 10 ounces, 280 g | English cucumber |
| 2 tablespoons | 1 ounce, 30 ml | Lemon juice |
| 1 tablespoon | $\frac{1}{2}$ ounce, 15 ml | White vinegar |
| 2 tablespoons | 1 ounce, 30 ml | Olive oil |
| 1 teaspoon | | Fresh mint, chopped fine |
| 2 teaspoons | | Fresh parsley, chopped fine |
| To taste | | Salt and fresh pepper |
| $\frac{3}{4}$ cup | 3 ounces, 84 g | Black olives, pitted |

PROCEDURE

1. Peel tomatoes and slice $\frac{1}{8}$ inch (.3 cm) thick; arrange in a row on platter.
2. Peel cucumber and slice $\frac{1}{8}$ inch (.3 cm) thick; arrange in a row on platter.
3. Combine lemon juice, vinegar, olive oil, mint, and parsley; correct seasoning.
4. Pour over tomatoes and cucumber. Chill 15 minutes.
5. Garnish platter with olives before serving.

# Havuc Plakisi Braised Carrots

SERVES 4

| AMOUNT | MEASURE | INGREDIENT |
| --- | --- | --- |
| $\frac{1}{4}$ cup | 2 ounces, 60 ml | Olive oil |
| 1 cup | 4 ounces, 112 g | Onions, cut in half lengthwise, then sliced into thin semicircles |
| 1 pound | 16 ounces, 448 g | Carrots, $\frac{1}{4}$ inch (.6 cm) diagonal slices |
| $\frac{3}{4}$ cup | 6 ounces, 180 ml | Water |
| 2 tablespoons | | Parsley, chopped |
| 1 teaspoon | | Granulated sugar |
| To taste | | Salt and freshly ground black pepper |
| 1 teaspoon | | Fresh lemon juice |

**PROCEDURE**

1. Heat oil over medium heat and sauté onions until transparent, 5 minutes.
2. Add carrots and cook 5 minutes, stirring frequently.
3. Add water, half the parsley and sugar. Season to taste, cover pan tightly, and simmer on low heat until carrots are tender, 15 minutes. Remove from heat, add lemon juice, and correct seasoning. Remove to serving dish to cool to room temperature.
4. Serve sprinkled with remaining parsley.

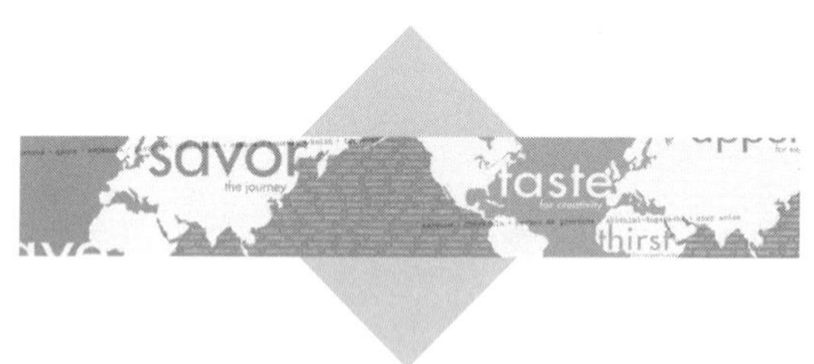

# Beyaz Pilave Plain Pilaf

SERVES 4

| AMOUNT | MEASURE | INGREDIENT |
| --- | --- | --- |
| 1 cup | 7 ounces, 196 g | Long-grain rice |
| 2 tablespoons | 1 ounce, 30 ml | Olive oil |
| $\frac{1}{4}$ teaspoon | | Turmeric |
| 1$\frac{3}{4}$ cups | 14 ounces, 420 ml | Chicken stock |
| To taste | | Salt |

**PROCEDURE**

1. Wash rice until water runs clean. Drain well.
2. Heat oil over medium heat and add turmeric; stir to incorporate.
3. Add rice and sauté for 5 minutes.
4. Add stock, salt to taste, and stir occasionally until boiling. Reduce heat, cover, and simmer 20 minutes or until firm to the bite but evenly tender.
5. Remove from heat and let stand, covered, for 5 minutes.
6. Fluff up with a fork and serve.

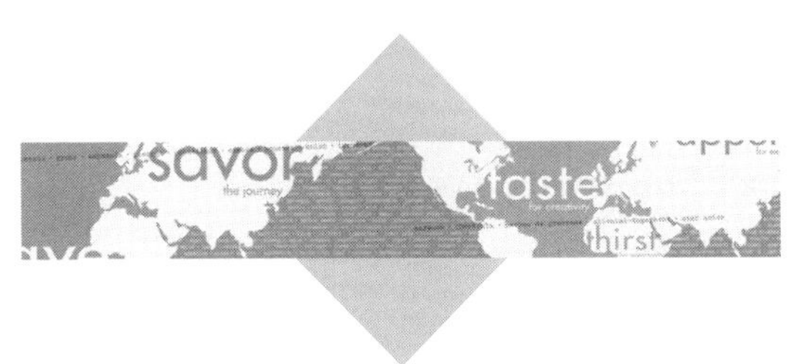

# Íncír Compostu Figs in Syrup

SERVES 4

| AMOUNT | MEASURE | INGREDIENT |
|---|---|---|
| | 12 ounces, 336 g | Dried figs |
| 3 cups | 24 ounces, 720 ml | Water |
| As needed | | Blanched almonds |
| $\frac{1}{2}$ cup | 4 ounces, 112 g | Granulated sugar |
| Thin strip | | Lemon rind |
| 2 tablespoons | 1 ounce, 30 ml | Fresh lemon juice |
| 3 tablespoons | $1\frac{1}{2}$ ounces, 45 ml | Honey |
| $\frac{1}{4}$ cup | 1 ounce, 28 g | Pistachios, almonds, or walnuts, chopped |
| $\frac{1}{2}$ cup | 4 ounces, 120 ml | Yogurt |

PROCEDURE

1 Wash figs and plump in cold water overnight, or simmer gently for 10 minutes. Drain and save liquid.

2 Insert almond in base of each fig; set aside.

3 Add sugar to water; heat to dissolve. Add lemon rind, juice, and honey; bring to a boil.

4 Add prepared figs and return to the boil. Simmer gently for 30 minutes, until figs are tender and syrup is thick. If necessary, remove figs and reduce cooking liquid. Remove lemon rind.

5 Arrange figs and pour syrup over, chill.

6 Sprinkle with chopped nuts and serve with yogurt.

# Africa

## The Land

The African continent is bordered by the Indian Ocean to the east, the Atlantic Ocean to the west, and the Mediterranean Sea to the north. It was once connected to Asia's land mass in the northeastern corner by the Sinai Peninsula, where the Suez Canal now exists. The Nile River in northeast Africa is the longest river in the world and has been a source of survival for many African people for thousands of years. The river and its tributaries run through nine countries and flow a total of 4,160 miles, providing food, fertile land, and a mode of transportation.

Northern Africa includes Algeria, Morocco, Tunisia, Libya, Egypt, and the Sudan. The Atlas Mountains run from Morocco to Tunisia, covering more than 1,200 miles and providing a route between the coast and the Sahara Desert. Both the High and Middle Atlas slopes have dense forests containing cedar, pine, cork, and oak trees. There are fertile valleys and tracts of pasture where livestock can feed. Within the mountain range, there is a wide variety of mineral deposits that have hardly been touched. The Sahara Desert separates northern Africa from the rest of the continent. All of the regions south of northern Africa are known as sub-Sahara.

Western Africa includes the countries Mali, Burkina Faso, Niger, the Ivory Coast (Cote d'Ivoire), Guinea, Senegal, Mauritania, Benin, Togo, Cameroon, Guinea-Bissau, Sao Tome and Principe, Cape Verde, Equatorial Guinea, Western Sahara, Liberia, Sierra Leone, Gambia, Ghana, and Nigeria. West Africa contains dense forests, vast expanses of desert and grassland, environmentally important wetland areas, and many large, sprawling cities. Virgin rain forests that once covered much of the West African coast have been drastically reduced by logging and agriculture. The southern regions' tropical rain forest grows some of the world's most prized hardwood trees, such as mahogany and iroko. The Niger River flows 2,600 miles and supports rich fish stocks.

Eastern Africa includes Ethiopia, Eritrea, Somalia, Djibouti, Rwanda, Burundi, Uganda, Kenya, Mozambique, Angola, and Tanzania. The Great Rift Valley dominates East Africa and includes Lake Victoria, the mountains of Kilimanjaro, and Mount Kenya. East Africa's coastline is among the finest in the world and includes an almost continuous belt of coral reefs that provide an important habitat for fish and other marine life. The vast expanses of savanna grassland that cover much of the rest of East Africa are home to many of the region's people and much of its rich wildlife. The Serengeti and the Masai Mara contain some of the greatest concentrations of wildlife in the world. In northern Kenya the savanna turns into a semiarid landscape where few people live and very little grows. Nairobi, Mombasa, Dar es Salaam, and Kampala are thriving modern cities in stark contrast to the vast savanna plains of Tanzania, the rain forests of western Uganda, and the remote deserts of northern Kenya. These cities reflect East Africa's relatively advanced development compared with other African countries.

Central Africa includes the Democratic Republic of the Congo (formerly Zaire), the Congo, Gabon, Chad, Central African Republic, Zambia, and Malawi. The great rain forest basin of the Congo River embraces most of Central Africa. Lake Chad is the fourth largest lake in Africa and is located in the Sahel zone of west-central Africa between Chad, Cameroon, Nigeria, and Niger. Lake Chad is a very important asset to the region, because of its contribution to the region's hydrology and because of the diversity of flora and fauna that it attracts. The Lake Chad region is known for its important role in trans-Saharan trade and for important archaeological discoveries that have been made here.

Southern Africa includes the countries of South Africa, Namibia, Lesotho, Swaziland, Botswana, as well as the islands of Madagascar, Mauritius, Seychelles, and Comoros. Like much of the African continent, this region is dominated by a high plateau in the interior, surrounded by a narrow strip of coastal lowlands. Unlike most of Africa, however, the perimeter of South Africa's inland plateau rises abruptly to form a series of mountain ranges before dropping to sea level. These mountains are known as the Great Escarpment. The coastline is fairly regular and has few natural harbors. Each of the dominant land features—the inland plateau, the encircling mountain ranges, and the coastal lowlands—exhibits a wide range of variation in topography and in natural resources, The interior plateau consists of a series of rolling grasslands (*veld* in Afrikaans), arising out of the Kalahari Desert in the north. The largest subregion in the plateau is the 1,200-meter to 1,800-meter-high central area known as the Highveld that stretches from Western Cape province to the northeast. In the north, it rises into a series of rock formations known as the Witwatersrand (literally, "Ridge of White Waters" in Afrikaans, commonly shortened to Rand). The Rand is a ridge of gold-bearing rock that serves as a watershed for numerous rivers and streams. It is also the site of the world's largest proven gold deposits and the country's leading industrial city, Johannesburg. North of the Witwatersrand is a dry savanna subregion known as the Bushveld, characterized by

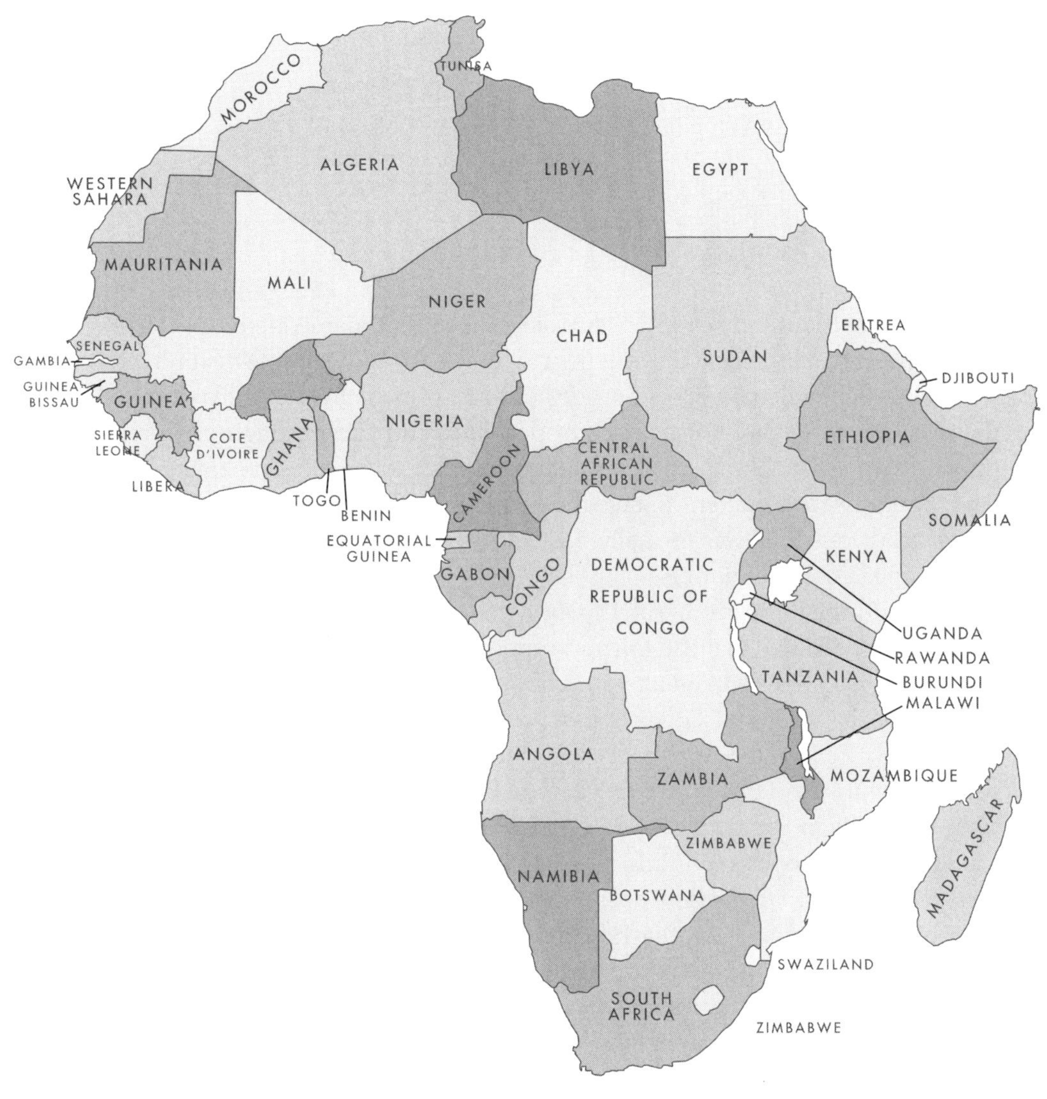
MOROCCO
TUNISA
ALGERIA
LIBYA
EGYPT
WESTERN
SAHARA
MAURITANIA
MALI
NIGER
CHAD
SUDAN
ERITREA
SENEGAL
GAMBIA
GUINEA
BISSAU
GUINEA
DJIBOUTI
SIERRA
LEONE
COTE
D'IVOIRE
GHANA
NIGERIA
ETHIOPIA
LIBERA
TOGO
BENIN
CAMEROON
CENTRAL
AFRICAN
REPUBLIC
SOMALIA
EQUATORIAL
GUINEA
GABON
CONGO
DEMOCRATIC
REPUBLIC OF
CONGO
KENYA
UGANDA
RAWANDA
BURUNDI
TANZANIA
MALAWI
ANGOLA
ZAMBIA
MOZAMBIQUE
MADAGASCAR
ZIMBABWE
NAMIBIA
BOTSWANA
SWAZILAND
SOUTH
AFRICA
ZIMBABWE

Africa

open grasslands with scattered trees and bushes. The Bushveld, like the Rand, is a treasure chest of minerals, one of the largest and best known layered igneous (volcanic) mineral complexes in the world. It has extensive deposits of chromium and significant reserves of copper, gold, nickel, and iron. South Africa is rich in diamonds and is the world's biggest supplier of platinum.

# History

Until about a thousand years ago, Africa was a land of many different tribes with a few larger kingdoms. It had little contact with the rest of the world. Over the next nine hundred years, it was slowly penetrated by other outside cultures, principally the Arabs of the Middle East and the seafaring nations of northwest Europe. These intruders brought their religions—Islam in the north and east, Christianity in much of the rest—and the slave trade. A few settled in the land, but most were content to take the continent's riches home with them. By the end of the 1800s, most of Africa was formally divided into European colonies, under the direct rule of the European colonial powers.

It was during this period, with the slave trade abolished and most of the continent explored, mapped, and divided, that the European powers began to govern Africa on a daily basis.

This colonial period ended, with a few exceptions, in the late 1950s and early 1960s. In the decade that followed Ghana's independence in 1957 (the first sub-Saharan country to gain independence), the British, French, and Belgians withdrew from almost all their African colonies. Only the Portuguese (in Angola, Mozambique, and Portuguese Guinea) and the white minority government of South Africa clung to colonial power.

After the European administrators went home, most of the newly independent countries set out to develop their economies along free enterprise lines and to establish systems of government. There have been some successes. A few economies have flourished, at least for a while, and there are signs that democracy has taken root in some countries. But mostly there have been failures. Over the last forty years, many African countries have succumbed to brutal dictators, and economic progress has been either minimal or nonexistent. As poverty and hopelessness have spread, violence has erupted both within and between states.

African countries are varied in their levels of economic development; however, the continent as a whole is considered to be a developing region. The most economically developed country is South Africa. Next are the Mediterranean countries in northern Africa as well as Nigeria. Zaire, Kenya, Cameroon, Ghana, Cote d'Ivoire, Zimbabwe, Gabon, Reunion, Namibia, and Mauritius are considered to be partly developed. The remaining countries are considered to be less developed.

# The People

The people of Africa belong to several thousand different ethnic groups. At the same time, over the centuries the different groups have also influenced one another and contributed to and enriched one another's culture. There are over fifty countries in Africa, and some have twenty or more different ethnic groups living within their boundaries.

While the majority of the countries in Africa are inhabited by people of African origin, some ethnic groups have been affected by the migration of Arab peoples into northern Africa. There are also Europeans whose families moved to Africa during the colonial period and have stayed on. In some parts of Africa, there are people of Asian origin, such as those from the Indian subcontinent. Some of the more widely known ethnic groups in Africa are Arabs, Ashanti, Bantu, Berbers, Bushmen, Dinka, Fulani, Ganda, Hamites, Hausa, Hottentot, Kikuyu, Luba, Lunda, Malinke, Moors, Nuer, Semites, Swahili, Tuareg, Xhosa, and Yoruba.

Although the majority of the people in Africa lead a rural life, the continent is urbanizing at a fast pace. Over a third of the population now lives in cities. Those who live and work in the major metropolitan areas live in ways similar to most people in the industrialized world. However, they may not always have all the advantages of those who live in the larger, more modern cities. Their schools may have fewer resources, the opportunities for earning a living may not be as varied, and the services available may not be as technologically advanced.

The lifestyle of those living in rural Africa has remained virtually unchanged for centuries. They have rich cultural heritages that they have passed down from generation to generation with very little influence from the outside world.

There is extreme poverty and vast wealth; there are people who suffer from droughts and famine and people who have plentiful food. There are vast, magnificent nature reserves with an abundance of wildlife and there are highly urbanized parts with major cities with high-rise buildings and modern amenities. Much of the economy is based on agriculture in most African countries; and yet only 6 percent of the land mass is arable, while 25 percent is covered with forests, and another 25 percent is used for pasture or rangeland. Approximately 66 percent of the available workforce is involved in farming. Most of the back-country communities practice subsistence farming, growing just enough to feed their villages.

# The Food

The prime characteristic of native African meals is the use of starch as a focus, typically accompanied by a stew containing meat or vegetables, or both. Starch filler foods, similar to the rice cuisines of Asia, are a hallmark. Yams, beans, lentils, millet, plantains, green bananas, and cassava are some of the essential foods in Africa. Meat is often used merely as one of a number of flavorings, rather than as a main ingredient in cooking. Other major foods, such as wheat and rice, are imported on a wide scale from Asia, Europe, and North America, especially in countries where the climate does not admit extensive cultivation.

The African taste and use of ingredients has changed a great deal. In the eastern part of the continent (especially in Kenya) Arab explorers brought dried fruits, rice, and spices and expanded the diets of the coastal farmers. They also brought oranges, lemons, and limes from China and India. The British imported new breeds of sheep, goats, and cattle, as well as strawberries and asparagus. Beans, cassava, groundnuts, corn, tomatoes, sweet potatoes, and seasonings like pepper, cinnamon, clove, curry, and nutmeg were introduced to Africa as a direct result of European exploration of the North American continent.

Traditional ways of cooking involve steaming food in leaf wrappers (banana or corn husks), boiling, frying in oil, grilling, roasting in a fire, or baking in ashes.

## NORTH AFRICA

The countries of North Africa that border the Mediterranean Sea are largely Muslim. As a result, their diet reflects Islamic traditions, such as not eating pork or any animal product that has not been butchered in accordance with the traditions of the faith. Each North African region has its signature seasonings. Morocco's *ras el hanout* (or "head of the shop") includes twenty-five to forty different ingredients, including cinnamon, black peppercorns, green cardamon, caraway, nutmeg, and rosebuds. As with curry powder, each vendor creates his or her own recipe. *Chermoula,* a Moroccan marinade, contains garlic, onions, mint, paprika, and almonds. Tunisia's *harissa,* a deep-red, hot table condiment with red chilies, cumin, garlic, tomatoes, vinegar, and olive oil is used even at breakfast. Morocco and Algeria have milder versions. Egyptians season meats with *baharat,* made with cinnamon, cumin, allspice, and paprika.

The national dish of Algeria and Tunisia is couscous, which is steamed semolina wheat, served with lamb or chicken, cooked vegetables, and gravy. This is so basic to the diet that its name in Arabic, *ta'am,* translates simply as "food." Common flavorings include onions, turnips, raisins, chickpeas, and red peppers, as well as salt, pepper, cumin, and coriander. Alternatively, couscous can be served sweet, flavored with honey, cinnamon, or almonds. Couscous presentation varies among regions. Algerians serve couscous, meat, and sauce in individual dishes, and mix them together at the table. Tunisians like it very moist with sauced meats or vegetables spooned over it. In Morocco, sauced meat or vegetables are served in a hole formed in a mound of couscous. Lamb is popular and is often prepared over an open fire and served with bread. This dish is called *mechoui.* Other common foods are *chorba,* a spicy soup; *dolma,* a mixture of tomatoes and peppers; and *bourek,* a specialty of Algiers consisting of minced meat with onions and fried eggs, rolled and fried in batter.

The most traditional dish in Morocco is a *tangine* (tanjine), named for the covered conical clay earthenware dish it is cooked in. It may be made with lamb, chicken, or other meat, and is a combination of sweet and sour flavors. It usually includes prunes, almonds, onions, and cinnamon. Pigeons are often included in dishes, particularly the *bastila*, a flaky pastry filled with meat, nuts, and spices and coated with sugar and cinnamon before it is baked. Popular vegetables include okra, *meloukhia* (spinachlike greens), and radishes. Fruits found in this region include oranges, lemons, and pears. Legumes such as broad beans (fava beans), lentils, yellow peas, and black-eyed peas are important staples. Mint tea and coffee are very popular beverages in this region.

The main crops in Egypt are barley and *emmer*, a type of wheat. Nuts such as pistachios, pine nuts, almonds, hazelnuts, and walnuts are cultivated. Apples, apricots, grapes, melons, quinces, figs, and pomegranates grow in this fertile region. Ancient gardens featured lettuce, peas, cucumbers, beets, beans, herbs, and greens. Pharaohs considered mushrooms a delicacy. Egypt has several national dishes. *Koushari* (lentils, macaroni, rice, and chickpeas) *kofta* (spicy, minced lamb), and *kebab* (grilled lamb pieces) are the most popular. *Ful* (pronounced "fool," bean paste), *tahini* (sesame paste), and *aish baladi* (a pitalike bread) are common accompaniments. Egypt's records indicate that bread was made in more than thirty different shapes. They included pita types made either with refined white flour called *aysh shami*, or with coarse, whole wheat *aysh baladi*. Sweet cakes were made by combining honey, dates and other fruits, spices, and nuts with the dough, which was baked in the shapes of animals and birds.

The main staple of the Sudanese diet is a type of bread called *kissra*, which is made of *durra* (sorghum, one of the most important cereal crops in the world) or corn. It is served with the many variety of stews. Dried okra is used in preparing stews like *waika*, *bussaara,* and *sabaroag*. *Miris* is a stew that is made from sheep's fat, onions, and dried okra. Vegetables like potatoes, eggplants, and others are used in preparing other stews with meat, onions, peanut butter, and spices. *Elmaraara* and *umfitit* are made of sheep lungs, liver, and stomach. To these are added onions, peanut butter, and salt; it is eaten raw. Soups are an important part of Sudanese cuisine; the most popular is *kawari'*, made of cattle's or sheep's hoofs with vegetables and spices. *Elmussalammiya* is a soup made with liver, flour, dates, and spices. These meals are accompanied with porridge (*asseeda*), which is made with wheat flour or corn, and served with *kissra*.

Due to climatic conditions and poor soils, Libya imports most foods. Domestic food production meets only about 25 percent of demand. Typically, grains such as wheat and barley, dates, and soft fruits provide the staple items, along with lamb and some fish.

## WESTERN AFRICA

This is the first part of Africa that Europeans explored. Prior to this, main staples included rice, millet, and lentils. Portuguese, British, Dutch, and other European traders introduced several foods that became staples, such as cassava and corn. Yams are an important crop in

West Africa and are served in a variety of dishes, including *amala* (pounded yam) and *egwansi* (melon) sauce. Millet is used for making porridge and beer. The plantain is abundant in the more tropical areas of West Africa. Dates, bananas, guava, melons, passion fruit, figs, jackfruit, mangos, pineapples, cashews, and wild lemons and oranges are also found here. Meat sources include cattle, sheep, chicken, and goat, though beef is normally reserved for holidays and special occasions. Fish is eaten in the coastal areas. Palm oil is the base of stew in the Gambia, southern, and eastern regions. In the Sahara area, peanut butter is the main ingredient for stew. All the stews in this territory are heavily spiced with chiles and tend to be based on okra, beans, sweet potato leaves, and cassava. Other vegetables are eggplant, cabbage, carrots, French beans, lettuce, onions, and cherry tomatoes.

Côte d'Ivoire is the world's leading producer of cocoa, and is the third largest producer of coffee in the world (behind Brazil and Columbia). It is also Africa's leading exporter of pineapples and palm oil. The people of Côte d'Ivoire rely on grains and tubers to sustain their diet. Yams, plantains, rice, millet, corn, and peanuts are typically an ingredient in most dishes. The national dish is *n'voufou* (called *fufu*), which is plantains, cassava, or yams pounded into a sticky dough and served with a seasoned meat (often chicken) and vegetable sauce called *kedjenou*. As with most meals, it is typically eaten with the hands, rather than utensils. *Kedjenou* is a meal prepared from peanuts, eggplant, okra, or tomatoes. *Attiéké* is a popular side dish. Similar to the tiny pasta grains of couscous, it is a porridge made from grated cassava. Habanero peppers are the most widely cultivated pepper. Fresh fruits are the typical dessert, often accompanied by *bangui*, a local white palm wine or ginger beer. Often the best place to sample the country's local cuisine is at an outdoor market, a street vendor, or a *maquis*, a restaurant unique to Côte d'Ivoire. These reasonably priced outdoor restaurants are scattered throughout the country and are growing in popularity. To be considered a *maquis* the restaurant must sell braised food, usually chicken or fish served with onions and tomatoes.

Nigeria has such a variety of people and cultures that it is difficult identify just one national dish. A large part of Nigeria lies in the tropics, where the popular fruits are oranges, melons, grapefruits, limes, mangoes, bananas, and pineapples. People of the northern region (mostly Muslim, whose beliefs prohibit eating pork) have diets based on beans, sorghum, and brown rice. The people from the eastern part of Nigeria, mostly Igbo/Ibo, eat *gari* (cassava powder) dumplings, pumpkins, and yams. The Yoruba people of the southwest and central areas eat *gari* with local varieties of okra and spinach in stews (*efo*) or soups. A common way coastal Nigerians prepare fish is to make a marinade of ginger, tomatoes, and cayenne pepper, and then cook the fish in peanut oil.

## EASTERN AFRICA

Extensive trade and migrations with Arabic countries and South Asia has made East African culture unique, particularly along the coast. The main staples include potatoes, rice, *matake* (mashed plantains), and a thick porridge made from corn. Beans or a stew with potatoes, or vegetables often accompany the porridge. Outside of Kenya and the horn of Africa, the stew is not as spicy, but the coastal area has spicy, coconut-based stews. The grain *teff* is used in this area and has a considerably higher iron and nutrient content than other grain staples found in Africa. In East Africa cattle, sheep, and goats are regarded as more a form of currency and status, and so are rarely eaten.

The cuisine of modern-day Somalia and Ethiopia is characterized by very spicy food prepared with chiles and garlic. In addition to flavoring the food, the spices also help to preserve meat in a country where refrigeration is rare. *Berbere* is the name of the special spicy paste that Ethiopians use to preserve and flavor foods. According to Ethiopian culture, the woman with the best *berbere* has the best chance to win a good husband. The national dish of Ethiopia is *wot*, a spicy stew. *Wot* may be made from beef, lamb, chicken, goat, or even lentils or chickpeas, but it always contains spicy *berbere*. *Alecha* is a less-spicy stew seasoned with green ginger. A soft white cheese called *lab* is popular. A common traditional food is *injera*, a spongy flat bread that is eaten by tearing it, then using it to scoop up the meat or stew. Although Ethiopians rarely use sugar, honey is occasionally used as a sweetener. A special Ethiopian treat is *injera* wrapped around a fresh honeycomb with young honeybee grubs still inside.

About half of the Ethiopian population is Orthodox Christian. During Lent, the forty days preceding the Christian holiday of Easter, Orthodox Christians are prohibited from eating any foods from animal products (no meat, cheese, milk, or butter). Instead they eat dishes made from beans, lentils, chickpeas, field peas, and peanuts called *mitin shiro*. The beans are boiled, roasted, ground, and combined with *berbere*. This mixture can be made into a vegetarian *wot* by adding vegetable oil and then shaped like a fish or an egg; it is eaten cold. During festive times such as marriage feasts, *kwalima*, a kind of smoked and dried beef sausage made with onions, pepper, ginger, cumin, basil, cardamom, cinnamon, cloves, and tumeric, is served.

Traditional Kenyan foods reflect the many different lifestyles of the various groups in the country. Staple foods consist mainly of corn, potatoes, and beans. *Ugali*, a corn porridge, is typically eaten inland, while the coastal peoples eat a more varied diet.

The Maasai, cattle-herding peoples who live in Kenya and Tanzania, eat simple foods, relying on cow and goat by-products (such as the animal's meat, milk, and blood). The Maasai do not eat any wild game or fish, depending only on the livestock they raise for food. The Kikuyu and Gikuyu grow corn, beans, potatoes, and greens. They mash all of these vegetables together to make *irio*. They roll *irio* into balls and dip them into meat or vegetable stews. In western Kenya, the people living near Lake Victoria (the second largest freshwater lake in the world) mainly prepare fish stews, vegetable dishes, and rice.

Swahili dishes reflect a history of contact with the Arabs and other Indian Ocean traders. Their dried fruits, rice, and spices expanded the Swahili diet. Here, coconut and spices are used heavily. Although there is not a specific national cuisine, there are two national dishes: *ugali* and *nyama choma*. Corn is a Kenyan staple and the main ingredient of *ugali*, which is thick and similar to porridge. *Nyama choma* is the Kiswahili phrase meaning "roasted meat." Huge chunks of meat are roasted over an open charcoal fire. Typically, the chunks consist of a whole leg, or the ribs making up one half of the chest. Special stoves are used so that the grill holding the meat can be raised or lowered depending on the conditions of the fire, and the temperatures needed to cook the meat. The *nyama choma* challenge is that after the countless raising and the lowering of the grill, the meat is well done but not dry. *Sukuma wiki* is a combination of chopped spinach or kale that is fried with onions, tomatoes, maybe a green pepper, and any leftover meat, if available. Fresh fruits include mangoes, papaya, pineapple, watermelon, oranges, guavas, bananas, coconuts, and passion fruit.

The Portuguese influence upon Angola and Mozambique is pervasive and subtle. They were the first Europeans to colonize Africa south of the Sahara in the fifteenth century. This relatively inconspicuous European country influenced African life more than the more direct and intrusive British, French, and Dutch. The Portuguese brought the European sense of flavoring with spices, and techniques of roasting and marinating to African foods. Catholicism also influenced Portuguese African cuisine in the sense of feast and fast days, and meatless Fridays. The Portuguese brought oranges, lemons, and limes from their Asian colonies. From South America they brought the foods of the new world: chiles, peppers, corn, tomatoes, pineapples, bananas, and the domestic pig. Mozambique is more fish based. Angola is reflective of the west side, with drier climate, and corresponding change in ingredients.

In addition to growing cashews, Mozambique is most known for its *piripiri*, or hot pepper dishes. Using the small, tremendously hot peppers of that country, sieved lemon juice is warmed and red freshly picked chiles are added and simmered exactly five minutes, then salted and pounded to a paste. This pulp is returned to heat with more lemon juice and served over meats, fish, and shellfish.

## CENTRAL AFRICA

Very little is known about central African cuisine, due partly to lack of documentation, as most central African languages were not written down until the colonial era of the eighteenth and nineteenth centuries. Slaves, ivory, rubber, and minerals interested most the Europeans and Arabs who went there.

One distinguishing characteristic of central African cooking is the use of edible leaves, collard greens, kale, and mustard greens. Often greens are the main ingredient in the daily stew, cooked with only a little onion, hot pepper, meat, fish, or oil for flavoring. Some of the greens consumed in central Africa are bitterleaf, cassava, okra, pumpkin, sorrel, sweet potato, and taro. People cultivate these greens as well as gather them from the wild. In many tropical areas of the world cassava is grown primarily for its tubers, but Africans have a long tradition of eating both the leaves and the tubers of this plant. Before cooking, women pound greens in a mortar and pestle, or roll them like giant cigars and use a sharp knife to shred them finely. *Saka-saka*, or *pondu*, is a dish made from cassava leaves, onion, and a bit of dried fish.

*Saka-madesu* contains cassava leaves cooked with beans. Another recipe, variations of which are found all over sub-Saharan Africa, calls for greens to be cooked with tomato, onion, and mashed peanuts.

One of the other distinguishing characteristics of central African cuisine is the use of red palm oil, obtained from the fruit of the African oil palm. Reddish and thick, it has a distinctive flavor for which there is no substitute. The oily pulp is cooked with chicken, onion, tomato, okra, garlic, or sorrel leaves, and chili pepper to produce a stew called *moambé* or *poulet nyembwe* (made with chicken). *Moambé* is also made with other meats.

One of the important central African cooking methods is steaming or grilling food wrapped in packets fashioned from the leaves of banana trees or other plants. This cooking method predates the use of iron and maybe even clay cooking pots. Certain leaves are especially favored because they give a particular flavor to food. *Maboké* (singular *liboké*, also called *ajomba* or *jomba*)—leaf-wrapped packets of meat or fish, with onion, tomato, and okra, seasoned with lemon juice or hot chile pepper—are grilled over hot coals or steamed in a pot. Crushed peanuts or *mbika* (seeds of a small gourd) are sometimes included. Filling the leaf packets with mashed beans (such as black-eyed peas) and sautéed peppers, then steaming, produces *koki* (also called *ekoki* or *gâteau de haricots*).

## SOUTH AFRICAN

The first people in South Africa, the San, were hunter-gatherers. The San have lived in Africa for nearly 30,000 years. About two thousand years ago, the Khoikhoi people moved into southern Africa from farther north. They settled in groups, raising sheep and cattle. Around A.D. 300, another group of people settled in what is now eastern South Africa. Known as the Bantu, they raised crops of corn, sweet potato, gem squash, and livestock.

Europeans first came to South Africa in 1488 when the Dutch East India Company established a food supply stop for the company's ships as they made their way around the Cape of Good Hope. Shortly after they arrived, the Dutch were joined by the Huguenots (Protestants from France) and the Germans. *Boerwors* is a homemade farmer's sausage evolved from recipes brought by German immigrants. In the fifteenth century, the Portuguese added traditional fish dishes. The South African waters, then as now, were rich in kingklip, snoek, red roman, hake, cod, and sole as well as abalone, oysters, mussels, calamari, shrimps, and crayfish. Cape Malay cuisine is one of the most flavorful in the country, characterized by a blend of styles and spices brought to South Africa by the Indonesian and Bengalese slaves. A mix of Asian, Indian, and European dishes is peppered with curry, cumin, ginger, and other exotic spices. Some of the best-known Cape Malay dishes include *sosaties* (traditional kebabs), *bobotie* (a curried one-pot meal made of minced meat cooked with brown sugar, apricots and raisins, milk-soaked mashed bread, and curry flavoring), and *bredies* (meat and vegetable casserole, much like a Shepherd's pie). Traditional dishes also include practical stews, such as *potjiekos*. The early hunters and trekkers stewed their game and whatever vegetables they could find from the land in a three-legged cast iron pot. As new animals were hunted, their meat was added to the pot, as were bones to thicken the stew. Today, *potjiekos* are just as popular and annual competitions to create the best are an important way of socializing around the campfire. Another typical South African food is *biltong*. Made of meat that has been dried, *biltong* is similar to meat jerky, made from any kind of meat, even ostrich, antelope, or crocodile.

The *braai* is the South African equivalent to the barbecue. Meat, fish, chicken, potatoes and onions are cooked over coals outdoors. The food may be *biltong* (jerky), *chilli-bites* (small balls of savory curried dough and vegetables deep fried) as a starter while waiting for the *sosaties* (kebabs), or *boerewors*. *Snoek braai* is a fish barbeque using snoek fish (a large game fish similar to a barracuda, a national delicacy, but very bony) caught off the Cape coast marinated in lemon juice, garlic, and herbs and cooked over coals.

*Mealies* are a very popular food in South Africa. Made from corn, *mealies* are either boiled or cooked over coals in the cob, or made into *mealie bread*. *Mealie pap*, a stiff cornmeal mix, is a staple food of the South African diet, accompanied by a variety of savory foods made from green vegetables and spiced with chili.

A dish called *umngqusho* is famous for being former President Nelson Mandela's favorite dish. It is made of *stamp mealies* (broken dried corn kernels) with sugar beans, butter, onions, potatoes, chiles, and lemons, then simmered. Another traditional dish is *mashonzha*. It is the Mopani caterpillar, cooked with chiles and often eaten with peanuts. *Melktert* is a typical South African dessert, a sour cream pastry filled with a mix of milk, flour, and eggs and flavored with cinnamon sugar.

# Glossary

**Agbono** This ground seed is used for its thickening properties. Like okra and baobab, it gives a sauce the slippery texture.

**Akara** Popular breakfast dish made from mashed black-eyed peas seasoned with salt, pepper, and onion, then deep-fried.

**Akassa** Ghanian porridge made from corn flour and hot water.

**Ana Ofia** Fresh meat from any forest animal. The meat is prepared by first singeing over an open fire, then washing and cutting as preparation for smoking, drying, or cooking. Most African meats are tough and stringy and therefore best prepared by marinating (in beer, wine, fruit juices, or soured milk), then cooking with moisture or used in soups and stews.

**Asida** Term used for a late morning meal usually consisting of *fufu* and relishes.

**Bajias** Small seasoned balls of cooked mashed potatoes or yams, flour-coated then deep-fried. A favorite of African Indians.

**Balila** Term used for the evening meal. In many areas care is taken to eat this before dark so as to avoid evil spirits.

**Bamia** Also called "ladyfingers." Both are names for okra.

**Baobab** The dried, powdered leaves of the Baobab tree, added to soups and stews for a slippery texture similar to okra.

**Baobab Tree** As functional as the coconut palm. Fruit and leaves are edible; ashes of the wood are used as salt; seeds and pods are roasted to make a drink or snack; the tree trunk is a source of water.

**Bastila** Flaky-crusted pigeon pie, a Moroccan specialty.

**Berbere** Red pepper spice paste used in Ethiopia.

**Biltong** Dried and salted raw meat similar to the beef jerky made in the United States. An older Afrikaner delicacy is made of ostrich, beef, kudu, or any other red meat.

**Bitterleaf (Ndole)** Variety of African greens used for medicinal as well as dietary purposes.

**Bobotie** A traditional South African dish of spicy-flavored ground lamb or beef (similar to meat loaf) topped with an egg custard; served with yellow rice.

**Boerewors** A traditional spicy South African sausage made of beef or lamb. Popular at open-air *braais* (barbecues).

**Bota** Thin gruel often prepared from millet and used as a supplementary food for infants.

**Braai** A barbecue featuring grilled meat, highly popular form of cooking (South Africa).

**Braaivleis** Afrikaans (a language derived from Dutch) for a barbecue.

**Breadfruit** A Malaysian evergreen timber tree (*Artocarpus altilis*) having large, round, yellowish, edible fruits. Breadfruit should be cooked as it begins to become ripe. Fully ripened, mushy breadfruit is not as good.

**Bredie** Traditional stews made from lamb or tomatoes and vegetables, cooked slowly over coals (South Africa).

**Callaloo** A casserole of vegetables, various fish, and seafood with meat and seasonings. A popular combination includes spinach, mixed seafood, and cubed lamb seasoned with garlic, chiles, and tomato paste. It thought that the Portuguese traders and explorers brought this recipe back with them. (This is also the name of a Caribbean soup named for the coarse green callaloo leaves from dasheen or taro plant.)

**Cardamom** Spice, the whole or ground dried fruit of *Elettaria cardamomum,* a plant of the ginger family indigenous to India and Sri Lanka. Used in curries, spiced tea, and coffee.

**Cassava** Also called manioc; the tuber from which manioc flour and tapioca are made. Slightly fermented and ground into flour, manioc is used to prepare the classic *gari.*

**Chapatis** Unleavened breads freshly made for a meal from almost any flour; they are rolled flat then deep-fried until they puff and brown. Well known in India and much favored by African Indians.

**Chenga** A thick milk soup made with rice or corn and thickened with corn flour (cornstarch). Considered one of the chief foods of East Africa.

**Cheese** The demand for cheese as a protein and vitamin-rich food supplement is growing in Africa, especially in light of an abundance of raw materials by way of cow's and goat's milk. Particular favorites are the Greek, Lebanese, and Italian styles of cheeses.

**Chihengi** Pineapple.

**Chin Chin** Deep-fried cookie leavened with Swahili yeast.

**Cocoyams** Variety of wild yams.

**Couscous** Cereal product made by moistening wheat flour and rolling it into small pellets, which are then steamed. A traditional staple food in North Africa.

**Daddawa** Black, fermented paste made from the flat beans of the locust tree. It has a very strong odor, but adds a wonderful flavor to sauces. Maggi sauce can be a substitute.

**Dendê oil** The Brazilian name for the densely rich palm oil brought to Brazil by West African slaves. Its reddish hue can be imitated by adding paprika to peanut or vegetable oil, though the flavor is not the same.

**Dovi** Paste of groundnuts (peanut butter).

**Duri** Mortar and pestle.

**Eguisi (Agusi, Agushi, Egushi)** Flour ground from seeds of various species of gourds, melons, pumpkins, and squashes, used as a thickener. In western Africa, the plants and seeds, as well as soups and stews made with them, are all called *egusi*.

**Fish** Dried, smoked, and salted. Drying and smoking were common methods of preservation before refrigeration. Used extensively in African cuisine.

**Fufu, Ugali, or Ampesi** Staple African food. Thick porridge-like mixture made by pounding then cooking any one of many starchy plant foods or mixtures of them. Corn, millet, rice, cassava, plantain, green bananas, or varieties of yams may be used. For eating, the mixture is formed into small balls with three fingers of the right hand then dipped into sauces or relishes made from fish, meat, or vegetables—almost always spicy hot.

**Futari Yams** Thick mixture of cooked potatoes flavored with groundnuts, tomatoes, and onions.

**Garden Eggs** Term for a small green-skinned African eggplants.

**Garri, or Gari** Slightly fermented cassava flour used in cooking. A favorite of many, especially Ghanians.

**Ghada** The midday meal.

**Groundnuts** Peanuts, a staple food.

**Guinea Pepper** Pepperlike spice made from the seed of a plant native to Africa, used in African cooking as a seasoning before the arrival of Asian black pepper.

**Gumbo** With a consistency between a soup and a stew, gumbo is derived from the African Bantu word for okra. Simmered gently with spicy seasoning, okra, and other vegetables, gumbos take their name from the main seafood or meat ingredient and are usually served over wild rice. In America, gumbos are a treasured part of Creole cuisine.

**Harira** Hearty soup with legumes, meat, and vegetables, important during Ramadan.

**Hovo or Hobo** Bananas.

**Lnjera** Classic Ethiopian bread prepared like a huge pancake from *teff* (fine millet flour).

**Ji Akwukwo** Very thick stew of many vegetables plus yams. Favorite in West Africa.

**Keuke** Corn bread prepared from wet fermented corn flour. Sour in East Africa, sweeter and whiter in West Africa.

**Kikwanga** Congo name for disc-shaped bread made from cassava flour. The same bread in Jamaica is called *bammy* and in the southern United States, pan bread.

**Kola Nuts** Brownish-orange, bitter nuts about the size of a chestnut. West Africans enjoy chewing them, and claim they give an extra burst of energy. These nuts contain two to three times the caffeine of coffee beans.

**Kuli-Kuli** Delicacy made from frying the residual groundnut paste after the oil has been extracted.

**Liboke (plural, Miboke)** Lingala word, meaning banana, used throughout the Congo region to describe food that is cooked, usually by steaming or grilling, in a packet made from banana leaves. Called *ajomba* or *jomba* along the Atlantic coast of central Africa.

**Madafu** Immature coconut water, a beverage.

**Maggi Cube or Maggi Sauce** Brand of bouillon cube and flavoring sauce, similar to soy sauce. Very popular in Africa.

**Maheu** Traditional drink for women and children; slightly alcoholic sweet liquid left from soaking cooked *fufu*.

**Mahshi** Almost any available variety of vegetable stuffed with a mix of ground meat or fish and rice and baked with tomato sauce.

**Manhanga** Term used to refer to many varieties of squash and pumpkin.

**Manioc or Cassava** General name given to any starch roots from which tapioca and other flours may be made.

**Manwiwa** Watermelon.

**Mealie** The South African name for cornmeal.

**Milioku Ngozi** Also called *blessing soup*. A hot West African soup usually made with a whole chicken and yams. Soup is served first, then sliced meat and vegetables are served afterward. Usually served at planting and harvest celebrations.

**Millet** The small grains of a cereal grass, used in preparation of some foods.

**Mseto** Swahili word for rice or lentils; usually cooked into a thick sauce, highly seasoned and served with meat or fish.

**Mudumbe** The succulent root fibers from the elephant ear plant.

**Muriwo** Relish or sauces accompanying *fufu*. These are an important part of the diet's nutrients, containing not only a wide variety of vegetables and seasonings (hot), but often meat and fish and bones, when available.

**Naarjes** South African tangerines, deep in color and rich in flavor.

**Nhopi** A *fufu* or porridge made from pumpkin.

**Niter Kibbeh** Clarified butter to which nutmeg, cinnamon, and cardamom seeds are added with turmeric for color, then browned, strained, and used as seasoning and cooking oil in Ethiopia.

**Ofe Nsala** A fiery pepper sauce made with a base of meat or fish. This is one of the most popular things served to women with new babies and may comprise the main part of the diet, diluted as a soup or gruel, or eaten with *fufu*.

**Ogbono** Seed kernel of the African wild mango, cooked and crushed to form a cake or powder used to thicken soups and stews.

**Ogede** Plantain.

**Oka Esiri Esi** A corn and milk soup.

**Okra** Generally thought to have originated in the wild in northern and northeastern Africa or western Asia, cultivated for its seedpod fruit.

**Olilie** One version of the seasoning paste made from dried, fermented, and cooked seeds, used for flavoring.

**Olele** A baked or steamed Nigerian pudding made from ground cowpeas (or blackeyed peas), onions, and salt.

**Palm Butter** Thick red paste made from palm nuts.

**Palm Oil** The reddish-orange oil extracted from the pulp of the fruit of the African palm. It's extremely high in saturated fat (78 percent) and has a distinctive flavor that is popular in West African and Brazilian cooking.

**Peanuts** Legumes, well suited to the West African climate and a staple food. Know by the English name of groundnuts.

**Periperi (Portuguese Hot Sauce)** A spicy hot-pepper sauce that goes on almost everything.

**Plantain** Tropical plant bearing a fruit similar to the banana. Plantains are more starchy than sweet and must be cooked before being eaten. They are staple crop in much of Africa. Used to make *fufu* and various beers or wines.

**Pombe** Beer made from plantains or bananas.

**Rupiza** Thin porridge or gruel made from powdered dried beans.

**Sabal Palmetto** The young sprouting leaves of cocoyams and sweet potatoes, cut and cooked as greens for relishes.

**Shea Butter** A fat extracted from the nut of the shea tree of West Africa. This butter is used to make margarine and chocolate.

**Sorghum** Cereal grass grown for grain or fodder, similar to corn, indigenous to Africa.

**Sorrel** Plant native to West Africa, the leaves have a strong acid flavor. In Africa the leaves and stalks are eaten as a cooked vegetables (greens).

**Sosaties** Barbecued pieces of meat on a stick, normally marinated in curry sauce (South African).

**Suya** Cut-up meats marinated in peanut oil then skewered and cooked.

**Swahili Yeast** Yeast made from the fermentation of ripe plantains, sugar, water, and wheat flour. Used as leavening agent for breads, buns, and fried cookies.

**Sweet Potato** Food plant, cultivated for its edible tuberous root and, particularly in Africa, for its leaves, which are eaten as greens.

**Tamarind** The fruit or pulp in the seedpods of *Tamarindus indica*, an evergreen tree native to Africa. It is the only spice of African origin cultivated and used world-wide, especially in Asian and Latin American recipes. The tamarind fruit is a seedpod, brown in color and several inches long, which contains a sour-tasting pulp.

**Taro** A tuber, similar to potatoes, cooked as a vegetable, and made into breads and porridges. Taro is especially well known as Polynesian Poi, which is made from fermented taro starch. It has a hairy outer skin, similar to a coconut's, which is removed. The large leaves (called *calalu* or *callaloo* in the Caribbean and in some parts of Africa) are cooked as greens. Some varieties of taro are highly toxic. Taro must be thoroughly cooked before it is eaten.

**Teff** Fine millet flour.

**Tomato** Native to the American tropics. Today, tomatoes and canned tomato paste are used to such an extent in African sauces, soups, and stews that many Africans might think that tomatoes were native to Africa.

**Trio** Swahili word for a combination of cooked vegetables, cubed or chopped and seasoned with oil and salt and pepper. Favorite in East Africa.

**Tseme or Nhembatemba** Special pot used for storing *dovi* (groundnut butter).

**Tuwo** Spicy okra sauce.

**Tuwonsaffe** In northern Ghana, the daily *fufu* is allowed to ferment in this "sourpot" and the *fufu* needed for meals is scooped from the *tuwonsaffe.*

**Ugali** Tanzanian staple cornmeal porridge of *fufu.*

**Wors (Vors)** Spicy sausages often sold by street vendors like hot dogs; essential at any *braai.* (South African)

**Yam** The nutritious white yam is a powerfully symbolic staple food frequently staving off malnutrition and starvation, particularly in West Africa. Often of immense size, one African yam can easily feed a family. Feast days are common and yams figure largely in any festive occasion. Because the egg symbolizes fertility and therefore eternity, eggs often accompany yams in these special dishes.

**Yassa** Traditional Senegalese (West African) marinade of lemon juice, onion, and mustard.

# Menus and Recipes from Africa

MENU ONE (NORTH AFRICA)

***Harira:* Lamb and Vegetable Soup**

**Fava Bean Salad**

**Tagine of Chicken, Preserved Lemon, and Olives**

**Couscous**

**Harissa**

**Fish Chermoula**

**Carrots with Black Currants**

***Mescouta:* Date Cookies**

MENU TWO

**Equsi Soup (Western Africa)**

***Akoho sy Voanio:* Chicken in Coconut Milk (Southern Africa)**

***Akara:* Black-Eyed Pea Fritters (Western Africa)**

***Mchuzi wa Biringani:* Eggplant Curry (Eastern Africa)**

**Boiled Plantains**

***Samaki wa Kupaka:* Grilled Fish (Eastern Africa)**

MENU THREE

***Kaklo:* Banana and Chile Fritters (Western Africa)**

***Muamba Nsusu:* Congo Chicken Soup**

***Sosaties* (South Africa)**

**Yellow Rice with Raisins (South Africa)**

**Grilled Tilapia**

***Irio* (Eastern Africa)**

# Harira Lamb and Vegetable Soup

SERVES 4

**This thick, peppery soup is a symbol of the Moroccan way of fasting. It is traditionally served after sundown during the month of Ramadan to break each day's fast.**

| AMOUNT | MEASURE | INGREDIENT |
|---|---|---|
| $\frac{1}{2}$ cup | 4 ounces, 120 ml | Ghee |
| 1 cup | 4 ounces, 112 g | Onions, $\frac{1}{4}$ inch (.6 cm) dice |
| $\frac{1}{4}$ cup | 8 ounces | Lean lamb, $\frac{1}{2}$ inch (1.2 cm) cubes |
| $\frac{1}{2}$ teaspoon | | Turmeric, ground |
| $\frac{1}{2}$ teaspoon | | Black pepper |
| $\frac{1}{4}$ teaspoon | | Cinnamon, ground |
| $\frac{1}{4}$ teaspoon | | Paprika |
| $\frac{1}{2}$ teaspoon | | Fresh ginger, minced |
| 3 cups | 24 ounces, 810 ml | White stock |
| $\frac{1}{2}$ cup | 2 ounces, 56 g | Celery, $\frac{1}{4}$ inch, (.6 cm) dice |
| To taste | | Salt |
| $\frac{1}{2}$ cup | 3 ounces, 84 g | Chickpeas, cooked, rinsed, and drained |
| $\frac{1}{4}$ cup | 2 ounces, 56 g | Lentils, red, soaked, and drained |
| 2 tablespoons | | Parsley, chopped |
| 1 teaspoon | | Cilantro, chopped |
| 1 cup | 6 ounces, 168 g | Tomatoes, peeled, seeded, $\frac{1}{4}$ inch (.6 cm) dice |
| $\frac{1}{4}$ cup | $\frac{1}{2}$ ounce, 14 g | Vermicelli (broken), orzo, or acini di pepe |
| 2 | | Beaten egg (optional) |
| To taste | | Lemon |

## PROCEDURE

1. Heat the ghee over medium heat and sauté the onion until soft, 3 to 4 minutes.
2. Add the lamb; cook 10 minutes or until lightly browned.
3. Add all the dry spices and ginger; cook 3 minutes, stirring constantly.
4. Add white stock, celery, salt, chickpeas, and lentils; simmer 45 minutes.
5. Add parsley, cilantro, and tomatoes; simmer 10 minutes.
6. Bring to a boil and add vermicelli; cook 1 minute or until pasta is just cooked.
7. Beat in egg, correct seasoning with lemon juice and serve.

# Fava Bean Salad

SERVES 4

| AMOUNT | MEASURE | INGREDIENT |
|---|---|---|
| 3 cups | 18 ounces, 504 g | Fava (or broad) beans, fresh or dried, shelled, or lima beans (lima beans may need to be cooked longer) |
| 1 | | Onion, cut in half |
| 1 teaspoon | | Salt |

**PROCEDURE**

1 Place the beans in water to cover to a depth of 2 inches (5 cm). Add the onion and salt; bring to a boil, reduce to a simmer, and cook 20 to 25 minutes. The beans should be very tender (creamy) but not mushy. Drain and discard the onion.

| AMOUNT | MEASURE | INGREDIENT |
|---|---|---|
| $\frac{1}{4}$ cup | 4 ounces, 120 ml | Olive oil |
| $\frac{1}{2}$ cup | 4 ounces, 120 ml | Fresh lemon juice |
| 1 $\frac{1}{2}$ teaspoons | | Cumin, ground |
| 1 tablespoon | | Garlic, minced |
| 6 tablespoons | | Fresh cilantro, leaves only, chopped |
| 6 tablespoons | | Flat-leaf parsley, chopped |
| To taste | | Salt and white pepper |
| $\frac{1}{2}$ cup | 2 ounces, 56 g | Green onions, white and green parts, thinly sliced |
| $\frac{1}{4}$ cup | 1 ounce, 28 g | Red radishes, thinly sliced |
| $\frac{3}{4}$ cup | 4 ounces, 112 g | Black olives, pitted |

**PROCEDURE**

1 Combine olive oil, lemon juice, cumin, and garlic; stir to mix. Add cilantro and parsley and correct seasoning.

2 Combine dressing and beans while the beans are still warm; toss.

3 Add green onions and radishes; toss well.

4 Plate and garnish with olives.

# Tagine of Chicken, Preserved Lemon, and Olives

SERVES 4

| AMOUNT | MEASURE | INGREDIENT |
|---|---|---|
| 1 tablespoon | | Garlic, minced |
| 1 tablespoon | $\frac{1}{2}$ ounce, 15 ml | Olive oil |
| $\frac{1}{2}$ teaspoon | | Black pepper |
| 1 | $2\frac{1}{2}$ pound, 1.12 kg | Chicken, cut into 8 pieces |

**PROCEDURE**

1 Combine the garlic, olive oil, and black pepper. Rub the chicken with the mixture and let set 2 hours.

| AMOUNT | MEASURE | INGREDIENT |
|---|---|---|
| 2 tablespoons | 1 ounce, 30 ml | Olive oil |
| $\frac{1}{4}$ teaspoon | | Black pepper |
| $\frac{1}{4}$ teaspoon | | Ginger, ground |
| Pinch | | Saffron |
| 1 teaspoon | | Cumin, ground |
| 1 stick | | Cinnamon |
| 1 teaspoon | | Coriander, ground |
| $1\frac{1}{4}$ cups | 5 ounces, 140 g | Onions, $\frac{1}{4}$ inch (.6 cm) dice |
| 2 cups | 16 ounces, 480 ml | Chicken stock |
| 1 cup | 5 ounces, 140 g | Green olives, pitted |
| $\frac{1}{2}$ cup | 3 ounces, 84 g | Preserved lemons, quartered strips (rinse lemons as needed under running water, removing and discarding pulp) |
| To taste | | Salt and pepper |
| As needed | | Couscous (recipe follows) |

**PROCEDURE**

1. Heat oil over medium heat and brown chicken on all sides, 8 to 10 minutes.
2. Add spices; cook 1 minute. Add onions and sauté over medium-high heat, 2 to 3 minutes.
3. Add stock and bring to a boil, reduce to a simmer, and cover, leaving lid ajar to allow steam to escape. Simmer 20 to 30 minutes or until chicken is tender.
4. Add olive and preserved lemons; cook 5 minutes. Remove chicken and reduce to sauce consistency, stirring. Correct seasoning.
5. Serve covered with sauce on couscous.

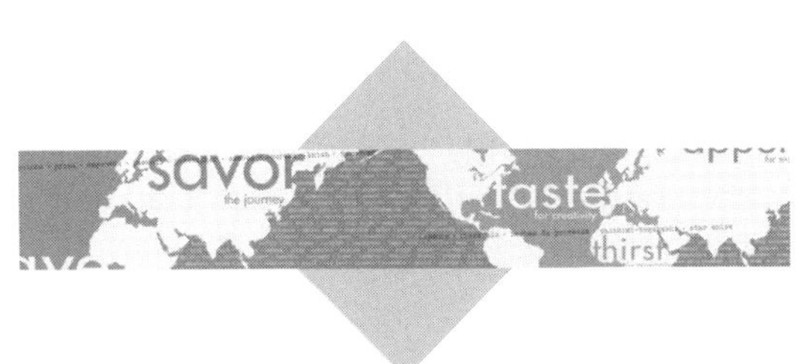

# Couscous

SERVES 4

**Real couscous is always steamed, not boiled. Precooked "instant couscous" cooked in this traditional method may result in mushy, overcooked pasta. If real (not "instant") couscous is not available, reduce the cooking time.**

| AMOUNT | MEASURE | INGREDIENT |
|---|---|---|
| 1 cup | 8 ounces, 240 ml | Warm water, mixed with 1 teaspoon salt |
| 3 cups | 18 ounces, 504 g | Couscous (not "instant couscous") |
| $\frac{1}{4}$ cup | 2 ounces, 60 ml | Olive oil |
| As needed | | Chicken stock |
| 2 tablespoons | 2 ounces, 60 ml | Butter |

PROCEDURE

1. Sprinkle half the salted water over half the couscous. Rub your hands with a little oil and sprinkle the remaining oil over the couscous. Use your hands to evenly distribute the oil and water into the couscous. Let the couscous form small pellets, but break any lumps. Add the remaining couscous and continue to process, adding more water to make the couscous uniformly damp, but not wet.
2. Place the couscous on a clean cloth; cover it with another cloth, and leave to rest 1 hour.
3. If not cooking over the tagine, bring the chicken stock to a gentle boil in the bottom part of a steamer. Place the couscous in the top part of a steamer; cover and steam couscous about 1 hour over the simmering broth.
4. Remove from the steamer and transfer to a bowl. Massage the butter into the couscous (careful not to burn yourself) and let cool 15 minutes.
5. Return the couscous to the steamer for an additional 30 minutes. Test for tenderness. The last two steps can be repeated.

# Harissa

**YIELD: 8 OUNCES**

| AMOUNT | MEASURE | INGREDIENT |
|---|---|---|
| 2 ounces | | Chile peppers, dried mixture of anchos, New Mexican, and guajillos |
| 2 ounces | | Cumin seeds |
| 1 teaspoon | | Paprika |
| $\frac{3}{4}$ cup | 4 ounces, 112 g | Onions, $\frac{1}{4}$ inch (.6 cm) dice |
| 3 tablespoons | | Flat-leaf parsley, chopped |
| 1 cup | 8 ounces, 240 ml | Olive oil |
| To taste | | Fresh lemon juice |
| To taste | | Salt |

**PROCEDURE**

1. Combine chile peppers, cumin seeds, and paprika over low heat, stirring constantly; toast 5 to 7 minutes. Cool.
2. Using a mortar and pestle, pulverize to a fine consistency.
3. Combine all ingredients and blend well.
4. Correct seasoning with lemon juice and salt

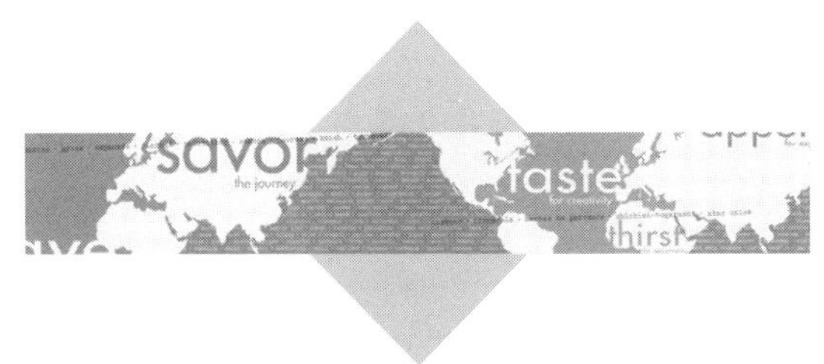

# Fish Chermoula

YIELD: $1\frac{1}{2}$ CUPS

| AMOUNT | MEASURE | INGREDIENT |
|---|---|---|
| **Chermoula Marinade** | | |
| 5 tablespoons | $\frac{1}{2}$ ounce, 14 g | Cilantro leaves, chopped |
| 5 tablespoons | $\frac{1}{2}$ ounce, 14 g | Flat-leaf parsley, chopped |
| 5 | 10 g | Garlic cloves, minced |
| 1 tablespoon | $\frac{1}{4}$ ounce, 7 g | Paprika, sweet |
| 2 teaspoon | | Cumin, ground |
| $\frac{1}{4}$ teaspoon | | Cayenne |
| 4 tablespoons | 2 ounces, 60 ml | Fresh lemon juice |
| 1 cup | 8 ounces, 240 ml | Olive oil |
| 1 teaspoon | | Salt |

**PROCEDURE**

1 Combine all ingredients in a food processor; pulse until thoroughly blended.

| AMOUNT | MEASURE | INGREDIENT |
|---|---|---|
| 4 | 5 ounce, 140 g each | Sea bass, scrod, flounder, or any firm white fish |
| 2 tablespoons | 2 ounces, 60 ml | Olive oil |
| As needed | | All-purpose flour |
| As needed | | Lemon wedges, for garnish |

**PROCEDURE**

1 Marinate the fillets in chermoula, 2 to 4 hours.
2 Heat oil over medium heat. Remove fillets from chermoula and pat dry.
3 Dredge in flour, shaking off any excess.
4 Sauté on both sides, turning only once, until golden brown on both sides, 2 to 3 minutes per side (depending on type of fish).
5 Serve with lemon wedges and flat bread.

# Carrots with Black Currants

SERVES 4

| AMOUNT | MEASURE | INGREDIENT |
|---|---|---|
| $\frac{1}{4}$ cup | 1 ounce, 28 g | Black currants |
| 4 tablespoons | 2 ounces, 60 ml | Butter |
| $\frac{1}{2}$ teaspoon | | Cinnamon, ground |
| $\frac{1}{4}$ teaspoon, or to taste | | Cayenne pepper |
| $2\frac{1}{2}$ cups | 15 ounces, 420 g | Carrots, peeled, $2\frac{1}{2}$ to 4 inch (6.25 to 7.5 cm) long julienne cut |
| $\frac{1}{2}$ cup | 4 ounces, 120 ml | Fresh orange juice |
| Garnish | | Flat-leaf parsley, chopped |

PROCEDURE

1 Soak currants covered in hot water 30 minutes. Drain and reserve $\frac{1}{4}$ cup (2 ounces, 60 ml) soaking liquid.

2 Heat butter over medium heat, add cinnamon, cayenne, and carrots; cook, stirring 2 to 3 minutes.

3 Add orange juice, currants, and reserved soaking liquid; bring to a boil, reduce to a simmer, and cook 3 to 5 minutes or until tender. If necessary, strain carrots, reduce the liquid to syrup consistency, and then recombine with carrots.

4 Correct seasoning; serve sprinkled with parsley.

# Mescouta

## Date Cookies

YIELD: 24 TO 30 BARS

| AMOUNT | MEASURE | INGREDIENT |
|---|---|---|
| $\frac{3}{4}$ cup | 3 ounces, 84 g | All-purpose flour |
| $\frac{1}{2}$ teaspoon | | Baking powder |
| 6 | | Eggs, well beaten |
| $\frac{1}{2}$ cup | 4 ounces, 112 g | Granulated sugar |
| 1 teaspoon | | Vanilla extract |
| $\frac{1}{2}$ cup | 4 ounces, 120 ml | Butter, melted |
| 1 cup | 4 ounces, 112 g | Dates, pitted, chopped |
| $\frac{1}{2}$ cup | 5 ounces, 140 g | Walnuts or almonds, finely chopped |
| 3 tablespoons | | Confectioner's sugar |

### PROCEDURE

1. Preheat oven to 350°F (176°C).
2. Sift flour with baking powder.
3. Combine eggs, sugar, vanilla, and melted butter, mix on medium or by hand until well-blended (3 minutes).
4. Gradually add flour mixture, a little at a time.
5. Add dates and nuts; mix well.
6. Put into a greased 8- or 9-inch (20 or 22.5 cm) square cake pan.
7. Bake 30 minutes or until a toothpick inserted in the center comes out clean.
8. While still warm, cut into rectangular bars about 1 inch (2.5 cm) wide.
9. Roll bars in confectioner's sugar.

# Equsi Soup (Western Africa) SERVES 4

| AMOUNT | MEASURE | INGREDIENT |
|---|---|---|
| 4 tablespoons | 2 ounces, 60 ml | Peanut oil or palm oil |
| 1 cup | 6 ounces, 168 g | Beef stew meat, $\frac{1}{2}$ inch (1.2 cm) cubes |
| 3 cups | 24 ounces, 720 ml | Beef or chicken stock |
| $\frac{1}{2}$ cup | 2 ounces, 56 g | Onion, $\frac{1}{4}$ inch (.6 cm) dice |
| 1 | | Green chile, seeded, chopped |
| $\frac{1}{4}$ cup | 1 ounce, 28 g | Okra, sliced $\frac{1}{4}$ inch (.6 cm) slices |
| 1 tablespoon | $\frac{1}{2}$ ounce, 15 ml | Tomato paste |
| 1 cup | 6 ounces, 168 g | Tomatoes, peeled, seeded $\frac{1}{4}$ inch (.6 cm) dice |
| $\frac{1}{2}$ cup | 1 ounce, 28 g | Dried shrimp |
| $\frac{1}{2}$ cup | 2 ounces, 56 g | Egusi, roasted and ground (or pumpkin seeds or pepitas) |
| 2 cups | 16 ounces, 180 ml | Beef or chicken stock |
| 3 cups | 8 ounces, 224 g | Spinach, washed and chopped |
| To taste | | Salt and cayenne pepper |

**PROCEDURE**

1. Heat oil over medium high heat. Pat meat dry and sauté until browned on all sides. Remove meat, reserve pan. Combine meat and first amount of beef stock; bring to a boil and reduce to a simmer.
2. Return pan to heat; when hot add onions and cook 3 to 5 minutes. Add chile and okra and cook 2 minutes stirring. Add tomato paste and cook 1 minute Add tomatoes and cook 3 to 5 minutes or until tomatoes are soft.
3. Add dried shrimp and ground seeds. Stir well.
4. Add onion-tomato mixture to the simmering meat and stir to combine. Add second amount of stock and cook until meat is tender.
5. Add spinach and cook until tender, 5 minutes.
6. Correct seasoning with salt and cayenne pepper.

# Akoho sy Voanio

## Chicken in Coconut Milk (Southern Africa)

SERVES 4

| AMOUNT | MEASURE | INGREDIENT |
|---|---|---|
| 1 | $2\frac{1}{2}$ pound, 1.12 kg | Chicken, cut into 8 pieces |
| 2 tablespoons | 1 ounce, 30 ml | Fresh lemon juice |
| 1 teaspoon | | Lemon zest |
| 1 teaspoon | | Salt |
| $\frac{1}{2}$ teaspoon | | Black pepper |
| $\frac{1}{4}$ teaspoon | | Cayenne pepper |
| $\frac{1}{4}$ cup | 2 ounces, 60 ml | Coconut oil or peanut oil |
| $1\frac{1}{2}$ cups | 6 ounces, 168 g | Onions, $\frac{1}{4}$ inch (.6 cm) dice |
| 1 tablespoon | | Garlic, minced |
| 1 cup | 6 ounces, 168 g | Tomatoes, peeled, seeded, $\frac{1}{2}$ inch (1.2 cm) dice |
| 1 teaspoon | | Ginger, minced |
| 1 cup | 8 ounces, 240 ml | Coconut milk |
| As needed | | Rice, cooked, hot |

**PROCEDURE**

1. Combine the chicken, lemon juice, zest, salt, black pepper, and cayenne; marinate 1 hour.
2. Heat oil over medium heat and sauté onions and garlic, 3 to 5 minutes. Add chicken and cook until chicken is almost cooked, 12 to 15 minutes.
3. Add tomatoes and ginger; stir well and cook 3 minutes.
4. Add coconut milk and simmer until chicken is completely cooked. Remove chicken pieces as they cook. Reduce sauce to desired consistency and serve over rice.

# Akara Black-Eyed Pea Fritters (Western Africa)

SERVES 4

| AMOUNT | MEASURE | INGREDIENT |
|---|---|---|
| 1 cup | 8 ounces, 224 g | Dried cowpeas (black-eyed peas) |
| $\frac{1}{2}$ cup | 2 ounces, 56 g | Onions, $\frac{1}{8}$ inch (.3 cm) dice |
| $\frac{1}{2}$ teaspoon | | Salt |
| $\frac{1}{4}$ cup | 1 ounce, 28 g | Green bell pepper, $\frac{1}{8}$ inch (.3 cm) dice |
| $\frac{1}{4}$ cup | 1 ounce, 28 g | Red bell pepper, $\frac{1}{8}$ inch (.3 cm) dice |
| 1 tablespoon | | Jalapeño, minced |
| $\frac{1}{2}$ teaspoon | | Ginger, grated |
| As needed | | Peanut oil, for frying |
| As needed | | African hot sauce (see recipe on page 541) |

**PROCEDURE**

1 Clean, pick over, and wash black-eyed peas. Soak, covered, in hot water 30 minutes. Drain and remove the skins by rubbing them between your hands. Rinse and drain well in a colander.

2 Crush or process the peas to a thick paste. Add enough water to form a smooth, thick batter that will cling to a spoon. Add remaining ingredients except oil; mix well and let stand 30 minutes.

3 Heat 2 inches (5 cm) oil over medium heat to 325°F (162°C).

4 Drop batter by the tablespoonful into the hot oil. Fry until golden, 2 to 3 minutes per side. Drain on paper towels. Serve hot with African hot sauce.

# Mchuzi wa Biringani

## Eggplant Curry (Eastern Africa)

SERVES 4

| AMOUNT | MEASURE | INGREDIENT |
|---|---|---|
| 5 cups | 16 ounces, 448 g | Eggplant, unpeeled, 1 inch (2.4 cm) cubes |
| 4 tablespoons | 2 ounces, 60 ml | Peanut oil |
| 1 cup | 4 ounces, 112 g | Onions, $\frac{1}{4}$ inch (.6 cm) dice |
| 2 teaspoons | | Garam masala (see recipe on page 567) or curry powder |
| 1 teaspoon | | Ginger, grated |
| 1 tablespoon | | Garlic, minced |
| 1 | | Green chile (serrano), seeded, minced |
| 1 cup | 6 ounces, 168 g | Tomato, peeled, seeded, $\frac{1}{2}$ inch dice |
| To taste | | Salt, pepper, and cayenne pepper |

**PROCEDURE**

1. Toss eggplant with a little salt; rub well and set aside 1 hour. Rinse and squeeze out as much liquid as possible from the eggplant cubes; pat dry with paper towels.
2. Heat oil over medium-high heat and sauté onions until soft, 3 minutes. Add garam masala, ginger, garlic and green chile. Cook, stirring continuously, 3 minutes.
3. Add eggplant; stir-fry until it begins to brown.
4. Add tomatoes and simmer until sauce is thickened and eggplant is tender.
5. Adjust seasoning.

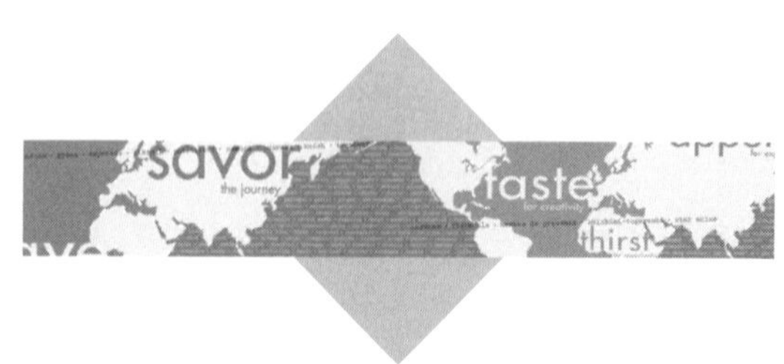

# Boiled Plantains

SERVES 4

**In Africa, boiled plantains are more common than fried plantains.**

| AMOUNT | MEASURE | INGREDIENT |
|---|---|---|
| 4 cups | 20 ounces, 560 g | Plantains, peeled, 2 inch (5 cm) pieces |
| To taste | | Salt and pepper |

**PROCEDURE**

1. Cover plantains with water and boil until tender.
2. Drain and serve in pieces or mash. Adjust seasoning.

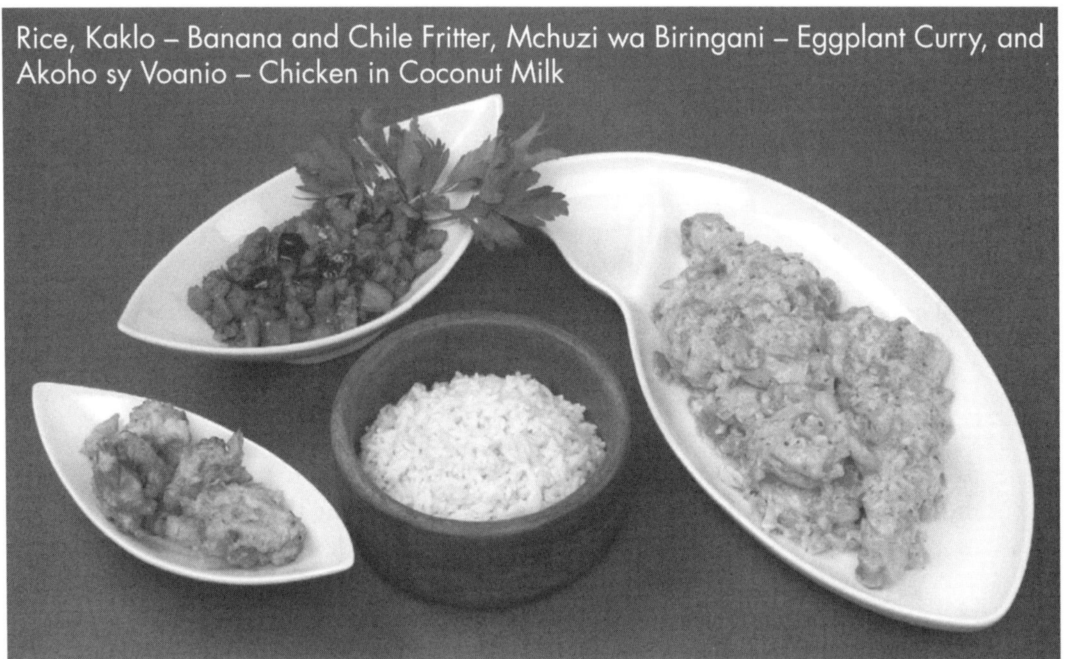

Rice, Kaklo – Banana and Chile Fritter, Mchuzi wa Biringani – Eggplant Curry, and Akoho sy Voanio – Chicken in Coconut Milk

# Samaki wa Kupaka

## Grilled Fish (Eastern Africa) SERVES 4

**One of many traditional Swahili fish dishes from Zanzibar, an African island in the Indian Ocean. *Samaki* is the Swahili word for "fish" and *mchuzi* means "curry" (or gravy, sauce, or soup).**

| AMOUNT | MEASURE | INGREDIENT |
|---|---|---|
| 2 teaspoons | | Ginger, grated |
| 2 tablespoons | | Garlic, minced |
| 1 | | Green chile (jalapeño), seeded, minced |
| As needed | | Salt |
| 1 | $2\frac{1}{2}$ to 3 pound, 1.12 kg to 1.34 kg | Whole fish (snapper, sea bass, sea perch, or other fresh white fish), gutted, scales and tail removed |
| 2 cups | 16 ounces, 480 ml | Coconut milk |
| 1 tablespoon | $\frac{1}{2}$ ounce, 15 ml | Tamarind paste |
| 1 teaspoon | | Garam masala (see recipe on page 567) |
| To taste | | Cayenne pepper |

PROCEDURE

1. Make a paste out of the ginger, garlic, green chile, and salt.
2. Make 4 shallow slashes on each side of the fish. With your fingers, work the paste into the slashes and cavity. Cover and let sit 1 hour.
3. Combine coconut milk, tamarind, garam masala, salt, and cayenne; simmer over low heat.
4. Heat a well-oiled grill or grill pan until very hot, then carefully lay the fish onto it. Cook the fish until a thin crust forms on the skin, which enables you to turn it with a spatula. After the fish has reached the half-cooked mark, begin spooning the sauce over the fish. Spoon more each time you turn it. Allow 3 to 4 minutes per side. The fish may be transferred to a 350°F (176°C) oven to finish cooking.

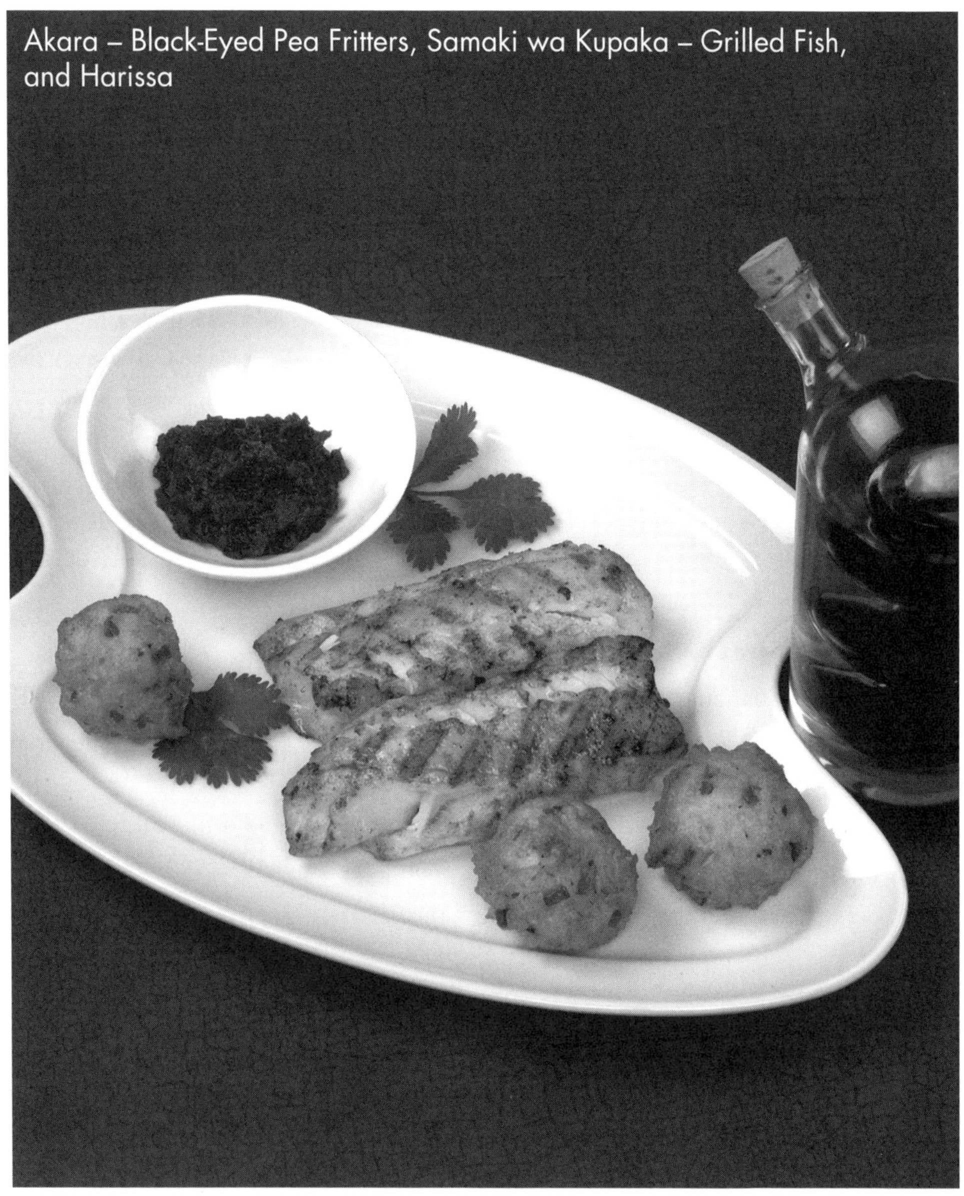

Akara – Black-Eyed Pea Fritters, Samaki wa Kupaka – Grilled Fish, and Harissa

# Kaklo Banana and Chile Fritters (Western Africa) SERVES 4

| AMOUNT | MEASURE | INGREDIENT |
|---|---|---|
| 2 cups | 8 ounces, 224 g | Bananas, peeled and mashed |
| $\frac{1}{2}$ cup | 2 ounces, 56 g | Onions, $\frac{1}{8}$ inch (.3 cm) dice |
| $\frac{1}{2}$ cup | 3 ounces, 84 g | Tomato, peeled, seeded, $\frac{1}{8}$ inch (.3 cm) dice |
| 1 tablespoon | | Green chile (jalapeño), seeded minced |
| $1\frac{1}{2}$ teaspoons | | Ginger, grated |
| $\frac{1}{2}$ teaspoon | | Salt |
| 1 cup | 4 ounces, 112 g | All-purpose flour |
| 2 tablespoons | 1 ounce, 30 ml | Water |
| As needed | | Peanut or coconut oil, for frying |

**PROCEDURE**

1 Combine bananas, onion, tomato, and chile; mash together.

2 Add ginger, salt, flour, and water to banana mixture and stir to combine; do not overwork. Let rest 30 minutes.

3 In a deep pan or fryer, heat 3 inches (5 cm) oil over medium heat to 375°F (190°C).

4 Deep-fry teaspoon-size portions; drain on paper towels.

5 Serve hot or cold as a snack or with a meal.

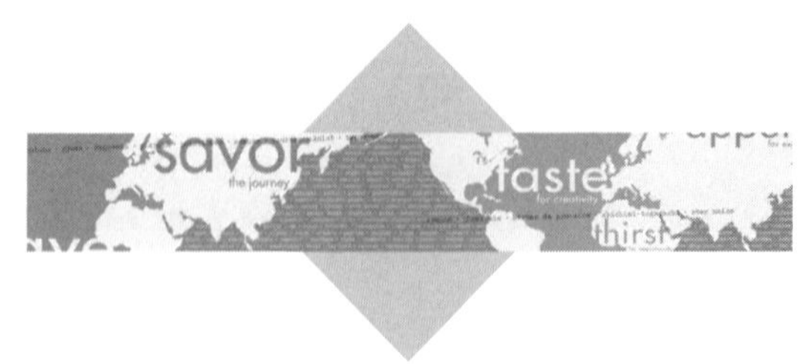

# Muamba Nsusu

## Congo Chicken Soup

SERVES 4

| AMOUNT | MEASURE | INGREDIENT |
|---|---|---|
| 1 | 2½ pound, 1.12 kg | Chicken, cut into 8 pieces |
| 1 quart | 32 ounces, 960 ml | Chicken stock |
| 2 tablespoons | 1 ounce, 30 ml | Palm oil |
| 1 cup | 4 ounces, 112 g | Onions, ¼ inch (.6 cm) dice |
| 1½ teaspoons | | Garlic, minced |
| ½ teaspoon | | Crushed red pepper flakes |
| 1 cup | 6 ounces, 168 g | Tomatoes, peeled, seeded, ½ inch dice |
| ¼ cup | 2 ounces, 60 ml | Tomato paste |
| ⅓ cup | 2½ ounces, 70 g | Peanut butter, containing only peanuts and salt |

PROCEDURE

1. Combine chicken and chicken stock; simmer until chicken is tender. Remove chicken from stock and retain stock at a simmer. Skin chicken and shred meat; set aside.
2. Heat oil over medium heat; add onions and garlic and sauté 3 to 5 minutes, until soft.
3. Add red pepper flakes and diced tomatoes; bring to a simmer.
4. Combine 1 cup (8 ounces, 240 ml) chicken broth from step 1 with tomato paste and peanut butter; stir until smooth.
5. Combine chicken meat, tomato mixture, chicken broth, and peanut butter mixture. Stir and continue to simmer unit the soup is thickened, 5 to 10 minutes; do not boil.
6. Serve hot.

# Sosaties (South Africa) SERVES 4

| AMOUNT | MEASURE | INGREDIENT |
| --- | --- | --- |
| 1 ½ cups | 8 ounces, 224 g | Dried apricots |
| ½ cup | 8 ounces, 240 m | Dry sherry |
| 1 pound | 16 ounces, 448 g | Lamb, lean, cut 1 inch (2.4 cm) cubes |
| | 8 ounces, 224 g | Pork, lean, cut ½ inch (1.2 cm) cubes |
| 6 | | Whole garlic cloves |
| To taste | | Salt and pepper |
| 3 tablespoons | 1 ½ ounces, 45 ml | Oil |
| ½ cup | 2 ounces, 56 g | Onions, ¼ inch (.6 cm) dice |
| 2 teaspoons | | Garam masala (see recipe on page 567) |
| 1 | | Garlic clove, minced |
| 1 tablespoon | ½ ounce, 14 g | Granulated sugar |
| 1 tablespoon | ½ ounce, 15 ml | Tamarind paste |
| 1 cup | 8 ounces, 240 ml | White vinegar |
| 1 tablespoon | ½ ounce, 15 ml | Apricot jam |
| 1 tablespoon | | Cornstarch |
| 1 tablespoon | ½ ounce, 15 ml | Red wine |

**PROCEDURE**

1. Combine apricots and sherry over medium heat; simmer until apricots are plump. Remove from heat and cool.
2. Combine the lamb and pork with the whole garlic cloves, season with salt and pepper, and toss.
3. Heat the oil over medium heat; add the onions and sauté 3 to 4 minutes. Add the garam masala and minced garlic. Sauté, stirring, 1 minute.
4. Add sugar, tamarind paste, vinegar, and jam; stir well and bring to a boil.
5. Dissolve the cornstarch in the red wine, add it to the pan, and cook until sauce has thickened, 2 to 3 minutes. Remove from heat and let cool.
6. Toss meat with half the sauce, reserve the other half. Marinate the meat 1 hour at room temperature or 3 hours under refrigeration.
7. Drain meat from marinade. Thread lamb, pork, and apricots on skewers.
8. Grill until browned on all sides, basting with marinade. Serve with heated sauce on the side.

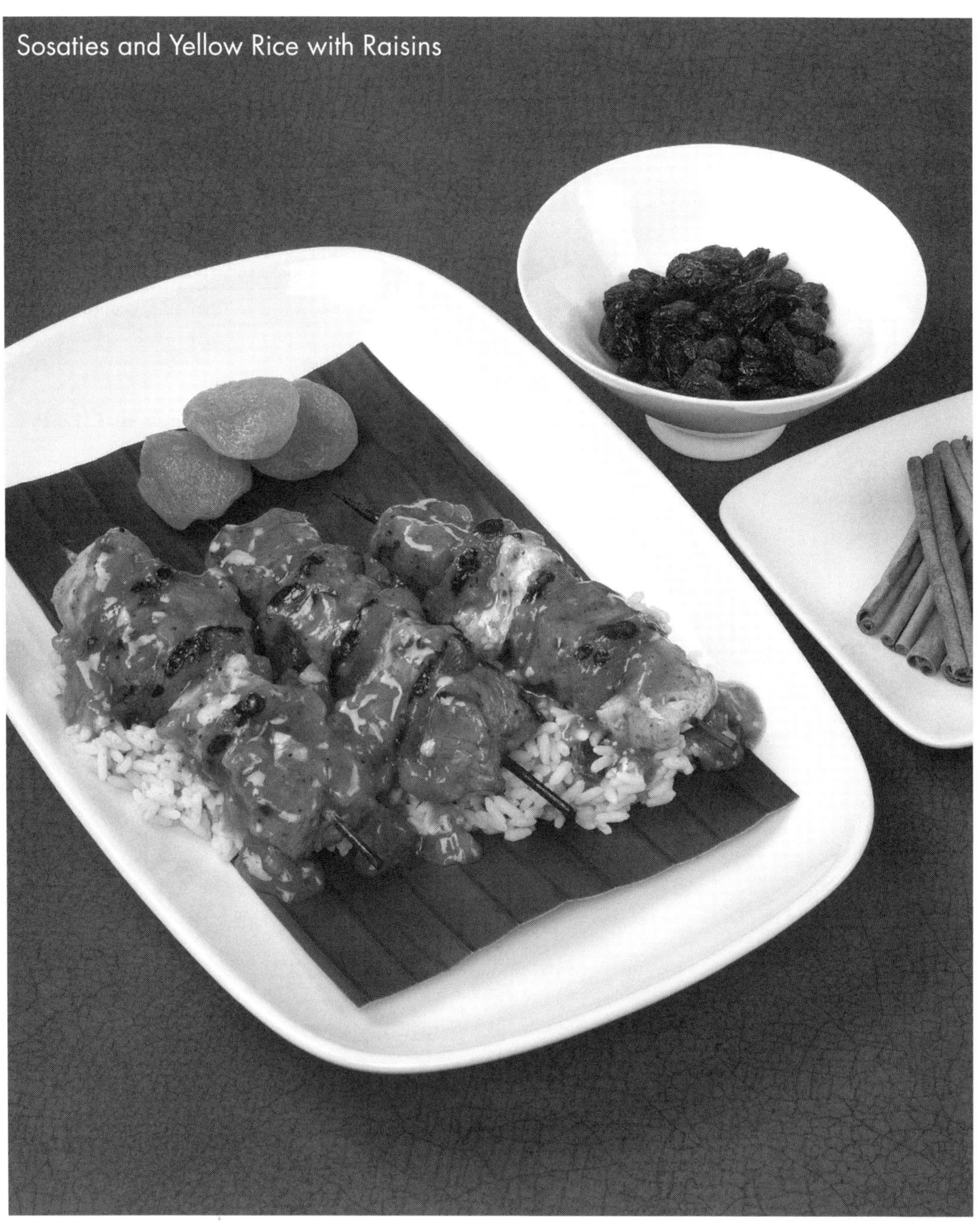

Sosaties and Yellow Rice with Raisins

# Yellow Rice with Raisins
## (South Africa) SERVES 4

| AMOUNT | MEASURE | INGREDIENT |
|---|---|---|
| $2\frac{1}{2}$ cups | 20 ounces, 600 ml | Water or chicken stock |
| 2 teaspoons | 9 g | Granulated sugar |
| $\frac{1}{2}$ teaspoon | | Turmeric, ground |
| 2 teaspoons | | Salt |
| 1 tablespoon | $\frac{1}{2}$ ounce, 15 ml | Butter |
| 1 | | Cinnamon stick, 2 inches (5 cm) |
| $\frac{1}{2}$ cup | 3 ounces, 84 g | Raisins |
| $\frac{1}{2}$ teaspoon | | Lemon, zest |
| 1 cup | 7 ounces, 196 g | Long-grain rice, washed twice |

**PROCEDURE**

1. Heat water to a boil, add all ingredients except rice, and stir to dissolve.
2. Add rice and return to a simmer; cover, reduce heat, and simmer about 20 minutes.
3. Remove cover and cook 5 minutes longer. Fluff the rice with a fork and serve.

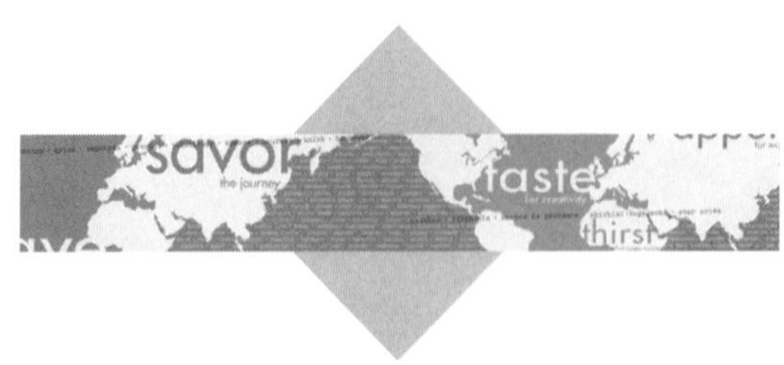

# Grilled Tilapia

SERVES 4

**Tilapia are native to the lakes and rivers of Africa, where it is called *ngege*. Outside of Africa, tilapia is called St. Peter's fish.**

| AMOUNT | MEASURE | INGREDIENT |
| --- | --- | --- |
| 4 5-ounce | 4 112–140 g | Boneless, skinless tilapia fillets |
| $\frac{1}{2}$ cup | 4 ounces, 120 ml | Vegetable oil |
| 1 cup | 4 ounces, 112 g | Onions, $\frac{1}{4}$ inch (.6 cm) dice |
| 1 cup | 4 ounces, 112 g | Green bell pepper, $\frac{1}{4}$ inch (.6 cm) dice |
| 1 tablespoon | $\frac{1}{2}$ ounce, 15 ml | Fresh lemon juice |
| 2 teaspoons | 10 ml | White vinegar |
| 1 teaspoon | | Cayenne |
| $\frac{1}{2}$ teaspoon | | Salt |
| | | African hot sauce (recipe follows) |

**PROCEDURE**

1. Combine all the ingredients except the tilapia. Mix well, add the fish fillets and marinate for 30 minute to 1 hour.
2. Remove from marinade, grill, broil or sauté.
3. Serve with African hot sauce.

## African Hot Sauce

SERVES 4

| AMOUNT | MEASURE | INGREDIENT |
| --- | --- | --- |
| 6 | | Chile peppers; dried mixture of anchos, New Mexican, and guajillos, or any hot red peppers |
| 1 cup | 4 ounces, 112 g | Green bell pepper, stemmed, seeded, chopped |
| 1 | | Garlic clove, chopped |
| $\frac{1}{2}$ cup | 2 ounces, 56 g | Onions, chopped |
| 10 tablespoons | 6 ounces, 168 g | Tomato paste |
| 2 tablespoons | 1 ounce, 30 ml | Water |
| $\frac{1}{2}$ teaspoon | | Granulated sugar |
| $\frac{1}{2}$ teaspoon | | Salt |

**PROCEDURE**

1. Remove stems and seeds from peppers. Combine all ingredients in a food processor, or process to a paste using a mortar and pestle.
2. Simmer over medium heat 1 hour. Cool and serve.

# Irio (Eastern Africa) SERVES 4

| AMOUNT | MEASURE | INGREDIENT |
|---|---|---|
| **2 cups** | **16 ounces, 480 ml** | **Water or chicken stock** |
| **1 cup** | **6 ounces, 168 g** | **Frozen, canned, or dried green peas, cooked and drained** |
| **3 cups** | **16 ounces, 448 g** | **Russet potatoes, peeled, quartered** |
| **$1\frac{1}{2}$ cups** | **9 ounces, 252 g** | **Corn kernels (3 ears, on the cob)** |
| **3 cups** | **6 ounces, 168 g** | **Greens or spinach, washed coarsely chopped** |
| **To taste** | | **Salt and pepper** |

**PROCEDURE**

1. Combine all ingredients and bring to a boil. Cover and simmer until tender, 15 to 20 minutes; longer if greens are used.
2. Mash with a potato masher until smooth and thick.

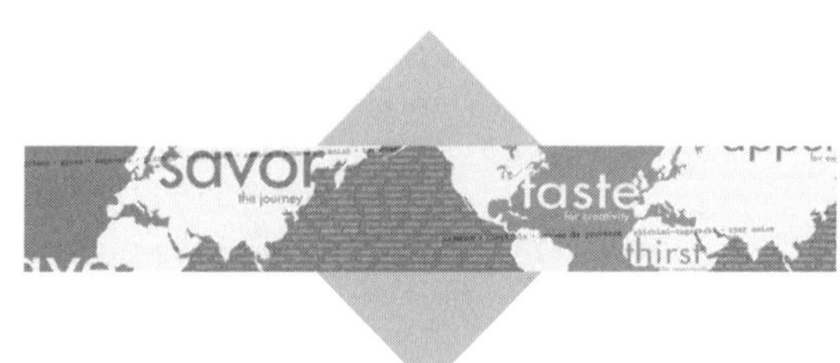

# India

## The Land

Set apart from the rest of Asia by the continental wall of the Himalayas, the Indian subcontinent touches three large bodies of water and is immediately recognizable on any world map. Between Africa and Indonesia, this thick, roughly triangular peninsula defines the Bay of Bengal to the east, the Arabian Sea to the west, and the Indian Ocean to the south. India's twenty-six states hold virtually every kind of landscape imaginable. From its northernmost point on the Chinese border, India extends nearly 2000 miles to its southern tip, off of which the island nation of Sri Lanka is located. India's northern border is dominated mostly by Nepal and the Himalayas, the world's highest mountain chain. Following the mountains to the northeast, India's border narrows to a small channel that passes between Nepal, Tibet, Bangladesh, and Bhutan, then spreads out again to meet Burma in an area called the Eastern Triangle. Apart from the Arabian Sea, its western border is defined exclusively by Pakistan.

India can be organized into north, south, east, and west regions. North India is the country's largest region, an area with terrain varying from arid mountains in the far north to lake country and forests. Along the Indus river valley, the north becomes flatter and more hospitable, widening into the fertile plains, the Himalayan foothills, and the Ganges river valley to the east. India's capital city, Delhi, is found in the north. Uttar Pradesh, the most populated state in the country, has beautiful monuments like Taj Mahal.

India reaches its peninsular tip with South India, which begins with the Deccan Plateau in the north and ends with Cape Comorin, where Hindus believe that bathing in the waters of the three oceans will wash away their sins. The southeast coast, mirroring the west, also rests beneath a mountain range, the Eastern Ghats.

East India is home to the sacred Ganges River and the majority of Himalayan foothills. East India also contains the Eastern Triangle, a small piece of land that extends beyond Bangladesh, culminating in the Naga Hills along the Burmese border.

West India includes the Thar Desert and the remarkable "pink city" of Jaipur. The coast is lined with some of India's best beaches. The land along the coast is typically lush, with rain forests reaching southward from Bombay all the way to into Goa. The long Western Ghats mountain chain separates the verdant coast from the Vindya Mountains and the dry Deccan plateau further inland.

Because of India's size, its climate depends not only on the time of year, but also the location. In general, temperatures tend to be cooler in the north, especially between September and March. The south is coolest from November to January. In June, winds and warm surface currents begin to move northward and westward, heading out of the Indian Ocean and into the Arabian Gulf. This creates a phenomenon known as the southwest monsoon, and it brings heavy rains to the west coast. Between October and December, a similar climatic pattern called the northeast monsoon appears in the Bay of Bengal, bringing rains to the east coast. In addition to the two monsoons, there are two other seasons, spring and autumn. Though the word *monsoon* often brings to mind images of torrential floods and landslides, the monsoon seasons are not all bad. Though it rains nearly every day, the downpour tends to come and go quickly, leaving behind a clean, glistening landscape.)

# History

The history of India can be traced in fragments to as far back as 700,000 years ago. The Indus Valley civilization, one of the oldest in the world, dates back at least 5,000 years. It is thought that the Aryans, a nomadic people possibly from Central Asia or northern Iran, migrated into the northwest regions of the Indian subcontinent between 2000 B.C. and 1500 B.C. Their intermingling with the earlier Dravidian cultures resulted in classical Indian culture that is known today.

The births of Mahavira (Jainism) and Buddhism around 550 B.C. mark the beginning of well-recorded Indian history. For the next 1500 years, India developed its civilization, and is estimated to have had the largest economy of the ancient world between the first and fifteenth centuries A.D., controlling between one-third and one-fourth of the world's wealth. It rapidly declined during European rule in the course of the Mughals Empire.

Incursions by Arab and Central Asian armies in the eighth and twelfth centuries were followed by inroads by traders from Europe, beginning in the late fifteenth century. By 1858,

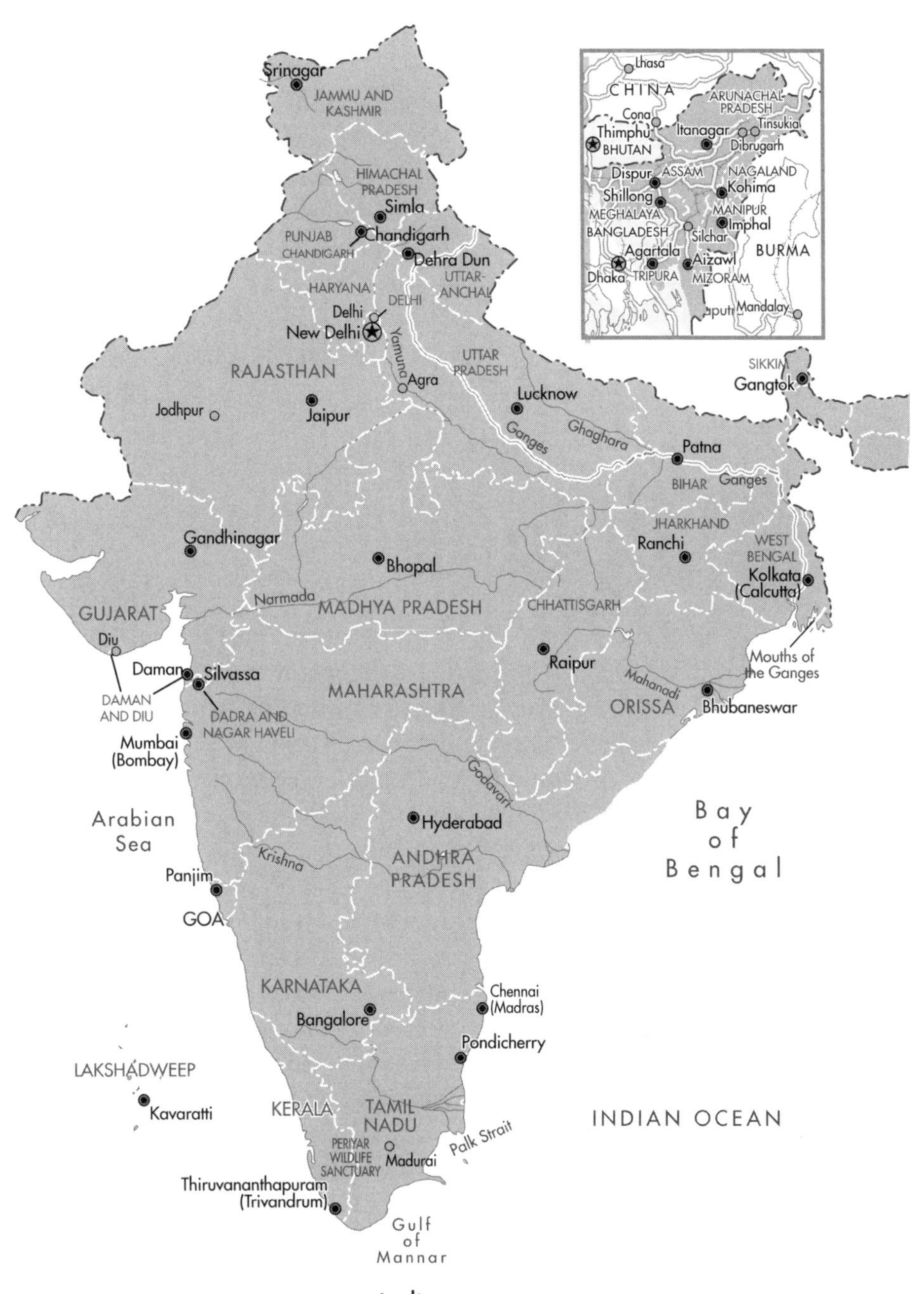
Srinagar
JAMMU AND KASHMIR
HIMACHAL PRADESH
Simla
PUNJAB
Chandigarh
CHANDIGARH
Dehra Dun
UTTAR-ANCHAL
HARYANA
DELHI
Delhi
New Delhi
Yamuna
RAJASTHAN
Agra
UTTAR PRADESH
Lucknow
Jodhpur
Jaipur
Ganges
Ghaghara
Patna
BIHAR
Ganges
SIKKIM
Gangtok
JHARKHAND
Ranchi
WEST BENGAL
Kolkata (Calcutta)
Gandhinagar
Bhopal
Narmada
MADHYA PRADESH
CHHATTISGARH
GUJARAT
Diu
Daman
Silvassa
DAMAN AND DIU
DADRA AND NAGAR HAVELI
Raipur
Mouths of the Ganges
MAHARASHTRA
Mahanadi
ORISSA
Bhubaneswar
Mumbai (Bombay)
Godavari
Arabian Sea
Hyderabad
Bay of Bengal
Krishna
ANDHRA PRADESH
Panjim
GOA
KARNATAKA
Chennai (Madras)
Bangalore
Pondicherry
LAKSHADWEEP
Kavaratti
KERALA
TAMIL NADU
INDIAN OCEAN
PERIYAR WILDLIFE SANCTUARY
Madurai
Palk Strait
Thiruvananthapuram (Trivandrum)
Gulf of Mannar
Lhasa
CHINA
ARUNACHAL PRADESH
Cona
Tinsukia
Thimphu
Itanagar
BHUTAN
Dibrugarh
Dispur
ASSAM
NAGALAND
Kohima
Shillong
MEGHALAYA
MANIPUR
Imphal
BANGLADESH
Silchar
Agartala
Aizawl
BURMA
Dhaka
TRIPURA
MIZORAM
Mandalay

India

the British Crown had assumed political control over virtually all of India. Indian armed forces in the British army played a vital role in both the World Wars.

Nonviolent resistance to British colonialism, led by Mohandas Gandhi (more commonly known as Mahatma Ghandi), Vallabhbhai Patel, and Jawaharlal Nehru, brought independence in 1947. The subcontinent was divided into the Secular Democratic Republic of India and the smaller Islamic Republic of Pakistan. A war between the two countries in 1971 resulted in East Pakistan becoming the separate nation of Bangladesh.

In the twenty-first century, India has made impressive gains in economic investment and output, and stands as the world's largest democracy with a population exceeding one billion. It is self-sufficient in terms of food, and is a fast-growing, economically strong country.

# The People

Birthplace of civilizations, cradle of world religions, India is home to almost a quarter of the world's population. India has dominated the world stage through most of human history, as the home of mighty empires, as a powerful trading nation, and as a hub of culture and civilization. Rumors of its empires and its wealth brought traders and travelers. Alexander the Great marched across Asia to India. Arab and Jewish traders sailed here. At one time Roman soldiers were barracked here. The ancient Greeks had trading colonies. Columbus wasn't looking for America; he hoped to find a new route to India. European history favored nations with an India connection.

India excelled in international trade. Five thousand years ago the thriving cities of the Indus Valley traded with Mesopotamia. Indian traders spread their goods and influence through Southeast Asia. Spices, gems, pearls, and silks flowed out of India into the rest of the world. Crafts, textiles, and exotic birds and animals were also traded. Hannibal's elephants came from India. So did many of the lavish fabrics craved by Roman nobility. At one point, so much gold was leaving Rome for India that the Roman economy was seriously weakened. Ideas and culture spread with trade goods. Philosophy, sciences, and medicine reached unrivaled heights, enriching the great scientific achievements of China and the Arab world. The influences of Indian thought can be found in early European culture, and still today, Indian philosophy influences modern global cultures.

The British colonial era brought new and different challenges to India, resulting in an independence movement that has left an indelible mark on nonviolent struggles for freedom and justice throughout the modern world. During this time in history, society in India wove an intricate web of relationships, rituals, and duties, yet remained astonishingly tolerant and diverse. Great religions developed and spread from India. Hindus, Buddhists, Jains, and Sikhs trace their roots to India.

English is the major language of trade and politics, but there are fourteen official Indian languages in all. There are more than twenty-four languages spoken by a million Indians, and countless other dialects. India has seven major religions and many minor ones, six main ethnic groups, and countless holidays.

# The Food

Throughout history India has been invaded and occupied by other cultures and each has left its own mark on Indian cuisine. Some of the predominant influences have been:

- During the Aryan period the cuisine of the great Hindu empires concentrated on the fine aspects of food and on understanding its essence and how it contributed to the development of mind, body, and spirit. After this period the cuisine was influenced by the following conquests from other cultures.
- Mongolians brought their hotpot cooking to India.
- The most notable later culinary influence in India was the influence of Persian rulers who established the Mughal Rule in India. They introduced their fondness for elegant dining and rich food with dry fruit and nuts. Muslims from western Asia brought their rich artistic and gastronomic culture to India. This influence lasted for more than four hundred years and is now part of the fabric of Indian culinary culture. The two cultures resulted in a magnificent cuisine called *Mughlai cuisine*. The lamb kebabs were laced with spices, the rice pilaf (*pilau*) of India was turned into *biryanis* (any number of layered rice, meat/vegetable, spice, and yogurt recipes) and lamb and meat roasts were flavored with Indian herbs, spices, and seasonings. Indian dishes were garnished with almonds, pistachios, cashews, and raisins. The Muslims also introduced leavened breads to India. The royal chefs created the cylindrical clay oven in which food is cooked over a hot charcoal fire known as the *tandoor*. The Indian *rotis* and the leavened breads were merged into *tandoori naans*. Meats were marinated in yogurt and spices and cooked in *tandoors*. Pork and beef were avoided to respect the traditions of both cultures. Since the Persian rulers loved sweets, sweetmeats were introduced.
- The Chinese introduced stir-fries to Indian and added a sweet taste to food. Their influence is mostly felt in western India.
- The tomato, chile, and potato, which are staple components of today's Indian cuisine, were brought to India by the Portuguese. The Indian *vindaloo* dish is a result of Portuguese influence.
- The British made ketchup and tea popular in India, but British food did not become popular in India. Although the British colonists mainly described Indian food as pungent, chile-spiked curries and rice and *rotis* were considered food for uncivilized pagans. Today, however, Indian food forms a staple diet of British food.

The essential ingredient that distinguishes Indian cooking from all other cuisines is the use of spices. Indian spices have an important place in all international markets and are even a commodity traded on the stock market. *Curry* is an all-purpose term devised by the English to cover the whole range of Indian food spicing. Indian cooks have at least twenty-five spices on their regular list and it is from these that they produce curry flavor. The spices are blended in certain combinations to produce specific dishes. *Garam masala,* for example, is a combination of cloves and cinnamon with peppercorns. Popular spices include saffron that is used to give *biryani* that yellow color and delicate fragrance. *Turmeric* also has a coloring property and acts as a preservative. Red and green chiles are ground, dried, or added whole to give a hot taste to curries. Ginger is considered to be good for digestion. Coriander is added to many *masalas* to cool the body. Cardamom is used in many sweet dishes and in meat preparations. Other popular spices are nutmeg, cinnamon, poppy seeds, caraway seeds, cumin seeds, fenugreek, mace, garlic, and cloves.

Indian dishes are cooked in three stages. The first stage is to prepare the base, or the gravy. This requires warming the oil with the spices and salt. The second stage involves adding the vegetables and stirring it into the gravy base. The third stage is to allow the dish to simmer until completely cooked. While this is the basic technique, the difference is in the blend of spices, which are broadly divided into two categories: powdered spices that have been freshly ground using a mortar and pestle, and the whole spices such as clove, cardamom, mustard seeds, nutmeg, and others.

A complete Indian meal would start with appetizers, which are usually fried or baked. This leads into the main course that comprises one or two vegetable dishes, along with pulses or a curry. Indian food has a number of side dishes to go with the main meal. The most popular is probably the *dahi,* or curd of yogurt. It cools the stomach after a very hot meal. Desserts such as *kulfi* (a kind of Indian ice cream), *rasgullas* (sweet little balls of rose-flavored cream cheese), and rice or milk puddings in sweet syrup are popular. An Indian meal finishes with *paan,* the name given to the collection of spices and condiments chewed with *betel* leaves. Found throughout eastern Asia, *betel* is mildly intoxicating and addictive, but after a meal it is taken as a mild digestive in small amounts. *Paan* sellers have a number of little trays and containers in which they mix the ingredients, which may include a part from the betel nut itself, lime paste, and various spices. Then they place it in the leaf, which is folded up and chewed.

To the western mind, India is perceived as a largely vegetarian cuisine, but this is not necessarily true. To a larger extent, religious beliefs (as compared to personal preference) dictate what a person cannot eat. For example, Islam forbids its followers from eating pork, while many Hindus do not eat beef. Followers of the Jain faith are strict vegetarians and take nonviolence to a very strict level, and respect life at any level, including plant life.

India can be very roughly divided into four culinary regions. Each region has several states in it and each state has its own unique food. Here's a brief look at the cuisines of north, west, east, and south India.

## NORTH INDIA

North India includes the states of Jammu and Kashmir, Himachal Pradesh, Punjab, Haryana, Delhi, Uttaranchal, Uttar Pradesh, Bihar, Madhya Pradish, Jharkhand, and Chattisgarh.

North India has extreme climates; summers are hot and winters are cold. There is an abundance of fresh seasonal fruit and vegetables. Its geographical position with relation to the rest of the subcontinent means that this region of the country has had strong Central Asian influences both in its culture and its food. *Mughlai* and *Kashmiri* styles of cooking are prevalent.

The food from north India traces its descent from Persian ancestors who started filtering into India from the eleventh century A.D. onward and then more markedly from the sixteenth century A.D., when the Mughals came to power. The Mughals brought with them Persian and Afghan cooks, who introduced rich and fragrant Persian rice dishes, such as *pilafs* and *biryanis*. Garnished with pounded silver (*vark*), these dishes along with spicy *kormas* (braised meat in creamy sauces), *koftas* (grilled spicy meatballs), and kebabs graced the tables of emperors.

A typical north Indian meal would consist of *pilafs*, thick, creamy *dals* (the Indian word for their many types of dried pulses), vegetables seasoned with yogurt or pomegranate powder, greens like spinach and mustard greens cooked with *paneer* (a fresh and delicate cottage cheese made from whole milk). North Indian pickles, fresh tomato, mint, cilantro chutneys, and yogurt *raitas*. North Indian curries usually have thick, moderately spicy and creamy gravies. The use of dried fruits and nuts is common even in everyday foods. Dairy products like milk, cream, cottage cheese, ghee (clarified butter), and yogurt play an important role in the cooking of both savory and sweet dishes. North Indians prefer breads to rice. This region is home to the stuffed *parathas* (flaky Indian bread with different kinds of vegetarian and nonvegetarian fillings), and *kulchas* (bread made from fermented dough). *Chappatis*, *parantha,* or *pooris* are their unleavened flat breads. Hot, sweet cardamom milk is commonly taken before going to bed. North Indian desserts and sweets are made of milk, *paneer*, lentil flour, and wheat flour combined with dried nuts and garnished with a thin sheet of pure silver. *Nimbu Pani* (lemon drink) and *lassi* (iced buttermilk) are popular drinks of the north.

In Jammu and Kashmir is found the tradition of *wazwan*, the fabulous aromatic celebratory banquet consisting of thirty-six delectable dishes. Most of the dishes are meat based and contain heavy dose of spices, condiments, and curds. *Rista* (meatballs in red gravy), *tabak maaz* (fried lamb ribs), and *rogan josh* (Indian lamb in spicy cream sauce) are just some of the dishes included in the *wazwan*.

Recipes from the hilly regions of Himanchal Pradesh and Uttaranchal are simple and nutritious, based on a huge variety of *dals* cooked slowly over fire. There is a lot of variety in cooking patterns in these areas as taste preference changes from one region to other.

The cuisine of Punjab and Haryana is rich in dairy products, grains, and most notably is the home of the *tandoori* (Indian clay oven) style of cooking. Favorites such as *tandoori chicken* and *naan* breads are all from this style of cooking. Food in Punjab and Haryana is rich in butter and ghee and contains many spices.

The *bawarchis* (cooks) of Awadh in Uttar Pradesh originated the *dum* style of cooking, or the art of slow cooking over a fire. *Dum pukht* refers to a slow method of cooking food. *Dum* means steam and *dum pukht* literally means to "choke off the steam." To do this the food is placed in a pot, usually made of clay, and dough is used to create a tight seal to prevent steam from escaping. The food is slowly cooked in its own juices and steam, allowing herbs and spices to fully infuse the meat or rice, while preserving the nutritional elements at the same time. The final result is rich in taste and aroma. *Korma* is a preparation of meat in gravy that is an essential item of the Awadh table. *Biryani* is cooked in *dum* style, as are *murg mussallam* (whole chicken) and *shami kebabs* (the "national" kebab of Awadh, made from minced meat heavily seasoned with *garam masala*). Mustard oil is a common cooking medium in north India, where the mustard plant grows extensively and is harvested in February and March. In Awadh the mustard oil is heated in large cauldrons till it smokes. Then it is passed through muslin cloth to remove any impurities. This oil is then collected and sealed in large earthenware pots or urns and buried in the earth, preferably under the shade of a tree or a cool place. It is left to mature for a period of nine to ten months, including through the rainy season, so that the oil is further cooled when the rainwater seeps into the ground. The long period of underground storage transforms the oil to a granular texture, which is used for cooking purposes.

In the vast plateau of Madhya Pradesh, the cuisine consists of both sweet and salty dishes. People of this part of the country do not have a distinct cuisine of their own, but they have combined the best of the food cultures from the neighboring states.

## WEST INDIA

The Arabian Sea guards the western region of India. West Indian states of Maharastra, Gujarat, Goa, and Rajasthan are regarded as the gateway to the western countries, particularly the Gulf region. The state of Maharashtra (which means "The Great State"), is one of the largest in India in terms of both size and population, and stands mostly on the high Deccan Plateau. It was the main historical center for the Maratha Empire, which defied the Mughals for almost 150 years, and which carved out a large part of central India as its domain. The capital of Maharashtra was once called Bombay, but the name of the city was changed to Mumbai by an act of the parliament in 1997. It acquired the nickname "Bollywood" because of its resemblance to the American film capital, Hollywood. Gujarat is one of India's wealthier states, with a number of important industries, particularly textiles and electronics, and it has the largest petrochemical complex in the country. Gujarat was the birthplace of Mahatma Gandhi, the father of modern India. The former Portuguese enclave of Goa has some of the world's most beautiful beaches. Almost 500 years of Portuguese rule have given Goa a unique culture, quite distinct from the rest of India, and includes a curious blending of cultures, from religion to architecture, cuisine to art. Rajasthan, literally "land of the kings," was once a group of princely kingdoms. The Rajputs, who ruled here for over a thousand years, were legendary for their chivalry.

The state is diagonally divided into the hilly and rugged southeastern region and the barren northwestern Thar Desert, which extends across the border into Pakistan.

Parts of Maharashtra are coastal and parts arid, and the food varies accordingly. Rice is the staple food grain and as in other coastal states, there is an enormous variety of vegetables, fish, and coconuts in the regular diet. Grated coconuts flavor many dishes, but coconut oil is not very widely used as a cooking medium. Rather, peanut oil is the main cooking medium and peanuts and cashew nuts are widely used in vegetable dishes. *Kokum*, a deep purple berry that has the same souring qualities as tamarind, is used to enhance coconut-based curries or vegetable dishes like potatoes, okra, or lentils. *Kokum* is especially used with fish curries, three or four skins being enough to season an average dish. It is also included in chutneys and pickles. The skins are not usually chopped but are added whole to the dish. Vegetables are steamed and lightly seasoned; there is little deep-frying and roasting. *Jaggery* (the traditional unrefined sugar in India) and tamarind are used in most vegetables or lentils dishes so that the food has a sweet-and-sour flavor, while the *kala masala* (special blend of spices) is added to make the food piquant. Powdered coconut is used for cooking in the inland regions. Among seafood, the popular delicacy is *bombil* (a very strong-smelling fish also known as Bombay duck or dak), which is normally served batter fried and crisp or dried and salted to be used in a curry. *Bangda,* or mackerel, is another popular fish in coastal Maharashtra is curried with red chiles and ginger. *Pomfret* is a fish eaten barbecued, stuffed, fried, or curried. *Pamphlet triphal ambat* is a traditional dish in which fish is cooked in creamy coconut gravy. Besides fish, crabs, prawns, shellfish, and lobsters are used.

In the vegetarian fare, the most popular vegetable is eggplant. A favorite style of cooking them is *bharlivangi,* or baby eggplant stuffed with coconut. Another typical dish is the *pachadi,* which is eggplant cooked with green mangoes and flavored with coconut and *jaggery*. All dishes are eaten with boiled rice or with *bhakris*, which are soft *rotis* made of rice flour. Special rice cakes called *vada* and *amboli* (a pancake made of fermented rice, *urad dal*, and semolina) are also eaten as a part of the main meal. Meals are not complete without *papads* (dried lentil chips), which are eaten roasted or fried. A typical feature is the *masala papad,* in which finely chopped onions, green chiles, and *chat masala* are sprinkled over roasted or fried *papads*. The most popular dessert of Maharashtra is the *puran poli,* which is *roti* stuffed with a sweet mixture of *jaggery* and *gram flour* (made from ground chickpeas, or chana dal) and is made at the time of the Maharashtrian New Year. Other popular sweets are the *ukdiche modak* (steamed rice flour dumplings), and the *shreekhand* (a thick yogurt sweet dish flavored with cardamom powder and saffron).

The state of Gujarat excels in the preparation of vegetarian dishes. The recipes are known for the subtle use of spices and rich texture. A selection of different dishes, usually served in small bowls on a round tray, is known as a *thali*. The *thali* consists of *roti, dal*, or *kadhi* (a "soup" made with chickpea flour, yogurt, water, lemon juice, and spices, along with fritters of chickpea flour and chopped vegetables that swell and soften), rice, and *sabzi/shaak* (a dish made up of different combinations of vegetables and spices, which may be stir-fried, currylike, or even dry-boiled).) Cuisine varies in taste and heat, depending on a given family. Gujarati food has been influenced by Chinese cuisine and is different from most all Indian cuisines in that the sweets are served with the meal. This is also a reason why there is more sweet and sour taste in their dishes. Other popular items include a vegetable preparation *Undhiu* (mixed winter vegetables), *gujarati kadhi*, a savory curry made of yogurt. Some common dishes include *khaman dhokla*, a salty steamed cake; *doodhpak*, a sweet, thickened milk confectionery; and *shrikhand*, a dessert made of yogurt, flavored with saffron and cardamom.

A particularly important part of the cuisine of the region is the unparalleled variety of snacks called *farsan*. *Farsan* means savory snack and usually refers to anything salty, fried, and crunchy. *Patra*, a famous *farsan*, is made from the long, black-stemmed *colocasia* (taro) leaves and Bengal gram flour. The leaves are spread with a batter of flour into which a pulp of tamarind and *jaggery* is mixed. Green chiles, ginger, sesame seeds, coriander seeds, mustard seeds, and salt are added. The leaves are placed one on top of the other and then folded from both sides. They are rolled tightly, the roll is tied with a thread, and then steamed for an hour. The rolls are then cut into half-inch-thick slices. These are sautéed in oil with mustard seeds and served hot, garnished with chopped coriander leaves and grated coconut.

As mentioned earlier, food in Goa has been influenced by the Portuguese. Local dishes like *vindaloo* (fiery hot and known as the "king of curries") and *xacut* (a curry, usually chicken, with white poppy seeds and red peppers) are evidence that Goa was a Portuguese colony until the 1960s. *Pork vindaloo* is a spicy concoction of red chiles, garlic, cooked with chunks of pork, Goa vinegar, and hard palm sugar served with plain boiled rice. Rice, fish, and coconut are the basic components of the typical Goan platter. The Goans make full use of their proximity to the sea coast by using fish, crabs, lobsters, and tiger prawns, which are cooked in a coconut, garlic hot sauce, or dry spices. An essential ingredient in Goan cooking is coconut milk made by grating the white flesh of a coconut and soaking it in a cup of warm water. Equally important is the *kokum* that gives it a sharp and sour flavor. The famous red Goan chiles are also a must for most dishes, as is tamarind. Goans make their own version of vinegar from toddy, which is distilled from the sap of coconut palm trees. Then there are the innumerable chutneys that are typical of the state.

Though there are two separate traditions in cuisine influenced by the respective religions of Hinduism and Christianity, there are some meeting points that present interesting harmony. While Hindus like lamb and chicken, Christians seem to prefer pork. However, both prefer fish and seafood to any other protein. Grinding spices is always part of the recipe and the nicer the dish the longer it takes to make. Although the styles of the various cultures, past and present, have had their effect on each other, the gravies of each style are at a complete variance. The names used are the same, as are the ingredients used, yet their aroma, flavor, taste, texture, and color can be completely different. The most commonly used spices are cumin, chiles, coriander, garlic, and turmeric. Subtle differences in ingredients or their use make the outcome of these similar recipes so different. The Christians prefer to use vinegar, while the Hindus use *kokum* and tamarind to get the tang in their respective cuisines. Northern

Goans grind their coconuts and masalas individually, while the southern Goans like to grind them together, and then pass it through a fine muslin cloth to retain flavor. Many times people vary the pork to mutton and chicken to make the various curries. The most famous Goan sweet meat is the many-layered *bebinca*. It is prepared by adding extract of coconut milk to flour, sugar, and other flavorings. Each layer is baked before adding the next one and the traditional version has sixteen layers. A soft jaggery-flavored fudge called *dodol* is made from palm-sap jaggery, rice flour, and coconut. *Rose-a-coque* is a flowerlike waffle that can be eaten alone or with cream or honey.

Cuisine from Rajasthan tells the tale of the struggle of its inhabitants who had to combat the harsh climate of the region. Historically food preparation in the royal kitchens was a very serious matter. Hundreds of cooks worked in the stately palaces and kept their recipes very closely guarded. Some recipes were passed on to their sons, while others were lost forever. The climate conditions, the lack of availability of vegetables, and the tradition of royal hunts all shaped the culinary traditions. Game cooking is considered a respected art form, largely because the skills required to clean, cut, and cook game are not easily acquired. With the Pathani invasions the art of barbecuing became highly regarded and some of the most popular dishes include *sula-smoked kebabs,* skewered boneless tender morsels of meat, such as lamb, that can be prepared eleven different ways. Perhaps the best-known Rajasthani food is the combination of *dal*, *bati*, and *churma—dal* is lentils, *bati* is a baked wheat ball, and *churma* is powdered sweetened cereal. Two meat dishes, *lal maans* (red meat), a fiery heavily spiced dish, and *safed maans* (white meat) cooked with almonds, cashew nuts, and coconut, are specialties in the region. In Rajasthan, *besan* is a major ingredient here and is used to make some of the delicacies like *gatte ki sabzi* (a popular curry), and *pakodi* (a curd-based curry with dal and red chiles). Also known as *gram flour* in many recipes, *besan* is a fine, pale yellow flour made from roasted *chana dal*. It is used as a batter for deep frying, such as vegetable fritters (*pakoras*), and in soups as a binding agent. Many Indian sweets are made from *besan*. It is to an Indian kitchen what eggs are to a Western kitchen.

The vegetarian cooking prepared by the Maheshwaris of Jodhpur is considered exceptional. And then there are the Jains, who are not only vegetarians, but who do not eat after sundown, and whose food must be devoid of garlic and onions. The region is also popular for the chutneys that are made out of local spices such as coriander, mint, garlic, and turmeric.

## EAST INDIA

The eastern region of India includes the states of Assam, Arunachal Pradesh, Manipur, Meghalaya, Mizoram, Nagaland, Orrisa, Sikkim, Tripura, and West Bengal. This is the least explored region of India for various reasons, including an underdeveloped infrastructure, the necessity of special permits, and the overall instablity of the whole region. The area is dominated by various tribes speaking many different languages and dialects. These states and union territories border with Myanmar, Bhutan, Tibet, and Bangladesh.

Fish and rice are a very important part of the diet of east India as a result of the many rivers and tributaries originating in the Himalayas. Centuries of silt carried from the Himalayan Plains and the shifting of river courses has resulted in uniquely fertile soil capable of producing a wide variety of crops and choice vegetables. The population is a balanced mix of vegetarian and nonvegetarian. The geographical location of this region means its food shows a strong influence of Chinese and Mongolian cuisine.

The eastern state of West Bengal is considered to be the cultural capital of India. Bengali food is coastal cuisine symbolized by rice and fish. The market is busy at all times with all sizes and shapes of carp, salmon, *hilsa*, *bhekti*, *rui*, *magur*, and prawns. Their *Macherjhol* (fish curry) is legendary all over India. Fish are also smoked, grilled, fried, made into *pakoras* (patties), stuffed into green coconuts, and then into burgers. Preparation is not elaborate and neither are most of the ingredients. Steaming and frying are popular methods of cooking. Mustard oil is used for cooking instead of ghee or peanut or coconut oil. The specialty of Bengali cuisine is the use of *panchphoron:* five basic spices of *nigella* (similar to black cumin or black caraway seed), fennel, cumin, mustard, and fenugreek. While sweets of north India are based on *khoya* (milk thickened slowly until it forms a sweet doughlike consistency), which is quite heavy, those of east India are based on *chena* (light cottage cheese) and are lighter on the palate and overall very delicate. The tradition of making cakes, locally known as *pitha*, flourishes. They are usually made from rice or wheat flour mixed with sugar, or grated coconut, then fried or steamed and served with a sweet syrup.

Sikkim has a completely different cuisine as compared to other states of east India. The food shows its apparent influence of food culture of neighboring countries, especially Tibet. *Momos* (steamed meat or vegetable filled wontons) are especially popular.

Rice is the staple diet in Assam and is eaten in various forms throughout the day. The Assamese eat a huge variety of rice-based breakfast cereals with milk, yogurt, or thick *cream akhoi* (puffed rice), *chira* (chura), *muri*, *komal chaul* (a specially processed rice which doesn't require cooking but just an hour's soak in cold water), and *hurum* to name but a few. Normally *jaggery* or sugar is added but for those who prefer savory items, salt can be added. Also there are the various kinds of *pitha* that are prepared from rice powder. Historically, Assam is the second commercial tea production region after southern China. Assam and southern China are the only two regions in the world with native tea plants. Assam tea revolutionized tea drinking habits in the nineteenth century since the tea, produced from a different variety of the tea plant, yielded a different kind of tea. Sold as "breakfast teas" the black tea is known for its body, briskness, malty flavor, and strong, intense color. Most recently, a home-grown chile pepper called *bhut jolokia*—known as "ghost chile"—became known officially in the Guinness World Records as the world's hottest chile. This thumb-sized red chile has more than 1,000,000 Scoville units (the level of a chile's heat measured by the content of capsaicin, the chemical that "heats" a chile) and is 125 times hotter than a jalapeño. The Meghalayan cuisine is based on meat, particularly pork. *Jadoh*—a spicy dish of rice and pork—is eaten almost any time. The city of Shillong is the source of authentic Chinese food. *Kyat*, the local brew is made from rice.

## SOUTH INDIA

The states within South India include Karnataka, Tamil Nadu, Kerala, and Andhra Pradesh. India's Great Divide is the Vindhya Mountains. They run from east to west, separating the fertile river valley of the Ganges River from the Deccan Plateau, which occupies much of the peninsula of India. South India's coastal plains are backed by the mountains rimming the wedge of the Deccan Plateau. On these plains lie the best beaches in South India. On the rimming mountains, the Western and Eastern Ghats, are the tea, coffee, and spice lands. Beyond these mountains are great old cities supported by rich farm lands. The south is gracious, graceful old India.

South India has hot, humid climate and all its states are coastal. Rainfall is abundant and so is the supply of fresh fruit, vegetables, and rice. South Indian cuisine is rice based. Rice are of three basic categories: the white long-grain rice is most commonly used; short-grain rice is used to make sweet dishes; and a round grain rice that is used for worship representing Health, Wealth, and Fertility. Steamed rice dumplings (*idlis*) and roasted rice pancakes (*dosais*) are paired with coconut chutneys for breakfast. The famous *masala dosai* is stuffed with spiced potatoes, vegetables, or even minced lamb.

A formal South Indian meal is divided into three courses of rice. The first is rice with *sambhar*, the everyday food of South India. Made from a handful of lentils or mung beans simmered in a pot of water until they disintegrate into a smooth, creamy mixture, *sambhar* is flavored with turmeric, sour tamarind, *asafetida* (a gum resin used for flavor and digestion), curry leaves, and toasted mustard seeds. The second course is rice served with *rasam*, a tangy, spicy tamarind and tomato-based soup with lentils. A small amount of one or two vegetables, fresh herbs, and spices are added. The third course is a cooling mixture of rice and buttermilk or yogurt. It may be served with nonspicy assorted vegetable dishes, namely the *aviyal* (mixed vegetable stew), *kari* (dry masala vegetables), and *kootu* (coconut and vegetable sauté).

South Indian *dals* and curries are soupier than north Indian *dals* and curries. South Indian chutneys are made of tamarind, coconut, peanuts, *dal,* fenugreek seeds, and cilantro. Coconut, either in a shredded, grated, or blended form, is found in most dishes here and coconut water is drunk for its cooling effect on the system. Meals are followed by coffee.

Before stainless steel became widespread, banana leaves were the plate of choice. There are specific dictates in India to serving food on a banana leaf, especially for celebratory feasts or religious offerings. From alternating dry vegetables with gravies to the exact corner for placing a sweet dessert, the order of up to twenty different foods follows a circular pattern that incorporates health, religion, and regional traditions.

Dishes are seasoned with toasted mustard seeds, red chiles, curry leaves, and oil. Coconut oil is most commonly used for cooking and frying. Vegetable oils like sunflower and canola are also used and ghee is poured over rice during daily meals or in special occasion dishes.

Andhra Pradesh produces fiery Andhra cuisine, which is largely vegetarian yet also includes a wide range of seafood. Fish and prawns are curried in sesame and coconut oils, and flavored with freshly ground pepper. Hyderabad, the capital of Andhra Pradesh, has a cuisine that is a direct result of the kitchens of the Muslim rulers, with the vibrant spices and ingredients of the predominantly local Hindu people. Its tastes range from the sour and the sweet to the hot and the salty, and foods are studded with dry fruits and nuts and exotic, expensive spices like saffron.

(Tamil Nadu has *Chettinad* cuisine, which consists of meat and poultry cooked in tamarind and roasted spices and is one of the most fiery of all Indian food. Oil and spices are used liberally and most dishes have generous amounts of peppercorns, cinnamon, bay leaves, cardamom, nutmeg, and green and red chiles. From Kerala comes *Malabari* cooking, with its seafood dishes; it is noted for its variety of pancakes and steamed rice cakes made from pounded rice.)

# Glossary

**Ajwain Seed** Carom seed, bishop's weed; resembles a small caraway seed but with the flavor of pungent thyme. Usually sprinkled on breads.

**Amchoor** Dried green mango powder used as a souring agent or to tenderize meats.

**Appam** Wafer-thin, round, flat bread, usually made of rice, potato, and/or various lentil flours.

**Asafetida** Known as *devil's dung* or *food of the gods*, it is a powdered gum resin that imparts a very strong onion-garlic flavor; a little goes a long way.

**Baghar, Tadka, or Chounk** The technique of adding spices and herbs all at one time to hot oil. This is done as a first step in the cooking process, or as the last, and then pouring the tempered oil over a cooked dish. The oil extracts and retains the sharp flavors of the spices, flavoring the entire dish.

**Balti** Means "pot" or "bucket." This stir-fried curry takes its name from the heavy, woklike dish in which the food is cooked and served. The dish is also known as a *karhai* or *karahi*.

**Barfi** A dessert made from milk that has been cooked slowly and reduced to a fudgelike consistency.

**Basmati Rice** Authentic Indian long-grained white rice with a unique nutty flavor.

**Belan** Rolling pin, about 12 inches long, with a long taper from the center toward each end.

**Biryani** A mixture of rice and spicy meat or vegetables arranged in layers, sprinkled with saffron and *ghee*. Traditionally the ingredients are tightly packed and sealed with *naan* dough. This method is also termed the *dum* style.

**Black Cumin Seeds (Kala Jeera, Saahjeers)** Darker and sweeter than ordinary cumin, used in curries and tandooris.

**Black Mustard Seeds** Preferred over the larger yellow mustard seeds common in the West.

**Bondas or Vadas** Round deep-fried savory snack made in different varieties usually from lentils or potatoes and eaten with a chutney.

**Chappati** The most common unleavened flat-bread in north India made with wheat flour, water, oil, and salt. Usually cooked on a *tava* or thick griddle and brushed with ghee. Similar to those prepared in Greece, the Middle East, and Mexico.

**Chutney** Fresh relishes made with fruits, vegetables, and herbs.

**Curry** The term "curry" means gravy or sauce. An authentic Indian curry is a combination of stir-fried wet masala (a mixture of onion, garlic, ginger, and tomato), various spices, and seasoning, to which other items are added and prepared as a stew-type dish.

**Dal, Daal** Dals are the primary source of protein in a vegetarian diet (especially in southern India). They include dried peas, beans, and lentils, plus split peas and other legumes. Ground powdered dal is used in crackers, unleavened breads, and spice mixtures.

**Dosas, Dhosas** Lentil flour-based pancakes, traditionally stuffed with mashed potatoes and onions, flavored with mustard seeds and turmeric, much like an Indian crepe or enchilada. A southern Indian delicacy, originally from Madras but now found all over India.

**Feni** A drink made from cashews or coconut is the perfect beach drink. It was originally a very basic and local drink; recently it has been commercialized.

**Fenugreek** Adds an earthy flavor to foods; available as seeds or powder.

**Ghee, or Desi Ghee** Clarified butter.

**Halva** Indian sweet made from a variety of finely grated vegetables, milk, and sugar, and flavored with cardamom. The consistency is that of a thick pudding.

**Jalfrezi** A style of cooking mixed vegetables or chicken in a tangy sauce.

**Kachumber** Indian salad usually made with cucumber, tomatoes, and onions flavored with salt, sugar, and lemon juice.

**Kadhai** A traditional Indian iron wok, much deeper and narrower than the Chinese wok. Used mainly for frying or braising. In authentic kadhai-style cooking, ingredients are cooked together in a thick, tomato-based sauce and seasoned with a savory garlic-ginger mixture.

**Kari Leaf or Curry Leaf (Kadi Patta)** Imparts an herbal, concentrated flavor of curry with a slight hint of lemon. Substitute chopped cilantro.

**Khoya** Also known as "mawa," it is made by reducing milk to a thickened consistency of soft cream cheese. Used widely in the making of many Indian desserts and sweet meats.

**Korma, Khorma** Indian braising, similar to Western braising. Indian cooks create rich thick braising liquids, as opposed to using a stock. Korma are generally made from yogurts, creams, and purees; spices are delicate and not usually hot or spicy. The meats are marinated in the braising liquid and then slow cooked.

**Kofta** Balls made of minced meat or mashed vegetables fried and mixed with a sauce or a curry.

**Kulchae** Flatbread often stuffed with onion or potatoes, seasoned with cilantro.

**Masala** Spices, herbs, and other seasonings ground or pounded together. When wet ingredients like water, vinegar, yogurt, and so on are added to the spice mixture, it is appropriately called a wet masala. Dry spice mixtures are also called garam masala or commonly known in the world as curry powder. Indian cooks generally don't use preprepared curry powder—originally a British invention to approximate Indian seasoning—but prefer making their own ever-changing blends.

**Muglai (Bawarchi)** Typical north Indian food named after the Mughal dynasty of Muslim rulers who ruled India for four hundred years.

**Naan** A traditional leavened bread, baked at very high temperatures against the wall of a tandoor oven.

**Pakora** Batter made of besan flour (ground chickpeas). Popular Indian crispy and spicy snack, served hot with coriander chutney, sometimes called *bhajias.*

**Papadam, Poppadum, or Paapar** Thin crisp discs, plain or flavored with spices and seasonings. A seasoned dough made from dried pulses that have been rolled, shaped, and dried in the sun. Papadam can be deep-fried, in which they puff up and turn airy, which also maximizes flavor. They can also be roasted over a flame, although these do not expand and are denser.

**Paratha** Whole-wheat flatbread, which has butter blended into the dough, and is then shallow-fried.

**Pasanda** A mild sauce prepared with mint leaves; adds aroma to dishes, in particular with paneer.

**Pomegranate Seeds (Anardana)** These serve as a souring agent in Indian cuisine.

**Pulao or Biryani** Indian basmati rice dish.

**Puri** Deep-fried whole-wheat flatbreads; they puff up when fried.

**Rahra** Lamb dishes with a partial stuffing of minced lamb.

**Raita** A traditional Indian side dish where the plain yogurt is combined with assorted items like dry fruits, or vegetables such as tomatoes, onions, or cucumbers.

**Roti** The word for bread in Hindi. *Tandoori roti* is bread baked in a tandoor; *rumali roti* (literally, "handkerchief bread") is a thin and flaky *paratha* made up of many layers.

**Samosa** A triangular deep-fried pastry appetizer.

**Seekh Kebab** The word *seekh* in Hindi means "skewer." Seekh kebab simply means kebabs on a skewer. Kebabs are usually made out of ground lamb mixed with various spices, cooked in a *tandoor* oven.

**Tikka** Tender pieces of poultry, meat, fish, prawns, and cottage cheese grilled in a tandoor.

**Tandoor** The traditional Indian oven made of special clay. All tandoori food is grilled on a charcoal at very high temperatures. Practically no fat is used in tandoori preparations.

**Tandoori Murgh** The bright red world-famous tandoori chicken. Chicken marinated with spices, red color, and yogurt is cooked in a tandoor.

**Tava** Traditional iron griddle used for making Indian breads and toasting spices.

**Tel (Oil)** Indian regional cooking is characterized by the use of different oils. Northern and central regions use peanut oil. Mustard oil is preferred in the eastern and some northern parts, while most southern regions prefer sesame and coconut oil. Sesame oil, peanut oil, and ghee are used in the western regions. Indian sesame oil is light and colorless, unlike the dark and aromatic Chinese type, which cannot be substituted.

**Varak** Fine thin edible silver foil used to decorate or garnish Indian desserts and *paan.* It is considered to be an aid to digestion.

**Vindaloo** An amalgamation of two Portuguese words: *vinho,* meaning "wine" (or vinegar) and *alho,* which means "garlic." A dish of Portuguese origin prepared with extra garlic, ginger, pepper, coconut (grated or milk), vinegar, and chiles to give a sharp, rich taste.

# Menus and Recipes from India

# Ananas Sharbat

## Pineapple Smoothie SERVES 4

| AMOUNT | MEASURE | INGREDIENT |
|---|---|---|
| $\frac{1}{4}$ cup | 1 ounce, 28 g | Pistachios, shelled, roasted, salted or unsalted |
| 4 cups | 32 ounces, 960 ml | Pineapple juice |
| $1\frac{1}{3}$ cups | 8 ounces, 224 g | Fresh pineapple, peeled, diced |
| 1 cup | 8 ounces, 240 ml | Buttermilk |
| $\frac{1}{4}$ cup | 2 ounces, 60 ml | Sour cream or plain yogurt |
| $\frac{1}{4}$ cup | 2 ounces, 56 g | Granulated sugar |
| 1 teaspoon | | Salt |

PROCEDURE

1. Add pistachios to blender and process until finely powdered.
2. Add remaining ingredients and process until mixed and frothy.

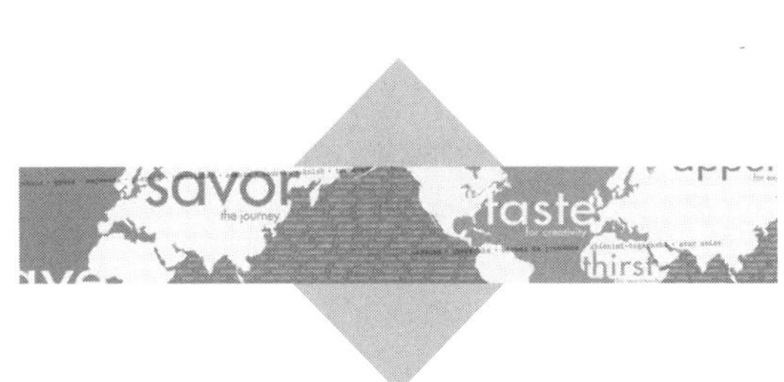

# Vegetable Samosas

YIELD: 16

| AMOUNT | MEASURE | INGREDIENT |
|---|---|---|
| **Pastry** | | |
| 2 cups | 8 ounces, 288 g | All-purpose flour |
| $\frac{1}{2}$ teaspoon | | Salt |
| 4 tablespoons | 2 ounces, 60 ml | Ghee, melted, or vegetable oil |
| 4 tablespoons | 2 ounces, 60 ml | Cold water |
| **Filling** | | |
| 4 tablespoons | 2 ounces, 60 ml | Vegetable oil |
| $\frac{1}{2}$ cup | 2 ounces, 56 g | Onion, $\frac{1}{4}$ inch (.6 cm) dice |
| 1 cup | 5 ounces, 140 g | Fresh or frozen green peas, cooked |
| 1 tablespoon | | Ginger root, grated |
| 1 | | Fresh hot green chile, seeded, minced |
| 2 tablespoons | | Cilantro, leaves only, minced |
| $1\frac{1}{2}$ cups | 9 ounces, 252 g | Potatoes, boiled until tender, peeled, cut into $\frac{1}{4}$ inch (.6 cm) cubes. |
| **Seasoning** | | |
| $\frac{1}{2}$ teaspoon | | Fennel seeds, ground |
| $\frac{1}{2}$ teaspoon | | Cumin seeds, ground |
| 1 teaspoon | | Turmeric |
| 1 teaspoon | | Garam masala (recipe follows) |
| 2 tablespoons | 1 ounce, 30 ml | Fresh lemon juice |
| As needed | | Vegetable oil, for frying |
| As needed | | Mint chutney, for serving |

## PROCEDURE

### Pastry

1. Sift the flour and salt into a bowl.
2. Add the melted ghee and rub it with your hands until the mixture resembles coarse bread crumbs.
3. Gradually add the cold water (more if necessary) and gather the dough into a stiff ball. Knead the dough for about 10 minutes, until smooth; make a ball, oil it, and wrap it up with plastic. Set aside 30 minutes.

**Filling**

1 Heat the oil over medium heat; add the onions and sauté until brown at the edges, 3 to 4 minutes.

2 Add peas, ginger, chile, cilantro, and 3 tablespoons ($1\frac{1}{2}$ ounces, 45 ml) water. Cover, lower heat to a simmer, and cook 3 minutes. Add more water if pan dries out.

3 Add diced potatoes and seasoning; stir to mix. Cook on low heat 2 to 3 minutes, stirring occasionally. Correct seasoning and balance with lemon juice and salt. Let cool.

**Filling the Pastry**

1 Divide dough into 8 balls. Roll each out into 6-inch (15 cm) circles and cut the circles in half.

2 Pick up one-half and form a cone, making a $\frac{1}{4}$-inch (.6 cm) wide, overlapping seam. Seal seam with a little water. You should now have a small triangular pocket.

3 Fill the pocket with 2 tablespoons (1 ounce, 30 ml) potato mixture. Close the top by sticking the open edges together with a little water. Press the seams down with the prongs of a fork. Repeat with the remaining dough.

**Cooking**

1 Fry the samosas until golden brown and hot; drain them on paper towels.

2 Serve hot, warm, or at room temperature, with mint chutney.

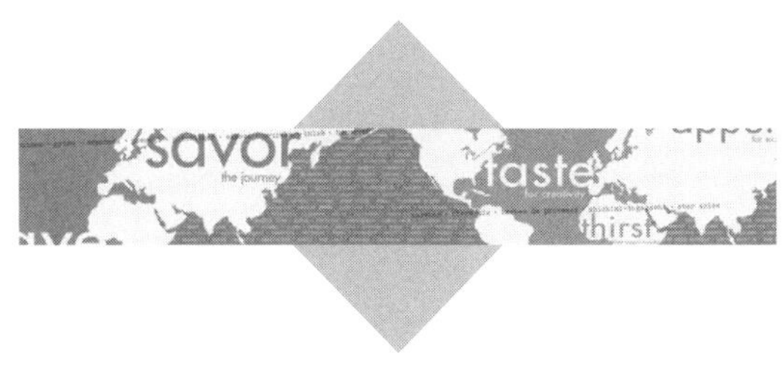

# Chicken Korma, Kashmiri Style

SERVES 4

| AMOUNT | MEASURE | INGREDIENT |
|---|---|---|
| 1 | $2\frac{1}{2}$ pound, 1.12 kg | Chicken |
| 4 | | Garlic cloves, minced |
| 2 tablespoons | | Fresh ginger, grated |
| 2 tablespoons | 1 ounce, 30 ml | Vegetable oil |
| $1\frac{1}{2}$ cups | 6 ounces, 168 g | Onions, cut in half lengthwise, then finely sliced |
| 2 tablespoons | 1 ounce, 30 ml | Ghee (clarified butter) |
| 2 inch (5 cm) | | Cinnamon stick |
| 6 | | Cardamom pods |
| 6 | | Cloves |
| 1 teaspoon | | Fennel seeds, ground |
| 1 tablespoon | | Sweet paprika |
| 1 teaspoon | | Coriander, ground |
| 1 teaspoon | | Cumin, ground |
| $\frac{1}{2}$ teaspoon | | Cayenne pepper |
| 1 teaspoon | | Turmeric |
| 2 teaspoons | | Salt |
| $1\frac{1}{2}$ cups | 9 ounces, 252 g | Tomatoes, peeled, seeded, $\frac{1}{4}$ inch (.6 cm) dice |
| $\frac{1}{4}$ cup | 2 ounces, 60 ml | Chicken stock or water |
| $\frac{1}{4}$ cup | 1 ounce, 28 g | Roasted unsalted cashews |
| 1 cup | 8 ounces, 240 ml | Plain yogurt, plain |
| As needed | | Cilantro sprigs, for garnish |

PROCEDURE

1. Cut chicken into 12 pieces as follows. Quarter chicken, remove skin, then cut each breast into four pieces and each leg into two pieces (between drumstick and thigh). Pat dry and reserve.
2. Using a mortar and pestle with a little water, make a smooth paste with the garlic and ginger.
3. Heat oil over medium heat; add the onion and cook, stirring often, until deep golden, 8 to 10 minutes. Remove from pan and set aside.

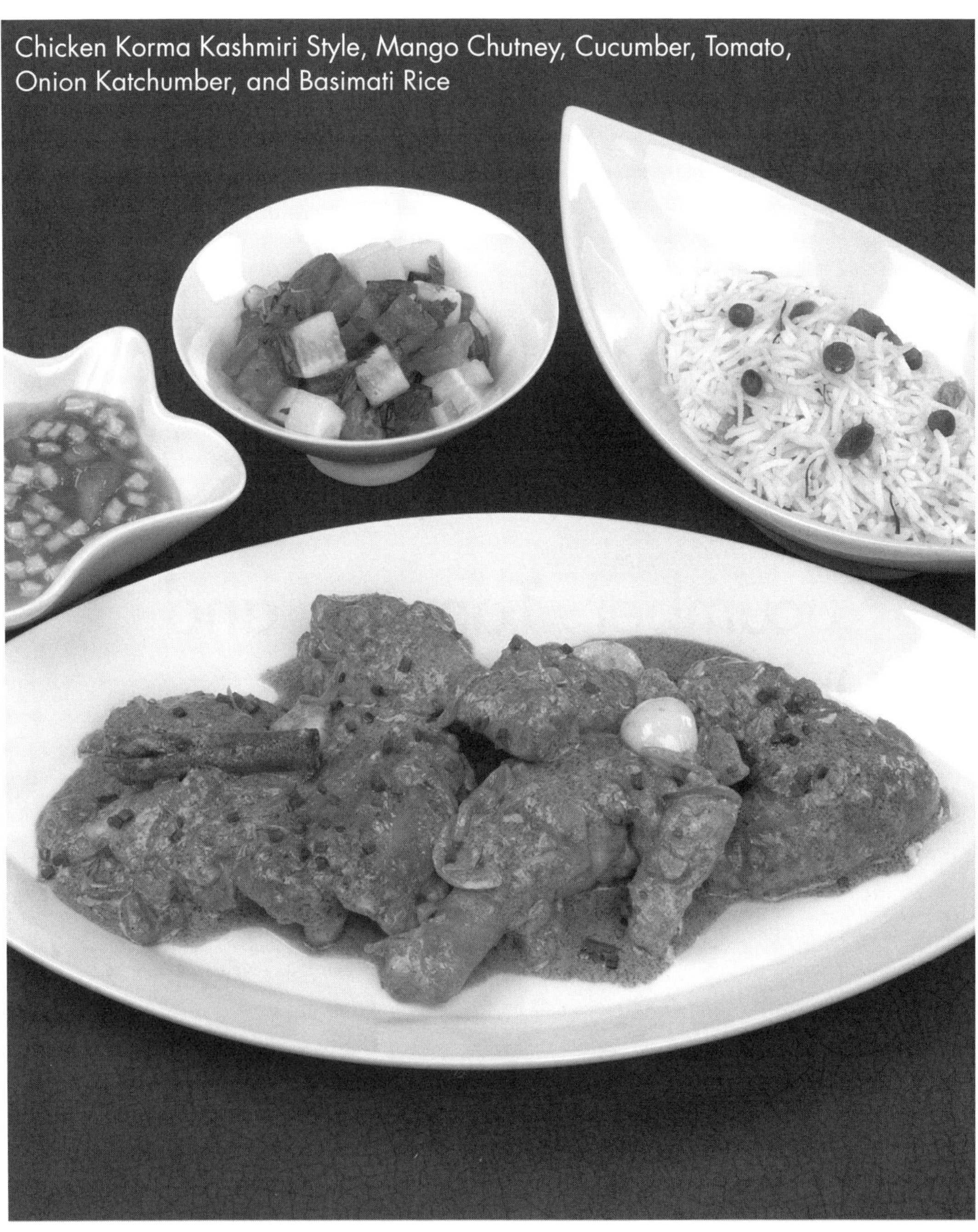

Chicken Korma Kashmiri Style, Mango Chutney, Cucumber, Tomato, Onion Katchumber, and Basimati Rice

4 Add ghee to the pan and when hot, add the ginger-garlic paste. Cook, stirring, until the mixture is fragrant and light brown, 2 to 3 minutes. Add cinnamon, cardamom pods, and cloves; stir for a few seconds. Add remaining dry spices and cook, stirring, until the mixture takes on an orange-red color and becomes fragrant, about 30 seconds.

5 Add chicken pieces and sear to light golden, about 3 minutes per side.

6 Add tomatoes with chicken stock and cook, stirring occasionally, unit tomatoes are very soft, 6 to 8 minutes.

7 As the tomatoes are cooking, combine the cashews with 2 tablespoons (1 ounce, 30 ml) water in a blender and process to a smooth paste, or use mortar and pestle. Add to the chicken mixture.

8 Whisk in the yogurt and stir to combine. Add reserved onions, bring to a boil, and reduce to a simmer. Cook, covered, until chicken is tender, approximately 15 to 20 minutes. Remove pieces as they cook completely; breast meat will cook before leg and thigh.

9 Serve chicken pieces covered with sauce and garnished with cilantro.

# Cucumber, Tomato, and Onion Katchumber

SERVES 4

| AMOUNT | MEASURE | INGREDIENT |
|---|---|---|
| $\frac{1}{2}$ cup | 2 ounces, 56 g | Red onion, $\frac{1}{4}$ inch (.6 cm) diced |
| 1 cup | 6 ounces, 168 g | Tomato, peeled, seeded, $\frac{1}{2}$ inch (1.2 cm) dice |
| 1 cup | 6 ounces, 168 g | Cucumber, peeled, seeded, $\frac{1}{2}$ inch (1.2 cm) dice |
| 2 tablespoons | | Cilantro, coarsely chopped |
| 1 teaspoon | | Green chile (jalapeño), minced |
| 3 tablespoons | $1\frac{1}{2}$ ounces, 45 ml | Fresh lime juice |
| 1 teaspoon | | Nigella seeds, toasted |
| To taste | | Salt and freshly ground black pepper |

PROCEDURE

1 Combine all ingredients, toss together, and let stand at least 1 hour before serving.

# Garam Masala Ground Spice Mixture

SERVES 4

| AMOUNT | MEASURE | INGREDIENT |
| --- | --- | --- |
| 1/2 | | Whole nutmeg |
| 3 tablespoons | | Cardamom seeds |
| 2 tablespoons | | Whole cloves |
| 2 tablespoons | | Whole cumin |
| 1 tablespoon | | Whole coriander |
| 2 tablespoons | | Whole black peppercorns |
| 3 inches | | Cinnamon stick |
| 4 | | Bay leaf |

PROCEDURE

1. Dry-roast all ingredients separately in a heated heavy skillet over medium heat until the spices emit a toasty aroma. Let cool.
2. Combine all ingredients except nutmeg in a clean spice grinder and grind them into a very fine powder or use a mortar and pestle. Finely grate nutmeg.
3. Store in a tightly closed jar until needed.

# Podina Chatni Green Chutney

SERVES 4

| AMOUNT | MEASURE | INGREDIENT |
| --- | --- | --- |
| 1 cup (firmly packed) | 2 ounces, 56 g | Mint leaves, picked |
| 1/3 cup | 1/3 ounce, 8 g | Cilantro leaves |
| 1 | | Green chile (jalapeño), seeded |
| 1 cup | 2 ounces, 56 g | Green onions, 1 inch (2.4 cm) lengths |
| 1 1/4 cups | 2 ounces, 60 ml | Jalapeño, seeded, minced |
| | | Lemon juice |
| 1 teaspoon | | Garam masala |
| 2 teaspoons | | Granulated sugar |
| 1 teaspoon | | Salt |
| 1/4 cup | 2 ounces, 60 ml | Water |

PROCEDURE

1. Place all ingredients in a food processor and purée, or pound in mortar and pestle a little at a time, until ground to a paste. If too dry, add a little oil and/or water. Chill.

# Palak Paneer Spinach with Curd Cheese

YIELD: 8 OUNCES; SERVES 4

**Paneer is a popular Indian soft cheese that is very similar to Ricotta cheese. It is high in protein and is substituted for meat in vegetarian dishes of Indian cuisine.**

| AMOUNT | MEASURE | INGREDIENT |
|---|---|---|
| **Curd Cheese** | | |
| 6 cups | 240 ml | Milk, whole or 2% low-fat |
| 1 cup | 8 ounces, 240 ml | Yogurt, at room temperature |
| 1 $\frac{1}{2}$ tablespoons | $\frac{3}{4}$ ounce, 20 ml | Fresh lemon juice |
| To taste | | Salt |
| As needed | | Ghee (clarified butter) |
| **Spinach** | | |
| 5 cups | 12 ounces, 336 g | Spinach, packed leaves, washed |
| 1 cup water | 8 ounces, 240 ml | Water |
| 2 tablespoons | 1 ounce, 30 ml | Ghee (clarified butter) |
| 1 teaspoon | | Cumin seeds |
| 1 cup | 5 ounces, 140 g | Onions, minced |
| 1 | | Green chile (jalapeño), slit lengthwise |
| 2 teaspoons | | Ginger, grated |
| 2 teaspoons | | Garlic, minced |
| 4 tablespoons | 2 ounces, 60 ml | Cream |
| As needed | | Salt, black pepper, and lemon juice |

## PROCEDURE

### Curd Cheese

1 Bring milk to a boil; be careful, because as soon as it boils it will start to froth. Remove from the heat; add yogurt and lemon juice. Reduce heat to medium and let mixture return to a boil, stirring gently, until the milk curdles and separates from the whey (the pale yellowish green transparent liquid), 6 to 8 minutes. The longer you cook the mixture, the firmer the final cheese. Turn off the heat and let stand, uncovered, to cool, about 15 minutes.

2 Line a colander with a double thickness of cheesecloth. Gently pour the contents of the pan into the colander. Gather the four corners of the cheesecloth and twist them together

Cascabel chile, on the cutting board clockwise from right: Red Fresno chiles, green chile de arbol, chipotle chile, dried chile de árbol, red chile de árbol, ancho chile, güero chile, serrano chile, santaka chile, jalapeno chile, habanero chile, pasilla chile. In the mortar, clockwise from left: bell pepper, sweet Italian pepper, mulato pepper, yellow wax hot pepper.

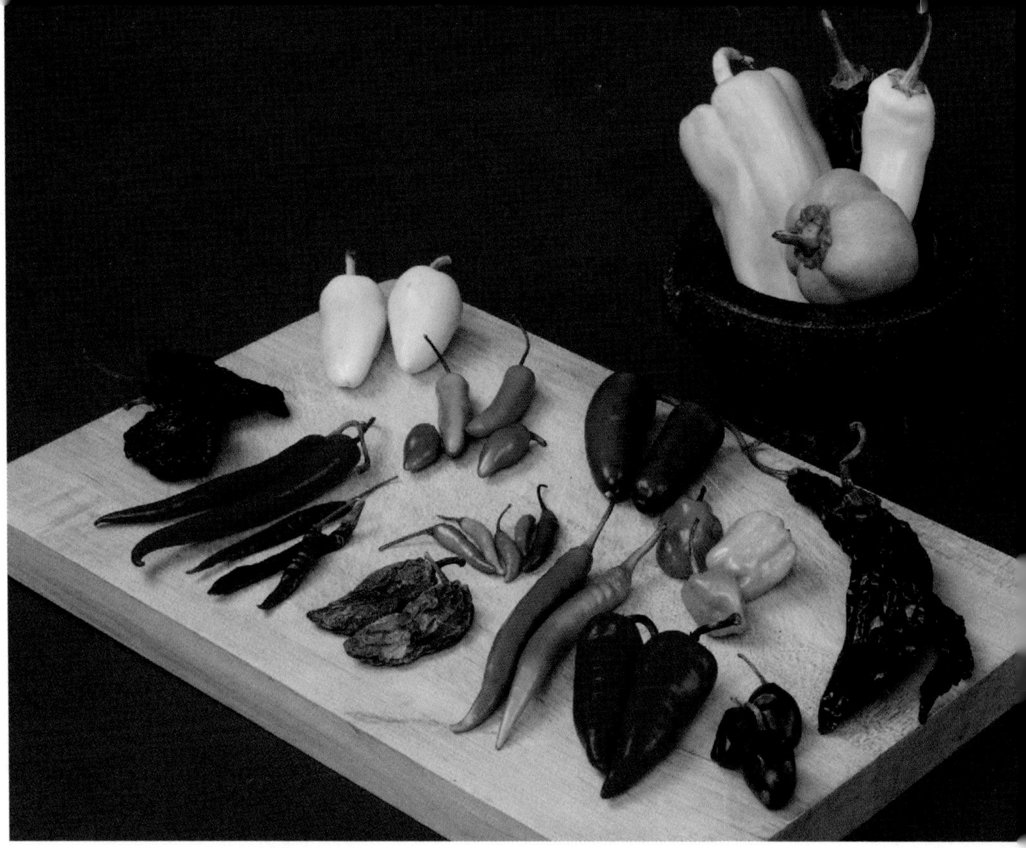

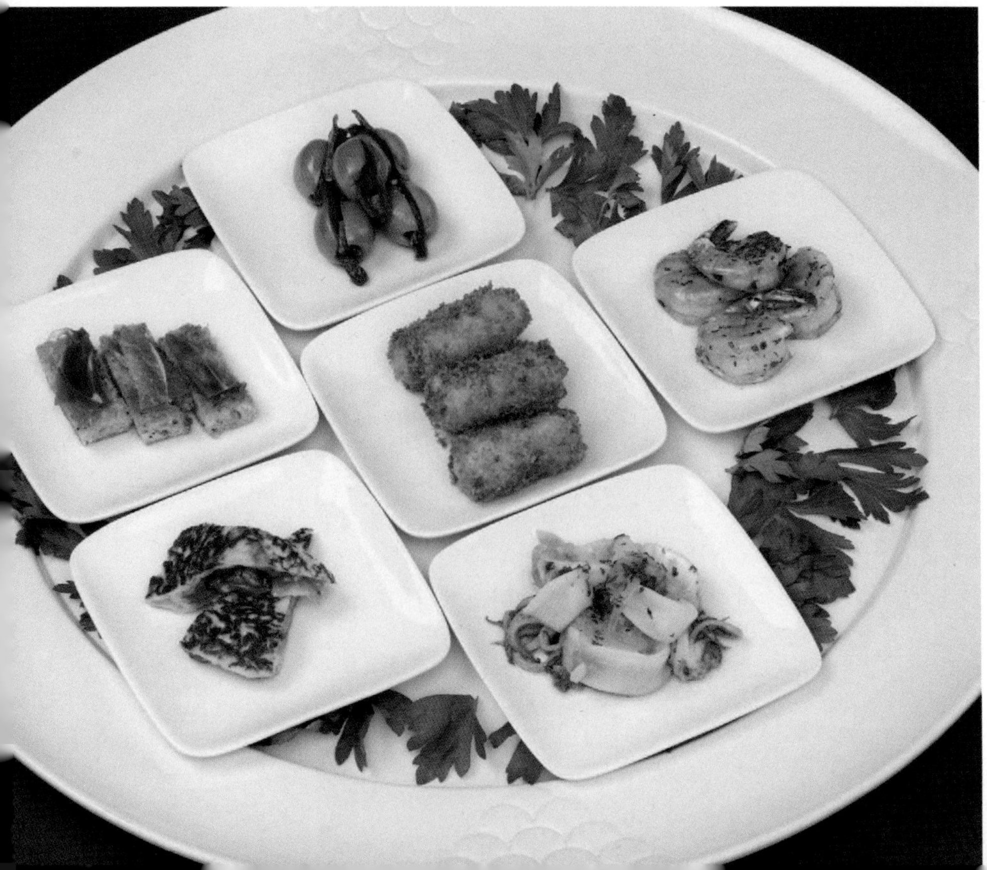

Tapas—in the middle, Croquetas de Jamón—Serrano Ham Fritters; clockwise, from bottom: Calamares encebollados—Squid with Caramelized Onions; Tortilla de Patatas—Potato Omelet; Pan Con Tomate—Tomato Toast; Aceitunas Verdes Rellenas de Pimiento y Anchoa—Green Olives Filled with Piquillo Peppers and Anchovy; Gambas Al Ajillo—Sizzling Garlic Shrimp (Spain)

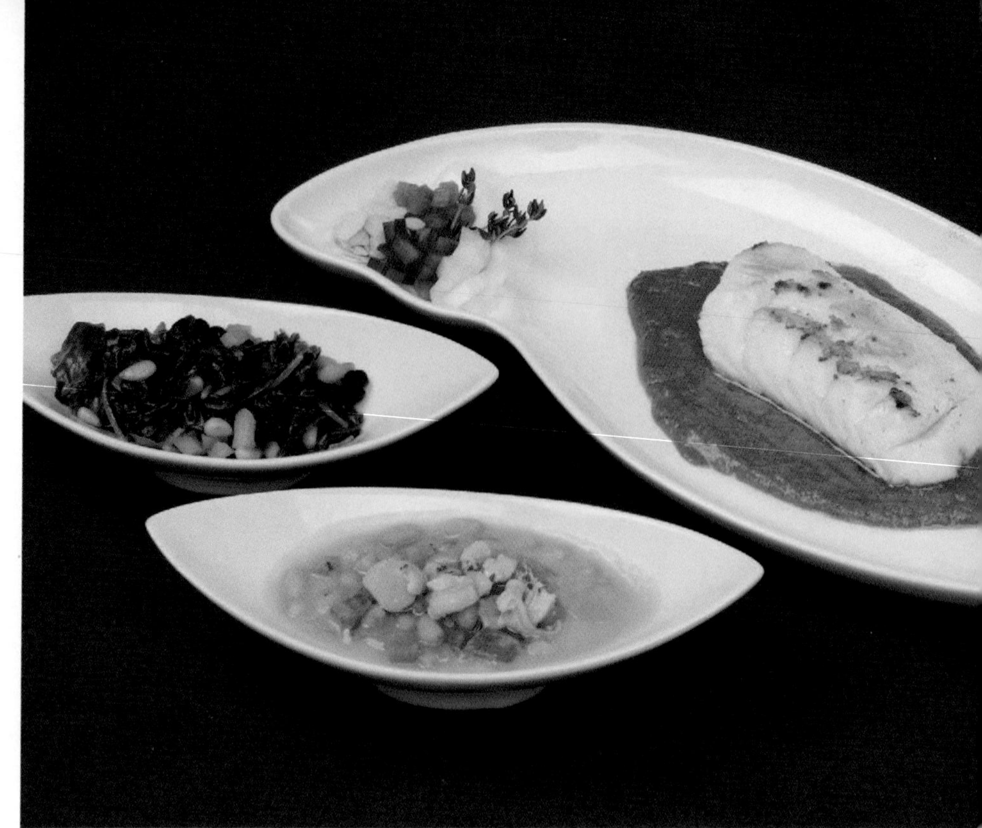

**Rape con Romesco—Monkfish with Romesco Sauce; Fabes con Almejas—Asturian Bean Stew with Clams; and Espinacas a la Catalana—Spinach, Catalan-Style (Spain)**

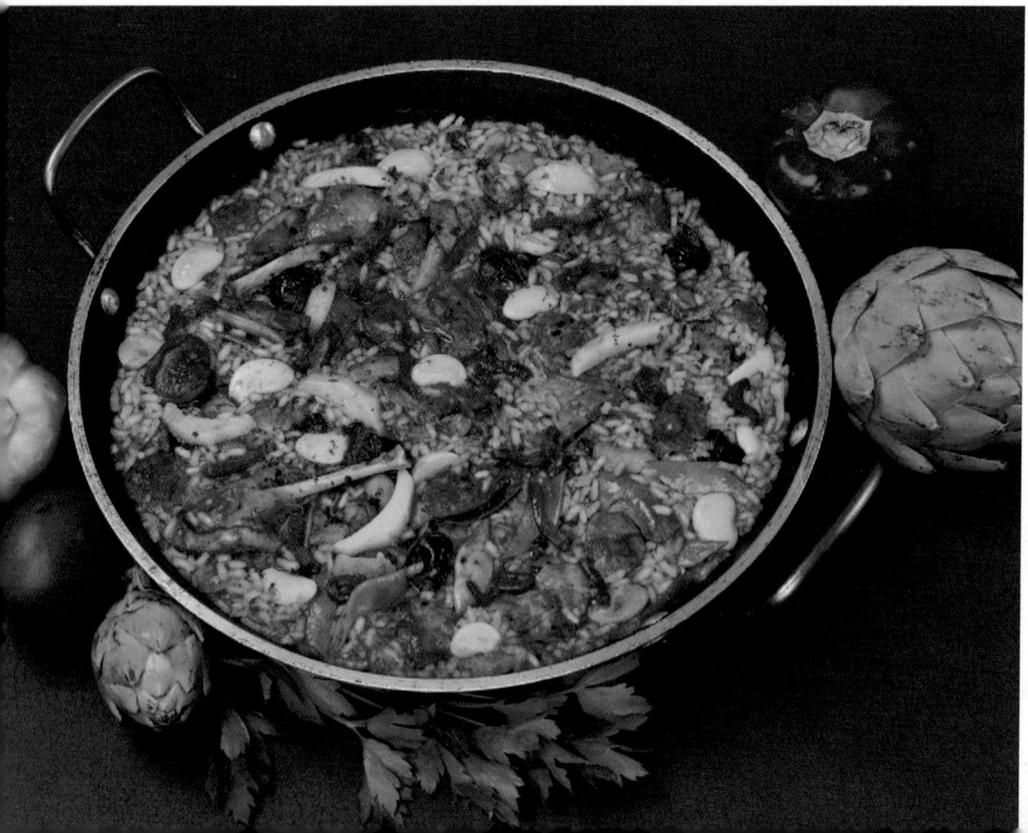

**Paella Valenciana (Spain)**

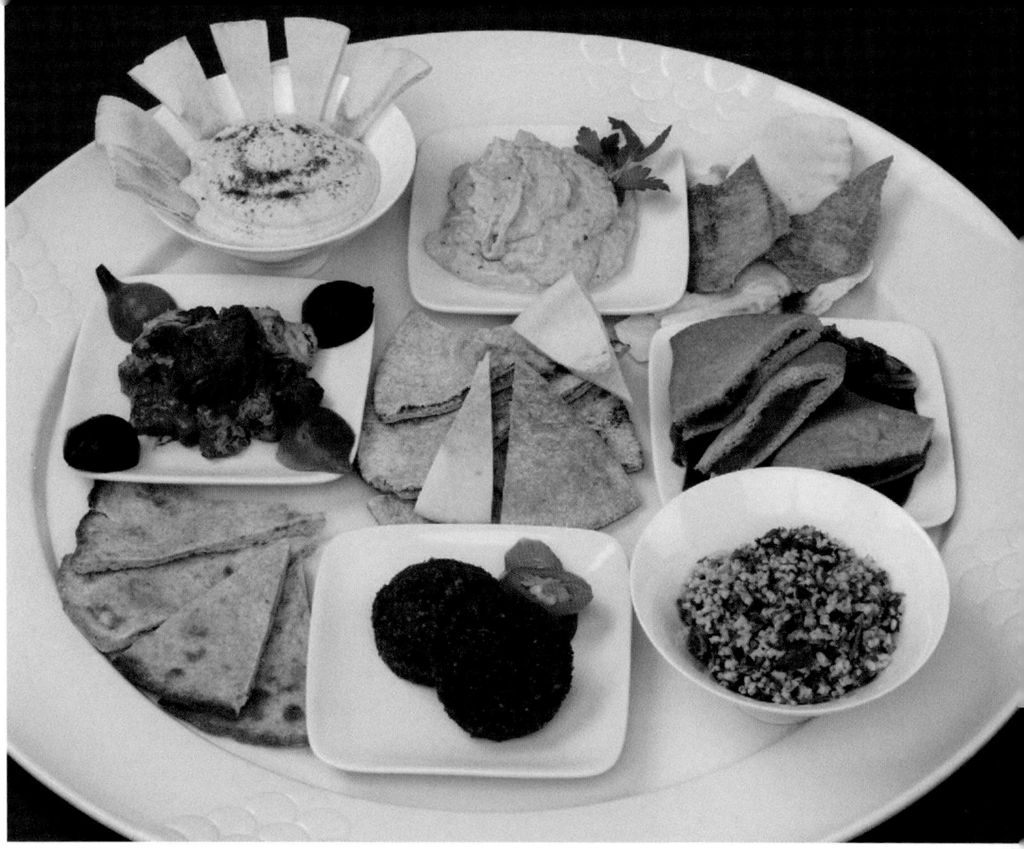

**Clockwise from the bottom: Falafel – Dried Bean Croquettes; Borani Chogondar—Beet and Yogurt Salad; Hummus Bi Tahini—Chickpea and Sesame Dip; Baba Ghannouj/ Moutabal—Eggplant Dip; Tabbouleh—Cracked Wheat and Herb Salad; assorted flat breads (Middle East)**

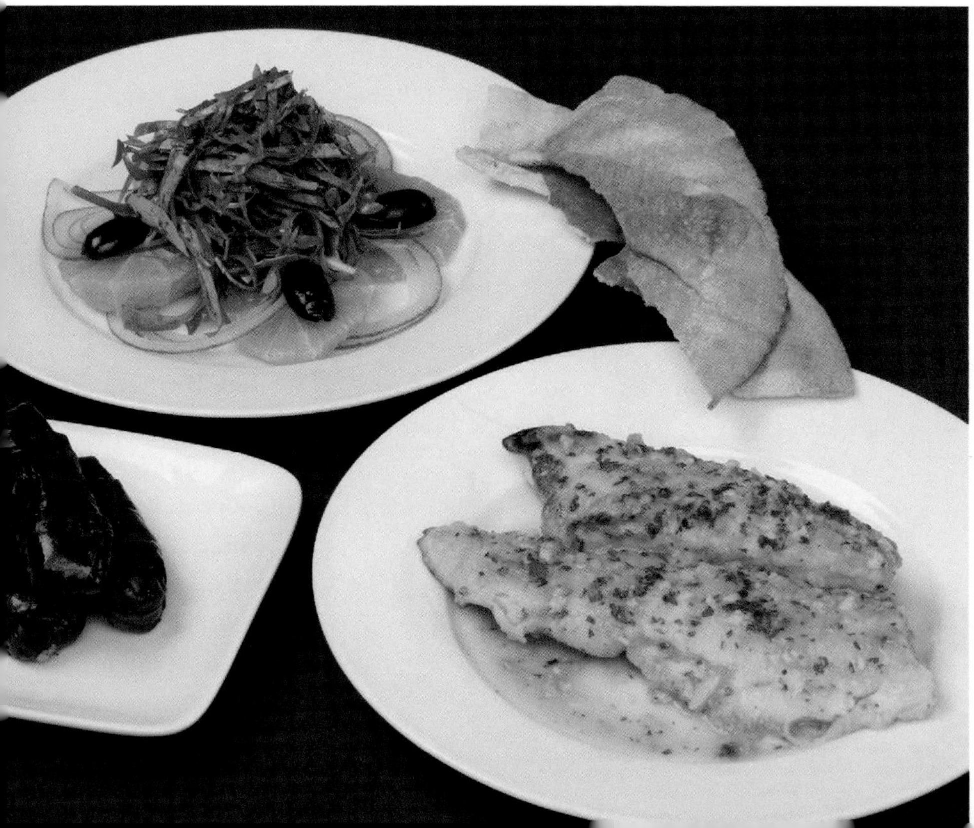

**Psari Savoro—Fried Fish with Rosemary and Vinegar; Dolmathakia Me Rizi—Stuffed Grape Vine Leaves; and Salata me Portokalia kai Elies—Orange and Olive Salad (Turkey, Greece, Crete)**

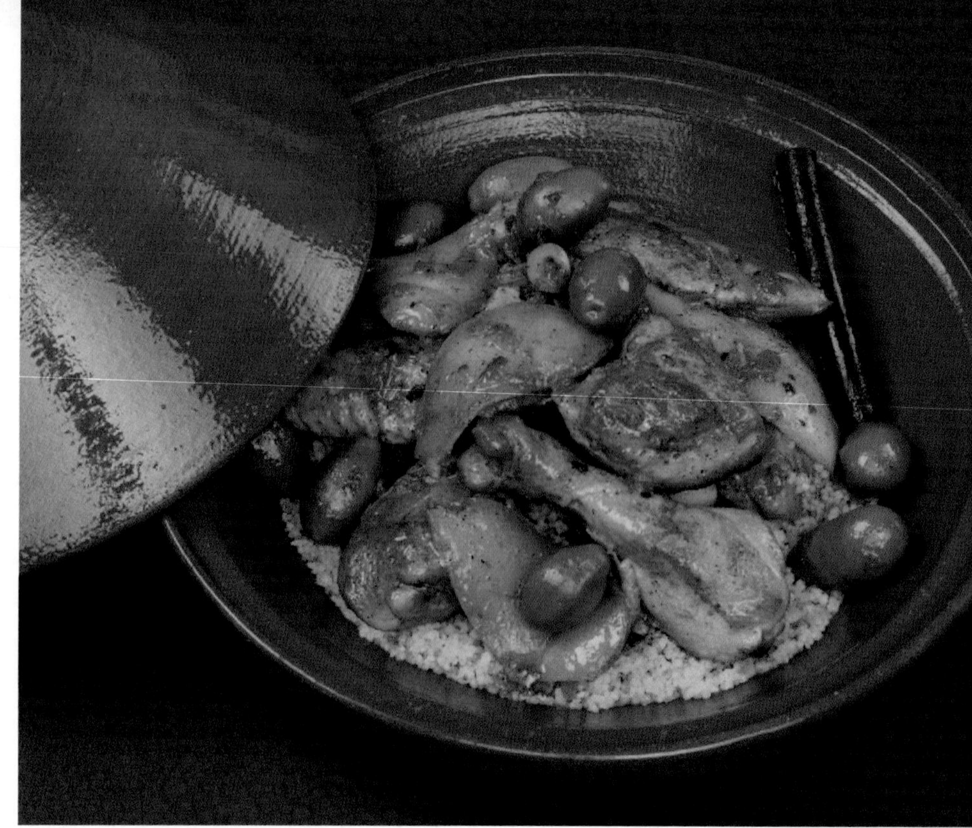

**Tagine of Chicken, Preserved Lemon and Olives (North Africa)**

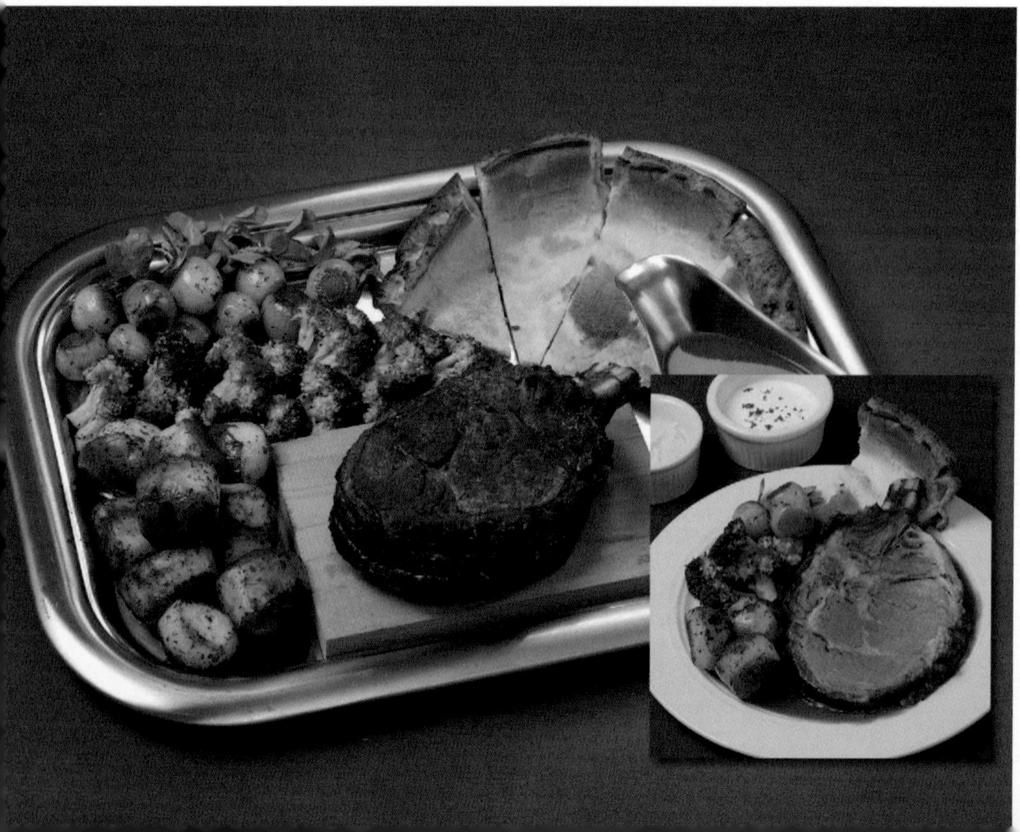

**Platter and plate, clockwise from bottom: Roast beef, roasted new potatoes, broccoli, glazed shallots, watercress, Yorkshire pudding, au jus (British Isles)**

Tomato Water Ice with Julienne of Smoked Salmon (British Isles)

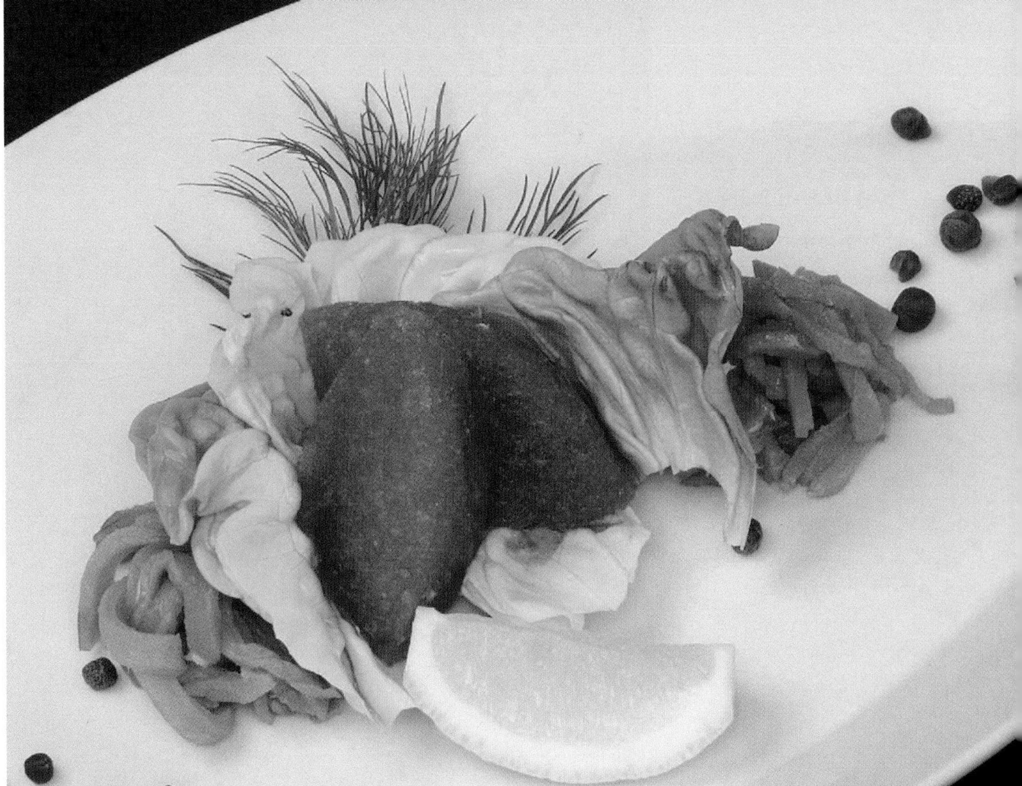

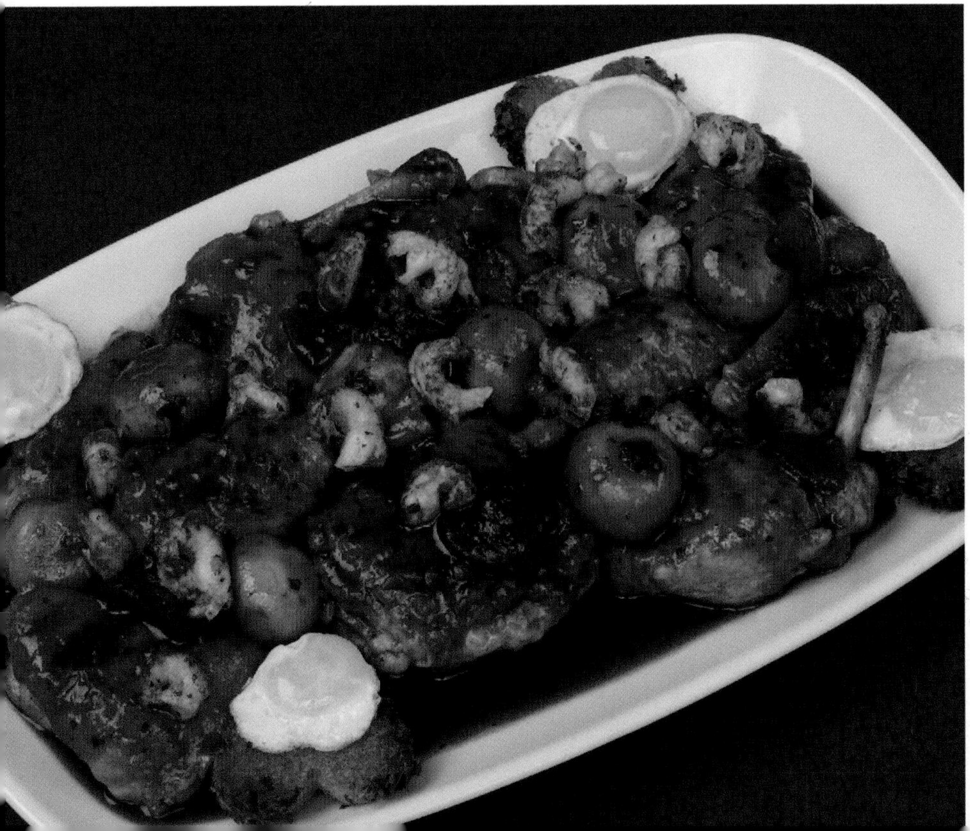

Poulet Sauté Marengo (France)

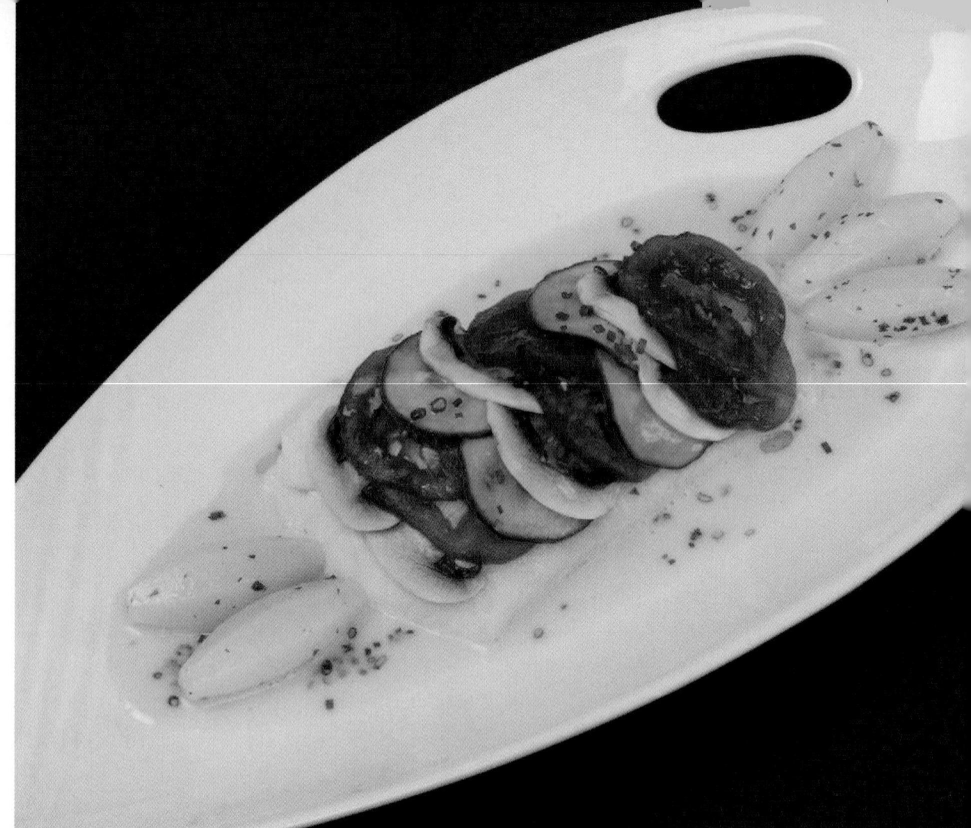

**Fillet of Fish Belle Mouginoise with Turned Potato (France)**

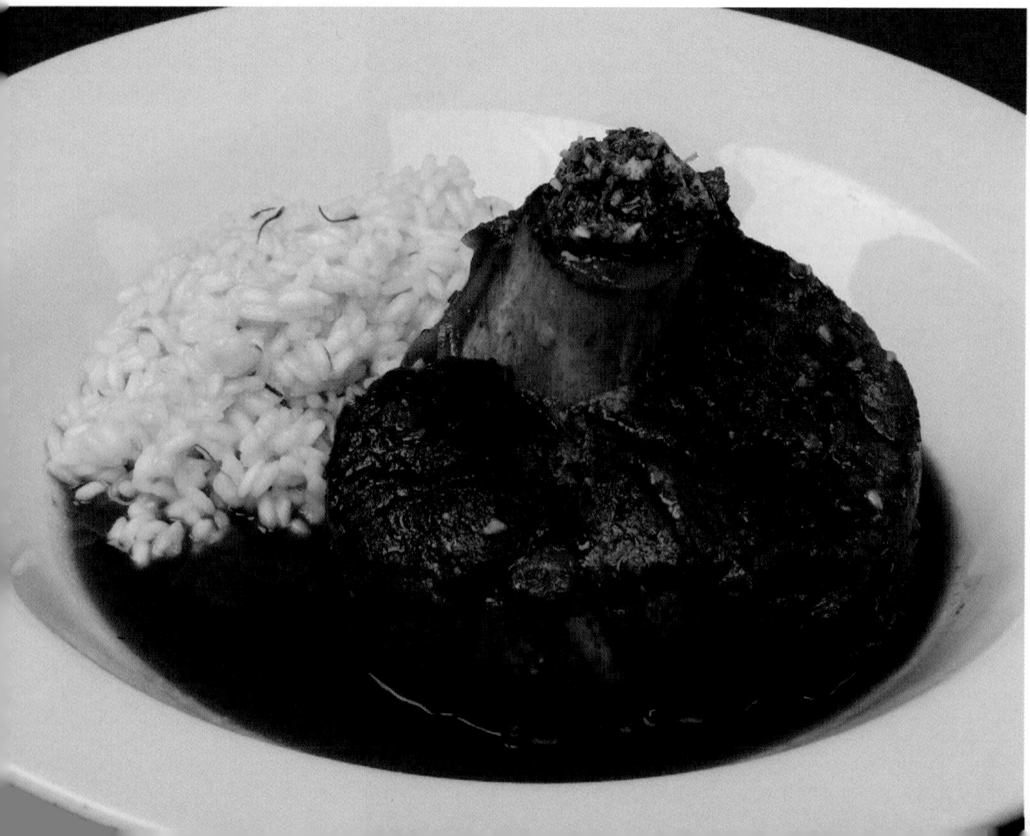

**Ossobuco Milanese and Risotto Alla Zafferano – Braised Veal Shanks and Risotto with Saffron (Italy)**

**Peperonata – Stewed Peppers (Italy)**

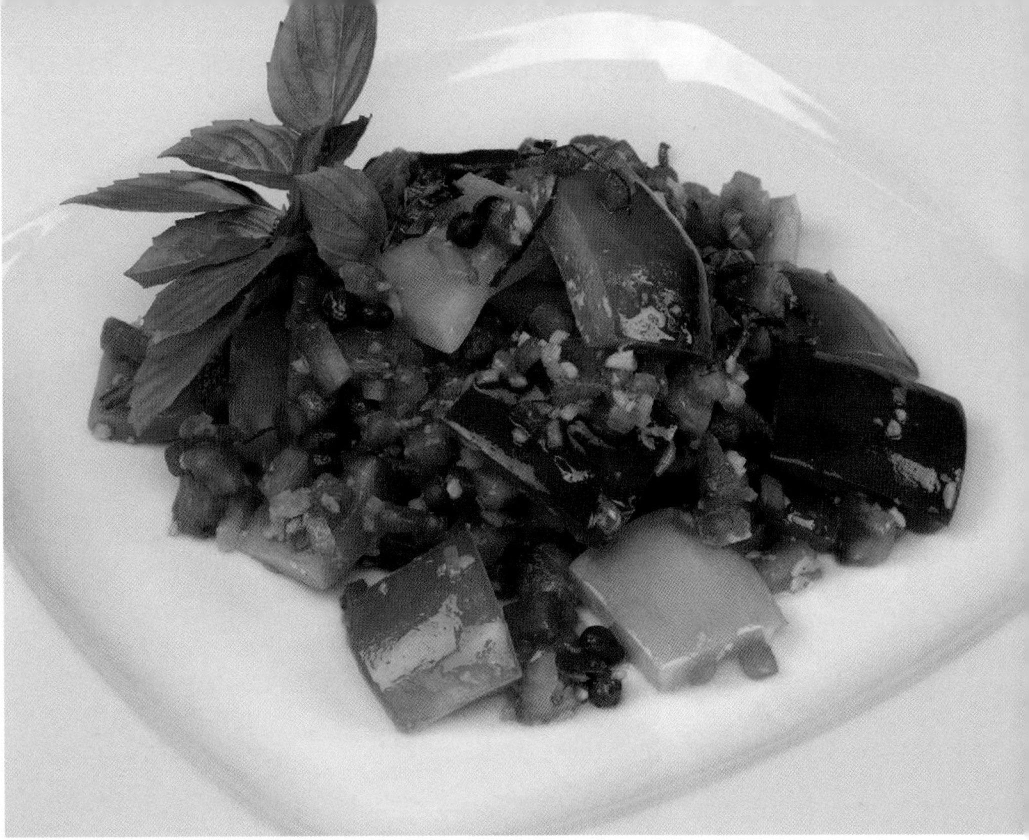

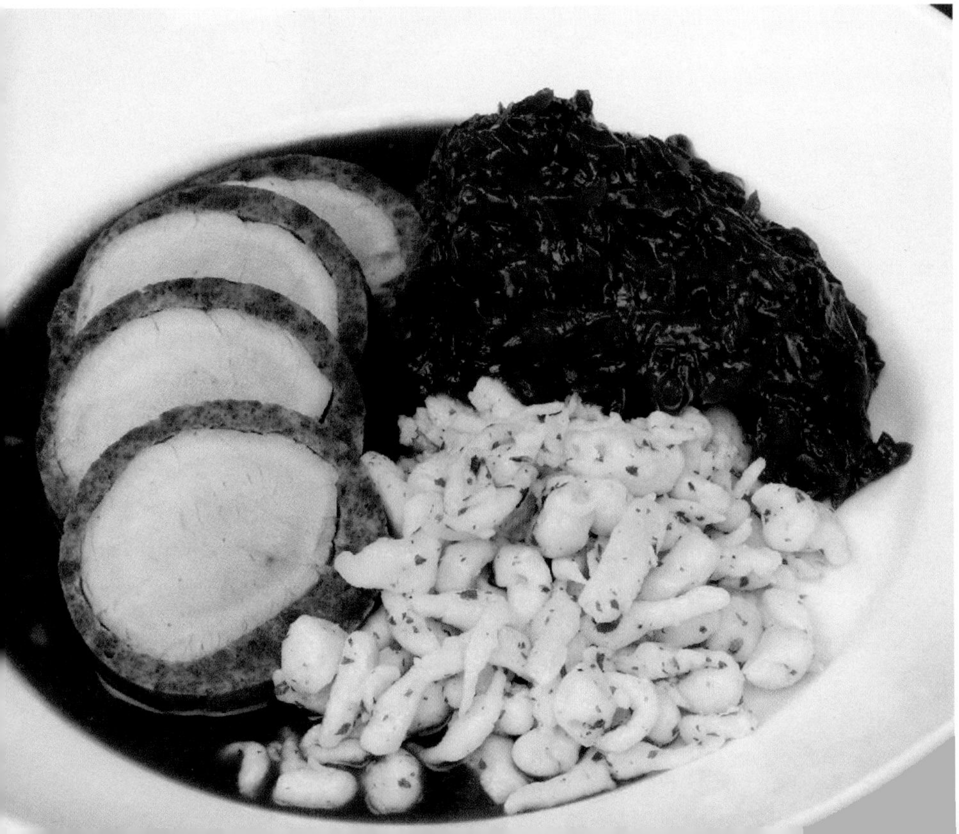

**Schweinelendchen im Schwarzbratmantel—Pork Tenderloin in a Dark Bread Crust; Rotkraut und Spätzle—Braised Red Cabbage and Spaetzle (Germany, Austria, Switzerland)**

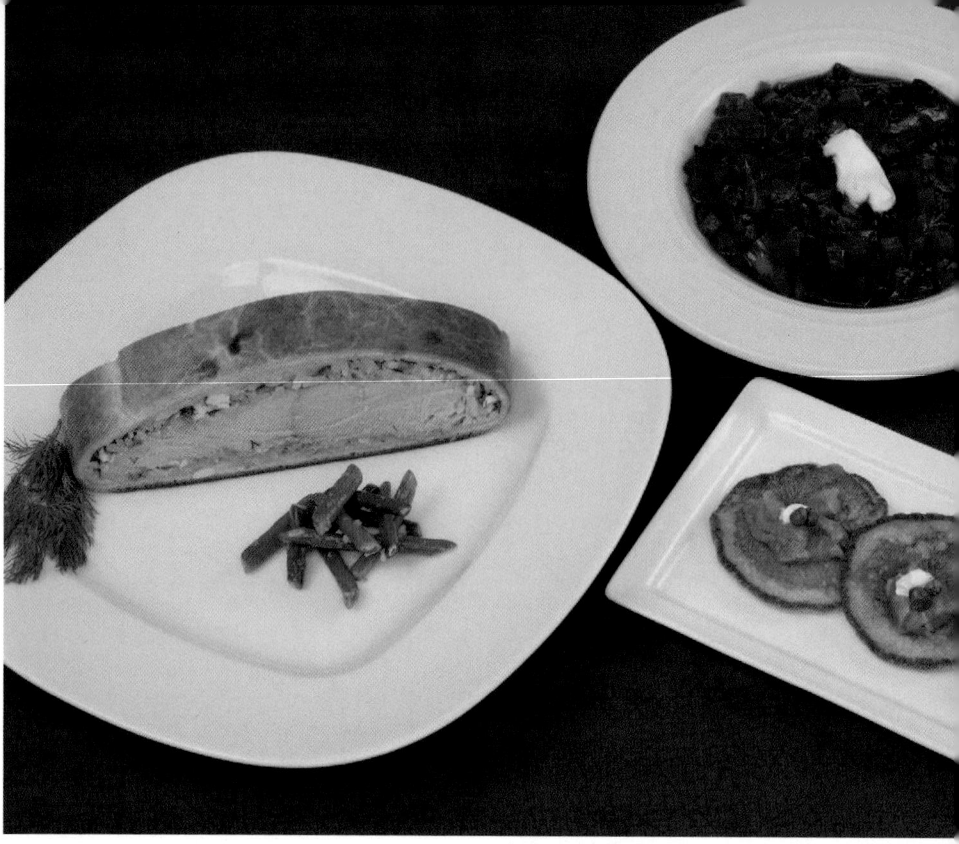

**Borshch Moskovsky—Moscow-Style Beet Soup; Blini—Buckwheat Pancakes; Kulebiaka—Salmon in Pastry (Scandinavia and Russia)**

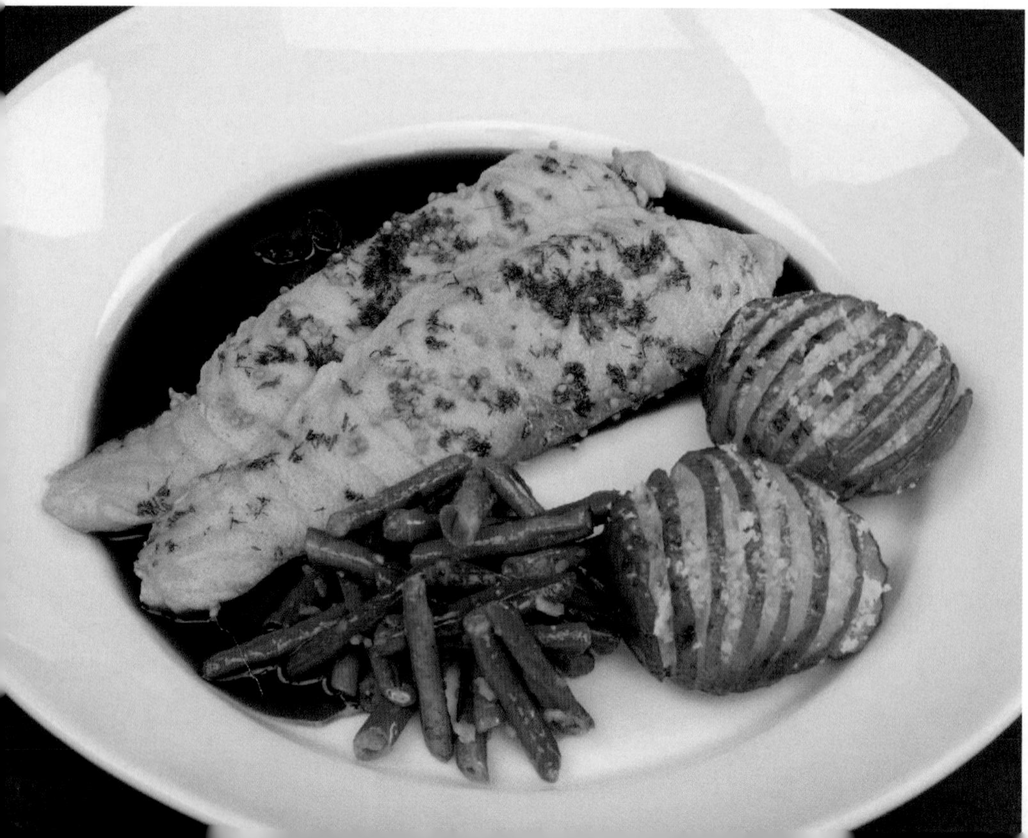

**Fried Dill-Cured Salmon with Sweet Sour Raisin Sauce, Hasselback Potatoes and Green Beans (Scandinavia and Russia)**

to pack the curds into a ball. Squeeze out as much liquid as possible by twisting the cheesecloth. Tie the corners and hang the cheese over a container to drain 2 to 3 hours.

3 When most of the liquid has drained, place the cheese on an upside-down plate. Put another plate or a sheet pan on top and 6 to 8 pounds of additional weight to squeeze the cheese further. Leave for an additional hour before unwrapping and using.

4 Unwrap and cut into 2-inch × $\frac{1}{2}$-inch × $\frac{1}{4}$-inch (2.4 cm × 1.2 cm × .6 cm) pieces.

5 Preheat the broiler. Brush about $\frac{1}{2}$ tablespoon (8 ml) ghee on paneer. Place on a lightly greased pan 4 to 6 inches (9.6 cm x 14.4 cm) from the heat source and broil until speckled with light brown spots, 2 to $2\frac{1}{2}$ minutes; watch closely, as it burns quickly. Brown both sides.

**Spinach**

1 Blanch the spinach in boiling salted water until wilted, 3 to 4 minutes. Immediately transfer to an ice water bath. Let cool completely; squeeze the spinach gently. Puree in blender or food processor, with $\frac{1}{2}$ cup (4 ounces, 120 ml) water or more if necessary. Process until smooth and velvety.

2 Heat the ghee and add the cumin seeds; let them splutter.

3 Add the onions and green chile; sauté until light brown, 3 to 5 minutes.

4 Add ginger and garlic, cook 2 minutes.

5 Add spinach and cook 2 to 3 minutes. Adjust consistency with additional water.

6 Add the browned paneer and cream; cook covered on low heat 3 minutes.

7 Adjust seasoning with salt, black pepper, and lemon juice.

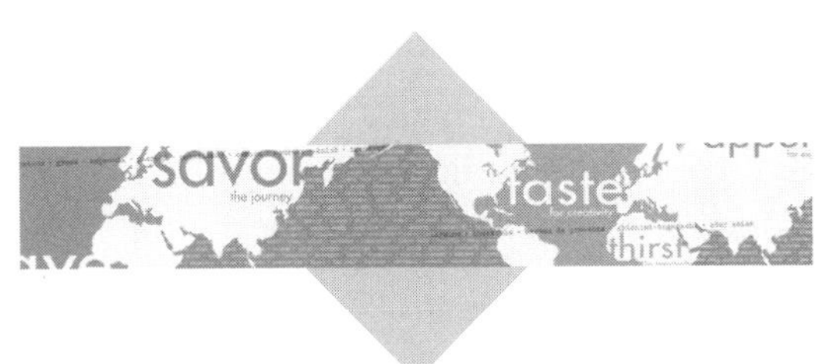

# Rajmah Red Kidney Bean Dal SERVES 4

| AMOUNT | MEASURE | INGREDIENT |
|---|---|---|
| $1\frac{1}{4}$ cups | 8 ounces, 224 g | Red kidney beans, picked over, washed, and drained |
| 6 cups | 48 ounces, 1.4l | Water |
| 3 | | Ginger slices, $\frac{1}{4}$ inch (.6 cm) thick |
| 1 tablespoon | | Salt |
| 3 tablespoons | $1\frac{1}{2}$ ounces, 45 ml | Fresh lemon juice |
| $\frac{1}{4}$ teaspoon | | Garam masala (p. 567) |
| $\frac{2}{3}$ cup | 5 ounces, 150 ml | Heavy cream |
| 3 tablespoons | $1\frac{1}{2}$ ounces, 45 ml | Ghee or vegetable oil |
| 1 teaspoon | | Cumin seeds |
| $\frac{1}{2}$ teaspoon | | Coriander seeds |
| 1 teaspoon | | Ginger, peeled, finely minced |
| 1 teaspoon | | Garlic, minced |
| $\frac{1}{2}$ teaspoon | | Cloves, ground |
| 2 | | Dried hot red chiles, split in half |

**PROCEDURE**

1. Bring beans and water to a boil, reduce to a simmer for 2 minutes. Turn off heat and let stand, uncovered, 1 hour.
2. Add 3 slices ginger and return to a boil; boil 10 minutes.
3. Reduce heat and simmer 1 hour with lid slightly ajar. Discard the ginger slices.
4. Mash half the beans or puree half in a blender. Add the salt, lemon juice, garam masala, and cream. Combine puree and whole beans, stir to mix, and adjust seasoning.
5. Heat ghee over medium heat. When hot, add cumin and coriander seeds; sauté two minutes. Add minced ginger and garlic; stir-fry until lightly browned. Add ground cloves and red chiles; stir once. Add spice mixture to beans.
6. Stir to mix.

# Mango Chutney

SERVES 4

| AMOUNT | MEASURE | INGREDIENT |
|---|---|---|
| $\frac{1}{4}$ | 2 ounces, 60 ml | Cider vinegar |
| 2 tablespoons | 1 ounce, 28 g | Granulated sugar |
| 2 tablespoons | 1 ounce, 28 g | Brown sugar |
| 1 | | Bay leaf, whole |
| 2 | | Whole cloves |
| $\frac{1}{8}$ teaspoon | | Cayenne pepper |
| $\frac{1}{8}$ teaspoon | | Turmeric |
| $\frac{1}{2}$ cup | 4 ounces, 120 ml | Water |
| 1 inch piece | 2.4 cm piece | Ginger, peeled, julienned |
| $\frac{1}{2}$ cup | 8 ounces, 224 g | Mango, peeled, cored, sliced |

**PROCEDURE**

1. In a nonreactive pan, bring vinegar, sugar, brown sugar, bay leaf, cloves, cayenne, turmeric, and water to a boil. Cook over medium heat until a light syrup forms, 8 to 10 minutes.
2. Add the ginger and cook another 5 minutes. Remove bay leaves and cloves.
3. Add the mango slices and cook, covered, over low heat until the fruit softens and absorbs the flavors, about 25 to 30 minutes.
4. If the chutney becomes too thick, add no more than 1 ounce of water at a time. The chutney should resemble preserves.

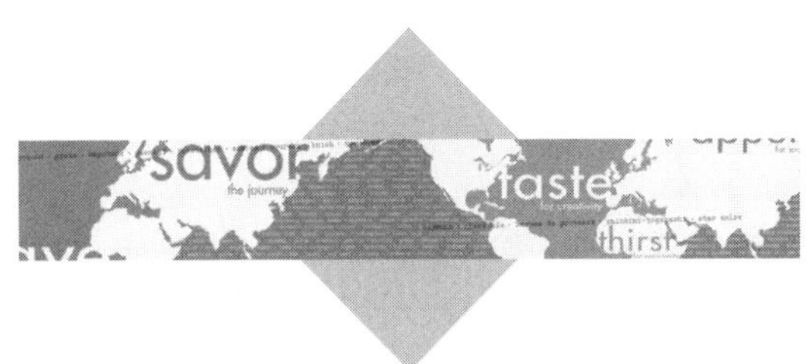

# Chapatis Flat Bread SERVES 4

| AMOUNT | MEASURE | INGREDIENT |
|---|---|---|
| $1\frac{1}{2}$ cups | 6 ounces, 168 g | Whole wheat flour |
| $\frac{1}{2}$ cup | 2 ounces, 56 g | All-purpose flour |
| 1 tablespoon | $\frac{1}{2}$ ounce, 15 ml | Oil |
| $\frac{1}{2}$ teaspoon | | Salt |
| $\frac{3}{4}$ cup plus 2 tablespoons | 7 ounces, 210 ml | Water |
| As needed | | Ghee |

**PROCEDURE**

1 In a mixer, food processor, or by hand, combine all ingredients except ghee to form a soft dough.

2 Knead the dough 6 to 8 minutes or until smooth. Cover and let rest 30 minutes.

3 Knead and divide into 10 equal parts. It will be somewhat sticky, so use flour to dust. Roll each into a ball on a floured surface. Press the ball into a patty. Roll patty out, dusting frequently, until it is about 3–4 inches (7.2 cm–9.6 cm) in diameter. Keep covered so they do not dry out.

4 Pick up to remove excess flour. Keep covered so they do not dry out.

5 Heat a tava, griddle, or skillet over medium-high heat. Cooking surface is hot enough when a little water sprinkled on bounces off the surface. Rub surface with a little oil.

6 Flatten a piece of dough with your palm, dust with flour, and roll the dough from the center outward into a circle 6–7 inches (14.4 cm–16.8 cm) across, $\frac{1}{16}$ inch (.15 cm) thick (don't be concerned if the finished shape is not perfect).

7 Pick up flatbread, slap it back and forth to shake off any excess flour, and gently slap it on to the pan. Make sure there are no creases, or use a spatula to spread it evenly. Cook until it starts to puff in places, then press the unpuffed portions very gently with the back of a spoon and guide the air to puff the whole chapatis. This process should take about 1 minute.

8 Drizzle 1 teaspoon ghee around the edges of the chapati. Use a spatula to turn over. The flatbread should start to balloon again; press gently and guide the air to parts that have not puffed so they fill with steam, about 30 seconds. Both sides should be lightly speckled brown.

9 Transfer cooked flatbreads to a cloth-lined basket and continue cooking the remaining pieces.

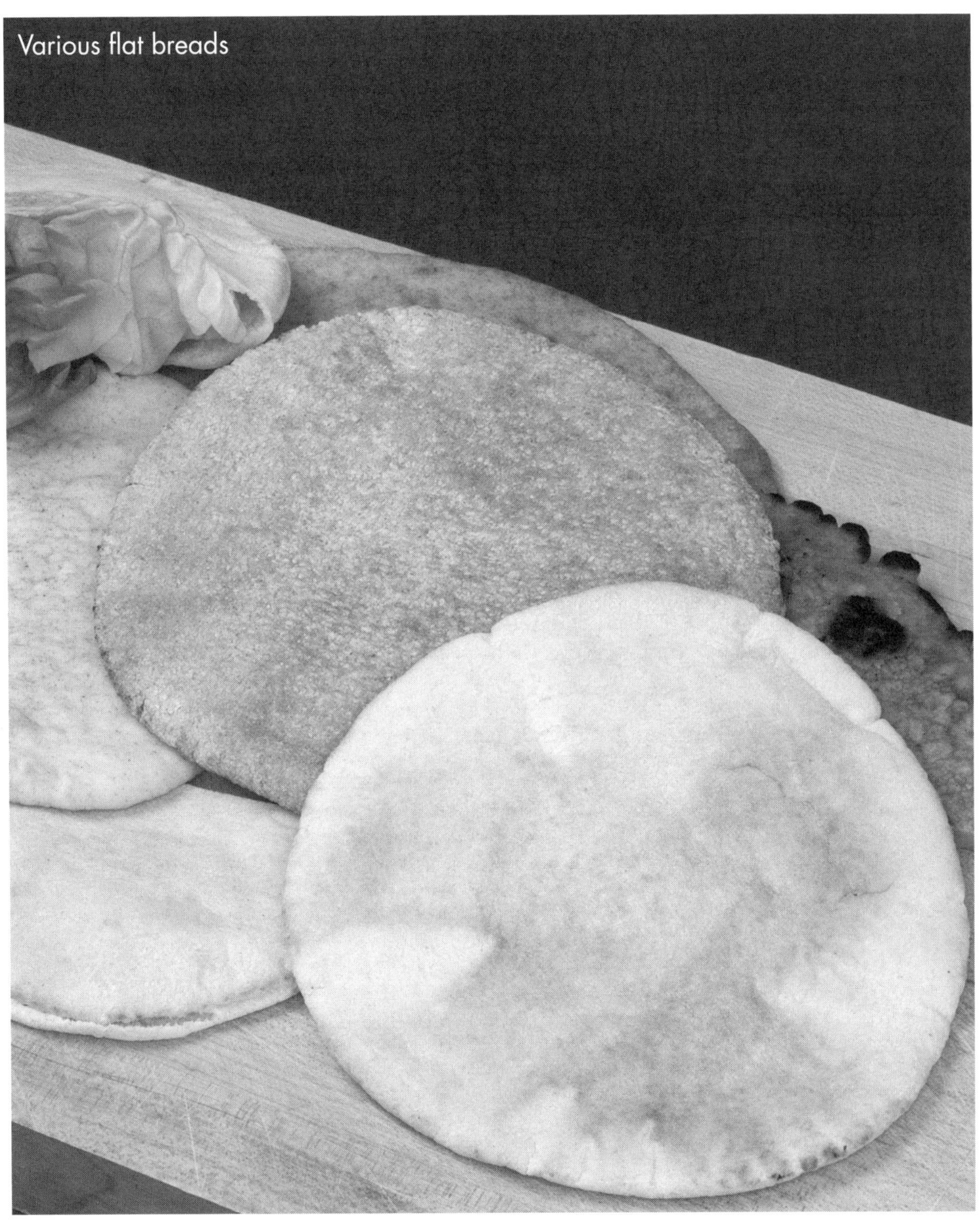

Various flat breads

# Khumbi Pullao Mushroom Rice

SERVES 4

| AMOUNT | MEASURE | INGREDIENT |
|---|---|---|
| 1 cup | 7 ounces, 196 g | Long-grain rice |
| 2 tablespoons | 1 ounce, 30 ml | Ghee or vegetable oil |
| $\frac{1}{2}$ cup | 2 ounces, 56 g | Onions, halved lengthwise, then finely sliced |
| 1 teaspoon | | Garlic, minced |
| 1 cup | 3 ounces, 84 g | Mushrooms, washed, cut $\frac{1}{8}$ inch (.3 cm) slices |
| $\frac{1}{4}$ teaspoon | | Ginger, minced |
| To taste | | Salt and garam masala (p. 567) |
| 2 cups | 16 ounces, 480 ml | Water |

PROCEDURE

1. Wash the rice in several changes of water and drain. Cover rice with cold water and let stand 30 minutes. Drain.
2. Heat ghee over medium heat; when hot, add onions and garlic and stir-fry 2 minutes or until onions are browning around the edges.
3. Add mushrooms and cook 2 minutes.
4. Add rice, ginger, salt, and garam masala; stir-fry two minutes.
5. Add water and bring to a boil. Cover tightly, turn heat to very low, and cook 25 minutes. Turn off heat and let sit, covered and undisturbed, 5 minutes.

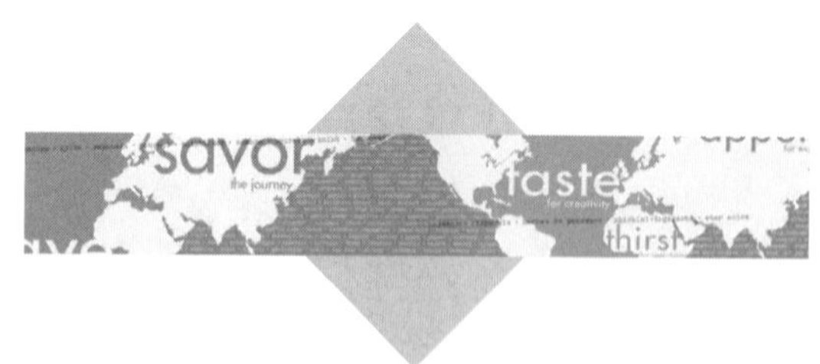

# Banana Erccherry

SERVES 4

| AMOUNT | MEASURE | INGREDIENT |
|---|---|---|
| 4 cups | 16 ounces, 114 g | Raw bananas, peeled, $1\frac{1}{2}$ inch (3.6 cm) pieces |
| $\frac{1}{2}$ cup | 4 ounces, 120 ml | Water |
| $\frac{1}{4}$ teaspoon | | Turmeric powder |
| To taste | | Salt |
| 1 cup | 6 ounces, 168 g | Fresh coconut scrapings or unsweetened flakes |
| 1 | | Whole red chile |
| $\frac{1}{2}$ teaspoon | | Cumin seeds |
| $\frac{1}{2}$ teaspoon | | Mustard seeds |
| 2 | | Green chiles, sliced (remove seeds to reduce hotness) |
| 4 | | Curry leaves |
| 1 tablespoon | $\frac{1}{2}$ ounce, 15 ml | Coconut oil |

**PROCEDURE**

1. Combine banana pieces, water, turmeric, and salt, cook until soft; mash.
2. Make a paste with $\frac{1}{2}$ the coconut, red chile and cumin seeds. Add to mashed bananas and set aside.
3. Heat coconut oil and add mustard seeds, green chiles, curry leaves, and remaining coconut and fry till golden. Mix in the banana mash and serve hot.

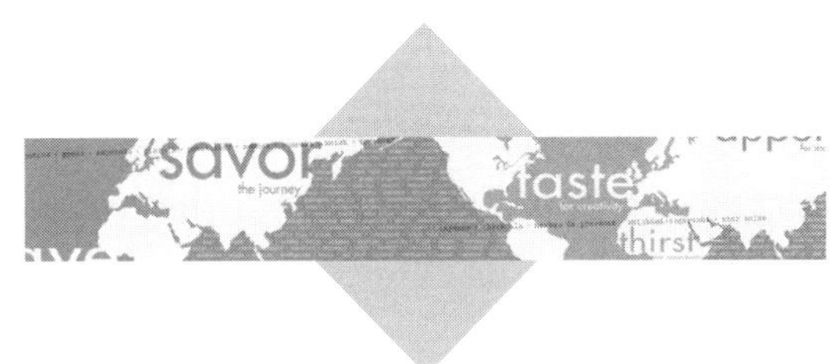

# Dosal Fermented Lentil Crepes with Potato Masala Stuffing SERVES 4

| AMOUNT | MEASURE | INGREDIENT |
|---|---|---|
| **Batter** | | |
| $\frac{3}{4}$ cup | 6 ounces, 168 g | Urad dal (black lentils) |
| $2\frac{1}{2}$ cups | $17\frac{1}{2}$ ounces, 490 g | Raw rice |
| 1 teaspoon | 5 gram | Fenugreek |
| **Masala Filling** | | |
| 2 tablespoons | 1 ounce, 30 ml | Ghee or vegetable oil |
| 1 teaspoon | 5 gram | Mustard seeds |
| 1 cup | 4 ounces, 112 g | Onion, $\frac{1}{4}$ inch (.6 cm) dice |
| 1 | | Green chile (jalapeño), seeded, minced |
| 4 | | Curry leaves |
| $\frac{1}{2}$ teaspoon | | Turmeric |
| 2 cups | 12 ounces, 336 g | Russet potatoes, cooked in their skins, peeled, and mashed lightly (chunky) |
| 1 tablespoon | $\frac{1}{2}$ ounce, 15 ml | Fresh lime juice |
| To taste | | Salt and white pepper |
| 2 tablespoons | | Cilantro, coarsely chopped |
| As needed | | Tamarind sauce (recipe follows) |

### PROCEDURE

**Batter**

1. Combine the dal and rice and soak 6 hours.
2. Drain and grind to a paste. Keep the liquid.
3. Let the paste ferment 4 hours.
4. Thin the paste to a crepe-batter consistency, using the retained soaking liquid.
5. Cook like a crepe and fill with masala filling.

**Masala Filling**

1 Heat ghee over medium heat, add mustard seeds, and sauté 30 seconds. Add the onion, jalapeño, curry leaves, and turmeric. Sauté until onions are transparent, 3 to 5 minutes.

2 Fold in the potatoes, heat the mixture through, and adjust seasoning with lime juice, salt, and white pepper. Finish by folding in the cilantro. Serve with tamarind sauce.

# Tamarind Sauce

**Frequently used in Indian cuisine, dark brown, crumbly palm sugar—also known as jaggery or *gur*—is made from the reduced sap of either the sugar palm or the palmyra palm. Substitute brown sugar only as a last resort.**

SERVES 4

| AMOUNT | MEASURE | INGREDIENT |
|---|---|---|
| 7 tablespoons | $3\frac{1}{2}$ ounces, 105 g | Tamarind paste |
| 10 tablespoons | 5 ounces, 150 g | Palm sugar |
| 2 cup | 16 ounces, 480 ml | Water |
| To taste | | Cayenne pepper |
| To taste | | Salt |

PROCEDURE

1 Combine tamarind, sugar, and water; bring to a boil, reduce to a simmer, and cook to a jamlike consistency.

2 Add salt and cayenne to taste.

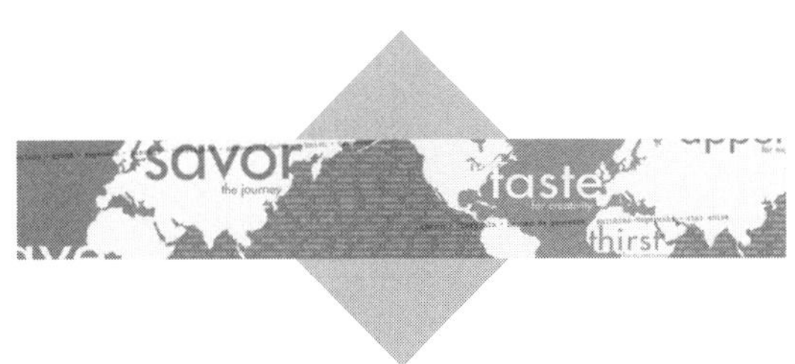

# Jhinga Kari Shrimp Curry SERVES 4

| AMOUNT | MEASURE | INGREDIENT |
|---|---|---|
| $\frac{1}{4}$ cup | 2 ounces, 60 ml | Ghee |
| 1 cup | 4 ounces, 112 g | Onions, cut in half lengthwise, then finely sliced |
| 2 | | Garlic cloves, minced |
| 1 teaspoon | | Ginger, minced |
| 2 teaspoons | | Coriander, ground |
| 1 teaspoon | | Turmeric |
| $\frac{1}{2}$ teaspoon | | Chile powder |
| $\frac{1}{2}$ teaspoon | | Cumin ground |
| 2 tablespoons | 1 ounce, 30 ml | White vinegar |
| 1 pound | 448 g | Shrimp (16 to 20 count), shelled and deveined |
| $\frac{3}{4}$ cup | 6 ounces, 180 ml | Water |

**PROCEDURE**

1. Heat ghee over medium heat and add the onions and garlic. Cook until soft and slightly brown, 10 to 12 minutes. Add ginger and cook 1 minute.
2. Make a paste out of the dry ingredients and vinegar.
3. Add paste to cooked onions and stir fry for 3 minutes, stirring constantly.
4. Add shrimp and toss to coat. Add water and cook until just cooked, 2 to 3 minutes.
5. Serve hot.

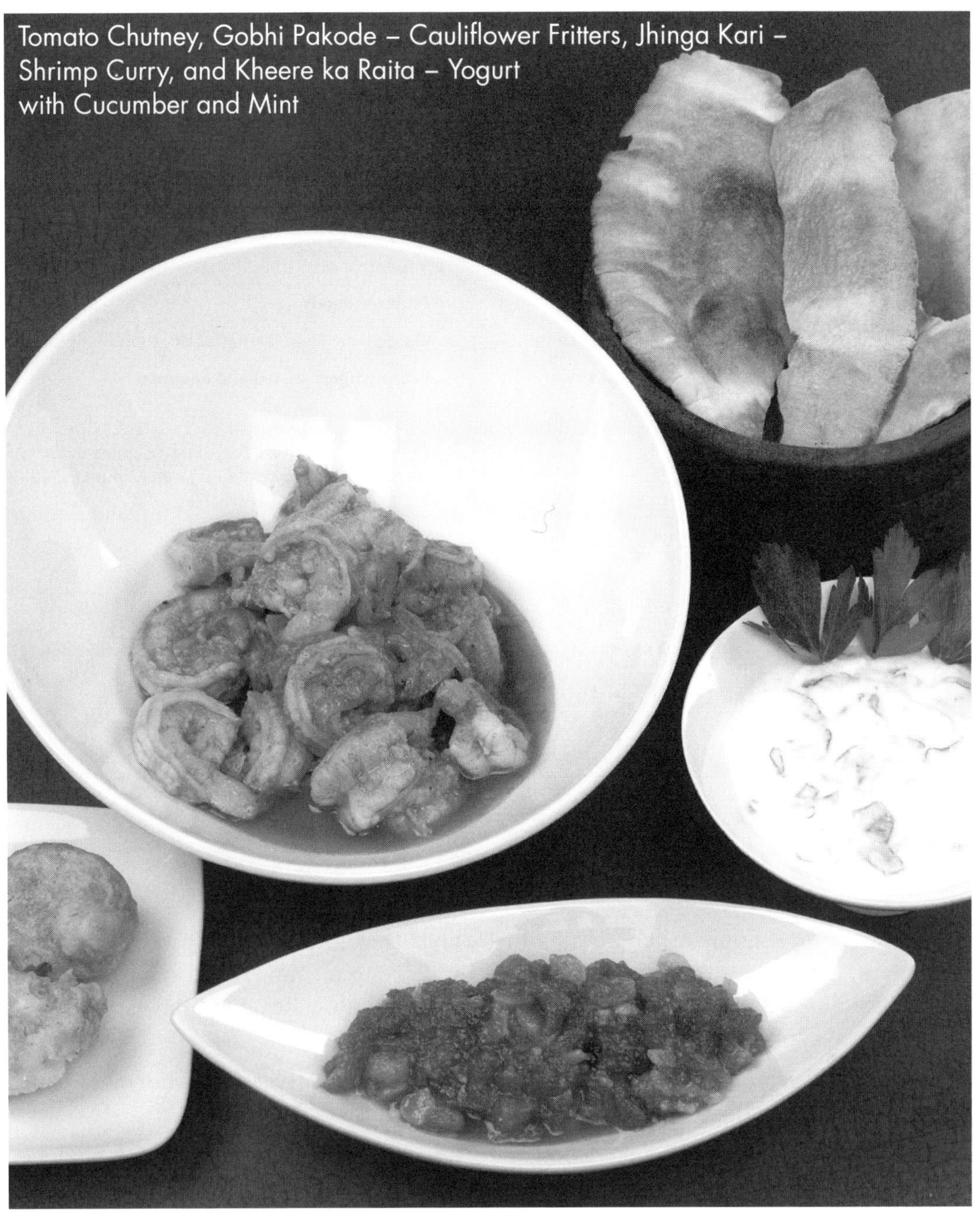

Tomato Chutney, Gobhi Pakode – Cauliflower Fritters, Jhinga Kari – Shrimp Curry, and Kheere ka Raita – Yogurt with Cucumber and Mint

# Eratchi Ularthiyathu

## Kerala-Style Lamb SERVES 4

| AMOUNT | MEASURE | INGREDIENT |
|---|---|---|
| 1 pound | 448 g | Boneless lamb shoulder, $\frac{1}{2}$ inch (1.2 cm) cubes |
| 3 tablespoons | $1\frac{1}{2}$ ounces, 45 ml | Vegetable oil |
| 1 teaspoon | | Mustard seeds |
| 2 cups | 8 ounces, 224 g | Onions, cut in half lengthwise, then finely sliced |
| 1 | 1 inch (2.4 cm) | Fresh ginger, peeled and chopped |
| 4 | | Garlic cloves |
| 3 | | Dried hot red chiles (cayenne or chiles de arbol), stemmed and softened in $\frac{1}{4}$ cup (2 ounces, 60 ml) water |
| 20 | | Curry leaves |
| 1 tablespoon | | Coriander, ground |
| $\frac{1}{4}$ teaspoon | | Black pepper, freshly ground |
| 2 cups | 12 ounces, 336 g | Tomato, peeled, seeded, chopped, with juice |
| 2 tablespoons | | Unsweetened flaked dried coconut |
| 1 teaspoon | | Fennel, ground |
| 1 teaspoon | | Salt |
| $\frac{1}{2}$ cup | 4 ounces, 120 ml | Water |

### PROCEDURE

1. Rinse the lamb pieces, combine with $1\frac{1}{2}$ cups (12 ounces, 360 ml) water over medium heat, and bring to a boil. Cover partially, reduce to a simmer, and cook until it is just becoming tender but is still chewy, 15 to 20 minutes. Remove from heat. Drain and discard cooking liquid.
2. Heat oil over medium heat; sputter mustard seeds and curry leaves in hot oil. Add onions and cook, stirring, until richly browned, 10 minutes.
3. Make a paste with the ginger and garlic, use a little water if necessary. Can be done in a blender or mortar and pestle.
4. Add paste to browned onions and cook until it begins to brown, 3 to 4 minutes.
5. Puree chiles and soaking water in blender. Add chile puree to onion mixture, add curry leaves, and cook 30 seconds or until fragrant.

6 Add coriander and black pepper and stir for 20 seconds. Add tomatoes with juice and cook, stirring, until very soft and the mixture starts to dry out, 7 to 9 minutes.

7 Add drained lamb cubes, coconut and stir until the meat is well coated with the masala.

8 Add fennel, salt, and water; bring to a boil and reduce to a simmer. Cook, stirring occasionally, until all the liquid is absorbed and lamb is tender, 25 to 35 minutes, adding additional water if necessary.

9 Serve hot.

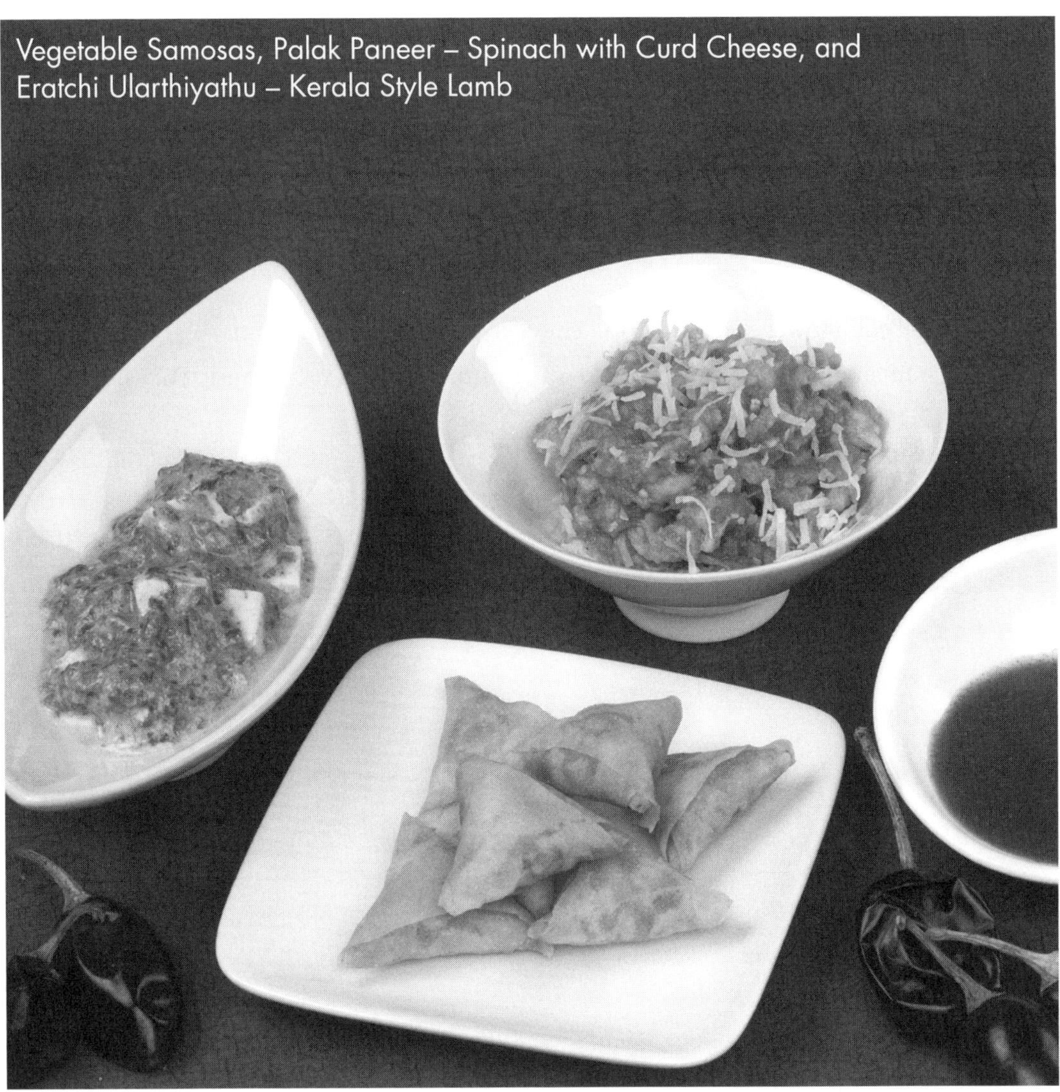

Vegetable Samosas, Palak Paneer – Spinach with Curd Cheese, and Eratchi Ularthiyathu – Kerala Style Lamb

# Gobhi Pakode Cauliflower Fritters

SERVES 4

| AMOUNT | MEASURE | INGREDIENT |
|---|---|---|
| 3 cups | 12 ounces, 336 g | Cauliflower florets |
| 1 cup | 7 ounces, 196 g | Besan (chickpea flour) |
| 1 tablespoon | | Coriander, ground |
| 1 teaspoon | | Turmeric |
| $\frac{1}{4}$ teaspoon | | Black pepper, freshly ground |
| $\frac{1}{8}$ teaspoon | | Cayenne pepper |
| 1 teaspoon | | Salt |
| 1 tablespoon | $\frac{1}{2}$ ounce, 15 ml | Vegetable oil |
| $\frac{3}{4}$ cup | 6 ounces, 180 ml | Cold water |
| As needed | | Oil for frying |

**PROCEDURE**

1. Parboil cauliflower, keeping firm. Transfer to ice water and drain.
2. Mix remaining dry ingredients; add water until a smooth nape consistency (coats the back of a spoon) is formed.
3. Let batter stand 30 minutes.
4. Heat frying oil to 375°F (190°C)
5. Coat cauliflower florets in batter; fry until golden brown. Drain on paper towels.
6. Serve hot or warm.

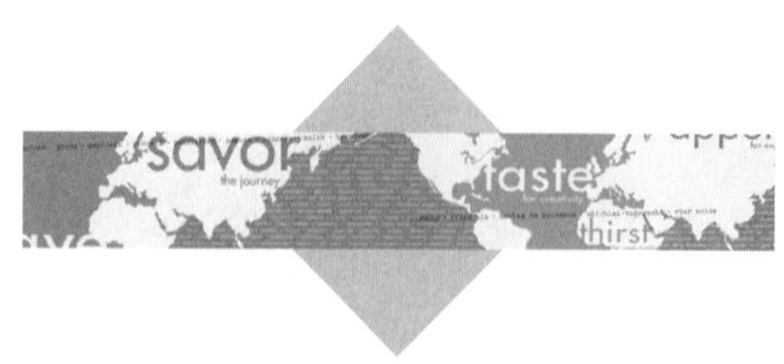

# Tomato Chutney

YIELD: 2 CUPS

| AMOUNT | MEASURE | INGREDIENT |
|---|---|---|
| 1 | 1 inch (2.4 cm) | Fresh ginger, peeled |
| 9 | | Garlic cloves |
| 1 teaspoon | | Caraway seeds |
| 1 cup | 8 ounces, 240 ml | Cider vinegar |
| 4 cups | 24 ounces, 672 g | Tomatoes, peeled, seeded, rough chopped |
| 3 | | Green chiles (serranos) seeded, chopped |
| $\frac{3}{4}$ cup | 5 ounces, 147 g | Granulated sugar |
| 1 tablespoon | | Golden raisins |
| 1 tablespoon | | Almonds, slivered, blanched |
| 1 | 2 inch, 4.8 cm | Cinnamon stick |
| 5 | | Whole peppercorns |
| $\frac{1}{4}$ teaspoon | | Cayenne pepper |
| 4 | | Whole cloves |

**PROCEDURE**

1. Grind ginger, garlic, and caraway with $\frac{1}{4}$ cup (2 ounces, 60 ml) vinegar to a paste.
2. Combine all ingredients and bring to a boil; reduce to a simmer. Cook until mixture thickens and turns dark, 1 to $1\frac{1}{2}$ hours.
3. Serve chilled or room temperature.

# Basmati Chaaval

## Plain Basmati Rice SERVES 4 TO 6

| AMOUNT | MEASURE | INGREDIENT |
|---|---|---|
| 2 cups | 15 ounces, 450 g | Long-grain rice |
| 1 teaspoon | | Salt |
| 1 tablespoon | $\frac{1}{2}$ ounce, 15 ml | Butter |
| $2\frac{2}{3}$ cups | 19 ounces, 570 ml | Water |

**PROCEDURE**

1. Wash rice in several changes of water. Drain.
2. Soak rice in 5 cups (40 ounces, 1.2 l) water 30 minutes. Drain thoroughly.
3. Combine rice, salt, butter, and water. Bring to boil. Cover with a tight-fitting lid, turn heat to low, and cook for 20 minutes.
4. Lift lid, mix gently but quickly with a fork, and cover again.
5. Cook additional 5 to 10 minutes or until rice is tender.

# Kheere ka Raita

## Yogurt with Cucumber and Mint SERVES 4

| AMOUNT | MEASURE | INGREDIENT |
|---|---|---|
| $1\frac{1}{2}$ cups | 12 ounces, 360 ml | Plain yogurt |
| $\frac{2}{3}$ cup | 4 ounces, 120 ml | Cucumber, peeled, coarsely grated |
| $1\frac{1}{2}$ tablespoon | | Fresh mint, chopped |
| $\frac{1}{2}$ teaspoon | | Cumin seeds, roasted and ground |
| $\frac{1}{4}$ teaspoon | | Cayenne pepper |
| To taste | | Salt and freshly ground black pepper |

**PROCEDURE**

1. Whisk yogurt until smooth and creamy.
2. Combine all ingredients and correct seasoning.

# Puris (Poori)

## Deep-Fried Puffed Bread

**YIELD: 12 POORI; SERVES 4**

| AMOUNT | MEASURE | INGREDIENT |
|---|---|---|
| 1 cup | 4 ounces, 112 g | Whole wheat flour, sifted |
| 1 cup | 4 ounces, 112 g | All-purpose flour |
| ½ teaspoon | | Salt |
| 2 tablespoons | 1 ounce, 30 ml | Vegetable oil |
| ½ cup | 4 ounces, 120 ml | Water |
| As needed | | Oil for frying |

**PROCEDURE**

1. Combine flours with salt.
2. Add vegetable oil and work with fingers until the mixture resembles coarse breadcrumbs.
3. Slowly add the water to form a stiff dough. Knead 10 to 12 minutes or until smooth. Rub with a little oil and set aside 30 minutes.
4. Work the dough again and divide into 12 equal pieces; round them into balls.
5. Keep them covered so they do not dry out.
6. Flatten and roll out into a 5-inch (12 cm) disk. Let disks set 5 minutes before frying.
7. Heat 1 inch frying oil to 350°F (176°C).
8. Place poori gently into the pan and use the back of a slotted spoon to push the poori gently into the oil with small swift strokes. Within seconds the poori will puff up.
9. Turn it over and cook an additional 30 seconds or until golden.
10. Remove with slotted spoon; drain on paper towels. Repeat until all are cooked.
11. Serve immediately.

# Chai Masala Spiced Tea SERVES 4

| AMOUNT | MEASURE | INGREDIENT |
|---|---|---|
| 1 cup | 8 ounces, 240 ml | Milk |
| 2 cups | 16 ounces, 480 ml | Water |
| 3 | | Cardamom pods |
| 2 | | Cloves |
| $\frac{1}{2}$ stick | | Cinnamon |
| $\frac{1}{4}$ teaspoon | | Fennel seed |
| To taste | | Granulated sugar |
| 4 | | Orange pekoe teabags |

PROCEDURE

1. Combine milk and water and bring to a boil. Stir in the spices and sugar to taste.
2. Turn off the heat, cover and let the spices steep 10 minutes.
3. Add the tea bags. Bring back to a boil, then turn off the heat and steep 3 minutes.
4. Strain and serve piping hot.

# Akhrote ka Raita Yogurt with Walnuts SERVES 4

| AMOUNT | MEASURE | INGREDIENT |
|---|---|---|
| $1\frac{1}{2}$ cups | 12 ounces, 360 ml | Yogurt |
| 2 tablespoons | | Fresh cilantro, chopped |
| 1 teaspoon | | Green chile, minced |
| 2 tablespoons | | Green onions, chopped fine |
| $\frac{1}{4}$ cup | 1 ounce, 28 g | Walnuts, chopped $\frac{1}{2}$ inch (1.2 cm) pieces |
| To taste | | Salt and pepper |

PROCEDURE

1. Whisk yogurt until smooth and creamy.
2. Fold in remaining ingredients and correct seasoning.

# Buttermilk Kadhi Soup

SERVES 4

| AMOUNT | MEASURE | INGREDIENT |
|---|---|---|
| 1 1-inch (2.4 cm) | | Fresh ginger, peeled |
| 3 | | Garlic cloves |
| 1 | | Green chile (serrano) stemmed |
| $\frac{1}{2}$ teaspoon | | Cumin seeds |
| $2\frac{1}{2}$ tablespoons | | Chickpea flour |
| 1 cup | 8 ounces, 240 ml | Water |
| 2 cups | 16 ounces, 480 ml | Buttermilk |
| 1 teaspoon | | Salt |
| 1 teaspoon | | Granulated sugar |
| 2 tablespoons | 1 ounce, 30 ml | Ghee |
| $\frac{1}{2}$ teaspoon | | Brown mustard seeds |
| 1 teaspoon | | Fenugreek seeds |
| 1 teaspoon | | Coriander seeds |
| $\frac{1}{2}$ teaspoon | | Turmeric |
| 15 | | Curry leaves or cilantro |
| Pinch | | Asafetida |

## PROCEDURE

1. Using a mortar and pestle or a food processor, pulverize the ginger, garlic, chile, and cumin seeds to a coarse-textured paste.
2. Combine the chickpea flour, half the water, the buttermilk, salt, sugar, and ginger-garlic paste. Bring to a low simmer, stirring to dissolve spices; cook uncovered 6 to 8 minutes. Correct seasoning with sugar and salt. Remove from heat.
3. Heat ghee over medium-high heat. Add mustard seeds, fenugreek seeds, and coriander seeds (if available). Cover with a spatter screen; cook until mustard seeds stop popping, about 30 seconds. Add turmeric, curry leaves, and asafetida; stir fry until leaves are crisp, 20 seconds.
4. Pour the seasoned oil over the soup. Serve hot.

# Sambhara Gujerati-Style Cabbage with Carrots, Eggplant, and Potato

SERVES 4

| AMOUNT | MEASURE | INGREDIENT |
|---|---|---|
| 4 tablespoons | 2 ounces, 60 ml | Ghee |
| 1 tablespoon | | Whole black mustard seeds |
| 1 | | Red hot chile, whole |
| 3 cups | 12 ounces, 336 g | Green cabbage, fine, long shreds |
| 1 cup | 4 ounces, 112 g | Carrots, peeled, coarsely grated |
| 1 | | Green chile (jalapeño), seeded, julienned |
| To taste | | Salt |
| To taste | | Granulated sugar |
| $\frac{1}{4}$ cup | | Cilantro leaves and some stems, chopped |
| 1 tablespoon | $\frac{1}{2}$ ounce, 15 ml | Fresh lemon juice |

PROCEDURE

1. Heat ghee; when hot, add mustard seeds; cook 5 seconds (seeds will start to pop). Add dried red chile and cook 10 seconds; chile should turn dark red.
2. Add cabbage, carrots, and green chile; toss to combine.
3. Reduce heat to medium and stir-fry 1 minute.
4. Add salt, sugar, and cilantro; stir and cook 5 minutes or until vegetables are just done but still crispy.
5. Add lemon juice and adjust seasoning. Remove red chile.

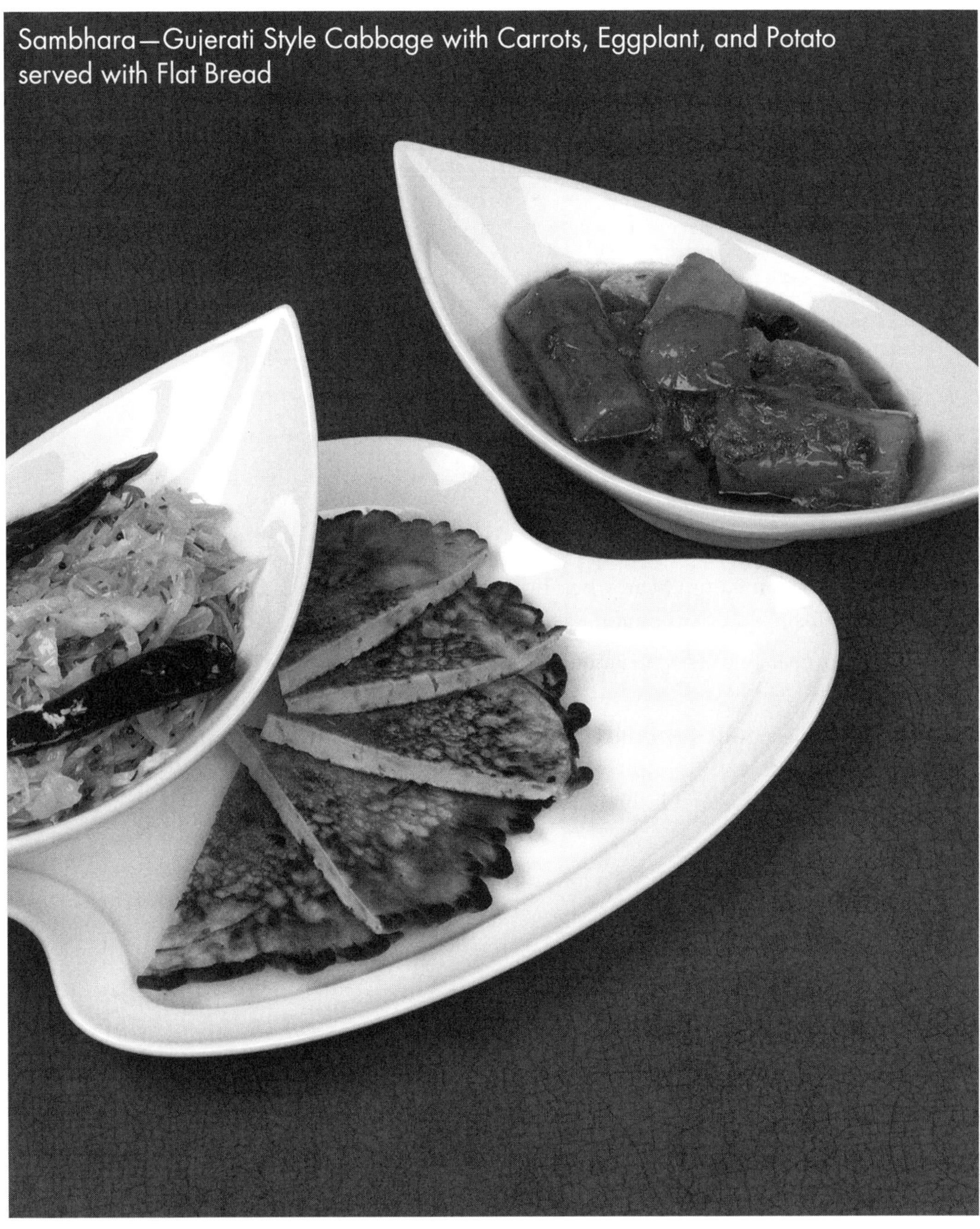

Sambhara—Gujerati Style Cabbage with Carrots, Eggplant, and Potato served with Flat Bread

# Eggplant and Potato

SERVES 4

| AMOUNT | MEASURE | INGREDIENT |
|---|---|---|
| $\frac{1}{4}$ cup | 2 ounces, 60 ml | Vegetable oil |
| $\frac{1}{2}$ teaspoon | | Black mustard seeds |
| 1 cup | 4 ounce, 112 g | Potatoes, cut $\frac{1}{2}$ inch (1.2 cm) dice |
| 1 cup | 4 ounces, 112 g | Eggplant, cut $\frac{1}{2}$ inch (1.2 cm) dice |
| $1\frac{1}{2}$ teaspoons | | Coriander seeds, ground |
| 1 teaspoon | | Cumin seeds, ground |
| $\frac{1}{4}$ teaspoon | | Turmeric |
| $\frac{1}{4}$ teaspoon | | Cayenne pepper |
| $\frac{1}{2}$ teaspoon | | Salt |

**PROCEDURE**

1 Heat oil over medium heat; when hot add mustard seeds, and as soon as they start to pop (5 seconds), add potatoes and eggplant.

2 Toss to coat and add coriander, cumin, turmeric, cayenne, and salt. Stir and sauté 2 minutes.

3 Add 3 tablespoons ($1\frac{1}{2}$ ounces, 45 ml) water, cover with tight-fitting lid, reduce heat to low, and simmer 10 minutes or until potatoes are tender. Stir occasionally. If vegetables stick to the pan, add a little more water.

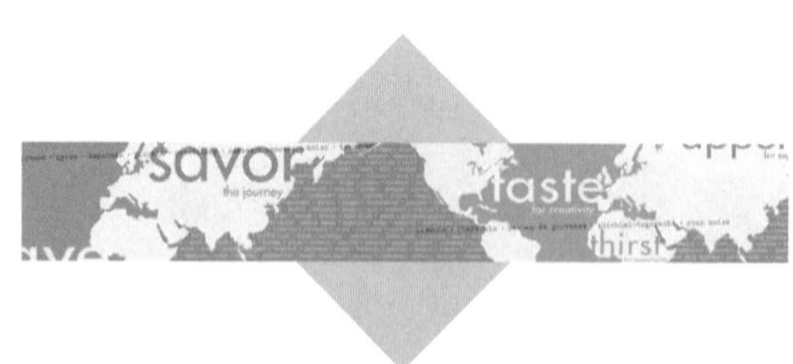

# Matira Curry

SERVES 4

| AMOUNT | MEASURE | INGREDIENT |
|---|---|---|
| 1 cup | 8 ounces, 240 ml | Watermelon juice; use cutting scrapes for puree |
| 1 teaspoon | | Chile powder |
| 1 teaspoon | | Turmeric |
| $\frac{1}{2}$ teaspoon | | Coriander seed, toasted |
| 2 | | Garlic cloves, minced |
| To taste | | Salt |
| $\frac{1}{4}$ teaspoon | | Cumin seeds, toasted |
| 1–2 tablespoons | $\frac{1}{2}$ to 1 ounce, (15 to 30 ml) | Fresh lime juice |
| To taste | | Granulated sugar |
| 4 cups | 16 ounces, 448 g | Watermelon, peeled, 1 $\frac{1}{2}$ inch (3.6 cm) cubes |
| 1 tablespoon | | Cilantro leaves, chopped |
| 1 tablespoon | | Mint, chopped |

**PROCEDURE**

1. Combine the juice, chile, turmeric, coriander, and garlic with a pinch of salt. Add toasted cumin seeds, bring to a boil, and reduce by $\frac{1}{3}$.
2. Season with lime juice and sugar to taste and continue to reduce to syrup consistency.
3. Add the melon cubes and cook over low heat until melon is heated throughout. Toss gently to coat all melon cubes with syrup.
4. Adjust the seasoning with salt, sugar, and lime juice. The final result should be tart.
5. Serve hot, garnished with cilantro and mint leaves.

# Pomfret Caldeen

## Fish in Coconut Sauce

SERVES 4

| AMOUNT | MEASURE | INGREDIENT |
| --- | --- | --- |
| 2 tablespoons | 1 ounce, 30 ml | Fresh lime juice |
| 1 teaspoon | | Salt |
| 1 teaspoon | | Turmeric |
| 4 | 5 ounces, 140 g portions | Skinless and boneless pompano fillets, or red snapper, grouper, bass, or cod |
| 3 | | Hot red chiles, stemmed and softened in $\frac{1}{4}$ cup water |
| 2 teaspoons | | Coriander seeds, toasted |
| 1 teaspoon | | Cumin seeds, toasted |
| $\frac{1}{2}$ cup | 3 ounces, 84 g | Coconut, freshly grated or unsweetened flakes |
| $1\frac{1}{2}$ cups | 6 ounces, 170 g | Onions, cut in half lengthwise, then finely sliced |
| 2 | | Garlic cloves |
| 1 teaspoon | | Tamarind concentrate, dissolved in $\frac{1}{4}$ cup (2 ounces, 60 ml) water |
| 1 cup | 8 ounces, 240 ml | Water |
| 2 tablespoons | 1 ounce, 30 ml | Vegetable oil |
| 1 cup | 6 ounces, 170 g | Tomato, peeled, seeded, $\frac{1}{4}$ inch (.6 cm) dice |

PROCEDURE

1. Combine lime juice, salt, and turmeric to make a marinade. Spread on fillets and let stand 30 minutes at cool room temperature or 1 hour under refrigeration.
2. Puree red chile, coriander seeds, cumin seeds, coconut, 1 cup onions, garlic, tamarind liquid and $\frac{1}{2}$ cup (4 ounces, 120 ml) water. Process until very smooth, adding more water if necessary.
3. Heat oil over medium-high heat; add remaining onions and cook, stirring, until deep golden brown, 6 to 8 minutes.
4. Add puree mix and continue to cook an additional 8 to 10 minutes.
5. Add tomato and remaining water; cook 8 minutes, stirring occasionally, until tomatoes are soft.
6. Correct seasoning and add the fish fillets. Simmer, turning once or twice if necessary, until the fish is just cooked.
7. Transfer fish to serving dish and correct consistency of sauce reducing or adding additional water. Correct seasoning and spoon sauce over fillets.

# Chana Dal Yellow Dal SERVES 4

**Chana dal is perhaps the "meatiest" tasting, with the slight sweetness of all the dals. Yellow split peas may be substituted; however, they are not the same.**

| AMOUNT | MEASURE | INGREDIENT |
|---|---|---|
| 1 $\frac{1}{2}$ cups | 9 ounces, 250 g | Chana dal (Indian yellow split peas) |
| 5 cups | 40 ounces, 1 l | Water |
| 1 | | Dried red chile, soaked and seeded |
| 3 | | Ginger, unpeeled, sliced $\frac{1}{4}$ inch (.6 cm) thin |
| $\frac{1}{4}$ teaspoon | | Turmeric, ground |
| $\frac{1}{4}$ teaspoon | | Garam masala (p. 567) |
| To taste | | Salt |
| 3 tablespoons | 1 $\frac{1}{2}$ ounces, 45 ml | Ghee |
| 1 teaspoon | | Cumin seeds |
| 2 | | Garlic cloves, chopped |
| $\frac{1}{2}$ teaspoon | | Red chile powder |

**PROCEDURE**

1. Pick over dal to remove small stones and discolored seeds. Put in a bowl of water, soak 15 minutes, and remove any that float. Wash well and drain thoroughly.
2. Combine dal and water, bring to a boil, and remove any surface scum.
3. Add red chile, ginger, and turmeric. Cover, leaving lid slightly ajar, and simmer gently 45 to 50 minutes or until the dal is tender. Stir every 5 minutes to prevent sticking. Remove ginger slices and chile. Add garam masala and salt; stir to mix.
4. Heat the ghee over medium heat. When hot, add cumin seeds; 10 seconds later add garlic. Cook until garlic is slightly brown. Add chile powder, stir to mix, and immediately add contents of pan to the dal. Stir to mix.

# Tarapori Patio Dried Bombay Duck Patio

SERVES 4

**Despite its name, Bombay duck is a lizardfish. Native to the waters between Mumbai (formerly Bombay) and Kutch in the Arabian Sea, they are also found in small numbers in the Bay of Bengal. Great numbers are caught in China Sea, too. The fish is often dried and salted before it is consumed. After drying, the odor of the fish is extremely powerful, and it must consequently be transported in airtight containers. The bones of the fish are soft and easily chewable.**

**Jaggery is the traditional unrefined sugar used in India.**

| AMOUNT | MEASURE | INGREDIENT |
|---|---|---|
| $1\frac{1}{4}$ tablespoons | 14 g | Jaggery, grated |
| $\frac{1}{4}$ cup | 2 ounces, 60 ml | Cider vinegar |
| 6 | | Dried Bombay ducks |
| 6 | | Garlic cloves |
| 4 | | Red chiles, dry |
| 1 teaspoon | | Cumin seeds |
| 1 tablespoon | $\frac{1}{2}$ ounce, 15 ml | Ghee |
| $\frac{1}{2}$ cup | 2 ounces, 56 g | Onions, cut in half lengthwise, then finely sliced |
| 1 teaspoon | | Salt |

PROCEDURE

1. Soak jaggery in $\frac{1}{2}$ the vinegar.
2. Remove head and tail from each Bombay duck and any finlike protrusions near the tail. Cut each Bombay duck into 4 pieces.
3. Grind to a paste garlic, red chiles, and cumin seeds with 1 tablespoon vinegar.
4. Heat ghee in a pan and fry the onion until brown.
5. Add masala paste and cook 5 minutes.
6. Add pieces of Bombay duck and mix well.
7. Add salt and remaining vinegar and cook 3 minutes.
8. Add vinegar and jaggery mixture and $\frac{1}{4}$ cup (2 ounces, 60 ml) water; cover and cook on low heat 10 minutes or till Bombay duck are soft.

# Hara Dhania Chatni

## Cilantro Chutney with Peanuts

YIELD: $1\frac{1}{4}$ CUP

| AMOUNT | MEASURE | INGREDIENT |
|---|---|---|
| 3 cups | 6 ounces, 168 g | Cilantro leaves and tender stems |
| 2 | | Green chiles (serrano), seeded |
| 1 teaspoon | | Cumin seeds |
| $\frac{1}{2}$ teaspoons | | Coriander seeds |
| 1 teaspoon | | Salt |
| $\frac{1}{4}$ cup | $1\frac{1}{2}$ ounces, 42 g | Unsalted peanuts, rough chopped |
| $\frac{1}{4}$ cup | 2 ounces, 60 ml | Fresh lime juice |
| $\frac{1}{4}$ cup | 2 ounces, 60 ml | Water |
| To taste | | Granulated sugar |

**PROCEDURE**

1 Combine all ingredients, using a mortar and pestle to make coarse chutney, or purée in a blender or food processor. Let stand 15 minutes.

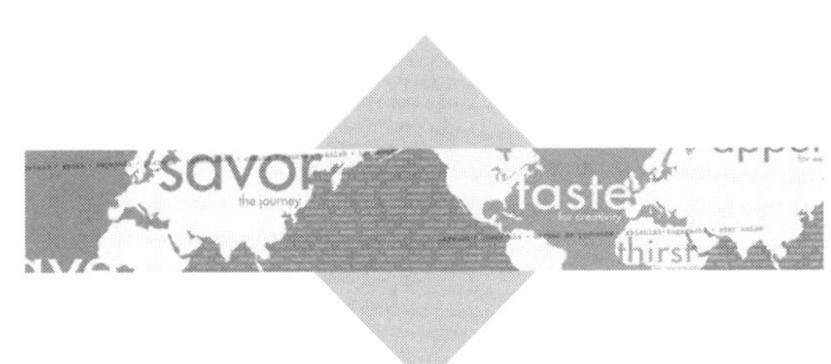

# Pork Vindaloo

SERVES 4

**Pork Vindaloo is the benchmark of Goan food. Goa is a tiny state on the west coast of India, famous for its distinctive cuisine.**

## MARINADE

| AMOUNT | MEASURE | INGREDIENT |
|---|---|---|
| 3 tablespoons | 1 ½ ounces, 120 ml | Malt vinegar |
| 1 ½ teaspoons | | Black peppercorns, crushed |
| 1 ½ teaspoons | | Brown sugar or jaggery |
| 8 | | Cardamom seeds, green |
| 8 | | Cloves |
| 3 | | Green chiles, seeded |
| To taste | | Salt |
| 1 ½ pounds | | Boneless pork shoulder, 1 inch (2.4 cm) cubes |

## PROCEDURE

1 Combine all ingredients except pork and mix well. Add pork, and marinate 1 hour.

## VINDALOO SPICE MIXTURE

| AMOUNT | MEASURE | INGREDIENT |
|---|---|---|
| 4 | | Garlic cloves, chopped |
| 2 tablespoons | ½ ounce | Ginger, peeled, chopped |
| 2 | | Red chiles, seeded |
| ½ teaspoon | | Mustard seed |
| ½ teaspoon | | Fenugreek seed |
| 1 teaspoon | | Cumin seeds |
| 2 teaspoons | | Coriander seeds |
| ½ teaspoon | | Turmeric |
| ½ teaspoon | | Cinnamon, ground |
| 2 tablespoons | 1 ounce, 30 ml | Malt vinegar |

### PROCEDURE

1 Using a mortar and pestle or blender, make a paste with the garlic, ginger, spices, and vinegar.

| AMOUNT | MEASURE | INGREDIENT |
|---|---|---|
| **3 tablespoons** | **$1\frac{1}{2}$ ounces, 45 ml** | **Oil** |
| **$1\frac{1}{2}$ cups** | **6 ounces, 168** | **Onions, $\frac{1}{4}$ inch (.6 cm) dice** |

**PROCEDURE**

1. Heat the oil over medium heat, add onions, and cook until golden brown, 6 to 8 minutes.
2. Add spice paste and cook over medium low heat, 10 minutes, or until the oil separates from the paste. Add up to 2 tablespoons (1 ounce, 30 ml) water, if necessary.
3. Remove pork cubes from marinade and add to pan. Cook 5 minutes over medium-high heat, stirring constantly. Add marinade.
4. Add 1 cup (8 ounces, 240 ml) warm water. Bring to simmer, cover, and lower heat. Cook 45 minutes or until pork is tender. Stir to prevent sticking.

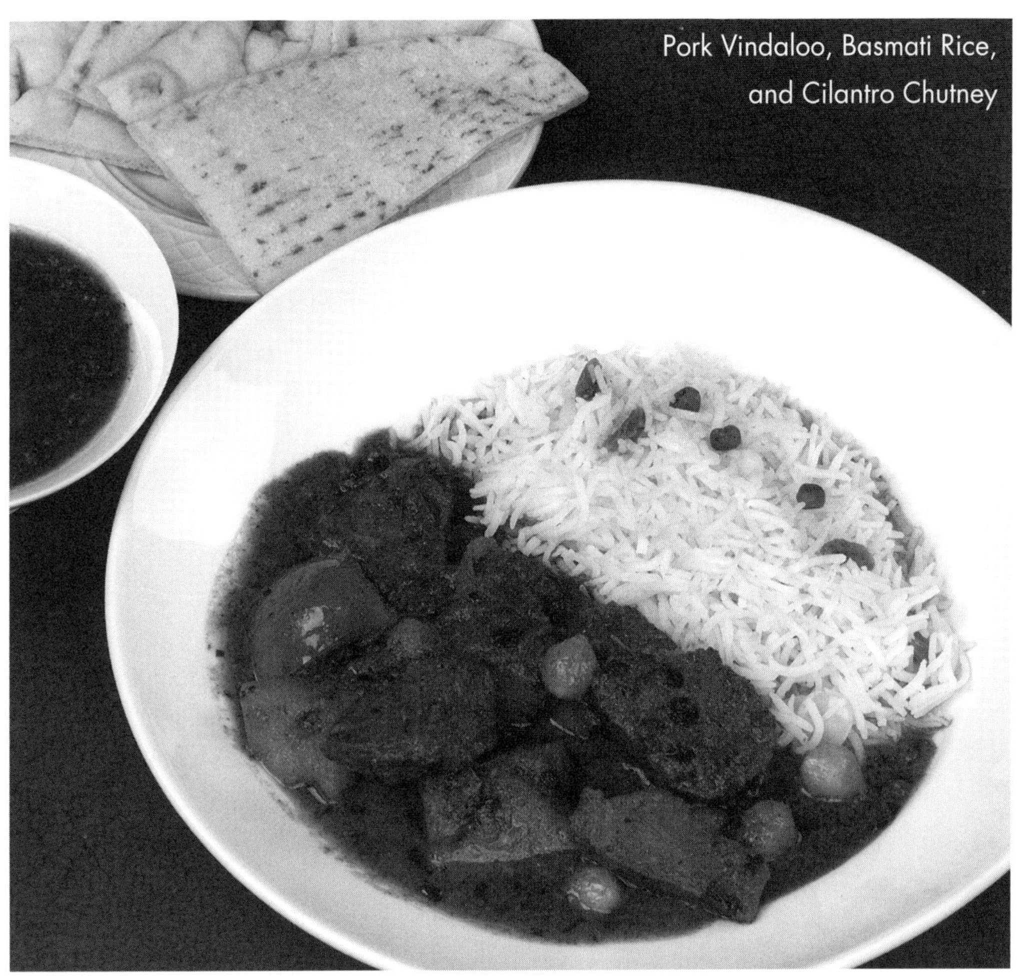
Pork Vindaloo, Basmati Rice, and Cilantro Chutney

# Naan

SERVES 4

| AMOUNT | MEASURE | INGREDIENT |
|---|---|---|
| 2 tablespoons | 1 ounce, 30 ml | Milk, 110°F (43°C) |
| 1 teaspoon | | Granulated sugar |
| 1 teaspoon | | Dry yeast |
| 2 cups | 8 ounces, 224 g | All-purpose flour |
| ½ teaspoon | | Baking powder |
| ¼ teaspoon | | Salt |
| ¼ cup | 2 ounces, 60 ml | Yogurt |
| ¼ cup | 2 ounces, 60 ml | Milk |
| 1 | | Egg yolk |
| 2 tablespoons | 2 ounces, 60 ml | Ghee |

**PROCEDURE**

1. Combine the milk and sugar; stir to dissolve. Sprinkle yeast over and let stand until the yeast begins to froth, about 10 minutes.
2. Sift together flour, baking powder, and salt.
3. In another container, mix together the yogurt, milk, egg yolk, and ghee.
4. Make a well in the center of the flour and add the liquid mixtures; work to form dough.
5. On a floured surface, knead the dough until it is smooth and elastic, 15 minutes.
6. Shape into a ball, cover, and let stand in warm area 1 hour.
7. Set a heavy baking tray (sheet pan) on the bottom rack of a preheated 500°F (260°C) oven. Preheat broiler.
8. Divide dough into 6 equal pieces and shape into balls. Flatten a piece of dough with your palm, dust with flour, and roll the dough from the center outward into a tear-shaped naan, about 8 inches (19.2 cm) long and 4 inches (9.6 cm) at its widest.
9. Remove the hot baking tray from the oven and slap the naan on to it. Immediately return the tray to the oven for 3 minutes; the naan should puff up.
10. Place the baking tray and naan under the broiler, about 3 to 4 inches (7.2–9.6 cm) away from the heat, for about 30 seconds or until the top of the naan browns slightly.
11. Wrap naan and serve hot.

# The British Isles

## The Land

The United Kingdom of Great Britain and Northern Ireland is a country in Western Europe and a member of the British Commonwealth and the European Union. Usually known as the United Kingdom, or UK, it is made up of four parts. Three of these parts—England, Wales, and Scotland—are located on the island of Great Britain and are considered nations in their own right. The fourth is Northern Ireland, which is located on the island of Ireland and is a province of the United Kingdom. The UK was formed by a series of Acts of Union, which united the countries of England (Wales already was a part of England), Scotland, and Ireland under a single government housed in London. The greater part of Ireland left the United Kingdom in 1922 to form a separate country when it became the Republic of Ireland, while the northeastern portion of the island, Northern Ireland, remains part of the United Kingdom. The UK is situated off the northwestern coast of continental Europe and is surrounded by the North Sea, the English Channel, the Celtic Sea, the Irish Sea, and the Atlantic Ocean.

England consists of mostly low hills and plains with a coastline cut into by bays, coves, and estuaries. Upland regions include the Pennine Chain, known as the "backbone of England," which splits northern England into western and eastern sectors. The highest point in England is Scafell Pike in the Lake District in the northwest, while the northeast includes the rugged landscape of the Yorkshire moors.

Wales has a varied geography with strong contrasts. In the south, flat coastal plains give way to valleys, then to ranges of hills and mountains in mid and north Wales.

Scotland is located in the north of Great Britain. The Scottish Lowlands and Borders are areas of gentle hills and woodland, contrasting dramatically with the rugged landscape of the Highlands in the north. A striking feature is Glen More, or the Great Glen, which cuts across the central Highlands from Fort William on the west coast northeast to Inverness on the east coast. A string of deep, narrow lochs (lakes) are set between steep mountains that rise past forested foothills to high moors and remote, rocky mountains.

Northern Ireland's northeast coast is separated from Scotland by the North Channel and is bordered by the Republic of Ireland in the west and south. The landscape is mainly low hill country. There are two mountain ranges: the Mournes, extending from South Down to Strangford Lough in the east, and the Sperrins in the northwest. Lough Neagh is the largest freshwater lake in the United Kingdom and one of the largest in Europe.

## History

The term *Celtic* is used rather generally to distinguish the early inhabitants of the British Isles from the later Anglo-Saxon invaders. After two expeditions by Julius Caesar in 55 and 54 B.C., contact between Britain and the Roman world grew, culminating in the Roman invasion in A.D. 43. Roman rule lasted until about 409, and its reach extended from southeast England to Wales and, for a time, the lowlands of Scotland.

When the Romans withdrew from the area, the lowland regions were invaded and settled by Angles, Saxons, and Jutes (tribes from what is now northwestern Germany). The last successful invasion of England took place in 1066 when Duke William of Normandy defeated the English at the Battle of Hastings and became King William I, known as William the Conqueror. Many Normans and others from France came to settle and French became the language of the ruling classes for the next three centuries. The legal and social structures of England were influenced by those across the Channel.

Scotland and England have existed as separate unified entities since the tenth century. Wales, under English control since 1284, became part of the Kingdom of England in 1536. In 1707 the separate kingdoms of England and Scotland, having shared the same monarch since 1603, agreed to a permanent union as the Kingdom of Great Britain. This was at a time when Scotland was on the brink of economic ruin and was ruled by a deeply unpopular monarch.

In 1800 the Kingdom of Great Britain united with the Kingdom of Ireland, which had been gradually brought under English control between 1169 and 1691 to form the United Kingdom of Great Britain and Ireland. This was an unpopular decision, taking place just after the unsuccessful United Irishmen Rebellion of 1798. The timing, when further Napoleonic

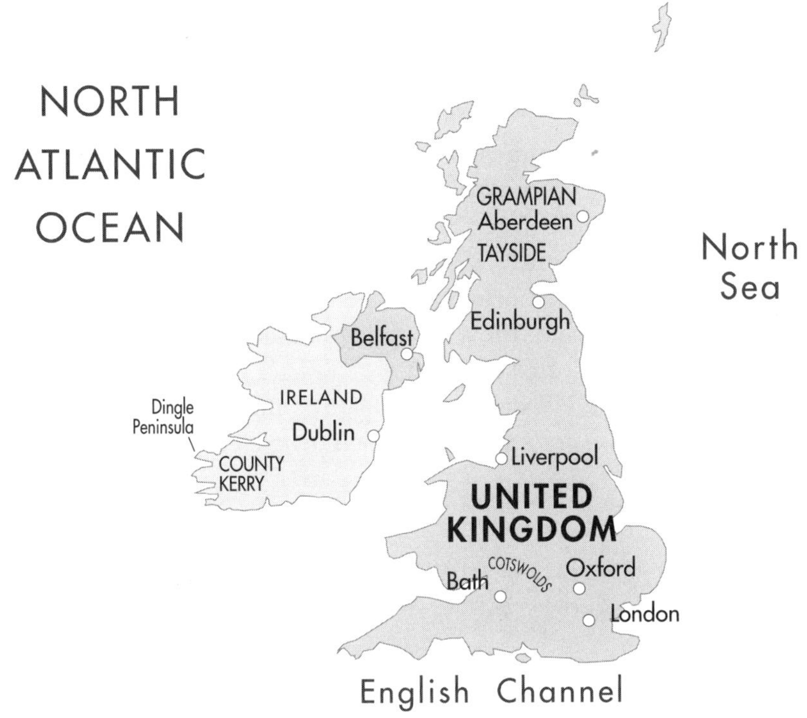


The United Kingdom

intervention or an invasion was feared, was predominantly due to security concerns. In 1922, after bitter fighting, the Anglo-Irish Treaty partitioned Ireland into the Irish Free State and Northern Ireland, with the latter remaining part of the United Kingdom. As provided for in the treaty, Northern Ireland, which consists of six of the nine counties of the Irish province of Ulster, opted out of the Free State and chose to remain in the UK. The nomenclature of the UK was changed in 1927 to recognize the departure of most of Ireland, and the name *United Kingdom of Great Britain and Northern Ireland* was adopted.

The United Kingdom, the dominant industrial and maritime power of the nineteenth century, played a leading role in developing Western ideas of property, liberty, capitalism, and parliamentary democracy as well as advancing world literature and science. At its zenith, the British Empire stretched over one-quarter of the earth's surface. The first half of the twentieth century saw the UK's strength seriously depleted in the two World Wars. The second half witnessed the dismantling of the empire and the UK rebuilding itself into a modern and prosperous nation.

# The People

A group of islands close to continental Europe, the British Isles have been subject to many invasions and migrations. Contemporary Britons are descended mainly from the varied ethnic stocks that settled there before the eleventh century. The pre-Celtic, Celtic, Roman, Anglo-Saxon, and Norse influences were blended in Britain under the Normans and Scandinavian Vikings who had lived in northern France. Although Celtic languages persist in Wales, Scotland, and Northern Ireland, the predominant language is English, which is primarily a blend of Anglo-Saxon and Norman French.

Since World War II the UK has absorbed substantial immigration, with Europe, Africa, and South Asia being the major areas from which people currently emigrate.

# The Food

Traditionally, England has been known as a country of "beefeaters," and roast beef and Yorkshire pudding has long been the country's usual Sunday dinner. Steak is also popular as an ingredient in hearty savory dishes such as steak and kidney pie or steak and mushroom pie. Being an island, Britain has always had a fresh supply of fish and seafood, both from the sea and from freshwater rivers. Salmon, Dover sole, turbot, mackerel, herring, oysters, eel, and shrimp are popular. Smoked fish is an English specialty, and smoked herrings, known as kippers, were once a very common breakfast dish. Fish and chips is traditional England takeaway food. Fish (cod, haddock, huss, plaice) is deep-fried in flour batter with chips (fried potatoes) and dressed in malt vinegar. England is renowned for its dairy products, particularly the rich clotted Devon cream from the country's southwest. There are also world-class cheeses produced in many counties, each fine variety bearing the name of its place of origin: Cheddar, Stilton, Cheshire, Derby, Lancashire, and Wensleydale, to name a few.

A traditional English breakfast provides a hearty start to the day. A typical menu may include several of the following: bacon, ham steak, homemade sage sausage, bratwurst, corned beef hash, scrapple, fried smelt, finnin haddie (smoked haddock), fried perch, home fries, baked stuffed tomato, fried green tomatoes, grilled whole mushrooms, roasted fresh garden vegetables, homemade baked beans, oven roasted potatoes, fried butternut or kabocha squash (a variety of winter squash), fried squash blossoms, and broiled baby zucchini. Pubs are popular for lunch and many still enjoy a typical "ploughman's lunch," consisting of bread, cheese, pickles, and sometimes cold meat, all washed down with a good glass of ale. Another simple and popular lunch item is the Cornish pasty, a pastry turnover filled with chopped meat, potatoes, and vegetables. It is said it had its origin in Cornwall, where it served both as a meal and "lunch box" for workers heading off to the mines. The pasty became the miners' meal of choice for many reasons. Not only was it a complete meal, but since arsenic was often found in the tin mines, the thick pastry crimp on the pasty allowed the miners to hold the pasty by this crust, then throw it away to avoid poisoning after they had eaten the body of the pasty.

For supper or "high tea," some favorite traditional English dishes include shepherd's pie, made with minced lamb and vegetables and topped with mashed potatoes; Gammon (ham) steak with egg; and Lancashire hotpot, a casserole of meat and vegetables topped with sliced potatoes. Bubble and squeak is made from cold vegetables and meat that have been leftover from a previous meal. This is fried in a pan together with mashed potatoes until the mixture is well cooked and brown on the sides. The name is a description of the sight and sound the ingredients make during the cooking process.

A sandwich has always been a very popular snack, but the first to eat one was the Earl of Sandwich (1718–1792). He was a dedicated gambler and refused to leave the gaming tables to eat. During one of his marathon gambling sessions he asked a waiter to bring him a piece of ham between two pieces of bread, and so invented the sandwich.

Afternoon tea was introduced in England by Anna, the seventh duchess of Bedford, in 1840. A tray of tea, bread, and butter was brought to her room during the late afternoon. This became a habit of hers and she began inviting friends to join her. This pause for tea became a fashionable social event. During the 1880s upper-class and society women would change into long gowns, gloves, and hats for their afternoon tea, which was usually served in the drawing room between four and five o'clock. Traditional afternoon tea consists of a selection of dainty sandwiches, scones served with clotted cream and preserves, cakes, and pastries. Tea grown in India or Ceylon is poured from silver teapots into delicate bone china cups.

Fruit desserts are popular, from pies and fruit crumbles to trifles and summer puddings made with fresh berries, as well as cakes flavored with spices or dried fruits, or filled with jam and cream. Dense steamed puddings such as plum pudding with brandy sauce are considered English Christmas traditions. French and Italian cooking are extremely popular in England, but it is Indian cuisine, first brought to Britain in the days of the Raj and further popularized with the arrival of Indian immigrants, that has become an important English food. In every city and town throughout the country there are Indian restaurants and "takeaways" serving a range of curries, chutneys, and Indian specialties.

The importance of agriculture to the Welsh economy as well as the availability of local products has created a cuisine and national diet that is based on fresh, natural food. In coastal areas fishing and seafood are important to both the economy and the local cuisine. While the Welsh national specialty is mountain lamb, it was the pig that was the basis of the diet in rural areas. Bacon remains an essential food, used today with the only two vegetables cultivated in Wales—leeks and cabbage. The national dish of Wales is *cawl,* a word for broth or soup that is a classic one-pot meal. Cooked in an iron pot over an open fire, it is made of bacon, lamb, cabbage, new potatoes, and leeks. The recipes vary from region to region and from season to season, based on what is available. Herring and mackerel are fried in bacon fat, roasted on a toasting fork, salted, or preserved. Oysters used to be prolific and one shellfish that remains plentiful is the cockle (a mollusk similar to a clam). Special traditional Welsh dishes include *laverbread* made from an edible seaweed known as laver. Also known as *bara lawr,* the *laverbread* is usually eaten sprinkled with oatmeal, then warmed in hot bacon fat and served with bacon for supper. Local markets and fairs usually offer regional products and baked goods. Wales is particularly known for its cheeses. Welsh rabbit, also called Welsh rarebit, a dish of melted cheese mixed with ale, beer, milk, and spices served over toast, has been popular since the early eighteenth century. Welsh cakes and breads include *bara brith,* the famous "speckled bread" with raisins and orange peel; *teisen lap,* a moist shallow fruitcake; and *teisen caraw,* a caraway seed cake. The type of food available in Wales is similar to that found in the rest of the United Kingdom and includes a variety of foods from other cultures and nations.

Scottish food is simple, with a heavy emphasis on meat. Roast lamb, roast beef, and steaks from Aberdeen-Angus cattle served with potatoes and bread make up the main meals. For many centuries Scottish cuisine centered on making use of every scrap of food available. This frugal attitude is seen in the Scottish national dish, a sausagelike concoction called *haggis.* It is made by chopping up the heart, liver, and lungs of a sheep, putting these ingredients in a bag made of the sheep's stomach, and boiling the bag and its contents. There are several types of breakfast foods and a full breakfast consists of fried eggs, bacon, sausage, tomatoes, and occasionally white or black pudding, which is a kind of blood sausage. Another Scottish breakfast dish is Arbroath smokies, known in England as kippers. They are lightly smoked herring served with butter. Oatcakes, known as *breed,* are made with oatmeal and bacon fat. The ingredients are mixed into a dough with warm water and then cut into rounds that are quickly fried on a griddle and then left to dry out. Traditional Scottish oatmeal is made with pinhead oats, or oats that have not been crushed or rolled. Scotch broth is a thick, wholesome soup made of various ingredients; the most important is barley, which is cooked with either lamb or beef as well as vegetables. This dish takes a lot of preparation and in the old days the Scotch broth pot never left the stove, with the last batch of broth forming the stock for a new pot of broth with a new set of ingredients.

*Mince and tattties* is similar to the English shepherd's pie. Minced beef, onions, and pinhead oatmeal are first fried and then mixed with vegetables and braised in gravy. The dish is served with boiled potatoes. *Cullen skink* is a thick stewlike soup made from smoked haddock, onions, and potatoes. *Stovies* are made from leftover cooked meat and potatoes, similar to corned beef hash. This is a very old dish with roots in the lives of the working poor. It is usually served with oatcakes and a glass of milk. *Clapshot* is not a main dish but an accompaniment to meat dishes; it is a mixture of mashed potatoes, turnips, and onions. Sweet puddings are popular and include *clootie dumping,* a mixture of fruitcake ingredients combined with spices, molasses, and suet wrapped in cloth and simmered in water for about four hours. *Cranachan* is the traditional harvest dish and is considered a very luxurious dessert. The table is laid with oatmeal, cream, honey, whisky, and raspberries. The family serves themselves with whatever combination of ingredients they choose. The traditional New Year's dessert is called *black bun* and is made from fruitcake baked inside a pastry case. The Scottish are also known for very fine shortbreads made with butter.

It is said when it comes to food there are three major periods in Irish history: before the potato arrived, after the potato arrived, and after the potato failed. Potatoes came to Ireland by way of South America, and by 1688 they were a staple of the Irish diet. The Irish population exploded in the first half of the nineteenth century, reaching about 8.5 million by 1845. The peasants were almost totally dependent on the potato for food—this crop produced more food per acre than wheat and could also be sold as a source of income. Unfortunately, it was particularly susceptible to potato blight, which could wipe out an entire crop very quickly. The crop regularly failed nationwide about every twenty years or so, but during the failure that began in 1845 and continued until 1849, at least a million people starved to death, while more than a million others emigrated to avoid starvation. Many peasants became too weak to work their tiny farms and were evicted from their homes because they could not pay rent. Meanwhile, unaffected crops such as corn sat in grain stores waiting to be shipped to England.

The diet changed dramatically after the famine. Potatoes continued to be important, but increasingly imports of cheap cornmeal, mainly from America, provided an alternative and cheap source of nutrition for the very poor. The fact that this cornmeal could also be fed to pigs and poultry made keeping them cheaper, which led to an increase in the availability of meat and eggs, both for consumption and as a means for farmers to earn cash. But most Irish people believed that pigs were all that this unpopular food was fit for, and by the end of the 1800s cornmeal was no longer eaten and had been replaced by locally grown oatmeal. Bread, potatoes, and oatmeal were staple foods and the people began to include bacon and eggs at breakfast time. The main meal was taken in the middle of the day and was usually meat, potatoes, and vegetables, usually cabbage, carrots, turnips, parsnips, or peas.

Historically the traditional Irish kitchen was the main living room of the house with a hearth built inside the chimney. Built into the wall of the chimney was a crane that could swing out over the fire or be pushed back against the wall when not in use. Whatever food had to be cooked was hung from this crane, usually in a large iron pot. The pot served as a saucepan and oven. When bread was baked it was put inside the pot and the lid placed firmly over it. Stew and potatoes were cooked in this same pot. Fish and mollusks were put into the stews on the coasts, while game, cattle, pig, goat, and sheep were available inland. Irish stew is a classic example, made from mutton, potatoes, onions, and flavored with parsley and thyme. Mutton is the dominant ingredient because the economic importance of sheep lay in their wool and milk produced and only old or economically nonviable animals ended up in the cooking pot, where they needed hours of slow boiling. Traditional foods include soda bread, originally made in the huge, black cooking pot and leavened with baking soda and sour milk. In the old days it served to use up milk left from the previous day. Another traditional food is *brack,* a cake made of dried fruit, eggs, lard, and flour. *Colcannon* is a dish made of potato and wild garlic, cabbage, or curly kale. *Champ* is a combination of mashed potato and egg, into which chopped scallions are mixed. *Carrageen moss* is another Irish delicacy, a seaweed that is collected and dried. The dried material is boiled and strained and the liquid left to cool, forming a jellylike substance said to be a very healthy food. Probably associated with Ireland more than other food or beverage is *stout* (black beer) originally produced by the Guinness brewery. It is an Irish success story of which all Irish people are proud.

During the 1980s and 1990s Ireland transitioned from an agricultural economy to a high-tech economy. The country, which has earned the nickname the Celtic Tiger, has one of the fastest growing economies in Europe. This has resulted in an increasingly sophisticated society. Dublin in particular has been transformed into an international city. By skipping the industrial revolution, it was necessary for everyone to rely on locally produced and home-grown foods from meat and seafood to dairy and vegetables, as there are few roads and factories to work in. Today, Ireland's chefs are taking advantage of international training, and a culinary renaissance is taking place producing dishes that are lighter and more sophisticated. The Irish Tourism Board has capitalized on this trend and coined the phrase "new Irish cuisine." Food today includes river oysters, grass-fed lamb, cows and pigs, and fresh or smoked salmon. Ireland's cheese-making tradition is developing, though Irish farmers have been making butter for hundreds of years. (Kerrygold butter is found around the world.) In the 1980s a group of small farmhouse cheese producers began making cheeses with milk from their own cows, goats, and sheep, and today artisan cheese makers are found all across the country. The farm-to-market movement is developing a great following, with its back-to-basics philosophy and emphasis on the true flavors of home grown, freshly prepared meals.

# Glossary

**Bangers** Sausages are called bangers in England and Ireland. They are traditionally made with pork, although beef bangers are now common. "Bangers and mash," the familiar pub meal, is made from mashed potatoes, good-quality sausages, and onion gravy.

**Bara Brith** A fruit bread made with raisins and orange peel.

**Barmbrack** A cross between fruitcake and bread, this round loaf is leavened with yeast, flavored with spices like allspice and nutmeg, and dotted with dried fruit such as raisins, currants, and candied citrus peel (Ireland).

**Biscuit** British term for a hard-baked product, such as a flat cracker or cookie.

**Black Pudding, Blood Pudding, or Blood Sausage** Sausage made of pork and seasoned pig's blood.

**Boxty** Potato cake that comes in three forms. *Pan boxty* consists of grated potatoes mixed with flour and fried in hot fat. *Pancake boxty* is grated raw potato mixed with cooked mashed potato, flour, and baking soda and fried on a griddle pan. Boiled boxty is grated raw and cooked mashed potatoes, but the dough is formed into a ball, boiled in water, allowed to cool, and then sliced and pan-fried (Ireland).

**Brawn** A coarse terrine, made using parts of a pig's head and sometimes pig's feet, it originated as a way to use every scrap of meat after the traditional village pig slaughter (Ireland).

**Bubble and Squeak** An old English dish, made from leftovers and named for the sounds the ingredients make while cooking.

**Carrageen Pudding** This milk and vanilla pudding is thickened with carrageen moss, a sea vegetable that contains natural gelatin. The dish dates back to the era when seaweed played a prominent role in the diets of coastal dwellers (Ireland).

**Cawl** A traditional Welsh soup made with lamb, chopped potatoes, leeks, carrots, swede (rutabagas), turnip, parsnips, and onions.

**Champs, or Poundies** Mashed potatoes with green onion, with a well of butter in the center. The mashed potatoes are eaten from around the outer edge of the well and dipped into the butter. To *champ* means to bruise, pound, or smash, hence the term *poundies.*

**Cheese**

**Ardrahan** Irish cheese with a semi-soft, smooth texture, a rich buttery flavor with a zesty tang, and an edible full-bodied rind from County Cork in South Ireland.

**Buxton Blue** A cousin of blue Stilton. It is lightly veined and has a deep russet coloring that hints at the very special tang of its flavor.

**Caboc** A rich, smooth, buttery cheese with a slight nutty flavor, due to being rolled in toasted pinhead oatmeal. One of Scotland's oldest cheeses, it is generally eaten when young, within five days of making.

**Caerphilly** The most famous of Welsh cheeses, a fresh, white, mild cheese with a delicate, slightly salty and lightly acidic flavor. Having a moderately firm, creamy, open texture, it was originally made a century and a half ago and eaten by hard-working Welsh miners.

**Cashel Blue** Soft-textured blue cheese from Wales.

**Cheddar** A hard cheese, its color can range from pale to deep yellow, depending on maturity. Produced in range of tastes from mild with a mellow flavor to vintage with a rich, strong flavor. Originating from the village of the same name in Somerset, though now produced worldwide, and falsely called Cheddar. It was originally made from ewe's milk, but by Tudor times it was also being produced from cow's milk.

**Cheshire** Its unique flavor derives from salt deposits in nearby pasturelands. Colored Cheshire does not differ in flavor from white Cheshire. Both have a slightly crumbly and silky texture and both have a wonderfully full-bodied, fresh flavor. The only difference is its color, produced by an ancient vegetable dye called annatto.

**Cornish Yarg** A semi-hard cheese that is creamy under the rind and slightly crumbly in the core. It has a young, fresh, slightly tangy taste and is made by hand in open round vats. After pressing and brining, the cheese is wrapped in nettle leaves.

**Crowdie** A Scottish cream cheese; the texture is soft and crumbly, the taste slightly sour.

**Derby** Has a smooth, mellow texture with a quite mild, buttery flavor. It is similar in taste and texture to Cheddar and ripens between one and six months.

**Double Gloucester** Pale orange in color, with a smooth, buttery texture and a clean, creamy, mellow flavor. Usually matured for around three or four months.

**Dovedale** A creamy soft, mild blue cheese. Most British cheeses are dry salted; however, Dovedale is brine-dipped to add the salt, giving it a distinctive appearance and flavor.

**Dubliner** Tastes like a mature Cheddar with the sweet aftertaste of Reggiano.

**Gubbeen, Smoked** Has a silky, pliable texture and a light smoked flavor.

**Lancashire** Creamy open-textured cheese with a mild flavor. Usually matured for two to three months. Creamy white in color.

**Laverbread** Cow's milk cheese, which is speckled with laverbread, an edible seaweed sometimes called Welsh caviar.

**Llanboidy** A Welsh cow's milk cheese, firm, smooth and silky in texture with a buttery, herby flavor.

**Sage Derby** Green-veined, semi-hard cheese with a mild sage flavor.

**Shropshire Blue** A British blue cheese invented in Scotland, made in a way similar to Stilton. The cheese is a bright red with blue veining, and a sharper taste than Stilton.

**Stilton** Known as the "King of English Cheeses." Smooth and creamy with complex, slightly acidic flavor. An excellent dessert cheese, it is traditionally served with Port.

**Warwickshire Truckle** Full-flavored, mature hard Cheddar-like cheese with a firm but creamy texture and nutty taste.

**Wensleydale** A moist, crumbly, and flaky-textured cheese with a mild buttermilk and slightly sweet flavor.

**Chips** Thickly cut French fries.

**Cockaleekie** A thick chicken, leek, and barley soup from Scotland.

**Colcannon** Typical country winter dish comprising mashed potato and chopped cooked kale or cabbage (Ireland).

**Cornish Pasty** The word "pasty" comes from "pasta." Originally made with a hard pastry that served as a container rather than something to be eaten, forming a sealed pastry envelope. Although it originally contained almost anything, the Cornish pasty now contains seasoned chopped root vegetables and minced beef. Also known as an *oggie* or *Bedforshire clanger.*

**Cruibeens** Salted pig's feet. Today, contemporary chefs who enjoy cruibeens' crisp skin and gelatinous meat stuff them with everything from sweetbreads to morel mushrooms (Ireland).

**Crumpet** A light and spongy small, round, unsweetened bread, cooked on a griddle, similar to an English muffin.

**Dingle Pies** A simple, filling, one-handed meal, these small meat pies traditionally fed farmers working the fields or fishermen out at sea. They consist of a "hot-water pastry"—a sturdy mixture made by boiling butter and water, then combining them with flour—with a filling of mutton, carrots, and onions.

**Double Cream** Very rich cream, containing 48 percent butterfat. Whipping cream in the U.S., by contrast, contains between 30 percent and 40 percent butterfat.

**Drisheen** Spectacularly strong-flavored sheep's-blood pudding, a specialty of Cork city, typically served with tripe (Ireland).

**Dublin Coddle** Dublin's contribution to the national cuisine, this simple stew of onions, bacon, and sausage was, like *cruibeens,* historically popular after a night of drinking (Ireland).

**Fadge** Also called potato bread, *fadge* is made from leftover mashed potatoes mixed with flour and butter, pressed into a thin disk, fried on a hot griddle (Ireland).

**Fish and Chips** Fish (cod, haddock, huss, plaice) deep fried in flour batter with chips dressed in malt vinegar. In northern English they often served with "mushy peas" (mashed processed peas). Not normally home cooked but bought at a fish and chip shop known as a *chippie.*

**Guinness Stout** A brand of strong dark beer that originated in the British Isles; made with dark-roasted barley and more fragrant of hops than other types of beer.

**Haggis** A Scottish pudding made of the heart, liver, and other parts of a sheep or lamb, minced with suet, onions, and oatmeal, highly seasoned and boiled in the stomach of the same animal.

**Hardtack** A large, hard biscuit made with unsalted, unleavened flour and water dough, baked and dried to give a longer shelf life. Hardtack has been used as a staple by sailors at least since the 1800s. Also known as ship biscuit or sea bread.

**Kedgeree** Originally known as *Khitcheri* in India; consists of boiled rice, fish, and eggs (cumin seeds and lentils are optional).

**Kippers** Split and smoked herring.

**Melba Toast** A very thinly sliced crisp toast, served warm.

**Mulligatawny** Curry-flavored soup, which reflects the British period in India.

**Mutton** Aged older lamb, with a very strong flavor and tougher texture than younger lamb.

**Pastie or Pastry** Individual pies filled with meats and vegetables. They should weigh about two pounds or more. The identifying feature of the Cornish pasty is the pastry and its crimping.

**Porridge** A simple dish of boiled oatmeal. It needs to be boiled slowly and stirred continuously with the traditional spirtle—a wooden stick about 12 inches long—to avoid lumps.

**Rarebit (Welsh Rarebit)** Cheese melted with ale or beer served over toast.

**Sandwiches** Said to have been invented by the fourth Earl of Sandwich so that he could eat conveniently at the gaming table. The first printed reference to it is from 1762. The cucumber sandwich is probably regarded as the typically English sandwich, although it is not very common. *Butties* and *sarnies* are slang for sandwiches.

**Scones** A Scottish quick bread said to have taken its name from the Stone of Destiny (or Scone), the place where Scottish kings were once crowned.

**Shepherd's Pie** Traditionally, minced lamb or mutton stew topped with mashed potatoes. Cottage pie is the beef version.

**Swede** The English name for rutabaga, a yellow root vegetable with a slightly sweet flavor. Mashed veggies like swedes, turnips, and potatoes are an important, although often maligned, part of British culinary history.

**Treacle** Molasses.

**Toad in the Hole** A large Yorkshire pudding cooked with sausages embedded in it.

**Trifle** A dessert typically consisting of ladyfingers, plain or sponge cake soaked in sherry, rum, or brandy, and topped with layers of jam or jelly, custard, and whipped cream.

**Yorkshire Pudding** A batter of egg, flour, and milk cooked in beef drippings. Originally served with gravy before the main course to reduce the appetite, today it is used as an accompaniment to beef roast.

# Menus and Recipes from the British Isles

MENU ONE

**Fennel and Red Onion Salad with Tarragon Dressing**

**Langoustine Soufflés**

**Glazed Shallots**

**Roast Beef and Yorkshire Pudding**

**Cheese and Herb Bread**

**Strawberry Shortbread**

MENU TWO

**Scotch Broth**

**Tomato Water-Ice with a Julienne of Smoked Salmon**

**Salad of Steamed Skate**

**Roast Belly of Pork with Black Pudding and Apples**

**Colcannon**

**Irish Soda Bread**

**Dundee Cake**

MENU THREE

**Baked Oysters with Bacon, Cabbage, and Guinness Sabayon**

**Crab and Champ Bake**

**Stuffed Shoulder of Lamb**

**Blue Cheese Potato Cakes**

**Whole Wheat Scones**

**Caledonian Cream**

# Fennel and Red Onion Salad with Tarragon Dressing

SERVES 4

| AMOUNT | MEASURE | INGREDIENT |
|---|---|---|
| 2 tablespoons | 1 ounce, 30 ml | White wine vinegar |
| 1 teaspoon | | Tarragon, chopped |
| $\frac{1}{2}$ cup | 4 ounces, 120 ml | Olive oil |
| To taste | | Salt and pepper |
| 1 cup | 4 ounces, 112 g | Red onion, sliced into thin rings ($\frac{1}{8}$ inch, .3 cm) |
| 3 cups | 12 ounces, 336 g | Fennel, sliced thin ($\frac{1}{8}$ inch, .3 cm) |

PROCEDURE

1 Mix vinegar, tarragon, olive oil, salt, and pepper.

2 Add red onions and fennel; toss to combine.

3 Cover and let stand 1 hour.

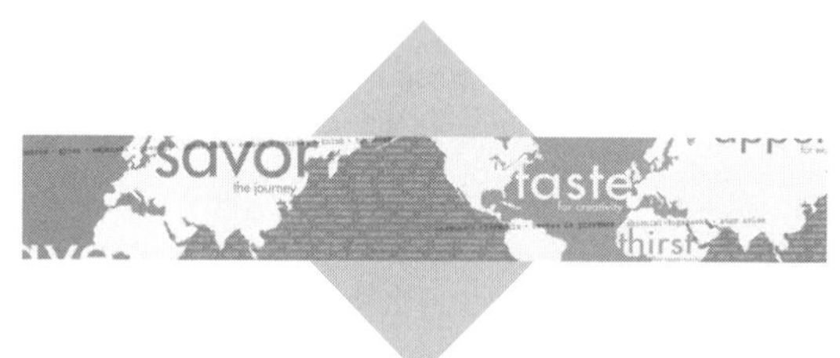

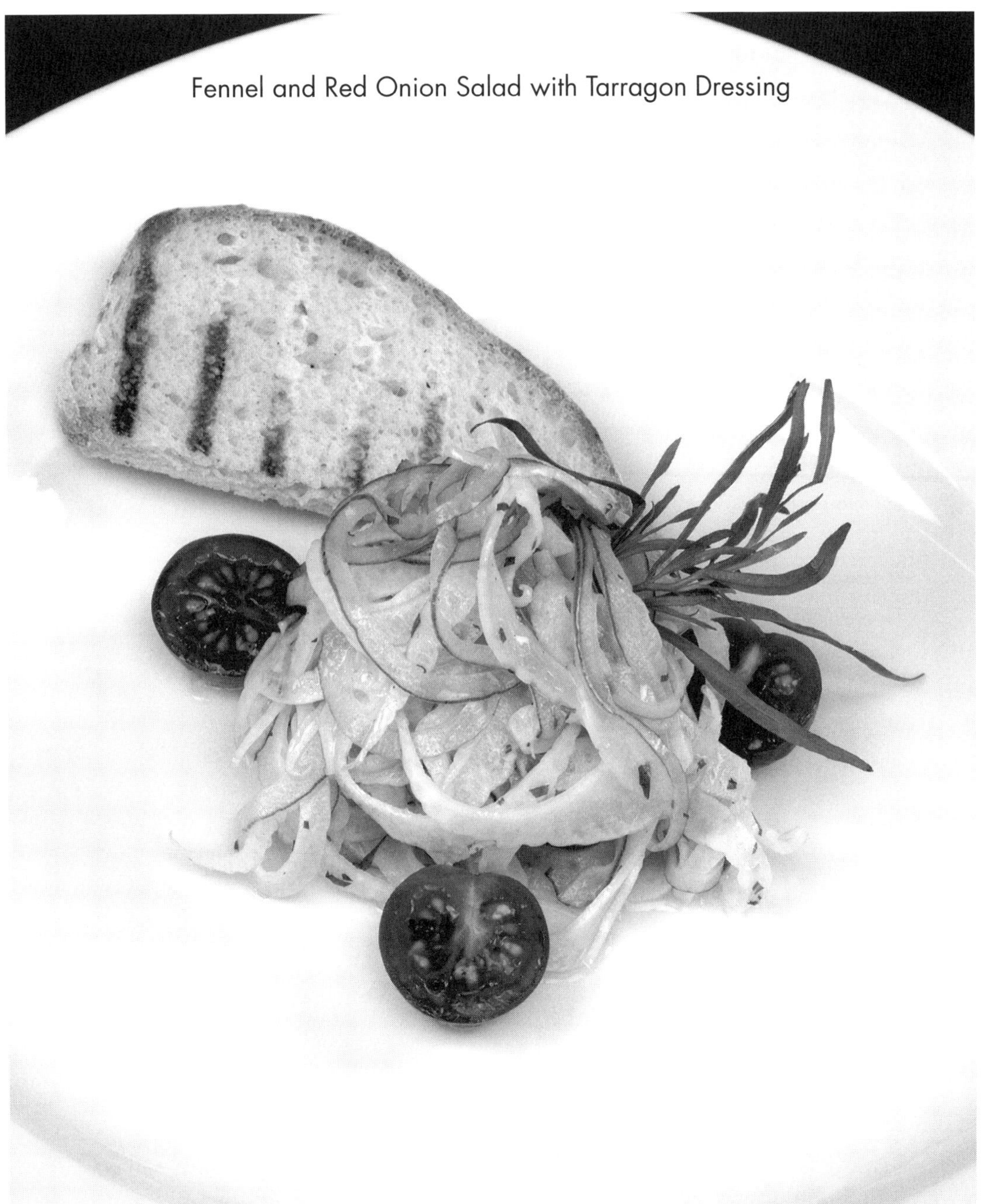
Fennel and Red Onion Salad with Tarragon Dressing

# Langoustine Soufflés

SERVES 4 TO 6

**The langoustine, also called Norway lobster, is available mainly from Brittany. It is a large prawn with a unique silky texture and succulent flavor.**

| AMOUNT | MEASURE | INGREDIENT |
|---|---|---|
| 3 tablespoons | $\frac{3}{4}$ ounce, 21 g | Bread crumbs, toasted |
| 1 cup | 8 ounces, 224 g | Raw shelled langoustine tails (substitute shrimp if langoustine are not available) |
| 1 cup | 8 ounces, 240 ml | Fish stock |
| 3 tablespoons | $1\frac{1}{2}$ ounces, 45 ml | Butter |
| 1 tablespoon | | Shallots, minced |
| 3 tablespoons | $\frac{3}{4}$ ounce, 21 g | All-purpose flour |
| 3 | | Egg yolks, beaten |
| $\frac{1}{8}$ teaspoon | | Cayenne pepper |
| 2 teaspoons | | Fresh lemon juice |
| 1 teaspoon | | Lemon zest |
| $\frac{1}{8}$ teaspoon | | Nutmeg |
| 3 | | Egg whites |
| Pinch | | Salt |

PROCEDURE

1. Preheat oven to 350°F (176°C).
2. Grease 4 to 6 individual 6- to 7-ounce (168 g to 196 g) ramekins and coat the insides with toasted bread crumbs. Chill.
3. Poach the langoustine tails in the fish stock about 2 minutes. Drain and roughly chop. Reserve the fish stock.
4. Melt the butter over medium heat; sauté shallots 2 minutes or until soft. Stir in the flour and cook 2 to 3 minutes.
5. Remove from heat; gradually stir in reserved fish stock. Return to heat and cook, stirring, 3 to 5 minutes, or until thick. Remove from heat and stir in egg yolks and langoustine tails. Season with cayenne, lemon juice, lemon zest, and nutmeg. Let cool slightly.
6. Whisk egg whites with the salt until stiff peaks form; fold into the langoustine mixture.
7. Spoon into prepared ramekins and bake 30 to 35 minutes. Soufflé should be puffed, browned, and fairly firm. Serve immediately.

# Glazed Shallots

SERVES 4

| AMOUNT | MEASURE | INGREDIENT |
|---|---|---|
| **4 cups** | **1 pound, 448 g** | **Shallots, peeled** |
| **4 tablespoons** | **2 ounces, 60 ml** | **Butter** |
| **2 tablespoons** | **1 ounce, 28 g** | **Granulated sugar** |
| **To taste** | | **Salt and pepper** |
| **1 tablespoon** | | **Parsley, chopped** |

**PROCEDURE**

1. Over medium-high heat, cover shallots with cold water. Bring to a boil and simmer 10 minutes. Drain.
2. In a saucepan, melt the butter over medium heat; add sugar and stir to dissolve. Add the shallots; season with salt and pepper. Cover and cook until the shallots are tender and well glazed, 5 to 8 minutes. Stir occasionally to prevent the sugar from burning. Sprinkle with parsley and serve.

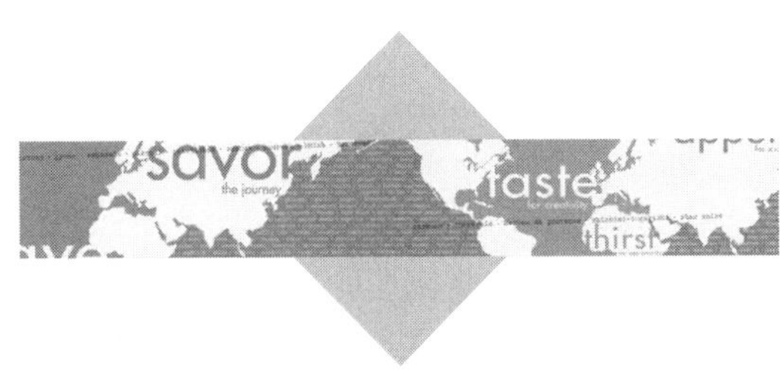

# Roast Beef and Yorkshire Pudding

SERVES 4

**Yorkshire pudding was originally cooked under the roast to catch the juices as the meat cooked and was then served as a first course with thick gravy. Mustard and horseradish sauce are the traditional accompaniments for roast beef.**

| AMOUNT | MEASURE | INGREDIENT |
|---|---|---|
| 3 pounds | 1.34 kg | Standing rib roast, or about a 2-pound (900 g) boneless sirloin-tip roast |
| Yorkshire Pudding | | |
| $\frac{3}{4}$ cup | 3 ounces, 84 g | All-purpose flour |
| Pinch | | Salt |
| $\frac{1}{2}$ cup | 4 ounces, 120 ml | Milk, room-temperature |
| $\frac{1}{2}$ cup | 4 ounces, 120 ml | Water, room-temperature |
| 1 | | Egg, room temperature |
| 1 tablespoon | $\frac{1}{2}$ ounce, 15 ml | Melted fat from the roasting pan |
| Gravy | | |
| 2 teaspoons | | All-purpose flour |
| $1\frac{1}{4}$ cups | 10 ounces, 300 ml | Beef stock |
| To taste | | Salt and pepper |

PROCEDURE

1 Sift the flour and salt together. Mix milk, water, and egg together and gradually beat into the flour; continue mixing until batter is smooth and lump free. Let stand 30 to 40 minutes.

2 Preheat oven to 425°F (218°C).

3 Place the beef on a rack in a roasting pan; season with salt and pepper.

4 Cook 15 minutes. Reduce the temperature to 350°F (176°C) and continue to roast until desired temperature is reached. Remove from oven and let rest 20 minutes before carving. Return oven to 425°F (218°C).

5 While the meat is resting, put the fat from the beef into a 9-inch-square (22 cm) 2-inch-deep (4.8 cm) pan. Return pan to oven, until fat is smoking hot. Immediately pour batter

into the hot pan. Bake in the hot oven until puffed and dry, 20 to35 minutes. Do not open the oven for the first 20 minutes. Cut into portions and serve with the roast.

6 To make the gravy, degrease the roasting pan. Sprinkle in the flour and stir well, scraping up the brown sediment. Cook, stirring, over high heat until flour has browned slightly. Add beef stock and stir well; bring to a boil and simmer 5 minutes. Add any juices from the resting meat and correct seasoning.

7 Serve with glazed shallots, steamed broccoli, and roasted new potatoes.

## Horseradish Sauce SERVES 4

| AMOUNT | MEASURE | INGREDIENT |
|---|---|---|
| **3 tablespoons** | **1 $\frac{1}{2}$ ounces, 45 ml** | **Fresh or prepared horseradish, grated** |
| **1 teaspoon** | | **White vinegar** |
| **2 teaspoons** | | **Fresh lemon juice** |
| **$\frac{1}{4}$ cup** | **2 ounces, 60 ml** | **Sour cream or double cream** |
| **2 tablespoons** | **1 ounce, 30 ml** | **Heavy cream** |
| **$\frac{1}{4}$ teaspoon** | | **Dry mustard powder** |
| **To taste** | | **Salt and white pepper** |

**PROCEDURE**

1 Combine all ingredients and mix well; correct seasoning.

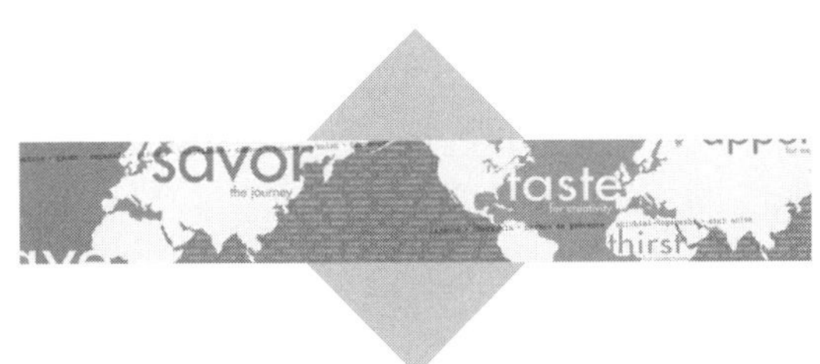

# Mustard Sauce SERVES 4

| AMOUNT | MEASURE | INGREDIENT |
|---|---|---|
| 2 tablespoons | 2 ounces, 30 ml | Butter |
| 2 tablespoons | $\frac{1}{2}$ ounce, 14 g | All-purpose flour |
| 1 cup | 8 ounces, 240 ml | Milk |
| $\frac{1}{4}$ cup | 2 ounces, 60 ml | Heavy cream |
| 1 tablespoon | $\frac{1}{2}$ ounce, 15 ml | White vinegar |
| 1 tablespoon | $\frac{1}{4}$ ounce, 7 g | Dry mustard |
| 1 tablespoon | $\frac{1}{2}$ ounce, 15 ml | Dijon mustard |
| 1 teaspoon | | Salt |
| $\frac{1}{2}$ teaspoon | | White pepper |

**PROCEDURE**

1 Over medium heat, thoroughly combine butter and flour. Cook 2 minutes.

2 Add milk, stirring constantly; bring to a boil. Reduce heat and simmer 3 minutes. Whisk in the cream, vinegar, mustards, salt, and pepper. Serve immediately.

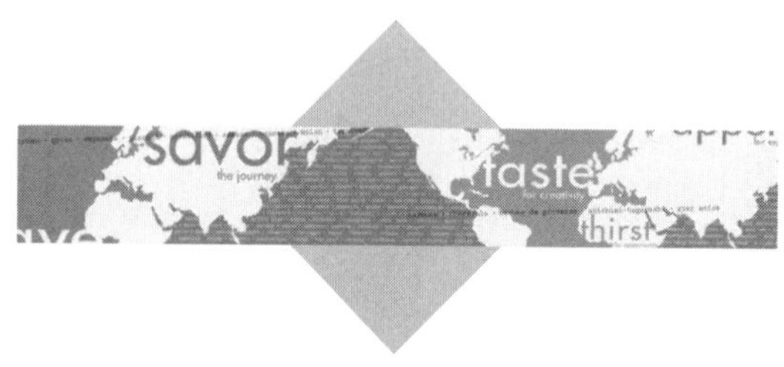

# Cheese and Herb Bread

SERVES 4

| AMOUNT | MEASURE | INGREDIENT |
|---|---|---|
| 1 teaspoon | | Granulated sugar |
| $1\frac{1}{4}$ cups | 10 ounces, 300 ml | Warm water (105°F, 40.5°C) |
| $2\frac{1}{4}$ teaspoons | $\frac{1}{4}$ ounce, 7 g | Active dry yeast |
| As needed | | Butter |
| 3 cups | 12 ounces, 336 g | All-purpose flour |
| $\frac{1}{2}$ cup | 2 ounces, 56 g | Bread flour |
| 2 teaspoon | | Salt |
| 1 teaspoon | | Dry mustard |
| $\frac{1}{2}$ teaspoon | | White pepper |
| 1 tablespoon | | Chives, minced |
| 2 tablespoons | | Parsley, chopped |
| 2 cups | 8 ounces, 224 g | Cheddar cheese, grated |

**PROCEDURE**

1. Preheat the oven to 375°F (190°C).
2. Dissolve the sugar in the water, and sprinkle in the yeast. Let stand 10 to 12 minutes, until frothy.
3. Butter $8\frac{1}{2} \times 4\frac{1}{2} \times 3\frac{3}{4}$-inch (20.4 × 10.8 × 6.6 cm) loaf pan.
4. Sift the flours, salt, mustard, and pepper into a bowl. Stir in the chives, parsley and three-quarters of the cheese. Add the yeast liquid to the dry ingredients and mix to a soft, smooth dough, 8 to 12 minutes using the hook attachment. Turn out onto a floured surface and round. Cover and let rise in a warm place about 1 hour, until doubled in size.
5. Turn the dough onto a floured surface and knead 2 to 3 minutes.
6. Fit into prepared loaf pan. Cover and let rise in a warm place 40 to 50 minutes.
7. Sprinkle the top with remaining cheese. Bake 45 minutes, until well risen and golden brown. Turn out and cool on a wire rack.

# Strawberry Shortbread

SERVES 4

| AMOUNT | MEASURE | INGREDIENT |
|---|---|---|
| 1 $\frac{1}{2}$ cups | 12 ounces, 360 ml | Strawberry coulis (pureed strawberries) |
| $\frac{3}{4}$ cup | 6 ounces, 168 g | Granulated sugar |
| As needed | | Fresh lemon juice |
| 4 cups | 16 ounces, 448 g | Strawberries |

PROCEDURE

1 Combine strawberry coulis and sugar; correct flavor with more sugar or a little lemon juice.

2 Wash strawberries, hull, and either half or leave them whole, depending on their size.

3 Toss with two-thirds of the strawberry coulis and set in the refrigerator.

## Shortbread Dough

| AMOUNT | MEASURE | INGREDIENT |
|---|---|---|
| 1 cup | 8 ounces, 240 ml | Butter |
| 1 cup | 3.75 ounces, 105 g | Confectioner's sugar |
| $\frac{1}{2}$ teaspoon | | Salt |
| 2 | | Egg yolks |
| 2$\frac{1}{4}$ cups | 9 ounces, 252 g | All-purpose flour, sifted |
| $\frac{1}{2}$ teaspoon | | Vanilla extract |
| | | Egg yolk, beaten with 1 tablespoon ($\frac{1}{2}$ ounce, 15 ml) milk |

PROCEDURE

1 Cut the butter into small pieces. Work the butter with your fingertips until very soft. Sift confectioner's sugar and add to the butter with the salt. Continue to work the mixture with the fingertips until the ingredients are thoroughly blended, then add the egg yolks, mixed with vanilla extract, and mix lightly.

2 Add the flour and mix evenly into the mixture.

3 Rub the pastry gently 2 or 3 times (only) using the palm of the hand. Do not overwork the short dough. Roll into a ball and flatten it out lightly. Wrap and chill 2 to 3 hours, until very firm. (When working with the dough later, it will soften very quickly.)

4 Preheat oven to 400°F (204°C).

5 On a lightly floured work surface, roll out the pastry to the thickness of about $\frac{1}{8}$ inch (.3 cm). Cut out 12 circles with a 4-inch (10 cm) scallop-edged pastry cutter and arrange on a baking sheet.

6 Brush with egg wash, and then draw lines with the back of a small knife or fork on the surface for decoration.

7 Bake 8 minutes; remove from oven, and let cool on baking sheet 1 to 2 minutes to firm. Then use a palette knife to transfer to a wire rack and cool.

8 To serve, place a shortbread disk on each plate. Over each spread a few prepared strawberries, then on top, balance a second layer of shortbread; garnish with more strawberries. Top with a shortbread dredged with confectioner's sugar. Spoon a little of the reserved coulis around and serve.

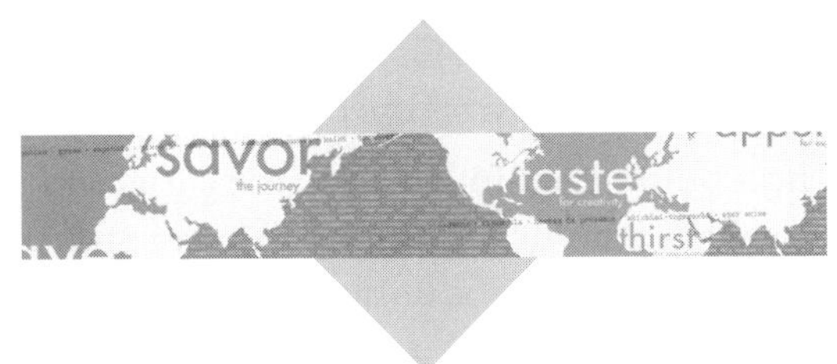

# Scotch Broth

SERVES 4

| AMOUNT | MEASURE | INGREDIENT |
|---|---|---|
| 12 ounces | | Mutton |
| $\frac{1}{4}$ cup | 1 ounce, 28 g | Pearl barley, soaked |
| 1 quart | 960 ml | Lamb, beef, or chicken stock |
| 2 tablespoons | 1 ounce, 30 ml | Butter |
| $1\frac{1}{2}$ tablespoons | | Garlic, minced |
| $\frac{1}{2}$ cup | 2 ounces, 56 g | Onion, $\frac{1}{4}$ inch (.6 cm) dice |
| $\frac{3}{4}$ cup | 3 ounces, 84 g | Leek, white and light green parts, $\frac{1}{4}$ inch (.6 cm) dice |
| $\frac{1}{2}$ cup | 2 ounces, 56 g | Celery, $\frac{1}{4}$ inch (.6 cm) dice |
| $\frac{1}{2}$ cup | 2 ounces, 56 g | Carrots, $\frac{1}{4}$ inch (.6 cm) dice |
| $\frac{1}{2}$ cup | 2 ounces, 56 g | Rutabaga, $\frac{1}{4}$ inch (.6 cm) dice |
| To taste | | Salt and pepper |
| 2 tablespoons | | Parsley, chopped |
| 1 tablespoon | | Fresh thyme, chopped |

PROCEDURE

1 Trim any excess fat from the mutton. Combine mutton, barley, and stock over medium heat and bring to a boil. Reduce to a simmer and cook 1 hour.

2 In a separate pan, heat butter until foamy. Add the garlic and onion and cook 2 minutes. Add the leeks and cook 2 minutes. Transfer to soup and add the celery, carrots, and rutabaga. Simmer 20 to 30 minutes or until vegetables are tender.

3 Remove meat, cut into $\frac{1}{2}$-inch (1.2 cm) cubes, and return to soup.

4 Skim off any fat, correct seasoning, and add parsley and thyme.

# Tomato Water-Ice with a Julienne of Smoked Salmon

SERVES 4

| AMOUNT | MEASURE | INGREDIENT |
|---|---|---|
| $1\frac{1}{2}$ pounds | 672 g | Ripe tomatoes, peeled, seeded, chopped |
| 2 tablespoons | 1 ounce, 30 ml | Fresh lemon juice |
| 1 teaspoon | | Worcestershire sauce |
| Few drops, to taste | | Tabasco |
| To taste | | Salt |
| $\frac{1}{2}$ teaspoon | | Granulated sugar |
| $\frac{1}{4}$ pound | 4 ounces, 112 g | Smoked salmon, julienned strips |
| Garnish | | Fresh dill sprigs |

PROCEDURE

1. Rub tomatoes through a sieve into a bowl. Stir in the lemon juice, Worcestershire sauce, Tabasco sauce, salt, and sugar.
2. Pour the mixture into a shallow container and freeze until frozen around the edges. Turn into a chilled bowl and beat to break up the ice crystals. Return to the container and freeze until hard.
3. To serve, chill serving plates. Scrape water-ice and shape into quenelles; place two onto each plate. Arrange 1 ounce (28 g) of smoked salmon on the plates and garnish with a dill sprig.

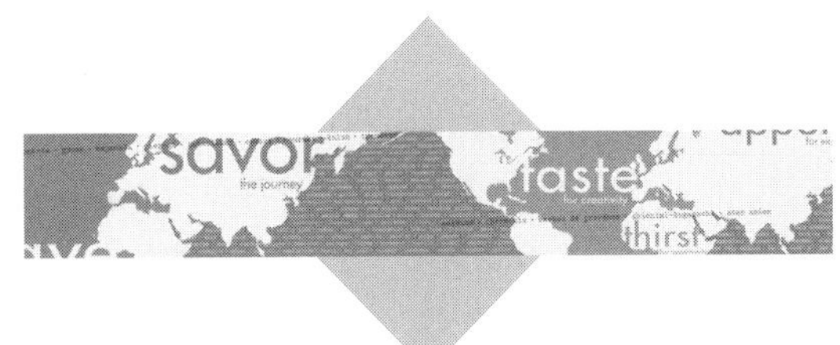

# Salad of Steamed Skate

SERVES 4

| AMOUNT | MEASURE | INGREDIENT |
|---|---|---|
| 1 | $1\frac{1}{4}$ pound, 20 ounces, 560 g | Skate wing, outer fins removed, washed |
| $\frac{1}{4}$ cup | 2 ounces, 60 ml | Butter, melted |
| 1 tablespoon | | Garlic, minced |
| 1 tablespoon | $\frac{1}{2}$ ounce, 15 ml | Fresh lemon juice |
| $\frac{1}{4}$ teaspoon | | Cayenne pepper |
| 1 tablespoon | | Tarragon, blanched in boiling water and chopped |
| $1\frac{1}{2}$ cups | 6 ounces, 168 g | Carrots, julienned |
| $1\frac{1}{2}$ cups | 6 ounces, 168 g | Zucchini, julienned, on seeds |

**PROCEDURE**

1 Combine the butter, garlic, lemon juice, cayenne pepper, and tarragon; correct seasoning. Brush the flavored butter over the skate wing.

2 Sprinkle the julienned vegetables over the perforated part of a steamer. Season the skate, place on top of the vegetables, brush with more butter.

3 Steam in a covered container 5 minutes on each side or until tender.

4 Remove; save the julienne to use in the salad.

5 Remove the skin from both sides and fillet the skate. Keep covered to retain the moisture.

## Salad

| AMOUNT | MEASURE | INGREDIENT |
|---|---|---|
| $\frac{1}{2}$ cup | 4 ounces, 120 ml | Fish stock |
| 1 tablespoon | | Shallots, chopped |
| 2 tablespoons | | Chives, chopped |
| 1 teaspoon | | Worcestershire sauce |
| 4 cups | 8 ounces, 224 g | Mixed baby greens |
| To taste | | Fresh lemon juice, salt, and black pepper |
| 1 cup | 6 ounces, 168 g | Tomato, peeled, seeded, $\frac{1}{4}$ inch (.6 cm) dice |

**PROCEDURE**

1 Warm fish stock.

2 Combine stock with 1 tablespoon ($\frac{1}{2}$ ounce, 15 ml) tarragon dressing, shallots, and chives. Add Worcestershire sauce and correct seasoning.

3 To serve, toss the salad greens with 4 to 6 tablespoons (2 to 3 ounces, 60 to 90 ml) of dressing and arrange in the center of 4 plates. Place the warm skate, cut in slices, around the edge of the greens. Season the fish with lemon juice and sprinkle the reserved julienne of carrot and zucchini over. Toss the diced tomato with a little dressing, and place a tablespoon on top of each serving.

4 Spoon the warm sauce over the skate and serve.

## Tarragon Vinaigrette

| AMOUNT | MEASURE | INGREDIENT |
|---|---|---|
| 1 tablespoon | | Shallots, chopped |
| 1 tablespoon | | Chives, chopped |
| 1 tablespoon | $\frac{1}{2}$ ounce, 15 ml | White wine vinegar |
| 1 tablespoon | $\frac{1}{2}$ ounce, 15 ml | Virgin olive oil |
| 1 tablespoon | $\frac{1}{2}$ ounce, 15 ml | Corn oil |
| 1 | | Garlic clove, flattened |
| $\frac{1}{2}$ teaspoon | | Granulated sugar |
| To taste | | Salt and black pepper |
| 1 tablespoon | | Tarragon, chopped |

**PROCEDURE**

1 Combine all ingredients and mix well.

# Roast Belly of Pork with Black Pudding and Apples

SERVES 4

| AMOUNT | MEASURE | INGREDIENT |
|---|---|---|
| 1 cup | 4 ounces, 112 g | Onions, $\frac{1}{4}$ inch (.6 cm) slices |
| 2 tablespoons | | Garlic, chopped |
| 1 tablespoon | | Fresh sage, minced |
| 3 pounds | 1.34 kg | Pork belly, rind removed |
| 2 cups | 16 ounces, 480 ml | Chicken stock |
| $\frac{1}{4}$ cup | 2 ounces, 60 ml | Cider |
| $\frac{1}{8}$ teaspoon | | Allspice |
| $\frac{1}{8}$ teaspoon | | Cinnamon |
| To taste | | Salt and pepper |
| $\frac{1}{4}$ cup | 2 ounces, 56 g | Brown sugar |

**PROCEDURE**

1 Preheat the oven to 325°F (163°C). In a roasting pan, place the onions in a single layer; sprinkle the chopped garlic and half the sage over the onions. Place the pork on top of the onions. Add the stock and pour the cider over the pork. Sprinkle the pork with the allspice, cinnamon, and remaining sage. Cover with aluminum foil and cook, basting every 20 minutes, for 3 hours or until the pork is tender.

2 Uncover and sprinkle with the brown sugar. Increase oven temperature to 400°F (204°C); return to the oven and cook, uncovered, 20 minutes or until glazed and golden brown. Correct seasoning and transfer to a platter and keep warm.

## Sauce

| AMOUNT | MEASURE | INGREDIENT |
|---|---|---|
| 2 cups | 16 ounces, 480 ml | Beef stock |
| 1 tablespoon | | Sage, chopped |

**PROCEDURE**

1 Combine stock and sage and reduce by half. Strain and keep warm.

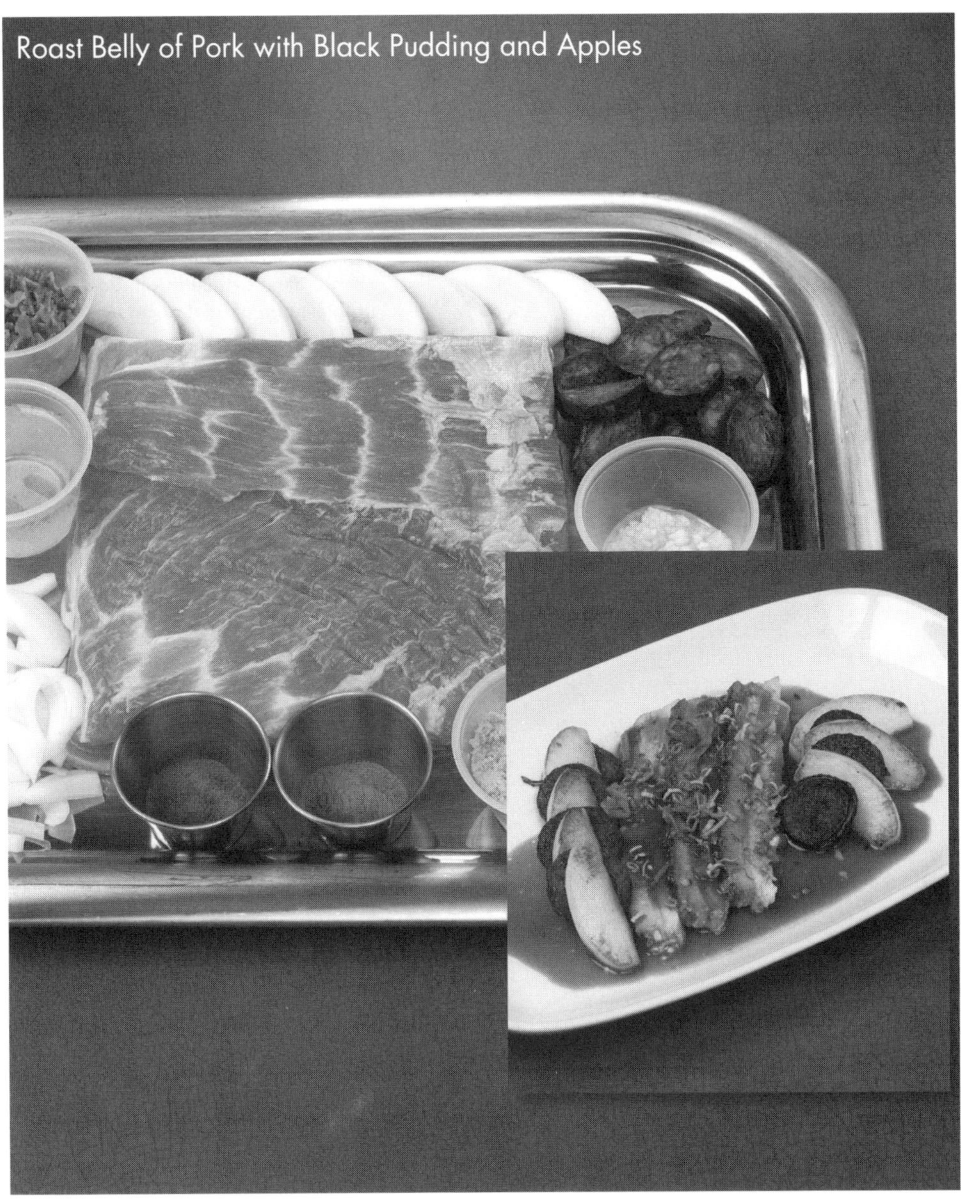

Roast Belly of Pork with Black Pudding and Apples

## Garnish

| AMOUNT | MEASURE | INGREDIENT |
|---|---|---|
| **1 tablespoon** | **$\frac{1}{2}$ ounce, 15 ml** | **Vegetable oil** |
| **4** | **2 ounces, 56 g** | **Black pudding slices, cooked crisp on each side** |
| **1** | | **Granny Smith apple, cut into 8 wedges, cooked in the same pan as the black pudding, until soft. Add 1 tablespoon of oil if necessary** |
| **4 each** | **1 ounce, 28 g** | **Bacon, cooked crisp, crumbled** |

**TO SERVE**

1. Slice pork thin; add any meat juices to the sauce.
2. Serve pork on a plate with sliced black pudding and apple. Spoon the sauce over and top with crumbled bacon.

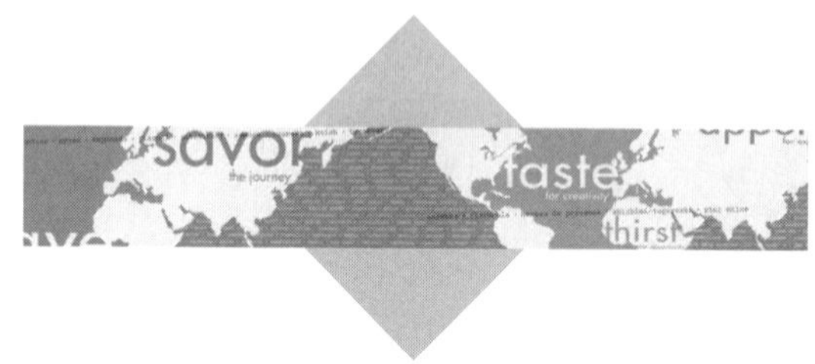

# Colcannon

SERVES 4

| AMOUNT | MEASURE | INGREDIENT |
|---|---|---|
| 2 cups | 8 ounces, 224 g | Cabbage, cored and shredded |
| 4 cups | 20 ounces, 560 g | Russet potatoes, peeled and cut into 2 inch (5 cm) pieces |
| 1 cup | 4 ounces, 112 g | Leeks, white and light green parts, washed and sliced |
| $\frac{1}{2}$ cup | 4 ounces, 120 ml | Milk |
| To taste | | Salt and pepper |
| $\frac{1}{4}$ teaspoon | | Mace |
| 5 tablespoons | $2\frac{1}{2}$ ounces, 75 ml | Butter, cut into small pieces |

**PROCEDURE**

1 Cook cabbage and potatoes separately in boiling salted water until tender, 10–12 minutes. Drain the cabbage and chop. Drain the potatoes and mash.

2 Combine the leeks and milk over medium heat. Bring to a simmer and cook 8 to 10 minutes or until tender. Add the potatoes, salt, pepper, and mace; stir to blend. Add the cabbage and butter; mix well until butter has melted and blended in. Correct seasoning and serve hot.

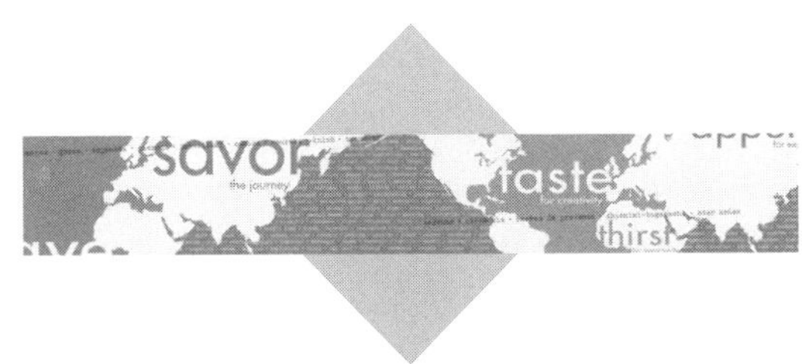

# Irish Soda Bread

SERVES 4

| AMOUNT | MEASURE | INGREDIENT |
|---|---|---|
| $1\frac{1}{2}$ cups | 6 ounces, 168 g | Whole wheat flour |
| 1 cup | 4 ounces, 112 g | All-purpose flour |
| 1 cup | 4 ounces, 112 g | Bread flour |
| $1\frac{1}{2}$ teaspoons | | Baking powder |
| 1 teaspoon | | Salt |
| $1\frac{1}{2}$ cups | 12 ounces, 360 ml | Buttermilk or plain yogurt |

PROCEDURE

1. Preheat oven to 450°F (232°C).
2. Sift together the flours, baking soda, and salt. Make sure to include any bran in the sieve. Stir to mix well.
3. Add the buttermilk, all at once, and mix to form a soft but not sticky dough.
4. Knead 2 minutes on a lightly floured surface, shape the dough into two small balls, and flatten slightly. Cut a deep cross in the dough with a sharp knife. Dust with flour and place on a floured cookie sheet.
5. Bake 10 minutes, then reduce the heat to 400°F (204°C). Bake an additional 25 to 30 minutes. When cooked, the loaf will be well browned and sound hollow when tapped on the bottom. Cool on a wire rack and serve the same day; it becomes stale quickly.

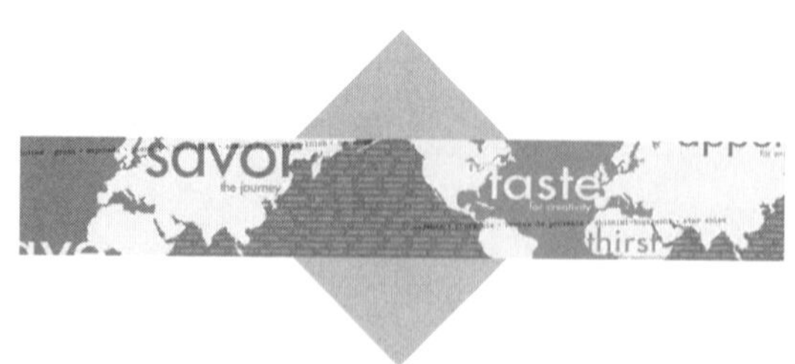

# Dundee Cake

SERVES 4

| AMOUNT | MEASURE | INGREDIENT |
|---|---|---|
| $\frac{3}{4}$ cup | 6 ounces, 168 g | Butter |
| $\frac{2}{3}$ cup | 5 ounces, 140 g | Granulated sugar |
| 4 | | Eggs |
| 2 cups | 8 ounces, 224 g | All-purpose flour |
| $\frac{1}{4}$ cup | 1 ounce, 28 g | Sliced blanched almonds |
| $\frac{1}{4}$ cup | $1\frac{1}{2}$ ounces, 42 g | Mixed candied citrus peel |
| $\frac{1}{2}$ cup | 3 ounces, 84 g | Currants |
| $\frac{1}{2}$ cup | 3 ounces, 84 g | Raisins |
| $\frac{1}{2}$ cup | 3 ounces, 84 g | Sultanas (seedless white raisins) |
| 2 tablespoons | 1 ounce, 30 ml | Fresh lemon juice |
| To taste | | Lemon zest |
| 1 teaspoon | | Baking powder |
| 2 tablespoons | 1 ounce, 30 ml | Irish whisky (optional) or milk |
| 2 tablespoons | 1 ounce, 30 ml | Hot milk |
| 1 tablespoon | $\frac{1}{2}$ ounce, 14 g | Granulated sugar |

PROCEDURE

1. Preheat the oven to 325°F (163°C).
2. Cream the butter and sugar until white and creamy.
3. Add the eggs, one at a time, with one tablespoon of flour with each addition; mix well after each.
4. Stir in the almonds, dried fruit, lemon juice, and lemon zest. Sift flour with baking powder and add. Mix well. Add the whisky or milk. If it is too stiff, add a little milk.
5. Place in an 8-inch (20 cm) greased and lined cake tin. Wet your hands and flatten the top. Cover with foil or parchment paper and bake at 325°F (163°C) 2 hours.
6. After 1 hour, remove the cover. Check the cake with a skewer toward the end of cooking; if it is still wet in the middle, return to the oven for an additional 5 to 10 minutes.
7. Combine the hot milk and sugar and brush top to create a dry glaze.
8. Keep in the pan 15 minutes, then turn out on a wire rack to cool.

# Baked Oysters with Bacon, Cabbage, and Guinness Sabayon

SERVES 4

| AMOUNT | MEASURE | INGREDIENT |
|---|---|---|
| 12 | | Oysters |
| 1 cup | 4 ounces, 224 g | Green cabbage, finely shredded |
| $\frac{1}{2}$ cup | 2 ounces, 56 g | Celery, peeled, finely julienned |
| 1 teaspoon | | Vegetable oil |
| 4 slices | 1 ounce, 28 g | Traditional Irish bacon or Canadian bacon, $\frac{1}{4}$ inch (.6 cm) dice |
| As needed | | Sabayon (recipe follows) |

**PROCEDURE**

1. Preheat oven to 450°F (232°C).
2. Open the oysters, saving the juice and reserving the deeper half of each shell.
3. Rinse the oysters and drain on a paper towel.
4. Rinse and dry the shells, then place on a bed of rock salt.
5. Strain oyster juice through a fine sieve.
6. Blanch cabbage and celery separately in salted boiling water 1 to 2 minutes, or until slightly wilted. Drain and immerse in ice water; drain well again.
7. Heat the oil over medium heat and cook the bacon until crisp. Remove and drain on paper towels. Remove most of the bacon fat from pan.
8. Add the cabbage and celery to pan and sauté just until warm.
9. Combine the oysters and their liquor and poach at a bare simmer until their edges begin to curl, about $1\frac{1}{2}$ minutes.
10. Divide the cabbage and celery mixture among the shells, put an oyster on top of each, and sprinkle the bacon over the oysters.
11. Spoon sabayon over each. Bake 5 minutes, or until the sabayon is just beginning to brown.
12. Grind pepper over the oysters and serve at once.

# Sabayon

| AMOUNT | MEASURE | INGREDIENT |
|---|---|---|
| **4** | | **Egg yolks** |
| **$\frac{1}{2}$ cup** | | **Guinness stout** |
| **$\frac{1}{2}$ teaspoon** | | **Kosher salt** |
| **To taste** | | **Black pepper** |

**PROCEDURE**

1 Combine the egg yolks, Guinness, salt, and pepper over simmering water and beat with a wire whisk until light, fluffy, and just beginning to set, 3 to 5 minutes. The sabayon must not get too hot during the cooking or it will become grainy; if it begins to feel warmer than body temperature, remove the pan briefly from the heat and beat continuously, until the mixture cools. Then return to the heat and continue cooking. When the sabayon has thickened into stable foam, remove from the heat and keep warm.

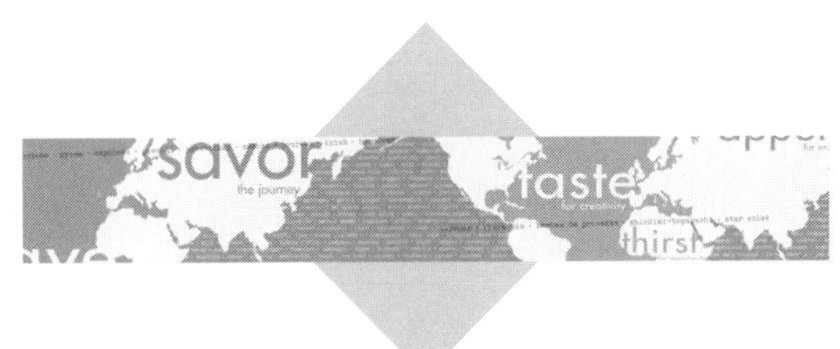

# Crab and Champ Bake

SERVES 4

## Tomato-Watercress Dressing

| AMOUNT | MEASURE | INGREDIENT |
|---|---|---|
| ½ cup | 3 ounces, 84 g | Tomato, peeled, seeded, ¼ inch (.6 cm) dice |
| 1 cup | 4 ounces, 112 g | Watercress, rinsed, stemmed, and coarsely chopped |
| ¼ cup | 2 ounces, 60 ml | Olive oil |
| 1 teaspoon | | Whole grain mustard |
| 1 teaspoon | | Granulated sugar |
| ¼ cup | 2 ounces, 60 ml | Cider vinegar |
| To taste | | Salt and fresh black pepper |

PROCEDURE

1 Combine all ingredients and stir to mix. Correct seasoning and chill.

## Champ

| AMOUNT | MEASURE | INGREDIENT |
|---|---|---|
| 5 cups | 1½ pounds, 672 g | Russet potatoes, peeled, quartered |
| ½ teaspoon | | Salt |
| ¼ cup | 2 ounces, 60 ml | Butter |
| 2 tablespoons | | Green onion, white part only, minced |
| Pinch | | Nutmeg |
| To taste | | Salt and pepper |

PROCEDURE

1 Cover the potatoes with cold water, add salt, bring to a boil, and simmer until tender, about 20 minutes.

2 Drain the potatoes and return to the pot. Cook over low heat about 3 minutes to allow them to dry.

3 Mash, grind, or rice the potatoes.

4 Heat the butter over medium heat; sauté the onion 1 minute, then mix into the potatoes. Season with nutmeg, salt, and pepper.

# Crab Filling

| AMOUNT | MEASURE | INGREDIENT |
|---|---|---|
| **1 ½ tablespoons** | **⅓ ounce, 10 g** | **All-purpose flour** |
| **½ cup** | **4 ounces, 120 ml** | **Fish stock** |
| **1 cup plus 2 tablespoons** | **9 ounces, 300 ml** | **Heavy cream** |
| **¼ teaspoon** | | **Lemon zest** |
| **1 cup** | **8 ounces, 224 g** | **Crabmeat, picked over for shells** |
| **To taste** | | **Salt, pepper, and Tabasco sauce** |
| **¼ cup** | **1 ounces, 56 g** | **Smoked Cheshire cheese or other smoked cheese, grated** |

**PROCEDURE**

1 Preheat oven to 400°F (204°C).

2 Combine the flour with ½ the fish stock; mix until smooth.

3 Over medium heat, combine cream, remaining fish stock, and lemon zest; reduce by ⅓. Mix in fish stock and flour slurry, and cook until thick, 3 to 5 minutes. Remove from heat, stir in the crabmeat, and season with salt, pepper, and Tabasco.

4 Butter four 6-ounce (180 ml) ramekins and place on a baking sheet. Fill halfway with mashed potatoes, fill the top half with crab filling.

5 Bake 15 minutes or until the filling is set. Sprinkle with cheese and brown under the broiler until tops are brown and the cheese bubbles.

6 Serve with a small amount of dressing drizzled around the ramekin and the remaining dressing on the side.

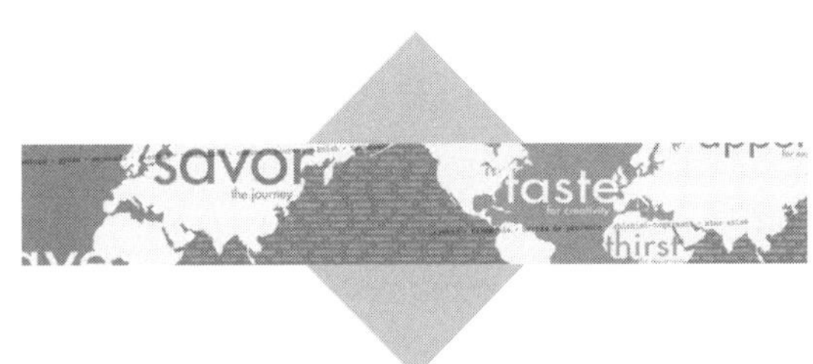

# Stuffed Shoulder of Lamb

SERVES 4

| AMOUNT | MEASURE | INGREDIENT |
|---|---|---|
| 4 cups | 8 ounces, 224 g | Spinach, fresh |
| $\frac{1}{4}$ cup | 2 ounces, 60 ml | Butter |
| 2 tablespoons | | Shallots, minced |
| 1 tablespoon | | Garlic, minced |
| $\frac{1}{4}$ cup | $\frac{1}{2}$ ounce, 14 g | Sun-dried tomatoes, chopped |
| $\frac{1}{4}$ cup | 1 ounce, 28 g | Dried apricots, soaked 15 minutes in warm water, chopped |
| To taste | | Salt and black pepper |
| 3 pounds | 1.36 kg | Lamb shoulder, boned |
| Two 6 x 3 inch strips | Two 15 x 7.5 cm strips | Pork fat |
| $\frac{1}{2}$ cup | 4 ounces, 120 ml | Port or good red wine |
| 1 cup | 8 ounces, 240 ml | Beef stock |
| 2 tablespoons | 1 ounce, 30 ml | Water |
| 1 tablespoon | | Cornstarch |

**PROCEDURE**

1. Blanch the spinach in boiling salted water 1 minute. Drain. Run under cold water and press to remove as much water as possible.
2. Heat the butter over medium heat; sauté the shallots and garlic 3 minutes. Add sun-dried tomatoes and apricots; cook 1 minute.
3. Add spinach and mix well; correct seasoning, remove from heat, and let cool.
4. Lay the lamb skin-side down on a flat surface. Score a cross, about 3 inches (7.5 cm) wide, in the center of the meat. Place stuffing in the center of the meat. Pull the edges of meat up and around the filling to make a neat roll.
5. Wrap the pork fat around the meat and tie tightly with string.
6. Roast at 350°F (176°C) 30 minutes per pound, basting occasionally or until desired doneness is achieved.
7. About 20 minutes before the end of the cooking time, remove the fat.
8. When cooked, remove lamb to a holding platter and let rest 15 minutes.
9. Pour off fat from the roasting pan. Add port and stir to dissolve pan juices. Add stock and reduce by half. Combine water and cornstarch and thicken the sauce if desired.
10. Adjust seasoning and serve sauce with meat.

# Blue Cheese Potato Cakes

SERVES 4

| AMOUNT | MEASURE | INGREDIENT |
|---|---|---|
| 2 cups | 10 ounces, 300 g | Russet potatoes, peeled and cut into 2 inch (5 cm) pieces |
| 2 tablespoons | 1 ounce, 30 ml | Butter |
| 1 tablespoon | | Chives, minced |
| 1 tablespoon | | Garlic, minced |
| 1/4 teaspoon | | Nutmeg |
| To taste | | Salt and fresh black pepper |
| 1 tablespoon | | Fresh dill, minced |
| 1 tablespoon | | Flat-leaf parsley, minced |
| 1/2 cup | 2 ounces, 56 g | Cashel blue cheese or other blue cheese, crumbled |
| 1 | | Egg yolk |
| 1 | | Egg, beaten |
| 1/4 cup | 2 ounces, 60 ml | Milk |
| 1/2 cup | 2 ounces, 56 g | All-purpose flour (breading station) |
| 1 cup | 4 ounces, 112 g | Fresh bread crumbs (breading station) |
| 1 cup | 8 ounces, 240 ml | Oil for pan frying |
| 1/2 cup | 4 ounces, 120 ml | Sour cream for topping (optional) |

PROCEDURE

1. Cook potatoes in salted boiling water until tender, 12 to 15 minutes. Drain and mash.
2. Melt butter over low heat; add chives and garlic and cook until soft, 1 to 2 minutes.
3. Add mashed potatoes, continue to stir; add nutmeg, salt, pepper, dill, and parsley. Remove from heat and cool.
4. When potato mixture is cool, add cheese and egg yolk. The cheese should remain in lumps; do not blend smooth. Shape the mixture into 8 cakes and refrigerate 30 minutes.
5. Combine egg and milk and set up a standard breading station (flour, egg wash, bread crumbs). Process potato cakes through the breading station.
6. Over medium-high heat, bring the oil to 350°F (176°C). Add the cakes and cook 3 to 5 minutes on each side, or until well browned on both sides. Serve hot with sour cream.

# Whole Wheat Scones

SERVES 4

| AMOUNT | MEASURE | INGREDIENT |
|---|---|---|
| $1\frac{1}{2}$ cup | 6 ounces, 168 g | Whole wheat flour |
| $1\frac{1}{2}$ cup | 6 ounces, 168 g | All-purpose flour |
| 2 teaspoons | | Baking powder |
| $\frac{1}{4}$ cup | 2 ounces, 60 ml | Butter |
| 2 teaspoons | | Warm corn syrup |
| $\frac{1}{2}$ cup plus 2 tablespoons | 5 ounces, 150 ml | Milk |
| Pinch | | Salt |

PROCEDURE

1. Preheat the oven to 375°F (190°C).
2. Mix dry ingredients.
3. Add butter and mix until it resembles coarse bread crumbs.
4. Stir in corn syrup and add enough milk to make a soft dough.
5. Turn out on a floured surface and roll out to about $\frac{1}{2}$ inch (1.2 cm) thick. Cut into small rounds with a cutter about $1\frac{1}{2}$ inch (3.8 cm) in diameter. Place the rounds on a floured baking sheet and cook in a preheated oven 10 to 15 minutes. Serve hot, spread with butter.

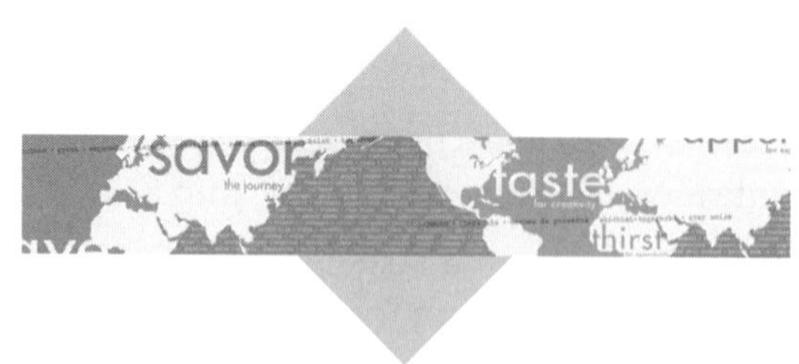

# Caledonian Cream

**Marmalade was developed in Dundee, Scotland, in 1797.**

SERVES 4

| AMOUNT | MEASURE | INGREDIENT |
|---|---|---|
| $\frac{1}{2}$ cup | 4 ounces, 112 g | Cream cheese |
| $\frac{1}{2}$ cup | 4 ounces, 120 ml | Double cream |
| 1 tablespoon | $\frac{1}{2}$ ounce, 15 ml | Bitter orange marmalade |
| 2 tablespoons | 1 ounce, 30 ml | Brandy or rum |
| 2 teaspoons | | Fresh lemon juice |
| To taste | | Granulated sugar |
| 4 | | Oranges, segmented, pith removed |
| 2 tablespoons | | Orange zest, blanched 30 seconds in boiling water and cooled |

PROCEDURE

1. In a blender, combine all ingredients except orange segments. Blend smooth; adjust sweetness with sugar.
2. Toss orange segments with additional brandy or rum, if desired.
3. Serve chilled, with cream on top of oranges. Garnish with orange zest.

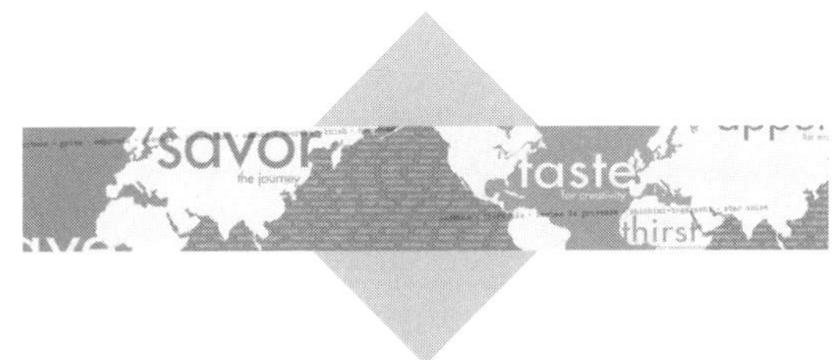

# France

## The Land

France is located in western Europe. It borders the English Channel and the Bay of Biscay to the west; the Mediterranean Sea to the south; Italy, Germany, Switzerland, and Belgium to the east; and Spain and Andorra to the southwest. The unique geography of France allows it to connect to all major western European nations by the land or the sea. France is connected to the UK by the English Channel Tunnel, and by land to Spain, Italy, Switzerland, Germany, and Belgium. The French coastline provides access by sea to northern Europe, America, and Africa via the North Sea, the Atlantic Ocean, and the Mediterranean.

France is the largest country in western Europe and the second largest country in Europe, with the fifth largest population in Europe. Over two-thirds of France is covered with mountains and hills, with the Alps, Pyrenees, and Vosges mountains the primary ranges. The Vosges mountains lie in northeast France, while the Pyrenees are sprawled along the Spanish border. Europe's highest peak, Mont Blanc, lies in the French Alps near the Italian and Swiss borders. Major rivers include the west-flowing Seine, the Loire, and the Garonne; the south-flowing Rhone that drains into the Mediterranean; and the Rhine River that forms the border with Germany. The topography chiefly comprises flat plains or gently rolling hills in the north and west, while the rest of the country is mountainous. It lies midway between the equator and the North Pole and enjoys a temperate climate. France generally has cool winters and mild summers, but the warm Gulf Stream current along the Mediterranean coast provides for mild winters and hot summers in the coastal region.

# History

The history of France is filled with tales of aristocrats, wars, and revolutions that have played a major role in its emergence as one of the most developed nations of the world.

In ancient times, France was a part of Celtic territory called Gaul. The Romans, led by Julius Caesar, captured Gaul in the first century B.C. During the second century A.D. Christianity gained a strong foothold in this region and thus became the major religion.

During the fourth century A.D., a German tribe called the Franks captured the eastern side of Gaul, along the banks of the River Rhine. By the seventh century, the entire region was taken over by the Franks. The Treaty of Verdun and the division of Charlemagne's Carolingian Empire into three parts (East Francia, Middle Francia, and West Francia) in 843 A.D. actually led to the emergence of France as a separate country. Over the years the country was ruled by the monarchy and royal dynasties like the Capetians, Valois, and finally the Bourbons.

The French monarchy reached its height in the seventeenth century during the reign of King Louis XIV. During his rule, the country became extremely powerful. Trade flourished and the country became a center for art and culture. The rule of the French monarchy, however, came to an end after the French Revolution of 1789, and the execution of the King Louis XVI and his wife, Queen Marie Antoinette. The French Revolution was a major event in the history of France and to the rest of the world. In 1799, Napoleon Bonaparte took control of France; he ruled from 1804 to 1814. After his defeat in the Battle of Waterloo in 1815, the monarchy was reestablished.

France had numerous colonial territories and it had the second largest holdings after those of the British Empire. France's ultimate victory in World War I and World War II after initially being invaded and partly occupied by German forces did not prevent the loss of the colonial empire, the comparative economic status, population, and status as a dominant nation state. Over the years the country has fought many wars, including the French Indochina War and a war with Algeria. France signed a peace declaration with Algeria in 1962 to bring an end to its colonial rule in that country.

In recent decades, France's reconciliation and cooperation with Germany have proved central to the political and economic integration of the evolving European Union, including the introduction of the euro in January 1999. France has been at the forefront of European Union member states seeking to exploit the momentum of the monetary union to create a more unified and capable European Union based on political, defense, and security apparatus. However, the French electorate voted against ratification of the European Constitutional Treaty in May 2005.

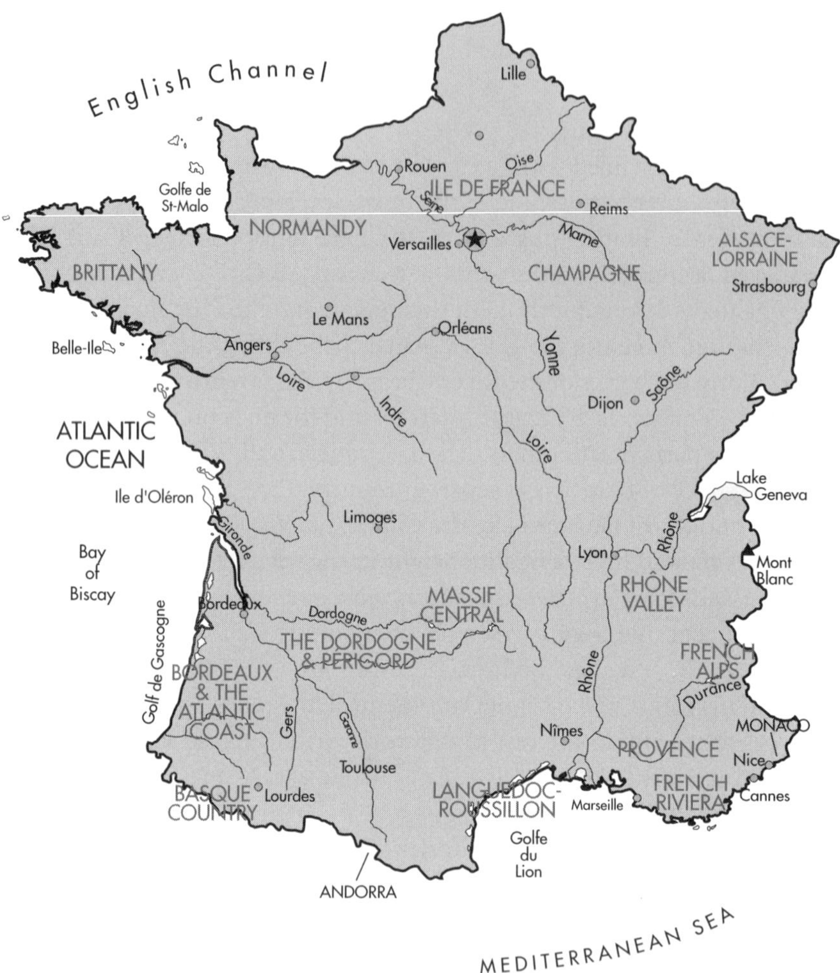


France

# The People

Until recently French culture has been characterized by tradition and continuity. Although much of the French identity comes from past glories and long-standing customs, the country has been faced in the last few decades with the realization that neither its history nor its traditional ways will be enough to keep the country peaceful and productive or a vital force on the international stage.

The twentieth century was a difficult one for France. The country that produced Charlemagne and Napoleon was occupied by Germany in two world wars, requiring rescue by nations it had seen as its cultural inferior. The country that had produced great humanitarians such as Voltaire and Rousseau was the only European nation to collaborate actively and officially with the Nazis. Its status after the war was questioned.

Though Charles de Gaulle was able to rekindle a sense of French pride, the post-WWII era was again a struggle. The student protests of 1968, which quickly grew to involve a wider range of people than had ever participated in protests before, raised issues that have not been fully resolved even today. Likewise, the dark side of French pride, the tolerance of intolerance, still has a negative impact on millions of French citizens. Yet France, according to historians and social scientists, seems more ready than ever to tackle its social issues, rather than assuming that the nation can continue as it always has.

# The Food

Since the sixteenth century, French cooking has been celebrated as the Western world's finest. Recipes prepared in the traditional style of haute cuisine, as developed by such renowned chefs as Jean-Anthelme Brillat-Savarin (1755–1826) or Georges Auguste Escoffier (1847–1935) are still featured in distinguished restaurants. This style features meats and fish prepared with sauces containing cream, egg yolks, sugar, brandy, flour, and other starches. Today's concern with dieting and health has produced a new style of cooking. Nouvelle cuisine, said to have been introduced by Paul Bocuse, emphasizes lighter, subtler tastes, requiring the best and the freshest raw ingredients. The term itself was created by two well-known food critics, Henri Gault and Christian Millau.

The diversity of French cuisine is due to the cultural influences and ingredients available in France's different regions. The French landscape is so varied that an accurate description requires breaking it down into nine separate geographic categories: the Paris Basin, northeastern France, the Rhone-Saone Valley, the Alps-Jura region, the Central Plateau, northwestern France, the Riviera, the Acquitaine Basin, and the Pyrenees Mountains.

## THE PARIS BASIN

The Paris Basin occupies north central France. This vast fertile plain is one of the world's richest farming areas. The city of Paris has played a unique role in French life. Ever since the Middle Ages, it has been not only the nation's capital, but also the leading center of culture, learning, the arts, fashion, commerce, and industry. Though there is no single culinary style, the area is referred to as "the garden of France." Numerous types of fruit and vegetables are grown, and fruit tarts are common—tarte tatin originated in the Loire River Valley in the south of the Basin. Game, from the Sologne forests in the east of the region, is a common ingredient in the region's excellent charcuterie.

Freshwater fish, particularly pike, shad, and eels, caught from the Loire and its tributaries are featured widely on menus. These are often accompanied by beurre blanc, an emulsified sauce made with a reduction of acid (which may be vinegar, wine, or citrus juice) and shallots into which cold, whole butter is blended.

Even better known as one of the world's premier wine-growing areas is the nearby province of Burgundy, east of the Loire valley. Few red wines produced anywhere are more cherished than Burgundirs. People eat well in Burgundy and the region boasts some of the best produce and meats. The cuisine is delicate without being overly fussy. Common components are pork, beef, chicken, onions, mushrooms, garlic, snails, and cream. Many of the traditional dishes are well known outside France, such as *coq au vin* (chicken in a red wine, mushroom, and onion sauce) and *bœuf à la bourguignonne* (beef stewed in red wine with mushrooms and onions). Other regional specialities include *marcassin farci au saucisson* (young wild boar with a sausage stuffing), *escargots à la bourguignonne* (snails raised on grape leaves, sautéed and served with parsley and garlic butter) and meat or fish dishes *en meurette* (in a red wine sauce). This region is also known for its wide variety of mustards; the city of Dijon is located in this region. Kir—blackcurrant liqueur mixed with white wine—is an aperitif from Burgundy.

Champagne is another province along Paris Basin's easternmost sections renowned for its vineyards. Its gently rolling terrain and chalky soil are ideal for cultivation of the grapes from which the celebrated sparkling wine is produced. The *méthode champenoise* for making champagne was invented by Dom Pérignon, a monk. Once the wine has been fermented and blended, a mix of cane sugar and yeast is added into the bottle to induce a second fermentation and produce the sparkle. It is left to mature for between one and five years, then the cork and any sediment is removed and the sweetness adjusted before being recorked and sold.

The Paris Basin's western region is along the Belgian border so there are also rich dishes of Flemish influence. The cooler climate lends itself to growing potatoes, cabbages, beets, watercress, endive, and leeks. *Flamiche* is a simple dish of leeks cooked with cream and eggs in a pastry crust. *Endive flamande* is made by wrapping endives in ham and serving them with a white sauce. *Carbonnade de boeuf* is another classic dish, where the beef is slowly braised in onions and beer. A stew called *chaudrée* (hence the word chowder) makes good use of the region's fish. The city of Lille is an important producer of charcuterie and beer. Pastries are quite basic, with *gaufres* (waffles eaten with sugar and fresh cream) being among the best known. In Champagne, *biscuits de Reims* are sweet, paper-thin macaroons.

## NORTHEASTERN FRANCE

Northeastern France consists mainly of the provinces of Alsace and Lorraine. Control of Alsace and Lorraine has gone back and forth between France and Germany over the centuries and this influence is evident in many of the local dishes. Pickled cabbage and pork are common. *Baeckeoffe* is a stew of marinated beef, pork, and mutton stewed with onions and potatoes in wine. *Choucroute alsacienne* is pickled cabbage flavored with juniper berries and served with sausages, bacon, or pork knuckle. The locals also enjoy all kinds of savory pies and tarts, the best-known being *tarte flambée* or *flammekuche,* which is a thin layer of pastry topped with cream, onion, and bacon and cooked in a wood-fired oven. The region is ideal for growing grains, which give Alsace a well-known reputation for the excellence and variety of its breads. Hops are also grown here and Alsace is the only region in France that brews beer. The fruit orchards, besides giving wonderful fruits, also foster the production of a variety of fruit-flavored brandies, known as *eaux-de-vie.*

From Lorraine comes the most famous of all, *quiche Lorraine*. Originally, this dish was made without cheese, but most recipes now include it and also add vegetables, seafood, or ham to the basic mix of eggs and cream.

## THE RHONE-SAONE VALLEY

Located in east central France, Lyons is this region's most important city. It dates back to the time of the ancient Gauls and today it ranks as France's second city. The Lyonnaise take pride in their city's reputation as a world capital of good eating and it is said that gastronomy is to Lyon what haute couture fashion is to Paris. The most obvious reason for Lyon's reputation as a leading gastronomic center of the world is that it is so well situated: it has access to the very best food supplies. It is near the Dauphine, one of the first regions of France where potatoes were successfully cultivated (in the seventeenth century). It is near the Charolais for beef, the farms of Bresse for poultry, the Auvergne for lamb, the lakes of the Dombes and Bourget for carp and frogs, Savoy for mushrooms, and innumerable rivers for fish.

It was a native of Lyons, the renowned chef Anthelme Brillat-Savarin, who said, "Tell me what you eat and I'll tell you who you are." Lyon's culinary fame is based on two main styles of cooking: hearty home cooking that uses seasonal vegetables and organ meats (offal, tripe, chicken gizzards, liver, and hearts), and the loftier traditional cuisine.

Classic bistros known as bouchons are an integral part of the gastronomic heritage of Lyon. *Bouchons* do not have the reputation of being fancy restaurants, though they offer a wide variety of meals, among which are the famous *pâté aux foies de volailles* (chicken liver pate), *quenelles* (light dumplings made of meat, fish, or cheese), *sauce nantua* (a crayfish butter béchamel), and *cervelle de canut* (traditionally, a farmhouse-style cheese would be used for this cream cheese spread/dip; the rather derogatory name translates as "silk weaver's brains," and is thought to reflect the poor regard in which the richer community held weavers). Bouchons offer a warm, convivial atmosphere, where customers sit elbow to elbow with a glass pot, the quintessential Lyon container filled with local wine.

### THE ALPS-JURA REGION

The mountainous Alps-Jura region is directly east of the Rhone valley. It borders on Switzerland and Italy. Rising to the south are the lofty French Alps. The Ognon and Doubs rivers, as well as the mountain lakes, provide a plentiful supply of fish, particularly salmon, and the forests are a good source of game. Fondue, and cheese in general, is common. For example, *brochette jurassienne* (pieces of cheese wrapped in ham and fried on a skewer) or *escalope de veau belle comtoise* (veal escalopes covered in breadcrumbs and baked with slices of ham and cheese) are classic dishes. Other specialities include *brési* (cured beef in thin slices) and *poulet au vin jaune* (chicken and morels in a creamy sauce flavored with the local wine).

### THE CENTRAL PLATEAU

Largest of the geographic regions, sprawling across south central France, is the forbidding, thinly populated Massif Central, or Central Plateau. It takes up one-sixth of the entire country. The province of Auvergne is a remote and rural region; its traditional cuisine is simple and filling. Dishes often feature a combination of pork, cabbage, potatoes, and cheese, such as *potée auvergnate,* a souplike stew of pork and cabbage with potatoes, onions, turnips, leeks, and garlic. A common accompaniment to meat is *truffade,* mashed potatoes made with cheese and then fried with bacon and garlic. A well-known local specialty is Roquefort cheese, made from sheep's milk. Roquefort-sur-Soulzon, the village where the cheese is produced, sits on top of a cliff. The cheese is aged in deep caves, noted for their high humidity and cool, even temperatures all year—46°F. A penicillin fungus that grows naturally in the caves is added to the cheese to produce its unique flavor. The process dates back to Roman times.

### NORTHWESTERN FRANCE

Northwestern France is dominated by the rocky Amorican Plateau. The area is largely taken up by the provinces of Normandy and Brittany. Each forms a peninsula protruding into the Atlantic Ocean.

Normandy is famous for raising fine brindled cattle. The milk of Norman cattle is unusually creamy, with a high fat content that is perfect for fatty cheese such as Camembert, as well as the rich, slightly salty Normandy butter. Normandy boasts extensive apple orchards. They produce a special variety of apple too small and bitter tasting for eating; instead, they are used for cider and calvados. Traditional dishes invariably feature creamy sauces laced with apples, cider, or calvados, such as *filet mignon de porc normande* (pork tenderloin cooked with apples and onions in cider and served with caramelized apple rings). The proximity of the sea means that fish and seafood feature commonly on menus. Favorites include *moules à la normande* (mussels in a cream and white wine sauce) and *sole normande* (Dover sole poached in cider and cream with shrimp). There are also some good meats. The lamb and mutton from the Cherbourg peninsula are rated very highly, as are the *andouilles from Vire* (smoked and cooked pork and tripe sausage, usually served cold as a starter). Rouen is known as the gastronomic capital of Normandy, famous for its duck dishes such as duck with cherries and *canard à la Rouennaise,* duck stuffed with its liver and cooked in red wine.

Brittany presents a bleaker landscape. Large areas are too rocky and barren for cultivation, though they do supply sparse grazing for cattle. Brittany tends to set itself apart from the rest of France, so it is surprising that it does not have its own distinctive style of cooking. Generally, Breton cuisine is simple, with little use of sauces, and features much fish and seafood. The only true Breton specialty is the pancake. *Crêperies* are a common sight, offering a range of savory and sweet pancakes (*galettes* and *crêpes,* respectively). The other regional dish is *cotriade,* a fish stew traditionally made from conger eel and the remains of the day's catch. Other specialties include *palourdes farcies* (baked clams stuffed with garlic, herbs, and shallots) or *pot au feu d'homard* (lobster, shrimp, scallop, mussel, and oyster stew). Brittany's young lambs, raised on the salt meadows, are also very good. Cider is the main drink associated with Brittany.

### THE RIVIERA

The best-known area within the Mediterranean region is the spectacularly scenic Riviera, with its mountains loping abruptly down to the coastal plain and the popular beaches. Nice and Cannes are the largest resort cities. Not far from the Italian border is glamorous Monte Carlo, capital of the tiny independent principality of Monaco.

France's busiest seaport, Marseilles, stands between the Riviera and the Rhone River. Marseilles is the main point of focus for trade between France, the Mediterranean region, and the vast world to the south and east. The mild Mediterranean climate ensures farmers a longer growing season than elsewhere in France. The lower valley of the Rhone is France's richest garden area, producing peaches, melons, strawberries, and asparagus. Olive and almond groves that are hundreds of years old are scattered across the region. West of the Rhone is an area devoted mostly to vineyards. They produce grapes suitable only for vin ordinaire, a good but inexpensive type of wine that is rarely exported.

Inland lies Provence, a region rich in history and tradition. Provençal cuisine is known for its use of herbs, olive oil, tomatoes, garlic, onions, artichokes, olives, and sweet and hot peppers. Dishes prepared *á la provençale* are made with tomatoes, garlic, olive oil, onions, herbs, and sometimes eggplant, while dishes made *á la niçoise* are similar but also include olives, capers, anchovies, and tarragon. It's not an area famous for its meat dishes, but a winter staple is *boeuf en daube* (beef stewed with red wine, onions, garlic, vegetables, and herbs). Fish and shellfish—sardines, red mullet, tuna, monkfish, sea bass, and anchovies—are commonly found on menus, even inland, and are often accompanied by *raï to* or *rayte* (red wine, tomato, garlic, and ground walnut sauce). Other fish dishes include *bouillabaisse* (stewlike soup with conger eel, scorpion fish, gurnet, and other fish; saffron, fennel, garlic, and bitter orange peel, served with garlic mayonnaise) and *soupe aux poissons* (smooth soup made from white fish and a chile and garlic mayonnaise). Slowly cooked stews such as *estouffade* and *daube* are based on beef or mutton. On the Côte d'Azur, Italian influences are noticeable, with wide use of pasta, especially ravioli and cannelloni, gnocchi, and *pistou* (similar to pesto).

Sharing the Mediterranean climate is the French island of Corsica about 120 miles to the southeast. This mountainous, heavily forested locale permits little farming. Its people fish and raise livestock.

## THE AQUITAINE BASIN

The gently rolling Aquitaine Basin occupies the area of southwestern France between the Central Plateau and the Atlantic. Fruit orchards and vineyards fill the river valleys. The region's primary river, the Garrone, flows in a northwesterly direction to the famous harbor of Bordeaux. It has given its name to the famous Bordeaux wines produced from the nearby vineyards. Grapes grown in the Cognac district to the north and the Armagnac district to the south are the raw material for well-known brandies. Bordeaux is known for its meat and its most celebrated dish is *entrecôte marchand de vin* (rib steak cooked in a rich gravy made from Bordeaux wine, butter, shallots, herbs, and bone marrow). Sweet treats include *cannelés* (caramelised brioche-style pastries) and the famous *marrons glacés* (candied chestnuts).

East of Bordeaux is a small agricultural district known as the Périgord. For such a rural region, the cuisine is surprisingly sophisticated. Two common ingredients are truffles (used in soups, sauces, pâtés, stuffing, and in meat preparations) and *foie gras* (enlarged liver of goose or duck that has been force-fed maize). Items on menus that are served *à la périgourdine* are stuffed with, accompanied by, or have a sauce of *foie gras* and truffles. *Ballottine de lièvre á la périgourdine* is hare stuffed with veal, rabbit, or pork, foie gras, and truffles, and flavored with brandy. *Cassoulet périgourdin* is a stew of mutton, haricot beans, garlic sausage, and goose neck stuffed with truffles and *foie gras*. Food is often cooked in goose fat, giving the cuisine its own distinctive taste. Walnut oil is a common salad dressing.

In the southernmost section of the Aquitaine, on the Atlantic coast and in the foothills of the Pyrenees, lives a unique culture, the Basques. They are a people apart from any in France or indeed any in Europe. Their place of origin is unknown. There are about a million Basques, but 90 percent of them live across the border in Spain. Languedoc-Roussillon, Gascony, and Basque country cooking use an abundance of olive oil, tomatoes, peppers, and spicy sausage; their food shares many similarities with that of Spain. *Cassoulet* (a casserole with meat and beans) is Languedoc's signature dish; Roussillon has a similar dish called *ouillade*. There are strong Spanish and Catalan influences in Roussillon too, with tapas-style dishes served in many wine bars. Gascon dishes are kept simple but hearty with lots of meat, fat, and salt. *Garbure* is a thick stew made with vegetables, herbs, spices, and preserved meats. *Poulet Basque* is a chicken stew with tomatoes, onions, peppers, and white wine; piperade is Basque comfort cooking (peppers, onions, and tomatoes cooked with ham and eggs). *Chipirones* (squid cooked in its own ink) is featured widely on menus along the coast. A common sweet is *gâteau basque* (black cherry pie). The locally prepared Bayonne ham is usually eaten sliced with bread but is also the basis of *jambon á la Bayonnaise* (ham braised in Madeira).

### THE PYRENEES MOUNTAINS

The Pyrenees Mountains loom south of the Aquitaine Basin. They form a range running nearly 280 miles in an east-west direction. With many peaks rising above 10,000 feet, the Pyrenees make a formidable barrier between France and Spain. Cattle and sheep graze along these hillsides. The cuisine, drawing on the wealth of local produce, has strong flavors. Particularly in the Pyrenees, Catalan dishes such as *boles de picoulat* (meatballs made with onions and olives in a sauce of tomatoes and herbs) and *saucisse à la catalane* (sausage fried with garlic, orange peel, and herbs) feature widely on menus. Game such as guinea fowl and partridge is common, as is trout from the mountain streams. Along the coast in the Mediterranean seacoast town of Collioure, dishes are served in a sauce of anchovy-and garlic-flavored mayonnaise.

# Glossary

**Aiguillettes** Long, thin strips of duck breast.

**Aioli** A sauce from Provence, similar to mayonnaise but heavily flavored with garlic; the Spanish version is called ali-oil (garlic oil).

**Allspice** A berry from the allspice tree. Pungent and aromatic, primarily used in pickling liquids, marinades, and spice cakes and fruitcakes.

**Americaine** Refers to a garnish of tomatoes and garlic, originally created for a lobster dish.

**Amoricaine** Refers to dishes that originated in Amorica, the Roman name for Brittany.

**Ancienne** Usually refers to dishes with a long history; often two or more garnishes are combined.

**Andalouse** Usually refers to a dish characterized by tomato paste, sweet peppers, and chipolata sausages.

**Anise** Sweet-smelling herb with feathery leaves producing aniseed; anise is the true taste of licorice.

**AOC** Appelation d'Origine Controlee, which roughly translates to "term of origin," is a certification granted to certain French wines, cheeses, butters, and other agricultural products by a government bureau known as the *Institut National des Appellations d'Origine* (INAO). Under French law, it is illegal to manufacture and sell a product under one of the AOC-controlled names if it does not comply with the criteria established by the AOC.

**Argenteuil** Refers to a dish that includes asparagus. The Argenteuil region (a suburb of Paris) has sandy soil in which the best asparagus used to grow.

**Aspic** Clear jelly used to coat cold foods.

**Attelets** Small skewers with ornamental heads used to decorate very elaborate dishes.

**Aurore (Sunrise)** A sauce or dish flavored with tomato paste or tomatoes.

**Babas** Small raisin-filled yeast cakes that are soaked in rum-flavored sugar syrup after baking.

**Batterie de Cuisine** French term for cooking equipment.

**Bavarian Cream (Bavarois)** A rich egg custard stiffened or set with gelatin and whipped cream added.

**Béchamel** A white sauce made from milk infused with flavoring and thickened with a roux.

**Beignets** Light French fritters made from choux pastry, or dipped in batter and deep-fat-fried.

**Bigarade** Means bitter.

**Bisque** A highly seasoned thick, creamy soup, classically of pureed crustaceans, thickened with rice.

**Blanquette** A stew of lamb, veal, chicken, or rabbit with a rich sauce made from the cooking liquid, often garnished with small onions and mushrooms.

**Bleu** A method of cooking trout in a vinegar-flavored court bouillon. Fresh-killed trout take on a bluish tinge.

**Bombe** A molded ice cream that is made in a traditional bomb-shaped mold, almost spherical with a flat bottom.

**Bonne Femme** Literally "good woman"; refers to traditional garnish of onion, bacon, and potato.

**Bordelaise** A dish containing red or white Bordeaux wine and beef marrow.

**Bouillabaisse** A Mediterranean fish stew that originated in Marseilles. Traditionally served in two dishes, one for the pieces of fish and the other containing slices of French bread with the broth poured on top.

**Boulangere** French for "baker"; refers to meat or poultry cooked on a bed of sliced potatoes. At one time, small houses in country districts of France had no ovens, so the Sunday lunch of leg of lamb was set in a dish with sliced potatoes and onions, which was left with the local baker to cook while the family was at church.

**Bourgeoise** Garnish of diced bacon, baby onions, and carrots cut to a consistent size.

**Bourguignonne** Cooked in the style of Burgundy, with mushrooms, onions, and red Burgundy wine.

**Braisiére** The traditional pan for braising, designed for kitchens that did not have an oven. The pan has an indented lid, in which live coals were placed so that the pan was heated from the top as well as from the bottom.

**Brandade** A mousse of salt cod (morue). *Brandade de morue* originally comes from Nimes in the Languedoc region of southern France.

**Bretonne** Cooked in the style of Brittany, on the northwest coast of France; beans are usually included in the dish.

**Brioche** Rich yeast dough; high egg and butter content give it a rich and tender crumb.

**Broche** To cook on a spit.

**Brochette (en)** Term for small pieces threaded on a skewer and broiled.
**Butter**

> **Beurre Blanc** White butter sauce.
>
> **Beurre Manie (Kneaded Butter)** A liaison of twice as much butter as flour worked together into an uncooked paste, added in small pieces to thicken a liquid at the end of cooking.
>
> **Beurre Noir** Also called black butter, it is heated until the solids turn a darker brown, then a few drops of vinegar are added.
>
> **Beurre Noisette** Literally, "hazelnut butter," this is melted butter that's cooked until the milk solids turn a very light brown, and the butter gives off a nutty aroma. When clarified at this point, this butter is called *ghee* in Indian cooking.

**Calvados** Apple brandy.

**Canape** Small open-faced, garnished pieces of bread or toast, they are always small (one or two bites) and served as an appetizer or with cocktails.

**Carbonade** Originally a dish that was simmered over coals (charbon), now it refers to a rich beef stew made with ale or beer.

**Cardinal** A dish characterized by a sauce with a red color; for savory dishes the sauce usually contains lobster coral (roe), tomato paste, or pimiento; and for sweet dishes a strawberry or raspberry sauce.

**Cassolettes** Containers made from pastry or vegetables such as cucumber.

**Cassoulet** A rich, slow-cooked bean stew or casserole originating in the southwest of France, typically containing pork sausages, pork, goose, duck, and sometimes mutton; pork skin (*couennes*); and white haricot beans.

**Celeriac (Celery Root)** Large knobby root resembling a turnip or rutabaga with a taste of celery.

**Cepes** Wild mushrooms; known as porcini mushrooms in Italy and *Steinpilzen* in Germany.

**Chasseur** Means "hunter-style"; refers to a mushroom garnish flavored with shallots and white wine.

**Chaudfroid** Means "hot-cold"; typically refers to a cold dish that is first coated with a cold velouté or béchamel-based sauce, then coated with a layer of aspic.

**Cheese**

**Abondance** Cow's milk cheese with both a fruity and nutty flavor and a unique aroma.

**Banon** Goat's milk cheese, a mild soft cheese with a nutty flavor and a firm supple texture. As it ripens, the surface of the cheese takes on the color of a leaf, and the odor of wet earth.

**Beaufort** Cow's milk cheese, aromatic, fruity, and vegetable-like.

**Bleu d'Auvergne** Cow's milk blue cheese with a spicy, nutty strong flavor.

**Bleu de Gex, Bleu du Haut-Jura** Cow's milk, blue cheese, soft and creamy, sometimes a bit crumbly; it is mild with a hint of hazelnut.

**Bleu des Causses** Cow's milk blue cheese; the flavor is spicy, nutty, and strong.

**Brie** The name is applied to big, round, soft cheeses with white mold. On average they have a diameter of 28 cm. The taste is aromatic, with mushroom and hazelnut overtones.

**Brie de Meaux** Cow's milk soft cheese with a hazelnut, herb, lightly acidic and fruity taste, known as "the cheese of kings."

**Brie de Melun** Known as the "little brother" of Brie de Meaux, it is small in size. Its aroma is much stronger, more robust, and saltier. It has a slightly bitter taste that, if left to unfold, develops into a completely soft, hazelnut and fruit flavor.

**Brillat-Savarin** Soft, bloomy-rind cow's milk cheese; it has a finely acidic taste with tender or creamy consistency.

**Brocciu** Ewe's and goat's milk cheese, with a very creamy and fresh taste.

**Cabecou du Perigourda** Raw goat's milk cheese; the taste is goaty and soft on the palate.

**Camembert de Normandie** Cow's milk soft cheese, fresh, lightly acidic, ripe, fruity, mushroom flavored. Camembert is perfectly ripe when the body is the same supple, butter-smooth texture throughout.

**Cantal** Firm cow's milk cheese with a taste of hazelnut and fresh milk.

**Chabichou** A whole-milk goat cheese and one of the best French goat cheeses. It has a light and goaty aroma. It is very creamy and soft.

**Comté** The very first cheese to gain French AOC status, protecting its manufacturing and maturing methods. It is a cow's milk, pressed, and cooked cheese, with a nutty and rich but clean flavor, with a fruity aftertaste.

**Crottin de Chavigol** Small cylindrical shaped cheese, the flavor is subtle and slightly nutty. Young cheese is solid and compact, as it ages it becomes crumbly and the mold on the rind matures into a bluish color.

**Emmental** Has been produced since at least the thirteenth century in the Rhône-Alpes region. It is a hard cheese made from cow's milk, cooked and pressed. There are many holes (also called eyes) inside it. A good Emmental must have at least three holes every 6 inches. Its taste is fruity with a subtle nutty core, and its aroma is very delicate.

**Fourme d'Ambert** A tangy representative of the French variety of blue mold cheeses. It has quite strong mold veins and a yellowish-gray rind. Its flavor is mild, with light nut and mushroom overtones.

**Laguiole** Pressed, uncooked cow's milk cheese with an aromatic, lightly acidic, herbal, strong, tangy-sour taste.

**Langres** Soft cheese, with red culture; the rind has an intense smell. The flavor is full but quite salty.

**Maconnais** Goat cheese, which becomes harder, saltier, and tangy with ripening. It has an ivory-colored rind which becomes brown with age. Soft cheese with a fresh milky flavor when young, becoming dry and crumbly with maturity.

**Morbier** Cow's milk cheese; melting, lightly fruity and aromatic are all characteristics of this sliced cheese with a beige-colored rind and ivory-colored dough.

**Neufchâtel** The slight tangy and sour soft cheese with white mold is available in six different shapes and sizes. Especially characteristic of Neufchâtel is the shape of a heart.

**Ossau Iraty** A ewe's milk cheese from the Basque region. Nutty, aromatic, vegetable-like taste.

**Pasteurized Camembert** Less strong and more neutral than Camembert de Normandie.

**Pélardon** Pélardon of the Cévennes is one of the oldest goat's milk cheeses in Europe; it has a goat's milk flavor, light and nutty.

**Pont-l'Eveque** This soft, washed-rind cow's milk cheese may be the oldest cheese variety from Normandy that is still produced today. It is a very flavorful cheese, with a lightly herbal taste.

**Pouligny Saint-Pierre** With a characteristic cone shape, this goat cheese has the nickname pyramid or Eiffel tower. It has a smooth goat's milk taste, a bit sour, and a nutty aroma.

**Reblochon** Cow's milk cheese, full-flavored, buttery, and creamy.

**Rocamadour** Goat's milk cheese, with a fresh, lightly acidic, heavy, ripe, and nutty taste.

**Roquefort** Ewe's milk cheese, from the south of France, characterized by its very white body pierced by blue-green mold veins. It is exceptionally smooth and rich on the palate. It has a ewe's milk flavor, tangy, salty, and strong. Even today, this cheese can only be ripened in the natural stone caves of Mont Combalou in the community of Roquefort-sur-Sulzon.

**Saint-Maure de Touraine** The most obvious way to identify this cheese is by the straw through its center. The straw is there to keep the roll-formed cheese together and to allow air through to the core. This goat's milk cheese has a subtle flavor with a slight hint of mushroom.

**Saint-Nectaire** The supple, white center melts in the mouth and unfolds a fine, bitter flavor with a touch of salt, walnuts, and spices.

**Salers** Cow's milk, pressed, uncooked cheese that is firm, very aromatic, and fruity.

**Tome des Bauges (or Tome de Savoie)** Cow's milk cheese, with a semisoft texture and a mild, creamy taste.

**Valencay** Goat's milk cheese, with a mild, lightly nutty taste.

**Chervil** Herb that is a member of the parsley family. It is sweeter and more aromatic than parsley.

**Clamart** A dish garnished with peas, often piled onto artichoke bottoms. Clamart is a suburb of Paris where peas used to be grown.

**Compote** Term for fresh or dried fruit poached in a thick simple syrup to which flavorings may be added.

**Coulis** French for a puree of any liquid pulp.

**Cream of Tartar** Juice from grapes that is pressed out after fermentation, then refined to powder. It is used as a leavening agent, to keep egg whites firm and to cut the grain of sugar syrup and prevent it from crystallizing.

**Crecy** A dish characterized by carrots.

**Crepe** A very thin French pancake that can be sweet or savory.

**Cressonniere** Refers to a dish garnished or made with watercress.

**Croissants** French pastries that are made into the shape of crescents.

**Croustade** A case made from pastry or bread that is filled with a savory mixture.

**Crudites** Raw vegetables that are arranged and served as an appetizer.

**Darne** "Slice" or "slab" in French; refers to the center cut of a large fish, usually salmon, cod, or haddock.

**Degorger** To remove impurities and strong flavors before cooking.

**Diable (à la)** Means "deviled"; refers to dishes flavored with spices and prepared hot sauces.

**Dieppose (à la)** Food prepared in the style of Dieppe, a French port on the northern coast, known for its shrimp and mussels, usually combined with mushrooms and white wine.

**Dijonnaise (à la)** A dish that includes Dijon-style mustard.

**Doria (à la)** A dish garnished with cucumber.

**Dubarry (à la)** Refers to cauliflower.

**Duglere** A dish that includes a velouté sauce with tomatoes and parsley.

**Duxelles** Finely chopped mixture of mushrooms, shallots, and herbs, cooked in butter and used to flavor soups, sauces, and stuffings.

**Entremet** Means "between dishes"; used to refer to all vegetables and salads served as the second course, except for the meat. Now *entremets* is used to refer to any dessert (served after the cheese in France).

**Espagnole** Basic brown sauce on which all other brown sauces are based.

**Financiere (à la)** Literally, "banker's style," referring to a rich garnish of kidneys, sweetbreads, mushrooms, and quenelles.

**Fines Herbes** A classic blend of chopped herbs that includes chervil, tarragon, and chives. Note that parsley is not considered a fine herb.

**Flamande (à la)** In the Flemish style, normally a garnish of braised root vegetables.

**Fleuron** Small crescents of cooked puff pastry used as a garnish.

**Florentine (à la)** A dish with spinach.

**Foie Gras** The liver of a goose that has been specially fattened.

**Frangipane** An almond, sugar, and butter mixture used in cakes and pastries.

**Frappe** Iced dessert.

**Fricassee** A stew of white meat, poultry, fish, or vegetables with a white or velouté sauce.

**Galantine** Boned chicken, turkey, duck, or game bird or a boned breast of veal, stuffed, rolled, tied, and poached. Served cold.

**Galette** Any sweet or savory mixture that is shaped in a flat round.

**Gateau** French for "cake"; refers to the classic French cakes with genoise base.

**Genoise** A sponge cake, richer and with a closer textured than regular sponge cake; made in the same manner but without fat.

**Georgette** Dishes with baked potato.

**Gougere** Savory choux pastry mixed with cheese, then baked plain or filled with a savory mixture.

**Grand'mere** Home-style dishes made with potatoes, onions, and bacon.

**Gratin (au)** To cook food covered in crumbs, butter, sauce, or grated cheese in the oven. *Gratiner* means to brown cooked food under the broiler.

**Grenadin** A small piece of veal resembling a tournedos steak, usually taken from the round.

**Hongrois** Dish using Hungarian paprika in a sour cream sauce.

**Jardiniere** French for "garden-style"; a garnish of small carrots, peas, string beans, button onions, and small potatoes.

**Jus (au)** The term used for meat served in its own natural cooked juices.

**Lyonnaise (à la)** Dishes made with onion and potato garnish.

**Macedoine** Either a mixture of diced or sliced cooked vegetables served in a dressing, or uncooked fruits in a syrup or liqueur.

**Madeleine** Shell-shaped light sponge cakes, made in special Madeleine pans that give the characteristic shape.

**Marmite** Stockpot; originally the name of the French pot used for making pot-au-feu. Petite marmite is a clear soup made in a marmite pot.

**Matelote** French name (meaning "sailor style") for a fish stew made with wine, the dish may be made with veal or poultry.

**Menagere (à la)** Means "housewife" and refers to simply prepared dishes like mashed potatoes or meat garnished with carrots, turnips, and potatoes.

**Meunière** The term used to describe sautéing fish in butter and completing the dish with meunière butter—butter cooked to a nut-brown color, flavored with fresh chopped herbs and lemon juice.

**Milanaise (à la)** In the style of Milan; dishes with macaroni, cheese, tomato, and ham.

**Morels (Morilles)** Wild mushrooms with a rich aromatic flavor.

**Mousse** A sweet smooth mixture, airy and rich. Savory mousses set with gelatin are always served chilled.

**Nantua (à la)** Name given to dishes that include a shrimp or crayfish puree or garnish.

**Navarin** A lamb stew cooked with root vegetables.

**Niçoise (à la)** A dish characterized by tomatoes, anchovies, tuna fish, garlic, and black olives.

**Nivernaise (à la)** Dish that includes carrots as a major ingredient.

**Normande (à la)** Refers to braised fish dishes with a cream (Normande) sauce. With meat or chicken it includes apple cider and Calvados (apple brandy).

**Orloff** A presentation for veal where the roasted meat is carved and each slice is coated with mornay or soubise sauce, and then reassembled.

**Orly** Fish or meat coated with a rich batter and fried crisp.

**Panada** A binding agent of choux pastry, thick béchamel sauce or bread crumbs used to thicken.

**Papillote (en)** French for "cocoon," it means to wrap in a buttered paper case, then cook and serve in the case.

**Parfaits** Rich iced dessert, with an egg mousse base and lightly flavored whipped cream. May be layered with meringues or ladyfingers.

**Parmentier** Dishes garnished with potatoes.

**Pâté** A savory mixture usually made from ground meat.

**Patisserie** A small pastry or pastry shop.

**Paupiette** A piece of meat, fish, or poultry that is filled with a stuffing, then rolled into a small cylinder and cooked.

**Paysanne** Peasant fashion or homey cooking style.

**Perigourdine (à la)** Dishes prepared with truffles.

**Petits Fours** Small pastries that are easy to eat, in one or two bites.

**Pilaf** Rice dish made from long-grain rice sautéed with onions in fat, and then cooked in stock.

**Piquante** A brown sauce flavored with capers and gherkins; also means a sharp or stimulating flavor.

**Poeler** Literally, "to cook in a frying pan."

**Princesse (à la)** Dishes garnished with asparagus tips.

**Printanier (à la)** Garnish of fresh spring vegetables.

**Provencale (à la)** Dishes using tomatoes, peppers, eggplants, garlic, olives, and other specialties of the Provence region of southern France.

**Quatre Epices (Four Spices)** A French spice mixture consisting of white pepper, ginger, nutmeg, and cloves.

**Quenelles** Oval dumplings made from fish, chicken, rabbit, or veal. A mousseline mixture with the addition of egg whites, seasoning, and cream, poached and served with sauce.

**Quiche** A savory egg custard. The most famous version is quiche Lorraine made with cheese, ham, or bacon and sometimes onions.

**Ragout** A slow-cooked stew that is not thickened.

**Reine (à la)** Sauce suprême with a puree of white meat chicken.

**Remoulade** Mayonnaise-based sauce.

**Ravenir** To fry lightly without really cooking.

**Rillette** Type of pork pâté made from unsmoked pork belly and goose, rabbit, chicken, or turkey.

**Rissoler** To brown slowly in fat.

**Rossini** A dish made with small cuts of meat, foie gras, and truffles served with a Madeira sauce.

**Salmis** A form of ragout (stew) made from feathered game or poultry that is lightly roasted, cut up, and gently simmered.

**Salpicon** Mixture of ingredients that have been cut into shreds or strips, often bound with a rich white or brown sauce.

**Shallot** A member of the lily family, closely related to the onion. Their small bulbs usually sport a papery, reddish-brown skin and a white interior flesh that has a sweeter flavor than even mild onions.

**Socle** Means "base" in French, name given to edible food that forms a platform on a serving dish.

**Sorrel** Dark green long, narrow, tender, succulent leaves with a slightly acid tang or lemony flavor.

**Soubise** Garnish or flavoring of pureed or finely sliced onions, normally mixed with rice.

**Souse** Food covered in wine vinegar or wine and spices, and cooked slowly; it is cooled in the same liquid. Sousing gives the food a pickled flavor.

**Supreme** All the white meat on the chicken from the breast down to the wing bone, removed from the bone in one piece.

**Tournedos** Steak cut from the filet. It can be as thick as 2 inches (5 cm), but should be completely trimmed of fat. Typically tied to keep their shape during cooking.

**Velouté** Basic French sauce made with a roux and white stock; enriched with an egg yolk and cream liaison.

**Veronique** Refers to a dish containing green grapes.

**Vol-au-vent** Round case of puff pastry.

# Menus and Recipes from France

MENU ONE

*Endives au Lait d'Amandes Douces:* **Braised Endive with Almond Cream**

*Consommé Brunoise:* **Beef Consommé with Vegetables**

**Tomato Clamart**

*Huîlres Chaudes aux Courgettes: Warm Oysters with Zucchini*

**Potatoes Parmentier**

*Poulet Sauté Marengo:* **Chicken Sauté Marengo**

*Salade Bigouden:* **Lettuce Salad**

*Crème Brulée*

MENU TWO

*Soupe à l'Oignon:* **French Onion Soup**

*Emincés de Rognons de Veau:* **Sliced Veal Kidneys**

*Navarin d'Agneau:* **Lamb Stew**

*Farcis de Blettes:* **Stuffed Swiss Chard**

**Watercress Salad with Endive and Cucumbers**

*Pannequets au Citron:* **Crêpes Stuffed with Lemon Soufflé**

MENU THREE

*Ratatouille*

*Soupe de Legumes aux Petits Coquillages:* **Vegetable Soup with Shellfish**

*Le Blanc de Poisson Belle Mouginoise:* **Fillet of Fish Mouginoise**

*Filet de Porc Farci Lyonnaise:* **Stuffed Pork Tenderloin**

*Salade de Poire:* **Pear Salad**

*Mousse au Chocolat:* **Chocolate Mousse**

# Endives au Lait d'Amandes Douces

## Braised Endive with Almond Cream

SERVES 4

| AMOUNT | MEASURE | INGREDIENT |
|---|---|---|
| 8 | | Small to medium Belgian endives |
| 2 tablespoons | 1 ounce, 30 ml | Vegetable oil or peanut oil |
| 1 teaspoon | | Granulated sugar |
| 1 tablespoon | $\frac{1}{2}$ ounce, 15 ml | Fresh lemon juice |
| To taste | | Salt |
| $\frac{1}{2}$ cup | $2\frac{1}{2}$ ounces, 70 g | Blanched slivered almonds |
| $1\frac{1}{4}$ cups | 10 ounces, 300 ml | Heavy cream |
| $1\frac{1}{2}$ tablespoons | $\frac{3}{4}$ ounce, 22 ml | Butter |

**PROCEDURE**

1. Preheat the oven at 350°F (175°C).
2. Trim the endives; discard any brown outside leaves. Trim $\frac{1}{8}$ inch (.3 cm) from the pointed end. Wash in cold water and drain well. Arrange them tightly in a oiled flameproof pan with oil, sugar, lemon juice, and salt. Add cold water to cover.
3. Place something on top to weight them; cover and bake 30 to 40 minutes or until tender. Check for doneness by piercing the base with a paring knife; the blade should go in easily. When cooked, raise the oven temperature to 400°F (205°C).
4. Drain the endives and pat dry.
5. Combine the almonds and cream and bring slowly to a boil. Simmer 6 to 8 minutes over low heat, making sure the cream does not boil over.
6. Puree the almonds and cream in a blender; strain through a fine sieve, stirring and pressing with a wooden spoon so that as much mixture as possible passes. Correct seasoning and keep warm.
7. Heat the butter over medium heat until it just begins to color. Add endive and sauté until golden-brown on both sides, 6 to 8 minutes.
8. Arrange in a gratin or baking dish, cover with almond cream, and bake 15 minutes or until the cream has thickened.

# Consommé Brunoise

## Beef Consommé with Vegetables

YIELD: $\frac{1}{2}$ GALLON

| AMOUNT | MEASURE | INGREDIENT |
|---|---|---|
| 1 pound | | Fresh beef shank meat (coarsely ground) |
| $1\frac{1}{2}$ cups | 8 ounces, 224 g | Mirepoix, coarsely ground ($\frac{1}{2}$ onion, $\frac{1}{4}$ carrot. $\frac{1}{4}$ celery) |
| 1 cup | 8 ounces, 240 ml | Egg whites, beaten |
| $\frac{3}{4}$ cup | 4 ounces, 112 g | Tomatoes, coarsely chopped |
| 1 cup | 4 ounces, 112 g | Leeks, chopped |
| $\frac{1}{2}$ cup | 4 ounces, 120 ml | Crushed ice |
| $\frac{1}{2}$ teaspoon | | Dried thyme leaves |
| 1 | | Bay leaf |
| 3 | | Parsley stems |
| 1 | | Garlic clove |
| 1 tablespoon | | Whole peppercorns |
| 1 | | Clove |
| $2\frac{1}{2}$ quarts | 80 ounces, 2.4 l | Beef stock, cold |
| $\frac{1}{2}$ cup | 2 ounces, 56 g | Onion brulé, chopped |
| To taste | | Salt |
| Garnish | | |
| $\frac{1}{3}$ cup each | | Brunoise carrot, turnip, celery, and leek |

PROCEDURE

1. Combine ground meat, mirepoix, egg whites, tomatoes, leeks, ice, and spices. Mix well, keep chilled.
2. Mix stock into above mixture. Agitate well to distribute ingredients evenly throughout stock to insure better clarification.
3. Place mixture in a heavy-bottomed stockpot.
4. Bring gently to a simmer; stir occasionally until raft forms. Do not stir after the raft has formed.
5. Vent the raft.
6. Simmer carefully for $1\frac{1}{2}$ hours.
7. In the last half hour, make a small hole in the raft and place the onion brulé in the consommé.

8 Strain carefully through several layers of cheesecloth.

9 Degrease, adjust salt.

10 Blanch garnish ingredients in boiling salt water until just cooked, then shock in an ice water bath. Heat in a little consommé and add to soup when serving; each portion requires 2 tablespoons garnish.

11 Add garnish just before serving, and serve hot.

# Tomato Clamart

SERVES 4

| AMOUNT | MEASURE | INGREDIENT |
|---|---|---|
| 4 | 5 x 6 (12.5 cm x 15 cm) | Tomatoes |
| To taste | | Salt and pepper |
| $\frac{1}{4}$ cup | 2 ounces, 60 ml | Butter |
| $1\frac{1}{4}$ cups | 8 ounces, 224 g | Peas, cooked |

PROCEDURE

1 Peel the tomatoes, cut off $\frac{1}{4}$ of the top, remove the seeds and juice, and season the inside with salt and pepper. Place in a 350°F (175°C) oven until half cooked.

2 Heat the butter, add the peas, season, and fill tomatoes with the peas.

3 Return to the oven and reheat.

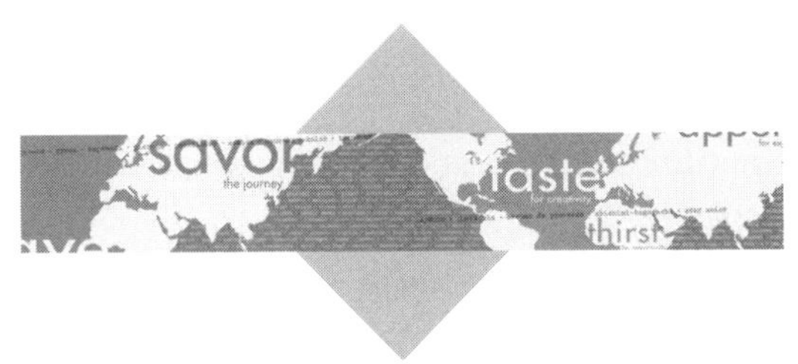

# Huîlres Chaudes aux Courgettes

## Warm Oysters with Zucchini

SERVES 4

| AMOUNT | MEASURE | INGREDIENT |
|---|---|---|
| 12 | | Large oysters |
| | | If needed, additional oyster liquor |
| 4 | | Nori sheets, for presentation |
| $1\frac{1}{2}$ cups | 9 ounces, 252 g | Zucchini, sliced into very thin rounds ($\frac{1}{8}$ inch, .3 cm), about 10 slices per oyster |
| $\frac{1}{2}$ cup | 4 ounces, 120 ml | Heavy cream |
| 1 cup | 8 ounces, 240 ml | Butter |
| 4 teaspoons | 40 ml | Fresh lemon juice |
| To taste | | Salt, pepper, and cayenne |

### PROCEDURE

1. Open the oysters, pour their liquor through a cheesecloth-lined strainer into a small heavy saucepan, and reduce over high heat to $\frac{1}{4}$ cup (2 ounces, 60 ml). Set oysters aside until ready to serve.
2. Arrange a sheet of nori on each of the four plates and put the deep halves of the oyster shell on the seaweed, 3 per order.
3. Blanch the zucchini in salted boiling water for 2 minutes and then drain.

### FINISHING AND SERVING

1. Bring reduced oyster liquor to a boil and add the cream. Reduce on high heat 1 minute, then whisk in 12 tablespoons (6 ounces, 180 ml) butter, bit by bit, still at a boil. When all the butter is absorbed, add the lemon juice, remove from the heat, and check seasoning.
2. Whisk the sauce 1 minute off the heat. This step is essential so the temperature is reduced or the sauce may separate.
3. Melt remaining butter over medium heat and add the zucchini. Season with salt, pepper, and cayenne to taste. Cook until the zucchini is just warm, then remove from heat.

4 Add the oysters to the butter sauce and heat over very low heat for 30 seconds, shaking the pan in a circular motion while heating the oysters.
5 Place one oyster in each shell.
6 Arrange the zucchini rounds on top of each oyster, overlapping them.
7 Lightly coat with sauce and serve.

# Potatoes Parmentier

SERVES 4

| AMOUNT | MEASURE | INGREDIENT |
|---|---|---|
| 2 tablespoons | 1 ounce, 30 ml | Vegetable oil |
| 4 tablespoons | 2 ounce, 60 ml | Butter |
| 3 cups | 16 ounces, 448 g | Russet potatoes, peeled, $\frac{1}{2}$ inch (1.2 cm) cubes |
| To taste | | Salt and pepper |
| 1 tablespoon | 4 g | Parsley, chopped |

**PROCEDURE**

1 Over medium heat, combine the oil and butter.
2 Add the potatoes and sauté 10 to 12 minutes, or until an even golden color and completely cooked.
3 When ready to serve, correct seasoning and toss with parsley.

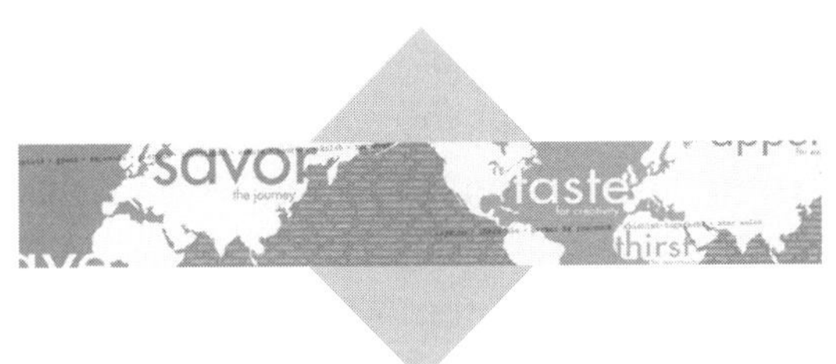

# Poulet Sauté Marengo

## Chicken Sauté Marengo

SERVES 4

| AMOUNT | MEASURE | INGREDIENT |
|---|---|---|
| 2 tablespoons | 1 ounce, 30 ml | Vegetable oil |
| 2 tablespoons | 1 ounce, 30 ml | Butter |
| 1 $2\frac{1}{2}$ to 3 pound | 1.12 kg to 1.34 kg | Chicken, disjointed, (drumstick cut at knuckle, thigh boneless, wing center, wing thick end, breast cut in half) |
| 1 tablespoon | | Shallot, minced |
| 1 tablespoon | | Garlic, minced |
| 1 tablespoon | $\frac{1}{2}$ ounce, 15 ml | Tomato paste |
| 1 cup | 6 ounces, 168 g | Tomato, peeled, seeded $\frac{1}{4}$ inch (.6 cm) dice |
| $\frac{1}{2}$ cup | 4 ounces, 120 ml | White wine |
| $1\frac{1}{2}$ cups | 12 ounces, 360 ml | Espagnole, demi-glaze or jus lié |
| 1 cup | 4 ounces, 112 g | Button mushrooms, washed and trimmed |
| As needed | | Salt and pepper |
| Garnish | | |
| 4 | | Crayfish tails or 4 large shrimp |
| 2 tablespoons | 1 ounce, 30 ml | Stock |
| 4 | | Eggs |
| 1 tablespoon | | Parsley, chopped |
| 4 | | Bread slices, cut into heart shapes |
| 4 tablespoons | 2 ounces, 60 ml | Butter |

### PROCEDURE

1 Heat oil and butter over medium high heat and brown the chicken pieces on all sides. Remove chicken from the pan; drain and reserve the fat.

2 In the same pan, return 2 tablespoons (1 ounce, 30 ml) reserved fat; add the shallot and garlic; cook 2 minutes or until soft.

3 Add tomato paste, cook 1 to 2 minutes. Add chopped tomato; cook gently, stirring 3 to 4 minutes.

4 Add wine and reduce by half. Add espagnole sauce, return chicken pieces, add mushrooms, and bring to a simmer. Cover and cook slowly 25 to 30 minutes or until the chicken is tender. Remove pieces as they cook.

5 To prepare the garnish, simmer the crayfish tails or shrimp in the stock until just cooked, 2 to 3 minutes; drain and keep warm.

6 Heat the reserved fat and French fry the eggs (cook egg in fat at 160 degrees, very slowly until the whites are creamy and the yolk is hot but still liquid.)

7 Heat the remaining butter and fry the heart-shaped bread slices.

8 Arrange the chicken on a platter, spoon the sauce over.

9 Dip the point of each crouton in the sauce, then into the chopped parsley, and arrange around the edge with the crayfish tails. Place a fried egg on each crouton and serve at once.

## Salade Bigouden Lettuce Salad SERVES 4

| AMOUNT | MEASURE | INGREDIENT |
|---|---|---|
| **2** | | **Boston lettuce heads, washed and dried** |
| **6 tablespoons** | **3 ounces, 90 ml** | **Cider vinegar** |
| **2 tablespoons** | **1 ounce, 28 g** | **Granulated sugar** |

**PROCEDURE**

1 When ready to serve, tear up the lettuce and toss with the vinegar.

2 Sprinkle the sugar over the lettuce and toss lightly again.

3 Serve as salad course.

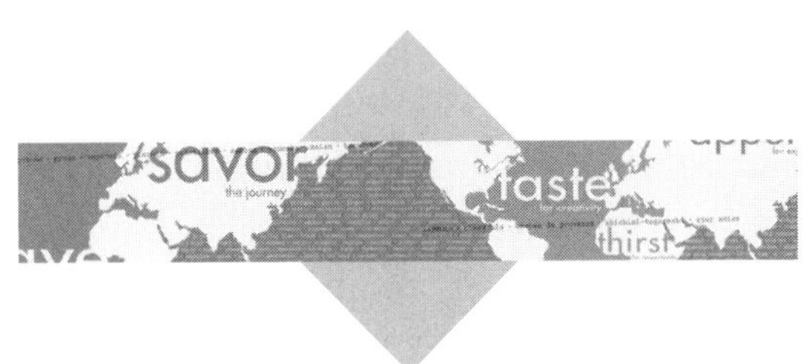

# Crème Brulée

SERVES 4

| AMOUNT | MEASURE | INGREDIENT |
|---|---|---|
| 2 cups | 16 ounces, 480 ml | Heavy cream |
| 6 | | Egg yolks |
| $\frac{1}{2}$ cup | 4 ounces, 112 g | Granulated sugar |
| 1 teaspoon, or to taste | | Vanilla |
| Pinch | | Salt |
| 4 tablespoons | 2 ounce, 56 g | Brown sugar |

**PROCEDURE**

1. Place cream in a nonreactive pan and heat to the scalding point; remove from heat.
2. Mix—do not whip—the egg yolks and sugar until combined. Gradually pour in a little of the hot cream to temper the eggs. Add remaining cream, stirring constantly; add vanilla and a pinch of salt; strain.
3. Pour the custard into 4 (5-ounce) ramekins; be sure to fill the forms to the top because, like any custard, it will settle slightly once it is cooked. Place forms in a hotel pan, or other suitable container, and add hot water around the forms to reach halfway up the sides.
4. Bake at 350°F (175°C) for about 30 minutes, or until the custards are set. Do not overcook or you will have a broken and unpleasant finished product.
5. Remove from the water bath and let cool slightly at room temperature, then refrigerate until thoroughly chilled.
6. Spread brown sugar over a sheet pan lined with paper, and dry in the oven for a few minutes. Let cool. Use a rolling pin or dowel to crush the sugar and separate the grains. Reserve.
7. For the presentation, sift or sprinkle just enough of the dry brown sugar on top of the custard to cover. Whip away any sugar that is on the edge of the form. Caramelize the sugar in a salamander or under a broiler or use a torch.
8. Serve plain or garnished with fresh fruit or berries.

# Soupe à l'Oignon

## French Onion Soup SERVES 4

| AMOUNT | MEASURE | INGREDIENT |
|---|---|---|
| $\frac{1}{4}$ cup | 2 ounces, 60 ml | Butter |
| 5 cups | 16 ounces, 448 g | Onions, peeled, thinly sliced |
| 2 tablespoons | $\frac{1}{2}$ ounce, 14 g | All-purpose flour |
| $\frac{3}{4}$ cup | 6 ounces, 180 ml | White wine |
| $1\frac{1}{4}$ quarts | 40 ounces, 1.2 l | Beef stock |
| 1 | | Bouquet garni (recipe follows) |
| 8 | | Slices French baguette |
| $\frac{1}{2}$ cup | 2 ounces, 56 g | Gruyère cheese, grated |
| Bouquet Garni | | |
| 2 | | Leek, green parts only, 4-inch (10 cm) pieces |
| 1 | | Bay leaf |
| 3 | | Fresh sprigs thyme |
| 4 | | Large fresh sprigs parsley |
| 1 | | Celery stalk |

PROCEDURE

1 To prepare bouquet garni, lay herbs on one piece of leek green and cover with remaining piece of leek. Tie securely with kitchen string, leaving a length of string attached so the bouquet garni can be easily retrieved.

2 Heat butter over medium heat. Add onions and cook until tender and golden brown, 15 to 20 minutes.

3 Add the flour and cook 2 minutes, stirring.

4 Add wine, bring to a boil, reduce heat, and simmer 2 minutes. Gradually add the stock. Add bouquet garni and bring to a boil. Reduce to a simmer; cover and cook 30 minutes.

5 To serve, add two slices of bread to each soup bowl and sprinkle with cheese. Pour the boiling soup over the bread and cheese. Or toast the bread slices and float on top of the soup and sprinkle with cheese. Broil unit the cheese melts.

# Émincés de Rognons de Veau

## Sliced Veal Kidneys

SERVES 4

**Veal kidneys have nothing in common with the taste of lamb, pork, or beef kidneys. Kidneys should be cooked a few minutes only at the highest possible heat. They should be pink in the middle. Drain the kidney in a sieve for a few minutes (pink liquid will run out of the kidneys and should be discarded). Veal kidneys must be served pink; if overcooked they become chewy and lose their delicate flavor.**

| AMOUNT | MEASURE | INGREDIENT |
|---|---|---|
| 2 each | 10 ounces, 280 g | Veal kidneys (total 20 ounces, 560 g), as clean as possible, in their own suet, which should be white and crumbly |
| To taste | | Salt and pepper |
| 10 tablespoons | 5 ounces, 150 ml | Butter |
| 20 each | | Shallots, peeled whole |
| 4 tablespoons | 2 ounces, 60 ml | Madeira wine |
| $\frac{3}{4}$ cup | 6 ounces, 180 ml | Beef stock |
| $\frac{1}{2}$ cup | 1 ounce, 28 g | Flat-leaved parsley |
| 2 each | | Garlic cloves, mashed whole |

**PROCEDURE**

1. Remove the outer membrane from the kidneys with the point of a paring knife. Butterfly the kidney into lengthwise halves and remove most of the strip of fat and gristle that runs through the middle. Season with salt and pepper.
2. Use a small cast-iron pan (if possible), heat over high heat 2 tablespoons (1 ounce 30 ml) butter to brown the kidneys. Brown on all sides and move to a 450°F (230°C) oven. Cook 10 to 15 minutes, turning frequently.
3. Remove from oven, set kidneys aside, and cover to keep warm. Pour out all the fat and replace with 4 tablespoons (2 ounces, 60 ml) butter, and then add the shallots.
4. Cook shallots in oven until soft. Crush to a puree using a fork. The sugar they contain will bind the kidney juices and caramelize slightly.

5 Stir in the Madeira and then add the stock, a little at a time. Reduce to sauce consistency, then strain. Whisk in 1 ounce (30 ml) butter and correct seasoning.

6 Discard any juices that have accumulated around the kidneys. Slice into medium to thin slices. Arrange on a plate and brush with a little melted butter.

7 Blanch the parsley in boiling salted water, then dry on a cloth. Melt 1 ounce (30 ml) of butter, sauté mashed garlic cloves for 30 seconds, and remove them. Add parsley, stirring continuously until just crisp.

8 Serve kidneys with sauce spooned over and parsley garnish.

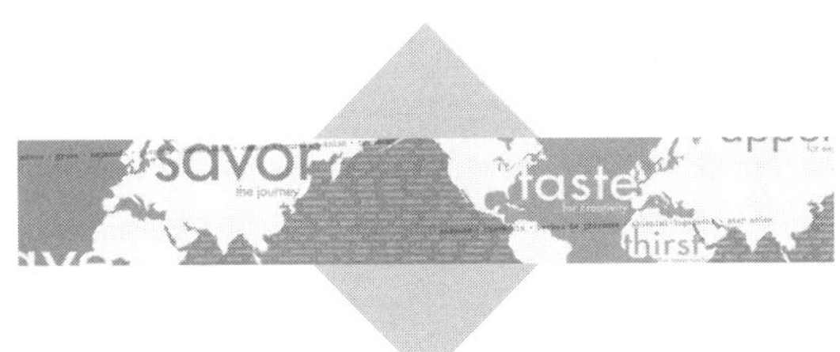

# Navarin d'Agneau Lamb Stew

SERVES 4

| AMOUNT | MEASURE | INGREDIENT |
|---|---|---|
| 2 pounds | 896 g | Lamb stew meat, 1 inch (2.4 cm) cubes |
| 2 tablespoons | 1 ounce, 30 ml | Olive oil |
| 2 tablespoons | 1 ounce, 30 ml | Butter |
| As needed | | All-purpose flour |
| 1 cup | 4 ounces, 112 g | Onions, $\frac{1}{4}$ inch (.6 cm) dice |
| 2 tablespoons | | Garlic, minced |
| 2 tablespoons | 1 ounce, 30 ml | Tomato paste |
| 1 cup | 6 ounces, 168 g | Tomatoes, peeled, seeded, $\frac{1}{4}$ inch (.6 cm) dice |
| $\frac{3}{4}$ cup | 6 ounces, 180 ml | White wine, dry |
| 2 cups | 16 ounces, 480 ml | White stock |
| 1 each | | Bouquet garni (see page 669) |
| 1 $\frac{1}{2}$ cups | 6 ounces, 168 g | Russet potatoes, peeled, $\frac{1}{2}$ inch (1.2 cm) dice |
| 1 cup | 4 ounces, 112 g | Carrots, peeled, $\frac{1}{2}$ inch (1.2 cm) dice |
| 1 cup | 4 ounces, 112 g | Turnips, peeled, $\frac{1}{2}$ inch (1.2 cm) dice |
| 1 cup | 4 ounces, 112 g | Pearl onions, peeled |
| $\frac{1}{2}$ cup | 2 ounces, 56 g | Green peas |
| To taste | | Salt and white pepper |
| 1 tablespoon | | Chervil, chopped |
| 1 tablespoon | | Parsley, chopped |

PROCEDURE

1. Trim the meat, removing any excess fat. Dry lamb cubes.
2. Heat the oil and butter over medium-high heat.
3. Dredge lamb in flour and shake to remove any excess; add to hot fat and sear on all sides; remove and set aside.
4. Add onions to pan and sauté onions 3 to 4 minutes or until soft. Add garlic and cook 1 minute.
5. Add tomato paste and cook 2 minutes or until fragrant. Add diced tomato and cook three minutes.

6. Add white wine and cook 2 minutes; scrape bottom of pan to get all the drippings.
7. Add stock and bouquet garni, and return meat to pan. Bring to a boil, reduce to a simmer, and cook 40 minutes or until meat is almost tender.
8. Remove meat and strain sauce; discard bouquet garni.
9. Add potatoes, carrots, turnips, and pearl onions to sauce and return meat; simmer until vegetables and meat are tender, 15 to 20 minutes.
10. Add green peas; simmer 3 minutes or until hot.
11. Adjust seasoning, stir in chervil, and sprinkle with chopped parsley when serving.

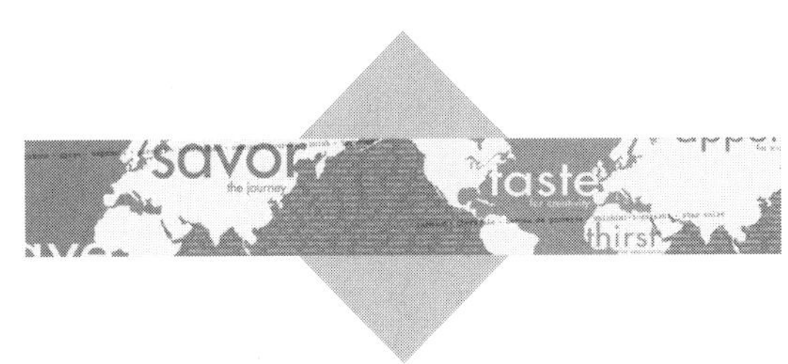

# Farcis de Blettes Stuffed Swiss Chard

**SERVES 4**

**Broad-stemmed Swiss chard tends to oxidize, so it should be cooked in a *blanc*.**

| AMOUNT | MEASURE | INGREDIENT |
|---|---|---|
| 1 tablespoon | $\frac{1}{4}$ ounce, 10 ml | Dried currants |
| 4 teaspoons | | Rice |
| 1 cup | 4 ounces, 112 g | Onions, $\frac{1}{4}$ inch (.6 cm) dice |
| $\frac{1}{2}$ cup | 4 ounces, 120 ml | Olive oil |
| 12 each | | Large Swiss chard leaves |
| 4 tablespoons | | All-purpose flour |
| 1 tablespoon | $\frac{1}{2}$ ounce, 14 g | Pine nuts |
| To taste | | Salt and pepper |

**PROCEDURE**

1. Preheat oven to 275°C (135°C).
2. Soak currants in warm water to cover for 10 minutes.
3. Parboil rice in salted water for 12 minutes; drain and cool under cold running water.
4. Over medium heat, sauté onions in 2 tablespoons (1 ounce, 30 ml) oil for 1 minute.
5. Prepare a *blanc*.
6. Wash and dry the chard, making sure not to damage the leaves. Run a knife along the stalk; separate the green from the white. Cut stalks into 2-inch (5 cm) lengths. Blanch leaves in a blanc for 1 minute, run under cold water and dry.
7. Cook chard stalks in a blanc until just tender, 10 to 15 minutes
8. Heat 4 tablespoons (2 ounces, 60 ml) olive oil over medium heat. Add the cooked chard stalks and sauté, stirring often, 5 minutes.
9. Combine sautéed stalks, currants, pine nuts, rice, and onions; correct seasoning.
10. Form stuffing into balls, 1 tablespoon each. Wrap each ball neatly in a Swiss chard leaf.
11. Arrange the balls tightly in a baking dish, smooth side up. Sprinkle with the remaining olive oil, add about $\frac{1}{4}$ inch (.6 cm) water, and bake 30 to 35 minutes.
12. Serve hot, in the baking dish.

# Blanc

| AMOUNT | MEASURE | INGREDIENT |
|---|---|---|
| **4 tablespoons** | **1 ounce, 28 g** | **Flour** |
| **3 quarts** | **96 ounces, 2.8l** | **Cold water** |
| **1 tablespoon** | **$\frac{1}{2}$ ounce, 15 ml** | **White vinegar** |
| **$\frac{1}{2}$ cup** | **$3\frac{1}{2}$ ounces, 98 g** | **Coarse salt** |

**PROCEDURE**

1. Hold a fine-mesh strainer over a deep pot and place the flour in the strainer.
2. Pour cold water in a slow stream through the flour, stirring with a whisk to make the flour disperse and pass through the strainer.
3. Add white vinegar and coarse salt.
4. Bring to a boil and add the chard stalks.
5. Cook 10 or 15 minutes or until just tender.
6. Drain stalks and chop coarsely.

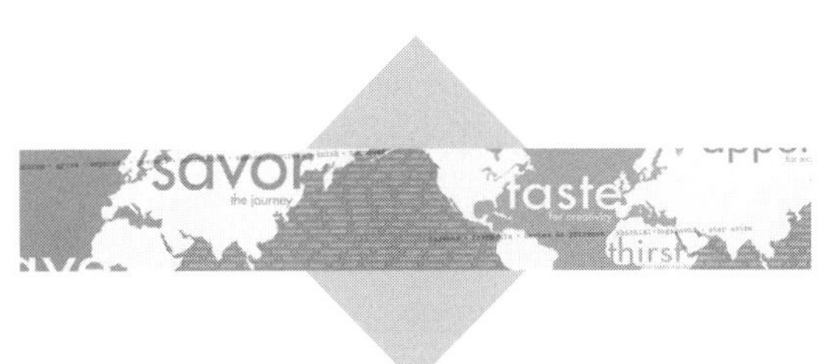

# Watercress Salad with Endive and Cucumbers

SERVES 4

| AMOUNT | MEASURE | INGREDIENT |
|---|---|---|
| 2 cups | 6 ounces, 168 g | Watercress (two bunches) |
| 1 cup | 6 ounces, 168 g | Cucumbers, peeled, seeded, thinly sliced |
| 2 | | Belgian endive |
| 1 teaspoon | | Dijon-type prepared mustard |
| 1 tablespoon | $\frac{1}{2}$ ounce, 15 ml | Fresh lemon juice |
| 4 tablespoons | 2 ounces, 60 ml | Olive oil |
| To taste | | Salt and pepper |
| 8 each | | Cherry tomatoes, for garnish |

**PROCEDURE**

1. Trim off tough stem from watercress; wash, spin dry, and refrigerate until needed.
2. Soak cucumbers in ice cold salt water until needed. When ready to make the salad, drain cucumbers and dry before serving.
3. Separate the leaves from the central stems of the endive and refrigerate.
4. Combine the mustard, lemon juice, and oil; whisk and correct seasoning.
5. At serving time, toss each ingredient separately in a little of the dressing; correct the seasoning for each.
6. Arrange on plates, endives first, like the spokes of a wheel, then make a bed of cress, and a topping of cucumber slices. Add a few halved cherry tomatoes.

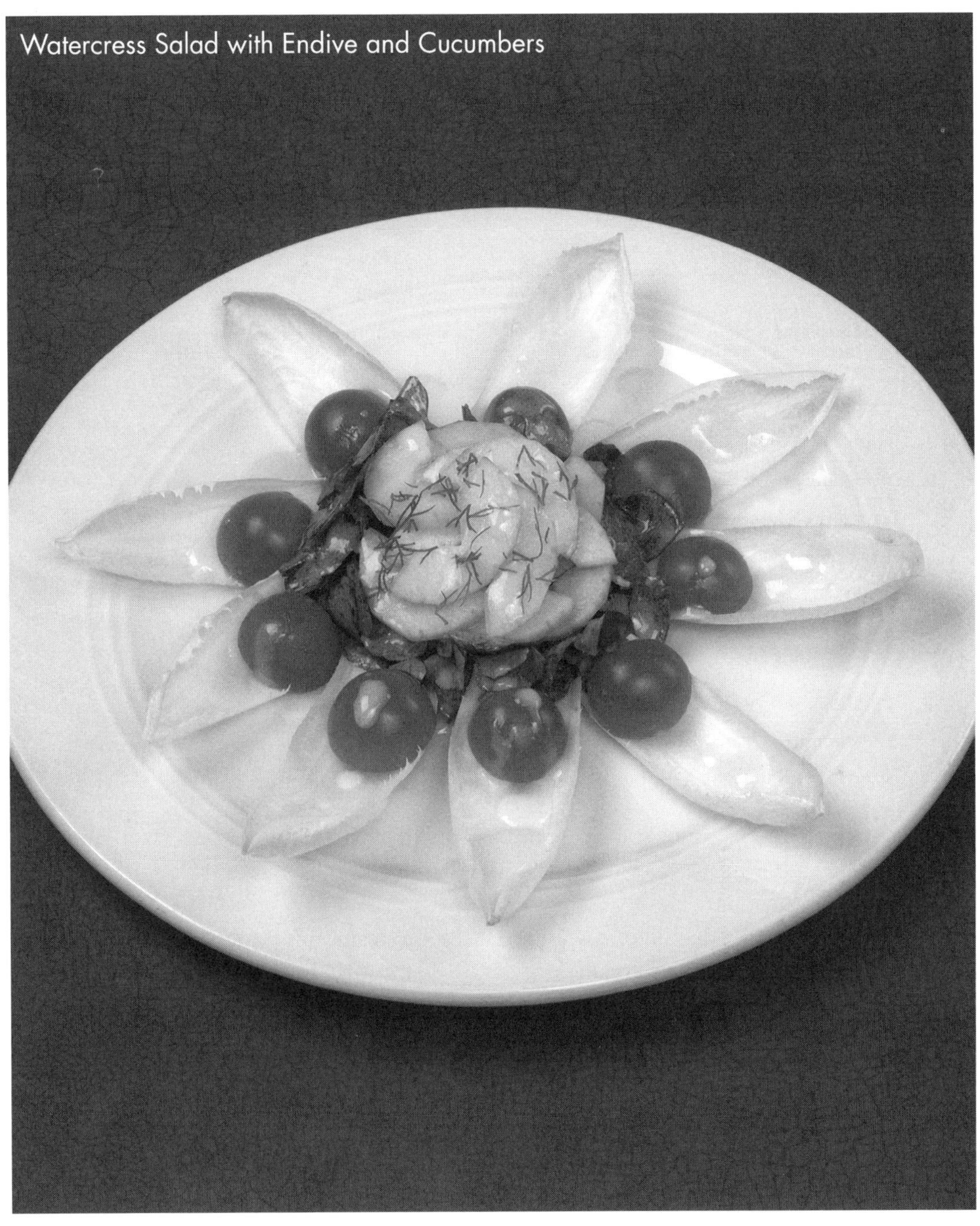

Watercress Salad with Endive and Cucumbers

# Pannequets au Citron

## Crêpes Stuffed with Lemon Soufflé

SERVES 4

| AMOUNT | MEASURE | INGREDIENT |
|---|---|---|
| **Crepe Batter** | | |
| 2 each | | Eggs |
| ½ cup | 4 ounces, 120 ml | Milk |
| 2 tablespoons | 1 ounce, 30 ml | Butter, melted |
| ½ cup | 2 ounces, 56 g | All-purpose flour |
| 2 tablespoons | 1 ounce, 28 g | Granulated sugar |
| Pinch | | Salt |
| 1 teaspoon | | Vanilla extract |
| **Raspberry Sauce** | | |
| 1 cup | 6 ounces, 168 g | Raspberries, fresh or frozen, pureed and strained |
| ¼ cup | 2 ounces, 56 g | Granulated sugar |
| **Soufflé Batter** | | |
| 1 cup | 7 ounces, 210 ml | Pastry cream (recipe follows) |
| 2 tablespoons | 1 ounce, 30 ml | Lemon juice |
| 1 teaspoon | | Lemon zest |
| 4 each | | Eggs whites |
| As needed | | Confectioner's sugar |

### PROCEDURE

1. Combine all ingredients for the crepe batter into a smooth paste; adjust the thickness to the consistency of heavy cream. Refrigerate 30 minutes before making crepes.
2. Over medium heat, preheat a crepe pan and brush with a little melted butter.
3. Place an enough batter to just coat the bottom of the pan with a thin layer.
4. Cook the crepes until almost dry; turn over and cook the other side. Make two per serving.
5. For the raspberry sauce, combine raspberry puree with the sugar and bring to a boil. If sauce is not thick enough, thicken with a little cornstarch slurry. Remove from heat; set aside to cool.
6. For the soufflé, combine pastry cream, lemon juice, and zest.

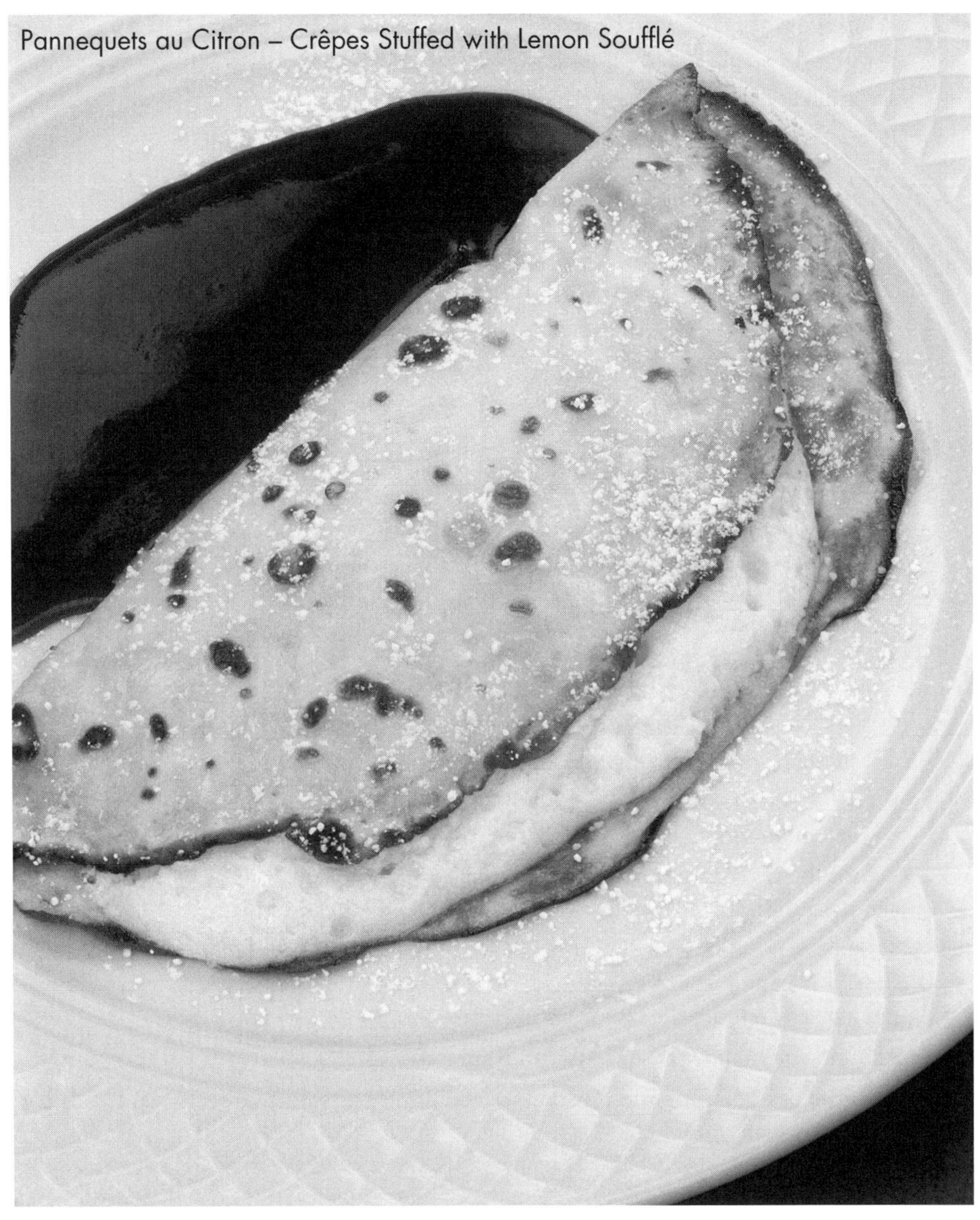

Pannequets au Citron – Crêpes Stuffed with Lemon Soufflé

7 Whip egg whites to a firm peak and gently fold into pastry cream.

8 Place 3 to 4 tablespoons of lemon soufflé mixture on one half of each crepe; fold the second half lightly over the soufflé mixture.

9 Bake at 375°F (190°C) on a well-buttered baking tray for 12 minutes.

10 Dust well with sugar and serve immediately, with raspberry sauce.

## Pastry Cream

YIELD: ABOUT 3 CUPS

| AMOUNT | MEASURE | INGREDIENT |
|---|---|---|
| **2 cups** | **16 ounces, 480 ml** | **Milk** |
| **2/3 cup** | **5 ounces, 140 g** | **Granulated sugar** |
| **$\frac{1}{4}$ cup** | **1 ounce, 28 g** | **Cornstarch** |
| **6** | | **Egg yolks** |
| **2 tablespoons** | **1 ounce, 30 ml** | **Butter, soft** |
| **2 teaspoons** | | **Vanilla extract** |

**PROCEDURE**

1 Combine $1\frac{1}{2}$ cups (12 ounces, 360 ml) of the milk and all the sugar in a saucepan. Stir to dissolve the sugar, then place over medium heat and bring to a boil.

2 Combine the remaining milk and the cornstarch, then the egg yolks.

3 Whisk about $\frac{1}{2}$ cup (4 ounces, 120 ml) boiling mixture into the yolk mixture. If there are any apparent lumps, strain the yolk mixture into another container.

4 Return the remaining milk to medium heat and bring to a boil. Begin whisking the milk and pour the yolk mixture into the boiling milk in a steady stream.

5 The pastry cream will begin to thicken immediately. Whisk until it comes to a boil; make sure you get all the corners and sides to prevent scorching. Continue to cook 1 minute. Immediately remove the pan from the heat.

6 Add the butter and vanilla; whisk until smooth.

7 Pour the pastry cream into a container and cover the surface directly with plastic wrap. Chill immediately until cold.

# Ratatouille

SERVES 4

| AMOUNT | MEASURE | INGREDIENT |
|---|---|---|
| 1 cup | 8 ounces, 240 ml | Olive oil |
| 1 cup | 4 ounces, 112 g | Onions, $\frac{1}{2}$ inch (.6 cm) dice |
| 1 cup | 4 ounces, 112 g | Green bell peppers, $\frac{1}{2}$ inch (.6 cm) dice |
| 1 cup | 4 ounces, 112 g | Zucchini, $\frac{1}{2}$ inch (.6 cm) dice |
| 2 cups | 8 ounces, 224 g | Eggplant, $\frac{1}{2}$ inch (.6 cm) dice |
| 2 cups | 12 ounces, 336 g | Tomatoes, peeled, seeded, $\frac{1}{2}$ inches (.6 cm) dice |
| 2 | | Garlic cloves, minced |
| To taste | | Salt and pepper |
| 2 tablespoons | | Fresh thyme |
| 2 | | Bay leaves |

**PROCEDURE**

1. Over medium heat, heat $\frac{1}{2}$ the oil and sauté the onions and green peppers, 4 to 5 minutes.
2. In a second sauté pan, heat the remaining oil and sauté the zucchini and eggplant, 10 to 15 minutes or until tender. Combine the onion mixture with the eggplant mixture.
3. Add the tomatoes, garlic, salt, pepper, thyme, and bay leaves. Cook, covered, on top of the stove, 30 to 40 minutes. Remove bay leaves. Serve warm or at room temperature.

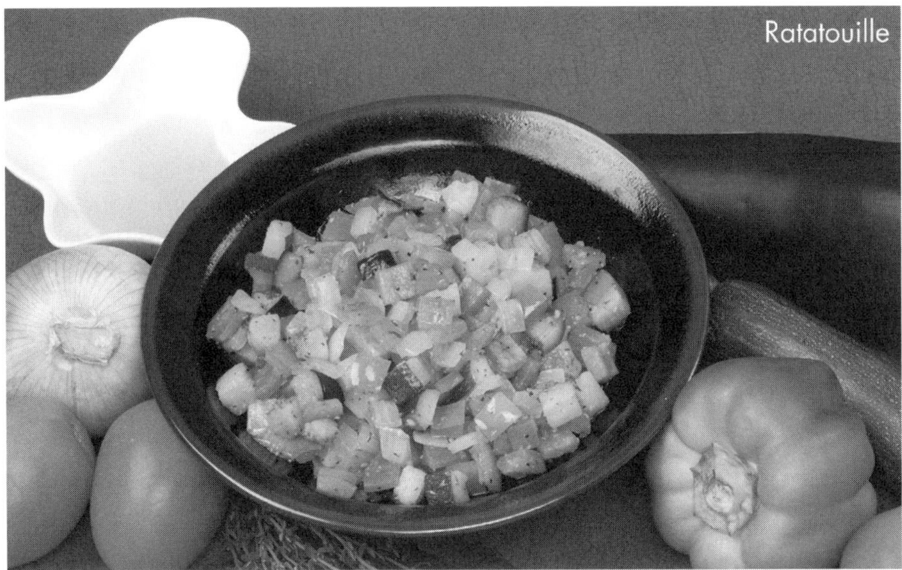

Ratatouille

# Soupe de Legumes aux Petits Coquillages Vegetable Soup with Shellfish

SERVES 4

**Paysanne cut: A flat, square, round or triangular cut with dimensions of $\frac{1}{2}$ inch × $\frac{1}{2}$ inch × $\frac{1}{8}$ inch (1.2 cm x 1.2 cm x .3 mm).**

| AMOUNT | MEASURE | INGREDIENT |
|---|---|---|
| 2 cups | 10 to 12 | Small mussels |
| 2 cups | 10 to 12 | Small clams |
| 4 | | Sea scallops |
| 3 tablespoons | $1\frac{1}{2}$ ounces, 45 ml | Olive oil |
| 1 cup | 8 ounces, 240 ml | Vegetable stock |
| $\frac{1}{4}$ cup | 2 ounces, 60 ml | White wine |
| $\frac{1}{4}$ cup | 1 ounce, 28 g | Green onion, minced |
| 1 each | | Garlic clove, minced |
| $\frac{1}{2}$ cup | 2 ounces, 56 g | Tender green part of leek, paysanne cut |
| $\frac{1}{2}$ cup | 2 ounces, 56 g | Turnip, paysanne cut |
| $\frac{1}{2}$ cup | 2 ounces, 56 g | Carrots, paysanne cut |
| $\frac{1}{2}$ cup | 2 ounces, 56 g | Zucchini, paysanne cut |
| $\frac{1}{2}$ cup | 2 ounces, 56 g | Savory cabbage, paysanne cut |
| $\frac{1}{2}$ cup | 3 ounces, 84 g | Tomato, peeled, seeded, $\frac{1}{4}$ inch (.6 cm) dice |
| $\frac{1}{4}$ cup | 2 ounces, 60 ml | Butter |
| To taste | | Salt and pepper |

## PROCEDURE

1. Wash the mussels and clams; remove the beards from the mussels.
2. Cut the scallops into 3 slices and cut each slice into 3 sticks.
3. Heat 1 tablespoon ($\frac{1}{2}$ ounce, 15 ml) olive oil and add the clams and $\frac{1}{2}$ cup vegetable stock. Simmer the clams only until they open; remove from the heat immediately as they open or they will become tough. Set aside and strain the cooking liquid through a cheesecloth-lined sieve into a saucepan. Save the cheesecloth; it will be used again.
4. Combine the remaining vegetable stock and white wine over low heat and add the mussels. Check the mussels and remove as they open. When all are open, strain the cooking liquid

and combine with the clam liquid. Reduce the mussel and clam liquid by half. Shell mussels and clams; reserve meat.

5 Heat the remaining olive oil over medium heat and add the onions and garlic; cook 1 minute; add to the shellfish cooking liquid and bring to a boil over high heat.

6 Add vegetables and cook 2 minutes. Remove from heat and stir in the butter.

7 Add the tomato dice and mussels and return to a boil; immediately remove from the heat and add the clams and scallops. Check seasoning and serve.

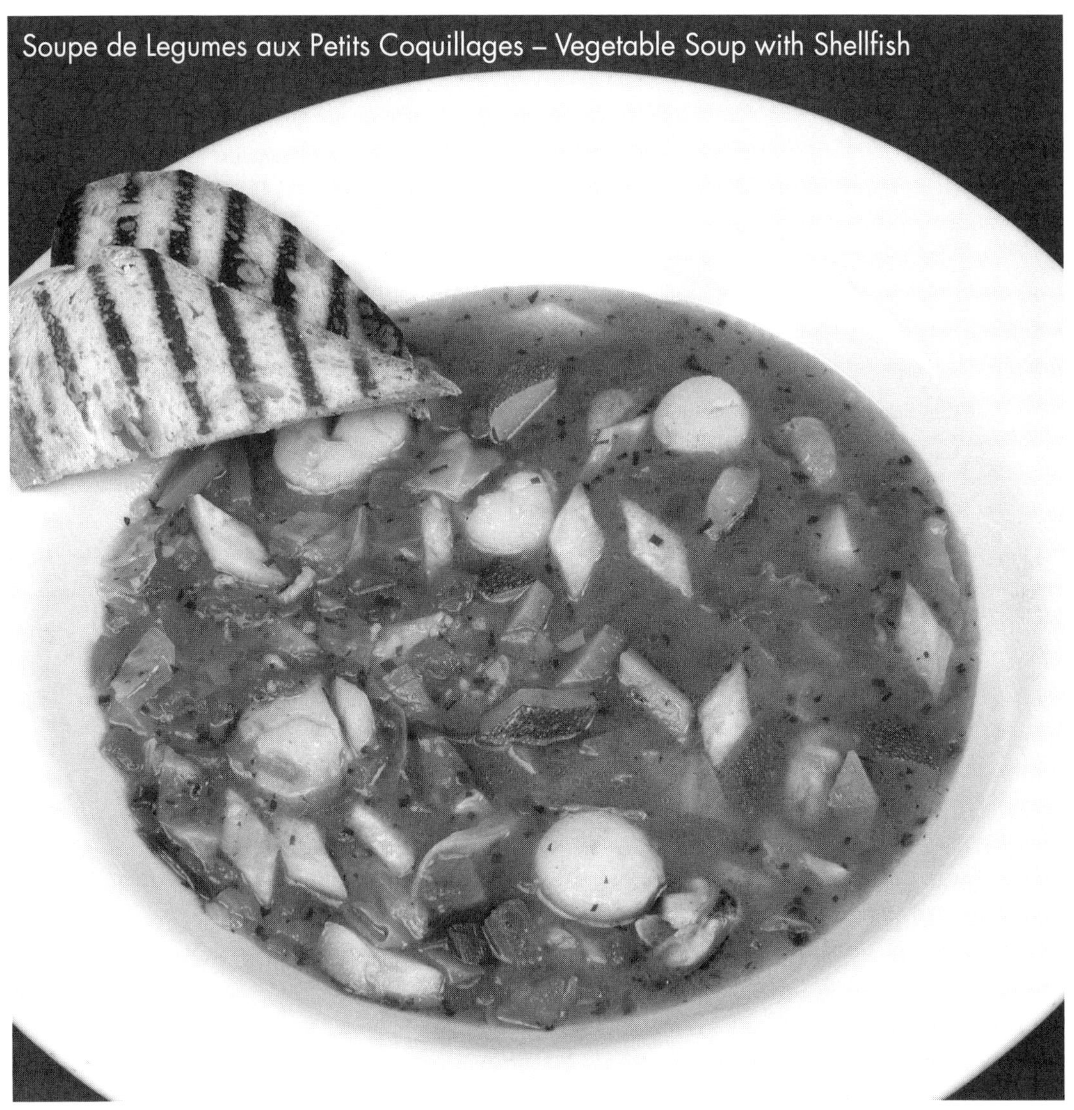
Soupe de Legumes aux Petits Coquillages – Vegetable Soup with Shellfish

# Le Blanc de Poisson Belle Mouginoise Fillet of Fish Mouginoise

SERVES 4

**Roger Verges' Moulin de Mougins restaurant is the inspiration for this recipe.**

| AMOUNT | MEASURE | INGREDIENT |
|---|---|---|
| 2 | 5 x 6 in (12.5 cm x 15 cm) | Firm red tomatoes, peeled |
| 1 each | | English seedless cucumber, unpeeled |
| 4 each | | Very large mushrooms, white as possible, more if large are not available |
| 4 each | 5 ounces, 140 g | Skinless and boneless fish fillet, $\frac{1}{2}$ inch (1.2 cm) thick (sea bass, red snapper, ling, turbot, orange roughie, or any firm white fish) |
| To taste | | Salt and pepper |
| Enough to grease pan | | Butter |
| 3 tablespoons | | Shallots, minced |
| 3 tablespoons | 1$\frac{1}{2}$ ounces, 45 ml | Vermouth |
| 6 tablespoons | 3 ounces, 90 ml | White wine |
| 2 tablespoons | 1 ounces, 30 ml | Chicken or fish stock, jelled |
| $\frac{1}{2}$ cup | 4 ounces, 120 ml | Heavy cream |
| 4 tablespoons | 2 ounces, 60 ml | Butter |
| 2 tablespoons | | Chives, minced |

## PROCEDURE

1 Finely slice ($\frac{1}{8}$ inch, .3 cm) tomatoes, cucumbers, and mushrooms.

2 Arrange the vegetables in 3 separate neat rows along the length of the fish fillets, with slices overlapping: mushrooms overlapped by tomatoes and cucumbers overlapping the tomatoes. Season with salt and pepper.

3 Butter a pan large enough to hold the fish. Spread the shallots on the bottom of the pan and the place the fish on top.

4 Add the vermouth and wine, place in a preheated 400°F (205°C) oven, and cook 4 to 6 minutes or until fish is just cooked; do not overcook.

5 Remove the fish from the cooking liquid; set aside and keep moist and warm.

6 Add fish stock and cream; reduce liquids to sauce consistency (coats the back of a spoon), 1 to 2 minutes. Whisking vigorously, add the butter, then the chives. Correct seasoning and remove from heat.

7 Sauce the base of each plate. With a pastry, brush the vegetables with a little melted butter to give them sheen.

8 Place fish on the sauced plate and serve hot.

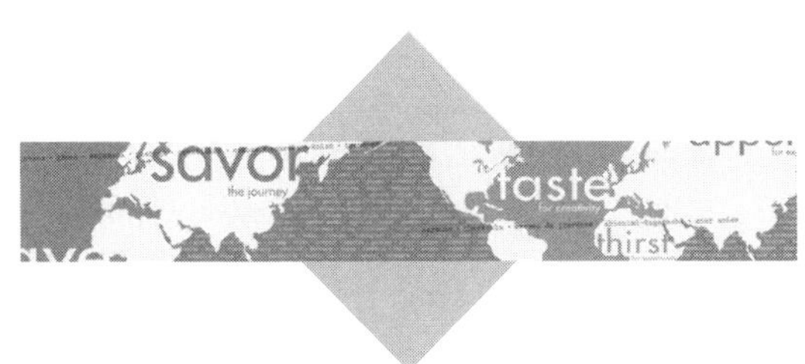

# Filet de Porc Farci Lyonnaise

## Stuffed Pork Tenderloin SERVES 4

| AMOUNT | MEASURE | INGREDIENT |
|---|---|---|
| **Stuffing** | | |
| $\frac{1}{2}$ cup | 2 ounces, 56 g | Onions, $\frac{1}{4}$ inch (.6 cm) dice |
| 1 tablespoon | $\frac{1}{2}$ ounce, 15 ml | Butter |
| $\frac{1}{2}$ cup | 2 ounces, 56 g | Ground pork |
| $\frac{1}{2}$ cup | 2 ounces, 56 g | Fresh white bread crumbs |
| 2 teaspoons | | Sage, chopped |
| 1 tablespoon | | Chervil, chopped |
| To taste | | Salt and pepper |
| 1 each | | Egg yolk |
| **Pork** | | |
| 1 pound | 448 g | Pork tenderloin (1 large) |
| 2 tablespoons | 1 ounce, 30 ml | Butter |
| 1 cup | 4 ounces, 112 g | Red onions, thinly sliced |
| $\frac{1}{2}$ cup | 2 ounces, 56 g | Celery, peeled, $\frac{1}{4}$ inch (.6 cm) |
| $\frac{1}{2}$ cup | 4 ounces, 120 ml | Brown stock |
| $\frac{1}{4}$ cup | 2 ounces, 60 ml | Heavy cream |
| 1 teaspoon | | Arrowroot, mixed to a paste with 1 tablespoon ($\frac{1}{2}$ ounce, 15 ml) water |

### PROCEDURE

1. Make the stuffing: sauté the onions in the butter over medium heat unit soft but not brown.
2. Off the heat, combine the onions, ground pork, bread crumbs, herbs, salt, pepper, and egg yolk. Mix well.
3. Make a slit down the length of the pork tenderloin and open the meat so it is flat. Tap to even out the thickness and flatten slightly.
4. Spread the stuffing, arranging neatly head to tail. Roll to shape and truss with string.
5. Preheat oven to 350°F (176°C).

6 Over medium heat, brown the pork in 2 tablespoons (1 ounce, 30 ml) butter on all sides; remove.

7 Add the sliced onions and celery; cook 7 to 8 minutes, stirring frequently. Place pork on top of onion mixture, add stock, cover pan, and braise in the oven 30 to 40 minutes, or until pork stuffing is cooked.

8 Remove pork; arrange onions and celery on a platter or plates.

9 Add the cream to the cooking pan, bring to a boil, and cook 2 minutes. Use slurry to adjust consistency. Correct seasoning.

10 Remove string and slice pork; arrange on top of onion/celery mixture. Spoon sauce over pork.

11 Serve with mashed potatoes.

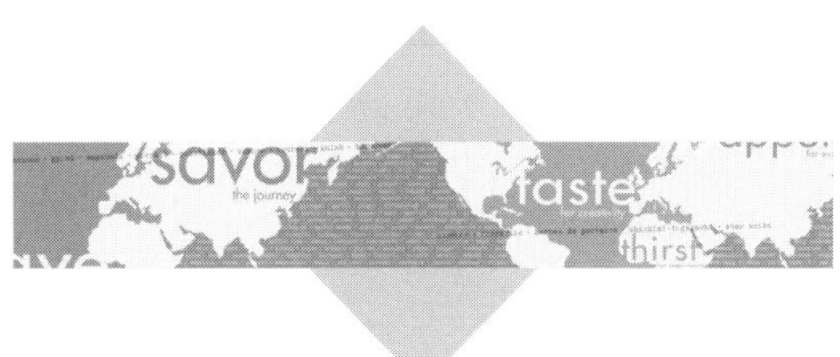

# Salade de Poire Pear Salad

SERVES 4

| AMOUNT | MEASURE | INGREDIENT |
|---|---|---|
| 1 cup | 4 ounces, 112 g | Carrots, peeled, julienned |
| 1 cup | 4 ounces, 112 g | Turnips, peeled, julienned |
| 2 tablespoons | 1 ounce, 30 ml | Sherry vinegar |
| 6 tablespoons | 3 ounces, 90 ml | Olive oil |
| 2 each | Medium size | Pears, peeled, cored, cut into 4 slices |
| 1 cup | 4 ounces, 112 g | Celery, peeled, $\frac{1}{4}$ inch (.6 cm) dice |
| 1 cup | 4 ounces, 112 g | Leeks, white part only, $\frac{1}{4}$ inch (.6 cm) dice |
| To taste | | Salt and pepper |
| Garnish | | Pomegranate seeds (optional) |

## PROCEDURE

1. Separately blanch carrots and turnips in salted water until crispy tender, 3 to 4 minutes. Drain, cool, and set aside.
2. Combine sherry vinegar and olive oil to make vinaigrette; correct seasoning.
3. Toss pears in vinaigrette as soon as they are peeled.
4. Moisten each vegetable with a little of the vinaigrette.
5. Arrange pears on 4 plates, surround with small heaps of each vegetable, and garnish with pomegranate seeds, if desired.

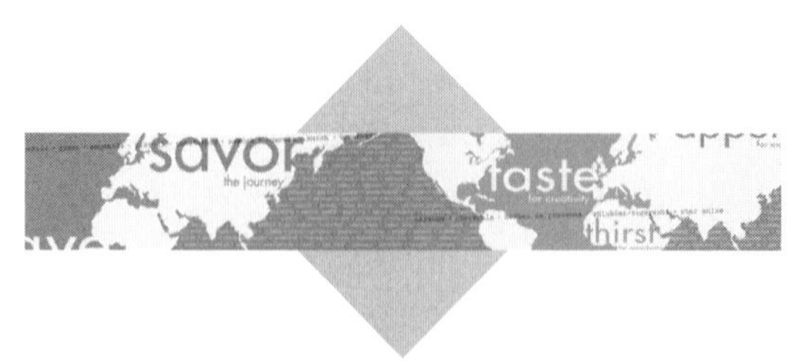

# Mousse au Chocolat

## Chocolate Mousse

YIELD: $1\frac{1}{2}$ QUARTS

| AMOUNT | MEASURE | INGREDIENT |
|---|---|---|
| **12 ounces** | **336 g** | **Bittersweet or semisweet chocolate, finely chopped** |
| **6 tablespoons** | **3 ounces, 90 ml** | **Butter, softened** |
| **$\frac{1}{2}$ cup** | **$3\frac{3}{4}$ ounces, 105 g** | **Granulated sugar** |
| **6 each** | | **Egg yolks** |
| **$\frac{1}{2}$ cup** | **4 ounces, 120 ml** | **Coffee** |
| **$1\frac{1}{4}$ cup** | **10 ounces, 300 ml** | **Heavy cream** |

**PROCEDURE**

1. Place chocolate over a hot water bath. After the chocolate begins to melt, stir with a rubber spatula. Continue stirring until the chocolate is $\frac{3}{4}$ melted. Remove the bowl from over the water and stir continuously to complete the melting.
2. To be sure that the butter is very soft, but not melted, divide the butter into 4 or 5 parts and whisk into the chocolate, until the butter has been completely absorbed. Set aside to cool to room temperature. If the butter is too cool it will set the chocolate. If the butter is too soft, the whey will release and cause the chocolate to seize.
3. Slowly whisk the sugar into the egg yolks in a stream. Whisk in the coffee and place the egg yolk mixture over the simmering hot water bath, whisking constantly until very thick. Transfer to a mixing bowl and whip by machine on medium speed until cool.
4. When mixture is cool, fold in the chocolate-butter mixture.
5. Whip cream to soft peaks; fold into the chocolate mixture.
6. Serve in small portions. Recommended accompaniments are Crème Chantilly, Crème Anglaise, or a flavored Crème Anglaise.

# Italy

## The Land

Italy is a long, thin peninsula that extends from the southern coast of Europe. Its immediate neighbors—France, Switzerland, Austria, and Slovenia—are in the north, where the Alps form a broad arc around the northern part of the country. Except in the north, Italy is surrounded by water. The country has a coastline of about 4,700 miles, bordered by the Adriatic Sea to the east, the Ionian Sea to the south, the Tyrrhenian Sea to the west, and the Ligurian Sea to the northwest. On a map, the Italian peninsula resembles a tall boot extending into the Mediterranean Sea toward the northern coast of the African continent, which at its closest point is only about 90 miles away. Italy includes a number of islands; the largest two are Sicily and Sardinia. And it has two small independent states within its borders: the Republic of San Marino (just 25 square miles in the Italy's northeast) and Vatican City (only 0.17 square miles within the city of Rome).

Italy's boot shape is formed around two ranges of mountains that form a T. The top crossbar is the Alps mountain range, which stretches from France to Slovenia. The north-south range is the Apennines, which twist along the length of the boot, leaving very little low coastal land.

Italy's northern region consists of the Alps and the Po valley. The largest city in the region is Genoa, the center of Italy's shipbuilding industry and the birthplace of Christopher Columbus. The Po valley contains Italy's most productive farmland, much of which is devoted to growing grain, especially rice, corn, and wheat.

The central southern region contains the nation's capital, Rome, and Tuscany's capital, Florence, historically two of the most influential cities in Europe. Much of the land to the south is dry and yields few agricultural products.

Southern Italy is characterized by the rugged terrain of the Apennine Mountains. Land in the central part of this region is not as fertile or as well-irrigated as in the north; however, the area has many small farms that grow beans, wheat, olives, and the grapes used to produce Chianti wines.

Sicily is the largest of all the Mediterranean islands. Most of its hilly terrain is used to grow wheat and beans and as grazing land for sheep. In the shadow of the active volcano Etna, tropical fruit trees thrive.

Sardinia has few good roads and a harsh, mountainous terrain that is mainly used for raising sheep and, where irrigation is possible, growing wheat, olive trees, and grapevines.

# History

Italy has been ruled by emperors, popes, monarchs, democratically elected presidents, and prime ministers. The country has experienced periods of astonishing development, from the grandeur of the Roman Empire and the beauty of the Renaissance to devastating wars in the nineteenth and twentieth centuries and an economic boom in the 1960s.

The migrations of Indo-European peoples into Italy probably began about 2000 B.C. and continued to 1000 B.C. Know as the Etruscans, this founding civilization ruled from about the ninth century B.C. until they were overthrown by the Romans in the third century B.C. By 264 B.C., much of Italy was under the leadership of Rome. For the next seven centuries, until the barbarian invasions destroyed the western Roman Empire in the fourth and fifth centuries A.D., the history of Italy is largely the history of Rome. From A.D. 800 on, the Holy Roman Emperors, Roman Catholic popes, Normans, and Saracens all fought for control over various segments of the Italian peninsula. Numerous city-states, such as Venice and Genoa, whose political and commercial rivalries were intense, as well as many small principalities, flourished in the late Middle Ages. The commercial prosperity of northern and central Italian cities, beginning in the eleventh century, combined with the influence of the Renaissance starting in the fourteenth century, reduced the effects of these medieval political rivalries. Although Italy's influence declined after the sixteenth century, the cultural Renaissance had strengthened the idea of a single Italian nationality. By the early nineteenth century, a nationalist movement developed and led to the reunification of Italy in the 1860s, except for Rome, which joined a unified Italy in 1870.

Followed by a monarchy, a dictatorship, and a new Italian government after World War II, Italy has maintained its unity. Today, Italy is officially the Italian Republic, with twenty regions that are based primarily on history and culture.

## The People

Italians trace their culinary heritage to Romans, Greeks, Etruscans, and other Mediterranean peoples who developed the methods of raising, refining, and preserving foods. Dining customs acquired local accents influenced both by culture and a land divided by mountains and seas. Additionally, independent-minded spirits developed among the regions during the repeated shifts of ruling powers that fragmented Italy throughout history.

Because of its geographical position, Italy has direct contact with and the influence of the main ethnic and cultural areas of old Europe (neo-Latin, Germanic, and Slavic-Balkan areas) as well as through North African countries, along with the world of Arab-Islamic civilizations. Consequently, while still anchored in the European and Western civilization, Italy can be considered a natural link to those African and western Asian countries that, bordering as they do on the same Mediterranean Sea, have shared historical events and cultural influences over many centuries.

## The Food

Italians are very proud of their cuisine since their food is renowned throughout the world. Italian cooking is still, however, very regional, with different towns and regions having their own traditions and specialties. The tomato, one of the signature ingredients of Italian cuisine, did not exist in Italy until Columbus brought some back from the New World. Olive oil is the principal cooking oil in the south. Butter is preferred in most of the north. Pasta in the south is normally tubular-shaped and made from eggless dough, while in the north it is usually flat, ribbon-shaped, and egg-enriched. Southern cooks season more assertively than northern ones, using garlic and lots of strong herbs. Northern cooks strive more for subtleties. Antipasto means "before the meal" and is the traditional first course of a formal Italian meal and may consist of many things. The most traditional offerings are cured meats, marinated vegetables, olives, peperoncini (marinated small peppers) and various cheeses. Other additions may be anchovies, bruschetta (toasted bread) upon which one may stack the meats or cheeses. The antipasto is usually topped off with some olive oil. Italians vie with the French for the title

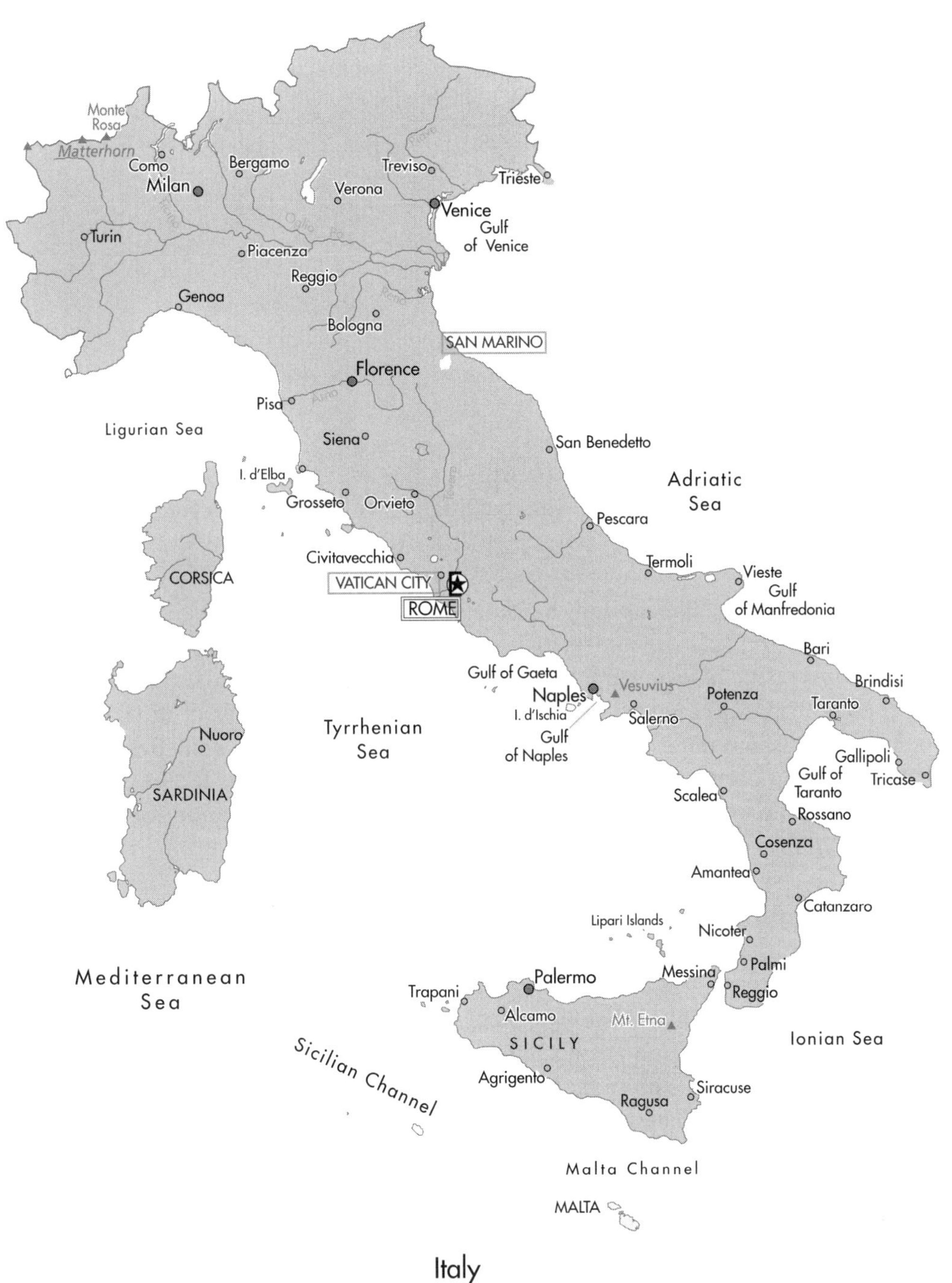

Monte Rosa
Matterhorn
Como
Milan
Bergamo
Verona
Treviso
Trieste
Venice
Gulf of Venice
Turin
Piacenza
Reggio
Genoa
Bologna
SAN MARINO
Florence
Pisa
Ligurian Sea
Siena
San Benedetto
I. d'Elba
Grosseto
Orvieto
Adriatic Sea
Pescara
CORSICA
Civitavecchia
VATICAN CITY
ROME
Termoli
Vieste
Gulf of Manfredonia
Bari
Brindisi
Gulf of Gaeta
Naples
Vesuvius
I. d'Ischia
Gulf of Naples
Salerno
Potenza
Taranto
Tyrrhenian Sea
Nuoro
SARDINIA
Gallipoli
Gulf of Taranto
Tricase
Scalea
Rossano
Cosenza
Amantea
Catanzaro
Lipari Islands
Nicoter
Palmi
Messina
Reggio
Mediterranean Sea
Trapani
Palermo
Alcamo
Mt. Etna
SICILY
Ionian Sea
Sicilian Channel
Agrigento
Siracuse
Ragusa
Malta Channel
MALTA


Italy

of the world's foremost wine drinkers. Italy, with a population of about 57 million, consists of twenty regions subdivided into ten provinces that take the names of prominent towns. Each province has its own distinctive foods and wines.

## NORTHERN ITALY

Northern Italy encompasses eight of the country's twenty regions:

- Emilia-Romagna
- Fruili-Venezia Giulia
- Liguria
- Lombardy
- Piedmont
- Trentino-South Tyrol
- Asota Valley
- Veneto

These eight regions boast the nation's highest standard of living and its richest diet in terms of both abundance and variety. The plains that extend along the Po and lesser rivers from Piedmont to the northern rim of the Adriatic proliferate with grain, corn, rice, fruit, livestock, and dairy products. Vineyards on slopes along the great arc formed by the Alps and Apennines mountains are Italy's prime sources of premium wine. Northern Italy also has a flourishing tourist trade on the Italian Riviera, in the Alps, and on the shores of its lakes.

The cuisine here is characterized by the use of butter (or lard), rice, corn (for polenta), and cheeses for cream sauces. An exception would be the olive oils of the Liguria and the Lakes regions. Pasta in the north is less popular than risotto and polenta. Seafood and shellfish are very popular on the coasts, and rivers and streams provide carp and trout. The eight northern regions produce about a third of Italian wine, though they account for more than half of the DOC/DOCG total.

**Emilia Romagna** Known as "Italy's Food Basket," this area produces some of the country's most famous foods, including Prosciutto de Parma, Mortadella, Parmigian-Reggiano, and balsamic vinegar. Cooks here are especially skilled at making stuffed pasta by hand, including the tortellini of Emilia and the cappelletti of Romagna, served with the famous Bolognese meat sauce (*Ragu*). Parmigiano-Reggiano is available around the world but its production is strictly enforced to ensure a continued tradition of quality. It takes about eight quarts of milk to make one pound of this delicacy, the so-called "king of cheeses." Aged for a minimum of twelve months and for as long as twenty-four months, Parmigiano-Reggiano is made according to the age-old traditions passed down from generation to generation. Pork products include Parma's famous *prosciutto* made from the meat of carefully raised local pigs, which is salted, cured with air descended from the Apennine mountains, then aged in special underground caves and closely tended to by Parma's *salumieri.*

Romagna is home to fish and seafood dishes, with eels being a favorite of Comacchio. Aceto balsamico, or balsamic vinegar, is produced exclusively in the province of Modena by the same time-honored method used for centuries. It is made from the must, or fresh juice, of wine grapes, most commonly from the Trebbiano grape. The grapes are left on the vine for the longest possible time to achieve maximum sweetness. The must is then cooked until it has reduced to a thick, sweet syrup. It then undergoes a fermentation process, poured into barrels made of ancient woods that impart their own distinctive flavor to the developing vinegar. When the vinegar is transferred to a smaller barrel, a bit of the old vinegar is left so the new vinegar comes into contact with the old. Time allows the vinegar to evaporate and become more deeply flavored, more richly colored, and more concentrated. It may be aged for years, decades, even centuries. By the time it is ready to bottle it is dark brown, slightly sweet, and highly concentrated. There is a panel of experts that approves a balsamic vinegar to be labeled as special after aging for twelve years and extra special after aging twenty-five years to ensure that the quality of these prized vinegars from Modena are maintained.

**Friuli-Venezia Giulia** Slavic, Austrian, and Hungarian influences make the cuisine of Friuli-Venezia Giulia unique. Trieste, the region's capital, straddles the Adriatic Sea and has long been the gateway to the East; the city's Viennese sausage, goulash, cabbage soups, and strudel pastries come from years under Austro-Hungarian rule. Particular to the cooking of the Friuli-Venezia Giulia is a pungent fermented turnip preparation known as *brovada,* served alongside spiced pork dishes. *San Daniele prosciutto* is considered one of the world's best hams, made only by twenty-seven small producers in the town of San Daniele. Free of additives and seasoned only with sea salt, San Daniele prosciutto has no more than 3 to 4 percent fat, and this is found only on the edges of the meat. The region is known for its vast cornfields, which feed the area's demand for *polenta.* For centuries, polenta, more than bread, was the staff of life for the frugal mountaineers of this region. Depending on the region and the texture desired, polenta is made with either coarsely, medium, or finely ground dried yellow or white cornmeal. Polenta derives from earlier forms of grain mush (known as *puls* or *pulmentum* in Latin, or more commonly as gruel or porridge) commonly eaten in Roman times and after. Early forms of polenta were made with such starches as the grain farro or chestnut flour, both of which are still used in small quantity today. When boiled, polenta has a smooth creamy texture, caused by the presence of starch molecules dissolved into the water.

**Liguria** Ligurian cuisine is called *cucina del ritorno,* or "homecoming" cooking, as a tribute to the sailors who would return home after months at sea. Fish dominates the menu, found in soups, stews, and salads. Liguria's best-known seafood specialty is *burida,* a seafood stew made with various fishes. The most famous of all culinary works from Liguria is its basil pesto sauce. Traditionally basil, olive oil, garlic, pine nuts, and Parmesan cheese are put in a mortar and pounded with a pestle to achieve a smooth sauce. The olive oil of the region is an exception to most of northern Italian cooking and plays an everyday role along this region's rocky coast. Because the salty air and humidity makes it difficult to bake good bread and keep it from spoiling quickly, *focaccia* was devised as a bread alternative that could be eaten hot out of the oven. This unleavened, thin, flat bread is usually topped with olive oil and salt, or with sage, cheese, or onions.

All cuisines have some type of dumpling and in Italy gnocchi recipes are recorded as far back as cookbooks of the thirteenth century. In some places gnocchi made of flour and water are considered "pasta" while dumplings made of different ingredients are called gnocchi. Gnocchi can be made with the most varied ingredients such as squash, bread, and semolina flour; and they can be flavored mixing the dough with spinach, saffron, and even truffles. They are boiled in water or broth, and like pasta, they can be dressed with many sauces such as pesto, tomato, butter and cheese. Today, gnocchi are primarily made with potatoes.

**Lombardy** The region's capital city of Milan is the most modern and cosmopolitan of cities and the cutting-edge fashion center of Italy. Lombardy occupies the central part of the Po Valley. It is known for its rice dishes including *minestrone alla Milanese,* made with vegetables, rice, and bacon. *Risotto alla Milanese* is a creamy dish of braised short-grain rice blended with meat stock, saffron, and cheese. Generous use of butter is a hallmark of Milanese/Lombard cooking. So is the preference for rice or polenta over pasta. Cream sauces are more popular here than in other regions. Being landlocked, Lombardy has few notable seafood specialties. Meat (especially veal) is most popular. The internationally renowned dish *osso buco* is veal shank braised with tomato, onion, stock, and wine, then topped with *gremolata,* a garnish made with parsley, garlic, and lemon rind. The choicest morsel in *osso buco* ("hole in bone") is the cooked marrow clinging to the hollow of the bone.

Regional Lombard cheeses include the blue-veined Gorgonzola, the creamy and mild Bel Paese, mascarpone, and the surface-ripened Taleggio. *Panettone* is the cherished Italian holiday bread. Jeweled with candied fruits (particularly citrus) and raisins, it first appeared in Milan about 1490 and was quickly adopted throughout Italy, from the Alps to Sicily. The traditional recipe calls for using nothing but white wheat flour, sugar, top-quality butter, eggs, and sultana raisins. In order to safeguard tradition and ensure that *panettone* is made in the time-honored, nonindustrial manner, efforts are currently underway to establish guidelines for ingredients and procedures that will serve as the basis for obtaining a special DOP (Protected Designation of Origin) certification from the European Union.

**Piedmont** Piedmont means "the foot of the mountains" in Italian. Although culinary influences from neighboring France can be seen in the regional cuisine, Piedmontese cookery is nonetheless distinct unto itself. The white Alba truffle is considered the most delicious and sought-after truffle in the world. An uncultivable mushroom, the valuable fungus can only be found between the months of November and February, in a few spots in France and Italy, including the Piedmont region. Gathering white truffles is a difficult process requiring a *trifulau,* or professional truffle hunter, and his trained dog or pig. The white truffle is found in five different varieties, determined by the species of tree on whose roots it originates. So depending on whether it is associated with the weeping willow, oak, poplar, linden, or vine plant, its color can range from white, sometimes veined with pink, to gray verging on brown. Italians eat them raw, shaved paper-thin over egg dishes, in plain pastas (dressed only with butter and cheese), fonduta (fondue), risotto, and other light foods. *Bagna cauda* is dipping sauce made with olive oil, chopped garlic, anchovies, butter, and sometimes sliced white truffles. Into this heated sauce the diner dips a wide choice of cold raw vegetables. Red wine is the traditional accompaniment. *Grissini* are thin and crispy breadsticks that have become popular throughout the country. Piedmonte produces about half of Italy's rice, and rice-based dishes like *panicia de Novara* (a vegetable soup with rice) and *risotto all Piedmontese* (risotto with meat stock, Parmesan, nutmeg, and truffle) are regional specialties. *Ribiola di Roccaverano* is a fresh cheese that is neither aged nor matured. Cylindrical in shape and high in fat, it is made from a combination of cow's, goat's, and sheep's milk, derived from two daily milkings. The texture is grainy and the color milky white. It has a delicate aroma and acidic flavor. The famous *Barolo* and *Barbaresco* wines are produced in this region. In addition to hunting truffles, fall is the time for hunting wild game, gathering nuts, and harvesting grapes.

**Trentino–South Tyrol** This region shares culinary traditions from both the Italian and German sides of the border. The cuisine combines Germanic, Hungarian, and Italian touches, and includes sauerkraut, beef goulash, and fruit-stuffed gnocchi with browned butter and breadcrumbs. Rather than pasta or risotto, cooks in this region prefer to prepare polentas made of cornmeal or buckwheat, or hearty soups garnished with bread dumplings. *Speck,* the region's prized smoked ham, flavors numerous dishes, from braised cabbage in red wine to long-simmered pork stews. *Speck* shares its name with a German pork product, but while German *speck* is basically lard, Italian *speck* has some similar characteristics to smoked bacon. Unlike American bacon that comes from the belly portion of the hog (same as *pancetta*), *speck* is made from hog legs. Speck originates from the Alto Adige region, where it is still a homemade process protected by a PGI designation. The meat is seasoned with salt and spices that include pepper, laurel, and juniper berries before being allowed to rest for about a month. *Speck* is then smoked using flavorful beech, ash, or juniper wood for ten days. Following that, the meat is aged for months to produce a smoky and slightly spicy product with a distinct pink/red interior with a small amount of fat. It is then used in pasta sauces, or with meat or eggs. Genuine *speck* must have a rind that is well marked, and should be slightly firm to the touch. *Canderlt,* made with bread and flour and served in a broth, is just one of several types of gnocchi (dumplings) popular in the region. The most popular cheeses include the fresh *Tosela, Spressa delle Giudicarie (DOP),* and *Puzzone di Moena.*

**Valle d'Osta (Asota Valley)** The traditional cooking of this region incorporates both French and Swiss influences. Stone-ground cornmeal is transformed into polentas. Traditionally polenta is prepared by constantly stirring cornmeal, water, and salt over heat for 40 to 45 minutes with a wooden stirring stick called a *mescola.* The resulting "mush" is then poured onto a wooden board to cool slightly and is cut with kitchen string while still hot. At one time, families would take "shifts" as stirrers; today, automatic stirring machines make the job easier. Fontina cheese, a semi-cooked, straw-yellow cheese with tiny holes and a soft texture, is used to make fonduta, or fondue, one of the region's famous dishes. Local bread is made of cold-hardy northern grains like rye or buckwheat. *Pane nero* (black bread) is a staple food made with rye and wheat flours that was once baked in the communal oven just once a year and dried to preserve it. Beef is the staple meat. *Carbonade* is a classic stew made with salt-cured or fresh beef, onions, red wine, butter, and nutmeg, often served with polenta.

**Veneto** In general, the cooking in this region is based on four basic foods: polenta, rice, beans, and vegetables along with wild fowl, mushrooms, or seafood. Traditional courses include *risi e bisi* (rice and peas), and *fegato alla Veneziana* (calf's liver fried with onions). *Radicchio di Treviso* is a bitter red chicory served as a salad but more often grilled and served with salt and olive oil. *Sopressa* is a finely ground pure pork sausage, traditionally made from pigs fed on chestnuts and potatoes. Veneto's contribution to Italy's pasta culture is a style of fresh pasta called *bigoli,* which gets its name from the traditional kitchen implement, a four-inch-wide bronze tube called a *bigolaro. Bigoli,* a long, spaghetti-style pasta with a hole in its middle, is made on a hand-operated press by forcing pasta dough through the bigolaro, then cutting the strands to the desired length. A typical preparation is *bigoli in salsa,* in which the pasta is tossed with a sauce of anchovies, olive oil, and cooked onions. This region is home to the city of Venice, known for its romantic canals and bridges. The main difference between the cuisines of Venice and other parts of Veneto is the availability of fresh seafood, ranging from prawns, shrimp, and clams to fresh fish and eels. *Baccala,* dried, salted codfish, is served throughout the area, often mixed with polenta into a "cream" that is served as an appetizer or first course.

### CENTRAL ITALY

Central Italy encompasses six of the country's regions:

- Abruzzo
- Latium
- Marches
- Molise
- Tuscany
- Umbria

The summers are hotter and longer than those in the north, and consequently tomato-based dishes are more common than they are further north. Braised meats and stews, grilled or roasted beef, lamb, poultry, pork, and game are popular. Central Italy has a rich farming tradition and cultivates many crops that are difficult to find elsewhere, including farro, an ancient grain domesticated by the Romans, and saffron. Miles of olive groves and vineyards dominate parts of the landscape. The cuisine is simple and rustic dishes are served with light sauces and seasonings.

**Abruzzo** This region is sparsely populated and geographically diverse. It is known for its livestock production and farming, the growing and production of the highly prized herb saffron, and an abundance of seafood specialties. Pasta, vegetables, and meat (especially lamb and pork) are the staples of this region. The pasta most often associated with Abruzzo is *maccheroni alla chitarra,* a square spaghetti so named because the device used in its production, made of a wooden box strung with steel wire, resembles a guitar. This is traditionally served with a lamb, tomato, and peperoncino sauce, sprinkled with local pecorino (sheep's milk) cheese. The red chile pepper peperoncino is known as *diavolino,* or little devil, and is a key ingredient in the cuisine of this area. The town of Sulmona is Italy's confectionary capital and is where the sugared almond was created 250 years ago. A blend of the best almonds and extra-fine sugar produce this traditional wedding candy *(confetti)*, which signifies the union of life through the bitterness of the almond and the sweetness of the candy of what matrimony and life may offer. The tradition is to give confetti candy to the guests at weddings; it is usually done in a group of five candies, each of which signifies Health, Wealth, Happiness, Longevity, and Fertility. The region's cheeses include a vast assortment of pecorino, and scamorza, a close relative of mozzarella. Three types of wine are predominant: *Montepulciano,* a robust red; *Cerasuolo,* a rosé; and *Trebbiano d'Abruzzo,* a crisp white.

**Latium** This rustic region is home to Rome, the capital of Italy, and much of its countryside remains as it must have been in the days of the Empire: quiet, dotted with sheep, the domain of farmers and shepherds who make a living in its hills and valleys. In Latium, milk-fed lamb is a favorite dish, usually baked and served with seasonal vegetables, and sheep's milk cheese is produced abundantly in small dairies and large cooperatives. Simple pastas made of flour and water are the basis of many famous pasta dishes that include *bucatini all'amatriciana,* with tomato, onion, bacon, and a dash of cognac; *spaghetti alla carbonara,* with bacon, eggs, butter, and cheese sauce dusted with black pepper "coal flakes"; and *spaghetti alla puttansesca,* which includes garlic, tomatoes, capers, olives, herbs, and anchovies. Over 90 varieties of artichokes are grown in Italy and are very popular in Rome where they are flattened and fried twice for *carcioif alla guidia* (Jewish style) or prepared *alla Romana,* stuffed with bread crumbs, parsley, anchovies, salt, and pepper. Meat dishes include *abbacchio al forno* (roast lamb) or *alla cacciatora* (lamb with an anchovy and rosemary sauce) and *saltimbocca* (a fillet of veal rolled in ham and flavored and served in a Marsala sauce).

**Marches** The food of Marches is a mix of rustic fare and seafood. *Brodetto* is a fish stew found along the Adriatic coast and varies in form from each coastal town. This regions' *brodetto* includes red and gray mullet, cuttlefish or squid (or both), oil, garlic, and saffron, served on either fried or toasted bread. Dried cod is used in a dish called *stoccafisso,* while sea snails cooked in fennel are a delicacy. The Marches signature dish is *porchetta,* where a roast suckling pig is either served whole, or is sliced into crispy bread rolls. Classic pastas include *papardelle alla papara,* a flat pasta with duck sauce, and *vincigrassi,* a lasagna containing cream, truffles, ragu, butter, Parmigiano-Reggiano, mozzarella, and various other ingredients. Other specialties include Ascolana olives stuffed with meat and lightly fried, pasta served with clams and mussels, risotto with farro grain, smoked trout from mountain streams, rabbit with fennel and sausage, and fava beans with fresh pecorino cheese. *Ciauscolo* salami is a specialty made by kneading very finely ground pork from the belly and shoulder of the pig with a good quantity of fat until the mixture is very soft. The meat is flavored simply with garlic, salt, and pepper, and it is often smoked. Given its soft consistency, much like a pâté, *ciauscolo* is meant to be spread onto bread rather than sliced. Casciotta d'Urbino cheese is pale yellow and is lightly perforated by characteristic little holes. Made from sheep's and cow's milk, it is eaten after maturing for twenty to thirty days.

**Molise** Because of their joint history, Molise shares many of the culinary traditions of the Abruzzo region, but there are also a few dishes unique to the region. One is *p'lenta d'iragn,* a white polenta made with potatoes and wheat and served with a tomato sauce. Another is *calconi di ricotta rustica*, ravioli stuffed with ricotta, provolone, and prosciutto, then fried in oil.

Traditionally, townspeople migrated to the area each year, bringing their sheep to Puglia. Because the animals were meant to be sold, not used for personal needs, meat was considered a luxury. As a result, very little meat is eaten. Vegetables, cheese, pasta, grains, and fresh fruit still dominate the diet today. Chile and garlic lace nearly every dish, as does Molise's golden olive oil. The cheeses of Molise include *scamorza, mateca,* and *burrino.* The interior of Molise is dotted with apple orchards of a very old type of tree that produces very aromatic fruit known as *mela limoncella.* Many families used to display these apples around their kitchen and living room doorframes because of their special scent. They have a green-yellow peel, a very strong scent, and a slightly acidic yet sweet flavor.

**Tuscany** The Etruscans, who likely hailed originally from Asia Minor, settled primarily in Tuscany around 1000 B.C., planting vines and olive groves and spreading their cultural and culinary influence as far as the islands of Corsica and Elba. It has been said that this is where Italian cooking was born—at the court of the Medici. The region is home to the extra-virgin Tuscan olive oil, an intense oil with a green to golden color. The white-hided cattle found in Tuscany's Chianna valley produce large cuts of meat that is low in fat. Florence offers its famous *alla fiorentina* steak and specialties that include *ribollita* (a thick vegetable soup), *fagioli all'uccelletto* (beans sautéed in garlic and sage with tomatoes), and *fagioli al fiasco* (beans with oil, onions, and herbs cooked in a round bottle—a *fiasco*—over a coal fire. Seafood dishes include *triglie* (red mullet) and a delicious fish soup known as *Cacciucco alla Livornese.* Known as "strong bread" and once considered an aphrodisiac, *panforte* is a cake containing almonds, honey, candied lemon and orange peel, flour, sugar, and spices. Tuscan wines are known worldwide, including *Chianti,* which comes in both red and white varieties.

**Umbria** Nicknamed "The Green Heart of Italy," Umbria is just southeast of Tuscany. Landlocked, it relies on pork for most of its classic preparations, and its pork butchers are said to be the best in Italy: every scrap of the pig is put to good use. Specialties like *guanciale* (the salted and cured meat from the pig's cheek) are added to pasta sauces and pots of fava beans or peas. Norcia in the Apennine foothills is the home of Italy's best black truffles (*tartufo nero*). Covered by a black skin with small wartlike bumps, the truffle has a purple-black flesh with distinctive white veins and a delicate scent. Unlike white truffles, which can only be eaten raw, black truffles can be heated and added to sauces and pastas without losing their flavor. Many types of handmade pasta like *strozzapreti* (priest stranglers) are not typically found outside Umbria. Besides homemade fresh egg pastas, the production of much of the dried pasta consumed throughout Italy occurs in Umbria. The wines of Umbria rank among Italy's finest. They include *Orvieto, Rosso di Montefalco, Sagrantino di Montefalco,* and vin santo, a sweet dessert wine often consumed with biscotti. Umbria is home to Perugina (now owned by Nestle), one of the major chocolate producers in Italy.

## SOUTHERN ITALY

Southern Italy, often referred to as the Mezzogiorno, encompasses four of the country's regions:

- Basilicata
- Campania
- Calabria
- Apulia (Puglia)

and the islands of:

- Sicily
- Sardinia

The symbol of southern Italian cooking is the tomato, although it arrived with peppers, beans, and potatoes from America in the 1500s. The eggplant was originally cultivated in Asia, although it now distinguishes the *parmigiana* classics of the Campania region and many other classic Italian dishes. The piquancy of southern cooking comes from herbs and spices, especially garlic and chile peppers. Italy's first pasta was produced in the south, though noodles were preceded by flatbreads called *focacce,* forerunners of pizza, which originated in Naples. Baked goods, including pastries, biscuits, and cakes, abound in the Mezzogiorno, though nowhere as evident as in Sardinia, where each village has its own style of bread making. Arab settlers in Sicily established a pasta industry during the Middle Ages, using durum wheat for the dried pasta types that still prevail in the south. Tubes and other forms of "short" pasta may be referred to generically as *maccheroni,* distinguished from "long" types such as spaghetti and vermicelli. Also popular are spiral-shaped fusilli, oblique tubes called penne, and larger tubes called ziti, or zite. Fresh pasta is also prized, sometimes, but not usually, made with eggs, in such familiar dishes as lasagna, fettuccine, and ravioli, with no shortage of local versions.

**Basilicata** Historically one of Italy's poorest regions, Basilicata is also one of its least populated. Today, the economic situation is much improved, but the cuisine remains anchored in peasant traditions. Along the region's coastline, seafood plays a major role in the diet, with favorites including mussels, oysters, octopus, red mullet, and swordfish. Vegetables include fava beans, artichokes, chicory, and various greens including *rucola* (rocket). Eggplants, peppers, *lampasciuoli* (a bitter type of onion), cauliflower, olives, and olive oil are all regional staples. Regional pastas include *orecchiette* and *bucatini,* both typically served with tomato sauce or with olive oil, garlic, and cauliflower.

**Campania** Best known around the world for its pizza, Campania's cuisine relies on vegetables and herbs, capers, dried pasta, and fresh farmhouse cheeses. In the nineteenth century, people living in the capital city of Naples were nicknamed *mangia maccheroni* (maccheroni eaters) and to this day, Neapolitans remain devoted pasta eaters. Their pasta is considered among the best and the most varied in all of Italy. Italian food would not be the same without spaghetti with *pommarola,* the famous tomato sauce. The volcanic soils of Campania grow some of the best produce in Italy, including San Marzano tomatoes, peaches, grapes, apricots, figs, oranges, and lemons. Campania's most famous cheese is *mozzarella di bufalo campania,* made from the milk of local water buffalos. Other popular cheeses include sheep's milk Pecorino, scamorza, ricotta (both cow and buffalo versions), and mascarpone. Parmigiano-Reggiano is popular in recipes of Campania, with meat and vegetable dishes served *alla Parmigiana.*

The region is also renowned for its fish and seafood specialties. Octopus is tenderized by stewing it in a sealed clay pot with olive oil, garlic, capers, olives, and parsley or with chiles and tomatoes. Squid and cuttlefish are boiled and served in salads, stuffed and baked, or fried into rings, while mussels and clams are cooked and tossed with handmade pasta or added to seafood salads. Salt cod, fresh sardines, and anchovies too are staples. Christmas is celebrated with a dish of eel marinated with vinegar and herbs or cooked with tomatoes and white wine.

Originating in Naples more than three hundred years ago, pizza is often thought of as "genuine" Italian food by non-Italians; but pizza was little known in Italy (outside of Naples) until the 1970s. Pizza came to the United States early in the twentieth century during the great migration of Italians from southern Italy. In 2004, Italy drew up a series of rules that must be followed to make a true Neapolitan pizza: the dough must rise for at least six hours and must be kneaded and shaped by hand; the pizza must be round and no more than 13.7 inches in diameter; and it may only be cooked in a wood-fired oven. And only three variations of pizza are permitted: *marinara* with garlic and oregano; *Margherita* with basil, tomatoes, and cheese from the southern Apennine Mountains; and the "extra" *Margherita,* which includes buffalo mozzarella from the Campania region.

**Calabria** Surrounded by the Tyrrhenian and the Ionian Seas, Calabria has 500 miles of coastline (the longest of any Italian region). Over the centuries, Greek, Arab, and Albanian influences have shaped the cuisine, where characteristic dishes are flavored with chile pepper;

sweet-and-sour preparations are popular; and desserts are often deep-fried and soaked in honey. *Melanzane alla parmigiana,* or eggplant Parmesan (eggplant that is fried, then baked in the oven with tomato and cheese), was created in Calabria, where the eggplant crop thrives. The dry climate, high temperature, and nearly calcium-free soil are ideal for growing eggplants because they prevent a buildup of the fruit's bitter juices and concentrate its sweet flavor. A popular breakfast in this region is called *murseddu.* It consists of a ragu made from pig and calf's liver that is cooked slowly in tomatoes, herbs, and hot red pepper, and then stuffed in the local *pitta bread.* Despite numerous attempts to export production to other areas in Italy and the world, *bergametto,* or bergamot oranges, thrive only in Calabria. Bergamot oranges have a smooth, thin peel, an acidic flavor, and an intense scent. They look like an orange, but their color ranges from green to yellow, depending on how ripe they are. Their essential oil is used to flavor liqueurs, tea (such as Earl Grey), sweets, and drinks.

**Apulia** Three staples are essential to the Apulian kitchen: wheat, vegetables, and olive oil. Semolina flour is turned into a variety of handmade pastas (some shaped like little ears, others like concave shells, others still like thick ropes), which are boiled with wild or cultivated greens, tossed with hearty meat ragus, or cooked into soups. Wheels of rustic bread are baked to be enjoyed as companions to daily meals and serve as the starting point for numerous appetizers, salads, soups, and simple desserts. The most interesting offering is *frisedda,* a twice-baked ring-shaped bread. And almost every dish is topped with olive oil—after all, Apulia is Italy's largest producer of olive oil. Fava beans are used to prepare thick soups, salads, and side dishes, and rice is baked with potatoes and seafood or vegetables to make an unusual main course called *tiella* (named after the pot in which it is cooked). The Apulians, shepherds by trade since ancient times, tend to prefer lamb, mutton, kid, and goat meat, which they cook simply with fragrant herbs, olive oil, and tomatoes or potatoes. Offal is popular in the area and lamb's hearts and intestines are skewered and cooked on a grill, then eaten with raw celery and sharp sheep's milk cheese. Pastries, cakes, and fritters are based on honey, nuts, and dried fruit, their origins in ancient Greece and echoes of the Orient. Apulians use a wide variety of wild and cultivated greens in the kitchen. Some, like sorrel, are relatively mild and astringent; others, like broccoli rabe and dandelions, can be bitter. Apulians tame the bitterness of these potent greens by lengthy cooking. They don't believe in undercooking vegetables; they prefer vegetables slippery soft, never crunchy. Bitter greens are typically boiled first in ample water, then sautéed slowly in olive oil.

**Sicily** The cuisine reflects the many invaders in this island's history and focuses on seafood (swordfish, tuna, mussels, prawns, sea bass, red mullet, anchovies, and more), eggplant, tomatoes, potatoes, beans and other vegetables, pecorino and many other cheeses, figs, capers, olives, almonds, pine nuts, fennel, raisins, lemons, and oranges. In parts of Sicily there are sweet-and-sour combinations like capers with sugar in *caponata,* a mix of eggplant, tomatoes, celery, olives, and capers cooked with vinegar and sugar. The *ceci,* or chickpea, has played an important role in Sicilian history and is well represented in the diet. *Panella* is a thin paste made of crushed *ceci* and served fried. *Maccu* is a creamy soup made from the same bean. Pasta is often served with a rich, spicy tomato sauce. Popular seafood dishes include grilled swordfish or snapper, *finocchio con le sarde* (fennel with sardines), and *sepia* (cuttlefish) served in its own black sauce with pasta. The best known Sicilian meat dish is *vitello al Marsala* (veal marsala) and is just one of many regional meat specialties that can also be made with lamb, kid, or rabbit. No other part of Italy has as many sweets and ices. Many desserts are derived from Arab and Greek influences and are made with almond pastes, candied fruits, ricotta, honey, raisins, and nuts. The best-known wine is Marsala, which is dark and strong.

**Sardinia** The island of Sardinia has been inhabited since the Neolithic age. Phoenician, Greek, Arab, Spanish, and French invaders have come and gone, marking the local language, customs, and cuisine. The mountainous inland terrain is home to wild animals (boar, mountain goat, and hare), which are transformed into pasta sauces, stews, and roasts. Lamb, the island's favorite meat, is often cooked with wild fennel, and sheep's milk cheese appears at nearly every meal. Spicy fish soups called *burrida* and *cassola,* along with lobsters, crabs, anchovies, squid, clams, and fresh sardines are all very popular along the Sardinian coast. Favorite Sardinian pasta dishes include *spaghetti con bottarga,* with dried gray mullet roe shaved on top, and *malloreddus,* gnocchi flavored with saffron and served with tomato sauce. *Culingiones* are round ravioli stuffed with spinach and cheese. Sardinia is known for its rustic sheep and goat cheeses like Pecorino Sardo and Fiore Sardo, which can be served either fresh or aged. The Sardinian interior produces some of the best lamb in all of Italy, known for being very lean. Sardinians enjoy their meats roasted and *porceddu* (the Sardinian version of porchetta), suckling pig, or kid (suckling goat) is roasted outdoors over aromatic woods.

# Glossary

**Agro** Foods may be referred to *agro/dolce. Agro* refers to the sour, often achieved through the use of vinegar. *Dolce* means sweet. Commonly found in some dishes from Sicily.

**Al dente** Literally "to the tooth," meaning cooked to the "point" or until just done but still crisp.

**Amaretti** Crisp almond macaroons sprinkled with coarse sugar.

**Amaretto** Almond liquor.

**Antipasto** Hors d'oeuvre; literally, "before the pasta."

**Apertivo** A beverage intended to awaken the palate and stimulate the appetite.

**Arborio Rice** Stubby, short-grain polished rice grown in Italy's Po valley. Its particular starch composition makes it the preferred rice for Italian risotto. It is perfect for dishes that are expected to absorb the flavor of the liquid in the recipe. *Carnaroli superfino* is the risotto rice most preferred by chefs due to its exceptional quality and structure, owing to high amylose starch content, which improves consistency, resistance to overcooking, and capacity for absorbing condiments and flavoring agents. The ideal rice for long-simmer, nonsticky risottos.

*Vialone nano* is another preferred risotto rice, with small, rounded grains, rich in amylose and very compact, allowing them to expand greatly during cooking. An ideal rice for no-stir risottos and rice salads, it is prized for its soft, light body.

**Arugula** Also known as rocket, garden rocket, rocket salad, rugola, or rucola; a type of leaf lettuce and a member of the mustard family. It is often served with air-dried beef Bresaola.

**Baccala** Cod that has been preserved with salt. In the Italian markets it's sold in slabs. It takes several soakings to remove the salt. Dry salt cod will keep indefinitely.

**Balsamic Vinegar *(Aceto Balsamico)*** An aged reduction of white sweet grapes (Trebbiano for red and Spergola for white sauvignon) that are boiled to a syrup. The grapes are cooked very slowly in copper cauldrons over an open flame until the water content is reduced by over 50 percent. The resulting "must" is placed into wooden barrels and older balsamic vinegar is added to assist in the acidification. Each year the aging vinegar is transferred to different wood barrels so that the vinegar can incorporate some of the flavors of the different woods. The only approved woods are oak, cherry, chestnut, mulberry, acacia, juniper, and ash. The age of the vinegar is divided into young (from 3 to 5 years maturation), middle (aged 6 to 12 years), and the highly prized very old (at least 12 years and up to 150 years old).

**Bianco** White, as in white sauce or white wine.

**Bollito Misto alla Piemontese** A rich and flavorful boiled dinner containing seven kinds of meat, seven vegetables, and seven condiments. The variety is important because each complements the others, producing a whole that is greater than the sum of the parts. Includes beef, veal, pork, chicken, tongue, *zampone,* or *cotechino* served with bagnet verde (green salsa made with parsley), bagnet ross (red salsa with tomatoes), mustard, horseradish, and salt.

**Bottarga** Sometimes called the poor man's caviar, bottarga is the roe pouch of tuna, grey mullet, or swordfish. It is massaged by hand to eliminate air pockets, then dried and cured in sea salt for a few weeks. The result is a dry hard slab, which is coated in beeswax for keeping. It is usually used sliced thin or grated. In Italy, it is best known in Sicilian and Sardinian cuisine; its culinary properties can be compared to those of dry anchovies, though it is much more expensive. Bottarga is often served with lemon juice as an appetizer or used in pasta dishes.

**Bresaola** Air-dried salted beef eye of round that has been aged about two to three months until it becomes hard and a dark red, almost purple color. It originated in the Valtellina valley in northern Italy's Lombardy region, with pieces of beef being strung up to cure in the cool Alpine air.

**Brodetto** Fish soup similar to the French bouillabaisse.

**Brodo** Broth, or stock, is a staple element in making good soups. In the Emilia Romagna region, stuffed pasta is often served in *brodo.*

**Bruschetta** A food originating in central Italy, typically made of grilled bread rubbed with garlic and topped with extra-virgin olive oil, salt, and pepper. It is usually served as a snack or appetizer. In Tuscany, bruschetta is called *fettunta,* meaning "oiled slice."

**Cacciatore** Chicken braised *alla cacciatora,* meaning "hunter's style," is a northern Italian preparation that usually includes onions, tomatoes, pancetta or lardo, and often mushrooms. In central Italy, garlic, rosemary, olives, and a touch of vinegar may be used.

**Caffe Latte** Espresso made with more milk than a cappuccino but only a small amount of foam. In Italy it is usually a breakfast drink.

**Cannoli** Italian pastry desserts. The singular is *cannolo,* meaning "little tube," with the etymology stemming from the Latin *canna,* or reed. Cannoli originated in Sicily and are an essential part of Sicilian cuisine.

**Capicola** Italian cold cut or salami.

**Cappuccino** Espresso with foamed milk and containing equal parts espresso, steamed milk, and foamed milk.

**Carpaccio** A dish of raw beef, veal, or tuna traditionally cubed and pounded thin, served as an appetizer. The name comes from the painter Vittore Carpaccio, who favored red colors reminiscent of raw beef. The dish was supposedly invented during 1950 in Venice when a famous actress of the day informed the owner of Harry's Bar that her doctor had recommended she eat only raw meat. Typically the thin slices are served with a dressing of olive oil and lemon juice plus seasoning, often with green salad leaves such as arugula or radicchio and thinly sliced Parmesan cheese.

**Cassata, Cassata Siciliana** A traditional sweet from the province of Palermo, Sicily, similar to the French gateau. It consists of pound cake moistened with kirshwasser or an orange liqueur and layered with a ricotta, candied peel, and chocolate filling, similar to cannoli cream. Most variants are also covered with a shell of marzipan or chocolate frosting.

**Coppa** A type of salami made from pork, salted, naturally aged, and stored raw. The finished product is cylindrical in shape and when sliced open it displays a homogenous interior of red meat flecked with pinkish-white spots.

**Fagato** Calf liver.

**Farro** *Grano farro* has a long and glorious history: it is the original grain from which all others derive, and fed the Mediterranean and Near Eastern populations for thousands of years; somewhat more recently it was the standard ration of the Roman legions that expanded throughout the Western world. Ground into a paste and cooked, it was also the primary ingredient in *plus,* the polenta eaten for centuries by the Roman poor. Important as it was, however, it was difficult to work and produced low yields. In the centuries following the fall of the Empire, higher-yielding grains were developed and farro's cultivation dwindled. By the turn of the century in Italy there were a few hundreds of acres of fields scattered over the regions of Lazio, Umbria, the Marches, and Tuscany. Often used in soups and salads.

**Frito Misto di Mare** Assorted deep-fried fish and seafood.

**Formaggi (Cheese)**

**Asiago d'allevo** A pressed, cooked cheese made from ewe's or cow's milk. It is a firm, strong table cheese after two to six months. Cheese ripened for longer periods of time are used for grating.

**Dolcelatte** A smooth, creamy blue cheese, milder than gorgonzola. Its name is officially registered and means "sweet milk."

**Fontina** A medium-hard cheese that melts easily. Made from full cream milk, it is ripened for about three months.

**Gorgonzola** A compact, creamy textured cheese with a strong flavor. A protected cheese, it is produced year round and is Italy's major blue-veined variety.

**Grana Padano** A cheese similar to Parmigiano-Reggiano but it ripens more quickly and is left to mature for one to two years

**Gruviera** A cheese with a sweet, nutlike flavor that is similar to Swiss Gruyère.

**Mascarpone** A cow's milk cheese that must be eaten very fresh. Its texture is like whipped butter or stiffly whipped cream. It is a delicious creamy dessert cheese.

**Montasio** A cow's milk cheese that is sold in one of three ways based on aging time of sixty days to up to ten months: fresh, middle, and aged. The fresh cheese is characterized as sweet. As it ages, the cheese takes on a certain piquancy.

**Mozzarella** A mild, white fresh cheese made by the special *pasta filata* process, whereby the curd is dipped into hot whey, then stretched and kneaded to the desired consistency. Fresh mozzarella, called *mozzarella di bufala* (buffalo mozzarella), has a soft texture and sweet, delicate flavor.

**Parmigiano-Reggiano** A finely grained hard cheese.

**Pecorino Romano** Made from sheep's milk, generally aged and classified as *grana* (hard, granular, and sharply flavored). A young, unaged ricotta pecorino is soft, white, and mild in flavor. The hard, dry cheeses are good for grating and may be used in recipes calling for Parmesan cheese, especially if a sharper flavor is desired.

**Provolone** Southern Italian cow's milk cheese with a firm texture and a mild, smoky flavor.

**Ricotta** Rich fresh cheese, slightly grainy but smoother than cottage cheese. It is white and moist and has a slightly sweet flavor.

**Stracchino** A fresh cow's milk cheese that contains about 50 percent milk fat. Its flavor is mild and delicate, similar to but slightly more acidic than cream cheese.

**Espresso** *Caffe* in Italy, strong in taste with a rich bronze froth known as a cream on top.

**Gelati** Italian ice creams.

**Grappa** Strong, clear Italian brandy made from the distilled remains of pressed grapes.

**Lardo** A type of *salumi.* It is made from the layer of fat directly under the skin of a pig, cured with salt and other spices, often pepper and garlic. This Italian specialty is often eaten raw in Italy as part of an antipasto. It is made from the back of the pig and is prepared by first cutting the meat and treating the individual pieces with salt and spices such as cinnamon. They are then immersed in brine and placed inside a vessel excavated from marble. So starts a slow process of seasoning in a unique microclimate at the end of which the meat achieves a distinctive smell and smooth consistency. Cut into slices at least 2 inches (5 cm) wide, the lardo can be white or slightly red. To serve, the meat is laid on hot toast. If it is produced well, the whole combination should just melt in the mouth.

**Limoncello** A lemon liqueur produced in southern Italy, mainly in the region around the Gulf of Naples and the coast of Amalfi and islands of Ischia and Capri, but also in Sicily, Sardinia, and the Maltese island of Gozo. It is made from lemon rinds, alcohol, water, and sugar. Bright yellow in color, sweet and lemony, but not sour since it contains no lemon juice.

**Marinara** Meatless tomato-based sauce.

**Minestrone** Italian vegetable soup.

**Mortadella** Bologna's most famous pork product, a softly flavored cooked sausage made from lean pork studded with small cubes of flavorful fat.

**Osso Buco** Braised veal shanks.

**Panettone** A typical cake of Milan, usually prepared and enjoyed for Christmas and New Year around Italy, and one of the symbols of the city. It is a delicate sweet yeast dough studded with golden raisins and jewel-toned glacéed citron.

**Panforte** A traditional Italian dessert containing fruits and nuts, and resembling fruitcake or *lebkuchen.* It may date back to thirteenth-century Siena, in Italy's Tuscany region.

**Pasta** In Italian the word *pasta* means "paste," and refers to the dough made by combining a durum wheat flour called semolina with a liquid, usually water or milk. The term *pasta* is used broadly and generically to describe a wide variety of noodles made from this type of dough.

**Agnolotti** Piemontese stuffed pasta; comes in a great many different varieties, some filled with cheese, others meat, and others still meatless. They are square and small, about an inch on a side, and are made using very thin sheets of pasta. They also are often made from cooked meat or leftovers.

**Angel Hair** "Fine hair" pasta, thinner and finer than spaghetti.

**Farfalle** Bow ties or butterfly-shaped pasta.

**Fettuccine** "Small ribbons" of pasta similar to spaghetti, but wider and slender, just like a ribbon.

**Fusilli** Pasta shaped like screws or springs.

**Lasagna** Thin, flat pasta with straight or rippled edges.

**Lumache** Large, conch shell–shaped pasta suitable for stuffing.

**Macaroni** A kind of moderately extended, machine-made dry pasta. Much shorter than spaghetti, and hollow, macaroni does not contain eggs.

**Manicotti** Long, plain tube-shaped pasta suitable for stuffing.

**Orecchiette** "Little ears" pasta shaped like tiny ears or bowls.

**Penne** Tubular pasta cut on the diagonal into pieces about an inch long.

**Ravioli** Square pasta dough that is stuffed.

**Spaghetti** A long, thin, slender pasta.

**Tortellini** A ring-shaped pasta typically stuffed with (but not limited to) a mix of meat (such as pork loin, prosciutto crudo, or mortadella) or cheese (such as Cheddar or Parmesan). Originally from the Italian region of Emilia (in particular Bologna and Modena), they are usually served in broth, with cream, ragu, or similar sauce.

**Tortelloni** A larger version of tortellini, usually stuffed with ricotta cheese and leaf vegetables, such as spinach

**Pesto** A puree of fresh herbs garlic, oil, and pine nuts.

**Polenta** Originating in Venice when maize was imported from America, polenta is made from coarsely ground cornmeal and is used in a variety of northern Italian dishes.

**Porcini** The same wild mushrooms known as *cepes* in French and *Boletus edulis* in Latin. Fresh porcini are fleshy, velvety, and earthy in flavor; dried porcini are highly aromatic, with an intense woodsy flavor.

**Primo Piatto** Literally, "first course."

**Prosciutto** Italian word for ham, usually referring to the raw cured hams of the Parma region. Prosciutto is seasoned, salt cured, and air dried. *Prosciutto cotto* means cooked and *prosciutto crudo* means raw.

**Risotto** Rice that has been toasted briefly in a *soffritto* and then cooked by gradually adding boiling stock or water and *mantecato* (adding butter and parmigiano). Rice suitable for risotto absorbs three times its weight in liquid. Risotto rice should be cooked al dente. The rice should be slightly moist but never sticky; each grain should be separate.

**Salumi** Italian meat products usually cured and predominantly made from pork. The term also encompasses bresaola, which is made from beef, and also cooked products such as mortadella and prosciutto cotto. It is equivalent to the French *charcuterie.*

**Sambuca** Clear, anise-flavored liqueur.

**Semolina** A yellow flour ground from high-protein durum wheat. Semolina is used in many brands of dried pasta because of its ability to stand up to kneading and molding. Semolina is also used to make gnocchi.

**Sformato** Derives from *sformare,* which means to unmold. The batter used to make a sformato typically contains beaten eggs (or white sauce), though what else goes into the preparation is up to the cook. Savory sformati can be made with vegetables, which are generally served as side dishes or light entrees, or they can be made with pasta, potatoes, or rice, set in ring molds and used to accompany stews. Sformati can also be sweet. In almost all cases they are served with sauces of one sort or another.

**Sopressate** Dry-cured salami, hung to dry for six to eight weeks. It loses 40 percent of its original weight.

**Zabaglione** Italian warm custard made with Marsala wine.

**Zampone** Stuffed pig's trotter. The foot and shin are boned and stuffed with ground pork snout and other ingredients. Zampone is traditionally eaten in Modena on New Year's Eve.

# Menus and Recipes from Italy

MENU ONE (NORTHERN ITALY)

*Zuppa alla Pavese:* **Pavia-Style Bread Soup with Cheese and Raw Egg**

*Gnocchi Di Patate in Salsa Di Parmesan Reggiano E Porie:* **Potato Gnocchi in Parmesan Cheese and Leeks**

*Vitello Tonnato:* **Chilled Veal in Tuna Sauce**

**Osso Buco Milanese**

*Cicorietta Saltata con Pancetta:* **Chicory Sautéed with Pancetta**

*Risotto allo Zafferano:* **Risotto with Saffron**

*Panna Cotta* **with Fresh Berries**

MENU TWO (CENTRAL ITALY)

*Tagliatelle al Peperoncino:* **Red Pepper Tagliatelle**

*Melanzane Involtino:* **Eggplant Roll**

**Tomato Bruschetta**

**Roasted Garlic Aioli**

*Pollo alla Toscana:* **Chicken Sautéed with Mushrooms**

**Basic Polenta**

*Asparagi al Parmigiano-Reggiano:* **Asparagus with Parmigiano-Reggiano**

**Tiramisu**

MENU THREE (SOUTHERN ITALY)

*Peperonata:* **Peppers Sautéed with Olive Oil and Capers**

*Braciole Calabresi:* **Stuffed Pork Bundles**

**Caponata**

**Fresh Tomato Sauce**

*Orechietti con Carciofi:* **Orechietti Pasta with Artichokes**

*Insalata di Seppie, Calamari, e Gamberi:* **Salad of Cuttlefish, Squid, and Shrimp**

**Focaccia Bread**

*Tunnu a Palirmitana:* **Tuna Fish, Palermo Style**

*Torta Caprese:* **Chocolate Almond Cake**

ADDITIONAL RECIPES

*Tagliatelle con Ragu Bolognese*

# Zuppa alla Pavese Pavia-Style Bread Soup with Cheese and Raw Egg

SERVES 4

| AMOUNT | MEASURE | INGREDIENTS |
|---|---|---|
| 1 | | Garlic clove, slit in half |
| 4 | | Bread slices, cut into 3 inch (7.6 cm) rounds |
| $\frac{1}{4}$ cup | 2 ounces, 60 ml | Butter |
| 4 | | Eggs |
| $\frac{1}{4}$ cup | 1 ounce, 28 g | Parmesan cheese, grated |
| 1 quart | 32 ounces, 960 ml | Clear chicken broth, boiling |

PROCEDURE

1. Rub garlic on both sides of bread slices.
2. Heat butter over medium heat until hot, but do not brown.
3. Add bread slices and cook until golden brown; remove from fat. If the bread soaks up all the butter, add more so the bread does not burn.
4. Place one crouton in each bowl.
5. Top each crouton with a raw egg and Parmesan cheese.
6. Add boiling chicken stock around egg, to poach the egg. Serve.

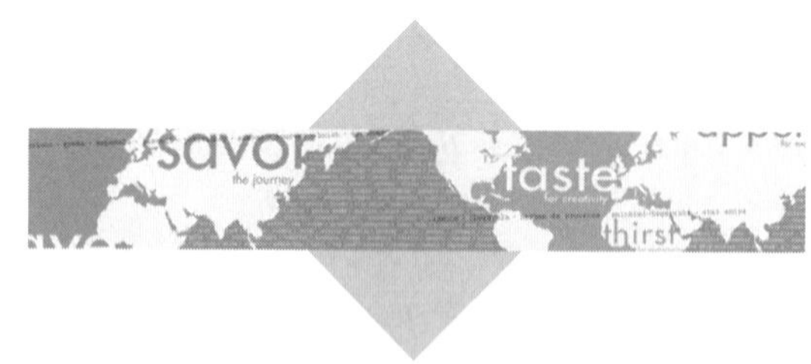

# Gnocchi Di Patate in Salsa Di Parmesan Reggiano E Porie

## Potato Gnocchi in Parmesan Cheese and Leeks

SERVES 4

| AMOUNT | MEASURE | INGREDIENTS |
|---|---|---|
| 4 cups | 1 $\frac{1}{5}$ pounds, 538 g | Russet potatoes, washed and dried |
| $\frac{3}{4}$ cup | 3 ounces, 84 g | All-purpose flour |
| 2 | | Egg |
| 4 tablespoons | 2 ounces, 60 ml | Butter, melted |
| $\frac{1}{2}$ cup | 2 ounces, 56 g | Parmesan cheese, grated |
| To taste | | Salt and white pepper |
| Sauce | | |
| 1 cup | 4 ounces, 112 g | Asiago, or Gorgonzola, or fontina cheese, grated |
| $\frac{1}{2}$ cup | 2 ounces 56 g | Parmesan cheese, grated |
| $\frac{1}{2}$ cup | 4 ounces, 120 ml | Heavy cream |
| 1 tablespoon | $\frac{1}{2}$ ounce, 15 ml | Olive oil |
| 1 cup | 4 ounces, 112 g | Leek, white part only, julienned |

PROCEDURE

1. With a fork make a few vent holes in the potatoes to allow the steam to escape. Bake in a 400°F (205°C) oven until tender, 45 minutes. While potatoes are still warm, peel and pass through a food mill or rices.
2. While still warm, mix in flour, egg, butter, Parmesan cheese, and a pinch of salt until dough is formed.
3. Roll the mixture into two rolls about 1 inch (2.4 cm) thick on a lightly floured surface; cut them into $\frac{3}{4}$ inch (1.8 cm) pieces. Roll the back of a fork across each piece. Place pieces on cheesecloth, dusted with flour.
4. To make sauce, melt Asiago and Parmesan cheese together with cream. Heat olive oil and sauté leeks until translucent; add to cheese sauce.
5. When ready to serve, place gnocchi in boiling salted water; cook until they rise to the surface. Drain well and serve with the sauce; grate additional cheese on top if desired.

# Vitello Tonnato Chilled Veal in Tuna Sauce

SERVES 4

| AMOUNT | MEASURE | INGREDIENT |
|---|---|---|
| 10 ounces | 280 g | Veal, eye round or top round |
| To taste | | Salt and pepper |
| 1 quart | 32 ounces | Veal stock |
| 1 cup | 8 ounces, 240 ml | Dry white wine |
| 1 | | Bouquet garni, with parsley, bay leaf, and oregano |
| Sauce | | |
| ½ cup | 4 ounces, 112 g | Tuna fish, canned in oil, drained |
| 2 | | Anchovy fillets, in oil, drained |
| 1 tablespoon | ½ ounce, 14 g | Capers in wine vinegar, drained |
| 2 tablespoons | 1 ounce, 30 ml | Olive oil |
| To taste | | Salt, pepper, and fresh lemon juice |
| Garnish | | |
| 1 | | Lemon, sliced thin |
| 1 tablespoon | ½ ounce, 14 g | Capers, rinsed |
| 8 | | Cetriolini (small pickled cucumbers), like cornichons |

PROCEDURE

1. Trim veal of all fat and silver skin, season with salt and pepper, wrap in cheesecloth, and tie like a salami.
2. Combine the stock, wine, and bouquet garni. Bring to a boil, add veal.
3. Reduce to a simmer and cover.
4. Poach 15 to 20 minutes; keep meat medium rare. Remove from heat and place pot in an ice bath. Let meat cool in liquid. Remove meat and discard bouquet garni.
5. Puree the tuna, anchovy, and capers in blender or food processor; drizzle in the olive oil. If too thick, thin with some poaching liquid. Season with lemon juice, salt, and pepper.
6. Remove string and cheesecloth from veal; cut into 12 thin slices.
7. Arrange veal on platter with a thin lemon slice between each slice of meat. Pour sauce over meat. Garnish with remaining lemon slices, capers, and cetriolini. Serve cold.

# Osso Buco Milanese

SERVES 4

| AMOUNT | MEASURE | INGREDIENT |
|---|---|---|
| 4 ($\frac{1}{2}$ inch thick) | 10 ounce, 280 g each | Veal shanks, bone and marrow in center |
| As needed | | All-purpose flour |
| 3 tablespoons | $\frac{1}{2}$ ounce, 45 ml | Olive oil |
| 3 tablespoons | $\frac{1}{2}$ ounce, 45 ml | Butter |
| 2 cups | 8 ounces, 224 g | Onions, $\frac{1}{4}$ inch (.6 cm) dice |
| 1 cup | 4 ounces, 112 g | Carrots, peeled, $\frac{1}{4}$ inch (.6 cm) dice |
| 1 cup | 4 ounces, 112 g | Celery, $\frac{1}{4}$ inch (.6 cm) dice |
| 2 | | Garlic cloves, minced |
| $\frac{1}{2}$ teaspoon | | Dried marjoram |
| $\frac{1}{2}$ cup | 4 ounces, 120 ml | Dry white wine |
| 2 cups | 12 ounces, 340 g | Tomatoes, peeled, seeded, $\frac{1}{4}$ inch (.6 cm) dice |
| $\frac{3}{4}$ cup | 6 ounces, 180 ml | Veal stock |
| To taste | | Salt and pepper |
| 1 | | Lemon peel, grated |
| Gremolata | | |
| 3 teaspoons | | Fresh parsley, chopped |
| 1 teaspoon | | Lemon zest |
| 2 | | Garlic cloves, minced |

PROCEDURE

1 Tie each piece of veal around the perimeter so that the meat does not separate from the bone during cooking. Lightly dust veal with flour.

2 Preheat an appropriate-sized cooking vessel in a 350°F (176°C) oven.

3 Add oil and butter to preheated cooking pan. Brown veal, remove from pan, and reserve in a warm place.

4 To the same pan, add onions, carrots, celery, garlic, and marjoram; cook over medium heat until soft.

5 Add wine, deglaze pan, and reduce by half. Add tomatoes and stock; simmer 10 minutes. Season with salt and pepper.

6 Return browned veal shanks to the mixture, add lemon peel, and braise in a 350°F (176°C) oven 1 hour or until tender.

7 When done, remove meat and degrease sauce. Adjust seasoning and return meat to sauce.

#### GREMOLATA

1. Combine parsley, lemon zest, and garlic; mix well.
2. Five minutes before serving, add the gremolata to the veal shanks and sauce, turning them gently from time to time so that they will take on the flavors.
3. Remove the string before serving. Place 1 shank on each place and serve with sauce.

# Cicorietta Saltata con Pancetta

## Chicory Sautéed with Pancetta

SERVES 4

| AMOUNT | MEASURE | INGREDIENT |
|---|---|---|
| 8 cups | 1 pound, 448 g | Chicory |
| 2 tablespoons | 1 ounce, 30 ml | Olive oil |
| $\frac{1}{4}$ cup | 2 ounces, 56 g | Pancetta, $\frac{1}{4}$ inch (.6 cm) dice |
| 2 | 1 tablespoon | Garlic cloves, minced |
| $\frac{1}{4}$ cup | $\frac{1}{2}$ ounce, 15 g | Parsley, chopped |
| $\frac{1}{2}$ cup | 4 ounces, 120 ml | Dry white wine |
| To taste | | Salt and pepper |

#### PROCEDURE

1. Clean and wash chicory at least 2 times. Blanch in boiling salt water, shock in ice water. Drain, removing as much moisture as possible.
2. Heat oil over medium heat, add pancetta, and cook until brown and crisp.
3. Add garlic; lightly brown. Add chicory; sauté until hot. Add parsley. Add wine and reduce until almost dry.
4. Correct seasoning and serve.

# Risotto allo Zafferano

## Risotto with Saffron SERVES 4

**Use a large-bottom pan so the flame can spread underneath.**

| AMOUNT | MEASURE | INGREDIENT |
|---|---|---|
| 1 tablespoon | $\frac{1}{2}$ ounce, 15 ml | Olive oil |
| 1 tablespoon | $\frac{1}{2}$ ounce, 15 ml | Butter |
| $\frac{1}{2}$ cup | 2 ounces, 56 g | Onions, $\frac{1}{8}$ inch (.3cm), dice |
| 1 cup | $6\frac{1}{2}$ ounces, 184 g | Medium-grain arborio rice |
| $\frac{1}{2}$ cup | 4 ounces, 120 ml | Dry white wine |
| 3 cups | 24 ounces, 720 ml | Chicken stock, hot |
| 1 pinch | | Saffron threads |
| $\frac{1}{4}$ cup | 1 ounce, 28 g | Parmesan cheese, grated |
| 2 tablespoons | 1 ounce, 28 g | Butter |
| To taste | | Salt and pepper |

### PROCEDURE

1. Heat first butter and olive oil over medium heat until it melts; cook onions until translucent.
2. Add the rice and cook until lightly toasted and fat has been absorbed, 1 to 2 minutes.
3. Add the white wine; stir until fully absorbed.
4. Add the chicken stock, $\frac{1}{4}$ at a time, stirring often. Allow stock to be completely absorbed before adding more stock.
5. Halfway through cooking (after 6 to 8 minutes), dissolve saffron in a little hot broth, let soak 3 minutes and add to the rice. Do not add at the beginning.
6. Stir the rice frequently, so it does not stick to the bottom of the pan. From start to finish, this dish should take 18 to 20 minutes.
7. When the rice is cooked al dente, turn off the heat. Vigorously beat in Parmesan cheese and butter off the heat. Correct seasoning and let stand, covered, for a few minutes, so the rice finishes cooking. Serve immediately.

# Panna Cotta with Fresh Berries

SERVES 4

| AMOUNT | MEASURE | INGREDIENT |
|---|---|---|
| 1 tablespoon | $\frac{1}{2}$ ounce, 14 g | Butter |
| $\frac{3}{4}$ tablespoon | | Unflavored gelatin |
| $\frac{1}{2}$ cup | 4 ounces, 120 ml | Milk |
| $\frac{1}{2}$ cup | 12 ounces, 360 ml | Heavy cream |
| $\frac{1}{4}$ cup | 2 ounces, 56 g | Granulated sugar |
| $\frac{1}{2}$ | | Vanilla bean, split, or 2 teaspoons vanilla extract |
| 1 cup | 3 ounces, 84 g | Assorted fresh berries |
| 2 tablespoons | | Spearmint, chiffonade |

PROCEDURE

1 Lightly butter the inside of four 6-ounce ramekins.

2 Sprinkle gelatin over $\frac{1}{4}$ cups (2 ounces, 60 ml) of milk. Let stand 3 to 4 minutes until soft.

3 Heat remaining milk, cream, sugar, and vanilla bean over medium heat, stirring occasionally, until simmering, about 5 minutes; remove from heat.

4 Combine softened gelatin with hot milk mixture; stir to completely dissolve, 1 minute. Strain through fine china cap; save vanilla bean.

5 Fill ramekins, cover with plastic wrap, and chill until set.

6 To unmold, fill a shallow pan with $\frac{1}{2}$ inch (1.25 cm) very hot water. One at a time, place ramekins in the hot water 15 seconds. Remove from water and dry the outside of the ramekins. Press the panna cotta around the edges to loosen and invert onto the center of 4 dessert plates.

7 Scatter berries and spearmint around the panna cotta and serve.

# Tagliatelle al Peperoncino

## Red Pepper Tagliatelle

SERVES 4

| AMOUNT | MEASURE | INGREDIENT |
|---|---|---|
| **2 teaspoons** | | **Red pepper flakes** |
| **$1\frac{1}{4}$ cups** | **6 ounces, 168 g** | **All-purpose flour** |
| **$\frac{1}{2}$ cup** | **$2\frac{1}{2}$ ounces, 70 g** | **Semolina flour** |
| **3** | | **Extra large eggs** |
| **2 teaspoons** | | **Olive oil** |
| **Pinch** | | **Salt** |
| **Sauce** | | |
| **1 cup** | **2 ounces, 56 g** | **Italian parsley, leaves only** |
| **To taste** | | **Coarse salt** |
| **$\frac{1}{2}$ cup** | **4 ounces, 120 ml** | **Olive oil** |

PROCEDURE

1. Coarsely grind the red pepper flakes with a mortar and pestle.
2. Prepare pasta: place flours in a mixing bowl with dough hook, add red pepper flakes. Combine eggs, oil, and salt, and beat together. Add egg mixture to dry ingredients while mixing on low; mix until well incorporated. Wrap dough and refrigerate 30 minutes.
3. Roll the dough through the pasta machine several times. Start at a thick setting and work down to almost the thinnest setting, a little more than $\frac{1}{16}$ inch (.2 cm). The red pepper specks should not break through.
4. Cut into tagliatelle (about $\frac{3}{8}$ inch wide); let stand until needed.
5. Chop parsley coarsely and set aside until needed.
6. Bring a large pot of salted water to a boil. Add coarse salt to taste.
7. Add pasta to boiling water and cook a maximum of 1 minute after the water has returned to a boil.
8. Drain and put in serving bowl.
9. Add oil and parsley; toss well. Serve immediately. No cheese should be added.

# Melanzane Involtino

## Eggplant Roll

SERVES 4

| AMOUNT | MEASURE | INGREDIENT |
|---|---|---|
| 1 | 16 ounces, 448 g | Large eggplant, in 8 thin slices |
| As needed | | Coarse salt |
| $\frac{1}{2}$ cup | 4 ounces, 120 ml | Olive oil |
| 8 | 4 ounces, 112 g | Ham, in 8 thin slices |
| 8 | 4 ounces, 112 g | Mozzarella cheese, 8 thin slices |
| 1 quart | 32 ounces, 960 ml | Fresh tomato sauce (see recipe on page 731) |
| $\frac{1}{4}$ cup | $\frac{1}{2}$ ounce, 42 g | Ricotta salata, crumbled |
| 1 tablespoon | | Fresh basil, chiffonade |

### PROCEDURE

1. Salt sliced eggplant and let sit 30 minutes. Rinse and pat dry.
2. Heat oil over medium-high heat and fry eggplant slices until nicely browned; add more oil if needed. Drain and blot excess oil.
3. Lay out eggplant, top with slices of ham and cheese, and roll up.
4. Place in hot oven to melt cheese.
5. Serve hot, topped with warm tomato sauce, ricotta salata, and basil.

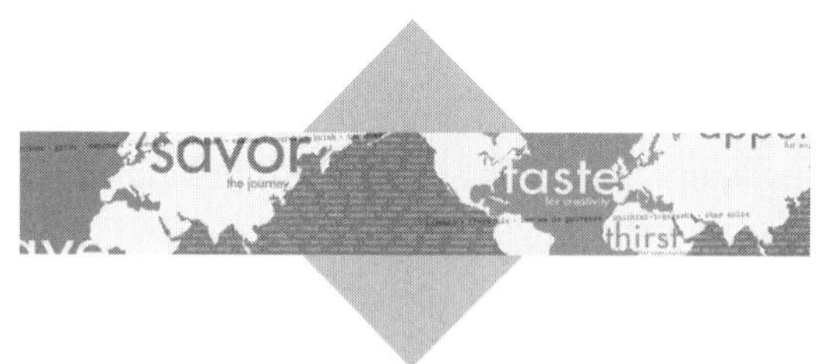

# Tomato Bruschetta

SERVES 4

| AMOUNT | MEASURE | INGREDIENT |
|---|---|---|
| $\frac{1}{3}$ cup | 2 ounces, 56 g | Red onions, shaved very thin |
| $\frac{1}{2}$ cup | 3 ounces, 84 g | Tomatoes, peeled, seeded, $\frac{1}{8}$ inch (.3 cm) dice |
| $\frac{1}{2}$ cup | 3 ounces, 84 g | Yellow tomato, peeled, seeded, $\frac{1}{8}$ inch (.3 cm) dice |
| $\frac{1}{4}$ cup | 1 ounce, 28 g | Shallot, finely diced |
| 1 | | Garlic clove, minced |
| 8 | | Basil sprigs |
| $\frac{1}{4}$ cup | 2 ounces, 60 ml | Olive oil |
| $\frac{1}{2}$ teaspoon | 8 ml | Red wine vinegar |
| 1 teaspoon | 5 ml | Balsamic vinegar |
| To taste | | Course salt and freshly ground pepper |
| 8 $\frac{1}{2}$-inch slices | 1.25 cm | Country bread |
| $\frac{1}{4}$ cup | 2 ounces, 60 ml | Roasted garlic aioli (recipe follows) |
| $\frac{1}{2}$ cup | 3 ounces, 84 g | Ricotta salata, crumbled |

**PROCEDURE**

1. Soak red onions in ice water 1 hour; drain and dry.
2. Combine tomatoes, shallots, and garlic; toss.
3. Remove 8 nice basil leaves for garnish. Finely chop remaining leaves and combine with tomato mixture.
4. Add the oil and vinegars; correct seasoning with salt and pepper. Let marinate at room temperature at least 30 minutes.
5. Lightly grill or toast the bread slices. Cool and spread with aioli.
6. Add red onions to tomato mixture and correct seasoning.
7. Set bread slices on plate and top with tomato mixture.
8. Garnish bruschettas with crumbled cheese and reserved basil leaves.

# Roasted Garlic Aioli

SERVES 4

| AMOUNT | MEASURE | INGREDIENT |
|---|---|---|
| 1 | 1 ounce, 28 g | Green onion, white part only |
| 1 | | Large egg yolk, at room temperature |
| 3 | | Garlic cloves, roasted and mashed to paste |
| $\frac{1}{4}$ teaspoon | | Dijon mustard |
| To taste | | Salt and pepper |
| $\frac{1}{2}$ cup | 4 ounces, 120 ml | Vegetable oil |
| $\frac{1}{4}$ cup | 2 ounces, 60 ml | Olive oil |
| $\frac{1}{2}$ teaspoon | | Fresh lemon juice |

**PROCEDURE**

1. Blanch green onion in boiling salted water 10 seconds. Transfer to a bowl of ice water. Drain and gently squeeze out excess water.
2. Chop onion.
3. Combine onion, egg yolk, garlic, mustard, and seasoning in a blender or small food processor fitted with metal blade. Process about 30 seconds until smooth and well combined.
4. With blender or processor running, slowly add the oils in a steady steam. Scrape down sides of bowl several times during blending. When the emulsion is thick and fluffy, season with lemon juice and correct seasoning. Refrigerate until needed.

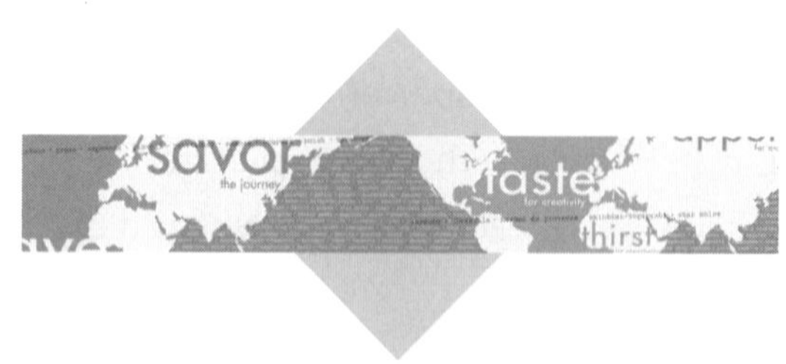

# Pollo alla Toscana

## Chicken Sautéed with Mushrooms

SERVES 4

| AMOUNT | MEASURE | INGREDIENT |
|---|---|---|
| 1 ounce | 1 ounce, 28 g | Porcini mushrooms, dried |
| 1 cup | 8 ounces, 240 ml | Chicken stock, warm |
| 1 3 to $3\frac{1}{2}$ pound | 1 1.36 kg to 1.58 kg | Chicken, cut into 8 pieces |
| $\frac{1}{4}$ cup | 1 ounce, 28 g | All-purpose flour |
| 4 tablespoons | 2 ounces, 56 g | Butter |
| $\frac{1}{4}$ cup | 2 ounces, 60 ml | Olive oil |
| 4 | | Fresh sage leaves |
| $\frac{1}{2}$ cup | 4 ounces, 120 ml | Dry red wine |
| 1 cup | 6 ounces, 180 ml | Tomatoes, peeled, seeded, passed through a food mill |
| To taste | | Salt and freshly ground black pepper |

**PROCEDURE**

1. Soak mushrooms in warm chicken stock 30 minutes; remove and reserve both. Check to make sure mushrooms are free of sand and strain stock through cheesecloth.
2. Lightly flour chicken and remove excess flour.
3. Heat butter and olive oil over medium heat.
4. Sauté chicken until light golden brown, about 10 minutes.
5. Add sage leaves and wine; reduce to almost dry over low heat.
6. Add mushrooms and chicken stock; reduce by half.
7. Add tomatoes; simmer 10 minutes. Check chicken to ensure it is cooked.
8. Correct seasoning, cook 1 minute, and serve.

# Basic Polenta

SERVES 4

**This ratio applies to soft polenta. For polenta that is to be baked, grilled, or used as a substitute for bread, use a 3:1 ratio of water to polenta, and the same amount of salt.**

| AMOUNT | MEASURE | INGREDIENT |
|---|---|---|
| 1 quart | 32 ounces, 960 ml | Water |
| $\frac{1}{2}$ teaspoon | 3 g | Salt |
| $1\frac{1}{3}$ cup | 8 ounces, 224 g | Yellow polenta, coarsely ground |

**PROCEDURE**

1. Bring water to a boil and add salt.
2. Reduce heat to low.
3. Add cornmeal, little by little, stirring constantly. Do not pour directly from the container, but use your hands, pouring a handful at time.
4. After all cornmeal has been added and incorporated, turn up heat to medium-high.
5. Cook 40 to 45 minutes, stirring constantly. The heat should be high enough to cause bubbles to rise and burst on the surface.
6. While stirring, pull the cornmeal off the sides and from the bottom up. Serve hot.

# Asparagi al Parmigiano-Reggiano Asparagus with Parmigiano-Reggiano

**SERVES 4**

| AMOUNT | MEASURE | INGREDIENT |
|---|---|---|
| **1 pound** | **448 g** | **Asparagus** |
| **As needed** | | **Salt** |
| **2 tablespoons** | **1 ounce, 28 g** | **Butter** |
| **$\frac{1}{2}$ cup** | **2 ounces, 56 g** | **Parmigiano-Reggiano, grated** |

**PROCEDURE**

1. Trim, peel, and blanch asparagus in salted boiling water until tender but not limp.
2. Preheat oven to 400°F (205°C).
3. Place asparagus lengthwise in buttered baking dish, staggering so the tips protrude.
4. Dot with remaining butter, sprinkle cheese on top, and bake until top forms a light brown crust.

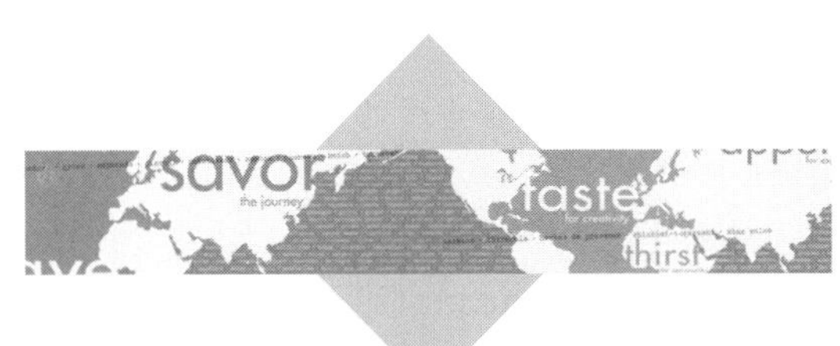

# Tiramisu

SERVES 4

**Tiramisu may be made with sponge cake instead of ladyfingers. Ladyfingers can also line the side of a mold instead of being placed in layers.**

| AMOUNT | MEASURE | INGREDIENT |
|---|---|---|
| 4 | | Eggs, separated |
| 1 $\frac{3}{4}$ cups | 12 ounces, 336 g | Granulated sugar |
| 2 cups | 15 ounces, 420 g | Mascarpone cheese |
| 3 tablespoons | $\frac{1}{2}$ ounce, 45 ml | Brandy |
| 18 | | Ladyfingers |
| 2 tablespoons | $\frac{1}{2}$ ounce, 14 g | Cocoa power |
| $\frac{1}{2}$ cup | 4 ounces, 120 ml | Strong espresso |
| 5 tablespoons | 1 $\frac{1}{4}$ ounces, 42 g | Pistachios, chopped fine |

**PROCEDURE**

1. Using the whisk attachment, beat on medium high speed the yolks with half the sugar until pale yellow and thick.
2. With mixer on medium speed, add cheese and whip until smooth.
3. Beat egg whites with half of the remaining sugar, and a pinch of salt to firm peaks.
4. Fold the egg whites into the egg yolk mixture.
5. Make a simple syrup with the remaining sugar and $\frac{1}{2}$ cup (4 ounces, 120 ml) water.
6. Add the espresso and brandy to simple syrup; mix well.
7. Moisten the ladyfingers or sponge cake with espresso mixture and make a layer in a deep serving dish.
8. Cover ladyfinger layer with a layer of mascarpone mixture, continue alternating layers of ladyfingers and the mascarpone mixture.
9. The last layer should be mascarpone, not ladyfingers.
10. Refrigerate 2 hours or more.
11. Just before serving, dust top with cocoa powder and sprinkle with chopped pistachios.

# Peperonata

## Peppers Sautéed with Olive Oil and Capers

SERVES 4

| AMOUNT | MEASURE | INGREDIENT |
|---|---|---|
| 1 cup | 4 ounces, 112 g | Red bell peppers, seeded, 1 inch (2.5 cm) wide strips |
| 1 cup | 4 ounces, 112 g | Green bell peppers, seeded, 1 inch (2.5 cm) wide strips |
| 1 cup | 4 ounces, 112 g | Yellow bell peppers, seeded, 1 inch (2.5 cm) wide strips |
| $\frac{1}{4}$ cup | 2 ounces, 60 ml | Olive oil |
| 1 cup | 4 ounces, 112 g | White onion, $\frac{1}{4}$ inch (.6 cm) dice |
| 1 | | Garlic clove, minced |
| $\frac{3}{4}$ cup | 4 ounces, 112 g | Tomatoes, peeled, seeded, $\frac{1}{4}$ inch (.6 cm) dice |
| 2 tablespoons | | Fresh basil, chopped |
| 1 tablespoon | | Capers, rinsed |

PROCEDURE

1. Seed, rib, and cut the peppers.
2. Heat half the oil over medium heat and sauté onions and garlic (*soffritto*) until golden brown.
3. Add tomatoes and basil, cook 10 minutes over low heat, and set aside.
4. Heat remaining oil and the add peppers. When peppers are just beginning to soften, add *soffritto* and capers.
5. Cook peppers until tender but still crisp. (If the skin begins to fall off, the peppers are overcooked.)
6. Remove from heat, correct seasoning, and serve.

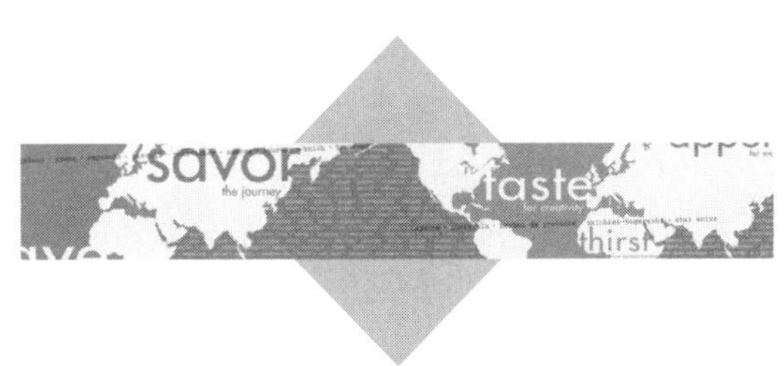

# Braciole Calabresi Stuffed Pork Bundles

SERVES 4

| AMOUNT | MEASURE | INGREDIENT |
|---|---|---|
| 2 | | Eggs, beaten |
| $\frac{1}{2}$ cup | 2 ounces, 56 g | Pecorino cheese, thinly sliced or slivered |
| 2 | | Garlic cloves, minced |
| 2 tablespoons | 10 g | Italian parsley leaves, chopped fine |
| $\frac{1}{2}$ cup | $\frac{1}{2}$ ounce, 42 g | Italian dried bread crumbs |
| As needed | | Salt and freshly ground pepper |
| | 16 ounces, 448 g | Pork loin, boned, cleaned of fat and silver skin, cut into 8 pieces |
| $\frac{1}{2}$ cup | 4 ounces, 120 ml | Olive oil |
| $\frac{1}{2}$ cup | 4 ounces, 120 ml | Fresh tomato sauce (recipe follows) |
| $\frac{1}{2}$ cup | 4 ounces, 120 ml | Chicken stock |
| $\frac{1}{4}$ cup | 2 ounces, 60 ml | Dry red wine |
| 2 | | Fresh rosemary sprigs |

PROCEDURE

1. Combine egg, cheese, garlic, and chopped parsley.
2. Slowly drizzle in the seasoned bread crumbs while mixing constantly. Use only enough bread crumbs to bring the mixture to a soft, spreadable paste. Correct seasoning. Be careful with the salt; consider the flavor of the cheese.
3. Tap the pork until the slices are about $\frac{1}{8}$ inch (.3 cm) thick and a rectangular shape.
4. Lightly brush the meat with olive oil. Season with salt and pepper.
5. Divided stuffing into 8 portions and spread each piece of pounded pork with stuffing, leaving $\frac{1}{4}$ inch (.6 cm) space around the edge of each piece.
6. Roll up and tie on each end and once in the middle.
7. Heat remaining oil over medium heat, brown bracioles on all sides. Place in an appropriate-sized ovenproof pan.
8. Combine tomato sauce, stock, red wine, and rosemary; mix well.
9. Pour liquid over the pork, bring to simmer, cover tightly, and cook for about 20 minutes just until tender. (Because the dish is made with loin it does not need to cook for a long period of time. Overcooking will dry and toughen the pork.)
10. When meat is tender, remove and reduce sauce. Serve 1 or 2 pieces, with braising liquid.

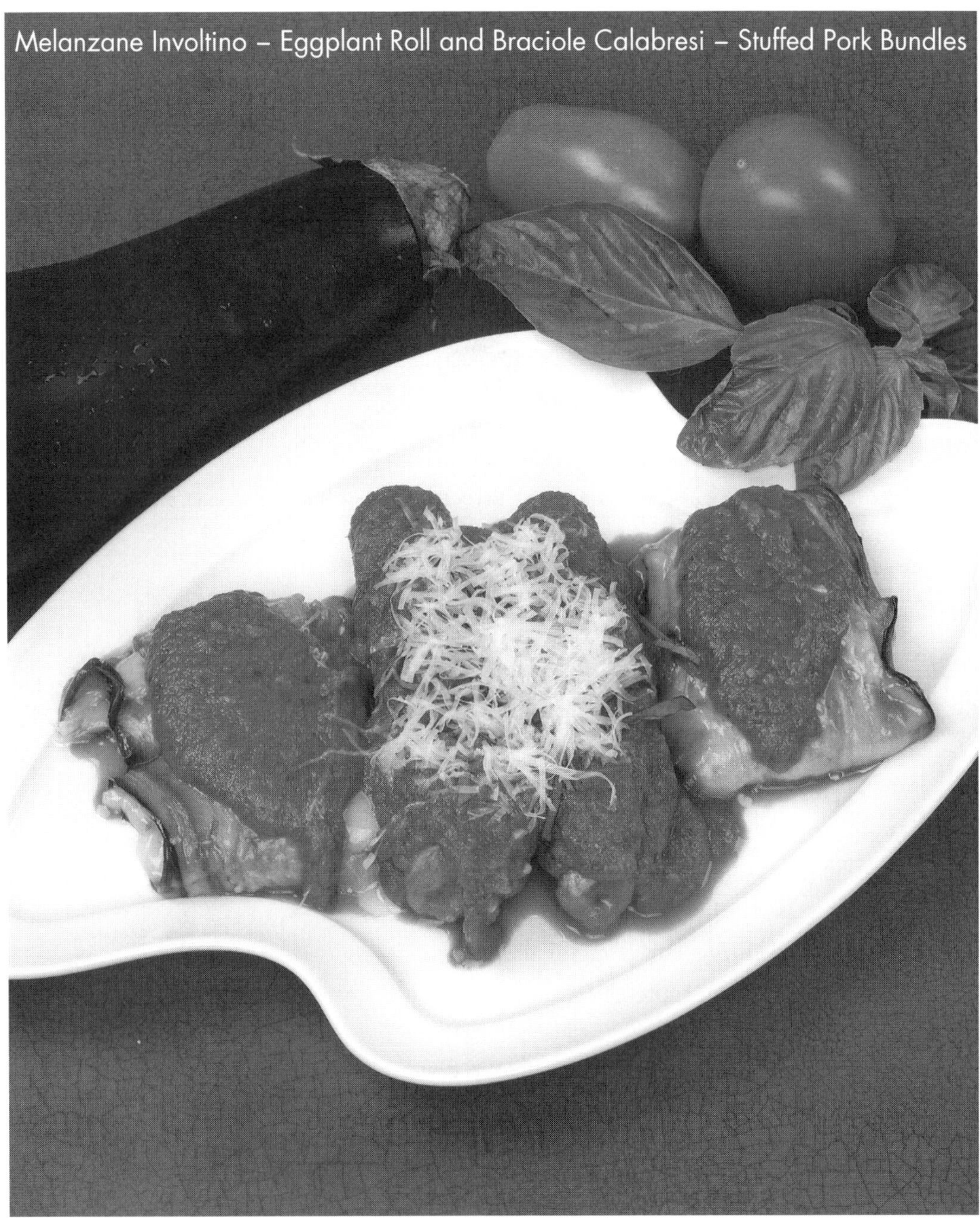

Melanzane Involtino – Eggplant Roll and Braciole Calabresi – Stuffed Pork Bundles

# Caponata

SERVES 4

| AMOUNT | MEASURE | INGREDIENT |
|---|---|---|
| 1 pound | 16 ounces, 448 g | Japanese eggplant (small, long eggplants), stems removed |
| 1 tablespoon | $\frac{1}{2}$ ounce, 15 g | Coarse salt |
| $\frac{1}{2}$ cup | 4 ounces, 120 ml | Olive oil |
| $\frac{1}{2}$ cup | 2 ounces, 56 g | Celery, $\frac{1}{4}$ inch (.6 cm), dice |
| $\frac{1}{2}$ cup | 2 ounces, 56 g | Red onion, $\frac{1}{4}$ inch (.6 cm) dice |
| 1 tablespoon | $\frac{1}{2}$ ounce, 28 g | Tomato paste |
| 2 teaspoons | 10 g | Granulated sugar |
| $\frac{1}{4}$ cup | 2 ounces, 60 ml | Red wine vinegar |
| $\frac{1}{4}$ cup | 2 ounces, 60 ml | Cold water |
| $\frac{1}{2}$ cup | 4 ounces, 112 g | Black Greek olives in brine, drained, pitted $\frac{1}{4}$ inch (.6 cm) dice |
| 3 tablespoons | 1 ounce, 28 g | Capers, rinsed |
| To taste | | Salt and pepper |

**PROCEDURE**

1. Wash eggplants and cut into 1 inch (2.5 cm) square cubes. (Do not peel the eggplant).
2. Place eggplant in a colander and sprinkle with coarse salt; toss well to coat eggplant evenly. Set colander in the sink and place dish inside the colander so it is in direct contact with the eggplant. Place a weight on top of the plate and let stand 1 hour.
3. Wipe off the eggplant to remove as much of the salt and clinging juices.
4. Heat oil over medium heat; add eggplant, and sauté 10 to 12 minutes or until completely cooked, stirring often.
5. Remove cooked eggplant from oil and reserve.
6. Over medium heat, sauté celery and onions in the same oil until soft, 5 to 10 minutes, stirring often.
7. In a bowl combine tomato paste, sugar, red wine vinegar, and cold water; blend well.
8. Remove cooked celery and onion mixture and combine with eggplant.
9. Add vinegar mixture to sauté pan, cook 5 minutes or until reduced by $\frac{2}{3}$.
10. Add olives to vinegar mixture; simmer 10 minutes.
11. Add vegetables and capers back to olive mixture and simmer together 10 minutes.
12. Correct seasoning and transfer to serving dish. This may be served warm, but it is better to let it marinate 1 hour in the refrigerator. Serve at room temperature or reheat.

# Fresh Tomato Sauce

SERVES 4

| AMOUNT | MEASURE | INGREDIENT |
|---|---|---|
| **2 tablespoons** | **1 ounce, 30 ml** | **Olive oil** |
| **$\frac{1}{4}$ cup** | **1 ounce, 28 g** | **Onions, minced** |
| **1** | | **Garlic clove, minced** |
| **2 tablespoons** | **1 ounce, 28 g** | **Tomato paste** |
| **2 cups** | **12 ounces, 336 g** | **Tomatoes, peeled, seeded, $\frac{1}{4}$ inch (.6 cm) dice** |
| **To taste** | | **Salt and white pepper** |

**PROCEDURE**

1 Heat oil over medium heat and sauté onion and garlic until onions are translucent, 3 minutes.

2 Add tomato paste and stir well.

3 Add tomatoes; simmer 10 to 15 minutes, until correct consistency is reached. Do not overcook or you will loose the fresh tomato flavor.

4 Correct seasoning.

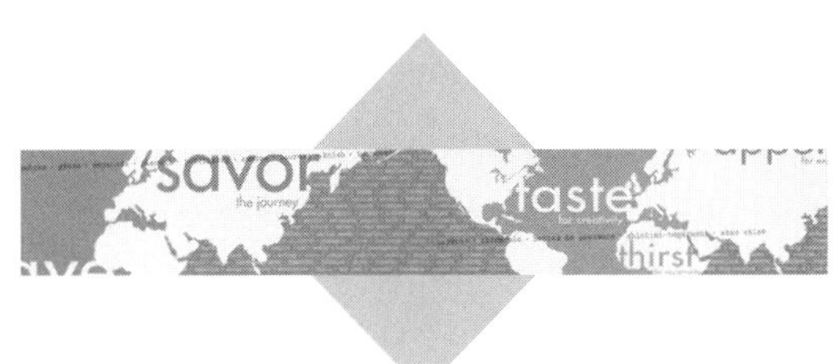

# Orechietti con Carciofi

## Orechietti Pasta with Artichokes

SERVES 4

| AMOUNT | MEASURE | INGREDIENT |
|---|---|---|
| 4 | | **Artichokes** |
| 1 | | **Lemon** |
| $\frac{1}{4}$ cup | 2 ounces, 60 ml | **Olive oil** |
| $\frac{1}{2}$ cup | 3 ounces, 84 g | **Pancetta, diced** |
| $\frac{1}{4}$ cup | 1 ounce, 28 g | **Onion, minced** |
| $\frac{1}{4}$ cup | 2 ounces, 60 ml | **Water or chicken stock** |
| $\frac{1}{4}$ teaspoon | | **Red pepper flakes** |
| | 16 ounces, 448 g | **Orechietti pasta, dried** |
| To taste | | **Salt and pepper** |
| 2 tablespoons | | **Parsley, chopped** |
| 1 cup | $4\frac{1}{2}$ ounces, 126 g | **Romano cheese, grated** |

**PROCEDURE**

1. Clean the artichokes, leaving on the tender parts of the heart; cut into very thin slices.
2. Squeeze the juice of the lemon over them.
3. Heat olive oil over medium heat and add pancetta. Sauté until crisp; add onions and cook 2 minutes.
4. Add sliced artichokes, water or chicken stock, and red pepper flakes. Cook until the artichokes are tender. Correct seasoning.
5. Cook pasta in boiling salt water; drain.
6. Toss pasta with artichoke sauce, herbs, and cheese. Serve.

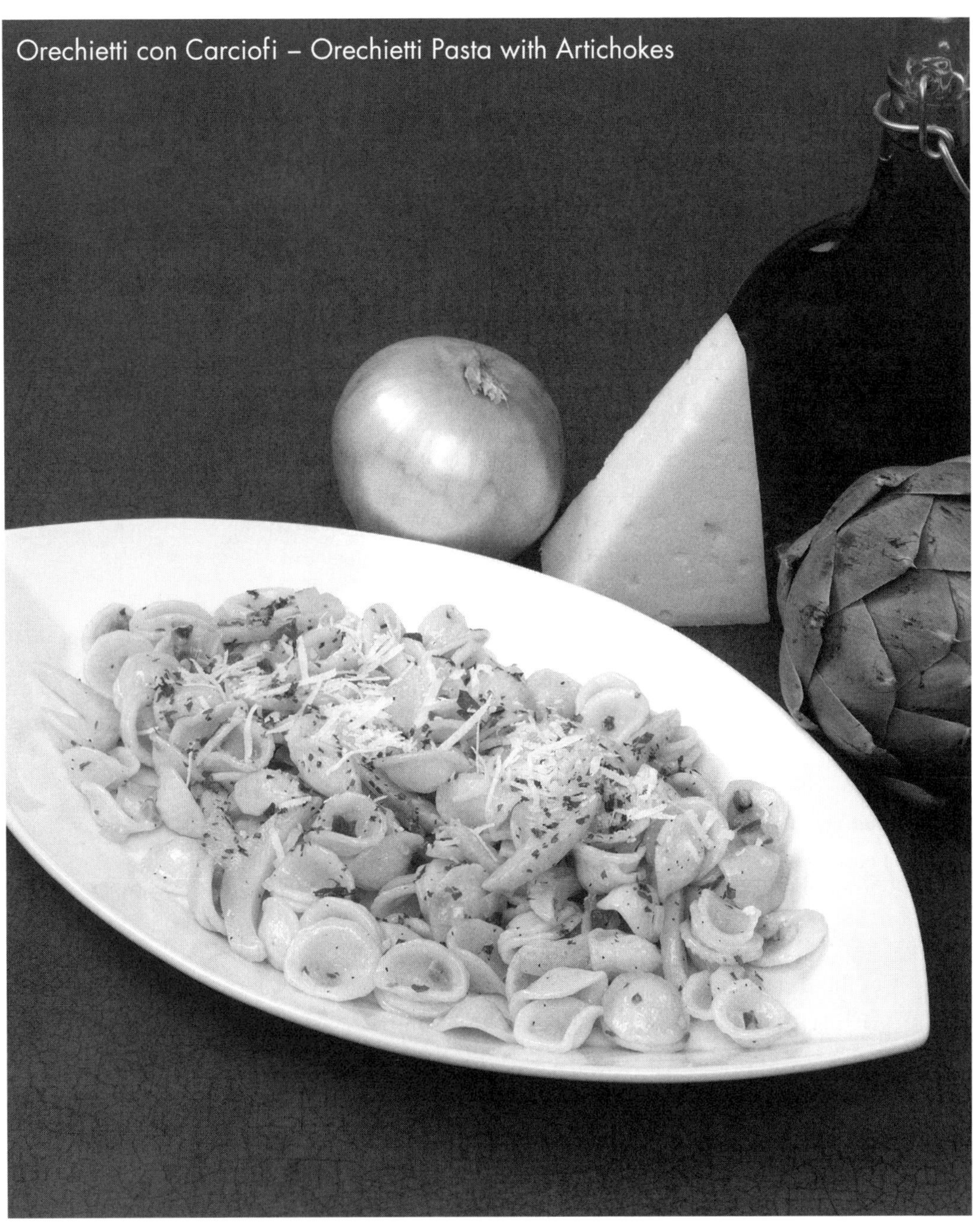

Orechietti con Carciofi – Orechietti Pasta with Artichokes

# Insalata di Seppie, Calamari, e Gamberi

## Salad of Cuttlefish, Squid, and Shrimp

SERVES 4

| AMOUNT | MEASURE | INGREDIENT |
| --- | --- | --- |
| 12 ounces | 12 ounces, 336 g | Cuttlefish, cleaned, cut into $\frac{1}{4}$ inch (.6 cm) strips |
| 12 ounces | 12 ounces, 336 g | Squid, cleaned, cut into $\frac{1}{4}$ inch (.6 cm) strips |
| 8 ounces | 8 ounces, 224 g | Shrimp, 31–35 count, peeled, cleaned, whole |
| | | Coarse salt |
| 1 cup | 8 ounces, 240 ml | Red wine vinegar |
| 3 cups | 15 ounces, 420 g | Boiling potatoes (but not new potatoes), 1 inch (2.5 cm) cubes |
| Sauce | | |
| 1 | | Garlic clove, minced |
| $\frac{1}{2}$ cup | 1 ounce, 28 g | Italian parsley, leaves only, coarsely chopped |
| 1 cup | 8 ounces, 240 ml | Olive oil |
| | | Salt and freshly ground black pepper |
| $\frac{1}{4}$ cup | $\frac{1}{2}$ ounce, 14 g | Basil leaves, coarsely chopped |
| $\frac{1}{4}$ cup | $\frac{1}{2}$ ounce, 14 g | Mint leaves, coarsely chopped |
| 2 tablespoons | 1 ounces, 30 ml | Fresh lemon juice |
| 1 tablespoon | $\frac{1}{2}$ ounce, 15 ml | Red wine vinegar |

### PROCEDURE

1. Combine cuttlefish and squid, cover with salted cold water; let stand 30 minutes. Drain.
2. Soak clean shrimp in salted cold water 30 minutes. Drain.
3. Bring a large pot of salted water to a boil with 1 tablespoon of red wine vinegar; add cuttlefish and squid, reduce to simmer, cover, and cook 20 minutes. Drain and cool.
4. Drain the shrimp and cook in boiling salted water, do not overcook. Drain and cool.
5. Cover potatoes with salted cold water and the remaining red wine vinegar; bring to a simmer. Simmer until tender. Drain and let cool at least 1 hour.
6. Combine all the ingredients for the sauce and mix well.
7. Combine cooked seafood and potatoes and toss with sauce.
8. Cool at least 1 hour before serving, for flavors to blend.

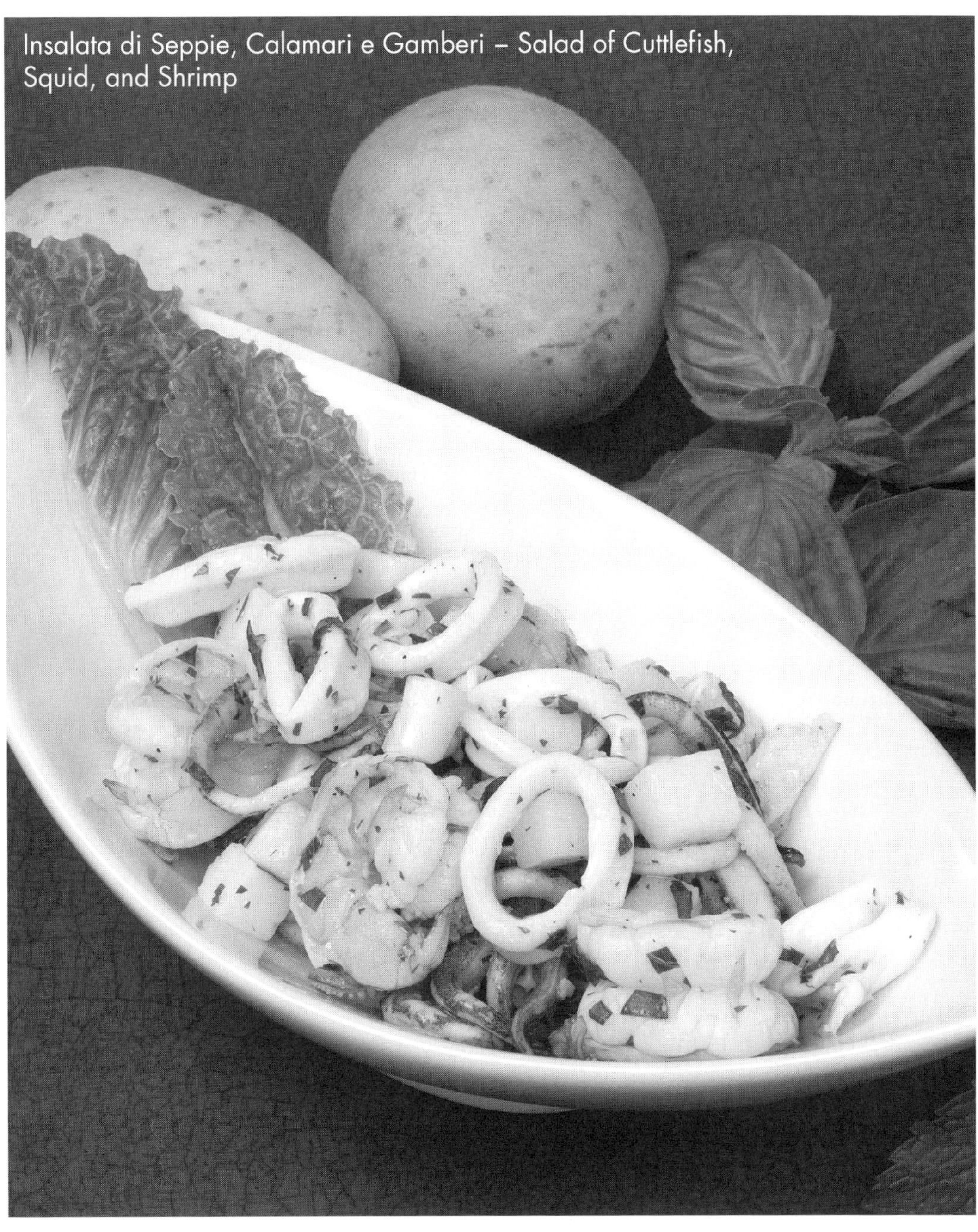

Insalata di Seppie, Calamari e Gamberi – Salad of Cuttlefish, Squid, and Shrimp

# Focaccia Bread

SERVES 4 TO 6

| AMOUNT | MEASURE | INGREDIENT |
|---|---|---|
| **Sponge** | | |
| 1 cup | 8 ounces, 240 ml | Warm water, 100°F (38°C) |
| 1 teaspoon | | Active dry yeast |
| 1 cup | 4 ounces, 112 g | All-purpose flour |
| **Focaccia** | | |
| $\frac{1}{2}$ cup | 4 ounces, 120 ml | Water |
| $\frac{1}{3}$ cup | 2.4 ounces, 72 ml | Dry white wine |
| $\frac{1}{3}$ cup | 2.4 ounces, 72 ml | Olive oil |
| 2 tablespoons | | Fine yellow cornmeal |
| $\frac{1}{2}$ teaspoon | | Kosher salt |
| $2\frac{3}{4}$ cups | 12 ounces, 336 g | All-purpose flour |
| 5 teaspoons | | Extra-virgin olive oil |
| 1 | | Garlic clove, minced |
| To taste | | Black pepper |
| $\frac{1}{2}$ teaspoon | | Rosemary, minced |
| To taste | | Kosher salt |

### SPONGE

1. Combine warm water and yeast and let stand 2 minutes; stir to dissolve.
2. Stir in flour until the mixture is smooth.
3. Cover and let stand at room temperature 24 hours.

### FOCACCIA

1. Preheat oven to 450°F (225°C).
2. Using a small mixer with dough hook attachment, mix sponge.
3. Slowly add the water, white wine, $\frac{1}{3}$ cup olive oil, cornmeal, and $\frac{1}{2}$ teaspoon salt. Mix until thoroughly incorporated.
4. Gradually add the $2\frac{3}{4}$ cups flour, mixing on low speed until the dough is formed.
5. Increase mixer to medium speed and work dough 5 minutes.
6. Remove from mixer to a greased bowl. Cover and let rise at room temperature about $\frac{1}{2}$ hours or until it doubles in size.

7 Grease a sheet pan with olive oil.

8 Transfer the dough to baking sheet and stretch it, using oiled fingers, until the dough completely fills the pan. Let the dough rest 5 minutes; the dough will shrink.

9 Restretch the dough to cover the pan completely. If it is still too elastic, let the dough rest longer and try again.

10 Let the dough rise in the pan at room temperature 1 hour.

11 Brush the focaccia with olive oil and sprinkle with rosemary and kosher salt to taste.

12 Bake for about 15 to 20 minutes or until nicely browned.

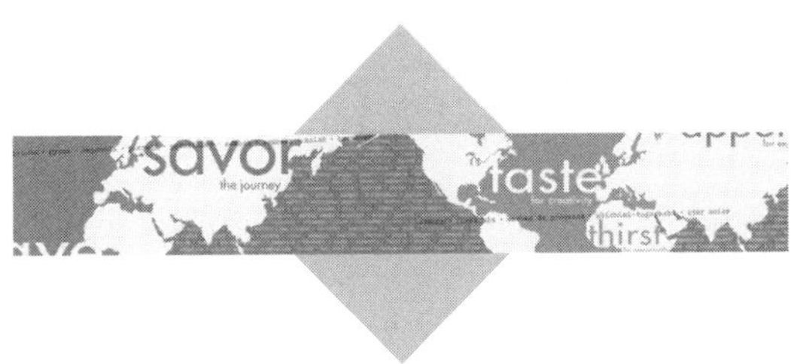

# Tunnu a Palirmitana

## Tuna Fish, Palermo Style

SERVES 4

| AMOUNT | MEASURE | INGREDIENT |
|---|---|---|
| 1 cup | 8 ounces, 240 ml | Dry white wine |
| 2 tablespoons | 1 ounce, 30 ml | Fresh lemon juice |
| 1 | | Sprig rosemary, fresh |
| 2 | | Garlic cloves, minced |
| 4 | 6 ounce (168 g) servings | Tuna loin |
| **Basting** | | |
| $\frac{1}{2}$ cup | 4 ounces, 120 ml | Olive oil |
| 3 | | Sardine fillets, oil packed |
| **Garnish** | | |
| 2 cups | 4 ounces, 112 g | Fresh arugula |
| $\frac{1}{2}$ cup | 4 ounces, 112 g | Lemon segments |
| $\frac{1}{2}$ cup | 2 ounces, 56 g | Red radish, julienned |
| $\frac{1}{4}$ cup | 2 ounces, 60 ml | Olive oil |
| To taste | | Freshly ground black pepper |

PROCEDURE

1. Combine wine, lemon juice, rosemary, and garlic; mix well.
2. Marinate tuna fillets in mixture 1 hour, turning at least once.
3. Heat $\frac{1}{2}$ cup olive oil in a pan until hot; remove from heat, add sardine fillets, and blend or mash together.
4. Remove tuna from marinade. Season with salt and pepper.
5. Grill until nicely marked and medium rare. Baste several times during process with sardine mixture; baste again when cooked.
6. Toss together arugula, lemon segments, radish, and olive oil; season.
7. Serve tuna fillet topped with arugula salad and fresh cracked black pepper.

# Torta Caprese

## Chocolate Almond Cake

SERVES 6 TO 8

| AMOUNT | MEASURE | INGREDIENT |
|---|---|---|
| **2 cups** | **8 ounces, 224 g** | **Semisweet or bittersweet chocolate, chopped** |
| **1 cup** | **8 ounces, 224 g** | **Butter, at room temperature** |
| **1 cup** | **7 ounces, 196 g** | **Granulated sugar** |
| **6** | | **Eggs, separated, at room temperature** |
| **$\frac{1}{2}$ cup** | **6 ounces, 168 g** | **Almonds, very finely ground** |
| **Pinch** | | **Salt** |
| | | **Unsweetend cocoa powder** |

**PROCEDURE**

1. Melt chocolate over hot water bath; stir until smooth. Let cool slightly.
2. Preheat oven to 350°F (176°C).
3. Grease and flour a 9-inch (22.5 cm) round cake pan. Tap out excess flour.
4. Using a paddle attachment, on medium speed beat $\frac{3}{4}$ cup (6 ounces, 128 g) of butter and sugar together until light and fluffy, about 3–5 minutes.
5. Add egg yolks, one at a time, beating well after each addition. With a rubber spatula, stir in the chocolate and the almonds; set aside.
6. Using beater attachment, whip egg whites and a pinch of salt until foamy.
7. Increase speed to high and beat in remaining sugar. Beat until egg whites are glossy and hold soft peaks when the beaters are lifted, about 5 minutes.
8. Fold $\frac{1}{4}$ meringue into chocolate mixture to lighten. Gradually fold in the remaining whites.
9. Scrape batter into the prepared pan.
10. Bake 45 minutes or until cake is set around the edges but soft and moist in the center and a toothpick inserted in the center comes out covered with chocolate.
11. Cool on rack 10 minutes.
12. Run thin metal spatula around the inside of pan, invert onto serving plate.
13. Let cool to room temperature, dust with cocoa powder, and serve.

# Tagliatelle con Ragu Bolognese

SERVES 4

**In and around Bologna each family may have their own particular recipe for ragu. Each feels theirs is the best, much like chili recipes in Texas, or gumbo in Louisiana. They are all based on a similar technique and similar ingredients, but the outcome of the dish has subtle yet distinct differences. Ragu Bolognese is usually composed of three meats: veal, pork fat back, and beef. The modern version presented here was given to Chef Joseph Bonaparte MHM, CCE, CCC, to cook for the Premio Internazionale Della Cucina Bolognese, a cooking contest conducted by the city of Bologna to promote its gastronomic heritage and the products produced in the region of Emilia-Romagna.**

| AMOUNT | MEASURE | INGREDIENT |
|---|---|---|
| 2 tablespoons | 1 ounce, 30 ml | Olive oil |
| 1 cup | 6 ounces, 168 g | Pancetta, $\frac{1}{4}$ inch (.6 cm) dice |
| 1 cup | 4 ounces, 112 g | Onions, $\frac{1}{4}$ inch (.6 cm) dice |
| $\frac{1}{2}$ cup | 2 ounces, 56 g | Carrots, $\frac{1}{4}$ inch (.6 cm) dice |
| $\frac{1}{2}$ cup | 2 ounces, 56 g | Celery, $\frac{1}{4}$ inch (.6 cm) dice |
| $1\frac{1}{4}$ cups | 10 ounces, 280 g | Lean ground beef |
| $\frac{1}{2}$ cup | 4 ounces, 120 ml | Italian white wine |
| 2 tablespoons | 1 ounce, 30 ml | Tomato paste |
| $\frac{1}{2}$ cup | 12 ounces, 360 ml | Beef stock |
| $\frac{1}{2}$ cup | 4 ounces, 120 ml | Milk |
| To taste | | Salt and pepper |
| 12 ounces | | Fresh tagliatelle |
| $\frac{1}{2}$ cup | 2 ounces, 56 g | Grana Pandano or Parmigiano-Reggiano |

PROCEDURE

1. Over low heat, combine the olive oil and pancetta. Cook until most of the fat has been rendered, 3 to 5 minutes; do not brown the pancetta.
2. Add the onion and cook 3 minutes. Add remaining vegetables and cook until evenly browned (caramelized), 5 to 7 minutes.
3. Add the ground beef and increase heat to medium. Cook, stirring frequently, until browned but not dried out; be sure to scrape the bits off the bottom of the pan.
4. Add the wine and cook 2 minutes.

5 Mix tomato paste and beef stock. Add to beef mixture and stir well. Bring to a low simmer.

6 Simmer sauce 1 to $1\frac{1}{2}$ hours. During the cooking process (15 mintues into the process), add the milk 2 tablespoons (1 ounce, 30 ml) at a time. After each addition stir well and let cook 5 to 10 minutes before the next addition of milk. The finished sauce should be rich and thick. Correct seasoning.

#### TO SERVE

1 Cook fresh taliatelle until al dente. Remove from the pasta cooking water directly into the hot ragu. The sauce is a condiment; it should accent the pasta, not overwhelm it.

2 Garnish with freshly grated Grana Pandano or Parmigiano-Reggiano.

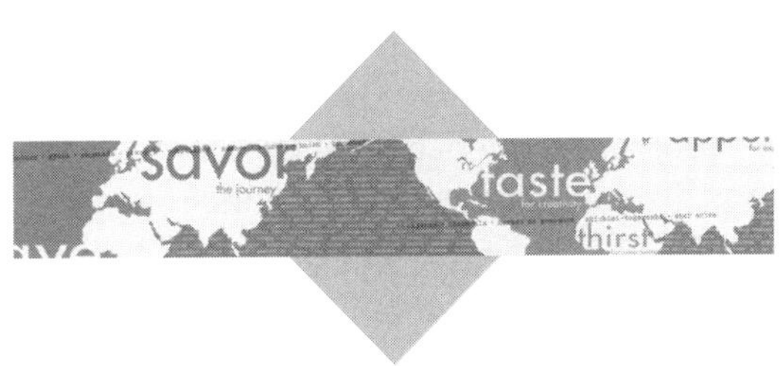

# Germany, Austria, and Switzerland

## The Land

Germany is surrounded by nine countries. To the north along the peninsula called Jutland, which lies between the North Sea and the Baltic Sea, is Denmark. To the west are France, the Netherlands, Belgium, and Luxembourg. Switzerland and Austria lie to the south. The Czech Republic and Poland lie to the east. With its irregular, elongated shape, Germany provides an excellent example of a recurring sequence of landforms found the world over.

From the north, a plain dotted with lakes, moors, marshes, and heaths retreats from the sea and reaches inland, where it becomes a landscape of hills crisscrossed by streams, rivers, and valleys. These hills lead upward, gradually forming high plateaus and woodlands and eventually climaxing in spectacular mountain ranges to the south.

While the Alps along the southern border of Germany are the largest of the European Alps, little Alpine terrain actually lies within Germany compared with Switzerland and Austria. The Black Forest, on the southwestern border with France, separates the Rhine River from the headwaters of the Danube River on its eastern slopes. The Danube cuts across the relatively flat land of central Bavaria, Germany's largest and oldest state, before curving to the southeast around the southern tip of the Bavarian Forest, another range on the border between Bavaria and the Czech Republic.

Austria borders eight countries. To the west are Switzerland and the tiny nation of Liechtenstein. Germany is to the northwest, the Czech Republic is to the north, Slovakia and Hungary are on the east, and Italy and Slovenia lie to the south. Mountains cover more than three-fourths of the Austrian landscape. The Alps, the great spine of Europe, rise in the western and southern half of the country. To the north is the Alpine Forelands, a sprawling valley studded by hills and low mountains. North of the Alpine Forelands is a separate mountainous area called the Granite Plate, made up of granite mountains and rich forests.

The Danube is Austria's major river and runs across the country from West to East. It is the only major river in Europe that follows this direction. The Alps act as a watershed and all major rivers north of the central mountains contribute to the Danube.

Austria is the most densely forested nation in central Europe. Woodlands and meadows cover more than two-thirds of the country. Huge wilderness areas are left undisturbed in Austria because the government has set them aside as national parks and nature areas. The law forbids building roads, houses, and factories in these preserves.

Switzerland is a landlocked country that shares its boundary with Austria and Liechtenstein in the east, France in the west, Italy in the south, and Germany in the north. The topography of Switzerland is mostly mountainous with the Alps in south and the Jura Mountains in the northwest. The central plateau consists of rolling hills, plains, and large lakes. Due to its steep hilly topography, Switzerland is the origin of many great European rivers, including the Rhine and the Rhone. Other rivers, such as the Po and the Danube, are fed by rivers originating here. Glaciers and high waterfalls are a common sight.

# History

Germany lies at the center of the continent and at the crossroads of Europe's business and cultural worlds. It also serves as the connection between western Europe and eastern Europe, as well as between Scandinavia and the Mediterranean world.

Germany was originally settled by numerous tribes, including the Ostrogoths, Visigoths, and Vandals, and later occupied by the Roman legions as far north as the Danube River. The country's history, however, really begins in A.D. 800, when various Germanic peoples came together under the rule of Holy Roman Emperor Charlemagne. After the division of Charlemagne's lands among his descendants, the easternmost German portion eventually gained the imperial title, and in ensuing centuries, German territory expanded eastward. Over time central authority weakened and local princes held most real power on the ground.

Growing conflicts between Catholics and Protestants resulted in the Thirty Years' War (1618–1648). The campaigns were fought for the most part in Germany; the countryside was laid waste, major towns were besieged and sacked, and the economy was ruined.

In the early nineteenth century the German states, as well as most of Europe, became part of Napoleon's French Empire. The Congress of Vienna, convened in 1814 after Napoleon's first defeat, instituted a German Confederation of thirty-five autonomous states and free towns. Germany became a unified nation in 1871 following the Franco-Prussian War.

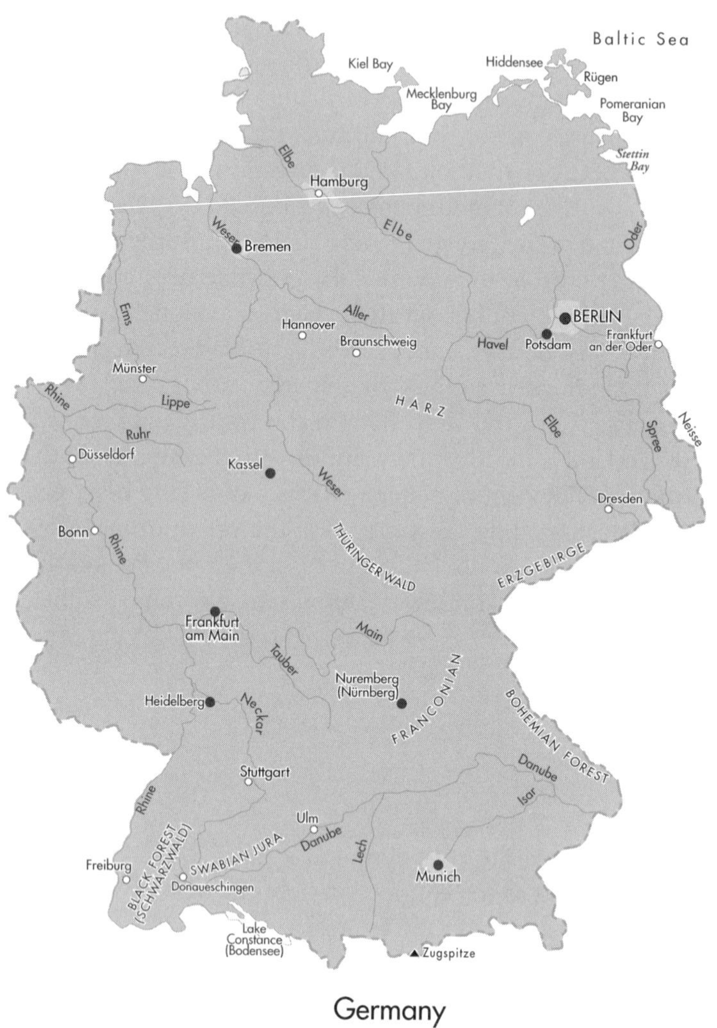


Germany

Twice during the twentieth century, Germany tried to expand outward from its central location to take control of its neighbors by force. World War I and World War II were the greatest conflicts of the century. On both occasions the scales were ultimately tipped against Germany and on both cases some of its original territory was lost.

After World War II, in addition to losing territory, the remainder of the country was occupied by foreign troops and divided into two countries, the democratic West Germany, occupied by the United States, England, and France, and Soviet-dominated communist East Germany. The line dividing Germany bristled with Cold War tension until 1989, when the

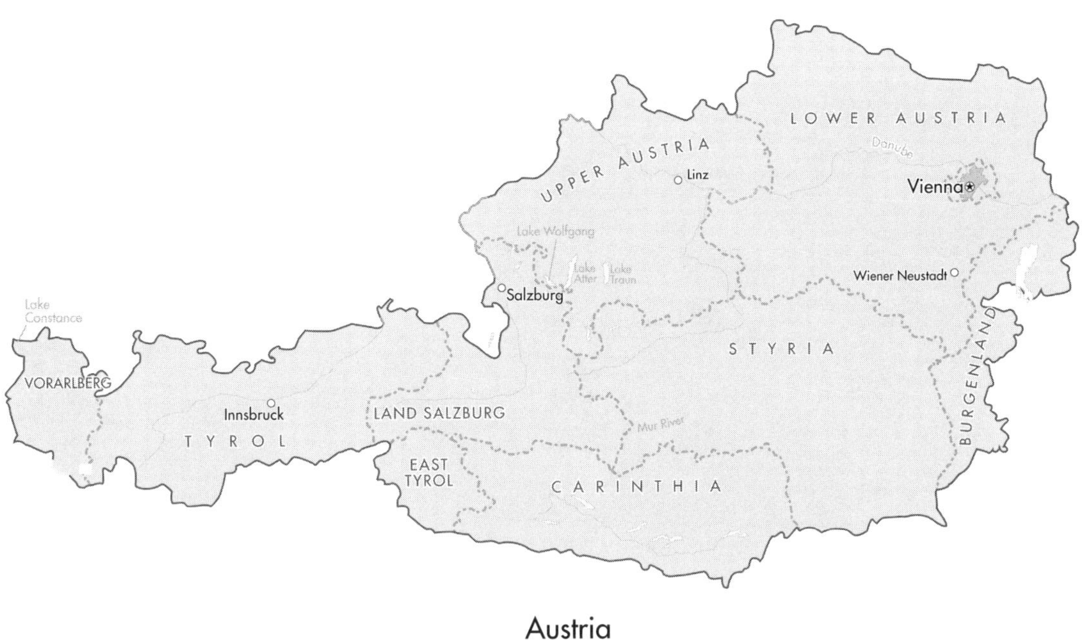


Austria

Berlin Wall fell. Reunification came late in 1990, when the two territories joined under West Germany's constitution became the united Federal Republic of Germany. Today Germany has risen to the status of a leading economic power and plays a fundamental role in the continuing development of the European Union.

The history of Austria begins amidst the reign of the Holy Roman Empire. The area that is now Austria was known as Noricum, a Celtic kingdom occupied by Rome. It went through a series of conquerors until it finally ended up back in the hands of the Roman Empire and stayed there until the end of the Empire in 476.

Under the Hapsburg dynasty Austria was one of Europe's dominating powers in the seventeenth and eighteenth centuries. The Empire of Austria was officially founded in 1805, and became Austria-Hungary in 1867. It split from Hungary following the end of World War I in 1918. At that time it was officially referred to as the Republic of German Austria; however, the name was changed in 1919 to the Republic of Austria. In 1938, Austria was annexed by Hitler's Germany and remained in that state until 1945 at the end of World War II. Following the war, the Allies occupied Austria until 1955, at which time the country signed the Austrian State Treaty, became a neutral independent republic, and joined the United Nations. In 1995, Austria joined the European Union, of which it is still a part.

Switzerland is situated in the heart of Central Europe and shares much of its history and culture with its neighbors Germany, France, Italy and Austria. By hard work, compromise,

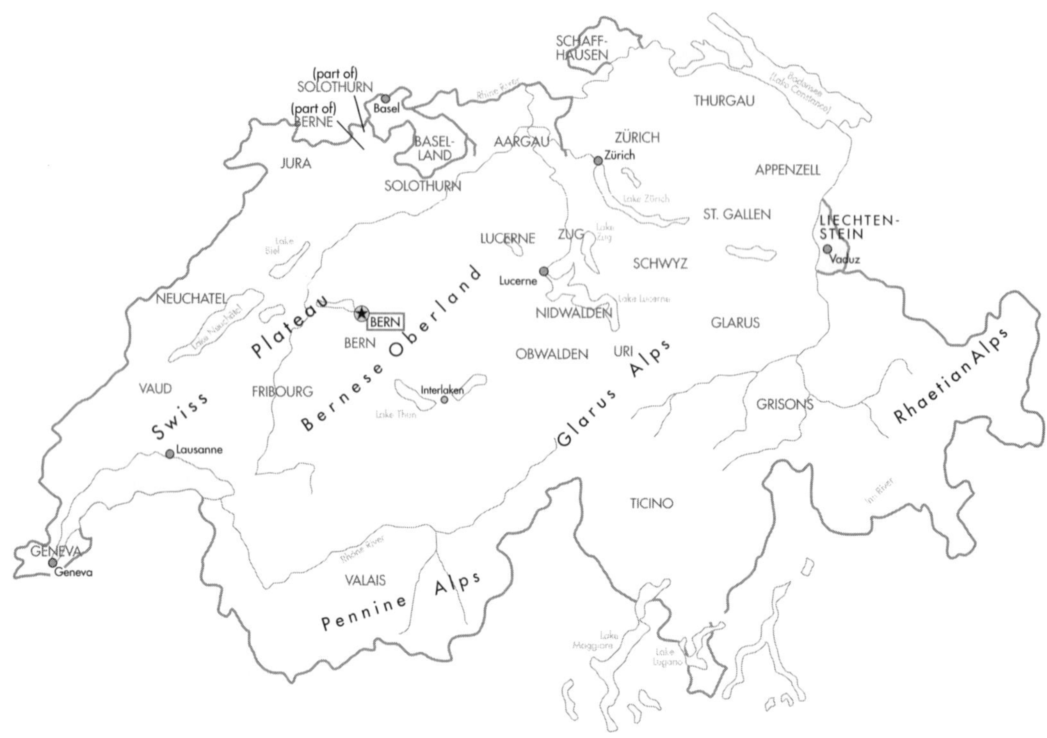


Switzerland

and a strong will to succeed, this small country has grown from a group of widely scattered settlements to one of the world's most prosperous nations.

Originally inhabited by the Helvetians, or Helvetic Celts, the territory comprising modern Switzerland came under Roman rule during the Gallic wars in the first century B.C. and remained a Roman province until the fourth century A.D. Under Roman influence, the population achieved a high level of civilization and enjoyed a flourishing commerce. Important cities, such as Geneva, Basel, and Zurich, were linked by military roads that also served as trade arteries between Rome and the northern tribes.

In spite of its location between nations that were frequently at war, Switzerland has stayed out of most of Europe's wars by using their diplomatic skills to keep neutral. Switzerland's mountainous terrain has been a natural barrier in times of conflict. Nowhere else do people speaking four different languages (German, French, Italian, and Romansh—closely related to Latin) and three major ethnic groups live in such harmony in so small a place (think of a circle with a radius of less than 71 miles). With a dedication to perfection and service, Switzerland is one of the wealthiest countries in the world, with a solid economic base.

# The People

Over the centuries, Germany has been a cradle of European music, literature, theater, and fine arts. From Beethoven and Bach to Goethe, Heine, and Schiller, Germany has produced some of the finest musicians and writers in the history of the civilized world. A strong cultural tradition remains in present-day Germany.

Germany does not celebrate any national festivals, not even a national day. They do, however, celebrate the country's reunification on October 3. What it lacks in national festivals, it makes up for in regional festivals. Each city and state in Germany celebrates colorful festivals that date back hundreds of years. Many of these festivals have been revived to preserve the local heritage. Every year since October 12, 1810, there has been a beer drinking festival in Munich. The Oktoberfest began as a horserace held in honor of the marriage of Bavarian Crown Prince Ludwig I and Princess Therese von Sachsen-Hildburghasen of Saxony. In the following years, the race was combined with the state agricultural fair, and booths serving food and drinks appeared. By the twentieth century these booths had developed into large beer halls. Today, the Oktoberfest lasts sixteen days. The festival is internationally famous and attracts tourists from every corner of the world.

Long ago, Austria was continental Europe's largest and richest empire. Over the ages, artists and architects from every corner of that empire traveled to its central cities to work their crafts. As a result, the towns of modern Austria are considered to be living museums, filled with art treasures and alive with history. The nation today is composed of dozens of ethnic groups, many a mixture of Germanic people from the north, Slavic people from the east, and Mediterranean people from the south. They are united primarily by the German language and the Roman Catholic faith. Austria is known as a storybook place of castles and kingdoms.

Switzerland has been described as a nation with no unity of ethnic heritage, language, or religion, but which is nonetheless united and prosperous. Although the culture could be described as a blend of German, French, and Italian influences, the distinct ethnic strands represent a considerable obstacle to the emergence of any homogeneous cultural identity.

# The Food

### GERMANY

German cuisine is famous the world over for its wurst, or sausages. There are over two hundred types of wurst. The most ordinary German sausage is bockwurst, made of fine ground meat and fat. Other original German sausages include the Bavarian white sausage *Weisswurst* (boiled and served with sweet mustard), *Bratwurst* (for frying), and *Blut* und *Leberwurste* (blood and liver). Germany is also well known for their hams. Great attention is paid to selecting top breeds of pigs that provide fine-flavored and succulent meat. All hams are first cured then either air-dried or cooked and often smoked. Brines and smoking bring individuality to each style, adding to the variety. The most famous German ham is the *Black Forest ham,* which has no bones and comes from the pig's back. Traditionally, this ham is cured with salt. Afterward, the ham is hung to dry and then smoked with cold smoke from fir wood. This gives the ham its distinguished taste. During this process, the ham will lose 30 to 40 percent of its original weight. *Westphalian ham* is produced from pigs raised on acorns in Germany's Westphalia forest. *Westphalian ham* is cured before being slowly smoked over a mix of beechwood and juniper branches. This results in a dark brown, very dense ham with a distinctive, light smoky flavor.

The heartiest German cuisine is from the state of Bavaria and is the cuisine most foreigners recognize as typically German. Pork remains the most popular meat, as exemplified by such dishes as *Jagerschnitzel,* grilled pork sausage topped with Swiss cheese and mushroom sauce, *Schweinebraten,* pork pot roast, and a Bavarian specialty known as *Beirbratl,* pork roasted in beer. Other meat favorites include *Rheinishcher Sauerbraten* (wine-stewed beef roast), roast knuckle of pork, and a host of recipes for goose, duck, and chicken. Bavarian flour dumplings are called *knoedel. Spaetzle* resembles Italian flat noodles, and both are typically served with meat or vegetables. Pickled radish is a popular accompaniment. Pickled cabbage, or sauerkraut, is found thought the country, prepared in different ways and used as both a vegetable and a garnish. White asparagus is one of those items that has cultural significance. It is a symbol of springtime with many local festivals dedicated to it. The official asparagus season in Germany, known as *Spargelzeit,* begins with the harvesting of the first crop in mid-April until June 24, the feast of St. John the Baptist. Sixty percent of asparagus produced in Germany is harvested during the month of May, the rest in April and June. During Spargelzeit, Germans eat asparagus at least once a day and, overall, consume on average a total of 72,000 tons per year.

The Rhineland, the land along the Rhine River, is known for potato-based dishes. Potato pancakes are a traditional Rheinland staple and go by many names, including Reibekuchen and Kartoffelpuffer. They are sometimes served with applesauce. *Kartoffelsalat* is a potato salad that is served warm. It is very similar to another German salad, *Kartoffel mit speck,* potatoes with bacon. The most famous dish of the region is *Sauerbraten,* which has become one of Germany's national dishes. *Sauerbraten* was originally made from horsemeat, but today beef is more commonly used. The meat is marinated in vinegar, a sweetening agent such as sugar beet syrup, apple syrup, or sugar, and seasonings containing juniper cones and cloves, and then braised. The sauce contains raisins and often a kind of gingerbread.

In northern Germany, seafood replaces pork as the popular protein due to the proximity to the North and Baltic seas. Particularly popular are *rollmopse*, rolled, pickled herring filets. Eel is often served smoked or as the principal ingredient of an eel soup-stew called *Aalsuppe.*

Many German cakes and cookies have their origins in a rich and colorful history going back many centuries. Cookies, cakes, and sweet rich yeast breads are crafted into complex patterns and shapes, often associated with ancient symbolic meanings. Two of the most famous are *Stollen* and *Lebkuchen. Stollen* is a breadlike cake with dried citrus peel, dried fruit, nuts, and spices such as cardamom and cinnamon, and is usually eaten during the Christmas season. The best-known *Stollen* is from Dresden. *Lebkuchen,* the most famous German gingerbread, is from Nuremberg. Known as the "king of cakes," the *Baumkuchen,* or "tree cake," is a kind of layered cake. When cut, the cake reveals the characteristic golden rings that give it its name. To get the ring effect, a thin layer of batter is brushed evenly onto a spit and allowed to bake until golden. The most skilled baker will repeat this process numerous times. Some bakers have been known to create three-foot-long Baumkuchens consisting of twenty-five layers and weighing over a hundred pounds. These layers are then covered with sugar or chocolate glaze.

The German beer industry has been heavily regulated since the sixteenth century. In most countries, a percentage of rice or corn is used in the fermentation process but Germany forbids this practice. The only ingredients allowed in German beers are barley, malt, hops, yeast, and water. Germany has over 1,500 breweries and offers more than 5,000 varieties of beer. Most beers in Germany are of the bitter variety and in the Alpine region malty lagers are dominant. *Weizen,* or "white beer," is a cloudy, effervescent, top-fermented beer.

## AUSTRIA

Austrian food is similar to German food, but with Hungarian and Slavic elements lingering from the days of the Austro-Hungarian Empire. The Eastern European influence is mainly Hungarian, and the cooking is characterized by the use of much paprika and the use of more beef than pork. Originally from Turkey, paprika was adopted into Austro-Hungarian cooking in dishes like *goulash* and creamy red chicken *paprikash.* The Turkish influence was also expanded by introducing coffee to Europe via Austria, and still today Austria has the best-developed coffee culture in all of Europe. Its extensive border with Italy made Austria a gateway for the migration of Mediterranean cuisines into northern Europe.

Vienna has a diverse yet harmonious range of dishes reflecting the city's mix of nationalities and food cultures through the centuries. One of the most famous culinary dishes is *Wiener Schnitzel.* A close relative of Italian *veal Milanese, Wiener Schnitzel* probably originated in Italy and then migrated to Austria. In Viennese restaurants, the dish is made with milk-fed veal cutlets that are pounded thin, coated with egg and bread crumbs, and then fried. Many Austrian home cooks prefer pork cutlets for their schnitzel.

Another more traditional Austrian meal is *Tafelspitz* (boiled beef). This national dish is both a general term for the dish and the most common cut of meat used, from the upper leg of the cow. Restaurant menus often offer this with more than 20 other cuts, including the *Kavalierspitz* ("gentleman's portion," from the shoulder) and the *mageres Meisel* ("part without fat," from the front shoulder). The meal begins with the cooking broth as a soup course, and then slices of the meat, accompanied by a chive sauce, horseradish, and sides like creamed spinach and potatoes. Other favorites include *Lungenbraten* (beef tenderloin stuffed with goose liver, served with cream sauce and dumplings), *Backhendl* (chicken dipped in a mixture of flour, breadcrumbs, and beaten egg, and then deep-fried and served with lemon wedges) was considered a symbol of prosperity in Vienna during the reign of Emperor Franz Joseph in the 1800s. *Schlutzkrapfen* are Austrian ravioli filled with cheese, potatoes, herbs, vegetables, or meats and then fried or boiled. Noodles are an integral part of Austrian cooking. Egg pastas, an import from Italy, are popular in the southern provinces of Carinthia and Tyrol, where they are served savory with cheese or pork, or sweet with fruit, nuts, or poppy seeds, butter, and sugar. Pumpkin seed oil is a specialty of the south central province of Styria. This striking dark green oil is pressed from the roasted seeds of squat pumpkins and has an intense, nutty flavor. Traditional in potato salad and drizzled over noodle, fish, egg, and meat dishes, it's also used in a cheese spread for bread.

Austria is famous for their pastries, including the *Linzer Torte,* a jam tart with a lattice of nut pastry, and *Sacher Torte,* a rich chocolate sponge cake glazed with apricot jam and iced in bittersweet chocolate. The Viennese usually serve *Sacher Torte* with unsweetened whipped cream, which complements the chocolate cake and reduces the sweetness. A third pastry, *strudel,* illustrates the diverse origins of Austrian food. Supposedly created by a Hungarian but inspired by Turkish baklava, *strudel* is a wafer-thin pastry rolled around either a sweet or savory filling. Pastry or cakes and coffee are nearly inseparable and are sold in establishments called *Konditorei.* Another sweet specialty is the *Salzburger Nockerl,* a soufflé known to be "as sweet as cream and as tender as a kiss." It is said that the *Nockerl* was invented for a well-known bishop in the early seventeenth century and is supposed to resemble three mountains of Salzburg: Kapuzinerberg, Monchsberg, and Gaisberg.

## SWITZERLAND

Though cuisine in Switzerland is influenced by the German, Italian, French, and Austrian cultures, Swiss food has traditionally been marked by important cultural and regional variations. Cheese dishes are typical of the Alpine regions. Switzerland produces a great variety of cheeses, particularly hard cheeses; among them are *Appenzeller* and *Emmenthaler. Emmenthaler* is so typically Swiss that in Germany it is simply called *Schweizerkase* (Swiss cheese). It is world-famous for the large holes that are a result of gases from the fermenting process. The national dish, *fondue neuchateloise,* is a mixture of melted *Emmenthaler* and *Gruyère* cheeses and wine into which bread cubes are dipped. The origins of fondue are thought to be the high valleys where, cut off during the long winter months, the foods that kept the longest were stale bread, cheese, and pickles. Fondues in different regions of Switzerland use the local cheeses, and meat fondues are a popular modern dish where chunks of meat (instead of bread) are dipped into hot oil (instead of cheese) and "deep fried," then dipped in various sauces. Another specialty is *raclette,* which refers to both a famous cheese as well as a meal. Raclette cheeses are typically round, weighing 13 to 17 pounds and are about 11 inches in diameter and 3 inches thick. The cheeses are made from cow's milk and have a creamy consistency, which easily melts but does not get too runny. The semi-firm cheese is normally aged about three or four months. In the Swiss tradition, raclette cheese is melted over an open fire very slowly. As the cheese melts it is scraped off the wheel and served with boiled potatoes, bread, cornichons, and other pickled vegetables. The name comes from the French verb *racler,* meaning to scrape, because of the way the melted cheese is scraped off the block.

The Swiss chocolate industry, which originally grew out of the need to utilize the abundant milk produced in the pre-Alpine dairying regions, is world famous. One of many chocolate making pioneers Rodolphe Lindt (1855–1909) opened a chocolate factory powered by a water-wheel. A born manufacturer, his inventions led him to a new process by which he produced the first melting, or fondant, chocolate. The refining effect, which is known today as "conching," was first noticed by Lindt while processing chocolate over several days in a narrow mixing trough. He incorporated this into his production methods and, at the same time, developed equipment on principles still in use today. The addition of cocoa butter to the chocolate, to give it the necessary melting quality, was another important discovery. These discoveries, and the invention of milk chocolate by Daniel Peter, were essential to the manufacture and success of the fine Swiss chocolate industry.

In Germanic Switzerland, *rosti* comes close to a national dish. Although *rosti* is made with few ingredients—potatoes, salt, cooking oil, and a little milk—it takes skill to make the potatoes brown and crisp in a golden circle without burning them. Sausages and sauerkraut are also popular dishes. Around the lakes of eastern Switzerland freshwater fish like the delicate zander (pike perch), saibling (lake trout), and felchen (whitefish) can be found on menus. Western Switzerland is influenced by French cuisine and culture, and in Ticono, pasta, polenta, and risotto are signs of a common culture with Italy.

Health foods, whole grains, and fresh vegetables were popular in Switzerland long before they caught on elsewhere. This health food movement started at the clinic of Dr. Max Bircher-Benner (1867–1939), which was founded in Zurich in 1897. Nearly a century later, many Swiss people still follow his advice and begin each meal with an uncooked food, limit meats in their diet, and preserve vitamins by cooking vegetables for just a short time. The most famous dish served at Dr. Bircher-Benner's clinic was a breakfast cereal called *Bircher Muesli.* This original muesli used oatmeal, water, lemon juice, milk, apples, and almonds.

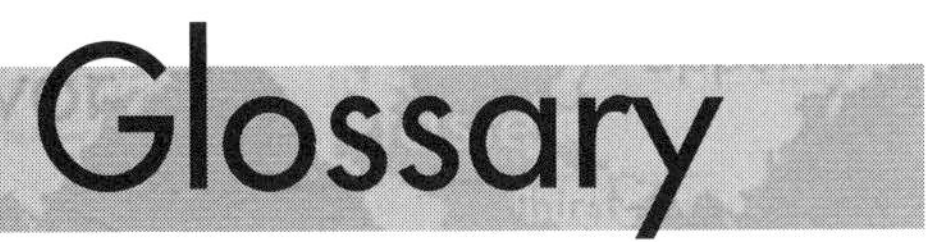

# Glossary

**Auflauf** Casserole.

**Beilagen** Side dishes.

**Bier** There are over 5,000 varieties of beer brewed in 1,500 breweries in Germany.

**Pils** A good all-around lager-style, bottom-fermented light beer, it has a strong hoppy aroma and flavor, with a long, dry finish.

**Altbier and Kölsch** Aromatic, hoppy, bitter beers. *Altbieris* is darker and *Kölsch* is lighter. Both are considered everyday drinking beer.

**Wheat Beers** Brewed from malted wheat and malted barley, there are three styles: Hefe (cloudy), for which the yeast is retained; Kristall (clear), when the yeast is removed; and dark wheat beer.

**Bockbier** "Big" flavor beers with a malty, aromatic, and lightly hoppy bitterness. Color ranges from light golden to dark.

**Black Forest Ham (Schwarzwälder Schinken)** A smoked and cured ham sold in wafer-thin slices. Made from a single boneless joint with a pronounced smoky flavor. Ideal for appetizers.

**Cheeses**

**Allgäuer Emmentaler** German hard cheese with a nutty flavor, similar in taste to Swiss cheese.

**Appenzeller** Product of northeast Switzerland, a hard cow's milk straw-colored cheese. It has a strong smell and a nutty or fruity flavor, which can range from mild to tangy; depending on how long it is aged.

**Bergader** German soft, smooth-textured cheese with large blue veins and a strong, piquant taste.

**Bergkäse** Austrian traditional hard cheese made from raw cow's milk and matured for six months. It is quite mild and creamy but melts well and is used in fondue.

**Blauschmimmelbrie (Bavarian Blue Brie)** Delicate blue-veined cheese with a creamy center and velvety-ripened skin.

**Bruder Basil** Bavarian semi-soft cow's milk cheese with a rich, creamy texture and smoky flavor.

**Butter Käse (Butter Cheese)** Fresh, creamy, flavor reminiscent of better cheddars similar to Parmesan.

**Cambazola** Creamy, blue cheese made from cow's milk. Texture is smooth and rich, with a spicy and slightly sweet-sour flavor.

**Doppelrhamstufel** Soft German cheese made with "double cream." It has a mildly lactic aroma and a slightly salty taste.

**Emmenthaler** Generally known in the U.S. as Swiss cheese, this is a yellow, medium-hard cheese, with characteristic large holes. It has a piquant but not too sharp taste.

**Esrom** A mild cheese when young, but becomes very robust as it ages, developing a stronger flavor similar to Limburger but with a sweeter edge and the consistency similar to Port Salut.

**Gruyère** A hard yellow cheese made from cow's milk, it is named after the town of Gruyères in Switzerland. The cheese is sweet but slightly salty, with a flavor that varies widely with age. It is often described as creamy and nutty when young, becoming more assertive, earthy, and complex with age.

**Kugelkase** An Austrian cheese made from cow's milk. It is a creamy, ball-shaped cheese with pepper, caraway seeds, and paprika added so that the curd becomes infused with their aroma.

**Limburger** A very strong-smelling German cheese. Made with cow's milk, it has a tangy, creamy, Brie-like flavor and pungent aroma. Most of the strong taste is found in the rind.

**Mondseer** Austrian cheese also known as Schachtelkase, close to Munster or Limburger despite its relative hardness. It has a slightly spicy aroma and sweet-sour taste.

**Sbrinz** Originated in Switzerland, it is a whole cow's milk cheese, aged two to three years. Sometimes this hard grating cheese is aged less and then it is called *Spalen.*

**Schloss** A milder form of Limburger, but with a stronger flavor. It has a white and golden color; the flavor is tangy, mild, and pungent, depending on how ripe it is. Schloss has a semi-firm and creamy texture.

**Steppenkäse** A mild cheese similar in taste to Tilsit, but lower in fat.

**Tilsit** A light yellow German and Swiss semi-soft cheese with a hearty flavor that becomes robust with age. It is often flavored with caraway seed and peppercorns.

**Cornichons** Pickled baby gherkins.

**Fondue** Probably the most famous Swiss dish. Traditional fondue is made out of melted cheese.

**Goulash** A type of beef stew from Hungary that always contains paprika.

**Gabelfruhstuck** Literally a "fork meal," referring to the traditional 10:00 A.M. snack in Austria, usually a small meat dish or sausage.

**Jause** Literally "gossip time;" refers to pastry and coffee taken in the late afternoon. May occasionally be an elaborate spread of small sandwiches, pastries, and tea (Austria).

**Katenspeck** *Katen* is the German word for "barn," meaning that this ham is made farmhouse style: cured, smoked, and cooked.

**Kartoffel, Kartoffelsalat** Potato, potato salad (served warm).

**Knödel** Dumplings.

**Kochwurst** Boiled sausages such as leberwurst (liverwurst), ready to eat without heating.

**Kuchen** Cake, either sweet or savory.

**Landbrot** Germany's daily bread, made from wheat with a little light rye flour for a moist texture. The name translates to "farm bread."

**Leberkäse** A high-quality meatloaf made from minced pork and beef that can be eaten hot or cold. Served on a bun, it is the Bavarian's answer to the burger.

**Lebkuchen** Honey-sweet, richly spiced ginger cake.

**Linzer Torte** Named for the Austrian town of Linz, this is more a flan than a torte; a rich nut pastry filled with fine raspberry preserves, crisscrossed with more nut pastry, baked, then served with whipped cream.

**Marzipan** Marzipan is an almond and sugar paste used to ice cakes and other pastries or sculpted into a variety of shapes to be eaten as candy or used as cake decorations. It is governed by strict food laws ensuring a blend of two parts ground almonds to one part sugar, with rose water the only flavoring permitted. After the ingredients are mixed, marzipan reaches a consistency of dough or soft rubber and can be rolled, shaped, cut, or molded.

**Muesli** A healthy, tasty mixture of raw or toasted grains (such as oats, wheat, millet, barley, and wheat germ), dried fruits, nuts, and seeds.

**Palatschinken** Thin, small pancakes, similar to crepes, usually served filled and rolled with preserves, sprinkled with nuts or crumbs, and topped with whipped cream (Austria).

**Paprika** Vivid red powder, ground from dried chile peppers, available in sweet and hot varieties. Originally from Turkey, paprika was adopted by Austro-Hungarians in dishes like goulash.

**Pumpernickel** Rich, dark 100 percent rye bread made by a unique method involving time, skill, and care.

**Pumpkin Seed Oil** A specialty of Austria's south central province of Styria, it is a striking dark green oil, pressed from the roasted seeds of pumpkins. It has an intense, nutty flavor.

**Quark** A thick, cultured dairy product similar to ricotta, but creamier with a tarter flavor.

**Raclette** A Swiss dish consisting of cheese melted and served on boiled potatoes or bread.

**Rathskellar** Generally, a restaurant in the basement of a city hall, serving classic dishes.

**Reibekuchen/Kartoffelpuffer** Potato pancakes.

**Roggenbrot** Rye bread.

**Rohwurst** Hard, dry sausages, such as salami, which don't require cooking.

**Rosti** May be considered Switzerland's national dish. It is made with potatoes, salt, cooking oil, and a little milk.

**Rotkohl** German pickled red cabbage.

**Sacher Torte** Two layers of a slightly bitter chocolate cake sandwiched together with apricot jam, glazed with chocolate, and served with of whipped cream on the side. The actual recipe is a closely guarded secret involving as many as thirty two steps. It was created by Franz Sacher in 1832 and continues to be served in the Hotel Sacher, opened in 1832 by Franz's son, Eduard.

**Sauerkraut** Thinly shredded white cabbage salted and left to ferment for weeks to develop a unique piquant flavor.

**Schlutzkrapfen** Austrian ravioli filled with cheese, potatoes, herbs, vegetables, or meats, and fried or boiled.

**Schnaps** Means "gulp" in old German, which is how it should be drunk. There are two main types: The first is *Korn,* a clear grain spirit, neutral liquor similar to vodka. The second is made from distilled spirits known collectively as *Obstwasse*r, produced from fruit juices, fermented naturally without the addition of sugar or alcohol. The most important is *Kirschwasser,* made from late-ripening black cherries.

**Senf** A mustard mixed with vinegar, salt, spices, and sugar. German mustards are very aromatic.

**Spätzle (Knodel, Nocker, Spaetzle)** Literally, "little sparrows," these are small noodles or dumplings made of flour, eggs, and water or milk.

**Stollen** A yeast loaf rich with candied fruits, raisins, and other flavorings.

**Strudel** Layers of flaky pastry wrapped around a fruit filling, often of apples and raisins.

**Süsser Senf** Unique to Germany, a gentle, piquant, sweet mustard dressing.

**Tafelspitz** This boiled beef dish is Austria's national dish.

**Wacholder** Dark blue juniper berries with a clean flavor, at first slightly bitter, then almost sweet. They are often substituted for bay leaf in the typical German "bouquet garni."

**Weinstube** A small local restaurant where the main beverage is wine.

**Weisser Spargel** Throughout Germany, white asparagus has a special stature; it symbolizes the beginning of spring, and many local festivals are dedicated to it.

**Westphalian ham** This ham is produced from pigs raised on acorns in Germany's Westphalia forest. It is cured before being slowly smoked over a mix of beechwood and juniper branches, resulting in a dark brown, very dense ham with a distinctive, light smoky flavor.

**Wiener Backhendle** A Viennese specialty of egg-dipped, crumbed fried chicken pieces that are then finished by oven baking.

**Wienerbrot** A Scandinavian term literally meaning Viennese bread, but which actually refers to pastries made from puff pastry; known elsewhere as Danish pastry.

**Wiener Schnitzel** Perhaps the most famous Viennese specialty; large thin (pounded) scallops of veal, egged and crumbed and crisply fried.

**Wurst** The term for any sausage. All types of German sausage are required by law to be 100 percent meat with no fillers.

**Zopf** Special bread, typically served on Sunday for breakfast in Switzerland.

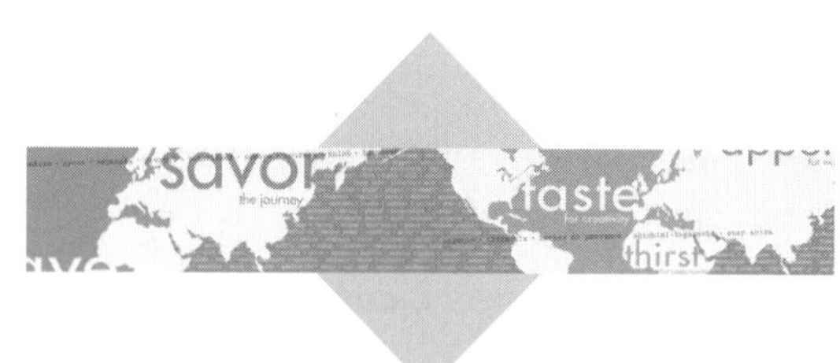

# Menus and Recipes from Germany, Austria, and Switzerland

MENU ONE (GERMANY)

***Rahmilinsen mit Salat:* Lentil Ragout with Greens**

***Kartoffelsuppe mit Miesmuscheln und Lauch:* Potato Soup with Mussels and Leeks**

***Kalbslebersteak mit Roter Zwiebelmarmelade und Senfesauce:* Calf's Liver with Red Onion Marmalade and Mustard Sauce**

***Schweinelendchen im Schwarzbratmantel:* Pork Tenderloin in a Dark Bread Crust**

***Rotkraut und Spätzle:* Braised Red Cabbage and Spaetzle**

***Mohncreme mit Rotweinbrinen:* Poppy Seed Cream with Pears in Red Wine**

MENU TWO (SWITZERLAND)

***Chindbettisuppe:* Childbed Soup**

***Filets de Rouget aux Herbettes:* Red Mullet Fillets with Herbs**

***Luzerner Chûgelipastete:* Puff Pastry with Meat Filling**

***Carnard Röti aux Endives:* Roast Duck with Chicory**

***Rosti:* Potato Cake**

***Zûrcher Öpfelbachis:* Shredded Dough Cakes with Apples**

MENU THREE (AUSTRIA)

***Bodenseefischsuppe mit Safran:* Fish Soup from the Bodensee with Saffron**

***Szegediner Gulasch:* Szeged Goulash**

***Gemischter Salat:* Mixed Salad**

***Wiener Schnitzel***

***Erdäpfelschmarrn:* Fried Potatoes**

***Salzburger Nockerl***

# Rahmilinsen mit Salat

## Lentil Ragout with Greens

SERVES 4

| AMOUNT | MEASURE | INGREDIENT |
|---|---|---|
| 1 cup | 7 ounces, 196 g | Green lentils |
| 2 tablespoons | 1 ounce, 30 ml | Olive oil |
| 2 tablespoons | $\frac{1}{2}$ ounce, 14 g | Bacon, minced |
| $\frac{1}{3}$ cup | 2 ounces, 56 g | Carrots, $\frac{1}{8}$ inch (.3 cm) dice |
| $\frac{1}{3}$ cup | 2 ounces, 56 g | Celery, $\frac{1}{8}$ inch (.3 cm) dice |
| $\frac{1}{3}$ cup | 2 ounces, 56 g | Onions, $\frac{1}{8}$ inch (.3 cm) dice |
| $\frac{1}{3}$ cup | 2 ounces, 56 g | Leeks, $\frac{1}{8}$ inch (.3 cm) dice |
| 2 | | Garlic cloves, minced |
| $\frac{3}{4}$ cup | 4 ounces, 112 g | Potatoes, $\frac{1}{4}$ inch (.6 cm) dice |
| $1\frac{1}{4}$ cups | 10 ounces, 300 ml | Chicken stock |
| $\frac{1}{2}$ cup | 4 ounces, 120 ml | Heavy cream |
| 3 | | Whole cloves |
| 2 | | Bay leaves |
| To taste | | Salt and pepper |
| 2 tablespoons | 1 ounce, 30 ml | Honey |
| 2 tablespoons | 1 ounce, 30 ml | Red wine vinegar |
| 3 cups | 6 ounces, 168 g | Mixed baby greens |
| 8 | | Tomato wedges, peeled, seeded |

PROCEDURE

1. Pick over lentils to remove small stones and discolored seeds. Put in a bowl of water and remove any that float. Wash lentils well and drain thoroughly.
2. Heat olive oil over medium heat, add bacon, and cook until slightly brown, 2–3 minutes. Add drained lentils, and stir to coat with oil.
3. Add carrots, celery, onion, leeks, garlic, and potatoes; sauté 3 to 4 minutes.
4. Add stock, cream, herbs, and spices. Simmer on low heat until lentils are soft, 30 to 45 minutes. Remove bay leaves and cloves.
5. Season with salt and pepper.
6. Just before serving, add honey and vinegar to warm ragout.
7. Plate the mixed baby greens with two tomato wedges, spoon the lentils over half the greens, and serve.

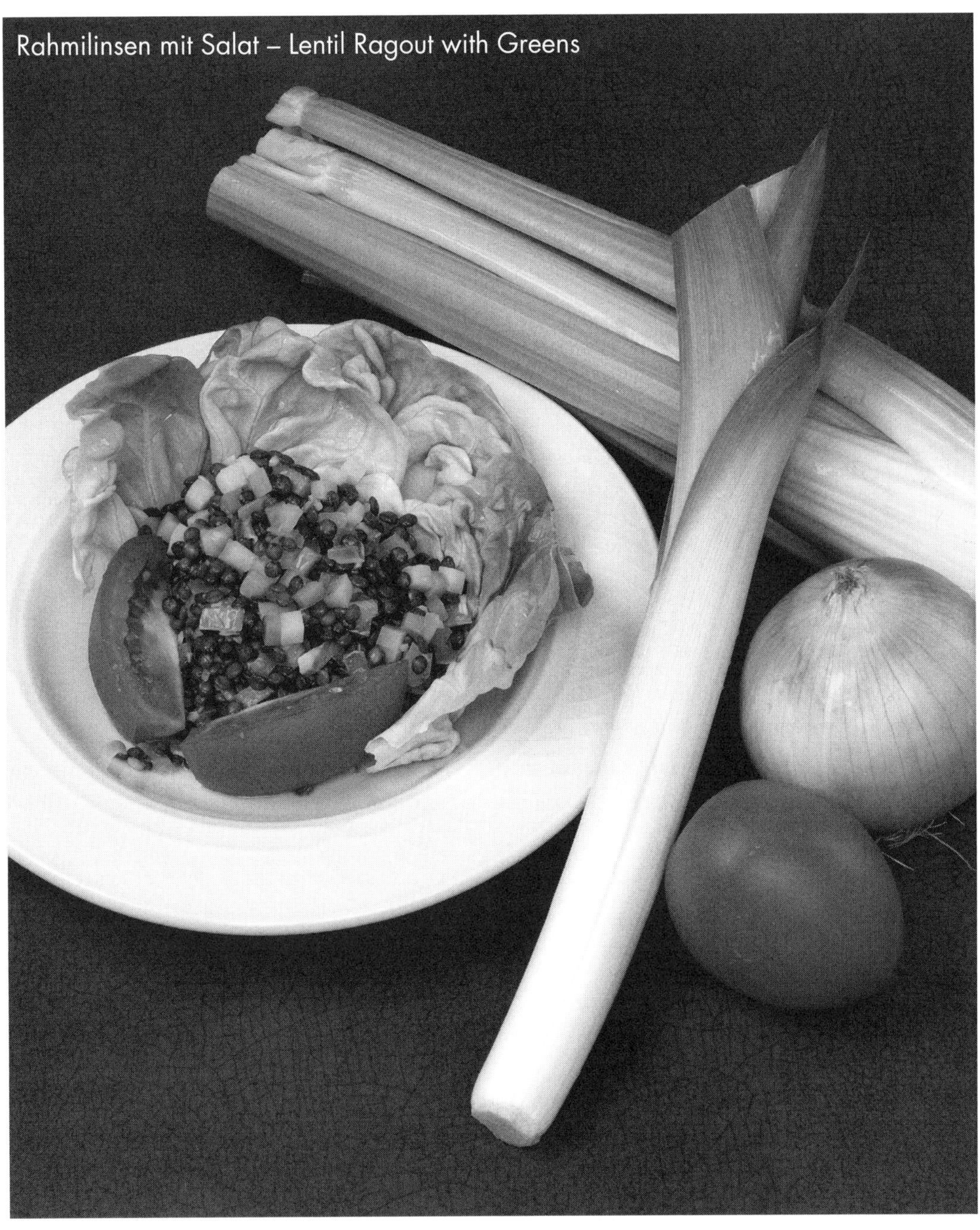

Rahmilinsen mit Salat – Lentil Ragout with Greens

# Kartoffelsuppe mit Miesmuscheln und Lauch

## Potato Soup with Mussels and Leeks

SERVES 4

| AMOUNT | MEASURE | INGREDIENT |
|---|---|---|
| **3 tablespoons** | **1 ½ ounces, 45 ml** | **Butter** |
| **2 tablespoons** | | **Shallots, minced** |
| **¾ cup** | **6 ounces, 180 ml** | **White wine** |
| **1 quart** | | **Mussels, washed, beards removed** |
| **¼ cup** | **2 ounces, 60 ml** | **Cold water** |
| **½ cup** | **2 ounces, 56 g** | **Leek, white and light-green parts, minced** |
| | **8 ounces 224 g** | **Potato, cooked, peeled, and pureed** |
| **To taste** | | **Salt, white pepper, and cayenne pepper** |

**PROCEDURE**

1. In a pan large enough to just hold the mussels, melt the butter over medium-low heat. Add shallot and soften for a minute without browning; add white wine and mussels.
2. Cover and raise the heat to medium-high; cook, shaking the pan from time to time, until the mussels open, 3 to 4 minutes. Do not overcook the mussels or they will become tough.
3. Strain the mussels and cooking liquid into another pan through a cheesecloth-lined strainer.
4. Remove mussels from the shells, set the meat aside, discard the shells, and reserve cooking liquid.
5. Combine cold water and cooking liquid, add leeks, and cook over medium heat, 3 to 4 minutes.
6. Add the potato puree to the soup $\frac{1}{3}$ at a time, whisking to mix well after each addition. If it is too thick after adding all the potato, thin with a little water.
7. Add mussels, bring back to a boil, remove from heat, and season with salt, pepper, and cayenne.
8. To serve, divide the mussels equally among 4 warm shallow bowls and pour a portion of the soup over.

# Kalbslebersteak mit Roter Zwiebelmarmelade und Senfesauce Calf's Liver with Red Onion Marmalade and Mustard Sauce

SERVES 4

| AMOUNT | MEASURE | INGREDIENT |
|---|---|---|
| **1 pound** | **16 ounces, 448 g** | **Calf's liver, trimmed** |
| **1 tablespoon** | **$\frac{1}{2}$ ounce, 15 ml** | **Butter** |
| **$\frac{1}{4}$ cup per serving** | | **Cooked egg noodles, hot** |
| **As needed** | | **Red onion marmalade (recipe follows)** |
| **As needed** | | **Mustard sauce (recipe follows)** |
| **Garnish** | | **Chopped parsley** |

**PROCEDURE**

1. Heat the butter over low heat, add liver, and cook about 1 minute on each side.
2. Turn off the heat and leave the liver to continue cooking in the pan 5 minutes. The liver should be pale pink all the way through.
3. Slice the liver thinly and arrange in overlapping slices on warm plates. Serve with red onion marmalade and mustard sauce, accompanied by noodles and topped with parsley.

# Red Onion Marmalade

| AMOUNT | MEASURE | INGREDIENT |
|---|---|---|
| 2 tablespoons | 1 ounce, 30 ml | Butter |
| 3 cups | 18 ounces, 504 g | Red onions, finely sliced |
| To taste | | Salt and pepper |
| 1 tablespoon | $\frac{1}{2}$ ounce, 15 ml | Wild-flower honey |
| 1$\frac{1}{2}$ cups | 12 ounces, 360 ml | Red wine (Lemberger, Cabernet, or Merlot) |
| To taste | | Fresh lemon juice |

**PROCEDURE**

1 Over medium heat, melt butter, add onions, and cook until transparent. Do not let them color. Season to taste with salt and pepper; stir in honey and wine.

2 Cover and transfer to a 300°F (150°C) oven. Cook 45 minutes, until the sauce has the consistency of marmalade. Check occasionally so it does not burn. Season to taste with lemon juice.

# Mustard Sauce

| AMOUNT | MEASURE | INGREDIENT |
|---|---|---|
| 1$\frac{1}{4}$ cups | 10 ounces, 300 ml | Brown stock or flavorful chicken stock |
| 1$\frac{1}{4}$ cups | 10 ounces, 300 ml | Heavy cream |
| $\frac{1}{2}$ cup | 4 ounces, 120 ml | White wine |
| 1 tablespoon | $\frac{1}{2}$ ounce, 15 ml | Medium-hot mustard |
| $\frac{1}{2}$ teaspoon | | Hot mustard |
| 2 tablespoons | 1 ounce, 30 ml | Cold butter, small cubes |

**PROCEDURE**

1 Combine all ingredients except butter and reduce until the mixture coats the back of a spoon.

2 Just before serving, whisk in the cold butter.

# Schweinelendchen im Schwarzbratmantel

## Pork Tenderloin in a Dark Bread Crust

SERVES 4

| AMOUNT | MEASURE | INGREDIENT |
|---|---|---|
| 2 tablespoons | 1 ounce, 30 ml | Vegetable oil |
| 1 pound | 16 ounces, 448 g | Pork tenderloin, cleaned |
| 12 ounces | | Lean ground pork |
| 2 | | Eggs |
| $\frac{3}{4}$ cup | 6 ounces, 180 ml | Heavy cream |
| To taste | | Salt and pepper |
| $\frac{1}{2}$ cup | 2 ounces, 56 g | Dark rye bread crumbs, dry |
| 1 cup | 8 ounces, 240 ml | Pork or beef demi-glace |

PROCEDURE

1 Heat the oil over medium high heat, sear the pork tenderloin, and set aside to cool.

2 In a food processor, process ground pork. Add eggs one at time, pulsing to incorporate. Scrape down sides and with machine running, add the cream in a steady stream. Scrape down sides; do not overprocess.

3 Remove mixture to a bowl over an ice bath. Poach or sauté a sample and adjust seasoning; add more cream if mixture is too stiff. Fold in bread crumbs.

4 Lay out a piece of plastic wrap large enough to wrap around the pork tenderloin two or three times. Spread the bread crumb mixture in an even layer just large enough to surround the pork tenderloin. Place the tenderloin in the middle of the bread crumb mixture; surround the tenderloin with the mixture. Wrap plastic around and tie ends so it is watertight. Poach in a 160°F (71.1°C) water bath 30 to 40 minutes or until an internal temperature of 155°F (68°C) is reached. Remove from water bath.

5 Let set 5 to 10 minutes, remove wrap, slice, and serve with demi-glace.

# Rotkraut und Spätzle

## Braised Red Cabbage and Spaetzle

SERVES 4

| AMOUNT | MEASURE | INGREDIENT |
|---|---|---|
| 1 pound | 16 ounces, 448 g | Red cabbage |
| 2 tablespoons | 1 ounce, 30 ml | Butter |
| $\frac{3}{4}$ cup | 4 ounces, 112 g | Onions, $\frac{1}{4}$ inch (.6 cm) dice |
| 5 | | Juniper berries |
| 4 | | Cloves |
| $\frac{1}{2}$ tablespoon | | Granulated sugar |
| 1 cup | 6 ounces, 168 g | Tart green apples, peeled, cored, $\frac{1}{4}$ inch (.6 cm) dice |
| $\frac{1}{4}$ cup | 2 ounces, 60 ml | Red wine vinegar |
| $\frac{1}{2}$ teaspoon | | Salt |
| 1 | | Bay leaf |
| 1 tablespoon | | Cornstarch |
| $\frac{1}{2}$ cup | 4 ounces, 120 ml | Dry red wine |
| As needed | | Spätzle (recipe follows) |

PROCEDURE

1 Trim the coarse outer leaves from the cabbage and discard; quarter the cabbage, remove the hard white core at the point of each quarter and discard, then slice each quarter very thinly.

2 Melt butter over medium high heat; add onions, juniper berries, cloves and sprinkle in the sugar, and cook to dissolve, 2 minutes.

3 Add apples, sauté 5 minutes or until soft and golden.

4 Add cabbage and sauté 5 minutes, until nicely glazed.

5 Add red wine vinegar and bring to a simmer. Add salt and bay leaf; toss to combine, push bay leaf down into the cabbage.

6 Cover and simmer 20 to 25 minutes, until cabbage is crisp-tender.

7 Sprinkle cornstarch over the cabbage and toss well to mix. Add the red wine. Heat to a strong simmer and cook, stirring, 3 to 5 minutes, until liquids are thickened. Remove from heat.

8 Discard bay leaf.

9 Simmer 5 minutes longer, uncovered. Serve with spaetzle.

# Spätzle

YIELD: 4 CUPS

| AMOUNT | MEASURE | INGREDIENT |
|---|---|---|
| 2 cups | 8 ounces, 224 g | All-purpose flour |
| $\frac{1}{8}$ teaspoon | | Freshly grated nutmeg |
| $\frac{1}{2}$ teaspoon | | Salt |
| 2 | | Eggs |
| $\frac{3}{4}$ cup | 6 ounces, 180 ml | Milk |
| 3 tablespoons | $1\frac{1}{2}$ ounces, 45 ml | Butter, melted |
| To taste | | Salt and pepper |

PROCEDURE

1. Sift together flour, nutmeg, and salt. Make a well in the center.
2. Whisk the eggs with the milk and pour into the well of dry ingredients.
3. Mix with a wooden spoon, then use a mixer or food processor to beat the mixture until it is bubbly and elastic.
4. Pour batter into a spätzle hex or use a colander with medium to large holes. Force the batter through the holes into boiling salted water. Let the dough fall into the slightly bubbling water; cook about 2 to 3 minutes. Generally, the dumplings will float on the surface when sufficiently cooked.
5. Remove from the top with a slotted spoon or skimmer, wash under cold running water to remove excess starch, and let drain.
6. Heat butter over medium heat, add drained spaetzle, and toss to heat, or sautée in butter until golden and crispy. Correct seasoning.

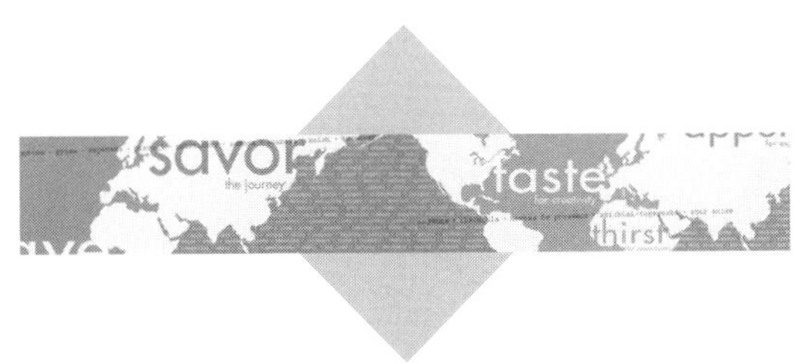

# Mohncreme mit Rotweinbrinen

## Poppy Seed Cream with Pears in Red Wine

SERVES 4

| AMOUNT | MEASURE | INGREDIENT |
|---|---|---|
| 1 cup | 8 ounces, 240 ml | Red wine |
| $\frac{1}{4}$ cup | 2 ounces, 56 g | Granulated sugar |
| 1 stick | | Cinnamon |
| | | Zest from 1 orange |
| 1 | | Vanilla pod or 1 teaspoon vanilla extract |
| 2 tablespoons | 1 ounce, 30 ml | Pear schnapps, such as Poire William (optional) |
| 2 | | Pears, peeled, cored, and thinly sliced |
| As needed | | Poppy seed cream (recipe follows) |
| 3 tablespoons | | Toasted almonds, sliced |
| $\frac{1}{2}$ cup | 4 ounces, 120 ml | Heavy cream, whipped |

### PROCEDURE

1. Heat red wine, sugar, cinnamon stick, orange zest, vanilla pod, and schnapps; stir to dissolve. Bring to a boil.
2. Pour hot syrup over pears and macerate 2 to 3 hours, so they take on color.

### PRESENTATION

1. Place two quenelles of poppy seed cream on dessert plates. Arrange pear slices attractively on the side, pour a little syrup around, and garnish with almonds and whipped cream.

# Poppy Seed Cream

| AMOUNT | MEASURE | INGREDIENT |
|---|---|---|
| $\frac{1}{4}$ cup | 1 ounce, 28 g | Poppy seeds |
| 2 tablespoons | 1 ounce, 30 ml | Red wine |
| 1 | | Egg |
| 1 | | Egg yolk |
| 2 | | Gelatin leaves, soaked in 4 tablespoons (2 ounces, 60 ml) water |
| | $3\frac{1}{2}$ ounces, 98 g | White couverture chocolate |
| 1 tablespoon | $\frac{1}{2}$ ounce, 15 ml | Honey |
| 1 cup | 8 ounces, 240 ml | Heavy cream, whipped to soft peaks |

**PROCEDURE**

1. Grind the poppy seeds with a spice grounder or mortar and pestle. Combine the poppy seed paste and red wine; bring to boil for 1 minute. (This tempers their harsh taste.) Strain and reserve the poppy seeds.
2. Combine whole egg and egg yolk.
3. Stir gelatin and soaking water over hot water to dissolve.
4. Melt white chocolate over simmering water.
5. Whisk eggs over hot water until they start to thicken. Add the softened gelatin, the melted chocolate, and honey. Stir in the poppy seeds (but not the red wine) and remove from heat.
6. When mixture has cooled down (do not wait for it to get cold and set), fold in whipped cream. Refrigerate until set.

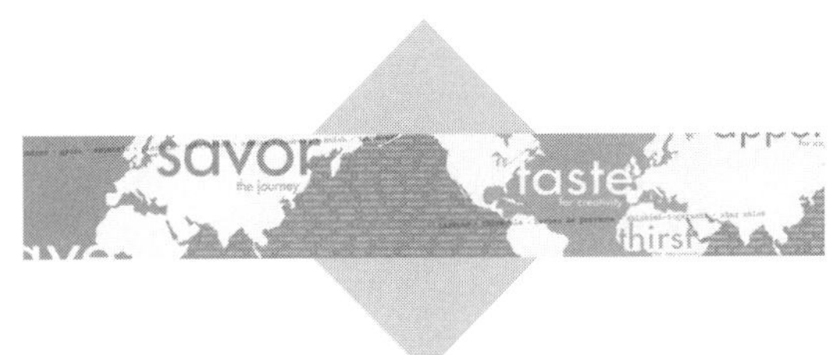

# Chindbettisuppe Childbed Soup

SERVES 4

| AMOUNT | MEASURE | INGREDIENT |
|---|---|---|
| 1 cup | 6 ounces, 168 g | Carrots, peeled, coarsely chopped |
| 1 cup | 6 ounces, 168 g | Celery, coarsely chopped |
| 1 | $2\frac{1}{2}$ pound, 1.12 kg | Whole chicken |
| 2 quarts | 64 ounces, 1.92 l | Chicken stock |
| 1 | | Bunch parsley |
| 3 | | Peppercorns, crushed |
| 1 | | Bay leaf |
| $\frac{1}{2}$ cup | 4 ounces, 120 ml | Milk |
| $\frac{1}{2}$ cup | 4 ounces, 120 ml | Heavy cream |
| To taste | | Salt and pepper |
| $\frac{1}{4}$ cup | $1\frac{1}{2}$ ounces, 42 g | Corn kernels |
| $\frac{1}{2}$ cup | 2 ounces, 56 g | Leek, trimmed, cut into thin slices |
| 3 | | Eggs |
| $\frac{1}{4}$ cup | $\frac{1}{2}$ ounce, 14 g | Chives, minced |

PROCEDURE

1. Combine carrots, celery, chicken, chicken stock, parsley, peppercorns, and bay leaf; bring to a boil. Reduce to simmer and cook 50 minutes.
2. Remove chicken, bone breast, cut into thin strips, and set aside.
3. Strain stock and reserve.
4. Add 3 cups (24 ounces, 720 ml) stock to a saucepan and reduce by two thirds over medium-high heat.
5. Add milk and cream to reduced broth, correct seasoning, and set aside.
6. Cook corn in boiling salted water until tender. Drain and reserve.
7. Steam leeks until tender.
8. Beat eggs together with a pinch of salt. Bring soup to a boil. Stir in eggs and remove from heat.
9. Arrange chicken meat, corn, and leeks in warm soup plates and cover with soup.
10. Sprinkle with chives and serve.

# Filets de Rouget aux Herbettes

## Red Mullet Fillets with Herbs

SERVES 4

**Rouget is a red-skinned fish with delicate meat, similar to the goatfish found around the Bahamas and the Florida Keys. When available, the Hawaiian moano or kumo goatfish can be substituted, or use red snapper.**

| AMOUNT | MEASURE | INGREDIENT |
|---|---|---|
| 3 tablespoons | 1 $\frac{1}{2}$ ounces, 45 ml | Olive oil |
| 1 $\frac{1}{2}$ tablespoons | $\frac{3}{4}$ ounce, 20 ml | Butter |
| 4 | 3 ounces, 84 g each | Boneless, skinless fillets of fish |
| To taste | | Salt, pepper, and cayenne |
| 3 tablespoons | $\frac{1}{2}$ ounce, 14 g | Shallot, minced |
| 2 teaspoons | | Garlic, minced |
| $\frac{1}{2}$ cup | 4 ounces, 120 ml | White wine |
| $\frac{1}{4}$ cup | 1 ounce, 28 g | Herbs, minced (chervil, parsley, tarragon, chives) |
| $\frac{1}{2}$ cup | 3 ounces, 84 g | Tomato, peeled, seeded $\frac{1}{8}$ inch (.3 cm) dice |

### PROCEDURE

1. Preheat oven to 525°F (274°C).
2. Put the oil in an ovenproof dish or sauté pan large enough to hold the fillets in one layer. Add the butter and melt over low heat.
3. Season fish with salt, pepper, and cayenne.
4. Arrange fillets in a single layer, not overlapping. Sprinkle the garlic and shallot over the fish and add the wine.
5. Cook in the preheated oven 2 minutes, turn the fillets, and continue cooking 1 minute more (depending on thickness). Remove fillets to warm plates.
6. Over medium heat, add herbs and diced tomatoes to cooking pan. Bring to a boil; check seasoning.
7. Pour the tomato-herb sauce around the fillets and serve.

# Luzerner Chûgelipastete

## Puff Pastry with Meat Filling

SERVES 4

**Puff Pastry**

| AMOUNT | MEASURE | INGREDIENT |
|---|---|---|
| As needed | | All-purpose flour |
| | 8 ounces, 224 g | Puff pastry |
| 1 | | Egg |
| Pinch | | Salt |

**PROCEDURE**

1. Preheat oven to 375°F (190°C).
2. Lightly flour a work surface and the dough. Press the dough in successive firm strokes in both directions with a rolling pin. Move the dough frequently to renew the flour under and on it. Roll out to $\frac{3}{13}$ inch (.5 cm) thick and place on a paper-lined pan. Allow dough to rest in refrigerator about 1 hour.
3. Remove dough from refrigerator, dock well, and cut into 8 heart shapes, using a cutter or knife. Place 4 of the shapes on a paper-lined pan.
4. Cut out the center of the other 4 hearts and discard them, leaving 4 heart shaped rings.
5. Whisk together the egg and salt and paint the hearts on the pan with the egg wash.
6. Center the heart-shaped rings on the heart bases and firmly press them into place.
7. Dock the rings with the point of a paring knife at $\frac{1}{2}$ inch (1.2 cm) intervals.
8. Bake in preheated oven about 25 minutes, until well risen and deep golden. Cool on rack.

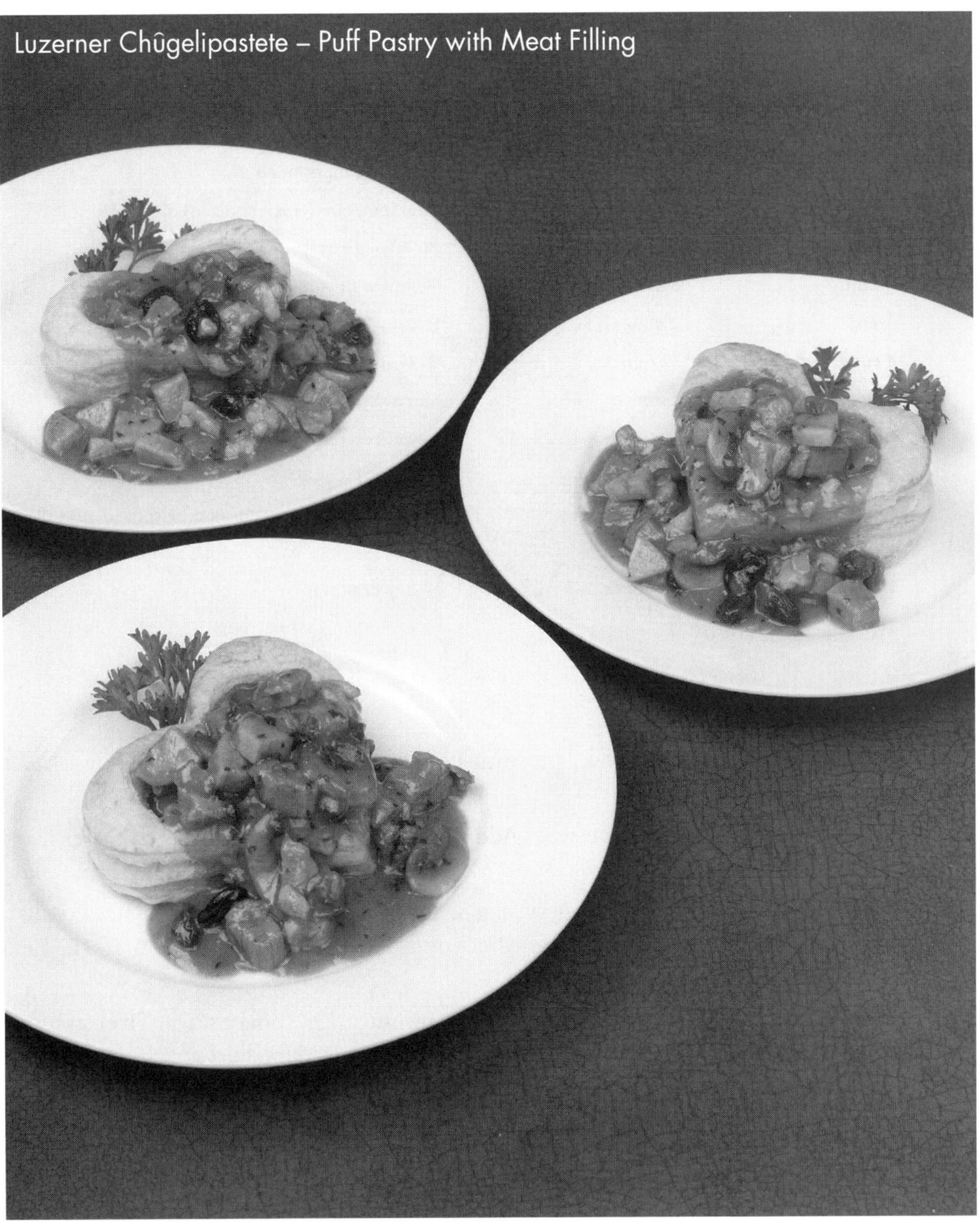
Luzerner Chûgelipastete – Puff Pastry with Meat Filling

**Filling**

| AMOUNT | MEASURE | INGREDIENT |
|---|---|---|
| 1 ½ tablespoons | 1 ½ ounces, 40 ml | Butter |
| ½ cup | 2 ounces, 56 g | Onion, cut ¼ inch (.6 cm) dice |
| 1 | | Garlic clove, minced |
| 1 cup | 6 ounces, 168 g | Veal loin, cut ½ inch (1.2 cm) dice |
| 1 cup | 6 ounces, 168 g | Pork loin, cut ½ inch (1.2 cm) dice |
| ¾ cup | 6 ounces, 180 ml | White wine |
| ⅓ cup | 2 ounces, 56 g | Raisins |
| 4 cups | 32 ounces, 960 ml | Beef stock |
| 1 cup | 6 ounces, 168 g | Uncooked veal sausage meat |
| 1 cup | 6 ounces, 168 g | Sweetbreads |
| 1 ½ tablespoons | ¾ ounce, 20 g | Butter |
| 1 cup | 3 ounces, 84 g | White mushrooms, cleaned, trimmed, and thinly sliced |
| 1 tablespoon | | Flour |
| 1 cup | 8 ounces, 240 ml | Heavy cream |
| To taste | | Salt, pepper, and nutmeg |

**PROCEDURE**

1. Heat first quantity of butter over medium-high heat; sauté onions and garlic until translucent, 2 to 3 minutes.
2. Add veal and pork and brown well. Add white wine and raisins and cook over low heat 10 minutes. Set aside.
3. Bring stock to a boil. Fill a pastry bag with sausage meat and press small balls into simmering stock. Remove pan from heat and allow sausage to cool in stock. Remove from pan and set aside.
4. Reheat stock, add sweetbreads, and poach 20 minutes. Let cool in stock. Trim sweetbreads and remove any filaments of fat, gristle, or tubes. Set aside; retain poaching stock.
5. Heat second quantity of butter over medium-high heat and sauté mushrooms, 3 minutes.
6. Dust with flour and stir well.

7 Add beef stock used to cook sausage and sweetbreads and bring to a boil. Remove mushrooms and set aside.

8 Add cream to stock and cook until it is reduced to sauce consistency (coats the back of a spoon).

9 Return meat, sausage balls, sweetbreads, and mushrooms to sauce; bring back to heat. Season to taste with salt pepper, and nutmeg.

10 Carefully reheat puff pastry to warm. Remove center and use as a lid if desired.

11 Divide 1 cup filling and sauce among the four puff pastry containers; serve remaining filling separately.

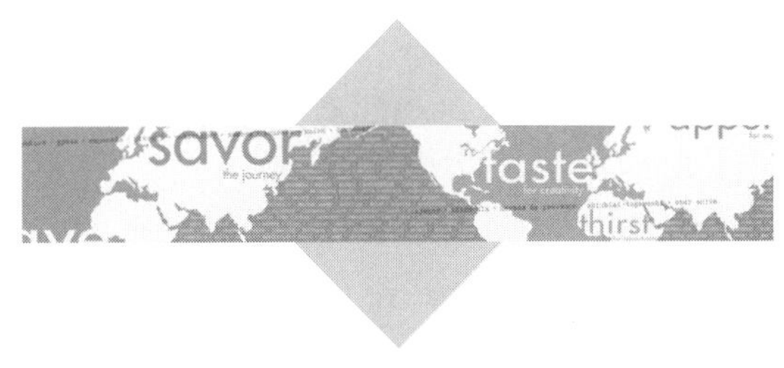

# Carnard Röti aux Endives

## Roast Duck with Chicory

SERVES 4

| AMOUNT | MEASURE | INGREDIENT |
|---|---|---|
| 1 | $3\frac{1}{2}$ to 4 pound, (1.58 to 1.81 kg) | Whole duck |
| To taste | | Salt and pepper |
| 1 tablespoon | $\frac{1}{2}$ ounce, 15 ml | Vegetable oil |
| 2 tablespoons | $\frac{1}{2}$ ounce, 14 g | Shallots minced |
| 1 | | Garlic clove, minced |
| 2 tablespoons | 1 ounce, 30 ml | Red wine vinegar |
| 2 tablespoons | 1 ounce, 30 ml | Port |
| $\frac{1}{2}$ cup | 4 ounces, 120 ml | Water |
| 3 tablespoons | $1\frac{1}{2}$ ounce, 45 ml | Cold butter, cut in small pieces |
| $\frac{1}{4}$ cup | 2 ounces, 60 ml | Butter, clarified |
| 8 | | Endive heads, small and dense |
| Pinch | | Granulated sugar |
| $\frac{1}{2}$ | | Lemon |
| To taste | | Orange zest |
| 1 tablespoon | ($\frac{1}{2}$ ounce, 15 ml) | Butter |

### PROCEDURE

1. Cut off the solid section at the base of each endive and separate the leaves, discarding any that are damaged.
2. Preheat oven to 450°F (232°C).
3. Cut wings off at the second joint. Reserve the heart and liver and chop into small pieces. Remove any excess fat and season inside and out with salt and pepper. Truss.
4. Heat oil in a roasting pan over high heat. Place duck on its side in the pan; sear 2 minutes. Turn to other side and sear 2 minutes. Leave on its side and put in preheated oven. Cook 20 minutes total (8 minutes on one side, 8 minutes on the other side, then 4 minutes on its back), or until desired doneness. Duck should be rare to medium rare. Remove from oven, untruss, and pour the cavity juices into a saucepan. Keep duck warm.
5. Pour off excess fat from the roasting pan. Place pan over low heat; add shallots and garlic, cook 2 minutes. Add vinegar and port, reduce by half, then add water. Stir to deglaze and bring to a boil. Add liquid from duck and return to a boil. Remove pan from the heat, then return it to the heat, so it reboils several times and reduces to 4 tablespoons. Strain into a new pan, correct seasoning, and whisk in cold butter to thicken. Strain and reserve.

6 Heat clarified butter in large frying pan; add endive leaves and fry about 1 minute until they begin to brown. Season with salt, pepper, and sugar and a squeeze of lemon juice. Grate the zest from the orange over endive, using a nutmeg grater.

7 Sauté duck liver and heart in remaining butter.

8 Cut duck into 4 servings. Arrange endive leaves in a circle around the edge of 4 heated plates. Place a quarter of the duck in the center, spoon sauce over duck, and sprinkle with the chopped liver and hearts. Serve remaining sauce on the side.

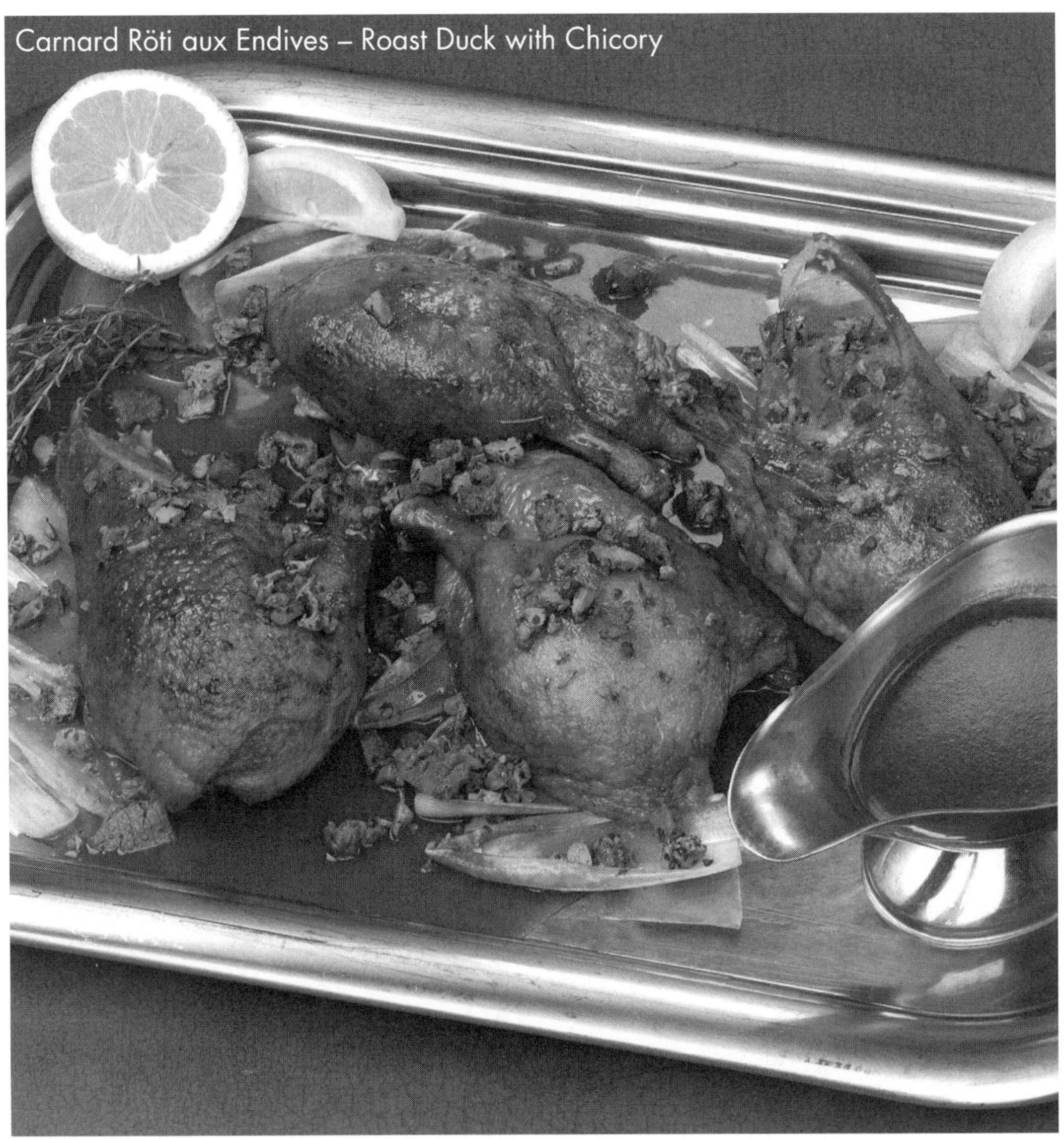
Carnard Röti aux Endives – Roast Duck with Chicory

# Rosti Potato Cake SERVES 4

| AMOUNT | MEASURE | INGREDIENT |
|---|---|---|
| 11 ounces, 308 g | | Idaho potatoes |
| 2 tablespoons | 1 ounce, 30 ml | Butter, clarified |
| To taste | | Salt |

**PROCEDURE**

1. Peel the potatoes and cut into thin sticks. Rinse off the starch, drain, and dry well.
2. Heat seasoned pan (so they will not stick) with half the butter and fry half the potatoes without stirring, pressing them down occasionally to form a cake. Season with salt.
3. When the bottom is cooked, about 10 minutes, turn over and fry the other side. The rosti should be cooked through with a golden-brown crust.
4. Keep warm and cook the other half of the potatoes.

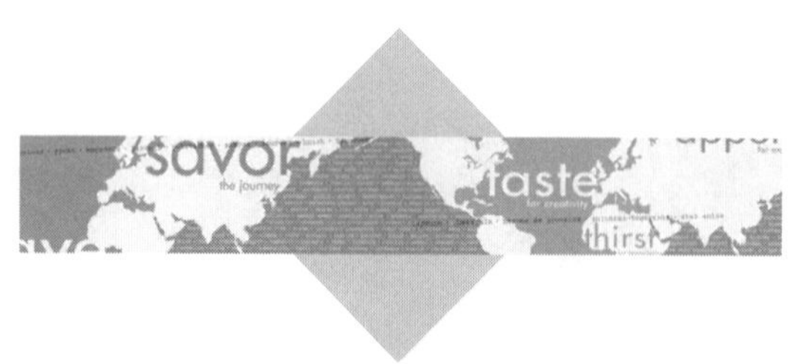

# Zûrcher Öpfelbachis

## Shredded Dough Cakes with Apples

SERVES 4

| AMOUNT | MEASURE | INGREDIENT |
|---|---|---|
| $\frac{2}{3}$ cup | 2.75 ounces, 77 g | All-purpose flour, sifted |
| $\frac{2}{3}$ cup | 5.25 ounces, 158 ml | Milk |
| $\frac{1}{2}$ cup | 4 ounces, 120 ml | Heavy cream |
| 3 tablespoons | 1.5 ounces, 42 g | Granulated sugar |
| $\frac{1}{2}$ | | Vanilla bean, seeds scraped |
| $\frac{1}{2}$ | | Grated lemon zest |
| Pinch | | Salt |
| 1 tablespoon | $\frac{1}{2}$ ounce, 15 ml | Kirsch |
| 3 | | Eggs |
| 2 tablespoons | 1 ounce, 28 g | Granulated sugar |
| 3 cups | 12 ounces, 336 g | Apples, tart, peeled, cored, $\frac{1}{4}$ inch (.6 cm) slice |
| 1$\frac{1}{2}$ tablespoons | $\frac{3}{4}$ ounce, 20 ml | Butter |
| 3 tablespoons | 1 ounce, 28 g | Dried currants |
| $\frac{1}{4}$ cup | 1 ounce, 28 g | Walnuts, toasted |
| 3 tablespoons | | Confection's sugar |
| 1 teaspoon | | Cinnamon |

PROCEDURE

1. Combine the flour, milk, cream, first quantity of sugar, vanilla seeds, lemon zest, salt, and kirsch. Mix to a smooth batter. Add eggs and mix well.
2. Over medium heat, caramelize second quantity of sugar until a light brown. Add apples and toss to coat; cook 1 minute.
3. Heat the butter in a well-seasoned pan (so it will not stick). Add batter and place pan in an oven preheated to 425°F (220°C), until it has turned golden-brown and the surface has dried, about 5 minutes. Shred the dough into small pieces.
4. Combine currants, walnuts, dough, and apple mixture; toss.
5. Sift together confectioner's sugar and cinnamon.
6. Place dough and apple mixture on 4 warm plates and dust with cinnamon-sugar to serve.

# Bodenseefischsuppe mit Safran

## Fish Soup from the Bodensee with Saffron

SERVES 4

| AMOUNT | MEASURE | INGREDIENT |
|---|---|---|
| $\frac{1}{4}$ cup | 1 ounce, 28 g | Carrots, $\frac{1}{4}$ inch (.6 cm) dice |
| $\frac{1}{4}$ cup | 1 ounce, 28 g | Onion, $\frac{1}{4}$ inch (.6 cm) dice |
| $\frac{1}{4}$ cup | 1 ounce, 28 g | Celeriac, $\frac{1}{4}$ inch (.6 cm) dice |
| $\frac{1}{4}$ cup | 1 ounce, 28 g | Fennel, $\frac{1}{4}$ inch (.6 cm) dice |
| 6 cups | 48 ounces, 1.44 l | Fish stock |
| 5 | | Peppercorns, crushed |
| $\frac{1}{2}$ teaspoon | | Mustard seeds |
| 1 | | Bay leaf |
| 1 tablespoon | | Fresh dill, chopped |
| 1 tablespoon | | Fresh chervil, chopped |
| 1 tablespoon | | Fresh parsley, chopped |
| $\frac{1}{4}$ teaspoon | | Pernod |
| 2 teaspoons | | Fresh lemon juice |
| To taste | | Salt, white pepper, cayenne pepper |
| | 5 ounces, 140 g | Lake trout fillets, or any mild fish |
| | 5 ounces, 140 g | Lake perch fillets |
| 8 | | Saffron strands, for garnish |
| 1 teaspoon each | | Fresh dill, chervil, and parsley, for garnish |

PROCEDURE

1. Combine all vegetables, stock, peppercorns, mustard seeds, and herbs.
2. Simmer, uncovered, 25 minutes. Strain, add Pernod and lemon juice, and correct seasoning.
3. Cut fish fillets into approximately $\frac{1}{2}$ ounce (14 g) spoon-size pieces.
4. Poach in salted water until just done, 3 to 4 minutes; remove to 4 warm soup plates.
5. Pour soup over fish. Garnish each with saffron, dill, chervil, and parsley.

# Szegediner Gulasch

## Szeged Goulash

SERVES 4

| AMOUNT | MEASURE | INGREDIENT |
|---|---|---|
| $\frac{1}{4}$ cup | 1 ounce, 28 g | Bacon, diced |
| $1\frac{1}{2}$ pounds | 680 g | Boneless pork, trimmed, 1 inch (2.4 cm) cubes |
| $1\frac{1}{2}$ cups | 8 ounces, 224 g | Onions, $\frac{1}{4}$ inch (.6 cm) dice |
| 2 | | Garlic cloves, minced |
| 1 tablespoon | | All-purpose flour |
| 2 tablespoons | | Sweet Hungarian paprika |
| 2 teaspoons | | Caraway seeds |
| 1 | | Bay leaf |
| 1 tablespoon | | Fresh sage, chopped |
| 1 tablespoon | | Fresh oregano, chopped |
| To taste | | Salt and pepper |
| 1 cups | 8 ounces, 240 ml | Apple juice or cider |
| 4 cups | 32 ounces, 960 ml | Chicken stock |
| 2 cups | 16 ounces, 480 ml | Sauerkraut, drained and rinsed |
| 4 cups | | Spätzle or egg noodles |
| $\frac{1}{2}$ cup | 4 ounces, 240 ml | Sour cream |

**PROCEDURE**

1. Render the bacon until crisp. Remove and set aside, leaving 1 to 2 tablespoons ($\frac{1}{2}$ to 1 ounce, 15 to 30 ml) fat in pan.
2. Over medium-high heat, add pork and brown the meat. (This step may be done in small batches.) Remove meat and set aside.
3. Add onions and cook 2 to 3 minutes. Add garlic and cook until onions are soft, 2 minutes longer.
4. Sprinkle flour, paprika, and all seasonings, stir to combine, and cook 1 minute (do not fry the paprika). Return the meat to the pan.
5. Add cider and stock, bring to a boil, and reduce to a simmer. Simmer 35 to 45 minutes or until meat is tender.
6. Add well-drained sauerkraut and mix well. Heat and serve with egg noodles. Garnish with sour cream and reserved bacon.

# Gemischter Salat Mixed Salad

SERVES 4

**Serve the cucumber, cabbage, and tomato salads as separate parts of an assorted salad.**

## Cucumber Salad

| AMOUNT | MEASURE | INGREDIENT |
|---|---|---|
| 1 cup | 6 ounces, 168 g | Cucumber, peeled, seeded, thinly sliced |
| 1 teaspoon | | Salt |
| 1 | | Garlic clove, minced |
| $1\frac{1}{2}$ tablespoons | $\frac{3}{4}$ ounce, 20 ml | Cider vinegar |
| 3 tablespoons | $1\frac{1}{2}$ ounces, 45 ml | Salad oil |
| 1 teaspoon | | Chopped dill |
| To taste | | Salt and pepper |

### PROCEDURE

1. Toss cucumbers with salt. Let sit 5 minutes, then rinse and drain cucumbers.
2. Add garlic, vinegar, oil, and dill, and correct seasoning.

## Krautsalat: Cabbage Salad

| AMOUNT | MEASURE | INGREDIENT |
|---|---|---|
| 3 cups | 12 ounces, 336 g | Green cabbage, shredded |
| $1\frac{1}{2}$ teaspoons | | Salt |
| 1 teaspoon | | Caraway seeds |
| $1\frac{1}{2}$ teaspoons | | Granulated sugar |
| $\frac{1}{4}$ cup | 2 ounces, 60 ml | Cider vinegar |
| $\frac{1}{2}$ cup | 4 ounces, 120 ml | Vegetable oil |

### PROCEDURE

1. Trim the coarse outer leaves from the cabbage and discard; quarter the cabbage, remove the hard white core at the point of each quarter and discard, then slice each quarter very thin.

2 Toss shredded cabbage with salt and let stand 15 minutes. Squeeze the cabbage, mix again. Let stand 15 minutes, and squeeze again.

3 Combine remaining ingredients and mix well. Toss with cabbage and let stand 30 minutes before serving.

# Tomato Salad

| AMOUNT | MEASURE | INGREDIENT |
|---|---|---|
| 1 tablespoon | | Fresh oregano, chopped |
| $\frac{1}{2}$ cup | 4 ounces, 120 ml | Vegetable oil |
| 3 tablespoons | 1 $\frac{1}{2}$ ounces, 45 ml | Red wine vinegar |
| 2 cups | 6 ounces, 168 g | Tomatoes, peeled, seeded, cut into wedges |
| 1 cup | 4 ounces, 112 g | Onions, very thinly sliced |
| To taste | | Salt and pepper |

**PROCEDURE**

1 Combine oregano, oil, and vinegar; toss with tomatoes and onions. Correct seasoning.

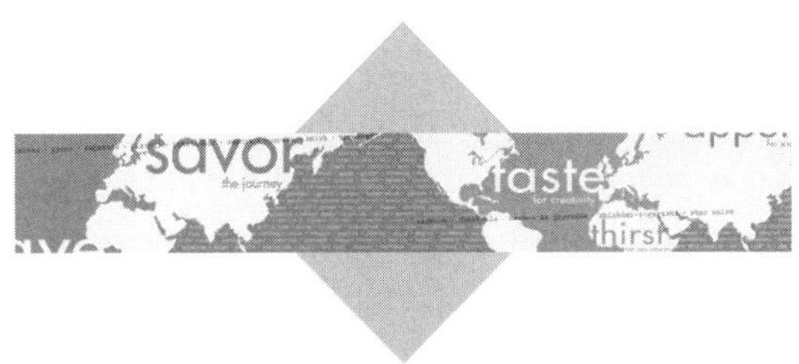

# Wiener Schnitzel SERVES 4

**For traditional Wiener Schnitzel, the veal is fried in lard. Pork, chicken, or turkey can be substituted and oil can be used for frying.**

| AMOUNT | MEASURE | INGREDIENT |
|---|---|---|
| 4 | 4–5 ounces, 112–140 g | Scallops of veal, pork, or turkey, tapped thin |
| As needed | | All-purpose flour |
| 2 | | Eggs whisked with a little water and pinch of salt |
| As needed | | Bread crumbs, dry or fresh (not panko) |
| As needed | | Vegetable oil, for frying |
| 4 | | Lemon slices |
| To taste | | Salt and pepper |

#### PROCEDURE

1. Season and dredge the meat in flour, egg wash, and bread crumbs, coating each scallop.
2. Heat oil and pan-fry over medium-high heat until golden brown on both sides. Remove and drain on paper towels. Correct seasoning.
3. Serve topped with one lemon slice, pressing it down with a fork to season the schnitzel. Serve with Erdäpfelschmarrn and vegetable of choice.

# Erdäpfelschmarrn Fried Potatoes SERVES 4

| AMOUNT | MEASURE | INGREDIENT |
|---|---|---|
| 1 pound | 16 ounces, 448 g | All-purpose potatoes |
| 1 teaspoon | | Salt |
| $\frac{1}{2}$ teaspoon | | Caraway seeds, crushed |
| $\frac{1}{4}$ cup | 2 ounces, 60 ml | Butter |
| $\frac{1}{2}$ cup | 2 ounces, 56 g | Onions, $\frac{1}{4}$ inch (.6 cm) dice |

#### PROCEDURE

1. Boil potatoes until just cooked; drain. While still hot, slice $\frac{1}{4}$ inch (.6 cm) thick. Sprinkle with salt and crushed caraway seeds.
2. Heat butter over medium-high heat and sauté onions until light brown. Add potatoes and fry until light brown, turning often.

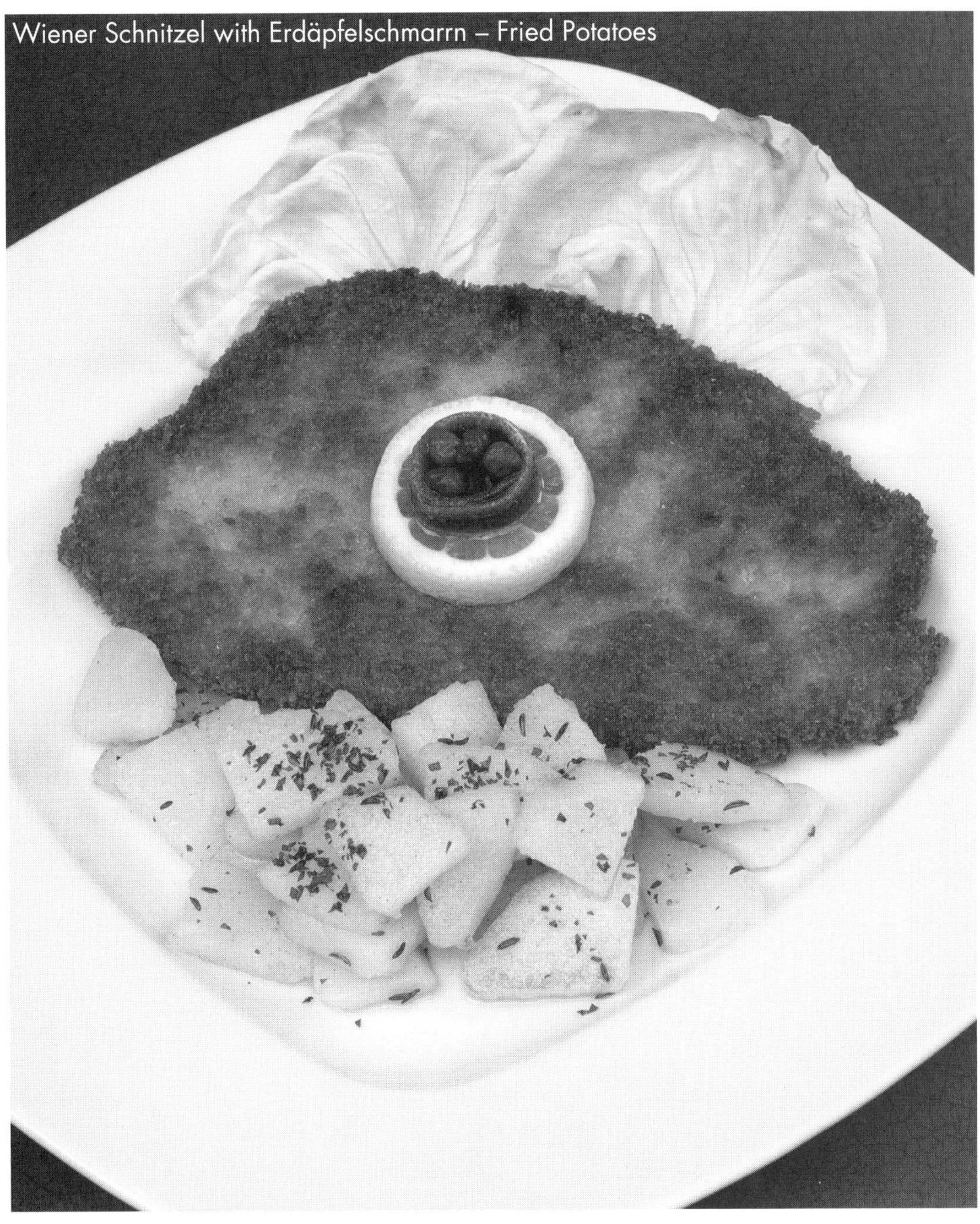

Wiener Schnitzel with Erdäpfelschmarrn – Fried Potatoes

# Salzburger Nockerl

SERVES 4

| AMOUNT | MEASURE | INGREDIENT |
|---|---|---|
| $\frac{1}{4}$ cup | 2 ounces, 60 ml | Butter, softened |
| 5 tablespoons | $2\frac{1}{2}$ ounces, 70 g | Granulated sugar |
| 5 | | Egg yolks |
| $\frac{1}{4}$ cup | 1 ounce, 28 g | All-purpose flour |
| 5 | | Egg whites, beaten to stiff peaks |
| $\frac{1}{2}$ cup | 4 ounces, 120 ml | Milk |
| As needed | | Vanilla-flavored powdered sugar |

PROCEDURE

1. Preheat oven 450°F (232°C).
2. Cream together butter and sugar until light. Add egg yolks in two additions, beating well after each addition until light and fluffy.
3. Fold in flour.
4. Fold in egg whites.
5. Bring milk to a boil in a 10-inch (25 cm) skillet and immediately pour batter into the hot milk.
6. Place pan in preheated oven, reduce heat to 400°F (204°C) and bake for 6 to 8 minutes until golden. Nockerl should be firm on the outside, but light and fluffy on the inside.
7. Cut into portions and place on warm plates dusted with vanilla powdered sugar. Serve immediately. Nockerl will not tolerate waiting; it will collapse.

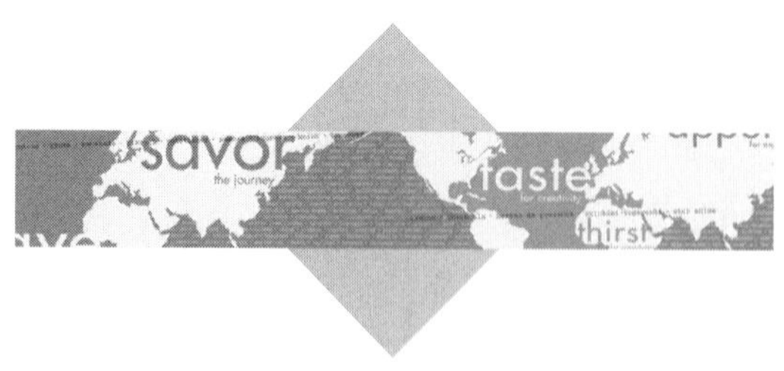

# Scandinavia and Russia

## The Land

Scandinavia is located in northern Europe and includes Denmark, Norway, and Sweden. Finland, Iceland, and the Faroe Islands are considered by some to be part of Scandinavia as well. Denmark borders the Baltic and North Seas, on a peninsula north of Germany. It is the smallest of the Scandinavian countries, even including the over four hundred islands, some of which are inhabited and linked to the mainland by ferry or bridge. The landscape consists mainly of low-lying, fertile countryside broken by beech woods, small lakes, and fjords. Greenland and the Faroe Islands are also under the sovereignty of the Kingdom of Denmark, although both have home rule. The Faroe Islands are a group of eighteen islands in the North Atlantic with a population of nearly fifty thousand, whose history dates from the Viking period. Fishing and sheep farming remain the two most important occupations on these islands.

Norway borders the North Sea and the North Atlantic Ocean, west of Sweden. The name Norway comes from *Nordweg,* meaning "way to the north." This country is well named, as almost half of it lies north of the Arctic Circle. Nearly two-thirds of it is mountainous and its mountain ranges extend almost the entire length of the country. From the inland mountains and mountain plateaus, the landscape falls sharply toward a coastline dotted with innumerable islands. The country has traditionally been divided into five principal regions: Nord Norge (North Norway), Trøndelag/Midt-Norge (Trondheim Region/Mid-Norway), Vestlandet (West Country), Østlandet (East Country), and Sørlandet (South Country).

Sweden borders the Baltic Sea and the gulfs of Bothnia, Kattegat, and Skagerrak, and is sandwiched between Finland and Norway. The terrain of Sweden is mostly flat or gently rolling lowlands, with mountains in the west.

Finland is the northernmost country on the European continent. Although other countries have points extending farther north, nearly one quarter of its total landmass lies north of the Arctic Circle. It is the fifth largest country in Europe, yet it is also one of the least populous, with five million people. It is heavily forested and contains thousands of lakes, numerous rivers, and extensive areas of marshland. Only 8 percent is cultivated land, and the rest is wasteland made up of swamps, arctic fells, and sand. Except for a small highland region in the extreme northwest, the country is a lowland that is less than 600 feet above sea level. An archipelago of 17,000 tree-covered islands and smaller rocky islands are scattered off its coast.

Iceland is an island that lies in the North Atlantic Ocean, east of Greenland, and just touches the Arctic Circle. It is one of the most volcanic regions in the world. More than 13 percent is covered by snowfields and glaciers, and most of the people live along the 7 percent of the island that is made up of fertile coastland.

Russia borders the Arctic Ocean, between Europe and the North Pacific Ocean. Due to Russia's immense size, its terrain varies greatly. The most pronounced characteristics are broad plains with low hills west of the Urals; vast coniferous forest and tundra in Siberia; and uplands and mountains (the Caucasus range) along the southern borders.

# History

From the Viking age (approximately 800–1066) onward, the Nordics have fought each other, formed unions with each other, and ruled over each other. Sweden ruled over Finland for over six hundred years, Denmark ruled over southern Sweden for over six hundred years (or, alternatively, Sweden has ruled over eastern Denmark for the past three hundred years), and over Norway for nearly five hundred years, while Iceland was ruled from Norway for some two hundred years and then from Denmark yet another five hundred years, and the list goes on. Finland is the only country not to have ruled over any of the others. Unavoidably, this has caused some antipathies, but it has also made the Nordic cultures more uniform.

Denmark, Norway, Sweden, and Iceland shared a more or less homogenous "Viking" culture in the Viking age, and Finland, while not strictly speaking a "Viking" country, did have a Viking age and a culture very close to its western neighbors, and at the close of this era was absorbed into the Swedish kingdom.

Scandinavian culture today could be described as a potpourri of this "original" culture, medieval German influence, French influence in the centuries that followed, and several other smaller sources, not forgetting local development and national romantic inventiveness. A

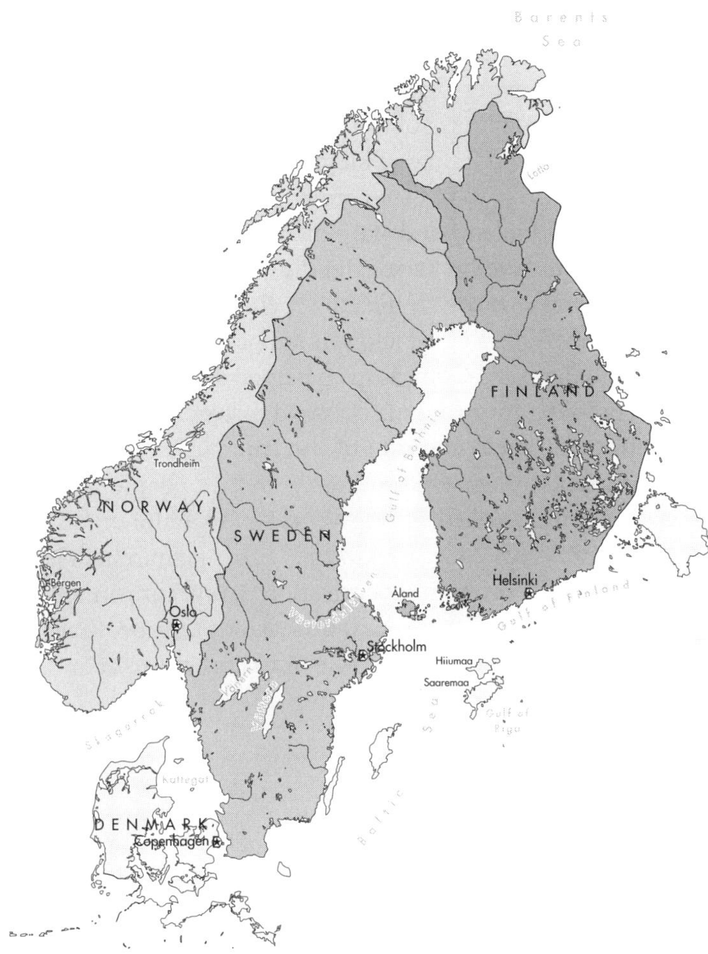


Scandinavia

significant factor is also the fact that the Nordic countries never had an era of feudalism to speak of; personal freedom has always been highly valued. One of the expressions of this freedom is the "everyman's right" in Norway, Sweden, and Finland, giving all residents free access to the forests, seas, and uncultivated land.

Russia's history extends back over a thousand years with the establishment by Vikings of a territory they named Rus. The Viking presence diminished through gradual absorption by the native Slavic peoples. Several hundred years later, the Mongols swept over Russia, remaining through the fourteenth century. A new ruler, Ivan the Great, brought Moscow to the fore and developed an empire based on his marriage to a Byzantine princess, Sophia, niece of the last Byzantine emperor Constantine XI. The expansion only continued over the next several hundred years and by the end of the seventeenth century, Tsar Peter the Great had made great strides toward transforming Russia into a true power. He devised a new capital called St. Petersburg, which became a glittering European center. But it was Catherine the Great, at the beginning of the eighteenth century, who entered into treaties and alliances with Prussia and Austria that solidified Russia's position as a true power in Europe. Alexander I, part of the group that successfully defeated Napoleon, held the title not only of tsar, but grand duke of Finland and king of Poland. The nineteenth century saw Russia begin to industrialize with development extending to the far reaches of the tsar's realm. In 1917, the tsarist regime fell to revolution led by socialists who intended to create a republican government. This first revolution failed and was supplanted by Bolshevik forces later that year, with Vladimir Lenin as chairman. Communism helped develop the country but it brought with it one of the most repressive governments in world history. Along with some not insignificant successes—modernization, becoming one of the true superpowers on the planet, the space race, athletics—the twentieth century for Russia and its people was marked by brutal wars (at least twenty million citizens died during World War II alone), disastrous participation in Afghanistan's civil war that was compared to the U.S. quagmire in Vietnam, and, for most of the population of the USSR, economic deprivation. Communism fell in 1992, following the collapse of communist governments throughout Eastern Europe. Russia continues to struggle with democracy but seems unlikely to ever return to communism.

## The People

People living north of the Arctic Circle are treated to two of the most amazing phenomena on earth. The Northern Lights, or aurora borealis, can be viewed there between November and February. These lights are caused when solar particles collide with the atmosphere of the Earth. And from mid-May through June in this region the sun does not set, while between mid-November and January, the sun does not rise.

The Sami people live in the far north of the Scandinavian peninsula. They are Europe's only indigenous people, and their origins are unknown. With one of the smallest populations in the world, these people, until the early decades of this century, were nomadic, following the reindeer up into the mountains, where they lived together during the summer months. The Sami people of today number about forty thousand in all, divided between Finland, Norway, Russia, and Sweden. In earlier times the Sami were called *Lapps* (as in Lapland and Lappmarken) and *Finns* (as in Finnmark and Finland).

Ethnically, the majority of Danes are of Scandinavian descent, a Germanic people who have occupied Norway, Sweden, and Denmark since pre-Viking times. The languages of the three countries are closely related. A small German-speaking minority lives in southern Jutland

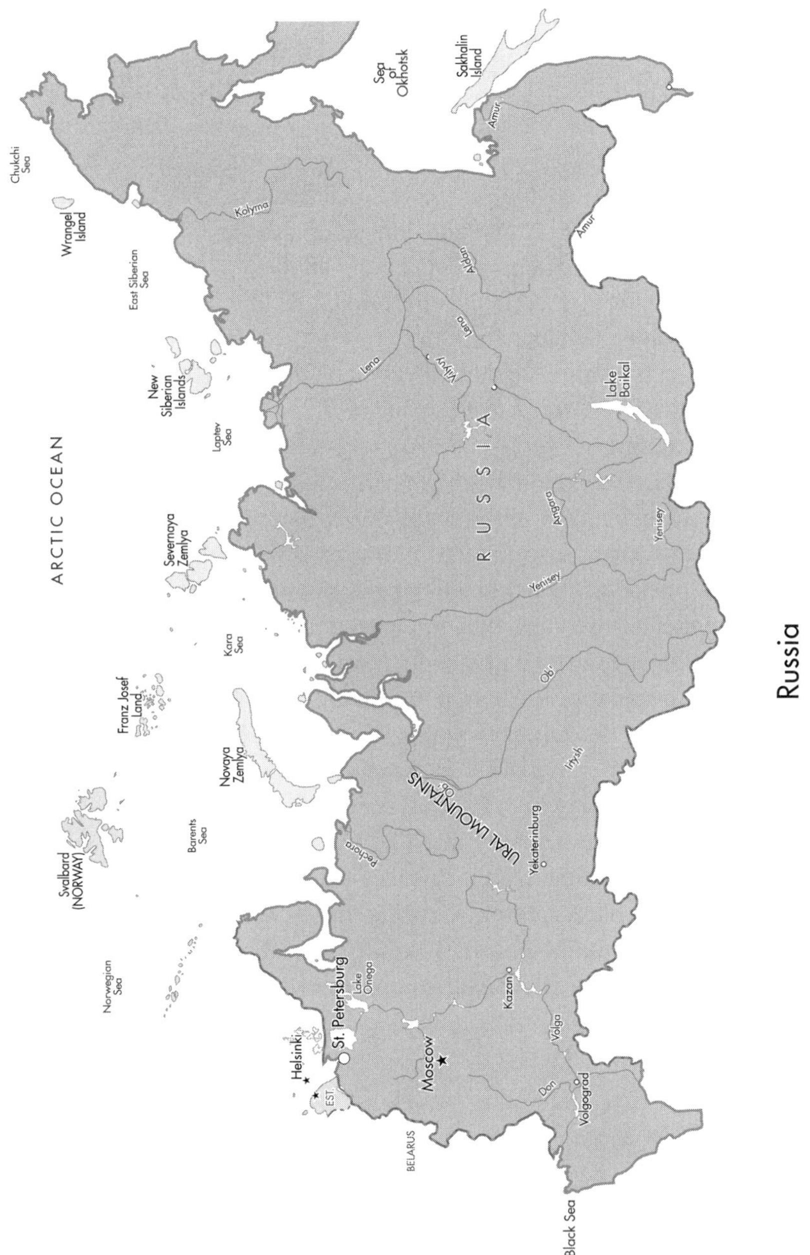
ARCTIC OCEAN
Chukchi Sea
Wrangel Island
East Siberian Sea
New Siberian Islands
Laptev Sea
Severnaya Zemlya
Kara Sea
Franz Josef Land
Novaya Zemlya
Svalbard (NORWAY)
Barents Sea
Norwegian Sea
Sea of Okhotsk
Sakhalin Island
Amur
Kolyma
Aldan
Lena
Vilyuy
Lake Baikal
R U S S I A
Angara
Yenisey
Ob'
Irtysh
URAL MOUNTAINS
Yekaterinburg
Pechora
Kazan
Volga
Don
Volgograd
Moscow
St. Petersburg
Lake Onega
Helsinki
EST
BELARUS
Black Sea

Russia

near the German border. An Inuit population inhabits the Danish territory of Greenland, and the Faroe Islands have a Nordic population, descendents of Viking colonizers.

The Norwegians are a remarkably homogenous people of Germanic origin. Apart from several thousand Sami and people of Finnish origin in the northern part of Norway, the country has no large minority groups. Norway is home to small numbers of Americans, Britons, Chileans, Danes, Iranians, Pakistanis, Swedes, and Vietnamese, among other groups.

Sweden's population consists mainly of Scandinavians of Germanic descent. Sweden's immigrant population and ethnic diversity have increased rapidly in recent decades. For many years, Sweden was a nation of emigrants. From 1860 to World War I, more than one million Swedes left the nation, mainly for the United States. Emigration declined significantly after 1930, as the nation industrialized and grew more prosperous. Sweden welcomed many refugees and displaced people after World War II. Since that time, immigration has accounted for nearly half of Sweden's population growth. Many immigrants have come to Sweden as guest workers or as political refugees. Today, approximately one-fifth of the people are immigrants or have at least one foreign-born parent.

The Finns are a people of unknown geographic origin. They have lived in Finland and in neighboring parts of Russia, Estonia, and Latvia for several thousand years.

Icelanders are one of the most homogenous peoples. They are predominantly of Nordic origin, descendants of hardy people who emigrated from Norway in the Middle Ages. There are also some Celtic influences from immigrants from the British Isles. Often in its history, Iceland has suffered major population losses from epidemics, volcanic eruptions, and earthquakes. From the mid-twentieth century, many rural Icelanders began moving to coastal towns and villages. Today, some 93 percent of the people now live in cities and towns. About 60 percent of Iceland's total population lives in Reykjavík. The overall population density is three people per square kilometer (7.8 per square mile).

Most of the roughly 150 million Russians derive from Eastern Slavic peoples, whose original homeland was likely present-day Poland. Russian is the official language and an official language in the United Nations. The language of writers such as Tolstoy, Dostoevsky, Chekov, Pushkin, and Solzhenitsyn has great importance in world literature.

# The Food

## DENMARK

The first half of the twentieth century was not a good period for Danish cooking. Though the cuisine was well developed, there was greater emphasis on nutrition, hygiene, and cost than on culinary art. At the same time, the food industry offered cheap substitutes such as margarine, stock cubes, flavor additives, and essences, and the result was an overstretched and heavy cuisine. The change started in the 1960s and the Danish cuisine of potatoes and gravy was rejected. The Danes turned to other countries for innovation, first the French bourgeois cuisine, and later Italy and other Mediterranean countries. The cuisine is now based on white bread and wine and therefore very different from the traditional Danish cuisine with its rye bread and beer. In the late twentieth century, the tendency to regard food as a means of expression and cooking as a lifestyle broke through. Being a chef became prestigious and chefs began to have their own television programs and restaurants at an ever younger age. International cuisines were explored, international trends came and went. After experimenting with fusion cuisine, most people returned to the idea that the best food came from the shortest and simplest trip from soil to table. This brought a focus on the primary produce that thrives best in the Danish climate, including apples, wild berries and fungi, vegetables such as cabbage and root vegetables, and fish, such as gurnard, hake, weever, lemon sole, and turbot, as well as shellfish from the Danish coast.

Danish cuisine still contains elements from the late 1800s, before industrialization. This was the age of what is called storage housekeeping, with a cuisine based on beer and rye bread, salted pork, and salted herring. Among the dishes from those days that are still eaten today are *øllebrød* (a dish made of rye bread, sugar, and nonalcoholic beer), *vandgrød* (porridge, usually barley porridge, made with water), *gule ærter* (split-pea soup), *æbleflæsk* (slices of pork with apples fried in fat), *klipfisk* (dried cod), *blodpølse* (black pudding), *finker* (similar to Scotland's haggis), and *grønlangkål* (thickened stewed kale). In the second half of the nineteenth century, the cooperative movement age, milk and potatoes played a prominent part and dishes such as roast pork and gravy, boiled cod with mustard sauce, consommé with meat, bread or flour dumplings, rissoles (also known as frikadellers, or any variation of meatball), minced beef patties, and other dishes based on minced meat. The same period saw the emergence of many fruit dishes such as *rødgrød* (thickened stewed fruit), *sødsuppe* (fruit soup), and stewed fruits. The range of vegetable dishes was expanded with boiled cabbage in white sauce, red cabbage, pickled beetroot, cucumber salad, and peas and carrots in white sauce.

## NORWAY

On the northernmost coast of Norway, cod is hung on poles and dried in the wind without salt. For more than a thousand years this product was sold to other European countries to acquire such rare commodities as wine, wheat, and honey. They called this fish "stockfish," or *stoccafisso* or *estocafix.* A French cookbook manuscript from 1393 explains how boiled *stofix* should be eaten with mustard or dipped in butter. However, the fish must first be pounded with a wooden hammer and then soaked in water for many hours. Adding wood ash lye to the water makes the fish particularly soft and flavorful. The result of this process is the celebrated lye fish (lutefisk), today a Norwegian and Swedish specialty, and as in certain areas of the United States, closely identified with Norwegian and Swedish immigrants. Salmon (fresh and cured), herring (pickled or marinated), trout, codfish, and other seafood balanced by cheeses, dairy products, and excellent breads (predominantly dark/darker) show the influence of long seafaring and farming traditions. *Lefse* is a common Norwegian potato flatbread, especially at Christmas. Game has always been a central ingredient in Norwegian cooking. Elk dominates in most inland areas, with venison served more in western regions. Reindeer is the specialty in the north, even though it is available throughout the country.

## SWEDEN

The Swedish culinary tradition is also one of food storage. During the brief harvest period, people gathered what they needed and saved it for future use. During the long, dark period of the year people would have to survive on the preserved foods. Fresh berries were a luxury, since most were cooked into jam for winter. Eating fresh vegetables was almost wasteful, since vegetables needed to be preserved or pickled. The same was true of potatoes and other root vegetables, which were stored in an earth cellar. The fruits that were available in winter were considered more precious than summer apples and August pears. Swedish bread was traditionally also baked with a long shelf life in mind. Rye bread was baked slowly into durable dark *kavring* loaves or dried into crispbread (*knäckebröd*) or rusks (*skorpor*) that could be stored for long periods. Similarly, drinking fresh milk or eating fresh butter and eggs was a pleasure when it occurred. Milk was fermented or otherwise preserved with the aid of bacterial cultures, becoming various yogurt-like soured milks (including *filmjölk* and stringy *lćngfil*), curdled milk (*filbunke*), or sour cream (*gräddfil*), or else it was made into cheese.

Surströmming, or fermented Baltic herring, is sold in cans, and when opened a strong, foul smell is released, the result of a fermentation process. This method of preservation was invented long ago, when brining food was quite expensive due to the costs of salt. When fermentation was used, on the other hand, just enough salt was required to keep the fish from rotting. *Surströmming* is served with boiled potatoes and onions and often rolled into a slice of *tunnbröd,* a type of thin, flat unleavened bread.

Today a wider variety of fresh Swedish ingredients are available, including seafood, poultry, lamb, beef, veal, and wild game. On the coast the specialties are shellfish, fresh mackerel, and cod. Modern chefs use lingonberries, cloudberries, root vegetables, Baltic herring, wild game, and Västerbotten cheese in new ways but traditional methods of smoking, fermenting, salting, drying, marinating, and poaching continue. The Swedish word *smorgasbord* has found its way into many other languages. *Smor* means butter, or spread, and *smorgas* has come to stand for bread that has been spread with something—an open-faced sandwich. *Bord* means table, or board, as in room and board. But it has come to mean much more, bringing thoughts of a large display of many foods set out on long tables. Fish dishes are grouped together—pickled herring, herring in cream, salmon with dill, marinated salmon, and oysters with mustard sauce. The cold dishes come next—a variety of cheeses, cottage cheese, a raw vegetable tray, pickled beets, and salads of fresh fruits. In the hot section, choices include stuffed pork loin, meatballs, sliced ham and turkey, rice and potatoes fixed several ways, brown beans, and vegetable casseroles. Several kinds of bread, plus butter are offered. The dessert table is filled with cookies, fruit bread, rice pudding, custard, cheesecake, and fruit tarts.

## FINLAND

The Finnish diet has been particularly functional throughout the ages. Their forefathers cultivated rye, oats, and barley and dried the crops for the long winter ahead, when they were used to make porridge or fermented bread. They picked berries in the woods in the summer, preserved lingonberries for the winter, and looked for cranberries under the melting snow in early spring. If the crops failed, pine bark was added to the bread or fresh new spruce shoots eaten in the spring. In the summer, milk was preserved by fermenting it.

## ICELAND

Icelanders faced a thousand years of tough times and general famine. Nothing would grow on the island (until they discovered that they could build greenhouses on volcanoes for warmth), and nothing would live there (except Arctic foxes and sheep). They had to subsist on whatever food they could find. As a result of this deprivation, Icelanders have an obsession with preserving food any way they can, and with eating almost anything. *Hákarl* is shark meat that has been buried for three to six months to allow it to putrefy; it is then eaten in small chunks. Icelandic lamb has a distinctively "wild" flavor, reportedly due to roaming the countryside and eating untainted herbs. Some of the most traditional dishes involve making full use of every part of the slaughtered sheep. Offal from a sheep is minced together with its blood and served in the sheep's stomach to make *slatur.* Another delicacy is pickled ram's testicles. Or *svið,* a sheep's head that's been burned to remove the wool, cut in two, boiled, and either eaten fresh or pressed into jelly. Salted, smoked, or slathered in curry sauce, Iceland's national bird, the puffin, is a popular dish. Today, fish pulled from unpolluted waters and lamb that feed on unfertilized fields make up the staples of Iceland's entirely organic cuisine. Lobster, ocean perch, cod, salmon, and trout are other basic elements of the cuisine. Fish is traditionally baked, salted, or combined with garlic and onion in a stew. Smoked salmon is a favorite, along with fish pâtés and pickled herring. For dessert, there's *skyr,* a rich curd best mixed with cream or topped with wild berries. Another national favorite is *randalín,* a cake layered with blueberry jam.

## RUSSIA

Peasant food is the foundation of traditional Russian cuisine. The long cold winters meant that the food consumed needed to provide warmth and energy to ensure survival during the very cold winter. Bread made from rye and kasha and various grains including barley, wheat, and millet became staples in the Russian diet. Rye was the ideal grain for planting during the short unpredictable growing season. Domestically produced meat included beef, pork, and mutton. Chickens, geese, and ducks made up domestic fowl. Game comprised just about every kind of available animal, from hares and squirrels, to deer and wild boar. Fish was a major staple, both because of its abundance and because of the numerous fast days in the Eastern Orthodox calendar in which all animal products were prohibited, including butter, milk, and cheese. The varieties of vegetables was limited and included cabbage, onions, garlic, and turnips and they were pickled, salted, boiled, stewed, baked, fried, braised, roasted, and broiled. The forests provided hazelnuts, mushrooms, and berries. Spices and seasonings used in Russian cooking were often imported from Byzantium and the East, including vinegar, cinnamon, mint, anise, pepper, linseed oil, salt, dill, and poppy seed. The principal sweetener was honey. Food preparation was determined by the peculiarities of the Russian oven: it had to be baked, simmered, stewed, or boiled; in other words, it must have consisted of stews, casseroles, pies, soups, but not (or very little) of poached, fried, sautéed foods—those that require an open flame.

Mongol and Tartar invasions in the thirteenth century brought new techniques, such as making sour milk, grilling meat, and the use of spices. Clotted sour milk became a staple diet to most Russians, and lasted well into the twentieth century. Due to Russia's close proximity to Persia and the Ottoman Empire, smoked meat, pastry cooking, green vegetables, salads, wines, and chocolate were introduced in the sixteenth to eighteenth centuries.

An important part of Russian cuisine is the *zakuski* (hors d'oeuvre) ceremony. *Zakuski* are the equivalent of a Scandinavian smorgasbord. By the early nineteenth century, it became fashionable in sophisticated homes to serve *zakuski* on a separate table in the dining room or in an adjacent room. Depending upon the occasion the *zakuski* menu included one or more fish dish, one or more meat dish, one or more salad and vegetable dish, one or more egg dish, marinated and/or salt-pickled vegetables and mushrooms, and marinated fruits (plums, apples, and others), condiments, including mustard, horseradish, and freshly ground pepper, and homemade dark breads.

Soup has always been vital to the Russian cuisine and can be divided into several different groups. Traditional soups ranged from *borsch, ukha, teur,* and *shchi.* Cold soups are based on *kvass,* light soups and stews feature water and vegetables, while noodle soups incorporate meat, milk, and mushrooms. Soups that are based on cabbage are called *shchi,* with thick soups such as *rassolnick* and *solynaka* being based on meat broth. Grain- and vegetable-based soups, as well as fish soups complete the traditional soup list.

One of the traditional meat dishes in Russian cuisine is *Studen,* or *Kholodets,* a dish that is made from jellied pork meat or veal. Spices and vegetables are added, and it is usually served with mustard or ground garlic, together with horseradish and *smetana* (a variety of sour cream similar to crème fraîche). *Pelmeni* are small stuffed dumplings traditional to Siberia, although they may have originated in northern China. Tribal groups in Siberia used these dumplings as portable food as they could be frozen and stored in quantity. Traditionally *pelmeni* are stuffed with a meat or meat mixture, potatoes with onions, *tvorog* cheese (farmer's cheese), or even bits of fish, shrimp, or crab. *Shashlik* is a form of shish kebab made of beef, pork, or lamb. These skewers are either all meat, all fat, or alternating pieces of meat and fat. Meats for *shashlik* (as opposed to other forms of shish kebab) are usually marinated overnight in a high-acidity marinade like vinegar, dry wine, or sour fruit/vegetable juice with the addition of herbs and spices. *Pejmen* is made from finely chopped meat in a thin dough made of flour and eggs, and possibly milk or water. According to the traditional Uralian recipe, the filling is made of 45 percent beef, 35 percent lamb, and 20 percent pork. Pepper, garlic, and onions are added to the meat. Beef Stroganoff is a combination of beef, mushrooms, and sour cream. Beef Stroganoff was the prize-winning recipe created for a cooking competition held in the 1890s in St. Petersburg, Russia. The chef who devised the recipe worked for the Russian diplomat Count Pavel Alexandrovich Stroganov, a member of one of Russia's grandest noble families. Russian blini are descended from one the most common prepared foods, fried flat bread. Russians, in fact, translate "blini" as "pancakes" when speaking English, although the ultra-thin, slightly tart Russian blini is more like the French crepe and German blintz.

Tea is the most popular drink in Russia. The Russian tea party is a social event where tea and biscuits are served. This tradition started back in 1638. The Russian samovar (teapot) is a cultural symbol of the Russian past. *Kvas* is a Russian national drink, a simple fermented drink with a low level of alcohol made from bread, apples, pears or other fruits.

# Glossary

**Aebleskiver** A waffle or a pancake dough formed like a tennis ball, with various fillings. Cooked in an *aebleskiver* pan, typically served sprinkled with powered sugar and raspberry jam. A Danish delicacy.

**Almond Potatoes** A special variety of potatoes grown in the Nordic countries. The Finnish variety, called *lapin puikula*, has been granted the Protected Designation of Origin label, the PDO, which is given by the European Union to regional foods in order to protect them from any usurpation or imitation. This potato variety is floury. Its tubers are small, long-oval, curved, and pointed, with a yellow-colored flesh and a buttery taste. Outside Scandinavia, the *lapin puikula* may be available under the name yellow Finn. Yukon gold potatoes or other similar varieties may be substituted.

**Anise Seeds** These tiny seeds, which smell and taste like licorice, are used to flavor breads, rusks, cookies, candies, and beverages. In some dishes, a little anise seed may be used to replace fennel seed.

**Aquavit (Akvavit)** Flavored distilled liquor, ranging in alcohol content from 42 to 45 percent. It is clear to pale yellow in color, distilled from a fermented potato or grain mash, and flavored with caraway or cumin seeds. Other preparations use lemon or orange peel, cardamom, aniseed, and fennel.

**Blini** A thin pancake often served in connection with a religious rite or festival in several Slavic cultures.

**Borscht (Borsch, Borsht, or Bortsch)** Vegetable soup, usually including beet roots.

**Caraway Seeds** A pungent aroma and a distinctly sweet but tangy flavor, besides the Arab countries and India, the strongly scented and highly aromatic caraway seeds are also widely used in Germany and Russia and in Scandinavian countries like Denmark and Finland.

**Caviar** Sturgeon eggs that have been salted and allowed to mature. Sold fresh or pasteurized, there are three types of Russian caviar, differentiated by size, color, and species of sturgeon. Caviars have specific grades: they refer to colors, not flavor or size. Grade 1 (000) is the lightest color, also called "royal caviar." Grade 2 (00) is medium dark with a gray tone. The darkest caviar is 0. The three different types of caviar come from three different species of sturgeon: beluga, osetra, and sevruga.

**Beluga** is the largest sturgeon; the female takes twenty years to mature, weighing up to a ton, and measuring up to fifteen feet long. It produces the largest and most fragile eggs and most expensive caviar. Beluga caviar ranges from light to dark pearl gray, smooth, with a mildly sweet flavor of delicate hazelnut.

**Osetra** are native to the Caspian Sea, and osetra caviar is usually the best quality available. The female osetra takes up to fifteen years to mature, weighs up to 500 pounds, and measures as much as six feet in length. Osetra produces an even roe, which has a golden hue, strong nutty flavor, and a mild taste.

**Sevruga** are native to the cold depths of the Caspian Sea. Sevruga is the smallest and most prolific of the caviar sturgeons. The female sevruga takes seven years to mature, and weighs no more than 200 pounds. Sevruga produces caviar that is dark gray or black in color and with a strong taste of mildly fruity flavor.

**Cheeses**

**From Denmark**

**Blue Castello** Soft-ripened, creamy blue Brie from Denmark. A good dessert cheese.

**Danablu** (Danish Blue) Flavorful blue cheese, slightly spicy with a moist marbled texture.

**Danbo** The cheese has a pale, elastic interior with a few small holes.

**Esrom** Creamy, semi-soft cheese made from cow's milk. Esrom has a greasy, yellow-brown rind and is buttery in texture. It has a mild, pleasant taste.

**Havarti** Has a buttery aroma and can be somewhat sharp in the stronger varieties, much like Swiss cheese. The taste is buttery, and from slightly sweet to very sweet, and it is slightly acidic. The texture, depending on type, can be supple and flexible.

**Mycella** A Danish version of Gorgonzola with a blue-green mold and mild aromatic taste. It is a traditional, creamy blue cheese made from cow's milk. The veins in the cheese provide an attractive contrast to the very pale, creamy, almost buttery interior.

**Saga** Original Saga is a cross between blue cheese and Brie, a creamy, blue-veined cheese with a white-mold rind. It is very mild for a blue-veined cheese. Saga is an excellent dessert cheese best served with fruit and wine.

### From Sweden

**Adelost** Creamy blue cheese made from cow's milk. Ripens in two to three months and has a fat content of 50 percent.

**Graddost** Similar to Gruyère, graddost has a mild nuttiness, somewhat tangy flavor. This cheese melts easily and keeps well.

**Hushallsost** Creamy, semi-soft cheese made from cow's milk. The flavor is mild and creamy, with a lemon-fresh finish. It is made with whole milk, rather than skimmed.

**Mesost** A caramelized cheese that looks like fudge and has a caramel flavor with a bitter aftertaste.

**Swedish Fontina** Milder and firmer than its Italian counterpart. Nutty and mild, it is made from partially skimmed cow's milk.

**Vasterbottenost** A slow-maturing cheese that ripens for eighteenth months, resulting in a pungent, bitter taste. This cheese is excellent for grilling and grating.

### From Norway and Finland

**Aura** Finnish blue cheese, made with cow's milk, it has a strong and piquant, fruity flavor and a creamy crumbly consistency.

**Gjetost** Cow's or goat's milk cooked to achieve a cheese with a slightly sour but sweet caramel taste with a smooth texture similar to fudge. Ekte or genuine Gjetost is made with goat's milk alone.

**Jarlsberg** Cow's milk cheese with large holes, a rich buttery texture and mild, sweet nutty flavor. Similar to Emmentaler with a slightly lower fat content and melts easily.

**Juustoleipa** A specialty cheese native to Finland and Lapland, the baking process produces a creamy and smooth texture under a browned, crusty surface. It is best served warm.

**Nokkelost** A spiced semi-soft cheese with caraway, cumin, and cloves.

**Turunmaa** This Finnish Havarti-type cheese has a smooth and lacy, creamy texture and a mild but full, slightly tangy flavor.

**From Russia**

**Arakadz** Made of sheep's milk, it is semi-hard with a nutty flavor.

**Brindza** Similar to feta cheese, its soft, milky flavor is made from sheep's or goat's milk.

**Chanakh** or **Klukh Panir** Salty soft cheese.

**Chilichil** A hard, sour, saltwater cheese that must be rinsed before eating.

**Yeghegnatzor** Soft cheese made with a mixture of sheep and goat milk, with leavening, herbs, seeds, and roots added.

**Cloudberries** Relative to the raspberry and blackberry, the cloudberry is the smallest of this group. The fruit is red when unripe, turning soft and orange at maturity.

**Coriander Seeds** Dried coriander seeds have a pleasant scent and a lemony flavor.

**Fćrikćl** Called the Norwegian national dish, it is lamb and cabbage stew using the neck, shank, and breast, together with the bones of the lamb. The fat and bones of the parts used for fćrikćl are the key to the flavor of this dish.

**Fruit soup** Dessert soup popular in Scandinavia, often made with dried fruits.

**Golubtsi** Cabbage rolls filled with millet.

**Gravlax (Gravlaks, Graavilohi, Graflax)** Salmon cured with salt, sugar, and dill.

**Herring** Small saltwater fish found mainly in the North Atlantic and the North Sea. Herring is an oily fish, containing many essential nutrients and healthy fatty acids. Herring is most commonly eaten salted or preserved. Herring preparations include:

**Bismarck** Fresh, marinated in white wine/vinegar brine with carrots, onions, and spices.

**Bloater** Ungutted, lightly salted, and mildly hot- or cold-smoked, similar to kipper.

**Buckling** Briefly pickled in brine and hot-smoked.

**Kipper** Deboned, split, and flattened, lightly salted, dried, and mildly cold-smoked.

**Matjes** Fresh or lightly salted herring, or cured in spiced sugar-vinegar brine; also called soused herring.

**Schmaltz** Mature, fatty herring, filleted and preserved in brine. (*Schmaltz* is Yiddish for rendered chicken or goose fat, whereas in German it means melted animal fat, usually pork or goose fat.)

**Kasha** In Russian, the word *kasha* is used in a broad sense for various cooked grains such as buckwheat, millet, and oats. In America, the term refers to roasted buckwheat groats, which have a toasty nutty flavor.

**Kissel** Common dessert, sweetened with juice or milk, thickened with corn or potato starch; red wine or dried fruits may be added. Served hot or cold, often considered a soup.

**Knedliky** Czech bread dumplings.

**Kringle** Oval, butter-layered Danish pastries; originally pretzel-shaped, almond filled coffee cakes.

**Kulebiaka, Koulibiaka, Koulibiac** Large, narrow pie filled with salmon or sturgeon, mushrooms, rice, and hard-boiled eggs.

**Kulich** Russian traditional yeast-leavened Easter bread containing candied and dried fruits, nuts, and liqueur.

**Kvas** Russian meaning "sour beverage," a low-fermented drink made from bread and fruit.

**Lapskaus** Traditional Norwegian dish of leftovers mixed together, cooked as a soup or stew.

**Lefse (Lef-suh)** A traditional Scandinavian flatbread made from potatoes and flour, similar to the tortilla.

**Lingonberries** Small, red, pea-sized berries with a delicious flavor combining sweetness and tartness, the taste resembling that of wild cranberry.

**Lutefisk** Scandinavian delicacy, made from air-dried whitefish (cod), prepared with lye, in a sequence of particular treatments.

**Malossol** A Russian term used to describe the amount of salt used in the initial curing process. Malossol means "lightly salted" in Russian; today the term has come to mean any high-quality caviar.

**Mämmi** A traditional Finnish Easter dessert, a baked malt porridge.

**Okroshka** A cold soup based on kvas; the main ingredients are vegetables that may be mixed with cold boiled meat or fish.

**Pelmeni** Russian-type ravioli filled with various fillings.

**Pirogi, *pierogi*** Slavic dumplings that are boiled and then fried.

**Piroshki** Small meat filled pastry.

**Rasstegai** Small open-topped pies.

**Rissoles** A shallow or deep-fried minced meat dish.

**Rømmegrøt** Norwegian Christmas pudding.

**Samovar** A classic Russian tea urn.

**Sharlotka** Charlotte Russe.

**Shashlyk** Russian version of shish kebabs, marinated meat grilled on a skewer.

**Sireniki** Cheese fritters.

**Smetana** Russian in origin, this thick, yellowish-white and slightly sour-tasting cream contains about 40 percent milk fat. It is made by curdling pasteurized cream. Smetana can be replaced with crème fraîche with a similar fat content, but smetana is usually more sour in taste.

**Smörgćsbord (Smorgasbord)** Swedish term meaning an abundant buffet meal set with several hot and cold dishes, from appetizers to desserts, laid out together on the table. The word *smörgćsbord* literally means "sandwich table" or "bread and butter table." It is known and served throughout the Nordic countries, enriched with local delicacies in each country. Known as *kolde bord* in Denmark, and as *seisova pöytä, noutopöytä*, or *voileipäpöytä* in Finland. The famous Russian appetizer buffet, zakuska table, has several characteristics similar to smorgasbord.

**Smørrebrød** Danish word for open sandwiches, a major part of the Scandinavian diet.

**Solyanka** Thick, spicy, and sour Russian soup.

**Surströmming** Literally "sour herring," an old, traditional Swedish preparation of fermented Baltic herring cured with dill, sugar, salt, and coarse peppercorns. The process produces lactic acid preserving the fish, similar to the development of sauerkraut.

**Syrniki** Fried curd fritters, garnished with sour cream, jam, honey, and/or applesauce.

**Vodka** A distilled drink, the name stemming from the Russian word *voda,* meaning water.

**Wallenberg Steak** Classic Swedish veal hamburger steak usually served with potato puree, boiled green peas, and sugared lingonberries or lingonberry jam.

**Zakouski (Zakuska, Zakuski)** Russian hors d'oeuvre presentation.

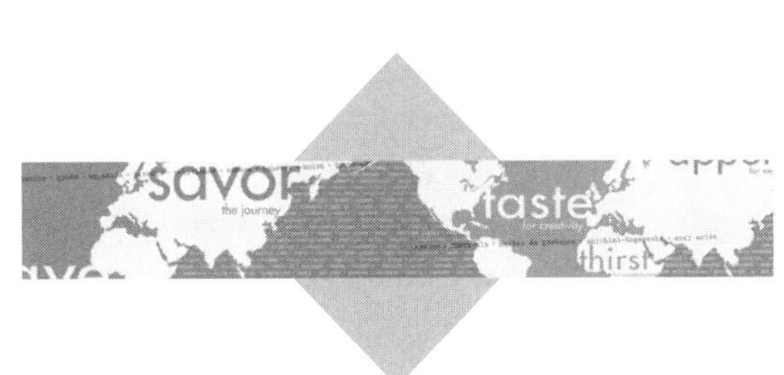

# Menus and Recipes from Scandinavia and Russia

MENU ONE (SCANDINAVIA)

***Sillsallad:* Herring and Beet Salad (Sweden)**

***Grønkćlsuppe:* Kale Soup with Poached Egg (Denmark)**

***Stekt Rimmad Lax med Korintsćs:* Fried Dill-Cured Salmon with Sweet-and-Sour Raisin Sauce (Sweden)**

***Hasselback Potatis:* Hasselback Potatoes**

***Lefse:* Potato Flatbreads (Norway)**

***Æblekage:* Apple Trifle (Denmark)**

MENU TWO (RUSSIA)

***Borshch Moskovsky:* Moscow-Style Beet Soup**

***Blini:* Buckwheat Pancakes**

***Grechnevaya Kasha:* Buckwheat Groats**

***Kulebiaka:* Salmon in Pastry**

***Chahohbili:* Georgian-Style Chicken**

***Loby:* String Beans in Sour Cream Sauce**

***Syrniki:* Sweet Cheese Fritter with Berry Kissel**

OTHER RECIPES

***Shchi:* Cabbage Soup**

***Vatrushki:* Pot Cheese Tartlets**

***Pelmeni:* Siberian Meat Dumplings**

***Frikadellen:* Meat Patties**

***Syltede Rodbeder:* Pickled Beets**

***Agurkesalat:* Marinated Cucumbers**

***Beef Stroganov:* Sautéed Beef in Sour Cream Sauce**

# Sillsallad

## Herring and Beet Salad (Sweden) SERVES 4

| AMOUNT | MEASURE | INGREDIENT |
|---|---|---|
| $\frac{1}{2}$ cup | 3 ounces, 84 g | Herring, pickled, $\frac{1}{4}$ inch (.6 cm) dice |
| $\frac{1}{2}$ cup | 3 ounces, 84 g | Red beets, boiled in skin, peeled, $\frac{1}{4}$ inch (.6 cm) dice |
| 3 tablespoons | 1$\frac{1}{2}$ ounces, 45 ml | Mayonnaise |
| 6 tablespoons | 3 ounces, 90 ml | Sour cream |
| 1 tablespoon, or to taste | $\frac{1}{2}$ ounce, 15 ml | Malt vinegar |
| 1 teaspoon | | Pickling brine from herring |
| $\frac{1}{2}$ cup | 2 ounces, 56 g | Golden Delicious apple, peeled, cored, $\frac{1}{4}$ inch (.6 cm) dice |
| $\frac{1}{2}$ cup | 3 ounces, 84 g | Red bliss potato, boiled in skin, peeled, $\frac{1}{4}$ inch (.6 cm) dice |
| $\frac{1}{4}$ cup | 1$\frac{1}{2}$ ounces, 42 g | Red onion, $\frac{1}{4}$ inch (.6 cm) dice |
| $\frac{1}{4}$ cup | 1$\frac{1}{2}$ ounces, 42 g | Sweet pickle, $\frac{1}{4}$ inch (.6 cm) dice |
| To taste | | Salt and pepper |
| 4 | | Green leaf lettuce |
| 1 tablespoon | | Capers, rinsed |
| 12 | | Thin red onion rings, soaked in ice cold water. |

### PROCEDURE

1. Set aside 1 tablespoon diced herring and 1 tablespoon diced beets for garnish.
2. Combine mayonnaise and sour cream and season with malt vinegar and pickling brine.
3. Combine apple, herring, potato, beets, onion, and pickle, fold into sour cream dressing, and let set 1 hour before serving.
4. Correct seasoning with salt, pepper, and additional vinegar.
5. Line plates with lettuce leaves and mound salad in center. Garnish with reserved diced herring and beets, capers, and red onion rings.

# Grønkćlsuppe

## Kale Soup with Poached Egg (Denmark)

SERVES 4

| AMOUNT | MEASURE | INGREDIENT |
|---|---|---|
| 1 pound | 448 g | Kale |
| 2 tablespoons | 1 ounce, 28 g | Butter |
| $\frac{1}{2}$ cup | 4 ounces, 112 g | Bacon, $\frac{1}{4}$ inch (.6 cm) dice |
| 1 cup | 4 ounces, 112 g | Onion, $\frac{1}{4}$ inch (.6 cm) dice |
| $\frac{3}{4}$ cup | 3 ounces, 84 g | Carrots, $\frac{1}{4}$ inch (.6 cm) dice |
| 2 cups | 8 ounces, 224 g | Leek, white and light green parts, $\frac{1}{4}$ inch (.6 cm) dice |
| 2 tablespoons, more if necessary | | Flour |
| $4\frac{1}{4}$ cups | 34 ounces, 1 liter | Chicken stock |
| To taste | | Salt and white pepper |
| 4 | | Eggs, poached |

**PROCEDURE**

1. Remove center ribs from kale leaves, wash carefully, blanch, drain well, and chop coarsely.
2. Heat butter over medium-low heat, add bacon, and cook until fat has been rendered; do not brown.
3. Add vegetables; sauté without coloring until soft, 5 to 8 minutes.
4. Add flour to make a roux; cook 3 minutes.
5. Add stock and cook 10 minutes.
6. Add kale; cook until kale is tender, 15 minutes or longer.
7. Adjust seasoning, and place a hot poached egg in the middle of each serving.

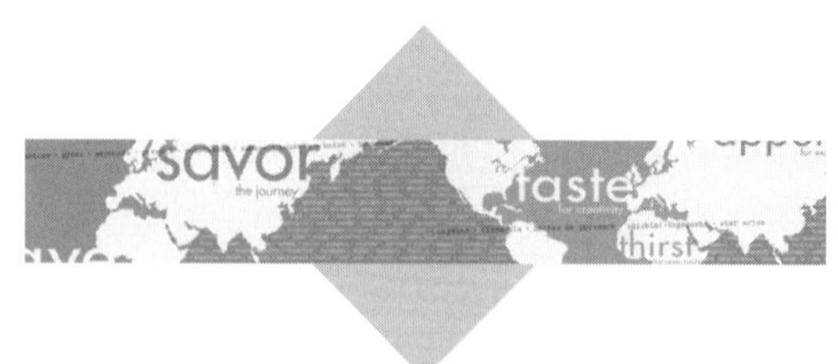

# Stekt Rimmad Lax med Korintsćs Fried Dill-Cured Salmon with Sweet-and-Sour Raisin Sauce (Sweden)

SERVES 4

| AMOUNT | MEASURE | INGREDIENT |
|---|---|---|
| 3 tablespoons | | Coarse salt |
| 2 tablespoons | | Granulated sugar |
| 1 teaspoon | | White peppercorns, cracked |
| 4 tablespoons | | Fresh dill, chopped |
| 8 | $2\frac{1}{2}$ ounce, 70 g | Skinless, boneless salmon, bias cut |
| 3 tablespoons | | Raisins |
| $1\frac{1}{2}$ cups | 12 ounces, 360 ml | Brown veal stock |
| 2 tablespoons | 1 ounce, 30 ml | Butter |
| 2 tablespoons | | Flour |
| 2 tablespoons | 1 ounce, 30 ml | Simple syrup |
| 2 tablespoons | 1 ounce, 30 ml | Malt vinegar |
| As needed | | Flour, for dredging |
| $\frac{1}{2}$ cup | 4 ounces, 120 ml | Clarified butter |

**PROCEDURE**

1. Combine coarse salt, sugar, peppercorns, and dill, sprinkle on both sides of salmon. Let cure 30 minutes. Rinse under cold water and dry well.
2. To make sauce, simmer raisins and veal stock until raisins are soft but not mushy, 10 minutes. Drain raisins; reserve stock and raisins.
3. Melt butter over medium heat and add flour to make roux; cook 2 minutes. Add stock and cook 15 minutes. Add simple syrup and vinegar, and correct with more of either to create a well-balanced sweet-sour taste. Add raisins and keep hot.
4. Season salmon with salt and white pepper, dredge in flour. Heat clarified butter over medium-high heat and pan-fry salmon pieces until crisp, about 1 minute on each side.
5. Serve with sauce, buttered green beans, and Hasselback potatoes.

# Hasselback Potatis

## Hasselback Potatoes YIELD: 4

| AMOUNT | MEASURE | INGREDIENT |
|---|---|---|
| 12 | | Red bliss potatoes, about 2 ounces (56 g) each |
| 4 tablespoons | 2 ounces, 60 ml | Butter, melted |
| $\frac{1}{4}$ cup | | Fresh bread crumbs |
| To taste | | Salt and white pepper |

PROCEDURE

1. Preheat oven to 400°F (204°C).
2. Put each potato in the bowl of a wooden spoon, like you would carry an egg in an egg-spoon race, and cut across at about $\frac{1}{4}$-inch (.6 cm) intervals. Cut each potato not quite through so they are still joined together at the bottom.
3. Heat butter over medium high heat and add cut potatoes; heat until sizzling.
4. Season with salt and pepper; roast 15 to 20 minutes, basting every 5 minutes.
5. Sprinkle with bread crumbs, baste with butter, and cook until bread crumbs are golden and potatoes are soft, 10 to 15 minutes.

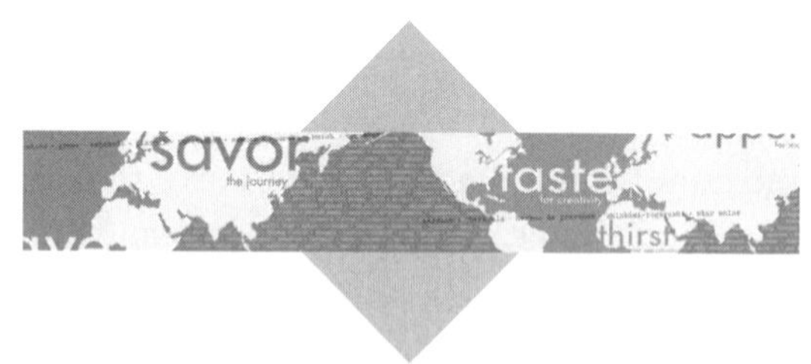

# Lefse Potato Flatbreads (Norway) YIELD: 4

**Lefse are also tasty sprinkled with sugar and cinnamon.**

| AMOUNT | MEASURE | INGREDIENT |
|---|---|---|
| $\frac{1}{2}$ cup | 4 ounces, 120 ml | Butter, melted |
| $\frac{1}{4}$ cup | 2 ounces, 60 ml | Milk, hot |
| $\frac{1}{2}$ teaspoon | | Granulated sugar |
| 2 cups | 12 ounces, 336 g | Russet potatoes, boiled in the skin, peeled and riced while hot |
| 1 cup, plus more for dusting | 4.4 ounces, 124 g | All-purpose flour |
| As needed | | Salt |
| As needed | | Butter |

**PROCEDURE**

1. Combine butter, milk, and sugar bring to a simmer.
2. Combine hot milk mixture with potatoes and mix.
3. Add flour and salt; stir to create soft, slightly sticky dough. Do not work the dough; handle as you would "short dough." Chill.
4. Roll out into a rope and cut 8 equal pieces, roll out (thin) to approximately 5-inch (12.5 cm) diameter rounds, like tortillas, dusting rolling surface with flour as needed.
5. Heat a heavy frying pan or flat griddle. Cooking surface is hot enough when a little water sprinkled on bounces off the surface. Lefse are cooked on a dry surface; do not add any fat to griddle.
6. Roll lefse onto the rolling pin, transfer lefse to hot griddle, and cook until brown "freckles" appear on the heated surface, 1 minute.
7. Flip and cook second side until freckled, 1 minute or until lefse looks cooked.
8. Stack between towels and cook remaining lefse. It is important to cool the lefses between towels so they do not dry out.
9. Restack lefses once or twice to remove moisture and to keep them from getting soggy.
10. Serve warm, spread with butter and rolled up like logs.

# Æblekage Apple Trifle (Denmark)

SERVES 4

| AMOUNT | MEASURE | INGREDIENT |
| --- | --- | --- |
| 3 cups | 18 ounces, 500 g | All-purpose cooking apple (such as Golden Delicious), $\frac{3}{4}$ inch (1.87 cm) dice |
| $\frac{1}{2}$ cup | $3\frac{1}{2}$ ounces, 98 g | Granulated sugar |
| $\frac{1}{2}$ teaspoon | | Vanilla extract |
| 3 tablespoons | $1\frac{1}{2}$ ounces, 45 ml | Water |
| $\frac{3}{4}$ cup | 3 ounces, 98 g | Fresh bread crumbs |
| $\frac{1}{4}$ cup | $1\frac{3}{4}$ ounces, 50 g | Granulated sugar |
| 5 tablespoons | $2\frac{1}{2}$ ounces, 70 g | Butter |
| 1 cup | 8 ounces, 240 ml | Whipping cream |
| $\frac{1}{4}$ cup | 2 ounces, 60 ml | Red currant jelly |

## PROCEDURE

1. Combine apples, first quantity of sugar, vanilla, and water; simmer, covered, over medium heat until apples are soft but not mushy; check after 10 minutes. Let cool.
2. In a sauté pan over medium heat, toast bread crumbs until golden. Add second quantity of sugar and cook 1 to 2 minutes until nicely browned.
3. Off the heat, add butter and stir until combined with bread crumbs; remove from pan and cool.
4. Layer apples and bread crumb mixture in serving bowl, starting with apples and finishing with bread crumbs.
5. Decorate trifle with whipped cream and jelly.

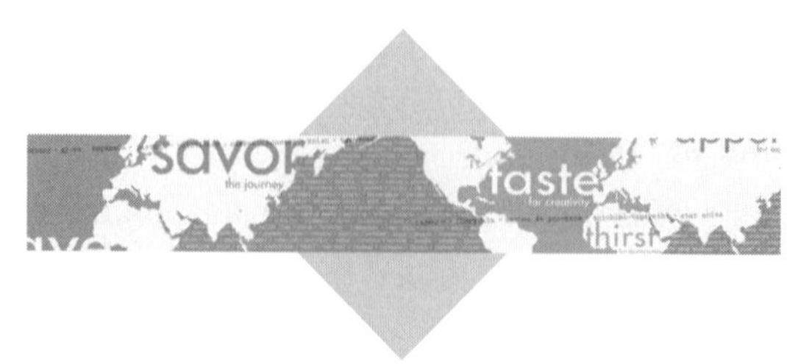

# Borshch Moskovsky

## Moscow-Style Beet Soup

SERVES 4

| AMOUNT | MEASURE | INGREDIENT |
|---|---|---|
| 1 tablespoon | $\frac{1}{2}$ ounce, 15 ml | Butter |
| 2 tablespoons | 1 ounce, 28 g | Bacon, $\frac{1}{4}$ inch (.6 cm) dice |
| 1 cup | 4 ounces, 112 g | Onions, $\frac{1}{4}$ inch (.6 cm) dice |
| 1 | | Garlic clove, minced |
| $\frac{1}{2}$ cup | 2 ounces, 56 g | Celery, $\frac{1}{4}$ inch (.6 cm) dice |
| $\frac{1}{2}$ cup | 2 ounces, 56 g | Carrots, $\frac{1}{4}$ inch (.6 cm) dice |
| 2 cups | 10 ounces, 280 g | Beets, peeled, $\frac{1}{4}$ inch (.6 cm) dice |
| 2 tablespoons | 1 ounce, 30 ml | Red wine vinegar |
| $\frac{1}{2}$ teaspoon | | Granulated sugar |
| 1 cup | 6 ounces, 180 ml | Tomatoes, peeled, seeded, $\frac{1}{4}$ inch (.6 cm) dice |
| To taste | | Salt and white pepper |
| 4 cups | 32 ounces, 960 ml | Chicken, beef, or vegetable stock |
| 1 cup | 4 ounces, 112 g | Green cabbage, cored and finely shredded |
| $\frac{1}{2}$ cup | 2 ounces, 56 g | Potatoes, peeled, $\frac{1}{4}$ inch (.6 cm) dice |
| 2 | | Parsley sprigs, tied together with 1 bay leaf |
| 2 tablespoons | | Fresh dill or flat-leaf parsley, finely diced |
| $\frac{1}{4}$ cup | 2 ounces, 60 ml | Sour cream |

### PROCEDURE

1. Heat butter over medium heat and render bacon; do not brown.
2. Add onions and cook, 3 minutes; add garlic and cook 2 minutes until both are translucent.
3. Add celery and carrots; cook 3 minutes.
4. Add beets, stir in red wine vinegar, sugar, tomatoes, 1 teaspoon salt, and white pepper to taste.
5. Add 1 cup stock and simmer, covered, 15 to 20 minutes.
6. Add remaining stock, the cabbage, and potatoes; bring to a boil. Reduce heat, submerge parsley and bay leaf, and simmer, partially covered, until potatoes and cabbage are soft but still hold shape.
7. Stir in dill and serve with sour cream as accompaniment.

# Blini Buckwheat Pancakes

SERVES 4

**Serve with sour cream or melted butter, topped with thin-sliced smoked salmon, red salmon roe, thin-sliced smoked sturgeon, black caviar, or pickled herring.**

| AMOUNT | MEASURE | INGREDIENT |
|---|---|---|
| 1 ½ teaspoons | 3 g | Active dry yeast |
| ¼ cup | 2 ounces, 60 ml | Luke warm water, 110–115°F (43.3–46.1°C) |
| ¼ cup | 1 ounce, 30 g | Buckwheat flour |
| 1 cup | 4 ounces, 112 g | All-purpose flour |
| 1 cup | 8 ounces, 240 ml | Lukewarm milk, 110–115°F (43.3–46.1°C) |
| 2 | | Egg yolks, slightly beaten |
| Pinch | | Salt |
| ½ teaspoon | | Granulated sugar |
| ¼ cup | 4 ounces, 120 ml | Butter, melted and cooled |
| 1 cup, plus more for serving | 8 ounces, 240 ml | Sour cream |
| 2 | | Egg whites |
| Garnish | | Caviar, smoked salmon, sturgeon, or herring fillets |

## PROCEDURE

1. Sprinkle yeast over lukewarm water, let stand 3 minutes, make sure it is active, and stir to dissolve. Let stand 3 minutes in a warm, draft-free area.
2. Combine half the buckwheat flour and half the all-purpose flour. Make a well in the center and add half the warm milk and the yeast mixture. Slowly work the flour into the liquid. Cover the bowl and set aside in a warm, draft-free area until the mixture has nearly doubled in size, 2 hours.
3. Beat in remaining flours; let rest 1 hour.
4. Gradually add remaining warm milk, egg yolks, salt, sugar, 1 tablespoon (½ ounces, 15 ml) melted butter, and 1½ tablespoons (¾ ounce, 20 ml) sour cream.
5. Beat egg whites to stiff peaks, fold into batter, and let rest 15 minutes.
6. Preheat oven to 200°F (93°C).
7. Heat a heavy frying pan or flat griddle. Cooking surface is hot enough when a little water sprinkled on bounces off the surface.

8 Grease the cooking surface and pour 3 tablespoons ($1\frac{1}{2}$ ounce, 45 ml) of batter for each pancake; cook 2 to 3 minutes, brushing the top lightly with butter. Turn pancake over and cook 2 minutes, or until golden brown. Keep warm in oven until remaining pancakes are cooked.

9 Serve hot, accompanied with remaining melted butter and sour cream. Garnish with caviar.

# Grechnevaya Kasha

## Buckwheat Groats

YIELD: 4

| AMOUNT | MEASURE | INGREDIENT |
|---|---|---|
| **1 cup** | **6 ounces, 168 g** | **Buckwheat groats** |
| **1** | | **Egg, beaten** |
| **1 teaspoon** | | **Salt** |
| **3 tablespoons** | **$1\frac{1}{2}$ ounces, 45 ml** | **Butter** |
| **$2\frac{1}{2}$ cups** | **20 ounces, 600 ml** | **Boiling water** |

PROCEDURE

1 Toss together buckwheat groats and egg until the grains are thoroughly coated.

2 Over medium heat in an ungreased pan, cook uncovered, stirring constantly, until groats are lightly toasted and dry.

3 Add salt, butter, and 2 cups (16 ounces, 480 ml) boiling water. Stir, cover tightly, reduce heat to low, and simmer, stirring occasionally, about 20 minutes. After 20 minutes check for tenderness; if necessary, add the additional water and continue cooking until tender and water is absorbed, and the grains are separated and fluffy.

4 Correct seasoning and serve.

# Kulebiaka Salmon in Pastry

SERVES 4

| AMOUNT | MEASURE | INGREDIENT |
|---|---|---|
| **Brioche Dough** | | |
| 3 tablespoons | $1\frac{1}{2}$ ounces, 45 ml | Milk |
| 1 tablespoon | $\frac{1}{4}$ ounce, 7 g | Granulated sugar |
| 1 tablespoon | $\frac{1}{4}$ ounce, 7 g | Active dry yeast |
| 2 cups | 14 ounces | Bread flour |
| 3 | | Eggs |
| 1 teaspoon | 2 g | Salt |
| 6 tablespoons | 3 ounces, 90 ml | Butter, melted |
| **Rice Filling** | | |
| **Step 1** | | |
| 2 tablespoons | 1 ounce, 30 ml | Butter |
| $\frac{1}{4}$ cup | 1 ounce, 28 g | Onion, $\frac{1}{4}$ inch (.6 cm) dice |
| 1 cup | 7 ounces, 196 g | Rice |
| $1\frac{1}{2}$ cups | 12 ounces, 360 ml | Chicken stock |
| **Step 2** | | |
| 2 tablespoons | 1 ounce, 30 ml | Butter |
| 3 cups | 8 ounces, 224 g | Mushrooms, diced |
| 2 tablespoons | 1 ounce, 30 ml | Fresh lemon juice |
| **Step 3** | | |
| $\frac{1}{4}$ cup | 2 ounces, 60 ml | Butter |
| $\frac{3}{4}$ cup | 3 ounces, 84 g | Onion, $\frac{1}{4}$ inch (.6 cm) dice |
| 1 | | Egg, hard-boiled, finely chopped |
| 1 | | Egg yolk |
| 1 tablespoon | | Fresh dill, chopped |
| To taste | | Salt and pepper |
| **Assembly** | | |
| $\frac{3}{4}$ pound | 12 ounces, 336 g | Boneless, skinless salmon fillet |
| As needed | | Egg wash |

### BRIOCH DOUGH

1. Over medium heat bring milk and sugar to 110–115°F (43.3–46.1°C).
2. Sprinkle yeast over warm milk and rehydrate 10 minutes.
3. Combine $\frac{3}{4}$ cup (3 ounces, 84 g) flour, 1 egg, and 1 teaspoon salt. Add yeast mixture, blend until a smooth soft dough, and cut a deep X across top. Cover with plastic wrap and let starter rise at room temperature, 1 hour.
4. Beat remaining eggs with butter.
5. Slowly work remaining flour and egg mixture into starter dough; knead the mixture by hand until the dough is smooth and shiny, 6 to 8 minutes.
6. Lightly butter a large bowl and scrape dough into bowl. Lightly dust dough with flour to prevent a crust from forming.
7. Cover bowl with plastic wrap and let dough rise at room temperature until more than doubled in bulk, 1 hour. Punch down dough and lightly dust with flour.

### FILLING

1. **Step 1.** Heat butter and sauté onions until translucent. Add rice and cook 1 minute.
2. Add stock and season. Bring to simmer, cover, reduce heat to low, and cook about 15 minutes. Remove cover and cook 5 minutes longer. Fluff rice.
3. **Step 2.** Heat butter over medium high heat, add mushrooms, and cook until moisture has evaporated. Add lemon juice and cook 30 seconds.
4. **Step 3.** Heat butter over medium high heat, add onions, and cook until translucent.
5. Combine cooked rice, cooked onion and mushroom mixture, hard-boiled egg, egg yolk, and dill. Correct seasoning and cool to room temperature before assembling.

### ASSEMBLY

1. Roll out dough to $\frac{1}{8}$ inch (.3 cm) thick and spread $\frac{1}{2}$ inch (1.2 cm) layer of rice mixture in the center of the dough, the size of the salmon fillet.
2. Place salmon fillet on top of rice; add another $\frac{1}{2}$ inch (1.2 cm) layer of rice mixture on top.
3. Brush egg wash over edges of pastry and fold dough over to completely cover the rice and salmon. Trim excess dough. Place seam side down on a parchment lined baking pan. Rest 30 minutes in refrigerator.
4. Brush with egg wash, poke vent holes, and bake at 375°F (190°C) until golden brown and salmon fillet is cooked, around 145°F (63°C). Let set 10 to 15 minutes before cutting.

# Chahohbili Georgian-Style Chicken

SERVES 4

| AMOUNT | MEASURE | INGREDIENT |
|---|---|---|
| 5 tablespoons | $2\frac{1}{2}$ ounces, 75 ml | Butter |
| 3 cups | 18 ounces, 504 g | Onions, $\frac{1}{2}$ inch (1.2 cm) dice |
| 3 pounds | 48 ounces, 1.3 kg | Chicken, cut into 12 pieces |
| 3 tablespoons | $1\frac{1}{2}$ ounces, 45 ml | Tomato paste |
| 1 cup | 6 ounces, 180 ml | Tomato, grated |
| $\frac{3}{4}$ cup | 3 ounces, 84 g | Sweet red pepper, minced |
| 1 teaspoon | | Hot pepper flakes |
| To taste | | Salt and pepper |
| 2 cups | | Italian parsley, rough chopped, packed |
| 1 cup | | Coriander greens, rough chopped, packed |
| 2 | | Garlic cloves, chopped |
| To taste | | Hot pepper flakes |

PROCEDURE

1 Heat butter over medium-low heat; add onions and cook until translucent and soft, 20 minutes.

2 Pat chicken dry, turn heat to medium, and add chicken to onions. Cook 2 to 3 minutes, turning often.

3 Add tomato paste, cook 1 minute, then add tomato, sweet pepper, and hot pepper flakes. Cover and simmer until chicken is cooked, 30 minutes.

4 In a mortar, add a pinch of salt to parsley, coriander, and garlic; crush to a coarse paste (this is essential).

5 Add herb mixture, and hot pepper to taste, to saucepan, mix well, and bring to a boil; remove from heat immediately.

6 Serve hot.

# Loby String Beans in Sour Cream Sauce

SERVES 4

| AMOUNT | MEASURE | INGREDIENT |
|---|---|---|
| 3 cups | 12 ounces, 336 g | Fresh string beans |
| 3 tablespoons | $1\frac{1}{2}$ ounces, 45 ml | Butter |
| 1 cup | 4 ounces, 112 g | Onions, thinly sliced |
| $\frac{1}{2}$ cup | 2 ounces, 56 g | Green bell pepper, $\frac{1}{4}$ inch (.6 cm) dice |
| 1 cup | 6 ounces, 168 g | Tomato, peeled, seeded, $\frac{1}{4}$ inch (.6 cm) dice |
| 2 teaspoons | | Fresh basil, chopped |
| $\frac{1}{2}$ cup | 4 ounces, 120 ml | Sour cream |
| To taste | | Salt and pepper |

PROCEDURE

1. Cook beans in boiling salted water just until done. Drain, shock in cold water, drain again, and set aside.
2. Heat butter over medium high heat and sauté onions until translucent, 3 minutes. Add green pepper and cook 3 minutes.
3. Add tomato and basil, raise heat to high, and cook 1 minute to remove excess moisture from tomato; cook longer if necessary.
4. Add green beans and sauté until heated completely.
5. Stir in sour cream, correct seasoning, and serve hot.

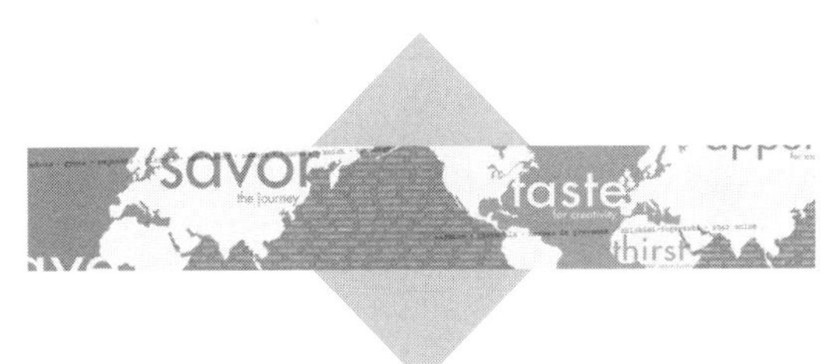

# Syrniki Sweet Cheese Fritter with Berry Kissel

SERVES 4

| AMOUNT | MEASURE | INGREDIENT |
|---|---|---|
| 2 cups | 16 ounces, 448 g | Cottage cheese or large-curd pot cheese |
| 4 | | Egg yolks |
| $1\frac{1}{3}$ cups | 5 ounces, 140 g | All-purpose flour |
| $\frac{1}{4}$ teaspoon | | Salt |
| 2 tablespoons | | Granulated sugar |
| $\frac{1}{2}$ cup | 4 ounces, 120 ml | Butter |
| Berry Kissel | | |
| $\frac{1}{4}$ cup | 2 ounces, 56 g | Granulated sugar |
| 2 tablespoons | | Cornstarch |
| Pinch | | Salt |
| 1 cup | 8 ounces, 240 ml | Water |
| 2 cups | 8 ounces, 224 g | Blackberries |
| 2 cups | 8 ounces, 224 g | Raspberries |
| $\frac{1}{2}$ teaspoon, or to taste | | Fresh lemon juice |

PROCEDURE FOR FRITTER

1. Set cheese in colander, cover with towel, and weigh it down. Let drain 2 to 3 hours.
2. With the back of a spoon, rub cheese through a fine sieve set over a bowl.
3. Beat egg yolks into cheese, one at a time, then gradually beat in the flour, salt, and sugar.
4. Shape into 4 equal portions. On a floured surface, form into 3- to 4-inch (7.2 to 9.6 cm) cylindrical links. Wrap and chill 30 to 45 minutes.
5. Cut into 1-inch (2.4 cm) pieces and fry in butter over medium-high heat 3 to 5 minutes on each side, or until golden brown. Serve hot fritters with berry kissel or sour cream.

**PROCEDURE FOR BERRY KISSEL**

1. Combine sugar, cornstarch, and salt.
2. Over medium heat combine water and $\frac{1}{4}$ of the berries, simmer 2 minutes. Drain mixture, reserving both liquid and berries.
3. Gradually whisk in reserved hot liquid to the sugar mixture and bring to a boil; stir and cook 3 minutes. Remove from heat and strain.
4. Add all berries and lemon juice to liquid. Chill.

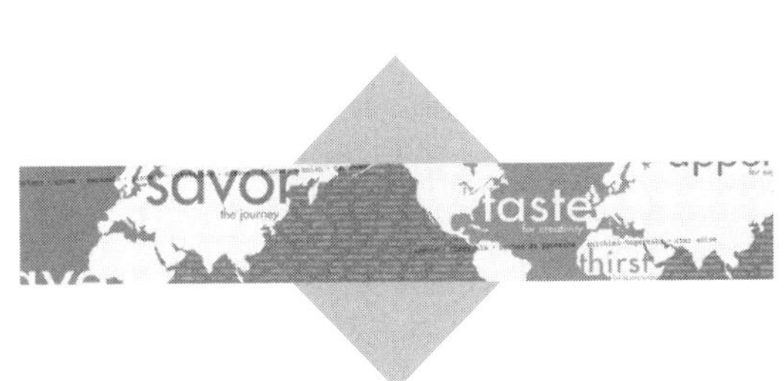

# Shchi Cabbage Soup

SERVES 4 TO 6

| AMOUNT | MEASURE | INGREDIENT |
|---|---|---|
| **Beef Stock** | | |
| | 8 ounces | Lean brisket of beef |
| $2\frac{1}{2}$ pounds | | Beef marrow bones, cracked |
| 2 quarts | 1.9 l | Water |
| 1 cup | 4 ounces, 112 g | Onion, peeled and quartered |
| 1 cup | 4 ounces, 112 g | Carrot, peeled, large rough chop |
| | | 2 celery tops, 6 sprigs parsley, 2 bay leaves tied with string |
| 1 tablespoon | | Salt |

PROCEDURE FOR STOCK

1 In a heavy to 6- to 8-quart pot, bring the beef, beef bones, and water to a boil over high heat, skimming off any foam and scum as they rise to the surface.

2 Add the onion, carrot, tied greens, and salt; partially cover, and reduce the heat to low. Simmer 1 to $1\frac{1}{2}$ hours, or until the meat is tender but not falling apart.

3 Remove meat, cut into small dice, and set aside. Continue to simmer the stock partially covered, 2 to 4 hours longer. Strain the stock through a fine sieve, discarding the bones and greens. Skim off and discard as much of the surface fat as possible.

| AMOUNT | MEASURE | INGREDIENT |
|---|---|---|
| **Soup** | | |
| 2 tablespoons | 1 ounces, 30 ml | Butter |
| 1 cup | 4 ounces, 112 g | Onions, thinly sliced |
| | 12 ounces | White cabbage, quartered, cored, coarsely shredded |
| 1 cup | 4 ounces, 112 g | Celery root, peeled, julienned |
| 1 cup | 4 ounces, 112 g | Parsnip, peeled, julienned |
| $1\frac{1}{4}$ cups | 8 ounces, 224 g | Boiling potatoes, peeled, $\frac{1}{4}$-inch (.6 cm) dice |
| 1 cup | 6 ounces, 168 g | Tomatoes, peeled, seeded, and chopped |
| 1 teaspoon | | Salt |
| To taste | | Freshly ground black pepper |

**PROCEDURE FOR SOUP**

1. Heat butter over medium heat, add onions, and sauté 7 to 8 minutes, or until soft.
2. Add cabbage, celery root, and parsnips; cover and simmer 15 minutes.
3. Add stock and reserved diced beef. Simmer, partially covered, 15 minutes. Add potatoes and cook until potatoes are tender, 10 minutes.
4. Add tomatoes, simmer 5 minutes, and correct seasoning.
5. Serve hot with vatrushki.

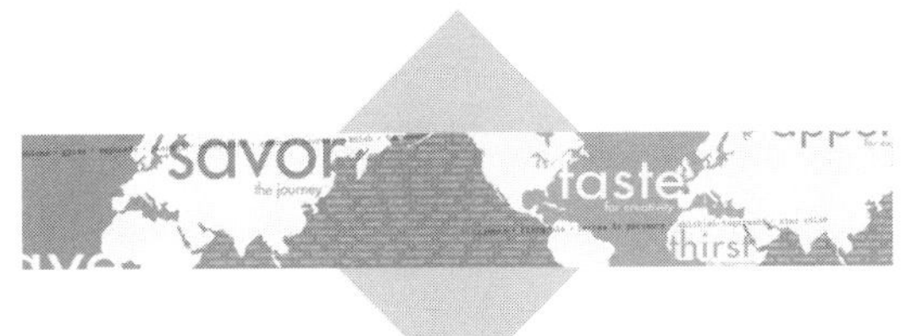

# Vatrushki Pot Cheese Tartlets SERVES 4

| AMOUNT | MEASURE | INGREDIENT |
|---|---|---|
| **Dough** | | |
| **1 $\frac{3}{4}$ cups** | **7 ounces, 196 g** | **All-purpose flour** |
| **$\frac{1}{2}$ teaspoon** | | **Baking powder** |
| **$\frac{1}{2}$ teaspoon** | | **Salt** |
| **1** | | **Egg** |
| **$\frac{1}{2}$ cup** | **4 ounces, 120 ml** | **Sour cream** |
| **4 tablespoons** | **2 ounces, 60 ml** | **Butter** |

**PROCEDURE**

1 Sift together the flour, baking powder, and salt. Make a deep well in the center of the flour and drop in the egg, sour cream, and butter. With your fingers, slowly mix the flour into the liquid ingredients, then beat vigorously with a wooden spoon until it forms smooth, moderately firm dough. Chill 30 minutes.

| | | |
|---|---|---|
| **Filling** | | |
| **1 cup** | **8 ounces, 224 g** | **Large-curd pot cheese (cottage cheese)** |
| **2 teaspoons** | **20 ml** | **Sour cream** |
| **1** | | **Egg** |
| **$\frac{1}{4}$ teaspoon** | | **Granulated sugar** |
| **$\frac{1}{4}$ teaspoon** | | **Salt** |
| **1** | | **Egg yolk, mixed with 1 tablespoon ($\frac{1}{2}$ ounce, 15 ml) water** |

**PROCEDURE**

1 Drain the cheese by placing it in a colander, covering it with a double thickness of cheesecloth or a kitchen towel, and weighting it with a heavy dish on top. Let it drain undisturbed 2 or 3 hours, then with the back of a large spoon, rub the cheese through a fine sieve. Beat into it the sour cream, egg, sugar, and salt. Chill at least 30 minutes.

**PREPARATION**

1 On a lightly floured surface, roll dough into a circle of about $\frac{1}{8}$ inch (.3 cm) thick. With a 4-inch (10 cm) cookie cutter, cut out 8 circles; there will be excess dough. Dough can be reworked and rerolled.

2 Make a border around each circle by turning over about $\frac{1}{4}$ inch (.6 cm) of the dough all around its circumference and pinch in decorative scalloped pleats.

3 Place $1\frac{1}{2}$ tablespoons of the filling into the center and flatten it slightly, leaving a border.

4 Using a pastry brush, coat the filling and borders with the egg yolk and water mixture, then prick the dough lightly with a fork.

5 Bake in the center of a 400°F (204°C) oven, 15 minutes or until pale golden in color.

6 Serve *vatrushki* as an accompaniment to a soup or alone as a first course.

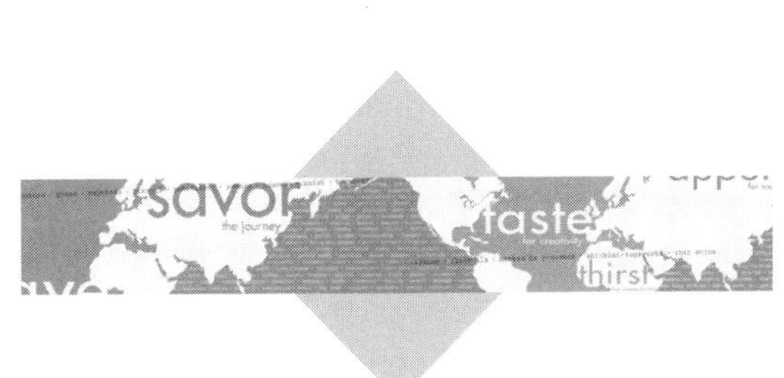

# Pelmeni Siberian Meat Dumplings

YIELD: 3 DOZEN

| AMOUNT | MEASURE | INGREDIENT |
|---|---|---|
| **Dough** | | |
| 2 cups | 8 ounces, 224 g | All-purpose flour |
| ½ teaspoon | | Salt |
| 2 | | Eggs |
| ½ cup | 4 ounces, 120 ml | Water |

**PROCEDURE**

1. Sift together flour and salt and make a deep well in the center. Beat eggs and water together and pour into well. With your hands or a large spoon, slowly mix the flour into the liquid ingredients until the mixture can be gathered into a compact ball.
2. Transfer the dough to a lightly floured surface and knead it by folding it end to end, then pressing it down and pushing it forward several times with the heel of your hand. Sprinkle the dough with extra flour when necessary to prevent it from sticking to the board. Knead about 10 minutes, or until the dough is smooth and elastic. Shape into a ball, cover, and rest 1 hour at room temperature.

| AMOUNT | MEASURE | INGREDIENT |
|---|---|---|
| **Filling** | | |
| 2 tablespoons | 1 ounce, 30 ml | Butter |
| 1 tablespoon | ½ ounce, 15 ml | Vegetable oil |
| ½ cup | 2 ounces, 56 g | Onions, minced |
| 1 cup | 8 ounces, 224g | Lean top round or beef chuck, ground twice |
| 1 cup | 8 ounces, 224 g | Fresh pork fat, ground twice |
| 1 teaspoon | | Salt |
| ½ teaspoon | | Black pepper, fresh ground |
| ½ cup | 4 ounces, 120 ml | Melted butter (optional) |

**PROCEDURE**

1. Melt the butter in the oil over high heat. When the foam has almost subsided, add the onions; cook over moderate heat, stirring frequently, 3 to 4 minutes, or until they are soft and lightly colored. Remove onions from pan, and cool.

2. To the cooled onions, add the meat, pork fat, salt, pepper, and $\frac{1}{2}$ cup (4 ounces, 120 ml) cold water and mix well until the ingredients are well combined and the mixture is smooth.
3. On a lightly floured surface, roll the reserved dough into a rough rectangle about $\frac{1}{8}$ inch (.3 cm) thick. Slide hands under the dough, stretch dough with backs of clenched fists, working from center in all directions until dough is paper thin. Cut out rounds of the dough with a $2\frac{1}{2}$- to 3-inch cookie cutter.
4. Place ground meat mixture in the lower half of each round. Make the dumplings as large as you can, but leave room to seal up the dough; run a finger lightly dipped in water around the edges and fold the exposed dough over the filling. Seal the edges by pressing firmly with the prongs of a fork. Dip your fingers in water again and lift up the two corners, pinching them together to form a round or triangular pouch.
5. Over high heat bring salted water to a vigorous boil, cook dumplings, uncovered, 5 to 7 minutes, or until they rise to the surface of the water. With a slotted spoon, transfer them to a double thickness of paper towels and let them drain while you cook and drain the remaining dumplings.
6. Serve hot with melted butter, if desired.

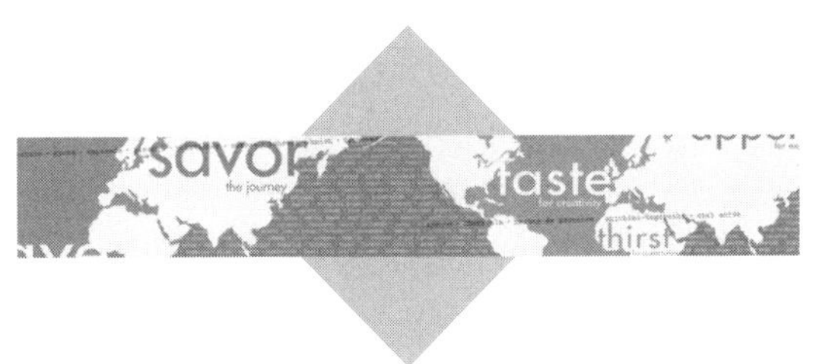

# Frikadellen Meat Patties YIELD: 8

| AMOUNT | MEASURE | INGREDIENT |
|---|---|---|
| 2 tablespoons | 1 ounce, 30 ml | Butter |
| $\frac{2}{3}$ cup | 3 ounces, 84 g | Onions, minced |
| 1 | | Bay leaf |
| 1 | | Fresh thyme sprig |
| 1 | | Garlic clove, minced |
| 2 teaspoons | | Caraway seeds, ground |
| 1 | | Egg |
| $\frac{1}{2}$ cup | 2 ounce, 28 g | Bread crumbs, fresh |
| $\frac{1}{4}$ cup | 2 ounces, 60 ml | Milk |
| 6 tablespoons | 3 ounces, 90 ml | Heavy cream |
| $1\frac{1}{2}$ cups | 12 ounces, 336 g | Veal, ground |
| $1\frac{1}{2}$ cups | 12 ounces, 336 g | Pork, ground |
| 2 tablespoons | $\frac{1}{4}$ ounce, 7 g | Parsley, chopped |
| 1 tablespoon | | Fresh dill, chopped |
| 2 teaspoon | | Lemon zest |
| To taste | | Salt and pepper |
| 2 tablespoons | 1 ounce, 30 ml | Vegetable oil |
| 2 tablespoons | 1 ounce, 30 ml | Butter |

**PROCEDURE**

1 Melt first quantity of butter over medium-high heat, add onions, bay leaf, and thyme, sauté 3 minutes or until onions are soft and translucent.

2 Add garlic, cook 1 minute; add caraway, cook 30 seconds, remove from heat, and cool.

3 Mix together bread crumbs, milk, and heavy cream, let sit 2 minutes.

4 Combine egg, bread crumb mixture, veal, pork, parsley, dill, lemon zest, and onion mixture (remove bay leaf and thyme sprig) until completely incorporated. Test a small portion for seasoning: sauté until done, taste, and adjust seasoning with salt and pepper. Form into oval patties and refrigerate at least 1 hour.

5 Heat pan over medium high heat, add the oil and remaining butter. When butter is melted, add patties. Sauté 3 to 5 minutes on one side, depending on size and thickness of

patties. Turn over and continue to cook an additional 3 to 5 minutes or until juices run clear. Patties can be finished in a hot oven.

6 Serve hot or cold, garnished with pickled beets and marinated cucumbers.

## Syltede Rodbeder Pickled Beets

YIELD: 2 CUPS

| AMOUNT | MEASURE | INGREDIENT |
|---|---|---|
| 2 cups | 12 ounces, 336 g | Beets, roasted, peeled, cooled, $\frac{1}{4}$ inch (.6 cm) half moon slices or any preferred cut |
| $\frac{1}{2}$ teaspoon | | Caraway, ground |
| 2 tablespoons | 1 ounce, 30 ml | Orange juice |
| 2 teaspoons | 20 ml | Red wine vinegar |
| $\frac{1}{4}$ teaspoon | | Coarse salt |
| To taste | | Black pepper, freshly ground |
| $\frac{1}{2}$ teaspoon | | Orange zest |

PROCEDURE

1 Combine all ingredients and marinate at least 1 hour.

## Agurkesalat Marinated Cucumbers

YIELD: $1\frac{1}{2}$ CUPS

| AMOUNT | MEASURE | INGREDIENT |
|---|---|---|
| 1 cup | 6 ounces, 168 g | Seedless cucumber, julienned |
| $\frac{1}{2}$ cup | 1 ounce, 28 g | Green onion, white and green parts, thinly sliced |
| To taste | | Salt and pepper |
| 1 teaspoon | | Sugar |
| 4 teaspoons | $1\frac{1}{3}$ ounces, 40 ml | Cider vinegar |
| 2 tablespoons | | Fresh dill, chopped |

PROCEDURE

1 Combine all ingredients and marinate 30 minutes before serving.

# Beef Stroganov

## Sautéed Beef in Sour Cream Sauce

SERVES 4

| AMOUNT | MEASURE | INGREDIENT |
| --- | --- | --- |
| $\frac{2}{3}$ tablespoon | 4 g | Dry mustard powder |
| $\frac{2}{3}$ tablespoon | 8 g | Granulated sugar |
| 1 teaspoon | 4 g | Salt |
| 1 tablespoon | 10 ml | Hot water |
| 4 tablespoons | 2 ounces, 60 ml | Butter |
| 1 cup | 4 ounces, 112 g | Onions, julienned |
| 3 cups | 9 ounces, 252 g | Mushrooms, thinly sliced lengthwise |
| $\frac{1}{4}$ cup | 2 ounces, 60 ml | Dry white wine |
| | 1 pound, 448 g | Beef, sirloin or filet, trimmed of all fat, cut across the grain into $\frac{1}{4}$ inch (.6 cm) slices, then sliced into $\frac{1}{4}$ inch (.6 cm) strips |
| To taste | | Salt and pepper |
| $\frac{1}{2}$ cup | 4 ounces, 120 ml | Sour cream, warm |

**PROCEDURE**

1. Combine mustard powder, sugar, salt, and hot water to form a paste.
2. Heat 2 tablespoons (1 ounce, 30 ml) butter over medium high heat, sauté onions until soft and translucent, 3 minutes. Add mushrooms and white wine; cook, stirring, until mushrooms are cooked and almost dry. Remove from heat and set aside.
3. Heat remaining 2 tablespoons (1 ounce, 30 ml) butter over medium-high heat and sauté beef until lightly browned. Meat may be cooked a half at a time to ensure sautéing and not stewing.
4. Add mustard mixture to meat and toss to combine.
5. Add mushroom onion mixture to beef; correct seasoning.
6. Add sour cream slowly, working to combine; heat to a simmer, do not boil.
7. Serve hot, with wide noodles, kasha, rice, or straw potatoes.

# References


**BOOKS**

Alford, Jeffrey, and Naomi Duguid. 2000. *Hot, Sour, Salty, Sweet.* Workman Publishing, Inc. New York, New York.
Andres, Jose. 2005. *Tapas A Taste of Spain in America.* Random House, Inc. New York, New York.
Blajekar, Mridula. 2000. *Secrets from an Indian Kitchen.* Pavilion Books, Ltd. London, England.
Burum, Linda. 1985. *Asian Pasta.* Harris Publishing Co. Berkeley, California
Hae-Jin Lee, Cecilia. 2005. *Eating Korean.* John Wiley and Sons, Inc. Hoboken, New Jersey.
Harris, Jessica B. 2003. *Beyond Gumbo.* Simon & Schuster. New York, New York.
Hazan, Marcella. 1986. *Marcella's Italian Kitchen.* Alfred A. Knopf. New York, New York.
Hiremath, Laxmi. 2005. *The Dance of Spices.* John Wiley and Sons, Inc. Hoboken, New Jersey.
Hom, Ken. 1996. *Asian Ingredients.* Ten Speed Press, Berkely, California.
———. 1994. *Chinese Kitchens.* Hyperion. New York, New York.
Ingram, Christine. 2002. *The World Encyclopedia of Cooking Ingredients.* Anness Publishing, Ltd. London, England.
Jaffrey, Madhur. 1999. *World Vegetarian Cuisine.* Random House, Inc. New York, New York.
Johnson, Margaret, M. 2003. *The New Irish Table.* Chronicle Books LLC. San Franscisco, California.
Kamman, Madeleine. 1989. *Savoie: The Land, People, and Food of the French Alps.* Macmillan Publishing Company. New York, New York.
Kennedy, Diana. 2000. *The Essential Cuisines of Mexico.* Clarkson Potter Publishing. New York, New York.
———. 2003. *From My Mexican Kitchen.* Clarkson Potter Publishing. New York, New York.
Lambert-Ortiz, Elisabeth. 1979. *The Book of Latin American Cooking.* Random House. New York, New York.
Law, Ruth. 1990. *Southeast Asia Cookbook.* Donald I. Fine, Inc. New York, New York.
Luard, Elisabeth. 2006. *Classic Spanish Cooking.* MQ Publishers, Inc. New York, New York
Read, Mark. 2001. *Lemongrass and Lime.* Ten Speed Press, Berkeley, California.
Shimbo, Hiroka. 2000. *The Japanese Kitchen.* The Harvard Common Press. Boston, Mass.
Sonnenfeld, Albert. 1999. *A Culinary History of Food.* Penguin Books. New York, New York.
Stow, Josie and Han Baldwin. 2005. *The African Kitchen.* Interlink Books. Northampton, MA.
Tropp, Barbara, 2001. *The Modern Art of Chinese Cooking.* HarperCollins Publishing, New York, New York.
VanAken, Norman. 2003. *New World Kitchen.* HarperCollins Publishers. New York, New York.
Von Bremzen, Anya. 2005. *The New Spanish Table.* Workman Publishing. New York, New York.
Wright, Clifford A. 2003. *Little Foods of the Mediterranean.* Harvard Common Press. Boston, Mass.
Zia Chu, Madame Grace. 1980. *The Encyclopedia of Asian Cooking.* Mandarin Publishers Limited. Quarry Bay, Hong Kong.

**WEBSITES**

www.Historycentral.com
www.NationbyNation.com
www.geographia.com
www.britannica.com
www.AsiaRecipe.com
www.foodbycountry.com

# Index

## B

## D

## H

## N

## O

## P

## T